Hazardous Materials Toxicology: Clinical Principles of Environmental Health

Hazardous Materials Toxicology
Clinical Principles of Environmental Health

Edited by

John B. Sullivan, Jr., M.D.
Medical Director, Arizona Poison Center
Diplomate, American Board of Medical Toxicology
Fellow
American Academy of Clinic Toxicology
Director, Clinical Toxicology Program
Associate Professor
Section of Emergency Medicine
University of Arizona Health Sciences Center
Tucson, Arizona

Gary R. Krieger, M.D., M.P.H., D.A.B.T.
Manager, Partner (Ltd.), Health Systems Group
Dames & Moore
Denver, Colorado
Adjunct Assistant Professor of Toxicology
Department of Environmental and Molecular Toxicology
University of Colorado
Boulder, Colorado

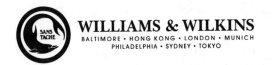
WILLIAMS & WILKINS
BALTIMORE · HONG KONG · LONDON · MUNICH
PHILADELPHIA · SYDNEY · TOKYO

Editor: Laurel Craven
Managing Editor: Marjorie Kidd Keating
Project Editor: Mary Kidd
Designer: Karen S. Klinedinst
Illustration Planner: Ray Lowman
Production Coordinator: Barbara J. Felton
Cover Designer: Karen S. Klinedinst

Accurate indications, adverse reactions, and dosage schedules for drugs are provided in this book, but it is possible that they may change. The reader is urged to review the package information data of the manufacturers of the medications mentioned.

Printed in the United States of America

Library of Congress Cataloging-in-Publication Data

Hazardous materials toxicology : clinical principles of environmental health / edited by John B. Sullivan, Jr., Gary R. Krieger.
    p.   cm.
  Includes bibliographical references and index.
  ISBN 0-683-08025-3
  1. Toxicology. 2. Environmental health. I. Sullivan, John B.
(Burke) II. Krieger, Gary R.
  [DNLM: 1. Hazardous Substances—toxicity. WA 465 H4285]
RA1211.H39   1992
615.9′02—dc20
DNLM/DLC
for Library of Congress   91-27784
                                             CIP

The publishers have made every effort to trace the copyright holders for borrowed material. If they have inadvertently overlooked any, they will be pleased to make the necessary arrangements at the first opportunity.

                        91 92 93 94 95
             1 2 3 4 5 6 7 8 9 10

To Kay, John, Katherine, and Sara Sullivan

and

To Larry, Jeanne, Taylor, and Lauren Krieger

for their patience

Foreword

Toxicology has a long history and a bright future! The evolution of hazardous materials into the workplace and the environment is a subject of great interest to health professionals. As can be seen from the scope and depth required in this text, the field of toxicology is interdisciplinary and intradisciplinary. The assessment of the potential for physical or chemical agents to produce effects on cells is enormous. A hazardous toxicology situation can begin in the workplace or as an acute toxic exposure of one individual and extend into our food, soil, air, and water. Primary care health professionals will be increasingly asked to make individual recommendations to patients as well as public policy decisions for our society concerning environmental health. This text will undoubtedly assist us by placing in one location the basic science, regulatory aspects, emergency response, and technical specificity for individual toxicants. The challenge to all health professionals is to utilize the information presented in this text so that we may make appropriate scientific decisions that aid individual patients and offer sound public policy that is cost-effective and health-protective.

Charles E. Becker, M.D.
Professor of Medicine, UCSF
Head, Division of Occupational Medicine and Toxicology
San Francisco General Hospital
Director, Center for Occupational and Environmental Health
University of California
San Francisco, California

Upon review of this book, I cannot help but reflect in awe on the long distance we have traveled in two decades in the field of toxicology and emergency medicine. In the early seventies when I first became involved in emergency medicine, there was essentially no access to information on the recognition, management, disposition, and outcome of most poisonings. The so-called poison centers were self-designated hospitals where a physician, usually a junior house officer, looked up the potential poisoning in an ancient textbook of toxicology. This made the house officer more expert than the caller, but it is frightening to remember the total ignorance of the system. One can only contemplate with horror the number of tragedies caused by mistreatment and undertreatment, and all due to overall ignorance.

In the late seventies when I was in Chicago, there was a chlorine spill from a Southside factory. At the emergency department at the University of Chicago, we received a phone call from a worried worker at the factory announcing the spill. He had no information about the gas, how many people were affected, and how many people would be affected. There were no physicians at the university who knew anything about chlorine gas, although one older physician remembered that it had been one of the poisonous gases in World War I. He thought he remembered that breathing through urine-soaked handkerchiefs might be protective.

Fortunately the prevailing winds blew the spill over Lake Michigan, but after the "dust had settled" it was estimated that there would have been over one million affected people and an unknowable number of deaths had the chlorine settled onto the populous Southside.

In the mid-eighties, there was a nitric acid spill in the city of Denver. Fortunately it occurred on a late Saturday night. Twenty-four hours later, it would have involved the Monday morning rush hour traffic. There were a small number of exposed people, and while the incident was frightening, it was controlled more by luck than by planning or wisdom.

Nevertheless, there was a significant difference between the possible responses to the two events—the involvement of the Rocky Mountain Poison Control Center as a resource. Five minutes after the spill was brought to my attention as the emergency physician on duty at Denver Health and Hospitals Emergency Department, the poison center specialist informed me of the potential medical problems, and the toxicologist on call provided a resource to utilize in advising the police and fire departments.

Bhopal and Chernobyl provided the world with the reality that industrial pollution of the environment is a very real possibility in any city. While these two tragic disasters may never be completely understood or duplicated and may never recur in the same fashion, what is frightening is the potential for occurrence. In trying to fathom a response, I have often been struck by the impossibility of the involved community to react to such a maxidisaster. I am also puzzled why it has not happened more often.

The present text is another example of the kind of resource that is developing as the medical community and the rest of society become more sophisticated and more interested in a response to the hazards of an industrial society. While I still wonder why it has taken so long to develop an appropriate response to emergencies, it is even more puzzling why there has been no general expertise in industrial hazards. Even with effective poison control centers, there is a paucity of information from within an industry, never mind from outside. The prehospital care and emergency medicine systems have to react rather than proact, and it is exciting to finally see an effort to bring some education and wisdom to this field before the disasters occur.

When I first looked at the Contents, I thought that it would require a special interest and background to appreciate this book. That this material would be beyond the general appreciation of the emergency physician, and even the toxicologist, seemed likely. But as I read the book, I found that the material covered things I had either encountered in the practice of emergency medicine, read about in disaster experiences from around the world, or wondered about in trying to understand the reactions to industrial pollution exposure.

The chapter on the psychologic stress syndrome induced by exposure is very timely since every emergency department frequently sees small clumps of workers who have been exposed to some noxious substance at work. If there is any public information about the exposure, such as radio or television announcements, one can confidently predict a small epidemic of psychosomatic presentation. The description of the syndrome would be valuable to every emergency physician.

This book will serve as an excellent resource, not only to the emergency department, but to the poison center as well. Every agency that has a role to play in the management of a disaster would profit from having the book as a resource to draw upon, both in the management of specific situations and in the preparations that go into disaster planning.

Even though this book is extensive, it is sure to miss some material that will be thought to be necessary. While this will be solved to some degree by future editions, the principles necessary for introduction to the topic and the specific management guidelines are well-presented in this first edition.

I still have anxiety about the form of industrial disaster that might occur within my own community, but just as the last two decades have produced the kind of information and training that makes it much more likely to survive a major life or limb threat, this book will provide a useful resource to help deal with the frightening and potentially overwhelming industrial disasters.

Peter Rosen, M.D.
Adjunct Professor of Medicine and Surgery
Department of Emergency Medicine
University of California, San Diego
San Diego, California

Preface

The medical toxicology of hazardous materials has become a major focus for an increasing number of health professionals. Emergency medicine physicians, poison centers, occupational medicine specialists, nurses, industrial hygienists, public health specialists, and emergency responders and planners are all intimately involved in the evaluation and analysis of hazardous materials exposures. The toxicology and potential health effects of these materials have linked this broad network of health professionals together. Over the last ten years, the scope and importance of hazardous materials toxicology has expanded beyond health professionals and impacts an enormous number of nonmedical groups such as financial institutions, city, state, and county planning boards, and private corporations.

Hazardous Materials Toxicology is an attempt to present the myriad actual and potential health implications of hazardous materials in a single reference textbook. The book is subtitled *Clinical Principles of Environmental Health* because we feel that there is an important synergy between environmental rules and regulations affecting hazardous materials and the medical evaluation of toxicity.

With hazardous materials toxicology, health professionals must have a dual perspective: (a) the direct health effects of a presenting individual, and (b) the ability to extrapolate from an affected individual patient to a potentially exposed group or population. Individual exposure requires a specific and immediate focus, while group and population effects can have serious public health implications.

Hazardous Materials Toxicology provides the individual perspective by initially presenting information on organ system toxicity and principles of immediate treatment and evaluation. The group or population viewpoint is organized in a series of sections on specific hazardous substances and general industries. While our primary focus has been directed toward North American rules and regulations, we have tried to provide and reference relevant international experience. We feel a dual approach will allow our readers an opportunity to explore the current toxicology of hazardous materials while simultaneously considering the broader environmental and public health issues of contamination and pollution.

Hazardous Materials Toxicology reflects our background with emergency medicine/poison centers and occupational/environmental medicine. While we are indebted to our co-authors, colleagues, and publisher, our primary appreciation is directed toward our families. With family support and patience, we have completed our goal.

John B. Sullivan, Jr., M.D.
Gary R. Krieger, M.D., M.P.H.

Robert Anderson, M.D., M.P.H.
Vice President, Science and Technology
Manville Sales Corporation
Denver, Colorado

John S. Andrews, Jr., M.D., M.P.H.
Assistant Director for Science
Agency for Toxic Substances and Disease Registry
Centers for Disease Control
Atlanta, Georgia

Marci Balge, R.N., M.S.
Occupational and Environmental Health Specialist
Program Director, Medical Surveillance
Dames & Moore
Denver, Colorado

Bryan Ballantyne, M.D., D.Sc., Ph.D., F.A.A.C.T., F.R.C.
Director of Applied Toxicology
Union Carbide Corporation
Danbury, Connecticut
Adjunct Professor of Pharmacology and Toxicology
West Virginia University
Morgantown, West Virginia

John R. Balmes, M.D.
Assistant Professor
Center for Occupational and Environmental Health
Lung Biology Center
Chest Service, San Francisco General Hospital
Department of Medicine
University of California, San Francisco
San Francisco, California

Donald G. Barceloux, M.D.
Associate Clinical Professor of Medicine
Department of Emergency Medicine
University of California at Los Angeles
Los Angeles, California

Gerry Bates, C.E.P.
Tucson Fire Department
Tucson, Arizona

Craig Beck, C.I.H.
International Health and Safety Manager
Dames & Moore
Denver, Colorado

John G. Benitez, M.D., F.A.C.E.P.
Clinical Toxicology Fellowship Director
Assistant Professor of Medicine
University of Pittsburgh
Pittsburgh, Pennsylvania

Neal L. Benowitz, M.D.
Professor of Medicine
Chief, Division of Clinical Pharmacology and Experimental
   Therapeutics
University of California, San Francisco
San Francisco

Alfred M. Bernard, Ph.D.
Research Associate of the Belgian Fund for Scientific
   Research
Unit of Industrial Toxicology and Occupational Medicine
Catholic University of Louvain
Brussels, Belgium

Jamie Blose, Pharm.D.
College of Pharmacy
University of Arizona
Tucson, Arizona

Ann Broderick, M.D.
Fellow in General Internal Medicine and Occupational
   Medicine
Department of Internal Medicine
The University of Iowa College of Medicine
Iowa City, Iowa

Alvin C. Bronstein, M.D., F.A.C.E.P., D.A.B.M.T.
Medical Director
Toxicology/Occupational Health Program
Boulder Community Hospital
Boulder, Colorado

Bradford O. Brooks, Ph.D.
Immunotoxicologist
Health Effects Research Department
IBM Corporation
Boulder, Colorado

William B. Bunn III, M.D., J.D., M.P.H.
Senior Director
Health Safety and Environment Department
Manville Sales Corporation
Denver, Colorado

Douglas Campbell, M.D.
Clinical Toxicology Fellow
University of Arizona Health Sciences Center
Tucson, Arizona

Dean E. Carter, Ph.D.
Professor
Department of Pharmacology and Toxicology
College of Pharmacy
University of Arizona Health Sciences Center
Tucson, Arizona

Gerald R. Chase, Ph.D.
Chief, Epidemiologist/Biostatistician
Manville Sales Corporation
Denver, Colorado

Kenneth H. Chase, M.D., F.A.C.P.M.
President
Washington Occupational Health Associates, Inc.
Washington, D.C.

Steven M. Chernow, M.D., F.A.C.E.P.
Assistant Professor of Surgery
Assistant Professor of Medicine
University of Colorado Health Sciences Center
Denver, Colorado

John J. Clary, Ph.D.
Bio Risk
Berkeley Heights, New Jersey

Marianne Cloeren, M.D., M.P.H.
Resident, Occupational Medicine
The Johns Hopkins School of Hygiene
Baltimore, Maryland

Elizabeth Criss, R.N.
Arizona Emergency Medicine Research Center
University of Arizona College of Medicine
Tucson, Arizona

Clifton D. Crutchfield, Ph.D., C.I.H.
Director
Industrial Hygiene and Environmental Health Services
University of Arizona
Tucson, Arizona

Steven C. Curry, M.D.
Department of Medical Toxicology
Good Samaritan Regional Medical Center
Phoenix, Arizona

Joseph Darcy, Ph.D., C.I.H.
Joe Darcy Associates
Kent, Washington

Richard C. Dart, M.D., Ph.D.
Assistant Professor
Section of Emergency Medicine
Associate Director, Arizona Poison Center
Co-Director, Clinical Toxicology Program
University of Arizona Health Sciences Center
Tucson, Arizona

Jou-Fang Dang, M.D.
Division of Clinical Toxicology
Department of Medicine
Veterans General Hospital
Taipei, Taiwan

Bradley Y. Dennis, M.D.
Medical Director
South Central Bell
Birmingham, Alabama

Heeten Desai, M.D., A.B.E.M., A.B.M.T., F.R.C.P.
Department of Emergency Medicine
St. Paul's Hospital
Vancouver, British Columbia, Canada

Samir M. Douidar, M.D., Ph.D.
Assistant Professor
Department of Pediatrics
Texas Tech University Health Sciences Center
Amarillo, Texas

Alan M. Ducatman, M.D., M.Sc.
Director, Environmental Medical Service
Massachusetts Institute of Technology
Cambridge, Massachusetts

Bill Durham
Fire Inspector
Hazardous Materials Unit
Tucson Fire Department
Tucson, Arizona

Jacek Dutkiewicz, Ph.D.
Institute of Agricultural Medicine
Lublin, Poland

Francis J. Farrell, M.D.
Adult and Pediatric Allergy
Watertown, New York

Christopher M. Filley, M.D.
Associate Professor of Neurology and Psychiatry
Department of Neurology
University of Colorado Health Sciences Center
Denver, Colorado

Don Fisher, M.D., M.S.
Medical Director
Occupational Health Network
Albuquerque, New Mexico

Gary Fujimoto, M.D.
Department of Occupational Medicine
Palo Alto Medical Foundation
Palo Alto, California

Lorne K. Garrettson, M.D., F.A.A.P.
Associate Professor of Pediatrics
Director, Section of Clinical Toxicology and Pharmacology
Emory University School of Medicine
Atlanta, Georgia

Edward C. Geehr, M.D.
Professor and Chairman
Department of Emergency Medicine
Albany Medical Center
Albany, New York

Robert J. Geller, M.D., F.A.A.P.
Diplomate, American Board of Medical Toxicology
Director and Medical Director
Georgia Poison Center
Assistant Professor of Pediatrics
Emory University School of Medicine
Atlanta, Georgia

David A. Gilmore, Jr., M.D.
Fellow, Clinical Pharmacology/Toxicology
University of Colorado Health Sciences Center
Denver, Colorado

Peter L. Goering, Ph.D.
Research Toxicologist
Center for Devices and Radiological Health
Food and Drug Administration
Rockville, Maryland

Harriet S. Goldman, D.D.S., M.P.H.
Chair, Department of Dentistry
Morristown Memorial Hospital
Morristown, New Jersey
Associate Professor of Clinical Dentistry
Columbia University School of Dental and Oral Surgery
New York, New York

Melissa Gonzales, M.S.
Industrial Hygiene
School of Health Related Professions
University of Arizona
Tucson, Arizona

William V. Gustin
Captain
Metro-Dade County Fire Department
Miami, Florida

Myron C. Harrison, M.D., M.P.H.
Medical Director
IBM Corporation
Purchase, New York

Gretchen Heins, B.S.
Senior Project Manager
Dames & Moore
Seattle, Washington

Thomas W. Hesterberg, Ph.D.
Senior Toxicologist
Manville Sales Corporation
Denver, Colorado

J. Michael Hitt, M.D.
Medical Director
Helian Occupational/Corporate Medical Center
Tucson, Arizona

Dana L. Hofstetter, B.S.E., M.A., S.D.
Associate, Holland & Hart
Boise, Idaho

John P. Holland, M.D., M.P.H.
Section of Occupational Medicine
Virginia Mason Medical Center
Seattle, Washington

L. D. Hooper, D.V.M.
Department of Pathology
Comparative Toxicology Laboratories
Kansas State University
Manhattan, Kansas

Katherine L. Hunting, Ph.D., M.P.H.
Research Assistant Professor
Division of Occupational and Environmental Medicine
The George Washington University Medical Center
Washington, D.C.

Katherine Hurlbut, M.D.
Fellow, Clinical Toxicology
Section of Emergency Medicine
Arizona Poison Center
University of Arizona Health Sciences Center
Tucson, Arizona

Richard D. Irons, Ph.D.
Professor
Molecular Toxicology and Environmental Health Sciences
    Program
School of Pharmacy
Professor
Department of Pathology
School of Medicine
University of Colorado Health Sciences Center
Denver, Colorado

James P. Kelly, M.D.
Instructor of Neurology and Psychiatry
Department of Neurology
University of Colorado Health Sciences Center
Denver, Colorado

James P. Keogh, M.D.
Associate Professor
Department of Occupational Medicine
University of Maryland School of Medicine
Baltimore, Maryland

Allen G. Kraut, M.D., F.R.C.P.C.
Assistant Professor
Department of Internal Medicine
Department of Community Health Sciences
University of Manitoba
Winnipeg, Manitoba, Canada

Edward P. Krenzelok, Pharm.D., D.A.B.A.T.
Director, Pittsburgh Poison Center
Children's Hospital of Pittsburgh
Professor
Schools of Pharmacy and Medicine
University of Pittsburgh
Pittsburgh, Pennsylvania

Gary R. Krieger, M.D., M.P.H., D.A.B.T.
Manager, Partner (Ltd.), Health Systems Group
Dames & Moore
Denver, Colorado
Adjunct Assistant Professor of Toxicology
Department of Environmental and Molecular Toxicology
University of Colorado
Boulder, Colorado

Donald B. Kunkel, M.D.
Medical Director
Samaritan Regional Poison Center
Department of Medical Toxicology
Good Samaritan Medical Center
Phoenix, Arizona

Jan A. Larson, B.A.
Environmental Health and Safety Manager
Ball Aerospace Systems Group
Boulder, Colorado

Robert R. Lauwerys, M.D., D.Sc.
Professor
Unit of Industrial Toxicology and Occupational Medicine
Catholic University of Louvain
Brussels, Belgium

Hon-Wing Leung, Ph.D., D.A.B.T., C.I.H.
Union Carbide Corporation
Danbury, Connecticut

Richard Lewis, M.D., M.P.H.
Occupational and Environmental Medicine
Cleveland, Ohio

Daniel F. Liberman, Ph.D.
Biohazard Assessment Officer
Massachusetts Institute of Technology
Cambridge, Massachusetts

Daniel C. Liebler, Ph.D.
Assistant Professor
Department of Pharmacology and Toxicology
University of Arizona College of Pharmacy
Tucson, Arizona

Christopher H. Linden, M.D.
Assistant Professor of Medicine
Division of Emergency Medicine
Director, Regional Poisoning Treatment Center
University of Massachusetts Medical Center
Worcester, Massachusetts

Michael Lipsett, M.D.
State of California
Department of Health Services
Berkeley, California

John A. Lowe, C.I.H.
Senior Environmental Scientist
Dames & Moore
Sacramento, California

Timothy C. Marrs, M.D.
Medical Division
Chemical Defense Establishment
Porton Down
Wiltshire, England

Melanie A. Marty, Ph.D.
Acting Chief, Air Toxicology Unit
California Department of Health Services
Berkeley, California

Michael A. McGuigan, M.D., C.M.
Associate Professor of Pediatrics and Pharmacology
Faculty of Medicine
University of Toronto
Medical Director
Ontario Regional Poison Information Centre
The Hospital for Sick Children
Motherisk Program
The Hospital for Sick Children
Toronto, Ontario

Geraldine C. Meinke, Ph.D.
Research Assistant Professor
Department of Microbiology and Immunology
University of Arizona Health Sciences Center
Tucson, Arizona

Jacqueline Messite, M.D.
Director, Office of Public Health
New York Academy of Medicine
Clinical Professor
Department of Environmental Medicine
New York University College of Medicine
New York, New York

Linda M. Micale, M.S.
Manager of Environmental Compliance
Dames & Moore
Tucson, Arizona

Linda H. Morse, M.D.
Chief, Division of Occupational Medicine and Employee
  Health Services
Santa Clara Valley Medical Center
San Jose, California

Larry L. Needham, Ph.D.
Chief, Toxicology Branch
Division of Environmental Health Laboratory Sciences
Center for Environmental Health and Injury Control
Centers for Disease Control
Atlanta, Georgia

Lee S. Newman, M.D.
Pulmonary Division and
Occupational and Environmental Medical Division
National Jewish Center for Immunology and Respiratory
  Medicine
Assistant Professor
Department of Medicine and
Department of Preventive Medicine and Biometrics
University of Colorado School of Medicine
Denver, Colorado

Frederick W. Oehme, D.V.M., Ph.D.
Department of Pathology
Comparative Toxicology Laboratories
Kansas State University
Manhattan, Kansas

Gary Pasternak, M.D., M.P.H.
Division of Occupational Medicine and Employee Health
  Services
Santa Clara Valley Medical Center
San Jose, California

Donald G. Patterson, Jr., Ph.D.
Chief, Dioxin and Related Compounds Laboratory
Toxicology Branch
Division of Environmental Health Laboratory Sciences
Center for Environmental Health and Injury Control
Centers for Disease Control
Atlanta, Georgia

Dennis J. Paustenbach, Ph.D., D.A.B.T., C.I.H.
McLaren Environmental Engineering
ChemRisk Division
Alameda, California

John M. Peters, M.D., Sc.D.
Professor and Director
Division of Occupational and Environmental Medicine
Department of Preventive Medicine
University of Southern California School of Medicine
Los Angeles, California

Karen K. Phillips, M.D., M.P.H.
Associate Medical Director
Barlow Occupational Health Center
Whittier, California
Clinical Instructor
Division of Occupational and Environmental Medicine
Department of Preventive Medicine
University of Southern California School of Medicine
Los Angeles, California

Paul D. Phillips, A.B., J.D.
Chairman, Natural Resources Department
Partner, Holland & Hart
Denver, Colorado

Steven Piantadosi, M.D., Ph.D.
Associate Professor of Oncology and Biostatistics
Director of Biostatistics
The Johns Hopkins Oncology Center
Baltimore, Maryland

Steven Pike, M.D., M.Sc.
President and Chief Executive Officer
EnviroMD, Inc.
Tucson, Arizona

Jacob L. Pinnas, M.D.
Associate Professor
Department of Internal Medicine
University of Arizona Health Sciences Center
Tucson, Arizona

Peter T. Pons, M.D., F.A.C.E.P.
Assistant Director, Emergency Department
Denver General Hospital
Assistant Professor of Emergency Medicine
Department of Surgery
University of Colorado Health Sciences Center
Denver, Colorado

William Powers, Jr.
Hines H. Baker and Thelma Kelley Baker Chair in Law
The University of Texas School of Law
Austin, Texas

Steven R. Radis
Senior Meteorologist
Dames & Moore
Santa Barbara, California

Ricardo E. Rodriguez, Ph.D.
Assistant Professor
Department of Chemistry
Texas Wesleyan University
Fort Worth, Texas

Neil L. Rosenberg, M.D.
Director, Center for Occupational Neurology and
    Neurotoxicology
Colorado Neurological Institute
Englewood, Colorado
Assistant Clinical Professor of Medicine
University of Colorado School of Medicine
Denver, Colorado

C. Ford Runge, Ph.D.
Director, Center for International Food and Agricultural
    Policy
Associate Professor
Department of Agricultural and Applied Economics
University of Minnesota
St. Paul, Minnesota

Richard F. Salluzzo, M.D.
Director
Department of Emergency Medicine
Albany Medical Center
Albany, New York

Lee M. Sanderson, Ph.D.
Center for Chronic Disease Prevention and Health Promotion
Centers for Disease Control
Atlanta, Georgia

Richard S. Schottenfeld, M.D.
Assistant Professor of Psychiatry
Yale University School of Medicine
New Haven, Connecticut

David A. Schwartz, M.D., M.P.H.
Assistant Professor of Medicine
Director, Occupational Medicine
Pulmonary Disease Division
Department of Internal Medicine
The University of Iowa College of Medicine
Iowa City, Iowa

Barbara Scolnick, M.D.
Medical Director of Corporate Care
Department of Occupational Medicine
Waltham Weston Medical Center
Waltham, Massachusetts

Donna L. Seger, M.D., F.A.C.E.P., A.B.M.T.
Assistant Professor of Medicine and Surgery
Division of Emergency Medicine
Department of Surgery
Vanderbilt University Medical Center
Acting Medical Director
Middle Tennessee Poison Control Center
Nashville, Tennessee

Caryl S. Shaver, M.D.
Section of Occupational and Preventive Medicine
Family and Community Medicine
University of Arizona Health Sciences Center
Tucson, Arizona

Peter G. Shields, M.D.
Laboratory of Human Carcinogenesis
Division of Cancer Etiology
National Cancer Institute
National Institutes of Health
Bethesda, Maryland

Dennis J. Shusterman, M.D., M.P.H.
California Department of Health Services
Berkeley, California
Division of Occupational Medicine
University of California, San Francisco
San Francisco, California

Claus-Peter Siegers, M.D.
Department of Pharmacology and Toxicology
Medical University of Lubeck
Lubeck, Germany

I. Glenn Sipes, Ph.D.
Professor and Head
Department of Pharmacology and Toxicology
University of Arizona College of Pharmacy
Tucson, Arizona

William M. Snellings, Ph.D.
Occupational Health and Product Safety Manager
Union Carbide Chemicals and Plastics Company, Inc.
Danbury, Connecticut

Wayne R. Snodgrass, M.D., Ph.D.
Associate Professor, Pediatrics and Pharmacology-
  Toxicology
Head, Clinical Pharmacology-Toxicology Unit
Medical Director, Texas State Poison Center
University of Texas
Medical Branch at Galveston
Galveston, Texas

Daniel Spaite, M.D.
Associate Professor
Section of Emergency Medicine
Medical Director, Air Care
University Medical Center
Arizona Health Sciences Center
Tucson, Arizona

Daniel A. Spyker, Ph.D., M.D., F.A.A.C.T.
Pilot Drug Evaluation Staff
Center for Drug Evaluation and Research
Food and Drug Administration
Rockville, Maryland

Charles E. Stewart, M.D., F.A.C.E.P.
Director of Research and Education
Spectrum Emergency Care, Inc.
Colorado Springs, Colorado

John B. Sullivan, Jr., M.D., D.A.B.T., F.A.A.C.T.
Medical Director, Arizona Poison Center
Director, Clinical Toxicology Program
Associate Professor
Section of Emergency Medicine
University of Arizona Health Sciences Center
Tucson, Arizona

F. William Sunderman, Jr., M.D.
Northeast Utilities Professor of Toxicology
Departments of Laboratory Medicine and Pharmacology
University of Connecticut Medical School
Farmington, Connecticut

Ana A. Taras, M.P.H.
Program Associate
Office of Public Health
New York Academy of Medicine
New York, New York

Douglas M. Templeton, Ph.D., M.D.
Department of Clinical Biochemistry
University of Toronto
Department of Biochemistry
The Hospital for Sick Children
Research Institute
Toronto, Ontario, Canada

David J. Thomas, Ph.D.
Assistant Professor
Department of Pediatrics
University of Nebraska Medical Center
Omaha, Nebraska

Theodore G. Tong, Pharm.D.
Professor, Pharmacy Practice and Pharmacology and
  Toxicology
College of Pharmacy
Executive Director
Arizona Poison Control Center
University of Arizona
Tucson, Arizona

Richard L. Urie, C.I.H.
Urie Environmental Health, Inc.
Golden, Colorado

Mark Van Ert, Ph.D., C.I.H.
Assistant Professor
Division of Community and Environmental Health
Director of Occupational Safety and Health Program
University of Arizona
Tucson, Arizona

Richard A. Versen, M.P.H., C.I.H.
Manager, Product Safety
Manville Sales Corporation
Denver, Colorado

George L. Voelz, M.D.
Laboratory Associate
Los Alamos National Laboratory
Los Alamos, New Mexico

Michael P. Waalkes, Ph.D.
Acting Chief, Inorganic Carcinogenesis Section
Laboratory of Comparative Carcinogenesis
National Cancer Institute-Frederick Cancer Research and
  Development Center
Frederick, Maryland

Zakaria Z. Wahba, Ph.D.
Food and Drug Administration
Division of Bioequivalence
Rockville, Maryland

Neill K. Weaver, M.D.
Consultant in Occupational and Environmental Medicine
Arlington, Virginia
Former Director, Medicine and Biological Science
American Petroleum Institute
Washington, D.C.

Larry Welch, Ed.D.
Assistant Professor of Psychiatry
Department of Psychiatry
Staff Neuropsychologist
Vanderbilt University Medical Center
Nashville, Tennessee

Laura S. Welch, M.D.
Associate Professor and Director
Division of Occupational and Environmental Medicine
The George Washington University Medical Center
Washington, D.C.

John A. Whysner, M.D., Ph.D.
Vice President
Washington Occupational Health Associates, Inc.
Washington, D.C.

Contents

Basic Science and Clinical Principles of Hazardous Materials Toxicology

Introduction to Hazardous Materials Toxicology

John B. Sullivan, Jr., M.D.
Gary R. Krieger, M.D., M.P.H.

HAZARDOUS MATERIALS AND HEALTH

It is estimated that 260 million tons of hazardous waste are produced yearly by approximately 14,000 generators in the United States alone (1). Over the last 20 years, the public, the government, and private producers of waste have initiated major efforts to address the myriad problems associated with hazardous materials and environmental pollution. These problems are local, regional, national, and global in terms of both generation and disposal. While the majority of significant hazardous materials exposures are occupationally related, the environmental exposure of populations has now become a major focus. Issues such as the location of waste treatment facilities, outdoor and indoor air pollution, the extensive environmental contamination by agricultural chemicals and pesticides, the disposal of chemical, medical, and radioactive wastes, and the health effects of hazardous waste sites have become targets of communities, politicians, environmental groups, and industries.

Environmental contamination and pollution of air, water, and soil in developing nations is recognized as a source of illness and mortality. As these nations struggle to modernize and apply technologies learned from the industrialized nations, pollution controls are being ignored. The extensive agricultural base of developing countries has been associated with widespread pesticide use and subsequent spread beyond points of application. Waste disposal practices in developing countries typically consist of dumping into rivers, water supplies, and landfills without proper waste containment or treatment. Third World and developing nations are also becoming the disposal sites of industrialized nations whose regulations and laws prohibit the disposal of some types of wastes.

Earlier approaches to solving contamination problems in the United States began with air and water pollution controls in the 1970s. Since the inception of antipollution programs, levels of air and water pollution have been drastically reduced. Industrial emissions of smoke, dust, and combustion products have been reduced to the point that acute health effects are now preventable. Carbon monoxide and lead emissions from automobiles have been reduced 80% in the air we breathe (2). However, environmental contamination involves much more than air and water pollution.

Hazardous materials must be viewed from the perspective of both the occupational and the environmental arena. The exposure of individuals as well as populations on a local, regional, and global scale must be a focus for the future. Government at all levels and businesses operating in national and international markets must be concerned with the effect of hazardous materials on the environment and on humans. The problems and consequences of hazardous material disposal, treatment, and generation have become economic, political, and social issues. Business and governmental policies relating to health effects, economics, and the ethics of hazardous waste generation, storage, and disposal on an international scale have to be formulated.

Hazardous materials and hazardous processes pose a present and future health risk. Health care providers at the community and national levels are frequently asked to comment and decide on the potential risk of a given chemical or industrial process. Traditionally, occupational medicine, toxicology, and environmental health have not received the high profile in medical colleges that is now becoming recognized as necessary. The vast majority of health care providers are ill-prepared to confront issues ranging from emergency medical response for hazardous materials releases to the potential for longterm health problems associated with hazardous materials exposure.

Since the advent of the Occupational Safety and Health Act in 1970, occupational injury from chemical exposures and other hazardous materials have become a focus of health care from the medical, legal, and regulatory standpoints. Occupational injuries and illness arising from exposures to chemicals are actually difficult to ascertain accurately. The Bureau of Labor Statistics indicates that the highest injury rates from all causes occur in the mining, agricultural, construction, and manufacturing industries (3). Most figures of injury from occupational sources are gross underestimates. In 1984, the Bureau of Labor Statistics estimated that 5.3 million work-related accidents and injuries occurred in the United States (3). Given the fact that workers switch jobs frequently and that a latency period is often involved in the development of an occupational illness, it is easy to understand why these injuries are underestimated.

In the 1980s, concern over environmental exposures to the public began to mushroom. Name recognition such as Love Canal, Three Mile Island, and Bhopal justifiably fed the fear that stored, used, produced, or disposed-of chemicals could have tremendous health and environmental effects. Even nature itself added to these fears with the eruption of Mount St. Helens and the disaster at Lake Nyos. These events gave way to more recent serious releases such as the Chernobyl nuclear disaster and the Alaska oil spill.

Agriculture, aerospace, mining, and chemical manufacturers have been targeted as industries that produce public exposure to a wide variety of pesticides, solvents, metals, and chemical waste sites around the country. Pollution of water with metals and solvents has increased the public's fear of cancer. Public and employee exposures and fears of toxic materials have inevitably led to a surging increase in toxic tort litigation.

For most physicians and other health care providers, the need to respond to, evaluate, and treat hazardous materials exposures represents their first introduction to this complex problem. For these reasons, we have organized this book around the basic knowledge of clinical toxicology and environmental health principles required to understand the issues of toxic exposure, prevention, treatment, and emergency response. An understanding of basic science concepts of toxicology, dose-response relationships, metabolism of chemicals to toxic intermediates, and antidotes is essential background. Principles of epidemiology, chemical carcinogenesis, target organ toxicology, and risk assessment are valuable guides to the health care provider in understanding the nature of chemical risks to humans. Environmental health and safety issues are presented to help the reader understand the complex relationship between the presence of a chemical in the environment and the potential health consequences. Since many problems confronting the physician arise from specific sites and specific chemicals, focused discussions keyed to these sites and chemicals are presented to aid in defining exposures, making diagnoses, managing the problems encountered, and preventing illnesses.

ENVIRONMENTAL LAW AND REGULATION

The history of regulation in the United States (Table 1.1) can be traced to public response and to the need for occupational and environmental response to increasing pollution, chemical spills, and a general fouling of the environment. Numerous laws have been enacted in response to concerns regarding hazardous materials and wastes. The sheer number of chemicals and hazardous substances is staggering. Health care providers, engineers, industrial hygienists, and environmental health specialists must be familiar with the alphabet of regulations: TSCA, RCRA, OSHA, SARA, FIFRA, CERCLA. These fundamental regulations cover hazardous materials from cradle to grave. Many of these distinct American laws have parallel foreign country equivalents, since American experience and scientific databases are used in the development of international safety and health regulations. The regulatory environment has seen the proliferation of a multitude of laws; however, the laws having the most impact regarding regulatory control over substances in the environment and disposal of hazardous materials are the following (4):

The Clean Air Act (CAA, 1970)
The Clean Water Act (CWA, 1972)
Safe Drinking Water Act (SDWA, 1974)
Federal Water Pollution Control Act (FWPCA, 1972)
Toxic Substances Control Act (TSCA, 1976)
Resource Conservation and Recovery Act (RCRA, 1976)

Table 1.1. Federal Laws Related to Exposures to Toxic Substances

Legislation	Administering Agency	Regulated Products
Food, Drug and Cosmetics Act (1906, 1938, amended 1958, 1960, 1962, 1968)	FDA	Food, drugs, cosmetics, food additives, color additives, new drugs, animal and feed additives, and medical devices
Federal Insecticide, Fungicide and Rodenticide Act (1948, amended 1972, 1975, 1978)	EPA	Pesticides
Dangerous Cargo Act (1952)	DOT, USCG	Water shipment of toxic materials
Atomic Energy Act (1954)	NRC	Radioactive substances
Federal Hazardous Substances Act (1960, amended 1981)	CPSC	Toxic household products
Poultry Products Inspection Act (1968)	USDA	Food, feed, color additives, and pesticide residues
Occupational Safety and Health Act (1970)	OSHA, NIOSH	Workplace toxic chemicals
Poison Prevention Packaging Act (1970, amended 1981)	CPSC	Packaging of hazardous household products
Clean Air Act (1970, amended 1974, 1977)	EPA	Air pollutants
Hazardous Materials Transportation Act (1972)	DOT	Transport of hazardous materials
Clean Water Act (formerly Federal Water Control Act) (1972, amended 1977, 1978)	EPA	Water pollutants
Marine Protection, Research and Sanctuaries Act (1972)	EPA	Ocean dumping
Consumer Product Safety Act (1972, amended 1981)	CPSC	Hazardous consumer products
Lead-Based Paint Poison Prevention Act (1973, amended 1976)	CPSC, HEW (HHS), HUD	Use of lead paint in federally assisted housing
Safe Drinking Water Act (1974, amended 1977)	EPA	Drinking water contaminants
Resource Conservation and Recovery Act (1976)	EPA	Solid waste, including hazardous wastes
Toxic Substances Control Act (1976)	EPA	Hazardous chemicals not covered by other laws, includes premarket review
Federal Mine Safety and Health Act (1977)	DOL, NIOSH	Toxic substances in coal and other mines
Superfund Amendments and Reauthorization Act (1986); Comprehensive Environmental Response, Compensation, and Liability Act (1981)	EPA	Hazardous substances, pollutants and contaminants at waste sites

Comprehensive Environmental Response, Compensation and Liability Act (CERCLA, 1980).

These laws regulate the environmental media of water, air, and soil, the health concerns of hazardous substances in the environment, and the generation, distribution, and use of toxic substances including pesticides (Table 1.2).

The Clean Air Act of 1963 provided guidelines and standards to control air pollution from vehicles as well as from stationary sources. National Ambient Air Quality Standards were established by the Clean Air Act, and states were given the authority and responsibility to carry out these regulations. The Environmental Protection Agency (EPA) also set standards for hazardous air pollutants from industrial sources and placed controls on automobile and truck emissions, as well as on gasoline content of lead and other additives.

The Federal Water Pollution Control Act of 1948 gave authority to the federal government to control improper discharge of hazardous wastes into rivers, lakes, and streams. This act eventually was extensively revised in 1972 to become what is known as the Clean Water Act. Standards for the direct discharge of industrial waste into water and for publicly held waste treatment facilities were set by the Clean Water Act. A federal permit system was devised to monitor these discharges. Costs of technologies to comply with pollution discharge regulations were also considered.

The Safe Drinking Water Act of 1974 set standards for piped drinking water quality. This act specifies minimal concentrations of identified contaminants such as arsenic, lead, mercury, cadmium, chromium, nitrates, bacteria, turbidity, and some chlorinated hydrocarbons, among others.

The Toxic Substances Control Act (TSCA) of 1976 provided laws to regulate the introduction of new chemicals into the market as well as those currently on the market in terms of health and environmental risks. TSCA specifies that the EPA must maintain an inventory of all chemicals manufactured or processed. This act is directed specifically at the inherent risk of the chemicals.

The Resource Conservation and Recovery Act of 1976 (RCRA) provided control over the disposal and generation of hazardous waste. It was basically an amendment to the Solid Waste Disposal Act of 1965. Whereas most of the other federal acts are oriented to control of pollutants in certain media such as water and air, RCRA is designed to regulate the actual problem of hazardous waste generation to its final disposal, including storage and transportation. RCRA is not specific for a certain environmental medium. RCRA actually was designed to regulate solid waste. However, due to the confining nature of the term "solid waste," the EPA broadened this definition to include hazardous waste.

The Comprehensive Environmental Response, Compensation and Liability Act of 1980 (CERCLA), also referred to as Superfund, became the basis for the cleanup of high priority hazardous waste dump sites around the nation. Under CERCLA, the EPA, other federal agencies, states, and private parties respond to hazardous materials releases, including oil spills in the framework of the National Contingency Plan. This plan calls for a ranking of toxic hazards, called the Hazard Ranking System (HRS). The HRS is required to accurately assess the relative risk of hazardous sites and facilities to human health and the environment.

The Federal Insecticide, Fungicide, and Rodenticide Act (FIFRA) regulates the manufacture, distribution, and use of pesticides. FIFRA requires registration of pesticides as either general use or restricted use. The EPA can recall or cancel pesticide registration for misuse, misapplication, adulteration, mislabeling, or adverse environmental impact.

Many of these regulatory acts have undergone changes from amendments through the years (Table 1.2). Occupational health and safety issues also have undergone many changes since the advent of the Occupational Safety and Health Act of 1970. Initially, the federal government focused on regulation and setting standards of exposure in the work environment. In the 1980s the emphasis for enforcement and worker protection was turned over to the voluntary compliance of the employer (6). The 1980s witnessed a reduction in funding for regulatory activities as well as a reduction in enforcement of regulations. In 1983, the Occupational Safety and Health Administration (OSHA) issued the Federal Communication Standard which required container warning labels and material safety data sheets for certain substances deemed to be toxic which are used in the work environment. Worker and environmental protection programs have been directed more by politics and litigation than by science and sound environmental health practices (5, 6). Right-to-know laws and federal regulations lost clarity because of the diverse number of agencies involved, jurisdictional conflicts, and overlapping responsibilities of different agencies.

On October 17, 1986, when President Reagan signed into law the Superfund Amendments and Reauthorization Act (SARA), this 5-year, $8.5 billion program provided the federal authority as well as the resources required to address the issues of hazardous waste site problems in the United States. Since the inception of the Superfund program in 1980, there have been more than 31,000 sites identified as potentially hazardous. Of these, approximately 9,000 sites have had completed investigations. A National Priorities List (NPL) has been established for sites with the greatest hazard potential.

However, as of 1989 only 1,224 sites had been placed on the National Priorities List. NPL sites are identified by their potential hazards to nearby populations, groundwater contamination, surface water contamination, or air pollution. It is estimated that there are 375,000 underground storage tanks that have been leaking that could contaminate ground water or have already done so (7). Since early 1989, the EPA has been able to begin remedial action on approximately 20% of the NPL sites (7). The time from site identification to start of clean-up operations averages 7–9 years (7). Superfund enforcement actions can require private parties to pay for or undertake activities at any Superfund site. The EPA and states can also recover from private parties costs associated with clean-up and monitoring. Superfund operated under a budget of $1.5 billion in 1989.

Removal actions are undertaken to stabilize or remediate hazardous waste sites. SARA allows up to $2 million and 12 months for such removal actions. However, the costs of remediation can be as high as $1 million an acre (5). Remediation activities have resulted in 18 NPL sites being removed from the list since 1988. Many of these waste sites require continuing monitoring, treatment of groundwater, and assessment. Remediation activities at hazardous materials sites could last decades, and costs could soar into the hundreds of billions of dollars (6).

HAZARDOUS SUBSTANCES AND WASTES

A hazardous substance has been broadly defined as a substance which upon exposure results or may result in adverse effects on health and safety of humans in an occupational setting (8).

Table 1.2. Summary of Environmental Health Laws and Regulations

Act	Authority, Enforcement, and Purpose
Clean Air Act, 1963 (CAA)	The EPA is charged with regulation of air pollutants from stationary and mobile sources. The CAA was passed in 1963 but had few enforcement provisions. The 1970 amendment to the CAA established National Ambient Air Quality Standards (NAAQS) to protect public health and welfare. The 1970 and 1977 amendments provided the legal authority and enforcement required. The individual states were given the responsibility to attain and maintain the standards set forth. Each state was required by the Act to submit an implementation plan to achieve NAAQS. The CAA 1970 amendment also set forth technology forcing provisions that set specific emissions limitations, this is known as New Source Performance Standards (NSPS). In 1977, the EPA set National Emission Standards for Hazardous Air Pollutants (NESHAPS) which was designed to set the standards for and regulate new as well as existing sources of designated hazardous air pollutants. The Clean Air Act prohibits the use of dispersion techniques or intermittent control devices for the control of air emissions. The CAA regulates vehicles that travel highways. The EPA insures compliance of automobile manufacturers for control of vehicle emissions and regulates the amount of lead and additives in gasolines.
Clean Water Act, 1972 (CWA)	Began as the Federal Water Pollution Control Act in 1948. It was revised in 1972 to introduce technology forcing effluent standards to make waters fishable and swimable. The CWA has as its purpose to provide federal assistance for construction of publicly owned sewage treatment plants, to regulate the discharge of pollutants from point sources, and to regulate spills of hazardous waste and oil. The 1972 amendment established standards (National Pollutant Discharge Elimination System, NPDES), for regulating direct discharge of pollutants into water in interstate as well as intrastate waterways. There were two deadlines for polluters, 1977 and a more stringent 1983 date. A 1977 amendment extended the 1977 deadline for industrial polluters if certain requirements were being met and extended the deadline for publicly owned treatment companies if noncompliance was the result of construction delays or lack of federal funding. Also, cost considerations regarding the best available versus the best conventional technology to employ to comply with standards was included. The CWA requires the EPA to set standards for the direct discharge of toxic pollutants into waterways, standards for pretreatment of waste that is discharged by a private company into publicly owned waste treatment facilities, and standards that regulate thermal pollution such as caused by power plants. A federal permit system was established to enforce water quality standards and effluent standards. Discharge without a permit or in violation of a permit could bring about sanctions.
Safe Drinking Water Act (SDWA), 1974	This Act provides for maximum contaminant levels in piped drinking water used for human consumption. Identified pollutants are: lead, arsenic, mercury, cadmium, barium, chromium, selenium, silver, nitrates, coliform bacteria, fluoride, turbidity, lindane, endrin, methoxychlor, trihalomethanes, toxaphene, radionuclides, 2,4-dichlorophenoxyacetic acid, and 2,4,5-trichlorophenoxyacetic acid. The SDWA is designed to protect human health from contaminated drinking water. Secondarily the Act is designed to protect the public by specifying the taste, color, odor, and other conditions of water for human consumption. Under the SWDA, individual states have the authority of regulation as well as enforcement. The EPA reserves the right to compel compliance through federal court if necessary. The EPA has emergency powers to take whatever necessary action to protect the public from contaminants that have entered the water system if the EPA finds that state authorities have not acted in a timely manner to relieve the threat to the public. Additionally, the EPA can employ what is termed, "Suggested No Adverse Response Levels," or SNARLS, to help guide regional EPA offices and states in setting levels of selected water contaminants. SNARLS are used as guidelines in determining imminent threats to human health.
Federal Insecticide, Fungicide, and Rodenticide Act (FIFRA, 1947)	FIFRA, amended in 1972, 1975, and 1978, regulates the production, use, and distribution of pesticides. Since 1970, the EPA has had the authority to regulate pesticides. Pesticide regulation first occurred in 1910 under the authority of the Insecticide Act. This Act protected the consumer against mislabeling and ineffective products. A pesticide is defined under FIFRA as any substance or mixture of substances that is intended for preventing, destroying, repelling, or mitigating any pest, and any substance or mixture intended for use as a plant regulator, defoliant, or dessicant. These include insecticides, fungicides, herbicides, dessicants, defoliants, nematocides, and rodenticides. FIFRA requires the registration of all pesticides with the EPA. Pesticides are classified as general use or restricted use. Restricted use pesticides can only be applied by licensed applicators. Along with the FDA, FIFRA establishes pesticide tolerance levels for agricultural products and foods. The EPA can force removal or discontinuation of a pesticide that is in violation of the Act. Individual states have the right, responsibility, and the authority to regulate pesticides under FIFRA. The EPA can always override the state if the state is not or cannot enforce the regulations.
Resource Conservation and Recovery Act, (RCRA), 1976	RCRA regulates the generation and disposal of hazardous waste. This is distinct from regulating an environmental medium such as air or water. RCRA grew out of amendments to the Solid Waste Act, 1965. RCRA gives a broad definition to the term solid waste and actually defines hazardous waste in terms of a waste or combination of wastes which may cause or contribute to an increase in mortality or an increase in illness or pose a present or potential hazard to human or environmental health. RCRA targets waste that is transported, stored, treated, or disposed of improperly. RCRA thus is a means to regulate the management of hazardous waste from generation to disposal. The EPA was required by RCRA to identify and list hazardous materials. In order to do so, RCRA provides a tracking system for the generators of hazardous wastes. Generators must keep records of their wastes and under RCRA are ultimately liable for the proper transport, storage, treatment, and disposal of these wastes.

Table 1.2.—*continued*

Act	Authority, Enforcement, and Purpose
Comprehensive Environmental Response, Compensation, and Liability Act, (CERCLA), 1980	Commonly referred to as Superfund, CERCLA was the result of federal legislation directed at compensation for cleanup of hazardous waste sites. CERCLA was designed to expedite remediation and reimbursement for cleanup activities. The Act created a fund to pay for the cleanup and remediation following the release of a hazardous substance that presents a public health threat. The Superfund consists of $1.6 billion dollars financed over a five-year-period by fees levied on petroleum (87.5%) and the remainder of the fund generated by tax revenue (12.5%). The concept of a "release" is central to CERCLA. A release of a hazardous material does not include occupational exposures, exhaust emissions, release of radioactive material from a nuclear accident, nor the normal application of pesticides. Governmental response is limited to six months or a sum of $1 million in expense, whichever comes first. Mandatory reporting is required for a release of any reportable amounts of hazardous materials. Fines exist if reporting does not occur.
Toxic Substances Control Act, (TSCA), 1976	TSCA regulates hazardous chemicals currently in existence as well as prevents chemicals from entering the market that may have an unreasonable risk to health or the environment. TSCA is directed at the inherent toxicity of the chemical. The Act mandates that the EPA maintain and publish a listing of chemicals manufactured or processed in the United States. Manufacturers are required to report to the EPA data concerning the uses, amounts produced, byproducts, number of exposed workers, and adverse effects of the chemical on the health of humans and the environment. Manufacturers and processors of new chemicals are required to give the EPA a 90-day notice prior to manufacturing or use. This notice must include data concerning health and environmental consequences and is also made available to the public. The EPA can require testing of chemicals. The EPA has the authority to prohibit use, production, processing, distribution, or disposal of a chemical. Labeling and proper recordkeeping are required.

Adapted and used by permission from: Castro, KM. Environmental health law, Chapt 8 in: Blumenthal D, ed. Introduction to environmental health. New York: Springer Publishing Company, 1985.

This definition ignores nonoccupational settings. The Environmental Protection Agency originally defined hazardous waste as a waste that poses a threat to human health or the environment when mismanaged (9). These definitions do not adequately cover the wide variety of circumstances and exposures that could potentially result in environmental contamination or health problems. Since the advent of these definitions as promulgated by the federal government, many states have expanded their definitions to include additional toxicity characteristics of wastes and substances and have named certain chemical hazards.

Title III of SARA established requirements for federal, state, and local governments to provide planning for chemical emergencies as well as for informing the public about chemicals stored, used, and released in communities. This law is known as the Emergency Planning and Community Right to Know Act (EPCRA). The law established structure at both state and local levels of government to assist communities in planning for chemical emergencies. This act requires business and other facilities in the community to provide information to the public on the variety of chemicals stored and requires release of information for over 300 chemicals. Businesses are required to report accidental releases and spills of extremely hazardous substances and hazardous substances regulated by the Comprehensive Environmental Response, Compensation, and Liability Act (CERCLA) to state and local response officials. Material Safety Data Sheets (MSDS) must be available to these officials. Inventories of these chemicals, as well as their location within the building structure, must be reported. EPCRA contains the following four main provisions with respect to a community's response and right to know concerning hazards:

1. emergency planning for chemical releases;
2. emergency notification of chemical accidents and releases;
3. reporting of hazardous chemical inventories; and
4. toxic chemical release reporting.

In addition, the law deals with trade secrets as well as disclosure of chemical information to the public and health care professionals.

There still remains a lack of basic preparation and education of health care agencies, hospitals, and providers with regard to toxic exposures, emergency medical response to hazardous materials releases, and management of the overall problem.

RISK

The intrinsic toxicity of a chemical is not as great an issue as the risk associated with its use or exposure. Actual risk and the perception of risk are a dichotomy that continues to fuel litigation as well as societal discontent and the public fear relating to hazardous materials. Assessment of risk to individuals and to society must account for potential harmful effects of chemicals to individuals, populations, and the environment. What constitutes an acceptable level of risk? What are the factors that must be considered in determining true risk and acceptable risk? Why is the public's perception of risk from chemical exposure at times at odds with commonly accepted scientific and medical views? For some individuals, risk is determined by the mere presence of a chemical or the perception of the presence of a chemical. The fear factor is a powerful force in the regulation of chemicals and constitutes an instigator of litigation. What will society accept as a reasonable level of exposure to some chemicals in order to enjoy a certain lifestyle? These are difficult questions. Considerations in assessing risk include benefits gained, availability of alternate chemicals, extent of public use, employment, economics, environmental effects, conservation of natural resources, and health effects on individuals as well as on populations.

It is important to realize that toxic chemicals and wastes are the products and ingredients of humans living and doing business. As compared with a natural disaster, toxic disasters can be either very visible, such as a chemical spill or an explosion, or can be as subtle, such as ground water contamination from chlorinated hydrocarbon solvents. Toxic disasters and chemical contamination are humanmade and usually derive from systems failure, human error, or faulty technology. Threats and fears concerning toxic hazards arise from a lack of understanding of the longterm effects of exposure and the extent of environmental contamination (10). Business managers must be aware of these fears as well as the source of these fears. The business manager thus has a true role in the education of workers and the public.

There is a widening difference between public opinion and science that is almost daily demonstrated in the lay press regarding environmental health issues. This treatment of the subject of risk sometimes drives a wedge between the public and the scientific community. Examples include the handling of asbestos in public buildings, the location of hazardous material treatment plants, and fear of a specific chemical substance in the environment. Scientists' and the public's perception of error is another example. Whereas a scientist is very concerned about hastily performed, unreplicated, uncontrolled experiments, the public seems to be more frightened of not detecting an effect. Thus the public has developed a general feeling that nothing should be introduced into commerce or the environment without first being proven to be absolutely safe. However, science is incapable of demonstrating absolute safety.

Fears of toxic exposure have escalated, and science, in the public's view, seems to be unable to resolve these fears adequately. Fear of illness following any exposure to a chemical, harmless or not, has increased the number of litigations and worker compensation claims. Fear of cancer, injury, and illness, even though no injury can be demonstrated or cause and effect found, can be compensated for with large monetary judgments.

As the public's perception of risk continues to clash with the scientific community's assessment of risk, emotion and perception will gain more credibility. Emotion and public perception are as real as scientific measurements but are certainly not as valid in describing the actual risk of a chemical.

THE ROLE OF TOXICOLOGY

A poison is an agent which has the capacity in and of itself, or when combined with another substance(s), or through metabolism to produce a deleterious effect in a biologic system. Almost any substance can be a poison or be toxic. There are many areas of toxicology which deal with poisons and hazardous substances, including the following:

clinical or medical toxicology
occupational toxicology
environmental toxicology
regulatory toxicology
biochemical toxicology
forensic toxicology
immunotoxicology
reproductive and genotoxicology
mutagenesis and carcinogenesis

Toxicologists cannot accurately predict the risk associated with an exposure to humans. Predicting human hazard using animal studies in the laboratory has been routinely accepted for years, but its validity is now being questioned (11). In vitro

alternatives to animal testing using tissue cultures are gaining in popularity. However, these in vitro methods are unlikely to replace the time-honored animal studies but instead will play an increasingly more important role (11).

The public demands certainty with little room for error from toxicology in determining health hazards (11). Toxicologists and other scientists are forced to extrapolate data to humans due to the obligation of regulatory agencies to act on populations at risk from exposures. Toxicology as a predictive science has developed because of the regulatory requirements imposed by society on society (11). Human risk data are gathered from many different sources including epidemiologic studies, animal studies, clinical cases of human exposure evaluation, and medical surveillance.

Human responses to toxic exposures may also help define certain disciplines of toxicology. The increased training in clinical toxicology and environmental health disciplines, along with the greater sophistication of laboratory assay methods and diagnostic techniques, has begun to allow for better definition and diagnosis of a toxic response or health effect in human exposures. These toxic responses can be biochemical, behavioral, carcinogenic, mutagenic, pathologic, physiologic, immunologic, or teratogenic.

Toxicology has the responsibility to be responsive to the needs of the individual and the public. Despite the fact that it does not and cannot have all answers and be precise in all tests, toxicology remains the discipline for the future anticipation of health and environmental effects.

THE YEAR 2000 AND BEYOND

What are the issues for the 21st century with regard to hazardous materials and health effects? In exploring past and present failures, a list of general areas deserving and in desperate need of attention from the government, business, academia, and the public sectors might read as such:

1. innovative technologies to reduce and further control wastes;
2. new disposal technologies;
3. global problems of generation and disposal of hazards;
4. better training for health care providers and environmental health professionals;
5. emphasis on prevention of exposures;
6. change in business policy regarding hazardous waste;
7. public policy changes regarding resource consumption;
8. changes in governmental policy regarding response to environmental contamination and human exposures in the work environment; and
9. revision of the toxic tort system.

The global expansion of population will continue. World population is now at 5 billion and is expected to double by the middle of the next century. The use of resources will continue to parallel population growth. Thousands of chemicals are in everyday use in industry and agriculture, and 500 to 1000 new chemicals are introduced each year into the market (2). While nations that are technologically advanced will continue to control and demand control of pollution and environmental contamination, developing nations will not. Traditional approaches to control are too expensive even for advanced nations. The expense associated with hazardous waste land disposal and incineration in the United States has risen from $250 per ton to $1500 per ton (2). The total cost of cleaning up hazardous waste sites on the Natural Priorities List in the United States is estimated to be in the billions of dollars. This is hardly affordable by any nation.

Many changes are required, not just in the developed nations, but globally. There must first be a willingness to conserve resources on an individual, community, and business scale (2, 5). Minimization of waste using innovative technologies to reduce waste production are needed within the business community. As economies become more global and nations develop economic interdependency, the business community must be willing to develop strategies that prevent or reduce the generation of waste, that allow recycling of materials, and that consume less resources. Business must also seek better ways to dispose of the hazardous waste generated. Land disposal and incineration technologies will have to be altered, and new methods such as biodegration of waste and the use of biodegradable disposable consumer products need to be developed. The current thinking of the business community must be reversed, and the mindset changed to focus on waste reduction, innovative disposal and waste reduction technologies, resource conservation, and changes in chemical content of raw materials. Also business will have to work more closely with communities and the government to address the health issues associated with global hazardous waste generation, control, and disposal. Innovative changes for social and economic reasons must be encouraged by business.

There is a need for better education of physicians, environmental health specialists, engineers, lawyers, and business managers. Educational changes at the primary, secondary, and graduate levels are needed in order to foster new habits. Innovative university curricula are needed that focus on environmental health and toxicology issues in a multidisciplinary fashion (3, 4). Development of cross-trained specialists in health policy, business management, and toxicology will allow knowledgeable individuals to be positioned at policy and decision-making levels of industry, government, and academia. Research in areas of pollution control, disposal, and waste minimization technologies should be encouraged and sponsored by private industry, citizen groups, and government. New methods in early identification of toxic exposures and disease prevention must receive attention from academic medical centers and universities. Development of a multidisciplinary team approach to occupational and environmental health problems for diagnosis and treatment can allow physicians, clinical toxicologists, industrial hygienists, and nurses to focus on health problems due to hazardous materials, control exposures, and prevent disease from occurring.

Governments of all countries will have to give status and authority to agencies which have the task of protecting the environment (2). The various responsible agencies within governments regarding energy production, economic development, agriculture, mining, and other resource development practices should be coordinated under a policy of environmental protection.

Opinions for reform in the litigation system with respect to toxic torts continue to circulate (12). Issues of medical causation have traditionally clashed with legal causation. Due to the uncertainty of toxicology, courts are forced to make decisions that science cannot regarding toxic exposures and presence or absence of disease.

Many changes are required in the manner in which we live and do business if we are serious about the control of hazardous materials in our environment and work.

REFERENCES

1. Simmons JE, DeMarini DM, Berman B. Lethality and hepatoxicity of complex waste mixtures. Environ Res 1988;46:74–85.

2. Cortese AD. Innovative approaches to protecting the environment in the 21st century. Toxic Substances J 1989;9:1, 1–9.

3. The cause for concern: an analysis of the problem. In: Role of the primary physician in occupational and environmental medicine. Washington, DC: Institute of Medicine, National Academy Press, 1988.

4. Wentz CA, Peters RW, Kavianian HR, Montemagno CD. The role of universities in hazardous waste management part I: teaching and research. Hazardous Waste and Hazardous Materials 1990;7:2, 211–221.

5. McCloskey M. Re-thinking how public interest organizations defend public health through pollution control in the United States. Am J Ind Med 1990; 17:755–760.

6. National Association for Public Health Policy; Council on Occupational and Environmental Health. Occupational safety and health legislative agenda, 1989. J Public Health Policy 1988;winter:544–555.

7. Abelson PH. Cleaning hazardous waste sites. Science 1989;246:4934.

8. U.S. Department of Labor, Occupational Safety and Health Administration. Hazardous waste operations and emergency response (29 CFR Part 1910). Fed Reg 1988;51:244.

9. Greer LE. Definition of hazardous waste. Hazardous Waste 1984;1:3, 309–322.

10. Erikson K. Toxic reckoning: business faces a new kind of fear. Harvard Business Review 1990;1:118–126.

11. Jackson SJ, Rhodes C, and Oliver GJA. Humane approaches to acute toxicity assessment of industrial chemicals. Toxic Substances J 1989;9:279–311.

12. Brennan TA. Would a federal judicial science board improve toxic tort litigation? Am J Ind Med 1990;17:761–771.

2

Basic Principles of Toxicology

Bryan Ballantyne, M.D., D.Sc., Ph.D.
John B. Sullivan, M.D.

INTRODUCTION

Toxicology and Hazard

Toxicology, essentially concerned with addressing the potentially harmful effects of chemicals, is a recognized scientific and medical discipline encompassing a very large number of basic and applied issues. Although only generally accepted as a specific area of knowledge and investigation for a few recent decades, its principles and implications have been widely appreciated. The Greek, Roman, and subsequent civilizations knowingly used certain substances and extracts for their lethality in hunting, protection, warfare, suicide, and homicide. Historical aspects of toxicology have been reviewed by Doull and Bruce (1980) and Dekker (1987) (1, 2). Currently, activity in toxicology is largely concerned with determining the biologic potential adverse effects from chemicals, both natural and synthetic, on biologic systems in order to assess hazard and risk to humans and lower animal forms, and thus define appropriate precautionary, protective, and restrictive measures. Substances of considerable practical or potential practical use in commerce, the home, the environment, and medical practice may present variable types of harmful effects. The nature of these effects is determined by both the physicochemical characteristics of the material and the pattern of exposure. For humanmade and human-used materials, a critical analysis may be necessary in order to determine the risk-benefit ratio for use in specific circumstances and what protective and precautionary measures are needed. Indeed, with drugs, pesticides, industrial chemicals, food additives, and cosmetic preparations, mandatory toxicology testing and governmental regulations exist.

Major and extensive rapid developments in the scientific basis and practice of toxicology have been obvious since the early part of the 1950s. These developments have resulted for a variety of reasons, principal among which are those listed in Table 2.1. Reflecting these developments has been a proliferation in the number of textbooks, monographs, and journals devoted to general and special aspects of toxicology; a proliferation of abstracting services related to toxicology information; the provision of courses at undergraduate and graduate levels dealing with general and specialized areas; and the establishment of a private industry devoted to toxicology testing and consultation. Along with these factors has been an increase in the number of professional organizations and certification boards specifically devoted to toxicology. As a consequence of the markedly expanded scope of toxicology, the number of differing subdisciplines, and the need

Table 2.1. Major Driving Forces for the Recent Expansion and Development of the Scientific Basis and Practice of Toxicology

- Exponential increase in the number of synthetically produced industrial chemicals
- Major increase in the number and nature of new drugs, pharmaceutical preparations, tissue-implantable materials, and medical devices
- Mandatory testing and regulation of chemicals used commercially, domestically, and medically
- Enhanced public awareness of potential adverse effects from xenobiotics (non-naturally occurring) to humans, animals, and the environment
- Litigation, principally as a consequence of occupation-related illness, unrecognized or poorly documented product safety concerns (including drugs), and environmental harm

for varying professional activities, the practice of toxicology may be subdivided and described by areas of major involvement and specialization; the major areas are shown in Table 2.2.

DEFINITION AND SCOPE OF TOXICOLOGY (Tables 2.1 and 2.2) (1, 2)

Toxicology is a discipline concerned with activities related to a study of the potential of chemicals, or mixtures of them, to produce harmful effects in living organisms. One overview definition proposed to cover the various facets of toxicology (3) is as follows:

Toxicology is a study of the interaction between chemicals and biologic systems in order to quantitively determine the potential for the chemical(s) studied to produce injury which results in adverse effects in living organisms, and to investigate their nature, incidence, mechanism of production, factors influencing, and reversibility of such adverse effects.

Within the scope of this definition, adverse effects are those that are detrimental to either the survival or the normal functioning of the individual or a biologic system. Inherent in this definition are the following key issues:

1. Chemicals, or metabolic products, must come into close structural and/or functional contact with tissue(s) or organ(s) for which they have a potential to cause injury.
2. When possible, the observed toxicity (or an endpoint reflecting it) should be quantitatively related to the degree of

Table 2.2.   Major Subspecialities of Toxicology

Specialty	Major Functional Components
Clinical	Causation, diagnosis, and management of established poisoning in humans
Veterinary	Causation, diagnosis, and management of established poisoning in domestic and wild animals
Forensic	Establishing the cause of death or intoxication in humans by analytical procedures and with particular reference to legal processes
Occupational	Assessing the potential of adverse effects from chemicals in the occupational environment and the recommendation of appropriate protective and precautionary measures
Product	Assessing the potential for adverse effects from commercially produced chemicals and formulations, and recommendation on in-use patterns, and protective and precautionary procedures
Pharmacologic	Assessing the toxicity of therapeutic agents
Aquatic	Assessing the toxicity on aquatic organisms of chemicals discharged into marine and fresh water
Toxinologic	Assessing the toxicity of substances of plant and animal origin, and substances produced by pathogenic bacteria
Environmental	Assessing the effects of toxic pollutants, usually at low concentrations, released from commercial and domestic sites into their immediate environment and subsequently widely distributed by air and water currents and by diffusion through soil
Regulatory	Administrative function concerned with the development of interpretations of mandatory toxicology testing programs and with particular reference to controlling the use, distribution, and availability of chemicals used commercially, domestically, and therapeutically
Laboratory	Design and conduct of in vivo and in vitro toxicology testing programs

exposure to the chemical (the exposure dose). Ideally, the influence of differing exposure doses on the magnitude and/or incidence of toxic effect should be investigated. Such dose-response relationships are of importance in confirming a causal relationship between chemical and toxic effect, in assessing relevance of the observed toxicity to practical (in-use) exposure conditions, and to allow hazard evaluations and risk assessment.

3. The primary aim of most toxicology studies is to determine the potential for harmful effects in the intact living organism, in many cases (and often by extrapolation) to humans.
4. Toxicologic investigations should ideally allow the following characteristics of toxicity to be evaluated:
   a. The basic structural, functional, or biochemical injury produced;
   b. Dose-response relationships;
   c. The mechanism(s) of toxicity, i.e., the fundamental chemical and biologic interactions and resultant aberrations that are responsible for the genesis and maintenance of the toxic response;
   d. Factors that may modify the toxic response, e.g., route of exposure, species, sex, formulation of test chemical, and environmental conditions;
   e. Development of approaches for recognition of specific toxic responses; and
   f. Toxic effect reversibility either spontaneously (healing) or by antidotal or other procedures such as treatment.

The word toxicity is used to describe the nature of adverse effects produced and the conditions necessary for their induction. Toxicity is the potential of a material to produce injury in biologic systems. For pharmacologically active and thera-

peutic agents (''drugs'') a description of the nondesired effects is most appropriately undertaken using the following specific terms:

Side effects: undesirable effects that result from the normal pharmacologic actions of the drug.
Overdosage: implication that toxicity, particular to the drug, will occur.
Intolerance: implication that the threshold dose to produce a pharmacologic effect is lowered; this may be a consequence of a genetic abnormality.
Idiosyncrasy: an abnormal reaction to a drug due to an inherent, frequently genetic, anomaly.
Secondary effects: those arising as an indirect consequence of the pharmacologic action of a drug.
Adverse drug interactions: adverse effects produced by a combination of drugs but not seen when the drugs are given separately at the same dose.

Toxicity (i.e., the potential to injure) evaluation must be clearly differentiated from the exercise of hazard evaluation, which is the evaluation of the likelihood that a given material will exhibit its known toxicity under particular conditions of use. The general approach used to assess hazards is by the following sequence for particular substances:

1. Search for all available health-related information on the substance and, if appropriate, substances of close chemical structure. This may include information on physicochemical properties, in vivo and in vitro toxicology, epidemiology, known occupational and domestic incidents, case reports, monitoring, and use patterns;
2. Detailed impartial review of information accessed, empha-

sizing those studies conducted by credible scientific standards and by relevant routes of exposure;

3. Interpretation of the credible and relevant literature in order to define toxicity, mechanism, dose-response relationships, and factors influencing toxicity.
4. Conclusions regarding potential adverse effects from the substance under specific conditions of use;
5. Definition of acceptable handling or use conditions and acceptable exposure to the substance with respect to immediate and longterm conditions of use;
6. Determination of the management of overexposure situations; and
7. Communication of the toxicology review, hazard evaluation, recommended protective and precautionary measures, and management of overexposures. Recommendations on additional information or investigations are desirable.

RISK ASSESSMENT

The process and understanding of hazard evaluation and of its scientific basis is now at a level where reliable interpretation and prediction can be made. Currently risk assessment is an important developing component of regulatory, environmental and occupational toxicology. It is the objective of risk assessment processes to assess the probability that adverse health effects will develop from known, or suspect, chemicals in the environment or workplace. Quantitative risk assessments are frequently conducted for worktime or lifetime exposure to low concentrations of chemicals. They are based on extrapolating dose-response relationships from animal studies or human data, to determine risk at known or anticipated range of occupational or environmental exposure dosages. The approaches are frequently employed to assess risk from carcinogens, teratogens, reproductively active substances, and genotoxic materials. At this time, there is insufficient information on mechanisms of toxicity for particular materials to allow scientifically valid, appropriate mathematical models to be developed for a specific toxic effect. The current method of extrapolation makes many assumptions which include: (a) the existence of thresholds for specific toxic endpoints, (b) linearity of dose-response relationships, (c) comparability of metabolism and pharmacokinetic parameters between species, (d) the interaction between xenobiotics and biologic systems at low concentrations, and (e) the statistical reliability and biologic variability resulting from the relatively small numbers of animals that may technically and ethically be incorporated into animal studies. Thus, with current mathematical approaches of data extrapolation, quantitative risk assessments should be regarded as "best guesses" for environmentally safe exposure dosages. The findings from quantitative risk assessment may result in risk management measures being undertaken. This involves the development and implementation of regulatory action, taking into account additional factors such as available control measures, cost-benefit analyses, and "acceptable" levels of risk.

DESCRIPTION AND TERMINOLOGY OF TOXIC EFFECTS

Before toxicity can develop, a substance must come into contact with a body surface such as skin, eye, or mucosa of the alimentary or respiratory tract; these are respectively, the percutaneous, transocular, oral, and inhalation routes of exposure (Fig 2.1). If harmful effects occur at the sites where a substance comes into initial contact with the body, they are referred to as local effects. If substances are absorbed from the sites of contact, they or their metabolites may produce toxic effects systemically. Many materials may produce both local and systemic toxicity. Also, since toxicity can depend on the number of exposures, an additional classification of toxic effects is those developing after a single (acute) exposure or after multiple (repeated) exposures. Repeated exposure can cover a wide time span; however, it is convenient to refer to shortterm exposure (not more than 5% life span), subchronic exposure (5–20% of life span), and chronic exposure (entire life span or a greater portion of it). Examples of toxic effects classified according to site and incidence of exposure are given in Table 2.3.

Toxicity also may be described as temporary (reversible or transient) or permanent (persistent). Latent (delayed-onset) toxicity exists when there is a period free from signs following an acute exposure. Cumulative toxicity involves progressive injury produced by successive exposures. Examples of toxicity by time scale are given in Table 2.4. Substances may also be classified and described by the primary tissue or organ that is the target for toxicity (hepatotoxic, nephrotoxic, neurotoxic, genotoxic, ototoxic, immunotoxic). A description of the toxicity of a material requires inclusion of whether effects are local, systemic, or mixed; nature and (if known) mechanism of toxicity; organs and tissues affected; and condition of exposure (including species, route, and number or magnitude of exposure).

NATURE OF TOXIC EFFECTS

The nature and magnitude of a toxic effect depends on the physicochemical properties of the substance, its metabolism, the conditions of exposure, and the presence of protective mechanisms. The latter factor includes physiologic mechanisms such as adaptive enzyme induction, DNA repair mechanisms, and phagocytosis. Some of the more frequently encountered types of morphologic and biochemical injury constituting a toxic response are tissue pathology (pathotoxicology), aberrant growth processes, altered biochemical pathways, or extreme physiologic responses such as the following:

Inflammation is a frequent local response to irritant chemicals or a component of systemic tissue injury. The inflammatory response may be acute, with irritant or tissue-damaging materials, or chronic, with repetitive exposure to irritants or the presence of insoluble particulate material. Fibrosis may occur as a consequence of the inflammatory process.

Necrosis, used to describe circumscribed death of tissues or cells, may result from a variety of pathologic processes induced by chemical injury, such as corrosion, severe hypoxia, tissue

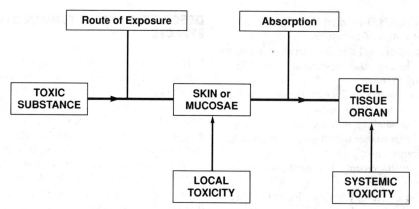

Figure 2.1. Basis for general classification of toxic effects.

Table 2.3. Examples of Toxicity Classified According to Time Scale and Site

Exposure	Site	Effect
Acute	Local	Skin corrosion
		Lung injury
	Systemic	Acute renal or hepatic injury
		Hemolysis
	Mixed	Lung injury and methemoglobinemia
	Local	Skin sensitization
		Lung sensitization
		Nasal septal ulceration
	Systemic	Neuropathy
		Liver injury
	Mixed	Respiratory irritation and neurobehavioral changes
Chronic	Local	Bronchitis
		Laryngeal carcinoma
	Systemic	Cancers of blood and solid tumors
	Mixed	Emphysema and kidney injury
		Pneumonitis and neuropathy

Table 2.4. Examples of Toxicity Classified According to Time Scale for Development or Duration

Time Scale	Effect Example
Persistent	Testicular injury
	Scarring (skin/eye)
	Pleural mesothelium
Transient	Narcosis
	Sensory irritation
Cumulative	Squamous metaplasia
	Liver fibrosis
Latent	Pulmonary edema
	Peripheral neuropathy
	Pulmonary fibrosis

damage, or reactive metabolite binding. With certain substances, differing patterns of zonal necrosis may be seen. In the liver, for example, chemicals may produce centrilobular necrosis or peripheral lobular necrosis (5, 6).

Enzyme inhibition by chemicals may affect biologic pathways, producing impairment of normal function. The induction of toxicity may be due to accumulation of substrate or to deficiency of product or function. For example, organophosphate anticholinesterases produce toxicity by accumulation of acetylcholine at cholinergic synapses and neuromuscular junctions. Cyanide inhibits cytochrome oxidase and interferes with mitochondrial oxygen transport, producing cytotoxic hypoxia.

Biochemical uncoupling agents interfere with the synthesis of high energy phosphate molecules, but electron transport continues, resulting in excess energy liberation as heat. Thus, uncoupling produces increased oxygen consumption and hyperthermia. Examples of uncoupling agents are dinitrophenol and pentachlorophenol.

Lethal synthesis occurs when foreign substances of close structural similarity to normal substances become incorporated into biochemical pathways are then metabolized to a toxic product. A classical example is fluoroacetate, which becomes incorporated in the Krebs cycle as fluoroacetyl coenzyme A, which combines with oxaloacetate to form fluorocitrate. The latter inhibits aconitase, blocking the tricarboxylic acid cycle, and results, particularly, in cardiac and nervous system toxicity (6).

Lipid peroxidation in biologic membranes by free radicals starts a chain of events resulting in cellular dysfunction and death. The complex series of events includes oxidation of fatty acids to lipid hydroperoxides, which undergo degradation to various products, including toxic aldehydes. The generation of organic radicals during peroxidation results in a self-propagating reaction (7). Carbon tetrachloride is metabolized by a hepatic cytochrome P-450-dependent monooxygenase system to trichloromethyl and trichloromethyl peroxy radicals; the former radical is probably involved in covalent binding to macromolecules, and the latter radical initiates the process of lipid

SCHEME	INITIATOR-PROMOTER RELATIONS	NEOPLASM
A	I	No
B	I P P P P P P P P	Yes
C	I P P P P P P P P P P	Yes
D	I P P P P P P P P P	Low/No
E	P P P P P P P P P P P P P P P	No
F	P P P P P P P P P P I	No
G	I I I I I I I I	Yes

Figure 2.2. Schematic representation of functional interrelationships between initiator and promotor in the two-stage mechanism of carcinogens. **A,** An initiating dose of a carcinogen is not by itself oncogenic. **B,** If initiator dose is followed by multiple applications of a promotor, neoplasia results (the classical initiator-promotor relationship). **C,** If promotion is delayed after initiation, a neoplastic response occurs, indicating persistent initiating process. **D,** If promotor dosing is infrequent or doses small, there may be neoplasia or a low tumor incidence, indicating a threshold for the promoting effect. **E,** Multiple applications of a promotor alone does not result in neoplasia. **F,** Initiation must precede promotion. **G,** A carcinogen may act as both initiator and promotor.

peroxidation leading to hepatic centrilobular necrosis. The zonal necrosis is possibly related to high cytochrome P-450 activity in centrilobular hepatocytes (8).

Covalent binding of electrophilic reactive metabolites to nucleophilic macromolecules may have a role in genotoxic, carcinogenic, teratogenic, and immunotoxic events. Important cellular defense mechanisms exist to moderate these reactions, and toxicity may not be initiated until these mechanisms are overwhelmed.

Receptor interaction, at a cellular or macromolecular level, with specific chemical structures may modulate the biologic effect (excitatory or inhibitory) mediated by the receptor.

Immune-mediated hypersensitivity reactions by antigenic materials are important considerations for skin and lung, which can result in allergic contact dermatitis and asthma.

Immunosuppression by foreign substances may result in altered host defense mechanisms, thus leading to infections.

Neoplasia is a major consideration in repeated exposure to carcinogens. Tumorigenesis and oncogenesis describe the development of neoplasms; the word carcinogenesis should be restricted to malignant neoplasms. In experimental and epidemiologic situations, oncogenesis may be exhibited as an increase in the total number of neoplasms, an increase in specific types of neoplasm, the occurrence of "rare" or "unique" neoplasms, or a decreased latency to detection of neoplasm.

Chemical carcinogenesis is a multistage process. The first and critical stage is a genotoxic event followed by other processes leading to the pathologic, functional, and clinical expression of neoplasia. One multistep model that has received considerable attention is the initiator-promotor scheme (Figure 2.2). The first stage, that of initiation, requires exposure to a genotoxic active material which results in binding of the ini-

tiator or reactive metabolite to cellular DNA. The second stage, that of promotion, permits the expression of the carcinogenic potential of the initiated cell. Promoting agents have the following characteristics:

- they do not need to be genotoxic;
- they are given by repeated exposure after initiation;
- they show some evidence for reversibility; and
- they may have a threshold for promoting activity.

Genotoxic initiators may also act as promoters after initiation. Substances causing or enhancing a carcinogenic process may cause DNA injury, and then exert oncogenic effects by mechanisms other than genotoxicity. Genotoxic materials acting directly with DNA are referred to as primary carcinogens; those requiring metabolic activation are procarcinogens, with the metabolically active electrophil being the ultimate carcinogen. Primary carcinogens include alkylene epoxides, sulfate esters, and nitrosoureas; procarcinogens include polycyclic aromatic hydrocarbons, aromatic amines, azo dyes, and nitrosamines.

Carcinogens include the following differing functional classes: promoters, cocarcinogens, hormones, immunosuppressives, and solid state materials. Cocarcinogens are materials which, when applied just before or with genotoxic carcinogens, enhance the oncogenic effect. Various mechanisms may be responsible for this enhancement, including increased absorption, increased metabolic activation of the procarcinogen, decreased detoxification, or inhibition of DNA repair. One particular group of carcinogens of considerable current interest are the peroxisome proliferators, which induce liver tumors in rodents. These materials characteristically produce hepatomegaly, cause hepatocyte peroxisome proliferation, and induce several liver enzymes including those of peroxisomal fatty acid β-oxidation system. Phthalate esters are one class of compound producing peroxisomal proliferation and experimental hepatocarcinogenesis (9). For genotoxic carcinogens, and for the purpose of risk assessment, it is usually assumed that a threshold for carcinogenesis does not exist.

Genotoxic chemicals which interact with DNA may be classified as clastogenic or mutagenic. Clastogenic effects occur at the chromosomal level and are visible by light microscopy. They may involve simple breaks, rearrangement of segments, or gross destruction of chromosomes. If severe, they may be incompatible with normal function, and cell death occurs. The relevance of chemically induced sublethal cytogenetic effects is not clearly understood but could lead to dysfunction of the reproductive system and tissues with rapid cell turnover rates.

Mutagenic effects are focal molecular events in the DNA molecule, which involve either substitution of a base-pair, or deletion or addition of a base. Base-pair transformations ("point mutations") may occur by direct chemical transformation, incorporation of abnormal base analogs, or alkylation. Addition or deletion of a base will result in a disturbance of the triplet code and, hence, alteration of the codon sequence distal to the addition or deletion ("frameshift mutation"). Intracellular DNA repair enzymes are present, but if the repair mechanism is exceeded abnormal coding will be transcribed into RNA and expressed as altered protein structure and possibly function, depending on the molecular segment affected. The relationship of chemically induced mutation to genetic abnormality is unclear. However, it is now generally accepted that in genotoxic carcinogenesis the molecular DNA event of initiation is fundamental to multistage oncogenesis. There is now considerable evidence showing a good correlation (with some test systems) between carcinogenic potential and mutagenic potential. Because of this, the use of certain mutagenicity test procedures has become widely accepted as a means of screening chemicals for their carcinogenic potential (10, 11).

Developmental and reproductive toxicity are, respectively, concerned with adverse effects on the ability to conceive and with adverse effects on the structural and functional integrity of the fetus up to and around parturition.

Adverse effects on reproduction may result from a variety of differing effects on reproductive organs and their neural and endocrine control mechanisms (12). Developmental toxicity deals with adverse effects on the fetus from the stage of zygote formation through the stages of implantation, germ layer differentiation, organ formation, and growth processes during intrauterine development and the neonatal period. The most extreme toxicity, death, may occur as preimplantation loss, embryo resorption, fetal death, or abortion. Nonlethal fetotoxicity may be expressed as delayed maturation, including decreased body weight and retarded ossification. Structural malformations (morphologic teratogenic effects) may be external, skeletal, or visceral. The preferential susceptibility of the fetus to chemical and other environmental insults in comparison to the adult state is related to: (a) small numbers of cells and rapid proliferation rates; (b) a large number of nondifferentiated cells lacking defense capabilities; (c) requirements for precise spatial and temporal interactions of cells; (d) limited metabolic capacity; and (e) immaturity of the immunosurveillance system (13). There is increasing awareness that functional, in addition to structural, malformations of development may occur. Malformation from chemicals may result from: (a) genotoxic injury; (b) interference with nucleic acid replication, transcription, or translation; (c) essential nutrient deficiency; and (d) enzyme inhibition. The most sensitive period for induction of structural malformations is during organogenesis: Functional teratogenic effects may be induced at later stages, particularly neurobehavioral malformations (14).

Pharmacologic effects may be induced by drugs and chemicals, and these may be significant as causes of temporary health problems as well as side effects of medication. For example, drowsiness or narcosis from acute overexposure to an organic solvent may clearly be of relevance in safe workplace considerations; such a reversible narcosis needs to be differentiated from central nervous system injury resulting from longterm low concentration exposure (15). Another important pharmacologic effect, particularly from airborne materials in the workplace, is peripheral sensory irritation. Materials having such effects interact with sensory nerve receptors in skin or mucosa, producing local discomfort and related reflex effects. For example, with the eye there is pain or discomfort, excess lachrymation, and blepharospasm; inhaled peripheral sensory irritants cause respiratory tract discomfort, increased secretions, and cough. Although many of these effects are warning and protective in nature, they are also distracting and can predispose to accidents. For this reason peripheral sensory irritant effects, along with other considerations, are widely used in defining exposure guidelines for workplace environments (16).

FACTORS INFLUENCING TOXICITY OF A CHEMICAL IN ANIMAL STUDIES

In animal studies the nature, severity, incidence, and probable induction of toxicity depend on a large number of exogenous and endogenous factors. Some of the more important are as follows:

Species and Strain. Species and strain differences in susceptibility to chemically induced toxicity may be due to differences in rates of absorption, metabolism, formation of toxic metabolites, and excretion. In some cases animal studies may give underestimates, and in other instances overestimates, for acute oral toxicity to humans. For example, the acute oral LD_{50} of ethylene glycol has been determined in several laboratory mammals to range 4.7–7.5 g/kg, and that for methanol to range 5.63–7.50 g/kg, both these chemicals have a greater toxicity to humans, with a minimal lethal dosage around 0.5–1.0 ml/kg (17, 18).

Age. With some substances age may significantly affect toxicity, probably mainly due to relative metabolizing and excretory capacities.

Nutritional Status. This may significantly influence the level of cofactors and biotransformation mechanisms important for the expression of toxicity. For example, diet may markedly influence the natural tumor incidence in animals and modulate carcinogen-induced tumor incidence (19). Khanna et al. (1988) studied the effect of protein deficiency on the neurobehavioral effects of acrylamide in rat pups exposed during the intrauterine and early postnasal stages. They found acrylamide more toxic in protein-deficient hosts (20). Feeding is an important factor in the design and interpretation of acute oral toxicity studies. For example acute oral toxicity of drugs may range significantly with a higher toxicity in starved animals. This greater acute toxicity in the starved animals may be due to accelerated gastric emptying and increased intestinal absorption. The importance of dietary factors in toxicity has been reviewed (21).

Time of Dosing. Diurnal and seasonal variations in toxicity may relate to circadian variations in biochemical, physiologic, and hormonal profiles.

Environmental Factors. A variety of environmental factors are known to influence the development of toxicity, including temperature, and relative humidity. The influence of temperature may vary between differing chemicals and the effects investigated. The influence of temperature on toxicity is clearly an important consideration in arctic and tropical areas.

Exposure (Dosing) Characteristics. The nature, severity, and likelihood of toxicity is influenced by the magnitude, number, and frequency of dosing. Thus, local or systemic toxicity produced by acute exposure may also occur by a cumulative process with repeated lower dosage exposures, and additional toxicity may be seen with the repeated exposure situations. For example, acute exposure to formaldehyde vapor causes peripheral sensory irritant effects and (with sufficiently high concentrations) injury and inflammatory change in the respiratory tract; shortterm repeated vapor exposure may result in the development of respiratory sensitization; longer term vapor exposure may cause squamous metaplasia and nasal tumors in animals (22). The relationships for cumulative toxicity by repetitive exposure compared with acute exposure may be complex, and the potential for cumulative toxicity from acutely subthreshold doses may not be quantitatively predictable. For example, the median lethal concentration (LC_{50}) for a 4-hour exposure to trimethoxysilane vapor is 47 ppm; by repeated exposure over a 4-week period (7 hr/day, 5 days a week) the LC_{50} is 5.5 ppm, with most deaths occurring during the first week and a 40% mortality at 5 ppm. Thus, the potentially lethal concentration for short-term repeated exposure is significantly lower than for acute exposure with trimethoxysilane. The irritant characteristics of the material would suggest this as a possibility, although the magnitude would not be accurately predictable. In contrast, exposure to benzene vapor for 26 hours (95 ppm) or 96 hours (21 ppm) produced severe bone marrow cytotoxicity, while a similar exposure dose given over a longer period of time (95 ppm for 2 hr/day for 2 weeks) produced little toxicity (23).

For repeated exposure, the precise profiling of doses may significantly influence toxicity. For example, with formaldehyde in a 4-week vapor inhalation study, it was determined that exposure of rats to 10 or 20 ppm by interrupted exposure over eight exposure periods produced more nasal mucosal cytotoxicity than did continual exposures (24).

Formulation and Presentation. For chemicals given orally or applied dermally, toxicity may be modified by the presence of materials in formulations that facilitate or retard the absorption of the chemicals. With respiratory exposure to aerosols, particle size significantly determines the depth of penetration and deposition in the respiratory tract.

Miscellaneous. A variety of other factors may affect the nature and exhibition of toxicity, depending on the conditions of the study, for example, housing conditions, handling, dosing volume. Variability in test conditions and procedures may result in significant interlaboratory variability in results of otherwise standard procedures.

BIOMETABOLISM AS A DETERMINANT OF SYSTEMIC TOXICITY

Systemic toxicity results from a complex interrelationship between absorbed chemical and metabolic products, distribution of parent compound and metabolites in body fluids and tissues, binding and storage characteristics, and excretion (Fig. 2.3).

Absorption. The absorption of a substance from the site of exposure may result from passive diffusion, facilitated diffusion, active transport, or the formation of transport vesicles (pinocytosis and phagocytosis). The process of absorption may be facilitated or retarded by a variety of factors. Elevated temperature increases percutaneous absorption by cutaneous vasodilation and surface-active materials facilitate penetration. The integrity of the absorbing surface is an important factor relevant to evaluation of hazards from chemicals contaminating the skin. Also, the concentration of the chemical in contact with the surface and the surface area of contact are important features relating to absorption.

Biodistribution. After absorption, materials circulate either free or bound to plasma protein or blood cells; the degree of binding, and factors influencing the equilibrium with the free form, may influence availability for metabolism, storage, or excretion. Within the tissues there may be binding, storage, metabolic activation, or detoxification; binding may produce a high [tissue]/[plasma] partition and be a source for slow redistribution into the circulation following the cessation of environmental exposure. Examples of storage sites include adipose tissue for lipophilic materials (including chlorinated pesticides), and bone for fluoride, lead, and strontium. The relationship between exposure dose and release rate may be complex; for example, volatile lipophilic materials are generally more rapidly released from tissues sites compared to nonvolatile lipophilic substances. Tissue permeability may be modified by tissue-specific barriers, such as the blood-stain barrier and placenta. (25).

Biotransformation. Metabolism of chemical substances is classified under two major transformation processes:

Phase I Reactions—A functional group is introduced into the molecule by oxidation, reduction, or hydrolysis.

Phase II Reactions—There is a conjugation of an absorbed chemical, or its metabolite, with an endogenous substrate.

For many materials there is an initial Phase I reaction to produce materials which are conjugated by Phase II processes. In other instances only a Phase II process may occur. Reactions of a Phase I type include oxidation, reduction, and enzymic hydrolysis; Phase II reactions include conjugation with glucuronic acid, sulfate, glycine, and glutathione, and acetylation and methylation. Phase I reactions may result in the formation of toxic metabolites from relatively innocuous precursors (metabolic activation). Phase II conjugates are generally more water soluble than parent compound or Phase I metabolites and hence more readily excreted. With toxic parent compounds or toxic metabolites, there may be conversion to less toxic products. Many activation reactions are catalyzed by a cytochrome P-450-dependent monooxygenase system in the liver. A major determinant of toxicity is the overall balance between absorption of a chemical, its metabolic activation and detoxification, and the excretion.

Excretion. Substances may be excreted as parent compound, metabolites, and/or Phase II conjugates. A major route of excretion is renal, and in some cases the urinary elimination of parent compound, metabolite, or conjugate may be used as a means for assessing absorbed dose. Some materials may be excreted in bile and feces; in such cases there may also be enterohepatic recycling of the parent compound or metabolite. Certain volatile materials and metabolites may be eliminated in expired air. The excretion of materials in sweat, hair, nails, and saliva is usually quantitatively insignificant, but these routes may be of importance for a forensic or occupational exposure diagnosis of intoxication (26, 27). Materials excreted in milk may be transferred to the neonate.

General Considerations. The probability of adverse effects developing in response to environmental chemical exposure depends particularly on the magnitude, duration, frequency,

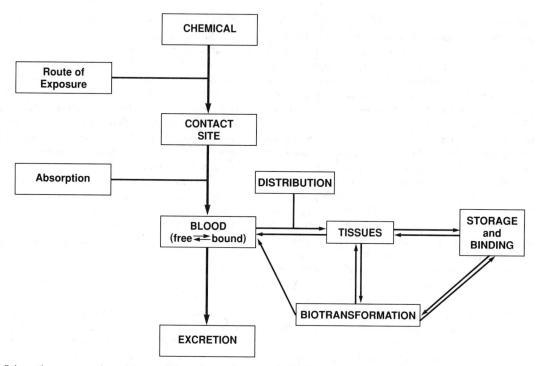

Figure 2.3.   Schematic representation of the possible pathways for a chemical absorbed from a primary contact site (route of exposure).

and route of exposure. These factors will determine the amount of material to which an organism is exposed (the environmental exposure dose) and hence the amount of material which can be absorbed (the absorbed dose). The latter determines the amount of material available for distribution and metabolite formation and thus the likelihood of producing a toxic effect. For a given environmental exposure the probability of inducing toxicity depends on the relationship between rate of absorption, metabolism (activation and detoxification), and elimination of parent compound and metabolites.

The amount of a chemical in contact with the absorbing surface is one of the principal determinants of absorbed dose. In general, the higher the concentration, the greater the absorbed dose. However, if mechanisms other than simple diffusion across a concentration gradient are operating, a simple proportionate relationship between concentration and absorbed dose may not exist. In such instances, a rate-limiting factor could result in proportionately smaller increases in absorbed dose for incremental increases in concentration at the absorption site. In particular when there is absorption by active transport, there may be saturation of the absorption process and a ceiling value.

When there is repeated exposure, the relative amounts of metabolites and the distribution and elimination of metabolites and parent compound may be different from that following an acute exposure. For example, repeated exposure may induce and enhance mechanisms of biotransformation of the absorbed material and thus alter the relative proportions of parent compound and metabolite. Also, if there is slow detoxification, storage, and/or slow excretion, repeated exposures may lead to the accumulation of toxic species and hence to a potential for cumulative toxicity.

ROUTES OF EXPOSURE

The primary route by which a material comes into contact with the body, and from where it may be absorbed in order to exert systemic toxicity, is the route of exposure. In the circumstances of environmental exposure the routes of exposure are by ingestion, inhalation, and dermal or eye contact. Also, for investigational, therapeutic, and certain forensic purposes, intramuscular, intravenous, and subcutaneous injections may be routes of exposure.

The relationship between route of exposure, biotransformation, and potential for toxicity may be complex and influenced by the magnitude and duration of the dose. Chemicals that undergo hepatic activation are likely to exhibit greater toxicity when given orally than if absorbed across the lung or skin, due to the high proportion of material passing directly via the portal vein following oral dosing. In contrast, chemicals that undergo hepatic detoxification are likely to be less toxic orally than when absorbed percutaneously or across the respiratory tract. However, in determining the influence of route of absorption on biotransformation and toxicity, both the magnitude and time scale for dosing should be considered. Thus, when a single large dose of a metabolically activated compound is given orally, its rapid metabolism may result in the development of acute toxicity. However, if the same material is given orally at much lower rates, then there will be slow and sustained absorption, and in such circumstances the rate of generation of the toxic species may approach that resulting from continuous exposure by other routes. With materials that are detoxified by the liver, a slow continuous alimentary absorption will result in an anticipated low toxicity, compared with other routes of exposure. However, an oral dose may result in the detoxifying capacity of the liver being overwhelmed, and unmetabolized material may enter the circulation to produce toxicity. Specific routes of exposure are as follows:

Oral. If a material is sufficiently irritative or corrosive, it will cause local inflammatory or corrosive effects on the upper alimentary tract. This can lead to fibrosis, dysphagia, and esophageal perforation with mediastinitis and/or peritonitis. Additionally, carcinogenic materials may induce tumor formation in the alimentary tract. The gastrointestinal tract is an important route by which systemically toxic materials may be absorbed.

Percutaneous Absorption. Skin contact is an important route of exposure in the occupational and domestic environment. Local effects may include acute inflammation and necrosis, chronic inflammatory responses, immune-mediated reactions, and neoplasia. The percutaneous absorption of materials can be a significant route for the absorption of toxic materials. Factors influencing the percutaneous absorption of substances include skin site, integrity of skin, temperature, formulation, concentration and, physicochemical characteristics such as molecular weight, hydrophilic and lipophilic characteristics of the material (28, 29).

Inhalation. The likelihood for toxicity from atmospherically dispersed materials depends on a number of factors, the most important of which include physical state, size, water solubility, concentration, and time and frequency of exposure. The water solubility of a gas or vapor influences the depth of penetration of a material into the respiratory tract. As water solubility decreases and lipid solubility increases, there is a more effective penetration toward the alveoli. Water-soluble molecules, such as formaldehyde, are deposited in the upper respiratory tract.

The penetration and distribution of fibers and particulates in the respiratory tract are determined principally by their size. Thus, in general, particles having a mass medium aerodynamic diameter greater than 50 μm do not enter the respiratory tract; those >10 μm are deposited in the upper respiratory tract; those having a range of 10–2 μm are deposited in the trachea, bronchi, and bronchioles; and only particles whose diameter is less than 1.2 μm reach the alveoli. Thus, larger insoluble particles are more likely to cause local reactions in the upper respiratory tract. The potential for alveolar injury and absorption is greater with smaller diameter particles (30, 31).

The likelihood that inhaled substances will produce local effects in the respiratory tract depends on their physical and chemical characteristics, solubility, reactivity with tissue components, and site of deposition. Dependent on the nature of the material, conditions of exposure, and biologic reactivity, the types of response produced include acute inflammation and injury, chronic inflammation, immune-mediated hypersensitivity reactions, and neoplasia. The degree to which inhaled gases, vapors, and particulates are absorbed, and their potential to produce systemic toxicity, depends on molecular weight, solubility in tissue fluids, metabolism by lung tissue, diffusion rate, and equilibrium state.

Eye. Local and systemic adverse effects may be produced by contamination with liquids, solids, and atmospherically dispersed materials. Local effects include transient inflammation, permanent injury, and hypersensitivity reactions. Penetration may lead to iritis, glaucoma, and cataract. Systemically active amounts of material may be absorbed from periocular blood vessels and/or nasal mucosa following passage down the nasolachrymal duct (32, 33).

EXPOSURE TO MIXTURES OF CHEMICALS

An evaluation of the hazards from exposure to multiple chemicals can be much more demanding than is the case for a single chemical. In assessing toxicity from mixtures it is important to consider: (a) chemical and/or physical interactions of the individual materials; (b) the effect that one chemical may have on the absorption, metabolism, and pharmacokinetic characteristics of another; and (c) the possibility for interaction between parent compound and metabolites (34). A convenient descriptive classification for effects produced by binary mixtures of chemicals is as follows:

Independent effect:	Substances qualitatively and quantitatively exert their own toxicity independent of each other.
Additive effects:	Materials with similar qualitative toxicity produce a response that is quantitatively equal to the sum of the effects produced by the individual constituents.
Antagonistic effect:	Materials oppose each others' toxicity, or one interferes with the toxicity of another; a particular example is that of antidotal action.
Potentiating effects:	One material, usually of low toxicity, enhances the expression of toxicity by another; the result is more severe injury than that is produced by the toxic species alone.
Synergistic effects:	Two materials, given simultaneously, produce toxicity significantly greater than anticipated from that of either material; the effect differs from potentiation in that each substance contributes to toxicity, and the net effect is always greater than additive.

In assessing the toxicity of mixtures, the following need to be taken into consideration:

- possible physical and chemical interactions—which may result in the formation of new substances or groupings or influence bioavailability;
- time relationships of the exposure for the various components;
- route and conditions of exposure;
- physical and physiologic factors affecting absorption;
- mutual influence of materials and metabolites on biotransformation, pharmacokinetic characteristics, and target organ doses of toxic species;

- relative affinities of the target sites; and
- potential for independent, additive, antagonistic, and interactive processes between the various chemical species.

Mixtures can be complex and in addition to parent materials, contain degradation products, contaminants and trace additives. It is important to be aware that small quantities of highly toxic materials may have equal or greater significance with respect to adverse health effects. For example, repeated exposure to small quantities of monomer residuals in polymeric materials, such as ethylene oxide, propylene oxide, vinyl chloride, and formaldehyde can produce serious health effects (3). The contribution to toxicity by trace materials is illustrated by the presence of trialkyl phosphorothioate or phosphorothionate impurities in organophosphate anticholinesterases and the presence of 2,3,7,8-tetrachlorodibenzodioxin in chlorophenols (35, 36).

Many instances of enhancement of toxicity by specific routes are known. Thus, on the skin the systemic toxicity of a material may be enhanced by other materials which facilitate percutaneous absorption. For example, the presence of a surface-active material may result in increased absorption; the presence of a primary irritant may produce local erythema resulting in increased skin blood flow, thus enhancing absorption and the presence of other materials may produce changes in ionization or solubility characteristics. If the viscosity of a material is increased, this may enhance local or systemic toxicity due to persistence on the skin.

The inhalation exposure of chemicals may be modified by the presence of sensory irritants, which can alter the rate and depth of breathing. Some substances may cause anosmia, and hence remove an olfactory warning for other inhaled materials. Particulates may adsorb other materials which can be inhaled. When trace quantities of highly volatile and toxic materials are present in a mixture, they may have significant influence on toxicity and hazard. For example, if materials containing trace amounts of acrolein are handled in stagnant air conditions, then potentially toxic air concentrations of acrolein may develop; in contrast, when there is free air flow the vapor components may be close to their relative concentration in a liquid mixture, and thus the acrolein air concentration may be low (37). Thus, the degree of ventilation of an area may significantly influence the toxicity of the atmosphere resulting from vaporization of the individual constituents of a liquid mixture.

The determinants of overall toxicity resulting from exposure to a mixture of chemicals can be very complex. Toxicity may be modified by prior or simultaneous exposure, resulting in enhancement or suppression of metabolic activation or detoxification pathways. Modification of toxicity may also result from alterations in pharmacokinetic characteristics, variation in the distribution of absorbed materials and metabolites, alterations in the elimination of the toxic species, and competition for binding sites or receptors. All the above factors will influence the relative and absolute concentration of toxic species at target sites (34, 38, 39).

NATURE, DESIGN, AND CONDUCT OF TOXICOLOGY STUDIES

Toxicology studies attempt to quantitate the potential for a chemical, or mixture of chemicals, to produce local and systemic adverse effects factors that may influence the nature, severity, and reversibility of effects. Specific features that any toxicology testing study should include are as follows:

- the nature of the adverse effects, or, the fundamental pathologic process (pathotoxicology);
- relationship of the adverse effects to use of the substance in normal and occupational situations;
- dose-response relationships (average, range, hyperreactive groups, no-effects and minimum effects doses);
- modifying factors;
- effects of acute overexposure;
- effects of repeated exposure (short- and longterm);
- recognition of adverse effects;
- definition of allowable and nonallowable exposures;
- definition of monitoring procedures;
- guidance on protective and restrictive procedures;
- guidance on first aid and medical management; and
- definition of "at-risk" populations (e.g., sex, preexisting disease, genetically susceptible.

Information necessary for the above can be obtained from carefully designed and conducted studies. In many cases, it may not be economically possible to undertake a complete spectrum of toxicology studies, and in such circumstances it is necessary to carefully consider the most appropriate studies based on known chemical properties, existing toxicology, and anticipated conditions of use. The relevance and credibility of a toxicology study can be no better than its design and conduct. For the purposes of hazard evaluation, there is a need to emphasize exposure conditions that may exist under practical conditions of use.

Toxicology testing generally begins with single exposure *in vivo* or *in vitro* studies and progress to evaluating the effects of long-term repeated exposures. Studies having specific endpoints, such as teratology and reproductive effects, are conducted as the emerging toxicology profile and end-use exposure patterns dictate. Toxicology testing procedures can be conveniently subdivided into general and specific. The general toxicology studies are those in which animals are exposed to a test material and are examined for a variety of toxic effects that the monitoring procedures permit. Specific toxicologic studies are those in which exposed animals, or *in vitro* test systems, are monitored for a defined endpoint.

General Toxicology Studies. Toxicology studies are usually conducted in the sequence of acute, short-term, subchronic, and chronic. Ideally, the protocol for general studies should include provision for some animals to be kept for a period after the end of dosing in order to determine the reversibility of toxic effects. Acute studies give information on toxicity produced by a single exposure, including the effects of massive overexposure; they also give information of use for setting exposure conditions for short-term repeated exposure studies. The type of monitoring employed in general toxicology studies will depend on the nature of the test material, its known toxicity, degree of exposure, and the rationale for conducting the test. In general, since multiple exposure studies are most likely to produce the widest spectrum of toxicity, it is usual to employ extensive monitoring in these studies. The monitoring employed to detect functional toxicity in the living animal, and for the detection of toxic injury in dead animals, may include the following:

- inspection, on a regular basis, for signs of toxic or pharmacologic effects;
- body weight before dosing and at appropriate intervals during the dosing phase;
- food and water consumption;
- hematology for assessment of peripheral blood and hematopoietic response;
- clinical (serum) chemistry and of specific enzyme activities and urinalysis;
- gross and microscopic pathology with organ weight measurement; and
- special pathologic or functional tests on a case-by-case basis.

Specific Toxicology Studies. Many of these procedures are directed at determining a particular toxic effect for hazard evaluation purposes, but others are employed as ''screening'' or ''short-term'' tests to assess the potential of a substance to induce toxic effects. Some of the most frequently employed toxicology methods are:

Primary Irritation. These studies are designed to determine the potential of substances to cause local inflammatory effects of the skin and eye. In order to reduce the use of animals for eye irritancy testing, a variety of alternative procedures have been proposed, which include the use of enucleated eyes, various in vitro cell or tissue cultures, and the measurement of corneal thickness (40, 41, 42, 43).

Peripheral Sensory Irritation. Methods to assess the potential of a chemical to cause eye or respiratory tract discomfort with associated reflexes are particularly useful in occupational toxicology (16).

Immune-Mediated Hypersensitivity. Allergenic materials may produce hypersensitivity reactions by skin contact or inhalation. There are many excellent resources describing tests to determine the potential for chemicals to produce allergic contact dermatitis or asthmatic reactions (44, 45, 46).

Neurologic and Behavioral Toxicity. To confirm the existence, nature, site, and mechanism of toxic injury to the central and/or peripheral nervous system, a variety of approaches with varying degree of sophistication are available. These include observational test batteries, light and electron microscopy, selective biochemical procedures, electrophysiologic, pharmacologic, tissue culture, and metabolism techniques (47–50).

Teratology. Most studies are currently directed at assessing the potential for chemicals to induce structural defects of development and essentially involve administering the test material to the pregnant animal during the period of maximum organogenesis (13, 51, 52). Recently, there has been increasing interest in the development of methods to assess for possible adverse functional effects resulting from exposure of the fetus in both early and late gestation (53, 54).

Reproductive Toxicity. Reproductive studies are conducted to assess the potential for adverse structural and functional effects on gonads, fertility, gestation, fetuses, lactation, and general reproductive performance. Exposure to the chemical may be over one or several generations. In view of the necessarily comparatively low doses used over these longterm stud-

ies, they may not be sufficiently sensitive to detect most potentially teratogenic materials (55–57).

Metabolism and Pharmacokinetics. These studies may be of considerable significance in the interpretation of conventional toxicology studies, determination of mechanism of toxicity, assessment of the relationship between environmental exposure concentration and target organ toxicity, and design of additional studies to elucidate mechanisms of toxicity. Metabolic studies should yield information on the biotransformation of a material, the sites at which this occurs, and the mechanism of biotransformation. Pharmacokinetic studies should allow a quantitative measurement of the rate of uptake, the absorbed dose, the biodistribution, tissue binding and storage, and routes and rates of excretion of test material and metabolites (58, 59).

Genotoxicity. A number of tests, both in vitro and in vivo, are available to assess the mutagenic or clastogenic potential of chemicals. A positive genotoxic result is not a directly usable endpoint, but it may assist in defining a potential for adverse health effects or be used in screening for potential toxicity. Thus, materials with clear mutagenic activity may be suspect of being genotoxic carcinogens, and appropriate further studies may be required. Clastogenic materials may be suspect of reproductive or hematologic toxicity.

The most widely used in vitro mutagenicity test has probably been that described by Ames which utilizes histidine-dependent mutants of *Salmonella typhimurium* (60). The bacteria are incubated in a medium deficient in histidine; if the added test chemical is genotoxic, it causes a reverse mutation to the histidine-independent state, which permits bacterial growth. Various mammalian cell culture preparations have been used to assess mutagenic potential. A commonly used test system is a forward gene mutation assay in Chinese Hamster ovary (CHO) cells with a strain that is deficient in the enzyme hypoxanthine-guanine phosphoribosyl transferase (HGPRT) and which confers resistance to toxic purine analogs such as 6-thioguanine and permits growth of the cells in a medium containing such substrates. The presence of a mutant chemical will restore sensitivity to the presence of purine analogs, and this may be used to assess mutagenic potential quantitatively. Clastogenic potential can be assessed in vitro by exposing cultured cells and subsequently examining them by light microscopy for chromosome damage. It is usual to conduct *in vitro* genotoxicity studies in the presence and absence of a metabolic activation system in order to assess the possible influence of metabolism on the mutagenic potential of the test chemical. Frequently employed is a homogenate of liver from animals given the polychlorinated biphenyl, Arochlor, which induces a broad spectrum of hepatic P-450-metabolizing enzymes.

In vivo genotoxicity studies can be conducted in a variety of ways. For example, the specific locus test in mice involves exposure of nonmutant mice to the test substance and subsequently mating them to multiple-recessive stock. Mutant offspring have altered phenotypes such as hair or eye color, ear length, or hair structure. Clastogenic potential can be assessed *in vivo* by exposure to the test chemical and subsequently examining mitotically active tissue, such as bone marrow, for chromosome injury.

Combustion Toxicology. This is an important practical aspect of the investigation of a substance, since it has been estimated that 50–75% of deaths occurring within a few hours of being exposed to a fire are the result of inhalation injuries and systemic toxicity (61). The primary aim of combustion toxicology is to determine the adverse effects produced as a result of heating or burning of materials. Although considerable emphasis has been placed on acute effects, there has been increasing concern about the longterm consequences of repeated exposure to the products of combustion in occupationally exposed individuals, such as firefighters. The design and interpretation of appropriate studies may be difficult because of the large number of variables that may affect the nature, concentration, and temporal characteristics of products of combustion. The major factors influencing the toxicity and hazard from a fire atmosphere include the nature of the materials available for heating or burning, the phase of the combustion process, temperature, air flow and oxygen availability, and potential for interaction between the combustion materials generated. All of these factors may be required to be investigated and considered in evaluating the continually changing hazard from a fire. Principal lines of investigation and sources of information about toxicity and hazards from fire atmosphere are as follows:

1. physicochemical studies to determine the nature of the products of combustion generated under differing conditions of temperature and oxygen availability;
2. animal exposure studies, in which the products of combustion, generated under differing conditions, are passed to inhalation exposure chambers and the animals examined for signs of toxic and pharmacologic effects, and appropriately monitored by physiologic, biochemical, hematologic, and pathologic techniques;
3. clinical and forensic observations on fire casualties to determine the nature and cause of morbidity and mortality from exposure to a fire atmosphere.

It is also necessary to be aware of the presence of materials that may produce sensory irritation or central nervous system depression. Irritant effects on the eye or narcosis may impede escape from a potentially hazardous situation. Polymers, which constitute a major component of commercial and domestic buildings, provide good examples of the generation of irritant, and neurobehavioral toxic chemical species on combustion (3).

Antidotal Studies. In addition to knowing the likelihood for spontaneous reversibility of toxic injury (i.e., biochemical and morphologic healing), it may be of practical importance to investigate the induction of reversibility of toxicity by antidotal procedures (62). Indications for such studies include high acute toxicity (including dose and time to onset of effects); serious but potentially reversible toxicity; indications that early treatment may reduce or abolish latent toxicity; suspicions of a potential for antidotal effectiveness based on mechanism of toxicity; and confirmation that antidotal treatment is effective for a similar chemical for which an antidote has already been established.

In addition to investigating specific antidotal therapy, it may also be necessary to confirm whether standard methods of management and support are effective in treating toxicity from particular substances or groups of materials.

REVIEW AND CRITICISMS OF TOXICOLOGY STUDIES

A critical review of particular toxicology studies requires detailed case-by-case considerations, but attention should be directed to the following:

- The laboratory or institution reporting the studies should have the necessary scientific and/or medical credibility, capabilities, experience, and expertise in the areas being investigated.
- The objectives of the investigation should be clearly stated, and the study protocol should reflect this in detail.
- The work should be reported in a clear and unambiguous manner, with all the necessary detail to allow the reader to perform assessment and conclusions about the study.
- Adequate quality control procedures and standards appropriate to good laboratory practices should have been followed.
- The material tested should be precisely defined, including stability, the nature and amounts of any impurities, conversion products, or additives.
- It should be confirmed that the methodology used for exposure and monitoring of the *in vivo* or *in vitro* studies is sufficiently specific and sensitive to allow the objectives and endpoints to be determined.
- Studies should be designed to allow a determination of the significance of the results and permit hazard and risk assessment procedures. The number of test and control animals should be sufficient to allow the detection of biologic variability in response to exposure, to allow trends to be appreciated, and to permit statistical analyses. There should be sufficient dose-response information to allow decisions on causal relationships and doses required to produce threshold effects and those not producing toxicity.
- Monitoring should allow a determination to be made of whether any injury produced is a direct consequence of toxicity or a secondary effect. A primary effect is one produced as a result of a direct toxic effect of a chemical, or metabolite(s), on a target organ or tissue. Secondary effects are those occurring, at another nontarget site, as a consequence of toxicity in the primary tissue or organ. For example, primary pulmonary injury produced by inhaled irritant materials may result in significant hypoxemia and secondary hypoxic injury to other organs including liver, kidney, or brain. The study should allow a conclusion to be made that the toxicity induced is a consequence of the action of parent material or metabolite.
- Detailed assessment is required to determine whether the numerical data have been appropriately and correctly evaluated. Although there may be a statistical significance between a test group and the controls, this may not be of biologic or toxicologic significance. Conversely, changes or trends, not of statistical significance, may be of biologic and toxicologic relevance. Quantitative information should be viewed against the study as a whole. Normal biologic

variability, quantitative changes which imply pathologic processes, and the magnitude of any changes as they may relate to an adverse effect should be accounted for.

The above considerations demand careful design of toxicologic studies, taking into account all factors inherent in the defined and inferred objectives of the investigation.

HAZARD EVALUATION AND RISK ASSESSMENT

Toxicology is concerned with defining the potential for a material to produce adverse effects, while hazard evaluation is a process to determine whether any of the known potential adverse effects will develop under specific conditions of use. Thus, toxicology is but one of the many considerations to be taken into account in the hazard evaluation process. The following are some of the other factors that need to be taken into account in defining whether a material will be hazardous.

- physical and chemical properties of the material;
- patterns of use;
- characteristics of handling materials;
- source of exposure and route of exposure, both normal and possible misuse;
- control measures;
- magnitude, duration, and frequency of exposure;
- physical nature of exposure conditions (solid, liquid, vapor, gas, aerosol);
- variability in exposure conditions;
- population exposed (number, sex, age, health status); and
- any experience and information derived from exposed human populations.

An approach to define the probability of adverse health effects developing from longterm, low-dose exposure is that of quantitative risk assessment. This approach attempts to quantitate the risk of adverse health effects developing in response to environmental exposure to chemicals and may result in the development and implementation of risk management programs (64). The quantitative information on which the mathematical analyses are based is commonly derived from laboratory animal studies and occasionally from epidemiologic studies. In deriving risk values for particular exposure situations many assumptions are made in calculating risks for human exposures. These include similarity between species in metabolism and pharmacokinetic characteristics and validity and relevancy of experimental conditions. In addition, the endpoint must be homogeneous in the population, and thresholds may not exist. Since many of these and other assumptions may be invalid, the calculated risk assessment values may only have partial scientific validity and as such are principally used for administrative purposes and guidelines by regulatory agencies. Clearly, the most reliable risk assessments are those based on information derived from both animals and humans with graded dose-response relationships and a knowledge of the comparative metabolism and pharmacokinetics of the material under consideration. Physiologically based pharmacokinetic modeling is being used, and becoming accepted, as a method for enhancing the scientific basis and facilitating the intelligent interpretation of data used for risk assessment purposes, thus allowing greater confidence in risk evaluation (65).

SPECIAL CONSIDERATIONS IN HUMAN HAZARD EVALUATION

Laboratory toxicology studies are conducted under highly controlled conditions using healthy animals of a particular weight range. The extrapolation of such information to a heterogeneous human population, with differing lifestyles and variable states of health, needs to be undertaken with considerable caution, taking into account all possible known and predictable variables.

Many personal habits, including diet and medications may influence response to a toxic chemical. Two factors that have received special attention are cigarette smoking and excessive alcohol consumption. In some instances, there are clear indications of significantly enhanced toxicity, for example, synergism between cigarette smoking and asbestos or radon (66, 67). Heavy alcohol consumption may lead to chronic progressive liver injury and thus increase susceptibility to hepatotoxic substances and impair detoxification pathways. Alcohol consumption may also interfere with metabolic transformation of certain chemicals such as toluene, xylene, and trichloroethylene.

Individuals with preexisting illnesses may be at greater risk from chemicals. For example, those with established cardiovascular disease may be at increased risk from exposure to carbon monoxide or methemoglobin-generating substances, since both may compromise available oxygen supply to the myocardium. Inhalation of irritant materials may aggravate chronic pulmonary disease.

Individuals with genetically determined biochemical variants may be at greater risk from certain chemicals. Persons with hereditary methemoglobinemia may generate significant amounts of methemoglobin at exposure doses of nitrites or aromatic amines which cause only minor methemoglobin concentrations in the normal population.

CONCLUSION

Knowledge of the basic concepts of toxicology is necessary to understand health effects secondary to hazardous materials exposure. In most occupational and environmental exposure situations, the dose of a substance is not known. In addition, there may be multiple exposures. Thus great difficulty may arise in predicting health effects. Defining the nature of these exposures is the critical first step in understanding medical causation from hazardous materials.

REFERENCES

1. Doull J, Bruce MC. Origin and scope of toxicology. In: Ed. Klaassen CD, Amdur MO, Doull J, eds. Casarett and Doull's toxicology. The basic science of poisons. 3rd ed. New York: Macmillan Publishing Co., 1980:3–10.

2. Dekker WJ. Introduction and history. In: Maley TJ, Berndt WO, eds. Handbook of toxicology. Washington, DC: Hemisphere Publishing Corporation, 1987:1–19.

3. Ballantyne B. Toxicology. In: Encyclopedia of polymer science and engineering, vol. 16. New York: John Wiley, 1989:879–930.

4. Clayson DB. The need for biological risk assessment in reaching decisions about carcinogens. Mutat Res 1987;1985:243–269.

5. Mehendale HM. Hepatoxicity. In: Haley TJ, Berndt WO, eds. Handbook of toxicology. Washington, DC: Hemisphere Publishing Corp., 1987:74–111.

6. Ballantyne B. The comparative short-term mammalian toxicology of phenarsazine oxide and phenoxarsine oxide. Toxicology 1978;10:341–361.

7. Horton AA, Fairhurst S. Lipid peroxidation and mechanism of toxicity. CRC Crit Rev Toxicol 1987;18:27–79.

8. Albano E, Lott KAK, Slater TF, et al. Spin-trapping studies on the free-radical products formed by metabolic activation of carbon tetrachloride in rat liver microsomal fractions. Biochem J 1982;204:593–603.

9. Rao MS, Reddy JK. Perioxisome proliferation and hepatocarcinogenesis. Carcinogenesis 1987;8:631–636.

10. Krisch-Volders M. Mutagenicity, carcinogenicity and teratogenicity of industrial pollutants. New York: Plenum Press, 1984.

11. Brusick D. Principles of genetic toxicology. New York: Plenum Press, 1985.

12. Barlow SM, Sullivan FM. Reproductive hazards of industrial chemicals. London: Academic Press, 1982.

13. Tyl RW. Developmental toxicity in toxicologic research and testing. In: Ballantyne B, ed. Perspectives in basic and applied toxicology. London: John Wright, 1988:206–241.

14. Rodier PM. Chronology of neuron development: animal studies and their clinical implications. Childh Neurol 1980;22:525–545.

15. World Health Organization. Chronic effects of solvents on the central nervous system and diagnostic criteria. Environmental Health Criteria Series No. 5. Copenhagen: World Health Organization, 1985.

16. Ballantyne B. Peripheral sensory irritation as a factor in the establishment of workplace exposure guidelines. In: Oxford RR, Cowell JW, Jamieson GG, Love EJ, eds. Occupation health in the chemical industry. Calgary: 1984:119–149.

17. Sweet DV, ed. Registry of toxic effects of chemical substances. Vol 3. U.S. Department of Health and Human Services. Centers for Disease Control, NIOSH, 1985:2360.

18. Sweet DV, ed. Registry of toxic effects of chemical substances. Vol 3. Ed. D.V. Sweet. U.S. Department of Health and Human Services. Centers for Disease Control, NIOSH 19:3060.

19. Graso P. Carcinogenicity tests in animals: some pitfalls that could be avoided. In: Ballantyne B, ed. Perspectives in basic and applied toxicology. London: John Wright, 1988:268–284.

20. Khanna VK, Husain R, Seth PR. Low protein diet modifies acrylamide neurotoxicity. Toxicology 1988;49:395–401.

21. Angeli-Greaves M, McLean AEM. Effect of diet on the toxicity of drugs. In: Gorrod AW, ed. Drug toxicity. London: Taylor and Francis, 1981:91–100.

22. Wartrew GA. The health hazards of formaldehyde. J Appl Toxicol 1983;3:121–126.

23. Toft R, Olofsson T, Tuneck A, et al. Toxic effects on mouse bone marrow caused by inhalation of benzene. Arch Toxicol 1982;51:295–302.

24. Wilmer JWGM, Wouterson RA, Appleman LM, et al. Subacute (4-week) inhalation toxicity study of formaldehyde in male rats: 8-hour intermittent versus 8-hour continuous exposures. J Appl Toxicol 1987;71:25–26.

25. Lu FC. Basic toxicology. Washington, DC: Hemisphere Publishing Corp., 1985.

26. Pashal DC, DiPietro ES, Phillips DL, Gunter EW. Age dependence of metals in hair in selected U.S. population. Environ Res 1989;48:17–28.

27. Randall JA, Gibson RS. Hair chromium as an index of chromium exposure of tannery workers. Br J Ind Med 1989;46:171–175.

28. Stuttgen G, Siebel T, Aggerbeck B. Absorption of boric acid through human skin depending on the type of vehicle. Arch Dermatol Res 1982;272:21–29.

29. Kemppainen BW, Reifenrath WG. Methods for skin absorption. Boca Raton, CRC Press, 1990.

30. Stanton MF, Layard M, Tegeris A, et al. Relation of particle dimension to carcinogenicity in amphobile asbestosis and other fibrous minerals. J Natl Cancer Inst 1981;67:965–975.

31. Asher IM, McGrath PV. Symposium on electron microscopy of micro-

fibers. Stock No. 017-012-002244-7. Washington, DC: U.S. Government Printing Office.

32. Shell JW. Pharmacokinetics of topically applied ophthalmic drugs. Surv Ophthalmol 1982;26:207–218.

33. Ballantyne B. Acute system toxicity of cyanides by topical application to the eye. J Toxicol Cut Ocul Toxicol 1983;2:119–129.

34. Ballantyne B. Evaluation of hazards from mixtures of chemicals in the occupational environment. J Occup Med 1985;27:85–94.

35. Hollingshaus JG, Armstrong D, Toia RF. Delayed toxicity and delayed neurotoxicity of phosphorothionate and phosphonothionate esters. J Toxicol Environ Health 1981;8:619–627.

36. Kimbrough RD, Falk H, Stehr P, et al. Health implications of 2,3,7,8-tetrachlorodibenzodioxin (TCDD) contamination of industrial soil. J Toxicol Environ Health 1984;14:47–93.

37. Ballantyne B, Dodd DC, Pritts IM, Nachreiner DS, Fowler EM. Acute vapor inhalation toxicity of acrolein and its influence as a trace contaminant 2-methoxy-dihydro-2H-pyran. Hum Toxicol 1989;8:229–235.

38. National Research Council. Principles of toxicological interactions associated with multiple chemical exposures. Washington, DC: National Academy Press, 1988.

39. World Health Organization. Health effects of combined exposures in the workplace. Technical Report Series No. 647. Geneva: World Health Organization, 1981.

40. Nardone RM, Bradlaw JA. Toxicity testing with in vitro systems: I. Ocular tissue culture. J Toxicol Cut Ocul Toxicol 1983;2:81–98.

41. Shopsis C, Sathe S. Uridine uptake inhibition as a cytotoxicity test: correlations with the Draize test. Toxicology 1984;29:195–206.

42. Borenfraund E, Borrero O. In vitro cytotoxicity assays. Potential alternatives to the Draize ocular allergy test. Cell Biol Toxicol 1984;1:55–65.

43. Ballantyne B. Applanation tonometry and corneal pachymetry for prediction of eye irritating potential. Pharmacologist 1986;28:173.

44. Goodwin RFJ, Crevel WRW, Johnson AW. A comparison of three guinea-pig sensitization procedures for the detection of 19 reported human contact sensitizers. Contact Derm 1981;7:248–258.

45. Maurer T, Weirich EG, Hess R. Predictive contact allergenicity influence of the animal strain used. Toxicology 1986;31:217–222.

46. Karol MH, Stadler J, Magreni C. Immunotoxicologic evaluation of the respiratory system: animal models for immediate and delayed-onset pulmonary hypersensitivity. Fundam Appl Toxicol 1985;5:459–472.

47. Gad SC. A neuromuscular screen for use in industrial toxicology. J Toxicol Environ Health 1982;9:691–704.

48. Spencer PS, Bischoff MC, Schaumburg HH. Neuropathologic methods for the detection of neurotoxic diseases. In: Spencer PS, Schaumburg HH, eds. Experimental and clinical neurotoxicology. Baltimore: Williams & Wilkins, 1980:743–757.

49. Abou-Donia MB, Lapadula DM, Carrington CD. Biochemical methods for the assessment of neurotoxicity. In: Ballantyne B, ed. Perspectives in basic and applied toxicology. London: John Wright, 1987:1–30.

50. Dewar AJ. Neurotoxicity testing. In: Gorrod JW, ed. Testing for toxicity. London: Taylor and Francis, 1987:199–218.

51. Tuchmann-Duplessis M. The experimental approach to teratogenicity. Ecotoxicol Environ Safety 1980;4:422–433.

52. Beckman DA, Brent RL. Mechanisms of teratogenesis. Annu Rev Pharmacol 1984;24:483–500.

53. Vorhees CV. Behavioural teratogenicity testing as a method of screening for hazards to human health: a methodological proposal. Neurobehav Toxicol Teratology 1983;5:469–474.

54. Zbinden G. Experimental methods in behavioural teratology. Arch Toxicol 1981;48:69–88.

55. Baeder C, Wickramarante GAS, Hummler H. Identification and assessment of the effects of chemicals on reproduction and development (reproductive toxicology). Food Chem Toxicol 1985;23:377–388.

56. Rao MS, Schwetz BA, Park CN. Reproductive risk assessment of chemicals. Vet Hum Toxicol 1987;23:167–175.

57. Mattison DR. Reproductive toxicology. New York: Alan R. Liss, 1983.

58. Oehme FW. Absorption, biotransformation, and excretion of environmental chemicals. Clin Toxicol 1980;17:147–158.

59. Gibaldi M, Perrier D. Pharmacokinetics. New York: Marcel Dekker, 1982.

60. Ames BN. The detection of environmental mutagens and potential carcinogens. Cancer 1982;53:2034–2040.

61. Ballantyne B. Inhalation hazards of fire. In: Ballantyne B, Schwabe PH, eds. Respiratory protection. London: Chapman and Hall, 1981:351–372.

62. Marrs TC. Experimental approaches to the design and assessment of antidotal procedures. In: Perspectives in basic and applied toxicology. London: Butterworth, 1988:285–308.

63. Tyler TR, Ballantyne B. Practical assessment and communication of hazards in the workplace. In: Ballantyne B, ed. Perspectives in basic and applied toxicology. London: John Wright, 1988:330–378.

64. Hallenbeck WH, Cunningham KM. Quantitative risk assessment for occupational and environmental health. Michigan: Lewis Publishing, 1986.

65. National Research Council. Pharmacokinetics in risk assessment. Washington, DC: National Academy Press, 1987.

66. Hammond EL, Selikoff JJ. Relation of cigarette smoking to risk of death of asbestos associated disease among insulation workers in the United States. In: Bogorski D, Timbrell JC, Wagner JC, Davis W, eds. Biological effects of asbestos. Lyon, France: IARC Scientific Publications, No. 8, 1973:312–317.

67. Archer VE, Wagner JR, Lurdin FE, Jr. Uranium mining and cigarette smoking effects in man. J Occup Med 1972;15:204–211.

68. Calabrese EJ, Moore GS, Williams P. The effect of methyl oleate ozonide, a possible oxone intermediate, on normal and G-6-PD deficient erythrocytes. Bull Environ Contam Toxicol 1987;29:498–504.

69. Doss MO, Columbi AM. Chronic hepatic porphyria induced by chemicals: the example of dioxin. In: Foa V, Emmett EA, Maroni M, Columbus A, eds. Occupational and environmental chemical hazards. Chichester: Ellis Horwood, Ltd., 1987:231–240.

3

Exposure-Dose-Response Relationships

Bryan Ballantyne, M.D., D.Sc., Ph.D.

INTRODUCTION

A fundamental concept in biology is that of variability. Individual members of the same species and strain differ to variable degrees with respect to biochemical, cellular, tissue, organ, and overall characteristics. Additionally, within a given individual there is a spectrum of variability in certain features, e.g., cell size and biochemical function within a particular cell series. A specific example, for erythrocyte diameter, is shown in Figure 3.1. The differences between individuals are usually a consequence of genetic factors. Since toxic effects are due to adverse effects on biologic systems or to modifications of defense mechanisms, it is not unexpected that the majority of toxic responses will also show variability between individuals. Also, because of genetic and biochemical variability, even larger discrepancies in response will be observed between species. It is axiomatic to the toxicologist that, within certain limits and under controlled conditions, there is a positive relationship between the amount of material to which given groups of animals are exposed and the toxic response. The response of a given animal may differ from that of other animals in the same dose group. As the amount of material given to a group of animals increases so does the magnitude of the effect and/or the number affected. For example, a specific amount of a potentially lethal material given to a group of animals may not kill all of them; however, as the amount of material is increased so does the proportion of animals dying. This reflects the variability in the studied population's susceptibility to the lethal toxicity of the test substance. Likewise, if an irritant material is applied to the skin, as the amount of material given epicutaneously is increased there will occur (a) an increase in the number of the population affected, and (b) for a given member,

the severity of the inflammation will increase as the applied dose increases. For the two examples given above, death is an "all-or-none" response (a quantal response), while inflammation may be considered from a dose-response viewpoint as having two elements: its presence and the degree of inflammation which represents a continuous (or graded) response. The above considerations, which reflect variability in biologic systems, form the basis for the fundamental concept of dose-response relationships in both pharmacology and toxicology. Usually there is a positive relationship between dose and response in vivo and in many in vitro test systems.

The amount of material to which an organism is exposed is a prime determinant of toxicity. The dose-response relationships for differing toxic effects produced by a given material in a particular species may vary. Thus dose-response relationships have to be carefully interpreted in the context of the effect and the particular conditions under which the information was obtained.

The word "dose" is most frequently used to denote the total amount of material to which an organism or test system is exposed; "dosage" defines the amount of material given in relation to a recipient characteristic (e.g., weight). Thus, dosage allows a more meaningful and comparative indication of exposure. For example, 500 milligrams of a material given as an oral dose to a 250-gram rat or a 2000-gram rabbit will result in respective dosages of 2 and 0.25 mg/kg. It follows that comparative dosing should be based on dosage units. Dose in most reports usually implies the "exposure dose." That is, the total amount of material given to an organism by the particular route of exposure. Another expression of dose is "absorbed dose," which is the amount of material penetrating into the organism through the route of exposure. Absorbed dose may show a closer quantitative relationship with systemic toxicity than exposure dose, since it represents the amount of material directly available for metabolic interactions and systemic toxicity. A further expression of dose is "target organ dose," which is the amount of material (parent or metabolite) received at the organ or tissue exhibiting a specific toxic effect. This should be expressed (if possible) in terms of the mechanistically causative toxin (parent chemical or reactive metabolite). Clearly target organ dose is a more precise quantitative indication of toxicity than exposure dose, since it is a measure of the amount of material at the site of toxicity, whereas exposure dose is total dose to the organism, and only a proportion of this (or metabolite) will ultimately gain access to the target site(s) for the toxic response. However, the estimation of target organ or tissue dose requires a detailed knowledge of the pharmacokinetics and metabolism of the material. For this reason, most information relates to the exposure dose. In most environmental and occupational settings, the exact dose of a chemical or chemicals remains unknown.

The exposure dose is of practical importance since it reflects the amount of material to which the organism is actually exposed and the likelihood of development of a particular toxic

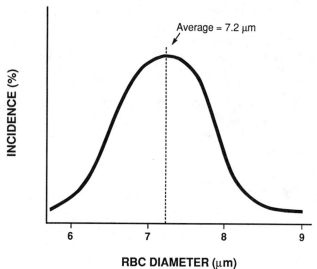

Figure 3.1. Frequency distribution curve for erythrocyte (RBC) diameter, showing a normal biologic distribution.

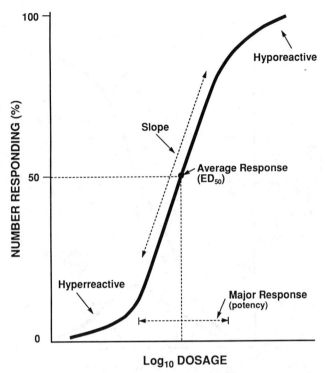

Figure 3.2. Typical sigmoid cumulative dosage-response curve for a toxic effect which is symmetrical about the average (50% response) point. The major response (potency) occurs around the average response. The slope of the curve is determined by the increase in response as a function of incremental increases in dosage. Hyperreactive and hyporeactive individuals are found at the extreme left and right sides of the curve, respectively.

endpoint. Absolute target organ doses allow a more detailed scientific evaluation of toxicity in relation to bioavailable chemical and, when related to exposure dose, may be used for rational risk assessment procedures.

If a material is capable of inducing several differing types of toxicity, the dose (or dosage) of material required to cause the individual effects may differ, with the more sensitive toxic effect appearing at the lower dosages. The first distinct toxicity, at lower dosages, may not necessarily be the most biologically significant effect. For example, with dermally applied materials, local inflammation may appear before systemic toxicity. Conversely, if the most significant toxicity occurs at lower dosages, then other toxicity at higher dosages may be overlooked.

NATURE OF THE DOSAGE-RESPONSE RELATIONSHIP

A given population has a quantitative variability in susceptibility to a chemical by individual members of that population. Thus, if groups of a genetically homogeneous population of animals of the same species and strain are given a particular material at different dosages, the proportion exhibiting a particular toxic effect will increase as the dose increases. This is shown schematically in Figure 3.2 as a cumulative frequency distribution curve, where the number of animals responding (as a proportion of the total in the group) is plotted as a function of the dosage given (as a $\log_{10}$ function). In many instances the resultant graph takes the form of a sigmoid curve, with a log normal distribution which is symmetrical about the mid-

point. This is typical dosage-response relationship, often referred to as a dose-response relationship. There are several important elements to this curve that require consideration when interpreting its toxicologic significance:

1. The majority of responding individuals do so symmetrically about the midpoint (i.e., the 50% response value). The position of the major portion of the dosage-response curve around its midpoint is sometimes referred to as the potency.
2. The midpoint of the curve (50% response point) is a convenient description of the average response and is referred to as the median effective dose for the effect being considered (ED_{50}). If mortality is the endpoint, then this is specifically referred to as the median lethal dose (LD_{50}). The median effective dosage is used for the following reasons: (a) it is at the midpoint of a log normally distributed curve; (b) the 95% confidence limits are narrowest at this point.
3. A small proportion of the population, at the left side of the dosage-response curve, responds at low dosages; this constitutes a hypersusceptible or hyperreactive group.
4. Another small proportion of the population, at the right side of the dosage-response curve, does not respond until higher dosages are given; this constitutes a hyposusceptible or hyporeactive group.
5. The slope of the dosage-response curve, particularly around the median value, gives an indication of the range of doses producing an effect. It indicates how greatly the response will be changed when the dosage is altered. A steep slope indicates that a majority of the population will respond over a narrow dosage range, while a flatter slope indicates that a much wider range of dosages is required to affect the majority of the population.

The shape of the dosage-response curve, and its extreme portions, depends on a variety of endogenous (as well as exogenous) factors, such as cellular defense mechanisms and reserves of biochemical function. Thus, toxicity may not be initiated until cellular defense mechanisms are exhausted or a biochemical detoxification pathway is near saturation. Also, saturation of a biochemical process which produces toxic metabolites may result in a toxicity plateau.

An important variant of the sigmoid dosage-response curve may be seen with genetically heterogeneous populations. In this situation, the presence of an usually high incidence in the hypersusceptible area could indicate the existence of a special subpopulation that has a genetically determined hypersusceptibility to the substance being tested (Fig. 3.3).

Data plotted on a dosage-response basis may be quantal or continuous. The quantal response is "all-or-none"; e.g., death. The graded, or variable, response is one involving a continual change in effect with increasing dosage, e.g., enzyme inhibition, degree of inflammation, or physiologic function such as heart rate. The dosage-response curve is often linearly transformed into a log-probit plot ($\log_{10}$ dose versus probit response) because it permits the examination of data over a wide range of dosages, and it allows certain mathematical procedures (e.g., calculation of confidence limits and slope of response) (Fig. 3.4). Quantal data can also be plotted as a frequency histogram or frequency distribution curve. This is done by plotting the percent response at a given dose minus the percent response at the immediate lower dose (i.e., response specific for the dosage). This procedure usually results in a gaussian distribution (Fig. 3.5), reflecting the differential biologic susceptibility of the test organism to the treatment. In such a normal

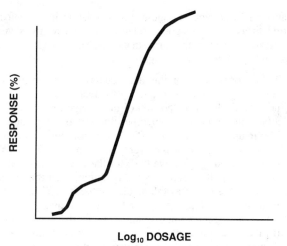

Figure 3.3.   Variant of the sigmoid cumulative dosage-response curve due to enhanced hyperreactive response; this may represent a genetic variant in a proportion of the population causing enhanced sensitivity to the toxic effect.

frequency distribution curve the mean ± 1 standard deviation (SD) represents 68.3% of the population; mean ± 2 SD represents 95.5%; and mean ± 3 SD is 99.7% of the population.

It is important to keep in mind that, with the exception of quantal responses, not only will the incidence of the effect of interest vary with dose and determine the dosage-response relationship, but the severity or magnitude of the effect will also change with varying dosage. Thus, for any given dosage producing a particular response incidence, those responding may show a difference in the magnitude of the effect.

Absence of a clear dosage-response relationship in a controlled experiment may indicate a nontoxic or nonpharmacologic action of the material. For example, an aminoalkyltrialkoxydisilane given by gavage to rats resulted in the following mortalities [expressed as (number dying)/(number dosed)]: 16 g/kg (4/5), 8 g/kg (0/5), 4 g/kg (3/5), and 2 g/kg (0/5). Clearly there was no dosage-response relationship in this study. Necropsy examination of rats that died showed that polymerization of the material had occurred in the stomach, producing a hard opalescent solid mass completely occluding the stomach. Thus, the cause of death was a consequence of

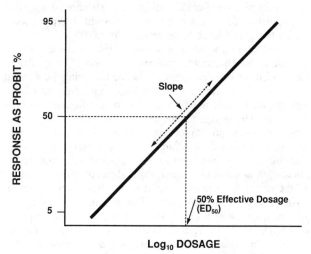

Figure 3.4.   Linear transformation of dosage-response data by log-probit plot.

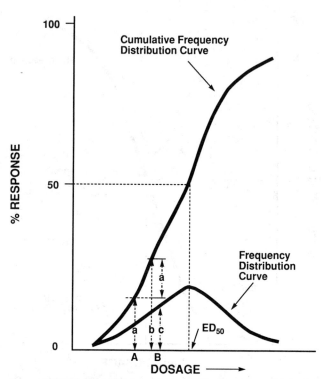

Figure 3.5.   Relationship between cumulative frequency distribution curve and normal frequency distribution curve for quantal data. The cumulative frequency distribution curve shows the proportion responding for each dosage and hence, the expected total response for any given dosage. The frequency distribution curve shows the response specific for that dosage compared with lower dosages. For the frequency distribution curve, the response, **c**, at any dosage (e.g., **B**) is obtained by taking the total response at that dosage, **b**, and subtracting the response, **a**, at the immediate lower dosage, **A**.

mechanical obstruction and nutritional deprivation, rather than of intrinsic toxicity.

For drugs, one convenient indication of "safety" often used is the ratio of the median effective dose causing death to that producing the desired therapeutic response (i.e., LD_{50}/ED_{50}); this is frequently referred to as the "therapeutic index" (TI_{50}). In general, the higher this ratio, the greater is the degree of safety with respect to lethality. However, considerable caution is needed in applying this information. For example, if the slopes of the dosage-response curves for drug effectiveness and lethality are parallel, then the assumption of an equal therapeutic ratio over a range of dosages and to a majority of the population is justified (Fig. 3.6). If, however, the dosage-response curve for lethality is shallower than that for the therapeutic response (Fig. 3.7), then there will be a decreasing therapeutic index at the lower dosages, and the hyperreactive groups may be at greater risk. One way to take into account differences in slopes is to calculate the ratio between that dosage causing a 1% mortality (LD_1) and that producing near maximum therapeutic efficacy (ED_{99}). This ratio, $[LD_1]/[ED_{99}]$ is referred to as the "margin of safety" (Fig.3.7). A complete appraisal of safety-in-use requires considerations of longterm and sublethal toxicity and, at the therapeutic dosages, the likelihood for side effects and idiosyncratic reactions.

The slope of the dosage-response relationship, particularly around the midpoint, can be of value for assessing hazard or potential for overdose situations. Thus, for lethality, a steep slope indicates that a large proportion of the population will

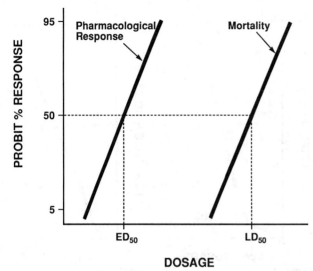

Figure 3.6. One simplistic method for assessing "safety ratios" for drugs is by comparing the ratio of the therapeutically effective dose (e.g., ED_{50}) and that mortality (LD_{50}); this ratio of $[LD_{50}]/[ED_{50}]$ is referred to as the therapeutic index (TI_{50}). For parallel pharmacologic effect and lethality dosage-response lines, the therapeutic index will be similar over a wide range of doses. However, nonparalled lines may give misleading conclusions if the TI_{50} is calculated (see Fig. 3.7).

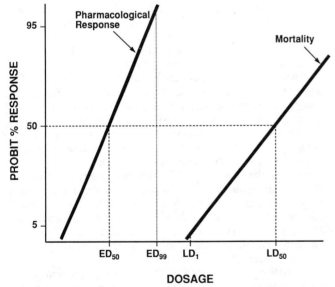

Figure 3.7. The TI_{50} may give a misleading index of drug safety if the dosage-response lines for pharmacologic and lethal effects are not parallel. In the example shown in this figure, there may be a reasonable margin based on LD_{50} and ED_{50}. However, due to the shallow slope of the mortality dosage-response line, the therapeutic index will be significantly lower at the 1% and 5% level, thus the hyperreactive group may be at greater risk. In this case a better index of safety will be the ratio of $[LD_1]/[ED_{99}]$, which is referred to as the "margin of safety."

be at risk over a small range of doses. Likewise, with a material producing central nervous system depression, a steep slope implies that a small incremental increase of dosage may result in coma rather than sedation.

In most cases of acute lethal toxicity, plotting the dosage-response information results in a log normal cumulative frequency distribution or gaussian frequency distribution. There may be two definite peaks in the frequency of distribution curve as opposed to an increase in hyperreactive groups at the left side of the dosage-response curve. Such a bimodal distribution may reflect different modes of lethality and latency. Earlier deaths at the lower dosages, producing the first phase of the bimodal distribution, represent a quantitatively more potent toxicity; those surviving the first phase toxicity may succumb to the higher dosage latent toxicity. One example of such a bimodal dosage-response for acute toxicity is provided by the anticholinesterase organophosphates: the first deaths are due to the cholinergic crisis resulting from acetylcholinesterase inhibition, and late deaths may result from delayed-onset peripheral neuropathy. In some cases log-probit plots will allow the determination of ED_{50} values for each subgroup in the bimodal distribution.

For many toxic effects, except genotoxic carcinogenesis, there is a dose below which no effect or response can be elicited; this corresponds to the extreme left side of the dosage-response curve. This dosage, below which no effect occurs, is referred to as the "threshold dose." The threshold concept, a corollary of the dosage-response relationship, is important in that it implies that it is possible to determine a "no-observable effect level" (NOEL), which can be used as a basis for assigning "safe levels" for exposure.

USE OF DOSAGE-RESPONSE INFORMATION

It is important to reiterate that conclusions drawn from dosage-response studies are valid only for the specific conditions under which the information was collected. Within this constraint, dosage-response information allows the following:

1. Confirmation that the effect being considered is a toxic (or pharmacologic) response to the chemical or therapeutic agent. Thus, a positive dosage-response relationship is good evidence that there is a causal relationship between exposure to the substance and the development of toxicity or pharmacologic effects.
2. Quantitative dose-response information allows the determination of an average (median) response, indicates the range of susceptibility in the population studied, and indicates where the dosage for hypersusceptible groups is expected.
3. The slope of the dosage-response curve gives information on the range of effective dosages and the differential proportion of the population affected for incremental increases in dosage. With a shallow slope the range of effective doses is widespread; the additional proportion of the population affected by incremental increases in dosage is small. In contrast, a steep slope implies the effective dose for the majority of the population is over a narrow range, and there will be a significant increase in the proportion of the population affected for small incremental increases in dosage.
4. The shape of the left side of the dosage-response curve may indicate the existence of an unusually high hypersusceptible proportion of the population. This may, for example, in-

dicate a genetically determined increased susceptibility to the chemical or pharmacologically active substance studied.

5. The data may allow conclusions on "threshold" or "no-effect" dosages for the response.

6. Quantitative comparison for a specific endpoint may be made between different materials with respect to average and range of response, particularly if the information has been collected under similar conditions.

The above considerations are illustrated in the following section devoted to lethality as the toxic endpoint for dosing.

DOSAGE-RESPONSE CONSIDERATIONS FOR ACUTE LETHAL TOXICITY

Since death is an "all-or-none" (quantal) response, it serves as a convenient example in discussing the collection, handling, interpretation, and use of dosage-response information. Death is an endpoint which has been incorporated as a major component of acute toxicity studies and is used for the calculation of LD_{50} values.

Acute lethal toxicity studies are conducted by giving differing dosages of the test material to groups of laboratory animals by a specific route of exposure and under controlled experimental conditions. Thus, animals of a particular species and strain, age, and weight are used; they are maintained under controlled conditions of diet, caging, temperature, relative humidity, and time of dosing. Following dosing, the number of mortalities at each dosage is recorded over a specified period of time, usually 14 days. When materials are given by dermal application, it is important to state the contact time with skin, and whether occluded or nonoccluded conditions are used. Clearly the degree of local injury and the potential for percutaneous systemic toxicity are functions of both the amount (or concentration) of test material applied and the duration of contact with the skin. For routes of exposure other than inhalation, the exposure dosage is usually expressed as mass (or volume) of test material given per unit of body weight; e.g., ml/kg^{-1} or mg/kg. For inhalation, the exposure dose is expressed as the amount of test material present for unit volume of exposure atmosphere; mg/m^3 or parts per million (ppm). It is also important for the inhalation route of exposure that the exposure time, as well as exposure concentration, be specified. The total inhalation exposure dose for a given atmospheric concentration of a specific material will depend on time. The longer the time, the greater the inhalation exposure dose and the higher the potential for adverse effects. Dose-response information collected for differing concentrations of an atmospherically dispersed material should be over similar periods of time in order to allow the most effective comparisons to be made. Alternatively, the effect of differing inhalation exposure doses can be made by exposing different groups to the same concentration of test substance for various exposure periods; this may allow the calculation of a median time to death (50% response rate) for the population exposed to a specific atmospheric concentration of test material (LT_{50}). By using both these approaches it is possible to reach conclusions on the differential sensitivity of a population to varying concentrations for a specified period of time or to differing exposure periods for a given concentration (LC_{50}).

Dosage-mortality data usually conform to the sigmoid cumulative frequency distribution curve (Fig. 3.8A). For comparative and statistical purposes, this may be converted to a

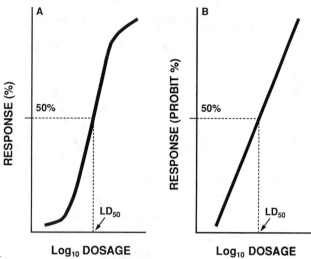

Figure 3.8.   Dosage-mortality data plotted as a cumulative frequency distribution curve (% response versus $\log_{10}$ dosage) in **A**, and linearly transformed by log-probit plot in **B**.

linear form using a log-probit plot (Fig. 3.8B). Lethal toxicity is usually initially calculated and compared at a specific mortality level; the most frequently used reference point is that dosage which causes 50% mortality in the population studied, since this represents the midpoint of the dosage range about which the majority of deaths occur and usually with a symmetrical distribution. This is referred to as the median lethal dose for 50% of the population studied (LD_{50}), i.e., that dose, calculated from the dosage-mortality data, which causes death of half of the population dosed under the specific conditions of the test. This concept of the LD_{50} was introduced by Trevan in 1927 (1). By inhalation, the reference is the lethal concentration$_{50}$ (LC_{50}) for a specified period of time (i.e., X-hour LC_{50}). Also, the contact time and whether the test conditions were occluded or nonoccluded should be stated for acute percutaneous LD_{50} values. The LD_{50} or LC_{50} values may be calculated by a variety of statistical procedures (2).

Other levels of mortality may be calculated such as the LD_5 and LD_{95}, which give statistical indications, respectively, of near-threshold and near-maximum lethal toxicity and the range of doses over which a lethal response may occur.

Since the LD_{50}, for economical and ethical reasons, is usually conducted with only small numbers of animals for each dosage group. There is an uncertainty factor associated with the calculation of the LD_{50} (or LC_{50}). This uncertainty is estimated by determining the 95% confidence limits; the dosage range over which there is only a 5% chance that the LD_{50} (or other LD value) lies outside. As shown schematically in Figure 3.9, 95% confidence limits are narrowest at the LD_{50}, which is an additional reason why this is an appropriate point for the comparison of acute lethal toxicity.

It should be stressed that the LD_{50}, by itself, is an insufficient index of lethal toxicity, particularly if comparisons are to be made between different materials. All dosage-response information should be examined, including slope of the dosage-response line and 95% confidence limits. Thus, two materials with differing LD_{50} values but overlapping 95% confidence limits should not be regarded as having significantly different lethal toxicity, since there is a statistical probability that the LD_{50} of one material will be within the 95% confidence limits of the other. However, when there is no overlap of 95% con-

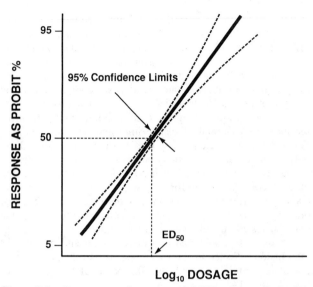

Figure 3.9. Dosage-mortality curve with 95% confidence limits. The limits are closest at the ED_{50} and diverge as the extremes of the dosage response are reached.

fidence limits, then the materials are considered to have significantly different lethal toxicity at the LD_{50} level (Fig. 3.10). A particularly important consideration is the slope of the dosage-response (Fig. 3.11). For example, if two materials have similar LD_{50} values with overlapping 95% confidence limits and identical slopes on the dosage-response lines (and therefore statistically similar LD_{10} and LD_{90} values), they are lethally equitoxic over a wide dosage range (A and B, Fig. 3.11). However, materials having similar LD_{50} values but differing slopes (and hence significantly different LD_{10} and LD_{90} values) may not be considered to be lethally equitoxic over a wide dosage range (A or B versus C, Fig. 3.11). Thus, materials having a steep slope (A or B, Fig. 3.11) may affect a much larger proportion of the population by incremental increases in dosages than is the case with materials having a shallow slope: Thus, acute overdose may be a more serious problem that

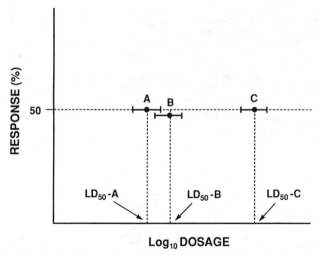

Figure 3.10. Comparison of the acute lethal toxicity of three compounds using LD_{50} data alone. Compounds **A** and **B** have overlapping 95% confidence limits and therefore have comparable acute lethal toxicity. Compound **C**, whose 95% confidence limits are separate from those of **A** and **B**, is significantly less toxic (higher LD_{50} dosage) than either **A** or **B**, based on LD_{50} values.

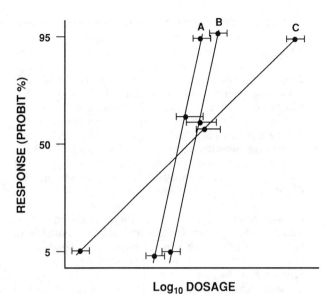

Figure 3.11. Influence of slopes of dosage-mortality data on the interpretation of LD_{50} data. All three materials (**A**, **B**, and **C**) have overlapping 95% confidence limits at the 50% response level and are therefore of comparable LD_{50}. Materials **A** and **B** have parallel dosage-response lines and overlapping confidence limits at 5% and 95%; therefore, these two materials are of comparable lethal toxicity over a wide range of doses. Material **C** with a shallower slope has significantly different LD_5 and LD_{95} values, and therefore over a wide range of doses has a differing lethal toxicity to materials **A** and **B**. With materials **A** and **B**, due to the steep slope of the dosage-response line, a much larger proportion of the population will be affected by small incremental increases in dosage. With material **C**, there may be a greater hazard for the hyperreactive groups, since the LD_5 lies at a much lower dosage than for **A** and **B**.

affects the majority population for materials with steeper slopes. In contrast, materials having a shallower slope (C, Fig. 3.11) may present problems for the hyperreactive groups at the left side of the dosage-response curve and may occur at significantly lower dosages than for hyperreactive individuals associated with the steep slope group. It follows from the above that a proper interpretation of acute lethal toxicity information should include examination of LD_{50}, 95% confidence limits, slope, and extremes of the dosage-response curve.

It should be emphasized that dosage-response information must be interpreted in terms of the conditions by which it was obtained. A multiplicity of factors may influence dosage-response relationships for a specific material, and the following few examples are used to illustrate the care necessary in interpreting LD_{50} information.

1. The numerical precision of the LD_{50} lies only in the statistical procedures by which it is attained. If an LD_{50} experiment is repeated at a later time, slightly different dosage-response data may be obtained because of biologic and environmental variability, resulting in a different numerical value for the LD_{50}. Therefore, LD_{50} values should be regarded as representing an order of lethal toxicity under the specific circumstances by which the information was collected.

2. An important consideration in interpreting the acute hazard from a chemical is the time to death. Thus, materials of similar LD_{50} but differing times to death may present different hazards. For example, with substances having similar LD_{50} values and slope values, those having more rapid times

to death can be considered as presenting a greater acute hazard. However, those substances with longer latency to effect may have a potential to produce cumulative toxicity by repeated exposure. For example, the acute oral LD_{50} of 2,4-pentanedione in the rat is 0.58 g/kg and that of 2,2-bis(4-aminophenoxy-phenyl) propane (BAPP) is 0.31 g/kg, with respective times to death of 2–5 hours and 13–14 days; on this basis 2,4-pentanedione would be regarded as presenting a greater potential hazard than BAPP (3).

3. A more complete interpretation of the significance of LD_{50} data may require a detailed consideration of the cause of death. If differing potentially lethal toxic effects are produced, it is important to know whether one or more are significant causes of death and whether this can lead to a bimodal dosage-response curve. Differing toxicities may lead to differing hazards by acute or latent mortality or morbidity. Clearly such a consideration is of importance in clinical toxicology for decisions on immediate medical management and observations for latent toxicity. For example, tert-butyl nitrite given by acute intraperitoneal injection to mice has a 30-minute LD_{50} of 613 mg/kg and a 7-day LD_{50} of 187 mg/kg. The earlier deaths were probably related to cardiovascular collapse and methemoglobin formation, whereas later deaths were due to liver injury (4).

4. Acute LD_{50} data may not be a guide to defining lethal toxicity by multiple exposures. Thus, with a material producing significant cumulative toxicity, the acute lethal dose (and dosage) may be significantly higher than that producing death by multiple smaller exposures. For example, the 4-hour LD_{50} for trimethoxysilane is 47 ppm (rat); when rats were given 20 exposures, each of 7 hours, over 4 weeks the LD_{50} was 5.5 ppm for that time period (5). Thus, the potentially lethal vapor concentration of trimethoxysilane for repeated exposure is significantly less than that for acute exposure.

The LD_{50} finds its principal applications as follows:

1. As a general index of extreme toxicity during routine toxicology testing and for comparison of the acute lethal toxicity of differing materials (within the constraints discussed above).
2. As a basis for classification of chemicals for regulatory purposes including manufacture, transport, use, and environmental considerations for chemicals and drugs.

The LD_{50} is not a biologic constant because of the influence of variability between strains and species and the modifying influence of many test and environmental conditions. Also, in

response to economic, scientific, and ethical demands, the LD_{50} procedure has been reevaluated and revised on many occasions (6, 7). By using fewer animals, approximate LD_{50} values can be calculated which give a reasonable order of acute lethal toxicity (8, 9). In one study an average of 6.8 rats was needed to determine an approximate lethal dose, compared with an average of 56.3 animals to determine the LD_{50} (10).

Any investigation into lethal toxicity should attempt to allow the maximum amount of usable information to be obtained. For this reason, acute toxicity studies should be designed not only to determine lethal toxicity but also to monitor for sublethal and target organ toxicity. This is possible by incorporating into the protocol observations for body weight, hematology, clinical chemistry, urinalysis, gross and microscopic pathology, and other specialized procedures as considered appropriate for the material tested. In this way a greater amount of relevant information can be obtained as well as useful and meaningful information collected to allow a comparative evaluation of acute toxicity, potential hazards, and the potential for cumulative toxicity (6, 11–13).

REFERENCES

1. Trevan JW. The error of determination of toxicity. Proc R Soc Lond 1927;101B:483–514.
2. Finney DJ. The median lethal dose and its estimation. Arch Toxicol 1985;56:215–218.
3. Tyler TR, Ballantyne B. Practical assessment and communication of chemical hazards in the workplace. In: Ballantyne ed. Perspectives in basic and applied toxicology, London Butterworth, 1988:330–378.
4. Maickel RP, McFadden DP. Acute toxicology of butyl nitrites and butyl alcohols. Res Commun Chem Pathol Pharmacol 1979;26:75–83.
5. Ballantyne B, Myers RC, Dodd DE, Fowler EH. The acute toxicity of trimethoxysilane (TMS). Vet Hum Toxicol 1988;30:343–344.
6. Zbinden G, Flury-Roversi M. Significance of the LD_{50} test for the toxicological evaluation of chemical substances. Arch Toxicol 1981;47:77–99.
7. Special Report. Van den Heuvel M. A new approach to the classification of substances on the basis of their acute toxicity. A report by the British Toxicology Society Working Party on Toxicity. Hum Toxicol 1984;3:85–92.
8. Lorke D. A new approach to practical acute toxicity testing. Arch Toxicol 1983;54:275–287.
9. Muller H, Kley HP. Retrospective study on the reliability of an "approximate LD_{50}" determination with a small number of animals. Arch Toxicol 1982;51:189–196.
10. Kennedy GL, Jr, Ferenz RL, Burgess BA. Estimation of acute oral toxicity in rats by determination of the approximate lethal dose rather than the LD_{50}. J Appl Toxicol 1986;6:145–148.
11. Sperling F. Quantitation of toxicology—the dose-response relationship. In: Sperling F, ed. Toxicology: principles and practice, Vol. 2. New York: John Wiley & Sons, 1984:199–218.
12. Tallarida RJ, Jacob LS. The dose-response relation in pharmacology. New York: Springer-Verlag, 1979.
13. Timbrell JA. Principles of biochemical toxicology. Chapter 2. London: Taylor and Francis, 1982.

4

Bioactivation: The Role of Metabolism in Chemical Toxicity

Daniel C. Liebler, Ph.D.
I. Glenn Sipes, Ph.D.

INTRODUCTION

Overview and Definitions

Biotransformation, which can be defined as metabolism by tissue enzymes, is the primary fate of chemicals in biologic systems. It represents the initial event in the clearance of most xenobiotics and typically yields innocuous products with little or no pharmacologic activity. In many cases, however, biotransformation yields *toxic metabolites*. This is called *bioactivation* and often leads to tissue damage. Bioactivation was first demonstrated in the late 1940s, when the Millers serendipitously discovered that yellow pigments in the livers of rats treated with hepatocarcinogenic azo dyes were actually dye molecules covalently bound to hepatic proteins (1). Subsequent work by many investigators has demonstrated that bioactivation is responsible for the toxic and carcinogenic effects of an extraordinarily diverse group of drugs, industrial chemicals, environmental pollutants, and even natural products (2–5).

A large and diverse group of enzymes catalyze bioactivation. Biotransformation enzymes are classified as *phase I* or *phase II* enzymes, depending on the reactions they catalyze. Phase I reactions modify lipophilic chemicals either by oxidation or hydrolysis to produce or expose polar functional groups. Phase II reactions add polar biomolecules to the substrate to produce very polar metabolites that often are excreted by specific mechanisms. The multiplicity and catalytic diversity of phase I and II biotransformation enzymes thus allow an organism to biotransform an extraordinarily diverse range of chemicals. On the other hand, this same metabolic versatility also results in bioactivation of a broad range of chemical toxicants.

Products of biotransformation whose formation can lead to toxicity are termed *toxic metabolites*. In many cases the toxic metabolites are transient, unstable products called *reactive intermediates* or *reactive metabolites*. Reactive metabolites are therefore the species that ultimately produce molecular damage. The common characteristic of virtually all reactive metabolites is that they have been rendered electron-deficient by metabolism. Such electron-deficient molecules, termed *electrophils*, tend to react preferentially with electron-rich molecules, termed *nucleophils*. In a cellular environment, the most prominent nucleophils are sulfur, nitrogen, and oxygen atoms found on important macromolecules such as proteins and DNA. Electrophils either add to nucleophils to produce *covalent adducts* or remove electrons from nucleophils to produce *oxidation products*. In either case, the structure and function of target nucleophils is changed. These changes amount to molecular damage and can lead to cell and tissue dysfunction.

Nevertheless, bioactivation does not necessarily result in injury for two reasons. First, toxic metabolites may undergo *detoxication*, a diminishing of chemical reactivity. Detoxication may involve enzyme-catalyzed biotransformation or nonenzymatic chemical reactions. Second, molecular damage to

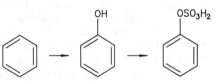

Figure 4.1. Metabolism of benzene to phenol and phenyl sulfate by phase I and phase II enzymes.

cell macromolecules often can be repaired, or the affected component can be replaced. Consequently, detoxication and repair are often as important as bioactivation in determining the susceptibility of tissues to chemical injury. Tissues in which bioactivation is efficiently balanced by detoxication and repair are resistant to injury. On the other hand, high doses, repeated exposures, or increased bioactivation due to enzyme induction may drive the relationship between bioactivation and detoxication to a threshold of imbalance and precipitate injury.

Biotransformation yields nontoxic metabolites as well as toxic metabolites, and nontoxic biotransformation may ultimately affect tissue responses to intoxication. Despite its potential significance, however, nontoxic biotransformation is beyond the scope of this review. The focus here is on enzymatic production of toxic metabolites, the properties and disposition of reactive metabolites, the properties and disposition of reactive metabolites, protection against reactive metabolites by detoxication, and the interplay between these factors that leads to selective tissue injury.

Concepts of Phase I and Phase II Metabolism

Phase I metabolism can be broadly defined as biotransformation that either adds polar functional groups or exposes latent functional groups in a substrate. Addition of polar groups is almost always achieved by introduction of oxygen into the substrate by oxidases. Exposure of latent polar groups can be accomplished either by oxidases or by hydrolases, which include esterases and amidases. *Phase II* metabolism is the biosynthetic conjugation of substrates with endogenous biomolecules such as glucuronic acid, sulfate, and glutathione. Specific transport systems for the conjugates direct their excretion from tissues. Together, phase I and II metabolism convert lipophilic chemicals to more hydrophilic products and direct them to specific excretion pathways. Biotransformation of the leukemogenic solvent benzene is an excellent example of the complementary roles of phase I and II metabolism (Fig. 4.1). Phase I metabolism first introduces polarity by adding a hydroxyl group to convert benzene to phenol. Phase II conjugation with the bulky, polar sulfate group amplifies the polar characteristics of phenol and produces a very water-soluble product that is readily excreted.

Organs of Biotransformation and Significance of Extrahepatic Bioactivation

The liver is the most important organ of biotransformation, due largely to its high content and great diversity of phase I and II enzymes. In addition, the splanchnic circulation carries all orally absorbed chemicals through the liver before they reach the systemic circulation. The leaky hepatic capillary network and the extensive surface area provided by hepatocyte micovilli promote efficient hepatic extraction of chemicals at the cellular level. The liver also is the major metabolite-releasing organ (Fig. 4.2). Phase I products released into the systemic circulation may then produce effects in other tissues (6). The liver also releases conjugate products of phase II metabolism into the blood, from which they may be extracted for renal metabolism, and into the bile, from which they may enter cycles of enterohepatic recirculation (7). Despite this dominant role of hepatic metabolism, other tissues may make critical contributions to bioactivation. The kidney and lung both contain relatively high levels of phase I and II enzymes. The kidney is particularly important because this organ has specific systems for the absorption and catabolism of phase II metabolite conjugates. These and other tissues, including the stomach, intestine, gonads, and skin, may play key roles in local generation of toxic metabolites despite their modest contributions to systemic metabolism (8).

Although hepatic metabolism plays a central role in biotransformation, extrahepatic bioactivation may nonetheless be of great importance in determining many toxic responses. When extrahepatic bioactivation plays a crucial role in toxicity, it does so by generating greater levels of reactive metabolites in the most susceptible tissues than does the liver (9). Some very reactive metabolites may not survive in the circulation at levels sufficient to induce critical injury in extrahepatic tissues, even when hepatic production of the reactive metabolite outstrips that in other tissues. Extrahepatic tissues also may either produce certain toxic metabolites more efficiently, or they may produce different metabolites of greater toxicity than does the liver. Finally, extrahepatic metabolism may be uniquely capable of converting nonreactive toxic metabolites from the liver to reactive metabolites (see below).

ENZYMES OF BIOACTIVATION: PHASE I ENZYMES

The remarkable variety of chemicals that undergo bioactivation is a consequence both of the diversity and catalytic versatility of phase I enzymes. Most biotransformation enzymes exist in multiple forms, called isozymes, each of which may accept many structurally diverse substrates. Phase I enzymes involved in bioactivation are grouped here by the types of reactions they catalyze and include: (a) the mixed-function oxidases: cytochromes P-450 (P-450) and flavin-containing monooxygenase (FMO), (b) prostaglandin synthetase-hydroperoxidase (PGS) and other peroxidases, (c) alcohol dehydrogenase and aldehyde dehydrogenase, (d) flavoprotein reductases, and (e) epoxide hydrase. Table 4-1 lists representative examples of bioactivation reactions that are catalyzed by phase I enzymes.

Mixed-Function Oxidases

P-450 and FMO both reside in the endoplasmic reticulum of cells and accept reducing equivalents from NADPH (Fig. 4.3). The P-450s are a large "superfamily" of enzymes that may be subdivided into several complex multigene families (10). Individual tissues frequently contain several different P-450 isozymes, and tissue-specific forms also occur. The expression of individual enzymes may be subject to genetic polymorphisms, and various isozymes may be induced by drugs, hormones, and environmental chemicals (11). P-450s are also subject to inactivation by suicide substrates and reactive metabolites (12). P-450 isozymes often display overlapping substrate specificities, so that more than one isozyme may contribute to biotransformation of a chemical, although one isozyme often predominates. P-450s accept electrons from NADPH via the intermediary flavoprotein NADPH-cytochrome P-450 reductase. P-450s are hemoproteins the levels of which are controlled in part by heme biosynthesis and thus related to iron metabolism. Metabolic alterations, such as starvation, that lower the $NAD(P)H/NAD(P)^+$ ratio can lower enzyme activity. Oxidations by P-450 dominate phase I biotransformation. P-450s catalyze the oxidation of virtually all classes of organic molecules (14). P-450 substrates range from simple one-carbon molecules such as chloroform to steroids and the complex heterocycle cyclosporin. P-450s also may catalyze the reductive bioactivation of a limited number of halogenated hydrocarbons, such as carbon tetrachloride and the anesthetic halothane, to

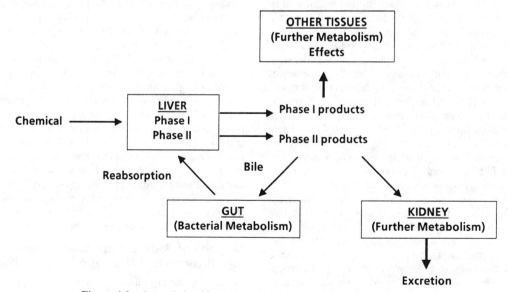

Figure 4.2. Interrelationships between organs involved in biotransformation.

Table 4.1. Examples of Reactive Intermediates Formed by Bioactivation: Phase I Processes

Parent Chemical	Reactive Intermediate	Generic Class	Enzymes Involved
$CHCl_3$ chloroform	O $\parallel$ $Cl\text{-}C\text{-}Cl$ phosgene [a]	acyl halide	P-450
$CH_2 = CH\text{-}CH_2OH$ allyl alcohol	O $\parallel$ $CH_2 = CH\text{-}C\text{-}H$ acrolein	α, β-unsaturated aldehyde	alcohol dehydrogenase
$ClCH_2CH_2Cl$ 1,2-dichloroethane	O $\parallel$ $ClCH_2C\text{-}H$ 2-chloroacetaldehyde	aldehyde	P-450
$(CH_3)_2N\text{-}N = O$ 1,1-dimethylnitrosamine	$CH_3\text{-}N_2{}^+$ methyldiazonium ion [a]	alkyl diazonium ion	P-450
$CH_3(CH_2)_4\,CH_3$ n-hexane	$O \quad\quad O$ $\parallel \quad\quad \parallel$ $CH_3\text{-}C\text{-}(CH_2)_2\text{-}C\text{-}CH_3$ 2,5-hexanedione	diketone	1. P-450 [b] 2. alcohol dehydrogenase
$ClCH = CH_2$ vinyl chloride	O $\diagup \ \diagdown$ $ClCH\text{-}CH_2$ chloroethylene oxide	epoxide	P-450
benzo[a]pyrene 	benzo[a]pyrene diol epoxide 	diol epoxide	1. P-450 [b] 2. epoxide hydrase 3. P-450 or peroxidase
benzene 	p-benzoquinone 	quinone	1. P-450[b] 2. peroxidase
CCl_4 carbon tetrachloride	$\bullet CCl_3$ trichloromethyl radical[a]	alkyl radical	P-450 (reduction)
paraquat 	paraquat 	cation radical	flavoprotein reductases
p-aminophenol 	p-benzoquinone imine 	quinone imine	peroxidase
thioacetamide S $\parallel$ CH_3CNH_2	thioacetamide-S,S-dioxide $O \ \ \ O$ $\diagdown S \diagup$ $\parallel$ CH_3CNH_2	S,S-dioxide	FMO, P-450

[a] Rearrangement of primary metabolite yields reactive intermediate
[b] Multiple enzymatic steps are represented in sequence

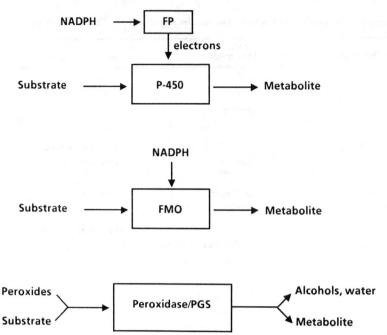

Figure 4.3.   Comparison of enzymes and cofactor requirements for phase I bioactivation by P-450 (top), FMO (middle), and peroxidases (bottom). FP, flavoprotein reductase; PGS, prostaglandin synthetase-hydroperoxidase.

produce reactive free radicals (see below (12)). This unusual reaction is favored under hypoxic conditions.

In contrast to the biochemical diversity of the P-450s, FMO occurs in tissues as a single enzyme form in a given species and is not inducible. FMO accepts electrons directly from NADPH and oxidizes a limited range of substrates, mainly basic nitrogen compounds (e.g., hydrazines, aryl amines) and thiocarbonyl compounds (e.g., thioacetamide, parathion)(13).

Prostaglandin Synthetase-Hydroperoxidase and Other Peroxidases

A diverse group of peroxidases catabolize hydrogen peroxide or other hydroperoxides to water and alcohols (Fig. 4.3). Oxidants generated as side products in these reactions may then produce reactive metabolites from many chemicals, including aromatic amines, phenols, hydroquinones, alkenes, and polycyclic aromatic hydrocarbons (15, 16). Peroxidases such as leukocyte myeloperoxidase, eosinophil peroxidase, and chloroperoxidase use hydrogen peroxide produced by the leukocyte respiratory burst. PGS, on the other hand, forms prostaglandin hydroperoxides from arachidonic acid as primary products. During the subsequent reduction of these hydroperoxides, other cosubstrates such as drugs and chemicals are oxidized. This mechanism, known as *cooxidation*, consumes arachidonic acid and a cosubstrate to produce prostaglandins and oxidized cosubstrates. The wide distribution of PGS in mammalian tissues suggests that it may be involved in a number of extrahepatic bioactivation reactions, particularly in tissues with low P-450 content, such as the renal inner medulla and the urinary bladder endothelium (15).

Dehydrogenases

Due to its high content of alcohol and aldehyde dehydrogenases, the liver is the major organ of alcohol metabolism. Al-

cohol dehydrogenases oxidize primary, secondary, and aromatic alcohols to aldehydes and ketones (17). Aldehyde dehydrogenases oxidize a variety of aldehydes to the corresponding carboxylic acids (18). Both enzymes use NAD+ as a cofactor. A specific formaldehyde dehydrogenase uses NAD+ and reduced glutathione together as cofactors to oxidize formaldehyde to formic acid. Both enzymes exist in multiple forms with overlapping substrate specificities and are ethanol-inducible. Rates of alcohol metabolism reflect not only enzyme levels, but also the disposition of inhibitory aldehyde products and cofactor levels (17). Substrates of major toxicologic significance are ethanol, methanol, ethylene glycol, and allylic alcohols, whose conversion to reactive aldehydes and ketones often results in tissue injury. Although it generally serves a detoxication role, aldehyde dehydrogenase may participate in bioactivation of ethylene glycol by oxidizing glycolaldehyde to oxalate (18).

Flavoprotein Reductases

The flavoprotein reductases NADPH:cytochrome P-450 reductase and NADH dehydrogenase bioactivate certain quinone-containing chemicals, nitroaromatics, and bipyridylium compounds through a single electron transfer to generate radicals (19). These radical intermediates may transfer an electron to molecular oxygen, which regenerates the parent compound and initiates an oxygen radical cascade that may ultimately damage cellular biomolecules (Fig. 4.4). The NAD(P)H-driven oxidation-reduction of chemicals, which gives rise to oxygen radicals, is termed "redox cycling" (20) and is largely dependent on the redox potentials of the enzyme and substrate, so not all quinones, nitroaromatics, and bipyridylium compounds are reduced. Chemicals whose bioactivation by this mechanism leads to oxygen radical formation include the bipyridylium herbicide paraquat, the antitumor agent Adriamycin, a variety of nitroar-

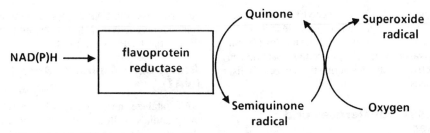

Figure 4.4. Oxygen radical production by flavoprotein-catalyzed redox cycling of a quinone.

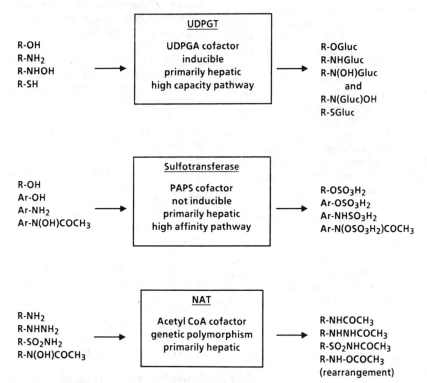

Figure 4.5. Reactions and characteristic features of phase II biotransformation reactions catalyzed by UDPGT (top), sulfotransferase (middle), and NAT (bottom).

omatic compounds, including the antibiotic nitrofurantoin, and some iron and copper chelates (19).

Epoxide Hydrases

Like the aldehyde dehydrogenases, epoxide hydrases serve both bioactivation and detoxication functions. Epoxide hydrase catalyze the hydrolytic opening of epoxides to trans-dihydrodiols (21). Microsomal and cytosolic forms of epoxide hydrase have been characterized; they require no cofactors or prosthetic groups. The leading example of bioactivation by the microsomal enzyme, hydrolysis of polycyclic aromatic hydrocarbon monoepoxides, would appear at first to be detoxication. However, the dihydrodiol products are then oxidized again by P-450 to reactive diol epoxides, which are poor substrates for epoxide hydrase and are much more carcinogenic than the monoepoxides (22).

Tissue Distribution of Phase I Metabolism

With the exception of peroxidases, the highest levels of all of the phase I enzymes are in the liver. P-450s are found in many

other tissues, including kidney, lung, intestinal mucosa, skin, adrenal cortex, and testis (8). FMO activity is restricted to liver and, to a lesser extent in humans, the lung (14). Peroxidases are widely distributed but probably are important bioactivation enzymes only in tissues where P-450 activities are relatively low, such as bone marrow, renal inner medulla, uterine endometrium, bladder epithelium, and skin (16). Bioactivation by dehydrogenases is limited largely to the liver (17, 18).

ENZYMES OF BIOACTIVATION: PHASE II ENZYMES

Most phase II biotransformation reactions produce inactive metabolites or result in detoxication. Nevertheless, phase II enzymes participate in the bioactivations of several classes of chemicals. Like phase I biotransformation, phase II processes operate on a structurally diverse range of substrates. This characteristic reflects the relatively broad substrate specificity of individual enzymes and the contributions of multiple enzyme forms to metabolism. Phase II enzymes are grouped here by category and include: (a) ester or amide-forming enzymes such as UDP-glucuronosyl transferases (UDPGT), sulfotransferases, and acetyl CoA: amine N-acetyltransferases (NAT), (b) the glutathione-S-transferases (GST), which catalyze the S-alkylation of glutathione, and (c) cysteine conjugate β-lyase (β-lyase), which cleaves certain cysteine conjugates to produce reactive metabolites during the renal catabolism of glutathione conjugates.

UDP-Glucuronosyl Transferases and Sulfotransferases

UDPGT catalyzes the transfer of glucuronic acid from the cofactor uridine diphosphate-glucuronic acid (UDPGA) to nucleophilic hydroxyl groups, amines, and thiols on substrates to form esters (O-glucuronides), amides (N-glucuronides), and thiolesters (S-glucuronides) (23) (Fig. 4.5). Although UDPGT are less inducible than P-450s, agents such as phenobarbital, polycyclic aromatic hydrocarbons, dioxin, and polyhalogenated biphenyls induce up to five-fold increases in selected enzyme activities. Different isozymes display relative specificity for planar aromatic substrates, bulky aliphatic substrates, bilirubin, and steroids (23). No selective inhibitors for UDPGT are known. Levels of the UDPGA cofactor are depleted by fasting, which may lower glucuronidation rates in vivo (24). UDPGT catalyze the formation of both N- and O-glucuronides from N-hydroxyarylamines. The former are the more stable but decompose to reactive products under mildly acidic conditions, such as are found in urine (25). This decomposition to reactive products is thought to explain, in part, the generation of bladder tumors by aromatic amines.

Several different sulfotransferase enzymes transfer sulfate from the cofactor 3'-phosphoadenosine-5'-phosphosulfate (PAPS) to alcohols, phenols, and hydroxysteroids to produce the corresponding sulfate esters (26) (Fig. 4.5). One of these enzymes, aryl sulfotransferase, mediates bioactivation of aryl hydroxylamines and arylhydroxamic acids. Although not inducible, the enzyme is inhibited by pentachlorophenol and 2,6-dichloro-4-nitrophenol (26). Sulfotransferases often display a higher substrate affinity than do UDPGT. The small hepatic PAPS cofactor pool may become depleted and produce a dose-dependent shift from sulfation to glucuronidation. Sulfation is therefore regarded as a ''highly affinity-low capacity'' system and glucuronidation as a ''low affinity-high capacity'' system.

Nevertheless, the PAPS cofactor pool and, consequently, sulfotransferase activity is less susceptible to dietary manipulation than is the UDPGA pool (24).

Acetyl CoA: Amine N-Acetyltransferase (NAT)

NAT catalyze the acetylation by acetyl CoA of aromatic primary amines, sulfonamides, hydrazines, and hydrazides (27) (Fig. 4.5). At least one enzyme catalyzes the rearrangement of arylhydroxamic acids to N-acetoxyarylamines (Ar-NHOCOCH$_3$), which are reactive alkylating agents (28). A genetic polymorphism in acetylation activity has been characterized in humans and rabbits. In the rabbit model, this polymorphism governs susceptibility to certain arylamine toxicants and carcinogens whose bioactivation involves N-acetylation (29). In addition to its role in arylamine and arylhydroxamic acid carcinogenesis, NAT initiates the bioactivation of hydrazine-containing drugs such as isoniazid (30). Nevertheless, the relationship between acetylator phenotype and susceptibility to isoniazid toxicity remains unclear despite numerous clinical and epidemiologic studies (31). This is perhaps due to the complicated role of N-acetylation, which can both generate and detoxicate reactive hydrazine metabolites.

Aryl sulfotransferase and UDPGT, along with NAT, complete the biotransformation of toxic and carcinogenic arylamines (Ar-NH$_2$) and N-acetylarylamides (Ar-NHCOCH$_3$) by converting their phase I metabolites [N-hydroxyarylamines (Ar-NHOH) and arylhydroxamic acids (Ar-N(OH)COCH$_3$)] to reactive esters (28) (Fig. 4.6). The N,O-esters produced by these enzymes differ in stability and in chemical reactivity toward proteins and DNA. The N,O-sulfates and N-acetoxy derivatives of arylhydroxamic acids are much more reactive than the N,O-glucuronides and N-hydroxy-N-glucuronides, which may serve as transport forms of the carcinogens. Consequently, sulfotransferase and NAT are critical mediators of hepatocarcinogenic bioactivation, whereas UDPGT-dependent bioactivation may contribute to extrahepatic carcinogenesis (28).

Glutathione-S-Transferases (GST)

GST catalyze conjugate formation between reduced glutathione (GSH) and electrophilic cosubstrates. Although GST are found

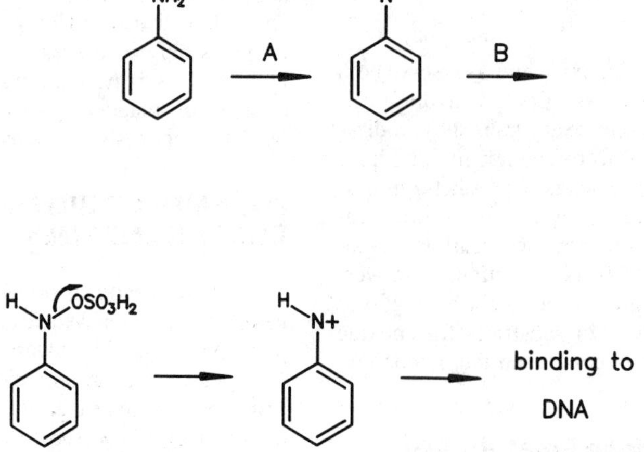

Figure 4.6. Formation of a reactive N,O-sulfate ester from an arylamine carcinogen by phase I N-hydroxylation, **A,** followed by phase II conjugation, **B.** The labile sulfate ester decomposes to produce a reactive *arylnitrenium ion*, which binds to DNA. Decomposition of analogous N-acetoxy and N,O-glucuronide derivatives also yields arylnitrenium ions.

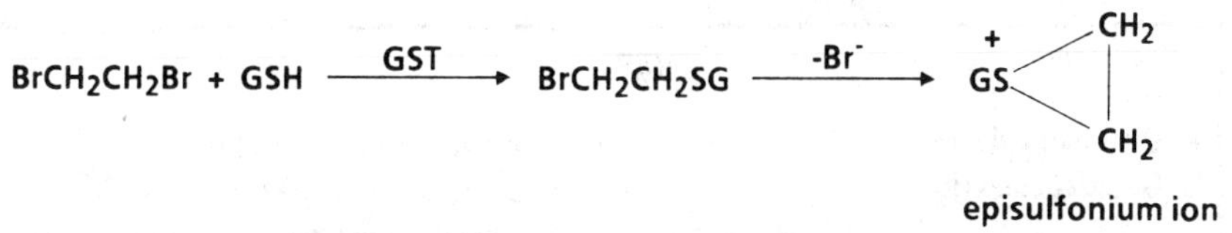

$$BrCH_2CH_2Br + GSH \xrightarrow{\text{GST}} BrCH_2CH_2SG \xrightarrow{-Br^-} GS\overset{+}{\underset{CH_2}{\diagup CH_2}}$$

episulfonium ion

Figure 4.7. Phase II bioactivation of the carcinogen 1,2-dibromoethane. The initial glutathione conjugate, called a "sulfur mustard," rapidly decomposes to a reactive episulfonium ion which alkylates DNA.

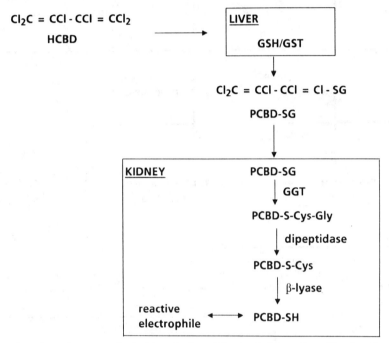

Figure 4.8. The roles of hepatic and renal enzymes in the bioactivation of the renal toxicant hexachlorobutadiene (HCBD). The pentachlorobutadienyl glutathione conjugate is formed in the liver and degraded by renal γ-glutamyltranspeptidase (GGT), dipeptidase, and β-lyase to the corresponding thiol derivative, which rearranges to a reactive electrophil.

in virtually all tissues, the liver contains the highest levels, where GST comprise up to 10% of the total hepatic cytosolic protein (32). GST comprise a large enzyme family in which expression of isozymes is often tissue-specific. Many xenobiotics induce GST, and the human enzymes display extensive polymorphism (32). Although GST primarily function as a versatile and effective enzymatic detoxication system, two types of GST-dependent bioactivation have been documented. In the first, GSH conjugation with 1,2-dihaloalkanes is followed by facile cyclization of the S-(2-haloethyl)glutathione intermediate to yield a reactive episulfonium ion (33, 34) (Fig. 4.7). In the second, glutathione conjugates of certain haloalkanes and haloalkenes give rise to cysteine conjugates, which are degraded to reactive metabolites by cysteine conjugate β-lyase in the kidney (35).

Cysteine Conjugate β-Lyase

Renal β-lyase is found both in cytosol and in mitochondria. This pyridoxal phosphate-containing enzyme, which is identical to glutamine transaminase K, cleaves cysteine-S-conjugates to pyruvate, ammonia, and a thiol fragment (36). Depending on the structure of the conjugated xenobiotic moiety, the thiol fragment may rearrange to a reactive electrophil (35). The activity of the enzyme is stimulated by α-keto acids, which regenerate the pyridoxal form of the enzyme from the pyri-

doxamine form. β-Lyase catalyzes the bioactivation of a limited number of halocarbon-cysteine conjugates, which are ultimately derived from glutathoine conjugation (35). This enzyme thus completes a bioactivation process begun by GST in the liver. The roles of GST and β-lyase in the bioactivation of the nephrotoxicant hexachlorobutadiene (HCBD) are summarized in Figure 4.8.

Tissue Distribution of Phase II Metabolism

Phase II enzymes occur in the principal organs of metabolism including liver, kidney, lung, gut, and skin. However, the liver contains the highest levels of UDPGT, sulfotransferase, and N-acetyltransferase activity and probably is the principal site of bioactivation by these enzymes (5). GST-catalyzed bioactivation is potentially important in any tissue where it occurs, because some of the products formed are reactive enough to cause damage at the site where they are formed. Indeed, chemicals such as halogenated aliphatic fumigants, whose bioactivation requires only GST often produce damage at the site of exposure (37, 38). β-Lyase activity is found in both liver and kidney, but cysteine conjugates that are substrates for this enzyme are generated exclusively in the kidney by renal catabolism of glutathione conjugates (35).

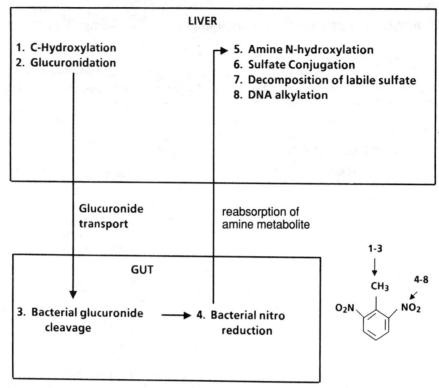

Figure 4.9. Interplay between hepatic and gut bacterial enzymes in the bioactivation of the hepatocarcinogen 2,6-dinitrotoluene. Hepatic metabolism to the glucuronide (steps 1 and 2) presents the molecule to gut bacteria, which reduce the nitro group to an amine (step 4). Reabsorption, hepatic N-hydroxylation, and conjugation (steps 5 and 6) produce a labile N,O-sulfate ester, which decomposes to a reactive intermediate that alkylates DNA.

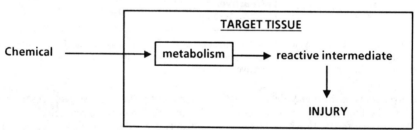

Figure 4.10.   Model 1.

Gastrointestinal Bacterial Enzymes

Metabolism of chemicals by bacteria in the gut may cleave phase II metabolites to release their precursors. This is accomplished by bacterial hydrolases that catabolize glucuronides and sulfates. Reabsorption of these completes the cycle of entero-hepatic recirculation (7). In addition, the anaerobic environment of the gut promotes reductive biotransformation of chemicals by bacteria. Bacterial reduction of nitroaromatic compounds yields amines that may be reabsorbed and undergo further hepatic bioactivation (39). Bacterial β-glucuronidase and nitro-reductases play an indispensible role in the multistep bioactivation of 2,6-dinitrotoluene (40) (Fig. 4.9).

FACTORS AFFECTING METABOLISM: THE METABOLIC BASIS OF INDIVIDUAL VARIATION

The ability of tissues to bioactivate chemicals depends on the variety, activities, and levels of biotransformation enzymes they contain. To a great extent, enzyme activities are an in-

trinsic characteristic for a given tissue and reflect genetic controls, age, and sex. Superimposed upon these restrictions are environmental factors that may dramatically alter enzyme content and activity. These extrinsic factors include enzyme induction and inhibition, nutrition, and disease.

Genetic Factors

Subtle differences in enzyme structure and content between different individuals may account for interindividual variation in susceptibility to chemical toxicity. Such differences may produce variations in enzyme activities in enzyme activities towards certain substrates. For example, some individuals in any given ethnic population display a decreased P-450-dependent metabolism of certain drugs (41). Recent studies suggest that certain hepatic P-450s in these "slow metabolizers" are structurally altered compared with the corresponding enzymes in normal individuals (42). Slow metabolizers may also lack the isozyme required to catalyze a particular reaction, as has been found in some rat stains that display genetic variation in drug metabolism (43). This structural alteration of the enzyme

Table 4.2. Classification of Toxic Chemicals According to the Role of Bioactivation: Model 1

Chemical Class: Examples	Target Tissue	Bioactivation Enzyme(s)	Ultimate Toxic Metabolites	Effect(s)	Reference(s)
Aromatic amines Benzidine, 2-naphthyl- amine	1. Bladder 2. Liver	Peroxidase NAT, P-450, NAT or sulfotransferase	Diimines, radicals? N,O-Acetoxy or N,O-sulfate deriva- tive	Carcinogenicity Carcinogenicity	16 3
Arylhydroxamic acids Acetylaminofluorene	Liver	P-450, sulfotransfer- ase	N,O-Sulfate ester	Carcinogenicity	3
Bipyridylium herbicides Paraquat, diquat	Lung, liver	Flavoprotein reduc- tases	Cation radicals, oxy- gen radicals	Toxicity	69
Furans 4-Ipomennol, 3-meth- ylfuran	Lung, liver, kidney	P-450	α,β-Unsaturated di- carbonyls, epox- ides?	Toxicity	70
Haloalkanes (a) CCl_4, CCl_3Br, halo- thane	Liver, lung, kidney	P-450	Radicals	Toxicity	71
Haloalkanes (b) $CHCl_3$, 1,1,2-trichlo- roethane	Liver, kidney	P-450	Acyl halides	Toxicity	71
Haloalkanes (c) 1,2-Dibromoethane, 1,2-dichloroethane, 1,2-dibromo-3- chloropropane	Respiratory tract, stomach, esopha- gus, testis	GST	Episulfonium ion	Carcinogenesis	32, 34
Haloalkenes 1,1-Dichloroethylene, trichloroethylene	Liver, lung, kidney	P-450	Acyl halides, alde- hydes, epoxides	Toxicity, carcinogen- icity	4
Haloaromatics Bromobenzene, chlo- robenzene, polyhal- ogenated biphenyls	Liver, lung, kidney	P-450	Arene oxides, qui- nones	Toxicity	9, 72
Hydrazines 1,2-Dimethyl hydra- zine	Colon, liver	P-450, FMO	Diazomethane	Carcinogenesis	73
1,1-Dimethyl hydra- zine	Liver (vasculature)	FMO	Methylradical, di- methyl diazenium ion	Carcinogenesis	73
Nitroaromatics Ronidazole, nitrofur- antoin	Lung, liver	Flavoprotein reduc- tases	Anion radicals, oxy- gen radicals	Toxicity	9, 74
N-Nitrosamines Dimethylnitrosamine	Liver, stomach, lung	P-450	Methyldiazonium ion	Carcinogenesis	75
Polycyclic aromatic hy- drocarbons Naphthanlene, benzo[a]pyrene	Lung, skin, mam- mary gland	P-450, epoxide hy- drase, peroxidase	Arene oxides, qui- nones	Toxicity, carcinogen- esis	76
Pyrrolines Monocrotaline	Liver	P-450	Pyrroles	Carcinogenesis	4
Thiono-sulfur com- pounds Thioacetamide, α- naphthyl thiourea, carbon disulfide	Liver, lung	FMO, P-450	S-Oxide;S,S-dioxide, atomic sulfur	Carcinogenesis, tox- icity	9, 77

probably reflects genetic alterations and could either enhance or suppress bioactivation, depending on the role of the enzyme involved. Polymorphisms in drug metabolism also have been observed for N-acetylation of aromatic amine-, aryl sulfon-amide-, and aryl hydrazine-containing drugs (44). Slow acetylators are more prone to develop drug-induced lupus erythematosus (44), whereas rapid acetylators more rapidly bioactivate aryl hydrazines (31). Extensive genetic polymorphisms in human P-450 and GST enzymes (32, 42), which are

the most extensively studied human biotransformation enzymes, suggest that genetic diversity in human populations could influence susceptibility to toxicants and carcinogens, although this view is certainly speculative.

Sex and Age

Large sex differences in monooxygenase activities have been reported in rats and mice and are a result of hormonal regulation

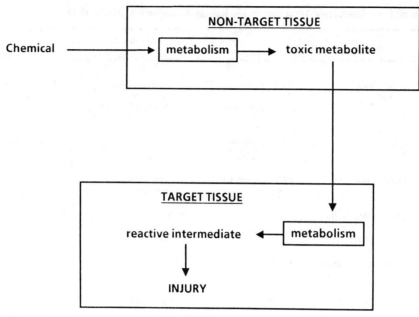

Figure 4.11.   Model 2.

Table 4.3.   Classification of Toxic Chemicals According to the Role of Bioactivation: Model 2

Chemical Class: Example	Initial Bioactivation Site: Enzyme	Primary Toxic Metabolite(s)	Target Tissue: Bioactivation Enzyme(s)	Ultimate Toxic Metabolite	Effect(s)	Reference(s)
Aromatic hydrocarbons						
Benzene	Liver: P-450	Phenol, hydroquinones, catechol	Bone marrow stem cells: myeloperoxidase	Quinones	Toxicity, leukemogenesis	78
Haloalkenes						
Hexachlorobutadiene	Liver: GST	Glutathione conjugate	Renal proximal tubule: 1. γ-Glutamyl transpeptidase 2. Dipeptidase 3. β-Lyase	Thionoacylhalide, thioketene	Toxicity	35, 79
Nitroaromatics						
2,6-Dinitrotoluene	1. Liver: a. P-450	a. Dinitrobenzyl alcohol	Liver: e. P-450	e. Hydroxylaminonitrobenzyl alcohol	Carcinogenesis	40
	b. UDPGT	b. O-Glucuronide	f. Sulfotransferase	f. N,O-Sulfate ester		
	2. Gut: c. Bacterial β-glucuronidase	c. Dinitrobenzyl alcohol				
	d. Bacterial nitroreductase	d. Aminonitrobenzylalcohol				

of some biotransformation enzymes (45). In humans, such differences are less apparent because sex-linked variation may be obscured by the superimposition of extensive genetic variation. Age-dependent variation in metabolism is most prominent in the fetus/neonate and in the elderly. It is well-known that underdeveloped biotransformation enzyme systems in neonates may predispose them to chemical toxicities. These toxicities result from the accumulation of a parent chemical or its toxic metabolites. This could also lead to fetal accumulation of some toxic chemicals from the maternal circulation, despite maternal contributions to clearance. However, to suggest that biotransformation is largely absent in the fetus and the neonate is an oversimplification. Unlike nonprimate species, the human fetus is capable of bioactivating foreign chemicals by the P-450 system (46). In addition, placental enzymes may contribute to bioactivation (47). Biotransformation in the fetus/neonate should therefore be regarded as a dynamic characteristic that reflects the variable states of development of several enzyme systems involved.

A decline in metabolism-dependent drug clearance is commonly observed in the elderly (48). Several factors are potentially implicated in these changes, including reduced hepatic blood flow and reduced biotransformation enzyme content. Decreased bioactivation also may reflect the effects of disease states on biotransformation (see below).

Enzyme Induction

Many drugs, environmental pollutants, and natural products share the ability to induce the synthesis of biotransformation enzymes. This phenomenon, called induction, has been extensively studied in animals and has important implications for bioactivation in humans. Induction requires increased de novo synthesis of new enzyme as a result of gene activation by the inducing agent (49). This is reflected by increased levels of mRNA that code for the induced proteins. Some inducers, such as the polycyclic aromatic hydrocarbons and 2,3,7,8-tetrachlorodibenzodioxin (TCDD, dioxin), and steroid hormones interact with cytosolic receptors in target cells (11). This complex migrates to the nucleus and activates genes for inducible proteins. Other inducers, such as barbiturates, apparently act through a different mechanism (50). Inducers may enhance the synthesis of some isozymes within an enzyme class yet suppress the synthesis of others. For example, both phenobarbital and the polychlorinated biphenyl mixture Arochlor 1254 induce several rat P-450s while concomitantly lowering the levels of some P-450s found in uninduced animals (51). Moreover, inducing agents often affect levels of more than one enzyme system, as illustrated by the ability of phenobarbital, polyhalogenated biphenyls, and polycyclic aromatic hydrocarbons each to induce not only P-450 but also UDPGT and GST. Concomitant induction of multiple phase I and II enzymes makes the overall effect of an inducer on bioactivation difficult to predict.

One consequence of enzyme induction is to increase enzyme activity in the principal tissues of bioactivation. This is observed, for example, with carbon tetrachloride (52) or bromobenzene (53) bioactivation in the liver. Following enzyme induction with phenobarbital, the bioactivation of these two chemicals is dramatically increased, as is the severity of the liver injury they produce. Alternatively, induction can produce such a disproportionate increase in bioactivation in another tissue that the locus of bioactivation shifts to that tissue. This was observed when animals induced with the polycyclic aromatic hydrocarbon 3-methylcholanthrene were subsequently treated with the toxic furan derivative, 4-ipomeanol (54). In induced animals, the locus of toxicity was shifted from lung to liver, due to increased bioactivation in the liver by induced enzymes. This increased hepatic metabolism lowered circulating levels of 4-ipomeanol enough to diminish pulmonary bioactivation to levels that did not produce pulmonary damage. On the other hand, phenobarbital pretreatment protected against both hepatic and pulmonary toxicity by inducing glucuronidation of 4-ipomeanol, a nontoxic biotransformation pathway (55).

In humans, induction may occur as the result of exposure to chemicals through chronic lifestyle habits (e.g., polycyclic aromatic hydrocarbon ingestion through smoking; alcohol consumption) or through acute treatment with therapeutic agents (e.g., barbiturates, rifampin). Certain environmental pollutants (polyhalogenated biphenyls, dioxins, halogenated insecticides) may induce biotransformation enzymes in humans, as they are potent inducers in animal models (5).

Enzyme Inhibition

Many clinically important drug interactions result when some drugs inhibit mixed-function oxidation, thereby inhibiting the biotransformation of other agents. Like inducers, inhibitors can potentially enhance or inhibit bioactivation. Bioactivation that involves a particular enzyme can be blocked by inhibiting the enzyme. On the other hand, inhibition may block nontoxic pathways of biotransformation and direct increased amounts of substrate through a toxic pathway, a phenomenon referred to ''metabolic switching.''

Different types of inhibitors include (4): (a) competitive inhibitors, such as alternate substrates; (b) noncompetitive inhibitors, such as alkylating agents that react with enzymes but do not compete with substrates; (c) suicide inactivators, which form enzyme-bound, reactive metabolites that destroy the enzyme during its catalytic cycle; and (d) reactive products that inactivate the enzymes where they were formed or other enzymes. Other inhibitors may block the synthesis of a prosthetic group or cofactor. Examples of this latter class include cobalt, which inhibits heme biosynthesis, upon which P-450 depends for activity (4), and agents that deplete GSH (56), which is required for GST-dependent conjugation. Inhibition of bioactivation also can occur with repeated low doses of a chemical that gives rise to reactive metabolites that destroy enzymes. Such low-dose pretreatment has been demonstrated effective in protecting laboratory animals against several toxic chemicals (9).

Nutrition and Disease

Biotransformation can be curtailed or altered under conditions of nutritional insufficiency and disease. In laboratory animals, 24–36-hour starvation lowers the NADPH/NADP+ ratio, depletes UDP-glucuronic acid for glucuronide synthesis, and depletes tissue stores of GSH and sulfur-containing amino acids necessary for GSH synthesis (57). Less severe dietary deficiencies, such as low protein diets, carbohydrate, vitamin, and mineral deficiencies all tend to reduce biotransformation in animals. Similar effects are postulated but not well-documented in humans (57). Hepatic diseases, including cirrhosis, hepatitis, and obstructive jaundice retard the hepatic clearance of many drugs and are expected to block the hepatic bioactivation of toxicants (58). Alternatively, hypothyroidism, hepatic, renal, pulmonary, or gastrointestinal disease may promote bioactivation and toxicity in other tissues by slowing or removing nontoxic clearance pathways.

REACTIVE METABOLITES AS ULTIMATE CHEMICAL TOXINS AND CARCINOGENS

A common misconception regarding reactive metabolites is that they react indiscriminately with cellular components. Due to their electrophilic nature, reactive metabolites either oxidize or form covalent adducts with cellular nucleophils. Selectivity in electrophil-nucleophil interactions results from mutually reinforcing chemical reactivities of both species (4). Electrophils preferentially modify nucleophils with whose chemical properties they are especially compatible. Consequently, reactive metabolites display a considerable degree of target selectivity in their reactions with biomolecules. For example, α,β-unsaturated carbonyl compounds and quinones bind almost exclusively to proteins, whereas carbocations (carbonium ions, R_3C+) and epoxides extensively modify DNA (4). Acylating agents such as isocyanates and acyl halides form stable adducts with lysine amines in proteins but are not known to react with DNA (4).

Free radicals comprise an important subgroup of reactive metabolites with unique properties (59). Although they undergo many of the same reactions as nonradical electrophils, free radicals are particularly important because they initiate radical chain reactions which, in effect, convert endogenous cellular constituents to reactive radicals. Some radical metabolites transfer electrons to molecular oxygen, which generates a cascade of reduced oxygen species (20). These vary considerably in reactivity, from the moderately reactive superoxide anion radical to the reactive nonradical hydrogen peroxide and the ultra-reactive hydroxyl radical. Free radicals attack and damage all classes of biomolecules, causing peroxidation of and fragmentation of proteins, DNA, and lipids.

Reactive metabolites may be classified on the basis of their stability, which dictates the distance they may migrate from their site of origin to react with a target (4). The most reactive are the intermediates formed by suicide inactivators, which, by definition, react with the enzyme during its catalytic cycle (12). Suicide inactivators of P-450 include vinyl halides, terminal olefins, acetylenes, dihydropyridines, and cyclopropyl compounds (12). Next are very reactive products that are released from the enzyme, but which react primarily with that protein. A reactive acyl halide metabolite of chloramphenicol (60) and electrophilic sulfur released from parathion (61) both are examples of reactive products that inactivate P-450. N-Acetoxy arylamine metabolites likewise inactivate the N-acetyl transferase isozyme that produces them (28). Less reactive are metabolites that may migrate to other compartments within a cell or tissue. This group may comprise the majority of electrophils generated by metabolism. These metabolites share the ability to cross biologic membranes, a characteristic that has been demonstrated for metabolites of several toxic or carcinogenic chemicals including benzo[a]pyrene, bromobenzene, dimethylnitrosamine, vinyl chloride, 1,1-dichloroethylene, and trichloroethylene (4). Less reactive still are those metabolites that may leave their tissue of origin to produce damage in other tissues. Examples of this class are 2,5-hexanedione, a hepatic hexane metabolite that causes peripheral neuropathy (62), pyrrolic metabolites of pyrrollizidine alkaloids, which migrate from liver to the lung, where they produce endothelial damage (9), and epoxides of 4-vinylcyclohexene, which produce ovarian toxicity (63).

DETOXICATION

Detoxication refers to all reactions, whether enzyme-catalyzed or not, that consume toxic metabolites without producing injury. The simplest of the nonenzymatic reactions is hydrolysis, which may be a major detoxication mechanism for very reactive electrophils, such as acyl halides, some epoxides, carbocations, isocyanates, and episulfonium ions (4). The most important nonenzymic detoxication of radicals is by reaction with biologic antioxidants, such as vitamin E and vitamin C, which react with free radicals to produce relatively unreactive antioxidant radicals that do not further propagate radical injury (64).

Enzyme-catalyzed detoxication of nonradical reactive metabolites is accomplished principally by GST and, to a lesser extent, by epoxide hydrase (65). Although GSH reacts nonenzymatically with many electrophils, GST catalysis greatly increases the rate and efficiency of the reactions. The multiplicity of GST enzymes with broad substrate specificities and their high content in many tissues make GST the most versatile detoxication system known (32, 65). In vivo, experimental inhibition of this system is accomplished by GSH depletion rather than by enzyme inhibition per se. Depletion of tissue GSH by starvation, by inhibition of GSH synthesis, or by chemical GSH depletion dramatically increases both covalent binding of reactive metabolites to tissue components and tissue injury (65).

The glutathione redox cycle provides GSH-dependent protection against injury (66). Hydrogen peroxide and other hydroperoxides are reduced to innocuous alcohols and water by GSH and the selenoenzyme glutathione peroxidase. The glutathione disulfide produced by this reaction is reduced back to GSH by the NADPH-dependent glutathione reductase. The glutathione redox cycle thus consumes one molecule each of hydroperoxide and NADPH. The cycle can be inhibited by antitumor nitrosoureas, whose isocyanate breakdown products inactivate glutathione reductase, or by severe GSH depletion (66). Dietary selenium deprivation lowers glutathione peroxidase levels and may increase tissue sensitivity to oxidant stress (67). Some GST express peroxidase activity and may participate in hydroperoxide metabolism.

Two other enzymes of great significance for free radical detoxication are superoxide dismutase and catalase. Superoxide dismutase catalyzes the dismutation of two superoxide anion radicals to produce one molecule each of oxygen and hydrogen peroxide (68). Found in all tissues, SOD isozymes relay on Cu-Zn or Mn centers for catalytic activity, but require no additional cofactor. Hydrogen peroxide is then further catabolized by the GSH redox cycle (see above) or by catalase, a peroxisomal enzyme found in many tissues. Catalase requires no cofactor and catabolizes only hydrogen peroxide.

MODELS OF TISSUE SUSCEPTIBILITY: CLASSIFYING TOXIC AND CARCINOGENIC CHEMICALS BY PATTERNS OF BIOACTIVATION

Many tissues are targets for injury by toxic metabolites of chemicals. Some of these tissues are capable of extensive biotransformation; others are not. Several enzyme-catalyzed metabolic steps, sometimes by enzymes in more than one tissue, are required to produce reactive metabolites from some chemicals. Others undergo simple, one-step bioactivation. Some toxic metabolites produce injury at the sites where they are formed, whereas others may migrate to produce effects at distant sites. Obviously, the sometimes complicated interplay between these factors dictates how and where bioactivation causes tissue injury. The following three models provide a framework for classifying chemical toxicants and carcinogens on the basis of how their bioactivation leads to tissue injury.

Model 1

The target tissue contains the necessary enzymes to bioactivate the parent chemical to a reactive metabolite, which produces

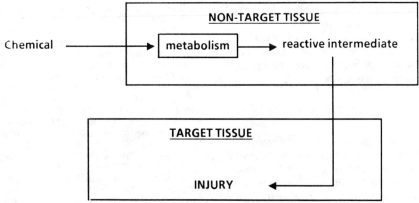

Figure 4.12. Model 3.

Table 4.4 Classification of Toxic Chemicals According to the Role of Bioactivation: Model 3

Chemical Class: Example	Bioactivation Site: Enzyme	Toxic Metabolite(s)	Target Tissue	Determinant of Susceptibility	Effect	Reference(s)

Alkanes
  Hexane
	Liver:
	  a. P-450
	  b. Alcohol dehydro-genase
		2,5-Diketone	Peripheral nerve	Binding to lysine residues in axonal neurofiliments	Toxicity	62, 80

Aromatic amines
  2-Naphthylamine
	Liver:
	  a. P-450 or FMO
	  b. UDPGT
		N-Glucuronide	Bladder epithelium	Hydrolysis of N-glucuronide in acidic urine yields reactive product	Carcinogenesis	25

Glycols
  Ethylene glycol
	Liver:
	  a. Alcohol dehydro-genase
	  b. Aldehyde dehydro-genase
		Oxalate	Renal tubules	Calcium oxalate, precipitate blocks, renal tu-bules	Toxicity	81

Haloalkenes Vinyl chloride	Hepatic paren-chymal cell: P-450	Epoxide	Hepatic endothelial cell	Deficient DNA re-pair in endothelial cell vs. parenchy-mal cell	Carcinogenesis	4
Hydrazines 1,2-Dimethyl-hy-drazine	Hepatic paren-chymal cell: P-450	Diazomethane	Hepatic endothelial cell	Deficient DNA re-pair in endothelial cell vs. parenchy-mal cell	Carcinogenesis	82
N-Nitrosamines Dimethyl nitrosa-mine	Hepatic paren-chymal cell: P-450	α-Hydroxy-N-ni-trosamine	Hepatic endothelial cell	Deficient DNA re-pair in endothelial cell vs. parenchy-mal cell	Carcinogenesis	82
Pyrrolines Pyrrolizidine al-kaloids	Liver: P-450	Pyrroles	Pulmonary endothe-lium	"First pass" clear-ance of reactive hepatic metabo-lites	Toxicity	4, 9

injury (Fig. 4.10). This is the simplest model and can be applied to many toxicants and carcinogens that produce their effects in tissues with significant bioactivation capacity, such as the liver, lung, and kidney (Table 4.2). This model applies best to chemicals whose toxic metabolites are very reactive and may not migrate far from the cells that produce them.

Model 2

The target tissue cannot biotransform the parent chemical to a reactive metabolite in situ but can further bioactivate a toxic metabolite produced by another tissue (Fig. 4.11). This model applies mainly to chemicals whose initial metabolism is in the liver (Table 4.3). However, other obligate biotransformation steps may take place in other tissues, such as the gut, where bacterial biotransformation may produce a toxic metabolite that is reabsorbed and causes toxicity elsewhere. The target tissues contain biotransformation enzymes that are not present in the liver, such as enzymes of glutathione conjugate catabolism in the renal proximal tubules, peroxidases in the renal inner medulla, lymphocyte myeloperoxidase in bone marrow, and extrahepatic tissue-specific forms of P-450. The primary metabolites are chemically unreactive, but the secondary metabolites are reactive enough to produce injury principally in the tissue where they are formed.

Model 3

The target tissue can neither completely nor partially bioactivate the parent chemical but is uniquely susceptible to a reactive metabolite produced by another tissue (Fig. 4.12). This model generally applies to chemicals that produce damage in tissues where bioactivation either does not occur or may occur to a minimal extent (Table 4.4). Target tissues in this model could range from peripheral nerves, which display little if any biotransformation capacity, to lung, which is active in biotransformation. Their common characteristic is that both lack the ability to bioactivate a given chemical yet are damaged by its metabolites from another tissue. The biochemical bases of susceptibility could involve exposure to high levels of a toxic metabolite, inadequate detoxication, a preponderance of targets compatible with a certain reactive metabolite, or inadequate repair. The assignment of a chemical to this model can be made with confidence only when the bioactivation of a chemical and the fate of its reactive metabolites are known. Uncertainty regarding either of these may lead one to incorrect classification under model 3 when a more proper classification would be model 1 or 2.

REFERENCES

1. Miller EC, Miller JA. The presence and significance of bound aminoazo dyes in the livers of rats fed p-dimethylaminoazobenzene. Cancer Res 1947;7:468–480.

2. Anders MW, ed. Bioactivation of foreign compounds. Orlando, FL: Academic Press, 1985.

3. Miller EC, Miller JA. Searches for ultimate chemical carcinogens and their reactions with cellular macromolecules. Cancer 1981;47:2327–2345.

4. Guengerich FP, Liebler DC. Enzymatic activation of chemicals to toxic metabolites. CRC Crit Rev Toxicol 1985;14:259–307.

5. Sipes IG, Gandolfi AJ. Biotransformation of toxicants. In: Klaassen CD, Amdur MO, Doull J, eds. Casarett and Doull's toxicology: the basic science of poisons. 3rd ed. New York: Macmillan, 1986:64–98.

6. Boyd MR, Statham CN. The effect of hepatic metabolism on the pro-

7. duction and toxicity of reactive metabolites in extrahepatic tissues. Drug Metab Rev 1983;14:35–47.

7. Duggan DE, Kwan KC. Enterohepatic recirculation of drugs as a determinant of therapeutic ratio. Drug Metab Rev 1979;9:21–41.

8. Rydstrom J, Montelius J, Bengtsson M, eds. Extrahepatic drug metabolism and chemical carcinogenesis. Amsterdam: Elsevier, 1983.

9. Boyd MR. Biochemical mechanisms of chemical-induced lung injury: roles of metabolic activation. CRC Crit Rev Toxicol 1980;7:103–176.

10. Nebert DW, Nelson DR, Adesnik M, Coon MJ, Estabrook RW, Gonzalez FJ, Guengerich FP, Gunsalus IC, Johnson EF, Kemper B, Levin W, Phillips IR, Sato R, Waterman MR. The P-450 superfamily: update on listing of all genes and recommended nomenclature of the chromosomal loci. DNA 1989;8:1–14.

11. Eisen HJ. Induction of hepatic P-450 isozymes: evidence for specific receptors. In: Ortiz de Montellano PR, ed. Cytochrome P-450: structure, mechanism and biochemistry. New York: Plenum, 1986:315–344.

12. Ortiz de Montellano PR, Reich NO. Inhibition of P-450 enzymes. In: Ortiz de Montellano PR, ed. Cytochrome P-450: structure, mechanism and biochemistry. New York: Plenum, 1986:277–314.

13. Wislocki PG, Miwa GT, Lu AYH. Reactions catalyzed by the cytochrome P-450 system. In: Jakoby WB, ed. Enzymatic basis of detoxication. Vol. 1. New York: Academic Press, 1980:136–182.

14. Ziegler DM. Flavin-containing monooxygenase: catalytic mechanism and substrate specificities. Drug Metab Rev 1988;19:1–32.

15. Marnett LJ, Eling TE. Cooxidation during prostaglandin biosynthesis: a pathway for metabolic activation of xenobiotics. In: Hodgson E, Bend JR, Philpot RM, eds. Reviews in biochemical toxicology. Vol. 5. New York: Elsevier, 1983:135–172.

16. O'Brien PJ. Radical formation during the peroxidase catalyzed metabolism of carcinogens and xenobiotics: the reactivity of these radicals with GSH, DNA and unsaturated lipid. Free Radic Biol Med 1988;4:169–183.

17. Bosron WF, Li TK. Alcohol dehydrogenase. In: Jakoby WB, ed. Enzymatic basis of detoxication. Vol. 1. New York: Academic Press, 1980:231–248.

18. Weiner H. Aldehyde oxidizing enzymes. In: Jakoby WB, ed. Enzymatic basis of detoxication. Vol. 1. New York: Academic Press, 1980:261–280.

19. Smith MT, Evans CG, Thor H, Orrenius S. Quinone-induced oxidative injury to cells and tissues. In: Sies H, ed. Oxidative stress. Orlando, FL: Academic Press, 1985:91–113.

20. Kappus H, Sies H. Toxic drug effects associated with oxygen metabolism: redox cycling and lipid peroxidation. Experientia 1981;37:1233–1241.

21. Siedegard J, DePierre J. Microsomal epoxide hydrase: properties, regulation and function. Biochim Biophys Acta 1983;695:251–270.

22. Levin W, Buening MK, Wood AW, Chang RL, Kedzierski B, Thakker D, Boyd DR, Gadaginmath GS, Armstrong RN, Yagi H, Karle JM, Slaga TJ, Jerina DM, Conney AH. An enantiomeric interaction in the metabolism and mutagenicity of (+)- and (−)-benzo[a]pyrene-7,8-oxide. J Biol Chem 1980;255:9067–9074.

23. Siest G, Antoine B, Fournel S, Magdalou J, Thomassin J. The glucuronosyltransferases: what progress can pharmacologists expect from molecular biology and cellular enzymology? Biochem Pharmacol 1987;36:983–989.

24. Mulder GJ. Sulfation: metabolic aspects. In: Bridges JW, Chasseaud LF, eds. Progress in drug metabolism. Vol. 8. Philadelphia: Taylor and Francis, 1984:35–100.

25. Kadlubar FF, Miller JA, Miller EC. Hepatic microsomal N-glucuronidation and nucleic acid binding of N-hydroxyarylamines in relation to urinary bladder carcinogenesis. Cancer Res 1977;37:805–814.

26. Jakoby WB, Duffel MW, Lyon ES, Ramaswamy S. Sulfotransferases active with xenobiotics: comments on mechanism. In: Bridges JW, Chasseaud LF, eds. Progress in drug metabolism. Vol. 8. Philadelphia: Taylor and Francis, 1984:11–34.

27. Weber WW, Glowinski IB. Acetylation. In: Jakoby WB, ed. Enzymatic basis of detoxication. Vol. 2. New York: Academic Press, 1980:169–186.

28. Hanna PE, Banks RB. Arylhydroxylamines and arylhydroxamic acids: conjugation reactions. In: Anders, MW, ed. Bioactivation of foreign compounds. Orlando, FL: Academic Press, 1985:376–402.

29. Weber WW. Acetylation pharmacogenetics: experimental models for human toxicity. Fed Proc 1984;43:2332–2337.

30. Timbrell JA, Mitchell JR, Snodgrass WR, Nelson SD. Isoniazid hepatotoxicity: the relationship between covalent binding and metabolism in vivo. J Pharmacol Exp Ther 1980;213:364–369.

31. Hein DW. Isoniazid toxicity as related to acetylator status. Fed Proc 1983;42:3087–3091.

32. Mannervik B and Danielson UH. Glutathione transferases: structure and catalytic activity. CRC Crit Rev Biochem 1988;23:283–337.

33. Rannug U. Genotoxic effects of 1,2-dibromoethane and 1,2-dichloroethane. Mutat Res 1980;76:269–295.

34. Peterson LA, Harris TM, Guengerich FP. Evidence for an episulfonium ion intermediate in the formation of S-[2-(N^7-guanyl)ethyl]glutathione in DNA. J Am Chem Soc 1988;110:3284–3291.

35. Anders MW, Lash LH, Dekant W, Elfarra A, Dohn DR. Biosynthesis and biotransformation of glutathione S-conjugates to toxic metabolites. CRC Crit Rev Toxicol 1988;18:311–341.

36. Stevens JL, Ayoubi N, Robbins JD. The role of mitochondrial matrix enzymes in the metabolism and toxicity of cysteine conjugates. J Biol Chem 1988;263:3395–3401.

37. Olson WA, Habermann RT, Weisburger EK, Ward JM, Weisburger JH. Induction of stomach cancer in rats and mice by halogenated aliphatic fumigants. J Natl Cancer Inst 1973;51:1993–1995.

38. Reznik G, Stinson SF, Ward JM. Respiratory pathology in rats and mice after inhalation of 1,2-dibromo-3-chloropropane and 1,2-dibromoethane for 13 weeks. Arch Toxicol 1980;46:233–240.

39. Goldman P. Role of the intestinal microflora. In: Jakoby WB, Bend JR, Caldwell J, eds. Metabolic basis of detoxication. New York: Academic Press, 1982:323–338.

40. Kedderis GI, Dyroff MC, Rickert DE. Hepatic macromolecular covalent binding of the hepatocarcinogen 2,6-dinitrotoluene and its 2,4-isomer in vivo: modulation by the sulfotransferase inhibitors pentachlorophenol and 2,6-dichloro-4-nitrophenol. Carcinogenesis 1984;5:1199–1204.

41. Idle JR, Smith RL. Polymorphism of oxidation at carbon centers of drugs and their clinical significance. Drug Metab Rev 1979;9:301–317.

42. Guengerich FP, Distlerath LM, Reilly PEB, Wolff T, Shimada T, Umbenhauer D, Martin MV. Human liver cytochromes P-450 involved in polymorphisms of drug oxidation. Xenobiotica 1986;16:367–378.

43. Larrey D, Distlerath LM, Dannan GA, Wilkinson GR, Guengerich FP. Purification and characterization of the rat liver cytochrome P-450 involved in the 4-hydroxylation of debrisoquine, a prototype for genetic variation in oxidative drug metabolism. Biochemistry 1984;23:2787–2795.

44. Uetrecht JP, Woosley RL. Acetylator phenotype and lupus erythematosus. Clin Pharmacokinet 1981;6:118–134.

45. Skett P. Hormonal regulation and sex differences of xenobiotic metabolism. In: Bridges JW, Chasseaud LF, Gibson GG, eds. Progress in drug metabolism. Vol. 10. Philadelphia: Taylor and Francis, 1987:86–140.

46. Rane A, Pacifici GM. Formation and metabolism of toxic metabolites in the human fetus. In: Soyka LF, Redmond GP, eds. Drug metabolism in the immature human. New York: Raven Press, 1981:29–35.

47. Pelkonen O. Xenobiotic metabolism in human placenta. In: Soyka LF, Redmond GP, eds. Drug metabolism in the immature human. New York: Raven Press, 1981:19–27.

48. Loi CM, Vestal RE. The effects of age on hepatic drug metabolism. In: Cutler NM, Narang PK, eds. Drug studies in the elderly. New York: Plenum Press, 1986:101–121.

49. Bresnick E. Induction of the enzymes of detoxication. In: Jakoby WB, ed. Enzymatic basis of detoxication. Vol. 1. New York: Academic Press, 1980:69–84.

50. Fonne R, Meyer UA. Mechanisms of phenobarbital-type induction of cytochrome P-450. Pharmacol Ther 1987;33:19–22.

51. Guengerich FP, Dannan GA, Wright ST, Martin MV, Kaminsky LS. Purification and characterization of liver microsomal cytochromes P-450: electrophoretic, spectral, catalytic, and immunochemical properties and inducibility of eight isozymes isolated from rats treated with phenobarbital or β-naphthoflavone. Biochemistry 1982;21:6019–6030.

52. Brodie BB, Reid WD, Cho AK, Sipes G, Krishna G, Gillette JR. Possible mechanism of liver necrosis caused by aromatic organic compounds. Proc Natl Acad Sci USA 1971;68:160–164.

53. Garner RC, McLean AEM. Increased susceptibility to carbon tetrachloride poisoning in the rat after pretreatment with oral phenobarbitone. Biochem Pharmacol 1969;18:645–650.

54. Boyd MR, Dutcher JS. Renal toxicity due to reactive metabolites formed in situ in the kidney: investigations with 4-ipomeanol in the mouse. J Pharmacol Exp Ther 1981;21:640–646.

55. Statham CN, Boyd MR. Effects of phenobarbital and 3-methylcholanthrene on the in vivo distribution, metabolism, and covalent binding of 4-ipomeanol in the rat. Biochem Pharmacol 1983;31:3973–3977.

56. Chasseaud LF. Role of glutathione and glutathione-S-transferases in the metabolism of carcinogens and other electrophilic agents. Adv Cancer Res 1979;29:175–274.

57. Guengerich FP. Effects of nutritive factors on metabolic processes involving bioactivation and detoxication of chemicals. Annu Rev Nutr 1984;4:207–231.

58. Howden CW, Birnie GG, Brodie MJ. Drug metabolism in liver disease. Pharmacol Ther 1989;40:439–474.

59. Pryor WA. Free radical biology; xenobiotics, cancer and aging. Ann NY Acad Sci 1983;393:1–23.

60. Halpert J. Covalent modification of lysine during the suicide inactivation of cytochrome P-450 by chloramphenicol. Biochem Pharmacol 1981;30:875–881.

61. Halpert J, Hammond D, Neal RA. Inactivation of purified rat liver cytochrome P-450 during the metabolism of parathion (diethyl-p-nitrophenylphosphorothionate). J Biol Chem 1980;255:1080–1089.

62. Kravasage WJ, O'Donoghue JL, DiVincenzo GD, Terhaar CJ. The relative neurotoxicity of methyl n-butyl ketone, n-hexane and their metabolites. Toxicol Appl Pharmacol 1980;56:433–441.

63. Smith BJ, Mattison DR, Sipes IG. The role of epoxidation in 4-vinylcyclohexene-induced ovarian toxicity. Toxicologist 1989;9:118.

64. Machlin LJ, Bendich A. Free radical tissue damage: protective role of antioxidant nutrients. FASEB J 1987;1:441–445.

65. Reed DJ. Cellular defense mechanisms. In: Anders MW, ed. Bioactivation of foreign compounds. Orlando, FL: Academic Press, 1985:71–108.

66. Reed DJ. Regulation of reductive processes by glutathione. Biochem Pharmacol 1986;35:7–13.

67. Sies H. Hydroperoxides and thiol oxidants in the study of oxidative stress in intact cells and organs. In: Sies H, ed. Oxidative stress. Orlando, FL: Academic Press, 1985:73–90.

68. Fridovich I. Superoxide dismutases. Adv Enzymol Relat Area Mol Biol 1986;58:61–97.

69. Bus JS, Aust SD, Gibson JE. Paraquat toxicity: proposed mechanism of action involving lipid peroxidation. Environ Health Perspect 1976;16:139–146.

70. Ravindranath V, Burka LT, Boyd MR. Reactive metabolites from the bioactivation of toxic methylfurans. Science 1984;224:884–886.

71. Macdonald TL. Chemical mechanisms of halocarbon metabolism. CRC Crit Rev Toxicol 1982;11:85–120.

72. Jollow DJ, Mitchell JR, Zampaglione N, Gillette JR. Bromobenzene induced liver necrosis. Protective role of glutathione and evidence for 3,4-bromobenzene oxide as the hepatotoxic intermediate. Pharmacology 1974;11:151–169.

73. Prough RA, Maloney SJ. Hydrazines. In: Anders MW, ed. Bioactivation of foreign compounds. Orlando, FL: Academic Press, 1985:433–449.

74. Josephy PD, Mason RP. Nitroimidazoles. In: Anders MW, ed. Bioactivation of foreign compounds. Orlando, FL: Academic Press, 1985:451–483.

75. Archer MC, Labuc GE. Nitrosamines. In: Anders, MW, ed. Bioactivation of foreign compounds. Orlando, FL: Academic Press, 1985:403–431.

76. Thakker DR, Yagi H, Levin W, Wood AW, Conney AH, Jerina DM. Polycyclic aromatic hydrocarbons: metabolic activation to ultimate carcinogens. In: Anders MW, ed. Bioactivation of foreign compounds. Orlando, FL: Academic Press, 1985:178–242.

77. Neal RA, Halpert J. Toxicology of thiono-sulfur compounds. Annu Rev Pharmacol Toxicol 1982;22:321–339.

78. Eastmond DA, Smith MT, Irons RD. An interaction of benzene metabolites reproduces the myelotoxicity observed with benzene exposure. Toxicol Appl Pharmacol 1987;91:85–95.

79. Lock EA. Studies on the mechanism of nephrotoxicity and nephrocarcinogenicity of halogenated alkenes. CRC Crit Rev Toxicol 1988;19:23–42.

80. Genter St Clair MB, Amarnath V, Moody MA, Anthony DC, Anderson CW, Graham DG. Pyrrole oxidation and protein cross-linking as necessary steps in the development of γ-diketone neuropathy. Chem Res Toxicol 1988;1:179–185.

81. Roberts JA, Seibold HR. Ethylene glycol toxicity in the monkey. Toxicol Appl Pharmacol 1969;15:624–631.

82. Swenberg JA, Richardson FC, Boucheron JA, Dyroff MC. Relationships between DNA adduct formation and carcinogenesis. Environ Health Persp 1985;62:177–183.

5

Principles in the Development of Antidotes to Toxic Materials

Timothy C. Marrs, M.D.

INTRODUCTION

Only in the case of a few poisons does an effective and specific antidote exist (Table 5.1) (1, 2). For the treatment of most other toxins, therapy is generally symptomatic.

Antidotes are, in many respects, similar to other drugs, but as a group, they have certain special features in common. In most circumstances the antidote is used once or a few times and then usually in life-threatening situations. Furthermore, the randomized clinical trial in human patients is not possible. Despite the fact that the aim of preclinical studies is to show safety and efficacy, reliance on animal efficacy studies for the assessment of effectiveness of antidotes is necessary.

Most antidotes have evolved after the discovery of an antidote that was less than optimal, a "lead" compound (3). Compounds that acted in the same manner, often chemically analogous to the "lead" compound, were then studied, the one with the best therapeutic index eventually becoming the accepted antidote. Examples of this type of evolution include dimercaprol (British anti-Lewisite, BAL). This drug, designed for use in World War II against the organic arsenical, lewisite, is a dithiol chelating agent. It has been extensively studied by Thompson and colleagues (4, 5). The subsequent introduction of 2,3-dimercaptosuccinic acid (DMSA) and dimercaptopropanesulfonic acid (DMPS) combined the same active dithiol chelating grouping within a more hydrophilic molecule, reducing the toxicity and rendering the drug orally active. The idea of using dithiol compounds in this way had its origin in the suspicion that arsenic was toxic by virtue of its ability to combine with sulfhydryl groups in biologic molecules. The "classical therapy" for cyanide, sodium nitrite combined with sodium thiosulfate, arose from the discovery of the usefulness of amyl nitrite

in cyanide poisoning. It was discovered that pralidoxime (2-PAM) minimized the effect of hydroxylamine in tetraethylpyrophosphate (TEPP) poisoning (7–9). Hydroxylamine was studied because it was similar to the substrate of the enzyme, acetylcholinesterase. With many "lead" compounds the origin of the antidotal mechanism has been discovered in the laboratory, while others have arisen from pharmacologic investigations.

In all cases, except those antidotes discovered by chance and those derived from screening large numbers of compounds, the genesis of the antidote has depended on an extensive knowledge of the mode of action of the toxin. It is important, when attempting to develop antidotal treatment of a novel poison, to gain in-depth knowledge of the toxicology of the toxin involved.

TOXICOLOGY OF THE POISON

Defining the mechanism of a toxic substance is necessary in order to develop an antidote. Acute lethality studies are an important first in these studies. Due to the fact that there can be major differences with respect to the effects of a toxin on different animal species, the careful selection of an appropriate animal model is crucial. Dimercaprol and pralidoxime were both developed from studies detailing the mode of action of specific toxins.

Acute lethality studies require the determination of the median lethal dose of the toxin (LD_{50}). The LD_{50} value has received much criticism regarding its usefulness (10, 11). The LD_{50} study does not define the mechanism of the toxin. However, when the LD_{50} study is conducted, the slope of the curve can be altered by antidotal therapy, and thus the study can have some utility in the investigation of a new therapy (12). Acute lethality studies should be conducted in several animal species. The route of exposure in the study should be similar to that in real human exposure situations.

The median effective dose (ED_{50}) is another measurement traditionally performed in toxicology investigations. The ED_{50} is used to study the potential reversal of nonlethal toxic effects, as opposed to those of acute lethality.

The subchronic toxicity of the poison is rarely of interest in design of experiments to test antidotal efficacy, but the delayed toxicity is of importance. Such poisons include carbon monoxide and organophosphorus anticholinesterases (13–15). In these cases, animals in acute lethality studies may have to be retained longer than usual, and the ED_{50} (lowest dose giving the delayed effect in 50% of the animals) may be required where the delayed effect of interest is nonlethal.

Some indication of organ-specific toxicity may be obtained during the LD_{50} test if the animals are autopsied. At other times it is necessary to study the effect of high sublethal doses of the poison. The reason for this is that death, rather than sacrifice,

Table 5.1. Poisons and Antidotes

Poison	Antidote
Heavy metals	Chelators
Cyanide	Sodium nitrite, sodium thiosulfate, dicobalt EDTA, hydroxocobalamin, 4-dimethylaminophenol
Hydrogen sulfide	Sodium nitrite, 4-dimethylaminophenol
Organophosphates	Atropine, pyridinium oximes
Carbamates	Atropine
Methanol	Ethanol, 4-methylpyrazole
Ethylene glycol	Ethanol, 4-methylpyrazole
Acetaminophen	N-acetylcysteine
Chlorates, nitrites	Methylene blue 1% solution
Opiates	Naloxone
Hydrofluoric acid	Calcium gluconate (gel and injectable)
Chlorine gas inhalation	Sodium bicarbonate/normal saline nebulized inhalation

of some of the animals during LD_{50} studies makes interpretation of the histology difficult. It may be necessary to study the effects of the toxin on specific cell types within the target organ to define the site of action at the cellular level.

It is important to know whether it is the poison itself or a metabolite which is toxic. This will profoundly influence the likely therapeutic strategy, since the biochemical pathway from poison to active metabolite may provide a possible site of action for an antidote. The pharmacokinetics of the toxin may be useful in designing animal efficacy studies and in the choice of animal model.

MECHANISM OF ANTIDOTAL ACTION

Mechanisms of antidotal action include: (*a*) antidotes that directly bind or chelate toxins; (*b*) antidotes that act indirectly to influence binding or metabolism of toxins via some activity with enzymes; (*c*) antidotes that bind or affect toxic metabolites; (*d*) antidotes that act as receptor antagonists of toxin or toxic metabolites.

ANTIDOTES THAT DIRECTLY BIND OR CHELATE TOXINS

Many antidotes bind directly to the toxin to produce a less toxic product or one which is readily mobilized, metabolized, and excreted. Such antidotes include calcium gluconate used in fluoride burns. Other examples include the chelating agents used in heavy metal poisoning as well as dicobalt edetate and hydroxocobalamin used in cyanide poisoning. The Fab fragments used in digoxin poisoning and monoclonal antibodies in soman poisoning react directly and nonenzymatically with toxins.

Metal Chelating Agents

These comprise a group of drugs which mobilize and enhance the elimination of metals by complexation. Disodium calcium ethylenediaminetetraacetate ($CaNa_2EDTA$) and its analogs chelate lead and zinc can be used in cadmium poisoning. Dimercaprol (British anti-lewisite, BAL (4, 5) is used for the treatment of arsenic poisoning. Newer, water-soluble analogs of dimercaprol, dimercaptosuccinic acid (DMSA) and dimarcaptopropane sulfonic (DMPS), are useful for the same purpose. Penicillamine is a monothiol chelator, which has been used for some years for the treatment of Wilson's disease and will mobilize a variety of metals. N-Acetyl DL-penicillamine and D-penicillamine are less toxic than the racemic mixture and are to be preferred. Deferoxamine is a compound that specifically binds iron.

Dicobalt Edetate and Hydroxocobalamin

There are many analogies between chelation therapy and other antidotes reacting directly with the poison. In the case of the cobalt cyanide antidotes, the stability of cobalt/cyanide complexes has been known for many years, but cobalt is a fairly toxic metal and was considered to be too toxic for clinical use. This view was changed by the discovery of the efficacy of hydroxocobalamin in the treatment of experimental cyanide poisoning of mice (16). Hydroxocobalamin is not a convenient antidote. Although a concentrated preparation is being developed in France (17), formulations available at present are for the treatment of pernicious anemia, and very large volumes would thus be necessary to treat cyanide poisoning, especially as one molecule of hydroxocobalamin only binds one molecule of cyanide. The introduction of dicobalt edetate, a cyanide antidote popular in Europe, was based on work carried out by Paule (18–22) which apparently aimed at finding a compound with the efficacy of inorganic cobalt and the low toxicity of hydroxocobalamin. Numerous cobalt compounds were studied: the chloride, acetate, gluconate, and glutamate. Among these compounds were two organic complexes of cobalt, cobalt histidine and dicobalt edetate. Both were effective and less toxic than the other compounds studied. The final choice between them was made on the basis of the apparently more favorable therapeutic index of dicobalt edetate.

Antibodies and Fab Fragments

In the case of many poisons, no antidote of acceptably low toxicity has been discovered. In such circumstances it is possible to adopt an immunologic approach. Fab antibody fragments have been used in poisoning by digoxin (23–25). The advantage of Fab fragments over whole antibodies is that the former are less immunogenic and can be eliminated by glomerular filtration (26). Despite the greater immunogenicity of whole antibodies, the use of monoclonal antibodies in poisoning by the organophosphorus nerve agent soman has been reported (27), and murine monoclonal antibodies against paraquat have been produced with the aim of eventual therapy (28). Immunotherapy for poisoning is a method of treatment that is of wide general applicability (29), and theoretically it can be used against any toxin to which antibodies can be made. Using antibodies as antagonists of toxins is supported by the high number of possible antibody combinations for antigens (which exceeds 1×10^{10}), the high resolution and specificity of antibodies, the use of Fab fragments, the use of hybridoma technology to produce monoclonal antibodies, and the ability of antibodies to behave as antiidiotypes to produce receptor site antagonism.

There are constraints on the general use of antibody therapy to reverse toxic effects of drugs and other toxins. Antibody efficacy depends on:

Obtaining high affinity, high titer immunoglobulin (IgG),
Isolating a highly purified IgG or Fab fragment,
A favorable mole to mole ratio between toxin and antibody,
Ability of the antibody to influence toxin pharmacokinetics,
Route and timing of administration, and
Immunogenicity and acute allergic reactions.

ANTIDOTES THAT ACT INDIRECTLY TO INFLUENCE BINDING OR METABOLISM

Sodium Nitrite, Sodium Thiosulfate, and Methylene Blue

Indirect mechanisms of antidotal action are exemplified by the present treatment for cyanide poisoning, using methemoglobin-forming agents, sodium nitrite or 4-methylaminophenol. These agents produce formation of methemoglobin by the oxidation of hemoglobin in the erythrocyte. Both cyanide and hydrogen sulfide have a higher affinity for methemoglobin, as compared to that of cytochrome oxidase enzymes. In the case of cyanide, the chelation with methemoglobin forms cyanmethemoglobin, thus trapping cyanide, the erythrocyte, and effectively lowering plasma cyanide concentrations (30–32). Following the administration of sodium nitrite, a sulfur donor, sodium thiosulfate, is administered intravenously. Since methemoglobinemia is reversible and will release cyanide back into plasma, thiosulfate administration to form a less toxic thiocyanate ion is crucial to successful therapy (33). There is evidence that the therapeutic combination of sodium nitrite and sodium thiosulfate therapy is synergistic (34).

Another indirectly acting antidote is methylene blue. Methylene blue, as a 1% solution, is used to reverse toxic methemoglobinemia produced by a variety of nitrites and nitro-containing compounds (41). Methylene blue acts as a nonenzymatic catalyst to increase the activity of NADH-linked methemoglobin reductase enzymes to reduce methemoglobin to hemoglobin (42). Methylene blue administered in excess can also cause methemoglobinemia (43).

Unlike most of the above antidotes, which react directly and nonenzymatically with the toxin, the administration of sodium thiosulfate exploits an endogenous enzymatically catalysed pathway. A number of routes of detoxification of cyanide exist, of which that catalysed by rhodanese is the most important. This enzyme catalyses the conversion of cyanide to the much less toxic thiocyanate ion. Since its activity is normally limited by the supply of sulfur donor, the whole process may be hastened by intravenous injection of sodium thiosulfate. In actual fact, it has long been recognized that sodium thiosulfate used alone is not a very effective cyanide antidote. Although it can accelerate cyanide transulfuration 13–30-fold (35, 36). A further important feature of thiosulfate treatment of cyanide poisoning is that the enzyme rhodanese is located in the mitochondrion, which is relatively inaccessible to sodium thiosulfate administered intravenously. Thus, the rather slow action of this antidote is readily explicable. In an attempt to improve sulfur treatment of cyanide poisoning, various other compounds, including sodium ethane and propane thiosulfonates and tetrathionate have been studied (37–40). In some respects they are superior to sodium thiosulfate in animal studies, but none has achieved clinical use.

OXIMES

The complexity of the action of the pyridinium oximes, pralidoxime chloride (2-PAM) and obidoxime (Toxigonin), in organophosphate poisoning is only now becoming apparent. It is clear that these drugs have a variety of actions, many of which, especially the newer ones such as HI-6, may contribute substantially to their beneficial activity in organophosphate poisoning. Therefore, to some extent, their action defies therapeutic classification. Nevertheless, as generally depicted, the target of the oxime antidote is the complex formed between the poison and the various cholinesterases. Dephosphorylation or dephosphonylation of the enzyme is accompanied by phosphorylation of the oxime. Salts of pralidoxime, the chloride (2-PAM),

methanesulfonate (P2S), or methylsulfate have become one component of the standard treatment of organophosphate poisoning. In chemical defense, the inefficacy of PAM salts against tabun is a major disadvantage. Some bis-pyridinium oximes are active against tabun and seem as effective or more effective than pralidoxime salts in organophosphorus pesticide poisoning. Therefore, in certain countries, for example Germany, obidoxime, a bis-pyridinium oxime, is used instead of 2-PAM. Although oximes are generally administered along with atropine in poisoning by organophosphate pesticides, their cholinesterase-reactivating potency varies against different organophosphate nerve agents and pesticides. It is known that they are relatively inactive against certain pesticides (44). However, the large number of organophosphate derivatives, together with the lack of information on the reactivating effects of oximes on their complexes with cholinesterases, means that it is often necessary to assume that oximes will be effective and proceed with treatment. Reported to be important with pesticides (45), ''aging,'' loss of an alkyl group from the phosphorylated or phosphonylated enzyme, renders it refractory to oxime reactivation (46). In chemical defense, the lack of effectiveness of 2-PAM or obidoxime against ''aged'' cholinesterase is responsible for poor results in the experimental treatment of soman poisoning. Newer pyridinium oximes, HI-6 and pyrimidoxime, have been studied in order to solve this problem, but it is likely that their efficacy in soman poisoning is due to extremely rapid reactivation of the enzyme or to noncholinesterase reactivating properties of these oximes (47–49).

ANTIDOTES THAT AFFECT TOXIC METABOLITES

When a poison exerts its action by the formation of a toxic metabolite it may be possible to treat the poisoning by inhibiting the metabolic pathway involved, by increasing the rate of metabolism or elimination of the toxic metabolite, or binding the metabolite.

ETHANOL AND 4-METHYLPYRAZOLE

Inhibition of metabolite formation can occur by competitive or noncompetitive inhibition, or by deprivation of a cosubstrate or cofactor of the reaction. An example is methanol poisoning where the toxic metabolites are formic acid and formaldehyde (50). Several substances are known to inhibit alcohol dehydrogenase, such as 4-methylpyrazole (51). In practice, however, ethanol, which is also a substrate for this enzyme, is used so that the metabolism of methanol is inhibited competitively. Ethylene glycol (15) is another alcohol giving rise to a metabolic acidosis, but with the formation of oxalic acid rather than formic acid. Poisoning by ethylene glycol can be treated analogously with ethanol (52, 53), while pyrazole and 4-methylpyrazole have been used experimentally (54, 55).

N-ACETYLCYSTEINE

A number of substances have been used in the treatment of poisoning with acetaminophen, including cystamine, methionine, and N-acetylcysteine. N-Acetylcysteine achieved widespread use. Its mode of action is, to some extent, controversial, but the most likely explanation is that it restores hepatic reduced glutathione, which detoxifies N-acetyl-p-benzoquinoneimine, a powerfully electrophilic metabolite of acetaminophen that produces hepatic necrosis (56–58).

Antidotes That Antagonize Effects at the Target Organ or Receptor Site

This type of antidote acts without any chemical alteration of the poison. Broadly this involves two types of processes: (a) antagonism at specific pharmacologically characterized receptors or other receptor macromolecules or (b) functional antagonism.

NALOXONE, OXYGEN, ATROPINE

True receptor antagonism is exploited in the treatment of narcotic poisoning by the antagonist naloxone, and in a number of other situations (59–61).

Oxygen is used in the treatment of carbon monoxide poisoning. Carbon monoxide is toxic because it has a very high affinity for hemoglobin, forming the pigment carboxyhemoglobin, which is not capable of carrying oxygen. 100% oxygen or, better still, hyperbaric oxygen can decrease the duration of coma and lessen overall mortality from this gas (62). There is also evidence that the prevalence of late sequelae is reduced (63–65). Oxygen competes with carbon monoxide for the hemoglobin molecule.

The relationship between carboxyhemoglobin and the partial pressure of oxygen in the blood is expressed by the Haldane equation:

$$\frac{COHgb}{O_2Hgb} = (m)\frac{PCO}{PO_2}$$

Due to the high affinity of CO for hemoglobin (240 times that of O_2), the higher the partial pressure of O_2, the faster the decline in COHgb. The mass effect of a very high PaO_2 as can be attained by hyperbaric oxygen is:

21% O_2 (room air) = PaO_2 100 mm Hg = 0.3 ml O_2/100 ml blood

100% O_2 = PaO_2 673 mm Hg = 2 ml O_2/100 ml blood

2 ATM (hyperbaric) = 4.3 ml O_2/100 ml blood

Since CO also binds to other heme-containing proteins, such as cardiac myoglobin and cytochrome enzymes, it is probable that the Haldane effect would also occur at these sites to displace CO.

The use of atropine in organophosphate and carbamate anticholinesterase poisoning is not true receptor antagonism. Atropine blocks the muscarinic receptors to prevent the effects of excess acetylcholine produced by the inhibition of cholinesterase. Somewhat analogously, physostigmine, used in atropine poisoning, promotes the accumulation of acetylcholine, which overcomes the anticholinergic effects of atropine.

The use of diazepam in toxin-induced seizures, such as organophosphates, is an example of clinical efficacy induced by receptor site occupation of a drug that does not directly antagonize the toxin (66). Other examples of functional antagonism include supportive therapies that lessen or control toxic effects (67–69).

DEVELOPMENT OF NEW DRUGS

Principles involved in new drug development are: (a) modification of an already existing drug (lead drug concept); (b) modification of naturally occurring substances such as antibodies; (c) random testing of a variety of organic compounds; (d) coincidental finding of an active compound. Unless such a compound already exists, the most difficult part of development of an antidote to a poison is the identification of a "lead" drug.

ASSESSMENT OF ANTIDOTAL EFFICACY

Studies in Vitro

Certain aspects of the action of antidotes can be studied in vitro. This is particularly so with direct-acting antidotes. However, there are always limitations on extrapolation of the data to the treatment of human poisonings. This is exemplified by the situation with metals and chelators. Here there is a body of knowledge that enables the prediction of efficacy of particular chelating drugs against particular metals on theoretical grounds (70–72). However, on occasions, stability constants of the metal-chelator complex can be misleading as Catsch and Harmuth-Hoene (73) found with penicillamine and diethylenetriamine pentaacetate in the treatment of mercury poisoning. These workers found that penicillamine was the more effective metal chelating agent, while the corresponding stability constants would suggest the reverse. Further to refine studies in vitro and hypothesizing that hydrophobicity of the chelator ligand complex was important in successful chelation therapy, Yokel and Kostenbauder (74) studied chelating agents for use in aluminum poisoning in an octanol/aqueous system and in rabbits poisoned with this metal. They concluded that the ideal chelator would have a high affinity for the metal of interest, be sufficiently water-soluble to take by mouth, and be sufficiently lipid soluble to distribute to sites of accumulation of the metal. If this is generally the case, partition studies would clearly improve the predictivity of in vitro studies of antidotes of this class. Nevertheless, the in vivo situation cannot be approximated in vitro, even with chelating agents, a group of antidotes where in vitro studies could be misleading.

The mechanism of action of other direct-acting antidotes can be studied without using animals, and the stability of antidote-poison complexes is a useful index of efficacy. With a family of antidotes having similar modes of action, the field may be narrowed without using animals. In vitro studies may also be useful with antidotes that are not direct-acting. Both sodium nitrite and 4-dimethylaminophenol form methemoglobin in vitro (75), Moreover, human blood can be used. However, even if species difference is avoided by the use of human blood, a major difficulty remains with this group of antidotes; the argument has been raised that sodium nitrite does not act primarily by producing methemoglobin. Obviously, if that is the case sodium nitrite and 4-dimethylaminophenol cannot validly be compared using relative speed of methemoglobin formation as the criterion of efficacy in vitro or even in vivo. By contrast, if a classical efficacy study is performed in vivo, with lethality as the endpoint, the mechanism of antidotal action is not important in interpretation of the results.

In the case of more complex chemical interactions between antidote and poisons, such as occur when the pyridinium oximes are used to treat organophosphate poisoning, many approaches using in vitro methodology can be used in the study of the antidote. Cholinesterase reactivation by pralidoxime salts or bispyridinium oximes was studied by Ganendrin and Balabaskaran (76) and Hibbiger and Vojvodić (77). Such studies are extremely valuable in evaluating the various oximes against different cholinesterases inactivated by different organophosphorous compounds. An additional advantage is that cholinesterases of human origin can be used. Furthermore, the in vitro approach has proven useful in the study of the precise mode of action of the pyridinium oximes at the cellular level and in the study of the noncholinesterase reactivating properties of these drugs (78–81). It must be recognized that, as with chelating agents in metal poisoning, there are major limitations to the information that can be obtained in vitro, because the situation in the whole animal can only be approximated.

Experiments in vitro can often be useful in receptor antagonism whether or not the antagonism is at pharmacologically characterized receptors. Receptor binding assays (82) are a particularly useful technique.

In the case of functional antagonism, in vitro studies tend to be less useful and more difficult to design. The limitations of the in vitro approach become apparent when attempts are made to compare two or more antidotes that work by different mechanisms. Here, problems of extrapolation to the in vivo situation make the experiments difficult to interpret (83).

Studies In Vivo

Having identified a possible antidotal mechanism and ascertained that a ''lead'' antidote works in vitro, it is necessary to conduct studies in animals. The aim of such experimental work is to study the efficacy of the potential antidote and to determine that it is sufficiently nontoxic to be clinically useful. Both efficacy and toxicity studies will require the choice of suitable experimental animals. There is no reason why the same species should be used for both purposes. Paule (19) chose between cobalt histidine on the basis of an efficacy study in dogs and a toxicity study in mice. The reasons that a species is a satisfactory model of human poisoning in efficacy studies (i.e., similar metabolic or pharmacokinetic handling) often render the same species suitable for toxicity studies.

CHOICE OF ANIMAL MODEL

The most difficult part of antidotal development is the choice of an animal species that adequately models the poisoning and the action of the antidote in humans. The choice of animal model depends on similarity in absorption, distribution, excretion, and metabolism, and target of the toxicant, and similar factors with the antidote. Other considerations influencing the choice may include the amount of information available on particular species, together with size, availability, and cost of

particular animals. The use of large or exotic animals will limit the numbers that may be studied. It is therefore necessary to make a balanced judgment on the basis of toxicologic considerations and factors such as expense and convenience. When considering pharmacokinetic and metabolic factors it must be remembered that the importance of these depends on the way the poison and antidote work. If they act without metabolic activation it is their rate of removal from their target which is the main factor to be considered; such removal may be by metabolism or urinary excretion. Consideration of pharmacokinetic properties, as well as the biotransformation of both the toxin and potential antidote, are important factors influencing selection of an animal model. In general, if the toxicity of the agent in question is due to a metabolite or distribution to a target organ, then clinical pharmacokinetic studies and knowledge of metabolism are crucial to successful antidotal therapy. Animal species must then be selected to allow such extensive investigations. If the toxin acts directly as the parent compound, then species selection is less critical.

Interspecies Differences in Absorption and Distribution

Major differences between an animal species and humans in absorption kinetics by the usual route of entry of the poison renders that species unsuitable as a model. Often human poisoning is by ingestion. When studying oral poisons it is essential to remember that species differences in gastrointestinal pH will considerably affect both rate and site of absorption of weak electrolytes by altering their ionization (84). Among compounds that are more slowly absorbed in humans than other animals following oral administration is pentobarbital (85). This drug is more slowly absorbed from the human stomach than that of dogs or cats. It is crucial that the animal study closely simulate the actual route of human exposure and absorption.

Most often, antidotes are given intravenously, in which case absorption rates after oral administration are irrelevant. Although pharmacokinetics after intravenous administration are important, major differences between the species occur less often by this route than by mouth. Oral antidotes include metal chelators such as 2,3-dimercaptosuccinic acid (DMSA), D-penicillamine, and N-acetylcysteine (86–88). The use of oral metal chelators as therapeutic agents allows for the outpatient management of metal poisonings. Also, the gastrointestinal absorption of these drugs is well understood. Oral N-acetylcysteine is commonly used for acetaminophen toxicity, but an intravenous form has been tested and is efficacious in preventing and blunting hepatotoxicity from acetaminophen in acute oral overdose.

Toxins absorbed from dermal or inhalational routes of exposure can be difficult to study and require sophisticated animal models and technologies. Monkey and pig skin most closely duplicate human skin in absorption dynamics and anatomy and are thus frequently used in dermatoxicity studies (87, 89). Inhaled toxins require complicated technologies including inhalation chambers to simulate the actual exposure scenario. Delivery of the toxin may be in the form of an aerosol, vapor, particle, or fiber. Nose-only exposures of animals eliminates other body contact and external contamination that could introduce error into the study (87–90).

A source of variability in toxic effects in inhalation studies is the differences in the rate and depth of ventilation of the animals being studied, which could deliver different exposure doses. The difference in ventilation is an important aspect in human toxicity since pulmonary exposure to a toxin is dependent on the rate and depth of ventilation in many situations of low level exposure. Other important parameters are the intrinsic toxicity of the chemical, its water solubility, and concentration in the breathing zone of the animal being studied. The influence of ventilation on the delivery of a highly toxic poison is best demonstrated by cyanide gas exposure. Variability in lethality following cyanide gas exposure in animal species is probably due to variations in ventilation since the poison is so toxic (91–96).

Another important role of the lung is in biotransformation of inhaled chemicals (92). Thus, error can be introduced in toxicity studies if this factor is not considered and the inhalation route not studied in terms of metabolite production by the lung. Choice of dose is complicated by the two variables of concentration and duration of exposure, as many poisonous gases do not obey Haber's law and the LCt_{50} (concentration $\times$ time killing 50% of the animals) is not constant. Doubtless for these reasons, the inhalation route is often not used for administration of toxicants that are primarily an inhalation hazard. In view of the role of the respiratory tract as a site of biotransformation of xenobiotics (92), this is to be deprecated. It is perhaps permissible to use a substitute route in certain circumstances, but such studies should be visualized as a preliminary to inhalation experiments. Particular problems arise where inhalation poisons, especially irritants, have local effects on the lungs. In such cases it is generally impossible to carry out antidotal studies after intoxication by any route other than inhalation. An alternative, the intratracheal route, was studied by Brown et al. (93), who concluded that the failure of intratracheally administered solutions to penetrate to the periphery of the lung resulted in significant pathologic differences and limited the usefulness of this route as a substitute for inhalation. As well as being unphysiologic and toxicologically unsatisfactory, the technique is not particularly easy.

Neither percutaneous nor inhalation routes are modes of administration for antidotes. An exception is the use of amyl nitrite in cyanide poisoning. This antidote was formerly believed to work by producing methemoglobin. However, while amyl nitrite can produce quite substantial quantities of methemoglobin in animals, it does not seem to do so in humans (19, 94, 95). There are possible reasons for this, such as a difference in absorption or in hemoglobin sensitivity, but it is more likely that healthy humans cannot be persuaded to inhale amounts comparable to those given to animals (96).

Another important point that may affect the behavior of both toxicants and antidotes is their extent of plasma protein binding. In many cases (e.g., cyanide) this affects activity. Plasma protein binding studies are often carried out using fairly simple procedures, such as equilibrium dialysis, and should be a preliminary to the choice of animal model. In many instances the extent of plasma protein binding can be determined in vitro. For example, Sturman and Smith (97) added salicylate to plasma

from humans and a number of animal species. Plasma from humans, rhesus monkeys, guinea pigs, and rabbits all showed high binding capacities, while lower protein binding was seen in the plasma of baboons, horses, dogs, rats, and mice. Conversely, protein binding with amphetamines is less in human plasma than that from many other mammals (98). Other important toxicants that are protein-bound include certain metals, cyanide, and morphine (99). There is evidence that the proportion of the toxicant not protein-bound tends to increase with higher concentrations, so that, with drug overdose, protein binding at therapeutic concentrations is not a reliable guide to overdose (100). A further consideration is binding within the erythrocyte. Some substances (e.g., arsenic) show considerable species variation in binding to red cell components, especially hemoglobin (101, 102).

Plasma protein binding of antidotes has been less studied, and where it has differences have generally not been great (103). Penicillamine and the opioid antagonists and partial agonists, naloxone, naltrexone, and nalorphine, all show a degree of protein binding (103–105). Dimercaptopropane sulfonic acid is reported to show a greater degree of plasma protein binding in humans than in dogs (88).

Differences in Metabolism

While species differences in metabolism may be an important cause of differing responses to toxicants, this is not always the case. With very quick-acting poisons, such as cyanide, concentrations at the target may be determined over the period of a few minutes. Drawbaugh and Marrs (106) concluded that hepatic levels of rhodanese, the enzyme generally believed to be responsible for catalyzing the major part of cyanide detoxification, did not determine interspecies differences in susceptibility to acute cyanide poisoning, simply because there was no time for any substantial amount of transsulfuration to occur. Furthermore, qualitative differences in metabolism may be less important than differences in the rate of metabolism, especially with direct-acting toxicants. Where substances are toxic by virtue of their metabolism to a metabolite, species differences influencing the conversion are most likely to affect choice of animal model. Metabolism of the toxic metabolite will have to be considered in addition, so that the situation is more complicated than that of the direct-acting toxicant.

Many species, strain, and sex differences in metabolism of common poisons have been described. Urinary metabolites and metabolites present in the plasma, are studied using radiolabeling techniques combined with high pressure liquid chromatography.

A number of important species differences have been reported among phase I and phase II metabolic processes. These differences affect the toxicity of the alcohols, methanol and ethylene glycol. With methanol, there is a major difference between humans and pigtail macaques, on the one hand, and rats, on the other. Differences in the specificity of alcohol dehydrogenase mean that the acidosis characteristic of human poisoning can only reliably be reproduced in the pigtail macaque (48, 107). Interestingly the rhesus monkey only sometimes develops acidosis. There is a considerable difference in toxicity of ethylene glycol in different species. This substance is more toxic to cats than to rabbits or guinea pigs; humans appear to resemble cats in susceptibility (108–109). There are major interspecies differences in p-hydroxylation of aromatic compounds (110). This is exemplified by the metabolism of amphetamine, which appears in the urine of humans predominantly unchanged but where a substantial proportion is p-hydroxylation in rats (111). Numerous species differences in metabolism of organophosphate pesticides have been recorded (112); thus the much greater degree of hepatic demethylation seen in dogs than rats renders the dog generally more resistant to certain organophosphates (113). There are also major interspecies differences in serum esterase activity toward organophosphates among mammalian species (114).

Species differences in phase II reactions are very common, but, since they often do not affect the concentration of the toxicant at its target, they are frequently unimportant. A major exception is the relative failure of the cat to form glucuronides, with phenol (115), acetaminophen (116), and morphine (117), an idiosyncrasy that seems to render cats rather susceptible to some of these compounds. Unless there is clear evidence that the behavior of blood levels of a toxicant are similar in humans and cats, the latter are generally unsuitable for the study of poisoning by aromatic compounds.

Species differences in metabolism of antidotes are less studied than those in toxicants. With the cyanide antidote, 4-dimethylaminophenol, there are major differences in excretion products in rats, dogs, and humans (118–121).

With poisons and antidotes, it is species differences that are the most important considerations, but the possibility of strain and age-related differences must be considered. Examples of the latter were described in beagles by Ecobichon and colleagues (122). With the cyanide antidote, 4-aminopropiophenone, which requires metabolism to an N-hydroxy metabolite before acquiring activity, both species (Wood, unpublished data) and sex differences in metabolism have been observed (123). Because the observed sex differences had a major effect on methemoglobin production, it would be expected to affect the efficacy of this antidote.

Species Differences in Excretion

With rapidly acting toxicants, such as hydrogen cyanide and hydrogen sulfide, differences in excretion are unlikely to affect the outcome of the poisoning. With more slowly acting poisons this is not the case, and species differences in both biliary and urinary excretion may be important. Biliary excretion is particularly important, and significant species differences often exist. Stein and others (124), found that guinea pigs and rabbits had lower excretion rates of methyl mercury than mice, rats, and hamsters. Abou-el-Makerem et al. (125) divided animals into good, intermediate, and poor excretors. Monkeys fall into the poor group, and there is some evidence that humans are similar (89).

Species Differences in Response at the Target

Major differences in target organ response can be a serious problem with toxicants regardless of the mechanism of toxicity. An example is provided by those compounds that are toxic by virtue of producing methemoglobin and also by the methemoglobin-producing cyanide antidotes. Small laboratory animals, particularly mice, are much less sensitive than either dogs or humans to this group of compounds. While some interspecies variation may be caused by differences in susceptibility of the hemoglobin to catalytic oxidation (75), most is due to difference in the level of erythrocytic methemoglobin reductase (126–128). Where antagonism occurs at pharmacologically characterized receptors, species differences in receptor specificity, density, and distribution will have to be considered.

Choice of Model—Other Considerations

In particular types of experiments the choice of model may be influenced by considerations other than metabolism and pharmacokinetics. Thus organophosphate-induced delayed neurotoxicity is often studied in hens (129) because of the great sensitivity of atropinized hens to the development of this phenomenon. Pigeons have been used to study T-2 trichothecene toxicity due to their propensity to vomit (130). Where behavioral endpoints are required, decisions on species are often difficult. Furthermore, the ability of the species in question to perform the test may be the determining factor. Attempts to study the more complex aspects of human behavior often require the use of primates.

Choice of Model Conclusion

Smith and Caldwell (131), who reviewed drug metabolism in nonhuman primates, stated that they generally had an advantage over nonprimate species as metabolic models for humans. In certain behavioral studies they also have advantages. Nevertheless there are instances in which they differ from humans. Moreover, the use of primates has major disadvantages from the animal welfare, cost, and husbandry points of view. Other species commonly used in studies of the effects of antidotes are the dog and rabbit and various rodent species. Larger animals, generally farm animals, may be used in the study of poisons and antidotes if they are the target species (132, 133). Birds and other nonmammals have only rarely been used because of major metabolic and physiologic differences from humans. Moreover, their response to toxicants is poorly documented. Ultimately the choice of model is made on similarity to the target species (usually humans) in pharmacokinetic and metabolism of both poison and antidote.

CHOICE OF MODEL IN ANTIDOTE TOXICITY STUDIES

The acute toxicity of the antidote is required for more than one purpose. The first is in the design of efficacy experiments, as a guide to maximum allowable dose, and the second is for regulatory submission. It is therefore convenient to carry out acute toxicity studies in two species, one not being rodents (i.e., rats and dogs or monkeys), as required by most regulatory authorities. If the species to be used in efficacy studies is not one of these three, additional toxicity studies should be carried out on that species.

Table 5.2. Design of Experiments to Assess Antidotal Efficacy

Animals	Species, strain, sex
	Numbers
	Controls
Poison	Dose
	Route
	Solvent, diluent, excipients
	Stability
	Dose volume
Antidote	Dose
	Route
	Solvent, diluent, excipients
	Stability
	Dose volume
Temporal factors	Time between poison and antidote administration
Outcome	Lethality
	Biochemical toxicity
	Hematologic toxicity
	Physiologic changes
	Behavioral toxicity
	Neurotoxicity
	Pathotoxicology

Design of Antidote Efficacy Studies in Vivo

Preliminary to the introduction of a novel antidote into clinical practice is the demonstration that it is effective in vivo experimental conditions. There are a number of reasons why it is impossible to move straight from a theoretical antidotal mechanism to treatment of human poisoning, both regulatory and scientific. In these respects, antidotes are similar to other drugs. However, there are some ways in which antidotes, as a class, differ from other drugs, and the main one is that the human clinical trial under controlled conditions is not possible. While case reports of the use of antidotes have great value, the advantage of animal experimentation is that the dose of poisoning, and the time relationship between the poisoning and administration of the antidote can be controlled.

In vivo efficacy studies share many features with other scientific experiments. It is important to design studies to obtain the maximum information. The study must be scientifically valid in terms of animal numbers and design; sources of observer bias should be eliminated, and aspects of the experiment such as diet, age, and sex of the animals, the time of day, and other points should be standardized. This is most suitably done by designing a detailed protocol. It must also be appreciated that the study has to be designed to demonstrate that the antidote will be effective in humans. A study in an unsuitable species, however well-designed, will not achieve this object. The general rule is that, a species with a similar response to the poison and the antidote to that in humans should be used. Furthermore, the experiment should be constructed so that the poisoning and treatment mimic, as closely as possible, the likely sequence of events in a human poisoning.

Because of the large number of aspects of efficacy studies which are open to variation (Table 5.2), a variety of different protocols have been employed.

ANIMALS

The number of animals used is determined by the overall experimental design. The other factor to be considered is the use of controls. While data from the literature may be helpful in the initial dosing schedules, failure to use controls will considerably diminish the scientific validity of the experiment. More debatable is the use of control groups receiving the treatment without the poison. With more toxic antidotes, it is desirable to know that the antidote is not contributing to the toxicity ascribed to the poison. Therefore, while the absence of a treatment-only group does not necessarily render a study invalid, its presence is recommended.

POISON

Important factors influencing the overall design of the study is the dose of poison to be used as the challenge and whether a variable or single dose regime is to be adopted. One of the designs most frequently adopted is that in which the LD_{50} of the poison is measured with and without treatment to give a protection ratio (also called dose reduction factor, potency ratio (132, 134), and protective ratio (135). The advantage of this type of design is that it exploits the known (or presumed) relationship between log dose and probit mortality (136), and it gives the result of the study as a single figure. The disadvantages are that large numbers of animals are necessary, not only for the LD_{50}, but also for the preliminary studies that are usually necessary. The protection ratio type of design has usually been adopted if small laboratory animals have been used in the study. Moreover, the desire to exploit log dose probit mortality relationships may have encouraged some workers to use animals that are unsuitable models of the human poisoning and its treatment. The result of doing this is that the efficacy of the toxicant and antidote may be established in mice with perfect confidence but no conclusions as to its likely usefulness in humans may be drawn. Another point that must be considered is that the single figure that results from protection ratio studies is not always as meaningful as appears. This is because the slopes of the log dose probit mortality lines for the treated and untreated animals may not be parallel. In that case the protection ratio only describes the antidotal efficacy in animals poisoned with a dose equal to the LD_{50}. Since the clinical toxicologist is usually interested in what happens at supralethal doses, the likely efficacy in clinical human poisoning may be underestimated or overestimated, depending on the direction of the deviation. It is even possible that the lines may cross, implying a therapeutic penalty at certain doses. Deviations from parallelism in protection ratio studies are common and suggest that either the cause of death has been changed or that the antidote contributes to lethality. Ways around the problem have been suggested (NL Cross, unpublished) that involve expressing the results in ways more relevant to the usual human high dose poisoning. If the LD_{50} protection ratio is retained, the LD_{90} ratio can be quoted in addition.

Protection ratio-type experimental designs have been widely adopted despite these problems. Thus, studying cyanide poisoning in mice, Smith (137) determined the effect of the experimental antidote, sodium cobaltinitrite, on the LD_{50} of sodium cyanide. In the same species the antidotal properties of sodium pyruvate and rhodanese have also been studied (34, 134). The same type of design was adopted by Heilbron and Tolagen (138), Hobbiger and Vojvodić (139), Berry and Davies (140), Gordon et al. (135), Inns and Leadbeater (141), and Cetković et al. (142), all studying the therapy and prophylaxis of organophosphate poisoning.

Although protection ratio-type designs have generally not been used in larger animals, there are a few examples of such use. For example, Burrows and Way (132) studied cyanide antidotes in sheep, while Dirnhuber et al. (143) investigated the protection afforded by pyridostigmine against soman poisoning in rhesus monkeys and marmosets.

The main alternative to dosing using the log dose probit mortality relationship is to use a single dose of toxicant and compare the outcome (e.g., survival) in an untreated group and a group treated with the antidote. In some studies the choice of dose of the poison may have been simply based on guesswork, but it should be more properly based on knowledge of the dose-response of the test species to the poison. Frequently the dose of toxicant is chosen on the basis of LD_{50} and the slope of the log dose probit mortality line. The goal is a dose of toxin that is lethal to untreated animals but which a proportion of the treated animals can be expected to survive. The advantage of this type of design over the protection ratio-type design is that fewer animals are required. On the other hand only a small degree of antidotal action is needed to produce a dramatic improvement in survival (137). Nevertheless, this type of design has been widely used. In the case of the treatment of cyanide poisoning with 4-dimethylaminophenol, Lörcher and Weger (144), Klimmek et al. (145), and Marrs et al. (146) all employed this type of design. It has also been used in the study of prophylaxis of the same poisoning (147). These studies were all performed in dogs, as was that of Weger and Szinicz (148), who evaluated various oxime antidotes to organophosphorus nerve agents. A similar experimental design was used by Pill et al. (149), working on poisoning by the cyanogenic antihypertensive drug, sodium nitroprusside, in mice and rabbits. Examples are also provided by the work of Klemm (150), on physostigmine antidotes in small laboratory animals, that of van Stee (51), who studied the experimental ethylene glycol antidote, pyrazole, in rats and dogs, and a study by Agoston et al. (151) in which the treatment of verapamil-poisoned cats with 4-aminopyridine was studied.

Ideally, the poison should be administered by the same route it usually enters to the body. Many poisons are ingested; in that case they would logically be administered by gavage. Alternatives such as the intramuscular and the intravenous route produce different pharmacokinetics, while intraperitoneal administration is not comparable to any human route of poisoning.

As has been discussed, inhalation poisoning, an important industrial route of exposure, raises particular problems, especially where local effects or metabolism occur in the lung. Moreover, there is both the total dose to be considered (Ct, concentration $\times$ time) and the concentration. In inhalation studies, the ideal of a pharmacologically acceptable study under realistic conditions tends to be more constrained than in experiments using other routes of administration. Similar difficulties exist in the evaluation of treatments for compounds toxic

to the skin. For example, with organophosphates, poisoning is frequently by several routes simultaneously. In such circumstances it is logical to use the preponderant one. The use of a single route can represent a deviation from the human situation. In all cases, it is essential to standardize variables such as the time over which administration takes place.

Diluents

It is essential that a diluent not contribute toxic actions of its own. This is usually achieved by using saline or distilled water, but sometimes other solvents, for example, dimethyl sulfoxide, are needed. The possibility of unexpected solvent effects must be controlled for in the study. The stability of the toxicant in solution is sometimes a problem, for instance, with cyanide (147); if so, the material should be made up as freshly as possible and assayed at the end of the study.

If large dose volumes are used in small laboratory animals, hemodynamic disturbances may occur. Unusual routes, such as the intratracheal one, as a substitute for inhalation severely limit the dose volume and may limit the dose of an insoluble toxin.

ANTIDOTE

The antidote dose depends on its acute toxicity and the anticipated effective dose, and pilot studies may be needed. Where there are inadequate data, a high dose is often used to show efficacy, and reduced stepwise. Sometimes the doses of both poison and antidote are systematically varied (16), but more usually the antidote is used at a constant dose. Where the effectiveness of a novel antidote is being compared with a clinically established antidote, the latter is often given at the human dose adjusted for the weight of the animal, but allowance must always be made for known interspecies differences in response.

The antidote should be given by the most clinically useful route of administration. In the vast majority of acute poisonings, this will be by intravenous injection. In subacute and chronic poisoning, and in heavy metal poisoning, a multiple dosing regime, perhaps with oral dosing, may be appropriate.

Generally, preparations of antidotes have to be suitable for intravenous injection. Ideally they should be given as the formulation eventually to be used clinically. This is often not practicable; indeed during initial studies experimental antidotes may not even be chemically pure. For these reasons it is essential to document the source and purity of antidote, the solvent used, and any other substances added. The results of not doing this can be seen in the published literature on dicobalt edetate. The preparation available in the United Kingdom and France (Kelocyanor) contains glucose as well as dicobalt edetate. In certain studies it is unclear if the commercially available Kelocyanor was used, or some other preparation, or pure aqueous dicobalt edetate. This makes comparison of studies very difficult. In addition, failure adequately to identify active ingredients, excipients, and impurities may create problems at the licensing stage.

With a few antidotes, stability is a problem. The main example of this is the otherwise promising organophosphorus antidote, HI-6 (41). While this is mainly a logistic problem affecting the practicality of clinical use of the antidote, the possibility of deterioration of an experimental antidote in the laboratory should be considered.

Protein Denaturation and Purity for Antibodies as Antidotes

The purification of IgG from whole antiserum may result in a loss of IgG that is specific for a toxin targeted for neutralization. Purification procedures may involve chemical precipitation of IgG from antisera with polyethylene glycol or ammonium sulfate which results in a mixture of endogenous and specific IgG. Some specific IgG may be lost, and it has been estimated that this may be up to 50% of specific IgG. Another procedure used to isolate specific antibody is immunoabsorbent affinity chromatography. This method relies on harsh conditions such as low pH of elution buffer to concentrate IgG and release it from the affinity column affinant. These acidic buffer elutions denature protein.

Efficacy testing of immunotherapies must include protein assays, affinity binding studies, and activity studies of the antibody. The route of administration as well as the overall protein load must be considered in any animal studies.

TEMPORAL FACTORS

One of the features of the efficacy study most difficult to solve is the time relationship between administering the poison and the antidote. This is particularly true of antidotes being used for rapidly acting poisons such as hydrogen cyanide and organophosphorus nerve agents. In these instances, the time relationship between poison and antidote may crucially affect the outcome. In various studies the antidote has been given before, simultaneously with or after the poison (152). The use of prophylactic protocols has been criticized as producing misleading results and only seems appropriate when evaluating antidotes to be used militarily in a chemical defense context (136).

The antidote can be given at a fixed time after administration of the poison or at the onset of a particular clinical sign. Thus Burrows and Way (132) gave antidotes 5 minutes after cyanide, and Klimmek et al. (145) gave it 1 or 4 minutes afterwards. Similarly, Kepner and Wolthuis (153) gave oximes 1.5 minutes after soman injection. The criticism of this approach lies in its implication for therapy.

The alternative is to administer treatment at the onset of poisoning, a procedure adopted by Lörcher and Weger (144) and Marrs et al. (146) studying cyanide antidotes. While this may be more realistic, a fairly dramatic sign must be used, and care must be taken to avoid observer bias. These problems can be avoided by using a change in a physiologic variable as the cue for treatment.

OUTCOME

In most of the experiments death or survival has been the endpoint of the study. A variety of physiologic or biochemical measurements have been carried out in antidotal studies. Sometimes these have been used alone, but they have also frequently been used as adjuncts to lethality, often to confirm that the antidote had the anticipated mechanism of action (38). Survival time should always be recorded in conventional lethality studies, and increased survival time can be used as a measure of success (27, 154).

Other endpoints that may be desirable in studying antidote efficacy include clinical pharmacokinetic parameters in half-life, volume of distribution, and elimination of both toxin and metabolites. This is particularly valuable for drugs that directly bind to toxins, drugs that either enhance metabolism or inhibit metabolism of the toxin. Generally, when the clinical pharmacokinetics of a toxin are altered, the toxicity will be altered. Examples of this are the alteration of plasma concentration and the volume of distribution of protein poisons or drugs by antibodies; the prevention of metabolism of ethylene glycol and methanol by ethanol or 4-methypyrazole; and the increased urinary elimination of lead by 2,3-dimercaptosuccinic acid. Thus efficacy of an antidote can be studied using pharmacokinetic endpoints, instead of lethality or pathological processes. An example of an undesirable change in tissue distribution is the observation by Aposhian et al. (155) that dimercaprol (BAL) increased the arsenic concentration in the brain after poisoning with arsenicals. Aaseth (156) stated that animal studies were essential in the evaluation of chelating agents. In these biologic studies, half-life decrease is often used to measure the success of treatment (157); however, decreased concentration of the toxicant in the target organ is better (156). Since the chelator might produce non-biologically active chelates, concentration of active toxicant might be the best endpoint. An exception to this is chelation of radioactive elements. In this case the goal is to rid the body of as much as possible in order to minimize the longterm effects of contamination with radionuclides (159).

Other biochemical endpoints can be used. In nitroprusside poisoning concentrations of cyanide, the toxic metabolite of sodium nitroprusside are appropriate (160), but it should be noted that some cyanide antidotes interfere with cyanide assays. The metabolic acidosis associated with methanol and ethylene glycol poisoning can be used to evaluate the success of therapy for toxicity of these alcohols. Clay and Murphy (52), when studying the effect of the alcohol dehydrogenase inhibitor 4-methylpyrazone in ethylene glycol poisoning, used change in plasma pH. Other types of biochemical endpoints that have been used include liver function tests. De Vries et al. (152) used such tests to evaluate acetylsalicylic acid against hepatotoxicity associated with acetaminophen. Investigating the effect of indomethacin and other treatment regimes on lung fibrosis produced by administration of butylated hydroxytoluene, Kehrer and Witschi (161) measured hydroxyproline. An essential feature of the use of a nonlethal endpoint in an antidotal study is that it is related to a reversal or diminished effect of the poisoning. The use of erythrocyte or plasma cholinesterase as an index of oxime therapy in organophosphate poisoning does not correlate closely with events at the neuromuscular junction or central nervous system, which are important in determining the outcome of the poisoning.

Prevention of red blood cell hemolysis is a useful endpoint for studying efficacy of a drug for treatment of arsine poisoning. Hemolysis is a clinical endpoint responsible for increased morbidity and mortality following arsine gas exposure.

Other useful physiologic and electrophysiologic parameters for studying antidote efficacy include the electrocardiogram and its various intervals, the electroencephalogram, or electromyography and nerve conduction velocities. The efficacy of an antidote in reversing effects of a cardiotoxin that affects the PR, QRS, or QT complexes of the electrocardiogram can be studied by appropriately monitoring these intervals. Other cardiotoxic effects can best be monitored by cardiac dynamics such as blood pressure, heart rate, cardiac chamber pressure changes, and contractility of the myocardium.

Anatomical pathology and tissue histopathology are always important in the efficacy studies of a treatment modality. This includes gross anatomical changes in organs as well as microscopic changes in target tissues. Both are necessary since gross organ examination may be normal, yet definite histopathology has occurred. In some instances electron microscopy may be necessary to study pathotoxicologic effects.

Histopathologic endpoints are used in a lethal context. Gross changes such as lung weight for poisons giving rise to pulmonary edema are sometimes used (162). More commonly, microscopic anatomical pathology is used. An example is the effect of oxygen on chemical lung injury, where fibrosis can be assessed (93). Visualization by an anatomic pathologist may be unreliable in detecting minor changes, but image analysis techniques are making this type of approach much more attractive. Furthermore, the use of pathologic studies has obvious advantages in the study of treatment of poisoning by drugs such as acetaminophen, where there is more than one target organ. It was shown by Jeffrey and Haschek (163) that dimethyl sulfoxide protected against the hepatic changes but not the respiratory toxicity induced by acetaminophen in the mouse.

Different from the above endpoints is the use of a behavioral outcome to determine success or failure. There are situations where the investigators have been more interested in the threshold for incapacitation. Generally, this has been because the casualty would be in a situation where incapacitation might disable them from protecting themselves. This is primarily of importance in a military context but is also important in the context of cyanide and carbon monoxide poisoning in fires. In other instances the reason for the use of behavioral endpoints is not so clear, and it may have been that there was a desire to reuse animals, a procedure not scientifically sound. Behavioral outcomes were used by D'Mello (164) in guinea pigs poisoned with organophosphates or cyanide and by Palfai and Felleman (165) in mice challenged with digitoxin.

ANTIDOTAL REGIMES

Some antidotes are given in combination with another one. Well-known examples include the methemoglobin-inducing cyanide antidotes, sodium nitrite and 4-dimethylaminophenol, which are followed by sodium thiosulfate and the oximes, pralidoxime chloride and obidoxime, which are accompanied by

atropine. The rationale, in both cases, is probable synergism (40, 166). Where antidotes are designed to be used in combination, it is logical to use them in efficacy experiments. This raises no particular problems except that it increases the complexity of the experiment and may complicate the choice of animal model and dosing schedule.

COMPARISON OF ANTIDOTAL REGIMES

Before moving on to clinical studies, the most useful step, after establishing the efficacy of the antidote in animals, is to compare the antidote with those already in use. With many treatment regimes this is simple because there is a generally accepted therapy. For some poisonings, however, there is no worldwide agreement on appropriate treatment. For example, in the United States sodium nitrite and thiosulfate are used in cyanide poisoning, while in the United Kingdom and France dicobalt edetate (Kelocyanor) is preferred. German-speaking countries use 4-dimethylaminophenol. Similar differences are found with oximes where the United States favors pralidoxime chloride; the United Kingdom, pralidoxime methanesulfonate; France, pralidoxime methylsulfate; and Germany, Poland, and Sweden, the bispyridinium oxime, obidoxime chloride. Possibly, international organizations such as the International Programme on Chemical Safety of the World Health Organization might sponsor studies to compare these antidotes in animals. Investigators tend to evaluate new treatments against those already in use in their own country.

Antidotes and Regulatory Toxicology

Regulatory requirements for antidotes are no different than for other drugs. It is, however, generally recognized that, as a class of drugs, antidotes are often relatively toxic. Some adverse effects are predictable on the basis of acute toxicity studies. For example the low LD_{50} of BAL as compared with dimercaptopropanesulfonic and dimercaptosuccinic acids suggests the latter two chelating agents might be safer than the first, a conclusion which clinical experiences support. Often toxic effects are closely related to desirable pharmacologic effects. Thus the toxicity of dimercaprol and other chelating agents has been related to interaction with essential trace elements and is caused by the lack of specificity of chelating agents (167). It has to be recognized that certain toxic effects, such as the occasional reactions seen in humans to dicobalt edetate (168) and N-acetylcysteine (169), are rarely observed in animals and only usually become apparent when the drug is introduced into clinical use.

In actual fact the degree to which the toxicity of antidotes has been studied before introduction varies. In some cases, e.g., 2-PAM (41, 170), acute, repeated dose and subchronic studies have been carried out in experimental animals. The cyanide antidote, sodium nitrite, has also been studied after repeated administration. Other aspects of toxicity such as reproductive toxicity and teratogenicity have been studied for some antidotes. Mutagenicity data are available on a few, for example, pralidoxime salts and HI-6 (170) and 4-dimethylaminophenol (171). Many will feel that such investigations are irrelevant to the use of drugs on single occasions and in life-threatening situations, and, in general, in the United States, they would not be requested (172).

CLINICAL STUDIES

Phase I testing of antidotes does not differ from other drugs. It is always a difficult and serious decision to introduce a novel chemical into a human. The decision involves balancing expectation of success and improvement in existing therapy against the work and money involved.

Much of the information gained during phase I studies is pharmacokinetic: protein-binding, clearance, volume of distribution, and plasma half-life, together with urinary excretion and identification of metabolites after single dose administration to human volunteers. At this point it may be possible to identify major differences and similarities to the animals previously used in toxicity and efficacy studies. It is in phase II studies that the special difficulties with antidotes become apparent. While it may be possible to design some sort of clinical trial, one that fully satisfies the criteria of Mahon and Daniel (173) is inconceivable. Probably for this reason many antidotes have been introduced after simple uncontrolled trials of efficacy, often organized as multicenter trials.

Conclusions

In many ways, antidotes are unattractive drugs to the pharmaceutical industry. The market is often small, while the drugs are expensive to develop. It is therefore not surprising that many have been developed under a military impetus.

REFERENCES

1. Sullivan JB: Poisonings, drug overdose, and toxic exposures. In: Kravis, T Warner C, eds: Emergency Medicine—A Comprehensive Review. 2nd ed. Aspen Publishers, Rockville, Maryland: 1987.
2. Virenque C. Antidotes et traitment specifique dans les intoxications aigües. Cah Anesthesiol 1983;31:371–376.
3. Burger A. Drug design. In: Hamner CE, ed. Drug development. Boca Raton, FL: CRC Press, 1982:53–72.
4. Stocken LA, Thompson RHS. British anti-lewisite 3. arsenic and thiol excretion in animals after treatment of lewisite burns. Biochem J 1946;40:548–554.
5. Thompson RHS. Therapeutic applications of British antilewisite. Br Med Bull 1948;5:319–324.
6. Pedigo LG. Antagonism between amyl nitrite and prussic acid. Trans Med Soc Va 1988;19:124–131.
7. Wilson IB, Ginsberg S. A powerful reactivator of alkylphosphate-inhibited acetylcholinesterase. Biochim Biophys Acta 1955;18:168–170.
8. Wilson IB. Acetylcholinesterase. XI. Reversibility of tetraethylpyrophosphate inhibition. J Biol Chem 1951;190:111–117.
9. Wilson IB. Molecular complementarity and antidotes for alkylphosphate poisoning. Fed Proc 1959;18:752–758.
10. Rumack BH, Lovejoy FH. Clinical toxicology. In: Klaasen CD, Amdur MO, Doull J, eds. Casarett and Doull's toxicology, the basic science of poisons. 3rd ed. New York: Macmillan, 1986:879–901.
11. Brown VKH. Acute toxicity testing. In: Balls M, Riddell RJ, Worden AN, eds. Animals and alternatives in toxicity testing. London: Academic Press, 1983:1–16.
12. Natoff IL, Reiff B. Quantitative studies of the effect of antagonists on the acute toxicity of organophosphates in rats. Br J Pharmacol 1970;40:124–134.
13. Garland H, Pearce J. Neurological complications of carbon monoxide poisoning. Q J Med 1967;36:445–455.
14. Werner B, Back W, Akerblom H, Barr PO. Two cases of acute carbon monoxide poisoning with delayed neurological sequelae after a "free" interval. J Toxicol Clin Toxicol 1985;23:249–266.
15. Aldridge WN, Barnes JM, Johnson MK. Studies on delayed neurotoxicity produced by some organophosphorus compounds. Ann NY Acad Sci 1969;160:314–322.
16. Muschett CW, Kelley KL, Boxer GE, Rickards JC. Antidotal efficacy of vitamin B_{12a} (hydroxo-cobalamin) in experimental cyanide poisoning. Proc Soc Exp Biol Med 1952;81:234–237.
17. Rousselin X, Garnier RL. Intoxication cyanhydrique: conduite à tenir en milieu de travail et aspect actuel du traitement de l'intoxication aigüe. Doc Méd Travail 1985;23:1–8.
18. Paulet G. Intoxication cyanhydrique et chélates de cobalt. J Physiol (Paris) 1958;50:438–442.
19. Paulet GL. L'intoxication cyanhydrique et son traitement. Paris: Masson SA, 1960.
20. Paulet G. Nouvelles perspectives dans le traitement de l'intoxication cyanhydrique. Arch Mal Profess 1961;22:120–127.
21. Paulet G. Au sujet du traitement de l'intoxication cyanhydrique par les chélates de cobalt. Urgence 1965:611–613.
22. Paulet G, Chary R, Bocquet P, Fouilhoux M. Valeur comparée du nitrite de sodium et des chélates de cobalt dans le traitement de l'intoxication cyanhydrique chez l'animal (chien-lapin) nonanesthesié. Arch Int Pharmacodyn 1963;127:104–117.
23. Smith TW, Haber E, Yeatman L, Butler VP. Reversal of advanced digoxin intoxication with Fab fragments of digoxin specific antibodies. New Engl J Med 1976;294:797–800.
24. Lloyd BL, Smith TW. Contrasting rates of reversal of digoxin toxicity with digoxin-specific IgG and Fab fragments. Circulation 1978;58:208–283.
25. Stolshek BS, Osterhout SK, Dunham G. The role of digoxin-specific antibodies in the treatment of digitalis poisoning. Med Toxicol 1988;3:167–171.
26. Cole PL, Smith TW. Use of digoxin-specific Fab fragments in the treatment of digitalis intoxication. Drug Intell Clin Pharm 1986;20:267–269.
27. Lenz DE, Brimfield AA, Hunter KW. Studies using a monoclonal antibody against soman. Fundam Appl Toxicol 1984;4:S156–S164.
28. Johnston SC, Bowles M, Winzor DJ, Pond SM. Comparison of paraquat-specific murine monoclonal antibodies produced by in vitro and in vivo immunization. Fundam Appl Toxicol 1988;11:261–267.
29. Sullivan JB. Immunotherapy in the poisoned patient overview of present applications and future trends. Med Toxicol 1986;1:47–60.
30. Vesey CJ. Letter. Clin Toxicol 1979;14:307–308.
31. Ballantyne B. Letter. Clin Toxicol 1979;14:311–312.
32. Marrs TC, Bright JE. Effect on blood and plasma cyanide levels and on methaemoglobin levels of cyanide administered with and without previous protection using PAPP. Hum Toxicol 1987;6:139–145.
33. Daunderer M. Klinische Erfahrungen mit dem Antidot 4-DMAP, einem Methamoglobinbildner zur Behandlung von Vergiftungen mit Blausäure und ihren Salzen, von Schwefelwasserstoff und von Stickstoffwasserstoffsäure und ihren Salzen. Dissertation for the appointment as Reader, University of Munich, Federal Republic of Germany, 1979.
34. Chen KK, Rose CL, Clowes GHA. Methylene blue, nitrites and sodium thiosulphate against cyanide poisoning. Proc Soc Exp Biol Med 1933;31:250–251.
35. Cristel D, Eyer P, Hegemann M, Kiese M, Lörcher W, Weger N. Pharmacokinetics of cyanide in poisoning of dogs and the effect of 4-dimethylaminophenol or thiosulfate. Arch Toxicol 1977;38:177–189.
36. Sylvester DM, Hayton WL, Morgan RL, Way JL. Effects of thiosulfate on cyanide pharmacokinetics in dogs. Toxicol Appl Pharmacol 1983;69:265–271.
37. Clemedson C-J, Hultman HI, Sörbo B. The antidote effect of some sulfur compounds and rhodanese in experimental cyanide poisoning. Acta Physiol Scand 1954;32:245–251.
38. Clemedson C-J, Hultman HI, Sörbo B. A combination of rhodanese and ethanethiosulfonate as an antidote in experimental cyanide poisoning 1955;35:31–35.
39. Frankenberg L. Enzyme therapy in cyanide poisoning: effect of rhodanese and sulfur compounds. Arch Toxicol 1980;45:315–323.
40. Baskin SI, Kirby SD. The interaction of sodium thiosulfate (NaS_2O_3) and 1,4(N,N-dimethysulfide) with guinea pig liver rhodanese. Toxicologist 1988;8:531.
41. Kiese M, Lörcher W, Weger N, Zierer A. Comparative studies on the effects of toluidine blue and methylene blue on the reduction of ferrihaemoglobin in man and dog. Eur J Pharmacol 1972;4:115–118.

42. Kiese M. Methemoglobinemia, a comprehensive treatise. Cleveland, OH: CRC Press, 1974.

43. Bright JE, Inns RH, Marrs TC. Methaemoglobin production and reduction by methylene blue and the interaction of methylene blue with sodium nitrite in vivo. Hum Toxicol 1989;8:359–364.

44. Bismuth C, Inns RH, Marrs TC. The efficacy and clinical use of oximes in anticholinesterase poisoning. In: Ballantyne B, Marrs TC, eds. Clinical and experimental toxicology of organophosphates and carbanates. Sevenoaks, England: Butterworth-Heinemann, 1991.

45. Gyrd-Hansen N, Kraul I. Obidoxime reactivation of organophosphate-inhibited cholinesterase activity in pigs. Acta Vet Scand 1984;24:86–95.

46. Hobbiger F. Reactivation of phosphorylated anticholinesterase. In: Koelle GB, ed. Handbuch der experimentelle Pharmakologie XV. Berlin: Springer-Verlag, 1963:921–980.

47. de Jong LPA, Wolring GZ. Reactivation of acetylcholinesterase inhibited by 1,2,2¹-trimethylpropylmethylphosphonofluoridate (soman) with HI-6 and related oximes. Biochem Pharmacol 1980;29:2379–2385.

48. Schoene K, Hochrainer D, Oldiges H, Krugel M, Bruckert HJ. The protective effect of oxime pretreatment upon the inhalative toxicity of sarin and soman in rats. Fundam Appl Toxicol 1985;5:S84–S88.

49. Kiffer D, Minard P. Reactivation by imidazo-pyridinium oximes of acetylcholinesterase inhibited by organophosphates. Biochem Pharmacol 1986;35:2527–2533.

50. Cooper JR, Kini MM. Biochemical aspects of methanol poisoning. Biochem Pharmacol 1962;1:405–416.

51. Clay KL, Murphy RC, Watkins WD. Experimental methanol toxicity in the primate: analysis of metabolic acidosis. Toxicol Appl Pharmacol 1975;34:49–61.

52. Peterson DI, Peterson JE, Harding MG. Experimental treatment of ethylene glycol poisoning. JAMA 1963;186:955–957.

53. Wacker EC, Haynes H, Fisher W. Treatment of ethylene glycol poisoning with ethyl alcohol. JAMA 1965;194:1231–1233.

54. van Stee EW, Harris AM, Horton MI, Back BC. The treatment of ethylene glycol toxicosis with pyrazole. J Pharmacol Exp Ther 1975;192:251–259.

55. Clay KL, Murphy RC. On the metabolic acidosis of ethylene glycol intoxication. Toxicol Appl Pharmacol 1977;34:49–61.

56. Huggett A, Blair IA. The mechanism of paracetamol-induced hepatotoxicity: implications for therapy. Hum Toxicol 1983;2:399–405.

57. Dawson JR, Norbeck K, Anundi I, Moldeus P. The effectiveness of N-acetylcysteine in isolated hepatocytes against the toxicity of paracetamol, acrolein and paraquat. Arch Toxicol 1984;55:11–15.

58. Flanagan RJ. The role of acetyl cysteine in clinical toxicology. Med Toxicol 1987;2:93–104.

59. Jeffreys DB, Volans GN. An investigation of the role of the specific opioid antagonist naloxone in clinical toxicology. Hum Toxicol 1983;2:227–231.

60. Prescott LF. New approaches in managing drug overdosage and poisoning. Br Med J 1983;287:274–276.

61. Bateman DN, Chaplin S. Antidotes to human toxins. In: Turner P, Volans ON, eds. Recent advances in clinical pharmacology and toxicity. Vol 4. Edinburgh: Churchill-Livingstone, 1989:173–195.

62. Matthieu D, Nolf M, Durocher A, Saulnier F, Frimat P, Furon D, Wattel F. Acute carbon monoxide poisoning risk of late sequelae and treatment by hyperbaric oxygen. Clin Toxicol 1984;23:315–324.

63. Ginsberg MD, Myers RE. Experimental carbon monoxide encephalopathy in the primate. I. Physiologic and metabolic aspects. Arch Neurol 1974;30:202.

64. Ginsberg MD, Myers RE, McDonagh BP. Experimental carbon monoxide encephalapathy in the primate. II. Clinical aspects, neuropathology and physiologic correlation. Arch Neurol 1974;30:209.

65. Barois A, Grosbuis S, Goulon M. Les intoxications aigües par l'oxyde de carbone et les gaz de chauffage. Rév Prat 1974;29:1211–1231.

66. Lipp JA. Effect of benzodiazepine derivatives on soman-induced seizure activity and convulsions in the monkey. Arch Int Pharmacodyn 1975;202:244–251.

67. Burrows G, Way JL. Antagonism of cyanide toxicity by phenoxybenzamine. Fed Proc 1976;35:533.

68. Ashton D, van Reempts J, Wauquier A. Behavioral, electroencephalographic and histological study of the protective effect of etomidate against histotoxic dysoxia produced by cyanide. Arch Int Pharmacodyn Ther 1980;254:196–213.

69. Dubinsky B, Sierchio JN, Temple DE, Ritchie DM. Flunarizine and

verapamil: effects on central nervous system and peripheral consequences of cytotoxic hypoxia in rats. Life Sci 1984;34:1299–1306.

70. Ringbom A. Complexation in analytical chemistry. New York: Wiley Interscience, 1963.

71. Pearson RG. Hard and soft acids and bases, HSAB, Part II. Underlying theories. J Chem Educ 1968;45:643–648.

72. Goyer RA. Toxic effects of metals. In: Klaasen CD, Amdur MO, Doull J, eds. Casarett and Doull's toxicology: the basic science of poisons. New York: Macmillan, 1986:582–635.

73. Catsch A, Harmuth-Hoene AE. New developments in metal antidotal properties of chelating agents. Biochem Pharmacol 1975;24:1557–1562.

74. Yokel RA, Kostenbauder HB. Assessment of aluminum chelators in an octanol/aqueous system and in the aluminum-loaded rabbit. Toxicol Appl Pharmacol 1987;91:281–294.

75. Bright JE, Marrs TC. A model for the induction of moderate levels of methaemoglobinaemia in man using 4-dimethylaminophenol. Arch Toxicol 1982;50:57–64.

76. Ganendrin G, Balabaskaran S. Reactivation studies on organophosphate inhibited human cholinesterase by pralidoxime (P-2-AM). SE Asian J Trop Med 1976;7:417–423.

77. Hobbiger F, Vojvodić V. The reactivating and antidotal actions of N,N¹-trimethylenebis (pyridinium-4-aldoxime) (TMB-4) and N,N¹-oxydimethylenebis (pyridinium-1-aldoxime (Toxogonin), with particular reference to their effect on phosphorylated actylcholinesterase in the brain. Biochem Pharmacol 1966;15:1677–1690.

78. Kuhnen H. Activation and inhibition of acetylcholinesterase by toxogonin. Eur J Pharmacol 1970;9:41–45.

79. Kuhnen H. Activating and inhibitory effects of bispyridinium compounds on bovine red cell acetylcholinesterase. Toxicol Appl Pharmacol 1971;20:97–104.

80. Schone K, Steinhanses J, Oldiges H. Protective activity of pyridinium salts against soman poisoning in vivo and in vitro. ArzneimForsch 1976;22:1802–1803.

81. Alkondon M, Rao KS, Albuquerque X. Acetylcholinesterase reactivators modify the functional properties of the nicotinic acetylcholine receptor ion channel. J Pharm Pharmacol 1988;245:543–556.

82. Dunn G, Koshikawa N, Durcan MJ, Campbell IC. An examination of experimental design in relation to receptor binding assays. Br J Pharamacol 1988;94:693–698.

83. Gee SJ, LeValley SE, Tyson CA. Application of a hepatocyte-erythrocyte coincubation system to studies of cyanide antidotal mechanisms. Toxicol Appl Pharmacol 1987;88:24–34.

84. Moffatt AC. Absorption of drugs. In: Gorrod JW, Becket AH, eds. Drug metabolism in man. London: Taylor and Francis, 1978:1–23.

85. Hume AS, Bush MT, Remick J, Douglas BH. Comparison of gastric absorption of thiopental and pentobarbital in rat, dog, and man. Arch Int Pharmacodyn Ther 1968;171:122–127.

86. Vale JA, Meredith TJ, Goulding R. Treatment of acetaminophen poisoning. Arch Int Med 1981;141:394–396.

87. Smith D, Ortiz L, Archuletta R. A method for chronic nose-only exposures of laboratory animals to inhaled fibrous aerosols. In: Leong B, ed. Inhalation toxicology and technology. Ann Arbor Science, Ann Arbor MI: 1981;89–105.

88. Hruby K, Donner A. 2,3-Dimercapto-1-propanesuphonate in heavy metal poisoning. Med Toxicol 1987;2:317–323.

89. Calabrese EJ. Principles of animal extrapolation. New York: John Wiley, 1983.

90. Papirmeister B, Gross CL, Petrali JR, Hixson CJ. Pathology produced by sulfur mustard in human skin grafts on athymic nude mice. 1. Gross and light microscopial changes. J Toxicol Cut Ocul Toxicol 1984;3:371–391.

91. McNamara BP. Estimation of the toxicity of hydrocyanic acid vapors in man. Edgewood Arsenal Technical Report No EB-TR-76023. Washington, DC: Department of Defense.

92. Baron J, Burke JP, Guengerich FP, Jakoby WB, Voigt JM. Site for xenobiotic activation and detoxication within the respiratory tract: implications for chemically-induced toxicity. Toxicol Appl Pharmacol 1988;93:493–505.

93. Brown RFR, Marrs TC, Rice P, Masek LC. The histopathology of rat lung following exposure to zinc oxide/hexachloroethane smoke or instillation with zinc chloride followed by treatment with 70% oxygen. Environ Health Perspect 1990;85:81–87.

94. Paulet G. Sur la valeur du nitrite d'amyle dans le traitement de l'intoxication cyanhydrique. CR Soc Biol 1954;148:1009–1014.

95. Bastian G, Meercker H. Zur Frage der Zweckmä βigkeit der Inhalation

von Amylnitrit in der Behandlung der Cyanidevergiftung. Naunyn Schmiede-berg's Arch Exp Pathol Pharmacol 1959;237:285–295.

96. Marrs TC. The choice of cyanide antidotes. In: Ballantyne B, Marrs T, eds. Clinical and experimental toxicology of cyanides. Bristol: John Wright, 1987:383–401.

97. Sturman JA, Smith MJH. The binding of salicylate to plasma protein in different species. J Pharm Pharmacol 1967;19:621–623.

98. Baggot JD, Davis LE, Neff CA. Extent of plasma protein binding of amphetamine in different species. Biochem Pharmacol 1972;21:1813–1816.

99. Baggot JD, Davis LE. Species differences in plasma protein binding of morphine and codeine. Am J Vet Res 1973;34:571–574.

100. Rosenberg J, Benowitz NL, Pond S. Pharmacokinetics of drug over-dose. Clin Pharmacokinet 1981;6:161–192.

101. Hunter FT, Kip AF, Irvine JW. Radioactive tracer studies on arsenic injected as potassium arsenite. J Pharmacol Exp Ther 1942;76:207–220.

102. Ducoff HS, Neal WB, Straube RL, Jacobson LO, Brues AM. Biological studies with arsenic II. Excretion and tissue localization. Proc Soc Exp Biol Med 1948;69:548–554.

103. Reuning RH, Malspeis L, Franks RE, Notari RE. Testing of drug delivery systems for use in the treatment of narcotic abuse. Natl Inst Drug Abuse Res Monog 1977;141:43–45.

104. Neugebauer G. Einfluβ hover iv Dosen von D-Penicillamin auf toxische Herzglykosidwirkungen am Meerschweinchen. Arzneim forsch 1977;27:2073–2074.

105. Misra AL, Pontani RB, Vadlamani NL, Mule SJ. Physiological dis-position and biotransformation of allyl-1, 3-14C naloxone in the rat and some comparative observations on nalorphine. J Pharmacol Exp Ther 1976;196:2257–2268.

106. Drawbaugh RB, Marrs TC. Interspecies differences in rhodanese (thi-osulfate sulfurtransferase, EC 2.8.1.1.) activity in liver, kidney, and plasma. Comp Biochem Physiol 1987;86B:307–310.

107. Tephly TR, Parkes RE, Mannering GJ. Methanol metabolism in the rat. J Pharmacol Exp Ther 1964;143:292–300.

108. Troisi FM. Chronic intoxication by ethylene glycol vapour. Br J Ind Med 1950;7:65–69.

109. Gessner PK, Parke DV, Williams RT. Studies on detoxication. Biochem J 1961;79:482–489.

110. Williams RJ, Caldwell J, Dring LG. Comparative metabolism of some amphetamines in various species. In: E Usden, SH Snyder, eds. Frontiers in catecholamine research. New York: Pergamon Press, 1978:927–932.

111. Dring LG, Smith RL, Williams RT. The metabolic fate of amphetamine in man and other species. Biochem J 1970;116:425–435.

112. Hathway DE, Brown SS, Chasseaud LF, Hutson DH. Foreign com-pound metabolism in mammals. Vol 1. London: Chemical Society, 1970.

113. Crawford MJ, Hutson DH, King PA. Metabolic demethylation of the insecticide dimethylvinphos in rats, in dogs and in vitro. Xenobiotica 1976;6:745–762.

114. Mendoza CE, Shields JB, Greenhalgh R. Activity of mammalian serum esterases towards malaoxon, fenitroxon and paraoxon. Comp Biochem Physiol 1977;56C:189–191.

115. Capel ID, French MR, Millburn P, Smith RL, Williams RT. The fate of (14-C)-phenol in various species. Xenobiotica 1972;2:25–34.

116. Savides MC, Oehme FW, Nash SL, Leipold HW. The toxicity and biotransformation of single doses of acetaminophen in dogs and cats. Toxicol Appl Pharmacol 1984;74:26–34.

117. Millburn P. Factors affecting glucuronidation in vivo. Biochem Soc Trans 1974;2:1182–1186.

118. Eyer P, Kiese M. Biotransformation of 4-dimethylaminophenol: reac-tion with glutathione and some properties of the reaction products. Chem Biol Interact 1976;14:165–178.

119. Eyer P, Gaber G. Biotransformation of 4-dimethylaminophenol in the dog. Biochem Pharmacol 1978;27:2215–2221.

120. Eyer P, Kampffmeyer E. Biotransformation of 4-dimethylaminophenol in the isolated perfused rat liver and in the rat. Biochem Pharmacol 1978;27:2223–2228.

121. Klimmik R, Krettek C, Szinicz L, Eyer P. Weger N. Effects and biotransformation of 4-dimethylaminophenol in man and dog. Arch Toxicol 1983;53:275–288.

122. Ecobichon DJ, D'ver AS, Erhart W. Drug disposition and biotrans-formation in the developing beagle dog. Fundam Appl Toxicol 1988;11:29–37.

123. Bright JE, Woodman AC, Marrs TC. Sex-differences in the production of mathaemoglobinaemia by 4-aminopropiophenone. Xenobiotica 1987;17:79–83.

124. Stein AF, Gregus Z, Klaassen CD. Species differences in biliary ex-cretion of glutathione-related thiols and methylmercury. Toxicol Appl Phar-macol 1988;93:351–359.

125. Abou-el-Makerem MM, Millburn P, Smith RL, Williams RT. Biliary excretion of foreign compounds. Biochem J 1967;105:12289–12293.

126. Malz E. Vergleichende Untersuchungen über die Methämoglobinre-duktion in kernhaltigen und kernlosen Erthrozyten. Folia Haematol (Leipzig) 1962;78:510–515.

127. Smith JE, Beutler E. Methemoglobin formation and reduction in man and various animal species. Am J Physiol 1965;210:347–350.

128. Stolk JM, Smith RP. Species differences in methemoglobin reductase activity. Biochem Pharmacol 1966;15:343–351.

129. Murphy SD. Toxic effects of pesticides. In: Klaasen CD, Amdur MO, Doull J, eds. Casarett and Doull's toxicology: the basic science of poisoning. 3rd ed. New York: Macmillan, 1986:519–581.

130. Fairhurst S, Marrs TC, Parker HC, Scawin JW, Swantson DW. Acute toxicity of T2 toxin in rats, mice, guinea pigs, and pigeons. Toxicology 1987;43:31–49.

131. Smith RL, Caldwell J. Drug metabolism in non-human primates. In: Parke DV, Smith RL, eds. Drug metabolism from microbe to man. London: Taylor and Francis, 1977:331–358.

132. Burrows GE, Way JL. Cyanide intoxication in sheep: enhancement of efficacy of sodium nitrite, sodium thiosulfate and cobaltous chloride. Am J Vet Res 1979;40:613–617.

133. Gupta RC. Acute malathion toxicosis and related enzymatic alterations in Bubalis bubalis: Antidotal treatment with atropine, 2-PAM, and diazepam. J Toxicol Environ Health 1984;14:291–303.

134. Schwartz C, Morgan RL, Way LM, Way JL. Antagonism of cyanide intoxication with sodium pyruvate. Toxicol Appl Pharmacol 1979;50:437–441.

135. Gordon JJ, Leadbeater L, Maidment MP. The protection of animals against organophosphate poisoning by pretreatment with a carbamate. Toxicol Appl Pharmacol 1978;43:2207–2216.

136. Way JL, Leung P, Sylvester DM, Burrows G, Way JL, Tamulinas C. Methaemoglobin formation in the treatment of acute cyanide poisoning. In: Ballantyne B, Marrs TC, eds. Clinical and experimental toxicology of cyanides. Bristol: John Wright, 1987:402–412.

137. Smith RP. Cobalt salts: Effects in cyanide and sulfide poisoning and on methemoglobinemia. Toxicol Appl Pharmacol 1969;15:505–516.

138. Heilbron E, Tolagen B. Toxogonin in sarin, soman and tabun poisoning. Biochem Pharmacol 1965;14:73–77.

139. Hobbiger F, Vojvodić V. The reactivating and antidotal actions of N,N¹-trimethylenebis (pyridinium-4-aldoxime) (TMB-4) and N,N¹-oxydimethylene-bis (pyridinium-4-aldoxime) (Toxogonin) with particular reference to their effect on phosphorylated acetylcholinesterase in the brain. Biochem Pharmacol 1966;15:1677–1690.

140. Berry WK, Davies DR. The use of carbamates and atropine in the protection of animals against poisoning by 1,2,2-trimethylpropyl methylphos-phonofluoridate. Biochem Pharmacol 1970;19:927–934.

141. Inns RH, Leadbeater L. The efficacy of bispyridinium derivatives in the treatment of organophosphate poisoning in the guinea pig. J Pharm Phar-macol 1983;35:427–433.

142. Cetković S, Cetković M, Jandrić D, Cosić M, Bosković B. Effect of PAM-2, HI-6, and HGG-12 in poisoning by tabun and its thiocholine-like analogs. Fundam Appl Toxicol 1984;4:S116–S123.

143. Dirnhuber P, French MC, Green DM, Leadbeater L, Stratton JA. The protection of primates against soman poisoning by pretreatment with pyridos-tigmine. J Pharm Pharmacol 1979;31:295–299.

144. Lörcher W, Weger N. Optimal concentration of ferrihemoglobin for the treatment of cyanide poisoning. Naunyn-Schmiedeberg's Arch Exp Pathol Pharmacol 1971;270:R88.

145. Klimmek R, Fladerer H, Weger N. Circulation, respiration and blood homeostasis in cyanide-poisoned dogs after treatment with 4-dimethylamino-pherol or cobalt compounds. Arch Toxicol 1979;43:121–133.

146. Marrs TC, Swanston DW, Bright JE. 4-dimethylaminophenol and di-cobalt edetate (Kelocyanor) in the treatment of experimental cyanide poisoning. Hum Toxicol 1985;4:591–600.

147. Marrs TC, Bright JE, Swanston DW. The effect of prior treatment with 4-dimethylaminophenol (DMAP) on animals experimentally poisoned with hy-drogen cyanide. Arch Toxicol 1982;51:247–253.

148. Weger N, Szinicz L. Therapeutic effects of new oximes, benactyzine and atropine in soman poisoning: part I effects of various oximes in soman, sarin and VX poisoning in dogs. Fundam Appl Pharmacol 1981;1:161–163.

149. Pill J, Engeser P, Höbel M, Kreye VAW. Sodium intorprusside (SNP):

comparison of the antidotal effect of hydroxocobalamin and sodium thiosulfate in mice and rabbits. Toxicol Lett 1980;SI1:156.

150. Klemm WR. Efficacy and toxicity of drug combinations in treatment of physostigmine toxicosis. Toxicology 1983;27:41–53.

151. Agoston S, Maestrone E, van Hezik EJ, Ket JM, Houwertjes MC, Uges DRA. Effective treatment of verapamil intoxication with 4-aminopyridine in the cat. J Clin Invest 1984;73:1291–1296.

152. de Vries J, de Jong J, Lock FM, van Bree L, Mullink H, Veldhuizen RW. Protection against paracetamol-induced hepatotoxicity by acetylsalicylic acid in rats. Toxicology 1984;30:297–304.

153. Kepner LA, Wolthuis OL. A comparison of the oximes HS-6 and HI-6 in the therapy of soman intoxication in rodents. Eur J Pharmacol 1978;48:377–382.

154. Hopff WH, Riggio G, Warner PG. Another approach to the treatment of organophosphate poisoning. Pharmacologist 1981;37:671.

155. Aposhian HV, Carter DE, Hoover TD, Hsu CA, Maiorino RM, Stine E. DMSA, DMPS and DMPA as arsenic antidotes. Fundam Appl Toxicol 1984;4:S58–S70.

156. Aaseth J. Recent advances in the therapy of metal poisoning with chelating agents. Hum Toxicol 1983;2:2257–2272.

157. Aaseth J. Mobilization of methyl mercury in vivo and in vitro using N-acetyl-DL-penicillamine and other complexing agents. Acta Pharmacol Toxicol 1976;39:289–301.

158. Stather JW, Stradling GN, Gray SA, Moody J, Hodgson A. Use of DTPA for increasing the rate of elimination of plutonium-238 and americium-241 from rodents after their inhalation as the nitrites. Hum Toxicol 1985;4:573–584.

159. Stradling GN, Moody JC, Gray SA, Ellinder M, Hodgson A. The efficacy of DTPA treatment after deposition of thorium nitrate in the rat lung. Human Exp Toxicol 1991;10:15–20.

160. Krapez JR, Vesey CJ, Adams L, Cole PV. Effects of cyanide antidotes used with sodium nitroprusside infusions: Sodium thiosulfate and hydrocobalamin given prophylactically to dogs. Br J Anaesth 1981;53:793–804.

161. Kehrer JP, Witschi H. The effect of indomethacin, prednisolone and cis-r-hydroxyproline on pulmonary fibrosis produced by butylated hydroxytoluene and oxygen. Toxicology 1981;20:281–288.

162. Fox RB, Harada RN, Tate RM, Repine JE. Prevention of thiourea-induced pulmonary edema by hydroxyl-radical scavengers. J Appl Physiol 1983;55:1456–1459.

163. Jeffrey EH, Haschek WM. Protection by dimethylsulfoxide against acetaminophen-induced hepatic but not respiratory toxicity in the mouse. Toxicol Appl Pharmacol 1988;93:452–461.

164. D'Mello GD. Drug treatment for organophosphate and hydrocyanic acid poisoning in the guinea-pig. Proceedings, International Symposium on Protection against Chemical Warfare Agents. Stockholm, Sweden, June 6–9, 1983:89–93.

165. Palfai T, Felleman VH. Effect of age, clonidine or propranolol on behavioral toxicity induced with digitoxin in mice. Pharmacol Biochem Behav 1982;17:399–404.

166. Litgenstein DA. On the synergism of the cholinesterase reactivating bis-pyridinium-aldoxime HI-6 and atropine in the treatment of organophosphate intoxications in the rat (Ph.D. thesis). Leyden, the Netherlands: Rijksuniversitet te Leiden, 1984.

167. Gabard B, Planas-Bohne F, Regula G. The excretion of trace elements in rat urine after treatment with 2,3-dimercaptopropane sodium sulfonate. Toxicology 1979;12:281–284.

168. Tyrer FH. Treatment of cyanide poisoning. J Soc Occup Med 1981;31:65–66.

169. Vale JA, Wheeler DC. Anaphalactoid reactions to acetylcysteine. Lancet 1982;2:998.

170. Marrs TC. Toxicology of oximes used in treatment of organophosphate poisoning. Adverse Drug React Acute Poisoning Rev 1991;10: (in press).

171. Lee CG, Webber TD. The mutagenicity of a cyanide antidote, dimethylaminophenol, in Chinese hamster cells. Toxicol Lett 1983;16:85–88.

172. Hoyle PC. Guidelines for non-clinical toxicology studies for chemical warfare agent (CWA) antidotes and pretreatments. Regul Toxicol Pharmacol 1988;8:367–375.

173. Mahon WA, Daniel EE. A method for the assessment of reports of drug trials. Can Med Assoc J 1964;90:565–569.

6

Epidemiology and Principles of Surveillance Regarding Toxic Hazards in the Environment

Steven Piantadosi, M.D., Ph.D.

INTRODUCTION

Epidemiologic investigation is based on the observation of natural differences in exposures and outcomes among subjects. Because these studies rely on natural exposures rather than on constructive experimental design, this has led to the use of the term "observational" when describing epidemiologic studies. This is not to say that all scientific studies are not based on observation; it is merely an attempt to characterize epidemiologic studies. The major distinction between true experimental studies and epidemiologic ones is in who or what controls the exposure (or treatment). In true experimental designs, the treatment or exposure is entirely under the control of the investigator. Although randomized methods may be used, the investigator also controls these. In contrast, epidemiologic studies do not control the exposure or treatment but instead control the selection of study subjects and the methods of analysis.

For this reason, epidemiologic studies cannot provide conclusive proof of cause-effect relationships and can only hypothetically control the kinds of biases that can influence all medical studies. In spite of the shortcomings of epidemiologic research, it has an extremely important role in the science of medicine and is particularly relevant to environmental surveillance. In fact, in this specific context, it is likely that epidemiologic methods will be the only ones useful. It is simply not feasible to consider conducting designed experiments in humans regarding exposures to toxic hazards in the environment.

TYPES OF SURVEILLANCE

Studies of exposure to toxic hazards in the environment can be loosely classified in three categories: (a) descriptive, (b) etiologic or analytic, and (c) intervention. Descriptive studies record the occurrence of illness or effects in individuals under different exposures. They are most frequently used for generating new hypotheses regarding cause-effect relationships between hazards and exposures but can also be used for identifying risk factors, identifying trends, and determining background levels. Etiologic or analytic studies attempt to establish causal relationships between hazards and diseases or toxic conditions. Several factors are necessary to strengthen cause-effect hypotheses. These are the proper temporal ordering of cause in effect, control of confounding factors, elimination of bias, and consistency with plausible mechanistic theories. Additionally, demonstration of a dose-effect relationship is helpful. Intervention studies can also support cause-effect inferences and are useful for establishing the success of programs designed to control toxic hazards. In rare circumstances, it may be possible to use true experimental designs for such studies.

In all of these types of studies, it is not possible to separate the information in epidemiologic inferences from true experimental research or other designed experiments. In any specific circumstance, it is not possible to say whether basic mechanistic toxicologic research or epidemiologic methods will provide the primary impetus for reliably detecting toxic hazards in the environment. Both kinds of studies must eventually be used to support causality.

BASIC EPIDEMIOLOGIC MEASURES

This section is a brief review of basic epidemiologic measures of association. It is not meant as a substitute for more extensive discussions in textbooks [e.g., (1–3)]. Surveillance of toxic hazards requires quantitative assessments of both absolute and relative risk.

Absolute Risk

The first distinction made is between a ratio and a proportion. Ratios of measured quantities can often be used as risk indices but are frequently not very informative. A true proportion, in which the denominator contains the numerator, is often more useful. These proportions are frequently called "rates," although time may not explicitly enter the proportion. For example, the infant mortality rate is described as the number of infant deaths in the first 28 days of life divided by the total number of live births.

$$IMR = \text{Infant deaths/total live births.}$$

This rate may be determined over any suitable interval of time.

Other basic descriptive epidemiologic measures are prevalence and incidence. Prevalence is a measure of existing cases in a defined population at some time. It is defined as:

$$\text{Prevalence} = \text{Number of existing cases/size of the population.}$$

In contrast, the incidence rate is a measure of new cases that arise in a population during a defined interval. The incidence rate is

$$\text{Incidence} = \text{Number of new cases/population at risk.}$$

The incidence rate is an estimate of a true rate of change. Its precision, in part, depends on the width of the time interval (and other factors).

There is an exact mathematical relationship between the incidence rate, the prevalence rate, and the survival of subjects with the condition; however, it is not simple and is frequently not exploited. This relationship is a convolution integral omitted here for simplicity. However, when the incidence rate and survival remain constant for a sufficiently long period of time, the prevalence of any condition is directly proportional to the incidence:

Table 6.1. Frequencies of Exposure among Cases and Controls in a Retrospective Study

	Cases	Controls	Total
Exposed	a	b	a+b
Not exposed	c	d	c+d
Total	a+c	b+d	T

Odds ratio = ad/bc

Prevalence = Incidence × average duration of disease.

Relative Risk

Epidemiologists are constantly attempting to estimate the increased risk that exposure to a toxic substance in the environment imparts to an individual. One common and useful measure of increased risk is the "relative risk" (or risk ratio or rate ratio), which is available from cohort studies. It is defined as the rate of an exposed group over the disease rate of a suitable reference or control group:

Relative risk = Risk in exposed subjects/
risk in unexposed subjects

= (number of events among exposed/
number exposed)/
(number of events among unexposed/
number unexposed).

If the relative risk is greater than 1.0, the risk of an event is greater in the exposed group. Relative risks as point estimates alone are seldom useful. Some estimate of their variability in the data or population being studied is essential. This is most commonly done by providing confidence limits for the estimated relative risk. Because of natural variability, confidence limits which overlap 1.0 do not provide evidence of increased (or decreased) risk.

Relative Odds

If a random sample of the population (e.g., cohort study) is not available, the relative risk can still be estimated under certain restrictions. Often, the odds ratio from a case-control study, calculated from summary data such as that presented in Table 6.1, accurately approximates the time relative risk.

Attributal Risk

The attributal risk (AR) is the proportion of events that can be attributed to the exposure in question. It is a useful concept when events can be caused by more than one factor. It is defined as:

AR = Number exposed with event/number exposed

− number unexposed with event/number unexposed

See Table 6.1:

AR = [a/(a + c) − b/(b + d)]/[1 − b(b + d)].

ADJUSTED RATES

Invariably, it is necessary to account for the effects of confounding variables when comparing event rates. The process of accomplishing this is termed "adjustment." Unadjusted, or crude, rates can be compared reliably only if the composition of the comparison groups with respect to influential factors is similar. When this is not the case, adjustment is necessary.

Standardization is a common method in which the rates of two or more populations are adjusted to correspond with a standard distribution. The method of the standardized mortality ratio (SMR) is most frequently used. This adjustment technique may be used whether or not the rates refer to mortality. To generalize the concept, we will refer to standardized event ratios (SERs). Basically, the SER is the rate in an exposed group compared with the rate that would be expected from the standard population. Mathematically,

Standardized mortality ratio = Observed rate/expected rate.

The expected rate or expected number of cases is obtained from the "average rate" operating on the standard population. Unfortunately, SMRs may not be directly comparable to one another, because adjustment is performed separately for each exposed group with its age distribution as the standard. In other words, two or more SMRs are not necessarily mutually standardized.

MULTIVARIATE REGRESSION

To correct deficiencies in standardization, and to adjust on more than one confounding factor at a time, multiple regression techniques are often used. The most common of these for epidemiologic applications is logistic regression. This procedure is described in detail elsewhere (4). In the dichotomous outcome case (diseased versus non-diseased), the outcome, coded as a 0 vs. 1, is modeled by a set of predictor variables, x, using the equation:

$$\text{Prob[outcome = 1]} = 1/(1 + e^{-\beta x}),$$

where β is a vector of parameter estimates, each of which is the logarithm of the odds ratio for that exposure factor. When the predictor variables are also dichotomous, the odds ratios can be interpreted directly as the odds of outcome given that characteristic divided by the odds of outcome without the characteristic. When the predictor variables are continuously distributed, the odds ratio is interpreted per unit change in the predictor variable. Thus, the technique is applicable when the predictor variables are not necessarily themselves categorical. Logistic regression methods are also applicable, with modification, when the design of a study incorporates matching and when outcomes have more than two ordinal levels.

INTERPRETATION OF EPIDEMIOLOGIC STUDIES

Because of the imperfect association between deterministic causes of disease (such as exposure to a toxin) and the ultimate development of a disease, epidemiologists have developed the concept of a "web of causation." This represents the interaction of factors that contribute to the occurrence of the disease. Although developed primarily for chronic diseases, it is a concept relevant to hazards from acute exposures as well. Firm scientific evidence that an exposure causes an outcome relies on five factors. These are strengths of association, replication, biologic plausibility, temporal sequencing, and dose response. Strength of association is important because strong effects are less likely to be the result of epidemiologic confounding or bias. The variability in bias which can enter epidemiologic studies is often about the same magnitude as the effects being examined. While bias and confounding can produce large effects, it is more likely that strong associations are due to an underlying causality.

Evidence of true causality is also increased when results of independent studies are qualitatively and quantitatively similar. This consistency can be expected whether the causality or link is a strong one or a weak one. Biologic plausibility is an important component of proof of cause. It is important that a biologic mechanism exists that produces the observed effect from a toxic exposure. This evidence may rely on data gathered in species other than humans.

It seems self-evident that a causal exposure should proceed the onset of symptoms or disease. However, there is often ambiguity about the precise time of exposure, and long latent periods may further confuse the issues. Also, long latent periods may provide an opportunity for other factors to influence the onset of disease. Finally, dose-response association is important but difficult to demonstrate epidemiologically. In the laboratory, dose-response relationships can usually be shown for causal factors. However, the natural variability in human populations and the imprecision of epidemiologic studies may not allow a clear evidence of dose response.

EPIDEMIOLOGIC DESIGNS

Observational studies can be constructed in a variety of ways. All have in common the fact that the investigator did not control the exposure of subjects to any particular treatment. However, the sampling, data collection, and analyses are all carefully planned, leading to several broad categories of design.

Case Series

The simplest, oldest, and causally weakest type of epidemiologic study is the case series or case report. When causal factors are extremely large compared with the bias of case selection and with the natural person-to-person variability in outcomes, case reports may convey very useful information about the hazards of toxic exposures. However, most often case reports generate hypotheses that must be tested and strengthened by more valid types of studies.

Case reports are most useful when outcomes are extremely rare and/or when there is detailed knowledge about mechanisms of disease. For example, the Centers for Disease Control was able to alert physicians to the appearance of acquired immunodeficiency syndrome because of a few cases of *Pneumocystis carinii* pneumonia in New York City, which was previously an uncommon event.

In general, case series cannot be relied on to yield convincing causal evidence. When events can be attributed plausibly to several factors, case reports can potentially mislead. For example, isolating the causative ''exposure'' in suspected cancer clusters may be impossible or misleading if the cluster really represents random variation.

Cohort Studies

For a comprehensive review of cohort studies, see Breslow and Day (5). A cohort study is a design in which a population or sample of subjects at risk of disease is followed through time to ascertain which individuals develop the outcome of interest. The design may be implemented in real time (prospectively) or may be reconstructed from existing records (retrospective). This design closely resembles a true experiment in which the investigator controls exposure or treatment. In fact, clinical trials are a type of cohort study in which exposure (treatment) is controlled by the investigator.

The cohort design allows estimation of both absolute risk and relative risk due to prognostic factors. However, it relies upon the outcome being relatively common. For example, a cohort study would be inefficient and unfeasible in a general population experiencing only a few events per thousand person-years of follow-up. Such a study might be useful in a high risk population (e.g., industrially exposed workers).

When cohort studies are performed prospectively, they have the advantage that many factors can be accurately determined on each subject at baseline. This can greatly limit selection bias. However, this design presupposes having a well-framed etiologic hypothesis when the study is started, i.e., it is not an exploratory tool.

Cross-Sectional Design

The cross-sectional design is also called a survey or prevalence design. It is based on random sampling of a population at a single point in time. Study subjects are characterized with regard to present, and perhaps past, factors, and a determination of outcome status is made in each.

This design is most useful for studying chronic diseases of relatively high frequencies. When the sampling is properly done, cross-sectional studies are useful for characterizing the population under study. Although the prevalence of outcomes can be determined, the cross-sectional study cannot estimate incidence, because it does not observe the transition from non-disease to disease status. Furthermore, certain factors may be seen to associate with prevalent cases, but the temporal and causal order of such associations cannot be determined from this study design.

Case-Control Designs

Case-control designs are primarily retrospective studies that compare previous exposure in subjects with disease to one or more groups of subjects without disease. The investigator plans and controls the selection of cases and noncases, but not the exposure. Cases may be prevalent or incident. Case-control studies are extensively dealt with in many sources (6, 7).

Because of the type of sampling employed, i.e., the cases are selected specifically because they have the outcome of interest, these designs allow estimation of the relative odds of exposure in cases and controls, but not absolute risk. In circumstances where the outcome is rare, the case-control design may be the only feasible one. These designs are further limited because information is obtained after the manifestation of disease, and cases and controls are often selected from different populations. Thus, this design is sometimes not suitable for exploring the consequences of an environmental exposure. Because these studies are inherently retrospective, they can be influenced by recall and other biases that arise from review of possibly incomplete documents.

Matching of cases and controls on one or more factors is often done to reduce the effects of confounders. For example, if age is related to outcome, controls may be selected to approximate within some interval the age of each case. In fact, matching *induces* confounding of a type (2), and its effects must be taken into account in the analysis. When there are too many confounders to make matching practical, an acceptable strategy is to match on only a few of the strongest confounders. Other examples of matching factors are gender, race, ethnic background, and other sociodemographic characteristics.

OTHER DESIGNS

Numerous other designs have been employed in epidemiologic and surveillance studies. Such designs are often useful for taking advantage of specific exposure and outcome situations in a population. Some examples are listed below.

Case-control studies can be nested within a cohort being followed for other purposes. In this setting, cases and controls are selected from the same defined population. Matching can also be employed.

Ecologic studies have groups rather than individuals as the unit of analysis. Often the grouping variable is a geopolitical boundary (e.g., state, county, or country) and the outcome is average disease rate. Invariably, the results of such studies, which take advantage of existing databases, are intended to refer to individuals. There are potential fallacies in these types of inferences, and such studies are probably only reliable for hypothesis generation (9).

Cluster studies examine outcome frequencies in groups defined by space, time, family, or other clustering. Special methods of analysis may be required to account for or detect nonindependence of outcomes.

Numerous other designs have been discussed in the epidemiologic literature. The interested reader is referred to Kleinbaum et al. (8, Chapter 5, 1982) for additional details.

SAMPLE SIZE FOR EPIDEMIOLOGIC STUDIES

There are few decisions in the study more important than the choice of sample size. Study requirements for a certain number of cases and controls influence the economic feasibility of the study, the strength of the epidemiologic effect that can be detected, and the chances that valid conclusions will be reached. Four quantities are relevant to the assessment of sample size; the study designer must choose the first three, and the mathematical formulation yields the fourth:

1. Type I error: the chance that random variation will yield spurious evidence of risk associated with exposure when no such risk exists.
2. Power: the chance that a true risk associated with exposure will be detected. Note that a negative conclusion places a premium on this quantity; assertions that there is no effect require a study with a high chance of finding an effect if there is one.
3. Relative risk: a measure of the strength of the smallest risk associated with exposure that is considered "worth" detecting: the study is not justified if the true risk is smaller, and the study is obligatory if the true risk is at least as large. Using P_r to denote the chance of exposure among cases and P_n to denote the same chance among controls, standard

epidemiologic theory indicates that the relative risk R is estimated by $P_r(1 - P_n)/P_n(1 - P_r)$.
4. C, the number of matched case-control sets (e.g., one case and two controls), needed to detect a true relative risk of R with given type I error and power. For this example with one case and two controls in each set, the study requires 3C subjects.

A review of the relevant calculations can be found in Breslow and Day (7, 1987, chapter 7). These can take into account matching which is justified only if matching factors have a very strong impact on the medical outcome, stratification (e.g., separate consideration of subjects in groups of similar age) and "dose" trend (e.g., possible increasing frequency of outcomes for those with longer exposure). In addition, assuming that those who cannot participate in the study or cannot be traced are similar to participants may not be correct. Because of losses and dropouts, inflation of the sample size is usually needed so that the desired number of subjects can actually be analyzed.

SUMMARY

Despite their limitations, epidemiologic studies are the only ones likely to be useful in examining the effects of toxic hazards in the environment on humans. When the effects of exposure are large, these studies will yield firm evidence of causality. However, when the effects of toxic hazards are small or become apparent only after a long interval, epidemiologic evidence must be supplemented by laboratory and other data to convincingly demonstrate causality. Similar evidence from independently conducted studies in different populations is very important in this regard.

Several types of effects are important when examining evidence for environmental hazards. Elevations in absolute rates, relative rates, incidence, prevalence, or shortened times-to-event may all be evidence of a toxic hazard. When comparing event rates, it is essential that rates be appropriately standardized or, preferably, adjusted for other factors that may produce the observed outcome. In the presence of multiple causal factors, the attributal risk is a useful measure of the effect of the exposure in question.

REFERENCES

1. Kahn HA. An introduction to epidemiologic methods. In: Lilienfeld AM, ed. Monographs in epidemiology and biostatistics. New York: Oxford University Press, 1983.
2. Rothman KJ. Modern epidemiology, Boston: Little Brown, 1986.
3. Salisburg DS. Statistics for toxicologists, New York: Dekker, 1986.
4. Cox DR, Snell EJ. Analysis of binary data. 2nd ed. Monographs on statistics and applied probability 32. New York: Chapman and Hall, 1989.
5. Breslow NE, Day NE. The design and analysis of cohort studies. Statistical methods in cancer research, Vol. 2. IARC Scientific Publications No. 82. Oxford University Press, 1987.
6. Schlesselman JJ. Case-control studies design, conduct, analysis. Monographs in epidemiology and biostatistics. New York: Oxford University Press, 1982.
7. Breslow NE, Day NE. The analysis of case-control studies. Statistical methods in cancer research, Vol. 1. IARC Scientific Publications No. 32, Oxford University Press, 1980.
8. Kleinbaum DG, Kupper LL, Morgenstern H. Epidemiologic research principles and quantitative methods. New York: Van Nostrand Reinhold Co., 1982.
9. Piantadosi S, Byar DP, Green S. The ecological fallacy. Am J Epidemiol 1988;127:893–904.

7

Risk Assessment for Toxic Hazards

L. D. Hooper, D.V.M., Ph.D.
Frederick W. Oehme, D.V.M., Ph.D.
Gary R. Krieger, M.D., M.P.H.

INTRODUCTION

There are innumerable potential hazards in every aspect of daily life. Many can be attributed to chemical exposure of one sort or another. People are exposed to a staggering array of chemicals and foreign substances (xenobiotics) known to be or suspected of being harmful. It is estimated that between 30,000 and 60,000 chemicals are used in industry, agriculture, and consumer products worldwide (1, 2). Over 1400 pesticides were in use in this country at the beginning of this decade (3). The Office of Toxic Substances is called upon to review approximately 2000 new chemical products each year (4). Many are candidates for evaluation and subsequent elimination or minimization. It would be impossible to totally eliminate risk arising from the manufacture and use of chemicals. Therefore, a method of determining the attendant human health risks involved in chemical exposure is necessary (5).

Intelligent, informed decisions are needed on which risks can and should be reduced, eliminated, or simply ignored. Such decisions require information about the likelihood and severity of the hazards (6). A foundation of understanding is necessary from which to make such decisions. This need has resulted in the evolution of the risk assessment process which has been developed to aid in identification, characterization, and quantification of risk (7).

Examining the general process of chemical risk assessment as it is currently practiced will lead to better understanding of true risk. The steps involved in risk assessment, as well as strengths and weaknesses of the process, will be examined.

HISTORICAL ASPECTS OF RISK ASSESSMENT

In biblical times Joseph recognized potential risk in facing the future without a stable food supply, so he stored grain for 7 years to manage the risk of famine. There is also an admonition in the bible against eating the meat of a diseased animal (8). Pliny the Elder in the first century A.D. advised fellow Romans to grow food in their own gardens to avoid unsafe food additives common in marketed food of the time.

Cancer risk assessment evolved in the 1950s as a result of concerns regarding the health effects of radioactive exposures (9). The Delaney Clause of the U.S. Federal Food, Drug, and Cosmetic Act established the regulation of exposures to hazardous substances in consumer goods in 1959 (10). Cancer risk assessment for toxic chemicals developed in the 1960s as a result of health concerns regarding a polluted environment (9). In 1961 the FDA proposed a risk assessment methodology previously published by Mantel and Bryan (11).

The Resource Conservation and Recovery Act (RCRA) of 1976 dealt with handling new solid waste as it is generated, transported, stored, or disposed (12). In 1980 the U.S. Supreme Court con-

firmed the need for quantitative risk assessment as a decision-making tool on which to establish legal footholds in litigation involving exposures to potentially hazardous substances (13). The Comprehensive Environmental Response, Compensation, and Liability Act of 1980 (CERCLA) addressed control, jurisdiction, and remediation of preexisting environmental contaminations not covered under RCRA (12, 14, 15, 81). CERCLA established a national program for responding to releases of hazardous substances into the environment. Superfund was instituted as a basis for undertaking environmental remediation when action by the U.S. government was deemed appropriate. The Superfund Amendments and Reauthorization Act (SARA) of 1986 addressed loopholes in CERCLA and reestablished the original legislation. Risk assessment today is an essential component of regulatory decision-making (16).

WHAT IS RISK ASSESSMENT?

Risk is the probability of harm or, more explicitly, the probability of injury, disease, or death under specific circumstances (17). Put another way, risk is the potential realization of unwanted consequences of an event (18). Risk assessment is the analysis of a risk situation. It is an evaluation of the probability of harm. Health risk assessment denotes a process of research and evaluation to quantify the probability of physical harm to humans attributable to a particular agent or agents (10). In the context of chemical exposure, risk assessment is an evaluation of the risk in human exposure to chemicals in the environment (8).

Quantitative risk assessment (QRA) in the use of experimental laboratory data and/or human epidemiologic data in a process to derive the probability of harm occurring to exposed human populations (13). It is a sophisticated process involving an array of techniques that can be used to identify potential risks to human health. These techniques include epidemiologic studies, laboratory studies involving whole animals or cultures of bacteria, cells or tissues, case studies of disease outbreaks, and longterm animal bioassays (8, 9). This deliberate process provides a basis for determining what we do know and what we don't know, allowing bounds to be set on the ranges of the unknown.

Quantitative risk values have been determined according to two operational schemes that arrive at one of two endpoints (19). Toxicities that affect body organs or systems without neoplasia and derive from substances which have a quantifiable dose level greater then zero, below which no toxic effects are seen, have been treated with the safety factor approach. This approach, which can be considered a threshold approach, yields a quantitative exposure level called an acceptable daily intake (ADI), a maximum contaminant level (MCL), or, more recently, a Reference Dose (RfD).

The ADI was defined by the Environmental Protection Agency (EPA) as the amount of a toxic agent in milligrams per kilogram of body weight/day which is not expected to result in any adverse effects after chronic exposure in the general population of humans, including sensitive subgroups (25). MCLs refer to the maximum chemical specific contamination allowed for human use in drinking water. RfDs are the EPA's preferred toxicity value for evaluating noncarcinogenic effects resulting from exposures at Superfund sites. The RfD is an estimate similar in concept to the ADI but is derived using a strictly defined methodology (87). RfD utilize a threshold approach but do not imply "acceptability." Toxicities that result in cancer, caused by exposure to a substance that has no threshold, no safe level above zero, have been treated by mathematical modeling to derive levels at which an increase in the incidence of cancer is at an acceptable level. This acceptable level has frequently been established at 1 excess cancer death in 1,000,000 lifetime exposures (1×10^{-6}); however, under site-specific circumstances, EPA guidance allows a risk range between 10^{-4} and 10^{-7} (11, 13, 14, 21, 22, 25). This second approach can be thought of as a nonthreshold methodology. The exposure level associated with this technique has been designated a virtual safe dose (VSD).

The specific area of regulatory risk assessment involves the establishment of the amount, level, or concentration of a chemical that may be considered safe or acceptable. MCLs, ADIs, RfDs and VSDs represent this type of risk value. These types of values are used by regulatory agencies in the United States, such as the EPA, in formulating regulations or legislation.

Site-specific risk assessment attempts to define the public health risk from a specific exposure circumstance, usually an environmental release. Current EPA regulations state that a site-specific baseline risk assessment (previously referred to as an endangerment assessment or public health evaluation by various government entities) is required to support all administrative and judicial enforcement actions under CERCLA and RCRA (21, 26, 81).

Recently, the EPA revised both the scope and content of the human health and ecologic baseline risk assessment protocol (21). These changes are incorporated into a new "Risk Assessment Guidance for Superfund; Part A—Human Health Evaluation, Part B—Ecological Evaluation" which replaces the previous EPA guidance, the Superfund Public Health Evaluation Manual (SPHEM) (14). When a site-specific risk assessment is being done, established risk values (ADIs, RfDs, or VSDs) will be compared with the site-specific exposure doses (ED) that the population at risk is expected to incur. Exposure doses are expressed with a variety of terms. Under the Superfund format, EDs are calculated as chronic daily intakes (CDIs). CDIs represent exposure expressed as mass of a substance contacted per unit body weight per unit time, averaged over a long period of time (e.g., 7 years to a lifetime). If regulatory risk assessment procedures have not previously established RfDs or VSDs, these values must be derived from available data for use in the ongoing QRA process. For chemicals examined under the threshold approach (noncarcinogenic chemicals), this comparison consists of establishing the ED or CDI to RfD ratio. This ratio has been designated a hazard index (HI). When the RfD (the presumed safe dose) is less than the CDI, the HI has a value greater than 1, and the risk associated with that exposure is presumed to be significant (21, 85, 86).

For a chemical examined under the nonthreshold approach (potential carcinogens), risks are estimated as probabilities. The CDI, the same value as if figured for the threshold approach but assumed to characterize a lifetime exposure, is multiplied by a carcinogenic potency factor which has been extrapolated

Table 7.1 Carcinogenic Risk Calculations

One-Hit Equation for Carcinogenic Risk Levels
$$\text{Risk} = 1 - \exp(-\text{CDI} \times \text{SF})$$
Where:
Risk = A unitless probability (e.g., 2×10^{-5}) of an individual developing cancer
exp = The exponential
CDI = Chronic daily intake averaged over 70 years mg/kg-day
SF = Slope factor or unit cancer risk in (mg/kg-day)$^{-1}$

Source: U.S. EPA 1989.

from relevant data. The carcinogenic potency factor, or slope factor (known as q*), is defined as the excess risk due to continuous lifetime exposure to 1 unit of carcinogen concentration (21). The product of the CDI and the carcinogenic potency factor yield a unitless risk value, which, if greater than that acceptable by the responsible authority, is deemed to represent a significant risk. The HI and carcinogenic risk calculations are summarized in Tables 7.1 and 7.2.

The VSD concept is merely a more convenient way of approaching the risk of cancer if risk analysis has already been accomplished for the chemical in question. That is, instead of starting with a CDI and applying the model to derive an actual cancer risk value, the CDI is simply compared with the VSD; if the CDI is greater, the risk of cancer has exceeded the tolerable limit established by the responsible authority.

The goal of the risk assessment process is to derive a quantitative or numerical value equating specific exposure conditions to the probability of the endpoint in question. The endpoint will be some form of adverse health effect, such as pulmonary fibrosis, cancer, or death. Ultimately, then, the QRA attempts to predict the future incidence of adverse health effects on a population under the exposure circumstances in question. The purpose of the risk assessment process is to provide a tool that will aid risk managers in making decisions about the environment, certain biologic populations, and ultimately human health (21). Risk assessment is the basis for most regulations and legislation concerning potentially hazardous substances (11, 81).

From a regulatory perspective, significant risk has not been well-defined. Unfortunately, there has not been a consistent level of cancer risk which triggers regulation within and between the various responsible federal and state agencies. Typically, risk is framed by two concepts: (a) *de manifestis* risk, a risk of obvious or evident concern, instantly recognized by a person of ordinary intelligence, and (b) *de minimis* risk, an acceptable level of risk that is below regulatory concern. This risk is derived from the legal principle, de minimis non curat lex, "the law does not concern itself with trifles." Travis et al. have carefully analyzed cancer risk management decisions by reviewing 132 federal regulatory decisions (22). Essentially,

Table 7.2. Non-Carcinogenic Risk Calculations

Noncancer Hazard Quotient = ED/RFD
Where:
ED = Exposure dose
RFD = Reference dose
Where ED and RFD are expressed in the same units and represent the same exposure period (i.e., chronic, subchronic, or shorter terms).

Source: U.S. EPA 1989.

Travis found several general guidelines: (a) there is a de manifestis individual lifetime risk level that is a function of population risk—10^{-5}–10^{-4} for small populations and 10^{-7}–10^{-6} for large populations; (b) regulatory action should be taken if the cost is below $2 million per life saved.

THE PROCESS OF RISK ASSESSMENT

The concept of risk assessment provides a basis for determining what we do know and what we don't, allowing us to set bounds on the ranges of uncertainty (18). Because of wide variability of conditions, there is no rigid cookbook approach that can be applied universally to all chemical exposure risk situations. However, there is a methodologic approach—a step-by-step process that can be used to ensure consistent and complete analysis of different situations. There are four components involved in the formalized risk assessment process (Fig. 7.1): (a) hazard identification; (b) toxicity assessment; (c) exposure assessment; and (d) risk characterization (17, 21, 23, 24, 79, 80, 83, 86). These four steps collectively address each of six key areas identified as essential in characterizing a risk situation involving a chemical exposure: (a) hazardous substances present in all media; (b) environmental fate; (c) magnitude and pathways of exposure; (d) populations at risk (e) toxicologic properties of substances present; and (f) extent and likelihood of expected health risk.

Hazard Identification and Evaluation

Hazard identification is a process that qualitatively and quantitatively evaluates whether there is a hazard present (12, 21). This process attempts to determine what substances or chemicals are present, sources, pathways by which they contact the

environment, and whether they have the ability to potentially produce adverse health effects in humans, animals, or the environment (Fig. 7.2). All data available on the substances present are collected, organized, and evaluated for toxic potential. Data are examined to determine whether there is evidence of carcinogenesis of toxic endpoints, such as functional, physiologic, biochemical, or pathologic alterations. A formal process known as indicator selection may be utilized if multiple chemicals are present; however, EPA has recently issued new guidelines that drastically revise previous methodology (14, 21).

Toxicity Assessment

The second step, toxicity assessment, is also referred to as dose response assessment (Fig. 7.3). This step defines the relationship between the dose incurred of the chemical and the potential development of adverse health effects (9, 12). The goal of this step is to determine where on the continuum of the dose-response curve an adverse human health effect is likely to occur. Standard slope factors and RfDs are utilized. If a compound does not have an EPA approved value, then special procedures may be employed to calculate these values. For example, an RfD can be calculated by dividing an experimentally derived safe exposure level by a safety factor. This value is available from experimental data on the chemical that most closely approximates a level or concentration at or below which no toxic effects were detected. This value is most commonly the *No Observed Adverse Effect Level* or (NOAEL). A safety factor makes allowances for uncertainties or knowledge gaps in the data available on the chemical under consideration. Safety factors are customarily established by the type of data available for the evaluation, as indicated in Table 7.3 (17, 23). Carcin-

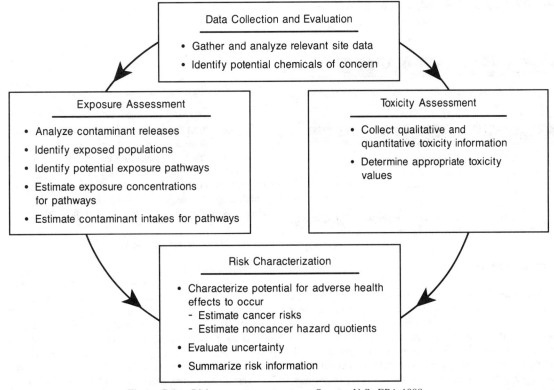

Figure 7.1.   Risk assessment summary. Source: U.S. EPA 1989.

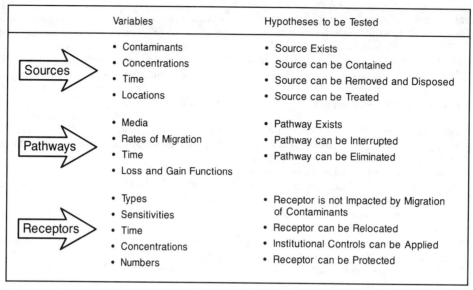

Figure 7.2. Elements of a conceptual evaluation model. Source: U.S. EPA 1989.

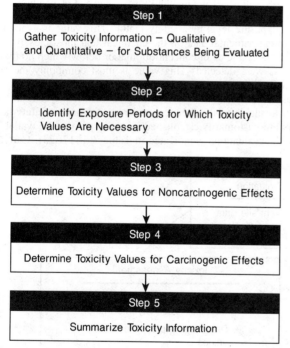

Figure 7.3. Steps in toxicity assessment. Source: U.S. EPA 1989.

ogenic slope factors can also be calculated; however, the choice of the dose-response model is critical.

Exposure Assessment

Exposure assessment is the quantification and evaluation of the dose of chemical incurred from the exposure situation under consideration (Fig. 7.4) (9). This step attempts to determine the type and magnitude of potential human exposures to chemicals (Figure 7.5) (15, 21). Monitoring data from air, soil, water, and biota are examined. Exposure assessment includes consideration of the population exposed and the magnitude, frequency, duration, and routes of exposure (21). The suscep-

Table 7.3. Safety Factors Used in Risk Assessment to Establish Reference Doses or Acceptable Levels of Exposure to Chemicals (21).

Safety Factor	Criteria for Application
10	Extrapolating data from longterm human exposure to allow for hypersensitive individuals in the population
10	Additional tenfold factor when extrapolating from chronic animal studies
10	Additional tenfold factor when less than chronic animal studies are available
1–10	Scientific judgment is used to establish any additional safety factor to account for uncertainties not addressed previously

tible population incurring exposure must be determined. The routes of exposure must be established, whether oral via ingestion from water or diet, inhalation, dermal contact, or any combination of these. Magnitude, frequency, and duration of exposures must be determined. Exposure doses are then calculated to give estimates of chronic daily and lifetime exposures, as in the enclosed example (Fig. 7.6).

Risk Characterization

Risk characterization is the final step in the QRA process. This step utilizes all information and assumptions acquired by the previous three steps (21); it provides qualitative conclusions regarding the likelihood that a chemical may pose a human health hazard. It also provides a quantitative risk value for exposure to the chemical(s) under consideration. Uncertainties in the data are pointed out and explained or rationalized if not addressed earlier in the process.

The target value of the risk characterization step is determined by the goal of the risk assessment. If the chemical under

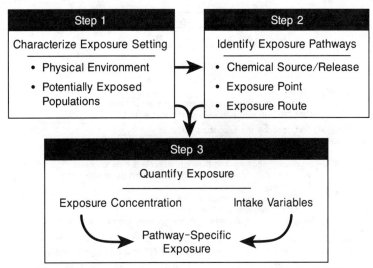

Figure 7.4. Exposure assessment process. Source: U.S. EPA 1989.

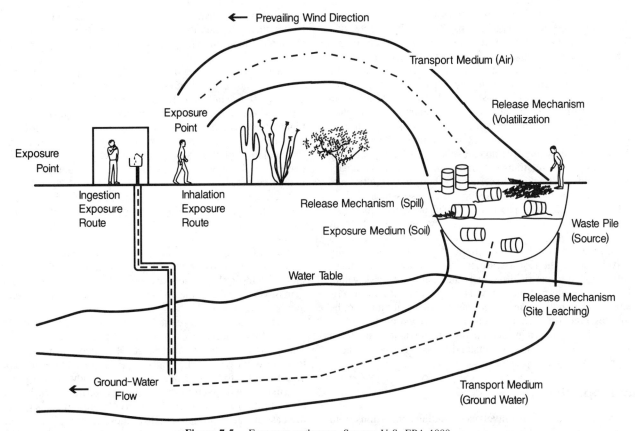

Figure 7.5. Exposure pathways. Source: U.S. EPA 1989.

consideration is a carcinogen, the target is a cancer risk value; that is, how many cases of cancer are expected beyond the background incidence in the unexposed population. If the chemical causes nonneoplastic toxic effects, the target value is a HI. In the case of a carcinogen, this allows a determination to be made if the number of excess cancer deaths likely to occur will be higher than acceptable. In the case of a substance with a toxic endpoint other than cancer, it allows a determination as to whether exposure will result in a significant likelihood of adverse toxic health effects. Both carcinogenic and noncarcinogenic effects can occur with the same substance

(e.g., arsenic, benzene); therefore, these effects are separately calculated and displayed.

STRENGTHS AND WEAKNESSES OF THE PROCESS

The process of risk estimation involves uncertainties because there are always gaps in knowledge or a lack in understanding of mechanisms (9). In every risk assessment procedure a large number of steps or decision points are involved where pieces of information are missing that make drawing conclusions un-

$$I = C \times \frac{CR \times EFD}{BW} \times \frac{1}{AT}$$

Where:

    I   = intake; the amount of chemical at the exchange boundary (mg/kg body weight-day)

- Chemical-related variable
  - C = chemical concentration; the average concentration contacted over the exposure period (e.g., mg/liter water)

- Variables that describe the exposed population
  - CR = contact rate; the amount of contaminated medium contacted per unit time or event (e.g., liters/day)
  - EFD = exposure frequency and duration; describes how long and how often exposure occurs. Often calculated using two terms (EF and ED):
    - EF = exposure frequency (days/year)
    - ED = exposure duration (years)
  - BW = body weight; the average body weight over the exposure period (kg)

- Assessment-determined variable
  - AT = averaging time; period over which exposure is averaged (days)

Figure 7.6.   Calculating chemical intakes. Source: U.S. EPA 1989.

certain. These crucial gaps in knowledge are filled with extrapolations, models, or assumptions (21, 23, 79, 80, 82, 85–87). The techniques used to fill these gaps are sources of uncertainty in the final product of the risk assessment process. These assumptions, extrapolations, or models can influence the outcome of the final risk value by negatively affecting the precision of the process. These procedures may result in an assessment that is based heavily on the unknown rather than predominantly on empirical data. In risk assessments in general, there are four general sources of uncertainty: (a) definition of the physical setting; (b) dose-response model applicability and assumptions; (c) transport, fate, and exposure parameter values; and (d) tracking uncertainty—how uncertainties are magnified through the various steps of the assessment.

The risk assessment process has been developed as a tool for decision-making. This tool is used by politicians, bureaucrats, and other government policymakers to make decisions concerning the health of the public. By using scientifically derived data in the risk assessment process, a certain authenticity is given to the final product, the quantitative risk value. However, because of the many data gaps present and unverifiable modeling techniques used, such authenticity may not be well-deserved. In fact, this authenticity may well be only a glossy veneer covering a confusing and invalid basis for a decision. It is important to understand some of the uncertainties inherent in the QRA process.

Extrapolation

The extrapolation process involves extending conclusions from what is known to exist in reproducible, experimental conditions to conditions that can be neither produced experimentally nor verified. Extrapolations in toxicologic risk assessment may be from one species to another (laboratory animal to human), from a high dose region on a dose-response curve to a low dose region, from one route of exposure in test animals to another in human exposure, or from continuous, static exposure conditions in the laboratory to uneven, discontinuous human exposures (33, 34). It is recognized that these extrapolations carried out directly use many assumptions that introduce uncertainties into the final risk value (35). It is also recognized that improved precision is needed to make extrapolations more reliable (31). Improved precision can only be achieved if more complete

knowledge of mechanisms of action, pharmacokinetics and toxicokinetics, and pharmacodynamics and toxicodynamics are available. Such knowledge is frequently unavailable for risk analyses.

Because carrying out individual laboratory experiments in sufficient numbers to demonstrate statistical differences as low as 1×10^{-6} would involve thousands of animals and many millions of dollars, such experiments are carried out at doses higher than would actually be experienced. This allows the numbers of test subjects per experimental group to be reduced. Extrapolation of the dose-response curve from the high dose experimental region to the low dose region of actual exposure is then necessary.

There are several mathematical models used to extrapolate data from high and low dose circumstances. It is not known which models are the best or even if any of them are close to reality. They all fit the data curve well in the high dose region but diverge from one another in the low dose region (13, 30). The further one extrapolates into the unknown region, the more the models diverge. There is no way to confirm or verify the accuracy of any of the models with currently available knowledge.

Extrapolation may take the form of extending experimental data from studies using a route of exposure that is not the same as that in actual circumstances. Frequently, this amounts to simply converting the concentration present in the exposure medium to a dose per unit body weight (54, 79, 80). Pharmacokinetic factors that may have profound influences on accurate risk values are frequently ignored. This is usually the case because no data exist on these factors. This results in significant uncertainty as pharmacokinetic parameters may be profoundly different when route of exposure is different.

Inappropriate Studies

Data from many studies may not be appropriately transferrable directly to risk assessment processes (37). Many times studies providing data on toxicity are devised and carried out with goals and objectives that may not be compatible or referable to risk analysis. Often these experiments are not designed to provide risk assessment data, and the use of said data for such purposes may be faulty.

Varying Protocols

Protocols for studies designed to provide risk assessment data can also lead to less than optimum data also (38). Potency of the chemical is not accounted for in carcinogenic studies. Endpoints of toxicity may be selected by circumstance instead of by biologic evaluation. Dosages tested in such studies use a maximum tolerated dose (MTD) that may have entirely different manifestations of pharmacokinetics at actual exposure doses.

Differing Mechanisms of Action

It has become widely accepted to place carcinogens in one of two mechanistic classifications (35). DNA-reactive carcinogens, those that react with nucleotides, are called genotoxic. Carcinogens that apparently act without evidence of a direct interaction with genetic material have been designated epigenetic (39, 40). The distinction between chemicals causing tumors via a genetic mechanism versus those causing tumors via an epigenetic mechanism is of great significance in risk assessment (41). The former may cause tumors at a very low level without a threshold while the latter must reach some saturation or threshold level before tumorigenesis and would, therefore, have some low level of safe exposure. Considering this implication, it is plausible—even probable—that human risk is not the same for different types of carcinogens (42).

Current theories of carcinogenesis recognize three distinct steps in development—initiation, promotion, and progression (43, 29). Initiators and promoters have loosely been characterized as genetic and epigenetic, as well as a mechanistic definition of the classification of different types of carcinogens. Currently used risk assessment techniques do not provide adequately for these distinctions in the process of carcinogenesis and do not account for differences in risk that may result.

Population Variabilities

QRA processes deal with the "typical individual" and it is well-recognized that this imaginary stereotype is typical of no one (4, 21, 79). Drawing conclusions about individual risks from processes and modeling techniques based on populations has questionable validity (44). Risk values are derived to apply to a population whose response to hazardous exposure is expected to lie on a normally distributed bell-shaped response curve. This provides little comfort to the individuals who may lie at the lower end of that normally distributed response curve. Averages, maximum likely values, or standardized values applicable only to general populations are all examples of assumptions that are used in risk assessments to characterize exposures to populations. These assumptions are sources of uncertainty that arise in exposure assessments.

Laboratory studies are done on severely inbred animals that lack genetic heterogeneity. Responses of test subjects lacking heterozygosity would not range as wide as in a natural, genetically heteregenous population, as is the human population (35). Applying conclusions drawn from studies using such test animal population would very likely undermine validity. Often such risk estimates do not accurately reflect the risk imposed on particularly susceptible subgroups of the population (45). Such subgroups may be more highly exposed, more prone to adverse effects because of other high risk factors, or physiologically more predisposed to adverse effects.

Safety Factors

The safety factor approach to determining an RfD or MCL gives the impression that there is a sharp, identifiable division between exposure that is safe and exposure that is unsafe (19). In fact, risk does not just disappear as exposure drops below some value. Risk can vary for different individuals under the same conditions. It can vary with inherent properties of the concentration level itself. An inhalation exposure at a level too low to be detected by smell is likely to have a higher risk associated with it than a greater exposure level that is noxious enough to discourage its inhalation. The point is that the safety factor scheme tends to be misinterpreted as providing a safe level of exposure where absolute safety may not always actually exist.

Variation in Exposure Assessment

Assessment of exposure is purported to be the weakest aspect of regulatory risk assessment (46) and particularly prone to widely variable estimates (4). Exposure values are usually derived from infrequent point measurements from sampling techniques prescribed by regulatory agencies such as the EPA (47). Average values are the norm. Human exposure levels derived in this manner are just estimates. Exposure doses are then figured using standard intakes for an average (70 kilograms) human (21, 48, 49, 79, 80), such as 2 liters of drinking water per day, 20 cubic meters of air breathed daily, or 100 milligrams of soil ingested per day. Such exposure values are likely to adequately characterize a small segment of the population and inadequately characterize a much larger segment. These techniques may lead to use of exposures that are widely divergent from actuality. The conditions of exposure may vary radically between the experimental conditions under which the data are collected and the actual exposure situation. Level, frequency, duration, and route of exposure differences are sources of uncertainty that make questionable the direct application of laboratory data to an actual exposure situation (19).

The source of exposure, such as contaminated media, often cannot be quantitated, characterized, for accurately placed in time or space. Average values or best guesses are often used. Diffusion models are frequently used to describe movement of chemicals in the environment. These models have improved significantly but can never precisely predict behavior of environmental contaminants.

Experimental Species Differences

Species differences in pharmacokinetic factors such as absorption, distribution, metabolism and excretion are factors that make extrapolations difficult. It is usually assumed, in the risk assessment process, that absorption in humans is equal to that in test species. This is usually due largely to lack of any evidence to the contrary. However, it is a rather broad assumption which is probably true in only a small minority of cases.

Use of Confidence Interval Limits

Laboratory test data provide a relatively small number of data points in a high dose range with which to draw conclusions about large populations in a very low dose range. Using the nonthreshold approach to estimate risk, extrapolations are used to derive a quantitative risk estimate. Extrapolation of the dose-response curve into the unknown low dose region makes use of various statistical models. Though the models used all vary in some way, one thing they have in common is the use of confidence limits or intervals. The accepted practice is not to use the best estimate (maximum likelihood or central tendency) of the linear extrapolation, but rather an upper limit of a confidence interval about that best estimate. Thus this type of quantitative risk estimate is generally expressed as an upper-bound estimate (21, 23). This is a statistical term that describes the degree of confidence that can be placed in the estimated risk value. In other words, the actual risk value would likely be less than the calculated upper bound an assigned percentage of the time. That percentage has been established by regulatory agencies which use the 95% upper confidence limit as the upper bound for cancer risk values (12, 21). Thus there is a 5% chance that the true risk is actually greater than the calculated risk. Using an interval as such gives the risk values obtained a margin of safety while at the same time giving them a degree of unreliability. That is, the projected risk is a less than precise estimator of the actual risk, and the less data available to make the projection, the less precise the final value. What may be more appropriate than using only the upper confidence limit would be to report the best estimate as well as the upper and lower confidence limits (21, 50). Information on the width of the confidence interval and the distance of the upper bound from the best estimate would enhance evaluation and interpretation of the risk value.

Environmental Factors

Environmental factors, such as heat, cold, humidity, airflow, noise, population density, nutrition, personal habits, activity, and pregnancy, may all have significant effects on biologic and physical parameters of xenobiotics. These factors may affect the exposure levels incurred by the population at risk. They may affect the pharmacokinetic processes of the exposed organism, absorption, distribution, metabolism, and excretion. These are factors not routinely accounted for in risk assessments, and they add unknown amounts of uncertainty to the process and undermine the precision and validity of the quantitative risk value obtained.

Risks Due to Multiple Exposures

Conservative assumptions and modeling techniques generally allow for a risk estimate to overstate the potential health hazard. One fact of environmental exposures that may result in an understatement of risk is that of multiple exposure (6). People are not exposed to a single chemical at one time under carefully defined ambient conditions as in the laboratory. Instead they are exposed to an infinite number of different mixtures which can never be duplicated experimentally. The question is, what effect do multiple exposures have on reliability of risk estimates? Are mixtures additive, synergistic, or antagonistic? Most likely all three are true in various situations. The risk assessment process does not adequately address this question.

Selection of Models

Model selection itself is a major source of uncertainty in the risk assessment process (51). Risk estimates derived from various high to low dose extrapolation models will usually fit the curve well in the high dose region but may vary by several

orders of magnitude in the low dose region (52). They may fit the experimental data well, but slopes may be drastically different in the low dose region (51, 53). In general, the choice of which model is best for a particular circumstance is not clear. More mechanistic knowledge is essential in choosing models. This is not currently the case largely because adequate mechanistic data do not exist for most chemicals.

Doses Based on Body Weight

Dose equivalency between species has long been based on body weight; however, it is now recognized that toxicities as well as pharmacokinetic parameters of many drugs do not vary linearly with body weight (36). The trend is slowly moving in the direction of using body surface area dose equivalencies.

Most Sensitive Species

The EPA chooses to consider the most sensitive species tested as being most like humans (51). This practice is consistent with the goal of estimating risk by erring on the side of safety. There is also evidence that humans are frequently the most sensitive species, at least as far as susceptibility to carcinogenic substances (56). Use of the most sensitive species, however, makes the assumption that humans are equal to that species. In reality, humans are probably only rarely equal in susceptibility to the most sensitive species tested. When not as sensitive, the risk estimate derived is overestimated and overprotection may result. When humans are more sensitive than the most sensitive species tested, the actual risk will be greater than what it is perceived to be, and harmful exposures may be incurred. This is another significant source of uncertainty that undermines reliability in risk assessment values.

Use of Epidemiologic Data

Epidemiologic studies are one of three major sources of information that are commonly used to determine qualitative and quantitative hazards. This type of data is frequently the only type of human exposure data available. However, because of insensitivity and a frequently poor record of exposure data, epidemiologic data are often of limited reliability and usefulness (19, 55, 57). Dose-response data are usually not recoverable from this type of study. Cause-effect relationships are difficult to establish in this type of study. Epidemiologic data are usually unable to detect small differences in effects. Environmental conditions, especially concurrent exposures or exposures to chemical mixtures, are unknown or uncontrollable. Observation patterns in epidemiologic studies often are random or irregular. Monitoring of exposures, body loads, and even disease incidence may be incomplete at best. Epidemiology is retroactive, taking place after exposures have occurred. Thus it is not available as a preventive tool initially. Long intervals between cause and effect are common, especially with carcinogens. Because of these reasons, reliability of epidemiologic data is questionable and should be critically examined before being included in the risk assessment process.

Use of Appropriate Assumptions

Assumptions are necessary in the risk assessment process to fill in gaps of knowledge regarding specific chemicals. As is often the case, there is insufficient evidence to decide what the most appropriate assumption is to fill in such a data gap. It has become the traditionally accepted procedure in such cases to apply the assumption that appears least likely to lead to an underestimate of the actual human health risks (12). This leads to a very conservative estimate of risk and may result in a very imprecise risk value, one which so overestimates the potential risk of a substance so as to make it unreasonable. The practice of deriving a conservative risk estimate does, however, result in what is probably the most beneficial advantage of using the quantitative risk assessment process. It provides a high degree of assurance that the actual risk will not exceed the estimate of risk (58). The cautiousness of current risk assessment techniques ensures more reliable protection of public health.

Transferring Data from Animals to Humans

It is widely assumed, to a greater or lesser extent, that toxicity or carcinogenicity data from experimental animals is transferable to humans. This practice of transferral of data between species is a subject of controversy in the scientific community. Almost all known human carcinogens have been demonstrated to be carcinogenic in some animal species (12). Arguments have been made against carrying this evidence to the conclusion that all proven animal carcinogens are probably human carcinogens. The fact that almost all human carcinogens are animal carcinogens does not prove that most animal carcinogens have the same potential in humans.

Laboratory animal bioassays used to test for toxicity or carcinogenicity may provide data that are not appropriate for application to humans. High doses used in animal studies, typically a MTD or some large fraction thereof, are not representative of the actual levels of human exposure. Species of laboratory animals may be so biologically different from humans that data are not valid at all (43). Some laboratory species are extremely sensitive to various toxic or carcinogenic substances which may not be the same in humans. Some species have naturally high background incidences of some tumor types. Occurrences of benign and malignant tumors are not distinguished between, but lumped together as total tumor incidence in most experimental protocols. These points may have a significant effect on validity of risk assessment if addressed.

NEW DIRECTIONS IN RISK ASSESSMENT

Low Dose Extrapolation

Modeling methods for performing risk assessments are becoming more numerous and more sophisticated. In modeling for low dose extrapolations, one attempts to relate exposure dose to response at doses exponentially lower than experimental data are available for. All the models in use today fit the high dose data well. They also tend to be essentially linear at low doses, and their numerical outcomes are not greatly different (13). Thus it is apparent that modeling techniques for low dose extrapolations are becoming more reliable. The obvious question is, "How reliable?"

Another question to address in the use of modeling for low dose extrapolation is that of variability (59). If there is more than one mechanism of carcinogenicity, as appears to be the case, then is it reasonable to think that one model will suffice to extrapolate dose-response curves for differing mechanisms? A model accounting for the multistage concept of carcinogen-

esis has been developed (43). It remains to withstand the test of scientific scrutiny and discussion but may have potential for significantly improving carcinogenic risk assessment.

Methods to Evaluate Relative Toxic Potencies

Comparative potency methods for assessing risks have been developed (35, 60, 61). These modeling methods utilize short-term mutagenesis and tumorigenesis data from other types of toxicologic or epidemiologic studies which can be applied to the risk assessment process. The concept behind these various methods is to determine, via some grading system, relative potency values for groups of toxic chemicals. In the absence of more definitive data, the comparative values are assumed to assign similar risks to chemicals having similar potencies. In this way, risks can be derived for chemicals with no or deficient data by using the data available from other chemicals. The opinion has been stated that none of the methods reviewed (61) were adequate for regulatory decision-making when used alone, but that all can make useful contributions to the process.

New Pharmacokinetic Models

Physiologically based pharmacokinetic models based on actual physiologic characteristics of organisms hold the potential for increasing the precision and reliability of chemical risk assessment. Such models are being developed and evaluated and have been demonstrated to enhance extrapolation of data across species and between routes of administration (62). These models have also shown the capability to predict the general behavior of toxicants in biologic systems (43). Pharmacokinetic studies are valuable for gaining a greater understanding of mechanisms, which will, in turn, allow for more precise risk assessment (55). The integration of knowledge of pharmacokinetics in assessing risks to chemical exposure is an important tool in improving estimates of risk (63). Laboratory studies aimed at answering the many questions regarding absorption, distribution, metabolism, and excretion of chemicals are providing valuable new data every day. The development of new models that specifically address the use of pharmacokinetic and toxicokinetic data in risk assessment is ongoing (12, 64). These improvements in the risk assessment methodology will improve the predictive power of risk assessment (34).

Precisely Defined Endpoints

The evaluation of a chemical can yield more specific knowledge if the endpoint examined is more specifically defined. By looking at more specific endpoints than general gross and micropathologic evidence of carcinogenicity or toxicity, a clearer picture of the health hazard present will develop. This is being addressed by tests being developed and used in the areas of mutagenicity, teratogenicity, reproductive toxicity, behavioral toxicity, neurotoxicity, and development toxicity (43). Cellular and molecular biology techniques, that are commonly being applied to toxicity studies, will yield more specific knowledge on which to base risk evaluations in the future. Measurement of a biologically effective dose for a carcinogen is a way of determining the amount of the chemical substance that has interacted with biologic targets (64). Such measurements are now possible and offer the possibility of more powerful tools in the conduct of QRA.

Identifying and Quantifying Uncertainty

Specific sources of uncertainty must be identified. The specific uncertainties can then be quantified for their influence on the risk assessment process (9). In this way, the unknown quantity is given limits, and greater confidence can be attributed to the quantitative risk values derived. A modeling method for conducting risk assessment for chemical exposure that incorporates uncertainty as a component of the process has been developed (65). This is an initial positive step that attempts to deal directly with the primary controversy undermining the reliability of QRA.

Structure-Activity Analysis

The use of structure-activity relationship analysis provides an additional tool in the scientist's bag of tricks with which to predict deleterious effects of a chemical (55). Chemical structure can be an accurate predictor, within limits, of potential toxicity or carcinogenicity (66). This tool can be used in selecting priorities for testing. It may also have the potential to predict mutagenicity or carcinogenicity of some classes of chemicals. The limiting factor in this instance is the same in most areas of risk assessment fraught with uncertainty—the lack of empirical data.

Incorporating New Methodologies in the Regulatory Process

Regulatory agencies, especially the EPA, are taking positive steps by incorporating new methods into their guidelines for performing QRA. The EPA has recently attempted to improve quality and appropriateness of QRA by developing guidelines on developmental toxicity, carcinogenicity, chemical mixtures, exposures, and mutagenicity (21, 67–71). Significant differences arise between risk assessments calculated using body surface area versus body weight. Body weight risk calculations can be several times lower using body weights (55). When extrapolating dose data between species, body surface area is the preferred method of equating doses (72). Recent EPA guidelines adopt surface area as the standard for dose calculation as opposed to body weight which has historically been used (32, 79, 80).

Improved Epidemiology

Epidemiologic data are frequently the only human-derived data available for risk evaluations. The science of epidemiology is becoming more well-known and widely accepted (10). The contributions epidemiology can make to safeguarding human health are becoming more well-enumerated. The conduct of epidemiologic studies is continually being refined. Probably most significant, the volume of epidemiologic data available for risk assessment application is continually expanding. Epidemiological data can be expected to play an expanded role in future risk evaluation.

Biologic Risk Assessment

The concept of biologic risk assessment has been introduced to the risk assessment process (73). This idea represents an aspect of risk assessment that directly addresses the relevance of specific animal results to the induction of human cancer. Biologic risk assessment is envisioned as improving the decision-making process wherein an experimentally identified animal carcinogen is determined to be an effective human carcinogen. It has the potential to provide a means of distinguishing between those animal carcinogens which are likely to pose a threat to humans and those which are not. This newly conceived process addresses three areas of risk assessment in need of refinement: (a) high to low dose extrapolation, (b) interspecies extrapolation, and (c) carcinogenic potency.

Balancing Qualitative and Quantitative Data

Risk assessment of carcinogens requires evaluation of qualitative as well as quantitative data. Evaluations must be made regarding weight of evidence when determining whether a chemical is actually carcinogenic or not. At the same time, determination of potency, the quantitative evaluation, must be accomplished. A method for assessing the carcinogenic hazards of chemicals that weighs both aspects in a two-way matrix classification has been devised (74). This method conceivably can provide a rational and reliable method for determining carcinogenic risk that balances quantitative and qualitative evidence, a positive move in refining the risk assessment process.

CONCLUSIONS

A decade ago the majority of the scientific community opposed risk assessment because of the inadequacies in the process. Quantitative risk assessment remains a subject of much debate today. The debate is a result of huge gaps in understanding of mechanisms of toxicity and assumptions made using inadequate data (75). The debate is over how to best perform risk assessment, how to improve the process, and how to apply the results (13). While discussion is taking place on the appropriateness of risk assessment, it will continue to be used to establish regulations and legislation and will probably assume an increasingly important role in product liability and tort litigations (12).

Risk assessment, especially for carcinogens, is not a clear-cut process (76). Many different models have been applied to the process. No single model has proven accurate; indeed, these models cannot be verified with current knowledge. The most glaring insufficiency in modeling is the lack of understanding of mechanisms of most toxic substances. It is recognized that improving the volume and quality of knowledge available is fundamental in improving the risk assessment process (32).

Extrapolation of toxicologic information between species of animals and humans remains a challenge. Considerations of dose administration, exposure data, routes of exposure, and pharmacokinetics are all areas that need to be addressed and improved (75). Consideration of heterogeneous exposure conditions and heterogeneous populations as well as exposure of complex chemical mixtures must be undertaken. Modeling techniques for extrapolations as well as for exposures, release migrations, and physiologic processes need to be improved (73).

Uncertainty is inherent in the risk assessment process. It must be addressed and evaluated during the process. The uncertainties involved in a risk estimate must be described quantitatively and qualitatively to provide a true picture of the reliability of the final risk value (77).

Modern strategies for risk assessment must include continual evolvement through newer, more informative and useful processes. Mechanistic studies must be more commonplace and more thorough before longterm whole-body studies are undertaken (38). Selection of species for testing must be made with more knowledge of mechanisms and pharmacodynamics to be more applicable to the human species. There is a need to develop risk assessment techniques and models that consider that many uncertainties in the process. Some of these are differences in species, tumor type, background incidence, sex, strain, mechanism of toxicity or carcinogenicity, and pharmacokinetics or toxicokinetics (50). To increase the precision and reliability of QRA, more and better information is necessary concerning mechanisms of toxicity, molecular targets, and pathways of metabolism, exposure, and dose, as well as characteristics of dose-response curves (1). Use of existing epidemiologic data in new ways, as well as contributing new data to that already in hand, will strengthen the QRA process and help lessen reliance on animal data (78).

The inadequacies of the risk assessment process are many. There is a large amount of uncertainty associated with quantitative risk values. Current QRA techniques result in only a range of risk at best, with the conservative approach assuring that the actual risk is probably much lower. Vast improvement is needed in the techniques applied to risk assessment, but at the present time there appears to be no acceptable alternative to its use (11). Risk assessment is the most systematic and proven method available to organize, analyze, and present information on environmental chemicals for the purpose of making decisions in the interest of public health (12).

A zero risk environment is impossible. It is important that the public understand the source and nature of risks to which they are subjected. It is desirable to identify and reduce health risks as much as possible. Every effort should be made to increase awareness of risks to allow individual choice for avoidance of those risks which cannot or should not be eliminated.

REFERENCES

1. Tarkowski S. Data base for risk assessment. Sci Total Environ 1986;51:19–25.
2. Brown HS, West CR, Bishop DR. Chemical health effects assessment methodology for airborne contaminants. Risk Anal 1987;7:389–402.
3. Oller WL, Cairns T, Bowman MC, Fishbein L. A toxicological risk assessment procedure: a proposal for a surveillance index for hazardous chemicals. Arch Environ Contam Toxicol 1980;9:483–490.
4. Moore JA. Problems facing the decision-maker in the risk assessment process. Teratogenesis Carcinog Mutagen 1987;7:205–209.
5. Indulski JA, Krajewski JA. Identification of priorities for chemical hazard control. Med Pr 1987;38:132–142.
6. Lave LB. Health and safety risk analyses: information for better decisions. Science 1987;236:291–295.
7. Slovic P. Perception of risk. Science 1987;236:280–285.
8. Borman SA. Origins of risk assessment. Anal Chem 1983;55:1438A–1440A.
9. Turturro A, Hart RW. Quantifying risk and accuracy in cancer risk assessment: the process and its role in risk management problem solving. Med Oncol Tumor Pharmacother 1987;4:125–132.
10. Whittemore AS. Epidemiology in risk assessment for regulatory policy. J Chronic Dis 1986;39:1157–1168.
11. Rodricks JV, Brett SM, Wrenn GC. Significant risk decisions in federal regulatory agencies. Regul Toxicol Pharmacol 1987;7:307–320.
12. ENVIRON Corporation. Elements of toxicology and chemical risk assessment. Washington, DC: ENVIRON Corp., 1988.
13. Flamm WG. Risk assessment policy in the United States. Prog Clin Biol Res 1986;208:141–149.
14. U.S. Environmental Protection Agency. Superfund public health evaluation manual. Washington, DC: Office of Emergency and Remedial Response, 1986.
15. U.S. Environmental Protection Agency. Superfund exposure assessment manual. Washington, DC: Office of Emergency and Remedial Response (OSWER 9285.5-1) 1988.
16. Cornfield J. Carcinogenic risk assessment. Science 1977;198:693–699.
17. U.S. Environmental Protection Agency. Risk assessment in Superfund student manual. Washington, DC: Office of Emergency and Remedial Response, 1987.
18. Rowe WD. Identification of risk. Prog Clin Biol Res 1986;208:3–22.
19. Rodricks JV, Tardiff RG. Conceptual basis for risk assessment. In: Rodricks JV, Tardiff RG, eds. Assessment and management of chemical risks. Washington, DC: American Chemical Society, 1984.
20. U.S. Environmental Protection Agency. Health effects assessment summary for 300 hazardous organic constituents in support of regulatory imposed analysis of the land disposal branch (LD13) and interim final incinerator regulations of the technical branch (TB) at the office of solid wastes. Washington, DC: Environmental Criterial Assessment Office, 1982.
21. U.S. Environmental Protection Agency. Risk Assessment Guidance for Superfund; Part A and Part B. Interim Final OSWER 9285. 701A, December 1989.
22. Travis CC, Crouch EAC, Klema ED. Cancer risk management. Environ Sci Technol 1987;21:415–420.
23. California Department of Health Services. California mitigation decision tree. California Department of Health Services, 1986.
24. Andersen ME. Quantitative risk assessment and occupational carcinogens. Appl Ind Hyg 1988;3(10):267–273.
25. Young FE. Risk assessment: the convergence of science and law. Regul Toxicol Pharmacol 1987;7:179–184.
26. U.S. Environmental Protection Agency. The endangerment assessment handbook. Washington, DC: Office of Waste Programs Enforcement, 1985.
27. Anderson EL. Quantitative approaches in the use in the United States to assess cancer risk. In: Vouk VB, Butler GC, Hoel DG, Peakall DB, eds. Methods for estimating risk of chemical injury: human and non-human biota and ecosystems. New York: John Wiley and Sons, 1985.
28. Alm AL. Introductory remarks. Toxicol Ind Health 1985;1:1–5.
29. Hart RW, Turturro A. Process and assumptions in risk assessment. Ann Clin Lab Sci 1986;16:353–357.
30. Brown CC: High to low dose extrapolation in animals. In: Rodricks JV, Tardiff RG, eds. Assessment and management of chemical risks. Washington, DC: American Chemical Society, 1984.
31. Flamm WG, Winbush JS. Role of mathematical models in assessment of risk and in attempts to define management strategy. Fundam Appl Toxicol 1984;4:S395–S401.
32. NRC. Risk assessment in the federal government, managing the process. Washington, DC: National Academy Press, 1983.
33. Hart RW, Fishbein L. Interspecies extrapolation of drug and genetic toxicity data. In: Clayson DB, Krewski D, Munro I, eds. Toxicological risk assessment, Vol 1. Boca Raton, FL: CRC Press, 1985.
34. Clewell HJ, Anderson ME. Risk assessment extrapolations and physiologic modeling. Toxicol Ind Health 1985;1:111–131.
35. Clayson DB. Problems in interspecies extrapolations. In: Clayson DB, Krewski D, Munro I, eds. Toxicological risk assessment, Vol. 1. Boca Raton, FL: CRC Press, 1985.
36. Withey JR. Pharmacokinetic differences between species. In: Clayson DB, Krewski D, Munro I, eds. Toxicological risk assessment, Vol 1. Boca Raton, FL: CRC Press, 1985.
37. Budiansky S. The risky business of assessing risk. Environ Sci Technol 1980;14:1281–1282.
38. Henschler D. Risk assessment and evaluation of chemical carcinogens—present and future strategies (editorial). J Cancer Res Clin Oncol 1987;113:1–7.
39. Williams GM, Welsburger JH. Chemical carcinogens. In: Klaassen CD, Amdur MO, Doull J, eds. Casarett and Doull's toxicology: the basic science of poisons. 3rd ed. New York: Macmillan, 1986.
40. Kroes R. Contribution of toxicology towards risk assessment in carcinogens. Arch Toxicol 1987;60:224–228.
41. Stott WT, Watanabe PG. Differentiation of genetic versus epigenetic mechanisms of toxicity and its application to risk assessment. Drug Metab Rev 1982;13:853–873.
42. Williams GM, Weisburger JH. Carcinogen risk assessment (letter). Science 1983;221:4605.
43. NRC. Drinking water and health. Washington, DC: National Academy Press, 1986.
44. Ashton JR. Risk assessment. Br Med J 1983;286:1843.
45. Van Ryzin J. Quantitative risk assessment. J Occup Med 1989;22:321–326.
46. Silbergeld EK. Risk assessment (letters). Science 1987;237:1399.
47. U.S. Geological Survey. Phase 11A remedial investigation of the Arkansas City dump site, Arkansas City, KS: 1986.

48. U.S. Environmental Protection Agency. Ambient water quality criteria documents. Washington, DC: Office of Water Regulations and Standards, 1980.

49. LaGoy PK. Estimated soil ingestion rates for use in risk assessment. Risk Anal 1987;7:355–359.

50. Park CN, Snee RD. Quantitative risk assessment: state-of-the-art for carcinogenesis. Fundam Appl Toxicol 1983;3:320–333.

51. Somers E. Making decisions from numbers. Regul Toxicol Pharmacol 1987;7:35–42.

52. Krewski D, Crump KS, Farmer J, Gaylor DW, Howe R, Portier C, Salsburg D, Sielken RL, Van Ryzin J. A comparison of statistical methods for low dose extrapolation utilizing time-to-tumor data. Fundam Appl Toxicol 1983;3:140–160.

53. Munro IC, Krewski DR. Risk assessment and regulatory decision making. Food Cosmet Toxicol 1981;19:549–560.

54. Pepelko WE. Feasibility of route extrapolation in risk assessment (editorial). Br J Ind Med 1987;44:649–651.

55. Perera FP. Quantitative risk assessment and cost-benefit analysis for carcinogens at EPA: a critique. J Public Health Policy 1987;8:202–221.

56. Crouch E, Wilson R. Interspecies comparison of carcinogenic potency. J Toxicol Environ Health 1979;5:1095–1118.

57. Crump KS, Allen BC, Howe RB, Crockett PW. Time related factors in quantitative risk assessment. J Chronic Dis 1987;40:101S–111S.

58. Rodricks J, Taylor MR. Application of risk assessment to food safety decision making. Regul Toxicol Pharmacol 1983;3:275–307.

59. Hoiel DG. Incorporation of pharmacokinetics in low-dose risk estimation. In Clayson DB, Krewski D, Munro I, eds. Toxicological risk assessment, Vol 1. Boca Raton, FL: CRC Press, 1985.

60. Lewtas J. A quantitative cancer risk assessment methodology using short-term genetic bioassays: the comparative potency method. Prog Clin Biol Res 1986;208:107–120.

61. Barr JT. The calculation and use of carcinogenic potency: a review. Regul Toxicol Pharmacol 1985;5:432–459.

62. Travis CC. Interspecies extrapolations in risk analysis. Toxicology 1987;47:3–13.

63. Dietz FK, Reitz RH, Watanabe PG, Gehring PJ. Translation of pharmacokinetic/biochemical data into risk assessment. Adv Exp Med Biol 1981;136 Part B:1399–1424.

64. Perera F. New approaches in risk assessment for carcinogens. Risk Anal 1986;6:195–201.

65. Lichtenberg E, Zilberman D. Efficient regulation of environmental health risks. The case of groundwater contamination in California. Sci Total Environ 1986;56:111–119.

66. Gottinger HW. HAZARD: an expert system for risk assessment of environmental chemicals. Methods Inf Med 1987;26:13–23.

67. U.S. Environmental Protection Agency. Guidelines for carcinogen risk assessment. Fed Reg 1986;51:33992–34003.

68. U.S. Environmental Protection Agency. Guidelines for exposure assessment. Fed Reg 1986;51:34042–34054.

69. U.S. Environmental Protection Agency. Guidelines for mutagenicity risk assessment. Fed Reg 1986;51:34006–34012.

70. U.S. Environmental Protection Agency. Guidelines for the health assessment of suspect developmental toxicants. Fed Reg 1989;54:9386.

71. U.S. Environmental Protection Agency. Guidelines for the health risk assessment of chemical mixtures. Fed Reg 1986;51:34014–34025.

72. Russell M, Gruber M. Risk assessment in environmental policy-making. Science 1987;236:286–290.

73. Clayson DB. The need for biological risk assessment in reaching decisions about carcinogens. Mutat Res 1987;185:243–269.

74. Brown HS, Bishop DR, West CR. A methodology for assessing carcinogenic hazards of chemicals. Toxicol Ind Health 1986;2:205–218.

75. Miya TS, Gibson JE, Hook JB, McClellan RO. Contemporary issues in toxicology, preparing for the twenty-first century: report of the Tox 90's Commission. Toxicol Appl Pharmacol 1988;96:1–6.

76. Stara JF, Mukerjee D, McGaughy R, Durkin P, Dourson ML. The current use of studies on promoters and cocarcinogens in quantitative risk assessment. Environ Health Perspect 1983;50:359–368.

77. Brown SL. Quantitative risk assessment of environmental hazards. Annu Rev Public Health 1985;6:247–267.

78. Enterline PE. A method for estimating lifetime cancer risks from limited epidemiologic data. Risk Anal 1987;7:91–96.

79. U.S. Environmental Protection Agency. Exposure factors handbook, Office of Health & Environmental Assessment. Washington, DC: 1990;600:8–90,043.

80. U.S. Environmental Protection Agency. Exposure assessment methods handbook, Draft. Washington, DC: Office of Health & Environmental Assessment, 1989.

81. U.S. Environmental Protection Agency. CERCLA Compliance with other laws manual. Parts I and II. OSWER 9234.1, 01 and 02.

82. U.S. Environmental Protection Agency. Proposed guidelines for exposure-related measurements. Fed Reg 1988;53:48830.

83. U.S. Environmental Protection Agency. Interim final guidance for soil ingestion rates. OSWER 1989;9850.4.

84. U.S. Environmental Protection Agency. Integrated risk information system (database). ORD 1989.

85. U.S. Environmental Protection Agency. Reviews of environmental contamination and toxicology 104. Cincinnati, OH: Office of Drinking Water Health Advisories, 1988.

86. U.S. Environmental Protection Agency. General quantitative risk assessment guideline non-cancer health effects. ECAP-CIN-538, 1989.

87. U.S. Environmental Protection Agency. Reference dose (RFD): description and use in health risk measurements. Appendix to A to Integrated Risk Information System, 1989.

8

Chemical and Environmental Carcinogenesis

Steven Piantadosi, M.D., Ph.D.
John B. Sullivan, Jr., M.D.

INTRODUCTION

Chemical carcinogens are toxic substances that produce cancer in animals or humans. Although these agents are absorbed, activated, metabolized, and excreted like drugs or toxins, they are unique in several ways. Chemical carcinogens have cumulative and delayed effects, chronic exposures of low levels are effective, and their chemical action on genetic molecules is unique (1).

Historically, the first evidence of chemical carcinogenesis came from the English physician, Percival Pott, who described in 1775 the occurrence of cancer in the scrotum in several of his male patients (2). These patients had a common environmental exposure as chimney sweeps which led Dr. Pott to conclude that the exposure to soot caused their cancer. It was not obvious that prevention of the exposure could be effective because, 100 years later high incidence of skin cancer was noted among German workers exposed to coal tar, a major ingredient in soot.

In the early 1900s, polycyclic hydrocarbons were shown to be the principle carcinogens in organic tars. The chemical structure of these agents is typified by benzo[a]pyrene and dibenz[a,h]anthracene, shown in Figure 8.1. In 1935, chemical carcinogenesis was demonstrated convincingly for a class of azo dyes. In 1937, aromatic amines (specifically 2-naphthylamine) were shown to be carcinogenic in dogs, reproducing the urinary bladder lesions noted in the late 1800s among workers exposed to some dyes. Subsequently, a sizable number of substances have been shown to be carcinogenic in animals and humans. Based on studies by the International Agency for Research on Cancer (IARC), at least two dozen substances seem to be strongly associated with the occurrence of cancer in humans (1). An updated summary is shown in Table 8.1.

Industrial processes strongly associated with carcinogenesis, even though the causative agent is not clearly identified, include

manufacture of amines (bladder cancer), chromatic (lung cancer), cadmium (prostate cancer), hematite mining (lung cancer), nickel (nasal cavity and lung cancer), and the rubber industry (lung cancer). The IARC lists 37 agents and processes that are probably carcinogenic and 147 that are possibly carcinogenic (Table 8.1).

CRITERIA FOR CHEMICAL CARCINOGENESIS

A chemical carcinogen is an agent which increases the occurrence of cancer compared to untreated controls when administered to animals. This definition is based on an increased relative rate of cancer, i.e., the absolute risk of a cancer in the population is irrelevant. Four types of increased neoplastic responses are accepted as evidence of carcinogenesis: (a) increased incidence of "naturally" occurring tumors, (b) development of new types of cancers, (c) a new multiplicity of cancers, and (d) a decrease in median time to tumor. These criteria tend to blur the distinction between initiation and promotion of cancers but are useful and conservative.

A wide variety of chemicals can produce one or more of these responses. Although these agents fall into several broad classes, the chemical structures and modes of action are diverse. In some cases, the term "promoter" or enhancer may be more appropriate than "carcinogen." In any case, the varying mechanisms of exposure that these different agents imply point to the need for specialized risk analysis and management.

Mechanisms of Action

The primary site of action of many chemical carcinogens is DNA. Current investigations focus on these nucleotides to which these carcinogens bind and the type of binding or adduct formation. Many details have been elucidated, such as the action of methylnitrosourea in producing carbonium ions and their binding to guanine. In humans, there is no direct evidence that DNA adducts other than those covalently bound can cause cancer. However, in bacteria, even intercalated binding of some chemicals is mutagenic, leading to the suspicion that covalent binding may not be required in other species.

The evidence in favor of DNA being the critical target of carcinogens can be summarized as follows:

1. Most cancers display some chromosomal abnormalities.
2. Most cancers display abnormal gene expression.
3. Many cancers display activated oncogenes.
4. Neoplasia is self-propagating, i.e., cancer is inherited at the cellular level.
5. Some genetic alterations predispose to cancer.
6. Carcinogens can be shown to react covalently with DNA.
7. Defective DNA repair predisposes to cancer.

Many carcinogens are activated by host metabolism. These

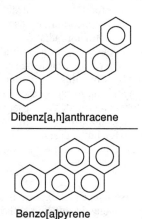

Dibenz[a,h]anthracene

Benzo[a]pyrene

Figure 8.1. Typical polycyclic hydrocarbon carcinogens.

Table 8.1. Chemicals and Processes Carcinogenic to Humans as Determined by the IARC

Aflatoxins
Aluminum production
4-Aminobiphenyl
Analgesic mixtures containing phenacetin
Arsenic and arsenic compounds*
Asbestos
Auramine, manufacture of
Azathioprine
Benzene
Benzidine
Betel quid with tobacco
N,N-Bis(2-chloroethyl)-2-naphthylamine (Chlornaphazine)
Bis(chloromethyl)ether and chloromethyl methyl ether (technical-grade)
Boot and shoe manufacture and repair
1,4-Butanediol dimethanesulfonate (Myleran)
Chlorambucil
1-(2-Chloroethyl)-3-(4-methylcyclohexyl)-1-nitrosourea (methyl-CCNU)
Chromium compounds, hexavalent*
Coal gasification
Coal-tar pitches
Coal-tars
Coke production
Cyclophosphamide
Diethylstilbestrol
Erionite
Furniture and cabinet working
Hematite mining, underground, with exposure to radon
Iron and steel founding
Isopropyl alcohol manufacture, strong-acid process
Magenta, manufacture of
Melphalan
8-Methoxypsoralen (Methoxsalen) plus ultraviolet radiation
Mineral oils, untreated and mildly-treated
MOPP (combined therapy with nitrogen mustard, vincristine, procarbazine, and prednisone) and other combined chemotherapy including alkylating agents
Mustard gas (sulfur mustard)
2-Naphthylamine
Nickel and nickel compounds*
Estrogen replacement therapy
Estrogen, nonsteroidal*
Estrogen, steroidal*
Oral contraceptives, combined[1]
Oral contraceptives, sequential
Rubber industry
Shale oils
Soots
Talc containing asbestiform fibers
Tobacco products, smokeless
Tobacco smoke
Treosulfan
Vinyl chloride

*Applies to the group of chemicals or process used and not necessarily to all individual chemicals.
[1]These agents have a *protective* effect against cancers of the ovary and endometrium.

reactive species bind covalently to DNA and other macromolecules. However, enzyme repair systems can replace damaged sections of DNA, allowing the cell to recover. If cellular reproduction occurs in the presence of DNA damage, point mutations, transpositions and other genetic alterations can occur. It is also plausible that binding and alteration of proteins that regulate gene expression can transform cells. Reproduction of damaged or transformed cells may produce preneoplastic lesions, some even perhaps clinically evident.

The different chemical classes of carcinogens typified in Figure 8.1 do not have common structural features. However, they have been shown to have common metabolic characteristics and tendencies to form reactants of a specific type. Much of the work demonstrating these pathways was accomplished by J.A. and E.C. Miller (3–5). During hepatocarcinogenesis, azo dyes were shown to become covalently bound to liver proteins (3). Similarly, benzo[l]pyrene became covalently bound to proteins in the skin of mice (4). Similar results were obtained in studies of other chemical carcinogens. The common metabolic pathway for the structurally dissimilar compounds appears to be conversion to electrophils (electron-deficient molecules) which then covalently bind to a variety of biologic macromolecules, most notably DNA.

In addition, for the electrophilic reactants, studies also suggest that free radicals are produced during metabolism (6). They carry no net change but do have an unpaired electron. The evidence in favor of this pathway is strengthened by observations that antioxidants, which inhibit free radical formation, can diminish the activity of some carcinogens (7).

These mechanistic explanations are satisfying for several reasons. They demonstrate and explain why metabolism of carcinogens is necessary for activation. Species differences in metabolism undoubtedly exist, which is consistent with other experimental evidence indicating that some carcinogens are species specific. Also, the genetic mode of action of most carcinogens may explain the long lead time between exposure to toxins and the appearance of cancer. However, not all carcinogens are activated by metabolism. A few, e.g., some chemotherapeutic drugs, do not require activation. Examples of carcinogens needing no direct activation are β-propiolactone, nitrogen mustard, and bis(chloromethyl)ether. Furthermore, there appear to be epigenetic and other mechanisms by which some other carcinogens act. These include the cytotoxic agents mentioned, plastics, hormones, and immune suppressants (1).

Cancer Initiation

The previous section emphasized the latency period between the application of a carcinogen and the ultimate appearance of the tumor. This delay is not due solely, or even principally, to the growth of neoplastic cells from micro- to macroscopic size. Instead, it is explained by the need for a second developmental stage in carcinogenesis for many chemicals. Such a latency period, with the same implication, is also seen for cancers induced by viruses and ionizing radiation.

Rous and Kidd (8) coined the term "initiation" to describe the application of tar to a rabbit's ear which could then be made to produce a tumor by wounding. Initiation alone is not sufficient to produce neoplasia in most cases, although host and environmental factors can provide the subsequent requirements discussed in the next section. Many chemical carcinogens can provide requirements for both stages.

The process of pure initiation has the following characteristics:

1. irreversibility,
2. cumulative effects of repeated exposures to initiator,
3. no morphologic changes in initiated cells,
4. dependency on metabolism and the cell cycle, and
5. no threshold dose or maximum response to the initiator

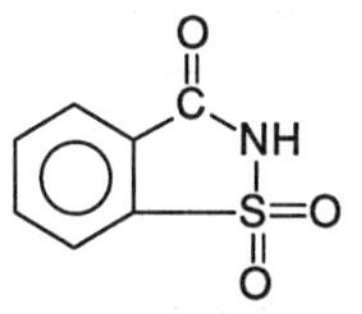

Figure 8.2. Chemical structures of some promoters.

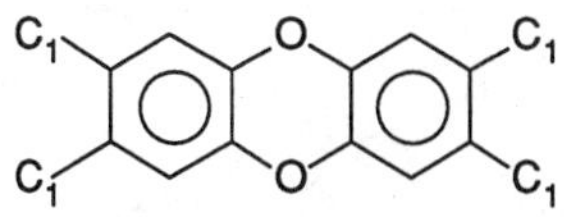

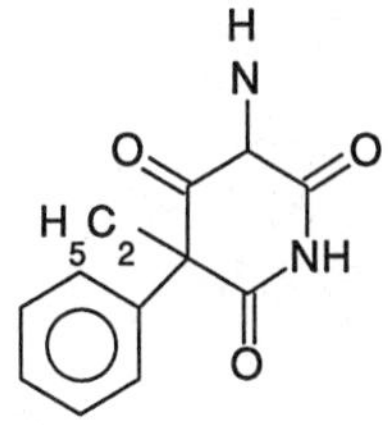

Cancer Promotion

Promotion is the process by which initiated cells complete the neoplastic transformation. In many cases, promotion requires the presence of an additional substance (promoter), which, by itself, may not be carcinogenic. The promoting agent probably alters gene expression with the subsequent manifestation of neoplasia in initiated cells. Promoters are often hormones, drugs, or plant products that react with cell membrane, nuclear, or cytoplastic receptors. Examples of some promoters are shown in Figure 2.

Most chemical carcinogens are both initiators and promoters (complete carcinogens) (Figure 8.3). A few are pure initiators, especially at low doses with promotion becoming manifest at higher doses. However, promoters cannot initiate a cancer but may transform neoplasms that were initiated by other environmental exposures or chance events.

Promotion is characterized by:

1. Reversibility and nonadditivity,
2. Morphologic changes in cells and gross appearance of neoplasia,
3. Noninitiation,
4. Modulation by environmental and lifestyle factors,
5. Threshold and maximal response.

A number of environmental factors are likely to be tumor promoters. In fact, human neoplasia may represent the effects of environmental and dietary promotion more than that of initiation. Environmental promoting agents probably include dietary fat, cigarette smoke, asbestos, halogenated hydrocarbons, alcohol, estrogens, and the substances in Figure 8.2.

HUMAN CARCINOGENESIS

Inferences regarding the carcinogenic action of toxins in human populations have come from two sources. These are epidemiologic investigations in small exposed populations and evidence from designed experiments in animals where sufficient knowledge is obtained to draw conclusions across species lines.

These latter types of studies are particularly important because it is extremely difficult to draw firm conclusions regarding carcinogenesis from epidemiologic studies alone. This is because of recall bias regarding exposure, low level and otherwise unknown exposures, and a long lag period between exposure and outcome. Because of the difficulty in firmly establishing carcinogenicity in humans, the IARC has adopted three categories for the strength of such evidence. These are:

1. Sufficient evidence indicating human cancer is definitely caused by exposure;
2. Limited evidence indicating that causality has not been proved because these studies have inadequately controlled confounders, bias, chance, or alternative explanations; and
3. Inadequate evidence, which means either no data available, weak epidemiologic data, or studies that showed convincingly no evidence of carcinogenicity.

There are large numbers of epidemiologic studies that demonstrate convincing carcinogenicity for lifestyle factors and dietary exposures in humans. These include alcohol, smoking, and aflatoxin.

Aflatoxin is associated primarily with liver cancer; high concentrations of this substance are found in the diet of some individuals in Africa and East Asia. In fact, the dose of aflatoxin ingested by certain individuals greatly exceeds the dose which has been proven carcinogenic in laboratory animals.

No discussion of chemical carcinogenesis in humans would be complete without mention of the leading human carcinogen, which is cigarette smoke. Current epidemiologic estimates indicate that approximately 90% of the lung cancer cases in the United States are a direct consequence of tobacco smoking. Considering the attributable risk of tobacco smoking in bladder cancer and gastrointestinal tract cancer, as much as 30% of the cancer deaths in the United States are a consequence of exposure to cigarette smoke.

A number of occupations are associated with higher incidence of cancer in humans. Most of these are listed in Table 8.1. In many cases, the precise mechanism by which cancers are produced is not known. For example, although there is considerable evidence that exposure to asbestos is carcinogenic, the exact mechanism is unknown. Fiberglass has been shown to be carcinogenic in rodents through an unknown mechanism but does not pose a detectable increase risk for humans.

Many of the manufacturing processes outlined in Table 8.1 involve exposure to a variety of chemicals such as dyes, benzene, cadmium, and pesticides. However, some industrial processes seem not to involve known carcinogens, indicating unknown mechanism of actions or interactions. The attributable risk due to occupational exposure for cancer deaths in the United States is under some dispute. Although estimates have been as high as 20%, it is more realistic to conclude that approximately 5% of cancer deaths in the United States can be contributed to occupational exposure.

QUANTITATIVE RISK ASSESSMENT OF CHEMICAL CARCINOGENS

In recent years, quantitative risk assessment for occupational and environmental exposures has become increasingly important because of the regulatory need to set acceptable standards for the release of an exposure to toxic substances in the environment. As evident from examining Table 8.1, many of these substances are important in common manufacturing proc-

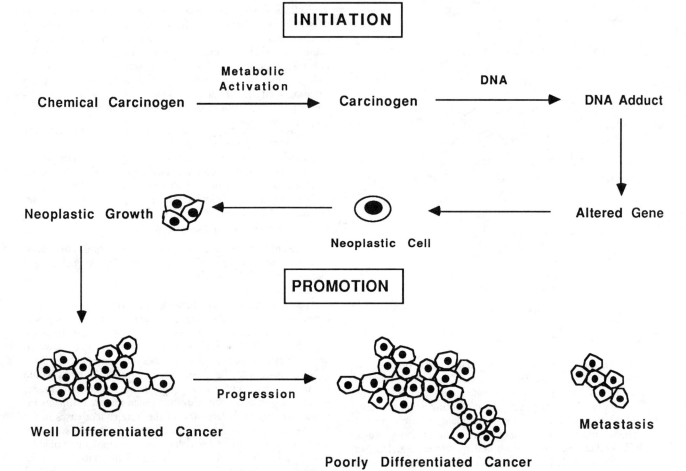

Figure 8.3. Carcinogenesis steps.

esses. However, not only must exposure to these substances be controlled, but any risk of developing cancer following exposure must be quantified. There is a body of mathematical, statistical, and regulatory knowledge which addresses this issue and is termed "quantitative risk assessment."

With regard to obtaining epidemiologic evidence, this is one area which has benefited from true experimental designs rather than observation only. These designs depend upon endpoints measured according to the definitions of chemical carcinogenesis provided earlier in this chapter. Statistical issues become important as a consequence of the Delaney Clause which was a component of the Food and Drug Act of 1958. This clause states, "No additive shall be deemed to be safe if it is found to induce cancer when ingested by man or animal, or if it is found after tests which are appropriate for the evaluation of the safety of food additives, to induce cancer in man or animal." As a consequence of the interpretation of this clause, statistical quantitative risk assessment is essential.

The principal question in quantitative risk assessment is an estimation of the risk imposed to individuals by low (environmental) doses of potentially carcinogenic agents. Accurate quantification of the low incidence of cancers in either humans or laboratory animals at such low doses would require the administration of these substances to huge numbers of experimental subjects. This is simply not feasible. As an alternative, the dose-response curves for carcinogens can be estimated at high doses (which are likely to yield increased incidence of

cancer) and mathematically extrapolated to the incidence at lower doses. Higher dose experiments can more easily be performed in smaller numbers of laboratory animals. However, the need for extrapolation of risk to low doses requires assumptions about the mathematical form of the dose response function and estimation of function parameters.

These kinds of data are almost never available from pure epidemiologic studies. When dose-response is demonstrated epidemiologically, studies never provide detailed information of the kind that could be extrapolated reliably to very low doses. Such studies are unplanned and undesigned, giving rise to the difficulties in forming causal links which are discussed elsewhere in this book. For this reason, laboratory experiments are usually conducted at doses higher than those expected in the environment. The Interagency Regulatory Liaison Group (1979) (9) recommended the following guidelines for such experiments: Lifetime studies on at least 50 animals of each sex in two different species with at least three dose groups (control, and two dose levels).

Dose-Response Models

The primary quantitative issues in dose-response modeling are the following:

1. The mathematical form of the dose-response function,
2. The incorporation of "background" in the model,

Table 8.2. Commonly Used Models for Assessing Risk from Chemical Carcinogens

Model	Mathematical Form
Log-probit	$F(d) = \phi[(\log(d) - \mu)/\sigma]$ $= \phi[a + b \log(d)]$ where $a = \dfrac{-\mu}{\sigma}$, $b = \dfrac{1}{\sigma}$, and $\phi(\cdot)$ is the cumulative normal distribution function.
Log-logistic	$F(d) = 1/[1 + e^{a - b\log(d)}]\ b > 0.$
One-hit	$F(d)\ 1 - e^{-\lambda d}.$
Gamma	$F(d) = 1 - e^{-(a_1 + b_1 d)\ (a_2 + b_2 d)\cdots}$
Multihit	$F(D) = 1 - e^{-\lambda_0 - \lambda_1 d - \cdots - \lambda_k d^k}, \lambda_i \geq 0.$
Weibull	$F(d) = 1 - e^{-bd^k}.$

3. The number of doses and animals per dose tested,
4. The method of estimation of model parameters.

It is quite likely that the probability of observing cancers of a specific type is greater than zero, even in the absence of a carcinogen, due to natural or environmental conditions. The statistical model attempts to predict the probability of cancer occurrence, p, as a function of dose, d. The observed effect may be death, weight loss, number of tumors, etc.

In the following formulas, we assume that P_0 is the background response or probability of cancer and $F(d)$ is the cumulative distribution of responses at a particular dose d. Two methods are commonly used to incorporate background into dose-response models. These are:

Equation 1 $\dfrac{Pd - P_0}{1 - P_0} = F(d)$

Equation 2 $Pd = F(d + d_0)$

The first formula assumes that background response independent of the response to the dose. This formula is most commonly used. One second formula assumes that the administered dose adds to the "baseline" dose already present. The form in which background is incorporated is often not critical, especially if the model is linear at low doses.

There are two general categories of models used for low dose extrapolation. These are termed tolerance and mechanistic. Tolerance models are not derived from biologic explanations of dose-response and are mainly statistically motivated. Commonly used tolerance models are the log-probit and log-logistic. In contrast, mechanistic models are derived from theories about carcinogenesis which give rise to quantitative probabilities of cancer incidence. Common mechanistic models are the one-hit, gamma multihit, multistage, and Weibull. Mechanistic models, for obvious reasons, are generally preferred over tolerance models. Several commonly used carcinogenic risk models are shown in Table 8.2.

The log-probit mode was first used in bioassay and was adopted in risk assessment primarily for convenience. The log-logistic model has a sigmoid curve very similar to the probit, because of the similarity between the logit and normal probability distributions. However, at low doses, the logistic model is more conservative. Because of its shape at low doses, the one-hit model was very conservative. In many instances, it does not provide a reasonable model for low dose extrapolation

in spite of its simplicity (10). The gamma model is intuitively appealing because of the assumptions underlying its derivation (11), but its practical implementation is difficult for computational reasons. The multistage model has the same mathematical form as the one-hit model with a polynomial in the exponent. It has been widely used recently. The Weibull model behaves similarly to the gamma, especially at low doses and is a special case of multistage model.

Estimation Procedures

Estimation procedures for the parameters of the dose-response function are similar in concept for all the models. They usually follow methods to obtain "maximum likelihood estimates" of the parameters. Simply stated, these procedures generate values for the parameters that were most likely to have produced the observed data if the model was correct. In some instances, mathematical transformation of the models can be used with alternative estimation procedures (such as weighted least squares) to produce estimates with the same or similar desirable properties as maximum likelihood estimates.

Following estimation of model parameters, low dose extrapolation is generally straightforward. Two techniques for extrapolation have been advocated: (a) direct mathematical extrapolation to low doses based on estimated parameters and (b) linear extrapolation back to the estimated background response from the lowest dose modeled, regardless of the dose-response model. The linear extrapolation technique has been discussed by Gaylor and Kodell (1980) (12). Linear extrapolation resembles the one-hit model which is linear at low doses.

A major endpoint of these analyses is the estimation of a virtually safe dose (VSD). This is a dose at which there is a small effect above control, usually in the range of 10^{-5}–10^{-8}. Because the VSD is outside the range of experimentally obtained data, its estimation is subject to many nuances and difficulties.

Because of the relatively small amount of data upon which model parameter estimates are based, there is often little difference between models in the observed range. However, when the incidence over background is small, as with VSD of 10^{-5} or less, the results can be quite different. In general, the predicted dose is smallest for the one-hit and multistage models and largest for the gamma multihit and log-probit models. Typically, the Weibull and log-logistic models are intermediate. This is a rough guideline and is not infallible for all data sets.

Other Considerations in Quantitative Risk Assessment

Other major issues in carcinogenic risk assessment are time-to-event analyses and pharmacokinetics. Time-to-event analyses attempt to model the incidence of tumors as a function of the interval between exposure and appearance of the cancer. Recall that shortening of median time to tumor is an indication of chemical carcinogenesis. In a commonly used form, the probability of observing a tumor at time t and dose d is given by the equation:

$$P(d, t) = 1 - e^{-g(d)H(t)}$$

where $H(t)$ is the cumulative hazard, and $g(d)$ is the dose function. The dose function, g, can be taken to be a polynomial. In a lifetime study, $H = 1$, and the model becomes equivalent to the multistage model.

Pharmacokinetic considerations become important because of a possible nonlinear relationship between administered dose and effective dose. Based on Michaelis-Menten kinetics, the effective and administered dose are related by:

$$E = \frac{aA}{(b + A)}$$

Where E is the effective dose and A is the administered dose. More complicated relationships between these two quantities are biologically plausible. However, the quantity and quality of data do not frequently support such modeling efforts.

In practice, pharmacokinetic information is frequently used to extrapolate across animal species, i.e., from rodent to human. This information can be used to correct for different routes of exposure, for example. In general, there are no widely accepted principles for utilizing data in this way.

In summary, chemical carcinogens are substances that increase the occurrence of cancer in humans. These substances act primarily by binding covalently to DNA. In many instances, this initiation must be accompanied by a second step (promotion) which can be produced by environmental or dietary substances, continued exposure to the carcinogen, or other factors. Many chemical substances are both initiators and promoters. Extensive studies and reviews by the IARC have determined that a sizable number of chemicals and processes are convincingly associated with human carcinogenesis. There are an even larger number of additional substances suspected of being carcinogenic, but less convincingly so.

For the toxicologist, it is important to assess quantitatively the risk associated with specific chemical carcinogens or other suspected carcinogens. The mathematical and statistical techniques for doing so represent a compromise between analytic rigor and sufficient experimental data. Risk assessment studies are typically performed at doses much higher than those experienced in an environmental setting. Mathematical techniques are used to extrapolate the results of such experiments back to the low levels of environmental exposure. Estimation of a "safe dose" also depends upon assumptions about background incidence of the cancers being observed.

CANCER CLUSTERS

A cluster is defined as a number of like or similar diseases occurring together in time and space. Clustering of disease can also apply to groups of cases linked by shared environments or exposures. The appearance of cancer cases within an occupational setting or in a community creates anxiety and fear among employees or members of a community. An environmental cause is usually thought to be the source of such a cancer cluster. The clustering of diseases such as cancer may be real or by chance. Investigation of a disease cluster can be very difficult depending on the disease, the multiplicity of chemical exposures, the size of the population in which the event occurs, and the ability to define the exposure. There are certain chemicals as well as occupational environments that have been identified as being causative of or associated with human carcinogenesis (Table 8.1). Fear of chemical carcinogenesis may be heightened by the presence of chemical hazards which may be suspected of being carcinogens. The public or employees find the presence of such a chemical to be unacceptable, even if they have not been linked to carcinogenesis.

Chemicals that have sufficient evidence for carcinogenicity in animals have been accepted as posing a hazard to humans. However, there are many problems associated with extrapolating evidence derived in animal models or in in vitro tests to humans. Also, the results of epidemiologic studies involving cancer incidence and prevalence in populations are often difficult to interpret. Establishing that a chemical or environment is associated with carcinogenicity requires the satisfaction of basic principles such as: (a) carcinogenesis is not explained by bias in the recording or detection involved in the study; (b) the cancer cannot be explained by chance alone; (c) the cancer is repeatedly found to be present in a variety of circumstances; (d) the cancer varies with dose and time of exposure.

The number of new chemicals introduced into commercial use each year add to the more than six million inorganic and organic chemicals registered by the Chemical Abstract Service of the American Chemical Society (13). However, only 20 or so of these chemicals are suspected of being human carcinogens. Attempting to apportion the cancer incidence and death to occupational exposures is quite difficult. It is estimated that 5% of occupationally related deaths are due to cancer. The attributable risk of chemicals to cancer causation is difficult to precisely estimate due to several factors: (a) a mobile work force makes tracking of exposures difficult; (b) latency periods and lengths of exposure are difficult to accurately ascertain; (c) employees may work several sites within the same company; (d) personal and prior health factors must be considered, such as smoking, illicit drug use, family history, and other habits; (e) employees may have multiple jobs; (f) the time of exposure may be difficult to document; (g) the clinical presentation of cancer may not occur for years following the exposure, and misdiagnosis can occur; (h) the exposure may be complex and involve multiple chemicals; and (i) over 60% of cancer-related deaths occur in people over 65 years of age.

The latency period from time of exposure to clinical signs of the disease is another critical feature to examine in any investigation of cancer clusters. For solid tumors, the latency period is typically 15 to 20 years. The latency period for hematologic tumors is 5–10 years. In some situations, an industry itself has been identified as being associated with a higher incidence of cancer. In these instances a single chemical causation has been impossible to document. Occasionally, in such occupational settings, certain jobs and tasks have been identified as being more hazardous and more likely to be associated with an increased risk of cancer.

Evidence that human exposure to a chemical or hazardous substance is carcinogenic is usually documented by epidemiologic studies, bioassays in animals, shortterm in vitro screening studies in mammalian cells, and mutagenicity studies in microorganisms. Extrapolating animal carcinogenesis studies to humans is difficult at best and involves many assumptions: (a) chemicals that may produce cancer in one or more species of animals may not cause cancer in humans; (b) the dose-response curve in the animal model is assumed to be the same for humans, and this may not be true; (c) a subthreshold dose or assumed "safe" level of a chemical carcinogen in animals cannot be assumed with certainty to be safe in humans; (d) a higher chemical dose may increase the incidence of carcinogenesis in animals or shorten the latency period but cannot be assumed to produce the same results in humans; and (e) the target organ in animals may not predict the target organ or cell type of cancer in humans (14, 15).

Table 8.3. Steps in the Investigation of a Cancer Cluster

1. Each case of cancer must be identified and confirmed. Histopathology and medical records should be reviewed for accuracy of diagnosis.

2. The time of occurrence of the cancer cases should be identified. Employees working for the company during this time should be evaluated. This step of the investigation can be affected by a changing workforce.

3. The observed number of cases should be compared to the expected number of cases. The expected number of cases may be obtained from cancer registries. This comparison should be age standardized, since the majority of cancer occurs in older individuals. Comparison of the observed number of cases to the expected number allows for the calculation of a standard mortality ratio (SMR). An SMR greater than one may indicate an excess of cancer.

4. After the types of cancer are identified, determination should be made as to whether a particular cell type or target organ is overrepresented in the population being studied.

5. The latency period must be evaluated. Latency is the time from the onset of exposure to a certain chemical or environment to appearance of clinical disease. The latency period for solid tumors is 15–20 years and for hematologic tumors, 5–10 years. If an individual is noted to have cancer after a recent exposure, then the latency period is too short to implicate the chemical or the environment as the cause.

6. Confounding and contributing factors must be evaluated. These include smoking, substance and drug abuse, a family history of cancer, multiple exposures to other chemicals or potential carcinogens, or employment in an industry that has been associated with carcinogenesis.

7. There may be a particular job or site in an area of industry that is over-represented in cases of cancer. The standard mortality ratio may not show an elevation of cancer cases in the industry overall, but specific jobs or sites may show an excess of deaths if separate SMRs are calculated for these sites and job descriptions.

8. If an excess of similar cases exists, then the issue of causation must be addressed. A chemical may be responsible, and further investigation is warranted. If there is a mixture of cancer types, then this is unlikely to be a true cancer cluster. If there is overrepresentation by a particular job, environment, or chemical exposure than a cluster may indeed be occurring. If there is no pattern of common exposures or job site locations, then the chances of a cluster are diminished.

9. An environmental assessment and industrial hygiene review is warranted to determine if exposures to potential carcinogens is occurring. Previous environment surveys should be reviewed and appropriate environmental monitoring conducted as needed.

10. The investigation should conclude that:
    (a) a cluster is not present;
    (b) a cluster may be present but is inconsistent with an occupational or environmental exposure cause;
    (c) a cluster is present and could be related to a chemical or environmental exposure; or
    (d) the cluster is definitely related to the exposure.

If an exposure or occupational setting is implicated, then aggressive corrective action must be undertaken.

Cancer Cluster Evaluation

The recognition of a clustering of cancer in a community or business heightens tensions and concerns leading to lengthy and expensive investigations. All too often, these investigations create further anxieties and tensions if the results are inconclusive. Too often, public demand instead of scientific discipline leads to inadequate studies being performed. Incidences of cancer are usually first recognized by employees or individuals in a community and are then brought to the attention of company management or the health department. Cancer cluster investigation begins with the disease and with attempts to find a cause instead of proceeding from a cause to an effect. The discovery of cases of cancer may be attributed to an environmental factor such as a chemical or to chance alone. However, it is very difficult to rationalize chance alone to concerned employees or members of a community. The approach to cancer cluster investigation should be methodical (Table 8.3) (15, 16).

The investigation and analysis of suspected cancer clusters begins with confirmation of the pathology and verification that the cancer cell type and histopathology is consistent with the diagnosis. Statistical methods have been devised for examining disease clusters. These statistical methods include: (a) direct survey of neighboring populations of potentially affected individuals and unaffected demographically controlled similar populations and (b) use of census tract data coupled with existing data contained in local, state, or federal registries. Disease registries are useful because they place given disease states in a framework of time and definable geographic boundaries.

The objective of the investigation is to determine if there is a real excess of cancer cases, if the cases are occurring independently or are related, if the cases are by chance alone, and if there is any environmental cause that can be identified. The use of many classical epidemiologic methods may not be applicable to cluster investigation due to the small numbers of people involved. Also, understanding how varieties of cancer are distributed in the population is important as well as understanding that cancer is the second leading cause of death in the United States. The cluster may thus represent normal carrier occurrences. No matter what the conclusion of a cancer cluster investigation, ongoing medical surveillance and environmental monitoring is important in order to address the concerns of employees, employers, and the public.

REFERENCES

1. International Agency on Research of Cancer. Overall evaluations of carcinogenicity. *IARC Monographs on The Evaluation of Carcinogenic Risks to Humans.* An Updating of International Agency on Research of Cancer Monographs Volumes 1 to 42, Suppl. 7, 1987.

2. Pott, P. Chirurgical observations relative to the cataract, the polypus of the nose, the cancer of the scrotum, the different kinds of ruptures, and the mortification of the toes and feet. London: Hawkes, Clarke, and Collins, 1775.

3. Miller EC, Miller JA. The presence and significance of bound amino azo dyes in the livers of rats fed p-dimethylaminoazobenzene. Cancer Res 1947;7:468.

4. Miller EC. Studies on the formation of protein-bound derivatives of 3,4-benzopyrene in the epidermal fraction of mouse skin. Cancer Res 1951;11:100.

5. Miller JA, Cramer JW, Miller EC. The n- and ring-hydroxylation of 2-acetylaminofluorene during carcinogenesis in the rat. Cancer Res 1960;20:950.

6. Nagta C, Kodama M, Ioki Y, Kimura T. Free radicals produced from chemical carcinogens and their significance in carcinogenesis. In: Floyd RA, ed. Free Radicals and Cancer. New York: Marcel Dekker, 1982:1.

7. Wattenberg LW. Inhibition of chemical carcinogenesis. J Natl Cancer Inst 1978;60:11.

8. Rous P and Kidd JG. Conditional neoplasms and subthreshold neoplastic states. J Exp Med 1941;73:365.

9. Interagency Regulator Liaison Group. Scientific bases for identification of potential carcinogens and estimation of risks. J Natl Cancer Inst 1979;63:241–268.

10. Food Safety Council. Quantitative risk assessment. proposed system for food safety assessment. Washington, DC: Food Safety Council, 1980b:137–160.

11. Rai K, Ryzin J Van. Risk assessment of toxic environmental substances using a generalized multi-hit dose response model. In: Breslow NE, Whittemore

AS. Energy and health. Philadelphia: Society for Industrial and Applied Mathematics, 1979:99–117.

12. Gaylor DW, Kodell RL. Linear interpolation algorithm for low dose risk assessment of toxic substances. J Environ Pathol Toxicol 1980;4:305–312.

13. Schottenfeld D. Chronic disease in the workplace and environment: cancer. Arch Environ Health 1984;39:150–157.

14. Sielken RL. Some issues in the quantitative modeling portion of cancer risk assessment. Reg Toxicol Pharmacol 1985;5:175–181.

15. Frumkin H, Kantrowitz W. Cancer clusters in the workplace: an approach to investigation. J Occup Med 1987;29:949–952.

16. Schulte PA, Ehrenberg RL, Singal M. Investigation of occupational cancer clusters: theory and practice. Am J Public Health 1987;77:52–56.

9

Principles of Medical Surveillance and Human Exposure Standards

Gary R. Krieger, M.D., M.P.H.
Marci Balge, R.N., M.S.

INTRODUCTION

Medical surveillance programs are designed to systematically collect and analyze health information on workers exposed to hazardous materials. This chapter describes the components involved in a comprehensive medical surveillance program and how these components interrelate. Components of a medical surveillance program include:

1. Biologic Monitoring;
2. Protocols for testing;
3. Determination of health hazards, exposures, and job-related risks;
4. Tracking systems;
5. Specific job descriptions, job duties, and job requirements; and
6. Exposure monitoring system:

Biologic monitoring is a key component which is designed to anticipate disease by sampling and analyzing solid tissues, secretions, or excretions. The end results of this monitoring are used to take both preventive and ongoing action in the workplace setting. To be effective, a medical surveillance program must meet all appropriate regulatory requirements and must be managed in a cost-effective and businesslike fashion.

This chapter will describe and analyze the components involved in a comprehensive medical surveillance program and how the components relate to current human exposure standards. The goals of a medical surveillance program can vary and are program and site specific.

PROGRAM GOALS AND EVALUATION

Ducatman cites several examples of program goals (3):

1. Establish epidemiologic surveys with the purpose of determining the frequency or natural history of a particular condition.
2. Protect the health of the public, for example, from communicable diseases.
3. Produce data which would meet regulatory and/or internal company exposure monitoring requirements. Regulatory exposure standards are not always available for all substances. Thus, many large companies have developed exposure standards for their internal use; however, most industrial based medical surveillance programs are regulatory-driven. The overall focus of this chapter is directed toward regulatory compliance issues for various hazards. Two recent journals have extensively reviewed medical surveillance programs in general and hazardous waste workers in particular (4, 5).

PROGRAM EVALUATION

To manage a successful program, internal evaluation criteria must be established. These criteria are based on several key issues:

1. The type of organization establishing the program (e.g., industrial, medical group practice);
2. The program administrators (e.g., funded versus internal vendor service);
3. Income source;
4. Internal audits; and
5. The employees in the surveillance program.

Within a program, the specific goals of the various managers and customers may not be the same. For example, the managers may view cost control within a context of minimum regulatory compliance as the primary goal, whereas, the worker's perspective of the program may focus on the desire to have maximum medical testing regardless of cost or effectiveness. Given this clear dichotomy, it is essential for the physician to balance these perspectives when developing overall program goals, objectives, and outcomes. Table 9.1 presents an example of specific program elements in the evaluation process (6). By using this model, it is possible, based on past efforts, to determine the direction of future program activities.

HUMAN EXPOSURE STANDARDS

Since September 1988, the Occupational Safety and Health Administration (OSHA) has indicated support for generic regulations in the areas of exposure monitoring and medical surveillance (7). If these proposed rule changes occur, they would have the effect of setting general examination requirements for all chemical exposures.

Unlike current requirements, the *proposed* generic requirements would have a broader scope:

1. Initial exposure monitoring of workers will be required of employers.
2. The frequency of follow-up monitoring will be specified.
3. The placement of air sampling techniques in terms of personal and/or environmental monitoring will be specified.
4. Procedures will be developed for employee observance of ambient sampling.
5. Medical surveillance requirements will be required for all employees exposed to one half the exposure limit.
6. The fact that employees will not be charged for the examinations will be emphasized.

Currently, OSHA regulations listed in 29 CFR 1910.120

Table 9.1. Model for Delineating Program Elements in the Evaluation Process

Preexisting Conditions	Program Components	Intervening Events	Impact	Consequences
Current state of the target group to be affected Organization implementing the program Degree of independence with other programs Larger environment in which both the target group and the organization function	Inputs: 1. Program objectives 2. Resources; activities	Factors which will affect how the program operates during the course of the evaluation; these factors may be either internal or external to the organization.	Extent to which operational indicators of objectives are attained.	Effects of attaining the objective.

Shortell, R. Health Program Evaluation. St. Louis, MO: Mosby, 1978.

require employers to implement medical surveillance programs in the following situations (8):

1. For employees who may be exposed to hazardous substances or health hazards at or above the permissible exposure limits (PELs) for 30 days or more per year.
2. In the absence of PELs, medical surveillance should be established for those employees working at limits above the published exposure levels for a given substance.
3. Employees who wear a respirator for 30 days or more per year must be examined.
4. HAZMAT employees, defined as employees who are designated to plug, patch, or temporarily control leaks from containers which hold hazardous substances, must be examined.
5. All employees who are injured due to overexposure from an emergency incident involving hazardous substances must be examined.

The large number of potentially hazardous materials and the frequency of their use virtually ensures that people will be exposed to hazardous substances at some time and to some degree.

Exposure refers to any contact of an organism with a chemical or physical agent. Exposure is quantified as the amount of the agent available at the exchange boundaries of the organism and available for absorption (Environmental Protection Agency) (9).

For the majority of the health effects, there is a general correlation between the amount of a toxic substance absorbed by the organism and the production of a physiologic response. This dose-response relationship implies that for many materials there are levels of exposure which can be tolerated without adverse health effects. Thus, it is important to accurately assess the magnitude, frequency, duration, and route of exposure. This exposure assessment generates a series of standards or limits that are considered safe for each material encountered.

Exposure limits vary from country to country, depending on the original data source. The United States, Western Europe, and Australia generally utilize health impairment data, while the Soviet Union (U.S.S.R.) frequently keys in on neurophysiologic changes in experimental animals. In addition, the safety factors applied to a data source can widely vary due to technical and socioeconomic factors. In the United States, exposure limits are statutory requirements, while in some countries exposure limits are included in labor agreements.

In the United States, one of the first groups to develop specific exposure guidelines was the American Conference of Government Industrial Hygienists (ACGIH). In 1941, ACGIH suggested maximum allowable concentrations (MACs) for use in industry. A list of MACs was compiled by ACGIH and published in 1946. In the early 1960s, ACGIH revised their recommendations and renamed them Threshold Limit Values (TLVs). TLVs are a registered trademark of the ACGIH and refer to the concept that there is a "threshold" dose or concentration below which there are no adverse effects. TLVs refer to air contaminants in the working environment. Broadly, a TLV refers to an airborne concentration and workplace condition under which it is believed that nearly all workers may be repeatedly exposed day after day without adverse effects (10). TLVs were formulated for use in the normal industrial workplace, not as general environmental standards. In addition, the notion of a TLV is not easily transferable to the situation found at chemical spills or at complex hazardous waste sites.

While the concept of TLVs has been adopted by many countries, there are other equally valued exposure limit systems:

1. *Dutch* — Maximum accepted concentration for noncarcinogenic substances;
2. *Soviet* — Maximum allowable concentration; and
3. *German* — Technical reference concentration.

The ACGIH system has been widely disseminated and is extremely influential both in the United States and internationally.

Compliance with regulations does not ensure corporate liability protection. The National Institute of Occupational Safety and Health (NIOSH) developed recommendations for medical surveillance covering over 400 chemicals. These recommendations differ from OSHA recommendations for more than 100 chemicals. It is quite common to discover that an exposure level is well below OSHA requirements but above NIOSH recommendations. In this situation, it may be prudent to monitor these exposures as part of the overall medical surveillance program.

EMPLOYEE SELECTION FOR MEDICAL SURVEILLANCE

Companies are constantly faced with a dilemma regarding who to actually include in their medical surveillance program (1–5). There are many employers who are involved with projects that require field work in areas where the exposures are not well-characterized and where the industrial hygiene database is incomplete. In addition, many employees with episodic exposures are in positions that involve contact with hazardous materials for less than 30 days per year. For example, supervisors and project managers go to hazardous job sites but rarely do any actual field work and have significantly decreased opportunity for exposures. Also, some employers hire temporary employees for large jobs that last fewer than 30 working days. Thus, there are a large variety of scenarios that can occur which create confusion for employers in determining whether an employee belongs in a medical surveillance program.

There are a variety of ways to approach this issue. One approach is to survey everyone in the company. The overall program is established with a preventive medicine focus, and exposure-specific protocols are provided for employees who perform hazardous materials work. A second possibility for defining participants is to include all employees, regardless of exposure length, who may at some point in the year perform work involving hazardous materials. A third and more job-specific way of selection is to include employees only on a project-by-project basis; however, there are operational problems associated with this method. Many jobs have quick starts that leave minimum time for performing an adequate baseline exam. Thus, employees can be sent to the field without appropriate medical evaluation and clearance.

In general, the current OSHA regulations direct the frequency of medical surveillance examinations for hazardous materials (11):

1. Depending on the prior job assignment and the potential of exposure to toxic substances,
2. At least once every 12 months unless the examining physician believes a longer interval (every 2 years) is appropriate,
3. The examining physician has the discretionary ability to initiate more frequent exam intervals,
4. At termination of employment or reassignment of job duties or location,
5. As soon as an employee states he/she has concerns related to signs and symptoms indicating overexposure to hazardous substances. In addition, if an unprotected employee has been exposed in an emergency situation, then an examination is required.

To facilitate the examination process, there is a standard set of information which ideally should be available to the physician or nurse:

1. The OSHA standards and surveillance requirements related to the hazardous substance,
2. The employees' job description, with emphasis on specific duties that may generate exposure,
3. Any exposure history and industrial hygiene monitoring data,
4. Use of personal protective equipment data from OSHA 1910.134, (12)
5. Data from prior exams.

HEALTH CARE PROVIDER SELECTION

Generally, the choice of physician(s) providing the medical surveillance examination is directed by the company. In many cases the company's human resources manager is responsible for the selection of services. There is specific criteria for physician selection recommended by the American Industrial Hygiene Association (AIHA) (13):

1. The physician should be board-certified in occupational medicine. If a board-certified physician is not available, either a board-eligible physician or a physician with experience and training in occupational medicine should be selected.
2. In the absence of a board-certified physician in occupational medicine, it is recommended that the examining physician provide employee medical records to a board-certified physician for review.
3. AIHA also recommends verifying state licensure, reviewing resumes, and performing a standard general employment interview and background check.

EXAMINATION CONTENT

OSHA's regulations state that the medical examination should include a medical and work history. Special emphasis is placed on possible symptoms related to the handling of hazardous substances, as well as overall fitness for duty. Fitness for duty includes the ability to wear personal protective equipment at any level as well as fitness for exposure to other hazards that may be expected at the work site. For example, due to temperature extremes, an individual may be medically fit to work as a driller in Level B in Colorado in January but not able to do the same work in Phoenix, Arizona, in July.

Unlike the general surveillance recommendations for most categories of workers, OSHA has specific rules for hazardous waste workers. The Federal Register of March 6, 1989, outlines the final rule related to 29 CFR 1910: Hazardous Waste Operations and Emergency Response (11). The section on medical surveillance includes specific provisions for baseline, periodic, and exit medical exams. The overall content of the exam is determined by the examining physician. After the exam and testing is complete, a formal written summary is required.

The physician's written opinion is specifically directed to include:

1. Recommended limitations or restrictions for the specific job duties,
2. Results of the medical exam and tests conducted; and
3. Statement that the employee has been informed of the exam results as well as of any conditions that require follow-up.

In addition, the written medical information sent to the employer should not reveal specific findings that are not work related (Appendices A and B).

RECORDKEEPING

According to CFR 1910.120, medical records of the medical surveillance program should be retained for a period of 30 years past the employee's termination date (4).

When an employee requests access to a record, the employer is responsible for assuring that access is provided within 15 days of the request by the employee or the employees designated representative. The designated representative should have written consent from the employe for access to the record. An example of such a consent form can be found in Appendix C. Upon receiving a request for medical records, the company physician may recommend that the employee: (a) consult with the examining physician to review the records, (b) accept a summary of the record in lieu of the entire record, or (c) recommend that the record be released only to a physician or other designated representative. If the physician believes that direct employee access to information contained in the records regarding a specific diagnosis of terminal illness or psychiatric condition could be detrimental to the employee's health, the employer may inform the employee that access will be provided to a designated representative with written consent. A physician maintaining the records may delete from the record identities of family members, personal friends, or fellow employees who have provided confidential information relative to the employee's health status.

Employers must provide the OSHA representative with immediate access to medical and exposure records upon request. Rules regarding OSHA access to records are covered in CFR 1910.20.

CLINIC SELECTION FOR MEDICAL SURVEILLANCE

The choice of examining physician and clinic has become highly competitive. Hospitals, clinics, and emergency departments all compete for this source of revenue. There are several variables that a company should consider in its selection criteria: location, proximity to the company, cost, local reputation among employees, access, turnaround time for results, ease of scheduling in a timely manner, physician specialties and certifications, and ability to comply with contractual arrangements established with laboratories.

Access and timely turnaround of exam results are critical. Ideally, an applicant is not placed in a position until the presence or absence of work restrictions has been medically determined. The physician performing the exam should have job descriptions as well as physical and psychologic job requirements per position so that an appropriate decision can be made regarding work restrictions specific to a position. Examples of job requirements are found in Appendix D.

Aside from logistical criteria, there are other equally important considerations:

1. Availability of ancillary services. Are ECG, pulmonary, x-ray, audiology, and laboratory services readily available? If an employee has to schedule appointments with several different services prior to the exam, it can become very time consuming and cumbersome;
2. Turnaround time for receipt of laboratory results;
3. Certification of technicians performing ancillary testing, specifically pulmonary functions and audiometrics;
4. Clinic personnel's knowledge of OSHA regulations pertaining to medical surveillance, medical record storage, and release of information; and
5. Ease of scheduling exams and meeting time constraints.

CONSULTING MEDICAL DIRECTOR

Employers without in-house medical departments generally select a physician consultant for the management of the medical surveillance program. This individual should be board-certified or eligible in occupational medicine and should perform the following tasks:

1. Oversee the selection of clinics and medical providers;
2. Provide quality assurance and quality control by reviewing all exam results and consulting with the physician who performed the exam when necessary;

3. Collaborate with industrial hygienists safety professionals and occupational health nurses in developing policies and protocols for the medical surveillance program;
4. Serve as a resource in toxicology; and
5. Conduct epidemiologic studies as indicated.

EXAM CATEGORIES

Preplacement — An examination designed to determine the medical appropriateness for a particular job placement.

Baseline — An examination conducted prior to work with hazardous materials or conditions; this exam establishes initial testing levels and determines the presence or absence of work restrictions for a particular position.

Periodic/annual — An examination conducted on an annual basis beginning 1 year after the baseline examination to monitor ongoing health status and determine the presence or absence of work restrictions.

Exit — An examination conducted when an employee terminates employment from a position requiring work involving hazardous materials or conditions.

Special — An examination conducted to determine health effects related to a specific exposure or event.

BASELINE EXAMINATIONS

If an applicant or employee has received an exit exam from his former employer within 6 months, the results can be obtained, reviewed for completeness and appropriateness, and used as the baseline for the current employer. If components are missing, only those missing should be ordered. Components of a baseline exam include:

1. Complete health history;
2. Physical exam;
3. Visual exam, with and without glasses;
4. Electrocardiogram; 12-lead resting ECG;
5. Chest x-ray, PA:
6. Audiometric testing to include 500, 1000, 2000, 4000, 6000, and 8000 Hz;
7. A complete and thorough health history.

Many questionnaires have been developed and are currently in use at many occupational medicine clinics; Appendix E is an example of a standard history form. Because of the importance of vision, with respect to job efficiency and safety, a detailed vision examination measuring visual acuity for near and distance, visual fields, color discrimination, and depth perception should be included.

PERIODIC/ANNUAL EXAMS

The components of an annual exam should be consistent with age, medical history, and job-related activities during the past year. An example of a testing protocol is shown in Appendix F. Periodic exams are usually done for employees with ongoing work activities involving hazards or exposures, but they are also useful in the monitoring of individuals with previous exposures to substances that can have long latency periods.

SPECIAL EXAMS

These exams are generally done to evaluate the effects of a specific hazardous material or general overexposure situation (e.g., fire, smoke exposure). Special exams are also conducted to obtain biologic exposure samples before and after shift.

SPIROMETRY

Routinely assessing pulmonary function with simple spirometry has become common practice in occupational medicine. When used in conjunction with the health history, physical exam, and chest x-ray results, spirometry results can identify preexisting pulmonary disease.

OSHA currently requires spirometry for employee exposure to asbestos, coke oven emissions, and cotton dust. NIOSH recommends spirometry for airborne substances including beryllium, cadmium, chlorine, formaldehyde, nitrogen dioxide, silica, sulfur dioxide, toluene diisocyanate, and wood dust.

There are several problems associated with spirometry:

1. Inadequate training of personnel conducting the tests,
2. Technically deficient spirometers,
3. Lack of standardization of test methodology, and
4. Lack of physician knowledge in interpreting test results.

In 1978, the American Thoracic Society (ATS) published standardization for spirometry (14). The ATS recently updated its recommendations (15). Spirometers do not need to perform all tests, but the ones they do perform should meet the specifications for that test. Equipment specifications have also been developed and are listed in Appendix G (16).

MONITORING PROTOCOLS

Two essential elements in the management of medical surveillance programs are the accurate evaluation of monitoring results and the development of monitoring protocols which are appropriate to the actual exposures encountered in the workplace.

Unlike employees in a stable manufacturing environment, hazardous waste workers encounter potential exposures to a variety of unidentified substances. Ambient monitoring and sampling data are generally not available prior to the initiation of work. Due to these unknown factors, these workers rely heavily on the use of personal protective equipment.

Biologic monitoring includes measurement of appropriate determinants in biologic specimens collected from the worker. Biologic Exposure Indices (BEIs) are references values intended as guidelines for the evaluation of potential health hazards (10). BEIs represent levels most likely to be seen in healthy workers exposed to chemicals to the same extent as workers with inhalation exposures to the Threshold Limit Value-Time Weighted Average (TLV-TWA). BEIs apply to 8-hour exposures, 5 days a week, and are not intended for use as a measure of adverse effects or for diagnosis of occupationally related illnesses. Utilizing human data, the BEI is based either on the relationship between intensity of exposure and biologic levels of the determinant or on the relationship between biologic levels and health effects. Biologic monitoring, which is complementary to air monitoring, should be conducted when it can (a) enhance or substantiate air monitoring, (b) test the efficacy of pre-placement examinations (PPE), (c) determine the potential for absorption, or (d) detect nonoccupational exposure.

While BEI offers a more direct measure of the exposure intensity, there are multiple confounding factors:

1. Physiologic and health status of the employee: body build, diet, sex, age, medication;
2. Exposure sources: intensity of the physical workload and fluctuations of exposure intensity, skin exposure;
3. Environmental sources: community and home air pollutants, water, and food contaminants;
4. Lifestyle variations: smoking, alcohol, personal hygiene; and
5. Methodologic sources involving specimen collection, storage, and analyses.

Urine, exhaled air, and blood specimens are used as biologic specimens. Quantitative collection of urine during a specific time period can be difficult due to the variability of urine output and concentration. Quality control over individual collection of a 24-hour urine specimen can also be difficult when employees are working in remote job sites.

In analysis of exhaled air, there are rapid changes of the concentration with time; in addition, the concentration is changing during expiration. Therefore, it is important to specify whether alveolar (end-exhaled air) or mixed-exhaled air is indicated. Workers with altered pulmonary function may not be suitable for exposure monitoring by exhaled air because it has been demonstrated that differences in metabolism can result in up to 100% variation.

In the analysis of data based on blood specimens, several factors should be considered. The plasma-erythrocyte ratio and the distribution of determinants among blood constituents can effect the outcome measurements. Unless indicated, the BEIs for volatile chemicals relate to venous blood, not capillary blood. A list of the Adopted Biologic Exposure Indices is presented in Appendix H (10).

Drugs can also affect the accuracy of biologic exposure indices because they alter the efficiency of specific metabolic pathways. Therefore, a careful medication history is critical (17).

LIVER FUNCTION STUDIES

Chronic alcohol consumption induces the hepatic metabolism of many chemicals. Studies have shown that blood ethanol levels between 5 and 15 mmol/l increase the internal exposure time as well as the concentration of toluene and styrene at TLVs. Exposure to chemicals can also increase the sensitivity to the effects of alcohol. Many possible mechanisms exist where alcohol can modify the disposition and kinetics of workplace chemicals. It is therefore essential in evaluating laboratory results during medical surveillance exams, to pay particular attention to the overall liver enzyme abnormalities. It is not uncommon to find mild transient abnormalities of liver function. Before conclusions are drawn, the tests should be serially repeated, and confounders such as alcohol, illness, and exercise should be controlled (4, 5, 17–20).

TRACKING

There are a variety of software systems available for managing a medical surveillance program. Medical clinics tend to focus on systems that store data while emphasizing tracking functions such as exam frequency and due dates. A well-integrated program offers the ability to track frequency, results, and the movement of an employee from one plant/location to another. This is important to prevent exam duplication, and unnecessary testing.

IMPLEMENTATION OF A PHYSICAL EXAM PROGRAM

Communication between the employer and physician regarding expectations is essential in implementing a successful medical surveillance program. Agreement on communication, protocols, and pricing is essential.

The physical exam is usually scheduled by the employee or the company's health and safety representative. To ensure efficiency, several steps should be followed.

When the exam is scheduled, all appropriate ancillary services should be completed within the same time. Thus, the entire exam is completed in a relatively short time period, and the physician has all results at the time of the physical. See Appendix I as an example of a routing schedule.

SUMMARY AND CONCLUSIONS

Medical surveillance is a critical cornerstone of any occupational medicine program. Successful programs combine state of the art science *with* high levels of managerial control. As OSHA moves toward a generic surveillance examination, the need for well-designed and managed programs will increase.

REFERENCES

1. Ashford NA. Policy considerations for human monitoring in the workplace. J Occup Med 1986;28:563–568.
2. Yodaiken RE. Surveillance, monitoring and regulatory concerns. J Occup Med 1986;28:570.
3. Ducatman AM. Medical surveillance programs (Postgraduate Seminar). Boston, Massachusetts: American Occupational Medicine Conference, May 1989.
4. Rempel D (Ed). Medical surveillance in the workplace. State of the Art Reviews—Occupational Medicine. Philadelphia: Hanley & Belfus, 1990;5(3).
5. Gochfield M, Favata EA (Eds). Hazardous waste workers. State of the Art Reviews—Occupational Medicine 5(1) Philadelphia: Hanley & Belfus, 1990;5(1).
6. Shortell R. Health program evaluation. St. Louis, MO: Mosby, 1978.
7. Code of Federal Regulations: 29 CFR 1910.120. Washington, DC: USGPO, 1988.
8. Code of Federal Regulations: 29 CFR 1910.120. Washington, DC: USGPO, 1988:82–89.
9. U.S. Environmental Protection Agency. Risk assessment guidance for superfund. Human health evaluation manual. Washington, DC: Environmental Protection Agency, December 1989.
10. American Conference of Governmental Industrial Hygienists: Threshold limit values and biological exposure indices, Cincinnati, OH: ACGIH, 1989.
11. Fed Reg. March 6, 1989:54(42):9386–9403.
12. Code of Federal Regulations; CFR 1910.134, Washington, DC: USGPO, 1988:360.
13. American Industrial Hygiene Association. Proposed criteria for the selection of appropriate medical resources to perform medical surveillance for employees engaged in hazardous waste operations, J Am Ind Hyg Assoc 1989;(Dec):A-820–872.
14. George RB, et al. American Thoracic Society Respiratory Care Committee—Position papers. ATS News 1978;4:6.
15. Gardner RM. Standardization of spirometry; a summary of recommendations from the american thoracic society, the 1987 update. Ann Intern Med 1988;108:217–220.
16. Horvath EP, Jr. Manual of spirometry in occupational medicine. National Institute for Occupational Safety and Health, Division of Training and Manpower Development, 1981.
17. Thomas V, F-B, Pierce J Thomas. Biological Monitoring V: Dermal Absorption, Appl Ind Hyg 1989;4(8):F-14–F-21.
18. Dossing M, Baesum J, Hansen S, et al. Effect of ethanol, cimetidene, and propanol on toluene metabolism in man. Arch Occup Environ Health 1984;54:309–315.
19. Favata EA, Gochfield M. Medical surveillance of hazardous waste workers; ability of laboratory tests to discriminate exposure. Am J Ind Med 1989;15:255–265.
20. Wallen M, Naslund PH, Nordquist MB. The effects of ethanol on the kinetics of toluene in man. Toxicol Appl Pharmacol 1984;76:414–419.

Appendix A

SUMMARY PROFILE

Employee Name: _____ Date of Exam: _____

Company: _____

Position: _____

The Examining Physician and/or Medical Consultant has reviewed the medical information regarding the afore-mentioned employee, and the following status has been established:

A (   ) There is no medical abnormality which will interfere with the duties of the individual.

B (   ) Medical condition exists which will not interfere with job responsibilities. The individual has been advised of this finding.

C (   ) The examination disclosed a medical abnormality which may require special consideration by the company.

_____

_____

_____

D (   ) Deferred pending further evaluation.

_____

_____

_____

E (   ) Clearance for respirator use, if applicable.
On the basis of the information obtained from the medical examination, the above named individual has been found medically:

(   ) qualified to use a respirator

(   ) not qualified to use a respirator

_____
Signature of Reviewing Physician

Appendix B

PHYSICIAN'S STATEMENT

Employer:

Employee:

Date of Exam:_____

Date of Birth: _____ Social Security Number: _____

1. On the basis of the information obtained from the medical examination of the above-named individual, this individual has been found medically:

    ( ) qualified for hazardous waste site work
    ( ) not qualified for hazardous waste site work*

2. On the basis of the information obtained from the medical examination of the above-named individual, as per OSHA (29 CRF 1910.134 (b) (10), this individual has been found medically:

    ( ) qualified to use a respirator
    ( ) not qualified to use a respirator*

Physician's Signature: _____

Printed Name of
Physician: _____

Physician's Address: _____

Physician's Phone No.: _____

Physician's State License No.: _____

OSHA 1910.134 (b) (10) states that persons should not be assigned to tasks requiring use of respirators unless it has been determined that they are physically able to perform the work and use the equipment. The local physician shall determine what health and physical conditions are pertinent. The respirator user's medical status should be reviewed periodically (for instance, annually).

*If it is the opinion of the examining physician that an examinee is unqualified to perform hazardous waste site work or to wear a respirator, the physician should append a further report to this statement which details reasons for the opinion.

DISCLOSURE AGREEMENT

I agree to allow my medical records to be given to and maintained by _____.
I agree to allow a copy of my medical record to be given to all physicians performing medical examinations on me as part of the medical surveillance program.

I acknowledge that my medical record will be used: to determine my suitability for work assignment, to determine my ability to wear respiratory protection, to fulfill the requirements of _____, and to comply with applicable local, state, or federal requirements.

I understand that I can obtain a copy of my medical records from the clinic and/or authorize a representative to receive these records.

I understand that if I have any questions regarding the medical surveillance program I can address these questions, to _____.

_____   _____
Print Name   Signature

_____ _____   _____
Date   Date of Birth   Social Security Number

_____   _____
Witness Name (Print)   Witness Signature

Appendix D

JOB RISKS/JOB REQUIREMENTS

Job Risks

1. Exposure to chemical vapors and/or dust
2. Exposure to carcinogen or teratogens (specify if known)
3. Skin contact with solvents or other chemicals (specify)
4. Exposure to humidity, temperature, and altitude changes (i.e., chamber clearance)
5. Exposure to ionizing radiation (i.e., x-ray exposure)
6. Exposure to laser equipment
7. Exposure to excessive noise
8. Work around hazardous machinery
9. Exposure to high voltage
10. Exposure to adhesives or bonding agents
11. None of the above applies
12. Other: _____

Job Requirements

1. Prolonged standing (More than 50%)
2. Excessive walking (More than 50%)
3. Kneeling or squatting repeatedly
4. Heavy pushing or pulling
5. Bending or stooping repeatedly
6. Working with arms above shoulder level
7. Lifting more than 25 pounds: Occasionally: _____
   Repeatedly: _____
8. Lifting more than 40 pounds: Occasionally: _____
   Repeatedly: _____
9. Having full use of both hands
10. Repetitive motion of hands and/or wrists
11. Prolonged Neck Flexion (i.e., microscope work)
12. Seeing with both eyes
13. Fine close work (i.e., small print and microscopic work)
14. Regular use of visual display units
    (days/week _____ hours/day _____)
15. Majority of job requires terminal work
    (days/week _____ hours/day _____)
16. Distinguish colors
17. Safety glass area
18. Operate power equipment and tools
19. Drive motor vehicle, specify: _____
20. Work on elevated levels (ladders, etc.)
21. Work alone (in isolated areas or at night)
22. Irregular work hours (evenings and nights)
23. Good voice discrimination (i.e., telephone work)
24. Excessive deadline responsibility
25. Requires respirator clearance
26. Cafeteria/food vending
27. None of the above applies
28. Other: _____

MEDICAL AND OCCUPATIONAL
HISTORY FORM
FOR BASELINE EXAMS

C-O-N-F-I-D-E-N-T-I-A-L
FOR MEDICAL USE ONLY

PART I: IDENTIFICATION

Name: _____ Date: _____
     (Last)   (First)   (M.I.)

Social Security Number: ____-___-____ Date of Birth: _____

Home Address: _____ Sex: M _____ F _____

_____

_____

        Ethnic Origin: Caucasian   Black   Hispanic   Other (Specify) _____

Marital Status: Married   Single   Separated   Divorced   Widowed

Home Telephone No.: (___) ___-_____

Emergency Contact: _____ Phone (___) ___-_____

Personal
Physician _____ Phone: (___) ___-_____

Job Title: _____ Date of Hire: _____

Name of person you report to for Hazardous Waste Operations:

_____

Regular Workplace Location: _____

Description of Responsibilities: _____

_____

_____

PART II: OCCUPATIONAL EXPOSURE HISTORY

A. Occupational Exposure Inventory

1. Please describe any health problems or injuries you have experienced in connection with any previous employment. _____

_____

Appendix E—*continued*

Name: _____ Social Security Number: _____

2. Have any of your coworkers also experienced health problems or injuries connected with the same jobs? If yes, please describe.

    _____

    _____

3. In general do you smoke ____ eat ____ on the job?

4. In your work, have you ever used a substance which caused you to break out in a rash? _____

    _____

    _____

5. Have you ever been off work for more than a day because of an illness or injury related to work? If yes, please describe.

    _____

    _____

6. Have you ever worked at a job which caused you to have breathing trouble such as coughing, shortness of breath, or wheezing? If yes, please describe. _____

    _____

7. Have you ever served in the military?   Yes ( )   No ( )
    If yes, amount of time spent in service ____ years.

8. Were you exposed to any toxic agents while in the military?   Yes ( )
    No ( )   If yes, please describe the substance and when you were exposed.

    _____

    _____

    _____

    _____

Appendix E—*continued*

Name: _____ Social Security Number: _____

B. OCCUPATIONAL PROFILE

Fill in the table below listing all jobs at which you have worked, including shortterm, seasonal, and part-time employment. Start with your present job and go back in chronologic order.

Workplace (Employer's Name and Address)	Dates Worked To	From	Full-Time or Part-Time	Type of Industry (Welding, Mining, Hazardous Waste, etc.)	Protective Equipment Used	Duration of Time Spent on Hazardous Site	Types of Material to Which You Were Potentially Exposed

C. Hazard Exposure List

Have you ever worked at a job or hobby in which you may have been exposed to any of the following substances or circumstances by breathing, touching, or ingestion? If you have, and know the specific substances, please circle the substance. If you only know the group and are unsure of the specific substance, check the box beside the group name.

A. Aerosols, vapors, gases _____
   Acetylene
   Carbon monoxide
   Ethylene oxide
   Formaldehyde
   Hydrogen cyanide
   Hydrogen sulfide
   Nitrogen dioxide
   Phosgene
   Sewer gas
   Smoke
   Sulfur dioxide
   Welding fumes

B. Biologic inhalants _____
   Bacteria
   Fungi
   Moles
   Spores

C. Corrosive substances _____
   Acids (hydrochloric, hydrofluoric, etc.)
   Alcohols, ammonias
   Alkalis
   Chlorine
   Phenol

Appendix E—*continued*

Name: _____   Social Security Number: _____

D. Inorganic dust and powders ____
   Asbestos
   Coal dust
   Fiberglass
   Fluoride
   Silica
   Talc

E. Insecticides, herbicides, pesticides ____
   Carbamates (Temik, Carbaryl, Aldicarb)
   Chlorophenoxy herbicides (Dioxin)
   Ethylene dibromide
   Ethylene dichloride
   Organochlorines (DDT, Aldrin, Endrin,
      Dieldrin, Chlordane, Lindane)
   Organophosphates (Parathion, Malathion,
      Diazinon)
   Pentachlorophenol (PCP)

F. Metals, metal fumes ____
   Aluminum
   Arsenic or arsine
   Beryllium
   Cadmium
   Chromium
   Cobalt
   Copper
   Iron
   Lead
   Manganese
   Mercury
   Silver
   Strontium
   Tin
   Uranium
   Vanadium

G. Petrochemicals ____
   Asphalt and tar
   Coal tar
   Naphthalene
   PAHs (polyaromatic hydrocarbons)
   PBB (polybrominated biphenyls)
   PCB (polychlorinated biphenyls)
   Petroleum distillates

H. Physical agents ____
   Heavy lifting
   Noise
   Heat stress
   Cold stress (hypothermia)
   Vibration

I. Plastics ____
   Vinyl chloride
   Fluorocarbons
   Epoxy resins
   Acrylonitrile
   Styrene

J. Radiation ____
   Radioactive materials
   Microwaves
   Ultraviolet rays
   X-rays
   Uranium

K. Solvents ____
   Benzene
   Carbon disulfide
   Carbon tetrachloride
   Chloroform
   Glycol ethers (Cellusolves)
   Ketones

L. Sensitizing agents ____
   Isocyanates, diisocyanates
   Nickel, platinum
   Proteolytic (detergent) enzymes
   Aliphatic amines
   Poison ivy, poison oak, poison sumac
   Insect stings

M. Miscellaneous ____
   Hydrazines
   Nonspecific dust exposure
   Picric acid
   Trinitrotoluene (TNT)
   Unexploded ordinances

Appendix E—*continued*

Name: _____ Social Security Number: _____

PART III: RESIDENTIAL INFORMATION

1. Do you use pesticides around your home or garden? ( ) Yes ( ) No

2. Have you ever changed your residence or home because of health problems? If yes, please describe.

3. Have you ever or are you currently living very near an industrial plant? If yes, please describe type of industry.

4. Does your spouse or any other household members have contact with dusts or chemicals at work or during leisure activities? ( ) Yes ( ) No

5. Do other members of your household use tobacco products? ( ) Yes ( ) No

PART IV: MEDICAL HISTORY

Do you have now or have you ever had any of the following illnesses or conditions?

____ Abnormal bleeding
____ Allergies, asthma, hayfever
____ Anemia
____ Arthritis, rheumatic fever
____ Chronic bronchitis, emphysema
____ Cancer, specify site _____
____ Cirrhosis of the liver
____ Coronary heart disease
____ Diabetes
____ Epilepsy
____ Fractured bones
____ Gall bladder
____ Glaucoma/cataracts
____ Gout
____ Hepatitis
____ Hernia/rupture
____ Hives or rashes

____ Hypertension (high blood pressure)
____ Jaundice
____ Kidney or bladder disease
____ Leukemia
____ Malaria
____ Migraine
____ Nervous or mental disorder
____ Piles or hemorrhoids
____ Phlebitis
____ Polio
____ Sinusitis
____ Skin disease (specify diagnosis) _____
____ Stomach disorders/ulcers
____ Stroke
____ Thyroid disease
____ Tuberculosis
____ Ulcer
____ Venereal disease
____ Other, specify _____

Medication: Are you now taking or have taken any of the following drugs?

( ) antibiotics ( ) antidepressants ( ) aspirin/Tylenol
( ) blood thinners ( ) birth control pills
( ) blood pressure medication ( ) cortisone/steroids
( ) insulin/diabetic medicine ( ) penicillin
( ) diuretic/water pills ( ) heart medication
( ) tranquilizers ( ) vitamins/minerals
( ) other prescription drugs ( ) other nonprescription drugs

List drugs taken regularly: _____

Known allergies: ( ) Medications (please specify _____)
( ) Pollens ( ) House dust ( ) Molds/spores
( ) Animal danders, feathers, or fur ( ) Sunlight or cold
( ) Foods ( ) Metal, jewelry ( ) Vaccines Other _____

Appendix E—*continued*

Name: _____ Social Security Number: _____

Hospitalization:

	Year	Operation or Illness	Name of Hospital
1st hospitalization			
2nd hospitalization			
3rd hospitalization			

Family History:

Indicate any blood relatives who had any of the following:

Disease	Mother	Father	Grandparent	Brother or Sister	Child
Anemia					
Arthritis					
Allergy (asthma, eczema, hayfever)					
Alcoholism					
Cancer					
Congenital malfunctions					
Diabetes					
Emphysema					
Epilepsy					
Glaucoma					
Gout					
Heart attack					
High blood pressure					
Kidney disease					
Gallbladder disease					
Mental or nervous disorder					
Stomach ulcers					
Stroke					
Thyroid disease					
Tuberculosis					

Appendix E—*continued*

Name: _____ Social Security Number: _____

	If Living Age	Age at Death	If Deceased Cause of Death
___ Mother			
___ Father			
___ Brother ___ Sister			
___ Brother ___ Sister			
___ Wife ___ Husband			
___ Son ___ Daughter			
___ Son ___ Daughter			

Vaccines, Immunizations and Tests:

Check vaccines/tests you have had. Enter the year you last were given the test or "shots." For tests, indicate if results were normal or abnormal.

Vaccines/Shots	Tests	Normal	Abnormal
( ) 19___ Tetanus	( ) 19___ GI Series	_____	_____
( ) 19___ Polio	( ) 19___ Electrocardiogram	_____	_____
( ) 19___ Influenza	( ) 19___ Colon X-ray	_____	_____
( ) 19___ Rubella	( ) 19___ Tuberculosis	_____	_____
( ) 19___ Measles	( ) 19___ Chest X-ray	_____	_____

Do you have a history of:

	Yes	No		Yes	No
Skin			**Pulmonary**		
Persistent skin trouble	___	___	Shortness of breath	___	___
New skin growths	___	___	Wheezing	___	___
Change in size or color of growth	___	___	Chronic cough	___	___
Growths that bleed	___	___	Blood streaked sputum	___	___
Growths that change in size	___	___	Chest pain	___	___
Athlete's foot	___	___	Pneumonia	___	___
			Pleurisy	___	___
Eyes			**Cardiovascular**		
Wear glasses	___	___	Chest pain	___	___
Eye inflammation	___	___	Chest pain with effort	___	___
Eye pain	___	___	Chest pain following food	___	___
Color blindness	___	___	Chest pain while walking or exercising	___	___
Difficulty with vision	___	___	Rapid heartbeat	___	___
(not corrected by glasses)			Skipped beats	___	___
			Fainting	___	___
Ears, nose, throat			Swelling of ankles	___	___
Hearing loss	___	___	Difficulty breathing while lying down	___	___
Deafness	___	___	Sleep on more than one pillow	___	___
Ringing in ears	___	___	Calf or leg pain with exertion	___	___
Ear infections	___	___	Varicose veins	___	___
Discharge from your ears	___	___	Elevated cholesterol	___	___
Perforated ear drums	___	___	Elevated triglycerides	___	___
Postnasal drip	___	___			
Nose bleeds	___	___			
Phlegm in throat	___	___			
Frequent colds or sore throats	___	___			
Hoarseness	___	___			
Difficulty swallowing	___	___			
Thyroid disorder	___	___			

Appendix E—*continued*

Name: _____ Social Security Number: _____

	Yes	No		Yes	No
Gastrointestinal			**Nervous system**		
Nausea	___	___	Recurrent headaches	___	___
Vomiting	___	___	Fainting	___	___
Indigestion	___	___	Dizziness	___	___
Heartburn	___	___	Loss of balance	___	___
Stomach pain	___	___	Visual disturbances	___	___
Recurring diarrhea	___	___	Speech difficulties	___	___
Frequent constipation	___	___	Seizures	___	___
Recent change in bowel habits	___	___	Muscle weakness	___	___
Blood in bowel movements	___	___	Muscle paralysis	___	___
Black bowel movements	___	___	Memory loss	___	___
Polyps	___	___	Blurred or double vision	___	___
Blood transfusion	___	___	Difficulty concentrating	___	___
Hemorrhoids	___	___			
Poor appetite	___	___			
Difficulty swallowing	___	___			

Do you have a history of:

	Yes	No		Yes	No
Orthopedic			**Urinary**		
Swollen joints	___	___	Blood in urine	___	___
Bursitis	___	___	Pus in urine	___	___
Tendonitis	___	___	Sugar in urine	___	___
Low back pain	___	___	Sense of bladder not empty after		
Neck pain	___	___	urination	___	___
"Slipped disc"	___	___	Burning or pain when urinating	___	___
Joint stiffness	___	___	Kidney infection	___	___
Calcium deposits	___	___	Bladder infection	___	___
Persistent numbness	___	___	Pass stone or gravel in urine	___	___
Tingling or weakness	___	___	Get up every night to urinate	___	___

For Women Only:	Yes	No
What was the date of your last menstrual period?	___/___/___	
Have you reached menopause or have you had a hysterectomy?	___	___
Do you menstruate regularly?	___	___
Do you have heavy bleeding or cramps with your periods?	___	___
Have you had bleeding between your periods?	___	___
Are you usually tense or jumpy prior to menstruation?	___	___
Do you examine your breast at least once a month?	___	___
Have you ever noticed any lumps or pain in your breast?	___	___
Have you had complications with any type of birth control?	___	___
Number of pregnancies?	___	___
Number of children born alive?	___	___
Number of premature births?	___	___
Number of miscarriages?	___	___

For Men Only:	Yes	No
Has a doctor ever told you that you have prostate trouble?	___	___
Have you had any burning or discharge from your penis?	___	___
Are there any swellings or lumps on your testicles?	___	___
Do your testicles get painful?	___	___

Appendix E—*continued*

Name: _____ Social Security Number: _____

PART V: PERSONAL HABITS

1. Over the past 6 months have you gained or lost more than 10 pounds? ( ) Yes ( ) No

2. If yes to Question 1, reason for weight change: _____

   _____

3. Have you ever smoked? Yes ( ) No ( ) If no, go on to Question 7.

4. Do you smoke now? Yes ( ) No ( ) If no, how long ago did you quit? _____

5. If yes, how long have you smoked? _____

6. Fill in the appropriate columns if you ever smoked.

	At Present	When You Stopped
Cigarettes (No./day)	_____	_____
Pipe (Pipefuls/day)	_____	_____
Cigars (No./day)	_____	_____

7. How many alcoholic drinks do you drink per day? _____

8. How many cups of coffee and/or tea do you drink per day?
   _____ cups coffee   _____ tea
   _____ cups decaffeinated coffee _____ decaffeinated tea

9. Do you have a regular exercise schedule? ( ) Yes ( ) No

10. If yes, your exercise is:
    ( ) strenuous (run, swim, aerobics) ( ) moderate (golf, bowling)
    ( ) mild (walking some distance)

11. Do you have difficulty falling or staying asleep? _____

12. Amount of hours you usually sleep? _____

13. Do you seem to feel exhausted or fatigued most of the time? ( ) Yes ( ) No

14. Do you have a craft or hobby which you do at home? _____

15. If so, please describe, particularly those involving use of chemicals or noise. _____

    _____

16. Check the words that best describe, in your opinion, the pressure or stress in the following areas of your life:

	None	Low	Medium	High
Job	_____	_____	_____	_____
Home	_____	_____	_____	_____
Finances	_____	_____	_____	_____
Social	_____	_____	_____	_____

Appendix F

PROTOCOL FOR TESTING

Test	Baseline	Annual	Exit	Remarks
		Testing Frequency		
Height and weight	X	X	X	
Blood pressure	X	X	X	
Pulse (resting)	X	X	X	
Temperature (oral) Fahrenheit	X	X	X	
Stool for occult blood	X	X	X	
Vision acuity (R&L)		X	X	
Vision titmus (R&L)	X			
Near-corrected and uncorrected				
Far-corrected and uncorrected				
Peripheral (visual field)				
Color				
Audiogram	X	X	X	
Pulmonary function test	X	X	X	
Chest X-ray	X	*See Remarks	*Note	Every 3 years for less than or equal to 40 years old. Every 2 years for more than or equal to 40 years old to less than or equal to 50 years old. Every year for more than 50 years old. *Note: For exit exams chest x-ray performed only if not performed in past year.
Cardiogram	X	*See Remarks	*Note	Every 3 years for less than or equal to 40 years old. Every year for more than 40 years old. *Note: For Exit exam, ECG performed only if not performed in past year.
Urinalysis (microscopic)	X	X	X	
Appearance				
Color				
pH				
Specific gravity				
Protein				
Acetone				
Glucose				
Occult blood				
WBC esterase				
WBC/HPF				
RBC/HPF				
Mucus				
Bacteria				
Epithelial cells				
Blood chemistry panel	X	X	X	
Calcium — Cholesterol				
Phosphorus — Triglycerides				
Sodium — T. Protein				
Potassium — Globulin				
Chloride — Albumin				
LDH — A/G ratio				
AST (SGOT) — BUN				
T. Bili — Creatinine				
GGT — Uric Acid				
ALT (SGPT) — Glucose				
Alk. Phos. — Iron				
HDL — T_4				
CBC count with differential	X	X	X	

Appendix G

MINIMAL SPIROMETRY STANDARDS SUMMARY

Test	Range/ Accuracy (BTPS liter)	Flow Range (liter/sec)	Time (sec)	Start Point	Resistance and Back Pressure	Test Signals
VC	7 liter/ ± 3% of reading or 50 ml, whichever is greater	0–12	30			Calibrated Syringe
FVC	7 liter/ ± 3% of reading or 50 ml, whichever is greater	0–12	10.0			(1) FVC = 5 liter T = 0.4 sec (2) FVC = liter T = 2.4
FEV$_t$	7 liter/ ± 3% of reading	0–12	t	Back extra polate or equivalent	Less than 1.5 cm H$_2$O liter/sec at 12.0 liter/sec flow	Same as FVC
FEV$_1$			1.0			
FEF 25–75%	7 liter/ ± 5% of reading or 0.1 liter/sec, whichever is greater	0–12	10.0	—	Same as FEV$_1$	Same as FVC
V	12 liter/sec ± 5% of reading or 0.2 liter/ sec, whichever is greater	0–12	10.0	—	Same as FEV$_t$	Manufacturer proof
MVV	Sine wave 250 liter/min 2 liter to ± 5% of reading	0–12 ±5%	12–15 ±3%	—	Pressure less than ± 10 cm H$_2$O at 2 liter TV 2.0 Hz	Sine wave pump 0–4 Hz ± 10% @ ± 12 liter/sec

Appendix H

ADOPTED BIOLOGIC EXPOSURE INDICES (10)

Airborne chemical [CAS #]

Indices	Timing	BEI	Notation
Benzene [71-43-2]			
Total phenol in urine	End of shift	50 mg/l	B, Ns
Benzene in exhaled air:	Prior to next shift		
mixed-exhaled		0.08 ppm	Cf
end-exhaled		0.12 ppm	Cf
Carbon monoxide [630-08-0]			Sc
Carboxyhemoglobin in blood	End of shift	Less than 8%	B, Ns
CO in end-exhaled air	End of shift	Less than 40 ppm	B, Ns
Ethyl benzene [100-41-4]			
Mandelic acid in urine	End of shift and end of workweek	2 g/l 1.5 g/g creat.	Ns
Ethyl benzene in end-exhaled air	Prior to next shift	2 ppm	Cf
n-Hexane [110-54-3]			
2,5-Hexanedione in urine	End of shift	5 mg/l	Ns
n-Hexane in end-exhaled air	During shift	40 ppm	Cf
Lead [7439-92-1]			Sc
Lead in blood	Not critical	50 μg/100 ml	B
Lead in urine	Not critical	150 μg/g creat.	B
Zinc protoporphyrin in blood	After 1 month exposure	250 μg/100 ml erythrocytes or 100 μg/100 ml blood	B
Phenol [108-95-2]			
Total phenol in urine	End of shift	250 mg/g creat. or 15 mg/hr	B, Ns
Styrene [100-42-5]			
Mandelic acid in urine	End of shift	1 g/l 0.8 g/g creat.	Ns Ns
Styrene in mixed-exhaled air	Prior to next shift	40 ppb	Cf
Phenylglyoxylic acid in urine	End of shift	250 mg/l 240 mg/g creat.	B, Ns
Styrene in mixed-exhaled air	During shift	18 ppm	Cf
Styrene in blood	End of shift	0.55 mg/l	Cf
	Prior to next shift	0.02 mg/l	Cf
Toluene [108-88-3]			
Hippuric acid in urine	End of shift	2.5 g/g creat.	B, Ns
	Last 4 hours of shift	3 mg/min	
Toluene in venous blood	End of shift	1 mg/l	Cf
Toluene in end-exhaled air	During shift	20 ppm	Cf
Trichloroethylene [79-01-6]			
Trichloroacetic acid in urine	End of workweek	100 mg/l	Ns
Trichloroacetic and trichloroethanol in urine	End of workweek and end of shift	300 mg/l 320 mg/g creat.	Ns
Free trichloroethanol in blood	End of shift and end of workweek	4 mg/l	Ns
Trichloroethylene in end-exhaled air	Prior to shift and end of workweek	0.5 ppm	Cf
Xylenes [1330-20-7]			
Methylhippuric acids in urine	End of shift	1.5 g/g creat.	
	Last 4 hrs of shift	2 mg/min	

Reprinted with permission, American Conference of Governmental Industrial Hygienists.

Appendix H—*continued*

NOTICE OF INTENT TO ESTABLISH

Airborne Chemical [CAS #]

Indices	Timing	BEI	Notation
Aniline [62-53-3]			
Total p-aminophenol in urine	End of shift	50 mg/l	Ns
Cadmium [7440-43-9]			
Cadmium in urine	Not critical	10 μg/g creat.	B
Cadmium in blood	Not critical	10 μg/l	B
Carbon disulfide [75-15-0]			
2-Thiothiazolidine-4-carboxylic acid			
(=TTCA) in urine	End of shift	5 mg/g creat.	
Dimethylformamide [68-12-2]			
N-Methylformamide in urine	End of shift	40 mg/g creat.	
Methyl Chloroform [71-55-6]			
Methyl chloroform in end-exhaled air	Prior to shift and end of work week	40 ppm	
Trichloroacetic acid in urine	End of workweek	10 mg/l	Ns, Cf
Total trichloroethanol in urine	End of shift and end of workweek	30 mg/l	Ns, Cf
Total trichloroethanol in blood	End of shift and end of workweek	1 mg/l	Ns
Methyl ethyl ketone (MEK) [78-93-3]			
MEK in urine	End of shift	2 mg/l	
Organophosphorus cholinesterase inhibitors			
Cholinesterase activity in red cells	Discretionary	70% of individual's baseline	B, Ns, Cf
Parathion [56-38-2]			
Total p-nitrophenol in urine	End of shift	0.5 mg/l	Ns, Cf
Cholinesterase activity in red cells	Discretionary	70% of individual's baseline	B, Ns, Cf
Pentachlorophenol (PCP) [87-86-5]			
Total PCP in urine	Prior to the last shift of workweek	2 mg/l	B
Free PCP in plasma	End of shift	5 mg/l	B
Perchloroethylene [127-18-4]			
Perchloroethylene in end-exhaled air	Prior to shift and end of workweek	10 ppm	
Perchloroethylene in blood	Prior to shift and end of workweek	1 mg/l	
Trichloroacetic acid in urine	End of workweek	7 mg/l	Ns, Cf

OCCUPATIONAL MEDICINE

Name: _____

Employer: _____

Please go to the following areas in the order designated in the left column.

_____	I. CVP Laboratory:	_____ Spirometry		
		_____ Bronchodilator		
		_____ EKG		
_____	II. Laboratory:	_____ CBC	_____ Urinalysis	_____ SMA$_{24}$
		_____ GGPT		
		_____ RBC chlorinesterase		
		_____ Other		
_____	III. Radiology:	_____ PA Chest		
		_____ PA and Lateral Chest		
_____	IV. Nursing:	_____ Visual screening		
		_____ Otoscopic exam		
		_____ Height		
		_____ Weight		
		_____ BP		
_____	V. Audiology:	_____ Audiometric screening		
_____	VI. Physician's exam			

10

Hepatotoxicity from Hazardous Chemicals

Samir M. Douidar, M.D., Ph.D.
Caryl S. Shaver, M.D.
Wayne R. Snodgrass, M.D., Ph.D.

INTRODUCTION

The liver, as the main organ responsible for the metabolism of xenobiotics, is particularly susceptible to injury from drugs and environmental toxins (1). A wide variety of substances which induce liver toxicity are recognized. These include natural hepatotoxins such as products of plants (fungal or bacterial metabolites) and minerals (2), products of chemical or pharmaceutical industry (3), or industrial byproducts and waste materials that, by polluting the environment, may gain access to humans (4, 5) (Table 10.1). Chemical-induced hepatic injury includes several forms but, in general, can be either cytotoxic or cholestatic. Cytotoxic injury which involves liver parenchyma producing necrosis, fatty change, cirrhosis, and carcinoma is a common manifestation of chemical-induced hepatic injury. Cholestatic injury can result in interference with bile secretion and in jaundice. Often liver injury is a mixture of both (6, 7). Drug- and chemical-induced liver disease may be so clinically subtle that estimates of incidence will be influenced by the method used to identify cases. Laboratory screening of all persons at risk will most certainly detect liver injury more often than will reliance on clinical symptoms or signs. However, this approach may be overly sensitive, and positive results may or may not be indicative of significant ''hepatotoxicity.'' On the other hand, routine tests may not be sensitive enough to detect other drug-induced liver disease (e.g., chronic methotrexate therapy) or toxic exposure-related liver disease (e.g., angiosarcoma due to vinyl chloride). Also, in some cases, these toxicities may appear gradually after several months or years of exposure, making detection difficult.

Medical screening and surveillance for hepatotoxicity due to environmental and occupational chemical exposure has become important for documenting workers' health and safety. Hepatic injury can be acute, subacute, or chronic. Fortunately, due to improved industrial hygiene monitoring of the most serious hepatotoxins, acute hepatotoxicity is rare. It is now more likely that hepatotoxicity will manifest as subacute and chronic hepatic injury. However, current laboratory methods of detecting hepatic damage remain best at detecting acute hepatotoxicity. Subacute or chronic hepatic disease is much more difficult to screen for because the methods used may not detect the damage done or may be overly sensitive, leading to unnecessary detection of false positive results (8) or, more importantly, may miss true subacute or chronic disease (high false negatives). Screening and surveillance programs must be structured with this in mind.

ANATOMY AND PHYSIOLOGY

Due to its anatomy and physiology, the liver is uniquely sensitive to xenobiotic damage.

First, the liver receives blood from two sources. The portal system brings venous blood from the gut. The liver also receives arterial blood from the hepatic artery. In addition, lymphatics from the gut travel to the liver. Toxins which are ingested, inhaled and then swallowed, or produced by gut bacteria enter the liver through portal blood. Inhaled gases and dermally absorbed toxicants enter the liver via the hepatic artery. The liver receives approximately 25% of the cardiac output. 25% of the total hepatic blood flow is arterial from the hepatic artery, and 75% is venous from the portal veins (and thus deoxygenated).

The hepatic artery and portal vein branch together with the lymphatics and sympathetic nerves to form the portal triad. The bile collecting system forms the last constituent of the portal triad. The blood travels from the portal triad through the hepatic sinusoids and is collected in the terminal hepatic vein. The endothelium has wide fenestrations in the sinusoids, and the hepatocytes have microvilli which increase surface area to absorb materials from the plasma. After percolating through the sinusoids, blood is collected into the terminal hepatic vein where it rejoins the systemic circulation (9).

The functional unit of the liver is the acinus. The area around the portal triad is called zone I, or periportal. The area surrounding the portal vein is termed zone III, or peripheral or centrilobular. Zone II is intermediate between zones I and III (10). Older descriptions of hepatic microanatomy were based on nonfunctional histologic patterns, while the zonal description of the acinus is based on the physiologic microstructure as described by Rappaport (Fig. 10.1).

The blood in zone I contains the highest concentration of oxygen, nutrients, hormones, and unmetabolized xenobiotics. Zone I cells have a higher concentration of glycogen synthesis enzymes as well as a high concentration of mitochondria involved in the Krebs cycle. More protein synthesis also occurs in zone 1 (10).

Zone III cells receive blood with a lower oxygen tension and are less active in glycogen and protein synthesis. However, the glucose/glycogen systems can vary in concentrations between zone I and zone III depending on nutritional status and other factors (11). Zone III is more active in glycogen storage and fat formation (10). Most important to toxicology is the high concentration of enzyme systems for biotransformation in zone III. Most notable is the cytochrome P450 system, also called the mixed function oxidase system (MFO) (12). Associated enzymes such as NADPH cytochrome c-reductase are also highest in zone III. MFO and NADPH cytochrome c-reductase are formed in and located on the endoplasmic reticulum (10). Agents which induce cytochrome P450 function also increase the smooth endoplasmic reticulum in zone III cells (13).

HEPATIC CELL METABOLISM OF XENOBIOTICS

Many organic xenobiotic agents are lipid soluble. In order to be excreted in the urine they must be made more polar or water soluble. A molecule can be made more polar by oxidation or

109

Table 10.1. Chemical Classes of Hepatotoxic Agents (Modified with permission from Zimmerman HJ. The adverse effects of drugs and other chemicals on the liver. New York, Appleton-Century-Crofts 1978:4.)

A. Inorganic agents:

Metals and metalloids: antimony, arsenic, beryllium, bismuth, boron, cadmium, chromium, cobalt, copper, iron, lead, manganese, mercury, gold, phosphorus, selenium, tellurium, thallium, zinc

Hydrazine derivatives

Iodides

B. Organic agents:

Natural

Plant toxins: albitocin, cycasin, icterogenin, indospicine, lantana, ngaione, nutmeg, pyrolidizine, safrole, tannic acid

Mycotoxins: aflatoxins, cyclochlorotine, ethanol, luteoskyrins, ochratoxins, rubratoxins, sterigmatocystins, and other antibiotics

Bacterial toxins: exotoxins (*C. diphtheria, Cl. botulinus, Str. hemolyticus*), endotoxins, ethionine

Synthetic

Nonmedicinal:
Haloalkanes and halolefins
Nitroalkanes
Organic amines
Azo compounds
Phenol and derivatives
Various other organic compounds

Medicinal agents:

Antibiotics: chloramphenicol, erythromycin estolate, erythromycin ethyl succinate, penicillins, cephalosporines, novobiocin, rifampicin, tetracyclines, sulfonamides, nitrofurans, clindamycin, spectinomycin, sulfones, and quinolones

Antifungal agents: amphotericin, 5-fluorocytosine, griseofulvin, ketoconazole, and saramycetin

Antimetazoal and antiprotozoal agents: emetine, amodiaquine, carbarsone, 8-hydroxyquinolines, metronidazole, thiabendazole, niclofan, hycanthone, and mepacrine

Antituberculous agents: cycloserine, isoniazid, rifampicin, p-aminosalicylic acid, and ethionamide

Antiviral agents: cytarabine, idoxuridine, vidarabine, and xenelamine

Endocrine agents: antithyroid drugs, oral hypoglycemics and steroids (e.g., oral contraceptives, anabolic C-17, glucocorticoids, and tamoxifen)

Anesthetic agents: halothane, methoxyflurane, ether, chloroform, nitrous oxide, and cyclopropane

Psychotropic agents: phenothiazines, thioxanthenes, butyrophenones, benzodizapenes, monoamine oxidase inhibitors, and tricyclic antidepressants

Anticonvulsants: phenytoin, phenobarbital, valproic acid, mephenytoin, and methadiones

Analgesics and nonsteroidal antiinflammatory drugs: acetaminophen, salicylates, indomethacin, diflunisal, ibuprofen, sulindac, phenylbutazone, naproxen, and fenoprofen

Cardiovascular agents: anticoagulants, antiarrhythmics (e.g., quinidine, procainamide, verapamil and nifedepine), antihypertensives (e.g., hydralazine, methyldopa and captopril), diuretic agents, antianginal, and antihyperlipidemic agents

Antineoplastic agents

Miscellaneous drugs: colchicine, allopurinol, cimetidine, disulfiram, vitamin A, iodide ion, thorotorast, ranitidine, BAL, penicillamine, dantrolene, zoxazolamine and others

hydrolysis. It can be made more polar by attaching another molecule which can facilitate excretion into the bile or kidney. The liver adds both types of groups to accomplish this excretion.

These reactions are divided into two sequential sets of reactions termed phase I and phase II. Phase I reactions make a compound more polar by oxidation, reduction, or hydrolysis (14). Phase II reactions modify components, generally by conjugation reactions, to make a compound more excretable and in some cases to make a product less toxic (15). The hepatic toxicity of most xenobiotics is due to phase I (or sometimes phase II) biotransformation (16). The metabolism of a toxic chemical can have three outcomes. It can become less toxic; it can be made to a more toxic intermediate which is subsequently detoxified; or it can be bioactivated to a more toxic metabolite, which can cause cellular damage (Fig. 10.2).

Phase I reactions occur predominantly in the hepatic smooth endoplasmic reticulum (SER) of zone III but are not limited to that location. The major reaction types and substrates are

1. *Flavin containing monooxygenase*—oxidation of tertiary and secondary amines, hydrazines, thioamides, thiols, disulfides, amino thiols, imines, and aryl amines.
2. *Epoxide hydrolase*—hydrates, arene oxides, and aliphatic epoxides.
3. *Esterases and amidases*—hydrolytic cleavage of esters, amides, and thioesters.
4. *Alcohol, aldehyde, ketone oxidation, and reduction systems*—oxidation, dehydrogenation or reduction of alcohols, aldehydes, and ketones.
5. *Mixed function oxidase (P450)*—Hydroxylation of aliphatic and aromatic structures, epoxidation of alkenes, oxidative deamination of aliphatic structures with a primary amino group, oxidative dealkylation of a carbon group attached to an O, N, S atom, oxidation of sulfur and nitrogen or desulfuration of sulfur containing organic compounds, and oxidative dehalogenation of halogenated compounds.
6. *Microsomal (P450)-mediated reductions*—Azo and aromatic nitro compounds and reductive dehalogenations.

Phase I reactions biotransforms many chemicals. The xenobiotic is biotransformed to a more reactive molecule by this metabolism, and a more chemically stable, as well as toxic, molecule can be formed. For example, a reactive, electrophilic molecule can be formed which can then alkylate proteins, DNA, or lipids. Free radicals can also be formed; these are very active molecules and participate in a self-propagating chain reaction of free radical transfer in the cell. Free radicals can cause peroxidation of lipid structures in the cell, inactive proteins, and DNA (17) (see chapter entitled Bioactivation and Metabolism of Chemical Toxicity).

Phase II reactions occur both in the endoplasmic reticulum and in the cytosol. They require energy, usually ATP, and add functional groups which increase molecular weight (17). In many cases they inactivate toxic intermediates formed in phase I reactions (14). Most also require cofactors. Major phase II reactions are as follows:

1. *Glucuronidation*—adds glucuronic acid to a wide variety of functional groups including aliphatic and aromatic alcohols, carboxyl acids, primary and secondary aromatic and aliphatic amines, and free sulfhydryl groups. Glucuronidation promotes excretion of the substrate by liver and kidney organic acid transport systems.

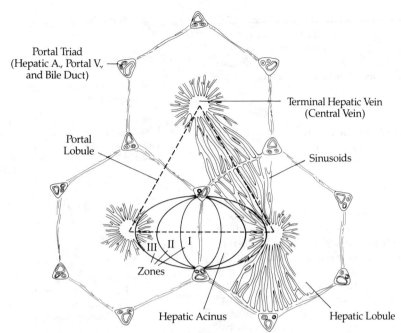

Figure 10.1. Hepatic Lobule and Hepatic Acinus. The acinus is the functional unit of the liver. Zone I is a microanatomically functional area around the portal triad in which the blood contains the highest concentration of nutrients, oxygen, hormones, and unmetabolized chemicals carried in the hepatic circulation. Zone III is the centrilobular area around the hepatic vein which contains cells that are less active in protein synthesis and glycogen synthesis. Zone III contains the highest concentration of biotransformation enzymes of mixed function oxidase (P450) system. Zone II is an intermediate functional area.

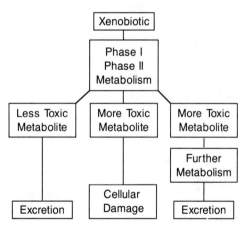

Figure 10.2. Possible outcomes of xenobiotic metabolism.

2. *Sulfotransferase*—transfer inorganic sulfate to hydroxyl groups, commonly aliphatic alcohols and phenols. Cysteine, required as a sulfur source, can be rate limiting. Sulfate conjugates are renally excreted (17).
3. *N-Acetyl transferases*—acetylates arylamines, hydrazines, hydrazides sulfonamides and primary aliphatic amines. The rate of acetylation can be genetically variable (17).
4. *Amino acid conjugation*—acts on groups containing a carboxylic acid group. The most common amine acids involved in conjugation are glycine, glutamine, and serine. Concentrations of these amino acids can effect the rate of conjugation (17).
5. *Glutathione S-transferase*—a very important phase II enzyme. It can detoxify highly reactive intermediates. It acts on electrophilic intermediates. Gluthione is also a cofactor for glutathione peroxidase which inactivates lipid peroxidation (14).

MORPHOLOGIC PATTERNS OF HEPATIC INJURY

Phase I and phase II reactions can contribute to the biotransformation of hazardous chemicals. These products of biotransformation are often the agents that ultimately cause hepatocellular damage. Regardless of the etiology of hepatocellular damage, the liver can only respond with a few pathologic responses. Hepatic injury from any source can manifest as steatosis, necrosis, cholestasis, fibrosis/cirrhosis, or cancer.

Steatosis

Steatosis, or fatty liver, often is an early sign of hepatotoxicity. It is associated with a decrease in the concentration of plasma lipids and plasma lipoproteins as demonstrated by studies with carbon tetrachloride. Carbon tetrachloride can interfere with the synthesis of the protein for triglyceride export from the liver. A similar mechanism likely is involved in other fatty liver damage (18).

Necrosis

Carbon tetrachloride has been extensively used to demonstrate possible mechanisms of hepatocellular necrosis. It seems likely that the final irreversible step in necrosis is disruption of calcium homeostasis. Calcium ions influx due to damage to the plasma membrane and other vital cell structures. This influx of calcium ions inactivates mitochondria, inhibits enzymes, and denatures structural proteins (19).

The cellular mechanism resulting in the disruption of calcium homeostasis is unclear. Studies on carbon tetrachloride demonstrate that inhibition of protein synthesis occurs prior to calcium homeostasis disruption via damage to ribosomes by carbon tetrachloride metabolites. Lipid peroxidation in the endoplasmic reticulum, which is involved with both calcium ion and triglyceride excretion, occurs in carbon tetrachloride-induced necrosis (17). How this explains necrosis for other hepatotoxins is unclear, but a similar mechanism is likely.

Cholestasis

Cholestasis is poorly understood but can be due to bile flow alterations, bile permeability, or dysfunction of microfilaments involved in bile transport (20).

Fibrosis and Cirrhosis

Fibrosis and cirrhosis are the end result of ongoing hepatic injury. Septae of collagen are deposited throughout the liver leading to distortion of the hepatic circulation. It is the disruption of circulation that leads to portal hypertension and the clinical syndrome associated with end-stage liver disease. It is associated most commonly with hepatitis and chronic ethanol use and has been observed in chronic carbon tetrachloride exposure (21). The mechanism is not clear, but increased collagen proline synthesis has been observed (20). Early fibrosis has also been demonstrated after exposure to organic solvents such as trichloroethylene and 1,1,1-trichloroethane (22, 23).

Hepatic Carcinogenesis

Hepatic carcinogenesis has been demonstrated for a number of naturally occurring and industrially produced chemicals. For many agents the mechanism of tumor production has not been determined. Carcinogenesis seems to involve a two-step process of induction, followed by a long latent period during which neoplasm develops. A promoter is required during this latent period to produce a cancer. Most chemical carcinogens act as initiators by causing structural damage to DNA (20). Several human hepatic carcinogens have been identified (see Table 10.2). Some are industrially produced chemicals, but many are naturally occurring biologic agents.

Occupationally induced liver disease is well described for many agents. For those at risk or with suspected exposure, certain laboratory methods are useful for diagnosis and screening and will be discussed later.

MORPHOLOGIC FORMS OF TOXIC HEPATIC INJURY

The main types of morphologic changes in the liver produced by chemicals, drugs, and other agents are listed in Table 10.3. Chemical hepatic injury can be acute or chronic. Acute injury may be cytotoxic or cholestatic. Cytotoxic injury may be manifested by necrosis, steatosis, or both. Cholestatic injury may be associated with hepatocanicular jaundice or canicular jaundice. Chronic hepatic injury includes several forms such as cirrhosis, chronic active hepatitis, steatosis, phospholipidosis, veno-occlusion, peliosis hepatitis, or hepatic neoplasms. (3).

Classification of Hepatotoxins and Mechanisms of Toxicity

Hepatotoxins are classified into two main categories: predictable (intrinsic) and unpredictable (idiosyncratic) (25). Predict-

Table 10.2. Some Proven or Suspected Liver Carcinogens
(Modified with permission from Davidson CS. Guidelines for hepatotoxicity due to drugs and chemicals. NIH Publication No. 79-313), Washington, DC, Dept. of Health, Education, and Welfare. 1979.)

A. Liver carcinogens in humans

Confirmed	Suspected
1. Vinyl chloride	1. Aldrin
2. Thorium dioxide	2. Carbon tetrachloride
3. Arsenic	3. Chloroform
	4. DDT
	5. Dieldrin
	6. Heptachlor
	7. PCBs
	8. Trichlorethylene

B. Liver carcinogens in animals

	Species
1. Azodyes or precursors, e.g., p-aminoazobenzene 4-dimethylaminoazobenzene O-aminoazatoluene	Rat, mouse
2. 2-Acetylaminofluorene (AAF)	Rat, mouse Hamster Rabbit, dog Fowl, cat
3. Nitroaromatic compounds Aromatic hydroxylamines, e.g., 4-nitroquinoline-1-oxide	Rat
4. Nitrosamines	Rat
5. Dialkyl or arylakyl Hydrazines	Rat
6. Urethane (ethyl carbamates)	Mouse
7. Thio compounds, e.g., thiourea throacetamide	Various rodents
8. Ethionine	Rat
9. Alkyl halides CCl_4 Chloroform Iodoform Benzyl chloride	Mouse, rat Hamster
10. Cycasin	Rat
11. Aromatic side chain derivatives, e.g., 1,1,1-trichloro-2,2-bis(p-chlorophenyl)ethane 1,1-dichloro-2,2-bis(p-chlorophenyl)ethylene	Mouse
12. Mold toxins, e.g., aflatoxin B, safrole	Rat

able hepatotoxicity is usually dose-related, can be produced in experimental animals, and usually affects a particular region of the hepatic lobule. Unpredictable or idiosyncratic hepatotoxicity occurs in unusually susceptible persons, cannot be reproduced in experimental animals, and is usually in a diffuse form (Fig. 10.3).

Table 10.3. Morphologic Types of Drug-Induced Liver Diseases (From Ockner RK. Drug-induced liver disease. In: Zakim D, Boyer T, eds. Hepatology. A textbook of liver disease. Philadelphia: W.B. Saunders Co. 1982:693, with permission.)

Type	Examples
Zonal necrosis	Acetaminophen, carbon tetrachloride
Nonspecific hepatitis	Aspirin, oxacillin
Viral hepatitis-like lesion	Isoniazid, methyldopa, halothane
Chronic active hepatitis	Methyldopa, dantrolene, isoniazid, propylthiouracil, sulfonamides, papaverine, clometacine
Cholestasis	
Hepatocanalicular	Chlopromazine, erythromycin estolate, organic arsenicals
Canalicular	Estrogens, anabolic steroids
Fatty liver	
Large globules	Ethanol, corticosteroids
Small droplets	Tetracycline, valproic acid
Vascular lesions	
Hepatic vein thrombosis	Oral contraceptives
Veno-occlusive disease	Certain antineoplastic agents
Peliosis hepatis	Anabolic steroids
Noncirrhotic portal hypertension	Vinyl chloride
Cirrhosis	Ethanol, methotrexate, chronic hepatitis-inducing drugs except glucocorticoids
Tumors	
Adenoma	Oral contraceptives, androgens
Focal nodular hyperplasia	Oral contraceptives
Carcinoma	Oral contraceptives, thorotrast vinyl chloride, anabolic steroids
Angiosarcoma	Thorotrast, vinyl chloride, arsenic, copper sulfate

Intrinsic Hepatotoxins

The mechanism by which intrinsic hepatotoxins and their metabolic products induce hepatic injury falls into two main categories: direct and indirect (21, 26). Direct hepatotoxins act by a physicochemical destruction of hepatocyte membranes through peroxidation with free radicals or activated oxygen formation. This membrane injury is the first step in direct hepatotoxicity which ends in either cell necrosis or steatosis. Few intrinsic hepatotoxins produce injury by a direct mechanism; examples are carbon tetrachloride (CCl_4), several other halogenated hydrocarbons, and yellow phosphorus (27). On the other hand, most of the intrinsic hepatotoxins produce injury by indirect mechanism. This injury results from a binding of the toxic agent or its products to cell membranes or molecules that leads to distortion of physiologic or biochemical pathways

essential for cell integrity. This binding may be covalent (e.g., acetaminophen, bromobenzene) or noncovalent (e.g., phalloidin) (28, 29, 30). Covalent binding appears to be the most important form of indirect hepatotoxicity. Protection against the toxic effects of covalent binding is provided by glutathione, which itself binds covalently to the reactive electrophilic metabolites of toxic agents (e.g., acetaminophen), converting them to nontoxic products which are readily excreted (31). Also, glutathione serves to reduce peroxides and so provides protection against the peroxidation by activated oxygen (32).

The hepatotoxic damage produced by indirect hepatotoxins may by either cytotoxic (expressed as steatosis or necrosis) or cholestatic (expressed as arrested bile flow).

Cytotoxic indirect hepatotoxins cause hepatic injury by interfering with metabolic pathways essential for parenchymal cell integrity. The biochemical and physiologic lesions induced by these agents lead to steatosis, necrosis, or both. Examples of agents that produce steatosis are tetracyclines (33), L-asparaginase (34), methotrexate (35), aflatoxin (21), and puromycin (36). Agents that cause necrosis include bromobenzene (37), 6-mercaptopurine (38), urethane (39), and thioacetamide (21). Some agents produce both steatosis and necrosis, such as toxins of amanita phalloides and tannic acid (21).

Ethanol can be classified as an indirect hepatotoxin. It leads to fatty metamorphosis by a number of adverse effects on hepatocyte metabolism (40). It also can lead to necrosis, perhaps by the necrogenic effects of acetaldehyde (41) or by increasing oxygen requirements of hepatocytes (42). Ethanol also potentiates the hepatotoxic effects of a number of known toxic agents through induction of the mixed function oxidase (MFO) system and consequent enhancement of biotransformation of these agents to toxic metabolites (43, 44). Of special clinical importance is the enhancement of the hepatotoxic effects of chlorinated hydrocarbons (45) and acetaminophen (46) by ethanol. Many cytotoxic indirect hepatotoxins are hepatocarcinogens, likely through alkylation or arylation of DNA (47).

Cholestatic indirect hepatotoxins, on the other hand, produce jaundice or impaired liver function by selective interference with hepatic mechanisms of excretion into the bile canaliculi, by injury to bile ducts or by inhibition of hepatocellular uptake from the blood of substances destined for biliary excretion (21). Cholestatic indirect hepatotoxins of clinical significance include methyltestosterone and some C-17 alkylated anabolic steroids such as ethinyl estrogen and progestrone derivatives used as oral contraceptives (38, 48, 49). The effect of these agents is dose related but modified by the individual susceptibility of the recipient. As an example, oral contraceptives are likely to produce jaundice in women who have had the benign cholestatic jaundice of pregnancy, a syndrome with a genetic basis (50). Most agents causing cholestatic disease are drugs rather than industrial or chemical hazardous materials (21).

The mechanism for the impaired function induced by these anabolic, progestational, and estrogenic steroids is unknown. There is evidence that indicates a precise structural requirement to induce injury, namely an alkyl group at C-17. Testosterone, which lacks this type of substituent, does not lead to impaired function, while methyl testosterone with the C-17 methyl substituent does (21).

There are several agents that produce cholestasis by selectively damaging the ductal system. 4,4-Diaminodiphenylmethane, a plastics hardener, led to an epidemic of cholestatic jaundice in England as a result of its presence as a contaminant of flour (19). A similar lesion has been reported in Spain as

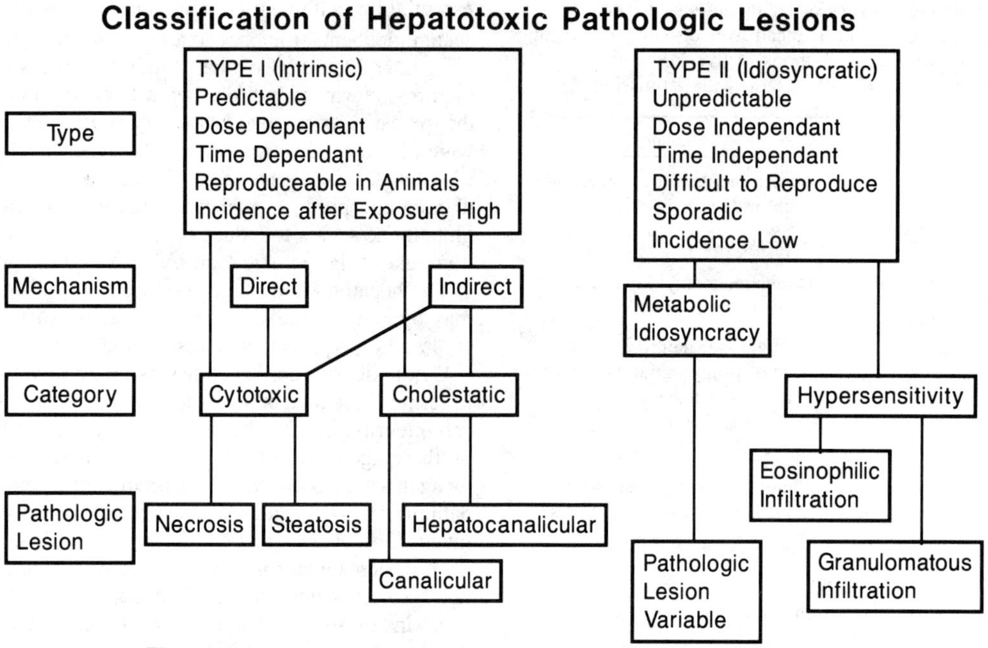

Classification of Hepatotoxic Pathologic Lesions

Figure 10.3.   Classification of pathologic lesions produced by hepatotoxins.

the result of ingestion of rapeseed oil contaminated with aniline (52). Paraquat poisoning also can produce ductal destruction (53). 5-Fluorouridine given by infusion through the hepatic artery in the treatment of metastatic carcinoma of the liver leads to an injury of the biliary tree resembling sclerosing cholangitis (54). Mycotoxins such as sporidesmin mainly cause ductal injury in some species (55).

Idiosyncratic Hepatotoxins

Many drugs unpredictably produce hepatic injury in a small proportion of recipients. Two mechanisms of idiosyncratic hepatic injury have been recognized: hypersensitivity and metabolic aberration.

Hypersensitivity-related hepatic injury develops after a relatively fixed "sensitization" period of 1 to 5 weeks and recurs promptly on readministration of the agent. It tends to be accompanied by systemic (fever, rash, eosinophilia) and histologic (eosinophil-rich or granulomatous inflammatory infiltrate in the liver) evidence of hypersensitivity. These hallmarks of hypersensitivity, especially when supported by a recurrence of the syndrome in response to a challenge dose, permit the inference that the hepatic injury is due to drug allergy and that the drug or a metabolite has acted as a hapten.

Lack of these hallmarks of hypersensitivity suggests that the idiosyncrasy may be the result of a metabolic aberration rather than of hypersensitivity. This is strongly supported by the observations of Speilberg and coworkers (56) who found that patients who had sustained hepatic injury in a hypersensitivity-type reaction to phenytoin had an apparent defect in converting the active metabolite (arene oxide) to the inactive dihydrodiol. The active metabolite probably acts as a hapten or may be cytotoxic.

Even among the agents that appear to produce hepatic injury related to hypersensitivity, there appear to be several catego-

ries. The circumstantial evidence for the role of hypersensitivity is most strongly suggestive for those drugs that produce hepatic injury only in association with systemic features suggestive of an allergic response, e.g., phenytoin (57). The role of hypersensitivity is somewhat less clear for drugs such as chlorpromazine, erythromycin estolate, and halothane, which produce hepatic injury that may or may not be accompanied by systemic features suggestive of drug allergy (48). On the other hand, drugs that cause systemic hypersensitivity do not necessarily cause hepatic injury, e.g., penicillin and procainamide (58). Furthermore, there are drugs that produce hepatic injury without clinical features of hypersensitivity. Some of these respond promptly to a challenge dose, e.g., tricrynafen-associated hepatic injury (59), while others do not, e.g., isoniazid and valproic acid.

It has been hypothesized that hypersensitivity leads to hepatic injury only when the respective drug has some intrinsic hepatotoxic potential. Those reactions that do not resemble serum sickness but are provoked by a challenge dose may be the result of hypersensitivity but by a different immunologic mechanism (3). Hypersensitivity and metabolic idiosyncratic reactions can also occur in occupationally induced liver injury.

CIRCUMSTANCES OF EXPOSURE TO HEPATOTOXINS

Hepatotoxins that may be encountered in the home include chemical toxins (e.g., CCl_4, yellow phosphorus, copper salts), botanical agents (e.g., mycotoxins) and large overdoses of ordinarily safe drugs (e.g., acetaminophen, ferrous salts, salicylates) (Table 10.4).

Poisonous mushrooms are still an important cause of acute hepatic necrosis injury (60). Food contaminated with aflatoxins has been implicated in the causation of acute hepatic disease as well as in etiology of hepatic carcinoma (61, 62). Pyrrolizidine alkaloid toxicity has been reported as a cause of hepatic disease in the United States and other parts of the world. Some

Table 10.4. Routes of Exposure to Hepatotoxic Agents (From Zimmerman HJ. Hepatotoxicity. The adverse effects of drugs and other chemicals on the liver. New York, Appleton-Century-Crofts, 1978:4, with permission).

Toxicologic
  Occupational
    Routine exposure to toxic agents
    Accidental exposure
  Domestic
    Accidental or suicidal exposure
    Ingestions of toxic contaminant food
    Exposure to euphoric toxic agents as a form of drug abuse
    "Autogenic" (synthesis in gastrointestinal tract of
      nitrosamines, ethionine, lithocholate)
  Environmental
    Pollution, food or water; pesticides, industrial pollution
    Pollution of atmosphere (hypothetical hepatotoxic hazard)
    Natural hepatotoxins

Pharmaceutical
  Iatrogenic
  Self-medication (drug overdose)

---

items obtained in "natural food" stores and some health remedies sold in pharmacies in the southwestern region of the United States have been reported to contain pyrrolizidine alkaloids (63). Exposure to these hepatotoxins can confuse evaluation of liver disease from industrially produced chemicals or occupational exposures to hepatotoxic agents.

Widely employed insecticides include a number of chlorinated aromatic hydrocarbons, some of which are hepatotoxic in large doses. Exposure of humans to these agents may be through contaminated food, occupational exposure, or accidental ingestion. Longterm storage in human tissues of DDT and other insecticides and their metabolites has been demonstrated (64). Nevertheless, there is no significant evidence of hepatic injury from sustained occupational exposure to the chlorinated insecticides (21). Accidental ingestion of large amounts of DDT (approximately 6 g) (65) and of paraquat (approximately 20 g) (66), however, has led to rare instances of centrilobular hepatic necrosis which has been fatal. Paraquat also has been reported to lead to destruction of intrahepatic bile ducts and cholestasis (53). In general, overt acute hepatic injury is a rare consequence of occupational exposure to toxic chemicals today.

IMPORTANT INDUSTRIALLY OCCURRING HEPATOTOXINS

To a large degree, the rate of overt, acute hepatotoxicity due to industrial agents has decreased due to the identification of a few agents which have been eliminated or hygienically controlled at the worksite. These agents include carbon disulfide, chloroform trichloroethylene, trichloroethane, toluene, halothane, and solvent mixtures (67). Other possible hepatotoxic agents including metallic and inorganic compounds have also been described (21). Agents which have been reported to cause occupationally induced hepatotoxicity in humans are included in Table 10.5.

Carbon tetrachloride and chloroform are known hepatotoxins. Carbon tetrachloride is metabolized to a free radical and interrupts protein synthesis leading to steatosis and necrosis (21). Chloroform acts by a different metabolite but causes steatosis and zone III necrosis (67).

Trichloroethylene hepatotoxicity was demonstrated by intentional "solvent sniffing." Elevations of alanine aminotransferase (ALT) and aspartate aminotransferase (AST) have occurred. Liver biopsy demonstrated centrilobular fibrosis with repeated exposures. Cardiac and neurologic effects were also noted (68).

1,1,1-Trichloroethane (a similar halogenated hydrocarbon to carbon tetrachloride and trichloroethylene) has been noted to cause acute hepatotoxicity in rare instances (69, 70). Liver biopsy after 1,1,1-trichloroethane overexposure has demonstrated eosinophilic infiltration in periportal cells and cholestasis. On electron microscopy proliferation of peroxisomes and smooth endoplasmic reticulum occurred. This case also had symptoms consistent with hypersensitivity, namely fever and urticaria (71). Cirrhosis has been described after recurrent episodes of exposure to trichloroethylene and 1,1,1-trichloroethane (72). However, a matched pair study was unable to demonstrate the effect of low level exposure to trichloroethylene on liver function laboratory tests (73).

Toluene has recently been demonstrated to cause mild pericentral fatty change with an elevation of ALT/AST ratio from occupational exposure in a print shop (74). Other investigations have not found associations of liver enzyme abnormalities and hepatotoxicity with toluene exposure (75, 76, 77).

Solvent mixtures have been investigated in the literature with conflicting results. Solvent mixture exposure is far more common than isolated solvent exposure. Car painters using solvent mixtures of toluene, xylene, butyl acetate, and white spirit, plus other alcohols and ketones showed no statistically significant elevation in liver function tests when compared with controls (78). House painters exposed to white spirit (which is a combination of aromatic and aliphatic hydrocarbons), paints and lacquers, and xylene, petroleum spirits, toluene, and methyl ethyl ketone, plus occasional use of industrial alcohols demonstrated elevated aminotransferases. Biopsy results included significant steatosis with focal necrosis, enlarged portal tracts, and fibrosis (79).

Carbon disulfide has caused fatty degeneration and hemorrhages of the liver in animals (80). It causes liver enlargement and periacinar degeneration and can inhibit drug-metabolizing enzymes (81).

Subacute or chronic exposure (82). Many other agents are suspected carcinogens (see Table 10.2).

FACTORS AFFECTING HEPATOTOXICITY

A variety of factors can influence both hepatic metabolism and hepatotoxicity of toxic chemicals, usually via modification of MFO or other phase I reaction. In many cases, induction of P450 mixed function oxidase system (MFO) can lead to the increased production of a toxic metabolite by favoring a biotransformation pathway which leads to that toxic product. The most notable inducer is ethanol, but other factors influence metabolism and toxicity as well.

MFO function can be modified in a number of ways. It can be induced by drugs like phenobarbital, but many xenobiotics also produce P450 enzyme system induction. Histologically, proliferation of the hepatic smooth endoplasmic reticulum occurs, predominantly in zone III when MFO induction occurs. Inducers of MFO include synthetic steroids, ethanol, 1,1,1-trichloroethane, polyhalogenated aromatics including DDT, polychlorinated or brominated biphenyls (PCB, PBBs), tetra-

Table 10.5.   Some Occupational Hepatotoxins or Possible Hepatotoxins.[a,b]

A. Aliphatic hydrocarbons
  1. Alicyclic hydrocarbons, e.g., cyclopropane
  2. n-Heptane
  3. Turpentine
B. Alcohols
  4. Allyl alcohol
  5. Ethyl alcohol
  6. Ethylene chlorohydrin
  7. Methyl alcohol
  8. Ethylene glycol ethers and derivatives
C. Ethers and epoxy compounds
  9. Dioxane
  10. Epichlorohydrin
  11. Ethylene oxide
  12. Ethyl ether
D. Acetates
  13. Methyl, ethyl, N-propyl, isopropyl, N-butyl, and amyl
  14. Ethyl silicate
E. Carboxylic acids and anhydrides
  15. Phthalic anhydride
F. Aliphatic halogenated hydrocarbons
  16. Carbon tetrachloride
  17. Chloroform
  18. Chloroprene
  19. Dibromochloropropane
  20. 1,2-Dibromoethane
  21. 1,2-Dichloroethane
  22. 1,2-Dichloroethane
  23. Ethylene dibromide
  24. Ethylene dichloride
  25. Methyl bromide
  26. Methyl chloride
  27. Methylene chloride
  28. Propylene dichloride
  29. Tetrachloroethane/tetrabromo
  30. Tetrachloroethylene
  31. 1,1,1-Trichloroethane
  32. 1,1,2-Trichloroethane
  33. Trichloroethylene
  34. Vinyl chloride
G. Aliphatic amines
  35. Ethanolamines
  36. Ethylene diamine
H. Cyanides and nitriles
  37. Acetonitrile
  38. Acrylonitrile
  39. Hydrogen cyanide
I. Aromatic hydrocarbons
  40. Benzene
  41. Diphenyl
  42. Naphthalene
  43. Styrene/ethyl benzene
  44. Toluene
  45. Xylene
J. Phenols and phenolic compounds
  46. Cresol
  47. Phenol
K. Aromatic halogenated hydrocarbons
  48. Benzyl chloride
  49. Chlorodiphenyls and derivatives
  50. Chlorinated benzenes
  51. Chlorinated naphthalenes
  52. Polychlorinated biphenyls
  53. Polybrominated biphenyls

L. Aromatic amines
  54. 2-Acetylamino-fluorene
  55. 3,3 Dichlorobenzidine and its salts
  56. 4-Dimethylaminoazobenzene
  57. 4,4-Methylenebis(2-chloroaniline)
M. Nitro compounds
  58. Dinitrobenzene
  59. Dinitrophenol
  60. Dinitrotoluene
  61. Nitrobenzene
  62. Nitroparaffins
  63. Nitrophenol
  64. Picric acid
  65. Tetryl
  66. Nitromethane
  67. Trinitrotoluene
  68. 2-Nitropropane
N. Miscellaneous organic nitrogen compounds
  69. Dimethylnitrosamine
  70. N,N-Dimethylformamide
  71. Ethylenediamine
  72. Hydrazine and derivatives
  73. Methylene dianiline
  74. N-Nitrosodimethylamine
  75. Pyridine
  76. N,N-Dimethylacetamide
O. Miscellaneous organic chemicals
  77. Beta-Propiolactone
  78. Carbon disulfide
  79. Dimethyl sulfate
  80. Mercaptans
  81. Tetramethylthiuram disulfide
P. Halogens
  82. Bromide/hydrogen bromides
Q. Metallic compounds
  83. Arsenic
  84. Arsine
  85. Beryllium
  86. Bismuth and compounds
  87. Boron and compounds (excluding the hydrides)
  88. Boron hydrides
  89. Cadmium and compounds
  90. Carbonyls (metal)
  91. Chromium and its compounds
  92. Copper
  93. Germanium
  94. Iron
  95. Naphthol
  96. Nickel and compounds**
  97. Phosphine
  98. Phosphorus and compounds (excluding phosphine)
  99. Pyrogallol
  100. Selenium and compounds
  101. Stibine
  102. Thallium and compounds
  103. Thorium dioxide (Thorotrast)
  104. Tin and compounds
  105. Uranium and components
R. Pesticides
  106. Bipyridyls
  107. Thallium sulfate
  108. Kepone
S. Physical hazards
  109. Ionizing radiation
  110. Vibration, whole body

[a]Early detection of occupational disease. World Health Organization, Geneva 1986.
[b]Davidson CS. Guidelines for hepatotoxicity due to drugs and chemicals. NIH Publication No. 79-313, Washington, DC, Dept. of Health, Education, and Welfare. 1979.

chlorodibenzodioxin (TCDD) (83), aldrin, hexachlorobenzene lindane, and chlordane (17).

The MFO system can be inhibited in a variety of ways as well. The activity of the MFO system can influence how a compound is metabolized, thus influencing the type of intermediate produced, therefore modifying the toxicity produced. Other factors which influence the P450 MFO systems:

1. *Nutritional state*: calcium, copper, iron, magnesium, and zinc deficiencies decrease MFO activities. Vitamin deficiencies (ascorbic acid, tocopherol, and B-complex) decrease MFO function, as does starvation. Low protein diets increase the toxicity of some xenobiotics.
2. *Age*: newborn and fetal animals are less able to biotransform xenobiotics by MFO. Old age increases toxicity of some agents; however, this may be due to factors other than the MFO system (i.e., decreased blood flow, uptake, or renal excretion).
3. *Genetic factors*: isozymes of MFO system exist (17), and the distribution of these can be genetically influenced. This will determine biotransformation products by favoring some reactions. Some phase II enzyme systems such as acetylases are also genetically variable (16).
4. *Gender* influences proportions of MFO isozymes in rats. This has not been reproduced in humans (17).
5. *Physical activity* and smoking *cigarettes* also influence the MFO system.

The ingestion of ethanol increases the toxicity of carbon tetrachloride and trichloroethylene (84). Ethanol and trichloroethylene are both metabolized by alcohol dehydrogenase, and concurrent administration of both competitively inhibit each other's metabolism and prolong the half-life of both agents (85). Methylene chloride toxicity was increased when chronically administered with ethanol for 5 days. However, when ethanol and methylene chloride were administered at high dose for 1 day the toxic effects were antagonized (86). Chloroform toxicity likewise is increased by coadministration with ethanol. Manganese and mercury toxicity may also be increased by ethanol (87). Blood concentrations of xylene, styrene, toluene, and trichloroethylene are all increased with concurrent ethanol administration (88).

Several toxins inhibit ethanol metabolism similar to the drug disulfiram. Disulfiram-like reactions are caused by the buildup of the metabolite acetaldehyde, which causes tachycardia, flushing, and throbbing headache, and can lead to cardiovascular collapse. Hepatic alcohol dehydrogenase is inhibited by some amides, pesticidal dithiocarbamates, thiurams, carbamates, cyanamides, nitroglycol, and some oximes (87), as do carbon disulfide, dimethylformamide (Table 10.6) (88). Solvents also influence the metabolism of other solvents. In most cases the longterm effects of the altered metabolism by ethanol and or solvent mixtures is unknown. However, ethanol may potentiate the angiosarcoma rate from vinyl chloride exposure (87).

CLINICAL EVALUATION OF HEPATOTOXICITY

Evaluation of hepatotoxicity from hazardous chemicals can be difficult. Investigation of acute liver injury is fairly routine, but the assessment of chronic hepatotoxicity is less obvious. Most of the tests for hepatotoxicity evaluation were developed to detect acute, severe liver damage. This section will first discuss the evaluation of acute hepatotoxicity. Then, the screening for chronic hepatotoxicity will be discussed, with the ap-

Table 10.6. Chemical: Ethanol Metabolic Interactions[a,b]

Disulfiram Reactions	Enhancement of Solvent Hepatotoxicity

Amides
  dimethyl formamide
	Halogenated hydrocarbons
	  Carbon tetrachloride
	  Trichloroethylene

Oximes
  N-Butyraldoxime
  Cyclohexanone oxime
  Methylethyl ketoxime
  Acetaidoxime
  Isobutylaldoxime
	Methylene chloride

Thiurams
  Disulfiram
	Metals
	  Manganese
	  Mercury

Carbamates
  Pyrazole
  Ziram
  Manam
	Vinyl chloride
	Xxylene
	Styrene
	Toluene

Sulfonureas	Carbon disulfide
Nitroglycol	

Cyanimide
  Calcium cyanamide
  N-Butyramide
  Isobutyramide	

Trichloroethylene	
Carbon disulfide	

[a]Hills BW, Venable HL. The interaction of ethyl alcohol and industrial chemicals. Am J Ind Med 1982;3:321–333.
[b]Dossing M. Metabolic interactions between organic solvents and other chemicals. In: Riihimaki V, Ulfvarson U, eds. Safety and health aspects of organic solvents. New York: Alan R. Liss, 1986:97–105.

plication of tests commonly used in acute hepatic function evaluation as applied to chronic or subacute liver damage.

Acute Hepatic Toxicity

Since chemical- or drug-induced liver disease may present initially with quite nonspecific symptomatology (e.g., fever or viral-like syndrome), a thorough and careful history regarding medication, alcohol intake, drug or chemical abuse, exposure to chemicals, and type of occupation is essential. Occupational and environmental toxic exposures can produce acute toxicity (Table 10.5). Past medical history of other diseases, particularly those involving the liver, should be explored. Personal and family history of allergy or hypersensitivity to food, medication, or chemicals is important in idiosyncratic mediated hepatitis.

When a patient presents with clinical or laboratory findings suggestive of impaired liver function, other diagnostic possibilities, which are not always easily distinguishable from chemical-induced liver injury, should be considered. These may include viral hepatitis (A, B, non-A, non-B), systemic bacterial, fungal, rickettsial or parasitic diseases, postoperative intrahepatic cholestasis, choleocholithiasis and/or acute pancreatitis, bile duct injury, congestive heart failure, cancer, and deterioration of preexisting liver disease. This broad differential diagnosis, together with the fact that the hepatotoxic potentials of most newly introduced agents are not known, makes it necessary for the clinician to remain constantly alert to the possibility that a seemingly nonspecific, unfavorable turn of events or change in liver function may represent chemical-induced liver injury.

The chemical and biochemical manifestations of chemical- or drug-induced hepatic disease reflect the histologic pattern of injury. Hepatocellular injury with necrosis usually resembles viral hepatitis in both clinical and laboratory findings. This type of injury is associated with malaise, nausea, and vomiting followed by jaundice. High levels of aminotransferase enzymes (AST, ALT) and depressed levels of plasma coagulation factors are characteristic findings. The most useful clinical clues to severity of necrosis are the prothrombin time and serum bilirubin concentration (89, 90).

Diffuse parenchymal degeneration with little necrosis, as in salicylate-induced hepatic injury, can lead to a syndrome resembling anicteric hepatitis (91). Toxic steatosis of the microvesicular type, as in tetracycline-induced hepatic injury, may lead to a syndrome resembling the fatty liver of pregnancy and Reye's syndrome (92) in its clinical, histologic, and biochemical features.

Cholestatic hepatic injury is clinically manifested by jaundice and pruritis. Laboratory findings include moderate elevations of aminotransferases, alkaline phosphatase, and cholesterol. The two types of cholestatic jaundice in humans (hepatocanalicular and canalicular) differ in their biochemical findings as they differ in their histologic findings. Levels of alkaline phosphatase are elevated more than threefold, and cholesterol values are increased in hepatocanalicular (e.g., chlorpromazine-induced) but not in canalicular (e.g., methyltestosterone-induced) hepatotoxicity (21). Fever, rash, and eosinophilia are usually associated with the hypersensitivity type of drug-induced hepatic injury. The "pseudomononucleosis" or serum sickness-like syndrome of fever, rash, lymphadenopathy, and lymphocytosis with "atypical" lymphocytes in the blood is a characteristic hypersensitivity reaction to a number of drugs (e.g., phenytoin, sulfonamides, aminosalicylic acid) (21, 48). Renal injury may occur as a result of nephrotoxic metabolites (methoxyflurane) (93) or as a manifestation of generalized hypersensitivity (48).

Toxic porphyria may be associated with several forms of hepatic injury. Hexachlorobenzene liver toxicity is associated with a form of porphyria resembling porphyria cutanea tarda (94). Griseofulvin-induced hepatic injury also may be accompanied by a similar defect in porphyria metabolism (95). Most cases of porphyria cutanea tarda are associated with alcoholism and alcoholic liver disease (96).

Several well-known hepatotoxins tend to present clinically in three distinct phases: (1) immediate, severe gastrointestinal or neurologic manifestations; (2) an asymptomatic period of relative well-being; (3) a phase of overt hepatic injury that often includes renal failure. This sequence is characteristic of poisoning due to CCl₄ (97), yellow phosphorus (98), hepatotoxic mushrooms (65), and, to some degree, acetaminophen hepatotoxicity (99).

Subacute and Chronic Hepatotoxicity

Acute hepatotoxicity is usually easy to recognize clinically and by laboratory means, particularly after large doses of toxic agents. Acute, occupationally induced hepatic injury has decreased due to control of certain hazardous agents. Hepatic damage, however, is not limited to acute toxicity but includes

Possible Outcomes of Hepatotoxin Exposures

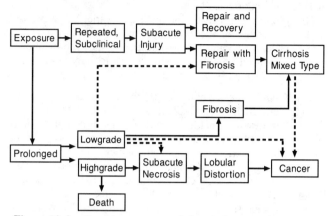

Figure 10.4. Possible outcomes of chronic hepatotoxin exposure. Modified with permission from Tamburro CH, Liss GM. Tests for hepatotoxicity: usefulness in screening workers. J Occup Med 1986;28:1034–1044.

subacute and chronic toxicity (21). Fig. 10.4 demonstrates how the dose and administration interval can have profound effect on eventual outcome. It is also evident why different tests are appropriate to detect the various outcomes of exposure to toxic agents. Vinyl chloride is an example of a hepatotoxin that causes damage from low level chronic exposure at doses below which acute toxicity is seen. Angiosarcoma and nonmalignant hepatocellular damage due to vinyl chloride is difficult to detect by current methods. Indeed, vinyl chloride has served as a model for developing surveillance methods for subacute and chronic hepatic damage from hazardous industrial chemicals (100). Through screening and surveillance, hepatotoxicity can be minimized and, hopefully, prevented.

An effective surveillance program for hepatotoxicity, as in all screening programs, needs to follow basic principles. It must be selective and tailored to the population at risk. It must detect disease before damage is evident. Treatment should be available for the condition. (In the case of occupational hepatotoxicity, eliminating or minimizing exposure is usually the only treatment.) The test itself must be valid and reliable. The risks and costs of the test should not outweigh the benefits. Finally, adequate follow-up is necessary (101).

HEPATOTOXICITY TESTING

Subclinical hepatic damage is more difficult to detect than acute hepatotoxicity. In terms of liver function tests, it is difficult to know what represents normal and abnormal in an asymptomatic population. In many cases abnormalities in standard liver enzyme batteries reflect late hepatotoxicity or hepatotoxicity from ethanol or other acute hepatotoxicity. It may also be that the pathogenesis of subacute or chronic hepatic injury is different from acute hepatotoxicity. In this case, tests designed to detect acute hepatotoxicity may be difficult to interpret. In an industrial setting the goal is to identify latent hepatotoxicity to prevent irreversible future liver damage.

Enzyme Levels

Hepatic enzymes are the most commonly obtained tests of liver function. Alanine aminotransferase and aspartate aminotransferase (ALT/AST) are often obtained as paired indicators of hepatocellular damage. They reflect changes in cellular permeability rather than cellular function and can be indicators of cellular necrosis. A variety of conditions including nutritional state, infection, and alcohol use can influence these levels (102). AST and ALT can also be found in heart, muscle, and lung (21). Obesity also elevates levels of AST/ALT. ALT is elevated to a somewhat greater degree in obesity (103).

Ratios of AST/ALT have been used to aid in diagnosis of liver injury. An elevated AST/ALT ratio has been associated with alcoholic liver disease (102). Elevation of the ALT/AST ratio greater than 1.6 has been associated with pericentral fatty change due to toluene (104).

Gamma glutamic acid transferase (GGT) is a sensitive indicator of liver injury and is specific to the liver. Elevation of GGT is associated with ethanol consumption and has a high false positive rate (102). Lactate dehydrogenase (LDH) likewise can be elevated with liver damage but is not specific for the liver since it is present in heart, muscle, lungs, and a variety of disease states (21).

Serum enzyme levels represent loss of hepatocyte cellular integrity and are accurate indicators of acute hepatic disease. They do not represent the metabolic function of the liver (48). In subacute or chronic hepatic injury, liver enzymes may only transiently elevate, then return to normal. Also, diminished functioning parenchyma will often not be reflected by serum enzymes and indeed, in end-stage liver disease, falling enzyme levels may reflect worsening disease due to loss of hepatic parenchyma. Overall, serum enzyme levels have lacked sensitivity for detecting early liver injury (100).

Usually accompanying hepatic enzyme testing are one or two tests that measure cholestatic functioning. Alkaline phosphatase (AP) and serum bilirubin (direct and indirect) are the most common tests for this. AP can also be present in bone and elevated with bone disease or damage. However, if bone disease is excluded, AP can be a very specific test of liver and biliary function (102). Bilirubin can be elevated in up to 5% of a population. This can be due to a congenital and benign disorder called Gilbert's disease. Usually bilirubin elevation reflects late changes of biliary injury or acute infection, so it is often not helpful in detecting damage from hazardous chemicals. 5'-Nucleotidase (5'NT) is specific to biliary tract disease. It has been used in evaluation of clinical disease, but not in screening for liver disease (102).

Functional Tests

Test of actual liver function rather than levels of circulating liver enzymes are also useful. Clearance tests have been proposed as being more sensitive and specific for detecting the functional ability of the liver (104).

Testing the functional ability of the liver has been demonstrated to identify early, subclinical disease. In the case of vinyl chloride, indocyanine green clearance (106) and serum bile acids (100) have detected early hepatic damage. Several other functional tests are currently possible. They include the aminopyrine breath test, antipyrine, caffeine, and phenacetin clearances. Serum bile acids and ionic dye clearances are also used.

The aminopyrine breath test is used to assess functional reserve of end-stage liver failure. Aminopyrine is oxidized by the MFO system and then demethylated. By radiolabeling aminopyrine and checking for expired $^{14}CO_2$, an indication of hepatic function is obtained. Due to the use of radiolabel, lack of data in an asymptomatic population, and uncertainties about interpretation of results, this is a difficult exam to use for detecting subacute or chronic hepatic disease caused by toxic chemicals (103). The test requires physical rest for 2 hours after administration of aminopyrine until sample collection. Measuring sequential radiolabel excretion rates during the 2 hours of study has enabled some authors to quantitate changes in microsomal enzyme function before and after exposure to inducers of the microsomal system. It is most useful for quantitating prognosis in known liver disease (106).

Antipyrine is a widely used index of microsomal enzyme activity. It is well absorbed from the GI tract. It is oxidized in phase I metabolism (MFO) to five metabolites which are conjugated in phase II and excreted. Antipyrine is eliminated in a linear fashion over time and is also distributed in total body water so samples of urine or saliva can be used to determine the clearance of antipyrine, giving an indication of microsomal function (107).

The test is limited due to its multiple metabolic pathways, any of which could be inhibited or turned on, making total clearance more complex than at first glance (102). It is best used for comparison of individuals rather than for screening populations. It also cannot be repeatedly used, because it is an inducer of its own metabolism. Its advantages are that the test is noninvasive and simple to administer (107).

Other tests of P450 (MFO) function are under study. These include caffeine and phenacetin breath tests (102). Also under study are d-galactose elimination capacity and 6-hydroxycortisol excretion. The advantage to the latter two methods are that both measure the metabolism of endogenous substances and are thus safer. Not enough is known about these tests to apply to a population for screening (107). In addition, not enough is known about the normal fluctuations of microsomal function to determine what is adaptive and harmless and what represents early toxicity.

Measurements of anionic dye clearances also have been used to detect subclinical liver disease. Bromosulfobromophthalene (BSP) clearance has been discarded due to its toxicity. Indocyanine green (ICG) has been studied, and at certain doses it shows great sensitivity to chemical-induced liver injury. It also shows dose-response correlation with vinyl chloride and vinyl monomer exposure, a known hepatocarcinogen and hepatotoxin (102).

Measurement of serum bile acids does not require administration of exogenous compounds. A single measure of fasting conjugated cholic acid (CCA) and cholylglycine (CG) can indicate the hepatic excretory function in a fashion similar to the way serum creatinine measurements indicate the excretory function of the kidney (102). CCA and CG are similar in sensitivity to GGT in detecting chemical-induced liver injury. CCA and AP are most specific for liver disease and correlate with portal tract changes in vinyl monomer disease. Serum bile acids correlate with ICG clearance in vinyl chloride liver disease. Serum bile acids may also be more sensitive to styrene-induced hepatotoxicity (108, 101).

Liver disease from chronic toxic exposure tends to demonstrate more fibrosis and evidence of chronic injury. Acute hepatotoxicity is more likely to show a cytotoxic response as seen in alcoholic, drug-related, and infectious acute hepatitis. This may explain why functional tests such as bilirubin and bile salt levels may correlate better with chronic or subacute hepatotoxicity, while serum enzyme levels are more useful in acute or non-chemically induced hepatic injury (100).

Hepatic Synthesis Tests

The liver is responsible for production of many circulatory proteins. Most commonly tested are serum albumin, protime, cholesterol, amino acids, and carrier protein molecules such as transferring. All are insensitive tests for screening for early liver toxicity. Prothrombin time, for example, indicates clotting factor deficiency. It is commonly used as a measure of severe acute hepatotoxicity due to the short half-life of the clotting factor activity measured. It is also useful in monitoring end-stage liver failure. It, like other tests for hepatic synthesis, is insensitive to mild or early liver injury. The liver has vast synthetic reserve, and only with extensive parenchymal loss will diminished tests of synthetic function be abnormal (102).

Structural Studies

Physical exam is a highly specific study, but with low sensitivity for evaluating early liver damage since hepatomegaly is a late effect of hepatotoxicity. Multiple radiologic studies, including computerized tomography, magnetic resonance imaging, isotope studies, and ultrasound studies, have not been helpful in screening an industrial population for hepatic injury. Up to 12% false positives and 35–40% false negatives have been demonstrated when using these methods in an industrial population (102).

Liver biopsy is highly sensitive and specific. It is obviously not indicated for screening purposes due to the risk of the procedure to an asymptomatic person. It is indicated for persistent abnormalities detected on screening evaluations, particularly when exposure to a possible hepatotoxin has occurred (102). Other etiologies for abnormal screening studies such as viral infections and therapeutic drugs should be ruled out prior to undertaking liver biopsy. Other indications for biopsy include unexplained hepatomegaly or splenomegaly, cholestasis of uncertain cause, suspected systemic or infiltrative disease, and suspected primary or metastatic liver tumor (109). In addition, liver biopsy results are difficult to interpret because the liver is limited in the types of pathology it can demonstrate (Table 10.3).

PROTOCOL FOR SCREENING FOR HEPATOTOXICITY IN A POPULATION EXPOSED TO HAZARDOUS CHEMICALS

Current testing methods for hepatotoxicity are not easily applied to screening programs. Up to 30% of asymptomatic workers subjected to a standard battery of serum liver chemistries had results in excess of laboratory normal subsets (110). Indeed, since elevated liver chemistries are so common, many physicians ignore abnormal liver chemistries unless greater than twice normal (103). This may lead to misdiagnosis and continuing indolent hepatic injury. Tests of low specificity are often used for screening. This is responsible for much of the difficulty, because as tests of low specificity they lead to high false positive results. The low sensitivity of other testing methods leads to high false negative results, particularly in a population with low disease prevalence. In addition, the range of normal for a laboratory is usually set to include 95% of the population it tests. Often a hospital lab is called upon to test people with other illness and known hepatic disease. The range of normal for this group may be different from the range of normal in the population being studied.

The risks of screening are also important to consider. If liver chemistries are passed as normal when they may represent early toxicity, a worker may be returned to a dangerous environment. If abnormal results are obtained on a nonspecific test, a worker may be removed unnecessarily from a worksite and be subjected to expensive, unnecessary, and sometimes risky evaluations or procedures.

These problems can be minimized by using the following guidelines:

1. Set normal levels for the population being screened. Setting the upper limit of normal to the 95th percentile with respect to the screened population has been shown to decrease the false positive results without increasing false negatives (110). A sample size of 150–250 will give adequate accuracy (111).
2. Use a wider range of normal if doing multiple tests. Multiple tests done on an individual increases the chance that an isolated false positive result will occur. If it is necessary to test using a panel of examinations, setting the normal range to include the 99th percentile will decrease false positives (111).
3. Screen with tests of high specificity first. Using a battery of tests of varying sensitivity and specificity will increase false positive results (102).
4. Follow tests of high specificity with tests of higher sensitivity to correctly identify true positives (102).
5. Follow-up positive results with more extensive diagnostic evaluations as the chance of a false positive is minimized (102).

A protocol studied recently used a sequence of alkaline phosphatase or serum bile acids as specific initial screens. The positives were followed with GGT or ICG (indocyanine green) tests. Positives in both the screen and subsequent testing require evaluation by a specialist as well as liver biopsy (See Table 10.7). This sequence decreased false positive occurrence and did not increase false negative occurrence (102). Further validation of this method is warranted before it can be recommended as a standard procedure.

Finally, workers assigned to a known or likely hepatotoxic environment should have adequate preplacement screening to rule out factors that would put them at increased risk. In this instance, it is wise to rule out preexisting damage to the liver from hepatitis, alcohol, or other causes. For this purpose, standard tests of hepatic disease such as enzyme levels and bile products are appropriate. An approach to testing workers in a hepatotoxic environment is provided in Table 10.7.

SUMMARY

Hepatotoxicity continues to be a major consequence of exposure to toxic chemicals. It is uniquely sensitive to their effects because of physiologic and anatomic factors that distribute absorbed chemicals to the liver. The liver metabolizes chemicals to facilitate excretion, but, in some cases, this biotransformation creates a more reactive or toxic compound which can produce hepatocellular damage insult to another organ.

Damage done to the liver can manifest in several forms, depending on the dose and frequency of exposures as well as on the severity of the toxin. A single, high dose of a chemical or small dose of an extremely toxic chemical can cause acute hepatitis and cytotoxic damage, which can lead to death.

Chronic exposure or frequent, subacute exposure to hepatotoxic chemicals can produce more indolent hepatic disease.

Table 10.7. Health Monitoring in a Hepatotoxic Environment[a,b,c]

Initial employee screening

Goal: rule out preexisting liver disease which would put employee at increased risk.

1. Medical history with specific questions about ethanol use, hepatitis, and previous liver disease.
2. Occupational history including previous worksite exposures and home or hobby exposures to hepatotoxins.
3. Medical exam directed towards the hepatobiliary system to detect hepatic enlargement or signs of chronic hepatic disease.
4. Urinalysis for urobilinogen and bile pigments.
5. Serum enzymes AST or GGT.
6. Serum bilirubin or alkaline phosphatase.
7. Follow-up or repeat abnormal exams.

Periodic surveillance

Goals: 1) rule out nonoccupational liver disease; 2) detect hepatic damage from hepatotoxic environment.

1. Same protocol as initial screening.
2. Tests more specific followed by test more sensitive to hepatic injury caused by the hepatotoxic agent. In the case of vinyl chloride, fasting bile salts followed by ICG clearance or GGT.
3. Follow-up abnormal values with further diagnostic tests.
4. Refer persistently abnormal screening studies or abnormal secondary studies to a specialist for consideration of biopsy and further diagnostic work-up.
5. Remove worker with abnormal screening tests from hepatotoxic environment until definitive diagnosis made. Follow abnormal tests after exposure ceases.

[a]Tamburro CH, Liss GM. Tests for hepatotoxicity: Usefulness in screening workers. J Occup Med 1986;28:1034–1044.
[b]Davidson CS, Leevy CM, Chamberlayne EC, eds. Guidelines for detection of hepatotoxicity due to drugs and chemicals. (NIH Publication No. 79-313), Washington, DC: Dept. of Health Education and Welfare. 1979.
[c]Early Detection of Occupational Diseases. Geneva: World Health Organization, 1986.

This may ultimately lead to fibrosis, scarring, and parenchymal loss. It may also induce or promote carcinogenesis.

Detection of acute hepatotoxicity is achievable with methods of testing commonly used today. In most cases, these methods were developed for detecting acute liver disease and end-stage liver failure. The challenge for the future is detecting chronic and subacute hepatic damage from toxic chemicals. In this way, liver disease from toxic chemicals in use today can be prevented.

REFERENCES

1. Zimmerman HJ. Hepatotoxic effects of oncotherapeutic agents. Prog Liver Dis 1986;8:621.
2. Kraybill HR. The toxicology and epidemiology of natural hepatotoxin exposure. Isr J Med Sci 1974;10:416.
3. Zimmerman HJ, Maddrey WC. Toxic and drug-induced hepatitis. In: Schiff L, Schiff ER, eds. Diseases of the liver. 6th ed. Philadelphia: J.B. Lippincott Co., 1987:591.
4. Anonymous. Drinking water: another source of carcinogens. Science 1974;186:809.
5. Ridder WE, Oehma FW. Nitrates as an environmental, animal and human hazard. Clin Toxicol 1974;7:145.
6. Rouiller CH. Experimental toxic injury of the liver. In: Rouiller CH, ed. The liver. New York: Academic Press, 1964:335.
7. Schaffner F, Raisfeld IH. Drugs and the liver: a review of metabolism and adverse reactions. Adv Intern Med 1969;15:221.
8. Tamburro CH, Liss GM. Tests for hepatotoxicity: usefulness in screening workers. J Occup Med 1986;28:1034–1044.
9. Campra JL, Reynolds TB. The hepatic circulation. In: Arias IM, Jakoby WB, Popper H, et al, eds. The liver: biology and pathobiology. 2nd ed. New York: Raven Press, 1988:911.
10. Rappaport AM. Physioanatomical basis of toxic liver injury. In: Farber E, Fisher MM, eds. Toxic injury of the liver. New York: Marcel Dekker, 1979:1–46.
11. Gumucio JJ, Chianale J. Liver cell heterogeneity and liver function. In: Arias IM, Jakoby WB, Popper H, et al., eds. The liver: biology and pathobiology. 2nd ed. New York: Raven Press, 1988:931.
12. Caldwell J. Biological implications of xenobiotic metabolism. In: Arias IM, Jacoby WB, Popper H, et al., eds. The liver: biology and pathobiology. 2nd ed. New York: Raven Press, 1988:355.
13. Nickels J. Effects of organic solvents on liver cell morphology. In: Riihimaki V, Ufvarson U. Safety and health aspects of organic solvents. New York: Alan R. Liss, 1986:115–119.
14. Jakoby WB. Detoxication: conjugation and hydrolysis. In: Arias IM, Jacoby WB, Popper H, et al., eds. The liver: biology and pathobiology. 2nd ed. New York: Raven Press, 1988:375.
15. Ziegler DM. Detoxication: oxidation and reduction. In: Arias IM, Jacoby WB, Popper H, et al., eds. The liver: biology and pathobiology. 2nd ed. New York: Raven Press, 1988:363.
16. Anders MW. Bioactivation mechanisms and hepatocellular damage. In: Arias IM, Jacoby WB, Popper H, et al., eds. The liver: biology and pathobiology. 2nd ed. New York: Raven Press, 1988:389.
17. Sipes IG, Gandolfi AJ. Biotransformation of toxicants. In: Klaassen CD, Amdur MO, Doull J, eds. Casarette and Doull's toxicology: the basic science of poisons. 3rd ed. New York: Macmillan, 1986:64.
18. Dianzani MU. Reactions of the liver to injury, fatty liver. In: Farber E, Fisher MM, eds. Toxic injury of the liver, Part A. New York: Marcel Dekker, 1979:281.
19. Farber JL. Reaction of the liver to injury, necrosis. In: Farber E, Fisher MM, eds. Toxic injury of the liver, Part A. New York: Marcel Dekker, 1979:281.
20. Plaa GL. Toxic responses of the liver. In: Klaassen CD, Amdur MO, Doull J, eds. Casarette and Doull's toxicology: the basic science of poisons. 3rd ed. New York: Macmillan Publishing Co., 1986:286–309.
21. Zimmerman HJ. Hepatotoxicity: the adverse effects of drugs and other chemicals on the liver. New York: Appleton-Century-Crofts, 1978.
22. Thiele DL, Eigenbrodt EH, Ware AJ. Cirrhosis after repeated trichloroethylene and 1,1,1-trichloroethane exposure. Gastroenterology 1982;83:926–929.
23. Baerg RD, Kimberg DV. Centrilobular hepatic necrosis and acute renal failure in solvent sniffers. Ann Intern Med 1970;73:713–720.
24. Williams GM, Weisburger JH. Chemical carcinogens. In: Klaassen CD, Amdur MO, Doull J, eds. Toxicology: the basic science of poisons. 3rd ed. New York: Macmillan Publishing Co. 1986:99–172.
25. Popper H. Drug-induced hepatic injury. In: Gall EA, Mostofi FK, eds. The liver. Baltimore: Williams & Wilkins, 1973:182.
26. Farber JL, Gerson RJ. Mechanisms of cell injury with hepatotoxic chemicals. Pharmacol Rev 1984;36:71s.
27. Recknagel RO. A new direction in the study of carbon tetrachloride hepatotoxicity. Life Sci 1983;33:401.
28. Mitchell JR, Jollow DJ. Metabolic activation of drugs to toxic substances. Gastroenterology 1975;68:392.
29. Mitchell JR, Nelson SD, Thorgeirsson SS, et al. Metabolic activation: biochemical basis for many drug-induced liver injuries. Prog Liver Dis 1976;5:259.
30. Kroker R, Hegner D. Solubilization of phalloidin binding sites from rat liver hepatocytes and plasma membranes by trypsin. Naunyn-Schmiedeberg's Arch Pharmacol 1973;279:339.
31. Mitchell JR, Thorgeirsson SS, Potter WZ, et al. Acetaminophen-induced hepatic injury: protective role of glutathione in man and rationale for therapy. Clin Pharmacol Ther 1974;16:676.
32. Aw TY, Hanna P, Petrini J, et al. Hepatic drug metabolism and drug-induced liver injury. In: Gitnick G, ed. Current hepatology, Vol 5. New York: John Wiley & Sons, 1985;113.
33. Schenker S. Pathogenesis of tetracycline-induced fatty liver. In: Gerog W, Sickinger K, eds. Drugs and the liver. Stuttgart: FK Schattauer-Verlag, 1975:179.
34. Pratt CB, Johnson WW. Duration and severity of fatty metamorphosis of the liver following L-asparaginase therapy. Cancer 1971;28:361.
35. Dahl MGC, Scheuer PJ. Methotrexate hepatotoxicity in psoriasis. Comparison of different dose regimens. Br Med J 1972;1:654.
36. Farber E. Biochemical pathology. Annu Rev Pharmacol Toxicol 1971;11:71.
37. Reid WD, Christie B, Krishina G, et al. Bromobenzene metabolism and hepatic necrosis. Pharmacology 1971;6:41.
38. Einhorn M, Davidson I. Hepatotoxicity of mercaptopurine. JAMA 1964;188:802.

39. Weiss DL, De Los Santos R. Urethane-induced hepatic failure in man. Am J Med 1960;28:476.

40. Leiber CS. Alcohol and the liver. Transition from adaptation to tissue injury. In: Khanna JM, Israel Y, Kalant H, eds. Alcoholic liver pathology. Ontario: Addiction Research Foundation, 1975:171.

41. Farber E. Some fundamental aspects of liver injury. In: Khanna JM, Israel Y, Kalant H, eds. Alcoholic liver pathology. Addiction Research Foundation, 1975:289.

42. Videla L. Increased oxidative capacity in the liver following ethanol administration. In: Khanna JM, Israel Y, Kalant H, eds. Alcoholic liver pathology. Ontario: Addiction Research Foundation, 1975:331.

43. Zimmerman HJ. Effects of alcohol on other hepatotoxins. Alcoholism Clin Exp Res 1986;10:3.

44. Strubelt O. Alcohol potentiation of liver injury. Fundam Appl Toxicol 1978;4:144.

45. Plaa GL. Toxic responses of the liver. In: Doull J, Klaassen CD, Amdur MO, eds. Casarett and Doull's toxicology: the basic science of poisons. 2nd ed. New York: Macmillan, 1980:206.

46. Soto C, Lieber CS. Increased hepatotoxicity of acetaminophen after chronic ethanol consumption in the rat. Gastroenterology 1981;80:140.

47. Miller EC, Miller JA. Hepatocarcinogenesis by chemicals. Prog Liver Dis 1976;5:699.

48. Zimmerman HJ. Clinical and laboratory manifestations of hepatotoxicity. Ann NY Acad Sci 1963;104:954.

49. Metreau JM, Dhumeaux D, Berthelot D, et al. Oral contraceptives and the liver. Digestion 1972;7:318.

50. Holzbach RT, Sanders JH. Recurrent intrahepatic cholestasis of pregnancy: observations on pathogenesis. JAMA 1965;193:542.

51. Kopelman H, Scheuer PJ, Williams R, et al. The liver lesion of the Epping jaundice. Q J Med 1966;35:553.

52. Solis-Herruzo JA, Castellano G, Colina F, et al. Hepatic injury in the toxic epidemic syndrome caused by ingestin of adulterated cooking oil (Spain 1981). Hepatology 1984;4:131.

53. Mullick FG, Ishak KG, Mahabir R, et al. Hepatic injury associated with paraquat toxicity in humans. Liver 1981;1:209.

54. Hohn D, Melnick J, Stagg R, et al. Biliary sclerosis in patients receiving hepatic arterial infusions of floxyuridine. J Clin Oncol 1985;3:98.

55. Slater TF, Strauli UD, Sawyer B, et al. Sporidesmin poisoning in the rat. Res Vet Sci 1964;5:540.

56. Spielberg SP, Gordon GB, Blake DA, et al. Predisposition to phenytoin hepatotoxicity assessed in vitro. N Engl J Med 1981;305:722.

57. Lee TJ, Carney CN, Lapis JL, et al. Diphenylhydantoin-induced hepatic necrosis. Gastroenterology 1976;70:422.

58. Davies GE, Holmes JE. Drug-induced immunological effects on the liver. Br J Anaesth 1972;44:941.

59. Zimmerman HJ, Lewis JH, Ishak KG, et al. Ticrynafen-associated hepatic injury: analysis of 340 cases. Hepatology 1984;4:315.

60. Rueff B, Benhamou JP. Acute hepatic necrosis and fulminant hepatic failure. Gut 1973;14:805.

61. Krishnamachari KAVR, Bhat RV, Nagarajan V, et al. Hepatitis due to aflatoxicosis: an outbreak in Western India. Lancet 1975;1:1061.

62. Wagon GN. Aflatoxins and their relationship to hepatocellular carcinoma. In: Okuda K, Peters RL, eds. Hepatocellular carcinoma. New York: John Wiley & Sons, 1976:25.

63. Ridker PM, Ohkuma S, McDermott WV, et al. Hepatic veno-occlusive disease associated with the consumption of pyrrolizidine-containing dietary supplements. Gastroenterology 1985;88:1050.

64. Bick M. Chlorinated hydrocarbon residues in human body fat. Med J Aust 1969;1:1127.

65. Smith NJ. Death following accidental ingestion of DDT: experimental studies. JAMA 1948;136:469.

66. Bullivant CM. Accidental poisoning by paraquat: report of two cases in man. Br Med J 1966;1:1272.

67. Klockars M. Solvents and the liver. In: Riihimaki V, Ufvarson U, eds. Safety and health aspects of organic solvents. New York: Alan R. Liss, 1986:139–154.

68. Baerg RD, Kimberg DV. Centrilobular hepatic necrosis and acute renal failure in "solvent sniffers." Ann Intern Med 1970;73:713–720.

69. Stewart RD, Andrews JT. Acute intoxication with methylchloroform. JAMA 1966;195:904–906.

70. Nathan AW, Towsland PA. Goodpastures syndrome and trichloroethane intoxication. Br J Clin Pharmacol 1979;8:284–286.

71. Halevy J, Pitlik S, Rosenfeld J. 1,1,1-Trichloroethane intoxication: a case report with transient liver and renal damage. Review of the literature. Clin Toxicol 1980;16:467–472.

72. Thiele DL, Eigenbrodt EH, Ware AJ. Cirrhosis after repeated trichloroethylene and 1,1,1-trichloroethane exposure. Gastroenterology 1982;83:926–929.

73. Kramer CG, Ott GM, Fulkerson JE, Hicks N, Imbus HR. Health of workers exposed to 1,1,1-trichloroethane: A matched-pair study. Arch Environ Health 1978;33:331–341.

74. Guzelian P, Mills S, Fallon HJ. Liver structure and function in print workers exposed to toluene. J Occup Med 1988;30:791.

75. Tahti H, Karkkainen S, Pyykko K, Rintala E, Kataja M, Vapaatalo H. Chronic occupational exposure to toluene. Int Arch Occup Environ Health 1981;48:61–69.

76. Brugnone F, Perbellini L. Toluene coma and liver function. Scand J Work Environ Health 1985;11:55.

77. Brugnone F, Perbellini L. Toluene coma and liver function. Scand J Work Environ Health 1985;11:55.

78. Kurppa K, Husman K. Car painters' exposure to a mixture of organic solvents. Scand J Work Environ Health, 1982;8:137–140.

79. Dossing M, Arlien-Soborg P, Petersen LM, Ranek L. Eur J Clin Invest 1983;13:151–157.

80. Magos L, Butler WH. Effect of phenobarbitone and starvation on hepatotoxicity in rats exposed to disulfide vapor. Br J Ind Med, 1972;29:95–98.

81. Bond EJ, DeMatteis F. Biochemical changes in rat liver after administration of carbon disulfide, with particular reference to microsomal changes. Biochem Pharmacol 1969;18:2531.

82. Wu W, Steenland K, Brown D, Wells V, Jones J, Schulte P, Halperin W. Cohort and case-control analyses of workers exposed to vinyl chloride: an update. J Occup Med 1989;31:518–523.

83. Reynolds ES, Moslen MT. Liver and biliary tree. In: Mottet NK, ed. Environmental pathology. New York: Oxford University Press, 1985:248.

84. Cornish HH, Adefuin J. Ethanol potentiation of halogenated aliphatic solvent toxicity. Am Ind Hyg Assoc J 1966;57–61.

85. Muller G, Spassowski M, Henschler D. Metabolism of trichloroethylene in man. Arch Toxicol 1975;33:173–189.

86. Balmer MF, Smith FA, Leach LJ, Yuile CL. Effects in the liver of methylene chloride inhaled alone and with ethyl alcohol. Am Ind Hyg Assoc J, 1976;345–352.

87. Hills BW, Venable HL. The interaction of ethyl alcohol and industrial chemicals. Am J Ind Med 1982;3:321–333.

88. Dossing M. Metabolic interactions between organic solvents and other chemicals. In: Riihimaki V, Ulfvarson U, eds. Safety and health aspects of organic solvents. New York: Alan R. Liss, 1986:97–105.

89. Clark R, Borirak-Chanyavat V, Davidson AR, et al. Hepatic damage and death from overdose of paracetamol. Lancet 1973;i:66.

90. Ritt DJ, Whelan G, Werner DJ, et al. Acute hepatic necrosis with stupor or coma: an analysis of thirty-one patients. Medicine 1969;48:151.

91. Zimmerman HJ. Aspirin-induced hepatic injury. Ann Intern Med 1974;80:103.

92. Hoyumpa AM, Jr, Greene HL, Dunn GD, et al. Fatty liver: biochemical and clinical considerations. Am J Dig Dis 1975;20:1142.

93. Elkington SG, Goffinet JA, Conn HO, et al. Renal and hepatic injury associated with methoxyflurane anesthesia. Ann Intern Med 1968;69:1229.

94. Schmid R. Cutaneous porphyria in Turkey. N Engl J Med 1960;263:397.

95. Hurst EW, Paget GE. Protoporphyrin, cirrhosis and hepatomata in the livers of mice given griseofulvin. Br J Dermatol 1963;75:105.

96. Lundvall O. Alcohol and porphyria cutanea tarda. In: Engel A, Larsson T, eds. Alcoholic cirrhosis and other toxic hepatopathies. Stockholm: Nordiska Bokhandelns Forlag, 1970:356.

97. Jennings RB. Fatal fulminant acute carbon tetrachloride poisoning. Arch Pathol 1955;59:269.

98. Rodriguez-Iturbe B. Acute yellow phosphorus poisoning. N Engl J Med 1971;284:157.

99. Harrison DC, Coggins CH, Welland FH, et al. Mushroom poisoning in five patients. Am J Med 1965;38:787.

100. Liss GM, Greenberg RA, Tamburro CH. Use of serum bile acids in the identification of vinyl chloride hepatotoxicity. Am J Med 1985;78:68–76.

101. Levy BS, Halperin WE. Screening for occupational disease. In: Levy BS, Wegman DH, eds. Occupational health: recognizing and preventing work-related disease. Boston: Little, Brown, 1988:75–82.

102. Tamburro CH, Liss GM. Tests for hepatotoxicity: usefulness in screening workers. J Occup Med 1986;28:1034–1044.

103. Hodgson MJ, Van Thiel DH, Lauschus K, Karpf M. Liver injury tests in hazardous waste workers: the role of obesity. J Occup Med 1989;31:238–242.

104. Guzelian P, Mills S, Fallon HJ. Liver structure and function in print workers exposed to toluene. J Occup Med 1988;30:791–796.

105. Brody DH, Leichter L. Clearance tests of liver function. Med Clin North Am 1979;63:621–630.

106. Tamburro CH, Greenberg RA. Effectiveness of federally required medical laboratory screening in the detection of chemical liver injury. Environ Health Perspect 1981;41:117–122.

107. Dossing M. Noninvasive assessment of microsomal enzyme activity in occupational medicine: present state of knowledge and future perspectives. Int Arch Occup Environ Health 1987;53:205–218.

108. Edling C, Tagesson C. Raised serum bile acid concentrations after occupational exposure to styrene: a possible sign of hepatotoxicity? Br J Ind Med 1984;41:257–259.

109. Isselbacher KJ, LaMont JT. Diagnostic procedures in liver disease. In: Petersdorf RG, Adams RD, et al., eds, Harrison's principles of internal medicine. 10th ed. New York: McGraw-Hill, 1983:1779–83.

110. Wright C, Rivera JC, Baetz JH. Liver function testing in a working population: three strategies to reduce false-positive results. J Occup Med 1988;30:693–697.

111. Reed AJ, Henry RJ, Mason WB: Influence of statistical method used on the resulting estimate of the normal range. Clin Chem 1971;17:275–284.

112. Davidson CS, Leevy CM, Chamberlayne EC, eds. Guidelines for detection of hepatotoxicity due to drugs and chemicals. (NIH Publication No. 79-313), Washington, DC: Dept. of Health Education and Welfare, 1979.

113. WHO. Early Detection of Occupational Diseases. Geneva: World Health Organization, 1986.

11

Pulmonary Toxicology

Lee S. Newman, M.D.

INTRODUCTION

The respiratory tract represents a unique, vast battleground. With its high surface area and rich vasculature, the lung exists in a delicately balanced state of siege. The upper respiratory tract is an important point of entry for toxins which may affect not only the lungs but other organs as well. The outcomes range from minor airway irritation to respiratory insufficiency to life-threatening systemic toxicities.

Inhalation is probably the most important route of exposure in the workplace and is an inescapable route of exposure to toxins in the general environment as well. The list of potential toxins is long, including air pollutants, herbicides, pesticides, cigarette smoke, and occupational hazards. Some exposures produce lung injury with a single inhalation, whereas others may act insidiously, taking effect only after many years of exposure. But however the toxic injury progresses, the pathologic and clinical sequelae can be expected to fall into one or more stereotypic patterns. These include: (a) reversible irritant effects on the lower and/or upper airway; (b) permanent damage to the airways; (c) damage to the gas exchange units of the lung; and (d) oncogenesis. Some agents produce multiple effects. For example, asbestos can cause not only pulmonary fibrosis but lung cancer as well. Cigarette smoke effects range from chronic bronchitis to emphysema and lung cancer. Hydrogen sulfide can produce everything from upper airway irritation to pulmonary edema to respiratory paralysis.

This chapter will focus on the principles of pulmonary toxicity and on the clinical approach to the diagnosis and assessment of injury to the respiratory system. This will be achieved by (a) examining anatomic and physiologic considerations, (b) reviewing the methods available for assessing the effects of chemical agents on the respiratory system, and (c) discussing examples of commonly encountered clinical scenarios.

RESPIRATORY TRACT ANATOMY

Deposition and retention of airborne substances is dictated in part by the anatomy of the respiratory tract. A useful, albeit simplified, approach divides the respiratory tract into three major regions: nasopharyngeal, tracheobronchial, and pulmonary (Fig. 11.1). These subdivisions of the respiratory tract are somewhat arbitrary. Although toxic agents may tend to affect one area more than others, the effects of inhaled agents are commonly detected in varying degrees throughout the respiratory tract. Furthermore, the respiratory tract is more than a series of interconnected tubes. More than 40 types of specialized cells are found in the respiratory tract, and they vary in their susceptibility to inhalation injury.

Nasopharynx

The nasopharynx begins at the anterior nares where air enters the nose in an upward direction and passes horizontally back-ward to join the pharynx. To do so it must negotiate two 90° bends before lining up with the pharyngolaryngotracheal path to the lungs. These bends in airflow with inspiration form the first barrier to the inhalation of airborne toxicants. The air turbulence created by the turbinates causes the larger particles (those in the 5–10 μg range) to be impacted and trapped in mucosa lined by highly vascular, mucous epithelium. The larynx lies in series with the nasopharynx, trachea, and conducting airways. Therefore laryngeal injury may result if the causative agent can successfully negotiate the nasopharynx.

Conducting Airways

Upon passing through the larynx, air enters the trachea where airway dimension is relatively more fixed. The trachea, bronchi, and bronchioles serve as the conducting airways. As the conduit to the gas exchange components of the lungs, these airways are the second major line of defense against inhaled toxicants. The conducting airways are lined by ciliated epithelium. Mucus-secreting cells, goblet cells, brush cells, Clara cells, and a number of other rare cell types produce a thin mucus layer. The cilia on the surface of the airways rhythmically beat to remove particles from the deeper recesses of the lung along the mucociliary escalator. Transport rates along the mucociliary escalator in the trachea and large bronchi can be as rapid as 1–4 cm/minute. Mucociliary transport is a major mechanism for clearing inhaled particles from the conducting airways and hence serves as a major method of pulmonary toxin removal.

The intrapulmonary airways can be subdivided into three major categories: cartilaginous bronchi, membranous or respiratory bronchioles, and the gas exchange ducts and sacs. The upper airway plus the cartilaginous bronchi are responsible for most of the airway's resistance and so-called "dead space" measured by physiologic methods as described below.

Respiratory bronchioles are 0.5-millimeter wide tubes which are short, numerous, and highly distensible. Respiratory bronchioles are lined by some ciliated epithelium and cuboidal epithelium, which flatten into alveolar epithelium as the bronchioles open into the gas exchange portions of the lung. They extend into the alveolar ducts and alveolar sacs, which are thin-walled tubes that serve both as conducting airways and in gas exchange. The sacs are clusters of several alveoli which terminate in one or more alveoli branching from alveolar ducts.

Pulmonary Parenchyma

The alveoli themselves are thin pouches which open at one end into either an alveolar sac or an alveolar duct or directly onto a respiratory bronchiole. Discrete fingers of several hundred alveoli sacs and ducts are referred to as terminal respiratory units (Fig. 11.2).

Gas exchange occurs principally in the alveoli. The barrier

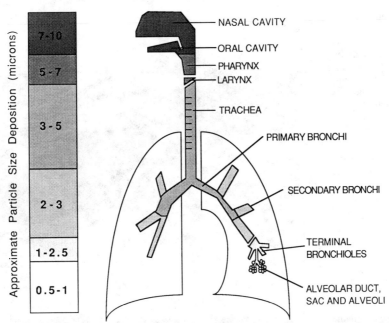

Figure 11.1. Schematic illustration of respiratory tract anatomy and approximate pattern of particle deposition.

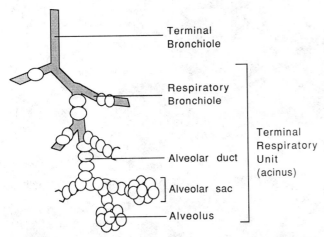

Figure 11.2. Gas exchange occurs starting at the level of the respiratory bronchiole. The terminal respiratory unit (or acinus) is composed of a respiratory bronchiole and the distal alveolar ducts, sacs, and alveoli.

to gas exchange consists of three main layers: the alveolar epithelium, a thin "interstitial" space, and the capillary endothelium (Fig. 11.3). The alveolar epithelium is composed principally of two cell types. Type I alveolar cells form thin sheets of cytoplasm to facilitate gas exchange. Type II alveolar cells are cuboidal and covered with microvilli with cytoplasm rich in lamellar bodies. These are intracellular storage sites for the surfactant which help maintain the pulmonary surface area. Type III alveolar cells are extremely rare but are also found lining the alveoli. Alveolar macrophages in the alveoli ingest foreign particles and play a key role in triggering inflammatory and immunologic reactions in the lung. They contain many lysosomes filled with digestive enzymes, especially acid hydrolases. The macrophages can transverse the alveolar unit via the airway, lymphatics, or pulmonary blood vessels.

The interstitial space normally consists of a few elastic fibers, collagen fibrils, and fibroblasts, among other cell types. Dis-

tortion of this space by fibrosis or inflammatory cell infiltration can produce devastating alterations in the gas exchange capabilities of the lung.

Pathologic processes which affect any part of the terminal respiratory unit—epithelium, interstitium, or vascular endothelium—can produce profound alterations in gas exchange. Denudation of epithelium may alter surface tension and produce intraalveolar exudation of cells and edema; interstitial fibrosis may alter gas diffusion properties; blood flow changes may lead to ventilation/perfusion mismatching, among other physiologic effects.

Pulmonary Circulation and Lymphatics

The pulmonary blood vessels parallel the airways. The bronchial (systemic) circulation provides for the metabolic needs of the airways as far distal as the terminal bronchioles. This bronchial circulation is composed of arteries branching from the aorta or intercostals, sending branches to the trachea and esophagus along the path of the mainstem bronchi and pulmonary vessels to the deep lung and to the visceral pleura. Bronchial capillaries interdigitate in the bronchial submucosa. Venous blood returns from the trachea and cartilaginous bronchi into bronchial veins draining into the azygous or hemiazygous. In the deeper lung, the bronchial blood anastomoses with pulmonary venules, returning to the left side of the heart in venous admixture.

The pulmonary arteries are responsible for carrying oxygen-poor blood to the lung's gas exchange units. They enter the lungs at the hilum adjacent to the main bronchi and travel in parallel with the branches as each airway generation subdivides to the level of the respiratory bronchiole. Venous return similarly parallels bronchi and pulmonary arteries but at some slight distance away from the airways. In the region of gas exchange, the pulmonary arteries branch out to supply each discrete terminal respiratory unit. The pulmonary veins drain parts of several such terminal respiratory units. This pulmonary vas-

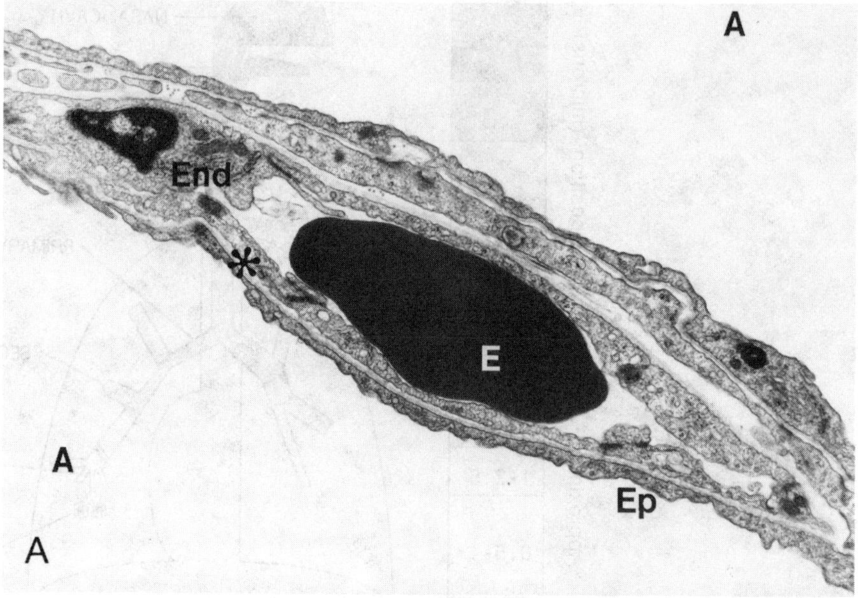

Figure 11.3a. Electron micrograph (12,000X magnification) of alveolar wall from normal lung. Alveolar air space (A) is separated from the alveolar capillary by attenuated epithelium (Ep) and basal lamina (*). An endothelial cell (End) containing an erythrocyte (E) completes the gas exchange unit. Photomicrograph by Sheryl Campbell.

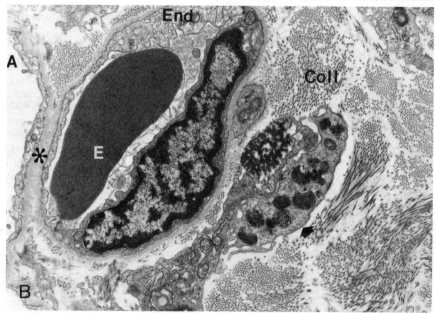

Figure 11.3b. In comparison with the normal alveolar wall in Figure 3a, marked alterations can be seen in this gas exchange unit from a patient with pulmonary fibrosis. The alveolar space (A) at far left abuts an alveolar epithelial cell with thickened basal lamina (*) separating it from the capillary endothelium (End). An erythrocyte (E) is contained within the capillary. Marked collagen deposition (Coll) can be seen to distort the alveolar capillary unit. Arrow indicates a mast cell in the fibrotic interstitium. (Magnification 12,000X) Photomicrograph by Jan Henson.

cular bed is extremely dynamic. The arteries are as distensible as veins in other parts of the body.

The capillary network is an extremely high volume bed where blood slows to allow gas exchange through the tripartite alveolar wall. Capillary networks cross several alveoli and then merge into venules.

The lungs have extensive lymphatics which help maintain the homeostasis of the lung both in terms of volume shifts and defense mechanisms. While most inhaled toxic compounds are carried up the airways by the mucociliary escalator, some are cleared via the lymphatics. The lymphatics can be divided into (a) capillaries, located in the connective tissue but not in the alveolar walls, and (b) collecting lymphatics, which are recognized by their smooth muscle cells and valves and carry lymph from the periphery of the lung to hilar lymph nodes. Anatomically there are interconnected superficial and deep plexuses. The two carry lymph to the hilum or to regional lymph nodes found around the major bronchi and trachea. Lymph ultimately flows into the right lymphatic duct or into the thoracic duct. Patches of lymphoid tissue are also found along the tracheobronchial tree, and such bronchus-associated lymphoid tissue (BALT) serves an important role in immune responses to antigen stimulation.

RESPIRATORY TRACT PHYSIOLOGY

A clinically relevant way to think about respiratory physiology is in terms of (a) ventilation, (b) gas exchange, and (c) nonventilatory functions. This section will discuss these aspects by placing the physiology in context with tests of pulmonary function.

Ventilation

Ventilation is the action of moving air through the nasopharynx and tracheobronchial tree into terminal respiratory units where gas exchange can occur. The ability to ventilate is dependent on mechanical factors such as the ability of the thoracic cage to enlarge and the diaphragm to move downward during inspiration. It is also dependent on the elastic properties of the lung, which include passive recoil of the lung during expiration.

Pathologic processes in the respiratory system may affect ventilation in one of several ways.

1. Mechanical/structural: Conditions that alter neuromuscular function or coordination or that prevent full expansion of the lung (distortion of the thoracic cage, pain, obesity) can limit the ability to fully inspire, thereby reducing ventilation. Such problems may be recognized on pulmonary function tests as a "restrictive" pattern of low lung volumes.
2. Airways: Alterations of the airways either due to acute injury and edema (e.g., alkali and acid burns) or chronic bronchial wall inflammation (e.g., chronic bronchitis from cigarette smoking or asthma from inhalation of sensitizing chemicals) will slow the rate at which air is expired. These abnormalities are recognized on pulmonary function tests as an "obstructive" pattern.
3. Elasticity: Alterations in the compliance properties of the lungs greatly affects ventilation. Increasing stiffness, as seen in fibrotic lung disease, is associated with low lung volumes and an inability to increase volumes upon demand. Airflow itself may be normal; however, the total volume of inspired air will be "restricted." Alternately, decreasing stiffness, as seen in emphysema, is associated with airflow obstruction.

Any of these alterations may be associated with abnormalities in gas exchange discussed below.

MEASUREMENT OF AIRFLOW AND LUNG VOLUMES

Appreciation of how inhalational exposures affect pulmonary performance requires an understanding of the lung capacities, volumes, and airflow as illustrated in Fig. 11.4.

Lung Volumes and Capacities

The amount of air that can be exchanged in and out of the lung with maximum inspiratory and expiratory effort is referred to as the vital capacity (VC). Even with the most complete expiration possible, the lung never completely collapses but retains a small volume referred to as the residual volume (RV). The sum of the vital capacity plus the residual volume is the total lung capacity (TLC). Under normal resting conditions, the amount of air that we breathe in and out of our lungs represents only a part of the vital capacity. This normal amount of air exchange is the tidal volume (TV). The air that is left in the lungs at the end of the tidal breath is the functional residual capacity (FRC). When exertion places greater demands on the body, normal individuals can improve ventilation and thereby improve gas exchange in two ways: by increasing lung volume and by increasing respiratory rate, as discussed below.

Lung volumes can be greatly altered by certain pathologic conditions induced by inhaled toxicants, as illustrated in Fig. 11.5. For example, the lung volumes and capacities can become exceedingly large due to air trapping, as is seen in asthma and chronic obstructive lung disease with emphysema. In such cases, the TLC increases, but a disproportionately great increase occurs in the RV and FRC. Conversely, conditions that produce an increase in lung stiffness (elastic recoil), such as the granulomatous diseases and interstitial fibrosis, cause the TLC and other volumes and capacities to decrease. The net effect is a decrease in the amount of air exchanged in and out of the alveoli. Under such circumstances, the body must rely less on recruitment of lung volume to meet the needs for improving ventilation and increasing gas exchange.

To investigate diseases that may have affected lung volume, it is necessary to perform pulmonary function tests which include the actual measurement of lung volumes, usually by the helium dilution method or the body plethysmograph.

Simple spirometry cannot be used to measure most lung volumes and capacities. Spirometry principally gives information about air flow, with the exception of measuring the vital capacity. But, as can be seen in Fig. 11.5, vital capacity

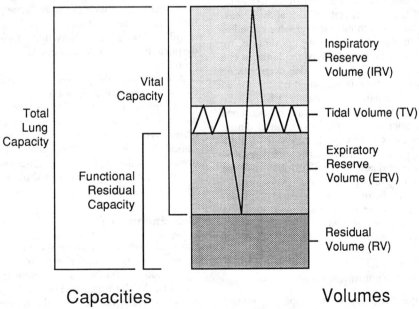

Figure 11.4. Lung volumes and capacities.

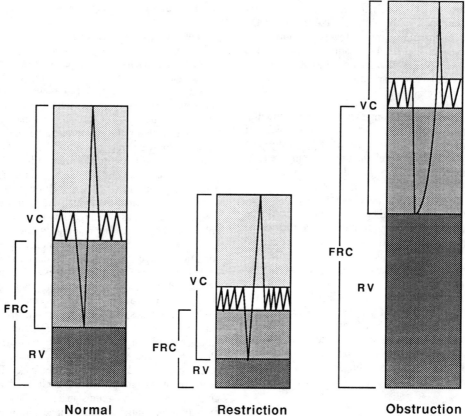

Figure 11.5.   Lung volumes and capacities in normal individuals and in restrictive and obstructive lung disease.

cannot be used alone to distinguish between restrictive disease and air trapping. It only gives a hint of the source of the abnormality.

Airflow

Airflow limitation is a common consequence of many inhalational injuries. Here the simple spirometer is the single most useful tool. With it one can generate a picture of the dynamics of air movement out of the lung. Specifically, it allows measurement of how much air has been moved over what period of time, which translates into air flow rates. By convention, we focus on the expiratory volume forced out of the lungs in one second (FEV_1). But airflow limitation can also occur during other parts of expiration, such as is measured by the forced expiratory flow in the middle half of expiration (FEF_{25-75}). To make the most out of the FEV_1, it should always be examined in relation to the total amount of air that was expired during the test, the forced vital capacity (FVC). The FEV_1/FVC ratio allows us to determine not only whether airflow is decreased but whether the decrease is due to a parallel decrease in the total amount of air in the lung or is a true obstruction of airflow.

By performing spirometry before and after the use of a bronchodilator, it is possible to detect whether airflow obstruction is fixed or whether there is an element of reversibility suggesting underlying bronchospasm and reactive airways disease (asthma).

Exercise Physiology and Ventilation

Since ventilation is a dynamic process, the simple assessment of resting lung volumes and resting airflow frequently does not

give a complete picture of the severity of an insult to the respiratory system. Exercise studies help to assess what ventilatory reserve the pulmonary system has following inhalational injury.

To maximize ventilation, an individual has two options: (a) increase respiratory rate and/or (b) increase the amount of air exchanged with each breath. Both increase when normal individuals exercise. Normal individuals can triple or quadruple their tidal volume with exercise. Some patients with interstitial lung disease have normal "resting" lung volumes but fail to recruit additional respiratory units during exercise, leading to dyspnea, high respiratory rate, and possibly even gas exchange problems.

A second type of ventilatory abnormality detected by exercise studies but which is not always obvious on resting studies is referred to as exercise-induced bronchospasm. Individuals with reactive airways disease develop nonspecific airways hyperreactivity, meaning that, even if one specific toxic agent caused the asthma, bronchospasm can now be triggered by a number of other irritants. Exercise itself can provoke bronchospasm, which can be detected by measuring airflow before and after exercise.

Gas Exchange

Gas exchange occurs along the entire alveolar surface, with oxygen moving by diffusion from the alveolar side into the blood, and carbon dioxide diffusing from the blood into the alveolus. As illustrated in Fig. 11.3a, the gases must diffuse across the pulmonary epithelial cell, the basement membrane, through the interstitial space, the basement membrane underlying the endothelial cells, and through the capillary endothelium. Oxygen must then exchange through the plasma and across the membrane of the red blood cell in order to combine with hemoglobin to form oxyhemoglobin.

Alterations in diffusion of gases can occur due to pathologic changes in any of these layers. The classic example is thickening of the interstitial space as seen in pulmonary fibrosis, or replacement of the normally attenuated alveolar epithelial cells by cuboidal shaped cells as seen in diffuse alveolar epithelial damage from chemical inhalation. Gas exchange abnormalities may also occur due to alterations in the matching between ventilation and perfusion, as seen in emphysema, where large regions of lung may be perfused but not adequately ventilated.

The major measurable physiologic effects of impaired gas exchange include: (a) abnormal ventilation due to increased respiratory rate and/or attempts to increase tidal volume; (b) hypoxemia at rest and/or with exercise; and c) exercise limitation, related to an early switch to anaerobic metabolism and subsequent lactic acidosis. These abnormalities can occur in association with lung diseases that produce restrictive, obstructive, or mixed patterns on pulmonary function testing. For example, both interstitial fibrosis and emphysema can cause gas exchange abnormalities.

DIFFUSING CAPACITY

In estimating the extent of gas exchange abnormalities, clinicians rely on several tests, including the use of the carbon monoxide diffusing capacity. In order to estimate the diffusing capacity of the lung, one must know the amount of gas that is diffusing across the barrier in some unit of time. One must also know the mean difference in the partial pressures of the gas between the alveolus and the capillary. The calculation of the actual mean difference in partial pressures for oxygen between alveolus and capillary is difficult, since the partial pressures vary across the course of the capillary. In contrast carbon monoxide has such high affinity for hemoglobin that the mean gradient is easier to estimate. This is the main reason that carbon monoxide is typically used to assess diffusing capacity of the lungs (DL_{CO}). The single breath technique, although easier to perform than the multiple breath (steady-state) technique, is performed under conditions of breathholding and therefore may not be as accurate a reflection of the true diffusion abnormality. When abnormal, the DL_{CO} is helpful, but it is a relatively late and insensitive indicator of gas exchange abnormalities in some disease states.

ARTERIAL BLOOD GAS ANALYSIS

To obtain an overall estimate of gas exchange, most clinical laboratories perform arterial blood gas analysis. The resting arterial blood gas provides information about the partial pressure of gases (oxygen and carbon dioxide) dissolved in the blood and can be used to estimate the alveolar-arterial oxygen difference $(A-a)DO_2$. In normal persons this A-a gradient is usually between 2 and 17 torr at room air but widens in pathologic states that affect gas exchange.

Patients can have normal resting arterial blood gases and still have significant gas exchange abnormalities. For this reason, the estimation of gas exchange during exercise can become especially important. If abnormalities in gas exchange are not evident during exercise, then there is not a clinically significant gas exchange problem. Whether performed on a cycle ergometer or on a treadmill, the information obtained about an individual's pulmonary impairment and gas exchange abnormalities is invaluable. If the study is performed correctly, it is one of the most sensitive indicators of underlying respiratory disease. Such studies provide information about the level of exercise which an individual can maximally tolerate and about how much of the exercise limitation is related to gas exchange, ventilatory disorders, or cardiovascular disorders. Although time-consuming and expensive, exercise tests play an important role in the long-term assessment and follow-up of patients with toxicologic lung injury.

Nonventilatory Functions of the Lung

Aside from ventilation and gas exchange, the respiratory system has several other important functions. These include the production and secretion of hormones and mediators, biotransformation of chemical compounds, and removal of vasoactive agents from the bloodstream. Examples of the ability of the lungs to metabolize foreign chemicals include the handling of basic amines. There are enzymes in the lung capable of transforming substances such as aromatic polycyclic hydrocarbons. However, compared with other organs such as the liver, the lung plays a small role in the biotransformation of drugs and toxic chemicals. It must be remembered, however, that the lung is capable of selective uptake of some compounds, such as paraquat, into agents that produce pulmonary toxicity. With regard to removal of vasoactive agents, the classic example is the conversion of the polypeptide angiotension I into angiotension II as the enzyme passes through the lung. The converting enzyme is found in pulmonary capillary cells. Major inactivation of 5-hydroxytryptine also occurs in the lung. A number of prostaglandins are inactivated or removed from circulation in the lung. As more is learned about these nonventilatory functions, it becomes clear that injury to the lung may have wide-ranging implications for the system as a whole.

DEPOSITION AND CLEARANCE OF INHALED SUBSTANCES

Toxic materials in inhaled air come in basically two forms: gases and aerosols. Aerosols are droplets of liquid or are particles suspended in gas.

The site of deposition for inhaled gases is largely determined by the solubility of the gas in the aqueous layer of the respiratory mucosa. Gases that are extremely water-soluble, such as ammonia and sulfur dioxide, will be deposited and removed predominantly by the upper respiratory tract. Thus they exert their main toxic effects on the upper airways and will only damage the peripheral air spaces when inhaled in high concentrations. Alternatively, gases that are of low water solubility, such as oxides of nitrogen and phosgene, may predominantly injure the pulmonary parenchyma. The less soluble the gas, the greater the potential for damage at the level of the terminal respiratory unit.

Many factors influence the deposition of particulate matter. Factors include: (a) the characteristics of the aerosol itself, (b) the anatomy of the respiratory tract, and (c) the breathing pattern of the individual. The size of the particle is usually the predominant factor affecting deposition, although particle density and shape also contribute to the pattern seen. The majority of particles greater than approximately 10 microns in diameter are successfully filtered out by the nasopharynx. Particles in the range of 0.5–3 microns are deposited predominantly in distal airways and alveoli. Particles less than approximately 0.5 microns in diameter

Table 11.1   Identifying Occupational and Environmental Causes of Lung Disease

---

Occupational history
  Chronologic job list
  Potential exposures from each job

Environmental history
  Dwelling location, heating and ventilation, furnishings, fabrics
  Chemicals: insecticides, herbicides, cleaning agents
  Hobbies and associated exposures
  Pets
  Habits: smoking, illicit drugs
  Other inhabitants and their exposures

Biologic monitoring
  Medical examination
  Lung tissue analysis for mineral content
  Arterial blood gas analysis (e.g., carboxyhemoglobin)
  Immunologic testing

Worksite or home evaluation
  Material Safety Data Sheet review for evidence of pulmonary irritants or sensitizers
  Discuss job exposures with plant foreman, supervisor, or health and safety personnel
  Review industrial hygiene data if available from company or from federal agency investigations
  Conduct walkthrough investigation
  Survey workforce and perform atmospheric analyses if indicated by walkthrough findings

---

are mainly exhaled without significant deposition (see Fig. 11.1). Details of the physics of particle deposition have been well reviewed elsewhere and are beyond the scope of this chapter.

Another major determinant of how inhaled agents affect the respiratory tract pertains to the types of lung cells found at the deposition site. Cells vary in their susceptibility to toxic agents. For example, not only is the upper airway and tracheobronchial tree the site of deposition of sulfur dioxide, but smooth muscle cells located there appear to be especially susceptible to toxic injury.

Clearance of particles is also of great importance in determining the toxic effects of inhaled agents. Particle clearance can refer to elimination of particles from the body or to their translocation to other organs following their initial deposition in the respiratory tract. In general, highly water-soluble particles and gases are absorbed through the epithelial layer into the bloodstream near where they have been deposited. The clearance of insoluble particles is dependent on where they impact. If they are deposited in the nasopharynx and tracheobronchial tree where there is ciliated epithelium and a layer of mucus, then most other particles will be transported up the mucociliary escalator where they are swallowed or expectorated. At the alveolar level, where there is no ciliated epithelium, the defense against foreign matter is largely in the hands of alveolar macrophages. These alveolar macrophages phagocytose particles, destroy microorganisms, and may then migrate up the tracheobronchial tree or into the lymphatics. Some particles engulfed by the macrophages are not successfully digested and may cause cell lysis. The fate of such particles is less certain. Some of the dead macrophages and associated particles are presumably removed by tracheobronchial clearance. Some are retained and become part of an ongoing pulmonary inflammatory reaction. The death of alveolar macrophages and the subsequent liberation of cellular products

may, in fact, trigger a number of pathologic responses, including fibrosis, emphysema, and granuloma formation. Neutrophils also play an important role in the handling of particles in the lung, especially after the inflammatory reaction has commenced. And some foreign particles in the alveolar space also may pass into the pulmonary lymphatics or eventually dissolve and diffuse into the capillary blood.

TOOLS IN ASSESSMENT OF PULMONARY TOXICITY

The past 20 years have seen significant advances in the tools available to clinicians for the assessment of toxic injury in the lung. In a field which has been largely dominated by the chest roentgenogram. the advent of computed tomography (CT) scans, radionuclide studies, the fiberoptic bronchoscope, and fiberoptic laryngoscope have been major advances. This section will review the application of these various tools and discuss some of their limitations as applied to the evaluation of toxic injuries. Subsequent sections will illustrate the clinical application of these tools in toxic injury evaluations.

Occupational and Environmental Exposure Assessment

HISTORY

One of the first steps in the evaluation of an individual with suspected pulmonary injury from injury from a toxic exposure is to determine the exposure. Sometimes it is easy, as when a worker gets sprayed in the face with ammonia and promptly develops respiratory symptoms. But more often it is not a trivial task. It requires a careful environmental and occupational history. When the disease onset is delayed or the suspected exposure is complex, the physician must generate a database that includes both the jobs that the individual has had as well as the types of exposures which he/she may have experienced on those jobs. The simplest and most systematic way of approaching the occupational history is to generate a chronologic list of all jobs. One can then elaborate on each of those jobs by asking specific questions about the exposures encountered. This can be a time-consuming task, but such detective work is often rewarding.

It is also important to obtain information about non-work-related exposures: medications, pets, hobbies, smoking habits. For example, a patient was diagnosed with occupational asthma due to the inhalation of toluene diisocyanate (TDI), a component of an automotive spray paint. He left his job, but continued to be exposed by doing spray painting in his garage as a "hobby." Part-time dental technicians may work out of basement shops producing amalgams that contain beryllium, which can induce chronic granulomatous disease. Weekend welders run some risk of developing metal fume fever which their clinician might erroneously call "the flu." Secondary or "passive" exposure to toxic substances can occur if carried home by family members. This occurred historically with asbestos fibers on the clothes of asbestos workers, causing asbestosis and cancer in family members. Smoking history should always be obtained. Cigarette smoke can sometimes cause the same symptoms as those seen with other exposures and can have additive or multiplicative effects when combined with toxicants.

MATERIAL SAFETY DATA SHEETS

Sometimes it is apparent that there is a hazard in the workplace which has caused pulmonary symptoms, but additional information is needed to help pinpoint the specific cause. Some investigative options are listed in Table 11.1. Workers frequently do not know all the chemicals that they come in contact with and cannot fully assess the associated risks. Material Safety Data Sheets (MSDS) form a crucial link between the exposures and the diagnosis. MSDSs are required by law to be present and available in the workplace. We routinely review MSDSs when patients present with possible work-related symptoms for indirect evidence of exposure to sensitizers and pulmonary irritants.

ON-SITE INVESTIGATION

In the occupational medicine clinic setting, one further step in linking a patient's disease and workplace involves on-site investigation. Walk-throughs of a plant can usually be arranged with the plant manager and commonly provide insights unobtainable in the doctor's examining room. In our own practice we work as a team with industrial hygienists. When needed, it is possible to do on-site atmosphere analysis and obtain information on the health of other workers. The clinician should inquire whether any federal agencies have investigated the workplace. On such occasions, additional information can be obtained by reviewing reports from Occupational Safety and Health Administration (OSHA) or National Institute of Occupational Safety and Health (NIOSH). Discussion of atmosphere analysis and survey methodology are beyond the scope of this chapter.

By doing additional homework and field work, the clinician has the opportunity to not only make a more firm diagnosis of the patient's condition, but can potentially help to prevent other individuals from developing disease in the workplace.

DETECTION OF MINERALS IN THE LUNG

Analysis of the dust content of tissue specimens can serve as another way of confirming exposure. If a large piece of material such as an entire lobe of lung or at least several grams of lung tissue can be obtained, the tissue can be treated chemically or ashed to remove organic material. Mineral content of the remaining inorganic matter is then analyzed. The inorganic particles can be measured for size and number, and their mineral content determined. Most of these methods destroy the tissue and therefore do not allow us to observe how the dust burden correlates with anatomy and pathology. There are numerous methodologic and standardization problems with digested tissue analysis for mineral/fiber content. These include potential sampling error and variability in digestion techniques, fiber extraction, counting, and analysis methods.

Alternatively, tissue can be sectioned for light microscopy or for scanning or transmission electron microscopy. Microscopy methods, while subject to significant sampling error due to the very small amount of tissue being studied, can yield a great deal of information about particle size, composition, and crystalling structure. Microscopy potentially gives critical information about the relationship of particle to pathology but provides a relatively poor estimate of the amount of mineral present.

Light Microscopy

The light microscope will detect only large particles which can be either identified by their polarization characteristics or staining properties. Some crystalling minerals such as talc and silica are birefringent, when examined under polarized light. Carbonaceous dusts such as graphite, carbon particles, and coal dust are readily seen using routine histologic staining methods, especially as they are ingested by alveolar macrophages. Asbestos bodies (ferruginous bodies) can be seen on routine hematoxylin and eosin stained sections, but are better seen using iron stains (e.g., Prussian blue) due to their ferritin coating. Unfortunately the light microscope only will detect particles greater than approximately 0.5 microns in size.

Electron Microscopy

The transmission electron microscope allows the pathologist to see the shadows of electron-dense materials as the electron beam is passed through the tissue specimen. The scanning electron microscope generates a three-dimensional image as the electron beam reflects off of the surface of the tissue. These methods can be linked with an electron probe, crystallographic deraction methods, and x-ray energy spectrometry to give more specific information about the actual mineral content of the particles being observed. Unfortunately these analyses are expensive, time-consuming, and subject to sampling error. Also, certain lightweight minerals are poorly detected. These tools are finding exciting research applications. In the future they may have greater clinical application in improving the specificity of our diagnoses of inhalationally induced lung disease.

Clinical Examination

The patient's symptoms should be carefully reviewed with at least three goals in mind: (a) identifying the level of the respiratory tract which has been affected, e.g., nasopharynx versus bronchial tree; (b) assessing the timing of onset, latency, and severity of the illness; and (c) guiding further diagnostic testing. Details of the signs and symptoms produced by various toxic injuries to the respiratory system are described in subsequent chapters.

The physical examination may provide a few crucial clues. Patients with asbestosis or other pneumoconioses may have dry rales heard at the lung bases upon inspiration. The patient with occupational asthma may have wheezing heard on auscultation; however, given the reversible nature of reactive airways disease there may be clinical examinations which are completely normal. An individual who has developed acute mucosal injury due to an alkali or acid burn may have stridor. However, none of these clinical findings is pathognomonic for a specific toxic insult.

In any case of suspected toxic injury, a complete exam—beyond just the respiratory tract—must be performed. Are there signs of chronic pulmonary insufficiency such as clubbing and cyanosis? Are there dermatitic changes that suggest a common sensitizer of lung and skin? Are other mucous membranes such as the conjuctivae affected as well? Is there blood in the stool due to an asbestos-related gastrointestinal malignancy? A thorough examination is essential.

Chest Imaging

RADIOGRAPHY

The chest radiograph is one of the cornerstones in the assessment of toxic injuries to the respiratory tract. Although evidence of obstructive lung disease can be found on chest radiograph, the greater application pertains to toxic injuries which produce interstitial infiltrates, such as the pneumoconioses. Table 11.2 lists the common radiographic findings in occupational and environmental lung diseases. Classically we look at (a) shape of opacities (e.g., irregular versus rounded); (b) size of opacities; (c) profusion (the number of opacities per unit lung); (d) the extent and location of the infiltrates (e.g., upper lobe versus lower lobe predominance); and (e) presence of ancillary findings such as pleural plaques, adenopathy, pulmonary hypertension, cardiac enlargement, and Kerley's lines. These five main observations form the basis of a formal reading system known as the International Labor Organization (ILO) 1980 Classification of Radiographs of the Pneumoconioses. Although designed for the systematic recording of radiographic changes caused by inhalation of mineral dusts, the principles can be applied in reading films from any of the diffuse interstitial diseases listed in Table 11.2.

By this classification, small opacities (less than 10 millimeters in diameter) are described as ''rounded'' as seen in diseases such as silicosis, or ''irregular'' as seen in asbestosis. The letters ''p,'' ''q,'' and ''r'' are used to subdivide rounded opacities according to size—up to 1.5, 1.5–3.0, and 3.0–10.0 millimeters, respectively. Similarly, the letters ''s,'' ''t,'' and ''u'' describe the predominant sizes of small irregular opacities. In the classification system each radiograph's opacities are classified according to the most common and next most common shape and size. For example, ''s/t'' indicates that the majority of opacities are size s, and the second most common size is t. Profusion, the number of small rounded or small irregular opacities per lung zone, is divided into four main categories from 0 through 3 and these are further divided along a 12-point scale ranging from 0/− to 3/+. To score the extent of involvement, each lung is arbitrarily divided into three zones by horizontal imaginary lines one third and two thirds of the distance between the apex of the lung and the dome of the diaphragm.

The ILO classification also systematically describes large opacities (greater than 10 millimeters) as well as pleural plaques and other abnormalities. A set of standard ILO reference films are routinely used by readers in judging the shape, size, and profusion of opacities on a given chest radiograph.

The opacity's shape (round versus irregular) is of limited utility. Most interstitial lung diseases can present with a range of opacities from pure round to reticular nodular to pure linear or irregular. Even in simple silicosis—the classic example of rounded opacities—the opacities can assume a more reticular appearance on the chest radiograph, depending on factors such as dust burden and duration of illness.

Distribution of diffuse infiltrates may be of slightly greater predictive value, although again there are many exceptions. Opacities are found throughout the lungs in most interstitial lung diseases. However, in a number of toxicant-induced diseases there is a lower lung predominance. Examples include nitrofurantoin-induced disease, metallic mercury embolism, interstitial pulmonary edema, pulmonary fibrosis, asbestosis, and talcosis. Relatively few of the diffuse interstitial lung diseases will show an upper lung field predominance, with two notable exceptions from the standpoint of toxic inhalation: silicosis and chronic beryllium disease.

Hilar adenopathy, with or without ''egg shell'' calcifications, is seen in silicosis as well as in some cases of coalworkers' pneumoconiosis and occasionally in chronic beryllium disease.

A pattern of acute pulmonary edema in a patient without trauma or heart disease raises the specter of chemical exposure. The typical pattern will be that of diffuse fluffy alveolar infiltrates but with a normal heart size. Drugs that can cause a noncardiogenic pulmonary edema pattern include amphotericin B, aspirin, hydrochlorothiazide, lidocaine, major tranquilizers, opiates, and sedatives as well as sympathomimetic agents. Alveolar hemorrhage is often indistinguishable from the pulmonary edema pattern on chest radiograph. This can result from a number of exposures including agents such as D-penicillamine and trimellitic anhydride.

The limitations of the chest radiograph need to be acknowledged. First, the chest radiograph often correlates poorly with the clinical activity of interstitial lung diseases. For example, the chest radiograph may be markedly abnormal in coal workers who have normal pulmonary function. A number of inhaled dusts may produce ''benign pneumoconioses.'' When dusts are radiodense, they produce radiographic changes but with little or no pathologic or physiologic abnormality upon further investigation. Conversely, some patients with significant pulmonary embarrassment have normal appearing chest radiographs. Radiographically inapparent clinical illness can occur in patients with farmers lung or other hypersensitivity pneumonitides, beryllium disease, and asbestosis.

A second major limitation of the chest radiograph is its lack of specificity. Many types of injury produce similar radiographic changes. This lack of specificity prevents us from relying too heavily on the chest radiograph in differential diagnosis of chest disease. For example, although it is classically taught that silicosis produces small rounded opacities predominantly in the upper and midlung fields, there are many cases described in which the disease may have lower lobe predominance with a more reticular appearance on chest radiograph. Asbestosis is classically credited with producing small irregular opacities in the lower lung fields; however, this disease can produce mid- and upper lung field predominant disease. Even the presence of pleural plaques, which many occupational medicine physicians equate with asbestos exposure, has limited specificity. There are many pulmonary diseases (related or unrelated to toxicologic insult) which can produce bilateral pleural disease, including silicosis, diatomaceous earth pneumoconiosis, and chronic beryllium disease. Previous chest surgery or chest trauma may also confound the assessment of pleural disease. However, in the proper clinical context, presence of plaques and infiltrates in an asbestos-exposed individual may be sufficient to diagnose asbestosis.

GALLIUM SCINTIGRAPHY

Gallium-67 imaging has been applied in the examination of inflammatory lung disease, but has relatively limited proven application. The limitations of this nuclear medicine technique are based on its lack of specificity, and the fact that the examination takes a long time to perform, with useful data obtainable at earliest 18–24 hours after injection of the gallium-67 tracer. In principle the gallium acts by binding to transferrin. In inflammatory lesions such as malignancies, infections, and chronic inflammation such as granulomatous disease, the gallium

Table 11.2. Common Radiograpic Findings in Occupational and Environmental Lung Disease

Radiographic Finding	Disease
Diffuse infiltrates, interstitial pattern (nodular, reticular, reticulonodular)	Aluminum lung (Shaver's disease) Asbestosis Bronchiolitis obliterans Chronic beryllium disease Chronic brucellosis Coalworker's pneumoconiosis Drug-induced disease (e.g., bleomycin, methotrexate, gold, busulfan) Extrinsic allergic alveolitis (hypersensitivity pneumonitis) Fuller's earth Hard-metal disease (cobalt) Histoplasmosis Kaolinosis (china clay) Mixed dust fibrosis Oxygen toxicity Paraquat poisoning Pneumoconiosis due to radiopaque dusts (siderosis, silver, stannosis, baritosis, antimony, rare earth pneumoconiosis, titanium, zirconium, chromite) Radiation pneumonitis Silo-filler's disease (oxides of nitrogen) (late phase) Talcosis Thesaurosis (hair spray) Vineyard sprayers' lung (copper sulfate) Zinc chloride
Diffuse infiltrates, acinar/alveolar pattern (including pulmonary edema)	Acetaldehyde Acrolein (acrylic aldehyde) Acute aspiration (water, alcohol, kerosene) Acute cadmium poisoning Acute beryllium disease Acute silicoproteinosis Adult respiratory distress syndrome Ammonia Burns Chlorine Cobalt Fire smoke Hydrocarbon pneumonitis Hydrogen chloride Hydrogen fluoride Hydrogen sulfide Hydrogen phosphide (phosphine) Hydrogen selenide Lithium hydride Manganese Mercury vapors Methyl bromide Nickel carbonyl Organophosphates Oxides of nitrogen (silo-filler's disease) Ozone Paraquat poisoning Phosgene Polymer fume fever Selenium Sulfur dioxide Titanium tetrachloride Toluene diisocyanate Trimellitic anhydride lung disease/anemia Zinc chloride
Diffuse infiltrates, "mixed" acinar and reticulonodular pattern	Chronic beryllium disease Drug-induced disease (methotrexate, bleomycin) Extrinsic allergic alveolitis (hypersensitivity pneumonitis) Pulmonary edema (many causes)
Segmental consolidation	Occupational infections (including brucellosis, tularemia, anthrax) Psittacosis-ornithosis Vanadium (heavy exposure)

continues

Table 11.2.   *Continued*

Radiographic Finding	Disease
Cystic or cavitary lesions	Coalworker's pneumoconiosis, complicated (large opacities)
	Caplan's nodules
	Coccididiomycosis
	Cystic bronchiectasis
	Histoplasmosis
	Silicosis, complicated (large opacities)
	Silicotuberculosis
Solitary or multiple pulmonary nodules	Coalworker's pneumoconiosis
	Progressive massive fibrosis
	Caplan's necrobiotic nodules
	Complicated (large opacities)
	Cryptococcosis
	Histoplasmosis
	Occupational or environmental lung malignancies
	Silicosis
	Complicated (large opacities)
	Rheumatoid silicotic nodules
Hyperinflation	Chronic obstructive lung disease
	Emphysema (tobacco exposure, possibly cadmium)
	Occupational asthma (many causes)
Hilar and mediastinal lymphadenopathy	Chronic beryllium disease
	Mushroom workers' lung (rare in other extrinsic allergic alveolitides)
	Occupational infections (including brucellosis, tularemia, histoplasmosis, coccidiodomycosis)
	Silicosis
Mediastinal widening	Aluminum lung (Shaver's disease)
	Anthrax
Pleural effusions	Asbestos exposure
	Asbestosis
	Mesothelioma
Pleural plaques	Asbestos exposure
	Chronic beryllium disease
	Diatomaceous earth lung (free silica)
	Extrinsic allergic alveolitis (chronic)

is transferred from transferrin to local iron-binding proteins such as lactoferrin. These proteins are found on the surface of macrophages or in the granules of leukocytes. The net effect is localization of gallium-67 at sites of cellular inflammation.

In practice, we have found gallium scanning to be useful when routine radiographic procedures have been unrevealing but the clinical scenario still suggests that there is an active pulmonary process. Under such circumstances, a positive gallium scan may help the clinician decide to proceed with more invasive and specific tests such as lung biopsy.

COMPUTERIZED TOMOGRAPHY

(CT scan) has become an indispensable tool for imaging the chest. It provides information not only about the pulmonary parenchyma but also about the mediastinum, pleura, and chest wall. Improvements in resolution, in particular the advent of "thin section" high resolution CT scanning, now allows visualization of even minute and subtle interstitial lung abnormalities. In some cases the CT scan's level of detection is far superior to that of the conventional chest radiograph. With it we visualize subtle plaques and effusions from asbestos, conglomerate masses from silicosis, and even small cavities from silicotuberculosis which would otherwise evade early detection. With high resolution CT scans it is now easy to diagnose bronchiectasis and to spot radiographically unapparent interstitial infiltrates. CT scans have also demonstrated great sensitivity in imaging the upper respiratory tract, including the sinuses, posterior pharynx, and tracheobronchial tree.

The role of CT scanning in comparison to the use of magnetic resonance imaging (MRI) has yet to be fully explored in relation to the respiratory tract. At its current level of development, the MRI has no advantages over CT of the lungs, mediastinum, and hilar regions. However, for the present, CT scans can be more rapidly performed, are more accessible to most clinicians, and provide better resolution of intrathoracic structures than MRI. Future work with magnetic resonance may change this status.

Physiologic Assessment

Pulmonary function tests provide clues to the type of toxicologic insult to the respiratory tract, as discussed above. Table 11.3 lists the common physiologic findings in a number of occupational and environmental lung diseases. But by and large the main value of pulmonary function tests and exercise physiology studies lies more in the assessment of degree of impairment and response to treatment than in diagnosis. Physiologic assessment is only a guide to determining the underlying diagnosis, and for that matter should also only be considered a guide in determining an individual's level of impairment and disability.

The clinician must be aware of the limitations of each test. Spirometry and measurements of lung volumes are greatly in-

Table 11.3. Examples of Physiologic Abnormalities In Occupational and Environmental Lung Disease

Airflow limitation (obstruction)
  Without bronchodilator response:
    Bronchiectasis (e.g., ammonia)
    Chronic bronchitis (e.g., irritant dusts and fumes, coal dust, tobacco smoke)
    Chronic obstructive lung disease (e.g., tobacco smoke)
    Emphysema (e.g., tobacco smoke, possibly cadmium, nitrogen dioxide)
    Upper airway obstruction (e.g., tracheal stenosis following chemical burn to airway; laryngeal malignancy due to asbestos)
  With bronchodilator response
    Reactive airway disease (asthma) (see Table 11.4).
    Reactive Airways Disease Syndrome (RADS) (e.g., high dose, single exposure to airways irritants)
Restrictive physiology
  Bronchiolitis obliterans (e.g., oxides of nitrogen, sulfur dioxide)
  Chronic beryllium disease
  Chronic extrinsic allergic alveolitis (e.g., avian proteins, fungal spores)
  Hardmetal disease (giant cell pneumonitis due to cobalt)
  Interstitial fibrosis (e.g., methotrexate, nitrofurantoin, oxygen toxicity)
  Pneumoconioses (e.g., asbestosis, silicosis)
  Talcosis
  Pleural disease (e.g., mesothelioma, diffuse pleural thickening)
Mixed disorder (obstructive plus restrictive physiology)
  Asbestosis
  Bronchiolitis obliterans
  Chronic beryllium disease
  Extrinsic allergic alveolitis
  Silicosis
  Tobacco smoke plus toxicant exposure

fluenced by factors such as: (a) patient effort and understanding of the testing procedure; (b) skill of the technician performing the testing; (c) the equipment and testing methods being used; (d) standardization and quality control of the equipment used in physiologic assessment; (e) variation in definition of physiologic abnormalities by various interpreters of pulmonary function tests. This is a large and complex subject; however, a few examples may help to clarify the major issues confronted in the application of pulmonary function testing.

SPIROMETRY

Simple spirometry is commonly used in industry and in clinical practice as a screening test. Unfortunately even with NIOSH-certified spirometry technicians, there is still a great deal of mediocre data being generated. Even with good quality spirometry, simple spirometry only gives the clinician a few key pieces of information: (a) low FEV_1/FVC ratio indicates airflow obstruction; (b) low flows during the middle half of expiration (the FEF_{25-75}) also help indicate airflow limitation; (c) improvement in FEV_1/FVC after bronchodilators indicates reversible airflow obstruction; (d) serial decrements in FEV_1/FVC ratio on annual examinations is a useful indicator of disease progression; (e) used pre- and postexposure, FEV_1/FVC can help to define the cause of airflow obstruction; (f) low FVC may imply restrictive physiology but cannot and should not be relied on as the sole indicator of lung volume status.

Normal spirometry does not exclude the possibility of significant, impairing lung disease. It does not give sufficient information about lung volumes, gas exchange, or response to specific triggers of asthma. Furthermore, a single set of normal spirometry values does not exclude possible asthma. Since airflow limitation can be completely reversible, serial measurements may be required.

A frequently encountered scenario is one in which an individual has inhaled a suspected toxic agent and presents with symptoms of shortness of breath, chest tightness, or wheezing. Spirometry is normal, with no bronchodilator response. The clinician might conclude erroneously that there is nothing physiologically wrong with the individual, on the basis of a single clinical interview. However, when evaluated during a time of significant symptoms, the patient's pulmonary function tests may show a dramatic airflow limitation. If the spirometry is still "normal," but symptoms persist, several options are available for ruling-out occult asthma. These include:

1. *Nonspecific inhalation challenge testing*, using methacholine or histamine as the challenge substance—individuals with airways hyperreactivity will develop transient bronchospasm and a concomitant drop in airflow upon inhaling these compounds.
2. *Peak flow meter recording*—measurements of peak flow can be conveniently performed by the individual during symptomatic and asymptomatic periods. If significant variation in peak flows is recorded by the patient, this serves as a clue to airways hyperreactivity. Furthermore, if used correctly, peak flows can help identify specific patterns of hyperreactivity as discussed below.
3. *Airways resistance and conductance measurement*—an increasing number of clinical pulmonary physiology laboratories have the capacity to detect airflow limitation both by flow measurements and by directly measuring airways resistance and airways specific conductance. The principle is simple: high airways resistance and low conductance imply narrowing of the conducting airways. The advantage of measuring specific conductance and airways resistance is that these tests are often more sensitive than FEV_1 in detecting airflow abnormalities. They are also more effort-independent than other measures of airflow. Like measures of airflow, they can be performed both pre- and postbronchodilator.

LUNG VOLUME ASSESSMENT

Measurement of the lung compartments (volumes and capacities) are generally made by one of several methods, including helium dilution, nitrogen wash, and body plethysmography. The latter is by far the fastest method. It is more expensive but only slightly more difficult to perform compared with inert gas methods. Some patients are unable to use the "body box" due to claustrophobia, obesity, or skeletal deformity. Again, the quality of results is dependent on patient understanding, effort, and technician skill. When assessing for the presence of either air trapping or restrictive lung disease, one of these methods should be used to generate an accurate picture of lung volumes. As in spirometry, normal lung volume alone does not fully exclude the possibility of significant underlying lung disease.

A common scenario in which lung volumes are normal but fail to identify serious underlying toxicologic injury is seen with interstitial lung diseases such as pneumoconioses. A patient with asbestosis may have "normal lung volumes," leading the clinician to conclude erroneously that this individual is unimpaired. However, individuals with pneumoconioses or other interstitial lung diseases may have normal lung volumes but severe derangement of gas exchange. When the clinical suspicion is high, the workup should not stop with lung volumes but should include tests designed to examine abnormalities of gas exchange.

GAS EXCHANGE

The ultimate task of the respiratory system is to regulate oxygen and carbon dioxide tension in the blood. As such, tests that measure abnormalities in gas exchange are critical to the assessment of respiratory damage. As discussed earlier in this chapter, gas exchange is evaluated clinically using the DL_{CO} and arterial blood gas determinations at rest and during exercise. The DL_{CO} provides a relatively good approximation of gas exchange abnormalities due to ventilation-perfusion mismatching, venous admixture (shunting), and barriers to diffusion of gases. But it does not separate among these causes. Simply put, the diffusing capacity is a measure of the ability of the respiratory system to conduct air from alveolus to capillary blood. The test is performed by either a single breath or steady-state technique. The latter is preferred because breathholding creates artificial conditions in which to measure diffusion and also may be more difficult for patients with lung disease. A number of theoretical considerations must be taken into account in such testing, including the hemoglobin, alveolar volume, and temperature. DL_{CO} has limited sensitivity and should not be singularly relied upon in the estimation of pulmonary gas exchange.

A resting room air arterial blood gas can be extremely useful and sometimes is the only clue to abnormal gas exchange even in the face of normal lung volumes and normal diffusing capacity. From the blood gas one should not only examine the absolute partial pressures of oxygen and carbon dioxide, but also calculate the A-a gradient. This alveolar-arterial gradient for PO_2 is an estimation of the differential passage of oxygen and carbon dioxide between the alveolus and the arterial blood. It is an indirect equivalent of DL_{CO} but can be abnormal even when DL_{CO} is not. Exercise physiology testing can be done either with continuous measurement of oxygen saturation by oximetry or by the use of an indwelling arterial catheter for the serial sampling of arterial blood gases. The latter is more invasive but gives more accurate and reliable information. When oximetry is used, blood gases should be drawn at rest and at peak exercise to confirm the correlation between PO_2 and oximetry. A maximum exercise study provides invaluable information about a patient's exercise capacity and about the degree of gas exchange abnormality. Normal individuals increase ventilation and improve oxygenation. Patients with interstitial lung disease suboptimally increase ventilation and desaturate during exercise. In our experience this test provides a wealth of practical information and is often more sensitive than DL_{CO}.

Endoscopy

Flexible fiberoptic scopes have had an important impact on the evaluation of the upper and lower respiratory tracts. Rhinoscopy is extremely useful in helping to examine alterations in the region of first line defense against inhaled toxicants. Direct laryngoscopy permits careful examination of the nasopharynx, including the larynx and proximal trachea. This can prove very useful when faced with suspected acute chemical burns or in assessing for chronic scarring of the upper respiratory tract.

The fiberoptic bronchoscope allows us to inspect the airway from the level of the posterior pharynx through four or five generations of bronchi and to obtain samples of lung tissue for histologic examination. Sometimes simple visual inspection of the airway can help clarify a confusing clinical picture. The small pieces of bronchial and parenchymal tissue obtainable with a biopsy forceps are often sufficient to make outpatient diagnoses of lung disease. For example, there is an extremely high yield on transbronchial biopsy for the diagnosis of granulomatous diseases such as beryllium disease and extrinsic allergic alveolitis (hypersensitivity pneumonitis).

Bronchoalveolar lavage, a technique in which aliquots of normal saline are instilled and suctioned from a small segment of peripheral lung, is still principally a research tool, with a few important exceptions. Examination and immunologic testing of the cells from lavage has helped to identify a number of inhalational injuries including beryllium disease and extrinsic allergic alveolitis. In these diseases, there is a marked increase in lavage lymphocytes, whereas a normal lavage contains mainly macrophages. There is good correlation between the high lymphocyte counts and the underlying granulomatous pathology. Furthermore, testing of cells obtained from lavage for their immunologic reactivity allows the clinician to make a specific diagnosis of beryllium disease, as discussed elsewhere in this text. With these few exceptions, bronchoalveolar lavage still has relatively limited clinical application in the evaluation of pulmonary toxic insults.

Immunologic Evaluation of Pulmonary Toxicity

An emerging area of intense research and new clinical application is the immunologic assessment of inhaled toxicant effects. Some offending agents have nonspecific inflammatory effects on cell populations. Others are antigenic, causing specific immune responses both within the lung and systemically. Normally the local immune system can handle the routine barrage to which the lung is subjected. But the response can go awry, producing harmful effects such as granuloma formation, pulmonary fibrosis, and bronchial hyperreactivity. This topic has been well reviewed elsewhere and will only be discussed briefly here. The main applications of immunology in assessment of occupational and environmental lung disease fall into several areas: (a) occupational asthma, (b) extrinsic allergic alveolitis (hypersensitivity pneumonitis), (c) pneumoconioses, and (d) occupational diseases caused by metal sensitization.

Most of the industrial agents that cause occupational asthma have known or suspected allergic properties although occupational and environmentally triggered asthma often occurs via multiple inflammatory, irritant, and pharmacologic mechanisms. While immunologic tests of hypersensitivity may help pinpoint a putative allergen, they generally will not prove causation, short of bronchoprovocation testing as discussed above.

The high molecular weight compounds such as those found in plant dusts, enzymes, animal dander, and urine can produce allergic bronchoconstriction by producing specific IgE and sometimes specific IgG antibodies. Therefore it is sometimes possible to use precipitins testing, radioallergosorbent tests (RAST), or enzyme-linked immunosorbent assays (ELISA) to detect responses to these agents. Low molecular weight compounds such as the anhydrides, plicatic acid, isocyanates, and metal salts may serve as protein-bound haptens, inducing humoral or cellular immune responses. Immunologic methods available for evaluating occupational asthma have been thoroughly reviewed elsewhere. The demonstration of specific antibodies indicates sensitization but may also be found in persons who have no asthma or allergic symptoms. Furthermore, some patients with allergen-induced asthma may be negative on immunologic tests, due to factors such as time since last exposure and methodologic flaws in assays. Therefore, results of immunologic tests must always be taken in the full clinical context. Major causes of occupational asthma are listed in Table 11.4.

Extrinsic allergic alveolitis is an immunologically mediated hypersensitivity reaction that occurs after exposure to a variety of organ dusts. Examples include: farmers' lung disease (involving an immune response to one or more bacterial or fungal antigens found in moldy hay), pigeon breeders' disease, bagassosis, and humidifier fever among others. A partial list of causes of extrinsic allergic alveolitis is found in Table 11.5. In the clinical setting of this hypersensitivity reaction, precipitins tests can help identify "new" antigens. They can also be used to confirm the clinical suspicion of hypersensitivity. However, because of the high rate of positive precipitins in asymptomatic exposed subjects as well as the variability of precipitins responses over time and the lack of a truly exhaustive battery of test antigens, precipitins testing should only be considered an adjunct to diagnosis. A positive precipitins test can support the clinical diagnosis of extrinsic allergic alveolitis but should not be relied on to either solely include or exclude this diagnosis.

With regard to the pneumoconioses, specifically coal workers' pneumoconiosis, silicosis, and asbestosis, a number of immunologic abnormalities in blood and in bronchoalveolar lavage have been identified. None of these has any specific diagnostic or prognostic value in the clinical setting at this time. Clearly, immune regulation itself is altered in these disease states as evidenced by the increased risk of mycobacterial infection and connective tissue disease in individuals with pneumoconioses.

Occupational lung diseases caused by sensitizing metals have served as the paradigm for interstitial lung disease involving cell-mediated immune responses. Perhaps the single best application of these principles has been in the diagnosis of chronic beryllium disease, in which immunologic evaluation has now become the pivot point in the diagnosis. Testing for cellular immunity has been preliminarily described in other metal-induced diseases such as aluminum induced granulomatosis as well as for titanium, chromium, nickel, and gold.

OCCUPATIONAL AND ENVIRONMENTAL RESPIRATORY DISORDERS

The list of agents that can induce lung injury is legion, ranging from minor irritants to carcinogens. Damage varies from reversible upper airway inflammation to permanent airway bronchoconstriction and from reversible hypersensitivity reactions to irreparable fibrosis. Table 11.7 outlines the principal types of pulmonary responses to toxic insults.

The remainder of this chapter will focus on several common classes of injurious agents and clinical presentations of respiratory disorders produced by inhaled toxicants, providing a diagnostic approach to such problems.

Table 11.4 Examples of Occupational and Environmental Causes of Asthma

Agent Source	Population at Risk
Animal products	
Laboratory animals	Laboratory workers
Sea squirt fluid	Oyster/pearl gatherers
Avian proteins	Bird fanciers
Insects	
Locusts	Laboratory workers
Mites	Grain, flour mill workers, bakers
Moths, butterflies	Environmental exposure
Fungi	
Alternaria species	Bakers
Aspergillus species	Bakers
Cladosporium spores	Farm workers
Mushroom spores	Mushroom cultivation
Grains, flour, plants	
Wheat	Millers
Grain	Farm workers, grain handlers
Flour	Bakers
Castor beans	Farmers, gardeners
Gum acacia	Printers
Tobacco dust	Cigarette factory workers
Spices	Spice factory workers
Coffee beans	Exposure to green and roasted beans
Western red cedar	Workers, miller, joiners, carpenters
Oak	Millers
Cocabolla	Wood finishers
Redwood	Carpenters
Cotton, hemp, sisal, flax, and possible bacterial contaminants, endotoxin (part of clinical spectrum of Byssinosis)	Textile manufacturing, carders, sorters, weavers
Metals	
Chromates	Chrome plating and polishing
Platinum salts	Platinum refining
Nickel sulfate	Nickle plating
Nickel carbonyl	Chemist
Vanadium and vanadium pentoxide	Boiler cleaners
Cobalt	Tungsten carbide grinding
Stainless steel	Welders (chromium and nickel exposure)
Chemicals	
Fluorine	Aluminum potroom workers
Formalin	Laboratory workers, resin molding, hospital personnel
Ethanolamines	Aluminum cable soldering
Paraphenylene diamine	Fur dyers
Ethylene diamine	Rubber, shellac workers
Isocyanates Toluene diisocyanate, hexamethylene diisocyanate, diphenylmethane diisocyanate, naphthalene diisocyanate	Isocyanate manufacturing, plastics, factory workers, polyurethane foam manufacturing, automobile painters, printers, rubber workers, chemists, laminators, boat construction, tinners, insulators
Phthalic anhydride	Paint manufacturing, plastics molding

continues

Table 11.4 *Continued*

Agent Source	Population at Risk
Chemicals (cont'd)	
Trimellitic anhydride	Chemical workers
Colophony (pine resin)	Electronics soldering
Polyvinyl chloride fumes	Meatwrappers
Tetrachlorphthalic anhydride	Epoxy resin manufacturing
Dyes	Dye manufacturing, hairdressers
Drugs	
Methyl dopa	Pharmaceutical manufacturing
Penicillins	Pharmaceutical manufacturing
Psllium	Pharmaceutical manufacturing
Tetracycline	Pharmaceutical manufacturing
Sulfathiazole	Pharmaceutical manufacturing
Chloramines	Pharmaceutical manufacturing
Enzymes	
Trypsin	Plastics manufacturing
Pancreatic extract	Manufacturing, parents of children with cystic fibrosis
Bacillus subtilis	Detergent manufacturing

Clinical Approach to Suspected Toxicant-Induced Asthma

In the workplace and home environment, the number of chemicals, metals, dusts, and animal products capable of causing asthma has been estimated at greater than 200. A partial list appears in Table 11.4. The diagnosis of asthma related to pulmonary toxicants is a two-part process. First, one must confirm the presence of airways hyperreactivity. Second, one must establish an association between the asthma and the suspected causative agent. Fig. 11.6 illustrates an approach to the diagnosis of toxicant-induced asthma.

Patients with environmental or occupational causes of asthma generally present as any asthmatic patient does. Symptoms may include chest tightness, episodic shortness of breath, and sometimes wheezing. Not infrequently the patient may present only with cough. At this point it is incumbent upon the clinician to take a careful occupational environmental history. The symptoms may or may not have coincided with doing particular jobs at work or in a hobby. Other exposed individuals might have similar complaints. Patients themselves may make the association between their symptoms and a particular exposure, if the provocative agent induces an immediate pattern of hyperreactivity. But frequently the temporal relationship is missed because many substances can cause a late asthmatic response without any evidence of immediate airways hyperreactivity. In those individuals the symptoms of cough, wheezing, shortness of breath, or chest tightness may only occur after work or even during sleep. In such cases, inquiry about weekend and holiday improvement and relapses upon returning to work may yield important clues.

As illustrated in Fig. 11.6, once the suspicion of reactive airways disease has been raised, the clinician must confirm the diagnosis of asthma. The exam may or may not reveal obvious wheezing and airflow limitation on forced expiration. Pulmonary function tests that confirm the presence of airflow limitation with improvement after bronchodilator are sufficient to make the diagnosis of asthma. But some patients with occupationally induced asthma have normal lung function at the time of presentation. In such individuals, we proceed with nonspecific bronchoprovocation testing with methacholine or histamine inhalation.

Having thus demonstrated the presence of hyperreactive airways, it is then necessary to obtain objective evidence that the asthma is related to a specific agent in the environment. In some cases this is helped greatly by reviewing material safety data sheets. These may reveal the presence of a known sensitizer or pulmonary irritant. But more often than not it will not be possible to pinpoint the specific agent without a great deal of additional testing. Even then this exercise is often futile. Several ways in which a more specific diagnosis can be made include: (a) skin and serologic tests, (b) pulmonary function tests at the time of exposure, and (c) specific bronchoprovocation tests.

Immunologic tests are one indirect method for making a causal link of exposure to illness. Skin and serologic tests are useful usually only if the particular agent in question is an allergen and if the specific allergen has been well-characterized. Where the agent causes the individual to mount specific antibodies, prick or patch skin testing, RAST or ELISA testing may be successful. But negative immunologic testing does not exclude the diagnosis.

Several methods of pulmonary function testing are used to obtain more compelling evidence of environmentally related asthma. As discussed earlier in this chapter, peak flow measurements are particularly useful if the individual is continuing to have frequent exposure. In our practice, individuals are asked to make peak flow readings using a Mini-Wright peak flow meter approximately six times a day, including measurements both in and out of the environment in question. Such records preferably should be kept for two or more weeks, both while in and out of exposure. If the workplace is suspected, peak flows are used during periods on and off work, preferably including both weekends off and at least one to two weeks completely off. Fig. 11.7 shows a typical pattern of peak flows in an individual with work-related asthma. There are drawbacks to peak-expiratory flow recordings. Some individuals will only have intermittent exposure and, hence, intermittent symptoms. The symptoms may last not simply minutes but up to days after a single exposure. If an individual's asthma is poorly reversible, removal from exposure might not lead to demonstrable improvement in peak flows. Concurrent treatment such as with corticosteroids or cromolyn sodium may confound results. Variation in the patient's technique and accuracy of record keeping may, in some individuals, be additional drawbacks. However, in conscientious patients, peak flows can be invaluable in helping to identify asthma triggers.

Another method of demonstrating the environmental link to asthma involves the measurement of lung function before and after exposure. In the occupational setting, for example, preshift and postshift spirometry can be performed. This can be time-consuming and requires on-site spirometry, as airways hyperreactivity may reverse very quickly after removal from exposure. However, documentation of a 20% fall in FEV_1 over the work shift and a progressive drop in lung function across the course of the work week can be compelling. Pre- and postshift spirometry will not necessarily provide clues to the specific agent in question, but can rule in or rule out workplace triggers in general. Again, this technique may miss late asthmatic responses that may occur hours after exposure.

A third pulmonary function method of assessing for an association between the environment and asthma is to remove the individual from exposures, monitor symptoms, medica-

Table 11.5 Examples of Agents Causing Extrinsic Allergic Alveolitis (Hypersensitivity Pneumonitis)

Agent	Source	Disease
Amebae		
Naegleria gruberi	Humidifier water	Humidifier lung
Acanthamoeba spp.	Humidifier water	Humidifier lung
Animal proteins		
Bovine, porcine	Pituitary snuff	Snuff taker's lung
Murine	Rat, mouse urine	
Avian proteins		
Pigeon serum protein	Pigeon droppings	Pigeon breeder's disease
Parrot serum protein	Parrot droppings	Budgerigar fancier's disease
Chicken proteins	Chicken products	Feather plucker's lung
Bacterial		
Bacillus spp.	Humidifier water	Humidifier lung
	Wood dust,	
	Detergent (enzyme)	
Chemicals		
Isocyanates	Chemical manufacturing	
Trimellitic anhydride	Chemical manufacturing	
Fungi		
Alternaria spp.	Moldy wood pulp	Pulp worker's disease
Aspergillus spp.	Moldy malt, barley	Malt worker's lung
	Moldy hay	Farmer's lung
Graphium spp.	Moldy redwood dust	Sequoiosis
Penicillium spp.	Cheese mold	Cheese washer's lung
	Humidifier water	Humidifier lung
	Moldy cork	Suberosis
Insects		
Wheat weevil	Grain contamination	Miller's lung
Plant products		
Ramin	Sawdust, coffee dust, dried grass	Sequoiosis, coffee worker's lung, thatched roof disease
Thermophylic actinomycetes		
Micropolyspora faeni	Moldy hay	Farmer's lung
	Mushroom waste	Mushroom worker's lung
Thermoactinomyces sacchari	Bagasse	Bagassosis
Thermoactinomyces vulgaris	Moldy hay	Farmer's lung
	Mushroom waste	Mushroom worker's lung

tions, and spirometry until he or she is stable. Then the patient is "rechallenged" to the environment in question and reassessed for changes in symptoms, medication use, and pulmonary function.

In rare instances it may be necessary to perform specific bronchoprovocation tests with suspected agents and placebo control. We strongly discourage the indiscriminate use of such challenge tests. They are potentially dangerous as well as time-consuming and costly. They should be performed by experienced personnel in an inpatient setting only. The clinician must be prepared to handle severe reactions which sometimes occur immediately and/or 8–24 hours after challenge.

One form of bronchoprovocation is the simple Pepys-type challenge where the individual is asked to simulate his or her normal activity. Pulmonary function testing is performed before, during, and after exposure. More sophisticated methods employ whole body exposure level chambers with accurate real-time measurement of the exposure level. This technology is crucial in challenges which involve highly toxic chemicals, such as isocyanates.

After challenge, the individual is monitored carefully for development of one of the three patterns of asthmatic reactions: immediate, late, or dual responses as shown in Figure 11.8.

We recommend that challenge testing be reserved for (a) the research setting, to study previously unrecognized causes of asthma; and (b) rare occasions when the patient may otherwise refuse to believe that the causative agent is causing his or her asthma and refuses to leave exposure. Challenge testing has been advocated for use for medico-legal purposes; however, this is rarely, in and of itself, a sufficiently good reason to perform potentially dangerous provocation testing.

Physicians are often taught that environmental causes of asthma can be expected to resolve with removal from exposure. Unfortunately, this is not always the case. Over half of the individuals who have developed asthma from compounds as diverse as isocyanates and plicatic acid from Western red cedar remain symptomatic and have persistent bronchial hyperreactivity for years after cessation of exposure. Some patients with environmentally induced asthma improve after removal from exposure but will not recover completely. Prognosis is linked to the duration of exposure, the severity of airflow limitation at the

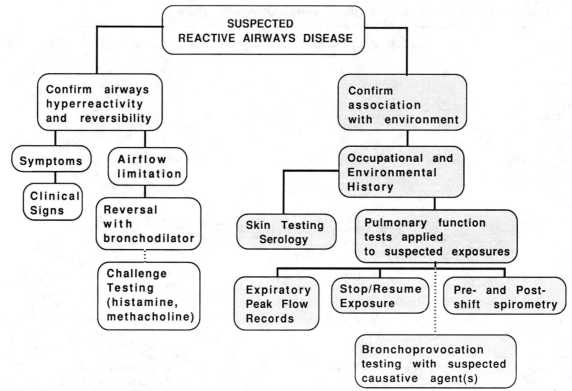

Figure 11.6.   Clinical approach to the evaluation of suspected reactive airways disease (asthma) related to environmental or occupational exposure. Dotted lines indicate tests less commonly employed in clinical evaluation. See text for explanation.

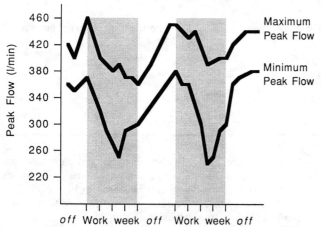

Figure 11.7.   Work-related patterns of airflow obstruction can be documented using an expiratory peak flow meter. One such work-related pattern is shown in which there is progressive decline in peak flow across the work week with weekend recovery of lung function.

time of diagnosis, and the specific causative agent, among other factors.

Reactive Airways Disease Syndrome (RADS)

We typically think of asthma as requiring a period of chronic antigen or irritant exposure prior to the development of clinical symptoms and signs. Recently researchers have described individuals who have developed the signs, symptoms, physiology, and pathology of reactive airways disease after a single, high level accidental exposure to irritating gases, fumes, or smoke, including chlorine and ammonia. The symptoms commonly occur within several hours of the initial exposure and resolve within several weeks, but with some individuals developing persistent airways hyperreactivity.

While the designation of reactive airways disease syndrome (RADS) as an entity separate from asthma has produced controversy, the take-home message is clear: airways hyperreactivity can be induced by a single high level exposure to irritants. This should be borne in mind at the time that patients present with acute accidental overexposures. For example, even if an individual with an acute inhalational injury has been successfully treated and released from the hospital, early pulmonary function assessment should be performed to exclude the possibility of persistent airways hyperreactivity.

Acute Inhalational Injury

Many mists, gases, and fumes can produce acute respiratory tract injury, as outlined in Table 11.6. Mechanisms include irritant, asphyxiant, and systemic toxicity.

As discussed earlier in this chapter, site of action is in part dependent on extent of exposure and solubility of the gas or size and structure of the particulate. Sometimes the specific agent is clearly identified, as in chemical tank accidents. But sometimes the agent may be a complex mixture of combustion and pyrolysis products as occurs in welding or in smoke inhalation injuries. Often the onset of symptoms is acute, as in sulfur dioxide and ammonia exposures, but may be delayed, as seen with nitrogen oxides and phosgene.

The irritant gases induce cellular injury in the airway by (a) forming acids (e.g., hydrogen chloride, sulfur dioxide); (b) depositing aklakis which produce deep, smoldering mu-

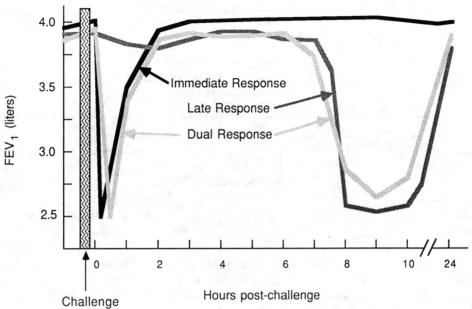

Figure 11.8. Three common patterns of airways hyperreactivity in response to inhaled agents are: (a) immediate airflow obstruction; (b) late occurrence of airflow obstruction; and (c) dual pattern with both an immediate and delayed response.

Table 11.6. Examples of Agents That Produce Acute Respiratory Tract Injury

Irritant gases, high solubility
Acetaldehyde (CH_3CHO)
Acrolein (acrylic aldehyde) ($CH_2:CHCHO$)
Ammonia (NH_3)
Hydrogen chloride (HCl)
Sulfur dioxide (SO_2)

Irritant gases, intermediate to low solubility
Chlorine (Cl_2)
Nitrogen oxides (NO_x)
Ozone (O_3)
Phosgene (carbonyl chloride) ($COCl_2$)

Asphyxiants
Carbon monoxide (CO)
Hydrogen cyanide (HCN)
Hydrogen sulfide (H_2S)

Systemic toxicants
Metal oxides (metal fume fever)
Tetrafluorethylene resin pyrolysis products (polymer fume fever)

cosal injury (e.g., ammonia); and (c) releasing oxygen free radicals (e.g., chlorine, ozone). The outcomes range from reversible conjunctival and upper airway irritation to airway hyperreactivity, laryngospasm, bronchiolitis obliterans, pulmonary edema, and death.

Asphyxiants interfere with the normal delivery of oxygen. Some do this by (a) blocking oxygen binding to hemoglobin, as seen with nitrogen dioxide and carbon monoxide; (b) blocking oxidative phosphorylation, as seen with hydrogen sulfide; or (c) displacing oxygen, as seen with carbon dioxide, methane, and helium.

Metal oxide fumes, such as zinc, magnesium, and copper, or heated polymers such as Teflon fluorocarbons can induce flu-like symptoms of fever, chills, chest pain, cough, and arthralgias, with negative chest radiographs. The mechanisms underlying polymer and metal fume fever are obscure. Neither is associated with prolonged symptomatology or permanent respiratory dysfunction.

The clinical approach to these acutely injurious agents is dependent on the specific chemical and its mechanism of injury and is discussed elsewhere in this text.

Upper Airway Inflammation (Rhinitis, Sinusitis, Tracheobronchitis)

Numerous agents can potentially injure the upper respiratory tract—our first line of defense. Symptoms are often immediate and obvious to the patient: burning sensation in the nose and throat, watery nasal discharge, epistaxis, hoarseness, sore throat, and cough which may be present acutely and even develop into chronic bronchitis. As discussed earlier, any or all of these symptoms may occur, depending upon the nature of the specific agent inhaled and its pattern of airway deposition.

Demonstration of upper airway irritant or allergic reactions to environmental agents is often problematic in that there are usually few objective findings. Diagnosis is clinical, and assigning cause is often conjectural. Abatement of symptoms with removal from exposure, and a temporal association between onset of symptoms and exposure serve as the best indicators of the causal link, especially if MSDSs or other data obtained from the workplace suggest patient contact with upper airway irritants. A nasal smear may help to identify irritant versus allergic reactions. Increased numbers of neutrophils on nasal smear may suggest an acute inflammatory response. Increased numbers of eosinophils may suggest allergic etiologies. Rhinoscopy and direct laryngoscopy can verify the degree of upper respiratory tract inflammation. Sinus radiographs may assist in assessing cases of longer duration where chronic sinusitis has occurred with or without secondary infection.

When cough is the predominant symptom, it is critical that cough-variant asthma be excluded by performing pulmonary function tests and even methacholine or histamine challenge. Industrial bronchitis is defined as persistent cough due to an

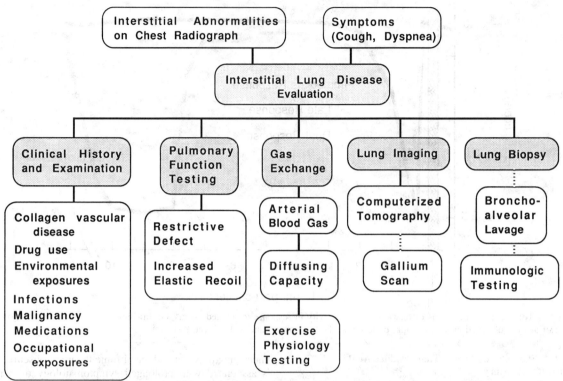

Figure 11.9.   Clinical approach to the diagnosis of interstitial lung disease caused by environmental or occupational agents. Dotted lines indicate tests which are less commonly employed but which may be useful in specific circumstances, as discussed in the text.

occupational exposure with no other apparent cause for cough. It usually occurs in the absence of airways hyperreactivity. In some cases of industrial bronchitis, we have proceeded to fiberoptic bronchoscopy to confirm and document the extent of the bronchial inflammation. But in most cases of upper respiratory inflammation from environmental agents, these more invasive tests are not performed. The cornerstone of treatment is removal from exposure. Symptomatic measures such as inhaled, insufflated, or oral corticosteroids or cromolyn sodium may be prescribed empirically.

Fortunately, most cases of environmentally induced rhinitis, sinusitis, and tracheobronchitis will resolve without significant longterm sequelae, unless there is concomitant airways hyperreactivity or deep lung injury. Another exception is in the case of chemical ''burns'' of either an acute or smoldering type as is seen with hydrochloric, nitric, or hydrofluoric acids. If severe injury occurs, secondary problems such as bronchiectasis, tracheal stenosis, or laryngeal dysfunction may result.

Assessment of Environmental Causes of Interstitial Lung Disease

Interstitial lung diseases represent a large portion of what pulmonologists see secondary to inhaled toxic agents. There are two common presentations. In one scenario, the patient obtains a routine chest radiograph which shows increased interstitial markings. This may occur as part of an annual physical, on a routine preoperative radiograph, or perhaps as part of an asbestos worker screening. Alternatively, the patient may present with unexplained symptoms of cough, dyspnea on exertion, and shortness of breath. Once suspected, the clinical evaluation of interstitial lung disease should have four goals: (a) to obtain sufficient information to make a firm diagnosis of the type of

interstitial disease; (b) to determine the causative agent; (c) to assess the severity of impairment from the disease; and (d) to determine a treatment plan.

Most pulmonologists start with the chest radiograph. It may provide important insights as discussed earlier in the chapter. Clues include the presence of associated findings such as adenopathy, which might be suggestive of sarcoidosis or beryllium disease, pleural plaques which, if the history is compatible, may be sufficient to confirm asbestos exposure, and cavitary lesions suggesting tuberculosis along with silicosis. More often than not, however, the findings on chest radiograph will not be sufficiently specific to allow the clinician to forego the further diagnostic evaluation outlined in Fig. 11.9.

The workup begins with a careful history, focusing on causes of interstitial disease, including medications, drug abuse, heart disease, malignancy, collagen vascular disease, fungal, viral, or bacterial infection, and occupational or environmental exposures. Table 11.7 lists some of the recognized environmental and occupational causes of the interstitial lung diseases. These are subdivided into those producing a principal pattern of (a) interstitial fibrosis, (b) granuloma formation, (c) bronchiolitis obliterans, (d) pulmonary edema, and (e) other, such as respiratory bronchiolitis and giant cell pneumonitis. Chronicity of symptoms and any temporal association of exposure to organic and inorganic agents may greatly help focus the diagnostic workup.

More often than not, additional testing including lung biopsy will be required to make a firm diagnosis. Transbronchial lung biopsy has proved extremely useful in diagnosis of granulomatous lung diseases. But because it is less accurate and less sensitive in the diagnosis of bronchiolitis obliterans and fibrosing lung disease, such cases may require open lung biopsies.

Table 11.7. Common Pathologic Changes Associated with Occupational and Environmental Causes of Interstitial Lung Disease

Diffuse interstitial fibrosis
(usual interstitial pneumonitis, desquamative interstitial pneumonitis, fibrotic nodules)
Aluminum
Asbestos
Beryllium (end stage)
Chronic extrinsic allergic alveolitis from fungal spores, avian proteins, isocyanates (see Table 11.5)
Chronic pulmonary edema (numerous causes, see Table 11.2)
Coal dust
Cobalt
Copper
Diatomaceous earth
Drugs (e.g., bleomycin, busulphan, cyclophosphamide, nitrofurantoin)
Ionizing radiation
Kaolin (china clay)
Mercury fumes
Mixed dust fibrosis
Nickel
Oil mists (lipoid pneumonia)
Paraquat
Silica
Talc

Granulomatous and/or mononuclear cell infiltration
(hypersensitivity and foreign body reactions)
Aluminum
Asbestos
Beryllium
Blastomyces dermititidis (North American blastomycosis)
Brucella abortis (chronic infection)
Coal dust
Cobalt
Coccidioides immitis
Copper (vineyard sprayer's lung)
Drugs (e.g., methotrexate, gold)
Extrinsic allergic alveolitis (see Table 11.5)
Histoplasma capsulatum
Oil mist (lipoid pneumonia)
Polyvinyl chloride (PVC) dust
Silicotuberculosis
Talc

Bronchiolitis obliterans
Ammonia
Cadmium oxide
Chlorine
Chloropicrin
Hydrogen fluoride
Hydrogen sulfide
Methyl sulfate
Oxygen toxicity
Oxides of nitrogen
Ozone
Phosgene
Sulfur dioxide
Trichlorethylene

Other
Giant cell pneumonitis due to cobalt (hard metal disease)

In certain instances, lung biopsy can be completely avoided. Examples include asbestosis. If an individual has a history of asbestos exposure, a typically long latency between first exposure and development of interstitial infiltrates, slow disease

Table 11.8. Occupational and Environmental Causes of Lung Cancer

Agent	Sources of Exposure
Asbestos	Insulators, brake repair, textile industry, asbestos mining, heating and ventilation, secondary exposures, non-industrial
Acrylonitrile	Chemical plants
Arsenates, arsenites, arsenic trioxide	Smelting, pesticide manufacturing, vineyard workers
Beryllium	Beryllium processing
Chloroethers Bis-chloromethyl ether, Chloromethyl methyl ether	Ion-exchange resin manufacturing, chemical plants (used for organic solvents, fungicides, bacteriocides)
Cadmium	Smelter, other industrial exposures
Chromium, chromates	Chromium, chromite ore extraction, pigment industry
Coal carbonization (agent unknown, possibly benzpyrene)	Coking plants, gas workers, steel carbonization
Ionizing radiation, radon daughters	Miners, potential home exposures
Mustard gas (bis[β-chloroethyl]sulfide)	Chemical warfare (workers and soldiers)
Nickel dust, fume	Nickel smelting, refining, calcining, nickel carbonyl processes
Tobacco smoke	Cigarette, cigar, pipe smoking
Vinyl chloride	Polymer industry

progression, and a typical x-ray pattern with irregular opacities and pleural plaques, further workup is probably unnecessary. This is sufficient information to make a presumptive diagnosis without proceeding to bronchoscopy or open lung biopsy. Similar principles apply to the noninvasive diagnosis of silicosis and coalworkers' pneumoconiosis. But if the clinical picture is not fully compatible with the physiologic and radiographic presentations of these diseases, biopsy will be needed to rule out other interstitial lung diseases.

A second example is the individual with clinical symptoms of acute extrinsic allergic alveolitis (hypersensitivity pneumonitis) in whom there is a readily identifiable etiologic agent—such as being a bird fancier or having pitched moldy hay. Such individuals can be given the clinical diagnosis of hypersensitivity pneumonitis, even without serum precipitins testing. Rather than proceeding immediately to additional diagnostic procedures such as lung biopsy, such patients can be treated by removing them from exposure and sometimes administering a short course of oral corticosteroids. If the clinical diagnosis was correct, one can anticipate a prompt reversal of symptoms, signs, pulmonary function, and x-ray abnormalities. If, however, the symptoms have been more chronic, the clinical diagnosis may be less clear-cut and lead ultimately to biopsy.

As discussed earlier in this chapter, bronchoalveolar lavage at the time of transbronchial lung biopsy may lend additional specificity to the diagnosis of interstitial lung disease, in the case of extrinsic allergic alveolitis, chronic beryllium disease, hard metal disease due to cobalt, and asbestosis. In fact, in some countries asbestos fibers in bronchoalveolar lavage are counted and used as an indication of underlying asbestosis.

Environmentally Induced Lung Cancer

The demonstration of respiratory tract malignancy secondary to toxic exposures is complicated by a number of factors. Tobacco smoke is the overwhelming respiratory carcinogen and confounds many studies of other suspected carcinogens. In some instances there is an additive or multiplicative risk when smoking is added to a cocarcinogen such as asbestos or ionizing radiation.

Much of what we know about carcinogens is predicated on animal studies which may or may not be pertinent to humans and on epidemiologic studies of cancer incidence in industrial cohorts where appropriate matching of control groups is sometimes a problem. This is a major topic which is beyond the scope of this chapter and has been well-reviewed elsewhere.

Table 11.8 lists the major known and suspected causes of occupational lung cancer, although some of these remain controversial despite decades of research.

SELECTED READINGS

Breeze R, Turk M. Cellular structure, function, and organization in the lower respiratory tract. Environ Health Perspect 1984;55:3–24.

Chan-Yeung M, Lam S. Occupational asthma—state of the art. Am Rev Respir Dis 1986;133;686–703.

Cherniack RM. Pulmonary function testing. Philadelphia: WB Saunders Co., 1977.

Cone JE. Occupational lung cancer. In: Rosenstock L, ed. Occupational pulmonary disease. Occupational medicine state of the art reviews. Philadelphia: Hanley and Belfus, 1987;2,273–295.

Daniele RP, ed. Immunology and immunologic diseases of the lung. Boston: Blackwell Scientific Publications, 1988.

King TE Jr. Bronchiolitis obliterans. In: Schwarz MI, King TE Jr eds. Interstitial lung disease. Toronto: BC Decker, 1988;325–342.

Murray JF, Nadal JA. eds. Textbook of respiratory medicine. Philadelphia: WB Saunders Co., 1988.

Newman L, Storey E, Kreiss K. Immunologic evaluation of occupational lung disease. In: Rosenstock L. ed. Occupational pulmonary disease. Occupational medicine state of the art reviews. Philadelphia: Hanley and Belfus, 1987;2,345–372.

Parkes WR. Occupational lung disorders. 2nd ed. London: Butterworth and Company, 1982.

Schwartz DA. Acute inhalational injury. In: Rosenstock L, ed. Occupational pulmonary disease. Occupational medicine state of the art reviews. Philadelphia: Hanley and Belfus, 1987;2,297–318.

Wasserman K, Hansen JE, Sue DY, Whipp BJ. Principles of exercise testing and interpretation. Philadelphia: Lea and Febiger, 1987.

12

Neurotoxicology

Neil L. Rosenberg, M.D.

INTRODUCTION

The nervous system comprises two major components: central nervous system (CNS) and peripheral nervous system (PNS). Structures that make up the CNS include brain, optic nerves, and spinal cord while the PNS is divided into somatic and autonomic divisions. Major components of the CNS and PNS are listed in Table 12.1. Any of the CNS and PNS sites represent potential targets for toxic assault, with the resulting clinical features reflecting the pattern of distribution of injury in the CNS, PNS, or both.

Two important concepts regarding toxic responses of the nervous system are that of the blood-brain and blood-nerve barriers. These barriers respectively protect the CNS and PNS from injury by toxins that may damage other organs or tissues. In addition, there exist blood-CSF (cerebrospinal fluid) barriers, which also can protect the CNS from certain toxins (1). However, several potential toxins do cross these barriers, and general anesthetics, analgesics, and organic solvents readily cross the blood-brain barrier. Common characteristics of those compounds that do cross the blood-brain barrier include being nonpolar and lipid-soluble. An additional factor related to susceptibility to toxic effects of compounds based on the blood-brain barrier is related to the maturity of the organism. In the immature brain, the blood-brain barrier is not fully developed, and some toxins may therefore accumulate in the immature brain, whereas in the fully developed, mature brain the same toxins are normally excluded. This concept is well-illustrated in the case of lead toxicity, where in children, lead may accumulate in the brain resulting in an acute encephalopathy, whereas lead encephalopathy is rare in adults since lead is normally excluded from the brain.

Three unique anatomic features exist that appear to contribute to the blood-brain barrier (1,2). The first is that capillary endothelial cells of the brain, in most areas, differ from the capillary endothelium elsewhere in the body. Those in the CNS are invested with glial (astrocytic) processes (Fig. 12.1). These astrocytic processes create a barrier to free access of substances to the other cellular elements which comprise the CNS. Areas of the CNS where the capillaries are not wrapped with these processes and theoretically not protected by this barrier include the median eminence of the hypothalamus (3), the median preoptic region (4), choroid plexus (5), and the area postrema around the fourth ventricle (5).

Additional features contributing to the blood-brain barrier are related to unique properties of CNS endothelial cells. One unique feature is the presence of tight junctions around the endothelial cells (Fig. 12.1) which do not allow many large molecules to enter the CNS. Small molecules, however, may penetrate these tight junctions or the cytoplasm of the endothelial and glial cells. An additional feature of CNS endothelial cells is that they lack pinocytotic vesicles in the cytoplasm and lack pores in the luminal surface of the endothelial membrane. Since these vesicles may transport some chemicals across the endothelial lining of capillaries, the absence of vesicles may also contribute to blood-brain barrier. Vesicles may appear on the endothelial cells of the CNS in pathologic states where the blood-brain barrier permeability is increased and may thus increase the susceptibility of the CNS to the effects of certain toxins.

The final anatomic feature which may contribute to the blood-brain barrier is the shared basement membrane between the endothelial cells of the capillaries and the astrocytic foot processes (Fig. 12.1). This basement membrane has an ordered fibrillar mucoprotein structure which may be able to transport molecules needed for cell nutrition while at the same time excluding other toxic substances.

A similar barrier exists in the PNS, the blood-nerve barrier, but like the CNS it also has areas which are permeable. In these areas, fenestrated epithelial cells allow even large molecules to be permeable and enter these areas of the CNS and PNS. Those areas of the PNS which have a different barrier include the dorsal root ganglia and the autonomic ganglia (6–9).

The cellular components of the nervous system and their subcomponents and functions are numerous and complex (10). However, in order to understand some basic principles of neurotoxic mechanisms, as well as to enable one to develop a reasonable classification of neurotoxic disease, some of the basic cellular components of both the CNS and PNS and their functions are important to understand. Cells of the nervous system can be divided among neurons, glial cells, and vascular endothelium. Endothelial cells of the nervous system are discussed above in relation to the blood-brain and blood-nerve barriers. Certain nervous system toxins act on the vasculature primarily, including lead (11, 12), cadmium (11, 13), and bismuth (11, 14).

Neurons are the basic functional element of the nervous system and are different from other cells in that they possess

Table 12.1.   Major Components of Central Nervous System and Peripheral Nervous System

Central nervous system
  Brain
  Spinal cord
  Optic nerves (cranial nerve II)

Peripheral nervous system
  Somatic division
    Cranial nerves (except optic nerves)
    Spinal nerves
    Dorsal root ganglia
    Peripheral nerves
      Motor-neuromuscular junction
      Sensory-special receptors
  Autonomic division
    Parasympathetic-cranial and sacral nerves and ganglia
    Sympathetic

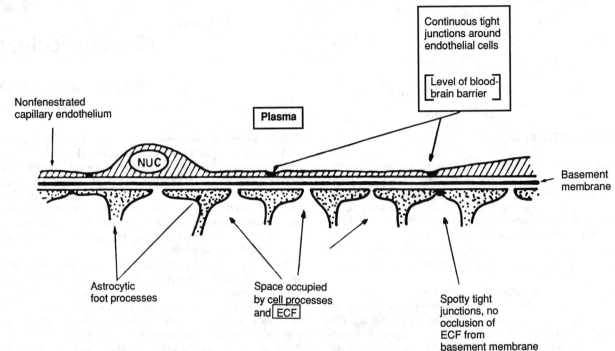

Figure 12.1. Reprinted with permission from Lewis AJ: Mechanisms of Neurological Disease, Little, Brown, 1976, p. 86.

dendrites and axons. Each neuron has multiple branching dendrites which may arise from any part of the neuron, including the entire surface of the cell body. Dendrites are modified elements of the cell which are involved primarily in signal reception and transduction. Dendrites form extensive structural networks which allow communication between neurons and integration of nervous system function. Unlike the numerous dendrites, a neuron produces only one axon, which is specialized for transmission of electrical signals, An axon is narrow at its origin, but then remains of uniform caliber until its terminal branches, which may vary in length from less than 1 millimeter up to 1 meter. Dendrites, by contrast, are rarely greater than 1 millimeter. Neurotoxins may affect either the neuronal cell body primarily (e.g., mercury, 1-methyl-4-phenyl-1,2,3,6-tetrahydropyridine), the axon (e.g., acrylamide, n-hexane), or the dendrite processes (e.g., monosodium glutamate). The sites of action of many other neurotoxin are not yet known, but may affect these components of the neuron or other elements of the nervous system specifically. Table 12.2 lists some of the neurotoxins affecting various structural components of the CNS and PNS.

Glial cells consist of astrocytes, oligodendrocytes, and microglia. Astrocytes are associated with neurons and may play a role in support of the neuron by maintaining a stable environment. Their probable role in maintaining a blood-brain barrier to certain toxins is discussed above. Oligodendrocytes in the CNS and Schwann cells in the PNS invest the axons of neurons and form myelin. Microglia are the CNS phagocytic cells whose role in relation to neurotoxins is not known.

Myelin, formed by oligodendrocytes in the CNS and Schwann cells in the PNS, can be damaged by a number of toxins (12). Myelin damage may occur by a primary effect of these toxins to the myelin without affecting the myelinating cell (i.e., oligodendrocyte and Schwann cell) such as hexachlorphene, triethyltin, and acetyl ethyl tetramethyl tetralin. Chemicals may

Table 12.2. Common Neurotoxins Affecting the CNS and PNS

CNS, neurons, cerebral atrophy	Thallium, organophosphates, organic solvents (styrene, trichloroethylene, toluene, 1,1,1-trichloroethane)
Basal ganglia	Carbon monoxide, methanol (putamen necrosis)
Cortical and cerebellar focal necrosis	Carbon monoxide
Neurobehavioral disorders, both acute and chronic,	Toluene, other solvents, organometals, ethylene oxide, lead, and other metals, CS_2
Axon degeneration and sensorimotor neuropathy	Metals (arsenic, mercury, thallium, organophosphates, CS_2, hexane, acrylamide, methylbutyl ketone, organic solvents, ethylene oxide
Motor neuropathy and myelin degeneration	Lead, hexachlorophene, tellurium, triethyl tin
Periperal neuritis and paresthesias	Thallium, arsenic, mercury
Trigeminal neuropathy	Trichloroethylene
Seizures and tremors	Ethylene oxide, organic solvents, metals, methyl bromide, sulfurylfluoride, organophosphates, chlorinated hydrocarbons
Weakness, fatique, headaches	Ethylene, oxide, organic solvents, carbon monoxide, organophosphates, lead
Ataxia and limb movement disorders	Manganese, ethylene oxide mercury, hexane
Autonomic ganglia and dorsal roots	Mercury, pyridoxine, doxorubicine

also produce myelin damage by causing primary damage to the myelinating cell and myelin such chemicals include: lead, cuprizon, and tellurium. Certain neurotoxins may also cause secondary damage to myelin by primarily damaging neurons (e.g., thallium), axons (e.g., n-haxane), or blood vessels (e.g., lead).

Our understanding of the organization of the nervous system, the blood-brain and blood-nerve barriers, and the specific cellular and subcellular components of the CNS and PNS is necessary in order to understand the basic mechanisms of neurotoxicity of various drugs and chemicals. Understanding these basic concepts is even more important since our understanding of basic biochemical mechanisms and of active metabolites of most neurotoxins is limited.

EPIDEMIOLOGY OF NEUROTOXIC INJURY

Incidence and Prevalence of Disease

Neither the incidence nor the prevalence of neurotoxic disease is known. There are several reasons for this complete lack of epidemiologic information. In general the overwhelming percentage of neurotoxin-induced disease is iatrogenic. The epidemiology of neurotoxicity of industrial and environmental agents has been reported primarily after an epidemic of neurotoxic illness occurs, and such epidemics are rare. In a large review of the epidemiology of neurologic disease, only a single instance of a neurotoxic illness was discussed (15). This neurotoxic disorder, subacute myeloopticoneuropathy (SMON), occurred in Japan from about 1956 to the mid-1970s, probably affected thousands of individuals, and was eventually linked to usage of clioquinol, an intestinal antiseptic and antidiarrheal agent (16). Removal of this agents from the market in Japan in the mid-1970s has been followed by a remarkable decrease of new cases. SMON therefore appears to be a large epidemic of an iatrogenic neurotoxic illness.

There have been occasional attempts to link occupational or environmental exposures to presumed idiopathic neurologic disorders. Most of these studies have major flaws and either have not been replicated, have been refuted in other studies, or have not been strongly linked to causation. Recent epidemiologic studies assessing occupational exposure to organic solvents have shown an increased risk of focal epilepsy (17) and multiple sclerosis (18), but no increased risk of development of Alzheimer's disease (19).

One of the major problems is the recognition of neurotoxic disease. In an individual with symptoms and an unclear or seemingly trivial history of chemical exposure, it can be difficult to decide whether the symptoms and/or signs related to neurotoxic disease or to an idiopathic, naturally occurring process. This apparent inability to decide whether or not a disease is related to neurotoxic mediated mechanisms obviously hinders the epidemiologic investigation of potential neurotoxic diseases.

Current epidemiologic studies are directed toward identifying links between degenerative neurologic disease and industrial and environmental toxins (20, 21) Additional epidemiologic studies are necessary to evaluate the incidence and prevalence of occupational neurotoxic illnesses, but this will not be feasible until markers for such illnesses are better defined.

The important chemical classes relative to occupational and environmental neurotoxicity are organic solvents, metals, pesticides, and gases. Table 12.3 lists those chemicals with major neurotoxic potential.

Table 12.3. Industrial Chemicals with Major Neurotoxic Potential

Organic Solvents	Pesticides
n-Hexane	Carbamates
Carbon disulfide	Organophosphates
Methyl ethyl ketone	Organochlorines
Methanol	Methyl bromide
Toluene	
Xylene	
Benzene	
Styrene	
Trichloroethylene	
1,1,1 - Trichloroethane	
Perchloroethylene	
Solvent mixtures	

Metals	Gases	Others
Aluminum	Carbon monoxide	Acrylamide
Antimony	Nitrous oxide	Strychnine
Arsenic	Hydrogen sulfide	Phenol
Barium	Hydrogen cyanide	
Bismuth	Ethylene oxide	
Gold	Methyl chloride	
Lead		
Lithium		
Manganese		
Mercury		
Selenium		
Thallium		
Silicon		
Tin		
Zinc		

BASIC MECHANISMS OF TOXICITY

The routes of exposure vary for the different neurotoxic chemicals. Most are absorbed with varying degrees of efficiency through more than one of the following routes: inhalation, ingestion, cutaneous. For example, toluene, an organic solvent, is primarily absorbed through the lungs (inhalation) and is absorbed to some degree through gastrointestinal tract (ingestion) and skin (cutaneous). Metals, such as lead and arsenic, are better absorbed through the gastrointestinal tract than through the lungs or skin, although some also occurs through these latter two routes. Elemental mercury vapor can be absorbed via inhalation. Pesticides can be readily absorbed through the skin as well as gastrointestinal tract, and gases clearly have their primary mode of absorption through the lungs.

There are, broadly speaking, two principal types of neurotoxicity, acute and chronic, which may involve the CNS, PNS, or both. Depending on the toxin and its neurotoxic potential, clinical syndromes may vary from acute CNS manifestations to chronic CNS manifestations, and/or peripheral neuropathy (Tables 12.4 and 12.5). Understanding some basic principles about these two categories will allow one to understand some of the basic mechanisms underlying neurotoxic disease.

Acute neurotoxic effects are commonly due to physiologic or biochemical changes in the nervous system and do not involve degeneration of neurocellular elements. These acute effects typically develop after a single, high level exposure and are usually rapidly reversible after the exposure is terminated, although in some cases, such as carbon monoxide, this may

Table 12.4. Central Neurologic Syndromes

Acute CNS Syndromes	Chronic CNS Syndromes
Dizziness	Mood changes
Gait disturbance	Depression
Incoordination	Irritability
Euphoria	Sleep disorders
Excitement	Difficulty concentrating
Obtundation	Memory lapse—short term
Seizures	Personality changes
Coma	Decreased attentiveness
	Dementia
	Parkinsonism
	Extrapyramidal and cerebellar signs

not be the case. Acute exposures are usually associated with behavioral changes (toxic encephalopathy) and are most often due to pharmacologic modification of excitable neuronal membranes or neurotransmitter function. In contrast, most chronic neurotoxic effects are due to repeated, lower level exposures and may not be completely reversible. Chronic neurotoxic effects are associated with pathophysiologic alterations of the structural elements of the nervous system. These structural elements include neurons, dendrites, axons, myelin, and myelin-forming cells. The effects are generally due to metabolic lesions of these elements or to production of cerebral hypoxia/ischemia. Chronic neurotoxic effects can involve both the CNS and the PNS.

The issue of cerebral hypoxia/ischemia is an important consideration in neurotoxicology. Cerebral hypoxia/ischemia can be either a primary effect of cellular metabolism, as in the case of cyanide intoxication (22), or may be secondary to systemic hypoxia secondary to cardiorespiratory insufficiency as can be caused by organic solvent-induced cardiac arrhythmias (23).

Cells that are at greatest risk from hypoxia/ischemia are neurons because of their high metabolic rates and oxygen consumption. Neuronal damage begins a few minutes after cessation of blood flow, and neuronal death will occur before complete cessation of oxygen or glucose transport (24). Other CNS cells are less sensitive to hypoxia/ischemia including oligodendrocytes, astrocytes, microglial cells, and capillary endothelial cells, and are in order of decreasing sensitivity to hypoxia/ischemia. In addition, white matter has lower oxygen requirements and therefore is less susceptible to the effects of hypoxia/ischemia than gray matter. Within the gray matter there are three areas most sensitive to the effects of hypoxia/ischemia: cerebral cortex (cell layer 4—small granule cells), cerebellar cortex (Purkinje cells), and the hippocampus (fields H1 and H3). In general, small cells with many dendrites are most

Table 12.5. Chronic Toxic Neuropathies

Involves long and large nerves of PNS and/or CNS

Polyneuropathy with distal involvement

Multifocal nerve pathologic changes

Peripheral denervation

Pathologic changes progress proximally toward the nerve cell body

PNS effects may predominate clinically

Behavioral changes may be present

susceptible, whereas motor cells (large neurons) with long axons and few dendrites are least sensitive to hypoxia/ischemia.

Three different pathophysiologic mechanisms can produce hypoxic/ischemic injury. *Anoxic anoxia* occurs when an inadequate supply of oxygen occurs in the setting of normal cerebral blood flow (e.g., carbon monoxide poisoning). *Ischemic anoxia* occurs when cerebral arterial blood flow is decreased to where oxygen is not adequately delivered (e.g., cardiac arrest from organic solvents). *Cytotoxic anoxia* occurs when something interferes with normal cellular metabolism, with normal cerebral blood flow, and systemic oxygenation (e.g., cyanide poisoning). Cerebral hypoxia/ischemia related to carbon monoxide is the most commonly identified mechanism of chronic neurotoxic illness which occurs in industry.

These descriptions of acute and chronic neurotoxicity are only generalizations, and many exceptions are known. For example, it is usually the case that chronic neurotoxic effects related to hypoxia/ischemia can result from a single incident. A single dose of certain organophosphates may also cause a chronic polyneuropathy. Also, compounds can exert both acute and chronic neurotoxic effects at different dose levels and by different mechanisms (25). For example, n-hexane will produce a nonspecific encephalopathy with acute, high level exposures, but with repeated, lower level exposures will produce a distal axonopathy.

A classification scheme of neurotoxic disease is needed. The major reason for difficulty in establishing one is that the basic mechanism of toxicity and primary cellular and subcellular targets are known for only a few neurotoxins.

DIAGNOSTIC STRATEGIES IN NEUROTOXICOLOGY

Recognition of overt neurotoxic disease is not difficult with a well-described clinical syndrome. What is more difficult is dealing with a symptomatic patient with an unclear or poorly defined history of chemical exposure. This is by far the most common clinical situation, and the question becomes, ''Does this represent neurotoxic disease or is this a naturally occurring (idiopathic) neurologic disease?'' If a naturally occurring disease is not obvious to the evaluating physician, there is great temptation to attribute the patient's illness to his or her neurotoxic exposure, even if it appears to be a trivial exposure. Understanding the following cardinal features of neurotoxic disease can assist in its diagnosis and management.

History

The key to the diagnosis of neurotoxic disease is through a focused history. Careful history taking can suggest or help establish the diagnosis of neurotoxic disease. Symptoms may not be particularly useful since they tend to be nonspecific and mimic those symptoms of other, naturally occurring neurologic diseases. The history should focus on the occupational and home environments as well as on the possibility that one is dealing with an iatrogenic or idiopathic disorder.

Occupational history taking is an often neglected or omitted portion of the medical and neurologic history (26, 27). The purpose of the occupational history related to a potential neurotoxic illness is to establish exposure or lack thereof to the suspected substance(s) or agents(s). It need not be detailed or time-consuming. The focus should be on the questions that will

Table 12.6. Occupational Exposure History

1. Where do you work and how long have you been employed?
2. What type of service or product is produced?
3. Describe specifically what you do while working.
4. What materials, chemicals, or process do you work with?
5. Are the materials vapors, liquids, or solids?
6. Do you have skin contact with the materials?
7. Do you inhale or breathe any vapors?
8. Do you use protective equipment such as gloves, repirators, barrier creams, or clothing?
9. Were you given training and instruction on proper use, maintenance, and cleaning of protective equipment?
10. What are the conditions of your work area with regard to ventilation and drainage?
11. Is there a temporal relationship between your symptoms and your workplace?
12. What happens to your symptoms before beginning work? During work? After leaving work? On weekends or prolonged times away from work?
13. Do others at work have similar problems?

yield the most productive information. In addition to the usual questions asked during the neurologic history taking, more direct questions related to the work environment are listed in Table 12.6. If the history fails to reveal an etiology in difficult cases, a workplace visit by the physician may be especially useful (28). A workplace visit by the physician and, in particular, the neurologist may be necessary given the large number of potentially neurotoxic chemicals (29).

Vigorous pursuit of nonworkplace neurotoxins should be undertaken if environmental or domestic exposure is suspected. Environmental contamination of potential neurotoxins is ubiquitous, but generally at such low levels that neurotoxic disease does not occur; however, rare epidemics of neurotoxic disease have been known to occur in communities where an industrial accident has occurred (30). Identification of these cases is not difficult, and a cause is usually readily apparent. More difficult are those cases where domestic poisoning or substance abuse is possible, and may require questioning of family and friends as well as home visits where hobby workshops, medicine cabinets, food and water sources, pesticide applications, and illnesses in pets and neighbors are investigated (25).

Physical Exam and Key Signs

Physical signs, like symptoms, mimic naturally occurring metabolic, nutritional, degenerative, and demyelinating neurologic diseases. Since neurotoxins cause either neuronal death or dysfunction, axonal degeneration or diffuse myelin dysfunction, it is rare that *focal* neurologic findings are seen. Since neurotoxins produce nonfocal syndromes, if an individual with a hemiparesis is being evaluated for neurotoxic exposure, a closer look at nontoxic etiologies should be pursued. It is evident that different clinical syndromes may be produced by the same toxin and that similar neurologic syndromes may be produced by dissimilar neurotoxins. The neurologic physical examination should be thorough, and key features of disease sought for. In

Table 12.7. Peripheral Nervous System Toxic Effects

Segmental Demyelination	Anonal Degeneration
Destruction of myelin sheath	Entire neuron may be involved
Axon may be spread	Distal axonal degeneration (distal axonopathy)
Results in decreased nerve condition velocity	Myelin sheath degeneration may occur
Recovery may be complete	Nerve conduction velocity is normal early, but amplitude of action potential may be decreased
	Distal muscle denervation
	Recovery is slow and may be incomplete

addition, pertinent positive as well as negative findings should be recorded.

Few clinical syndromes are diagnostic of neurotoxic disease; however, certain clinical features have on occasion strongly suggested a toxin. For instance, in an individual with a distal axonopathy, who has associated gastrointestinal disturbances, hair loss, and Mees lines, the diagnosis of metal-induced polyneuropathy, particularly arsenic, is obvious (31). An irregular tremor and opsoclonus is an unusual clinical presentation for a naturally occurring neurologic disease but was commonly seen with an outbreak of chlordecone (kepone) poisoning. However, these symptoms are not seen with other organochlorine pesticides (32). The neurologist must therefore be alert to the occurrence of some of these specific clinical syndromes, while in most instances the clinical findings will be nonspecific.

Clinical Syndromes

Toxic neuropathies can manifest as PNS effects, CNS effects, or both. Toxic neuropathies have been classically subdivided into segmental demyelination and axonal demyelination (Table 12.7) (33, 34). Toxic neuropathies commonly present with clinical patterns of symmetrical polyneuropathy, mixed sensorimotor symptoms affecting distal nerves early on, and anatomically multifocal areas of axonal degeneration (33, 34) (Fig. 12.2). Paresthesias of the hands and feet are some of the earliest clinical manifestations of toxic neuropathies. The clinical progression of toxic neuropathies will usually continue unless the individual's exposure is terminated (Fig. 12.3). Severe, permanent disability can result from toxic exposures which can be manifested clinically as central and peripreal neuropathies and dementia. Autonomic dysfunction is uncommon.

In some neuropathies, motor function may be more predominantly involved, as in the case with lead poisoning. Trichloroethylene is known to cause focal trigeminal neuropathy as well as facial anesthesia and cerebral atrophy. Chronic arsenic poisoning can cause painful neuritis and polyneuropathy in extremities. A particularly interesting form of neuropathy is the delayed toxic neuropathy which can occur 1–3 weeks following toxic exposures to organophosphate insecticides. Organophosphate-related neuropathy usually presents with painful, crampy muscles and distal paresthesia. Lower extremity weakness occurs and becomes progressive along with depression of the reflexes. Flaccid weakness of distal muscles may occur along with muscle wasting. The pathophysiology of organophos-

Pathological Features of Toxic Neuropathies

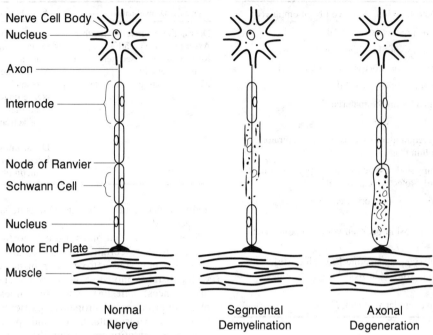

Figure 12.2.   Pathologic features of toxic neuropathies.

CLINICAL PROGRESSION OF TOXIC NEUROPATHY

Intermittent Numbness

Increased Sensitivity of Feet

Painful Neuritis of Hands and/ or Feet

Paresthesias of Hands and/ or Feet

Motor Weakness in Feet or Hands

Difficluty Grasping Objects

Ataxic Gait

Proximal Muscle Weakness of
Extensors then Flexors

Muscle Atrophy

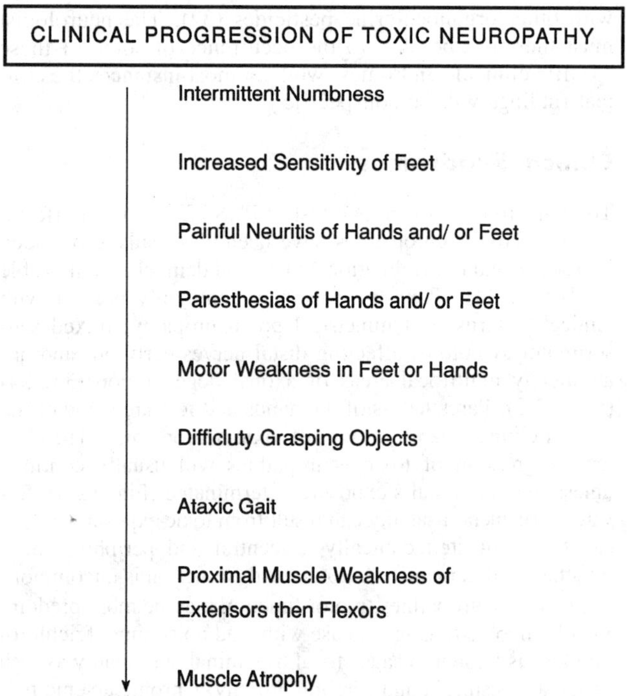

Figure 12.3.   Clinical progression of toxic neuropathy.

phate-induced neuropathy is thought to be secondary to phosphorylation of neurotoxic esterase enzyme present in nervous tissue.

Clinical pathologic correlation has revealed that multifocal changes have occurred in distal portions of the longest and largest axons following a toxic exposure (33, 34). Degenerative changes do not always begin in the terminal part of the axon. Clinically,

paresthesias of the hands and feet may occur at this stage. As exposure continues, these degenerative changes progress proximally toward the neuronal cell body (Fig. 12.4). As this proximal spread occurs, motor weakness and sensory changes become evident. CNS fibers may also be affected. The long and large pathways, such as the corticospinal tract and spinocerebellar tract, are usually the earliest area of the CNS involved in toxic neuropathies (33, 34). Both CNS and PNS changes in these sensitive, long and large tracts may be detected concurrently. The shorter and smaller diameter nerve tracts are usually the last to be involved following chronic neurotoxic exposures.

With progression of the clinical syndrome, abnormalities of motor nerve conduction and electromyography may become evident, the patient may develop extremity weakness with a mixed sensorimotor pattern, and the gait may become altered and ataxic. Peripheral nervous system signs may predominate in the clinical picture. The cerebral spinal fluid protein content is usually normal on examination. Following termination of the toxic exposure, clinical recovery may be gradual. Axonal regeneration may take months with the growth rate of 1 mm/ day. Painful neuritis may be present for months in some cases.

SPECIAL DIAGNOSTIC TESTS

Imaging

Neurodiagnostic tests are generally normal or nonspecific in most cases of neurotoxic illness (25). Neuroimaging studies, including computed tomography (CT) and magnetic resonance imaging (MRI), are usually normal and primarily useful in ruling out other conditions. The main reason that neuroimaging studies are usually normal is that neurotoxic injury is generally at a microscopic level and does not produce enough structural

Symptomatic Progression of Toxic Neuropathy

Insidious Onset	**Chronic Low Level Exposure Distal Portions of Scattered, Selected Fibers are Affected, Patient May Function Normally**

Lower Extremities Are Affected First	**Large and Long Axons Show Early Involvement**

Stocking-Glove Sensory Loss	**Clinical Signs Occur in the Feet and Hands Early in the Course as Degenerative Changes Are Occuring**

Loss of Achilles Muscle Stretch Reflex	**Fibers to the Muscles in the Calf May Show Early Involvement**

Motor Nerve Conduction Slowing	**Axonal Degeneration** **Scattered Motor Nerve Fibers May Be Intact and NCS May Appear Normal or Slightly Decreased Despite the Presence of Parasis** **Demyelinating Degeneration** **Motor Nerve Roots Are Diffusely Affected**

Clinical Recovery	**Axonal Degeneration Recovery is Slow (1 mm Per Day) and Regeneration May Take Months to Years**

Residual Disability	**There may be CNS degeneration Which May Not Be Apparent as Well As PNS Pathology. Residual Lesions May Include Ataxia, Spasticity, Cerebral Atrophy, Dementia, Permanent Neuropathies.**

Figure 12.4 Symptomatic progression of toxic neuropathy.

damage to be imaged. Some exceptions include anoxic brain injury related to carbon monoxide (35, 36) or cyanide (22) where macroscopic lesions of the basal ganglia have been described. CT imaging in cases of severe methanol intoxication has also occasionally revealed lesions of the basal ganglia (37, 38). In one instance, chronic toluene abuse, MRI has revealed a consistent pattern of white matter changes in individuals with persistent neurologic abnormalities (41). Other methods of neuroimaging such as positron emission tomography (PET) and

single photon emisson computed tomography (SPECT), which are methods of imaging different cerebral metabolic pathways, may become sensitive methods of studying neutotoxic effects but thus far have not been widely used (22).

Nerve Conditions Studies and Electromyography

Electrodiagnostic studies of the PNS, such as quantitative sensory testing and nerve conduction studies (NCS), have generally demonstrated nonspecific axonal dysfunction. Nerve conduction studies and electromyography can provide quantitative information to identify focal lesions and discern axonal degeneration from segmental degeneration. NCS can also be used to check the progression of neuropathy or the regeneration of nerve fibers. Conduction velocity of nerves can be normal or only slightly reduced when the pathology is predominantly axonal degeneration (33, 34). Thus in the majority of toxic neuropathies, even with clinically evident findings, the NCS will be normal. NCS is usually abnormal in segmental demyelination. A normal nerve condition velocity or EMG study does not rule out toxic neuropathy.

Due to the fact that there is a reduction in the number of functional axons in many toxic neuropathies, electromyography (EMG) studies may show abnormalities of the muscles supplied by the affected nerves (33, 34). Thus, the EMG will be helpful as an adjunct to NCS in determining axonal degeneration. The EMG may show abnormal spontaneous activity, such as fibrillation and high frequency potentials, in resting muscles of affected nerves. Upon active muscle contraction, the overall number of motor units is reduced in axonal toxic neuropathies. In clinical practice, the neuropathology pattern is usually one of a mixed axonal and segmental degeneration. Both EMG and NCS may be abnormal in organophosphate-induced neuropathy. Both NCS and EMG are usually normal early in the clinical course of toxic neuropathy.

Occasionally, sural nerve biopsy can provide a more definitive pathotoxicologic diagnosis for toxic effects and help corroborate EMG and NCS investigations.

Evoked Potentials

Other electrophysiologic tests which have been used in studying neurotoxic disease include auditory and visual evoked potentials, which have been found to be abnormal in cases of chronic toluene abuse (41). Evoked potentials are noninvasive electrophysiologic studies that can measure sensitive effects of toxins on the CNS. Properly performed, sensory evoked potentials can provide reliable information on the integrity of the sensory pathways from the periphery to the cortex (42). Evoked potentials can be visual or auditory in stimuli and are electrical manifestations of multisynaptic pathway activity from the distal axon and synapses involved in transmission of nerve activity to the CNS. Evoked potentials are thought to be an important tool for detection of subclinical or early neurologic disorders from toxic exposures. Evoked potential measurements use electrodes affixed to the scalp to record brain activity similar to electroencephalograms.

Both evoked potentials can be found to be abnormal in disorders affecting the myelin sheath (43). Auditory evoked potentials use sounds to measure brainstem responses. Visual evoked potentials use stroboscopic lights or light patterns. Evoked potentials are being studied as a sensitive screening tool for early neurotoxicity detection.

Neuropsychologic Studies

Other neurodiagnostic tests, such as neuropsychologic tests, though useful in defining the type and extent of CNS injury, have not proven to be of definitive value in differentiating neurotoxic disease from naturally occurring neurologic disease and even, in some instances, purely psychologic disorder. With rare exceptions, therefore, special neurodiagnostic studies have

helped neither in our understanding of the pathophysiology of neurotoxic disease nor in the specific diagnosis. Their primary value is in ruling out other conditions.

Neuropsychologic alterations following toxic exposures have been extensively reviewed in terms of a variety of occupational toxic exposures, including organic solvents, metals, and certain gases such as carbon monoxide. However, many factors can interfere with neuropsychologic evaluation of patients, such as: personality, cultural background, prior disease states, drug and alcohol abuse, premorbid IQ. Also other causes of disease must be ruled out.

The common neuropsychologic parameters stated to be affected by toxins include intelligence, language abilities, reasoning, visuospatial skills, attention, cognitive tracking, motor abilities, memory, sensory abilities, memory and learning, and personality (44).

Much has been written on the chronic exposure to solvents in working environments and the neuropsychologic disorder termed "solvent syndrome" (45, 46). Complaints of headache, behavioral changes, confusion, emotional dysfunction, fatigue, paresthesias, memory deficits, and depression have been attributed to this chronic exposure. Certain neuropsychologic parameters are important to test in diagnosing neuropsychologic effects from solvents. Neuropsychologic evaluation of toxic exposures is still in its infancy in terms of actually making toxic disease diagnoses.

REFERENCES

1. Lewis AJ. Functions of supporting cells. In: Lewis AJ, ed. Mechanisms of neurological disease. Boston: Little, Brown and Co., 1976;77–93.
2. Norton S. Toxic responses of the central nervous system. In: Klassen CD, Amdur MO, Doull J, eds. Casarett and Doull's toxicology: the basic science of poisons. New York: Macmillan, 1986;359–386.
3. Reese TS, Brightman MW. Similarity in structure and permeability to peroxidase of epithelia overlying fenestrated cerebral capillaries. Anat Rec 1968;169:4414.
4. Brightman MW, Reese TS. Junctions between intimately apposed cell membranes in the vertebrate brain. J Cell Biol 1969;40:648–677.
5. Olsson Y, Hossman KA. Fine structural localization of exudated protein tracers in the brain. Acta Neuropathol (Berl) 1970;16:103–116.
6. Brierly JB. The sensory ganglia—recent anatomical, physiological and pathological contributions. Acta Psychiatr Neurol Scand 1955;30:553–576.
7. Olsson Y. Topographical differences in the vascular permeability of the peripheral nervous system. Acta Neuropathol (Berl) 1968;10:26–33.
8. Jacobs JM, MacFarlane RM, Cavanaugh JB. Vascular leakage in the dorsal root ganglia of the rat, studied with horseradish peroxidase. J Neurol Sci 1976;29:95–107.
9. Jacobs JM. Penetration of systemically injected horseradish peroxidase into ganglia and nerves of the autonomic nervous system. J Neurocytol 1977;6:607–618.
10. Lewis AJ. Cells of the central nervous system. In: Lewis AJ, ed. Mechanisms of neurological disease. Boston: Little, Brown and Co., 1976;25–53.
11. Goyer RA. Toxic effects of metals. In: Klaasson CD, Amdur MO, Doull J, eds. Casarett and Doull's toxicology: the basic science of poisons. New York: Macmillian, 1986:582–635.
12. Duncan ID. Toxic myelinopathies. In: O'Donoghue JL, ed. Neurotoxicity of industrial and commercial chemicals, Vol. I. Boca Raton, FL: CRC Press, 1985:15–50.
13. Katz GV. Metals and metalloids other than mercury and lead. In O'Donoghue JL, ed. Neurotoxicity of industrial and commercial chemicals, Vol. I. Boca Raton, FL: CRC Press, 1985:171–191.
14. Goetz CG, Klawans HL. Neurologic aspects of other metals. In: Vinken PJ, Bruyn GW, eds. Intoxication of the nervous system, Part I. Amsterdam: Elsevier North-Holland, 1979:319–345.
15. Kurtzke JF, Kurland LT. The epidemiology of neurologic disease. In: Joynt RJ, ed. Clinical neurology. vol. 4. Philadelphia: JB Lippincott, 1983;66:1–143.
16. Tsubaki T, Honma Y, Hoshi M. Neurological syndrome associated with clioquinol. Lancet 1971;1:696.
17. Littorin ME, Fehling C, Attewell RG, Skerfving S. Focal epilepsy and

exposure to organic solvents: a case-referent study. J Occup Med 1988;30:805–808.

18. Amaducci L, Arfaioli C, Inzitari D, Marchi M. Multiple sclerosis among shoe and leather workers: an epidemiological study in Florence. Acta Neurol Scand 1982;65:94–103.

19. Shalat SL, Seltzer B, Baker EL Jr. Occupational risk factors and Alzheimer's disease: a case-control study. J Occup Med 1988;30:934–936.

20. Calne DB, McGeer E, Eisen A, Spencer PS. Alzheimer's disease, Parkinson's disease, and motoneurone disease: a biotropic interaction between aging and environment? Lancet 1986;2:1067–1070.

21. Spencer PS, Nunn PB, Hugon J, Ludolph AC, Ross RM, Roy DN, Robertson RC. Guam amyotrophic lateral sclerosis-parkinsonism-dementia linked to a plant excitant neurotoxin. Science 1987;237:517–522.

22. Rosenberg NL, Myers JA, Martin WRW. Cyanide-induced parkinsonism: clinical, MRI and 6-fluorodopa PET studies. Neurology 1989;39:142–144.

23. Reinhardt CF, Azar A, Maxfield ME, Smith PE JR, Mullin LS. Cardiac arrhythmias and aerosol "sniffing". Arch Environ Health 1971;22:265–279.

24. Lewis AJ. Disorders of energy supply: hypoxemia, hypoglycemia, and ischemia. In: Lewis AJ, ed. Mechanisms of neurological disease. Boston: Little, Brown and Co., 1976:235–254.

25. Schaumburg HH, Spencer PS. Recognizing neutotoxic disease. Neurology 1987;37:276–278.

26. Lee WR, McCallum RI. The occupational history. In: Raffle PAB, Lee WR, McCallum RI, Murray R, eds. Hunter's diseases of occupation. Boston: Little, Brown and Co., 1987;229–236.

27. Imbus HR. Clinical aspects of occupational medicine. In: Zenz C, ed. Occupational medicine. Chicago: Year Book Medical Publishers, 1988:107–119.

28. Allen N, Mendell JR, Billmaier DJ, Fontaine RE, O'Neill J. Toxic polyneuropathy due to methyl n-butyl ketone. Arch Neurol 1975;32:209–218.

29. Anger WK. Workplace exposures. In: Annau Z, ed. Anurobehavioral toxicology. Baltimore: Johns Hopkins Press, 1986;331–347.

30. McCabe LC, Clayton GD. Air pollution by hydrogen sulfide in Poza Rica, Mexico. Arch Ind Hyg Occup Med 1952;6:199–213.

31. Chhuttani PN, Chopra JS. Arsenic poisoning. In: Vinken PJ, Bruyn GW, eds. Intoxication of the nervous system, Part I. Amsterdam: Elsevier North-Holland, 1979:199–216.

32. Taylor JR, Calabrese VP, Blanke RV. Organochlorine and other insecticides. In: Vinken PJ, Bruyn GW, eds. Intoxications of the nervous system, Part I. Amsterdam: Elsevier North-Holland, 1979:391–455.

33. Schaumburg H, Spencer P. Toxic neuropathies. Neurology 29:429–431.

34. Lotti M, Becker C, Aminoff M. Occupational peripheral neuropathies. West J Med 1982;137:493–498.

35. Klawans HL, Stein RW, Tanner CM, Goetz CG. A pure parkinsonian syndrome following acute carbon monoxide intoxication. Arch Neurol 1982;39:302–304.

36. Schwartz A, Hennerici M, Wegener OH. Delayed choreoathetosis following acute carbon monoxide poisoning. Neurology 1985;35:988–99.

37. Choi IS. Delayed neurologic sequelae in carbon monoxide intoxication. Arch Neurol 1983;40:433–435.

38. Aquilonius S-M, Bergstrom K, Enoksson P, Hedstrand, Lundberg PO, Mostrom U, Olsson Y. Cerebral computed tomography in methanol intoxication. J Comput Assist Tomogr 1980;4:425–428.

39. Rosenberg NL. Methylmalonic acid, methanol, metabolic acidosis and lesions of the basal ganglia. Ann Neurol 1987;22:96–97.

40. Rosenberg NL, Kleinschmidt-DeMasters BK, Davis KA, Dreisbach JN, Hormes JT, Filley CM. Toluene abuse causes diffuse central nervous system white matter changes. Ann Neurol 1988;23:611–614.

41. Rosenberg NL, Spitz MC, Filley CM, Davis KA, Schaumburg HH. Central nervous system effects of chronic toluene abuse—clinical, brainstem evoked response and magnetic resonance imaging studies. Neurotoxicol Teratol 1988;10:489–495.

42. Arezzo J, Simson R, Brennan N. Evoked potentials in the assessment of neurotoxicity in humans. Neurobehavioral Toxicol Teratol 1985;7:299–304.

43. Starr A: Auditory brainstem potentials: their theory and practice in evaluating neural function. In: Halliday A, Butler S, eds. A textbook of clinical neuropsychology. New York: John Wiley and Sons, 1987.

44. Hartman DE. Neuropsychological toxicology—identification and assessment of human neurotoxic syndromes. New York: Pergamon Press, 1988.

45. Baker E, Smith T, Landrigan P. The neurotoxicity of industrial solvents: a review of the literature. Am J Ind Med 1985;8:207–217.

46. Grasso P, Sharratt M, Davies D, Irvine D. Neurophysiological and psychological disorders and occupational exposure to organic solvents. Food Chem Toxicol 1984;22:819–852.

13

Neurobehavioral Toxicology

James P. Kelly, M.A., M.D.
Christopher M. Filley, M.D.

INTRODUCTION

Neurobehavioral toxicology, a discipline in its early infancy, is the study of the adverse effects of toxic substances on brain function. As will become apparent, the clinical data on neurobehavioral syndromes related to toxins are fragmentary and largely inconclusive. Some agents, such as lead, toluene, and the organophosphate compounds, cause relatively distinct clinical syndromes, but for many others, information is seriously lacking. Neuropathologic studies have usually been limited. It is clear that extensive clinical studies, using standardized psychologic testing, carefully selected control groups, and neuropathologic information whenever possible, are needed to clarify the prevalence, nature, severity, and pathophysiology of toxic neurobehavioral syndromes. Neurologic, neuropsychologic, electrophysiologic, and neuroimaging studies will all play a prominent role in these investigations.

Research in the field of neurobehavioral toxicology suffers from several significant problems. First, human experimentation with substances known or suspected of posing toxic risks cannot be performed for obvious ethical reasons. Second, the results of even the most carefully controlled animal experiments do not necessarily apply to humans. Third, most existing knowledge about toxic effects on humans has been derived from accidental acute exposures when little or no data for comparison exist regarding low level chronic exposure, let alone the premorbid functioning of the exposed individuals. Fourth, most toxic exposures occur with a mixture of substances. Rarely can the effects of one substance be isolated from the other chemical constituents or the products of their metabolism. Fifth, physiologic correlates of toxic neurobehavioral effects, such as blood and urine levels of suspected agents, vary considerably and often unpredictably. Data collection is confounded by unpredictable timing between exposure and sample acquisition, individual differences in the metabolism of substances, varying degrees of exposure to the substance given variable concentrations, and duration of exposure. Finally, there exists a methodologic diversity inherent in the use of different neuropsychologic tests and test batteries which themselves often suffer from problems of uncertain validity and reliability.

Authors of current textbooks of neuropsychology and behavioral neurology offer limited discussions of issues related to toxicology (1, 2), confine their reviews to the effects of drug and alcohol abuse (3, 4), or exclude the subject altogether (5, 6). Other sources (7–9) address the topic directly and provide more in-depth reviews of assessment measures in neurotoxic disturbances.

The aim of this chapter is to provide an overview of existing knowledge regarding neurobehavioral toxicology. In general, syndromes related to neurobehavioral toxins take one of two forms: acute confusional state, characterized by rapidly evolving deficits in arousal and attention (10), and dementia, a persistent disorder of cognitive and emotional functioning (11). Most toxic agents can in fact cause either syndrome, the clinical picture depending on the degree or duration of exposure. The major portion of the chapter will focus on toxins with known neurobehavioral effects, emphasizing the most typical clinical presentations. We will briefly explore the problems related to assessing the harmful effects of neurotoxic substances and will attempt to elucidate the known adverse effects of a short list of substances on mental functions and behavior.

EPIDEMIOLOGY OF TOXIC INJURY

Incidence and Prevalence

Our industrialized society places certain portions of the population at risk for exposure to a wide variety of pollutants and chemicals, most of which have been introduced without full awareness of their toxicity. Modern industry often demands that workers labor in settings where potential hazards from neurotoxic substances exist, and the number of new compounds which may have adverse neurobehavioral effects is increasing at an alarming rate. Even so, an epidemiology of neurobehavioral toxicity has not evolved for the following reasons. First, the exposure-effect relationship is seldom easily established between a given substance and a behavioral disturbance. Second, only recently has there been a call for mandatory reporting of occupational diseases where a high risk of toxic exposure exists. The reporting of toxic exposure in the general population is inconsistent and incomplete owing to a lack of systematic surveillance comparable to the reporting mechanism for communicable disease (12).

Common Chemicals and Toxins Involved

Table 13.1 lists substances that are known to be associated with neurobehavioral toxic syndromes and which will be reviewed individually below. This list is not intended to represent an exhaustive review, but rather to provide a distillation of documented reports of neurotoxicity which have often been corroborated by postmortem pathologic changes.

The routes of exposure and absorption as well as the mechanisms of toxicity are agent-specific and will be covered here. As the focus of this text is on the toxicology of hazardous materials, we have intentionally excluded discussions of neurobehavioral syndromes related to prescription medications, alcohol, and drug abuse.

METALS

Lead—Lead encephalopathy is the best known metal intoxication with neurobehavioral effects. Children are particularly vulnerable, and in older buildings, where deteriorating leaded

Table 13.1.   Toxic Substances Associated with Neurobehavioral Dysfunction

Metals
    Lead
    Mercury
    Arsenic
    Manganese
    Thallium
    Aluminum
Gases
    Carbon monoxide
    Nitrous oxide
Solvents
    Toluene
    Styrene
    Xylene
    Methyl alcohol
    Carbon disulfide
    Trichlorethylene
    Perchloroethylene
    n-Hexane
    Ethylene oxide
    Ethylene glycol
    Carbon tetrachloride
    Methylene chloride
    Methyl chloride
    Acrylamide
Pesticides
    Organophosphates
    Organochlorines
    Paraquat

paint may be compulsively ingested by young children (pica), a severe, sometimes fatal syndrome may ensue (13). Adults may also develop acute or chronic encephalopathy, although peripheral neuropathy is the more typical neurologic manifestation; common sources of exposure are inhalation of tetraethyllead in gasoline (14) and ingestion of inorganic lead from contaminated "moonshine" whiskey (15). Lead intoxication may also occur in industry and especially involves paints, printing, pottery glazing, lead smelting, and storage battery manufacturing. Inattention, poor memory, hallucinations, delusions, and irritability are features of the acute syndrome, and patients may have seizures and signs of increased intracranial pressure (15). Fatal cases typically show cerebral edema as well as neuronal loss in the hippocampus and cerebellum, and astrocytic gliosis (14). Dementia occurs in cases of severe or untreated poisoning. Diagnosis can be difficult, particularly in cases complicated by alcohol or inhalant abuse, but a blood lead level in excess of 80 μg/100 ml has usually been necessary to produce clinical effects (16). Chelation therapy with ethylenediaminetetraacetic acid (EDTA) or penicillamine may reverse the acute toxic manifestations (17), but irreversible dementia may result despite treatment (14, 15, 18).

Low level exposure to lead, particularly in children, has been a disputed cause of neurobehavioral impairment. Several studies have shown an inverse relationship between blood lead concentration in children and cognitive development (19–22). Another study showed an increase in hyperactive behavior among children with chronically increased lead absorption (23). The effect of confounding factors on childhood development remains difficult to exclude (22), and these data, although suggestive, require further confirmation.

Mercury—Intoxication with mercury occurs either with the inorganic form of the metal, absorbed through the skin and respiratory mucous membranes of workers involved in the manufacture of thermometers, mirrors, incandescent lights, x-ray machines, and vacuum pumps (24), or from organic mercury ingested with contaminated water or fish (16). Inorganic mercury poisoning formerly afflicted workers in the hatting industry, and it is believed that the phrase "mad as a hatter" may reflect the neuropsychiatric manifestations of mercury intoxication (25). Irritability, social withdrawal, poor concentration, and memory disturbance characterize the syndrome (24), which may have a strongly psychiatric presentation.

Organic mercury poisoning causes a more severe encephalopathy, often accompanied by blindness and ataxia if prolonged. This devastating syndrome came to be known as Minamata disease after organic mercury entered the food chain in Japan's Kyushu Island during the 1950s. Pathologic changes involve the insular cortex, calcarine cortex, and cerebellum primarily, where neuronal degeneration, small hemorrhages, and gliosis are seen (26). The diagnosis is supported by elevated mercury levels in urine and blood, and treatment with penicillamine may be effective (27).

Arsenic—In the past, when syphilis was treated with arsenicals, arsenic poisoning was more common than at present, but occasional cases are encountered among individuals exposed to certain insecticides and disinfectants and among those employed in the manufacture of paints, prints, and enamels. Delirium has been described as in initial syndrome, with agitation, disorientation, and hallucinations (28); gastrointestinal symptoms and peripheral neuropathy may be prominent. Dementia has been regarded as rare, although it has been documented (29). Fatal cases disclose a hemorrhagic white matter encephalopathy at autopsy. Arsenic levels in affected patients are elevated in the urine and in the hair, where they may remain present for years. Chelation therapy with dimercaprol has had variable results (28, 29).

Manganese—This element is a rare cause of toxicity, but its propensity to produce a parkinsonian syndrome is notable. Exposure may occur through ingestion or inhalation of manganese by miners of the ore. A confusional state heralds the onset of the movement disorder, and features irritability, hallucinations, and compulsive acts. Dementia can progress in association with parkinsonism and may include euphoria and aggressiveness in addition to poor concentration and memory (30). Neuropathologic studies have consistently found degeneration in the basal ganglia (31). Urine and blood levels of manganese are elevated. Treatment with EDTA is beneficial in some cases (32), and levodopa may help with the movement disorder.

Thallium—Thallium is used in the manufacture of sulfuric acid, as a rodenticide, and as a depilatory. An acute confusional state with irritability or agitation, hallucinations, memory impairment, and confabulation can be seen (33), often with gastrointestinal symptoms and alopecia. Dementia may also be seen (34), accompanied frequently by neuropathy, ataxia, tremor, and seizures. Persistent neuropsychologic deficits have been documented in one case (35). Edema of the white matter is found postmortem in fatal cases. Urinary measurements of thallium can be helpful, and treatment with potassium oxide to enhance thalliuresis has been proposed (36). Chelation has no established value.

Aluminum—Interest in aluminum has recently increased after the discovery that this metal is putatively the cause of dialysis encephalopathy (37). A progressive confusional state does appear in dialysis patients who cannot adequately clear aluminum because of uremia. As dementia advances, dysarthria, myoclonus, seizures, and electroencephalographic abnormalities become prominent. Autopsy studies in fatal cases demonstrate significantly greater amounts of aluminum in gray matter than in dialysis patients without encephalopathy (37).

The relevance of these findings to the causation of Alzheimer's disease (AD) remains uncertain. Laboratory animals exposed to aluminum can develop neurofibrillary tangles (38), but aluminum levels in brain (39), cerebrospinal fluid (40), and serum (41) may be normal in AD patients. It appears unlikely that neurobehavioral toxicity from aluminum affects any individuals other than uremic patients exposed to aluminum in the process of dialysis.

Other metals—Numerous other metals have occasionally been noted to produce neurobehavioral impairment, which may take the form of an acute confusional state or dementia. Gold (42), used in the treatment of arthritic conditions, tin (43), and bismuth (44) have been implicated, as have iron, antimony, barium, copper, and silver.

GASES

Carbon monoxide—Exposure to carbon monoxide (CO) can cause changes ranging from mild confusion to coma and death. Suicide attempts or accidental exposures can be causative, or individuals may be exposed to the exhaust from inefficient motorized machinery in poorly ventilated areas (45). Headache and cherry-red skin occur with lower levels of exposure, and at carboxyhemoglobin (COHb) levels over 30%, confusion begins. Higher COHb levels may lead to dementia, characterized by aphasia, apraxia, agnosia, and amnesia (46). Neuropathologically, changes are similar to those of anemic anoxia, since the CO molecule deprives the brain of oxygen delivery by virtue of its very high affinity for hemoglobin. Laminar neurosis in the second and third cortical layers, neuronal loss in the hippocampus, and degeneration in the basal ganglia are all seen, reflecting the most oxygen-dependent regions of the brain (47). A delayed syndrome of postanoxic dementia may follow apparent recovery by days to weeks and is thought to be due to extensive cerebral demyelination (48). Treatment consists of removal from the source of CO and administration of oxygen. The benefit of hyperbaric oxygen therapy remains controversial.

Nitrous oxide—This anesthetic agent has long been a drug of abuse and is known to cause peripheral neuropathy as well as myelopathy after longterm abuse. Neuropsychologic testing after acute exposure demonstrates psychomotor slowing (49). Trace amounts comparable to those found in hospital operating rooms were found in one study to produce deficits of vigilance on audiovisual tasks (50), but these results could not be replicated (51).

SOLVENTS

Organic solvents are ubiquitous in our society. In 1984, approximately 49 million tons of industrial solvents were produced in the United States, and these chemicals found use in paints, adhesive, glues, coatings, degreasing and cleaning agents, dyes, polymers, plastics, textiles, printing inks, agricultural products, and pharmaceuticals (41). As many as 9.8 million workers were exposed to organic solvents over one year in these industries (52). The question of neurotoxicity, especially

neurobehavioral in nature, is critical because many individuals complain of memory, cognitive, and emotional disturbances. During the past 10 years, a substantial literature, mostly from Scandinavian countries, has developed on the neuropsychologic effects of solvent exposure in the painting industry. As will be seen, controversy exists over the validity of studies purporting to show that brain damage results from this kind of exposure.

A more compelling literature is also available concerning the effects of high dose exposure to solvents, mostly through the unfortunate but common practice of inhalant abuse (53). In many of these studies, the neurotoxic effects of highlevel intoxication are obvious, although the question of lowlevel effects remains unresolved. In this section, we will summarize data from major solvent studies, both those examining workplace levels and those evaluating exposure through abuse.

Toluene—Acute encephalopathy from toluene abuse may involve lethargy, hallucinations, or even coma, but ordinarily these resolve completely with abstinence (54). Persistent encephalopathy may also occur in chronic abusers (55) and may involve cerebrum, brainstem, optic nerve, and cerebellum (56). Neuropsychologic impairment has also been reported (57). The solvent is inhaled as a euphorigenic intoxicant, usually in the form of spray paint; it is the most commonly abused organic solvent. Toluene, like other solvents, is highly lipophilic, and therefore readily enters the lipid-rich central nervous system.

Our own studies have shown that the dementia syndrome is characterized by apathy, inattention, poor memory, and the absence of aphasia (58); this profile distinguishes the syndrome from the dementia of AD, for example, and suggests that cortical gray matter is not primarily involved. Indeed magnetic resonance imaging (MRI) studies and one pathologically verified case disclose that cerebral white matter is primarily, if not exclusively, involved (59). The clinicopathologic correlations are so striking that toluene abuse appears to form a prototype example of "white matter dementia" (60).

Less convincing are studies from Scandinavia in which workers in the painting industry have been diagnosed as having chronic cerebral damage as a result of longterm lowlevel exposure to solvents (61). This syndrome has been termed the "chronic painters' syndrome" (62) or the "psycho-organic syndrome" (63) and manifests symptoms including fatigue, irritability, depression, and memory loss. Many studies, however, have been poorly controlled (64), and the determination of solvent neurotoxicity has not been rigorously established. In addition, the effects of alcohol have not been carefully excluded (65). Most recently, one of the Danish groups that initially supported the validity of the chronic painter's syndrome reanalyzed test data on solvent-exposed workers and concluded that previous impressions of significant intellectual impairment could not be confirmed when proper control groups were used (66).

Styrene—This solvent is used in the manufacture of plastics, latexes, resins, and glues. Human toxicity is rare, but in a study of controlled exposure normal volunteers experienced inebriation and ataxia at high levels (67). Longterm deficits in neuropsychologic function have also been documented (68).

Xylene—Employed in the painting industry, xylene can cause an acute confusional state or even death (69). Chronic exposure is less well understood, and reports of "neurasthenic" or "astheno-autonomic symptoms" (70) must be interpreted very cautiously.

Methyl alcohol—Methanol toxicity causes a well-known acute syndrome of confusion, headache, gastrointestinal complaints, and visual symptoms ranging from blurriness to blindness (71). The toxicity does not relate to methanol itself, but to its metabolites, formic acid and formaldehyde. Methanol poisoning occurs in alcoholics who use the agent as an inexpensive or temporary alternative to ethanol, but industrial exposure through ingestion, inhalation, or absorption through the skin may occur in the paint, rubber, synthetic textile, linoleum, and dye industries. Postmortem studies show variable edema and petechiae in the third ventricular region, ischemic necrosis in the cerebellar cortex, and cystic necrosis of the putamen (71). Treatment involves ethanol, bicarbonate, and in severe cases, hemodialysis.

A dementia syndrome has not been described, although blindness may be permanent. One case of parkinsonism has been reported, and treatment with levodopa was beneficial (72).

Carbon disulfide—Inhalation of carbon disulfide may occur in workers in the agricultural industry who are exposed to various insecticides, and in the rubber and viscous rayon industries. Peripheral neuropathy and parkinsonism are known to occur (73), but encephalopathy may also complicate the picture. Usually neurobehavioral changes develop insidiously in exposed individuals and involve inattention, irritability, forgetfulness, and mood changes. Neuropsychologic deficits have been documented (74). Limited autopsy material has shown a diffuse small vessel occlusive process and signs of infarction due to thrombosis; the speculation has been made that carbon disulfide may predispose to cerebral atherosclerosis (73).

Trichloroethylene—This widely used solvent is employed as an anesthetic in European countries but in the United States finds application in dry cleaning, in degreasing metal parts, as a rubber solvent, as an adhesive in the shoe industry, and as an ingredient in printing ink, paper, lacquer, and varnish (75). It is also used in the extraction of oils and fats from vegetable products, such as removing caffeine from coffee (75). An acute syndrome and a chronic encephalopathy may each result from trichloroethylene inhalation (76), and a particularly specific neurologic sign is trigeminal anesthesia (75). Peripheral neuropathy may also be encountered.

Perchloroethylene—This solvent is used extensively in dry cleaning and in fabric finishing and metal degreasing. Acute syndromes are apparently rare, but one recent case of longterm exposure resulted in a dementia syndrome resembling AD; after removal from the source of exposure, the patient recovered to normal (77).

n-Hexane—This aliphatic hydrocarbon is well-known as a cause of peripheral neuropathy, but it is also known to enter the central nervous system. n-Hexane is used as an industrial solvent in many settings, and it can be inhaled from glue vapors in inhalant abusers. Peripheral changes include a well-documented axonal neuropathy (78), but subclinical damage to central axons has also been shown by visual and auditory evoked potentials (79).

Ethylene oxide—Data on the neurobehavioral effects of this solvent are rare, although a sensory neuropathy has been described (80). High level exposure to ethylene oxide has resulted in acute encephalopathy (81), and a recent case of chronic low level exposure documented a partly reversible dementia, with impaired concentration, poor memory, cognitive slowing, and emotional lability (82). Neuropathologic data are lacking.

Ethylene glycol—Often ingested in the form of antifreeze for its intoxicating effects, this agent has a variety of neurologic effects, including acute confusional states, with drowsiness, hallucinations, and even coma, and late personality changes.

Exposure may also occur in industrial settings. Neuropathologic studies have reported brain edema, calcium oxalate crystal deposition, widespread neuronal damage, small hemorrhages in cortex, white matter, and brainstem, and perivascular encephalitis (83).

Carbon tetrachloride—This solvent finds use in the home as a cleansing agent and in rubber processing, paint manufacture, fabric cleaning, and degreasing of metal parts. The organ system most vulnerable to carbon tetrachloride poisoning is the nervous system, and acute as well as chronic neurobehavioral effects can be seen (84). Ataxia and peripheral neuropathy can also be encountered. Autopsy studies have shown demyelination and necrosis in the cerebrum and neuronal cell loss in the cerebellar cortex.

Methylene chloride—Metabolism of this solvent after its inhalation produces CO, and effects on behavior may relate to the solvent itself or its metabolite. Acute effects on vigilance, mood, and reaction time have been noted, but no longterm central nervous system injury has been observed (70).

Methyl chloride—Inhalation of methyl chloride, or absorption through the skin, may occur in the production of silicones, butyl rubber, and tetraethyllead and in the process of molding polystyrene and polyurethane foams. Acute effects include confusion, lethargy, and drowsiness; rare chronic syndromes involving amnesia, mental slowing, and incoherent speech have been reported (85). Autopsy studies have been very limited and inconclusive.

Acrylamide—This agent is a polymer precursor used in the production of flocculators and grouting agents. Like many solvents, it has peripheral neurotoxic effects, causing an axonal neuropathy with primarily sensory involvement (86). Acrylamide is inhaled or absorbed, and acute central neurotoxicity can also occur, with confusion, poor concentration, and hallucinations (87). Subacute intoxication may cause drowsiness, inattention, and ataxia (86). Although the axonal neuropathy is recognized, no studies of brain alterations in acrylamide toxicity are available.

PESTICIDES

This group of chemicals is manufactured to destroy some form of life, and all produce at least some toxicity in humans. Insecticides, herbicides, rodenticides, fumigants, and fungicides are the major classes of pesticides. Workers involved in the preparation and use of these compounds may develop toxic syndromes, many of which involve organs outside the nervous system.

With regard to neurobehavioral toxicity, the organophosphate insecticides stand foremost among the pesticides, and these will be discussed in detail. Organochlorine compounds also have some adverse effects upon behavior, although their use has now become quite limited. One group of herbicides, the bipyridyl compounds, will be discussed, and thallium, a potent rodenticide, has been covered above. Cyanide, a commonly used fumigant, usually results in rapid death, but cyanide-induced parkinsonism without dementia has recently been described (88). Fungicides have not been shown to be particularly hazardous to the nervous system.

Organophosphate compounds—These chemicals, of which approximately 50,000 have been synthesized, act in the brain by irreversibly binding acetylcholinesterase. Widely used in agriculture and also available to home owners, these agents primarily affect the nervous system. During World War II, extremely potent forms of organophosphates were used as "nerve gases" (tabun, sarin, soman), and diisopropylphosphorofluoridate (DPF) became the best studied of the entire group (89). Parathion, malathion, diazinon, tetraethylpyrophosphate, and triorthocresylphosphate (TOCP) are also members of this large class (88). Organophosphates cause the majority of pesticide poisonings in this country (90). They can be inhaled, ingested, or absorbed through the skin. A peripheral neuropathy has been ascribed to TOCP poisoning in Jamaicans who consumed an extract of contaminated Jamaica ginger ("ginger jake paralysis") (91), and a more delayed neuropathy has been reported recently (92).

Neurobehavioral effects may be acute or chronic. An acute confusional state is due to excessive stimulation of central cholinergic receptors, and peripheral manifestations are also prominent (89). Muscarinic effects may dominate the early picture, with miosis, nausea, vomiting, diaphoresis, diarrhea, and bradycardia; later, nicotinic manifestations of weakness and fasciculations occur. The confusional state is characterized by restlessness, headache, poor concentration, impaired memory, dysarthria, and apathy. Seizures are common. With treatment, which involves atropine and pralidoxime, most patients recover completely, but several reports suggest that deficits may persist for months to years after exposure (93–95). Common features in these studies appear to be impaired concentration, anxiety, and disturbed memory, but these conclusions must be interpreted cautiously because of methodologic concerns (90). Neuropathologic studies have been quite limited, although studies in exposed animals reveal edematous changes (88).

Organochlorine compounds—This group of compounds contains a number of agents that have achieved some recent notoriety: chlorophenothane (DDT), chlordecone (Kepone), aldrin, dieldrin, heptachlor, and endrin. After evidence documenting adverse effects of fish-eating birds' egg shells by DDT, this agent was banned in 1972 for all but very limited uses. The other organochlorine compounds have been largely replaced by organophosphates which do not persist in the environment.

Few data on neurobehavioral toxicity are available, but DDT does act as a central nervous system stimulant, causing anxiety, irritability, dizziness, and seizures acutely (96). The only member of the organochlorine group to cause prolonged neurotoxicity appears to be chlordecone, which resulted in several exposed workers experiencing tremor and opsoclonus for up to 18 months. Confusion, irritability, hallucinations, and memory loss were seen in some individuals for an undetermined period (97).

Paraquat—This is the most important member of the bipyridyl herbicides from a toxicologic standpoint. Pulmonary toxicity has been most publicized (paraquat lung) and may be quite severe, but a recent case of suicide due to ingestion of paraquat disclosed significant brain damage as well. Anoxic changes were present, not unexpectedly, but in addition there were diffuse changes in cerebral white matter, possibly due to a direct toxic effect of the chemical (98).

ROUTES OF EXPOSURE AND ABSORPTION

Since the route of toxic exposure is specific to each substance, a brief description of the known mechanisms has been mentioned with each individual agent above. These primarily include inhalation, ingestion, and transdermal absorption. Firm evidence of exposure is sometimes available through physiologic testing for the presence of the substance itself or its metabolites in blood, urine, or both.

Regardless of the mechanism of exposure, all substances toxic to the brain must be blood-borne in order to produce their effects. They must penetrate complex barrier systems in and around the brain. These include the blood-brain barrier, the blood-cerebrospinal barrier, and the arachnoid barrier layer, each comprising specialized membrane components for selective permeability and "tight junctions" between adjacent cells (99).

BASIC TOXICITY MECHANISMS

The nervous system may be affected at many levels by toxic substances, and as a general rule resultant syndromes are diffuse in their manifestations. Because of their nonfocal presentations, neurotoxic disorders may be confused with metabolic, degenerative, nutritional, or demyelinating diseases (100). In addition, toxic syndromes rarely have specific identifying features on diagnostic tests such as computed tomography (CT), (MRI), or nerve conduction studies. As a result, subtle cases of intoxication may be very difficult to diagnose.

The neurotoxicity of a given substance may produce its effect at the level of intracellular processes, within the axon, at the presynaptic or postsynaptic membrane, or within the synaptic cleft or indirectly by affecting the glial cell and its myelin surrounding neuronal projections. In the discussions of individual toxins above, specific mention has been made of documented evidence of sites of pathologic changes. A mixed picture of central and peripheral nervous system abnormalities is not unusual, and it would be erroneous to classify toxins as affecting one or the other exclusively. For example, even though clinical reports of central nervous system toxicity reaching symptomatic levels may be rare, it is noteworthy that n-hexane has been known to enter the central nervous system (80). The possibility of central toxicity due to this and other known peripheral nervous system toxins should stimulate awareness that any lipophilic agent may have potential neurobehavioral toxicity.

DIAGNOSTIC STRATEGIES AND DEFINITION OF TOXIC EXPOSURE

History

Obtaining a detailed history regarding the presence of known or presumed toxic agents, as well as the nature and duration of exposure, is critical to the establishment of an exposure-effect relationship. Due to the mental status alterations frequently observed, this historical information may not be reliably obtained from the exposed individual. If any doubt about the accuracy of the history exists, every effort should be made to corroborate facts by obtaining results of pertinent environmental tests as well as interviewing others directly involved in the incident (coworkers, paramedics, etc.). It may also be helpful to consider the use of questionnaires or inventories designed specifically for toxic exposures and their neurobehavioral manifestations (101).

A standard medical history for premorbid physical or psychiatric problems must be documented. Current medication lists as well as alcohol or other drug use should be included. The use of drugs, legitimate or otherwise, by workers is a major

Table 13.2. Commonly Used Drugs Associated with Neurobehavioral Toxicity

Prescription
  Anticholinergic compounds
  Sedative/hypnotics
  Antipsychotics
  Lithium
  Antidepressants
  Anticonvulsants
  Levodopa
  Antihypertensives
  Steroids
  Digitalis
Recreational
  Alcohol
  Cocaine
  Amphetamines
  LSD
  PCP
  Marijuana
  Opiates
  MPTP

Table 13.3. Neuropsychologic Tests

Attention and Concentration
  PASAT (Paced Auditory Serial Attention Test)
  Digit Span
Memory
  Wechsler Memory Scale
  Benton Visual Retention
Psychomotor performance
  Finger tapping
  Grip strength
  Santa Ana Dexterity Test
Sensation and perception
  Tactual Performance Test (TPT)
  Seashore Rhythm Test
  Speech Sounds Perception Test
  Reitan-Klove Sensory Perceptual Examination
Sequencing, planning, and efficiency
  Trail Making Tests A and B
  Digit Symbol Test (Subtest of WAIS-R)
Abstraction and cognitive flexibility
  Halstead Category Test
  Wisconsin Card Sorting Test
  Stroop Color-Work Interference Test
Language skills
  Reitan Indiana Aphasia Screen Test
  Boston Diagnostic Aphasia Examination (BDAE)
Personality and emotional state
  Minnesota Multiphasic Personality Inventory (MMPI)
  Taylor Manifest Anxiety Scale
Intelligence and academic skills
  Wechsler Adult Intelligence Scale—Revised (WAIS-R)
  Wechsler Intelligence Scale for Children—Revised (WISC-R)
  Peabody Individual Achievement Test (PIAT)

consideration in the evaluation of possible neurobehavioral toxicity. A great many prescription drugs have wellknown acute and chronic neurobehavioral effects, and the recreational or illicit drugs have an obvious impact on cerebral function as well. Table 13.2 lists some of the more common drugs which may be implicated in neurobehavioral dysfunction.

A wide variety of medications used in neurologic, psychiatric, and medical practice have neurobehavioral effects. In general, the syndromes are familiar: a subacute or acute confusional state in cases with limited exposure to the drug, or dementia in patients with long-standing or inappropriate dosing. These toxic syndromes are more likely to appear in the elderly (102). Of particular concern are the anticholinergic drugs (103) and the sedative/hypnotics (104), but antipsychotics, lithium, antidepressants, and a number of other drugs may be implicated as well (11). Documentation of a careful drug history is critical in establishing the validity of a supposed toxic syndrome. As with the drugs of abuse, medications taken in excessive amounts can complicate the issue of neurobehavioral toxicity in a suspected case.

Although many toxins in the environment are capable of producing neurobehavioral toxicity, in many cases patient complaints represent psychiatric disturbances. These syndromes, which are perhaps related to stress, but not to a given toxin or toxins, are a major source of uncertainty to clinicians and investigators. It is not a simple matter, for example, to determine whether an individual who has noticed irritability and poor concentration after exposure to solvent vapor has a neurobehavioral syndrome or a psychiatric disorder exacerbated by stress.

Physical Exam

Unfortunately, the physical term is not typically helpful in the diagnosis of toxic neurobehavioral syndromes. Nevertheless, a detailed neurologic and mental status (105) examination may uncover signs of damage to cranial or peripheral nerves which could point to mixed peripheral and central toxic effects. Coordination and balance are less commonly affected. Signs of delirium (agitation, disorientation, fluctuating level of con-

sciousness) or dementia (intellectual decline, memory dysfunction) should be evident on mental status examination (106).

Laboratory Tests

The toxic substances or its metabolites may be detected in blood or urine. These are obviously specific to the agent involved and have been noted above. Routine screening of organ system disease with blood count, electrolytes, renal function tests, and liver function tests is appropriate. In addition, if dementia is a clinical concern and has not been evaluated, thyroid function tests, vitamin B12 level, and serology should be ordered. Spinal fluid studies for evidence of inflammatory or infectious conditions may be necessary if clinical suspicion is high.

Special Diagnostic Tests

In most cases, the need for quantified evaluation in neurobehavioral syndromes dictates that formal neuropsychologic testing be performed. The wide variety of psychologic tests available today makes standardization of neuropsychologic toxicology extremely difficult (8). A thorough neuropsychologic evaluation tests cognitive and emotional domains in detail. It is typical that the pattern of results over a broad spectrum of tests provide a clinical impression of toxic effect that no single test can provide. Table 13.3 provides a sample of widely accepted neuropsychologic tests along with the mental functions they test.

CT scans of the brain may detect atrophy in cases of toxic encephalopathy, but more often the information obtained is unconvincing and not supportive. However, CT scans should be considered to rule out other neuropathology such as tumor or hydrocephalus. As noted above, MRI scans have documented evidence of neurotoxic change in solvent abusers (59) and should be considered the neuroimaging technique of choice in toxic neurobehavioral syndromes.

Visual evoked potentials (VEP) and auditory evoked potentials (AEP) have been shown to detect subclinical dyfunction (79), but these tests are difficult to perform properly and do not offer a high yield of positive results in this setting. Electroencephalography (EEG) rarely adds to the clinical picture, with normal activity or minimal diffuse slowing the most common findings. Its usefulness seems to be in ruling out alternative diagnoses. Brain mapping of EEG activity and evoked potentials may provide valuable diagnositic information in the future, but at present it must be considered a research instrument (107).

DIAGNOSTIC STRATEGY SUMMARY

History
  Factual evidence sought regarding suspected exposure
  Documentation of premorbid level of functioning
  Preexisting neurologic or psychiatric disorders
  Occupational and social history
  Family history

Neurologic Exam
  Detailed mental status examination
  Cranial nerves including funduscopic exam
  Motor function
  Sensory function
  Coordination, gait, and reflexes

Laboratory Tests
  Toxin tests (or metabolites) in blood, urine, hair, and nails
    as appropriate
  Liver and kidney functions
  Thyroid functions
  Vitamin B12
  Serology
  Erythrocyte sedimentation rate
  Spinal fluid analysis

Neuropsychologic Consultation
  Thorough battery of cognitive and emotional tests
  Comparison with prior level of functioning or test data when
    available

Special Tests
  MRI scan or CT scan (if MRI not available)
  Evoked potential testing (if symptoms dictate)
  Nerve conduction studies and electromyography

Acknowledgment

The authors are grateful to Jonathan Filley, Ph.D., for his assistance in the preparation of this review.

REFERENCES

1. Lezak MD. Neuropsychological assessment. 2nd ed. New York: Oxford, 1983.
2. Strub RL, Black FW. Neurobehavioral disorders: a clinical approach. Philadelphia: FA Davis, 1988.
3. Heilman KM, Valenstein E, eds. Clinical neuropsychology. 2nd ed. New York: Oxford, 1985.
4. Grant I, Adams KM, eds. Neuropsychological assessment of neuropsychiatric disorders. New York: Oxford, 1986.
5. Mesulam M-M. Principles of behavioral neurology. 3rd ed. New York: Oxford, 1985.
6. Pincus JH, Tucker GS. Behavioral neurology. 3rd ed. New York: Oxford, 1985.
7. Gilioli R, Cassitto MG, Foa V, eds. Neurobehavioral methods in occupational health. Advances in the biosciences, Vol. 46. Oxford: Pergamon Press, 1982.
8. Hartman DE. Identification and assessment of human neurotoxic syndromes. In: Neuropsychological toxicology. New York: Pergamon Press, 1988.
9. Johnson BL, ed. Prevention of neurotoxic illness in working populations. New York: John Wiley & Sons, 1987.
10. Strub RC. Acute confusional state. In: Benson DF, Blumer D, eds. Psychiatric aspects of neurologic disease, Vol. 2. New York: Grune & Stratton, 1982.
11. Cummings JL, Benson DF. Dementia: a clinical approach. Boston: Butterworths, 1983:1–14.
12. Chorba TL, Berkelman RL, Safford SK, Gibbs NP, Hull HF. Mandatory reporting of infectious diseases by clinicians. JAMA 1989;262:3018–3026.
13. Albert JJ, Breault HJ, Friend WK, et al. Prevention, diagnosis, and treatment of lead poisoning in children. Pediatrics 1969;44:291–298.
14. Valpey R, Sumi SM, Copass MK, Goble GJ. Acute and chronic progressive encephalopathy due to gasoline sniffing. Neurology 1978;28:507–510.
15. Whitfield CL, Ch'ien LT, Whitehead JD. Lead encephalopathy in adults. Am J Med 1972;52:289–298.
16. Goetz CG, Klawans HH, Cohen MM. Neurotoxic agents. In: Baker AB, Baker LH, eds. Clinical neurology. New York: Harper and Row, 1981:1–84.
17. Graef JW. Clinical aspects of lead poisoning. In: Vinken PJ, Bruyn GW, eds. Intoxications of the nervous system. Part 1, vol. 36. Handbook of clinical neurology. New York: North Holland, 1979:1–34.
18. Perlstein MA, Attala R. Neurologic sequelae of plumbism in children. Clin Pediatr 1966;5:292–298.
19. Bellinger D, Leviton A, Waternaux C, Needleman H, Rabinowitz M. Longitudinal analyses of prenatal and postnatal lead exposure and early cognitive development. N Engl J Med 1987;316:1037–1043.
20. Needleman HL. Lead at low dose and the behavior of children. Acta Psychiatr Scand 1983;303 (suppl):38–48.
21. Dietrich KN, Krafft KM, Bornschein RL, et al. Low-level fetal lead exposure effect on neurobehavioral development in early infancy. Pediatrics 1987;80:721–730.
22. McMichael AJ, Baghurst PA, Wigg NR, Vimpani GV, Robertson EF, Roberts RS. Port Pirie cohort study: environmental exposure to lead and children's ability at the age of four years. N Engl J Med 1988;319:468–475.
23. Baloh R, Sturm R, Green B, Gleser G. Neuropsychological effects of chronic asymptomatic increased lead absorption. Arch Neurol 1975;32:326–330.
24. Vroom FQ, Greer M. Mercury vapor intoxication. Brain 1972;95:305–318.
25. Hunter D. The diseases of occupations. Boston: Little Brown, 1955.
26. Kurland LT, Faro SN, Siedler H. Minamata disease. World Neurol 1960;1:370–392.
27. Kark RAP, Poskanzer DC, Bullock JD, Boylen G. Mercury poisoning and its treatment with N-acetyl-D,L-penicillamine. N Engl J Med 1971;285:10–16.
28. Beckett WS, Moore JL, Keough JP, Bleecker MR. Acute encephalopathy due to occupational exposure to arsenic. Br J Ind Med 1986;43:66–67.
29. Freeman JW, Couch JR. Prolonged encephalopathy with arsenic poisoning. Neurology 1978;28:853–855.
30. Abd El Naby S, Hassanein M. Neuropsychiatric manifestations of chronic manganese poisoning. J Neurol Neurosurg Psychiatry 1965;28:282–288.
31. Yamada M, Ohno S, Okayasu I, et al. Chronic manganese poisoning: a neuropathological study with determination of manganese distribution in the brain. Acta Neuropathol 1986;70:273–278.
32. Mena I, Marin O, Feunzalida S, Cotzias GC. Chronic manganese poisoning. Neurology 1967;17:128–136.
33. Prick JJG. Thallium poisoning. In: Vinken PJ, Bruyn GW, eds. Intoxications of the nervous system. Part 1, vol. 36. Handbook of clinical neurology. New York: North-Holland, 1979:239–278.
34. Domnitz J. Thallium poisoning. A report of six cases. South Med J 1960;53:590–593.

35. Thompson C, Dent J, Saxby P. Effects of thallium poisoning on intellectual functioning. Br J Psychiatry 1988;153:396–399.

36. Bank WJ, Pleasure DE, Suzuki K, et al. Thallium poisoning. Arch Neurol 1972;26:456–464.

37. Alfrey AC, Legendre GR, Kaehny WD. The dialysis encephalopathy syndrome: possible aluminum intoxication. N Engl J Med 1976;294:184–188.

38. Klatzo I, Wisniewski H, Stretcher E. Experimental production of neurofibrillary degeneration. I. Light microscopic observations. J Neuropathol Exp Neurol 1965;24:187–199.

39. McDermott JR, Smith AI, Iqbal K, Wisniewski HM. Aluminum and Alzheimer's disease. Lancet 1977;2:710–711.

40. Delaney JF. Spinal fluid aluminum levels in patients with Alzheimer disease. Ann Neurol 1979;5:580–581.

41. Shore D, Milloon M, Holtz JL, King SW, Bridge TP, Wyatt RJ. Serum aluminum in primary degenerative dementia. Biol Psychiatry 1980;15:971–977.

42. McAuley DLF, Lecky BRF, Earl CJ. Gold encephalopathy. J Neurol Neurosurg Psychiatry 1977;40:1021–1022.

43. Foncin JF, Gruner JE. Tin neurotoxicity. In: Vinken PJ, Bruyn GW, eds. Intoxications of the neuron system. Part 1, vol. 36. Handbook of clinical neurology. New York: North-Holland, 1979:279–290.

44. Buge A, Supino-Viterbo V, Rancurel G, Pontes C. Epileptic phenomena in bismuth toxic encephalopathy. J Neurol Neurosurg Psychiatry 1981;44:62–67.

45. Gilbert GJ, Glaser GH. Neurologic manifestations of chronic carbon monoxide poisoning. N Engl J Med 1969;261:1217–1220.

46. Winter P, Miller J. Carbon monoxide poisoning. JAMA 1976;236:1502–1504.

47. Brierly JB. Cerebral hypoxia. In: Blackwood W, Corsellis JAN, eds. Greenfield's neuropathology. Chicago: Year Book Medical Publishers, 1976:43–85.

48. Plum F, Posner JB, Hain RF. Delayed neurological deterioration after anoxia. Arch Intern Med 1962;110:18–25.

49. Greenberg BD, Moore PA, Letz R, Baker EL. Computerized assessment of human neurotoxicity: sensitivity to nitrous oxide exposure. Clin Pharmacol Ther 1985;38:656–660.

50. Bruce DL, Bach MJ. Effects of trace concentrations of anesthetic cases on behavioral performances of operating room personnel. Cincinnati: National Institute for Occupational Safety and Health, 1976, NIOSH Technical Report No. 76–169.

51. Smith G, Shirley W. A review of the effects of trace concentrations of anesthetics on performance. Br J Anaesth 1978;50:701–710.

52. Organic solvents in the workplace. MMWR 1987;36:282–283.

53. Ron MA. Volatile substance abuse: a review of possible long-term neurological, intellectual, and psychiatric sequelae. Br J Psychiatry 1986;148:235–246.

54. Streicher HZ, Gabow PA, Moss AH, Kono D, Kaehny WD. Syndromes of toluene sniffing in adults. Ann Intern Med 1981;94:758–762.

55. Knox JW, Nelson JR. Permanent encephalopathy from toluene intoxication. N Engl J Med 1966;275:1494–1496.

56. Lazar RB, Ho SU, Melen O, Daghestani AN. Multifocal central nervous system damage caused by toluene abuse. Neurology 1983;33:1337–1340.

57. Hormes JT, Filley CM, Rosenberg NL. Neurologic sequelae of chronic solvent vapor abuse. Neurology 1986;36:698–702.

58. Fornazzari L, Wilkinson DA, Kapur BM, Carlen PL. Cerebellar, cortical, and functional impairment in toluene abusers. Acta Neurol Scand 1983;67:319–329.

59. Rosenberg NL, Kleinschmidt-DeMasters BK, Davis KA, Dreisbach JN, Hormes JT, Filley CM. Toluene abuse causes diffuse central nervous system white matter changes. Ann Neurol 1988;23:611–614.

60. Filley CM, Franklin GM, Heaton RK, Rosenberg NL. White matter dementia: clinical disorders and implications. Neuropsychiatry Neuropsychol Behav Neurol 1988;1:239–254.

61. Orbaek P, Gun N. Neurasthenic complaints and psychometric function of toluene-exposed rotogravure printers. Am J Ind Med 1989;16:67–77.

62. Arlien-Soborg P, Bruhn P, Gyldensted C, Melgaard B. Chronic painters' syndrome: chronic toxic encephalopathy in house painters. Acta Neurol Scand 1979;60:149–156.

63. Flodin U, Edling C, Axelson O. Clinical studies of psychoorganic syndrome among workers with exposure to solvents. Am J Ind Med 1984;5:287–295.

64. Errebo-Knudsen ED, Olsen F. Solvents and the brain: explanation of the discrepancy between the number of toxic encephalopathy reported (and compensated) in Denmark and other countries. Br J Ind Med 1987;44:71–72.

65. Juntunen J, Matikainen E, Antti-Poika M, Suoranta H, Valle M. Nervous system effects of long-term occupational exposure to toluene. Acta Neurol Scand 1985;72:512–517.

66. Gade E, Mortenson EL, Bruhn P. "Chronic painter's syndrome." A reanalysis of psychological test data in a group of diagnosed cases, based on comparisons with matched controls. Acta Neurol Scand 1988;77:293–306.

67. Stewart RD, Dodd HC, Baretta ED, et al. Human exposure to styrene vapor. Arch Environ Health 1968;16:656–662.

68. Gamberale F, Hultengren M. Exposure to styrene: II. Psychological functions. Work Environ Health 1974;11:86–93.

69. Morley R, Eccleston DW, Douglas CP, et al. Xylene poisoning: a report on one fatal case and two cases of recovery after prolonged unconsciousness. Br Med J 1970;3:442–443.

70. Grasso P, Sharratt M, Davies DM, Irvine D. Neurophysiological and psychological disorders and occupational exposure to organic solvents. Food Chem Toxicol 1984;22:819–852.

71. Schneck SA. Methyl alcohol. In: Vinken PJ, Bruyn GW, eds. Intoxications of the nervous system. Part 1, vol. 36. Handbook of clinical neurology. New York: North-Holland, 1979:351–360.

72. Guggenheim MA, Couch JR, Weinberg W. Motor dysfunction as a permanent complication of methanol ingestion. Presentation of a case with a beneficial response to levodopa treatment. Arch Neurol 1971;24:550–554.

73. Vigliani EC. Carbon disulphide poisoning in viscose rayon factories. Br J Ind Med 1954;11:235–241.

74. Hanninen H, Nurminen M, Tolonen M, Martelin T. Psychological tests as indicators of excessive exposure to carbon disulfide. Scand J Psychol 1978;19:163–174.

75. Feldman RG. Trichloroethylene. In: Vinken PJ, Bruyn GW, eds. Intoxications of the nervous system. Part 1, vol. 36. Handbook of clinical neurology. New York: North-Holland, 1979:457–464.

76. Feldman RG, Mayer RM, Taub A. Evidence for peripheral neurotoxic effect of trichloroethylene. Neurology 1970;20:599–606.

77. White RF, Feldman RG, Travers PH. Neurobehavioral effects of toxicity due to metals, solvents, and insecticides. Clin Neuropharmacol 1990;13:392–412.

78. Schaumburg HH, Spencer PS. Degeneration in central and peripheral neurons systems produced by pure n-hexane: an experimental study. Brain 1976;99:183–192.

79. Chang Y-C. Neurotoxic effects of n-hexane on the human central nervous system: evoked potential abnormalities in n-hexane polyneuropathy. J Neurol Neurosurg Psychiatry 1987;50:269–274.

80. Kuzuharas S, Kanezama I, Naleanishi T, Egashire T. Ethylene oxide polyneuropathy. Neurology 1983;33:377–380.

81. Gross JA, Haas ML, Swift TR. Ethylene oxide neurotoxicity: report of four cases and review of the literature. Neurology 1979;29:978–983.

82. Crystal HA, Schaumburg HH, Grober E, Fuld PA, Lipton RB. Cognitive impairment and sensory loss with chronic low-level ethylene oxide exposure. Neurology 1988;38:567–569.

83. Berger JR, Ayyar DR. Neurological complications of ethylene glycol intoxication. Report of a case. Arch Neurol 1981;38:724–726.

84. Stevens H, Forster FM. Effect of carbon tetrachloride on the nervous system. AMA Arch Neurol Psychiatr 1955;30:635–649.

85. Repko JD. Neurotoxicity of methyl chloride. Neurobehav Toxicol Teratol 1981;3:425–429.

86. LeQuesne PM. Clinical and morphological findings in acrylamide toxicity. Neurotoxicology 1985;6:17–24.

87. Igisu H, Goto I, Kawamura Y, Kato M, Izumi K, Kuroiwa Y. Acrylamide encephaloneuropathy due to well water pollution. J Neurol Neurosurg Psychiatry 1975;38:581–584.

88. Rosenberg NL, Myers JA, Martin WRW. Cyanide-induced parkinsonism: clinical, MRI, and 6-fluorodopa PET studies. Neurology 1989;39:142–144.

89. Koller WC, Klawans HL. Organophosphorus intoxication. In: Vinken GW, Bruyn PJ, eds. Intoxications of the nervous system. Handbook of clinical neurology, Part 1, vol. 36. New York: North-Holland, 1986:541–562.

90. Sharp DS, Eskenazi B, Harrison R, Callas P, Smith AH. Delayed health hazards of pesticide exposure. Annu Rev Public Health 1986;7:441–471.

91. Morgan JP. The Jamaica ginger paralysis. JAMA 1982;248:1864–1867.

92. Senanayake N, Karulliede L. Neurotoxic effects of organophosphate insecticides. N Engl J Med 1987;316:761–766.

93. Gershon S, Shaw FH. Psychiatric sequelae of chronic exposure to organophosphate insecticides. Lancet 1961;1:1371–1374.

94. Tabershaw IR, Cooper WC. Sequelae of acute organophosphate poisoning. J Occup Med 1966;8:5–20.

95. Metcalf DR, Holmes JH. EEG, psychological and neurological alterations in humans with organophosphate exposure. Ann NY Acad Sci 1969;160:357–365.

96. Murphy SD. Toxic effects of pesticides. In: Klaassen CD, Andrew MO, Doull J, eds. Casarett and Doull's toxicology: the basic science of poisons. New York: Macmillian, 1985.

97. Taylor JR, Selhorst JB, Houff SA, Martinez AJ. Chlordecone intoxication in man. I. Clinical observations. Neurology 1978;28:626–630.

98. Hughes JT. Brain damage due to paraquat poisoning: a fatal case with neuropathological examination of the brain. Neurotoxicology 1988;9:243–248.

99. Nolte J. The human brain: an introduction to its funcitonal anatomy. 2nd ed. St. Louis: CV Mosby, 1988:81.

100. Schaumburg HH, Spencer PS. Recognizing neurotoxic disease. Neurology 1987;37:276–278.

101. Hogstedt C, Andersson K, Hane MA. A questionnaire approach to the monitoring of the early disturbances in central nervous functions: In: Aitio R, Riihimaki K, Vainio H, eds. Biological montioring and surveillance of workers exposed to chemicals. Washington, DC: Hemisphere, 1984.

102. Drugs that cause psychiatric symptoms. Med Lett 1986;28:82–86.

103. Blazer DG II, Federspiel CF, Ray WA, Schaffner W. The risk of anticholinergic toxicity in the elderly: a study of prescribing practices in two populations. J Gerontol 1983;38:31–35.

104. Bergman H, Borg S, Holm L. Neuropsychological impairment and exclusive abuse of sedatives or hypnotics. Am J Psychiatry 1980;137:215–217.

105. Juntunen J. Neurological examination and assessment of the syndromes causeed by exposure to neurotoxic agents. In: Gilioli R, Cassitto MG, Foa V, eds. Neurobehavioral methods in occupational health. Advances in the biosciences. Vol 46. Oxford: Pergamon Press, 1982.

106. Strub RL, Black FW. The mental status examination in neurology. Philadelphia: FA Davis, 1977.

107. Genta P, Bruni I. Electroencephalographic spectral analysis. In: Gilioli R, Cassitto MG, Foa V, eds. Neurobehavioral methods in occupational health. Advances in the biosciences. Vol. 46. Oxford: Pergamon Press, 1982:55–69.

14

Renal Toxicity from Hazardous Chemicals

Alfred M. Bernard, Ph.D.
Robert R. Lauwerys, M.D., D.Sc.

INTRODUCTION

The unusual susceptibility of the kidney to toxic injury mainly stems from its function of regulating the volume and composition of body fluids. The two organs weigh around 300 grams in humans and receive 25% of the cardiac output. This blood flow is distributed to the nephrons, which constitute the functional and morphologic unit of the kidney (10^6 nephrons/kidney).

Each nephron is composed of a vascular part, the glomerulus, followed by an epithelial part, the tubule, which is divided into several segments as illustrated in Fig. 14.1.

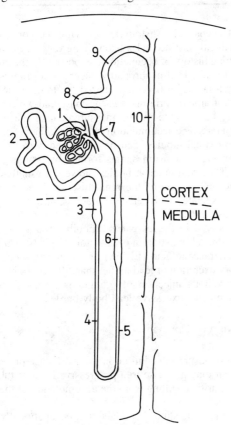

Figure 14.1. Schema of a nephron.
1. Glomerulus surrounded by the Bowman's capsule
2. Proximal convoluted tubule
3. Proximal straight tubule
4. and 5. Respectively, the thin descending and ascending limbs of the loop of Henlé
6. Distal straight tubule (also called the thick ascending limb of the loop of Henlé)
7. Macula densa
8. Distal convoluted tubule
9. Connecting tubule
10. Collecting duct

The glomerulus functions as a charge and size-selective filter, efficiently retaining vascular compartment proteins with a molecular weight higher than 40,000 (i.e., most plasma proteins) and allowing the passage of small molecules including the waste products of the organism. In humans, approximately 20% (i.e., 180 l/day) of the renal plasma flow are filtered by the glomeruli. From this copious filtrate, the tubule then recovers water, sodium chloride, and numerous other solutes. If this procedure is highly effective in removing toxic waste products, it implies, however, various physiologic processes which may concentrate toxic chemicals in some regions of the nephron or the interstitium.

Since most of the transport systems are localized in the proximal tubule, that part of the nephron is the most frequent target of nephrotoxic chemicals. In addition, because of its high energy and substrate requirements, the proximal tubule is also very sensitive to ischemia.

The loop of Henlé enables the kidney to concentrate urine by a countercurrent mechanism. Substances like urea which are not reabsorbed by the proximal tubule progressively concentrate in the loop of Henlé and can reach high concentrations in the deep medulla or the papilla (e.g., analgesics).

Sodium chloride and water can be further reabsorbed by the distal tubule and the collecting duct, the latter under the influence of the antidiuretic hormone. These two segments can also acidify urine through the secretion of H^+ and NH_4^+ (1).

EPIDEMIOLOGY

A substantial proportion of the human population is exposed to potentially nephrotoxic chemicals as a result of drug treatment, living or working in a contaminated environment, and accidental or intentional poisonings. The exact contribution of these various sources of exposure to the occurrence of acute or chronic nephropathies is largely unknown.

For the occupational exposure only, it is estimated that in the United States nearly four million workers are potentially exposed to nephrotoxic chemicals (3).

The annual incidence of acute renal failure is approximately 2 per 100,000. According to some authors (4, 5) up to 20% of the cases of acute renal failure might be ascribed to a toxic injury, mostly by drugs.

With respect to chronic renal failure, available data concern only the analgesic abuse nephropathy, which could be responsible for about 3% of end-stage renal failure cases in Europe. In some countries (Switzerland, Belgium) up to 20% of patients on renal dialysis have been analgesics abusers. It must be stressed, however, that about 50% of the cases of chronic renal failure are of uncertain etiology (6).

It is thus possible that some widespread occupational or environmental pollutants (heavy metals, solvents) or drugs other than analgesics (antibiotics, lithium, etc.) are involved in the development of chronic renal failure. Several observations tend to support this hypothesis: the well-documented occurrence of subclinical nephropathies in subjects occupationally exposed to nephrotoxicants such as lead or cadmium (7), the excess of mortality from renal diseases in cohorts of workers with previous exposure to these two heavy metals, and, more recently (8, 9), the demonstration that subclinical renal effects caused by the occupational exposure to cadmium are the forerunner signs of an accelerated and irreversible decline of the renal function (10).

ROUTES OF EXPOSURE AND ABSORPTION

The types of exposure to nephrotoxic chemicals may be domestic, occupational, environmental, therapeutic, or intentional. Heavy metals and solvents are widely used in industry. Solvents are also components of a number of chemical products used by the general population, such as paints, cleaning agents, glues, paint strippers, pesticides, etc.

The routes of entry of nephrotoxins may be inhalation, ingestion, or skin contact. In industry, inhalation represents the major route of exposure to metal fumes or dusts. Some ingestion of dusts may also occur either by the swallowing of inhaled particles cleared from the lungs or as a result of bad hygiene habits (e.g., smoking at the workplace or eating with contaminated hands or clothes). Inhalation is also the main route by which workers absorb solvents, although in some circumstances skin absorption may be very important (e.g., in cleaning or degreasing operations). For the general population, metals are usually absorbed via contaminated foods or drinks, whereas hydrocarbons may be absorbed by inhalation, skin contact, and accidental or deliberate ingestion. Children may ingest high amounts of heavy metals through pica or mouthing when playing on contaminated surfaces (e.g., in the vicinity of a smelter, in old houses with crumbling lead-based paints, etc.).

NEPHROTOXICANTS

Chemicals can affect the renal function or structures through a direct toxic action or through various systemic effects such as intravascular hemolysis, rhabdomyolysis, or cardiac failure. Only those chemicals producing specific effects on the kidney are considered here. The types of renal effects may vary from subclinical proteinuria to acute tubular necrosis or chronic renal failure, depending on the conditions of exposure (dose and duration) and the toxicologic properties of the chemical.

Table 14.1 lists occupational or environmental toxins that may cause acute or chronic renal diseases in humans. The list of drugs with possible side effects on the kidney is still longer, including more than 300 compounds (11). We briefly describe hereafter the nephrotoxic effects caused by chemicals that have been shown to be nephrotoxic in humans.

Metals

LEAD

Lead has been a very common cause of acute or chronic renal failure in the past. Acute tubular necrosis has been described following accidental or intentional absorption of high doses of lead. Cases of chronic renal failure have been reported in adults who had ingested high amounts of leaded paints during child-

Table 14.1. Examples of Industrial Chemicals Which May Cause Acute or Chronic Renal Damage in Humans

Metals	Hydrocarbons and Organic Solvents
Arsenic	Carbon tetrachloride
Bismuth	1,2-Dichloroethane
Chromium	Trichloroethylene
Cadmium	Chloroform
Copper	Toluene
Gold	Styrene
Lead	Methanol
Lithium	Ethylene glycol
Mercury	Diethylene glycol
Platinum	Ethylene glycol ethers
Silver	Hexachloro-1,3-butadiene
Thallium	Dichloroacetylene
Uranium	Carbon disulfide
	Dioxane

Miscellaneous
Paraquat
Mycotoxins
Silicon

hood (Queensland, Australia), following the consumption of alcohol illicitly distilled in lead-containing vessels, and in workers with a long history of occupational exposure. In the chronically exposed adult, lead nephropathy occurs as a progressive tubulointerstitial nephritis characterized by the absence of proteinuria or albuminuria in its early phase and which presently can only be detected by the measurement of the glomerular filtration rate. The accumulation of lead in kidneys, particularly in the proximal tubules, can be associated with the presence of intranuclear inclusion bodies formed by protein lead complexes. These intranuclear bodies, however, usually disappear with the progression of the renal disease. Lead nephropathy may be associated with heme synthesis disturbances, gout, and hypertension (9).

Lead stored in tissues can be mobilized and eliminated in urine by the administration of chelators (e.g., Na_2Ca ethylenediaminetetraacetic acid (EDTA) or dimercaptosuccinic acid). A urinary excretion of lead higher than 800 μg/24 hr following the intravenous injection of 0.5 grams Na_2Ca EDTA is an indication of an excessive lead body burden.

CADMIUM

Chronic exposure to cadmium in the workplace or general environment may give rise to a progressive form of tubulointerstitial nephritis resulting from the accumulation of the metal in renal cortex.

Epidemiologic studies conducted in occupationally exposed workers or in inhabitants of cadmium-polluted areas in Japan have demonstrated that the earliest subclinical manifestation of cadmium nephropathy consists of an increased urinary excretion of specific plasma proteins, particularly of low molecular weight proteins such as β_2-microglobulin or retinol-binding protein. The concentrations of cadmium in urine and renal cortex from which this subclinical proteinuria is likely to develop in 10% of exposed adults are estimated at 10 μg/g creatinine and 200 ppm, respectively (8). No efficient chelation therapy is available for chronic cadmium poisoning; $CaNa_2$ EDTA has been successfully used in cases of acute poisoning.

MERCURY

Acute exposure to certain inorganic or organic forms of mercury can cause an acute tubular necrosis and renal failure. It has been known for a long time that patients treated with mercurial compounds can develop a glomerulonephritis usually associated with proteinuria and occasionally with nephrotic syndrome. Cases of glomerulonephritis have also been reported following the chronic exposure to high levels of mercury in industry (12). At lower levels of exposure, mercury vapors or salts can cause various subclinical renal disturbances such as an increased urinary excretion of enzymes or of high molecular weight plasma proteins.

The concentration of mercury in urine from which these manifestations of nephrotoxicity may occur is estimated at 50 µg/g creatinine (13). Various chelating agents can be used in cases of acute or chronic mercury poisoning [dimercaprol, D-penicillamine, or dimercaptosuccinic acid (DMSA)].

ARSENIC

Acute arsenic poisoning may cause tubular necrosis. Acute or severe chronic poisoning is usually treated with the chelating agent BAL (2,3-dimercaptopropanol). Inhalation of arsine may also produce an acute tubular necrosis as a result of intravascular hemolysis.

Hydrocarbons and Organic Solvents

A number of solvents used in industry or in home products (halogenated hydrocarbons, ethylene glycol, petroleum distillates, toluene, etc.) are direct tubular toxins. Acute exposure to these solvents by inhalation or ingestion can produce tubular effects which, depending on the dose and the solvent, vary from a mild proteinuria or enzymuria to an acute tubular necrosis (14). For instance, glue, paints, or toluene sniffing may cause various signs of tubular dysfunction consistent with Fanconi's syndrome (aminoaciduria, glucosuria, tubular-type proteinuria, renal tubular acidosis, etc). Several case reports and epidemiologic studies suggest that subacute or chronic exposure to hydrocarbons (e.g., gasoline, paints, solvents) may lead to various types of glomerulonephritis, particularly the Goodpasture's syndrome (15). The latter is a rapidly progressive glomerulonephritis characterized by recurrent lung hemorrhages and by the presence of antibodies directed against the glomerular basement membrane.

Depending on the type of solvent, organs other than the kidney may be damaged, for example, the liver (halogenated hydrocarbons) and the central nervous system.

Paraquat, a dipyridilium herbicide, is a tubular toxin which can produce acute renal failure. Some plant or animal toxins (venoms or mycotoxins) can also produce renal damage. For instance, the causal agent of the endemic Balkan nephropathy might be the mycotoxin, ochratoxin A.

MECHANISMS OF NEPHROTOXICITY

The mechanisms leading to nephrotoxicity may be biochemical, immunologic, or hemodynamic.

Biochemical Mechanisms

Biochemical mechanisms are too numerous to be reviewed in detail here (16). With respect to tubular lesions, the mechanism frequently follows the same pattern: entry of the chemical into the tubular cell via the luminal or basolateral site by an active or passive transport system, accumulation of the chemical in one or several cellular compartments (lysosomes for aminoglycosides, cytoplasm for cadmium), and binding of the chemical or its metabolites to target macromolecules (membrane components, enzymes, etc.). Nephrotoxicity usually developes in a dose-dependent fashion from a certain concentration in the tubular cell (the so-called critical concentration).

For most organic nephrotoxins, the binding to cellular targets requires the activation of the substance into electrophilic metabolites. Reactive oxygen species are involved in the nephrotoxicity of some compounds (cephaloridine, puromycin aminonucleoside).

Immunologic Mechanisms

Immune-type nephritis may result from two basic processes: (a) the deposition of circulating immune complexes in the glomerular structures (granular deposits by immunofluorescence) or (b) the in-site formation of immune complexes between a circulating antibody and glomerular antigens or antigens "planted" in the glomerulus. In the latter case, the immunofluorescence pattern appears linear or granular depending on the distribution of the antigens. Immune complexes formed or deposited in renal structure may cause tissue lesions in a sequence of events involving, namely, the activation of the complement, the recruitment of leukocytes, and the release by the latter of proteases, reactive oxygen species, prostaglandins, etc.

Immunologic mechanisms of nephrotoxicity may lead to a glomerulonephritis (e.g., membranous glomerulonephritis induced by gold salts, mercurials, or D-penicillamine) or an acute interstitial nephritis (penicillin derivatives). The exact mechanisms by which chemicals trigger the hypersensitivity reaction are usually unknown. The chemical might in some cases behave as an hapten (e.g., methicillin), modify a self-antigen, or else release into the circulation normally hidden tissue antigens. In the gold-, D-penicillamine-, or mercury-induced glomerulonephritis, the immune reaction might be the consequence of a polyclonal activation.

The gold- and D-penicillamine-induced membranous glomerulonephritis are more frequently observed in patients with the HLA DR4 and DR3 antigen, respectively (12).

Hemodynamic Mechanisms

Hemodynamic alterations are frequently involved in the initiation or progression of toxic nephropathies.

In acute tubular injury, the renal function can be impaired by casts and cell debris obstructing the tubular lumen, by a back flow of glomerular filtrate across disrupted tubular epithelium, or by vasoconstricting substances such as thromboxane, endothelin, or the renin-angiotensin system. Nonsteroidal antiinflammatory drugs inhibit the synthesis of prostaglandins and may precipitate renal failure in subjects with circulatory impairment.

Once the glomerular filtration rate has been reduced to about 30% of normal as a result of toxic injury or renal disease, the evolution to end-stage renal failure becomes unavoidable, probably because remnant nephrons are progressively destroyed by the compensatory increase in the single nephron glomerular filtration rate (elevation of glomerular pressure and flow) (17).

DIAGNOSIS

The main clinical manifestations that may reflect renal injury are (1):

- hematuria, which denotes the presence of blood in urine and damage to the glomerular capillary wall.
- proteinuria (>0.5 g/24 hr). A proteinuria higher than 3.5 g/24 hr is characteristic of the nephrotic syndrome. The proteinuria may be of glomerular type composed mainly of high molecular weight proteins (i.e., with a molecular weight >40,000) or of tubular type with a predominance of low molecular weight proteins (molecular weight <40,000). The latter usually results from a proximal tubule injury, whereas the former is indicative of a loss of the glomerular barrier function.
- oliguria (urine output of less than <600 ml/day).
- azotemia i.e., the elevation of the serum concentration of small molecules such as urea, creatinine, or low molecular weight proteins (e.g., β_2-microglobulin).
- generalized edema, which in the absence of cardiac failure or cirrhosis is characteristic of the nephrotic syndrome (hypoalbuminemia).
- hypertension, which may develop as a consequence of glomerulosclerosis.

These manifestations often occur in groups or syndromes. The main clinical syndromes which may be induced by acute or chronic exposures to nephrotoxins are (17):

- acute renal failure, which is the acute suppression of the renal function with azotemia and often oliguria.
- chronic renal failure, which is the permanent loss of renal function with azotemia, acidosis, anemia, hypertension, and various other disturbances.
- tubulointerstitial nephritis (chronic or acute) with various signs of tubular dysfunction (tubular type proteinuria, urine acidification and concentration deficits, salt wastings, etc.).
- nephrotic syndrome characterized by heavy proteinuria (>3.5 g/24 hr), hypoproteinemia, edema, hyperlipidemia, and hyperlipiduria. Nephrotic syndrome can be due to several types of glomerulonephritis (membranous, minimal change, etc.).
- rapidly progressive glomerulonephritis, a syndrome with hematuria and oliguria leading to renal failure within weeks (e.g., Goodpasture's syndrome).

The diagnosis of specific types of nephropathies rests on various clinical tests or investigations such as urine analysis and microscopy; estimation of the glomerular filtration rate on the basis of serum creatinine or urea, or of the clearance of creatinine, inulin, or of labeled compounds; assessment of the tubular function (urine concentration and acidification ability, phosphate clearance, etc.); radiographic and radioisotopic investigations; and examination of renal biopsies by immunofluorescence, light, or electron microscopy.

Hygiene improvements in modern factories have considerably decreased the prevalence of acute or rapidly progressive renal diseases. The nephrotoxic action of industrial chemicals manifests more frequently through various biologic renal anomalies such as slight proteinuria or enzymuria. These renal effects, which are detectable only by the use of sensitive screening tests, might, however, reflect in some cases an incipient renal disease.

The diagnosis of a toxic nephropathy rests essentially on the patient history. It consists of questioning in order to determine whether the patient has or could have absorbed high doses of nephrotoxins either in the preceding hours or days for a nephropathy of acute onset or during lifetime for a long-standing renal disease. This search must be conducted by considering all possible sources of exposure: diseases or affections requiring prolonged treatment with potentially nephrotoxic drugs (e.g., antibiotics, analgesics); exposure in the home or work environment to nephrotoxic chemicals (solvents, heavy metals); ingestion of contaminated foods or drinks (e.g., by heavy metals, ethylene glycol); exposure to environmental pollutants (e.g., lead for children); drug addiction (e.g., glue sniffing), etc. One must be also aware of the possibility of synergisms between chemicals and that the absorption of relatively low doses of a nephrotoxin may in some cases cause severe renal damage. For instance, a moderate exposure to carbon tetrachloride vapors may produce an acute hepatorenal failure in subjects taking barbiturates (18).

Toxic nephropathies can be differentiated from other types of renal diseases on the basis of clinical or biochemical signs which are highly suggestive of a certain type of intoxication e.g., heme synthesis deficits in case of chronic lead poisoning, neurologic and hepatic symptoms for acute inhalation of halogenated hydrocarbons, or central nervous system disturbances in case of chronic poisoning by mercury.

The diagnosis of a toxic nephropathy is also greatly facilitated if the suspected chemical is found in high concentrations in biologic materials such as urine, blood, tissue biopsy, or gastric fluid. The maximum time that can elapse between the exposure and the sample collection for a reliable estimation of the absorbed dose depends on the kinetics of the chemicals in the analyzed compartment. It may range from a few hours for rapidly eliminated toxins up to years for cumulative toxins such as lead (EDTA mobilization test) or cadmium. A definitive diagnosis of a toxic nephropathy can be made only after having excluded all other possible causes such as infections, systemic disorders with renal involvements (diabetes, hypertension, amyloidosis, vasculitis, gout, metabolic diseases, etc.), hereditary nephritis, and malignancy.

SCREENING TESTS FOR NEPHROTOXICITY

At the present time, most clinicians rely on the use of serum creatinine for an indirect assessment of renal function. Although this test has the advantage of being simple, it is not sufficiently sensitive to be used for a screening purpose.

Because of its nonlinear relationship with the glomerular filtration rate, serum creatinine rises significantly only when the glomerular filtration rate has been decreased by 30–50%. A direct estimate of the glomerular filtration rate based on the clearance of endogenous creatinine, inulin, or labeled compounds permits a more sensitive assessment of the renal function, but such tests are not suitable for routine or large scale screening of populations at risk. Furthermore, these tests fail to detect early renal effects because of the extensive reserve of the kidneys, which masks the toxic injury until a considerable amount of renal parenchyma (up to 50%) is irreversibly lost. The prevention of renal diseases caused by occupational or environmental nephrotoxins requires the use of more sensitive tests capable of detecting renal effects at a stage when they are still reversible or at least not so advanced as to trigger a progressive renal disease. The following tests are presently the most sensitive for that purpose (19).

Proteinuria

An increased urinary output of proteins is frequently an early and sensitive indicator of renal damage. Since pathologic processes may at an early stage enhance the urinary excretion of individual plasma proteins without significantly affecting that of total proteins, it is preferable to measure specific urinary proteins with appropriate immunoassays. In practice, one usually recommends the determination in urine of two proteins, a high molecular weight protein such as albumin for the early detection of glomerular involvement and a low molecular weight protein such as retinol-binding protein or β_2-microglobulin for the early screening of proximal tubular damage. The ratio between the urinary excretion of β_2-microglobulin or retinol-binding protein and the albumin permits a differentiation of tubular, glomerular, or mixed type proteinuria.

Enzymuria

Injury to the kidney and particularly to the proximal tubule can be detected by measuring the urinary activity of kidney-derived enzymes. Of all the urinary enzymes that have been proposed as a nephrotoxicity index, so far the lysosomal enzyme β-N-acetylglucosaminidase has proven to be one of the most valuable. Advantages of this enzyme include its stability in urine, its high molecular weight (excluding a plasmatic origin), and its high activity in the kidney.

Urinary Excretion of Renal Antigens

Destruction of renal tissue can also be detected by measuring in urine kidney components which, when they are quantitated by immunochemical methods, are referred to as renal antigens. Renal antigens which have been proposed as urinary markers of nephrotoxicity include ligandin, carbonic anhydrase, alanine aminopeptidase, and adenosine deaminase-binding protein. It is possible that renal antigens, like kidney-derived enzymes, are mainly markers of the active phase of renal tissue destruction and may be less appropriate than assays relying on plasma protein excretion for detecting inactive phases of chronic renal diseases.

These various markers of nephrotoxicity can be measured on spot urine samples provided a correction is made for diuresis on the basis of urinary density or creatinine. Numerous epidemiologic studies have successfully used these markers to identify potentially nephrotoxic industrial chemicals or to establish dose-response-effect relationships (13). The tests which have proven the most useful in these studies are those measuring the urinary excretion of specific plasma proteins (e.g., β_2-microglobulin, retinol-binding protein, and albumin).

In a health surveillance program, it is also useful to examine the urine with a classical reagent strip, a test which is simple to perform and which can detect urinary anomalies such as glucosuria or hematuria. The microscopic examination of urine may be a useful additional test, but it is usually not applicable during routine monitoring of populations.

It is important to stress that none of the above described screening tests has an "ex officio" unfavorable prognosis. In some situations, they may merely reflect physiologic changes which do not necessarily imply a loss of functional or structural integrity of the renal tissue (e.g., orthostatic, febrile, or exercise proteinuria), whereas in other situations, they may reveal transient and reversible renal effects. This frequently applies to the acute tubulotoxic effects, not accompanied by a decline of glomerular filtration rate, which may be observed in a number of situations such as short treatment with antibiotics, surgery, or acute poisonings.

By contrast, when markers of nephrotoxicity become increasingly abnormal over months or years, they may suggest the development of a progressive and irreversible nephropathy with a less favorable prognosis.

REFERENCES

1. Leaf A, Cortran RS. Renal pathophysiology. 3rd ed. Oxford: Oxford University Press, 1985.
2. The Renal Commission of the International Union of Physiological Sciences. A standard nomenclature for structures of the kidney. Kidney Int 1988;33:1–7.
3. Landrigan PJ, Goyer RA, Clarkson TW, Sandler DP, Smith JH, Thun MJ, Wedeen RP. The work-relatedness of renal disease. Arch Environ Health 1984;39:225–230.
4. Anderson RJ, Linas SL, Berns AS, Henrich WL, Miller TR, Gabow PA, Schrier RW. Non-oliguric acute renal failure. N Engl J Med 1977;296:1134–1138.
5. Hou SH, Bushinsky DA, Wish JB, Cohen JJ, Harrington JT. Hospital acquired renal insufficiency: a prospective study. Am J Med 1983;74:243–248.
6. Gregg NJ, Elseviers MM, DeBroe ME, Bach PH. Epidemiology and mechanistic basis of analgesic-associated nephropathy. Toxicol Lett 1989;46:141–151.
7. Wedeen RP. Occupational renal disease. Am J Kidney Dis 1984;4:241–257.
8. Bernard A, Lauwerys R. Effects of cadmium exposure in man. In: Foulkes EC, ed. Cadmium toxicology, handbook of experimental pharmacology. Berlin, Heidelberg, New York: Springer-Verlag, 1986;136–177.
9. Bennett WM. Lead nephropathy. Kidney Int 1985;28:212–220.
10. Roels H, Lauwerys R, Buchet JP, Bernard AM, Vos A, Oversteyns M. Health significance of cadmium-induced renal dysfunction: a five-year follow-up. Br J Ind Med (in press).
11. Hamel JD, Biour M, Cheymol G. Nephrotoxicité médicamenteuse. Fichier bibliographique des atteintes rénales et des médicaments responsables: "nephrotox." Therapie 1988;43:211–217.
12. Druet P. Contribution of immunological reactions to nephrotoxicity. Toxicol Lett 1989;46:55–64.
13. Bernard A, Lauwerys R. Epidemiologic application of early markers of nephrotoxicity. Toxicol Lett 1989;46:293–306.
14. Lauwerys R, Bernard A, Viau C, Buchet JP. Kidney disorders and hematotoxicity from organic solvent exposure. Scand J Work Environ Health 1985;11 (suppl 1) 84–90.
15. Churchill DN, Fine A, Gault MH. Association between hydrocarbon exposure and glomerulonephritis: an appraisal of the evidence. Nephron 1983;33:169–172.
16. Ford SM, Hook JB. Biochemical mechanisms of toxic nephropathies. Semin Nephrol 1984;4:88–106.
17. Brenner BM, Meyer TW, Hostetter TH. Dietary protein intake and the progressive nature of kidney diseases: the role of hemodynamically mediated glomerular injury in the pathogenesis of progressive glomerulosclerosis in aging, renal ablation and intrinsic renal disease. N Engl J Med 1982;307:652–659.
18. Mahieu P, Geubel A, Rahier J, Scailteur V, Dieryck JP, Lauwerys R. Potentiation of carbon-tetrachloride hepato-nephrotoxicity by phenobarbital in man. Int J Clin Pharmacol Res 1983;3:427–430.
19. Lauwerys R, Bernard A. Preclinical detection of nephrotoxicity: description of the tests and appraisal of their health significance. Toxicol Lett 1989;46:13–29.

15

Cardiac Toxicology

Neal L. Benowitz, M.D.

INTRODUCTION

Approximately 50% of deaths in the United States result from heart disease or stroke. While many cardiovascular deaths may be accounted for by the known risk factors of hypertension, diabetes, cigarette smoking, hyperlipidemia, and genetic factors, many other cardiovascular deaths are not explained by these risk factors. Exposure to toxic chemicals both in the workplace and in the general environment may be responsible for a significant number of cases of cardiovascular disease.

Toxins can affect the cardiovascular system at a variety of sites (see Table 15.1). The heart may be injured by ischemia (atheromatous or nonatheromatous coronary artery disease), asphyxia, direct myocardial injury, and/or disturbances in electrical impulse formation or conduction. Blood vessels can be affected diffusely, by systemic vasoconstriction (resulting in hypertension) or by focal obstruction (arterial occlusive disease). This chapter discusses toxic cardiovascular disease from the perspective of the types of injury, with discussion of the epidemiology, mechanisms of toxicity, and clinical features for specific toxins within each class of injury. The scope of the chapter is limited to industrial and environmental chemicals. Medications, food poisoning, and plant poisoning, while important causes of acute cardiovascular disease, are not discussed. The reader is referred elsewhere for detailed discussion of cardiovascular complications of drug intoxication (1).

CAUSATION OF CHEMICAL-INDUCED CARDIOVASCULAR DISEASE

Cardiovascular disease is common in all industrialized countries, and causation of such disease by chemical exposures is often difficult to establish. Occasionally massive exposures to carbon monoxide or cyanide produce acute injury, and clear causation. Cardiovascular disease is seen in the context of low dose, repeated exposure. It is difficult to establish the cause of cardiovascular disease for several reasons. (a) Cardiovascular disease is common even in the absence of toxic exposures. Thus, in the typical workplace many workers will have cardiovascular disease, and it is difficult to spot clusters or epidemics. (b) There is often nothing specific, either clinically or pathologically, to establish toxic cardiovascular disease. If present, other risk factors are usually assumed to be the cause of cardiovascular disease. (c) It is rarely possible to document high tissue levels of suspected toxicants. (d) It is difficult to establish the level of exposure of a worker to industrial chemicals over the many years it may take to develop cardiovascular disease. (e) Cardiovascular toxicants are likely to interact with other risk factors or preexisting disease in causing or manifesting cardiovascular disease.

For the most part our ideas on causation of toxic cardiovascular disease are based on epidemiologic studies. Establishing causation through such studies is difficult because of the generally small increases in relative risk and potential confounding

Table 15.1. Chemical Toxins and Cardiovascular Disease

Atherosclerotic ischemic heart disease
  Carbon disulfide (1)*
  Carbon monoxide (3)
  Combustion products (3)
  Environmental tobacco smoke (2)
  Arsenic (3)

Nonatheromatous ischemic heart disease
  Organic nitrates (1)

Myocardial asphyxiants
  Carbon monoxide (1)
  Cyanide (1)
  Hydrogen sulfide (1)

Direct myocardial injury
  Cobalt (3)
  Arsenic (1)
  Arsine (1)
  Lead (3)
  Antimony (2)
  Organic solvents (3)

Arrhythmias
  Halogenated hydrocarbons (1)
  Organophosphates (1)
  Antimony (2)
  Arsenic (2)
  Arsine (1)

Hypertension
  Lead (2)
  Cadmium (3)
  Carbon disulfide (2)
  Organic solvents (3)

Peripheral arterial occlusive disease
  Arsenic (2)
  Lead (2)
  Carbon disulfide (2)

*Probability of Causation
  (1) = Definite
  (2) = Probable
  (3) = Possible

Adapted from Kristensen TS. Cardiovascular disease and the work environment. A critical review of the epidemiologic literature on chemical factors. Scand J Work Environ Health 1989;15:245–264.

with cardiovascular risk factors, including lifestyle and diet. In only a few cases has it been shown that removing a person or a population from a toxic exposure reduces the risk of cardiovascular disease.

Epidemiologic studies on chemical-induced cardiovascular disease must be viewed considering these limitations. The epidemiologic literature on chemical factors in causing cardiovascular disease has been comprehensively reviewed elsewhere (2). An attempt was made in that review to evaluate methodologic quality of studies that support causation for particular toxins. Based on the number of studies, the number of subjects studied, and the quality of the research design, the probability of causation by chemical risk factors was judged as summarized in Table 15.1. Selected epidemiologic studies or specific toxic exposures will be mentioned in the section on cardiovascular diseases caused by specific chemicals.

CARDIOVASCULAR DISEASES CAUSED BY SPECIFIC CHEMICALS OR TOXINS

Atherosclerotic Vascular Disease

There is substantial evidence for accelerated development of atherosclerotic coronary artery disease after exposure to carbon disulfide, combustion products, and arsenic. Nitroglycerin and carbon monoxide have also been associated with an increased incidence of coronary heart disease. These associations are weaker and are discussed briefly when these toxins are discussed in subsequent sections.

CARBON DISULFIDE

Epidemiology

Chronic exposure to carbon disulfide is well-documented to increase mortality from ischemic heart disease. Research has primarily been conducted on viscose rayon workers. A 2.5-fold excess in mortality from coronary heart disease in workers exposed to carbon disulfide was first reported in 1968 (3). Subsequently, a prospective study from Finland demonstrated a 5.6 relative increase in coronary heart disease mortality and a threefold increased risk of first nonfatal myocardial infarction in carbon disulfide-exposed workers (4). Interventions that reduce carbon disulfide exposure have been shown to reduce the risk of cardiovascular disease to control levels (5). This observation, along with findings of another recent study showing that ischemic heart disease mortality was increased with increasing exposure in the previous two years, while the increased risk did not persist in workers who had left the industry (6), suggests that carbon disulfide may also produce an acute reversible effect on the cardiovascular system.

Exposure

Carbon disulfide is primarily used as a solvent in the manufacturing of viscose rayon but is also used as solvent for rubber, fats, oils, resins, and the synthesis of other chemicals. Inhalation of the vapors is the major route of exposure, although carbon disulfide can also be absorbed through the skin.

Exposure to levels of 2000 ppm carbon disulfide results in narcosis; 1000 ppm has been associated with severe neuropsychiatric disturbance; 300–400 ppm produces mild poisoning after several hours. The concentration of carbon disulfide in workers with increased coronary heart disease who have been exposed is reported at 20–60 ppm. The current threshold limit value (TLV) is 10 ppm.

Mechanisms of Toxicity and Pathophysiology

Carbon disulfide-induced cardiovascular disease has been clearly demonstrated, and several likely mechanisms have been described. Carbon disulfide reacts with amines or amino acids in the body to form dithiocarbamates, which in turn complex trace metals (particularly copper and zinc) and chemically react with certain enzymatic cofactors such as pyridoxine (7, 8). The chelation of metals that are cofactors for enzymes, as well as direct inactivation by carbon disulfide, results in inhibition of many enzyme systems (including dopamine β-hydroxylase). Carbon disulfide may also interfere with normal inhibition of elastase activity, resulting in excess elastase activity with disruption of blood vessel walls and formation of aneurysms. Carbon disulfide has also been proposed to decrease fibrolytic activity with a resultant enhancement of thrombosis.

Inhibition of enzymatic processes is thought to produce a number of metabolic disturbances including abnormalities of lipid metabolism and thyroid function that can lead to hypercholesterolemia and hypothyroidism (7, 9). Inhibition of dopamine β-hydroxylase, an enzyme that converts dopamine to norepinephrine, may be responsible for hypertension as well as for some of the neuropsychiatric features of carbon disulfide intoxication. Inhibition of aldehyde dehydrogenase may result in a disulfiram-like reaction to alcohol, with flushing and hypotension.

Accelerated atherosclerotic vascular disease may occur as a consequence of carbon disulfide effects on blood pressure, lipids, thyroid function, glucose tolerance, and/or fibrolytic activity. The risks of carbon disulfide exposure remained after adjusting for hypertension and serum cholesterol, indicating that carbon disulfide may have other toxic effects on the cardiovascular system (10).

The resultant pathology includes atherosclerotic vascular disease involving the coronary, cerebral, and peripheral arteries. Renal vascular hypertension has also been reported. Microaneurysms and atrophic changes of the retina are seen in the eyes of workers chronically exposed to excessive amounts of carbon disulfide (11).

Clinical Features

Acute intoxication may produce symptoms and signs of encephalopathy or polyneuropathy, including fatigue, headaches, dizziness, disorientation, paresthesias, psychoses, and/or delirium. After chronic exposure patients may present with hypertension and/or manifestations of atherosclerotic vascular disease such as angina or myocardial infarction. It is noteworthy that the typical patient demonstrates one or more of the known risk factors for coronary artery disease, and only by an occupational history will the role of carbon disulfide be suspected. Work in rayon or rubber manufacturing, chemical manufacturing, or chemistry laboratories should prompt further inquiry into possible exposure to carbon disulfide.

An early sign of chronic carbon disulfide poisoning on physical examination is abnormal ocular microcirculation, characterized by microaneurysms and hemorrhages resembling those of diabetic retinopathy.

Laboratory findings may include a decrease in serum thyroxine levels and an increase in serum cholesterol levels, particularly those of the beta very low density lipoproteins. There are no practical methods for measuring concentrations of carbon disulfide in biologic fluids.

Other diagnostic studies that may be of use include fluorescein angiography of the retinal blood vessels which may show delayed filling of retinal arteries as an early sign of vascular disease. The electrocardiogram (ECG) sometimes shows evidence of ischemia or previous myocardial infarction. The presence of coronary artery disease may be confirmed by exercise stress testing and coronary angiography.

The vascular findings in patients with chronic carbon disulfide poisoning are similar to those seen in any patient with atherosclerotic vascular disease. The most specific finding is that of an abnormal ocular microcirculation in the absence of diabetes. The diagnosis is based on the clinical picture of premature vascular disease and history of exposure to excessive levels of carbon disulfide for more than 5–10 years.

COMBUSTION PRODUCTS (INCLUDING ENVIRONMENTAL TOBACCO SMOKE)

Combustion of organic materials produces a complex mixture of particulates and gases that include polycyclic aromatic hydrocarbons, nitrosoamines, aldehydes, hydrogen cyanide, nitrogen oxides, carbon monoxide, and, according to the source, certain trace metals including cadmium, arsenic, and lead. The fact that exposure to combustion products can cause atherosclerotic heart and vascular disease has been suggested by the strong association between cigarette smoking and atherosclerotic vascular disease. While the mechanism of disease is unknown, carbon monoxide, polycyclic aromatic hydrocarbons, and, in cigarette smokers, nicotine and certain glycoproteins, have been suspected as contributing to the process.

Epidemiology

Acute carbon monoxide poisoning can cause myocardial injury or aggravate underlying vascular disease. High level chronic exposures (carboxyhemoglobin [COHB] 20–30%) have been reported to produce a severalfold increase in the incidence of coronary artery disease in tatami mat makers in Northern Japan (12). These workers heated their buildings with charcoal braziers while tightly sealing windows and doors to conserve heat during cold winter weather.

Chronic carbon monoxide exposure at levels more relevant to occupational exposure (COHB 5–15%) has been suggested to place workers at increased risk of coronary artery disease. This observation is based on studies of carbon monoxide in animals (which have had conflicting results) and the association between COHB level and coronary artery disease risk in cigarette smokers (13, 14). The latter is difficult to interpret, because carbon monoxide exposure is strongly associated with exposure to other toxic substances in cigarette smoke. Epidemiologic studies of carbon monoxide exposure in humans report conflicting results. One study reported a dose-related association between carbon monoxide exposure and angina symptoms but not ECG abnormalities in foundry workers (15). A recent study found excess mortality from atherosclerotic heart disease in New York City tunnel officers (exposed to carbon monoxide from auto exhaust) with a standardized mortality ratio of 1.35 (95% confidence intervals of 1.09–1.68) (16). No relationship between duration of exposure and risk of disease was found; however, the excess risk did appear to decline after improvements in ventilation of the tunnels and declined after workers were no longer exposed. On the other hand, other studies in firefighters and foundry workers found no association between the level of carbon monoxide exposure and coronary heart disease risk (2). Thus the relationship between chronic carbon monoxide and atherosclerotic vascular disease remains uncertain.

Significantly excess mortality for ischemic heart disease has been reported in chimney sweeps and aluminum reduction workers who are exposed to combustion products (17, 18). A role for polycyclic aromatic hydrocarbons has been suggested.

Exposure to environmental tobacco smoke has been of considerable recent concern, particularly in regard to the risk of lung cancer, respiratory infection in children, and abnormal pulmonary function (19). There is, however, also evidence that environmental tobacco smoke may increase the risk of coronary artery disease. Seven studies have been reported, nearly all of which have found an increased relative risk for ischemic heart disease among nonsmokers married to smokers compared to nonsmokers married to nonsmokers (2, 20). The overall relative risk is small (on average 1.3) but, considering the large number of people exposed, may account for a significant number of cases of ischemic heart disease.

The biologic plausibility of a relative risk of 1.3 for passive smokers compared with a risk of 2 for active smokers has been questioned. However, the relative risk of smoking is based on comparisons with a groups of nonsmokers which includes passive smokers who appear to have a higher risk of ischemic heart disease than nonexposed nonsmokers. As a result the relative risk of coronary artery disease in smokers may have been underestimated.

Exposure

Exposure to combustion products is primarily by inhalation. Exposure to carbon monoxide may occur whenever there are combustion engines or other types of combustion, such as in foundries and in firefighting. Carbon monoxide poisoning may also occur with the use of faulty furnaces or heaters. Typical workplace exposure results in carboxyhemoglobin concentrations of 2–8%, while cigarette smokers commonly have concentrations of 5–15%. Studies of environmental tobacco smoke exposure using levels of cotinine (a metabolite of nicotine) in the blood and urine indicate that environmental tobacco smoke exposure may result in an intake equivalent of one-fourth to one cigarette per day (23). It is noteworthy, however, that the composition of sidestream smoke that is released into the environment is different from that of mainstream smoke that is inhaled by the smoker, owing to differences in heat of combustion and oxygen concentrations at the burning end. Consequently, compared with mainstream smoke, the concentrations of some toxic chemicals including polycyclic aromatic hydrocarbons, nitrosoamines, and formaldehyde in sidestream smoke are substantially enhanced over those of nicotine. In addition, with aging of environmental tobacco smoke, nicotine vaporizes, and nicotine concentrations in the air decline more quickly than do particulate concentrations. For these reasons measurement of nicotine-based markers in nonsmokers to derive cigarette-equivalents of exposure underestimate the exposure to other toxic constituents of tobacco smoke.

Mechanisms of Toxicity

Carbon monoxide might contribute to atherosclerosis in several ways. Carbon monoxide exposure may alter lipid metabolism and/or increase the permeation of lipids into blood vessel walls and may enhance platelet aggregation. High levels of carbon monoxide exposure accelerate atherosclerosis in hypercholesterolemic animals. Carbon monoxide could contribute to angina pectoris ischemic heart disease mortality by aggravating coronary ischemia by reducing the amount of oxygen carried by and released from hemoglobin. The effects of carbon monoxide on patients with preexisting coronary artery disease is discussed in detail in the section on myocardial asphyxiants.

The possible role of polycyclic aromatic hydrocarbons in accelerating atherogenesis is suggested by a hypothesis that the atherosclerotic plaque may derive from single smooth muscle cells that have been mutated (24). Chemical carcinogens such as the polycyclic aromatic hydrocarbons are known to cause mutations in various types of cells. High levels of exposure to benzo-a-pyrene or other polycyclic aromatic hydrocarbons enhance the development of atherosclerotic lesions in some experimental animals.

Clinical Features

A history of exposure to combustion engines, fire, or foundry work in association with atherosclerotic vascular disease should suggest the possible role of carbon monoxide and/or other combustion products. Patients may present with any manifestation of atherosclerotic vascular disease including angina pectoris, myocardial infarction, sudden death, or occlusive peripheral vascular disease. The risk of death from ischemic heart disease declines after cessation of exposure in cigarette smokers and similarly seems to decline with cessation of some occupational exposures, such as in tunnel officers (16). Laboratory studies may show increased concentrations of carboxyhemoglobin at the end of work, but levels will be back to normal within 12–24 hours of the last exposure. Elevation of hemoglobin concentrations is commonly seen in cigarette smokers and has been reported in some but not all studies of chronic carbon monoxide exposure.

ARSENIC

Epidemiology

Three epidemiologic studies have reported positive (although of small magnitude) associations between arsenic exposure (arsenic trioxide) and cardiovascular disease in copper smelter workers (25–27). One of these, a case-control study, reported dose-related increases in ischemic heart disease risk, with a standardized mortality ratio of 2.8 for ischemic heart disease among the more heavily exposed workers (27).

Exposure

Occupational toxicity has been of concern primarily in workers in smelters, where ore containing large amounts of arsenic are processed. Arsenical insecticides have been used in vineyards, and chronic arsenic poisoning has been reported in vintners. Exposure may be by inhalation of contaminated dusts or plant debris or may be by ingestion of contaminated foods (especially wine or beer).

Clinical Features

The clinical features are those of atherosclerotic vascular disease as discussed previously. Specific signs and symptoms of chronic arsenic poisoning—gastrointestinal disturbances, dermatitis and/or hyperpigmentation of the skin, and peripheral neuropathy—should be sought, but one does not usually find these with chronic low level exposures.

Nonatheromatous Ischemic Heart Disease

Ischemic heart disease may result from coronary vasospasm in the absence of athrosclerosis. Occupational exposure to nitrates, particularly nitroglycerin and ethylene glycol dinitrate, have been associated with such toxicity.

ORGANIC NITRATES

Epidemiology

In the 1950s, epidemics of chest pain and sudden death in munition workers were observed. These events typically occurred 36–72 hours after withdrawal from exposure to organic nitrates and were felt to be part of a nitrate withdrawal syndrome (28–30). Initial reports described workers with ischemic heart disease symptoms in the absence of or with only minimal atherosclerotic coronary artery disease. Subsequent epidemiologic studies have confirmed the association with a relative risk of 2.5 for cardiovascular mortality in workers exposed for 20 or more years (30). Epidemiologic studies have also suggested that nitrate exposure might contribute to accelerated atherosclerosis as well (31).

Exposure

Nitroglycerin and nitroglycol (ethylene glycol dinitrate) exposures occur in the munitions and explosives industries and among construction workers who handle dynamite. Dynamite is composed of about 60% organic nitrates, 25% blasting oil, and 10% dinitrotoluene, with a small amount of nitrocellulose and fillers. Blasting oil is 80% nitroglycol and 20% nitroglycerin and is the source of the volatile nitrates. Exposures tend to be greatest during explosive-mixing and cartridge-filling operations. Nitrates are highly volatile and are readily absorbed through the skin and lungs. Nitrates can permeate the wrapping material of dynamite sticks, so workers who handle dynamite should be advised to wear cotton gloves. Natural rubber gloves should not be used because they become permeated with nitrates and the gloves may enhance cutaneous nitrate absorption.

With current automated processes in explosives manufacturing, direct handling of nitrates by employees is minimized. However, levels of nitrates in the workplace environment must be controlled by adequate ventilation and by air conditioning during periods of hot weather. The current Occupational Safety and Health Administration (OSHA) exposure limit is 0.2 ppm for nitroglycerin, but even at lower levels (0.02 ppm or above) personal protective gear is recommended to avoid headache. Although there are no readily available biochemical measures to detect excessive nitrate exposure, findings of progressively decreasing blood pressure and increasing heart rate during the workday are suggestive of excessive exposure. Monitoring for these signs in employees may help prevent adverse effects of exposure to nitrates.

Blood concentrations of nitroglycerin have been measured in the workplace during production of gunpowder (32). Plasma concentrations of nitroglycerin in workers in the roll mill area were as high as 98.1 nmol/l (median) as compared with 5.7 nmol/l after taking 1.0 milligram nitroglycerin sublingually. Thus occupational exposures produce manyfold greater blood levels of nitroglycerin than does nitroglycerin in therapeutic doses.

Mechanisms and Pathogenesis

The occurrence of the nitrate withdrawal syndrome requires prolonged exposure to nitrates or nitrites. Initially workers experience the vasodilatory effects of nitrates, including flushing, headaches, and palpitations. These reactions tend to diminish over time, particularly over the course of the work week. With prolonged exposure, usually a year or longer, symptoms of nitrate withdrawal develop. The pathogenesis is thought to involve adaptation of physiologic systems to the vascular actions of nitrates. Nitrates directly dilate blood vessels, including those of the coronary circulation. With prolonged exposure, compensatory vasoconstriction, believed to be mediated by sympathetic neural responses, and activation of the renin-angiotensin system develops. If exposure to nitrates is stopped, compensatory vasoconstriction becomes unopposed, and coronary vasospasm with angina, myocardial infarction, or sudden death may result. Chest pain occurring during nitrate withdrawal has been termed "Monday morning angina" because it typically occurs 2 or 3 days after the last day of nitrate exposure. Mechanisms by which nitrates may promote atherosclerotic vascular disease are unknown.

Clinical Features

Workers exposed to excessive levels of nitrates typically experience headaches and may demonstrate hypotension, tachycardia, and warm, flushed skin. With continued exposure these symptoms and signs become less prominent. After 1–2 days without exposure to nitrates—generally occurring on weekends—signs of acute coronary ischemia, ranging from angina at rest to myocardial infarction or sudden death, may occur.

During episodes of pain, the ECG shows evidence of ischemia: either ST segment elevation or depression, with or without T-wave abnormalities. At other times, the ECG may be perfectly normal. Typical findings of myocardial infarction on ECG or an elevation of serum concentrations of the MB isoenzyme creatine phosphokinase (CPK). Results of exercise stress testing and coronary angiography when the patient is asymptomatic may be normal.

Treatment of myocardial ischemia due to nitrate withdrawal should include the administration of cardiac nitrates (such as nitroglycerin or isosorbide dinitrate) and calcium blockers. Case reports indicate that ischemic symptoms may recur, indicating a persistent tendency to coronary spasm, for weeks or months (33, 34). Therefore, longterm cardiac nitrate or calcium block therapy may be needed. The worker should be removed from sources of organic nitrate exposure.

OTHER CHEMICALS EXPOSURE

Acute myocardial infarction in the absence of coronary artery disease has occurred after acute exposures to solvents, presumably due to arrhythmias, and after acute intoxication with myocardial asphyxiants.

Myocardial Asphyxiants

Acute intoxications with asphyxiant chemicals can produce myocardial as well as generalized tissue injury. Such chemicals include carbon monoxide, cyanide, and hydrogen sulfide. Acute myocardial necrosis, including papillary muscle necrosis and pulmonary edema, have been observed (35,36). Severe intoxication with altered levels of consciousness would be expected to accompany asphyxia severe enough to produce myocardial injury.

CARBON MONOXIDE

Exposure

The major problem from asphyxiants occurs from carbon monoxide exposure in patients with preexisting coronary artery disease. Sources of exposure to carbon monoxide were described in the discussion of combustion products. Levels of carbon monoxide should be monitored if there are sources of combustion such as combustion engines or furnaces in the workplace. The current 8-hour threshold limit value is 35 ppm, which at the end of an 8-hour workday results in a carboxyhemoglobin concentration of 5%. This concentration is tolerated well by healthy individuals but not by people with cardiovascular or chronic lung disease. Workplace monitoring is easily done with a portable carbon monoxide meter. Biologic monitoring of workers involves measuring either the carboxyhemoglobin concentration in blood or the level of expired carbon monoxide, which is directly proportionate to the carboxyhemoglobin concentration. Elevated carbon monoxide levels should be anticipated in cigarette smokers.

Mechanisms and Pathogenesis

The pathogenesis of carbon monoxide poisoning occurs as a result of the high affinity of carbon monoxide for hemoglobin. The affinity of carbon monoxide for hemoglobin is more than 200 times that of oxygen. Binding of carbon monoxide and hemoglobin to form carboxyhemoglobin reduces delivery of oxygen to body tissues because the oxygen-carrying capacity of hemoglobin is decreased and because less oxygen is released to tissues at any given oxygen tension (i.e., there is a shift in the oxygen dissociation curve). Thus, a carboxyhemoglobin concentration of 20% represents a greater reduction in oxygen delivery than a 20% reduction in erythrocyte count. Other heme-containing proteins (e.g., myoglobin, cytochrome oxidase, and cytochrome P-450) bind 10–15% of the total body carbon monoxide, but the medical significance of their binding at usual levels of exposure to carbon monoxide is unsettled.

In healthy individuals exposed to carbon monoxide, the decrease in delivery of oxygen to tissues causes the cardiac output and coronary blood flow to increase to meet the metabolic demands of the heart. Although these compensatory responses allow healthy individuals to perform at normal work levels, their maximum exercise capacity is decreased. If, on the other hand, compensatory responses are limited, as in patients with coronary artery disease, carbon monoxide exposure may cause angina or myocardial infarction.

Clinical Features

Reduced exercise thresholds for the development of angina have been reported when carboxyhemoglobin concentrations are as low as 2.0% (37). Carbon monoxide decreases the ventricular fibrillation threshold in experimental animals and may do the same in humans (38). Severe carbon monoxide poisoning may cause acute myocardial infarction or sudden death, particularly in people with underlying coronary heart disease (39, 40).

In patients with angina pectoris, peripheral arterial occlusive disease, or chronic obstructive lung disease, low levels of carbon monoxide (blood carboxyhemoglobin 4% or less) reduce exercise capacity to the point of angina claudication or dyspnea, respectively (37, 41, 42). Low level carbon monoxide exposure may reduce maximum exercise capacity even in healthy workers (43).

Symptoms of carbon monoxide poisoning include headache (at carboxyhemoglobin concentrations as low as 10%) and nausea, dizziness, fatigue, and dimmed vision at higher concentrations.

The only specific laboratory finding is elevation of carboxyhemoglobin concentration. When arterial blood gases are measured the arterial oxygen tension is usually normal or slightly reduced while the venous partial pressure of oxygen (P_{O_2}) and oxygen content are substantially reduced. Although respiratory alkalosis due to hyperventilation is commonly observed, respiratory failure complicates the most severe poisonings. When there is marked tissue hypoxia, lactic acidosis develops.

Carbon monoxide is eliminated from the body by respiration, and the rate of elimination depends on ventilation, pulmonary blood flow, and inspired oxygen concentration. The half-life of carbon monoxide in a sedentary adult breathing air is 4–5 hours. The half-life can be reduced to 80 minutes by giving 100% oxygen by face mask, or it can be reduced to 25 minutes by giving hyperbaric oxygen (3 atmospheres) in a hyperbaric chamber.

Direct Myocardial Injury

Several chemicals are of concern as potential causes of myocardial injury.

COBALT

Epidemiology

Concern with cobalt has arisen from epidemics of cardiomyopathy first seen in the 1960s in drinkers of beer containing cobalt added to stabilize the foam (44, 45). The mortality rate in people affected with cobalt-induced cardiomyopathy was as high as 50% in some series. The importance of cobalt as an industrial cardiac toxin is uncertain. A recent study of tungsten carbide workers exposed to cobalt-containing dust found no overt systolic left ventricular dysfunction as tested by radionuclide ventriculography (46). However, there was a weak but statistically significant inverse correlation between resting left ventricular ejection fraction and duration of exposure, supporting a possible role for cobalt in causing myocardial disease. Workers with abnormal chest x-rays, presumably due to metal-induced interstitial lung fibrosis ("hard metal pneumoconiosis"), did show a reduced right ventricular ejection fraction, felt to be an early stage of cor pulmonale. While there is no other convincing epidemiologic evidence to indicate that cobalt is a risk factor for cardiovascular disease, there are case reports of cardiomyopathy in cobalt-exposed workers, including one case in which high levels of cobalt in the heart were measured at autopsy (47, 48).

Exposure

Cobalt is used along with tungsten carbide in the production of metal alloys used especially in the manufacturing of drills and bits. Exposure is primarily to cobalt powder and dust. Cobalt-60 is used medicinally for radiotherapy. Human exposure can be assessed by measuring urinary cobalt concentrations.

Pathophysiology

Cobalt depresses oxygen uptake by mitochondria of the heart and interferes with energy metabolism in a manner biochemically similar to the effects of thiamine deficiency (49). Because cobalt-exposed beer drinkers, but not individuals receiving high doses of cobalt for medical therapeutic reasons, develop cardiomyopathy, it has been speculated that cobalt, excessive alcohol consumption, and/or malnutrition act synergistically to produce myocardial injury. Most affected people have been heavy drinkers for many years, but the cardiomyopathy itself appeared within 1 year of the time that cobalt was added to the beer. The pathology in those who have died from cobalt-induced cardiomyopathy included myocardial necrosis with thrombi in the heart and major blood vessels.

Clinical Features

The clinical picture is that of a congestive cardiomyopathy with low cardiac output, venous congestion, pericardial effusion, and polycythemia. The electrocardiogram typically showed low voltage, ST segment depression, T-wave inversions, and in some cases Q-waves suggestive of myocardial infarction.

ARSENIC/ARSINE

Subacute arsenic poisoning caused by ingestion of arsenic-contaminated beer has been associated with cardiomyopathy and cardiac failure. In one epidemic in Manchester, England, 6000 people were affected, with 70 deaths (50). Arsenic poisoning can cause electrographic abnormalities and in one case was reported to cause recurrent ventricular arrhythmias of the torsades de pointe type (51). Little is known of the mechanism of arsenic-induced myocardial injury.

Arsine gas causes red blood cell hemolysis and, in some cases, death, from cardiac failure. Massive hemolysis which may persist for several days produces hyperkalemia, which can result in cardiac arrest. Electrocardiographic manifestions of acute arsine poisoning include high, peaked T-waves, conduction disturbances, various degrees of heart block, and asystole (52). Arsine may also directly affect the myocardium, causing a greater magnitude of cardiac failure than would be expected from the degree of anemia.

LEAD

The major cardiovascular concern for lead is its association with hypertension. Lead poisoning has also been associated with myocarditis and ECG abnormalities in children (53, 54). Case reports of "myocarditis" manifested as sinus bradycardia, ventricular ectopy, and diffuse ST-T wave changes on ECG, or sinus bradycardia with or without first degree atrioventricular block in lead-exposed workers have been reported (55, 56). In rats chronic exposure to lead produces degeneration of myofibrils with impairment of electrical and contractile function (56–58).

ANTIMONY

The therapeutic use of antimonial compounds for treatment of parasitic infections produces ECG abnormalities—primarily T-wave changes and QT interval prolongation—and has caused sudden death in some patients. An epidemic of sudden death and ECG abnormalities in workers exposed to antimony trisulfide in one factory has been described (59). When use of anitmony was stopped, no further deaths occurred, although ECG abnormalities persisted in some of the exposed individuals. Studies in animals confirm that chronic exposure to antimony can produce myocardial injury, although the mechanism has not been elucidated.

ORGANIC SOLVENTS

The major cardiovascular concern with solvent exposure is cardiac arrhythmias. However, several reports of myocardial failure in solvent exposed individuals have appeared in recent years (60–63). Dilated cardiomyopathy with severe cardiac failure developed in several people who were occupationally exposed to solvents (toluene or 1,1,1-trichlorethylene). In two of these cases there was biopsy evidence of myocarditis, while in one case there was no evidence of myocarditis at autopsy. One man developed an acute toxic myocarditis while painting in an unventilated room with a methyl cellulose-based paint. While these case reports should raise concern about excessive solvent exposure, the possibility of coincidental viral myocarditis must also be considered.

Arrhythmias

Arrhythmias are a common complication of ischemic heart disease and congestive cardiomyopathy but also may be precipitated by chemical exposures, particularly to halogenated hydrocarbons.

HALOGENATED HYDROCARBONS

Epidemiology

Numerous cases of cardiac arrhythmias or sudden death (presumably due to arrhythmias) in people abusing solvents or occupationally exposed to high levels of organic solvents or fluorocarbons have been described (64–67). Epidemiologic studies in general have not supported an overall increase in cardiovascular mortality in solvent-exposed workers, other than that with carbon disulfide as discussed previously. The primary cardiovascular risk from solvents appears to occur during acute intoxication. A study of hospital pathology residents showed an association between exposure to freon-22 and palpitations and arrhythmias as documented by ambulatory ECG monitoring (68). However, two recent studies of ambulatory ECGs in refrigerator repairmen exposed to fluorocarbons found no relationship between exposure and arrhythmias (69, 70).

Exposure

Exposure to solvents is widespread in industrial settings such as dry cleaning, degreasing, painting, and chemical manufac-

turing. Fluorocarbons are used extensively as refrigerants and as propellants in a wide variety of products. Solvent abuse, including sniffing of glue, spray paints, shoe polish, and typewriter correction fluid, most commonly occurs among adolescents and young adults. A variety of hydrocarbons have been implicated in sudden deaths. These include toluene, 1, 1, 1-trichloroethane, benzene, and fluorocarbons (freons). Assessment of exposure is most easily done by making workplace air measurements, although concentrations of some hydrocarbons may be measured in the expired air or in the blood of intoxicated patients.

Pathogenesis

Halogenated hydrocarbons have complex effects on the heart. At low levels of exposure solvents "sensitize" the heart to effects of catecholamines. Experimental studies have shown that the dose of epinephrine required to produce ventricular tachycardia or fibrillation is reduced after solvents are inhaled (71). Catecholamine release is induced by euphoria and excitement due the central nervous system effects of the solvents and also by exercise. Sensitization of the myocardium to effects of catecholamines and enhanced catecholamine release, in combination with asphyxia and hypoxia, is believed to be the cause of the arrhythmias, which can result in sudden death. At higher levels of exposure solvents may depress sinus node activity and thereby cause sinus bradycardia or arrest. Solvents may also depress atrioventricular nodal conduction and cause atrioventricular block. Bradyarrhythmias may then predispose to escape ventricular arrhythmias or, in cases of more severe intoxication, to asystole. The arrhythmogenic action of solvents may be enhanced by alcohol or caffeine.

The cardiac pathology in death cases is usually unremarkable, consistent with a sudden arrhythmic death, although acute myocardial infarction secondary to solvent intoxication has also been described. The finding of a fatty liver suggest chronic exposure to high levels of solvents or to ethanol.

Clinical Features and Treatment

The presence of symptoms of acute hydrocarbon exposure preceding the onset of arrhythmias or collapse should be ascertained. Symptoms of intoxication with hydrocarbon solvents or fluorocarbon propellants include dizziness, lightheadedness, headaches, nausea, drowsiness, lethargy, palpitations, or syncope. Physical examination may reveal ataxia, nystagmus, and/or slurred speech. The heart rate and blood pressure are usually normal except at the time of arrhythmias, when a rapid or irregular heartbeat is present and may be accompanied by hypotension.

Convulsions, coma, or cardiac arrest may occur after severe intoxication. Workers who have heart disease or chronic lung disease with hypoxemia may be more susceptible to the arrhythmogenic actions of solvents. Arrhythmias induced by solvents or propellants are expected to occur only at work while the worker is exposed to these agents. Arrhythmias may include premature atrial or ventricular contractions, atrial fibrillation, ventricular tachycardia or fibrillation, and asystole.

Solvent-exposed workers who report palpitations, dizzy spells, or syncopal episodes should be evaluated by 24-hour ambulatory ECG monitoring, including while at work. Workers with heart disease—especially those with chronic arrhythmias, should be advised to avoid exposure to potentially arrhythmogenic chemicals.

Since arrhythmias from hydrocarbons are related to sensitization of the heart to the actions of catecholamines, the use of beta-adrenergic-blocking drugs is most rational in treating solvent-induced arrhythmias. For workers who experience episodic arrhythmias in the workplace, the worker should be removed from the exposure or advised to use protective respiratory equipment. If a worker collapses and resuscitation is required, the use of epinephrine or other sympathomimetic drugs should be avoided if possible, since these agents may precipitate further arrhythmias.

ORGANOPHOSPHATES

Epidemiology

Acute intoxication with organophosphates and carbamate insecticides can produce diverse cardiovasular disturbances including hypotension, sinus tachycardia, sinus bradycardia, varying degrees of heart block, prolonged Q-T interval, ventricular premature beats, and ventricular tachycardia, often of the torsade de pointes type (72, 73). In one series 41% of patients with severe organophosphate poisoning had one or more cardiac arrhythmias (72). Chronic exposure to organophosphates has been associated with an increased prevalence of ECG abnormalities, although the significance of these abnormalities with respect to clinical cardiovascular disease is unknown.

Exposure

Organophosphate and carbamate insecticides are widely used in agriculture. They can be applied to crops be aerial spraying or by hand. Agricultural workers may therefore absorb insecticide by inhalation of mist or via cutaneous absorption. Continuing exposure may occur from contact with contaminated clothing or hair. The presence of some of the organophosphates may be measured in the blood or gastric fluid. Some organophosphates such as parathion have metabolites that may also be measured in the urine.

Pathophysiology

Organophosphates and carbamates inhibit acetylcholinesterase. The result is accumulation of acetylcholine at cholinergic synapses and myoneural juctions. The cardiovascular effects may vary over the time course of organophosphate poisoning. Early in acute poisoning, acetylcholine stimulates nicotinic receptors at sympathetic ganglia and causes tachycardia and mild hypertension. Later, when acetylcholine acts at muscarinic receptors or blocks ganglionic transmission by hyperpolarization, it causes bradycardia and hypotension. As a consequence of autonomic imbalance and asynchronous repolarization of different parts of the heart, there may be Q-T interval prolongation, and polymorphous ventricular tachycardia (torsades do pointe) has been reported (73).

The excess of acetylcholine at the myoneural junctions initially causes muscle paralysis, including paralysis of the diaphragm, which results in respiratory arrest. Other consequences are described with clinical findings below. As organophos-

phates act on autonomic neurotransmission there are no specific pathologic findings.

Clinical Findings and Treatment

Typical symptoms of mild organophosphate and carbamate poisoning include weakness, headache, sweating, nausea, vomiting, abdominal cramps, and diarrhea. Moderate poisoning may be associated with chest discomfort, dyspnea, inability to walk, and blurred vision. Physical signs are those of cholinergic excess and include small pupils, diaphoresis, salivation, lacrimation, an increase in bronchial secretions (which may resemble pulmonary edema), and muscle fasciculations. Early cardiovascular manifestations include tachycardia and hypertension. Later there may be bradycardia and hypotension. There is sometimes frank muscular weakness or, in severe poisoning, paralysis accompanied by respiratory failure, convulsions, or coma.

The failure of usual doses of atropine, a competitive antagonist of acetylcholine at muscarinic receptors, to reverse cholinergic signs strongly supports the diagnosis of organophosphate or carbamate poisoning.

The diagnosis is confirmed by the finding of a markedly depressed level of cholinesterase in red blood cells. Depression below 50% of normal is usually seen in patients with symptoms, and depression to less than 10% of normal is usually seen in patients with severe poisoning. Plasma cholinesterase activity is usually depressed also, but this correlates less well with clinical manifestations. Arterial blood gases may show carbon dioxide retention, hypoxia, or both.

Delayed repolarization with delayed Q-T interval prolongation on the ECG and episodes of ventricular tachycardia may be seen for up to 5–7 days after acute intoxication (73). The ECG also commonly shows nonspecific ST- and T-wave changes. As noted previously, a variety of arrhythmias have been observed. The chest x-ray may resemble pulmonary edema.

The differential diagnosis of signs and symptoms of cholinergic excess includes treatment with cholinesterase inhibitors, such as pyridostigmine, for myasthenia gravis. Small pupils may also be seen following ingestion of narcotics, clonidine, phenothiazines and sedative drugs, and in patients with pontine brain infarction or hemorrhage.

General treatment measures include decontamination (removal of clothing and thorough cleaning of skin and hair), support of respiration (including mechanical ventilation for respiratory failure), and support of circulation. Specific measures include the use of pralidoxime (2-PAM) to reverse muscular paralysis and other manifestations of excess acetylcholine, and the use of atropine to reverse bronchorrhea and bradycardia.

Intensive cardiac and respiratory monitoring of patients for several days after exposure is recommended, with particular attention to the possible late development of arrhythmias or respiratory failure. Heart block and polymorphous ventricular tachycardia with a prolonged Q-T interval are optimally treated by cardiac pacing. The use of antiarrhythmic drugs (such as quinidine, procainamide, and diisopyramide) that depress conduction or calcium channel blockers should be avoided.

OTHER CHEMICALS

Antimony has been associated with ECG abnormalities and an increased risk of sudden death presumably due to arrhythmias (59). Acute arsenic poisoning can cause ECG abnormalities;

in one case recurrent ventricular tachycardia of the torsades de pointe type has been described (51). Arsine exposure production disturbance including various degrees of heart block and asystole, probably related in part to hyperkalemia resulting from hemolysis (52).

Hypertension

As chronic hypertension is a major risk factor for premature atherosclerotic coronary vascular disease and stroke, the possibility that occupational and environmental factors can induce or aggravate hypertension is of concern. There is evidence that nonchemical factors such as work stress and noise may increase the prevalence of hypertension, but this chapter will focus on chemical factors, for which there is also evidence.

LEAD

Epidemiology

Epidemiologic studies suggest that low level lead exposure can chronically elevate blood pressure, at least in some populations (74). Such exposures can occur in the workplace or from other environmental sources. Several studies in large unselected populations, such as the NHANES study in the United States, have reported a positive relationship between lead concentration and systolic blood pressure, with an average 5-mmHg rise per 15 μg/dl lead blood concentration increment (75). Over the range of commonly observed blood lead concentrations (0.8–35 μg/dl), a blood pressure elevation of 10–15 mmHg would be predicted. A case-control study comparing 135 hypertensive patients and a similar number of age- and sex-matched normotensive controls supports the relationship between blood lead and diastolic blood pressure, and suggested even a greater quantitative contribution of lead to blood pressure elevation (76). Several mortality studies of lead-exposed workers have reported significant associations between blood pressure, the risk of cererovascular disease, and the extent of lead exposure, although not all studies have confirmed that relationship (2, 74).

It is noteworthy that chronic lead exposure increases the risk of chronic renal disease. Chronic renal disease may be contributed to by and/or may cause or aggravate hypertension. Several workplace epidemiologic studies have found increased mortality from chronic renal disease in lead-exposed workers (77).

Exposure

Environmental sources of lead include inhalation of automobile exhaust from gasolines containing alkyl lead additives, from ingestion of dust contaminated with lead paint, and from drinking water that had passed through lead piping. Occupational exposures to lead-containing dust or fumes occur in lead smelters, foundries, and in industries such as battery manufacturing, construction work, demolition, and vehicle radiator repair, where lead compounds are used.

Lead exposure can be assessed by measuring blood lead concentration. The average blood lead concentration in adults in the United States not exposed to lead is about 10 μg/dl (75). The "normal" range is up to about 35 μg/dl. Even within this range there is evidence of an increase in blood pressure with increasing concentrations of lead. Workplace exposures may result in levels that are much higher. Lead concentrations above 40–50 μg/dl are considered to be excessive. Erythrocyte protoporphyrin concentration, a biochemical test the correlates with blood lead concentration, begins to increase at blood lead levels of 25–30 μg/dl.

Pathophysiology

Low level chronic lead exposure increases blood pressure in animals (74). The major hemodynamic effect appears to be increased vascular resistance. Lead may increase vascular resistance by increasing plasma renin activity, increasing responsiveness of vascular smooth muscle to the pressor effects of endogenous vasoconstrictors such as norepinephrine or angiotensin II, and/or by direct contraction of vascular smooth muscle. The importance of increased plasma renin has been questioned because angiotensin II levels are not correspondingly increased, suggesting that lead may also inhibit angiotensin-converting enzyme. Furthermore, in people chronically exposed to lead, plasma renin activity is normal or low. Increased vascular tone and reactivity may result from increased intracellular calcium. Lead exposure increases calcium levels in various tissues, possibly due to inhibition of sodium potassium-ATPase and effects on calmodulin-mediated calcium transport.

Clinical Features

The clinical features of lead-induced hyertension are similar to those from hypertension of any cause. Other features of lead intoxication at low levels include slowed nerve conduction, impaired biosynthesis of hemoglobin (related to inhibition of δ-aminolevulinic acid and ferrochelatase) with an increase in erythrocyte protoporphyrin concentration, and hyperuricemia (due to increased tubular reabsorption of uric acid). At higher lead levels evidence of frank toxicity including anemia, peripheral neuropathy, and renal failure is seen.

CADMIUM

In animal studies low level cadmium exposure elevates blood pressure (78). Many epidemiologic human studies on hypertension and cardiovascular disease have examined the relationship to cadmium, and the results are generally inconclusive (2). Those studies reporting positive associations tend to be more methodologically flawed. Overall the evidence that exposure to cadmium in the workplace increases the risk of hypertension or cardiac vascular disease is unconvincing.

OTHER CHEMICALS

As noted previously carbon disulfide exposure may be associated with hypertension, possibly mediated by inhibition of dopamine β-hydroxylase. Exposure to organic solvents during pregnancy has been recently reported to increase the risk of hypertension and of preeclampsia (i.e., hypertension with edema and proteinuria) (79). In a case-referent study of 90 exposed American women, relative risks of 3.0 (95% CI 0.9–9.9) and 3.9 (2.5–5.4) for hypertension and preeclampsia, respectively, were observed. Of note was that the level of exposure to solvents was moderate, in most cases barely exceeding one-third of the TLV. This study is provocative but requires replication with a large number of patients.

Peripheral Arterial Occlusive Disease

There are few modern studies on chemical exposures and peripheral arterial occlusive disease. The older literature suggests that chronic high level exposure to carbon disulfide, arsenic, and lead are associated with an increased prevalence of peripheral vascular disease. For example, arterial disease with gangrene of the lower extremities due to chronic arsenic poisoning was historically called "black foot disease" (50). The pathophysiology of chemically induced peripheral vascular disease, with the possible exception of carbon disulfide as discussed previously, is unknown. In modern times cigarette smoking is the major risk factor for peripheral vascular disease, but environmental tobacco smoke has not yet been implicated. Once a person has peripheral arterial occlusive disease with intermittent claudication, exposure to carbon monoxide, even at low levels, significantly reduces exercise tolerance (41).

CONCLUSION

A number of chemicals have been implicated in the causation of cardiovascular disease. While there has been considerable scientific investigation, there are still many unanswered questions about causation for chemicals that have been discussed. A survey of the probability for causation for various chemicals is presented in Table 15.1. A problem in the evaluation of any particular patient is that cardiovascular disease is very common in the general population, and the clinical manifestations are generally nonspecific, so that causality for a specific toxic exposure is difficult to establish.

However, the data reviewed in this chapter may be of use in occupational and environmental medicine in several ways.

1. Knowledge of the potential cardiovascular toxins and associated diseases makes it possible for health care personnel to intelligently monitor exposed workers for early evidence of cardiovascular disease. An example of this is the use of funduscopy to assess early cardiovascular toxicity from carbon disulfide.
2. Knowledge of interactions between chemical toxins and medical diseases provides a basis for health care personnel to advise workers about safe workplace exposures. For example, a patient with angina pectoris should be advised not to work on a job where he or she is exposed to significant levels of carbon monoxide.
3. Knowledge of cardiovascular toxicology allows for more rational preemployment screening. Patients with underlying cardiovascular disease should not be placed in workplaces where they are exposed to chemicals that may aggravate their diseases.
4. Specific epidemiologic data have been used to improve workplace conditions and decrease occupation-related cardiovascular disease. For example, control of carbon disulfide exposure has reduced the incidence of ischemic heart disease in viscose rayon workers (5). Reduction of nitrate exposure in explosives manufacturing has reduced the incidence of sudden death in those workers. Similar controls are indicated for other known toxic exposures, including environmental tobacco smoke.

REFERENCES

1. Benowitz NL, Goldschlager N. Cardiac disturbances in the toxicologic patient. In: Haddad LM, Winchester JF, eds. Clinical management of poisoning and drug overdose. 2nd ed. Philadelphia: WB Saunders, 1990.
2. Kristensen TS. Cardiovascular diseases and the work environment. A critical review of the epidemiologic literature on chemical factors. Scand J Work Environ Health 1989;15:245–264.
3. Tiller JR, Schilling RSF, Morris JN. Occupational toxic factor in mortality from coronary heart disease. Br Med J 1968;4:407–411.
4. Hernberg S, Partanen T, Nordman CH, Sumari P. Coronary heart disease among workers exposed to carbon disulphide. Br J Ind Med 1970;27:313–325.
5. Nurminen M, Hernberg S. Effects of intervention on the cardiovascular mortality of workers exposed to carbon disulphide: a 15-year follow-up. Br J Ind Med 1985;42:32–35.
6. Sweetnam PM, Taylor SWC, Elwood PC. Exposure to carbon disulphide and ischaemic heart disease in a viscose rayon factory. Br J Ind Med 1987;44:220–227.
7. Tolonen M. Vascular effects of carbon disulfide. A review. Scand J Work Environ Health 1975;1:63–77.
8. Coppock RW, Buck WB. Toxicology of carbon disulfide: A review. Vet Hum Toxicol 1981;23:331–336.
9. Cavalleri A. Serum thyroxine in the early diagnosis of carbon disulfide poisoning. Arch Environ Health 1975;30:85–87.
10. Nurminen M, Mutanen P, Tolonen M, Hernberg S. Quantitated effects of carbon disulfide exposure, elevated blood pressure, and aging on coronary mortality. Am J Epidemiol 1982;115:107–118.
11. Karai I, Sugimoto K, Goto S. A fluorescein angiographic study on carbon disulfide retinopathy among workers in viscose rayon factories. Int Arch Occup Environ Health 1983;53:91–99.
12. Goldsmith JR. Carbon monoxide research: recent and remote. Arch Environ Health 1970;21:118–120.
13. Weir FW, Fabiano VL. Reevaluation of the role of carbon monoxide in production as aggravation of cardiovascular disease processes. J Occup Med 1982;24:519–525.
14. Wald N, Howard S, Smith PG, Kjeldsen K. Association between atherosclerotic diseases and carboxyhaemoglobin levels in tobacco smokers. Br Med J 1973;1:761–765.
15. Hernberg S, Kärävä R, Koskela R-S, Luoma K. Angina pectoris, ECG findings and blood pressure of foundry workers in relation to carbon monoxide exposure. Scand J Work Environ Health 1976;2 (suppl 1):54–63.
16. Stern FB, Halperin WE, Hornung RW, Ringenburg VL, McCammon CS. Heart disease mortality among bridge and tunnel officers exposed to carbon monoxide. Am J Epidemiol 1988;182:1276–1288.
17. Theriault GP, Tremblay CG, Armstrong BG. Risk of ischemic heart disease among primary aluminum production workers. Am J Ind Med 1988;13:659–666.
18. Hansen ES. Mortality from cancer and ischemic heart disease in Danish chimney sweeps; a five-year followup. Am J Epidemiol 1983;177:160–164.
19. Fielding JE, Phenow KJ. Health effects of involuntary smoking. N Engl J Med 1988;319:1452–1460.
20. Kawachi I, Pearce NE, Jackson RT. Deaths from lung cancer and ischaemic heart disease due to passive smoking in New Zealand. NZ Med J 1989;102:337–340.
21. Willett WC, Green A, Stampfer MJ, et al. Relative and absolute excess risks of coronary heart disease among women who smoke cigarettes. N Engl J Med 1987;317:1303–1309.
22. Matsukura S, Tomohiko T, Norikazu K, et al. Effects of environmental tobacco smoke on urinary cotinine excretion in non-smokers: evidence for passive smoking. N Engl J Med 1984;311:828–832.
23. The Surgeon General. The health consequences of involuntary smoking. Rockville, MD: U.S. Department of Health and Human Services, 1986.
24. Bond JA, Gown AM, Yang HL, Benditt EP, Juchau MR. Further investigations of the capacity of polynuclear aromatic hydrocarbons to elicit atherosclerotic lesions. J Toxicol Environ Health 1981;7:327–335.
25. Pinto SS, Enterline PE, Henderson V, Varner MO. Mortality experience in relation to a measured arsenic trioxide exposure. Environ Health Perspect 1977;19:127–130.
26. Lee-Feldstein A. Arsenic and respiratory cancer in humans: follow-up of copper smelter employees in Montana. J Natl Cancer Inst 1983;70:601–609.
27. Axelson O, Dahlgren E, Jansson CD, Rehnlund SO. Arsenic exposure and mortality: a case-referent study from a Swedish copper smelter. Br J Ind Med 1978;35:8–15.
28. Morton WE. Occupational habituation to aliphatic nitrates and the withdrawal hazards of coronary disease and hypertension. J Occup Med 1977;19:197–200.

29. Carmichael P, Lieben J. Sudden death in explosive workers. Arch Environ Health 193;7:424–439.

30. Lange RI, Reid MS, Tresch DD, Keelan MH, Bernhard VM, Coolidge G. Nonatheromatous ischemic heart disease following withdrawal from chronic industrial nitroglycerin exposure. Circulation 1972;46:666–678.

31. Levine RJ, Andjelkovich DA, Kersteter SL, et al. Heart disease in workers exposed to dinitrotoluene. J Occup Med 1986;28:811–816.

32. Gjesdal K, Bille S, Bredesen JE, et al. Exposure to glyceryl trinitrate during gun powder production: plasma glyceryl trinitrate concentration, elimination kinetics, and discomfort among production workers. Br J Ind Med 1985;42:27–31.

33. Klock JC. Nonocclusive coronary disease after chronic exposure to nitrates: evidence for physiologic nitrate dependence. Am Heart J 1975;89:510–513.

34. Przybojewski JZ, Heyns MH. Acute coronary vasospasm secondary to industrial nitroglycerin withdrawal. A case presentation and review. S Afr Med J 1983;63:158–165.

35. Corya BC, Black MJ, McHenry PL. Echocardiographic findings after acute carbon monoxide poisoning. Br Heart J 1976;38:712.

36. Middleton GD, Ashby DW, Clark F. Delayed and long-lasting electrocardiographic changes in carbon-monoxide poisoning. Lancet 1961;1:12.

37. Allred EN, Bleecker ER, Chaitman BR, et al. Short-term effects of carbon monoxide exposure on the exercise performance of subjects with coronary artery disease. N Engl J Med 1989;321:1426–1432.

38. Aronow WS, Stemmes EA, Zweig S. Carbon monoxide and ventricular fibrillation threshold in normal dogs. Arch Environ Health 1979;34:184–186.

39. Atkins EH, Baker EL. Exacerbation of coronary artery disease by occupational carbon monoxide exposure: a report of two fatalities and a review of the literature. Am J Ind Med 1985;7:73–79.

40. Scharf SM, Thames MD, Sargent RK. Transmural myocardial infarction after exposure to carbon monoxide in coronary artery disease: report of a case. N Engl J Med 1974;15:409.

41. Aronow WS, Stemmer EA, Isbell MW. Effect of carbon monoxide exposure on intermittent claudication. Circulation 1974;49:415–417.

42. Calvery PMA, Leggett RJ. Carbon monoxide and exercise tolerance in chronic bronchitis and emphysema. Br Med J 1981;283:878.

43. Horvath SM, Raven PB, Dahms TE, et al. Maximum aerobic capacity at different levels of carboxyhemoglobin. J Appl Physiol 1975;38:300–303.

44. Bonenfant JL, Miller G, Roy PE. Quebec beer-drinkers' cardiomyopathy: pathological studies. Can Med Assoc J 1967;97:910–916.

45. Kesteloot H, Roeland J, Willems J, Claes JH, Joosens JV. An enquiry into the role of cobalt in the heart disease of chronic beer drinkers. Circulation 1968;37:854–864.

46. Horowitz SF, Fischbein A, Matza D, et al. Evaluation of right and left ventricular function in hard metal workers. Br J Ind Med 1988;45:742–746.

47. Barborik M, Dusek J. Cardiomyopathy accompanying industrial cobalt exposure. Br Heart J 1972;34:113–116.

48. Kennedy A, Dornan JD, King R. Fatal myocardial disease associated with industrial exposure to cobalt. Lancet 1981;1:412–414.

49. Alexander CS. Cobalt and the heart. Ann Intern Med 1969;70:411–413.

50. National Research Council. Biologic effects of arsenic on man. In: Arsenic. Washington, DC: National Academy of Sciences, 1977;173–191.

51. Goldsmith S, From AHL. Arsenic-induced atypical ventricular tachycardia. N Engl J Med 1980;303:1096–1098.

52. Josephson CJ, Pinto SS, Petronella SJ. Arsine: electrocardiographic changes produced in acute human poisoning. Arch Ind Hyg 1951;4:43–52.

53. Kline TS. Myocardial changes in lead poisoning. Am J Dis Child 1960;99:48.

54. Silver W, Rodriguez-Torres R. Electrocardiographic study in children with lead poisoning. Pediatrics 1968;41:1124.

55. Read JI, Williams JP. Lead myocarditis: report of a case. Am Heart J 1952;44:797–802.

56. Myerson RM, Eisenhauler JH. Atrioventricular conduction defects in lead poisoning. Am J Cardiol 1963;11:409–412.

57. Asokan SK. Experimental lead cardiomyopathy: myocardial structural changes in rats given small amounts of lead. J Lab Clin Med 1974;84:20–25.

58. Williams BJ, Hejtmancik MR, Abreu M. Cardiac effects of lead. Fed Proc 1983;42:2989–2993.

59. Brieger H, Semisch CW, Stasney J, Piatnek DA. Industrial antimony poisoning. Ind Med Surg 1954;23:521–523.

60. Mee AS, Wright PL. Congestive (dilated) cardiomyopathy in association with solvent abuse. J R Soc Med 1980;73:671–672.

61. Weissberg PL, Green ID. Theophylline poisoning in adults. Br Med J 1979;1114.

62. McLeod AA, Marjot R, Monaghan MJ, Hugh-Jones P, Jackson G. Chronic cardiac toxicity after inhalation of 1, 1, 1-trichloroethane. Br Med J 1987;294:728–729.

63. Wiseman MN, Banim S. ''Glue sniffer's'' heart? Br Med J 1987;294:739.

64. Bass M. Sudden sniffing death. JAMA 1970;212:2075–2079.

65. Kleinfeld M, Tabershaw IR. Trichloroethylene toxicity: report of five fatal cases. Arch Ind Hyg Occup Med 1954;10:134–141.

66. Wright MF, Strobl DJ. 1, 1, 1-Trichloroethane cardiac toxicity: report of a case. J Am Osteopath Assoc 1984;84:285–288.

67. May DC, Blotzer MJ. A report of occupational deaths attributed to fluorocarbon-113. Arch Environ Health 1984;39:352–354.

68. Speizer FE, Wegman DH, Ramirez A. Palpitation rates associated with fluorocarbon exposure in a hospital setting. N Engl J Med 1975;292:624–626.

69. Antti-Poika N, Heikkilä J, Saarinen L. Cardiac arrhythmias during occupational exposure to fluorinated hydrocarbons. Br J Ind Med 1990;47:138–140.

70. Edling C, Ohlson C-G, Ljungkvist G, Oliv Ä, Söderholm B. Cardiac arrhythmia in refrigerator repairmen exposed to fluorocarbons. Br J Ind Med 1990;47:207–212.

71. Kobayashi S, Hutchenon, DE, Regan J. Cardiopulmonary toxicity of tetrachloroethylene. J Toxicol Environ Health 1982;10:23–30.

72. Finkelstein Y, Kushnir A, Raikhlin-Eisenkraft B, Taitelman U. Antidotal therapy of severe acute organophosphate poisoning: a multihospital study. Neurotoxicol Teratol 1989;11:593–596.

73. Ludomirsky A, Klein HO, Sarelli P, et al. Q-T prolongation and polymorphous (''torsade de pointes'') ventricular arrhythmias associated with organophosphorous insecticide poisoning. Am J Cardiol 1982;49:1654–1658.

74. Sharp DS, Becker CE, Smith AH. Chronic low-level lead exposure: its role in the pathogenesis of hypertension.. Med Toxicol 1987;2:210–232.

75. Pirkle JL, Schwartz J, Landis JR, Harlan WR. The relationship between blood lead levels and blood pressure and its cardiovascular risk implication. Am J Epidemiol 1985;121:246–258.

76. Beevers DG, Erskine E, Robertson M, et al. Blood lead and hyertension. Lancet 1976;1:1–3.

77. Landrigan PJ. Toxicity of lead at low dose. Br J Ind Med 1989;46:593–596.

78. Schroeder HA. Cadmium, chromium, and cardiovascular disease. Circulation 1967;35:570–582.

79. Eskenaza B, Bracken MB, Holford TR, Grady J. Exposure to organic solvents and hypertensive disorders of pregnancy. Am J Ind Med 1988;14:177–188.

16

Teratogenesis and Reproductive Toxicology

Michael A. McGuigan, M.D.

INTRODUCTION

Human reproduction involves a complex, integrated series of neurophysiologic events. Toxins may adversely affect successful reproduction at any level, from sexual maturation and function of the individual in question to the growth, development, and reproductive capacity of the offspring (Table 16.1). The complexity of the entire reproductive process makes it particularly susceptible to toxic injury. Adding to the difficulties in understanding "reproductive toxicity" is the fact that adverse consequences may result from a toxic insult to the mother, the father, or the fetus. In order to begin to understand reproductive toxicology, it is necessary to be familiar with both the female and male reproductive systems as well as fetal growth and development.

Female The female reproductive organ system consists of four anatomic components, the functions of which are regulated by steroids and hormones secreted from the pituitary gland and the ovaries.

The *ovaries* are two almond-shaped organs located on either side of the uterus. Physiologically, the ovaries are responsible for steroid and hormone secretion and for oogenesis, the production of female gametes (ova or oocytes).

The *fallopian tubes* (or oviducts) are tubular structures that connect the surface of each ovary with the uterine lumen. The fallopian tubes have two functions: they are the conduit by which the ovulated ovum (or oocyte) is transported to the uterus, and they are the location where fertilization of the ovum occurs. Thus, the most important function of the fallopian tubes is to provide an environment conducive to fertilization and subsequent transportation of the fertilized ovum to the uterus for implantation.

The *uterus*, located in the pelvic cavity, is a pear-shaped organ with thick walls and a single central lumen. Anatomically, it is divided into four regions (fundus, corpus, isthmus, and cervix) and is composed of three layers—the endometrium (the lining in which the fertilized ovum implants and grows, and in which the placenta develops and attaches), the myometrium (the muscular tissue responsible for the expulsion of the fetus), and the peritoneum.

The *vagina* is a fibromuscular tube that connects the lower part of the uterine cervix with the outside environment.

Male The male reproductive organ system consists of three anatomic components, the functions of which are regulated by steroids and hormones secreted from the pituitary gland and the testes.

The *testes* are two ovoid structures located in the scrotal sac. Physiologically, the testes are responsible for steroid and hormone secretion and for spermatogenesis, the production of male gametes (spermatozoa).

The *epididymis* is a convoluted tubular structure that connects each testis with the vas deferens (the tube that carries the spermatozoa to the prostatic urethra). The function of the epididymis is to provide an environment conducive to the maturation of the spermatozoa.

The *urethra* is divided into two sections: the prostatic and the penile urethra. The urethra is the conduit between the vas deferens and the outside environment.

Fetus Conceptions occurs within the fallopian tube, and the fertilized ovum is transported to the uterus where implantation occurs and placentation begins. This takes about 2 weeks, and the fertilized ovum is not usually susceptible to teratogenic insults during this period because it is relatively isolated from the maternal circulation. If major abnormalities or a critical loss of cells occurs during this period, the embryo is usually spontaneously aborted early enough so that the pregnancy is rarely identified. Once implantation into the uterine lining is established, the embryonic stage is begun and lasts for about 6 weeks. It is during this period that susceptibility to toxins is high, and major morphologic abnormalities occur (Fig. 16.1). Following the embryonic stage, the fetus grows and develops for the balance of the gestation. During this period, the susceptibility of developing organ systems to toxic injury varies. Each organ system has a critical time frame during which it is particularly susceptible to the development of morphologic abnormalities (Fig. 16.2). Organogenesis is largely limited to the first trimester, but genital development continues until near term, and central nervous system development continues throughout the gestation and into the postnatal period.

Table 16.1. Scope of Reproductive Toxicology

Preconception
    Sexual maturation
    Libido
    Genetic structure
    Gamete formation
    Gamete transport

Conception
    Fertilization
    Implantation
    Placentation
    Fetal loss

Pregnancy
    Embryo development
    Embryo teratogenicity
    Embryo fetotoxicity
    Fetal maturation

Birth
    Delivery
    Neonatal transition
    Lactation

Growth and development
    Altered reproduction of offspring
    Impaired intellectual function
    Transplacental carcinogenesis

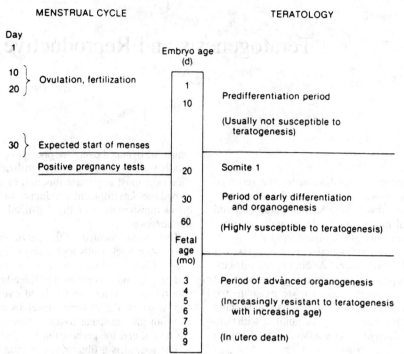

Figure 16.1. Relationship of adult female ovulation cycle to teratogenic susceptibility. From: Harbison RD, Evans MA. Teratogenic aspects of drug abuse in pregnancy. In: Rementeria JC, ed. Drug abuse in pregnancy and neonatal effects. St. Louis, MO: CV Mosby Co., 1977:191.

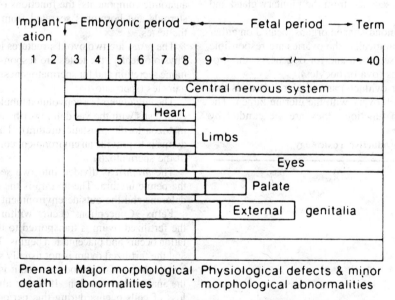

Figure 16.2. Critical periods of embryonic development. Copyright 1981, *The Medical Journal of Australia*, reprinted with permission.

EPIDEMIOLOGY OF TOXIC INJURY

Reproductive toxicology is the study of the adverse effects of environmental agents on the process of human reproduction. The incidence and prevalence of reproductive disorders caused by toxic injury depends on the particular outcome that is measured and the methods of the data collection. All information must always be compared with the normal background rates of fetal loss and spontaneous malformations.

Measured outcomes One commonly recorded outcome is fertility. Fertility, strictly speaking, measures the ability of a woman to conceive or become pregnant. True fertility measures only preimplantation events and does not distinguish between toxic injuries that occurred to the male or to the female reproductive system.

Another measurable reproductive outcome is fecundity. Fecundity is the ability to bear liveborn offspring and measures overall reproductive function. It does not distinguish between male and female toxic insults or normal and abnormal births, nor does it identify infants that are born prematurely or die shortly after birth. Term gestation is a reflection of a woman's ability to carry the fetus to term (38–40 weeks of gestation) and measures postimplantation events.

Fertility and fecundity (the so-called reproductive rates) are not

Table 16.2. Probabilities of Spontaneous Abortion

Time from Ovulation		Probability of Fetal Death in Gestation Interval (%)
1–6	days	54.6
7–13	days	24.7
14–20	days	8.2
3–5	wks	7.6
6–9	wks	6.5
10–13	wks	4.4
14–17	wks	1.3
18–21	wks	0.8
22–25	wks	0.3
26–29	wks	0.3
30–33	wks	0.3
34–37	wks	0.3
38+	wks	0.7

Modified from: Kline J, Stein Z. Very early pregnancy. In: Dixon RL, ed. Reproduction toxicology. New York, NY: Raven Press, 1985:259.

Table 16.3. Causes of Malformation in Humans

Unknown	65–70%
Genetic defects	20%
Drugs/environmental chemicals	4–6%
Chromosomal abnormalities	3–5%
Maternal infections	2–3%
Maternal metabolic imbalances	1–2%
Maternal reactions	<1%
Potentiative interactions	?

Modified from: Wilson JG. Teratogenic effects of environmental chemicals. Fed Proc 1977;36:1698–1703.

accurate ways of measuring the teratogenic potential of a substance. First of all, it is not always easy to diagnose an early pregnancy or to establish when conception occurred. Groups of women who are being studied prospectively may be more aware of pregnancies. The identification of fetal loss depends on the accurate diagnosis of pregnancy, and any suspected increases in fetal loss rates may be lost within the normal background of spontaneous postconceptual loss rate, estimated to range from 20–56% (3–5). The calculated estimates of the likelihood of spontaneous abortion at any given period of gestation are presented in Table 16.2. The causes of spontaneous abortions are heterogeneous, made up of chromosomally abnormal fetuses (30–50%) and chromosomally normal conceptions (7).

A third commonly measured outcome is malformations. Malformations may be observable at birth (congenital) or may not be noticed until much later. The specific malformation is traditionally anatomic or structural in nature, but malformations may also include physiologic (metabolic) or behavioral (psychologic) abnormalities. Human malformations are a common occurrence. Some type of detectable malformation is present in approximately 5–15% of all births, and the malformation is serious enough to need medical treatment in 2% of all births. The most common minor malformations not associated with major defects include abnormalities of hand creases, ears, and skin color. Malformation rates are, in general, a poor measure of the teratogenic potential of a substance. In fact, individual malformations resulting from toxic exposures may occur so rarely as to be statistically undetectable against the high baseline rate of malformations. While the incidences of malformations are well-established, the etiologies are not. In fact, for the majority of malformations the cause is unknown (Table 16.3).

Establishing the particular outcome to be monitored is difficult when trying to assess reproductive toxicity. The results of an acute exposure might not be expressed until weeks, months, or even years later. For example, the timing of the spermatogenic cycle may delay the expression of a toxic effect on spermatocytes until the cells have matured into spermatozoa and been ejaculated, a process which takes months. Toxic effects may also occur after longterm lowlevel exposure, especially if the toxic molecular insults are cummulative. Such effects could hasten menopause or alter sexual performance and behavior (9).

Data collection methods There are a number of different types of study methods used to collect data regarding the association of occupational exposure to adverse reproductive consequences (10). Correlative studies of groups of subjects compare (or correlate) the frequencies of occurrence of a particular disorder among different "at-risk" groups with the levels of exposure of these groups to the toxin in question. Results suggesting than an exposure is teratogenic are those demonstrating that the particular defect or malformation is more common in those groups with higher degrees of exposure.

Retrospective studies of individuals compare cases of a disorder with controls, with respect to the extent of exposure to possible toxins. These studies are also known as case-control studies, a very common type of report in which controls are selected to match the subjects. When an exposure is recalled more often by parents of children with defects than by control subjects, the results are considered suggestive that the exposure was teratogenic. Because these studies rely on individual recall, they are subject to a considerable amount of bias.

Prospective studies of individuals compare those exposed to a possible toxin with those who were not exposed (or who were exposed to a greater or lesser degree) with respect to the frequency of an adverse reproductive effect. These studies are also known as cohort studies, in which the identified exposed and control groups are followed over a period of time. Results suggesting than an exposure was teratogenic occur when the defects were found to be especially common in infants whose parents were known to have been exposed. These studies are also subject to bias, and they are incapable of detecting rare outcomes.

Intervention studies try to establish the frequency with which a disorder occurs in a control group (exposed to a possible toxin) compared with a group in which action has been taken to prevent or reduce exposure to the same toxin. If malformations occur less commonly after intervention, then the results suggest that exposure is teratogenic.

Case reports of adverse consequences of an exposure often serve as the initial basis for implicating specific compounds. These reports are common but are not initially helpful unless the results are rare or unique (e.g., thalidomide). The hypotheses generated by case reports need to be tested systematically before they can be regarded as conclusive.

Randomized trials are those in which subjects are exposed to a potential toxin at random. These studies are generally not subject to much bias but are almost never available.

The discovery of the teratogenecity of many chemicals and the suspicions and allegations directed against others have fostered the view that the chief cause of congenital malformations are environmental or workplace chemicals (11). This view is not correct (see Table 16.3). The identification of substances that have potentially deleterious effects of human reproduction is difficult. While a great deal of work has been done in animals, little has been established with respect to the dangers of industrial chemicals on human reproduction. Factors that make it difficult and problematic to extrapolate from animal data to humans include genetic susceptibility, intrinsic sensitivity of the developing tissues to the particular toxin, and interspecies variability in pharmacokinetic processes (including metabolism) which affects the magnitude and duration of exposure relative to the developmental stage (and metabolic capabilities) of the fetus (12).

It is clear from animal experiments and human epidemiologic studies that many industrial chemicals have the potential to be reproductive toxins. A recent estimate is that more than 2800 chemicals have been tested for teratogenicity and about 62% are not teratogenic (11). As more substances are tested and the sophistication of the evaluation process improves, more substances will be added to the reproductive toxicity list. Some of the substances that are believed to have adverse reproductive effects in humans are presented in Tables 16.4 and 16.5.

ROUTES OF EXPOSURE AND ABSORPTION

For the worker, the routes of exposure and absorption for most industrial chemicals are inhalation and dermal. Once the substance has been absorbed, it will be distributed throughout the mother's body. Pregnancy alters a number of pharmacokinetic parameters which modify the distribution (decreased protein binding, increased volume of distribution) and renal excretion (increased glomerular filtration rate) of toxins. The activities of maternal phase I and II metabolic pathways are reduced compared with the nonpregnant state. Toxic substances may be metabolized by the placenta (predominantly glutathione conjugation) or may cross the placenta unchanged. Once the toxic substance reaches the fetal circulation, it is distributed throughout the body of the fetus. The capabilities of fetal hepatic metabolism are limited and variable (15). Smooth endoplasmic reticulum appears at approximately 40–60 days of gestation. By midgestation, fetal phase I reactions function at 20–40% of adult values. Fetal phase II reaction activities are variable; glucuronidation capabilities are low, but enzyme systems for sulfate, glycine, and glutathione conjugation exist. The major pathways and maternal-fetal interrelationships are depicted in Figure 16.3. The variability of the fetotoxic effects resulting from this distribution depend on the timing of the exposure (Fig. 16.2): not only are different organ systems forming at different times and rates, but the activities of the fetal enzyme systems that may make a substance more toxic or less toxic are changing throughout the gestational period.

Breast milk may also serve as a source of xenobiotic chemicals in the broad sense of reproductive toxicology. Such things as metals (mercury, lead), halogenated hydrocarbons [tetrachlorethylene, polybrominated biphenyls (PBBs), polychlorinated biphenyls (PCBs)], and pesticides [dichlorodiphenyltrichloroethane (DDT) residues, dieldrin, heptachlorepoxide] may be transferred to the infant in significant quantities (17).

BASIC TOXICITY MECHANISMS

The reviews of published reports of reproductive toxicity document that slightly less than half of the reports deal with male and the rest with female reproduction (18, 19). About 45% of the reports on female reproduction are concerned with toxicity to the embryo/fetus or placenta, which results in spontaneous

Table 16.4.   Agents Reported to Affect Female Reproductive Capacity

Steroids
Androgens (natural and synthetic), estrogens, progestins

Antineoplastic agents
Alkylating agents, antimetabolites

CNS drugs
Anesthetic gases/vapors (halothane, enflurane, methoxyflurane, *chloroform*)

Metals and trace elements
Arsenic, beryllium, cadmium, lead (inorganic and organic), lithium, mercury (inorganic and organic), molybdenum, nicke, *selenium*, thallium

Insecticides
Benzene hexachlorides (lindane), carbamates (carbaryl), chlorobenzene derivatives (DDT, methoxychlor), indane derivatives (aldrin, chlordane, dieldrin), phosphate esters (parathion), miscellaneous (chlordecone, ethylene oxide, hexachlorobenzene, mirex)

Herbicides
Chlorinated phenoxyacetic acids (2,4-dichlorophenoxyacetic acid, 2,4,5-trichlorophenoxyacetic acid)

Food additives and contaminants
Cyclohexylamine, diethylstilbestrol, dimethylnitrosamines, monosodium glutamate, nitrofuran derivatives, nitrosamines, sodium nitrite

Industrial chemicals and processes
Formaldehyde, chlorinated hydrocarbons (PCBs, PBBs, *trichloroethylene*, tetrachloroethylene), ethylene dibromide, *ethylene dichloride*, ethylene oxide, ethylene thiourea, epichlorohydrin, aniline, plastic monomers (caprolactam, styrene, vinyl chloride, *vinylidene chloride*, chloroprene), phthalic acid esters, polycyclic aromatic hydrocarbons (benzo(a)pyrene), solvents (benzene, carbon disulfide, ethanol, glycol ethers, hexane, toluene, *xylene*), carbon monoxide, methylene chloride, *nitrogen dioxide*, miscellaneous (cyanoketone, hydrazines), aniline

Consumer products
Ethanol, tobacco smoke, flame retardants [tris-(2,3-dibromopropyl)phosphate]

N.B.: *Italics* indicate substances for which there is marked species differences but no adequate human data to allow risk assessment.
Modified from: Dixon RL. Toxic responses of the reproductive system. In: Klaassen CD, Amdur MO, Doull J, eds. Casarett and Doull's toxicology: The basic science of poisons. 3rd ed. New York: Macmillan, 1986:432–477. Zalstein E, Koren G. Occupational exposure to chemicals in pregnancy. In: Koren G, ed. Drug, chemical, and radiation exposure in pregnancy. The clinical approach. New York: Marcell Rekker, 1989:191–204.

abortion or pregnancy toxicity; 40% of the reports focus on the hypothalamic-pituitary-ovarian-uterine axis (20).

The conditions that must be met before a teratogenic agent can act are that a susceptible organism must come in contact with the required amount of an appropriate toxin at a vulnerable period in development. The basic mechanism of action of any toxin is the interruption of normal function. In order to accomplish this, the toxin must be absorbed and distributed within the body. Once at its target site, the toxin exerts some type of measurable effect. There are many mechanisms by which toxins exert their effects (21). Understanding the ways in which teratogenesis can be induced and the mechanisms through which chemicals act may allow the anticipation of risk to the fetus and a more accurate extrapolation from controlled animal data to random human exposures.

Mutations consist of a change in the sequence of nucleotides on the DNA molecule. The altered DNA code is responsible

Table 16.5. Agents Reported to Affect Male Reproductive Capacity

Steroids
Androgens (natural and synthetic), estrogens, progestins

Antineoplastic agents
Alkalating agents, alkaloids, antimetabolites, antitumor antibiotics

CNS drugs
Alcohols, anesthetic gases/vapors

Metals and trace elements
Aluminum, arsenic, boranes, *boron, cadmium*, cobalt, lead (inorganic and organic), manganese, mercury (inorganic and organic), molybdenum, nickel, silver, uranium, zinc

Insecticides
Benzene hexachlorides (lindane), carbamates (carbaryl), chlorobenzene derivatives (DDT, methoxychlor), indane derivatives (aldrin, chlordane, dieldrin), phosphate esters (dichlorvos, hexamethylphosphoramide), miscellaneous (chlordecone)

Herbicides
Chlorinated phenoxyacetic acids (2,4-dichlorophenoxyacetic acid, 2,4,5-trichlorophenoxyacetic acid, yalane) quaternary ammonium compounds (diquat, paraquat)

Rodenticides
Metabolic inhibitors (fluoroacetate)

Fungicides, fumigants, and sterilants
Apholate, captan, carbon disulfide, dibromochloropropane, *ethylene dibromide*, ethylene oxide, thiocarbamates, triphenyltin

Food additives and contaminants
Aflatoxins, cyclamate, diethylstilbestrol, dimethylnitrosamine, gossypol, metanil yellow, monosodium glutamate, nitrofuran derivatives

Industrial chemicals
Chlorinated hydrocarbons (hexafluoroacetone, *PBBs*, PCBs, TCDD), hydrazines (dithiocarbamoylhydrazine), monomers (vinyl chloride, chloroprene), polycyclic aromatic hydrocarbons (dimethylbenzanthracene, *benzo(a)pyrene*), solvents (*benzene*, carbon disulfide, glycol ethers, *epichlorohydrin* hexane, thiophene, toluene, xylene), toluene diisocyanate

Consumer products
Ethanol, flame retardants (tris-(2,3-dibromopropyl) phosphate), plasticizers (phthalate esters)

Miscellaneous
Physical factors (heat, light, hypoxia), radiation (α-, β-, γ-radiation; x-rays)

N.B.: *Italics* indicate substances for which there is marked species differences but no adequate human data to allow risk assessment. Modified from Dixon RL. Toxic responses of the reproductive system. In: Klaassen CD, Amdur MO, Doull J, eds. Casarett and Doull's toxicology: the basic science of poisons. 3rd ed. New York: Macmillan, 1986:432–477. Zalstein E, Koren G. Occupational exposure to chemicals in pregnancy. In: Koren G, ed. Drug, chemical, and radiation exposure in pregnancy. The clinical approach. New York: Marcel Rekker, 1989:191–204.

for the generation of abnormal cell proteins. Examples of substances that cause mutations include ionizing radiation, some cancer chemotherapy agents (alkylating agents), and some carcinogens.

Chromosome mechanisms include breaks or nondisjunction (failure to separate properly). Chromosomal abnormalities occur normally with increasing maternal age but also result from viral infections and irradiation. *Mitosis* consists of a complex of various processes by which two daughter cells normally receive identical complements of chromosomes. Many cancer chemotherapy agents (e.g., cytosine arabinoside, colchicine,

vincristine) interfere in mitosis. *Nucleic acid* integrity or function can be adversely affected by toxins. Improperly functioning nucleic acids result in abnormal production of cellular proteins and, thus, malfunction of the cell. Examples of substances that interfere in nucleic acid function include cancer chemotherapy agents (e.g., 6-mercaptopurine, actinomycin D, 5-fluorouracil) and antibiotics (e.g., lincomycin, streptomycin). *Biosynthesis* precursors or substrates may be utilized incorrectly if specific substances are deficient in the fetus due to maternal dietary deficiency or failure of absorption through the maternal gut or if the toxin interferes with placental transport of essential fetal nutrients. *Energy sources* within the cells may be inhibited and lead to teratogenesis or fetal death. For example, dinitrophenol or cyanide may interfere with the cellular electron transport system.

Although the exact etiology and mechanism of teratogenesis for the largest group of congenital anomalies is listed as "unknown," the probable causes include polygenic mechanisms (involvement of multiple genes), multifactorial mechanisms (interaction between the genes and one or more exogenous agents) synergistic interaction of toxins, and spontaneous errors of development.

Once the toxin has exerted its effects, it is metabolized (usually a processes of detoxification) and excreted. The final step is that of repair of damage (22). The alteration in enzyme function by toxins may result in teratogenesis (e.g., hydroxyurea, folic acid antagonists) or in mutagenesis due to inhibition of the enzymes that repair damaged DNA. In reproductive toxicology, this basic approach is made more complex because the process may involve an adult (female or male) only or an adult female and a developing fetus separated by a metabolically active placenta. Thus, damage to the fetus may arise from the toxin's effects on the mother, on the placenta, or on the fetus itself.

Substances that have been reported to cause ovarian toxicity following occupational exposure work in a number of ways. Indirect acting toxins are substances that either change the physiologic controls mechanisms of the organism or are metabolized (activated) to form molecules that then act in a direct fashion. Examples of indirect acting toxins include natural or synthetic sex steroids (e.g., androgens, oral contraceptives) which compete with endogenous sex hormones, pesticides which interact with estrogen receptors (e.g., organochlorine and organophosphate insecticides) or alter the rate of steroid production or clearance (e.g., DDT, PCBs), and metals (e.g., lead, mercury) which alter endogenous hormonal control (23).

Other examples of indirect acting toxins are those that affect the hepatic metabolism of gonadal hormones in the neonatal period [e.g., tetrachlorodibenzo-p-dioxin (TCDD), PCBs, chlordane] (24). PCBs alter the hepatic metabolism of gonadal hormones and, therefore, have the potential to alter the reproductive characteristics of the affected individual. PCBs administered to neonatal rats exerted longlasting effects on hepatic function (25), resulting in altered circulating levels of gonadal hormones. These data suggest that prenatal exposure to PCBs may result in compromised fertility later in life as a result of altered function not only in the genital organ system but also in extragenital organs (e.g., liver) (24).

Direct acting toxins may be structurally similar to a normal endogenous compound (e.g., diethylstilbestrol) or be chemically reactive (e.g., alkylating agents, cadmium) (23). Other examples of direct acting toxins include such compounds as cyclophosphamide, dibromochloropropane, and the polycyclic

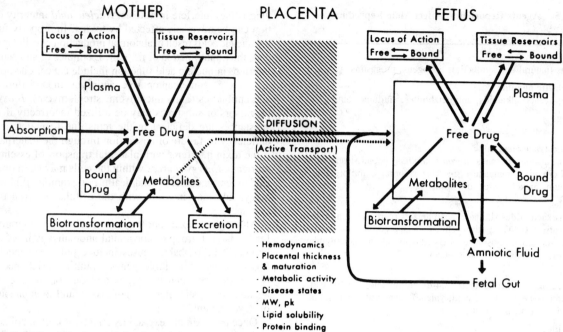

Figure 16.3. Maternal–placental–fetal pharmacokinetic relationships. From: Chow AW, Jewesson PJ. Pharmacokinetics and safety antimicrobial agents during pregnancy. Rev Infect Dis 1985;7:288–313.

aromatic hydrocarbons. For other substances such as carbon disulfide and organic compounds (e.g., hydrocarbons) the mechanism of action is not clear (20).

In order to put the above theories into perspective, it is useful to review the existing data on specific compounds.

Mercury compounds are practically uniformly teratogenic in animals, but this has not been the case in humans. Mercuric chloride has been related to abortion, but transplacental transfer of inorganic mercury has not been associated with congenital anomalies (26). Elemental mercury is absorbed by inhalation and may cause menstrual disturbances (26). Elemental mercury crosses the placenta and has been found in increased concentrations in the placenta and fetal tissues of dental workers (27).

Methyl mercury has been associated with Minamata disease, a syndrome produced by the dietary ingestion of various forms of methyl mercury. The sources of the methyl mercury included chemically polluted fish, contaminated flour or pork, and fungicide-treated grain.

Methyl mercury causes extensive damage to the fetal brain, with neural degeneration and glial proliferation occurring throughout the cerebral and cerebellar cortices (28). The clinical characteristics and the severity of the fetal disorder are related to the age of fetal exposure, namely, the second or third trimester. Although some of the effects of fetal methyl mercury exposure are recognizable at birth, others may not be identified until several months later. The manifestations of fetal exposure consist primarily of cerebral palsy (spasticity, hypotonia), mental retardation, microcephaly, abnormal eye movements (nystagmus, strabismus), and abnormal dentition (11). Absence of ingested dose data has precluded establishing a dose-response relationship for fetal damage.

Polychlorinated biphenyls (PCBs) are a group of more than 100 chemicals that have been used commercially as insulating fluids, heat exchanges, and chemical additives for several decades. Commercial formulations of PCBs are usually mixtures

of PCB isomers with contamination by the more toxic dibenzofurans.

The halogenated biphenyls generally have been teratogenic in laboratory animals. In humans, maternal ingestion of cooking oil containing 1000–1500 ppm of PCBs (which was contaminated with large amounts of dibenzofurans and quaterphenyls) during the first trimester has resulted in congenital abnormalities. Reported findings included stillbirths, intrauterine growth retardation, exophthalmos, dark brown skin discoloration, gingival hyperplasia, and spotted calcifications of the skull. Follow-up of the children revealed that the growth disturbances resolved over a few years but that the children tended to be apathetic and listless, with "soft" neurologic signs (29, 30). PCBs are transferred through breast milk, and this may be a significant source for infants of mothers exposed to these compounds.

In none of the reported cases was there a clear relationship between the degree of fetal toxicity and the maternal dose of PCB mixture (31). The specifics of these dietary exposures preclude direct extrapolation to occupational exposures.

Lead is teratogenic in the laboratory and has been known to be a reproductive hazard for more than a century. Lead begins to cross the placenta as early as 12–14 weeks of gestation. As maternal exposure continues, lead accumulates in fetal tissues so that fetal concentrations tend to rise throughout the balance of the pregnancy. The potential for cumulative toxicity is of special concern.

Among the major effects associated with maternal lead exposure are a higher incidence of miscarriage, abortion, preterm births, and perinatal mortality (32). There are also reports of poorer neurobehavioral performance in the children of women with blood lead levels above 10 mg/dl (0.5 mmol/l) (33). The ability of lead to induce major physical malformations in a human fetus has not been established.

Paternal lead exposure has been claimed to be associated with adverse fetal effects, but it is not clear whether this is due to direct lead effects on sperm (chromosomal aberrations or abnormal sperm number, shape, or activity) or to maternal exposure to the lead dust brought home by her spouse.

Cases of fetal lead exposure need to be followed carefully. The newborns of such pregnancies need to be evaluated at birth for biochemical evidence of lead poisoning (levels of blood lead and free erythrocyte protoporphyrin). Because lead is transferred in breast milk, periodic biochemical screening should be carried out through infancy. As the children grow and develop, they should be screened periodically for subtle neurologic deficits.

Industrial (organic) solvents generally have the potential to be reproductive hazards under the appropriate laboratory circumstances and are considered to be teratogenic in experimental animals.

Exposure to organic solvents during pregnancy has been associated with a number of congenital anomalies including sacral agenesis, central nervous system malformations, and cleft lip (11). These studies are suggestive, but suffer from significant methodologic problems. Other studies suggest that exposure to organic solvents is related to decreased libido, impotence, sperm abnormalities, menstrual irregularities, decreased fertility, spontaneous abortions, premature births, low birth weights, and neonatal problems.

In summary, none of the associations claimed concerning the induction of birth defects by industrial solvents has been convincing (11). However, because of their potential to induce adverse reproductive effects in animals, caution should be used in exposing women of childbearing age to this class of chemicals in the workplace.

Cancer chemotherapy agents have teratogenic potential in the human when exposure occurs in early pregnancy. Proven teratogens include alkylating agents (busulfan, chlorambucil, cyclophosphamide, mechlorethamine) and antimetabolites (aminopterin, azaserine, azathioprine, azauridine, cytarabine, 5-fluorouracil, methotrexate) (11). Women who receive chemotherapeutic agents for the treatment of cancer have a significant risk of bearing malformed infants, ranging from 1:10 to 1:50, depending on the agent and the exposure. Exposure to these drugs has been associated with spontaneous abortion, stillbirth, and neonatal mortality. The types of malformations attributed to cancer chemotherapy agents include multiple anomalies as well as defects in the central nervous system, skull and face, kidney and ureter, and the extremities and digits (11).

Nurses who had miscarriages were 2.6 times more likely to have been exposed occupationally to these drugs than nurses who bore live children (34). Also, increased rates of chromosomal abnormalities have been found in the nurses who were chronically exposed to these drugs (34).

On the other hand, there is no evidence that paternal exposure to cancer chemotherapy agents before or around the time of conception carries an increased teratogenic risk. Although the numbers in the study group were small, the incidence of birth defects in children fathered by 27 men treated for testicular cancer did not differ from that in the general population (35).

Radiation exposure in dosages less than 10 rads is not associated with any increase in congenital malformations. In the dose range of 10–15 rads, there may be a barely discernable increase, but this is uncertain. With dosages over 15 rads, there is a two- to threefold increase in the incidence of major malformations (36). The classic effects of high doses of radiation include embryonic or fetal death, congenital anomalies (mi-crocephaly, eye malformations, genital and skeletal malformations), mental retardation, and intrauterine growth retardation. These findings may occur following an acute exposure of more than 50 rad (36). An increase in chromosomally abnormal abortuses has been reported from fathers who were occupationally exposed to x-rays (37). Maternal radiation exposure has been associated with an increase in childhood cancer (e.g., leukemia) in the offspring (38).

Women of childbearing age working regularly with radiation must be monitored if there is a reasonable possibility of receiving more than a quarter of their maximum quarterly recommended limit of 1.25 rem. The National Council on Radiation Protection and Measurements recommends that the maximum permissible dose equivalent to the embryo and fetus from occupational exposures of the pregnant woman should be 0.5 rem during the entire pregnancy (39). The Nuclear Regulatory Commission suggests that women who are or expect to become pregnant and whose fetus could receive 0.5 rem or more before birth should seek ways to reduce their exposure within their present job or delay having children until they change job locations.

Preconception radiation may cause reduction or obliteration of gamete (ova or spermatozoa) production and also a decrease in the production of ovarian hormones (40). The sensitivity of the ovary appears to be greater in older women (40). Preconception radiation has not been demonstrated to lead to significant genetic hazards or subsequent fetal malformations in children. A study of a limited number of women who had been exposed to high levels of radiation before conception demonstrated normal offspring (41). Radiotherapy may cause temporary or permanent amenorrhea, depending on the dose and age of the woman. It may be advisable for patients receiving more than 25 rads to the gonads to wait for several months before conceiving (36).

Cadmium has quite a variable teratogenic potential in the laboratory which seems to depend on the particular salt used as well as the species of animal, the gestational exposure time, and the route of administration (11). These factors make it highly problematic to extrapolate from animal experiments to human occupational exposures. Based on animal data, the mechanism of cadmium teratogenesis appears to be through carbonic anhydrase inhibition. In addition, cadmium is concentrated in the placenta, and placenta malfunction has been noted.

In humans, the picture is less convincing. Reports of cadmium-induced testicular damage, impaired reproduction, and teratogenicity appear to be confined to high level exposure in animals (42). No fetal damage has been reported in women with Itai-Itai disease, a syndrome associated with high cadmium exposure (43). Other than an association of infants with lower birth weights with material occupational exposure to cadmium (44), cadmium does not appear to have any causal relationship to the induction of birth defects.

DIAGNOSTIC STRATEGIES—DEFINING TOXIC EXPOSURE

All substances are poisons; there is none which is not a poison. The right dose differentiates a poison and a remedy.

Paracelsus
(1493–1541)

Any approach to establishing diagnostic strategies for the evaluation of reproductive risks and defining what constitutes a toxic exposure must be based on the above quotation. Because there are no chemicals that are completely safe under all circumstances, a very important aspect of the diagnosis is trying to establish the degree of exposure. There is always a recognizable dose-response relationship that must be rationally applied to the particular individual. However, reliable use of a dose-response curve is difficult (45). It is likely that the dose-response relationship will be different for each chemical and the characteristics of the curve will depend on the gestational timing of the exposure and the reproductive outcome (response) observed. To improve reliability, more than one outcome should be followed, such as fertility, fetal loss, and malformation rates.

The past medical history of the exposed woman provides the background against which the risks of the occupational exposure must be interpreted. Important aspects of the general history include the patient's age and her race or ethnic background. The last two personal items are important because certain races or ethnic groups may have a predilection for the development of certain inherited abnormalities (e.g., neural tube defects). These data must be known in order to counsel accurately. If the woman is pregnant, information must be gathered about the types of birth control methods used, whether any ovulatory drugs were used, when her last menstrual period was, and what her estimated date of delivery is. In addition, her prepregnancy and current weights must be documented. Because certain chronic disease conditions or their treatment are associated with an increased risk to the fetus, questions must be asked about the existence of heart disease, hypertension, renal disease, diabetes mellitus, thyroid disease, epilepsy, and cancer. Intercurrent acute disease states (e.g., infections) and therapy need to be documented. Rubella, toxoplasmosis, and cytomegalovirus infections have been associated with congenital malformations. Also, details of the patient's dietary history should be explored, including such things as caffeine intake or special diets.

The "symptoms" or reasons for concern about reproductive toxicity will vary considerably, and these reasons will dictate the approach to managing the case. First, a worker may ask for information about toxic substances before she or he starts working in a particular area. In this case, no search for symptoms is required. Second, a worker may be concerned about a real (or imagined) exposure and want information on his or her personal reproductive risk. In this type of case, the details of the exposure (see below) and the symptoms need to be obtained. All symptoms associated with the exposure should be carefully documented along with their sequence of development, intensity, duration, and treatment. Even those symptoms that might be attributed to other causes (e.g., nausea and vomiting from "morning sickness") should be recorded. Any symptoms reported by coworkers should be noted as well. Third, a couple may present with a complaint of infertility and question the role of toxic exposures. For these cases, the physiologic causes should be explored in an appropriate setting by a qualified individual. Toxicologic causes must be included as part of the evaluation. Fourth, parents may be asking for information in order to make a retrospective causal judgment regarding existing malformations in their child.

Consideration must be given to the worker's "secondary" toxins, those nonoccupational substances to which the woman may be exposed. Information must be obtained regarding the use of ethanol, tobacco, and illicit drugs. Exposure to heat (hot tubs, saunas) and radiation must be asked about. Hobbies (e.g., lead or solvents from painting or ceramics), gardening (e.g., fertilizers, pesticides), or home renovations (e.g., paint removers, solvents, lead dust) may expose a pregnant woman to potentially toxic chemicals. One report claimed that 28% of a small study population had household exposure to chemicals during their pregnancies, primarily to paints, solvents, oven cleaners, hair dyes, and laboratory chemicals (46).

If the patient is a pregnant woman, similar information must be obtained concerning her partner: his age, race or ethnic background, occupation, history of disease, use of medications, and use of ethanol, tobacco, and drugs of abuse. Mumps infection in an adult male may be associated with reduced fertility.

The retrospective evaluation of potentially toxic exposures is difficult because recall bias is a significant problem. Individuals with reproductive failures are much likely to recall exposures than couples with successful outcomes. The establishment of the time of an exposure relative to the pregnancy depends on the method used for establishing when conception occurred. The most commonly used method, recollection, is notoriously inaccurate. The critical periods of fetal organ development make accurate timing very important in trying to determine the type of malformations that might be expected.

Of primary importance is the identification of the chemicals in question and the extent of the exposure. Chemicals should be identified by the appropriate Material Safety Data Sheet. A detailed description of the work performed by the patient should be obtained, including the frequency and duration of exposures and the types of protection used (ventilation system, respirator, protective clothing, etc). Documentation of the extent of the exposure in industrial settings is often lacking, and almost everyone has had multiple episodes of exposures to more than one substance. Certain maternal occupations (e.g., those involving exposure to anesthetic gases, cancer chemotherapy agents, ethylene oxide) have been associated with an increase in spontaneous abortion rates (7).

Certain disease states tend to run in families and may not necessarily be present in each generation. For this reason, questions should be asked about the presence of the following diseases in members of the paternal and maternal extended families: heart disease, hypertension, renal disease, diabetes mellitus, thyroid disease, epilepsy, and cancer. It is particularly important to establish the presence or absence of genetic diseases or malformations in the extended family. Common major malformations that tend to be familial include anencephaly, spina bifida aperta, club foot, cleft lip/palate, congenital dislocation of the hip, and pyloric stenosis (47).

The physical examination of the pregnant woman exposed to a toxic substance should be complete and thorough. The examination should include a thorough evaluation of the fetus including its movements, heart rate, and size.

A wide range of measures are available to estimate the degree of exposure or dose of a toxic substance, including estimates of emissions, limited monitoring information, direct monitoring of ambient conditions, analysis of concentrations present in blood or other body tissues, and identification of biologic responses that are indicators of exposure. Most often, however, these data are not available. In some cases, the best information available is that the worker was "exposed" or "not exposed." This type of classification is not optimal, because it reduces the probability of identifying changes in response occurring

Table 16.6. Methods Used for Prenatal Diagnosis

Visualization of the Fetus	Analysis of Fetal Tissues
Noninvasive	Amniocentesis
Ultrasonography	Chorionic villus sampling
Radiography	Fetoscopy
Invasive	Fetal blood sampling
Fetoscopy	Fetal skin biopsy
Fetography	Fetal liver biopsy
Amniography	

Table 16.7. Disorders that May Be Diagnosed by Ultrasonography in the Second Trimester

Miscellaneous
  Hydros fetalis
  Oligohydramnios
  Polyhydramnios
CNS
  Anencephaly
  Encephalocele
  Hydrocephalus
  Meningomyelocele
Chest
  Congenital heart disease
  Diaphragmatic hernia
  Pulmonary hypoplasia
  Small thoracic cavity
Abdomen/Gl
  Duodenal atresia
  Esophageal atresia
  Gastroschisis
  Omphalocele
Renal/GU
  Cystic kidneys
  Renal agenesis
  Hydronephrosis
Skeletal
  Digital anomalies
  Fractures
  Limb reduction deformities
  Skeletal dysplasias

with exposure and may limit the ability to recognize the effects of exposure. The best measure of exposure is the actual measured level of the toxin (preferably in biologic fluids, or in the environment). Even with accurate exposure data, undependable results may occur if the appropriate reproductive outcome (e.g., malformations or spontaneous abortions) is not recorded. A reasonable approach to categorizing exposure is to group the exposures into rational biologically appropriate categories (however they are defined). Whatever measure of exposure is used, it is critically important to consider the measured outcome in terms of the gestational timing of the exposure (45).

Biologic markers can provide accurate estimates of the human dose and uptake of hazardous chemicals. With respect to reproductive effects, biologic markers might be sought in semen, vaginal fluid, breast milk, and urine (9, 13), but these types of tests are not widely available. The values obtained from biologic and environmental monitoring are useful for helping to establish the dose or quantity of a chemical to which a woman was exposed. Biologic or environmental values that are considered as normal, safe, or acceptable for a worker cannot be assumed to be normal, safe, or acceptable for the fetus.

Potentially useful measures of male reproductive toxicity include body weight, testicular size and weight, semen analysis (including sperm count, motility, and morphology), and endocrine function (levels of luteinizing hormone, follicle-stimulating hormone, testosterone, and gonadotropin-releasing hormone).

Potentially useful measurements of female reproductive toxicity include body weight, endocrine function (levels of cyclicity of gonadotropin-releasing hormone, luteinizing hormone, follicle-stimulating hormone, prolactin, chorionic gonadotropin, estrogen, and progesterone), and evaluation of cervical mucus and cytology/histology.

There are a number of tests that are potentially useful for making a prenatal diagnosis of congenital disorders (Table 16.6). The procedure that is used will depend on the type of defect being sought. Ultrasound is the procedure of choice for the visualization of fetal body parts. Examples of the disorders that may be diagnosed by ultrasonography in the second trimester are presented in Table 16.7. Examinations repeated at intervals may be useful in diagnosing some conditions. Ultrasonography is a very low risk procedure, and there is no convincing evidence of any adverse effects on the mother or the fetus as a result of exposure to ultrasound.

Radiographic studies have been used to evaluate the fetus. Plain radiography will provide information about fetal skeletal ossification and may be useful in diagnosing some forms of bone dysplasias. Fetography and amniography utilize the introduction of a contrast material into the amniotic cavity. These techniques are used to visualize the contour of the fetal body and, because some of the contrast material is swallowed by the fetus, the outline of the fetal gastrointestinal tract. Radiographic techniques have, for the most part, been replaced by ultrasonography because of the risks associated with exposure to ionizing radiation and with the introduction of a catheter into the amniotic cavity.

Fetoscopy and amniocentesis are also invasive techniques. Fetoscopy is used to visualize fetal body parts and to obtain fetal tissue samples (e.g., blood, skin, liver) for analysis. Amniocentesis is used to obtain amniotic fluid for cell and biochemical analysis. All the above invasive procedures carry the risks of inducing spontaneous abortion, amnionitis, blood loss, and Rh isoimmunization.

Chorionic villus sampling is a safe and effective technique for the early prenatal diagnosis of cytogenetic abnormalities (48). The primary advantage to this technique is that it can be done substantially earlier than amniocentesis.

Continuous monitoring or surveillance of adverse consequences, another method for identifying reproductive hazards in the workplace, can serve many purposes (49). Reproductive defects monitoring systems can be used to monitor newborns and identify as quickly as possible an increase in the prevalance of specific malformations or groups of malformations. Surveillance systems also may be used to identify cases (infants born with a specific type of birth defect) for a case-control study. If the defect in question is a relatively rare one, without a registry system, it may be difficult to identify a large enough number of cases to make study worthwhile, especially if one does not want to trace cases too far back in time and risk jeopardizing the quality of the retrospectively collected information. Reproduction monitoring systems also can be used to look at the outcome of deliveries of a specific cohort of women (identified by occupation, degree of exposure, or other characteristics). In order to be useful, this type of service needs to be coupled with a registry of all births (to give a denominator) and include such data as the number of births in the area, the maternal age distribution, and birth weight and gestational age of the infants. The last function of a birth defects monitoring system is to compare trends in overall malformation rates in the general population with the trends in specific exposure populations.

Criteria have been suggested by which approaches to monitoring for mutations might be evaluated. (48, 50).

Relevance: Identified defects must be either clinically significant in themselves or be positively correlated with significant fetal pathology. There are arguments for and against the monitoring of common and less severe malformations. Minor dysmorphologic aberrations of the face, hands, or feet may be important signs for detection of new teratogens. Multiple malformations may be of great importance because many of the known human teratogens have produced malformation complexes rather than an increase in only one type of malformation.

Speed of detection and identification of malformations: Defects should be identifiable shortly after birth. Since defects observable in the neonatal period are likely to be due to fetal insults in the first 3–4 months of gestation, the effect of a teratogen would be apparent 5–9 months after its introduction into the environment. However, for behavioral abnormalities, internal organ malformations, and complicated birth defects, it may be a long time before enough details are known to permit an accurate diagnosis.

Sensitivity to a small increase in incidence rate: Moderate increases in rates (e.g., doubling or less) should be identifiable. Detecting a change in the prevalence of a specific malformation requires a knowledge of the preexisting prevalence in that population. Such baseline data must be established over a sufficiently long period of time and be collected in the same way as those data collected during the monitoring period.

Likelihood of identifying cause of increase: An increase in the incidence of an observed effect could be due to (a) variations in diagnosing or finding cases (change in ascertainment); (b) shifts in the population relating to variables (such as parental age, socioeconomic status) which may indirectly affect the incidence of a defect (e.g., Downs syndrome is associated with high maternal age and gastroschisis is associated with low maternal age); and (c) changes in teratogens or mutagens in the environment, either introduction of a new factor or an increase in a previously existing one. Once an increase has been identified, the primary conclusion that has to be drawn is whether the increase is real. Random excesses of observed versus expected cases occur commonly, at a rate which depends on the significance limits used in the statistical tests. An important contribution to the conclusion concerning whether an increase is real is a detailed analysis of the cases. If the increase is restricted to a specific combination of malformations or to a specific subtype of a malformation, the probability is great that the increase is real. On the other hand, decreases in malformation rates occur also and should not be ignored. Decreases may help to estimate the effects of preventive measures or may indicate the removal of a teratogenic factor from the workplace.

Sensitivity to multiple causes: The majority of malformations appear to be multifactorial in origin, and these traits may be more sensitive to abrupt changes in relevant gestational environmental factors than to pregestational environmental mutations in multiple genes. An observed abrupt rise in the incidence of a multifactorial trait is highly likely to have a single specific environmental cause. On the other hand, exposure to two (or more) known teratogens may result in a pattern of malformations that is not consistent with either teratogen. When working in a multifactorial system, it is extremely difficult to identify a specific environmental cause.

Comparability: The ability to compare data from different sources or reporting centers is important. The level of precision in describing and diagnosing abnormalities depends on many things, but above all on the qualifications of the examiner. Different information of variable degrees of accuracy will be reported by different sources (delivery rooms, nurseries, pediatric wards, operating specialties, and pathology departments).

Cost: The cost of monitoring for occupational related birth defects will depend on the number of individuals to be evaluated, the number of trained evaluating staff, and type of data collected and analysis.

DIAGNOSTIC STRATEGY SUMMARY

1. GATHER accurate patient and exposure information.
2. ESTABLISH the patient's intervention options.
3. COLLECT available literature information regarding pertinent human and animal exposures.
4. EVALUATE the patient and literature data for medical and statistical quality. Review the data critically!
5. ESTIMATE the risk based on the nature, extent, and timing of the exposure.
6. COMPARE the estimated risk *realistically* to baseline risks.
7. WEIGH the benefits of exposure versus the estimated risks of exposure.
8. DETERMINE the present condition of the fetus.
9. ASK for expert help, if needed.
10. HELP the patient make a realistic decision.
11. SUPPORT the patient's choices.
12. FOLLOW and document the patient's course and the outcome of the pregnancy. Follow-up may continue as the newborn infant grows and develops.

CONCLUSIONS

The evaluation of the reproductive risks to women and men from occupational exposure to chemicals is a complex and emotional issue. Unfortunately, the knowledge of the reproductive toxicity of industrial chemicals in humans is often incomplete or nonexistent. While many chemicals are potentially reproductive toxins, many are not. Similarly, many malformations are caused by toxins, but most are not.

Suspicions are justified, perspicacity is necessary; but it is not wise to present suspicions and beliefs as facts, lest we create modern superstitions. Let us be specific about dangers and not condemn all drugs and chemicals as fetotoxic, let us not confuse suspicions with facts, or we do great harm to our fellow man (J. Warkany, 1972).

REFERENCES

1. Harbison RD, Evans MA. Teratogenic aspects of drug abuse in pregnancy. In: Rementeria JL, ed. Drug abuse in pregnancy and neonatal effects. St. Louis MO: CV Mosby Co. 1977:191.

2. Stanley FJ. Fetotoxic chemicals and drugs. Med J Aust 1981;1:688–693.

3. Edmonds DK, Lindsay KS, Miller JF, et al. Early embryonic mortality in women. Fertil Steril 1982; 38:447–453.

4. French FE, Bierman JM. Probabilities of fetal mortality. Public Health Rep 1962; 77:835–847.

5. Whittaker PG, Taylor A, Lind T. Unsuspected pregnancy loss in healthy women. Lancet 1983; 1:1126–1127.

6. Kline J, Stein Z. Very early pregnancy. In: Dixon RL, ed. Reproductive toxicology. New York: Raven Press, 1985:251–265.

7. Kline JK. Maternal occupation: effects on spontaneous abortions and malformations. Occup Med—State of the Art Rev 1986; 1:381–403.

8. Wilson JG. Teratogenic effects of environmental chemicals. Fed Proc 1977; 36:1698–1703.

9. Dixon RL, Nadolney CH. Assessing risk of reproductive dysfunction associated with chemical exposure. In: Dixon RL, ed. Reproductive toxicology. New York: Raven Press, 1985:329–339.

10. Leck I. Teratogenic risks of disease and therapy. Contr Epidemiol Biostatist 1979;1:23–43.

11. Schardein JL. Chemically induced birth defects. New York: Marcel Dekker, 1985.

12. Nau H. Species differences in pharmacokinetics and drug teratogenesis. Environ Health Perspect 1986; 70:113–129.

13. Dixon RL. Toxic rewsponses of the reproductive system. In: Klaassen CD, Amdur MO, Doull J, eds. Casarett and Doull's toxicology. The basic science of poisons. 3rd ed. New York: Macmillan, 1986:432–477.

14. Zalstein E, Koren G. Occupational exposure to chemicals in pregnancy. In: Koren G, ed. Drug, chemical, and radiation exposure in pregnancy. The clinical approach. New York: Marcel Dekker, 1989:191–204.

15. Manson JM. Teratogens. In: Klaassen CD, Amdur MO, Doull J, eds. Casarett and Doull's toxicology. The basic science of poisons. 3rd ed. New York: Macmillan, 1986:195–220.

16. Chow AW, Jewesson PJ. Pharmacokinetics and safety of antimicrobial agents during pregnancy. Rev Infect Dis 1985; 7:288–313.

17. Wolff MS. Occupationally derived chemicals in breast milk. In: Mattison DR, ed. Reproductive toxicology. New York: Alan R. Liss, 1983:259–281.

18. Barlow SM, Sullivan FM. Reproductive hazards of industrial chemicals. New York: Academic Press, 1982.

19. Pruett JG, Winslow SG. Health effects of environmental chemicals on the adult human reproductive system. A selected bibliography with abstracts, 1963–1981. Federation of American Societies for Experimental Biology (FASEB) Special Publication NLM/TIRC-82/1 Bethsda, MD: Federation of American Societies for Experimental Biology.

20. Mattison DP. Clinical manifestations of ovarian toxicity. In: Dixon RL, ed. Reproductive toxicology. New York: Raven Press, 1985; 109–130.

21. Wilson JG. Current status of teratology. In: Wilson JG, Fraser FC, eds. Handbook of teratology, volume 1. New York: Plenum Press, 1977:47–73.

22. Steinberger E, Lloyd JA. Chemicals affecting the development of reproductive capacity. In: Dixon RL, ed. Reproductive toxicology. New York: Raven Press, 1985:1–20.

23. Mattison DP. Effects of biologically foreign compounds on reproduction. In: Abdul-Harim RW, ed. Drugs during pregnancy. Philadelphia: George F. Stickley, 1981:101–125.

24. McLachlan JA, Newbold RR, Korach JC, et al. Transplacental toxicology: prenatal factors influencing postnatal fertility. In: Kimmel CA, Buelke-Sam J, eds. Developmental toxicology. New York: Raven Press, 1981:212–232.

25. Lucier GW, McLachlan JA, Davis GJ. Transplacental toxicology of the polychlorinated and polybrominated biphenyls. In: Mahlum DD, Sikov MR, Hackett PC, Andrew FD, eds. Developmental toxicology of energy-related pollutants. Technical Information Center, United States Department of Energy; Washington, DC: 1978:188–203.

26. Barlow SM, Sullivan FM. Reproductive hazards of industrial chemicals. New York: Academic Press, 1982:386–406.

27. Wannag A, Skajaerasen J. Mercury accumulation in placenta and fetal membranes: a study of dental workers and their babies. Environ Physiol Biochem 1975; 5:348–352.

28. Matsumoto H, Koya G, Takeuchi T. Fetal Minamata disease. J Neuropathol Exp Neurol 1965; 24:563–574.

29. Harada M. Intrauterine poisoning. Clinical and epidemiological studies and significance of the problem. Bull Inst Const Med Kumamato Univ 1976; 25 (suppl): 1–60.

30. Yamashita F. Clinical features of polychlorobiphenyls (PCB)-induced fetopathy. Paediatrician 1977; 6:20–27.

31. Rogan WJ. PCBs and cola-colored babies: Japan, 1968, and Taiwan, 1979. Teratology 1982; 26:259–261.

32. Rom WN. Effects of lead on the female and reproduction: a review. Mt Sinai J Med 1976; 43:542–552.

33. Bellinger D, Leviton A, Waternaux C, et al. Longitudinal analyses of prenatal lead exposure and early cognitive development. N Engl J Med 1987; 316:1037–1043.

34. Selevan SG, Lindbohm M-L, Hornung RW, Hemminki K. A study of occupational exposure to antineoplastic drugs and fetal loss in nurses. N Engl J Med 1985; 313:1173–1178.

35. Senturia YD, Peckham CS, Peckham MJ. Children fathered by men treated for testicular cancer. Lancet 1985; 2:766–769.

36. Brent RL. The effect of embryonic and fetal exposure to x-ray microwaves, and ultrasound. Clin Perinat 1986; 13:615–648.

37. Boue J, Boue A, Lazar P. Retrospective and prospective epidemiological studies of 1500 karyotyped spontaneous abortions. Teratology 1975; 12:11–26.

38. Diamond EL, Schmerler H, Lilienfeld AM. The relationship of intrauterine radiation to subsequent mortality and development of leukemia in children: a prospective study. Am J Epidemiol 1973; 97:283–313.

39. National Council on Radiation, Protection and Measurement. Publ No 53, Washington, DC: 1977.

40. Mettler FA, Moseley RD. Medical effects of ionizing radiation. Orlando, FL: Grune & Stratton, 1985:126–191.

41. Horning SJ, Hoppe RT, Kaplan HS, Rosenberg SA. Female reproductive potential after treatment for Hodgkin's disease. N Engl J Med 1981; 304:1377–1382.

42. Webb M. Cadmium. Br Med Bull 1975; 31:246–250.

43. Thueraut J, Schaller KH, Engelhardt E, Gossler K. The cadmium content of the human placenta. Int Arch Occup Environ Health 1975; 36:19–27.

44. Sullivan FM, Barlow SM. Congenital malformations and other reproductive hazards from environmental chemicals. Proc R Soc Lond 1979; 205:91–110.

45. Selevan SG, Lemasters GK. The dose-response fallacy in human reproductive studies of toxic exposures. J Occup Med 1987; 29:451–454.

46. Hill RM, Craig JP, Chaney MD, et al. Utilization of over-the-counter drugs during pregnancy. Clin Obstet Gynecol 1977; 20:381–394.

47. Fraser FO. The epidemiology of the common major malformations as related to environmental monitoring. In: Hook EB, Janerich DT, Poter IH, eds. Monitoring birth defects and environment. The problem of surveillance. New York: Academic Press, 1971: 85–96.

48. Rhoads GG, Jackson LG, Schlesselman SE, et al. The safety and efficacy of chrionic villus sampling for early prenatal diagnosis of cytogenetic abnormalities. N Engl J Med 1989; 320:609–617.

49. Kallen B, Hay S, Klingberg M. Birth defects monitoring systems. Accomplishments and goals. In: Kalter H, ed. Issues and reviews in teratology, volume 2. New York: Plenum Press, 1984:1–21.

50. Hook EB. Some general considerations concerning monitoring: application to utility of minor defects as markers. In: Hook EB, Janerich DT, Porter IH, eds. Monitoring birth defects and environment. The problem of surveillance. New York: Academic Press, 1971:177–197.

17

Immunotoxicology

Bradford O. Brooks, Ph.D.
John B. Sullivan, Jr., M.D.

INTRODUCTION

The immune system consists of a complex and well-distributed network of both blood and lymphatic vessels through which course a myriad of immunocompetent cells (Figure 17.1). These elements, together with lymphoid organs (Table 17.1), work in concert to accomplish but one goal: to discriminate between "self" and "non-self." This "reconnaissance" network accomplishes its task using a stepwise strategy: (a) initial concentration of foreign or "non-self" elements into a few lymphoid organs; (b) rapid circulation of the lymphocyte population (immunologically specific components of the immune system) through these lymphoid organs so that the foreign agent (antigen) is exposed to the full repertoire of antigen-specific lymphocytes; and (c) dissemination of the products of the immune response (cells and humoral factors) to the blood and tissues. The manifestations of these responses may be localized or systemic, acute or chronic, reversible or irreversible, obvious or subtle and insidious.

There are a variety of in vitro and in vivo immunologic assay systems available to investigate the effects of chemicals and drugs on the immune system. Information concerning immunotoxic effects of drugs and chemicals can be used to extrapolate risk to humans in some instances. The sensitivity of the immune system to xenobiotics is a function of its complexity. The immune system is highly regulated, and many of the cells undergo rapid proliferation. Therefore, any toxic injury or dysfunction will be amplified as an alteration and inspected within an established assay. Immune alterations can be expressed as an enhancement or suppression of the immune function or no demonstrable effect. Immune enhancement could result in autoimmunity, hypersensitivity disease, or allergy states. Immune depression can result in increased incidence of infections or decreased surveillance of neoplasia. The immune cells can be easily isolated and their functions studied with in vitro assay systems. Antibodies can be isolated and quantitated.

ANATOMICAL CONSIDERATIONS OF THE IMMUNE SYSTEM

The Spleen

The spleen is the major filter for blood-borne antigens and infections as well as the major site of the immune response to foreign antigens. In addition to performing these tasks, the spleen also functions as a site of extramedullary hematopoiesis. The two basic anatomical components of the spleen are the capsule and trabeculae. The trabeculae form poorly demarcated areas within the spleen. These demarcated areas contain splenic nodules (white pulp) and splenic sinuses (red pulp). These areas are named due to their appearance in a freshly sectioned organ. The two histologic regions of the spleen, red pulp and white

pulp, represent functional immune areas. Most of the splenic pulp is red. The white pulp is irregularly scattered throughout the organ. Red pulp contains reticular cells, phagocytic cells, and circulating blood elements. White pulp consists of a dense population of lymphocytes. The spleen has no afferent lymphatics; thus, any antigen entering the spleen must do so through the blood vessels.

Thymus

Not a true lymphatic organ, the thymus is bilobular and located in association with the great vessels at the base of the heart. The thymus reaches a size of 10–15 grams at birth and 30–40 grams by puberty. After puberty, it involutes. Each of the two lobes of the thymus is subdivided into several smaller lobules. Each lobule consists of an outer cortex and an inner medulla. Thymocytes are concentrated in the cortical areas. The thymus also produces thymic humoral factor (THF) necessary for regulation of lymphoiesis in all lymphoid tissues.

Lymph Nodes

There are 500–600 lymph nodes in the body. They may be individually located or occur in certain anatomical groups along the course of blood vessels. Lymph nodes produce lymph and lymphocytes. Lymph nodes are divided into three structural histologic areas: cortex, paracortex, and medulla. Lymph flow arrives into the nodes by afferent vessels which also carry foreign antigens to the nodes. Efferent lymph vessels carry lymph-containing antibodies, lymphokines, and lymphocytes produced in response to antigenic stimulation. The cortex, site of B-cell depot, is usually a thin rim of tissue and lymphocytes. Upon antigenic stimulation, the cortex proliferates into germinal sensors containing dense populations of lymphocytes which differentiate into antibody-producing cells. In the dense portion of the germinal centers, the lymphocytes are actively dividing. The paracortex, between the cortex and medulla, is a T-cell site and a major area of T-cell and macrophage interaction. The medulla of the node is composed of cords and sinuses which serve to filter particulate matter from lymph. The medullary cords also contain lymphocytes, and, upon antigenic stimulation, these lymphocytes produce antibody.

Liver

The normal adult liver weighs between 1400 and 1600 grams and consists of a left lobe, a right lobe, and two rudimentary lobes: the caudate and quadrate. The right lobe makes up the majority of the liver's mass. Histologically, the liver consists of lobules. Each lobule has a central hepatic vein from which cords of hepatocytes concentrically radiate as spokes from a wheel. The outer boundaries of these lobules are demarcated

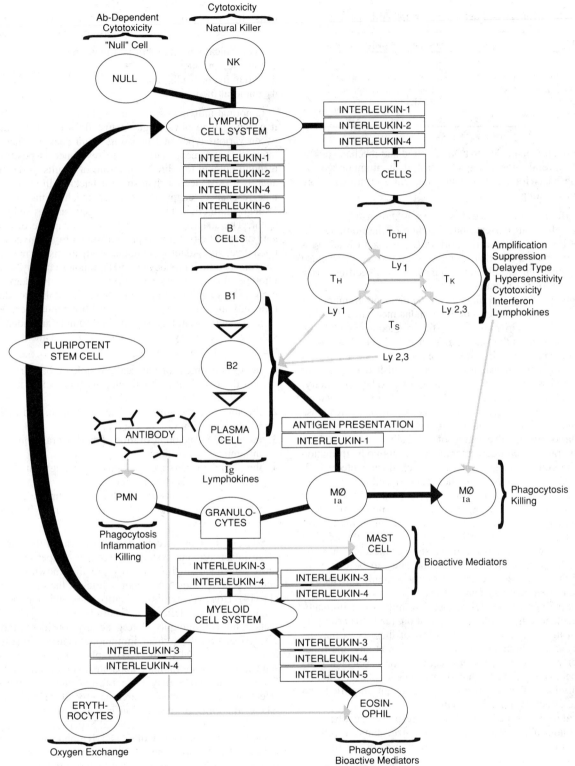

Figure 17.1. The immune system.

by a combination of hepatic artery, portal vein, and bile duct. This combination is referred to as the portal triad. The walls of hepatocytes which form the masses of liver lobules are penetrated by vascular sinusoids lined by endothelial cells and special reticuloendothelial cells, Kupffer cells, which have immune system function. Intrahepatic circulation of blood is bas-

ically through both the portal vein system and the hepatic artery. Sixty percent of hepatic blood flow is through the portal vein. The liver thus plays a pronounced role in host resistance mechanisms and antigen detection.

The past three decades have seen a virtual explosion in our understanding and exploitation of the immune apparatus (1–

Table 17.1.   Primary and Secondary Lymphoid Organs

Primary Lymphoid Organs	Secondary Lymphoid Organs
Thymus	Spleen
Bursa of fabricius (avian)	Lymph nodes
Fetal liver (mammal)	Gut-associated lymphoid tissue (GALT)
Adult bone marrow	

7). Although much is left to be discovered and mechanistically defined, several known characteristics of the immune system form the basis for an important paradigm and are therefore worth mentioning.

1. **Specificity**—Resistance to disease was known to be specific long before our current understanding of the immune system. Because of the early work of Landsteiner (8) and others, we now know that immune reactions can distinguish between even closely related molecules. Specificity is a hallmark of the immune response.
2. **Memory**—Once an antigen has elicited an immune response, certain elements of the immune mechanism are forever changed. In most cases, future encounters with the same antigen result in an augmented or "adaptive" response (positive memory). In certain cases, a second encounter with the same antigen can result in a diminished response or acquired tolerance (negative memory). Like specificity, memory is a hallmark of the immune response. Together, they may be used as criteria to decide whether a response is immunologic or nonimmunologic.
3. **Collaboration**—The nature of cell-cell and cell-cytokine (humoral cell product) interactions in antibody formation and in cell-mediated responses is well documented (5, 9, 10). The interaction of lymphocytes with cell products such as antibody or cytokines and nonlymphoid cells allows for an optimized and maximally effective immune response.
4. **Mobility**—Immunocompetent cells and their modulator/effector molecules must be able to circulate through the body. Both innate and adaptive resistance mechanisms must be able to disseminate through the body to be effective. Cell mobility also accounts for local immune interactions which often cause systemic effects.
5. **Clonal Expansion**—While there are millions of immunocompetent cells, sessile or in circulation, ready to participate in an immune response, only a few of these cells may be capable of recognizing a specific antigen at any one time. After recognizing a specific antigen, these selected cells immediately advance into a blastogenic phase, cloning themselves. This expansion allows for an amplified and more effective immune response.
6. **Regulation**—An effective immune response must be carefully controlled as to time of onset, size, humoral/cellular participants, and duration. Most responses of the immune apparatus represent a balance between up-regulatory and down-regulatory circuits. Immunopathologic mechanisms of hypersensitivity (Table 17.2) are thought to involve defects in immune regulation.

Immunocompetence

Immunocompetence is a state of functional immunity that provides for effective resistance to infectious agents and neoplastic cells. It depends on both innate and adaptive (acquired) resistance mechanisms. Innate defense mechanisms include:

1. mechanical barriers (skin and membranes),
2. secreted products,
3. inflammatory cells, and
4. humoral mediators.

In normal individuals, innate resistance is always operative; it depends upon physiologic status, does not distinguish between various types of "non-self," and does not increase its intensity upon reexposure. Innate resistance is positioned to respond quickly to a broad spectrum of insults; it depends on adaptive resistance mechanisms for backup. In contrast to innate resistance, adaptive resistance mechanisms are usually "silent" until elicited by specific antigen, such as an infectious agent. The adaptive immune response is capable of exquisite antigen specificity even when confronted by a universe of antigen diversity. Adaptive immune mechanisms are mediated by antigen-specific lymphocytes and antibodies via a hypothesized idiotype (up-regulatory)/antiidiotype (down-regulatory) network (7). Adaptive components have the ability to alter significantly their intensity and response time upon reexposure to "recall" antigen. Integration of both innate and adaptive resistance is necessary for maintaining a fundamental state of immunocompetence, consisting of

1. the establishment of physical/physiologic barriers to maintain the body's functional integrity and isolate it from the hostile environment in which it exists;
2. the ability to recognize, isolate, neutralize, and reject that which is foreign or "non-self";
3. the initiation and orchestration of diverse granulomatous and inflammatory reactions;
4. the ability to generate "adaptive" or augmented immune responses to "recall" antigens; and
5. the ability to deactivate or "turn-off" immune responses when foreign or "non-self" elements have been cleared from the body.

Some of the most forceful demonstrations of the importance of an intact immune system are seen in "experiments of nature." Included in this category are the known human and animal genetic/congenital abnormalities of the immune system (11–14). However, until the identification and diagnosis of the acquired immune deficiency syndrome (AIDS) (15–17), defects in human immunity were generally considered rare (14). The effect that the human immunodeficiency viruses (HIV) have upon the CD4 (helper) T-lymphocyte (18, 19) and subsequently the entire immune apparatus, is profound and lethal. Patients with AIDS may have life-threatening opportunistic infections and/or Kaposi's sarcoma (16, 20–23). Taken as a whole, the clinical presentation is that of severe cellular immunodeficiency, absence of delayed hypersensitivity, lymphopenia (absolute deficiency of CD4 T-lymphocytes), reversal of CD4 and CDB (suppressor) T-lymphocyte ratio, depressed mitogen responsiveness, and impaired natural killer (NK) cell function. In aggregate, the AIDS epidemic is a dramatic example of the importance of an intact and functional immune apparatus for health and quality of life (24).

IMMUNOTOXICITY

Immunotoxicity may be defined as the adverse effects of an unsuitable immune response caused by the direct or indirect

Table 17.2. Categories of Immunopathology

	Immunologic Constituent	Mediators	Immunopathology
Antibody Mediated			
1) Homocytotropic	IgE or IgG4	Histamines, Leukotrienes, & Cytokines	Asthma Anaphylactic Shock
2) Cell Surface Reactive	IgM, IgG, IgA Cell Surface-bound Ag	Complement, F_c receptors Cytokines, Lysosomal enzymes Granulocyte enzymes	Hemolytic Disease of the Newborn Graves' Disease Myasthenia gravis
3) Immune Complex	Ag-Ab complexes in circulation & in tissues	Immune complexes, Complement Cytokines, Lysosomal enzymes Oxygen radicals	Hypersensitivity Pneumonitis Rheumatoid arthritis
Cell Mediated			
4) Delayed Type Hypersensitivity	Macrophages Helper T-Cells Class II MHC Ags	Lymphokines, monokines, NK Cells	Allergic Contact Sensitivity
5) Cytotoxic	Suppressor T-Cells Class I MHC Ags	Cell-bound Ag, Lymphokines	Hepatitis B Cytopathology Graft *vs.* Host reactions

action of a xenobiotic. It may also result from an immunologically mediated host response to a xenobiotic, its metabolites, or host antigens altered by these substances.

Both clinical and research data reveal that chemicals and drugs may induce selective immunotoxicity, particularly if the toxicant exerts its effect during active growth periods of immunocompetent cells. Defects can occur at one or more points during maturation of the immune apparatus or deployment of an immune response (Figure 17.1). These abnormalities range from stem cell defects to changes in cytokine production or receptor density. Defects may be quantitative (e.g., loss of cell numbers due to selective cytotoxicity) or qualitative (e.g., functional impairment of cells or cell receptors). In addition, injury to other organs, malnutrition, or simple aging can also include alterations in immunity (25). Furthermore, a specific lesion of the immune apparatus can induce damage of organ systems to an extent that compromises the general health of the entire host (26). Therefore, immunotoxicity must always be viewed broadly, because of its ability to cause nonlymphoid pathology.

If immunocompetence represents an optimally "balanced" immune response, then profound immunosuppression and overt hypersensitivity represent undesirable/adverse extremes of immunotoxicity (Figure 17.2). The clinical significance of immunotoxicity is illustrated by examining the causes and consequences of the principal classes of immunotoxicity:

1. immunosuppression,
2. autoimmunity, and
3. hypersensitivity.

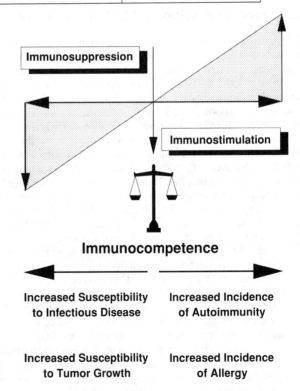

Figure 17.2.

IMMUNOSUPPRESSION

The clinical sequelae of immunosuppression can range from profound and life-threatening (11, 12, 21, 27) to academic curiosities. Pharmaceuticals (28), abused drugs (29), pesticides (30), and other environmental chemicals (31–33) may destroy or inhibit innate and acquired resistance mechanisms in humans and animals (Table 17.3). In addition to these gross immunotoxic effects, subtle immunosuppression may alter immunocompetent cell capabilities, such as differentiation (34), major histocompatibility complex (MHC) antigen expression/restriction (10, 35), and delays in the immunoglobulin M IgM to IgG antibody production shift in plasma cells (36). The clinical relevance of these subtle changes is difficult to assess. Ongoing studies involving patients exposed to polybrominated biphenyls (PBB) (32) or polychlorinated biphenyls (PCB)-adulterated cooking oils (37) reveal that the immunosuppressive effects of xenobiotics can be significant and persistent. Initial data indicate an increased incidence of cancer in PBB-exposed patients with immune alterations. Patients exposed to PPB with normal immune status have a tumor incidence of 0.5%, while PBB-exposed patients with confirmed immune alterations have a tumor incidence of 10.7% (38). Continued longitudinal follow-up of these individuals may reveal additional clinical consequences of the specific immune alterations described. Because the immune system is a multifaceted network that maintains a level of functional reserve, a toxic effect upon a particular immune cell or circuit may not necessarily lead to a detectable clinical manifestation. The clinically significant consequence of immunosuppression in humans is likely to be infectious disease (external assault) and neoplasia (internal assault).

Immunosuppression and Infectious Disease

Opportunistic infections are common in immunocompromised hosts (11, 12, 14, 20, 31). In fact, recurrent opportunistic infections are often the harbingers of an underlying immunodeficiency (11, 14). Many immunosuppressive chemicals and drugs also decrease host resistance (31). More omnious is the finding that exposure to common air pollutants such as ozone (O_3), nitrogen dioxide (NO_2), and sulfur dioxide (SO_2) increase most susceptibility to infection (39, 40). Multiple mechanisms are deployed by the immune apparatus to deal with different infectious diseases (41): both innate and acquired immunity are involved. For example, the clearance of extracellular pathogens (most bacteria, most metazoans, some viruses, and certain protozoa) depends upon the interaction of antibody, various leukocytes, and complement. The clearance of intracellular pathogens (some bacteria, most viruses, certain protozoa) involves cellular (altered self/cytotoxic) mechanisms. Because of our current understanding of immunity to microbes, groups of infectious agents can be associated with broad classifications of immune alterations (Table 17.4) and can be clues to the underlying mechanism of the immunologic defect in patients.

In addition to their clinical significance as consequences of human immunosuppression or immunodeficiency, infectious diseases, used as experimental probes, are highly effective tools for studying potential immunotoxicants (31, 42). Several infectious disease models have been exploited for screening xenobiotics for immunotoxic potential in animal prototypes of host resistance; *Listeria monocytogenes* (43), *Streptococcus pneumoniae* (43), *Trypanosoma muculi* (44, 45), *Plasmodium yoelii* (43), influenza virus (46), encephalomyocarditis virus

Table 17.3.   Selected Immunotoxicants and Associated Immunotoxicity

Chemical	Immune Alteration			
Environmental immunotoxicants	IS[a]	HY[b]	AI[c]	GR[d]
Ametryne	+	−	−	−
Asbestos	+	+/−	+	+
Benzene	+	−	−	−
Benzo(a)pyrene	+	−	−	−
Beryllium	−	+/−	−	+
Beryllium chloride	+	−	−	−
Beta-propiolactone	+	−	−	−
Cadmium	+	−	+	−
Cadmium chloride	+	−	−	−
Calcium cyanamide	+	−	−	−
Carbaryl	+	−	−	−
Carbon monoxide	+	−	−	−
Chlorine	+	−	−	−
Chloroform	+	−	−	−
Chlorophos	+	−	−	−
Chromium	−	+	−	−
Chromium chloride	−	+	−	−
Cobalt chloride	+	−	−	−
DDT	+	−	−	−
Dibromochloromethane	+	−	−	−
Dibutyltin dichloride	+	−	−	−
Dichlorophos	+	−	−	−
Diethyltoluamide	−	+	−	−
Dimethyl benzanthracene	+	−	+	−
2,4-Dinitrochlorobenzene	−	+	−	−
Dioctyltin dichloride	+	−	−	−
1,4-Dioxane	+	−	−	−
Epichlorohydrin	+	−	−	−
Ethanol	+	−	−	−
Ethylenediamine	−	+	−	−
Ethylenimine	+	−	−	−
Formaldehyde	−	+	−	−
Gallium	+	−	−	−
Gold	−	+	+	−
Halothane	−	−	+	−
Hexachlorobenzene	+	−	−	−
Hexamethylenediamine	+	−	−	−
Hydrazine	−	+	−	−
Lead	+	−	−	−
Lindane	+	−	−	−
Lithium	−	−	+	−
Magnesium	+	−	−	−
Malathion	+	−	−	−
Mercury	+	−	+	−
Methylcholanthrene	+	−	+	−
Methylmercury	+	−	−	−
Naphthalene	+	−	−	−
Nickel	−	+	−	−
Nickel chloride	+	−	−	−
Nitrogen dioxide	+	−	−	−
Nitrosomethylurethane	+	−	−	−
o-Benzyl-p-chlorophenol	+	−	−	−
o-Phenylphenol	+	−	−	−
Ozone	+	−	−	−
p-tert-Amylphenol	+	−	−	−
Parathion	+	−	−	−
Peroxyacetyl nitrate	+	−	−	−
Phthalic anhydride	−	+	−	−
Piperazine	+	−	−	−
Piperidine	+	−	−	−
Platinum	+	+	−	−

continues

Table 17.3. *Continued*

Chemical	Immune Alteration			
Polybromobiphenyl compounds	+	−	−	−
Polychlorobiphenyl compounds	+	−	−	−
Potassium dichromate	−	+	−	−
Silica	+	−	−	−
Sodium arsenite	+	−	−	−
Sodium bisulfite	−	+	−	−
Sodium cyanate	+	−	−	−
Sulfur dioxide	+	−	−	−
TCDD	+	−	−	−
TCDF	+	−	−	−
Tetrachlorophthalic anhydride	−	+	−	−
Tetraethyl lead	+	−	−	−
Thorium	+	−	−	−
Titanium	+	−	−	−
Tobacco	+	−	−	−
Toluene	+	−	−	−
Toluene diisocyanate	−	+	−	−
Tribufon	+	−	−	−
Tributyltin oxide	+	−	−	−
Trimellitic anhydride	−	+	−	−
Vinyl chloride	−	+/−	−	−
Wood, grain, and other organic dusts	−	+	−	−
Xylene	+	−	−	−
Immunosuppressive drugs				
Azathioprine	+	−	−	−
Cyclophosphamide	+	−	−	−
Cyclosporin A	+	−	−	−
Glucocorticosteroids	+	−	−	−
Pharmaceuticals				
β-Lactam antibiotics	+	+	−	−
Chlorpromazine	−	−	+	−
Diphenylhydantoin	+	−	−	−
Diethylstilbestrol	+	−	−	−
Griseofulvin	−	+	+	−
Hydralazine	−	−	+	−
Isoniazid	−	−	+	−
Methyldopa	−	−	+	−
Primidone	−	−	+	−
Procainamide	−	−	+	−
Quinidine	−	+	+	−
Streptomycin	−	+	+	−
Sulfonamides	−	−	+	−
Tetracyclines	−	+	+	−
Drugs of abuse				
Cannabinoids	+	−	−	−
Ethanol	+	−	+	−
Opiates	+	−	−	−

a IS, immunosuppression.
b HY, hypersensitivity.
c AI, autoimmunity. d GR, granuloma.

(46), and herpes simplex virus (46). All of these infectious agents require effective orchestration of most of the major elements of the immune apparatus for their successful elimination. In prospective immunotoxicty testing, the elegance of the host-resistance models arises from their ability to "test" functionally several entire circuits of the immune apparatus during a single experiment. The time required for this type of testing is 2–3 weeks. An example of a well-defined experimental host-parasite model for use in immunotoxicologic screening of xenobiotics is the *Trypanosoma musculi* mouse model. *T. musculi* is a nonpathogenic extracellular hemoflagellate. Murine infection with this parasite (Figure 17.3) is initially controlled by innate resistance mechanisms, or phagocytes. Later in the infection (10 days post infection), the logarithmic increase in parasitemia is brought under control by two separate antibody responses, one of which is thymus-dependent the other thymus-independent. Final elimination of this parasite, 18–20 days post infection, depends upon a combination of antibody and cellular immunity. In a single experiment, much of the immune repertoire can be tested functionally by *T. musculi* (Figure 17.3). Xenobiotic-induced alterations in phagocytosis, antibody production, or cell-mediated immunity are identified by significant rises in parasitemia at mechanism-dependent points in the infection. Because of their "real-life" simulation, host-resistance models are a sensitive and effective approach to the screening of potential immunotoxicants.

Immunosuppression and Cancer

Innate and adaptive resistance mechanisms are thought to participate in the immune response to tumors. Specifically cytotoxic T-lymphocytes and nonspecific natural killer cells (NK) are thought to perform crucial roles in limiting tumor growth (2, 6, 47). In addition, the macrophage plays a dual role: functioning as an effector, nonspecifically through phagocytosis, or specifically through lymphokine activation in acquired immune responses (2, 48).

The weight of evidence gathered to date demonstrates a relationship between disruptions in the immune apparatus (immunosuppression/immunodeficiency) and the development of certain types of neoplasia (27–29, 47, 49–51). The arguments for this association are convincing. Human and animal data demonstrate: (a) the occurrence of significantly greater numbers of diverse tumor types in immunosuppressed patients, such as lymphomas (52), cancers of the skin and lips (53), and leukemias; and (b) the association of a variety of immunosuppressive treatments such as irradiation, thymectomy, and immunotoxic chemical exposure with decreased tumor resistance and increased tumor growth rates and metastasis in experimental animal models (54). A particularly intriguing finding is that many known carcinogens also induce immune alterations. Illustrating this is a comparison of selected immunologic parameters in mice treated with benzo[a]pyrene (human carcinogen) and its noncarcinogenic congener, benzo[e]pyrene (Figure 17.4).These findings agree with a popular theory that the immune system, particularly those elements mediating delayed hypersensitivity are responsible for anticancer reconnaissance or immune surveillance (6, 55, 56). This hypothesis is based on two premises: (a) that neoplastic and normal cells generally have different antigenic portraits and (b) that the immune system responds to the antigenically modified (non-self) cells in essentially the same way it responds to infectious agents. Recent suggested refinements to this hypothesis suggest that lymphoid cells not only mediate immune responses against non-self, but also assist in regulating the differentiation of an assortment of normal (self) cells (56). Lymphoid cells accomplish this task by recognizing self rather than foreign or modified (non-self) antigens. By selectively driving the turnover of normal tissue cells, lymphoid cells impede the accumulation of small phenotypic/karyotypic abnormalities in the tissues. One prediction derived from this new concept of immune surveillance is that tumor escape from surveillance may be more

Table 17.4. Infectious Agents Associated with Immune Alterations

	B-Lymphocyte Defects	T-Lymphocyte Defects	Granulocyte Defects
Virus	Hepatitis B Echovirus	Rubeola Varicella Epstein-Barr Cytomegalovirus Herpes simplex Poxvirus	
Bacteria	*Pseudomonas* spp. *Hemophilus* spp. *Streptococcus* spp. *Meningococcus* spp. *Neisseria* spp.	*Mycobacterium* spp. *Listeria* spp. *Legionella* spp. *Salmonella* spp.	*Staphylococcus* spp. *Klebsiella* spp. *Nocardia* spp.
Yeast & Fungi		*Candida* spp. *Histoplasma* spp. *Cryptococcus* spp.	*Candida* spp. *Aspergillus* spp.
Parasite	*Giardia lamblia* *Pneumocystis carinii*	*Pneumocystis carinii* *Toxoplasma gondii* *Entamoeba histolytica* *Cryptosporidium* spp.	

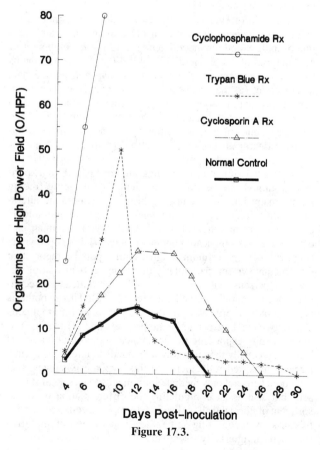

Figure 17.3.

significant consequences of immunosuppression, but, when studied in well-defined animal models, they also prove to be remarkably effective probes for the study of relevant immunotoxic effects of chemicals and drugs (54). In vivo tumor resistance models consist of either transplantable (42) or virus-induced (57) tumors that have been well characterized as to their behavior in specific inbred strains of mice or rats. Endpoints for in vivo assays of tumor resistance may include tumor size, mean survival time, response to secondary tumor challenge, or quantitation of metastases (54). In vivo tumor resistance assays are sensitive and extremely well-adapted to the screening of immunotoxic compounds for immunosuppressive activity (42, 43). In fact, ample evidence demonstrates that exposure to immunotoxicants can diminish natural and/or acquired tumor resistance in well-defined tumor models such as PYB6 sarcoma (nonmetastatic), B26F10 melanoma (metastatic), and murine sarcoma virus tumors (54). In addition, certain in vitro assessments of tumor resistance are useful adjuncts to in vivo tumor models. Both natural (NK cell) or acquired (cytotoxic T-lymphocyte) tumor resistance mechanisms can be studied in vitro. Each of the assays involve the quantitation of target tumor cell lysis via the release of chromium 51 label. These in vitro techniques have the advantage of refined control and manipulation of variables, the ability to use either human or animal cell systems, and significantly reduced time requirements (days). The combined use of both in vivo and in vitro tumor resistance assays provide sensitive endpoints for detecting biologically relevant immunotoxicity. However, like host-resistance models that utilize infectious agents, the sensitivity of in vivo tumor resistance assays results from the multiple mechanisms that control the in vivo immune response. These parameters cannot be sufficiently addressed by a single, stand-alone, in vitro assay system.

Xenobiotic-induced alterations of immune responsiveness are demonstrable in both humans and animals. Xenobiotic suppres-

accurately described as an escape from regulatory differentiation pressures.

As with infectious diseases, not only are tumors clinically

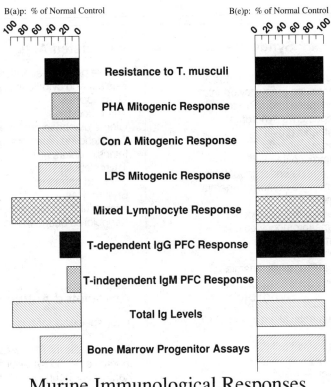

Murine Immunological Responses

Post Treatment

Figure 17.4.   Murine immunologic responses post treatment.

sion of immune responsiveness can lead to increased susceptibility to infectious disease, cancer or both. Even more portentous are the findings that even commonly encountered xenobiotics are capable of inducing immunosuppression.

AUTOIMMUNITY

One of the most profound riddles that the immune system must solve is how to respond to foreign antigen without responding to self. Basic immunologic research provides the basis for our understanding of the major histocompatibility gene complex (MHC) and its role in regulation of immune responses (2, 10, 35, 58). Recognition and response to non-self is MHC-restricted (requires recognition of self) (59, 60). From this understanding an apparent paradox arises; the immune system must recognize self in order to respond to something foreign. Despite our fragmentary understanding of how self-reactivity, or autoimmunity, is modulated, it is obvious that failure to regulate autoimmunity can have grievous consequences (4, 61, 62). Self-recognition is vital, but uncontrolled self-reaction is perilous. Perpetuating self-recognition while preventing deleterious self-reaction is a task of immune regulation. Since the turn of the century when Paul Ehrlich first coined *horror autotoxicus*, many associations between reactivity to self components and disease have been identified (61–67). Early investigations into the etiology of autoimmune responses favored a single agent, usually infectious (68). However, research of the past 15 years has revealed a new conceptual framework for comprehending autoimmune disease (2, 66, 69, 70). Although a thorough mechanistic understanding of the etiology

and pathogenesis of most autoimmune diseases is still incomplete, the progression from enigma to understanding continues. Inexorably, autoimmunity is attracting the attention of the clinician; physicians increasingly encounter diseases and syndromes in which autoimmune phenomena apparently contribute to symptoms, diagnosis, or prognosis.

Today, we know that autoimmunity is the basis for both normal immune reactivity and immune regulation (4, 67, 71, 72). Autoimmune disease results from quantitative abnormalities such as the amount of stem cell proliferation, amount of autoantibody production, and the quantity of antibody-antigen complex (immune complex [IC] formation. In addition, autoimmune disease is thought to occur through a multifactorial mechanism involving a combination of polygenic predisposition, environmental triggers, and defects in immune regulation. Evidence for genetic predisposition comes from numerous studies in which human lymphocyte antigens (HLA) associations and family studies indicate predisposition to produce autoantibodies. For example, close relatives of Hashimoto thyroiditis and pernicious anemia patients are found to produce significant titers of autoantibody to thyroid tissue and thyroglobulin (70). Immune response genes may also be important; many human autoimmune disorders are associated with the HLA-DRw3 phenotype (58, 61, 73). Furthermore, germline genotypic/phenotypic variations and defects in T-lymphocyte maturation are both hypothesized to contribute to impaired immune regulation (66), setting the stage for later development of autoimmune disease (Table 17.5). Several reports have documented defects in the suppressor circuits and other immunoregulatory circuits in autoimmune animal models (70). It is noteworthy

Table 17.5. Autoimmune Disease

	Syndrome	Associated Antigens (Ags)
Antibody-mediated Pathology	Systemic lupus erythematosus Autoimmune granulocytopenia Autoimmune thrombocytopenia Goodpasture's syndrome Myasthenia gravis Pernicious anemia Autoimmune thyroiditis Autoimmune endocrinopathies Autoimmune hemolytic anemia Pemphigus Immune granulocytopenia Immune thrombocytopenia Serum sickness Anaphylaxis Immune hemolytic anemia	Double or single-stranded DNA Nuclear and cytoplasmic Ags Granulocytes Thrombocytes Glomerular basement membrane Acetylcholine receptors Intrinsic factors Thyroglobulin Selected hormones Erythrocytes Intracellular epidermal Ags Xenobiotics bound to self-Ags " " " "
	Syndrome	**Associated Antigens (Ags)**
Cell-mediated Pathology	Experimental allergic encephalomyelitis Experimental arthritis Contact dermatitis	T-cell specificity for basic protein of myelin T-cell specific for *Mycobacterium tuberculosis* and synovial tissue Xenobiotics bound to self-Ags

that all the "ingredients" for an autoimmune response are likely present in normal individuals. Self antigens are accessible to circulating lymphocytes (58, 67, 70). There is also evidence that autoreactive lymphocytes are demonstrable in most normal subjects (4). Autoimmune diseases may be organ specific or non-organ specific, antibody mediated or cell mediated, and involve self antigens or environmental agents bound to self antigens.

Because xenobiotics influence lymphocyte activation, antibody synthesis production of cytokines, and other cellular interactions, it is not surprising that they may also induce autoimmune responses and autoimmune disease (Table 17.5). Numerous drugs have been implicated in the induction of autoimmunity (58, 61, 62). Mercury (66), dieldrin (64), and methylcholanthrene (74) are examples of chemicals known to elicit autoimmune responses. Xenobiotics may induce autoimmunity by at least four hypothesized mechanisms.

1. **Direct effects on the immune system**—xenobiotics may cause autoimmunity by direct effects on lymphocytes and/or macrophages (66). These effects may be demonstrated as reductions in T-lymphocyte suppressor activity, increases in T-lymphocyte helper activity, or polyclonal activation of B-lymphocytes (70). Direct evidence of methyldopa interference with T-suppressor function in human autoimmune hemolytic anemia has been demonstrated (75). Furthermore, procainamide is capable of affecting immune regulation by inhibiting cyclic AMP generation and stimulating T-helper cells (76). Metals such as mercury are reported to cause polyclonal B-lymphocyte stimulation (77).
2. **Release of autoantigens**—certain xenobiotics may disrupt and release tissue antigens into the general circulation, a qualitative effect. Alternatively, these chemicals may simply increase the quantity of autoantigens normally present

in the circulation. Autoimmune responses following chronic exposure to metals such as gold and mercury may be clarified by an understanding of these mechanisms (78).

3. **Alteration of autoantigens**—xenobiotics may alter autoantigens in such a manner as to no longer be recognized as self. Interactions with chemicals may either expose "hidden" determinants or furnish new determinants or autoantigens. An example of this type of interaction is hydralazine's ability to complex with deoxyribonucleoprotein.
4. **Cross-reactions between xenobiotics and autoantigens**—theory would suggest, but there is no evidence to support, possible shared antigenic determinants between xenobiotics and autoantigens. Accordingly, it is noteworthy that autoantibodies induced by procainamide, methyldopa, penicillamine, and hydralazine do not cross-react with these drugs.

There is no doubt that autoimmunity, as well as autoimmune disease, can be induced by chronic exposure to common xenobiotics. Human and animal data reveal that autoimmune phenomena are caused by multifactorial mechanisms that involve both immunogenetic and pharmacogenetic factors. Individuals charged with the prevention, diagnosis, and treatment of autoimmune disease should be aware of the role that xenobiotics may play in the development of these disorders.

HYPERSENSITIVITY

In spite of evidence that certain controlled hypersensitivity reactions can be beneficial (e.g., IgE response to parasites), most manifestations of hypersensitivity are unpleasant. In fact, hypersensitivity disorders are currently the most prominent form of immunotoxicity recognized in humans. Hypersensitivity is best portrayed as an exaggerated response to an antigenic stimulus, commonly distinguished by a reduced threshold to antigen. Regardless of their type, all hypersensitivity reactions are induced by "recall" antigens in or on a host who has become sensitized, i.e., who has previously effected an immune response to the antigen. It is estimated that more than 40 million Americans suffer from some form of hypersensitivity disease (79) and approximately 9% of all patients seeking medical care do so for treatment of hypersensitivity disorders.

Certain terms used by clinicians and researchers to describe hypersensitivity appear to overlap each other and therefore should be clarified:

1. The term **anaphylaxis** was introduced by Porter and Richet in 1902 to indicate adverse reactions to horse serum injected for therapy of infectious disease. The term suggests a reaction that is the opposite of prophylaxis. In the context of immunotoxicology, anaphylaxis has taken on the implication of an acute reaction involving both immunologic and inflammatory mechanisms.
2. The term **atopy** was introduced by Coca in the 1920s to describe a multiplicity of curious reactions then thought to be unique to humans. This word is derived from the Greek word *atopia*, meaning strangeness. Those curious reactions are now known to be allergies. In the context of immunotoxicology, atopy implies a constitutional or hereditary tendency to develop chronic hypersensitivity states, such as hay fever or asthma, especially to antigens that provoke no adverse reactions in "normal" subjects.
3. The term **allergy** was introduced by von Pirquet in 1906 to indicate altered reactivity as a result of a previous exposure. Today, the term allergy is often used to describe either atopic or anaphylactic reactions.

In addition to being the most predominant form of immunotoxicity, hypersensitivity disorders are certainly the most problematic form. Allergic disorders tend to be more "individualized" than most other forms of toxicity. Exposure conditions that elicit an allergic response in certain individuals may have no effect on others similarly exposed. Thus, the prospect of genetic predisposition is raised. Because hypersensitivity reactions are elicited by a diversity of antigens and occur in or on numerous organ systems of the body, they arise in what appears to be a bewildering array. In the 1950s Gell and Coombs devised a classification of hypersensitivity disorders based on the immunopathologic mechanism involved (modified in Table 17.2). While this classification is useful, it is particularly important to realize that more than one of these mechanisms can operate simultaneously in a patient. This begs consideration of those factors that determine what form of hypersensitivity (Table 17.2) is manifest. Most potentially toxic agents are of low molecular weight and may act as haptens. The type of hypersensitivity an agent elicits in a susceptible host depends on its route of exposure as well as on the nature of host constituent with which it interacts (Table 17.6). Most of our understanding of hypersensitivity has come from reactions to natural antigens such as pollens, house dust, or danders. It is now apparent that occupational exposure to chemicals and other xenobiotics (Table 17.3) is an important and growing cause of hypersensitivity disorders. With regard to occupational settings, most threshold limit values (TLV, registered trademark of the American Conference of Government Industrial Hygienists) are quantitatively determined by irritant and toxic effects of chemicals rather than by their sensitizing effects (80). Workers can become sensitized after exposure to concentrations well below the "allowable" threshold limit (80). From a pulmonary context, chemicals in

Table 17.6. Immune Interactions in Hypersensitivity

Host Constituent	Immune Interaction	Hypersensitivity
PROTEIN	Antibody (IgE or IgG) Response to hapten Sensitization of Mast Cells	Asthma or Allergic Rhinitis
	Antibody (IgM or IgG) Response Ag-Ab Complex formation Complement activation	Hypersensitivity pneumonitis
CELL	Antibody (IgG) Response to Ag-altered host cell	Autoimmune Hemolytic Anemia
	T-lymphocyte Response to Ag-altered host cell	Contact Dermatitis

the air may irritate the airways and lower the threshold for airway responsiveness. These same irritants may also be allergens for susceptible individuals.

The limitations of this chapter do not allow a thorough review of all aspects of hypersensitivity. Rather, examples of immediate hypersensitivity, immune complex reactions, and delayed hypersensitivity and their relationship to xenobiotics will be reviewed.

Immediate Hypersensitivity

Examples of immediate hypersensitivity (IH, Type I, Table 17.2) include allergic rhinitis, asthma, and atopic dermal reactions such as hives. Asthma and allergic rhinitis are the most common forms of IH (81) and are certainly the most important in an immunotoxicology context. These diseases are produced as the result of a two-step inflammatory reaction initiated by mediators, shown in Table 17.2, that are released by reaction of multivalent antigen with mast cells and basophils passively sensitized with cytophilic antibody on the surface. Effector cells release an arsenal of biologically active substances including histamine, heparin, serotonin, and arachidonic acid (Figure 17.5). The early phase of IH is characterized by two events. The first is smooth muscle contraction or dilatation of arterioles, mediated by histamine via H-2 receptors, typified by a wheal and flare skin reaction. The second is immediate smooth muscle contraction in pulmonary bronchi, resulting in bronchospasm and asthma. The late phase of IH is characterized by painful, indurated skin lesions on the one hand or compromised airway flow rate on the other. Late phase reactions are mediated by leukotrienes and prostaglandins, which are cellular metabolites of arachidonic acid. Evidence suggests that histamine also is capable of "switching off," or down-regulating delayed hypersensitivity responses by interaction with histamine receptors on T-lymphocytes which participate in these reactions (82). Multiple factors influence human capacity to mount an immediate hypersensitivity response. Included are genetic makeup, dose, duration, and route of exposure to allergen, antigen type, age, and lifestyle/habit. Of these factors, the most important is genetic makeup. Data suggest that the atopic state exhibits a defect in T-lymphocyte (T-suppressor) function (82, 83). Even animal models of sensitization demonstrate "high" and "low" responder strains (82). In addition, exposure to soluble, high molecular weight antigens including peptides, proteins, glycoproteins, and polysaccharides tends to select for IH (72).

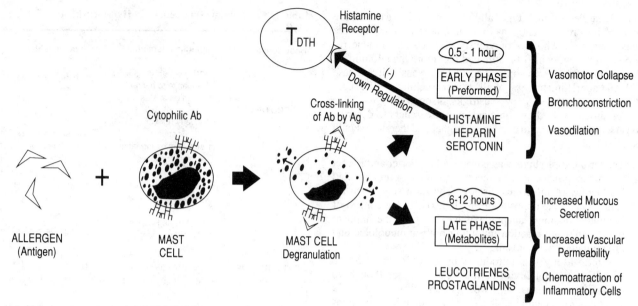

Figure 17.5. Mechanisms of early and late onset Type I hypersensitivity.

However, when combined with host carrier proteins, even low molecular weight haptens can become complete antigens and elicit an IH response. Furthermore, characteristics of the chemicals or other xenobiotics that sensitize an individual may not necessarily be the same as those that elicit an allergic response (58, 72). From an occupational perspective, it is the atopic worker who is most likely to suffer an allergic response to chemicals in the workplace. It is obvious that there is potential exposure to known sensitizers in the workplace (Table 17.3). Eventually, susceptible individuals will be identified by specific screening procedures before being exposed to occupational allergens.

Immune Complex Reactions

There is mounting evidence that injury to tissue caused by antigen-antibody complexes (type III, Table 17.2) is more common than initially supposed (84–87). Arthus reactions (local) and serum sickness (systemic) are the archetypes of this type of hypersensitivity. However, for this discussion, a description of a specific clinical counterpart of the arthus reaction, hypersensitivity pneumonitis, will suffice. Hypersensitivity pneumonitis, HP, is a phrase that includes a group of hypersensitivities caused by inhalation of numerous organic dusts and simple chemicals (Table 17.7). Typically, patients given histories of multiple bouts of dyspnea, fever, cough, and malaise (86). These symptoms start 4–6 hours following exposure to the causative antigen and may last for 12–24 hours. Chest roentgenograms during the acute phase show interstitial edema and, occasionally, patchy infiltrates (86). HP disorders exhibit several common features: (a) predominant involvement of the peripheral airways without systemic organ involvement; (b) lesions characterized by mononuclear cell, alveolar filling, interstitial infiltrates (T-suppressor/cytotoxic lymphocytes and macrophages) that progress to granulomas; (c) T-cells and alveolar macrophages present are markedly activated; (d) disease is associated with high levels of precipitating antibody against offending particulate antigens, with bronchial washes showing

elevated levels of IgG, IgA, IgM, and T-cell lymphokines. Pathology may involve both cell-mediated and immune complex mechanisms within the lungs. Experimental animal models suggest that interleukins 1 and 2 as well as leukotrienes and prostaglandins are involved in the progression of the disease (4, 88). As with most forms of immunotoxicity, ultimate modulation of this pulmonary granulomatous inflammatory response is determined by a series of genetically determined immunoregulatory events that are now being studied and identified.

Delayed Hypersensitivity

Cell-mediated immunity plays a critical role in resistance to many infectious agents (Table 17.4) and tumors, as well as a role in the pathogenesis of tissue injury in a number of diseases (type IV, Table 17.2). Whether cell-mediated reactions produce immunity or hypersensitivity, both are mediated by specifically sensitized T-cells. The reaction is manifest by infiltration of lymphocytes and monocytes at the site of antigen deposition. Only a few of the infiltrating cells are antigen specific (2, 88). Reaction of these few cells with antigen causes the release of cytokines which induce and maintain an inflammatory response and "recruit" large numbers of other cell types into the area. Tissue destruction may be caused by either antigen-specific T-(cytotoxic) lymphocytes or by lymphokine-activated macrophages. As the number of specifically reactive cells increases, many leave the local site of reaction and eventually migrate to the general blood circulation (2, 89). The hypersensitive state thus disseminates as a result of the distribution of these effector T-cells to various parts of the lymphoid system and other tissues, particularly the skin.

There are two archetypes of cell-mediated hypersensitivity: allergic contact dermatitis (ACD) and the tuberculin skin reaction. A classical manifestion of ACD is the rash of "poison ivy." Plant catechols, such as urushiol and toxicodendrol, are the causative allergens in this disorder. A variety of synthetic chemicals and natural products may cause ACD

Table 17.7. Hypersensitivity Pneumonitis

	AGENTS	DISORDERS
BACTERIAL & FUNGAL Ags	Thermophilic actinomycetes	Farmer's lung disease, Bagassosis, Mushroom worker's disease, Humidifier lung, Ventilation pneumonitis
	Penicillium spp.	Suberosis, Cheese washer's disease
	Pullularia spp.	Sauna lung
	Bacillus spp. (and derived enzymes)	Familial hypersensitivity pneumonitis, Detergent worker's disease
	Aspergillus spp.	Malt worker's lung
	Alternaria spp.	Wood pulp worker's disease
	Cephalosporium spp.	Basement pneumonitis
ANIMAL PROTEIN Ags	Avian Proteins	Pigeon breeder's disease, Duck fever, Turkey handler's disease, Feather plucker's disease
	Bovine and Porcine Proteins	Pituitary snuff taker's lung
	Rodent Proteins	Animal handler's pneumonitis
REACTIVE CHEMICALS	Toluene diisocyanate	TDI hypersensitivity pneumonitis
	Trimellitic anhydride	TMA hypersensitivity pneumonitis
	Diphenylmethane diisocyanate	MDI hypersensitivity pneumonitis
	Epoxy resins	Epoxy resin lung

in susceptible individuals. Ingredients in antibiotics, ointments, clothing, cosmetics, solvent mixtures, dyes, inks, and jewelry may be associated with ACD. Sensitization occurs after one or more dermal exposures to antigen; prolonged exposure, perhaps years, may be required. Antigens involved in such responses are often highly reactive chemicals, usually lipid soluble, capable of conjugating with host dermal proteins, the resulting complex recognized as foreign by the host. Langerhans cells (epidermal macrophages) are thought to play a pivotal role in antigen processing and presentation to T-lymphocytes (90). Early signs of ACD include erythema and edema. Intercellular edema progresses to vesicle formation, rupture, and oozing dermatitis. Severity of the dermal response may increase for several days without further contact with allergen; healing usually takes 2–4 weeks. It is noteworthy that, once developed, sensitization persists long after healing; subsequent exposure to even small amounts of

allergen will trigger a recrudescence of the entire ACD process. Systemic administration of allergen may induce severe generalized dermal reactions in previously sensitized individuals.

Pseudoallergic Reactions

The intersection of immunotoxicity and hypersensitivity is sometimes complex and puzzling. Multiple etiologies and mechanisms may induce similar signs and symptoms. An example of this concept is the bronchoconstrictive disorder, asthma, which may be induced by irritant, pharmacologic, toxic, or immunologic mechanisms (79, 82, 83). There are situations in which patients may present symptoms characteristic of immune-mediated hypersensitivities, ranging from skin rashes to anaphylaxis, in which it is not possible to establish that any immunologic mechanism is involved. The molecular basis of such phenomena is not completely understood. Certain chemicals and other xenobiotics have the ability to bypass the regular two-stage mast cell triggering process and act directly to cause degranulation (2, 82, 83). One mechanism is by direct liberation of mediators through cytolysis of the mast cell (cytotoxicity). Recent evidence also suggests the possibility of direct, but noncytotxic mast cell degranulation which does not involve immune mechanisms (91). Other agents are postulated to initiate pseudoallergic reactions via the formation of anaphylatoxic complement subcomponent (82, 82, 91). One of the most intriguing aspects of pseudoallergy is the very small number of patients involved in such reactions. Limited understanding notwithstanding, it is obvious that the mechanisms of pseudoallergy are varied despite similarities in the clinical manifestations.

The inclusion of hypersensitivity reactions in any discussion of immunotoxicology is valid and essential. Advances in our understanding of immunogenetics and the development of more sensitive and specific diagnostic tools should further promote efforts directed toward both prevention and accurate diagnosis of this common form of immunotoxicity.

PREDICTIVE TESTING AND DIAGNOSIS OF IMMUNOTOXICITY

The ability of chemicals and other xenobiotics to induce hypersensitivity responses has been known for many years (61, 79, 80). The scientific community has also recently developed an appreciation for the variety of substances that can suppress the immune system and diminish host resistance to infections and tumors. Through insightful planning and research, laboratory techniques have been developed and validated for evaluating the effects of chemicals on the immune system. These procedures include in vivo systems where the entire immune repertoire is intact, as well as in vitro ones which detect a chemical's effect on isolated circuits of the immune system. The diagnostic criteria for the identification of hypersensitivity disorders is in a more advanced state than that for the identification of other immunotoxic disorders. However, much effort is now being invested in developing and validating animal and human procedures to diagnose immunosuppressive, hypersensitivity, and autoimmune disorders. Significantly, these tests can help distinguish those chemicals for which the immune system is the primary target; immunotoxicity is probably most important when it occurs in the absence of other toxic effects.

Tiered Approach to Predictive Immunotoxicity Testing

The principal strategy of immunologists and toxicologists trying to determine potential immunotoxicity usually include a tiered panel of assays to measure immune function. No single immune function assay can be used to evaluate comprehensively all possible adverse effects of chemicals on the immune system. Historically, immunotoxicity assessments have been performed using laboratory animals, particularly rodents. Many different panels have been proposed (31, 33, 42, 92–94), but only recently has an effort been made to refine, compare, and validate these assays for predictive testing purposes (43). We present a two-tiered panel for the screening of chemicals for immunotoxicity (Table 17.8) that differs only slightly from that recommended by the National Toxicology Program (NTP) of the National Institute of Environmental Health Sciences (43). Our modifications include

the use of T-independent antigen probes (95) in addition to T-dependent antigens (tier 1) and the substitution of *Trypanosoma musculi* host resistance model (44, 45) instead of a *Plasmodium yoelii* model (tier II). These modifications are included because of the increased sensitivity they add to each of their respective tiers. The remainder of the two tiers is essentially the same as that of the NTP testing regimen. Assays of tier I are limited and positioned to serve as an initial screen for the assessment of potential immunotoxicants. Tier I assays readily detect potent immunotoxicants; the probability of detecting weak immunotoxicants is presumably less. That notwithstanding, no compound has been identified to date that can affect a tier II assay without also exhibiting an effect in some tier I assessment (43). Tier II is a more penetrating evaluation of immune function that is positioned to elucidate mechanisms employed by immunotoxicants identified by tier I assays. Because the most relevant endpoint for immune dysfunction is altered host resistance to infectious agents and tumors (96), emphasis is placed on developing sensitive models that correlate immune alterations with diminished host resistance. Typically, a 14-day repeat-dose regimen is used, although 30- and 90-day exposure regimens can be utilized when deemed appropriate. Other details regarding protocol design, methodology, and data analysis can be obtained from NTP's Guidelines for Immunotoxicity Evaluation in Mice (43). This type of approach should not only improve our ability to predict immunotoxicity but also provide a better understanding of relevant immune effector mechanisms involved in host resistance and other important immune functions.

Methods similar to those described above (Table 17.8) have also been successfully applied to the diagnosis of immunotoxicity in humans (32, 37, 51, 97). However, to be useful, interpretation of changes in human immune function must take into account: (a) normal variation of parameter measured; (b) toxicant effects (specific to the immune apparatus?); (c) confounding variables (age, health, medications, etc.); (d) clinical relevance of alteration; and (e) reversibility of alteration.

APPROACHES TO PREDICTIVE AND DIAGNOSTIC HYPERSENSITIVITY TESTING

Developing, validating, and standardizing methods for the diagnosis of hypersensitivity disorders is an important public health consideration due to the extensive prevalence of these diseases. Guidelines have been recently issued for both old and new technologies used in the diagnosis and treatment of hypersensitivity disorders (98). Because the guidelines are authoritative and serve as an excellent review of clinical diagnostic techniques and their respective foibles, recommendations will not be reiterated in this chapter. The availability, sensitivity, and reproducibility of in vivo and in vitro tests have provided clinicians with an important armamentarium in the modern practice of allergy. Certain tests and approaches have been found to be unreliable, and their use is highly questionable (99).

Predictive testing for potential sensitizing agents is usually done in animal models; the guinea pig is the animal of choice. There are three variations of predictive allergenicity testing in current use: (a) the Draize test (100), (b) the Buehler occluded-patch test (101), and (c) the Magnusson and Kligman Guinea Pig Maximization test (102). These tests vary with regard to route of exposure (intradermal versus cutaneous versus sub-

Table 17.8. Two-Tier Immunotoxicity Panel

PARAMETERS		PROCEDURES
TIER I (SCREEN)	IMMUNOPATHOLOGY	**Hematology -** Complete blood work up and differential count **Weights -** Body, spleen, thymus, kidney, liver and lungs **Cellularity -** Spleen **Histology -** Spleen, thymus, lymph nodes
	HUMORAL-MEDIATED IMMUNITY	Enumeration of IgM antibody plaque forming cells to T-dependent (SE) and T-independent (PVP) antigens & LPS mitogen response
	CELL-MEDIATED IMMUNITY	Con A mitogen response & mixed leukocyte response (MLR) against allogeneic leukocytes
	NON-SPECIFIC IMMUNITY	Natural killer (NK) cell activity (spleen)
TIER II (MECHANISM)	IMMUNOPATHOLOGY	Quantitation of splenic B- and T-cell numbers
	HUMORAL-MEDIATED IMMUNITY	Enumeration of IgG antibody plaque forming cells to T-dependent Ags
	CELL-MEDIATED IMMUNITY	Cytotoxic T-lymphocyte (CTL) function & delayed hypersensitivity (DTH) responses
	NON-SPECIFIC IMMUNITY	Enumeration of peritoneal macrophages & analysis of their phagocytic capacity
	HOST RESISTANCE MODELS (endpoints)	**Syngeneic Tumor Models** PYB6 Sarcoma (tumor incidence) B16F10 Melanoma (lung burden) **Bacterial Models** *Listeria monocytogenes* (mortality) *Streptococcus spp.* (mortality) **Parasite Models** *Trypanosoma musculi* (parasitemia) *Plasmodium yoelii* (parasitemia) **Virus Models** Influenza (mortality)

cutaneous, respectively), use of adjuvant, and timing of interval between sensitization and challenge. Of the three, the Magnusson and Kligman variation has been found to be a more rigorous test for experimentally determining the allergenic potential of a substance (28).

CLINICAL IMMUNOTOXICOLOGY

Despite the vast amount of information documenting immunotoxic effects of many chemicals and drugs in animal models, extrapolation from this animal data to humans remains difficult. There are common examples of chemicals such as beryllium, platinum, chromium, cadmium, chloromethyl ethers, ethylene oxide, formaldehyde, polyhalogenated aromatic hydrocarbons, epoxy resins, trimellitic anhydride, isocyanates, and glycol ethers known to produce human health effects via hematologic or immunologic mechanisms.

Detection of immune system effects and documenting causation of an immune alteration following chemical exposure requires careful analysis of the exposure circumstances, a thorough history and physical examination, and immunologic laboratory testing. Not all patients will present with easily documented end organ immunotoxicity such as glomerulonephritis, pneumonitis, asthma, dermatologic lesions and exanthems, or hepatitis from clearly defined exposure sources. Clinical evaluation of the immune system can be expensive and may lead to unnecessary and costly testing if not properly planned. The evaluation of the patient should include a thorough history and physical examination with particular attention to the classical signs and symptoms of immune disorders. Sophisticated

laboratory tests can provide detailed evaluation of humoral-mediated immunity (HMI), cell-mediated immunity (CMI), complement, and phagocyte functioning. However, these tests are not required in the vast majority of clinical immunologic evaluations of patients. It is possible to have insight into immune lesions by use of screening tests. However, the ultimate endpoint in determining proper functioning of the immune system is the presence of an intact host defense. Due to the dynamic nature of the immune system, results of tests will provide information only about a particular area of the immune system at one particular point in time. Also, it may be difficult to discern immune dysfunction resulting from some primary disease or poor nutritional status from disease resulting from a primary immune lesion.

Clinical Immunologic Screening

Eight immunologic tests have been recommended by the World Health Organization's Immunology Section for screening patients with suspected immune dysfunctions (103). These tests should be performed before other more elaborate and expensive tests are conducted in the diagnostic evaluation of the immune system (Figure 17.6). There are a variety of other in-depth confirmatory immunologic tests which can be performed beyond this initial screening (Figures 17.7 and 17.8). The judicious use of these tests and their proper interpretation are essential in the evaluation of possible immune disorders (104).

Immunoglobulin quantitation and protein electrophoresis provide direct information concerning the absence of an immunoglobulin class or the presence of a monoclonal or poly-

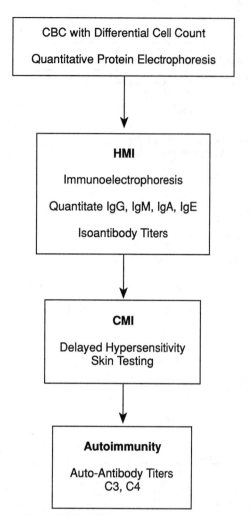

Figure 17.6.   Clinical immunotoxicology screening tests.

clonal gammopathy. The three major immunoglobulins quantitated are IgG, IgM, and IgA. IgE can be measured if allergies are part of the clinical syndrome; however, IgE may or may not be elevated. The detection of antigen-specific IgE and IgG requires more sophisticated testing such as by enzyme-linked immunosorbent assays. Hypogammaglobulinemias are usually the result of a secondary immune deficiency. The most frequent immunoglobulin deficiency is IgA, and in 50% of these cases the patient is clinically asymptomatic (105). Secretory IgA is a mucosal barrier defense mechanism, and its assay is separate from the measurement of regular IgA. Examination of the protein electrophoretic pattern can quickly indicate if a patient has normal concentrations of immunoglobulins, hypogammaglobulinemia, or a dysgammaglobulinemia.

Defects is cell-mediated immunity may be recognized by clinical symptoms of infections associated with common CMI functions. These functions are related to killing of intracellular pathogens, delayed hypersensitivity reactions to recognized antigens, tumor cell rejection, contact dermatitis, and tissue injury from autoimmunity. Diagnostic evaluation of cell-mediated immunity involves in vivo and in vitro testing procedures (Figure 17.8). Defects usually present as an increase in infections with agents such as viruses, intercellular pathogens, and fungi.

Any significant decrease in the number of T-lymphocytes will result in a lymphopenia in peripheral blood smears since

they make up approximately 75–85% of the peripheral blood lymphocyte population. Determination of the number of T-cells in peripheral blood is also performed by using the sheep erythrocyte rosette formation method (104). Another method for enumerating T-cells involves the use of fluorescent labeled monoclonal antibodies directed against mature T-cells (104).

Skin tests for delayed hypersensitivity can be performed using common antigens such as *Trichophyton*, *Candida albicans*, PPD, and mumps antigen. An erythematous dermal reaction and induration greater than 10 millimeters in diameter at 24, 48, or 72 hours after intradermal injection of 0.1 milliliter of the antigen into the volar surface of the forearm indicates that a complex series of cell-mediated events occurred: the antigen was recognized by lymphocytes and appropriately processed, helper/inducer T-cells were activated, lymphokines were secreted, and recruitment of nonsensitized lymphocytes to the antigen deposition area occurred (104). Development of a positive skin test is dependent on previous antigen exposure. A positive skin test result for delayed hypersensitivity indicates a normally functioning cell-mediated immune system, and 95% of the normal population will react to three out of five skin tests (106). Standardization of skin test antigens has been a problem, and lack of standardized reagents may complicate the skin test. This should be checked before applying any skin tests. Also, a negative result may indicate an improperly administered test and not an immune defect. A positive delayed hypersensitivity skin test indicates an intact and normally functioning cell-mediated immune system.

Measurement of autoantibodies can be useful in diagnosing mixed connective tissue disease, chronic active hepatitis, and systemic lupus. The commonly measured autoantibodies are antibodies against nuclei, smooth muscle, DNA, and thyroid tissue (104). Autoimmune diseases and chronic inflammatory states may be misdiagnosed as an immunotoxicity from xenobiotics. Antinuclear antibodies (ANA) can be present in healthy individuals, in patients with rheumatic and nonrheumatic disease, in family members of persons with autoimmune disease, and in the elderly (61). The finding of low titer autoantibodies in an individual is of little significance in making a diagnosis of an immune dysfunction. About 35% of normal people will have a positive ANA titer if their serum is checked at dilutions less than 1:10, and 4% will be positive at dilutions greater than 1:10 (104). Approximately 38% of persons greater than 60 years of age will be positive for ANA (104).

Normally, humans have antibodies against common antigens to which everyone is exposed. These antibodies occur as a normal response and can be quantitated: isohemagglutinins, antistreptolysin-O, antibodies to measles, mumps, polio, and tetanus toxoid immunizations (103, 104). The primary and secondary immune response to an antigen can be determined in some situations. Evaluation of the primary immune response requires an antigen to which the person has never been exposed. This can produce some problems and introduce risk to the patient. The secondary immune response is easier to evaluate and can be as easy as administration of tetanus toxoid and measuring antibody titers. However, the primary immune response is usually the most sensitive to immunosuppressants.

Complement system function can be screened for by quantifying C3 (alternate complement pathway), C4 (classical pathway), and CH_{50} (total complement). The measurement of CH_{50} is more useful for monitoring immune complex diseases like glomerulonephritis or systemic lupus (103, 104). Deficiencies in selected complement components can present with different

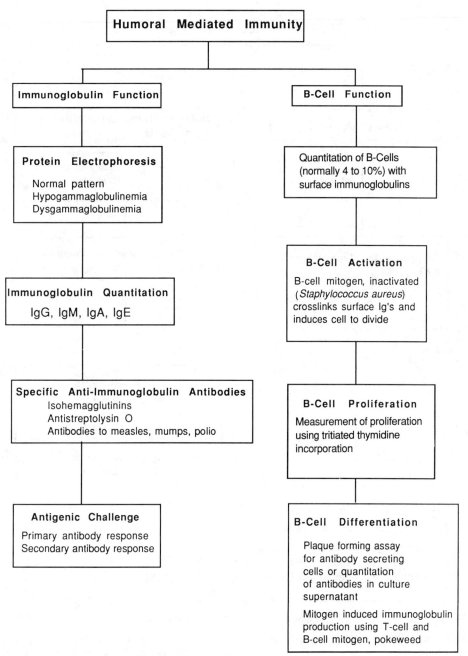

Figure 17.7. Humoral-mediated immunity.

disease patterns. Indications for assaying complement function are repeated infections by pyogenic bacteria, systemic bacterial infections, or suspected autoimmune disease. Some of the clinical syndromes associated with inappropriate activation of complement include recurring angioedema, chronic urticaria, palpable purpura, arthralgias, cutaneous vasculitides, unexplained fever, nephritis, and arthritides (107).

Reduced serum concentrations of the C4 is a sensitive indicator of a low level activation of the complement system. C3 usually has a high serum concentration, and its measurement provides information about the alternate complement pathway. A normal C4 with a low concentration of C3 indicates alternate pathway activation of the complement system (108). Low C3, C4, and CH_{50} is associated with classical pathway activation.

Normal C3 and C4 with a low CH_{50} suggests a deficiency of one of the other complement components.

Activation of the complement system and the presence of autoantibodies indicates immune complex diseases and autoimmunity. Positive results for immune complexes, the presence of certain autoantibodies, and complement system activation should encourage the clinician to search for end organ pathology in specific organ systems involved in the clinical syndrome. Negative results in the immune complex assays for complement and autoantibodies is helpful in ruling out a humoral-mediated cause of clinical defense.

Complete and detailed testing of the immune system can be entertained if an abnormality is demonstrated in the initial screening. However, these detailed tests are uncommonly re-

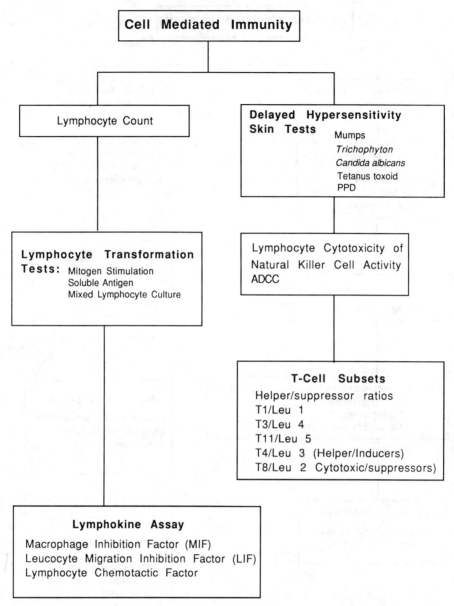

Figure 17.8. Cell-mediated immunity.

quired if sound clinical judgment is employed in evaluating a suspected immune dysfunction.

Other Immunology Tests

In some situations, quantitation of T-cell subpopulations may be indicated. This can be accomplished using monoclonal antibodies directed against specific T-cell surface receptors (104). Helper and suppressor cells can be enumerated in peripheral blood using monoclonal antibody assays which are commercially available. The most common monoclonal antibodies for the identification and quantitation of T-cell subsets are the Leu and OK series (107). T-helper cells, which comprise about 50–60% of the T-lymphocyte population, have surface membrane receptors for the Fc portion of IgM antibody. T-suppressor cells have receptors for the Fc region of IgG antibody, and these cells make up 25–35% of the T-lymphocyte population. Helper T-cells also have OKT4 and Leu-3 antigens, whereas cytotoxic/

suppressor T-cells have OKT8 and Leu-2 surface antigens (114). The normal helper:suppressor ratio is 1.8:2.2. Patients with acquired immunodeficiency syndrome may have helper/suppressor ratios less than 1.0 (108); however, a low ratio is not diagnostic of AIDS and can occur in other conditions.

For proper functioning of the immune system, especially the HMI, the participation of nonimmune cells and complement is critical to effectively protect the host against infectious agents. Both the complement system and phagocytes must function normally for antibody to provide host defense. Phagocytes are divided into neutrophils and macrophages (monocytes). A complete evaluation of phagocyte functions includes the following tests:

neutrophil count in peripheral blood;
nitroblue tetrazolium reduction;
chemotaxis;
phagocytosis;
killing ability.

However, not all of these tests are needed in screening for abnormalities. The absolute neutrophil count should be obtained by Wright's stain of a peripheral blood smear. This may reveal any neutrophil morphologic abnormalities. A polymorphonuclear cell (PMN) count less than $1000/mm^3$ is associated with an increased risk of infection. There are many etiologies of neutropenia including infections, drugs, and heredity. Neutropenia that is drug or chemical induced may be due to peripheral polymorphonuclear neutrophil (PMN) destruction from an autoimmunity or to depression of granulocyte formation in the bone marrow.

Critical functions of neutrophils are chemotaxis, phagocytosis, and killing of ingested microbial agents. Interference with any one of these functions can produce clinical disease. Ingestion and oxidative killing functions of neutrophils can be measured using the nitroblue tetrazolium reduction test. It is a limited test and is most useful for the diagnosis of chronic granulomatous disease. Another test of phagocytosis is the elic tation of chemiluminescence measured by scintillation counter.

Lymphocyte transformation tests can be conducted using a combination of mitogen stimulation (Con-A, pokeweed mitogen, or phytohemagglutinin [PHA]), soluble antigen to which lymphocytes are exposed in culture, or a culture of mixed lymphocytes.

METALS

Human exposure to metals is primarily occupationally related. Some metals are known immunotoxicants in animals as well as in humans (110, 111). Inorganic arsenic, lead, mercury, cadmium, chromium, nickel, and beryllium are present as contaminants from a variety of occupational and industrial processes. Exposure to inorganic lead, mercury, and cadmium has been known to produce glomerulonephritis secondary to glomerular basement membrane (GBM) deposition of anti-GBM antibodies (110–112). Clinical manifestations include proteinuria and occasionally a nephrotic syndrome. Metal-induced glomerulonephritis does not appear to be dose related. An immune glomerulonephritis may occur in up to 10% of patients receiving gold salt therapy for rheumatoid arthritis (112).

Cadmium is reported to produce renal tubular lesions as well as glomerulonephritis (112). Animal studies have demonstrated IgG glomerular deposits in the basement membrane as well as antibodies directed against GBM glycoproteins following chronic cadmium exposure. Cadmium has been shown to suppress antibody formation in animals and has been epidemiologically linked to respiratory cancer (110–113).

While lead can reduce host resistance to infection as well as interfere with reproductive functions, (110, 114) lead-induced immunotoxicity in humans has not been well documented. One study, which examined the effect of lead on 12 children documented to have measurable blood lead concentrations, did not demonstrate any significant effect on major immunoglobulin concentrations, total complement, C3 component of complement, or the antigenic response to tetanus toxoid (115, 116).

Metals can produce dermal and respiratory problems ranging from rashes to occupationally induced asthma. Chromium, beryllium, and platinum are particularly potent sensitizing metals and produce a variety of hypersensitivity pulmonary diseases as well as dermal lesions following human exposure (117, 118). Hexavalent chromium compounds can produce both corrosive and irritating effects following dermal exposure which consists of skin ulceration, dermatitis, and nasal septum ulceration (119). Chromium, a shiny white metal, is nontoxic in the elemental state. Chromium salts, trioxides, and chromic acid are strong irritants and oxidants which can produce immune-mediated glomerulonephritis (112, 119). Chronic inhalation of chromium dust can produce asthma and reactive airway disease (120).

Beryllium can cause pulmonary disease in milligram and microgram amounts. Controlling environmental air concentrations of beryllium has been demonstrated to control acute pulmonary disease in workers; however, chronic pulmonary disease is not dose related, and minute exposures can be a definite risk factor. Beryllium in all forms can cause human disease, usually via inhalation. Acute beryllium inhalation can cause tracheobronchitis and necrosis of the mucous membranes of the tracheobronchial area as well as conjunctivitis and rashes. Berylliosis may be delayed for several years post exposure. Chronic beryllium disease is characterized by granulomatous lesions in the lungs, skin, spleen, liver, lymph nodes, and kidneys. Acute exposure to beryllium dusts can produce inflammatory pneumonitis. Immunotoxicity from beryllium exposure is thought to occur through an antibody-mediated sensitization process (121, 122). Blastogenic transformation of lymphocytes occurs in the presence of beryllium sulfate in tissue cultures from patients with chronic berylliosis, but not in human controls (121, 122). A specific lymphocyte transformation test can be performed on blood and lung lavage lymphocytes of persons exposed to beryllium. This blood lymphocyte transformation testing is recommended as a specific and sensitive screening tool for exposed workers (see chapter on beryllium). Nodular granulomatous, noncaseating lesions have been documented in workers with inhalational exposure only. Direct skin contact with beryllium can cause hypersensitivity dermatitis. Beryllium is a potent sensitizing metal which can produce pulmonary and dermal disease via immunologic mechanisms not fully understood. Epidemiologic data also suggest an association between beryllium and lung cancer.

Nickel and nickel compounds (nickel, nickel carbonyl, nickel sulfate, nickel hydroxide, and nickel carbonate) can induce dermal as well as pulmonary disease. Nickel is associated with both lung and nasal cancer in exposed human populations (123). Workers who chronically inhale high concentrations of nickel dust may develop asthma. In addition, high environmental nickel exposure can cause nasal septum necrosis (124). Nickel carbonyl, a potent toxin the toxicity of which can be delayed hours after exposure, can produce a severe, delayed pulmonary distress syndrome consisting of pneumonitis and cerebral edema. Nickel carbonyl is metabolized in the body to Ni^{++} and carbon monoxide (124). Nickel carbonyl is an animal teratogen. Nickel is also a cause of allergic contact dermatitis (124). Nickel has been reported to be a stimulus for lymphocyte blastogenesis transformation in human lymphocytes and has been shown to bind directly to lymphocyte cell surface membranes (123).

Chronic exposure to manganous compounds can result in increased pulmonary infections as well as neurologic effects similar to parkinsonism (124). Manganese dioxide inhalational exposure can reduce host defense mechanisms of the lungs and result in pulmonary inflammation and impairment of pulmonary macrophages (124).

Chronic arsenic toxicity can produce hematologic effects with resulting disturbance of erythropoiesis, thrombocytopenia, granulocytopenia, and other blood dyscrasias (110, 111). Lymphatic cancers and leukemia have been associated with chronic arsenic exposure (110, 111). Arsenic-related dermatologic lesions include eczematous dermatitis, follicular dermatitis, and hyperkeratosis. Arsenic is also associated with basal cell and squamous cell skin cancers. Arsenic-related increased incidence of respiratory cancers has been reported in epidemiologic studies of smelter workers (125, 126). Selenium is a unique metal in that it may enhance the immune response. This immune enhancement has been demonstrated in animal models.

It is of interest to note that the metals that are considered to be primary irritants and human sensitizers are also those associated with human carcinogenesis (127).

Halogenated Polyaromatic Hydrocarbons

These compounds include polychlorinated biphenyls (PCBs), phenols, chlorinated dibenzo-*p*-dioxins, dibenzofurans, hexachlorobenzene, pentachlorophenol, and polybrominated biphenyls (PBBs) (128). PCBs were produced in the United States under the name Aroclor, a mixture of 209 congeners of PCBs (129). Following reports of animal and human toxicity, the production of PCBs in the United States was suspended in 1977. About half of the PCBs produced between 1966 and 1974 were used in electrical transformers (129). Even though PCBs in transformers are being replaced, a significant number still contain large amounts to which maintenance and repair personnel are still at risk for exposure. PCBs are inert and are resistant to environmental degradation and thus tend to accumulate in the environment. Human exposure occurs via inhalation or ingestion. The high lipid solubility of these compounds allows for them to accumulate up the food chain (130). Disposal of PCBs has taken place in hazardous waste sites and thus human exposures will continue to occur. These chemicals are classified as polychlorinated biphenyls, polybrominated biphenyls, polychlorinated dibenzo-*p*-dioxins (PCDD), and polychlorinated dibenzofurans (PCDF).

Toxic effects of PCBs include chloracne, ocular irritation, arthritis, gastrointestinal symptoms, and hepatotoxicity. One of the most intensely studied PCB compounds is 2,3,7,8-tetrachlorodibenzo-*p*-dioxin (TCDD), a contaminant of the herbicide 2,4,5-trichlorphenoxyacetic acid (2,4,5-T) (130). In 1973 an incidence in Michigan involving the contamination of dairy cattle feed with PBBs highlighted the concern over these compounds (131). Local farmers and Michigan residents who consumed these contaminated dairy products were found to have PBBs in the plasma. Immunologic investigations demonstrated that 34% of farm residents and 59% of PBB manufacturing workers had a reduction in T-lymphocyte numbers (132). B-cell and T-cell lymphocyte blastogenesis was reduced in exposed farmers and workers as compared with controls. In the Michigan population overall, T-cells and B-cells were normal as compared with controls (132). Two occurrences of rice oil contamination with human consumption of contaminated food have been extensively studied. These human exposures occurred in Japan in 1968 and in Taiwan in 1979 (130). In addition, PCDFs were found to be contaminants of PCBs. Animal immunotoxicology studies have demonstrated potent effects of these chemicals on the thymus, host resistance, cell-mediated immunity, and humoral-mediated immunity.

In humans, the immunologic health effects of PCBs has been difficult to demonstrate. Chloracne, a recognized dermatologic effect of PCB exposure, is probably the best described toxicity of the compounds along with hepatotoxicity (130). Although animal studies have proven the carcinogenicity of PCBs, there is no conclusive evidence that exposure to PCBs results in an increased incidence of cancer in humans (130). Small short-term epidemiologic studies of capacitor manufacturing workers exposed to PCBs have not indicated increased incidence of cancer (129). Other epidemiologic studies have also failed to demonstrate an increased incidence in cancer rates of exposed humans (133–135). In the 1979 incident in Taiwan, over 200 people were exposed to PCBs as a contaminant in rice oil. Chang studied the delayed immune response in 30 patients from the Taiwan incidence and compared their response with 50 controls (130). His findings documented that dermal lesions appeared to correlate with whole blood PCB concentrations. He also demonstrated decreases in IgM and IgA, but no effect on IgG. In addition, there was a decrease in the percentage of T-lymphocytes and T-lymphocyte helper cells as well as a suppression of delayed hypersensitivity to antigens (130).

Health effects from longterm exposure to TCDD have been reported following spills or contaminations which resulted in human exposure. In 1971, sludge oil contaminated with TCDD was sprayed on dirt roads at various sites in eastern Missouri (136). Twelve years later, in 1983, one of the nine residential sites where TCDD spraying had occurred became the focus of health effects investigation. The area chosen had TCDD concentrations in surrounding soil ranging from 39–1100 ppb. The mobile homes in the area had inside dust concentrations above 1 ppb. The study included 155 exposed individuals. There was no documented increase in the number of medical complaints above the control population in the study nor any incidences of chloracne or increased incidence of cancer. Nor was there any increased incidence of spontaneous abortions, reproductive problems, or congenital malformations. Basic liver function tests of all exposed individuals were normal. However, subclinical hepatotoxicity was suggested by some of the assays, particularly higher mean urinary uroporphyrin concentrations in exposed persons and correlation of serum levels of five liver enzymes (aspartate aminotransferase [AST], alanine aminotransferase [ALT], γ-glutamyltranspeptidase [GGTP], alkaline phosphatase, and alanine aminopeptidase) with years of residence at the contaminated site. Immunologic evaluation of the exposed individuals revealed an elevated incidence of anergy and relative anergy compared with controls. T-cell surface marker analyses demonstrated statistically significant decreases in percentages of T3, T4, and T11 cells in exposed groups. The number of non-T-lymphocytes in peripheral blood samples was elevated in the exposed group. There was no significant difference in T-lymphocyte proliferative response to mitogen stimulation nor cytotoxic T-cell activity in either of the groups. Overall, the exposed group had a nonstatistically significant increased frequency of abnormal T-cell subsets as well as a nonstatistically significant abnormality in T-cell function (136). The presence of in vitro immune alterations in the exposed population with the absence of overt clinical signs and symptoms of immune deficiency points to a subclinical immunotoxicity from TCDD following prolonged exposure.

Another study on individuals exposed to TCDD for 10 years who lived or worked near contaminated areas in Missouri showed no difference in the study population as compared with the control group in delayed hypersensitivity, T-cell subsets, and cytotoxic T-cell proliferation assays (137). A separate study reported health effects of TCDD in children following an environmental accident near Sevso, Italy, in 1976 (138). The exposed children totaled approximately 1500 and ranged in age from 6–10. Immunologic parameters were not studied, but liver function tests showed alterations in alanine aminotransferase and γ-glutamyltransferase.

An immunologic investigation of 55 transformer repairmen with high adipose concentrations of PCBs has been reported (129). These workers were predominantly exposed to Aroclor 1260 and some to Aroclor 1242. Physical examinations as well as immunologic evaluations were performed. Delayed hypersensitivity, evaluated with an intradermal injection of mumps and trichophytin antigens, was no different than in the nonexposed controls. There was no incidence of chloracne in this study.

While animal studies have supported the immunotoxicity of PCBs, human studies to date have been questionable in terms of immunologic health effects. The spectrum of dioxin toxicity is currently under evaluation by the EPA.

Pesticides and Insecticides

Pesticide exposure occurs mainly in agricultural workers, pesticide producers, and consumers of agricultural products. These include cholinesterase-inhibiting as well as noncholinesterase-inhibiting compounds along with a wide variety of pyrethroids, phenolic derivatives, and organic solvents. Defined immunotoxicity of pesticides in humans is limited to a few studies. However, animal studies have demonstrated wide-ranging immunologic dysfunctions including atrophy of lymphoid tissues as well as cell-mediated immunity and humoral-mediated immunity (HMI) immunosuppression induced by a variety of pesticides. Prenatal exposure of mice to chlordane has resulted in depressed cell-mediated immunity.

Bioaccumulation of chlorinated pesticides in adipose tissue of humans is documented by fat biopsy. These pesticides can be detected in serum as well as adipose tissue in a range of parts per million concentrations (139). Dichlorodiphenyltrichloroethane (DDT) and its metabolite DDE are detected in adipose tissue and serum of nonexposed individuals due to bioaccumulation through the normal food chain. Other pesticides found in adipose and serum of the general population include benzene hexachloride and its isomers, lindane, chlordane, heptachlor, heptachlor epoxide, and dieldrin. These organochlorine pesticides can be assayed for in adipose tissue as well as serum. Their presence in the general population creates a confounding factor. The presence of these pesticides and their metabolites in adipose tissue and serum at low parts per million and parts per billion do not appear to constitute an immunologic health risk in terms of altered host defense in the general population. Again, their presence indicates exposure and not disease.

Contact dermatitis from pesticide exposure is probably the most commonly recognized health effect and can occur from dermal exposure to organophosphates as well as a wide variety of fungicides, fumigants, and pyrethroid compounds. Autoimmunity in humans exposed to pesticides has been suggested (140). Studies of human leukocyte functions in vitro have demonstrated alterations following pesticide exposure (141). Cultures of human lymphocytes undergoing PHA mitogen blastogenic stimulation in the presence of pesticides demonstrated inhibition (141). Carbamates inhibited lymphocyte PHA stimulation by 10%, organophosphates by 11–18%, organochlorine pesticides (BHC, endrin, DDT) by 11–17% in this study. Lymphocyte stimulation in response to PHA as well as rosette formation of sheep RBCs when exposed to human lymphocytes are characteristics of T-lymphocytes. DDT was a potent inhibitor of in vitro human erythrocyte rosette formation.

In the same study, DDT did not alter neutrophil chemotaxis. However, methyl parathion and benzyl benzoate did inhibit PMN chemotaxis (141).

Studies with lindane have shown inhibiting effects on human lymphocyte PHA mitogenesis. Lindane was found to alter T-lymphocyte membrane-associated events leading to mitogen activation by PHA (142). Other studies have shown defects in chemotaxis, nitro blue tetrazolium (NBT) reduction by phagocytes, and phagocytosis in occupationally exposed workers (140). In addition, the incidence of infectious episodes was higher in these workers (143). In contrast, children exposed to DDT did not show alteration in antibody titers to diphtheria immunization (144).

Allergic and Hypersensitivity Pulmonary Disease

Between 2 and 15% of all asthma in industrialized countries is due to occupational chemical exposure (145). Allergic-mediated asthma has been documented to occur from sources including chemicals, vegetable matter, and proteins. Repeated exposure to the offending agent is required to produce sensitization. Once this IgE-mediated problem occurs, any exposure to minute amounts can precipitate bronchospasm. Sensitizing environmental contaminants and chemicals act as haptens by combining with proteins present in mucosal surfaces or to albumin and other serum proteins. Following repeated exposure, IgE antibodies can form directed against this hapten complex.

Occupationally related immunologic lung disease may present as asthma, hypersensitivity pneumonitis, or fibrotic lung disease. Reactive hypersensitivity of the airways that is nonimmunologically mediated can also be a result of exposure to irritant chemicals. Bronchospasm and cough to some degree is the usual clinical outcome. Stimulation of subepithelial vagal receptors by chemicals inhaled as vapors, aerosols, or dusts can induce this clinical syndrome (146). Many common chemicals and respiratory irritants can produce reactive airway dysfunction.

Allergenic metals can cause dermal and pulmonary lesions. There are 15 metals with the properties of both allergenicity and carcinogenicity. Arsenic, beryllium, chromium, and nickel are accepted as both animal and human carcinogens as well as potent sensitizing agents. Metals that are carcinogenic in animals or humans are also allergenic (146).

Trimellitic anhydride, a component of resin curing agents, toluene diisocyanate (TDI), methylene diphenyl diisocyanate (MDI), and phthalatic anhydrides (plasticizers) are well known precipitators of allergic asthma (146, 147). Trimellitic anhydride may produce an asthmatic syndrome, an irritant syndrome, and a sensitivity pneumonitis syndrome. The biotechnology industry is an occupational source of exposure to a variety of proteins, peptides, and chemicals that can result in IgE-mediated asthma. This includes enzymes such as papain, pepsin, alkaline phosphatase, glucosoxidase, peroxidase, ribonuclease; acrylamide monomers and aliphatic amines; and chemicals used to haptenize drugs to albumin molecules such as carbodiimides, toluene diisocyanate, glutaraldehyde, and phenylenediamine.

Nickel sulfate exposure has been demonstrated to produce a positive inhalational challenge test as well as antibody formation (148). Platinum workers can experience not only pulmonary sensitization with development of specific IgE and asthma, but also conjunctivitis and rhinitis (148).

Formaldehyde exposure is widespread due to its presence in multiple commonly used products including fabrics, wood products, particle board, and carpets. Formaldehyde is a direct upper airway and respiratory irritant at concentrations ranging from 1–3 ppm (149). Recognition of the health effects from low level formaldehyde exposure has recently resulted in a lowering of the previous OSHA standard of 3 ppm to 1 ppm. A variety of health effects including respiratory irritation, ocular irritation, headache, and cough can occur at formaldehyde concentrations between 0.05 and 1 ppm. Antibodies to the hapten complex of formaldehyde and human albumin have been demonstrated (109). Asthma secondary to formaldehyde exposure has been demonstrated; however, formaldehyde-induced asthma remains rare (150). Instead, due to its high water solubility, formaldehyde deposits mainly in the moist mucous membranes of the upper airway and produces a direct, nonimmunologic irritant effect on the respiratory system.

Hypersensitivity pneumonitis can be acute or chronic. The acute form of chemically induced hypersensitivity pneumonitis presents with fever, chills, nonproductive cough, chest pain, and dyspnea and usually resolves in 24 hours (148). Chronic pneumonitis from an immunologic etiology may occur following a chronic or subchronic exposure to low concentrations of chemicals. Fever, cough, fatigue, weight loss, and shortness of breath are the clinical manifestations. Permanent pulmonary fibrosis can occur unless the exposure is terminated. Chemicals known to produce hypersensitivity pulmonary disease include anhydrides, beryllium, and a variety of isocyanates, particularly toluene isocyanate (148).

A one-time exposure or multiple inhalational exposures to certain irritant chemicals can result in reactive airway disease manifested by chronic cough, broncospasm, chest tightness, and shortness of breath on reexposure to the same or other irritating chemicals (151). Chemicals that produce direct effects on the pulmonary airways usually do so via release of histamine from mast cells instead of an immunologic mechanism. Dust and cotton are known to produce a nonantigenic release of histamine that can result in cough and bronchospasm.

Immunologic Fibrotic Pulmonary Disease

Fibrotic pulmonary disease associated with immunologic abnormalities can occur as a result of the chronic inhalation of dusts and humanmade fiberogenic materials including asbestos, mica, graphite, silica, and beryllium. The release of lysosomal enzymes from macrophages occurs as a result of the phagocytosis of these humanmade fiberogenics. Pulmonary fibrosis, or chronic granulomatous disease in the case of beryllium, is a result of exposure. In addition, there are other immunologic abnormalities which occur as a result of human exposure to these fibers.

Patients with silicosis have been found to have elevated circulating immune complexes, including antinuclear antibody and rheumatoid factor (152). No direct correlation between severity of disease and the presence of immune complexes is documented. In addition, patients with silicosis have documented increased immunoglobulins with increased secretory IgA (148).

Asbestos-related lung disease has immunologic features. Asbestos fibers activate both classical and alternate complement pathways (148). Activity of natural killer cells and antibody-dependent cellular cytotoxicity (K cells) has been demonstrated to be depressed in patients with asbestosis (152–154). In ad-

dition, asbestosis is associated with a decrease in the number of T-cells, increased immune complexes, and increased serum immunoglobulin concentrations (148).

Chemical Dermatitis

Dermatitis from environmental exposures can be immunologic or nonimmunologic. Dermatitis secondary to contact from irritant and sensitizing chemicals is the most commonly seen occupational injury and is caused by a variety of chemical agents. Exposures occur by: (a) direct contact with chemicals in vapor phase, liquids, or solids; examples are chemicals containing formaldehyde, phenols, amines, metals, acids, alkalis, ethylene oxide, and other irritant chemicals; (b) systemic exposure via inhalation of airborne chemicals either volatilized or carried on particles of dust via contaminated ventilation systems, such as nickel dermatitis and berylliosis.

Rashes may appear in a variety of areas including exposed surfaces of the neck, arms, legs, face, and hands and nonexposed areas as well. Frequently, chemicals or fiberogenic materials such as fiberglass accumulate in work clothes and are in chronic contact with the skin. Soluble chemicals in a vapor phase may dissolve in the sweat present on skin surfaces. Clinical symptoms of airborne dermal irritants are itching, burning sensation, and ocular irritation. Rashes may be evident, and their clinical picture may vary from true urticarial lesions, papillar lesions, or maculopapular lesions. These airborne dermatoses have been subdivided into allergic contact dermatitis, nonimmunologic urticarial rash, phototoxic contact dermatitis, photoallergic contact dermatitis, nonallergic contact dermatitis, and acne venenata (155). The more commonly recognized contact urticarial rashes are to formaldehyde and nickel in occupational environments (155, 156). Nickel dermatitis can occur either by direct dermal exposure or via systemic exposure (157). Patients with sensitivity to nickel may develop a chronic course of eczema.

Contact dermatitis from corrosive chemicals such as cement, acids, and alkalis can be both a chemical burn from chromates and a contact dermatitis. Carbonless paper has recently been recognized as a source of human health effects including dermal and pulmonary irritation (158). Carbonless paper products contain a variety of irritating inks as well as formaldehyde.

Making a diagnosis of contact dermal allergy can be difficult, since many chemicals produce dermatitis via direct contact, nonimmunologic methods. Patch testing to prove the existence of cell-mediated immunologic dermatitis should be performed only by dermatologists with competence in this area. False-negative and false-positive results of patch testing are frequent (159).

Chemical Alteration of Phagocyte Function

Macrophages responsible for removing or neutralizing particles that invade the lungs are found in interstitial tissues of the alveoli or are free in the alveolar luminal surface. The effectiveness and efficiency of the phagocytosis and lysis functions by pulmonary macrophages dictate the ultimate level of pulmonary protection. Any chemical or particulate matter that interferes with either the absolute macrophage number or basic functions can produce pulmonary susceptibility to damage. Macrophage elimination of particulates involves (160):

1. chemotaxis;
2. opsonization by complement and antibody;

3. attachment of particle to phagocyte;
4. phagocytosis of particle;
5. formation of primary lysosome;
6. fusion with secondary lysosome; and
7. destruction of particle.

Interruption of normal pulmonary host defense can occur if any one event is interfered with by a pollutant. A variety of environmental pollutants stimulate increased numbers of macrophages in the pulmonary environment; these include lead oxide (PbO), nickel chloride ($NiCl_2$), nickel oxide (NiO), cadmium chloride ($CdCl_2$), carbon monoxide, quartz crystals, tobacco smoke, and a variety of environmental dusts (160). Some environmental contaminants such as silica, chrysotile asbestos, cadmium, acrolein, manganese dioxide, some lead oxides, and antimony reduce the absolute number of free pulmonary macrophages (160). Acute exposure of macrophages to ozone (O_3) or nitrogendioxide (NO_2) can decrease phagocytic activity and ability (160, 161). Other chemicals directly impairing phagocytic functions include nickel chloride ($NiCl_2$), cadmium, nickel, copper, mercury, zinc, platinum, vanadium oxides (V_2O_5), and cadmium oxide (CdO). The shape, size, chemical composition and surface area of the inhaled particles determine ultimate macrophage dysfunction.

The ultimate fate of the macrophage that ingests particles entering the respiratory system depends on whether the cell can destroy the particle or whether the particle destroys the cell. If the macrophage is killed, the toxin is then released into the lung environment to promote further damage. In some situations, the macrophage viability is effected, but cell lysis does not occur.

Interferon production by macrophages is depressed after exposure to ozone, automobile exhaust, and NO_2 (160). Alteration of macrophage lysosomal enzymes and release of these enzymes as well as other biologically active substances is promoted by certain environmental contaminants including release of prostaglandins, collagenase, elastase, plasminogen-activating factor, and lytic enzymes. Asbestos and silica particles stimulate the release of lysosomal enzymes which subsequently elicit inflammatory processes with tissue destruction and fibrosis of the lungs. Macrophage contents are then released to repeat the cycle (160, 161).

EXPOSURE VERSUS DISEASE

Dermatitis, asthma, and reactive airway disease are common clinical problems seen in occupational exposures involving sensitizing and irritant chemicals. Allergy and hypersensitivity can be caused by numerous chemicals used in occupational settings through direct contact with the chemical on the skin or through inhalation (Table 17.9). Pathotoxicology can also occur in liver, kidneys, and blood-forming organs secondary to altered immunologic responses. Detecting an immune system response and differentiating this response from adverse effects and disease secondary to a chemical exposure requires careful evaluation of the exposure circumstances, a thorough history and physical examination, and clinical immunologic laboratory testing. In addition, other disease states must be ruled out as a possible cause. Exposure to a chemical with a subsequent normal immune response must not be equated with disease. The normal immune response involves antigen encounter, lymphocyte activation, amplification of the immune response, and regulation of response (Table 17.10). So the presence of ac-

Table 17.9. Mechanisms Responsible for Chemically-Induced Hypersensitivity

Chemicals and/or metabolites are directly antigenic by themselves.

Chemicals or metabolites may haptenize with serum proteins to form new immunogens and autoantigens.
Chemicals or metabolites covalently bind to macromolecules present in the target organ areas of the lung, gastrointestinal tract, or skin.
Chemicals directly effect the immune system with activation of T-cell lymphocytes, activation of B-cell lines, and an increase in helper to suppressor T-cell ratio.

Autoantigens are released following tissue damage by chemical exposures.

There are shared antigen determinants between the chemical and tissue of the organism.

tivated lymphocytes indicates a normally responding immune system.

Exposure to a wide variety of chemicals occurs from occupational as well as home environments. Background chemical analysis of the air in both the home and occupational environment has revealed a complex mixture of volatile organic solvents to which individuals are exposed. Since most individuals spend the majority of their time indoors, chronic and long-term exposure to these chemicals occurs. As an example, concerns have arisen over exposure to low air concentrations of formaldehyde below the permissible occupational exposure limit of 1 ppm set by the Occupational Safety and Health Administration. Human health effects from exposure to low concentrations of compounds such as formaldehyde, trimellitic anhydride, diisocyanates, and organic hydrocarbon vapors can result in a variety of symptoms including ocular irritation, dermal irritation, chest tightness, cough, and severe headache. Misapplication of home pesticide spraying can also be a source of exposure to indoor air contaminants and a source of recognized illness from poor indoor air quality. Multiple low level chemical exposure is a fact of modern daily living, and health complaints arising from exposure to multiple chemicals are becoming more common.

In the process of deciding toxic causation, the clinician must account for the difference between exposure to a chemical with a resulting normal immune response and actual disease which may result from end organ damage or altered immune status. An example of this is the presence of antibodies to the conjugate of formaldehyde and human serum albumin. The presence of such IgG and IgM antibodies has been demonstrated in some individuals exposed to formaldehyde (109). The presence of these antibody titers means that haptenization of human serum proteins has occurred and that a normal immune response recognized the new immunogen. The presence of specific circulating IgG and IgM antibodies to formaldehyde-human serum albumin haptens demonstrates that exposure to formaldehyde can result in immune system stimulation to a neoantigen. How-

Table 17.10. Normal Response of The Immune System

1. Encounter of lymphocyte with antigen
2. Antigen recognition by the immune system
3. Activation of lymphocytes
4. Amplification of the immune response
5. Immune discrimination between self and non-self
6. Regulation and control over the immune response

ever, the clinician must be careful not to interpret this normal immune relapse as disease.

FUTURE DIRECTIONS

Future research in immunotoxicology will be spent in further development and refinement of relevant host resistance models; evaluation of in vitro models; refinement of reversibility modules in current assays; and, finally, a vigorous effort to identify those genetic elements that play a role in predisposition to certain immunotoxicities. As more data are gathered, immunotoxicology will undoubtedly remain both an important and difficult subdiscipline of toxicology. The useful intersections of immunotoxicology with occupational medicine and environmental health are only now being realized.

REFERENCES

1. Cavagnaro J. Immunotoxicology and the new biotechnology. Immunol Today 1987;8:102–104.
2. Sell S. Immunology, immunopathology and immunity. New York: Elsevier, 1987:1.
3. Talmage DW. The acceptance and rejection of immunological concepts. In: Paul WE, Fatham CG, Metzger H, eds. Annual review of immunology. Palo Alto: Annual Reviews, 1986:1–12.
4. Cohen IR. The self, the world and autoimmunity. Sci Am 1988;258:52–60.
5. Torok-Storb B. Cellular interactions. Blood 1988;72:373–385.
6. Kripke ML. Immunoregulation of carcinogenesis: past, present, and future. J Natl Cancer Inst 1988;80:722–727.
7. Jerne NK. Idiotypic networks and other preconceived ideas. Immunol Rev 1984;79:5–24.
8. Chase MW. Specificity of serological reactions: Landsteiner centennial. Ann NY Acad Sci 1970;169:9–10.
9. Platzer E, Gramatzki M, Rollinghoff M, Kalden JR. Lymphokines and monokines in the clinic. Immunol Today 1986;7:185–187.
10. Katz DH. Genetic control of cell-cell interactions. Pharmacol Rev 1982;34:51–62.
11. Purtillo DT, Linder J, Seemayer TA. Inherited and acquired immunodeficiency disorders. In: Colvin RB, Bhan AK, McCluskey RT, eds. Diagnostic immunopathology. New York: Raven Press, 1988:121–150.
12. Webster ADB. Immunodeficiency disease. In: Holborow EJ, Reeves WG, eds. Immunology in medicine: a comprehensive guide to clinical immunology. New York: Grune & Stratton, 1983:223–241.
13. Shultz LD, Sidman CL. Genetically determined murine models of immunodeficiency. In: Paul WE, Fathman CG, Metzger H, eds. Annual review of immunology. Palo Alto: Annual Reviews, 1987:367–404.
14. Buckley RH. Immunodeficiency diseases. JAMA 1987;258:2841–2850.
15. Stahl RE, Friedman-Kline A, Dubin R, Marmor M, Zolla-Paznev S. Immunologic abnormalities in homosexual men. Am J Med 1982;73:171–171.
16. Gallo R. The AIDS virus: Sc Am 1987;256:38–48.
17. Barre-Sinoussi F, Chermann IC, Rey F, et al. T-Lymphotrophic retrovirus from a patient at risk for acquired immune deficiency syndrome (AIDS). Science 1983;220:868–871.
18. Weber JN, Weiss RA. HIV infection: the cellular picture. Sci Am 1988;259:81–87.
19. Fauci AS. The human immunodeficiency virus: infectivity and mechanisms of pathogenesis. Science 1988;239:617–622.
20. Redfeild RR, Burke DS. HIV infection: the clinical picture. Sci Am 1988;259:70–79.
21. Glatt AE, Chirgwin K, Landesman LH. Treatment of infections associated with human immunodeficiency virus. N Engl J Med 1988;318:1439–1448.
22. Chiampi NP, Sundberg RD, Klompus JP, Wilson AJ. Cryptospiroidal enteritis and pneumocystis pneumonia in a homosexual man. Hum Pathol 1983;14:734–737.
23. Pitchenik AE, Fertel D, Bloch AB. Mycobacterial disease: epidemiology, diagnosis, treatment and prevention. Clin Chest Med 1988;9:425–441.
24. Fineberg HV. The social dimensions of AIDS. Sci Am 1988;259:106–112.
25. Shoham J. Vulnerability to toxic or therapeutic immunomodulation—as two complementary aspects of age and nutrition dependent immunodeficiency. In: Berlin A, Dean J, Draper M, Smith E, Spreafico F, eds. Immunotoxicology. Boston: Martinus Nijhoff Publishers, 1987:389–410.
26. Zbinden LC. A toxicologist's view of immunotoxicology. In: Berlin A, Dean J, Draper M, Smith E, Spreafico F, eds. Immunotoxicology. Boston: Martinus Nijhoff Publishers, 1987:1–11.
27. Heise ER. Diseases associated with immunosuppression. Environ Health Perspect 1982;43:9–19.
28. Dean JH, Murray MJ, Ward ED. Toxic responses of the immune system. In: Klassen CD, Amdur MO, Doul J, eds. Toxicology: the basic science of poisons. New York: Macmillan Publishing Company, 1986:245–285.
29. Gordon-Smith EC. Immune drug-induced blood dyscrasias. In: Gibson GG, Hubbard R, Parke DV, eds. Immunotoxicology. New York: Academic Press, 1983:161–170.
30. Cornacoff JB, Lauer LD, House RV, et al. Evaluation of the immunotoxicity of B-hexachlorocyclohexane (B-HCH). Int J Immunopharmacol 1988;10:293–299.
31. Bradley GS, Morahan PS. Approaches to assessing host resistance. Environ Health Perspec 1982;43:61–69.
32. Bekesi JG, Roboz J, Fischbein A, Roboz JP, Solomon S, Greaves J. Immunological, biochemical, and clinical consequences of exposure to polybrominated biphenyls. In: Dean JH, Luster MI, Munson AE, Amost H, eds. Immunology and immunopharmacology. New York: Raven Press, 1985:393–406.
33. Dean J, Luster M, Murray M, Lauer L. Approaches and methodology for examining the immunological effects of xenobiotics. In: Gibson GG, Hubbard R, Parke D, eds. Immunotoxicology. New York: Academic Press, 1983:205–218.
34. Burchiel SW, Hadley WM, Barton SL, Fincher RH, Lauer LD, Dean JH. Persistant suppression of humoral immunity produced by 7,12-dimethylbenz(a)anthracene (DMBA) in B6C3F1 mice: correlation with changes in spleen cell surface markers detected by flow cytometry. Int J Immunopharmacol 1988;10:369–376.
35. Simpson E. Function of the MHC. Immunol Suppl 1988;1:27–30.
36. Teal JM, Abraham KM. The regulation of antibody class expression. Immunol Today 1987;8:122–126.
37. Chang KJ, Hsieh KH, Lee TP, Tang SY, Tung TC. Immunologic evaluation of patients with PCB-poisoning: determination of lymphocyte subpopulations. Toxicol Appl Pharmacol 1981;61:58–63.
38. Berlin A, Dean J, Draper M, Smith E, Spreafico F. Synopsis, conclusions and recommendations. In: Berlin A, Dean J, Draper M, Smith E, Spreafico F, eds. Proceedings of the International Seminar on the Immunological System as a Target for Toxic Damage—present status, open problems, and future perspectives. Boston: Martinus Nijhoff Publishers, 1987:XI–XXVII.
39. Bates DV. The health effects of air pollution. J Respir Dis 1980;1:29–37.
40. Graham JA, Gardner DE. Immunotoxicity of air pollutants. In: Dean J, Luster MI, Munson AE, Amos H, eds. Immunotoxicology and immunopharmacology. New York: Raven Press, 1985:367–380.
41. Rook GAW. Immunology of infectious disease. In: Holborow EJ, Reeves WG, eds. Immunology in medicine: a comprehensive guide to clinical immunology. New York: Grune & Stratton, 1983:159–178.
42. Dean JH, Luster MI, Boorman GA, Leubke RW, Lauer LD. Application of tumor, bacterial and parasite susceptibility assays to study immune alterations induced by environmental chemicals. Environ Health Perspect 1982;43:81–88.
43. Luster MI, Munson AE, Thomas PT, et al. Development of a testing battery to assess chemically-induced immunotoxicity: national toxicology program's guidelines for immunotoxicity evaluation in mice. Fundam Appl Toxicol 1988;10:2–19.
44. House RV, Dean JH. *Trypanosoma musculi*: characterization of the T-lymphocyte dependency of immunity by selective immunomodulation of the mouse. *Mus musculus.* Exp Parasitol 1988;67:104–115.
45. Brooks BO, Reed ND. The effect of trypan blue on early control of trypanosoma nusculi parasitemia in mice. J Reticuloendothel Soc 1979;25:235–238.
46. Dempsey WL, Morahan PS. Immune mechanisms of host resistance to viruses and assessment of immunotoxicologic effects. In: Dean JH, Luster MI, Munson AE, Amos H, eds. Immunotoxicology and immunopharmacology. New York: Raven Press, 1985:55–68.
47. Harris G. Immunosuppressive drugs and carcinogenesis. In: Gibson GG, Hubbard R, Parke DV, eds. Immunotoxicology. New York: Academic Press, 1983:391–399.
48. Herberman RB. Immunological mechanisms of host resistance to tumors. In: Dean JH, Luster MI, Munson AE, Amos H, eds. Immunotoxicology and immunopharmacology. New York: Raven Press, 1958:69–78.
49. Gatti RA, Good RA. Occurrence of malignancy in immunodeficiency disease: a literature review. Cancer 1971;28:98–99.
50. Penn I. Development of cancer in transplant patients. Adv Surg 1978;12:155–191.

51. Bekesi JG, Roboz JP, Fischbein A, Selikoff IJ. Clinical immunology studies in individuals exposed to environmental chemicals. In: Berlin A, Dean J, Draper MH, Smith EMB, Speafico F, eds. Immunotoxicology. New York: Raven Press, 1988:347–361.

52. Penn I. Lymphomas complicating organ transplantation. Transplant Proc 1983;15:2790–2797.

53. Penn I. The occurrence of cancer in immune deficiencies. Curr Probl Cancer 1982;6:1–64.

54. Murray MJ, Kerkvliet NI, Ward EC, Dean JH. Models for the evaluation of tumor resistance following chemical or drug exposure. In: Dean JH, Luster MI, Munson AE, Amos H, eds. Immunotoxicology and immunopharmacology. New York: Raven Press, 1985:113–122.

55. Burnet FM. The concept of immunological surveillance. Prog Exp Tumor Res 1970;13:1–27.

56. Grossman Z, Herberman RB. ''Immune surveillance'' without immunogenicity. Immunol Today 1986;7:128–131.

57. Kervliet NI, Baecher-Steppan LG, Schmitz JA. Immunotoxicity of pentachlorophenol (PCP): increased susceptibility to tumor growth in adult mice fed technical grade PCP-diets. Toxicol Appl Pharmacol 1982;62:55–64.

58. Parker CW. Allergic reactions in man. Pharmacol Rev 1989;34:85–103.

59. Kolb H, Toyka KV, Gleichman E. Histocompatibility antigens and chemical reactivity in autoimmunity. Immunol Today 1987;8:3–6.

60. Rolink AG, van der Meer WGK, Melief CJM, Gleichman E. Intra-H-2 requirements for the induction of maximal positive and negative allogeneic effects in vitro. Eur J Immunol 1983;13:191–197.

61. Condemi JJ. The autoimmune diseases. JAMA 1987;258:2920–2929.

62. Smith HR, Steinberg AD. Autoimmunity—a perspective. In: Paul WE, Fathman GC, Metzger H, eds. Annual review of immunology. Palo Alto: Annual Reviews, 1983:175–210.

63. Daniell WE. Occupational solvent exposure and glomerulonephritis. JAMA 1988;259:2280–2283.

64. Hamilton HE, Morgan DP, Simmons A. A pesticide (dieldrin)-induced immunohemolytic anemia. Environ Res 1978;17:155–164.

65. Michaelson JH, McCoy JP, Hirszel P, Bigazzi PE. Mercury-induced autoimmune glomerulonephritis in inbred rats. I. Kinetics and species specificity of autoimmune responses. Surv Synth Pathol Res 1985;4:401–411.

66. Bigazzi PE. Autoimmunity induced by chemicals. J Toxicol Clin Toxicol 1988;26:125–156.

67. Smiley JD, Moore SE. Molecular mechanisms of autoimmunity. Am J Med Sci 1988;295:478–496.

68. Venables P. Epstein-Barr virus infection and autoimmunity in rhematoid arthritis. Ann Rheum Dis 1988;47:265–269.

69. Koffler R, Dixon FJ, Theofilopoulos AN. The genetic origin of autoantibodies. Immunol Today 1987;8:374–378.

70. Cooke A, Lydyard PN, Roitt IM. Mechanisms of autoimmunity: a role for cross-reactive idiotypes. Immunol Today 1983;4:170–175.

71. Feldman M, Londei M, Kissonerghis M, et al. Regulation of HLA class II expression and the pathogenesis of autoimmunity. Concepts Immunopathol 1988;5:44–56.

72. Parker CW. Hapten immunology and allergic reactions in humans. Arthritis Rheum 1981;23:1024–1036.

73. Burek CL, Rose NL. Autoantibodies. In: Colvin RB, Bhan AK, McCluskey RT, eds. Diagnostic Immunopathology. New York: Raven Press, 1988:87–120.

74. Bigazzi PE. Mechanisms of chemical-induced autoimmunity. In: Dean JH, Luster MI, Munson AE, Amos H, eds. Immunotoxicology & Immunopharmacology. New York: Raven Press, 1985:277–290.

75. Kirtland HH, Mohler DN, Horowitz DA. Methyldopa inhibition of suppressor-lymphocyte function: a proposed cause of autoimmune hemolytic anemia. N Engl J Med 1980;302:825–832.

76. Miller KB, Salem K. Immune regulatory abnormalities produced by procainamide. Am J Med 1982;73:487–492.

77. Druet P, Hirsch F, Sapin C, Druet E, Bellon B. Immune dysregulation and autoimmunity induced by toxic agents. Transplant Proc 1982;14:484–484.

78. Pelletier L, Pasquier R, Hirsch F, Sapain C, Druet P. Mercury-induced lymphocyte auto-reactivity. In: Gibson GG, Hubbard R, Parke V, eds. Immunotoxicology. New York: Academic Press, 1983:437–442.

79. Kaliner M, Eggleston PA, Matthews KP. Rhinitis and asthma. JAMA 1987;258:2851–2873.

80. Salvaggio JE. Overview of occupational immunologic lung disease. J Allergy Clin Immunol 1982;70:5–10.

81. Chan-Yeung M, Lam S. Occupational asthma. Am Rev Respir Dis 1986;133:696–703.

82. Stanworth DR. Mechanisms of hypersensitivity. In: Gibson GG, Hubbard R, Parke DV, eds. Immunotoxicology. New York: Academic Press, 1983:71–86.

83. Stanworth DR. Current concepts of hypersensitivity. In: Dean JH, Luster MI, Munson AE, Amos H, eds. Immunotoxicology & immunopharmacology. New York: Raven Press, 1985:91–98.

84. Fink JN, deShazo RD. Immunologic aspects of granulomatous and interstitial lung diseases. JAMA 1987;258:2939–2944.

85. Larsen GL. Hypersensitivity lung disease. In: Paul WE, Fathman CG, Metzger H, eds. Annual Review of Immunology. Palo Alto: Annual Reviews, 1985:59–86.

86. Salvaggio JE. Hypersensitivity pneumonitis. J Allergy Clin Immunol 1987;79:558–571.

87. Schleuter DP. Infiltrative lung disease hypersensitivity pneumonitis. J Allergy Clin Immunol 1982;70:50–55.

88. Kaplan A, Buckley RH, Mathews KP. Allergic skin disorders. JAMA 1987;258:2900–2909.

89. Duijvestijn A, Hamann A. Mechanisms and regulation of lymphocyte migration. Immunol Today 1988;10:23–28.

90. Goh CL. Immunologic mechanism in contact allergy—a review. Ann Acad Med Singapore 1988;17:243–246.

91. Goetzl EJ, Chernov T, Renold F, Payan DG. Neuropeptide regulation of the expression of immediate hypersensitivity. J Immunol 1985;135 (suppl) 802–805.

92. Dean JH, Padarthsingh ML, Jerrellis TR. Assessment of immunobiological effects induced by chemicals, drugs or food additives. I tier testing and screening approach. Drug Chem Toxicol 1979;2:5–17.

93. Dean JH, Luster MI, Boorman GA. Methods and approaches for assessing immunotoxicity: an overview. Environ Health Perspect 1982;43:27–29.

94. Dean JH, Luster MI, Boorman GA, Lauer LD. Procedures available to examine the immunotoxicity of chemicals and drugs. Pharmacol Rev 1982;34:137–148.

95. Brooks BO, Neuman EM, Reed ND. Differential recovery of antibody production potential after sublethal whole-body irradiation in mice. J Leuk Biol 1986;40:335–345.

96. Schwetz BA. Immunotoxicology: an important new subdiscipline of toxicology. Fundam Appl Toxicol 1988;10:1–1.

97. Bekesi JG, Roboz JP, Fischbein A, Selikoff IJ. Clinical immunology studies in individuals exposed to environmental chemicals. In: Berlin A, Dean J, Draper M, Smith E, Spreafico F, eds. Immunotoxicology. Boston: Martinus Nijhoff Publishers, 1987:347–361.

98. Bernstein IL. Proceedings of the Task Force on Guidelines for Standardizing Old and New Technologies Used for the Diagnosis and Treatment of Allergic Diseases. J Allergy Clin Immunol 1988;82 (suppl) 487–525.

99. Sullivan-Fowler M, Austin T, Hafner AW. Alternative therapies, unproven methods, and health fraud. Chicago: American Medical Association, 1988:1–47.

100. Klecak G. Identification of contact allergens: predictive testing in animals. In: Marzulli FN, Maibach HI, eds. Dermatoxicology. New York: Hemisphere Publishing Corp, 1983:143–236.

101. Ritz HL, Buehler EV. Planning, conduct, and interpretation of guinea pig sensitization patch tests. In: Drill VA, Lazar P, eds. Current concepts in cutaneous toxicity. New York: Academic Press, 1980:25–40.

102. Magnusson B, Kligman AM. The identification of contact allergens by animal assay: the guinea pig maximization test. J Invest Dermatol 1969;52:268.

103. Report of an IUIS/WHO Working Group. Use and abuse of laboratory tests in clinical immunology: critical considerations of eight widely used diagnostic procedures. Clin Exp Immunol 1981;46:662–674.

104. DeShazo RD, Lopez M, Salvaggio JE. Use and interpretation of diagnostic immunologic laboratory tests. JAMA 1987;258:3011–3031.

105. Virella G. Diagnostic evaluation of humoral immunity. In: Virella G, Goust JM, Fudenberg HH, Patrick CC, eds. Introduction to medical immunology. New York: Marcel Dekker, 1986:247–265.

106. Patrick CC, Goust JM, Virella G. Diagnostic evaluation of cell-mediated immunity. In Virella G, Goust JM, Fudenberg HH, Patrick CC, eds. Introduction to medical immunology. New York: Marcel Dekker, 1986:265–283.

107. Rosenfeld SI. Interpretation of complement and immune complex assays. In: Grieco MH, Meriny DK, eds. Immunodiagnosis for clinicians: interpretation of immunoassays. Chicago: Year Book Medical Publishers, 1983:161–187.

108. Katz P. Clinical and laboratory evaluation of the immune system. Med Clin North Am 1985;69:453–464.

109. Thrasher JD, Madison R, Broughton A, Gard Z. Building-related illness and antibodies to albumin conjugates of formaldehyde, toluene diisocyanate, and trimellitic anhydride. Am J Ind Med 1989;15:187–195.

110. Koller LD. Review/commentary: immunotoxicology of heavy metals. Int J Immunopharmacol 1980;2:269–279.

111. Koller LD. Effects of environmental contaminants on the immune system. Adv Vet Sci Comp Med 1979;23:267–295.

112. Druet P, Bernard A, Hirsch F, Weening JJ, Gengoux P, Mahieu P, Birkeland S. Immunologically mediated glormerulonephritis induced by heavy metals. Arch Toxicol 1982;50:187–194.

113. Koller LD, Exon JH, Roan JG. Antibody suppression by cadmium. Arch Environ Health 1975;30:598–601.

114. Cullen MR, Kayne RD, Robins JM. Endocrine and reproductive dysfunction in men associated with occupational inorganic lead intoxication. Arch Environ Health 1984;39:431–440.

115. Reigart JR, Graber CD. Evaluation of the humoral immune response of children with low level lead exposure. Bull Environ Contam Toxicol 1976;16:112–117.

116. Sachs HK. Intercurrent infection in lead poisoning. Am J Dis Child 1978;132:315–316.

117. Lam S, Chang-Yeung M. Occupational asthma: natural history evaluation and management. In: Rosenstock L, ed. Occupational Medicine State of the Art Reviews. Vol. 2. Philadelphia, PA: Hanley and Belfus, 1987:373–381.

118. Grammer LC. Occupational immunologic lung disease. In: Patterson R, ed. Allergic diseases: diagnosis and management. J.B. Lippincott Co, 1985:691–708.

119. Royle H. Toxicity of chromic acid in the chromium plating industry. Environ Res 1975;10:141–163.

120. Luster MI, Dean JH. Immunological hypersensitivity resulting from environmental or occupational exposure to chemicals: a state-of-the-art workshop summary. Fundam Appl Toxicol 1982;2:327–330.

121. Sprince NL, Kazemi H. Beryllium disease. In: Rom WN, ed. Environmental and occupational medicine. Boston: Little, Brown and Co, 1983:481–490.

122. Wilber CG. Beryllium in man. In: Wilber CG, ed. Beryllium: a potential environmental contaminant. Springfield, IL: Charles C. Thomas, 1980:77–92.

123. Sunderman FW. A review of the metabolism and toxicology of nickel. Ann Clin Lab Sci 1977;7:377–398.

124. Smith TJ, Blough S. Chromium, manganese, nickel, and other elements. In: Rom WN, ed. Environmental and occupational medicine. Boston: Little, Brown and Co, 1983:491–510.

125. Enterline PE, March GM. Cancer among workers exposed to arsenic and other substances in a copper smelter. Am J Epidemiol 1982;116:895–911.

126. Pershagen G. Lung cancer mortality among men living near an arsenic-emitting smelter. Am J Epidemiol 1985;122:684–694.

127. Eisenbud M. Carcinogenicity and allergenicity. Science 1987:1613.

128. Luster MI, Rosenthal GJ. The immunosuppressive influence of industrial and environmental xenobiotics. Trends Pharmacol Sci 1986:408–412.

129. Emmett EA, Maroni M, Schmith JM, Levin BK, Jefferys J. Studies of transformer repair workers exposed to PCBs: 1. Study design, PCB concentrations, questionnaire, and clinical examination results. Am J Ind Med 1988;13:415–427.

130. Kimbrough RD. Human health effects of polychlorinated biphenyls (PCBs) and polybrominated biphenyls (PBBs). Annu Rev Pharmacol Toxicol 1987;27:87–111.

131. Bekesi JG, Holland JF, Anderson HA, Fischbein AS, Rom WN, Wolff MS, Selikoff IJ. Lymphocyte function of Michigan dairy farmers exposed to polybrominated biphenyl. Science 1978;199:1207–1209.

132. Descotes J. Biphenyls: 1. Polybrominated biphenyls. In: Descotes J, ed. Immunotoxicology of drugs and chemicals. Amsterdam: Elsevier 1986:342.

133. Evans RG, Webb KB, Knutsen AP, Roodman ST, Roberts DW, Bagby JR, Garrett WA, Andrews JS. A medical follow-up of the health effects of long-term exposure to 2,3,7,8-tetrachlorodibenzeno-p-dioxin. Arch Environ Health 1988;43(4):273–278.

134. Stehr-Green PA, Burse VW, Welty E. Human exposure to polychlorinated biphenyls at toxic waste sites: investigations in the United States. Arch Environ Health 1988;43:420–424.

135. Brown DP. Mortality of workers exposed to polychlorinated biphenyls—an update. Arch Environ Health 1987;42:333–339.

136. Hoffman RE, Stehr-Green PA, Webb KB, Evans RG, Knutsen AP, Schramm WF, Staake JL, Gibson BB, Steinberg KK. Health effects of long-term exposure to 2,3,7,8-tetrachlorodibenzeno-p-dioxin. JAMA 1986;255:2031–2038.

137. Webb K, Evans RK, Stehr P, Ayres SM. Pilot study on health effects of environmental 2,3,7,8-TCDD in Missouri. Am J Ind Med 1987;11:685–691.

138. Mocarelli P, Marocchi A, Brambilla P, Gerthoux P, Young DS, Mantel N. Clinical laboratory manifestations of exposure to dioxin in children. A six-year study of the effects of an environmental disaster near Seveso, Italy. JAMA 1986;256:2687–2695.

139. Hayes WJ. Pesticides studied in man. Baltimore: Williams & Wilkins, 1982:202.

140. Descotes J. Biphenyls: 1. Polybrominated biphenyls. In: Descotes J, ed. Immunotoxicology of drugs and chemicals. Amsterdam: Elsevier, 1986:314–332.

141. Lee TP, Moscati R, Parks BH. Effects of pesticides on human leukocyte functions. Res Commun Chem Pathol Pharmacol 1979;23:597–609.

142. Roux F, Treich I, Brun C, Desoize B, Fournier E. Effect of lindane on human lymphocyte responses to phytohemagglutinin. Biochem Pharmacol 1979;28:2419–2426.

143. Hermanowicz A, Nawarska Z, Borys D. The neutrophil function and infectious disease in workers occupationally exposed to organochlorine insecticides. Int Arch Occup Environ Health 1982;50:329.

144. Costa M, Schvartsman S. Antibody titers and blood levels of DDT after diphtheric immunization in children. Acta Pharm Toxicol 1977;41:249.

145. Luster MI, Dean JH. Immunological hypersensitivity resulting from environmental or occupational exposure to chemicals: state of the art workshop summary. Fundam Appl Toxicol 1982;2:237–330.

146. Aaronson DW, Rosenberg M. Occupational immunologic lung disease. In: Patterson R, ed. Allergic Diseases Diagnosis and Management. Philadelphia: S.B. Lippincott Co, 1985:253–303.

147. Zeiss CR, Wolkonsky P, Chacon R, Tuntland PA, Levitz D, Prunzansky JJ, Patterson R. Syndromes in workers exposed to trimellitic anhydride. Ann Intern Med 1983;98:8–12.

148. Grammer LC. Occupational immunologic lung disease. In: Patterson R, ed. Allergic Diseases Diagnosis and Management. Philadelphia: J.B. Lippincott Co., 1985:691–708.

149. Alexandersson R, Kolomodin-Hedman B, Hedenstierna G. Exposure to formaldehyde: effects on pulmonary function. Arch Environ Health 1982;37:279–284.

150. Furge PS, Harries MG, Lam WK, O'Brien IM, Patchett PA. Occupational asthma due to formaldehyde. Thorax 1985;40:255–260.

151. Brooks SM, Weiss MA, Bernstein IL. Reactive airway dysfunction syndrome (RADS): persistent asthma syndrome after high level irritant exposure. Chest 1985;88:376–384.

152. Doll NJ, Stankus RP, Highes J, Weill H, Gupta RC, Rodriguez M, Jones RN, Alspaugh MA, Salvaggio JE. Immune complexes and autoantibodies in silicosis. J Allergy Clin Immunol 1981;68:281–285.

153. Kubota M, Kagamimori S, Yokoyama K, Okada A. Reduced killer cell activity of lymphocytes from patients with asbestosis. Br J Ind Med 1985;42:276–280.

154. Barbers RG, Oishi J. Effects of in vitro asbestos exposure on natural killer and antibody-dependent cellular cytotoxicity. Environ Res 1987;43:217–226.

155. Lachapelle JM. The concept of industrial airborne irritant or allergic contact dermatitis. In: Maibach HI, ed. Occupational and industrial dermatology. Chicago, IL: Yearbook, 1987:179–189.

156. Lindskov R. Contact urticaria to formaldehyde. Contact Derm 1982;8:333–334.

157. Nenne T, Kaaber K, Tjell JC. Treatment of nickel dermatitis. Ann Clin Lab Sci 1980;10:160–164.

158. LaMarte FP, Merchant JA, Casale TB. Acute systemic reactions to carbonless paper associated with histamine release. JAMA 1988;260:242–243.

159. Calnan CD. The use and abuse of patch tests. In: Maibach HI, ed. Occupational and industrial dermatology. Chicago, IL: Yearbook, 1987:28–31.

160. Gardner DE. Alterations in macrophage functions by environmental chemicals. Environ Health Perspect 1984;55:343–358.

161. Descotes J. In: Descotes J, ed. Immunotoxicology of drugs and chemicals. Amsterdam: Elsevier, 1986:359–362.

18

Multiple Chemical Sensitivities

John B. Sullivan, Jr., M.D.
Bradford O. Brooks, Ph.D.

CHEMICAL SENSITIVITY AND PUBLIC PERCEPTION OF RISK

Over the past several years a phenomenon known as multiple chemical sensitivity (MCS) has attracted the attention of health care providers as well as the courts. This phenomenon has been described as an environmental illness by some and as a perception of illness produced by amplification of fears and anxieties by others. Individuals diagnosed as having MCS report health problems ranging from minor discomforts to severe incapacitation due to a sensitivity to a variety of common environmental chemicals. The term multiple chemical sensitivities has been used to describe the syndrome experienced by these individuals (1). MCS has been called an acquired disorder characterized by recurrent syndromes referable to a variety of different organs. Neurobehavioral and immunologic disorders are commonly expressed by individuals diagnosed as having MCS. Symptoms are said to occur upon exposure to many different chemicals at doses far below those established as causing harmful effects in the general population. Debate continues to rage in the scientific community as well as in the courts regarding the validity of MCS as a disease entity and regarding the medical subculture in which this diagnosis is established.

Partially responsible for the increase in litigation and worker compensation claims involving chemical exposure and the development of multiple chemical sensitivity is the perception of risk shared by the public. Toxicology, as the discipline that studies the adverse effects of chemicals on living organisms, has the responsibility of predicting safety to individuals as well as the public. The public's concern regarding the health risk associated with a toxic hazard is legitimate. However, the perception of risk by society has changed dramatically in the last two decades. Entire scientific disciplines have evolved to assess risk. However, the perception of risk and the resulting emotions of individuals and the public at large is not controlled by scientific facts. The perception of most citizens in the United States is that they face a greater risk from toxic hazards today than in the past despite the fact that life spans have increased and medical care and diagnosis have advanced tremendously. This increased awareness of toxic hazards is fueled partly by the lay press, and the public has difficulty in discerning the credibility of the various information sources. In addition, non-peer-reviewed trade journals add to this confusion. Thus, the public's perception of risk is affected more by the lay press than by highly regarded medical and scientific journals.

There is a growing dichotomy between public opinion and science that is frequently demonstrated in the popular press regarding environmental health issues. This treatment of the subject of risk has driven a wedge between the public and the scientific community. An example of this is the handling of asbestos in public buildings. Scientists and the public's perception of error is another example. Whereas a scientist is very concerned about hastily performed, unreplicated, uncontrolled experiments with results which show an effect when in truth there is no effect (type I error), the public seems to be more frightened of not detecting an effect when in truth there is an effect (type II error). Thus the public has developed a general feeling that nothing should be introduced into commerce or the environment without first being proven to be absolutely safe. The public does not realize that true science is incapable of demonstrating absolute safety. To compound this matter, results of animal experimentation are sometimes loosely extrapolated to the human condition without a scientific basis or reason.

Fears of toxic exposure have escalated, and science, in the public's view, seems to be unable to resolve these fears adequately. Fear of illness following any exposure to a chemical, harmless or not, has increased the number of toxic tort litigations and worker compensation claims in the courts beyond reason. Fear of cancer, injury, and illness, even though no injury can be demonstrated or cause and effect found, can be compensated for in this manner with large monetary judgments (2). As the public's perception of risk continues to clash with the scientific community's assessment of risk, emotion and perception will gain more credibility. Emotion and public perception are as real as scientific measurements, but are certainly not as valid in describing the actual risk of a chemical.

MULTIPLE CHEMICAL SENSITIVITY AND DISEASE

Individuals diagnosed with MCS share common features: (a) The syndrome is initially acquired in relation to some type of environmental exposure to one or more chemicals. (b) Symptoms involve multiple organ systems. (c) Symptoms are reproduced by exposure to low levels of multiple, diverse chemicals instead of a single chemical. (d) Symptoms may recur in response to predictable chemical stimuli or environments. (e) The syndrome is elicited by very low level exposures which have no effect on the majority of the population. (f) No test of organ function or clinical evaluation can account for the symptoms (1, 3).

Most patients diagnosed as having MCS have no specific pathotoxicology or disease that is identifiable by clinical or laboratory evaluation. Any laboratory abnormality found can be readily explained by an alternative cause or recognized disease entity. Despite these facts, individuals with a diagnosis of MCS cling to the concept that they are ill and that their illness is environmentally induced. Many MCS-diagnosed individuals are involved in some sort or litigation of worker compensation claim and account for increased medical and legal costs. Precipitating factors may be occupational exposures, exposures at home, or some new environment in which someone becomes ill. In any event, the triggering factor may be unknown in a large majority of cases.

Medical evaluations of MCS patients can be difficult. These individuals are convinced that their health is permanently impaired by the environment in which they live and work. Many times they leave familiar surroundings and move into the mountains or desert in an attempt to be rid of contaminating chemicals in their environment. Their illness is at times incapacitating, and they may wear face masks to filter out impurities. Further complicating the evaluation of patients with MCS is their seemingly absolute dependence and reliance on a group of medical practitioners, termed clinical ecologists, from whom they receive the diagnosis.

CLINICAL ECOLOGY

Multiple chemical sensitivities is a proclaimed disease entity associated with a medical philosophy termed clinical ecology (3). Clinical ecology originated in the 1930s and 1940s from expanded concepts of food allergy and disease. It was believed that food allergies were causative of chronic diseases of unknown etiologies (3). The term allergic tension fatigue syndrome was introduced in 1954 by Spear (3). It was felt that food allergies caused behavioral and cognitive changes in some people. In the 1950s, Randolph introduced theories that organic chemicals can produce cognitive and multisystem disorders following very low level exposure (3). Randolph introduced the concept of multiple systems disease said to be produced by chemicals in the environment, resulting in unusual sensitivities (4, 5).

Clinical ecology has developed to include multiple practitioners around the United States, professional societies, journals devoted to the subject, and textbooks. Many individuals who believe that their multiple somatic problems are a result of some chemical exposure come to the attention of clinical ecologists. A diagnosis of multiple chemical sensitivity is offered to these individuals as a means to explain their symptoms. Clinical ecology is a form of medical practice based on the concept that there is a range of environmental chemicals that can be responsible for an illness. Clinical ecologists believe that the immune system is functionally interfered with or depressed by chemicals and that multiple chemical sensitivities result from an adverse immune reaction or an intolerance to environmental agents. The clinical ecology movement initially placed an emphasis on food sensitivity as a cause of chronic pain, fatigue, depression, and behavioral disorders; now chemicals have been implicated (3). A list of the chemicals said to be causative of multiple chemical sensitivity include petrochemicals, pesticides, a variety of detergents, alcohol-related products such as perfumes, vehicle exhaust fumes and vapors, natural gas, dental amalgam, and a wide range of many other industrial and domestic chemicals.

Environmental illness is said to be a result of the failure of human beings to adapt to the chemicals in their environment. Once these individuals are sensitized, they would react to very, very low concentrations of the causative agent, and their syndrome would be characterized by multiple symptoms referable to multiple organ systems. Eventually, the chemical ecology movement theorized that environmental chemicals formed haptens which induced neoantigens producing antibody formations to these chemicals and that these circulating immune complexes would activate the complement system and also result in inflammatory conditions.

In reality, the majority of patients given the diagnosis of MCS have no immune alteration when sufficiently evaluated by standard accepted laboratory and medical techniques. Some MCS patients may actually have disease, unrelated to any chemical exposure, that may go untreated due to the insistence by clinical ecologists that their problem is due to environmental exposures.

MCS AS AN ENVIRONMENTAL ILLNESS

Clinical ecologists do not describe the disease state of multiple chemical sensitivity in terms of traditional signs or symptoms or clinical laboratory features. Clinical ecologists have postulated that MCS results from a disturbed immune regulation caused by environmental chemicals which affect classes of lymphocytes, particularly T-suppressor cells (CD8 T-cells). A deficiency of the suppressor cell activity is said to produce an excessive immune response to many chemicals (4–6). Other theories state that environmental illness is a result of the release of inflammatory mediators by lipid peroxidation due to the toxic action of free radicals induced by chemicals (4–6). The cause of disease from these free radicals is said to be due to a deficiency of antioxidants such as ascorbic acid, glutathione, selenium, beta-carotene, and vitamin E (4–6).

There is no clear definition of multiple chemical sensitivity as a disease in the classic terms of pathologic, immunologic, biochemical, laboratory, and clinical abnormalities. Multiple chemical sensitivity as a disease syndrome does not have readily recognizable pathotoxicology, immune dysfunction, pathophysiology, or typical manifestations of allergy (6). However, to these patients, their syndrome is real, and efforts to confront them with facts is for the most part futile.

Clinical ecology as a medical discipline has been evaluated by the California Medical Association, the Ontario Minister of Health, and the American Academy of Allergy and Immunology. Reports from all three organizations, in 1986, found no evidence to support the concept underlying clinical ecology or its methods of diagnosis and treatment (3). The Ontario Ministry of Health, following the recommendation of a committee on environmental hypersensitivity disorders, established a definition based on interviews with clinical ecologists and their patients. This definition stated that,

Environmental hypersensitivity is a chronic condition continuing for more than three months, a multi-system disorder usually involving symptoms of the central nervous system. Affected persons are frequently intolerant to some foods and they react adversely to some chemicals and to environmental agents, singly or in combination, at levels generally tolerated by the majority of people. Affected persons have varying degrees of morbidity, from mild discomfort to total disability. Upon physical examination, the patient is normally free of any abnormal objective findings. Although abnormalities of complement and lymphocytes have been reported, no single laboratory test, including serum IgE, is consistently altered. Improvement is associated with avoidance with suspected agents and symptoms occur with re-exposure (4).

Literature reports and medical evaluations of patients suspected of multiple chemical sensitivity indicate that the diagnosis of environmental illness is applied to patients with chronic multiple symptoms who have an absence of objective physical findings and have no abnormal laboratory results. Terr has reviewed 50 clinical ecology cases, 46 of which were involved in worker compensation claims or litigation of some nature. Of these patients, 31 had multiple subjective symptoms, al-

Table 18.1. Chemicals Said to Be Detectable in the Blood of MCS Patients in Concentrations of Nanograms per Milliliter

2-Methylpentane
3-Methylpentane
n-Hexane
n-Pentane
2,2-Dimethylbutane
Cyclopentane
Ethylbenzene
1,1,1-Trichloroethane
Tetrachloroethane
Toluene
Xylene

though there were no abnormal physical or laboratory findings in any of these patients (6).

DIAGNOSIS OF MCS

The diagnosis of multiple chemical sensitivity is based on a history of exposure to some chemical or chemicals in the past and a response of the patient to provocation neutralization testing and challenge testing procedures. These testing procedures also include eliciting symptoms by exposing patients to chemicals in specifically constructed booths or chambers. However, clinical ecologists give very little attention to any physical signs, physiologic measurements of change, or actual measurement of air concentrations of chemicals during this testing. The most common symptomatic complaints of patients with multiple chemical sensitivities are fatigue, headache, nausea, malaise, pains in different organ systems, mucosal irritation, disorientation, dizziness, difficulty concentrating, and feelings of numbness and tingling in the extremities. Certainly, it is difficult to separate out these symptoms from stress reactions and amplification of fears and anxieties following chemical exposures.

Immunologic tests are sometimes performed and blood concentrations of a variety of volatile organic chemicals are obtained. Table 18.1 is a list of volatile organic chemicals said to be commonly present in the blood of some of these patients. Personal experience with evaluation of MCS patients has demonstrated that these chemicals are said to be found in the blood of patients with totally different chemical exposure histories in nanogram per milliliter concentrations. These same chemicals are commonly found as background indoor air contaminants in new buildings and as general indoor air contaminants. Many times, clinical ecologists will assay for pesticides and metabolites of pesticides found in lipid tissue and serum of patients. Pesticides commonly assayed for are heptachlor epoxide, trans-nonachlor, oxychlordane, gamma-BHC, and DDE. These chemicals are commonly found in the lipid tissues and serum of the majority of the United States population, and this prevalence invalidates the claim that they are causative of MCS.

Clinical ecology evaluations concentrate on patients' subjective assessment of their environment in producing symptoms. Extensive questionnaires are used to emphasize details of the patient's diet and exposure to substances at home and at work, even though the exposure to these substances cannot be documented. Much of the examination and history is a recall of the patient's subjective feelings in a variety of environments. Provocation testing is used to elicit these symptoms. During provocation testing, the appearance of any symptom at all is said to constitute a positive test to that substance. This type of provocation testing may include intradermal testing by injections of different materials such as extracts of food and other substances as well as chemicals. Sublingual provocation or the use of environmental control units for introducing the substance into the air of the patient is sometimes employed.

Treatment of MCS syndrome revolves around the use of elimination diets, the use of "neutralizing doses" of the offending substance in order to build up antibodies so that disease symptoms will not occur, and avoidance therapy (4). Avoidance of environmental chemicals, elimination diets, and symptom neutralization are the three main treatment regimens practiced. Avoidance therapy can be very difficult for the patient because the aim of this therapy is to achieve a natural environment devoid of toxic and/or synthetic chemicals. Specific chemicals which patients are told to avoid include formaldehyde, ethanol, phenol, a large variety of hydrocarbons, deodorants, pesticides, cosmetics, and vehicle fumes. Many of these individuals resort to construction of self-contained air filtered chambers within their home environments, and some move to less populated areas such as a mountain community, desert, or sea environment. Drastic measures are followed by some individuals at large expense.

The elimination diet is another important treatment recommended. Lists of foods to avoid are based on the patient's history. Neutralization therapy uses the administration of "antigens" to treat or prevent symptoms. These antigens are food extracts, chemicals, hormones, histamine, beta-carotene, and serotonin (4).

IMMUNE THEORIES OF MCS

Environmental chemicals are regarded as immunotoxins, and in many cases this has been substantiated in animal and human studies. Multiple chemical sensitivity is also said to be secondary to immune derangements or immune system alterations. Clinical ecologists feel that chemical exposure can result in the formation of haptens or neoantigens in the plasma of exposed individuals and that these neoantigens induce the production of antibodies. These antibodies are said to result in tissue damage and immune complexes which activate the complement system and generate mediators of inflammation (4, 6). Some clinical ecologists feel that the T-suppressor cells are more sensitive to damage from environmental chemicals as compared to other T-cells. They state that patients with environmental illness will have a higher than normal ratio of T-helper cells to T-suppressor cells and that this would enhance B-cell activity which could lead to excessive antibody production (3, 4). The measurement of inflammatory mediators has been used by clinical ecologists as an argument to prove chemical damage (3, 6).

Recent evaluations of patients exposed to low levels of formaldehyde have corroborated the existence of human serum albumin-IgG antibodies (7). However, it is reasonable to assume that this response to formaldehyde-albumin neoantigens is a normal antibody response and not an abnormal response that results in a disease process. The presence of antibodies is consistent with exposure, not disease. Aldehydes such as formaldehyde and glutaraldehyde are highly reactive with the amine groups of plasma proteins and will easily bind to these proteins to form haptens. Glutaraldehyde is commonly used to haptenize small chemicals to proteins in the laboratory.

An independent analysis of 50 cases of environmental illness by Terr showed that circulating levels of immune globulins, complement components, and lymphocyte subsets were normally distributed in the majority of cases. Some of these patients had elevated IgA and elevated B-cell count, but they also had a prior history of respiratory or cutaneous infections (6).

Many individuals suffer from true allergic disorders triggered by low level chemical or environmental exposures that cannot be easily identified. Patients presumed to have a diagnosis of MCS can be found to have other diseases, such as autoimmune disorders or allergies. Evaluation of MCS patients involves a careful search to rule out these disease states. The medical evaluation includes a careful history exploring exposure as well as prior disease states. Laboratory evaluation should focus on the specific complaints (8).

The use of a battery of extensive immunologic tests as commonly performed on these individuals is not justified. Certain basic tests can be used to determine the integrity of the immune system. In addition, extensive immune system testing will sometimes identify positive results in various antinuclear antibody titers that can be expected for certain populations of people tested. Clinical ecologists will attempt to use these positive antinuclear antibody tests to assert that an individual's immune system has been altered by a chemical exposure. However, positive antinuclear antibody tests (ANA) can be found in many normal human subjects and should never alone be used to argue the existence of MCS. Positive ANAs have been found to occur in 4% of individuals with a variety of general disease states, in 24% of individuals with some form of collagen vascular disease, in 33% of relatives of individuals with systemic lupus, in 6% of individuals with miscellaneous medical disease, in 14% of patients with a variety of arthritic disorders, in 88% of blood donors from age 25–45 at titers under 1:8, and in 17% of all hospitalized patients without rheumatologic disease (9). At serum dilutions up to 1:10, 35% of the general population will have a positive ANA; at dilutions greater than 1:10, this incidence falls to 4% (9). Individuals older than 60 years can be positive for ANA's in up to 38% of cases (10). Certain drugs such as procainamide, hydralazine, beta-receptor blockers, phenytoin, and methyldopa can produce drug-induced lupus with significant elevation of ANA titers for months and even years (11).

The frequency of false positive test results in a generally healthy population of patients screened for ANAs varies from 0–7%, based on the influence of disease prevalence on the predictive power of the test (9). The presence of a variety of antinuclear antibodies does not constitute the existence of an environmental disorder. Results of these immunologic tests must be interpreted not in terms of a test result, but in terms of the total clinical picture, the predictive value of the test, specificity and sensitivity of the test, and presence of true disease.

Many chemicals have been shown to produce immune alterations in laboratory animals at subclinical dosing, but these alterations have not been extrapolated to humans in terms of disease or detectable immune alterations (8). Hypersensitivity disease states and autoimmunity have been claimed by clinical ecologists to be the result of low level chemical exposures. Some chemicals can produce immune responses, such as formaldehyde, glutaraldehyde, isocyanates, and beryllium. Allergy and hypersensitivity can be the result of many chemical exposures, but there is also recognizable pathotoxicology such as asthma, nephritis, pulmonary disease, and rashes (8). Mechanisms responsible for chemically induced hypersensitivity include formation of neoantigens by haptenization with serum proteins, tissue damage releasing autoantigens, shared antigenic determinants existing between the chemical and target organ tissue, or chemicals directly affecting the immune system (8).

MCS as an environmental illness cannot be defined as a disease state using commonly accepted clinical criteria or laboratory documentation in the majority of cases. Documenting pathotoxicology is very difficult in most of these patients and is not present in the majority. There are exceptions to this, and these individuals are found to have verifiable symptomatology and/or disease that explains their symptoms. MCS is mainly a history of environmental exposure and a behavioral disturbance relating to this exposure. Presently, there is no experimental or clinical laboratory support for illness in the majority of MCS patients that are examined and stated to have immune deficiencies from multiple exposures to chemicals in the environment.

BEHAVIORAL AND PSYCHIATRIC ASPECTS OF MCS

Due to the disparity between the severity of symptoms in patients with MCS and the lack, or general paucity, of actual pathophysiologic findings in these individuals, some professionals have suggested that this disorder be classified as a psychiatric or somatoform disorder. The usual symptoms expressed by individuals with MCS are the kinds of symptoms that are relatively common throughout the general population. One study from the National Center for Health Statistics found that 78% of Americans reported being bothered by at least one of 12 common symptoms such as headaches, dizziness, and palpitations (12). The amplification of symptoms by individuals suffering from MCS may play a large part in the genesis of the disorder. A multitude of personality factors can predispose individuals to dwell on and amplify bodily sensations and somatic symptoms related to certain environments. Behavioral reinforcement and amplification of this cognitive process through detection of an odor or perception that an exposure to a chemical has occurred can culminate in an illness that is more behavioral than physical.

Multiple chemical sensitivity may also represent a form of posttraumatic stress disorder. This type of stress reaction secondary to toxic exposures has been well-described and is not uncommon (8). Individuals react to suspected or real toxic exposures in a variety of ways. Amplification of these fears can lead to somatic complaints and belief that toxic injury has occurred.

MANAGEMENT OF MCS PATIENTS

Treatment of MCS patients can be very difficult. Most MCS patients mistrust conventional medical methods and approaches to disease diagnosis and treatment. Many MCS patients are evaluated by independent medical examiners in the course of worker compensation litigation and come to resent traditional medical therapy. The overall goal of treatment should be to reintroduce the patient into a normal environment. How this is accomplished can vary, but must include general medical evaluation, psychiatric assessment, neuropsychologic evaluation, and behavioral modification. The individual must first be found to be free of a disease state that can be treated and then be willing to undergo further therapy. Since these individuals have received intense reinforcement to be mistrustful of traditional medical practice, gaining their trust and confidence is the first step to a successful treatment.

The essentials of therapy are multidisciplinary and center around: (a) reducing or eliminating a patient's avoidance behavior; (b) reducing or eliminating dependence on desensitization injections, diets, and medications prescribed by clinical ecologists; (c) demonstrating improvement in one or more specific areas to gradually reduce symptoms severity; (d) establishing success criteria that are visible to patients to allow them to build on to achieve the next goal; (e) developing a trusting relationship with the patient; (f) using behavior modification techniques and psychotherapy to achieve success in reducing and eventually eliminating anxieties and fears.

Some patients who are being treated by clinical ecologists are so disabled that they cannot live in normal environments. They are forced to sell their homes and move into "clean" rooms, or into other isolated environments in order to avoid chemicals. Their disability is mainly psychologic and behavioral. They are told to avoid exposure to everything from newspapers and detergents to vehicle fumes and to air of urban cities. Given the public's perception of risk from chemicals along with the placing of severe constraints and limitations on patients' lives, clinical ecology cannot be looked on as a benign patient-oriented discipline.

REFERENCES

1. Cullen MR. The worker with multiple chemical sensitivities: an overview. Occup Med State of the Art Reviews 1987;2:655–661.
2. Maskin A. Cancerophobia: an emerging theory of compensable damages. J Occup Med 1989;31:427.
3. Brodsky CM. Allergic to everything: a medical subculture. Psychosomatics 1983;24:731–742.
4. American College of Physicians. Clinical ecology. Ann Intern Med 1989;111:168–178.
5. Kahn E, Letz G. Clinical ecology: environmental medicine or unsubstantiated theory. Ann Intern Med 1989;111:104–106.
6. Terr AI. Multiple chemical sensitivities: immunologic critique of clinical ecology theories and practice. Occup Med State of the Art Reviews 1987;2:683–693.
7. Thrasher JD, Madison R, Broughton A, Gard Z. Building-related illness and antibodies to albumin conjugates of formaldehyde, toluene diisocyanate, and trimellitic anhydride. Am J Ind Med 1989;15:187–195.
8. Sullivan JB. Immunological alterations and chemical exposure. J Toxicol Clin Toxicol 1989;27:311–343.
9. Richardson B, Epstein W. Utility of the fluorescent antibody test in a single patient. Ann Intern Med 1981;95:333–338.
10. deShazo RD, Lopez M, Salvaggio JE. Use and interpretation of diagnostic immunologic laboratory tests. JAMA 1987;258:3011–3031.
11. DeSwarte RD. Drug allergy. In: Patterson R, ed. Allergic diseases: diagnosis and management. Philadelphia: J.B. Lippincott Co, 1985:505–661.
12. Scottenfeld RS. Workers with multiple chemical sensitivities: a psychiatric approach to diagnosis and treatment. Occup Med State of the Art Reviews, 1987;2:739–753.

Regulatory, Health, and Safety Aspects of Hazardous Materials

19

Introduction to Hazardous Materials Health and Safety Issues

Steven Pike, M.D., M.Sc.

Hazardous wastes and hazardous materials can generally be divided into the three broad categories of chemical, radioactive, and infectious or biologic. The Office of Technology Assessment estimates that between 255 to 275 million tons of wastes are produced annually in the United States (1). Although each state generates hazardous wastes, 10 are responsible for 65% of all hazardous waste produced. These are California, Illinois, Indiana, Louisiana, Michigan, Ohio, Pennsylvania, Tennessee, Texas, and West Virginia (1, 2). Most hazardous waste is a byproduct of manufacturing processes and industries involving organic chemicals, metals, electroplating, and electronics.

Wastes have traditionally been disposed of by landfill techniques or incineration. Controlling generation, disposal, and release of hazardous wastes into the environment has been addressed by the federal government in multiple legislative acts. In 1976 Congress passed the Resource Conservation and Recovery Act (RCRA) which established a regulatory program for hazardous waste management designed to regulate waste from the point of generation through disposal. RCRA includes the components of identification of a hazardous waste, a tracking system, waste facility management standards, and a system for issuing permits to handle, store, and dispose of wastes (1, 3). The Environmental Protection Agency (EPA) was designated as the authoritative body to regulate hazardous waste under RCRA for the protection of public health and the environment. Under original RCRA guidelines, hazardous waste referred only to solid wastes; however, the definition of what constitutes a hazardous waste has been broadened.

DEFINING HAZARDOUS WASTES

Defining what constitutes a hazardous waste can be difficult under RCRA guidelines and is different from defining a hazardous material in general. Wastes can vary from a single chemical to complex multiple mixtures of chemicals in varying concentrations. The RCRA definition of a hazardous waste includes solid waste, liquid and semiliquid waste, and gaseous material generated from industrial, commercial, mining, agricultural, and community activities which when improperly stored, transported, treated, or disposed of could present a potential human health and/or environmental hazard (1, 3). The potential hazard is actually judged by the proper or improper management techniques applied to the waste handling and disposal. The EPA identifies a waste as hazardous using two main criteria: (a) if by its characteristics it is toxic, carcinogenic, mutagenic, or teratogenic and it is on one of four EPA lists of chemical hazards; or (b) if it exhibits one or more of the following toxic hazards (1, 4):

Ignitability: These wastes could be ignited by routine handling. Included in this category are oxidizers and combustible gases as well as any spontaneously combustible substance or a substance that could support a fire if ignited.

Corrosivity: Corrosives may result in penetration and leakage of containers and produce health hazards to waste workers.

Reactivity: These are wastes that may explode or release gases that could be health hazards under normal conditions. This includes explosives, substances that react violently with water and air such as the alkali metals of sodium and potassium, substances that release toxic gases when exposed to water and/or acidic conditions (cyanide, hydrogen sulfide, phospine, arsine), or materials that are explosive when mixed with water or air.

Toxicity: This is the ability of the waste to leach out specified toxic concentrations of chemicals by an EPA-designed extraction procedure. If a certain concentration is able to be released during the testing of the waste, then the chemical waste is designated as hazardous. EPA standards exist for these chemical extract concentrations.

There are many exemptions to the EPA definition of hazardous wastes. However, this does not mean that these exempted wastes are not human health hazards. Examples of exemptions include industrial waste water discharge, home generated wastes, domestic sewage, mining wastes, agricultural wastes, wastes generated by fossil fuel combustion, small generators under 1000 kg/month, wastes associated with exploration for energy sources, and nuclear wastes which are regulated by the Department of Energy (DOE) (1–3). The individual states may define and regulate wastes differently than the EPA does and may apply more liberal or conservative controls to these wastes. In fact, millions of tons of hazardous waste not controlled by the EPA are produced by small generators. These wastes can contain toxic metals, organic compounds, pesticides, agricultural and mining wastes, and biologics. In many instances, the estimated amounts of hazardous wastes generated by the states is much higher than the federal estimates of those states.

Cleaning up waste sites designed by the EPA as health or environmental hazards is embodied in the Comprehensive Environmental Response, Compensation, and Liability Act of 1980 (CERCLA). This act, referred to as Superfund, defines liability in relation to reimbursement for hazardous waste site cleanup activity, requires detailed record keeping by facilities that store hazardous wastes, and requires immediate notification to the EPA if a release occurs (3, 5). Superfund was created by a combination of revenues generated over a 5-year period by fees levied against petroleum companies (87.5%) with the remainder from general tax revenues (12.5%) (3). These funds are to be used for the immediate cleanup of a chemical release which creates a health hazard. After the immediate cleanup the EPA seeks reimbursement of the fund from responsible parties involved in the transportation and disposal of the waste and, if necessary, initiates legal action against the responsible parties (3, 5). Pivotal to the use of these funds for cleaning up a waste site is the concept of a release of a hazardous material into the environment. This definition excludes occupational exposures as well as radioactive releases during a nuclear accident (3). Funding and scope of CERCLA were examined by the 1986 Superfund Amendment and Reauthorization Act (SARA).

Existing waste sites in the United States have been ranked according to their hazard, size, location, toxicity, and danger to the public and the environment. Once a waste site has been identified, it is placed on a National Priorities List, if the toxic hazard is ranked high enough. A remedial study of the site is then conducted to characterize the waste in terms of quantity, types of hazards, and environmental and public health risks. The decision to clean up a hazardous waste site is based on factors relating to health hazards to surrounding communities, environmental risks, the type of hazard present and its toxicity, the quantity of material present, the location of the site, the likelihood of spread versus containment of the hazard, and the potential for human health effects if the site is left untouched (6). If it is determined that the site will be cleaned up, then worker health and safety becomes a top priority.

The cleanup of the several thousand identified hazardous waste sites in the United States requires worker exposure to a variety of potential health hazards. Controlling exposures to toxic substances at hazardous waste sites requires a combination of three broadly focused efforts: (a) hazard identification and evaluation, (b) exposure assessment, and (c) worker, community, and environmental protection.

HAZARD IDENTIFICATION AND EVALUATION

The first step in controlling worker exposures at hazardous waste sites is the identification of existing hazards as well as of the forms of exposure that may occur to workers. The historical use of the site, characterization of the site relative to the chemical hazards present, and a site survey are important steps to identifying the presence of specific hazardous materials. This is often a difficult task because the history of the site may be poorly understood and the types of waste and quantities that were deposited are usually unknown. The manner in which waste was deposited may also be unknown. Waste may be deposited in containers or directly into the soil. The types of containers may vary and can include metal drums, plastic bags, boxes, or crates. Waste may be deposited and mixed with debris, may be partially incinerated, and may have undergone physical and/or chemical transformation. The physical form of the waste may vary. It may exist as liquids, solids, gases, slurries, and other mixtures. The different types of wastes that were deposited may have formed complex mixtures resulting in different hazards from those present in the original waste. Hazards may be potentially flammable or explosive. Site activities may release toxic gases, mists, fumes, or dusts when the waste is disturbed. Thus characterizing and identifying the toxic and physical hazards at waste sites is a critical first issue before any cleanup can begin.

Site History: The hazard identification process begins with thorough reviews of the site history regarding site operations, activities, waste disposal practices, and previous cleanup activities that can be obtained from interviews with employees, managers, and neighbors. Additional details can be obtained by reviewing company records, old photographs, shipping records, newspaper articles, legal documents, business licenses, and geologic surveys.

Site Characterization: Armed with information obtained from interviews and published sources, the site characterization can then provide more specific information regarding waste composition, concentration, and specific location on site. This requires an engineering, industrial hygiene, and analytical approach embodying properly conducted environmental surveys and environmental monitoring by trained professionals.

Site Control: Hazards often exist as complex mixtures which can be difficult to analytically characterize. A component of site control is proper use of environmental monitoring with strategies designed to detect hazards at site perimeters as well as within the breathing zone areas of site workers. Protection of the surrounding community from site releases as well as protection of site workers is a key issue of site control.

Hazards Evaluation: Having identified the hazards present as well as their composition, the site investigation team must then evaluate the hazard that each component poses and the hazard of the combination of components. Although, for the most part, the components emphasized will be chemical, hazards exist to personnel that go beyond the materials present. Hazards that pose an immediate danger to life or health (IDLH), are rapidly acting poisons, caustics, gases, explosives, oxygen deficiency, confined spaces, and ionizing radiation. Sometimes hazards are not obvious or identifiable and are unanticipated storage tanks, residues of chemicals, and low-lying areas where chemical vapors may accumulate. Hazards vary by site as the cleanup or evaluation progresses; the hazards may change both in degree of potential risk and ability to control them. Toxicity resulting from chemical exposure may be local, as in the case of acids and caustics, or may be systemic, as is the case with gases such as carbon monoxide, hydrogen sulfide, hydrogen cyanide, arsine, and phosphine.

EXPOSURE ASSESSMENT

The next major effort after hazard identification is exposure assessment. Exposure assessment develops from the information obtained from the site history and characterization data, the hazard identification process, environmental monitoring, and a knowledge of the operations to be performed by workers at the waste site. Risk of exposure and the assessment of exposure must take into account potentially harmful effects to the individual, the community, and the environment. Exposures can be classified as follows:

Acute exposure—A single, rapid exposure which may or may not be of high enough concentration to produce toxicity;
Subacute exposure—Multiple single exposures over a relatively short period of time measured in days or weeks;
Chronic exposure—Long duration, usually low level, exposure over a period of months and years with variation in the frequency; and
Longterm exposure—A continuous exposure over a period of years usually of a low concentration.

Workers must not only be protected from the relatively easily recognized and dramatic acute effects of chemicals but also from the delayed effects which are insidious and often have long periods of latency, but just as surely cause injury or death. Health effects must be prevented or reversed, but reversible effects must be recognized early and intervention initiated to prevent permanent damage. This forms the basis for determining the interval for periodic medical and surveillance examinations.

Some special problems exist that create the need for extending and supplementing the human sensory system to allow the worker to recognize danger. Hazards may be odorless and colorless, such as the gases carbon monoxide and methane, or may numb the sense of smell, thereby eliminating the warning odor of its presence, exemplified by the olfactory fatigue caused by hydrogen sulfide. Other hazards may cause damage at concentrations well below the odor threshold and preclude the nose as part of a warning system.

Other hazards besides the chemicals at a waste site that can result in injury or illness to site workers may be encountered during environmental conditions of extreme heat or cold which act as complicating factors. Workers having to wear bulky and heavy protective clothing and equipment are also at risk for added heat stress and motor skills difficulty.

Biologic hazards should be mentioned because waste sites may also have been used to dump not only chemicals but animal and human sewage, decaying vegetable matter, or hospital and medical waste. Infectious agents may pose hazards that are indigenous to the soil. In the San Joaquin Valley and Sonora desert the presence of coccidioidomycosis spores may pose a hazard as the ground is disturbed and dust is generated.

Responses to toxic materials can vary depending on the material, route of exposure, intensity and duration of exposure, and preexisting health status of the exposed person. Toxic responses can range from none to subclinical to overtly clinical. Toxic responses can be conveniently categorized according to the target organ affected. Thus the existence of medical surveillance programs to monitor worker exposures to hazardous materials is important to protect health.

PROGRAM DESIGN FOR WORKER PROTECTION

Once the hazards have been identified and anticipated, the route of exposure for each must be identified, and the program to protect the workers and prevent exposure is designated. The combination of hazard identification and exposure assessment leads to the final major effort, program design for worker protection as well as for chemical containment to protect the surrounding community and environment.

Program design comprises all the means and procedures used to ensure the safe working conditions for the workers decontaminating a hazardous waste site as well as the implementation of controls to prevent release of substances into the environment and surrounding community. There are six main elements of a program designed to protect workers: limiting or eliminating exposure, worker assessment, environmental monitoring, biologic monitoring, medical surveillance, and emergency response.

Limiting or eliminating exposure: Designing the health and safety program to anticipate the types of exposures that are likely to take place and implementing means of limiting or eliminating the exposure may take the form of:

1. Administrative controls on site access, time on site, training, work practices, and procedures;
2. Engineering controls on technology used to disturb the site, contain waste, transport, dispose, and incinerate wastes;
3. Personal protective equipment to minimize contact by skin, puncture, ingestion, or inhalation via respirators, gloves, boots, goggles, and overalls; and

4. Process controls such as limiting the amount of material disturbed at one time.

Worker assessment: Assessing the ability of the worker to perform under stressful conditions caused by protective clothing, heat, cold, and strenuous physical efforts is important. Forms of medical evaluations useful in this regard include preplacement medical evaluations, periodic medical evaluations for continued placement, performance-oriented evaluations, and termination medical evaluations.

Environmental monitoring: Environmental monitoring is needed to ensure that the engineering controls, administrative controls, and process controls are effective. This takes the form of:

1. Monitoring of ambient concentrations of hazardous chemicals as well as changes in ambient conditions;
2. Monitoring of ambient thermal conditions, heat and cold;
3. Monitoring of noise levels;
4. Monitoring of changing site conditions that may require modifications of techniques for site remediation or changes in respiratory protection or protective clothing;
5. Health physics monitoring of sites where radioactive waste is or may be present.

Biologic monitoring: Biologic monitoring is not only limited to measuring chemicals in biologic fluids and tissues, but also may include determining individual sensitivities and genetic susceptibilities. There are many ethical and legal issues associated with the use of any biologic monitoring technology as well as uncertainty as to how to interpret results. Caveats concerning the use of biologic monitoring are:

1. It is not ethical or desirable to use the human as an instrument for exposure assessment.
2. The presence of measured chemicals or metabolites in body fluids or tissue indicates exposure and does not necessarily indicate disease.
3. Negative information is useful to confirm the adequacy of protective measures.
4. Positive information is useful to attempt to quantify delivered dose in circumstances in which protective measures have been breached or have failed.
5. The use of a qualified laboratory is essential.

Medical surveillance: Medical surveillance is often the most emphasized of all the techniques used to protect the worker (7). However, physical examinations are becoming less useful as the overall state of health of the working population has improved. Manifestations of effects from hazardous materials are preceded in most cases by alterations in parameters that require measurement in the laboratory. Even the basic laboratory parameters traditionally measured may not be sensitive enough to define the occurrence of toxic exposures to working populations at these sites (8). Generally, toxic effects of substances may be categorized as physiologic, behavioral, biochemical, carcinogenic, or mutagenic. Sensitive indicators of toxicity are generally biochemical and/or physiologic alterations not identified on routine physical or laboratory examination. The ability of laboratory testing alone to discern exposures to chemical hazards remains poor. Basic hematologic and general blood chemistry screening is not sensitive or specific enough to identify an exposed worker population (8). More specific and sensitive laboratory measurements are needed. Examples

DISEASE RESULTING FROM HAZARDOUS MATERIALS EXPOSURE

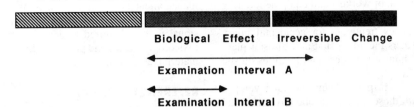

Figure 19.1. This figure schematically illustrates the development of a biologic effect resulting from a continuing exposure to a hazard. After a period of time the biologic effect becomes irreversible if not detected and treated. Examination interval **A** is too long because the next examination occurs when the biologic effect has undergone the irreversible change. The prior examination occurred before the biologic effect could be detected. The prior examination for interval **B** also occurred before the effect could be detected, but, because the interval is shorter than the latency between the first possible detection of the biologic effect and the development of the irreversible change, the next examination for interval **B** still occurs during the reversible period. If the occupational physician knows the latency between the first detectable biologic effect and the development of an irreversible change, the interval for the next examination can be set to a lesser interval, ensuring detection at an optimal time for the specific hazard.

of these include monitoring red blood cell cholinesterase as a response to organophosphate exposure, monitoring β-*n*-acetylglucosaminidase in urine as an early marker of nephrotoxicity, or the detection of abnormalities on nerve conduction studies, and electromyography as early evidence of toxic peripheral neuropathy.

The medical surveillance program is therefore less dependent on the physical examination and more dependent on the laboratory for the early detection and evaluation of biochemical and physiologic changes, yet the commonly used laboratory screening tests may not effectively define exposure. In all instances, the well-designed medical surveillance program should be tailored to the specific chemicals to which the workers are exposed. It should be designed to detect evidence of disease that is known to be causally linked to specific exposures and to detect unanticipated disease due to known or unknown exposures.

Medical surveillance attempts to provide a means of detecting subtle changes in organ function of a cohort that may be dismissed as part of normal human variation when examined on an individual basis. The proper approach to a medical surveillance program should be on the basis of the target organs affected. The main organ systems monitored include skin, nervous system, liver, renal system, pulmonary system, cardiovascular system, and blood. The physical examination should be designed with the specific job requirements in mind. A longitudinal follow-up is essential for adequately protecting and monitoring members of hazardous waste teams because of the latency effects of some exposures. Parameters should be defined to trigger further investigation.

Essentially, then, the individuals and the cohort should have normal values defined based on their own unique baseline values and should be monitored to detect cohort abnormalities as well as individual abnormalities. As the cohort grows, the group norms can be stratified by age, weight, sex, and exposure, and the trigger values can be adjusted accordingly.

The boundaries for the trigger values should be defined by the cohort average and also by specifying a value, i.e., one or two standard deviations away from the mean, for alerting the occupational physician of the possibility of some perturbation in the health of the cohort that requires further evaluation and definition. Likewise, the individuals in the cohort should also have trigger values identified based on their unique averages that would provoke further inquiry stemming from perturbations of the individual's normal or average parameters.

A thorough history of the individual workers assigned to the site is mandatory. The history will identify past exposures of the individuals and the doses if possible, unique sensitivities of the individuals based on genetic factors or allergic reactions, and past or existing medical conditions that modify the risk of one individual over another.

The physical examination should focus on the organ systems and be reported out by organ system. There should be an effort to identify and define risk factors for each individual, not only with regard to hazardous exposures, but with a view toward enhancing and promoting the health and well-being of the waste worker member. The physical examination must also be performance-oriented, i.e., demonstrating the ability to wear a respirator, carry a backpack, and carry equipment at the same time.

Interval or periodic examinations: The periodic evaluation of the worker is a form of biologic monitoring designed to identify physical manifestations of changes in physiology due to hazardous substance exposures. Early identification is desired in order to intervene at a point in time that will prevent injury and permanent impairment. This periodic evaluation will oftentimes require environmental monitoring to link exposure with effects, and this should be done with the guidance of a certified industrial hygienist. Fig. 19.1 illustrates the importance of the proper interval for periodic examinations in order to detect reversible changes before permanent impairment can occur.

The health and safety program must also be designed to provide for management of acute injury and illness resulting from hazardous materials exposures. There should be a previously identified medical center with the resources to handle the special needs of the hazardous materials patient.

Initial and periodic physical evaluations and the data generated should be reviewed, coded, and entered into an information system. Management of the individual's medical problems, if any, should be the responsibility of the occupational physician if related to any toxic exposure. The information system will link the data in the cohort and permit the compiling of statistical summaries. Evaluation of the group data will permit the occupational physician to identify subtle changes which might otherwise be missed in one or two individuals but which need observation and tracking. The information system should not only have such parameters established, but should have defined limits to trigger further investigation.

Decontamination and emergency response: Provisions must be made for decontamination of workers and equipment during egress from the waste site, and a disaster or emergency response plan is required. Emergency treatment for accidental injury encompass many parameters including first aid, disaster planning, and assessment of human resources and facilities on site and off site.

The hazardous materials response team should develop a working relationship with those physicians and environmental health professionals capable of providing toxicologic, industrial hygiene, emergency, and clinical management information relating to hazardous or toxic incident containment and control. This may involve sampling, protective measures for on-scene personnel, evacuation recommendations, and medical treatment.

CONCLUSION

Overall, hazardous materials management has increasingly required a multidisciplinary effort involving health professionals, specialized legal counsel, and management information systems. Given the legal requirements of "cradle-to-grave" accountability for hazardous materials, it is clear that health and safety issues will continue to receive significant attention. This trend is not confined to the United States. Hazardous waste management is a major issue in Western Europe as well as other industrialized countries. The health and safety professional will be required to demonstrate knowledge of medical toxicologic, legal, and public health issues involving hazardous materials and wastes.

REFERENCES

1. Travis CC, Cook SC, eds. Composition of hazardous waste. In: Hazardous waste incineration and human health. Boca Raton: CRC Press, 1989:1–15.

2. Carden JL. Hazardous waste management. In: Blumenthal DS, ed. Introduction to environmental health. New York: Springer Publishing Co, 1985:179–213.

3. Casto KM. Environmental health law. In: Blumenthal DS, ed. Introduction to environmental health. New York: Springer Publishing Co, 1985:215–247.

4. Code of Federal Regulations, 40 CFR, 261.10, 1985.

5. Barnard TH. Remedies. In: Northstein GZ, ed. Toxic torts-litigation of hazardous substance cases. Colorado Springs: Shepard's/McGraw-Hill, 1984:337–364.

6. Nelson N, Baker S, Levine S, et al. Cleanup of contaminated sites. In: Lave L, Upton A, eds. Toxic chemicals, health, and the environment. Baltimore: Johns Hopkins University Press, 1987:205–279.

7. Monroe C. Medical surveillance. Appl Ind Hyg 1989;4(4):F10–F14.

8. Favata E, Gochfeld M. Medical surveillance of hazardous waste workers: ability of laboratory tests to discriminate exposure. Am J Ind Med 1989;15:255–265.

20

Generation and Disposal of Hazardous Wastes: The Resource Conservation and Recovery Act

Linda M. Micale, M.S.

The generation and disposal of hazardous wastes represents a critical subset of the broader topic of hazardous materials toxicology. The manufacture, use, processing, or accidental release of hazardous materials may result in wastes which are considered hazardous under the Resource Conservation and Recovery Act, or RCRA (15). Passed in 1976, this federal law and its associated regulations seek to reduce public health risks and environmental impacts by controlling hazardous wastes from the time they are generated to their ultimate disposal.

This chapter summarizes the regulatory programs initiated by the Congress and developed by the Environmental Protection Agency (EPA) to implement RCRA. The chapter has three sections: Background, Basic Regulatory Requirements, and Conclusions. The first section discusses the primary issues surrounding the passage, amendment, and reauthorization of RCRA. Basic Regulatory Requirements covers the definition of hazardous wastes and identifies requirements applicable to hazardous waste generators; transporters; and treatment, storage, and disposal facilities. The final section discusses some of RCRA's impacts on industry, including process and waste management, worker exposure to hazardous wastes, and environmental issues.

BACKGROUND

Hazardous wastes are so designated due to the physical, biologic, or chemical characteristics of the wastes that may present risks to public health or environment. Shortterm health risks associated with hazardous wastes include immediate health impacts from inhalation, ingestion, or skin absorption (6). Environmental impacts on this time frame may include risks of fire, explosion, production of noxious gases, and polluted discharges to land or surface waters. Longterm health risks associated with chronic exposure to low doses of hazardous wastes include central nervous system problems, cancer, and birth defects (6, 13). These health risks may be tied to longterm environmental impacts. Hazardous wastes improperly disposed of on land may accumulate in and contaminate subsurface soils; soil contaminants may ultimately migrate to drinking water supplies (8).

Hazardous wastes are generated from a wide range of sources. Large generators include chemical and electronics manufacturers, while small quantity generators may include automobile repair shops and dry cleaners. The EPA reported the five most prevalent types of hazardous wastes generated in the United States in order of occurrence: corrosive wastes; mixtures of general waste types; mixtures of wastes which may be ignitable, corrosive, reactive, or toxic; chromium wastes; and mixtures of certain industrial wastes (9). According to this study, nearly half of all hazardous wastes are corrosive.

Estimates on the quantities of wastes generated have varied over the last several years, but all indicate the physical extent of the problem (8). At the time that RCRA was enacted, the EPA estimated that there were 50,000 hazardous waste sites nationwide, containing approximately 60 million tons of wastes (16). The same study estimated that more than 750,000 facilities generated hazardous waste. Studies completed by the Conservation Foundation in 1987 and the EPA in 1989 nearly quadrupled the estimate of waste quantities to more than 250 million tons (4, 9). Over 80% of this total was generated in the Northeast, Southeast and Gulf Coast states (9). Most of these wastes result from major operations; the EPA estimated that less than 5% of generators accounted for more than 95% of hazardous wastes generated in the United States in 1985 (9).

Health and environmental risks from improper waste handling and disposal are difficult to quantify. Although severe impacts are associated with these activities, most studies do not conclusively attribute human illness to longterm exposure to hazardous wastes (8, 13). In a 1987 risk analysis prepared by the EPA's Office of Policy Analysis, experts ranked a variety of risks from hazardous wastes (not including worker exposure) as medium to low (12). Some researchers suggest that the short time frame and reliability of available data is inadequate to establish health risks from longterm exposures. Another reason for such findings may include the difficulty of testing effects from mixtures of chemicals which interact in wastes, rather than from single chemicals with known toxicities (8, 13).

Study findings and government reports notwithstanding, a public opinion poll reviewed by the EPA at the time of the analysis rated risks from hazardous waste disposal as high (12). In the 1970s, public concern was fueled by the discovery of dumped chemical wastes at Love Canal, New York, and the images of children burned by chemicals oozing into their playground (13). In the 1980s, government reports of widespread groundwater contamination and the costs and complexities of remediation jolted the American populace. Thus, the magnitude of wastes produced and public perceptions about risks from hazardous wastes precipitated government regulations on waste management.

Solid Waste Disposal Laws

RCRA and the hazardous waste management program it triggered are relatively recent federal phenomena with statutory roots in the Solid Waste Disposal Act of 1965. Solid waste is generally described as municipal garbage; this act focused on the closing of open dumps and the development of "sanitary" landfills, where risks were presumably controlled. This act was amended in 1970 and 1973 by the Resource Recovery Act, which authorized the federal government to provide assistance and guidance aimed at improving solid waste management systems (14). The amendments did not establish strict requirements, unlike other acts passed during this era, for example, the Clean Air Act and Clean Water Act. EPA required only federal facilities to follow solid waste guidelines to build a model for industry and other levels of government. The guidelines were published in Title 40 *Code of Federal Regulations* (CFR), Parts 240 and 241; 243 through 247.

These early laws contained provisions to study hazardous waste management practices throughout the United States. One source suggests, however, that these provisions were basically ignored by the new EPA. Instead, the agency focused on air and water quality problems nationwide (16).

The Passage of RCRA

In the mid-1970s the U.S. Congress responded to growing public concerns over disposal of solid and hazardous wastes by drafting a comprehensive new law. Prior to its passage, the Congress held one year of public hearings on relevant waste management issues. The Senate enacted its version of the RCRA during the summer of 1976, but so many bills were introduced in the House that it was difficult to select one. The version that passed in October 1976 reflected major concepts of those various bills (14).

The original text of RCRA broadly encompassed solid waste management and recycling—perhaps this is why the act is titled "Resource Conservation and Recovery" instead of the "Hazardous Waste Management Act" (14, 16). This act's objectives were to reduce waste, conserve energy and natural resources, reduce or eliminate generation of hazardous waste as much as possible, and to protect human health and the environment. RCRA maintained the solid waste program of 1970, added a major hazardous waste regulatory program, prohibited open dumping, and provided grants for state and regional solid waste management planning. RCRA superseded the 1965 and 1970 acts (15).

Although RCRA contains a wide range of waste management provisions, EPA implementation clearly focused on Subtitle C management of hazardous wastes to prevent release to the environment. This subtitle mandates regulations to determine what wastes are hazardous (Section 3001); to notify EPA of hazardous waste activity, and to establish requirements for hazardous waste generators and transporters (Sections 3002, 3003); and for treatment, storage, and disposal facilities (sections 3004 and 3005). RCRA also allows for enforcement of standards through compliance orders, administrative orders, and consent decrees. Fines range from up to $25,000 per day for compliance violations to $250,000 for knowing endangerment of others through their handling of hazardous wastes (Section 3007/3008). Penalties for certain violations include imprisonment.

RCRA rulemaking has been a lengthy process, primarily due to the breadth and controversy surrounding many of RCRA's provisions. The original law stipulated that EPA develop regulations within 18 months in order to curb agency procrastination exhibited in the first solid waste amendments (16). Although proposed rules were published in 1978, finalization was difficult because EPA received a profusion of public comments. Comments from industry at this time claimed that the agency was placing severe burdens on American business. Other commenters were displeased that the agency took too few steps to prevent future Love Canals (16). EPA was sued to meet a court-ordered schedule to issue final hazardous waste regulations by December 31, 1979. The agency was unable to meet this deadline; final rules for hazardous waste lists; generators; transporters; and treatment, storage, and disposal facilities were issued by May 1980.

The Hazardous and Solid Waste Amendments (HSWA)

The Hazardous and Solid Waste Amendments were enacted in 1984. Unlike RCRA, HSWA's objectives emphasized hazardous waste. The Congress also added a section (1003b) which declared the national policy to be the reduction or elimination of hazardous waste generation as soon as possible. The policy also stated that present and future danger to the environment would be minimized by sending hazardous wastes to treatment, storage, and disposal facilities operating under the law. Despite strict deadlines for EPA, HSWA included a statutory hammer—its provisions would take effect whether or not EPA issued regulations (15).

HSWA broadened the scope of RCRA along a number of regulatory fronts. Some of its provisions, like the restrictions on land disposal of hazardous wastes, present the most difficult compliance challenges for industries under this federal program. In addition to the land disposal ban, HSWA sets minimum technology requirements for certain land disposal units, regulates underground storage tanks and the use of hazardous waste for fuel, and requires corrective action for all releases of hazardous wastes at permitted facilities. Other provisions include objectives for waste minimization, increased citizen suit capabilities, and a required inspection and permitting schedule. Given the scope of this law, the Congressional Budget Office expected that HSWA would double the costs of hazardous waste compliance by 1990 (16). At this time (1991), however, the regulated community appeared to favor reauthorization through HSWA and continued development of regulations (8). Standards set by Congress and the EPA allow many significant generators to reduce their liability under RCRA by implementing acceptable waste management or minimization strategies.

Reauthorization Issues

Despite the amendments and some 1500 pages of EPA regulations, hazardous and solid waste issues will arise again as Congress reauthorizes RCRA. RCRA was expected to be reauthorized in 1989 (2). As of this writing Congress did not succeed in reauthorization, but did debate several issues that indicate the maturation of this law. For example, Congress argued about the applicability of RCRA to federal facilities, particularly those at Department of Energy (DOE) sites. The DOE has earned a reputation in recent years as a poor steward of hazardous waste sites. In addition, Congress is reviewing the adequacy of solid waste regulations. Some sources indicate that the definition of solid and hazardous wastes will not change; however, solid waste management is expected to closely parallel hazardous waste requirements (2, 7). EPA estimates that municipal landfills now contain a significant percentage of the nation's hazardous wastes. Municipal ash from incinerators has been found to contain toxic levels of metals (11). Congress is attempting to close loopholes in solid and hazardous waste management by once again broadening the scope of the law.

RCRA's Relationship to Other Selected Laws

RCRA is related to a number of other environmental and worker safety laws. Four examples are:

- Comprehensive Emergency Response, Compensation and Liability Act of 1980 (CERCLA; also known as "Superfund");
- Emergency Planning and Community Right-to-Know Act of 1986 (EPCRA);
- Occupational Safety and Health Act of 1970; and
- Pollution Prevention Act of 1990.

Under CERCLA, the federal government is authorized to remediate inactive or abandoned disposal sites that pose a threat to public health or the environment (14). By contrast, RCRA generally focuses on proper management and corrective action at active waste sites.

EPCRA, Title III of the Superfund Amendments (SARA), requires three types of annual reporting by certain facilities that store or use hazardous chemicals in excess of regulatory thresholds. One requirement involves reporting releases of listed toxic substances to air, water, and land. EPCRA reports are accessible to the public and are expected to instigate waste reduction and improved management among reporting industries.

SARA also required the Department of Labor, through the Occupational Safety and Health Administration (OSHA), to develop standards for workers exposed to hazardous wastes. The regulations specify levels of training, contingency planning, medical surveillance, and hazard assessment aimed at maintaining good health at the work site. As noted earlier, RCRA regulations deal directly with hazardous wastes as they affect the environment and the general public, rather than with worker exposure to wastes.

The Pollution Prevention Act of 1990 is a first step toward reducing the quantity and toxicity of wastes generated in this country. It focuses on "source reduction" or changes in production, operation, and raw materials used as a means to prevent pollution and reduce the high cost of controlling pollution. The law requires facilities that file an annual toxic substances release report under EPCRA to file a source reduction report beginning in 1992.

In addition to the laws listed above, many of RCRA's requirements grew out of environmental laws in place at the time of enactment, including the Federal Water Pollution Control Act and the Clean Air Act (8).

BASIC REGULATORY REQUIREMENTS

This section continues by summarizing basic requirements of RCRA regulations contained in Title 40 CFR Parts 260 through 280. Requirements are typically more complex than they are presented in this section. The purpose of the regulations is to reduce risks attributed to hazardous wastes through specified management procedures.

This section does not discuss RCRA programs developed by states, although the EPA may grant states authority to do so. State RCRA programs must be at least as strict as the federal program. Many states have joint enforcement authority with EPA or may be fully authorized to implement RCRA and HSWA. State programs may completely adopt or add requirements to those discussed below.

Most of the federal requirements focus on the type of facility that deals with hazardous wastes: generators; transporters; and treatment, storage, and disposal facilities. Requirements begin with generators and become stricter and more comprehensive as facilities treat, dispose of, or store hazardous wastes for more than 90 days. These facilities must obtain a RCRA permit

to operate legally, as well as comply with certain permit conditions (5). Existing facilities in the process of obtaining a RCRA permit are considered "interim status" and must also comply with regulatory requirements. Such facilities maintain RCRA status until they undergo clean closure, a site decontamination and investigation process through which most hazardous wastes are removed and potential migration of residual wastes is prevented. In keeping with the cradle-to-grave philosophy of the RCRA, certain facilities are required to provide postclosure maintenance and monitoring.

This section also discusses the EPA's definition of hazardous wastes and selected regulations developed under HSWA aimed at reducing the potential for public or environmental exposure to these wastes.

Characterizing Solid and Hazardous Wastes

RCRA requires that waste generators must be able to "characterize" their wastes in accordance with the definitions provided in 40 CFR Part 261. When characterizing wastes, facility operators must first determine whether the material they generate is indeed a waste by EPA definition. A waste is a material that has served its original intended use and is discarded, intended to be abandoned, recycled, or "inherently waste-like". Materials that can be directly reused are not considered wastes by the EPA (1).

Next, facility operators must determine whether the waste they generate is solid waste. Solid wastes may be liquid, contained gaseous, semisolid, or solid; the category covers almost all wastes, including hazardous wastes and municipal garbage. Some materials are excluded from the definition of solid waste and, thereby, from RCRA regulations. These include point sources of pollution regulated under the Clean Water Act, an irrigation return flow, domestic sewage, in situ mining waste, or an Atomic Energy Commission Source. Although they are not regulated by RCRA, these wastes may still be "hazardous" from a chemical, physical, or biologic perspective. Beyond these and other exclusions identified in the regulations, two types of materials clearly are not solid waste: products or intermediary products of a manufacturing or mining process; and materials other than garbage, refuse, or sludge which are always used (14).

Once identified as a solid waste, facilities must determine whether their wastes are hazardous by RCRA definition. As noted above, hazardous wastes are a subset of solid wastes. Hazardous wastes may be specifically listed within the regulations or exhibit one or more of four characteristics outlined by EPA. The waste may be a mixture of a hazardous and solid waste, with some exceptions. Exclusions from RCRA hazardous wastes currently include household wastes, agricultural wastes used as fertilizers, mining overburden, and oil and natural gas exploration drilling waste, among others (40 CFR 261.4). While many recycling activities are exempt from RCRA Subtitle C, wastes that exhibit a hazardous waste characteristic when they are recycled are subject to hazardous waste regulations.

EPA's basis for defining listed and characteristic hazardous wastes is their toxicity. The CFR (Part 261.10) explains that characteristic hazardous wastes were identified as those which:

- cause or significantly contribute to mortality or irreversible illness;
- pose a substantial present or potential hazard to human health or environment during waste management.

40 CFR Part 261.11 indicates that listed hazardous wastes may also:

- be fatal to humans in low doses or meet specific lethal dose criteria in animals;
- contains certain toxic constituents listed in the regulations (Subpart B, Appendix VIII), unless specific circumstances are reviewed by EPA with the finding that substantial risk is not present.

LISTED HAZARDOUS WASTES (40 CFR Part 261.30)

EPA has established four waste lists. The "F" list contains wastes from nonspecific sources. The list is broadly used by industry because it includes spent solvents like toluene and methylene chloride. The "K" list contains hazardous wastes from specific sources, such as petroleum refining or the production of pigments and certain chemicals. The "U" list identifies discarded commercial chemical products and all off-specification containers and spill residues of the products. The "P" list parallels the "U" list by identifying "acutely" hazardous discarded commercial chemical products. Listed wastes that will be recycled, reused, or reclaimed must adhere to applicable hazardous waste regulations prior to these activities. Several hundred hazardous wastes are currently listed in the regulations. EPA has authority to list additional wastes based on toxicity factors listed above.

Mixtures of listed hazardous waste and solid waste are regulated as hazardous unless they can be successfully "delisted" through a comprehensive testing and reporting process. The process is intended to demonstrate that the specific waste stream in question is not hazardous by EPA definition. The EPA publishes industry proposals to delist wastes in the *Federal Register* and allows for public comment before making a final decision. Successfully delisted wastes and the facility that was granted the petition are identified in corresponding Appendix IX at 40 CFR 261.

CHARACTERISTIC HAZARDOUS WASTES (40 CFR Part 261.21)

In addition to listed wastes, RCRA allows EPA to identify hazardous wastes by characteristics that make them harmful to human health or the environment. There are four characteristics, each with specific definitions:

- **ignitability**—most common definition is the flashpoint below 140°F;
- **corrosivity**—most commonly a pH equal or less than 2 or equal to or greater than 12.5;
- **reactivity**—extremely unstable, tends to react violently or explode during management;
- **toxicity**—specific standards for certain metals, volatile organics, and pesticides based on a test that extracts these constituents from a waste. The method assumes a dilution factor that corresponds to the constituent concentration necessary to leach from a municipal solid waste landfill to ground water.

Mixtures of characteristic and solid wastes are hazardous only if the entire mixture exhibits one of the four characteristics.

Generator and Transporter Requirements

RCRA requirements applicable to generators and transporters of hazardous waste are found in 40 CFR Parts 262 and 263,

respectively. These requirements are aimed at reducing risks primarily through shortterm handling, sound waste management practices, and recordkeeping and reporting.

EPA's definition of generator refers to the specific site where waste is produced. Consequently, a company with many facilities at different locations must meet generator requirements at each individual site. Small quantity generators (SQGs) and "conditionally exempt" SQGs are offered some leniency by the regulations, primarily because EPA found it unfeasible to regulate the anticipated 125,000 SQGs. SQGs are those which generate between 100 and 1000 kilograms of hazardous waste per month. "Conditionally exempt" SQGs generate less than 100 kg per month.

RCRA regulates anyone who transports hazardous wastes with standards closely tied to Department of Transportation (DOT) regulations under the Hazardous Materials Transportation Act. Transporter standards apply to anyone who moves a hazardous waste off the site where it is generated or treated, stored, or disposed, even if it is brought to another facility owned by the same company in the same town. On-site movement is not covered. Transporters are subject to both EPA and DOT enforcement.

With the exception of a conditionally exempt SQGs, facilities must notify EPA that they manage hazardous wastes. Notification must be filed for each site or plant where waste activity occurs. Generators and transporters must obtain an EPA identification number before waste is transported, treated, stored, or disposed.

Both transporters and generators must comply with labeling, marketing, and placarding requirements for containers holding wastes. EPA approved the use of DOT regulations regarding packaging, marking, and placarding for transport purposes. Containers must also be compatible with the wastes they hold.

Most generators are allowed to store hazardous wastes on-site for up to 90 days without a permit. Accumulation times increase to 180 days or less for SQGs as long as no more than 6000 kilograms are accumulated. The regulations allow for an optimal 270 days for SQGs that send their wastes more than 200 miles. Conditionally exempt generators are allowed to accumulate not more than 100 kilograms waste on-site. The accumulation limits are reduced for acutely hazardous wastes from the "P" list.

Generators must follow tank and container rules established for treatment, storage, and disposal facilities if used to store hazardous wastes. Generators must also dispose of wastes at approved facilities in accordance with HSWA land disposal restrictions. Generator requirements on containers and accumulation limits may apply to transporters if they accumulate wastes or mix wastes of different DOT descriptions to consolidate them.

Generators have a number of reporting and recordkeeping requirements under RCRA, including a biennial report to EPA which indicates waste quantities and where they were stored, treated, or disposed. All test results or other rationale used to characterize the waste must be kept on file for three years from the date the waste was last sent to on-site/off-site treatment, storage, and disposal facilities (TSDs). Most generators must keep records that identify quantity, constituents, and disposition of wastes and furnish waste information to transporters and to TSDs that accept the waste. Conditionally exempt SQGs must self-regulate by ensuring that waste is sent to an appropriate facility or is legitimately recycled.

With one exception, generators must use an EPA manifest

to ensure proper disposal at a permitted facility and to designate ultimate destination. Manifests must be kept for 3 years; the generator receives a signed copy from TSD after that facility obtains the waste. SQGs need not use a manifest where waste is reclaimed under contractual agreement. In this case the transport vehicle must maintain a copy of the contract.

Transporters may only accept manifested wastes, and the manifest must be kept with waste at all times. When waste is delivered to another facility or the destination listed on the manifest, the transporter must date it, obtain the signature of the person delivered to, and retain a copy for records. The remaining copies are given to the person receiving wastes. Eventually, the generator receives a signed copy of the manifest after the waste has been delivered to its final destination. If the transporter is unable to deliver waste to the listed destination, he/she must contact the generator for further instructions. Like generators, the transporter keeps a copy of the manifest for 3 years.

Generators are responsible for controlling and cleaning spills of hazardous wastes at their facility. If the spill is expected to threaten human health or the environment, the generator must notify the National Response Center. Transporters are responsible for cleaning up spills during transport, regardless of who generated the initial waste. They are required to take immediate action to protect health and environment. Subsequently, transporters must give applicable verbal and written notification in the event of a spill.

Treatment, Storage, and Disposal Facilities

The strictest RCRA requirements apply to "TSD" facilities. In addition to basic management and recordkeeping, these requirements attempt to reduce risks of exposure through design and siting requirements, permitting, contingency planning, and facility closure. These facilities must be constructed and managed to prevent escape of hazardous wastes or their constituents to the environment. Increased regulation of TSDs results in part from the intensified waste handling activities and the extended timeframe of waste placement. The EPA reported that in 1985 there were 4944 TSD facilities managing 238 million tons of hazardous wastes (16).

RCRA regulations provide definitions for these facilities in 40 CFR 260.10(a). Each of these definitions is quite broad and has been subject to much interpretation by industry and the EPA. The regulations also specify two categories of TSDs, permitted and interim status for those existing facilities applying for a permit. Regulations for interim status facilities are found in 40 CFR Part 265; for permitted in 40 CFR Part 264. The regulations are similar for both categories.

RCRA applies to hazardous waste activities at TSDs occurring after the effective date of Subtitle C regulations on November 19, 1980, and not to abandoned sites or past disposal activities. Facilities rendered inactive on that date avoid RCRA standards. A number of other facilities are exempt from requirements (40 CFR 265.1), including certain publicly owned treatment works, solid waste management facilities that accept wastes only from conditionally exempt SQGs, recycling facilities, and totally enclosed treatment facilities. Like the exemptions for hazardous wastes, exemption from TSD requirements signifies fewer applicable requirements rather than an inherently nonhazardous activity.

WASTE MANAGEMENT REQUIREMENTS

A number of general requirements apply to all TSDs. Operators must have an EPA identification number and they must have detailed knowledge of a waste's chemical and physical characteristics before handling it at the facility. Operators must analyze wastes coming into facilities periodically to ensure that they are the same as listed on the manifest. A general waste analysis must be repeated as necessary for accuracy, and the operator must develop a waste analysis plan to describe facility procedure for waste identification.

TSDs must implement a number of activities to prepare for emergencies and prevent environmental accidents. Security measures are critical to preclude unauthorized entry. Operators must prepare and implement an inspection plan around the facility. Personnel conducting inspections and routine work at the facility are required to have expertise in their duties. Ignitable, reactive, and incompatible wastes must be handled carefully. Routine preparedness efforts must be augmented by a detailed contingency plan. Permitted facilities sited in floodplains or areas prone to seismic activity must be designed to reduce additional risks due to location.

TSDs must comply with land disposal regulations under HSWA which generally prohibit placement of hazardous wastes in a wide range of facilities unless they meet strict treatment standards (40 CFR Part 268). These standards may be technology based and/or may involve concentration limits for a specific constituent in a wastewater or non wastewater media. Treatment standards based solely on technologies are used typically where EPA cannot establish a concentration limit, in part, because appropriate analytical test methods do not exist.

Standards are based on an EPA determination that contaminants will not leach from the waste upon land placement and migrate to groundwater. Affected facilities include waste piles, surface impoundments, injection wells, land treatment facilities, and landfills, among other facilities. The requirements have been phased in over several years, with limited exemptions and case-by-case variances.

Facilities where hazardous waste is purposely placed on or into the land must conduct groundwater monitoring to assess the impact on the uppermost aquifer. Monitoring must be conducted in accordance with a written plan during operation and after facility closure (15, 16).

In addition to general requirements, the regulations set specific standards for ten types of facilities:

- containers
- tanks
- surface impoundments
- waste piles
- land treatment units
- landfills
- incinerators
- thermal treatment units
- chemical, physical, and biologic treatment units
- underground injection wells

Each of the requirements focuses on preventing and containing releases of hazardous wastes.

RECORDKEEPING AND REPORTING

TSDs must comply with a variety of reporting requirements. In addition to EPA notification and obtainment of an ID number, permitted facilities must document compliance with management of ignitable, reactive, or incompatible wastes. TSDs must immediately sign and date manifests, then return a copy to the generator within 30 days. They must maintain a complete operating record until closure, with specific requirements. Other basic reports include submittals for unmanifested waste within 15 days of receipt and reports for hazardous waste releases. The owner must obtain liability insurance during the operating life of the facility for claims arising from hazardous waste operations. Finally, suspicious findings of groundwater monitoring must be reported to EPA; monitoring records must be kept for the life of the site.

PERMITTING UNDER RCRA

As noted above, every owner of a TSD must obtain a permit to operate. EPA has a two-step approach to permitting, Parts A and B. Part A permit applications provide basic information about the facility and are conditions for qualifying for interim status. Information required in the Part B application includes:

- contingency plans for emergencies
- waste analysis procedures
- inspection schedules
- operating procedures to prevent environmental contamination at the site
- facility design and layout
- groundwater protection
- closure/post-closure plans
- list of containers, tanks, incinerators at site

Rules on issuing RCRA permits are in 40 CFR Parts 122, 123, 124, and 270. The permitting process can cost hundreds of thousands of dollars in preparation time for large, complex facilities. Facilities may need one or more years to address agency or public concerns, particularly if the siting of a new TSD near a population center is at issue. Permit issuance is based on an agency finding that the facility complies with RCRA. Once issued, permits are effective for 10 years, but may be reviewed, revoked, or modified by EPA if necessary. HSWA requires permit review by EPA every 5 years and a facility inspection every 2 years.

Under HSWA, EPA had 4 years to issue permits for land disposal, 5 years for incinerators, and 8 years for all other types of waste facilities. Interim status will expire and the facility must be closed if the deadlines are missed. Interim status terminated for land disposal facilities in November 1985 unless Part B was submitted at that time. The status terminated for incinerators in November 1989 unless a Part B was submitted in November 1986, and for all other facilities it will terminate in 1992 unless a Part B was submitted in November 1988. As of November 1988, only 168 final permits were issued for land disposal (5).

The RCRA Part B permit constitutes a detailed operating manual which prepares a facility to manage risks from hazardous wastes. Through the RCRA permitting process, TSDs are required to identify problem areas at their facilities which may pose a threat from storage of hazardous wastes, etc. The permit also requires certain conditions of operation which are audited through EPA or state RCRA inspections. The internal inspection program is one means that companies can use to reduce their environmental liability.

FACILITY CLOSURE AND POST-CLOSURE

All TSD facilities must have a written closure plan which includes an inventory of maximum wastes during active life; a description of steps to remove or decontaminate all facility containment systems, equipment, structures, and soils; a schedule for closure activities; and a cost estimate and financial assurances. The plan is reviewed by the public and must be amended as required by EPA or state authority. Disposal facilities must also prepare a post-closure plan which includes groundwater monitoring. This plan prepares for maintenance 30 years after the closing of the site.

RCRA regulations take into account the fact that preventing environmental harm at TSDs over the long term is costly. Financial responsibility requirements were established to ensure that funds for closure and post-closure are available.

SUMMARY AND CONCLUSIONS

Through the passage of RCRA and its amendments, the Congress instituted strict controls on hazardous waste management to reduce environmental and public health risks. The EPA developed RCRA regulations which define solid (nonhazardous) and hazardous wastes and set requirements for waste transporters and facilities that actively generate, treat, store, or dispose of hazardous wastes. RCRA contains provisions that allow the EPA to enforce regulations through administrative orders to comply, civil and criminal penalties, and injunctive relief against violators. In addition, amendments to RCRA increased the level of requirements applicable to regulated facilities, including bans on land disposal and minimum technology standards.

RCRA requirements are encyclopedic and require regulated industries to have a thorough knowledge of the inclusive definitions as well as of the standards in order to comply. The scope of these requirements can translate into significant implementation costs for the regulated industries. While it is difficult to place a cost figure on the wide range and size of facilities which implement RCRA requirements, it is generally accepted that the cost of preventing environmental releases is far overshadowed by the costs of corrective action or Superfund cleanups. The costs of implementation roughly increase from a few thousand dollars to hundreds of thousands annually as one moves from small quantity generator requirements through TSD compliance. Further, the slow rate of RCRA Part B permitting and the land disposal bans limit available storage, treatments, and disposal options, adding to the burden of handling hazardous wastes.

Given the high costs and difficulties of compliance, regulated industries are wise to evaluate their activities and find efficient, responsible means with which to implement RCRA requirements. A number of recommendations are offered to help regulated industries (6, 8, 10) reduce the costs of compliance and the risks of handling hazardous wastes.

First, facilities should perform a thorough audit of processes, wastes generated, and raw materials used in order to identify opportunities for reducing the quantity and toxicity of wastes. Process modifications or material substitutions may help reduce the potential for release of hazardous materials and exposures to facility workers. The audit may also consider the potential for reuse, reclaiming, or recycling hazardous wastes. The need for treatment and disposal of certain waste streams may be significantly diminished as a result.

Second, regulated industries which transport their hazardous wastes for storage, treatment, or disposal off-site should assess the integrity and compliance status of those facilities. The regulatory history may be evaluated, for example, by identifying the number of reported releases or corrective actions at the TSD. Common sources of information include hazardous waste management periodicals, regulatory agencies, and the EPA's SARA database. Other assessment safeguards may include technical evaluations through facility audits and a review of the facility's financial status and liability insurance. One source suggests that the costs of facility assessments may be reduced if several waste generators perform these studies jointly (6).

Finally, all of these activities should be part of a hazardous waste management plan that balances longterm benefits and risks (6, 10). Factors to consider include more than facility processes and TSD integrity. Regulated industries must also develop management programs that respond to public perceptions. From this perspective RCRA hazardous waste controls may, as suggested by the EPA Office of Policy Analysis, deal less with quantifiable risks than with response to perceptions of environmental and public responsibility.

REFERENCES

1. Buchanan MW. Recycling issues. In: The resource conservation and recovery Act (RCRA): the teenage years. Scottsdale, AZ: State Bar of Arizona, 1989.

2. Bureau of National Affairs, Inc. House staff member predicts little action on RCRA this Session, no house bill this year. Environmental reporter, current developments 1989; 20(5): 193.

3. Code of Federal Regulations. Title 40, Parts 260–280.

4. The Conservation Foundation. State of the environment: A view toward the nineties. Washington, DC: The Conservation Foundation, 1987.

5. Curry JS. Outline of RCRA permit requirements for hazardous waste treatment, storage and disposal facilities. In: The resource conservation and recovery act (RCRA): the teenage years. Scottsdale, AZ: State Bar of Arizona, 1989.

6. Goldman BA, Hulme JA, Johnson C. Hazardous waste management reducing the risk. Washington, DC: Island Press, 1986.

7. Kelley KP. Regulations force changes in environmental strategies. Hazmat world 1989; 2(7).

8. Krag BL. Hazardous wastes ad their management. Hazardous Waste and Hazardous Materials 1985; 2(3):251–308.

9. McCoy and Associates, Inc. "EPA releases report on 1985 hazardous waste generation and management. The Hazardous Waste Consultant 1989, 7(5):1–1 to 1–5.

10. McCoy and Associates, Inc. "GE develops method for determining true costs of waste management—including future liability. The Hazardous Waste Consultant 1988; 6(2):1–1 to 1–3.

11. McCoy and Associates, Inc. Municipal incinerator ash studied. The Hazardous Waste Consultant 1988; 6(2):1–22.

12. McCoy and Associates, Inc. Risk analysis shows hazardous waste problems overrated. The Hazardous Waste Consultant 1987; 5(3):2–26 to 2–28.

13. Paigen B. Goldman LR, Highland JH, Magnant MM, Steegman AT, Jr. Prevalence of health problems in children living near Love Canal. Hazardous Waste and Hazardous Materials, 1985;2(1):23–44.

14. Sullivan TFP. Resource conservation and recovery act. In: Environmental law handbook. 7th ed. Rockville, MD: Government Institutes, 1983.

15. U.S. Congress. Resource Conservation and Recovery Act of 1976. Public Law 94–580, October 17, 1986, as amended.

16. Worobec, MD. RCRA. In: Toxic substances controls primer. Washington, DC: Bureau of National Affairs, 1986.

21

The Toxic Substances Control Act

Paul D. Phillips, A.B., J.D.
Dana L. Hofstetter, B.S.E., M.A., J.D.

The Toxic Substances Control Act (TSCA) was enacted by Congress in 1976 (1). TSCA was designed to "fill the cracks" in environmental and health protection that remained despite the prior promulgation of numerous environmental and health statutes (2). The Federal Clean Air Act, the Clean Water Act, the Insecticide, Fungicide, and Rodenticide Act, the Food and Drug Act, and the Safe Drinking Water Act offered protection from certain substances or from certain pollutants in specific media. TSCA regulates the manufacture and use of chemical substances and mixtures that present an "unreasonable risk of injury to health or the environment" but remain unregulated by these more focused statutes (3). Conversely, because foods, drugs, pesticides, nuclear materials, tobacco, ammunition, water pollutants, and air pollutants were regulated under other laws, these materials were excluded from the scope of TSCA (4). Nevertheless, thousands of chemical substances are subject to TSCA's requirements.

TSCA imposes detailed reporting and recordkeeping requirements on manufacturers, processors, and commercial distributors of chemical substances or mixtures. Where there is insufficient existing information, TSCA allows the United States Environmental Protection Agency (EPA) to require that health and environmental tests be conducted on such substances. EPA, based on the reports it receives or based on other available information, can impose regulatory requirements on the distribution, use, and disposal of chemical substances. Simply put, TSCA provides EPA the authority to gather information on chemical substances and to regulate human and environmental chemical exposure based on that information.

Since information gathering is the hub of EPA's TSCA program, this chapter will first address the Act's reporting, testing, recordkeeping, and notification requirements. Then, the legal restrictions imposed upon the production or distribution of chemical substances under TSCA will be discussed. Finally, a description of TSCA enforcement measures will complete this overview.

INFORMATION GATHERING

EPA, under TSCA, administers numerous information gathering programs. These programs include: (a) inventory reporting, (b) premanufacture and significant new use notification, (c) chemical-specific data recording and reporting, (d) health and safety study reporting, (e) health and environmental effects testing, (f) substantial risk notification, and (g) significant adverse reaction recording. These information-gathering authorities enable EPA to identify chemical substances that pose unreasonable risks from which human health and the environment may need to be safeguarded.

Chemical Substances Inventory

TSCA directs EPA to compile an inventory of chemical substances manufactured, imported, or processed for commercial

purposes in the United States (5). In 1977, EPA promulgated regulations requiring manufacturers, processors, and importers of chemical substances for commercial purposes since January 1, 1975, to file reports for the purpose of compiling the inventory (6, 7). The initial inventory, based on the first reports received, was published in May 1979 (8). New chemical substances are added to the inventory as EPA receives notices of commencement of manufacture or import (9). Currently, the inventory contains over 63,000 chemical substances (10) and is available on commercial database systems such as DIALOG (11). The TSCA Inventory Update Rule requires that production information for certain chemical substances be updated every 4 years (12).

The main purpose of the inventory is to define what are new chemical substances requiring premanufacture notification (13). If a substance is not on the inventory, it is a new chemical substance, and the manufacturer or importer must, prior to commencing production or importation, submit premanufacture notification to EPA (14).

New Substance Premanufacture Notification and Significant New Use Notification

Manufacturers or importers of new chemical substances and manufacturers, processors, or importers of chemical substances for significant new uses must provide premanufacture or significant new use notice to the EPA at least 90 days before the manufacturing, processing, or importation begins (15, 16). While "new chemical substances" are any chemical substances not on the TSCA Chemical Substances Inventory, significant new uses for specific chemical substances are identified in EPA regulations (17). For example, EPA regulations provide that for 11-aminoundecanoic acid, a significant new use is "any use other than as an intermediate in the manufacture of polymers in an enclosed process when it is expected that the 11-aminoundecanoic acid will be fully polymerized during the manufacturing process, or a component in photoprocessing solutions (18)."

Some categorical exemptions from these premanufacturing and significant new use notification requirements exist (19). Substances manufactured in quantities less than 1000 kg/year, chemical substances produced in small quantities solely for research and development, and chemical substances produced for test marketing purposes are among the categories of exemptions available (20). However, for these exemptions to apply, certain conditions, including labeling and supervision requirements, must be fulfilled (21).

For new chemical substances, the premanufacture notice submitted to EPA must provide: chemical identity information, including chemical name, molecular formula, Chemical Abstracts Service registry number, structural diagram, anticipated impurities and byproducts; production, import, and use information, including estimated maximum production quantities, estimated quantities dedicated to each category of use and the percentage of the new substance present in each planned formulation; and human exposure and environmental release information, including process descriptions, worker exposure information, and environmental control technology identification (22, 23). Additionally, available health and environmental effects data should accompany the premanufacture notice submitted to EPA (24). EPA Form No. 7710-25 is the appropriate form to use for the submission of a premanufacture notice and the required accompanying information (25). Reporters of significant new uses also use this form and are generally required to provide the same information (26).

Chemical-Specific Reporting Requirements

Section 8(a) of TSCA provides EPA authority to promulgate chemical-specific recording and reporting requirements for substances in production. Under this authority EPA may require the recording and reporting of manufacturing, safety, use, and exposure information (27). The substances subject to these reporting requirements and the information required for each of these substances can be found at 40 *Code of Federal Regulations* (CFR) Parts 704 and 712. Recently, EPA has attempted to standardize the submission of chemical-specific reporting (28).

Health and Safety Study Reporting

TSCA authorizes EPA to require manufacturers, processors, and distributors to submit lists or copies of health and safety studies (29). This authority enables EPA to gather existing information about chemical substances; however, it does not authorize EPA to require manufacturers, processors, or distributors to perform health and safety studies. The list of substances subject to the health and safety reporting requirements is found at 40 CFR § 716.120 (1988).

The Act broadly defines "health and safety study" to include "any study of any effect of a chemical substance or mixture on health or the environment or on both . . ." (30). In its regulations promulgated pursuant to this authority, EPA has further indicated that it intends to broadly interpret the scope of health and safety data that must be reported (31). Studies of certain specified physical and chemical properties are required to be reported if the studies were conducted for the purpose of evaluating a substance's environmental or biologic fate (32). Similarly, monitoring data, if analyzed to measure human or environmental exposure to a listed substance, must be reported (33).

EPA exempts studies published in the scientific literature from the health and safety reporting requirements (34). Lists of ongoing studies, initiated studies, studies which are known to but are not in possession of the reporter, and studies previously sent to federal agencies without confidentiality claims may be provided in lieu of submission of actual copies of the studies (35). Copies of ongoing or initiated studies, however, must be submitted once they are completed (36). EPA may also request or subpoena the underlying data for any reported study (37).

Health and Environmental Effects Testing

In addition to being able to require the submission of existing health and safety studies or lists of such studies, EPA can require the performance of health or environmental testing of chemical substances (38, 39). EPA can require such testing when a chemical substance or mixture may present unreasonable risks and there is insufficient information about these effects, or when substantial quantities of a chemical substance will be produced, substantial environmental or human exposure is expected, and health and environmental effects information is insufficient (40). Upon occasion, where consensus among EPA, manufacturers, processors, and other interested parties is achieved, EPA will enter into testing consent agreements instead of promulgating a chemical-specific testing rule (41).

The testing rules EPA has promulgated for specific chemical substances can be found at 40 CFR Part 799 (1988). Monochlorobenzene, 1,2- and 1,4-dichlorobenzenes, 1,2,3- and 1,2,4-trichlorobenzenes, 9,10-anthraquinone, ortho-cresol, meta-cresol, para-cresol, and 1,1,1-trichloroethane are examples of the substances subject to EPA testing requirements. For example, manufacturers and processors of 1,2,3- and 1,2,4-trichlorobenzene are required to conduct environmental effects testing including marine invertebrate acute toxicity testing, marine fish acute toxicity testing, freshwater fish acute toxicity testing, freshwater invertebrate acute toxicity testing, and mysid shrimp (*Mysidopis bahia*) chronic toxicity testing, as well as health effects testing involving oncogenicity studies of two rodent species (42).

EPA has promulgated "good laboratory practice" standards as well as extensive chemical fate, environmental effects, and health effects testing guidelines (43). These detailed guidelines specify laboratory equipment requirements; laboratory protocol requirements; and data collection, reporting, and evaluation requirements. Manufacturers and processors conducting tests pursuant to one of EPA chemical testing rules are required to submit study plans including test protocol, supporting reasons for the selected protocol, test schedules, and summaries of the professional backgrounds of those conducting the study to EPA for approval (44).

Manufacturers or processors subject to a testing rule may obtain an exemption from testing requirements where duplicative data already have been or are going to be submitted to EPA by another manufacturer or processor in accordance with the testing rule (45). An exempt manufacturer or processor, however, may be required to partially reimburse the costs of those manufacturers or processors conducting the test (46).

Substantial Risk Notification

Section 8(e) of TSCA requires manufacturers, processors, or distributors to notify EPA upon obtaining information indicating that a commercial substance presents "a substantial risk of injury to health or the environment" (47, 48). These notices typically report the results of toxicity, teratology, and other health effects tests (49). EPA reviews the notices and issues a status report containing questions for the submitter, referrals to other agencies, and EPA follow-up actions (50). Copies of Section 8(e) notices and status reports are available from EPA (51).

Significant Adverse Reaction Recording

Section 8(c) of TSCA requires that manufacturers, processors, or distributors of chemical substances or mixtures "maintain records of significant adverse reactions to health or the environment . . . alleged to have been caused by the substance or mixture'' (52, 53). Additionally, Section 8(c) requires that, upon request, these records be made available for inspection by EPA (54). Allegations of significant adverse reaction may be made by any person, including employees, consumers, neighbors of the manufacturing or processing facility, or organizations on behalf of their members (55). However, ''known human effects,'' defined as ''a commonly recognized human health effect of a particular substance or mixture as described . . . in scientific articles or publications abstracted in standard reference sources [or] the firm's product labeling or material safety data sheets,'' need not be recorded (56). Section 8(c) requirements can significantly impact an internal company medical department or an occupational medicine clinic representing chemical producers or distributors.

HAZARDOUS CHEMICAL REGULATION AND CONTROL

Several provisions of TSCA provide EPA authority to regulate the manufacture, processing, distribution, use, or disposal of hazardous chemicals. TSCA, Section 6, specifies numerous means by which EPA can regulate hazardous chemicals posing unreasonable risks. These means include: prohibiting or limiting the manufacture, processing, or distribution of a substance; prohibiting or limiting the manufacture, processing, or distribution of a substance for a particular use; requiring the provision of adequate warnings and instructions; requiring the retention of processing records; requiring monitoring; prohibiting or regulating the manner or method of commercial use; prohibiting or regulating disposal; requiring notice of unreasonable risks to distributors, possessors, and the public coupled with replacement or repurchase of the hazardous substance; and requiring manufacturing and processing quality control procedures (57). For example, on July 12, 1989, EPA issued a rule under Section 6 of TSCA prohibiting in three scheduled stages the manufacture, importation, processing, and distribution of most asbestos-containing products (58). EPA has also restricted the manufacture of aerosol propellants containing fully halogenated chlorofluoroalkanes (CFCs) under its TSCA Section 6 authority (59).

Sections 5(e) and 5(f) of TSCA are intended to provide EPA the authority to control the manufacture, processing, distribution, use, or disposal of substances for which premanufacturing or significant new use notification has been submitted but before the manufacture of the new substance or the significant new use occurs (60). EPA has 90 days from the receipt of a complete premanufacture or significant new use notice to review the notice and determine whether regulatory action is necessary (61). Upon a determination of good cause EPA may extend this notice review period (62). If the notice review period expires and EPA has taken no restrictive regulatory action, importation or manufacture of the new chemical substance or significant new use chemical substance may begin (63, 64).

If EPA finds that insufficient information is available to assess health and environmental effects and the new substance or new use may present an unreasonable risk of injury to health or the environment or may result in substantial human or environmental exposure, EPA may issue an order or seek an injunction limiting the manufacture, processing, distribution, use, or disposal of the substance in question pending development of more information (65, 66). If EPA finds that the new substance or new use ''presents or will present an unreasonable risk of injury to health or the environment'' before a

formal rule can be promulgated preventing such unreasonable risk, EPA must publish an immediately effective proposed rule, issue an order effective upon expiration of the notice period, or apply for an injunction to restrict the manufacture, processing, or distribution of the substance at issue (67). For example, such immediately effective rules have been issued prohibiting the addition of nitrosating agents and requiring notification of customers and machine shop workers of potential health hazards of three metal-working fluids (68).

Additionally, TSCA provides two special regulatory authorities for imminent hazards and for substances posing ''significant risk of serious or widespread harm to human beings from cancer, gene mutations, or birth defects'' (69). TSCA's imminent hazard authority allows the EPA to initiate judicial proceedings for seizure of an ''imminently hazardous chemical substance or mixture or any article containing such a substance or mixture'' and for relief from any manufacturer, processor, distributor, user, or disposer of an imminently hazardous chemical substance (70). Imminent hazard relief includes risk notification to purchasers, risk notification to the public, recall, and replacement or repurchase of the imminently hazardous substance (71).

When EPA receives information indicating that a chemical substance may pose a significant human health risk of cancer, gene mutations, or birth defects, EPA must act within 180 days to prevent or reduce the risk or, alternatively, establish that the risk is not unreasonable (72). Methylene chloride, 4,4'-methylenedianiline, construction materials and fabrics containing formaldehyde-based resins, and 1,3-butadiene have been subject to this accelerated 180-day review (73).

TSCA PROVISIONS APPLICABLE TO SPECIFIC SUBSTANCES

TSCA has special provisions specifically applicable to polychlorinated biphenyls (PCBs), asbestos, and indoor radon (74). TSCA's PCB provisions prohibit the manufacture, processing, or distribution of PCBs in other than a totally enclosed manner except where the EPA finds that it will not present unreasonable risks (75). TSCA's PCB provisions also require EPA to regulate the disposal of PCBs and to regulate that PCBs be marked with warnings.

TSCA's asbestos provisions, which are lengthy and detailed, provide for the inspection of asbestos in schools and the implementation of necessary response actions required to afford protection from asbestos-containing material in schools (78). TSCA's indoor radon provisions provide for the development of a citizen's radon guide, the development of model construction standards for controlling radon, technical and financial assistance to state radon programs, and radon surveys of federal buildings and schools (77).

TSCA ENFORCEMENT MEASURES

Violators of TSCA are subject to civil penalties of up to $25,000 for each violation and criminal penalties of up to $25,000 for each day of violation and imprisonment of up to one year (78–80). Violations of TSCA include the failure to comply with any of TSCA's provisions or any EPA rules, orders, or requirements authorized by TSCA (81). Also, the commercial use of a chemical substance by one who knows or has reason to know that the substance was manufactured, processed, or distributed in violation of the premanufacturing and significant new use requirements, or in violation of an EPA rule or order limiting manufacture, processing, or distribution, is illegal (82). In addition to seeking civil or criminal penalties, EPA can initiate civil judicial actions in federal court to restrain violations of TSCA or to compel any action required by TSCA (83).

TSCA also provides for citizens' civil actions and citizens' petitions. After giving notice to EPA, members of the public can initiate actions against violators of TSCA (84). Additionally, members of the public can bring suit against the EPA administrator to compel the administrator to perform acts required by TSCA (85). TSCA also empowers private citizens to petition the administrator to issue, amend, or repeal rules (86).

CONCLUSION

TSCA provides EPA comprehensive authority to gather information about commercial chemical substances. It also empowers EPA to protect human health and the environment from perceived "unreasonable risks" posed by these commercial chemical substances. Relative to its potentially far-reaching applications, TSCA is a statutory "sleeping giant" whose regulatory authorities have only begun to be utilized. Because of its potential scope, TSCA is a statute that is likely to assume ever greater importance in the realm of hazardous materials regulation.

ENDNOTES

1. Public Law 94-469, 90 Stat. 2003, codified as amended at 15 United States Code, Section 2601, *et seq.*

2. S. Rep. No. 698, 94th Cong., 2nd Sess. 1 (1976).

3. The term "unreasonable risk of injury to health or the environment" is not defined in TSCA. TSCA's legislative history suggests that unreasonable risks are determined by weighing the likelihood and severity of harm against the substance's social benefits:

> During the hearings, a number of witnesses recommended that the bill include a definition of unreasonable risk. Because the determination of unreasonable risk involves a consideration of probability, severity, and similar factors which cannot be defined in precise terms and is not a factual determination but rather requires the exercise of judgment on the part of the person making it, the Committee [House Committee on Interstate and Foreign Commerce] did not attempt a definition of such risk. In general, a determination that a risk associated with a chemical substance or mixture is unreasonable involves balancing the probability that harm will occur and the magnitude and severity of that harm against the effect of proposed regulatory action on the availability to society of the benefits of the substance or mixture, taking into account the availability of substitutes for the substance or mixture which do not require regulation, and other adverse effects which such proposed action may have on society.

H.R. Rep. No. 1341, 94th Cong., 2d Sess. 13-14 (1976).

4. 15 U.S.C. § 2602(2) (B).

5. 5 U.S.C. § 2607(b).

6. 42 Fed. Reg. 64,572 (December 23, 1977); 40 C.F.R., Part 710 (1988).

7. Chemical substances manufactured or processed in small quantities solely for research, experimentation or chemical analysis purposes are excluded from the inventory. 15 U.S.C. § 2607(b).

8. 47 Fed. Reg. 25,767 (June 15, 1982).

9. 40 C.F.R. § 720.102 (1988).

10. 51 Fed. Reg. 21,483 (June 12, 1986).

11. DIALOG is an outline collection of informational databases that is available from Dialog Information Services, Inc., Palo Alto, California.

12. 51 Fed. Reg. 21,438 (June 12, 1986), codified at 40 C.F.R. Part 710, Subpart B (1988). These regulations require that importers and manufacturers producing at any single site 10,000 pounds or more of a chemical substance listed on the inventory and subject to update reporting provide information about production volume and production sites every four years.

13. 40 C.F.R. § 720.3(v) (1988).

14. 40 C.F.R. § 720.22 (1988).

15. 40 C.F.R. §§ 720.22 and 721.5 (1988).

16. Bioengineered microorganisms can be new substances subject to TSCA's premanufacture notification requirement. 51 Fed. Reg. 23,313 (June 26, 1986).

17. 40 C.F.R. Part 721, Subpart E (1988).

18. 40 C.F.R. § 721.350(a) (2) (1988).

19. 40 C.F.R. §§ 720.36, 720.38, 721.19, 723.50, 723.175 and 723.250 (1988).

20. 40 C.F.R. §§ 720.36, 720.38, and 723.50 (1988).

21. 40 C.F.R. §§ 720.36, 720.38, 721.19, 723.50, 723.175 and 723.250 (1988).

22. 40 C.F.R. § 720.45 (1988).

23. Upon approval by EPA, confidential business information submitted as part of a premanufacture notice will not be released to the public. 40 C.F.R. §§ 720.80–720.95.

24. 40 C.F.R. § 720.50 (1988).

25. 40 C.F.R. Part 720, Appendix A (1988).

26. 40 C.F.R. § 721.10 (1988).

27. 15 U.S.C. § 2607(a) (2).

28. *See* 53 Fed. Reg. 51,698 (December 22, 1988).

29. 15 U.S.C. § 2607(d).

30. 15 U.S.C. § 2602(6).

31. "It is intended that the term 'health and safety study' be interpreted broadly. Not only is information which arises as a result of a formal, disciplined study included, but other information relating to the effects of a chemical substance or mixture on health or the environment is also included. Any data that bear on the effects of a chemical substance on health or the environment would be included. Chemical identity is part of, or underlying data to, a health and safety study." 40 C.F.R. § 716.3.

32. 40 C.F.R. § 716.50 (1988).

33. 40 C.F.R. § 716.3 (1988).

34. 40 C.F.R. § 716.20(a) (1) (1988).

35. 40 C.F.R. § 716.35 (1988).

36. 40 C.F.R. § 716.60(b) (2) (1988).

37. 40 C.F.R. § 716.40 (1988).

38. 15 U.S.C. § 2603.

39. EPA has developed a computer database of testing submissions under TSCA, sections 4 and 8. The database (TSCATS) is available from Chemical Information Systems.

40. 15 U.S.C. § 2603(a).

41. 40 C.F.R. § 790.24(a).

42. 40 C.F.R. § 799.1053 (1988).

43. 40 C.F.R. Parts 792, 795, 796, 797, and 798 (1988).

44. 40 C.F.R. § 790.50 (1988).

45. 40 C.F.R. § 790.87(a) (1988).

46. 40 C.F.R. Part 791 (1988).

47. 15 U.S.C. § 2607(e).

48. "Substantial risk" is not defined in TSCA.

49. U.S. Environmental Protection Agency, Office of Toxic Substances. TSCA Chem-in-Progress Bull 1988;9(5):8,12.

50. *Id.*

51. *Id.* at 12.

52. 15 U.S.C. § 2607(c).

53. EPA has provided some guidance as to what constitutes a "significant adverse reaction." Significant adverse reactions of human health include but are not limited to:

> (1) Long-lasting or irreversible damage, such as cancer or birth defects;
> (2) Partial or complete impairment of bodily functions, such as reproductive disorders, neurological disorders, or blood disorders;
> (3) An impairment of normal activities experienced by all or most of the persons exposed at one time;
> (4) An impairment of normal activities which is experienced each time an individual is exposed.

40 C.F.R. § 717.12(a) (1988). Significant adverse reactions of the environment include but are not limited to:

> (1) Gradual or sudden changes in the composition of animal life or plant life, including fungal or microbial organisms, in an area;
> (2) Abnormal number of deaths of organisms (e.g., fish kills);
> (3) Reduction of the reproductive success or the vigor of a species;
> (4) Reduction in agricultural productivity, whether crops or livestock;
> (5) Alterations in the behavior or distribution of a species;
> (6) Long-lasting or irreversible contamination of components of the physical environment, especially in the case of ground water, and surface water and soil resources that have limited self-cleansing capability.

40 C.F.R. § 717.12(c) (1988).

54. *Id.*

55. 40 C.F.R. § 717.10(c) (1988).

56. 40 C.F.R. §§ 717.12(b) and 717.3(c) (1) (1988).

57. 15 U.S.C. § 2605.

58. 54 Fed. Feg. 29,442 (July 12, 1989).

59. 40 C.F.R. Part 762 (1988).

60. 15 U.S.C. §§ 2604(e) and (f).

61. 40 C.F.R. §§ 720.75(a) and 721.10(c) (1988).

62. 40 C.F.R. § 720.75(c) (1988).

63. 40 C.F.R. §§ 720.75(d) and 721.10(d) (1988).

64. Although EPA decides during the notification period not to regulate a new substance, EPA may initiate regulation of it after manufacture or import begins. 40 C.F.R. § 720.75(d).

65. 15 U.S.C. § 2604(e).

66. As of August 4, 1989, about 226 of these orders covering approximately 400 substances have been issued by EPA. Some of these orders are mutually agreed upon by EPA and the premanufacture notice submitter. Others are unilaterally imposed by EPA. August 4, 1989 telephone interview with L. Szelsman, TSCA, Section 5 Docket Officer, United States Environmental Protection Agency.

67. 15 U.S.C. § 2604(f).

68. 40 C.F.R. Part 747 (1988); 49 Fed. Reg. 36,846 (September 20, 1984); 49 Fed. Reg. 24,658 (June 14, 1984); 49 Fed. Reg. 2,762 (January 23, 1984).

69. 15 U.S.C. §§ 2606 and 2603(f).

70. ''Imminently hazardous chemical substance or mixture'' is defined as ''a chemical substance or mixture which presents an imminent and unreasonable risk of serious or widespread injury to health or the environment. Such a risk to health or the environment shall be considered imminent if it is shown that the manufacture, processing, distribution in commerce, use, or disposal of the chemical substance or mixture, or that any combination of such activities, is likely to result in such injury to health or the environment before a final rule under § 2605 of this title can protect against such risk.'' 15 U.S.C. § 2606(f).

71. 15 U.S.C. § 2606(b).

72. 15 U.S.C. § 2603(f).

73. 50 Fed. Reg. 42,037 (October 17, 1985) (methylene chloride); 50 Fed. Reg. 27,674 (July 5, 1985) (4,4'-methylenedianiline); 49 Fed. Reg. 21,898 (May 23, 1984) (construction materials and fabrics containing formaldehyde-based resins); 49 Fed. Reg. 845 (January 5, 1984) (1,3-butadiene).

74. 15 U.S.C. § 2605(e); 15 U.S.C. §§ 2641–2655; and 15 U.S.C. §§ 2661–2671.

75. 15 U.S.C. § 2605(e) (2).

76. The Asbestos Hazard Emergency Response Act of 1986, P.L. 99-519, 100 Stat. 2970, added these specific asbestos provisions to TSCA. Congress has also passed other asbestos-specific legislation, the Asbestos School Hazard Abatement Act of 1984, P.L. 98-377, 98 Stat. 1287, and the Asbestos Information Act of 1988, P.L. 100-577, 102 Stat. 2901, that have not been incorporated as part of TSCA.

77. The Indoor Radon Abatement Act of 1988, P.L. 100-551, 102 Stat. 2755, added indoor radon provisions to TSCA.

78. 15 U.S.C. § 2615.

79. EPA sometimes enters into consent agreements with violators and agrees to reduced fines in consideration of other factors. For example, EPA entered into a settlement agreement with Schnee-Morehead Company of Irving, Texas, where the company agreed to pay a civil penalty of almost $600,000 for manufacturing four new chemical substances without providing premanufacture notification. While the violations could have resulted in a fine of $4.7 million, EPA noted that the company voluntarily disclosed the violations and that the company would be unable to pay the higher fine and stay in business. U.S. Environmental Protection Agency, Office of Toxic Substances. TSCA Chem-in-Progress Bull 1989;10(1):3.

80. Criminal convictions in connection with TSCA violations have occurred. For example, Patrick Perrin, Martha C. Rose Chemical's former plant manager, is serving a 2-year federal prison sentence in connection with the company's illegal handling of PCBs. U.S. Environmental Protection Agency, Office of Toxic Substances. TSCA Chem-in-Progress Bull 1989;10(2):7.

81. 15 U.S.C. § 2614(1).

82. 15 U.S.C. § 2614(2).

83. 15 U.S.C. § 2616.

84. 15 U.S.C. § 2619(a) (1).

85. 15 U.S.C. § 2619(a) (2).

86. 15 U.S.C. § 2620.

22

Hazard Communications and Material Safety Data Sheets

Craig Beck, C.I.H.
Gary R. Krieger, M.D., M.P.H.

INTRODUCTION

Incidence involving chemicals and other hazardous materials annually result in thousands of injuries. An earlier report indicated that there were more than 125,000 chemical-related illnesses and injuries from 1976 through 1978 in the United States alone (1). Most injuries involve lack of understanding of the hazard that a chemical or material represents. Examples include: (*a*) flammable liquids and their vapors which can explode due to vapor migration to an ignition source, (*b*) the dermal absorption of organophosphate insecticides, (*c*) solvent vapors that displace oxygen in a confined environment, and (*d*) the generation of deadly gases following the reaction of two materials.

The occupational Safety and Health Administration (OSHA) reported in the *Federal Register* of August 24, 1987 (2), that at least 575,000 chemical products are used in businesses throughout the United States. Due to the extreme length of time required for OSHA to promulgate new health and safety standards for specific individual chemicals, it became apparent that a general standard was necessary. This general standard must include essential information concerning a chemical and must be transmitted to both employee and employer. Based on this information, employers could design and implement effective safety and health programs, and employees could better understand the hazards associated with the products they used. It was felt that, if the hazards were understood, employees would better appreciate and comply with the health and safety programs initiated by the employers.

GENERAL OVERVIEW

The Hazard Communication Standard, 29 Code of Federal Regulations (CFR) 1910.1200(a) states:

The purpose of this section (of 29 CFR) is to ensure that the hazards of all chemicals produced or imported by chemical manufacturers or importers are evaluated, and that information concerning their hazards is transmitted to affected employers and employees.

An additional purpose of this standard was to provide a program which was consistent throughout the United States. The OSHA regulation specifically preempted states, cities, towns, or other political subdivisions of a state from adopting or enforcing their own different forms of hazard communication programs. The only exemption to this preemption was for states with federally approved OSHA programs. These programs would be required to submit their hazard communication program to OSHA for approval prior to adoption by the states. In effect, this allowed OSHA to approve a state's hazard communication program and ensure consistency between the states and within the federal system.

OSHA published its original Hazard Communication Stand-

ard on November 23, 1983. The standard directed chemical manufacturers or importers to assess the hazards of chemicals they manufacture or import and to provide this information to those companies in the manufacturing sector, SIC Codes 20 through 39, which used the product. The companies were then required to transmit this information to their employees through the use of a comprehensive hazard communication program. This program involves the use of container labeling and other forms of warning, material safety data sheets, and employee training.

On August 24, 1987, OSHA's Hazard Communication Standard was revised to require nonmanufacturing employers, including agriculture, forestry, fishing, mining, construction, wholesale and retail trade, finance, insurance, real estate, and service groups, to provide their employees with similar hazard communication programs. Due to legal challenges by portions of the construction industry, the revised Hazard Communication Standard did not become final for the construction industry until February 15, 1989.

Manufacturing and nonmanufacturing laboratories are only required to comply with limited aspects of the standard. Labels must remain on the chemical containers and not be defaced; material safety data sheets received from the distributor must be maintained and accessible to the employees; employees must be informed of the chemical hazards and trained in the proper methods of handling these materials.

The standard covers a wide variety of chemicals which could cause adverse health effects:

Physical hazards include:	*Example:*
1. Flammable liquids	acetone, hexane
2. Flammable solids	magnesium
3. Combustible liquids	mineral spirits
4. Compressed gases	nitrogen, helium
5. Explosives	gunpowder, nitroglycerin
6. Organic peroxides	methyl isobutyl ketone peroxide
7. Oxidizers	oxygen, (95% nitric) acid
8. Pyrophoric materials	phosphorus, butyl-lithium
9. Unstable materials	picric acid
10. Water reactive materials	sodium metal

Examples of health hazards include carcinogens, irritants, sensitizers, corrosives, and specific organ system toxicants.

The appendix gives detailed definitions of each physical and health hazard, per the OSHA standard.

There are many materials which are not included under this standard: (*a*) hazardous wastes regulated by the U.S. Environmental Protection Agency; (*b*) tobacco and tobacco products; (*c*) wood or wood products; (*d*) manufactured items; and (*e*) food, drugs, or cosmetics intended for personal consumption by employees.

The Hazard Communication Standard consists of five major components: (*a*) hazard determination; (*b*) material safety data sheets (MSDSs); (*c*) a written hazard communication program; (*d*) labels and other forms of warning; and (*e*) employee information and training.

HAZARD DETERMINATION

Chemical manufacturers and importers must evaluate their materials and determine if they are considered hazardous. Employers may rely on the hazard evaluations conducted by the chemical manufacturers or importers, or they may choose to perform their own hazard evaluations on the chemicals used in their businesses. In general, due to both cost and the technical skills required to perform a hazard determination, the majority of employers rely on the evaluations of the manufacturers or importers.

At a minimum, all chemicals listed in the Occupational Safety and Health Administration Regulations 29 CFR Part 1910, Subpart Z, Toxic and Hazardous Substances or in the *Threshold Limit Values for Chemical Substances and Physical Agents in the Work Environment* published by the American Conference of Governmental Industrial Hygienists (ACGIH, latest edition) must be considered as hazardous. In addition, the following sources must be reviewed to determine whether a chemical is carcinogenic or potentially carcinogenic:

1. National Toxicology Program (NTP) *Annual Report on Carcinogens* (latest edition);
2. International Agency for Research on Cancer (IARC) *Monographs* (latest edition);
3. 29 CFR 1910, Subpart Z, Toxic and Hazardous Substances, Occupational Safety and Health Administration.

Mixtures of chemicals involve several complex issues compared with single component materials when attempting to determine the mixture's hazards; a hazard determination on a chemical mixture must be performed, however. Initially, a mixture can be tested as a whole to determine its physical and health hazards. For example, a given mixture could be submitted to a toxicology testing laboratory for health hazard evaluation. The same material could also be submitted to a chemical laboratory for determination of its physical properties. Generally, it is extremely time consuming and costly to evaluate a chemical mixture for potential health hazards, and many chemicals may be evaluated using an alternative procedure. As an example, if the mixture is not tested as a whole, the mixture is considered to have the health hazards exhibited by those components comprising 1% or more, by weight or volume, of the mixture. If one of the components is a carcinogenic hazard, the mixture is considered a carcinogen if the carcinogenic component is present in concentrations of 0.1% or greater. Finally, if the employer has evidence that a given component present in the mixture in concentrations less than 1% (or less than 0.1% for carcinogens) could reasonably be expected to be released in concentrations which would exceed an established OSHA permissible exposure limit or an ACGIH Threshold Limit Value, the mixture is assumed to pose a health hazard.

The evaluation procedures used by the chemical manufacturer, importer, or employer must be documented in writing and should describe the health and physical hazards which were evaluated for the chemical. The written procedures need only describe the general process used to perform the evaluations and are not required to describe in detail the procedures used for individual chemicals. However, some companies have described their specific hazard determination procedures in order to better document the evaluation process. This strategy has proven useful when the health hazard determination was challenged by a regulatory agency. It could also be used to limit future product liabilities.

The Hazard Communication Standard requires additional information which should be provided in the evaluation procedures:

- the person(s) responsible for the evaluation process;
- the information sources to be used;
- the criteria to be used to evaluate the studies or sources, e.g., statistical significance, number of positive results, whether conducted according to commonly accepted scientific principles; and
- a plan for reviewing and updating the hazard evaluations and MSDSs.

MATERIAL SAFETY DATA SHEETS

A MSDS is defined in the OSHA Hazard Communication Standard as "... written or printed material concerning a hazardous chemical ...". This form of information transfer was intended to be a cornerstone of an employer's hazard communication program in that the MSDS details the types of hazards associated with that material and the proper methods of protecting personnel from these hazards. A properly prepared MSDS should provide employers and employees sufficient information so that the product can be used in a safe manner.

The exact form or layout of the MSDS was not specified in the Hazard Communication Standard; however, in 1985 OSHA released its concept of a generic MSDS form (Fig. 22.1). An MSDS must be written in English and contain, at a minimum, this information: identity of the compound; chemical and common names; exposure limits; physical and chemical characteristics; physical hazards; health hazard data; carcinogenic potential; routes of entry; methods for controlling employee exposure; and precautions for safe handling and use.

Identity of the Compound

The identity of the material specified on the MSDS should be identical to the label on the materials container. In some cases this identity could be a product name, e.g., "Product XYZ," or it could be a very specific chemical name, e.g., ethylene glycol monomethyl ether.

Chemical and Common Names

If the material is composed of a single chemical, the MSDS must list its chemical and common names. In many cases the chemical's unique Chemical Abstract Service (CAS) identification number will also be included. If the material is a mixture, the MSDS must identify each component contributing to a known hazard by its chemical and common name, but the exact percentage of each component is not required to be listed. Those mixtures that have not been tested as a whole to determine the specific hazard must list those components considered to be health hazards (see **Hazard Determination**) by comprising more than 1% of the materials or more than 0.1% for those

Material Safety Data Sheet

May be used to comply with
OSHA's Hazard Communication Standard,
29 CFR 1910.1200. Standard must be
consulted for specific requirements.

U.S. Department of Labor

Occupational Safety and Health Administration
(Non-Mandatory Form)
Form Approved
OMB No. 1218-0072

IDENTITY *(As Used on Label and List)*	Note: *Blank spaces are not permitted. If any item is not applicable, or no information is available, the space must be marked to indicate that.*

Section I

Manufacturer's Name	Emergency Telephone Number
Address *(Number, Street, City, State, and ZIP Code)*	Telephone Number for Information
	Date Prepared
	Signature of Preparer *(optional)*

Section II — Hazardous Ingredients/Identity Information

Hazardous Components (Specific Chemical Identity; Common Name(s))	OSHA PEL	ACGIH TLV	Other Limits Recommended	% *(optional)*

Section III — Physical/Chemical Characteristics

Boiling Point		Specific Gravity (H$_2$O = 1)	
Vapor Pressure (mm Hg.)		Melting Point	
Vapor Density (AIR = 1)		Evaporation Rate (Butyl Acetate = 1)	
Solubility in Water			
Appearance and Odor			

Section IV — Fire and Explosion Hazard Data

Flash Point (Method Used)	Flammable Limits	LEL	UEL
Extinguishing Media			
Special Fire Fighting Procedures			
Unusual Fire and Explosion Hazards			

(Reproduce locally)   OSHA 174, Sept. 1985

Figure 22.1.   Generic MSDS.

Section V — Reactivity Data

Stability	Unstable		Conditions to Avoid
	Stable		

Incompatibility (*Materials to Avoid*)

Hazardous Decomposition or Byproducts

Hazardous Polymerization	May Occur		Conditions to Avoid
	Will Not Occur		

Section VI — Health Hazard Data

Route(s) of Entry: Inhalation?   Skin?   Ingestion?

Health Hazards (*Acute and Chronic*)

Carcinogenicity: NTP?   IARC Monographs?   OSHA Regulated?

Signs and Symptoms of Exposure

Medical Conditions
Generally Aggravated by Exposure

Emergency and First Aid Procedures

Section VII — Precautions for Safe Handling and Use

Steps to Be Taken in Case Material Is Released or Spilled

Waste Disposal Method

Precautions to Be Taken in Handling and Storing

Other Precautions

Section VIII — Control Measures

Respiratory Protection (*Specify Type*)

Ventilation	Local Exhaust		Special
	Mechanical (*General*)		Other

Protective Gloves	Eye Protection

Other Protective Clothing or Equipment

Work/Hygienic Practices

☆ U.S.G.P.O.: 1986-491-529/45775

Figure 22.1. *Continued*

components considered to exhibit carcinogenic potential. Those components of a mixture which are considered physical hazards must also be listed by their chemical and common names when the mixture has not been tested as a whole.

Exposure Limits

OSHA permissible exposure limits (PELs), ACGIH Threshold Limit Values (TLVs), National Institute for Occupational Safety and Health recommended exposure limits (NIOSH RELs), or other employee exposure limits recommended by the manufacturer, importer, or employer should be completed for each component listed by chemical and common name. If the mixture has been tested as a whole and a recommended exposure limit determined, this value should also be listed. It should be noted that this form of exposure limit technically is not considered a ''Threshold Limit Value'' or ''TLV,'' as these terms are trademarks of the ACGIH.

Physical and Chemical Characteristics

Certain physical and chemical characteristics will assist in evaluating the potential hazards posed by the material. Boiling point and vapor pressure are important in determining the ease with which a liquid will evaporate. Generally, those liquids with low boiling points and high vapor pressures will evaporate quickly. For example, acetone quickly evaporates; it has a boiling point at 133°F (56°C) and a vapor pressure of 226.3 mmHg at 25°C (3). In contrast, malathion has a boiling point at 156°C at 0.7 mmHg and a vapor pressure of 0.00004 mmHg at 20°C (4) and slowly evaporates. If the material is a flammable liquid, an increased fire hazard may result. An inhalation exposure could occur due to the evaporation of a toxic liquid. Vapor density is another important physical characteristic typically listed on an MSDS. Vapor densities less than 1.0 indicate that a gas or vapor is lighter than air and tends to rise; in contrast, a gas or vapor with a vapor pressure greater than 1.0 tends to concentrate in low areas and creates potential health or physical hazards, e.g., oxygen deficiency or a flammable environment. Appearance and odor of the material are other characteristics commonly included on the MSDS. It is important to remember that odor should not be relied on to determine potential exposure or overexposures to a material, as the minimum odor detection concentration can be well above the OSHA PEL or the ACGIH TLV. Two other important physical and chemical characteristics are water solubility and specific gravity. These parameters are useful in the determination of proper spill and fire control methods. For example, a material's specific gravity determines whether a material will float on water, e.g., specific gravity less than 1.0, or if it will sink in water, e.g., specific gravity greater than 1.0.

Physical Hazards

Fire and reactivity are physical hazards of a material. The fire-related characteristics listed on the MSDS would include: (a) flashpoint, the minimum temperature at which a liquid gives off sufficient flammable vapors to ignite in the presence of an ignition source; (b) lower flammable limit (LFL) and upper flammable limit (UFL), which indicate the ability of a material to pose a fire hazard. The LFL is the lowest concentration of the material in air which will produce a fire when an ignition source is present, while the UFL is the highest concentration of the material in air which will produce a fire when an ignition source is present. The concentration of material in air between the LFL and UFL is considered the flammable range and defines where a fire can be initiated or sustained provided sufficient fuel and oxygen are present. Below the LFL the mixture is too lean to burn, and above the UFL the mixture is too rich to burn. Other information that may be contained in this section of the MSDS includes: (a) fire-extinguishing media, water, foam, or dry chemical; (b) special firefighting procedures—use of self-contained breathing apparatus or other special forms of personal equipment; and (c) unusual fire and explosion hazards exhibited by the material when involved in a fire, e.g., the potential production of phosgene and hydrogen chloride in fires involving carbon tetrachloride or other chlorinated solvents.

Reactivity refers to a material's tendency to undergo chemical reactions with a subsequent release of energy. Information typically provided in an MSDS related to this hazard includes stability, chemical incompatibilities, hazardous decomposition products, or hazardous polymerization. For example, mercury fulminate is an unstable material that is explosive when dry. This would be noted on the MSDS under ''Conditions to Avoid.'' When potassium cyanide comes in contact with a strong acid such as sulfuric acid, the resulting reaction can release toxic hydrogen cyanide gas. This type of reactivity hazard would be included under a heading of ''Incompatibility.''

Health Hazard Data, Carcinogenic Potential, and Routes of Entry

This section of the MSDS will inform the reader about the type of health hazard associated with exposure to the material. Typically, the three primary routes of exposure in an industrial setting are inhalation, ingestion, and dermal. To ensure that proper personal protective equipment or other forms of control measures are used, it is important for employees and employers to know the routes by which a material could enter the body.

Acute and chronic health hazards associated with exposure to a chemical will be listed on the MSDS, as will a material's carcinogenic potential. If a material is listed in the National Toxicology Program, in the IARC *Monographs*, or by OSHA as a carcinogen, this must be noted in the MSDS. As required by the Standard, additional information must be included to assist physicians or other emergency medical personnel in determining whether a person has been, or may be, seriously injured from exposure to the material. This information includes signs and symptoms of exposure, medical conditions that could be aggravated by exposure, and emergency and first aid procedures.

Methods for Controlling Employee Exposure

After reviewing the hazard data, a logical regimen of measures is recommended to reduce employee exposure levels to the material. Control measures could include general dilution or local exhaust ventilation, proper work or personal hygiene practices, the use of personal protective equipment, or a combination of all these measures. If personal protective equipment is to be used, the specific type of protective equipment should be specified on the MSDS. For example, if an employee is exposed to airborne dusts containing lead, then a half-face or full-face respirator with a high efficiency particulate air (HEPA) filter cartridge may be specified. In some cases, a supplied air respirator may be specified in the MSDS. The specific types of glove material, eye protection, and other types of personal protective equipment may also be included in this category. Work or hygienic practices that might be recommended include: washing hands prior to eating, drinking, or smoking; not smoking in the area; not using high pressure air to clean work surfaces.

This portion of the MSDS must be evaluated very closely by the employer or employee, as the contents may be of limited use. For example, when describing the type of gloves to use, the MSDS might state, "Use impermeable gloves" or "Use of gloves recommended," rather than specifying a particular glove material such as butyl rubber, viton, or polyvinyl chloride (PVC). Liability concerns may cause a chemical manufacturer or importer to recommend the use of a supplied air respirator when an air-purifying respirator would be adequate.

Precautions for Safe Handling and Use

Information required to be included in this section details four areas: (a) the proper methods of handling and storing the materials; (b) measures needed to properly handle the material in the event of a release or spill; (c) disposal of the waste materials following a cleanup; and (d) other special precautions recommended by the importer, distributor, or employer preparing the MSDS. Disposal requirements can significantly vary from state to state and within given municipalities; therefore, information in this section may be of limited use. Thus, a typical recommendation on an MSDS would be, "Dispose of in accordance with federal, state, or local regulations."

OTHER REQUIREMENTS FOR MSDSs

The MSDS must list the name and address of the manufacturer, importer, or employer who prepared the MSDS. In addition, an emergency telephone number must be included so that employers or emergency medical personnel can obtain additional information on the material. The date of the latest preparation or revision of the MSDS must also be included.

All portions of the MSDS must be filled out; no blanks are permitted on the MSDS. If relevant information concerning some aspect of the material required on the MSDS could not be ascertained, then a "N/A" or other designation must be indicated.

Occasionally, new information concerning a chemical becomes available. When this occurs, the chemical manufacturer, importer, or employer must then revise the MSDS within 3 months to reflect this change. Manufacturers and importers must supply the employer with the revised MSDS with the first shipment of the material after the revised MSDS was prepared.

While there are many obvious advantages to a well-prepared MSDS, there are several problems associated with the current system. For example, there is no required or specified format for an MSDS, only types of information required to be included in the MSDS. This may increase the difficulty of an individual in identifying desired information. In addition, the technical nature of this document may increase the potential of its misrepresentation by personnel unfamiliar with its terminology. Another difficulty related to MSDSs is that they are typically written only in English. Many employees in the United States are recent immigrants from non-English-speaking areas of the world such as Southeast Asia and Central or South America. This type of employee may understand or speak limited English and subsequently may not comprehend the technical portions of the MSDS. Therefore, training in these alternative languages

and utilization of effective (multilingual) container labeling is essential to ensure that non-English-speaking employees comprehend the chemical's hazards.

One aspect related to the MSDS program which may create a serious difficulty, especially under emergency conditions, is a provision of the Standard which allows a chemical manufacturer, importer, or employer to designate a product as a "Trade Secret." Under this designation, the specific chemical name is not required to be included on the MSDS, provided the MSDS contains information regarding the specific properties and hazards associated with the material. In the case of medical emergencies, the Standard does contain an additional provision permitting physicians and nurses to request the specific identity of a hazardous chemical; this information must be immediately provided by the chemical manufacturer, importer, or employer. Under nonemergency situations, the specific chemical identity may be requested in writing by physicians, industrial hygienists, toxicologists, or other health personnel in order to assist them in the determination of toxicity. If the information is provided, a strict confidentiality agreement can be required by the manufacturer or importer. In difficult situations, OSHA can be contacted to resolve release-of-information issues.

LABELS AND OTHER FORMS OF WARNING

An integral portion of a facility's overall hazard communication program is the use of labels or other forms of warnings on chemical containers. Compliance with this portion of the Hazard Communication Standard is divided between those individuals who manufacture and distribute the chemicals and those who utilize the chemicals in the workplace. There are some chemical containers which do not require labeling by this Standard:

- Pesticides regulated by the Federal Insecticide, Fungicide, and Rodenticide Act which are labeled in accordance with those regulations;
- Foods, food additives, color additives, drugs, cosmetics, or medical or veterinary devices, regulated by the Food, Drug, and Cosmetic Act which are labeled in accordance with those regulations;
- Distilled spirits, wines, or malt beverages (beer) intended for nonindustrial use regulated by the Federal Alcohol Administration Act which are labeled in accordance with those regulations; and
- Consumer products regulated by the Consumer Product Safety Act which are labeled in accordance with those regulations.

Chemical Manufacturers and Distributions

Chemical manufacturers, importers, or distributors of chemicals covered by the Hazard Communication Standard must label each chemical container, e.g., 55-gallon barrel, 1-gallon bottle, with its identity, appropriate hazard warnings, and the name and address of the manufacturer or other responsible party. If the chemical is regulated by OSHA within 29 CFR 1910.1001 through 29 CFR 1910.1047 as a carcinogen, e.g., asbestos, arsenic, vinyl chloride, the container must be labeled with the appropriate hazard warning as required by the applicable standard. Warnings of other hazards posed by these materials should also be listed on the label.

Employers and the Workplace

Employers are required to ensure chemical containers used in their workplaces are properly labeled. If a container arrives from the chemical manufacturer or distributor with an appropriate label affixed to it, e.g., identity of the hazardous chemical(s) and appropriate hazard warnings, the employer is not required to add additional labeling. If the employer wants to place additional warning information on the container, he may do so, provided he does not remove, deface, or make illegible the original hazard label. The hazard warning can be of any type which conveys the appropriate hazards of the chemical, e.g., words, pictures, or symbols.

One alternative hazard warning system commonly used in industry to label containers is the Hazardous Material Identification System (HMIS) devised by the National Paint and Coatings Association (5). This system provides information concerning a material's health, flammability, and reactivity hazards, and also the proper types of personal protective equipment to be utilized while handling this material. The severity of each hazard is denoted using a numerical rating system, with a scale of "0" to "4." A rating of "0" indicates a minimum hazard while "4" denotes a severe hazard. The following is a summary of the HMIS ratings:

HEALTH HAZARD RATING ____________

FLAMMABILITY HAZARD RATING ____________

REACTIVITY HAZARD RATING ____________

PERSONAL PROTECTIVE EQUIPMENT REQUIRED ____________

____

Figure 22.2. HMIS-type label. From *National Paint and Coatings Association's HMIS Hazardous Materials Identification System's Revised Raw Materials Rating Manual.*

I. Health Hazard Rating

- **0 Minimal hazard** — No significant risk to health
- **1 Slight hazard** — Irritation or minor reversible injury possible
- **2 Moderate hazard** — Temporary or minor injury may occur
- **3 Serious hazard** — Major injury likely unless prompt action is taken and medical treatment is given
- **4 Severe hazard** — Life-threatening, major, or permanent damage may result from single or repeated exposures

II. Flammability Hazard Rating

- **0 Minimum hazard** — Materials that are normally stable and will not burn unless heated
- **1 Slight hazard** — Materials that must be preheated before ignition will occur. Flammable liquids in this category will have flashpoints (the lowest temperature at which ignition will occur) at or above 200°F (93.3°C) (NFPA Class IIIB)
- **2 Moderate hazard** — Material that must be moderately heated before ignition will occur, including flammable liquids with flashpoints at or above 100°F (37.7°C) and below 200°F (93.3°C) (NFPA Class II & Class IIIA)
- **3 Serious hazard** — Materials capable of ignition under almost all normal temperature conditions, including flammable liquids with flashpoints below 73°F (22.8°C) and boiling points above 100°F (37.7°C) as well as liquids with flashpoints between 73°F (22.8°C) and 100°F (37.7°C) (NFPA Class 1B and 1C)
- **4 Severe hazard** — Very flammable gases or very volatile flammable liquids with flashpoints below 73°F (22.8°C) and boiling points below 100°F (37.7°C) (NFPA Class 1A)

III. Reactivity Hazard Rating

- **0 Minimum hazard** — Materials that are normally stable, even under fire conditions, and will not react with water
- **1 Slight hazard** — Materials that are normally stable but can become unstable at high temperatures and pressures. These materials may react with water, but they will not release energy violently
- **2 Moderate hazard** — Materials that, in themselves, are normally unstable and will readily undergo violent chemical change but will not detonate. These materials may also react violently with water
- **3 Serious hazard** — Materials that are capable of detonation or explosive reaction but require a strong initiating source or must be heated under confinement before initiation, or materials that react explosively with water
- **4 Severe hazard** — Materials that are readily capable of detonation or explosive decomposition at normal temperatures and pressures

The HMIS and its variation also identify the types of personal protective equipment which should be used by personnel when handling a given material. Fig. 22.2 is a facsimile of an HMIS label which could be used on a chemical container. For example, a facility could state that the use of safety glasses and gloves is required by employees, which would be indicated on the HMIS under Personal Protective Equipment Required as

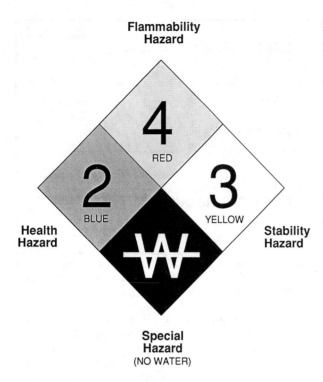

Figure 22.3.   NFPA 704 hazard warning symbol.

''A.'' The use of gloves and full-face respirator with organic vapor cartridges could be labeled as ''B.''

The manufacturer or importer of the material may provide the HMIS numerical ratings, listing those on the chemical's MSDS, or enough information should be included on the MSDS for the employer to develop the numerical ratings. If the proper information is not provided on the MSDS, the manufacturer should be contacted.

For employees to utilize the HMIS properly, wall posters summarizing the hazard information and personal protective equipment designations should be placed within the work areas for easy reference. Wallet cards are also available for distribution to employees. An adequate training program explaining the system is also required (see ''Employee Information and Training'' later in this chapter).

Another example of an alternative hazard warning system is the National Fire Protection Association (NFPA) 704 System (6). This system was designed to provide basic information primarily for firefighting personnel during fire emergencies. It utilizes a diamond-shaped figure divided into four sections (Fig. 22.3). Each section has a numerical rating of ''0'' through ''4'' to depict the chemical's health hazard (blue diamond), flammable hazard (red diamond), stability hazard (yellow diamond), e.g., water reactive, radioactive, oxidizers, or etiologic agents.

The general explanation of the numerical ratings for the health hazard portion of the symbol is given in Table 22.1.

Although the NFPA 704 system is very useful for properly trained firefighting personnel, it may be very confusing and could lead to misinterpretations. For untrained personnel, the system provides minimum information regarding the material's hazards and should be used in conjunction with the OSHA labeling requirements.

To assist employees in better understanding the NFPA 704 system, signs could be posted in the work areas which describe what each number means from a health, flammability, and stability hazard viewpoint. Although acceptable for use on chemical containers used in the workplace, the NFPA 704 system could be mistaken for shipping labels required by the Department of Transportation due to the similarity in the label's designs. Therefore, the NFPA labels cannot be placed on containers during shipment.

One other method that relates potentially harmful effects from contact with a hazardous chemical is the use of pictorial depictions (Fig. 22.4). These pictorial descriptions are placed on chemical containers based in Germany, Switzerland (7, 8), and other European countries to provide a quick reference to a chemical's hazard(s). In addition to using these pictograms on labels, they could be used on signs posted in specific areas of a workplace to graphically remind workers of the hazards. Personal protective equipment can also be adequately depicted through the use of pictures (Fig. 22.5).

As previously discussed, all containers of hazardous chemicals must be properly labeled. One exception to this requirement concerns stationary containers within a work area which have similar contents and hazards. In these circumstances, it is sufficient to place signs or placards which display the hazard information in the area of the containers. Standard operating procedures, process sheets, batch or blend tickets, or similar written materials can be posted on stationary containers in lieu of labels if they provide the required information and are readily available to the employees. Pipes and piping systems are not required to be labeled, although this generally is a good practice to follow, as it provides quick information in the event of a leak or a break in the piping system.

The only other exception to the labeling requirement is for portable containers which have materials transferred into them from labeled containers and which are intended for the immediate use of the employee who makes the transfer. Caution should be used under these conditions. It is very easy to visualize empty, portable, nonlabeled containers left on a workbench by one employee and picked up by another employee to use for a different chemical. Combining of incompatible materials could occur, resulting in serious injuries to unsuspecting employees. Thus, in order to standardize operations and reduce potential labeling problems, it may be more prudent to label all containers.

EMPLOYEE INFORMATION AND TRAINING

The Hazard Communication Standard requires that all employers provide each potentially exposed employee with certain information and training. This training should cover both normal work assignments and the accidental exposures from spills or leaking containers. Training must be hazard-specific. For example, if the information and training program initially covered flammables and the employee will now be exposed to a corrosive, additional specific information and training related to corrosive hazards must be provided.

Each affected employee must be informed of:

- the existence of the hazard communication standard and what the standard requires of the employer;
- the operations within the facility where hazardous substances are present and employee exposure could occur; and

Table 22.1. Explanation of Numerical Ratings for the Health Hazard Portion of Symbols

Identification of Health Hazard Color Code: BLUE		Identification of Flammability Color Code: RED		Identification of Reactivity (Stability) Color Code: YELLOW	
Signal	Type of Possible Injury	Signal	Susceptibility of Materials to Burning	Signal	Susceptibility to Release of Energy
4	Materials which on very short exposure could cause death or major residual injury even though prompt medical treatment were given.	4	Materials which will rapidly or completely vaporize at atmospheric pressure and normal ambient temperature, or which are readily dispersed in air and which will burn readily.	4	Materials which in themselves are readily capable of detonation or of explosive decomposition or reaction at normal temperatures and pressures.
3	Materials which on short exposure could cause serious temporary or residual injury even though prompt medical treatment were given.	3	Liquids and solids that can be ignited under almost all ambient temperature conditions.	3	Materials which in themselves are capable of detonation or explosive reaction but require a strong initiating source or which must be heated under confinement before initiation or which react explosively with water.
2	Materials which on intense or continued exposure could cause temporary incapacitation or possible residual injury unless prompt medical treatment is given.	2	Materials that must be moderately heated or exposed to relatively high ambient temperatures before ignition can occur.	2	Materials which in themselves are normally unstable and readily undergo violent chemical change but do not detonate. Also materials which may react violently with water or which may form potentially explosive mixtures with water.
1	Materials which on exposure would cause irritation but only minor residual injury even if no treatment is given.	1	Materials that must be preheated before ignition can occur.	1	Materials which in themselves are normally stable, but which can become unstable at elevated temperatures and pressures or which may react with water with some release of energy but not violently.
0	Materials which on exposure under fire conditions would offer no hazard beyond that of ordinary combustion material.	0	Materials that will not burn.	0	Materials which in themselves are normally stable, even under fire exposure conditions, and which are not reactive with water.

Reprinted with permission from NFPA 704-1990, *Identification of the Fire Hazards of Materials*, Copyright© 1990, National Fire Protection Association, Quincy, MA 02269. This reprinted material is not the complete and official position of the National Fire Protection Association, on the referenced subject which is represented only by the standard in its entirety.

- the location(s) within the facility where the written hazard communication program, the written procedures used for the hazard evaluation determinations, the lists of hazardous chemicals used in the facility, and the copies of MSDSs for the hazardous chemicals are maintained.

One of the most important aspects of the training is the hazard recognition and specificity. For example, if the facility uses materials which only exhibit the hazards of flammability and corrosivity, the employees should be trained only in those hazards; discussion of the other types of hazards which would not be encountered at the facility is not required. Training can be done by individual chemical or by categories of hazards. If only a small number of different chemicals are used in the facility, the training may be more meaningful if each chemical is discussed individually. If there are a large number of chemicals or if the types of chemicals change on a regular basis, the training program may be based on general hazard categories. When training is based on general hazard categories, it is essential that the discussion groups the facility's chemicals into their respective hazard categories.

The format of the training program has been left to the discretion of the employer. It can involve the use of videotapes, classroom lecture, slides, movies, hands-on training, or combinations of these.

The correct interpretation of MSDSs and container labels is essential for the employee's knowledge and understanding of the hazards with which he or she works. Because much of this information may be very technical in nature, the training program must present this information in a manner that is easy to comprehend. This also may involve the use of a multimedia presentation of the material. For example, the explanation of flashpoint and lower and upper flammable limits may be presented with a visual demonstration followed by a verbal discussion of these physical properties.

Employee training must include the methods such as color or odor which can be utilized to detect the presence of a chemical in the workplace which could create a hazard. Monitoring systems used by the employer to determine employee exposures, including personal monitoring or continuous monitoring instruments, should also be discussed in the training sessions.

Other aspects of the training would include the means by which employees can be protected from the chemical hazards. This could include a discussion of ventilation controls presently used at the facility to reduce the hazard potential, a discussion of the proper work practices that employees can use to reduce their exposure, or a discussion of the use of any personal protective equipment used by the employees, e.g., gloves, respirators, safety glasses. If emergency equipment is located in the facility, such as emergency showers or eyewashes, fire blankets, or fire extinguishers, this equipment should also be included in the discussion of protective equipment.

Other specific training which may be required involves nonroutine operations such as reactor vessel cleaning, work on charged piping systems, and clean-up of spills or other releases

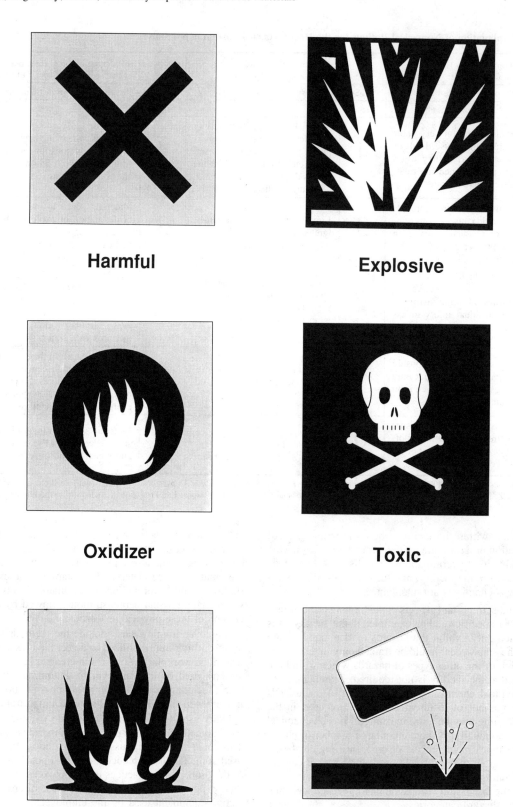

Figure 22.4.   Chemical hazards pictorial descriptions. Modified after Kuhn-Birett: *Merkblatter Gefahrliche Arbeitsstoffe: and Toxler Wegleitung durch die Arbeitssicherheit.*

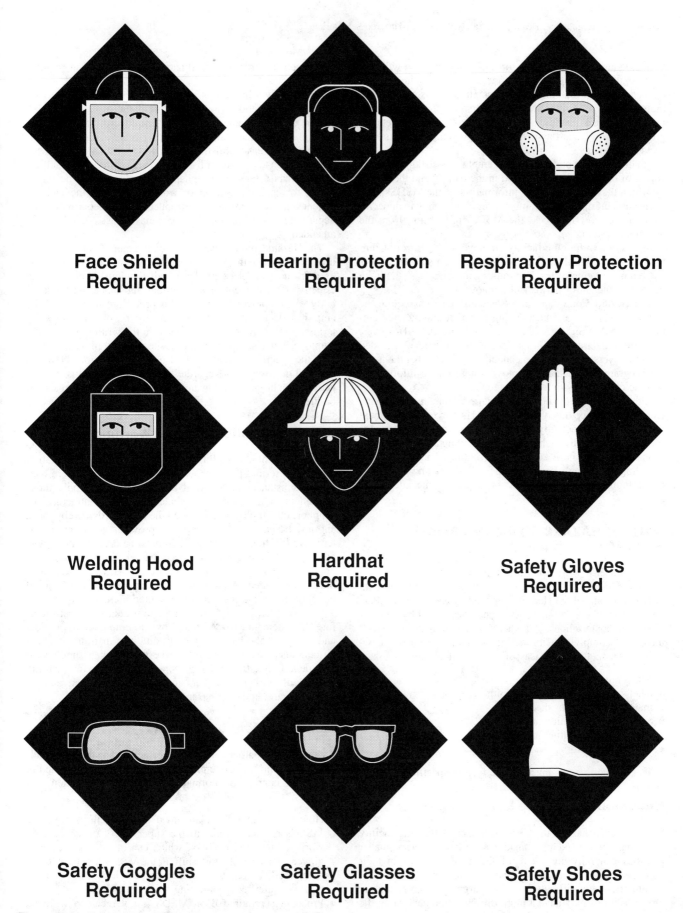

Figure 22.5. Personal protective equipment pictorial descriptions. Modified after Kuhn-Birett: *Merkblatter Gefahrliche Arbeitsstoffe: and Toxler Wegleitung durch die Arbeitssicherheit.*

of hazardous substances. This form of work situation will typically expose an employee to more hazards than those experienced during normal day-to-day operations. This may require more detailed training in the use of personal protective equipment, simulated hands-on demonstrations, or more detailed information on hazard assessment and preventive measures to prevent accidents.

Finally, it is important for the employees to know where copies of the MSDSs are retained in the facility and the means by which they can access this information. If the MSDSs have been computerized, the training program should include instruction on how to access the MSDS information from the computer system.

In addition to training facility employees, the Hazard Communication Standard requires the training of on-site contractors and temporary employees. The training must be consistent with the requirements for permanent employees.

The Hazard Communication Standard does not require the use of formal pre- and post testing means to monitor the employee's understanding of the presented materials. However, since the standard is performance-oriented, it is recommended that employers utilize some mechanism to ensure that the training program provided the employees appropriate information and the employer with adequate feedback.

Although the standard does not require training records, many employers do keep this type of record. These records document that the employee actually received the training. An attendance sheet signed daily by each employee attending a training course should be used, and a copy should be placed in each of the attending employee's personnel files. The data and content of the training course should also be a part of the attendance record.

WRITTEN HAZARD COMMUNICATION PROGRAM

The employer's written hazard communication program is a document which describes how the employer complies with the requirements of the Hazard Communication Standard. Many nonspecific or generic plans have been developed by consultants, trade organizations, and other groups to provide an "easy" method of complying with the Standard's requirements; however, it is essential that at least six specific items are discussed:

- hazardous substance list
- labels and other forms of warning
- material safety data sheets
- employee information and training
- hazards of nonroutine tasks
- on-site contractors

Thus, generic plans must still be facility-specific.

Hazardous Substance List

A list of each hazardous substances used within the facility must be generated and maintained in an orderly manner. Smaller facilities generally are aware of the materials used in their processes, and the generation of the hazardous substance list should not be too difficult; however, large, complex manufacturing facilities may have a more difficult time generating the initial hazardous substance list. The use of departmental questionnaires, facility walk-throughs, and reviews of purchasing

department records may facilitate this recordkeeping requirement.

The facility's hazardous substance list should include four areas of information: (a) the product name of each material; (b) the common name used by the employees; (c) the manufacturer of the material; and (d) for larger facilities, the departments or areas within the facility where the material is used.

In addition to the master list maintained for the entire facility, smaller lists arranged in alphabetical order should be maintained for each department or work area within the facility. Whenever a new product is introduced into a department, the department's list and the facility's master list could then be amended.

The Hazard Communication Standard requires that the method used to determine the hazard(s) posed by a material or chemical used in the workplace be described. Obviously, prior to the effective development of a hazardous substance list for a facility, the employer must have this procedure in place. If the employer decides to use the manufacturer's or importer's determination, this should be so stated in the written plan. If the employer's decision is to evaluate the material himself or herself, the specific procedures used for the evaluation should be outlined or described. Regardless of which method is used to perform the hazard determination, the responsible person should be identified.

Labels and Other Forms of Warning

This section of the facility's written hazard communication program describes the methods used to label containers of hazardous substances properly. If the employer uses only those containers of materials as provided by the manufacturer or supplier, the employer can rely on the labels provided by those entities. If, however, the employer provides additional or alternative labeling, then the system must be described. If alternative methods of labeling are used in the facility (batch tickets or warning signs posted in work areas), written descriptions must be provided. A copy of each alternative method should be included in this section of the written plan.

Clearly, chemical hazard information data changes; therefore, a system must be initiated by the employer for review and update of the hazard warnings and information contained on container labels. In addition, the written plan should also include a designation of the person(s) responsible for ensuring labeling of in-plant containers and shipping containers and for reviewing and updating hazard labels.

Material Safety Data Sheets

As one of the cornerstones of an effective hazard communication program, the dissemination of information contained in the MSDS is critical. Information required in the written plan includes:

- How the MSDSs are maintained in the facility, e.g., the MSDSs are maintained in the supervisor's office of each work station in a notebook which can be accessed by employees during each work shift; or the MSDSs are transferred to the facility's computer system and employees have access to a computer terminal during their work shift.
- Procedures required if an MSDS is not received with the initial shipment of a hazardous substance, e.g., the supplier and manufacturer of the hazardous substance will be sent a

letter stating that an MSDS was not received and the employer is now formally requesting an MSDS for that material; this letter would be followed by a registered letter within one month if an MSDS has still not been received.

- Description of alternative methods used in the work place other than MSDSs, e.g., use of written standard operating procedures or an MSDS which covers groups of chemicals used in a specific manufacturing process. These methods must also be available to employees at all times. The written plan should address this requirement.
- If the employer prepares his or her own MSDSs, a written procedure for updating an MSDS should be included in the plan, e.g., available hazard data will be reviewed and evaluated and upon the positive determination of new and significant information, the MSDS will be changed within 30 days, etc.
- The name of the person(s) responsible for obtaining and maintaining MSDSs.

Employee Information and Training

This section of the written hazard communication program discusses the means by which the facility will provide its employees with:

1. The identity of chemical workplace hazards;
2. Schedule of training and retraining;

3. An outline of the training program;
4. Location of the written hazard communication plan; and
5. The person(s) responsible for conducting the training program.

Hazards of Nonroutine Tasks

Some tasks at a facility may not be done on a routine basis and may present their own specific hazards. For example, cleaning or repair of a freon degreasing tank may pose an asphyxiation hazard if personnel are required to enter the tank. The written hazard communication plan must address these nonroutine tasks in a systematic fashion.

CONCLUSION AND SUMMARY

The OSHA Hazard Communication Standard provides for a systematic transfer of information from manufacturers of chemicals to the users of these materials. Through the utilization of material safety data sheets, training sessions, and written hazard communication programs, employers and employees are made aware of the safety and health hazards associated with the materials used in the workplace and the methods to protect against those hazards. Proper utilization and implementation of a facility's hazard communication program should assist in the reduction of chemically related occupational injuries and illnesses.

Appendix
(Excerpted from 29 CFR 1200)

A. Physical Hazards

"Combustible liquid" means any liquid having a flashpoint at or above 100°F (37.8°C), but below 200°F (93.3°C), except any mixture having components with flashpoints of 200°F (93.3°C), or higher, the total volume of which make up 99 percent or more of the total volume of the mixture.

"Common name" means any designation or identification such as code name, code number, trade name, brand name, or generic name used to identify a chemical other than by its chemical name.

"Compressed gas" means:

(i) A gas or mixture of gases having, in a container, an absolute pressure exceeding 40 psi at 70°F (21.2°C); or

(ii) A gas or mixture of gases having, in a container, an absolute pressure exceeding 104 psi at 130°F (54.4°C) regardless of the pressure at 70°F (21.1°C); or

(iii) A liquid having a vapor pressure exceeding 40 psi at 100°F (37.8°C) as determined by ASTM D-323-72.

"Explosive" means a chemical that causes a sudden, almost instantaneous release of pressure, gas, and heat when subjected to sudden shock, pressure, or high temperature.

"Flammable" means a chemical that falls into one of the following categories:

(i) "Aerosol, flammable" means an aerosol that, when tested by the method described in 16 CFR 1500.45, yields a flame projection exceeding 18 inches at full valve opening, or a flashback (a flame extending back to the valve) at any degree of valve opening;

(ii) A "Gas, flammable" means:

(A) A gas that, at ambient temperature and pressure, forms a flammable mixture with air at a concentration of thirteen (13) percent by volume or less; or

(B) A gas that, at ambient temperature and pressure, forms a range of flammable mixtures with air wider than twelve (12) percent by volume, regardless of the lower limit; or

(iii) "Liquid, flammable" means any liquid having a flashpoint below 100°F (37.8°C), except any mixture having components with flashpoints of 100°F (37.8°C) or higher, the total of which make up 99 percent or more of the total volume of the mixture;

(iv) "Solid, flammable" means a solid, other than a blasting agent or explosive as defined in 190.109(a), that is liable to cause fire through friction, absorption of moisture, spontaneous chemical change, or retained heat from manufacturing or processing, or which can be ignited readily and when ignited burns so vigorously and persistently as to create a serious hazard. A chemical shall be considered to be a flammable solid if, when tested by the method described in 16 CFR 1500.44, it ignites and burns with a self-sustained flame at a rate greater than one-tenth of an inch per second along its major axis.

"Organic peroxide" means an organic compound that contains the bivalent -O-O-structure and which may be considered to be a structural derivative of hydrogen peroxide where one or both of the hydrogen atoms has been replaced by an organic radical.

"Oxidizer" means a chemical other than a blasting agent or explosive as defined in 1910.109(a), that initiates or promotes combustion in other materials, thereby causing fire either of itself, or through the release of oxygen or other gases.

"Physical hazard" means a chemical for which there is scientifically valid evidence that it is a combustible liquid, a compressed gas, explosive, flammable, an organic peroxide, an oxidizer, pyrophoric, unstable (reactive) or water-reactive.

"Pyrophoric" means a chemical that will ignite spontaneously in air at a temperature of 130°F (54.4°C) or below.

"Unstable (reactive)" means a chemical which in the pure state, or as produced or transported, will vigorously polymerize, decompose, condense, or will become self-reactive under conditions of shocks, pressure or temperature.

"Water-reactive" means a chemical that reacts with water to release a gas that is either flammable or presents a health hazard.

(3) The chemical manufacturer, importer, or employer evaluating chemicals shall treat the following sources, as establishing that the chemicals listed in them are hazardous:

(i) 29 CFR Part 1910, Subpart Z, Toxic and Hazardous Substances, Occupational Safety and Health Administration (OSHA); or

(ii) *Threshold Limit Values for Chemical Substances and Physical Agents in the Work Environment*, American Conference of Governmental Industrial Hygienists (ACGIH) (latest edition).

B. Health Hazards

1. **Carcinogen:** A chemical is considered to be a carcinogen if:

   (a) It has been evaluated by the International Agency for Research on Cancer (IARC), and found to be a carcinogen or potential carcinogen; or,

   (b) It is listed as a carcinogen or potential carcinogen in the *Annual Report on Carcinogens* published by the National Toxicology Program (NTP) (latest edition); or,

   (c) It is regulated by OSHA as a carcinogen.

2. **Corrosive:** A chemical that causes visible destruction of, or irreversible alterations in, living tissue by chemical action at the site of contact. For example, a chemical is considered to be corrosive if, when tested on the intact skin of albino rabbits by the method described by the U.S. Department of Transportation in Appendix A to 49 CFR Part 173, it destroys or changes irreversibly the structure of the tissue at the site of contact following an exposure period of four hours. This term shall not refer to action on inanimate surfaces.

3. **Highly toxic:** A chemical failing within any of the following categories:

   (a) A chemical that has a median lethal dose (LD_{50}) of 50 milligrams or less per kilogram of body weight when administered orally to albino rats weighing between 200 and 300 grams each.

   (b) A chemical that has a median lethal dose (LD_{50}) of 200 milligrams or less per kilogram of body weight when

252

administered by continuous contact for 24 hours (or less if death occurs within 24 hours) with the bare skin of albino rabbits weighing between two and three kilograms each.

(c) A chemical that has a median lethal concentration (LC_{50}) in air of 200 parts per million by volume or less of gas or vapor, or 2 milligrams per liter or less of mist, fume, or dust, when administered by continuous inhalation for one hour (or less if death occurs within one hour) to albino rats weighing between 200 and 300 grams each.

4. **Irritant:** A chemical, which is not corrosive, but which causes a reversible inflammatory effect on living tissue by chemical action at the site of contact. A chemical is a skin irritant if, when tested on the intact skin of albino rabbits by the methods of 16 CFR 1500.41 for four hours exposure or by other appropriate techniques, it results in an empirical score of five or more. A chemical is an eye irritant if so determined under the procedure listed in 16 CFR 1500.42 or other appropriate techniques.

5. **Sensitizer:** A chemical that causes a substantial proportion of exposed people or animals to develop an allergic reaction in normal tissue after repeated exposure to the chemical.

6. **Toxic:** A chemical falling within any of the following categories:

(a) A chemical that has a median lethal dose (LD_{50}) of more than 50 milligrams per kilogram but not more than 500 milligrams per kilogram of body weight when administered orally to albino rats weighing between 200 and 300 grams each.

(b) A chemical that has a median lethal dose (LD_{50}) of more than 200 milligrams per kilogram but not more than 1000 milligrams per kilogram of body weight when administered by continuous contact for 24 hours (or less if death occurs within 24 hours) with the bare skin of albino rabbits weighing between two and three kilograms each.

(c) A chemical that has a median lethal concentration (LC_{50}) in air of more than 200 parts per million but not more than 2000 parts per million by volume of gas or vapor, or more than two milligrams per liter but not more than 20 milligrams per liter of mist, fume, or dust, when administered by continuous inhalation for one hour (or less if death occurs within one hour) to albino rats weighing between 200 and 300 grams each.

7. **Target organ effects:** The following is a target organ categorization of effects which may occur, including examples of signs, symptoms, and chemicals which have been associated with these effects. These examples are presented to illustrate the range and diversity of effects and hazards found in the workplace, and the broad scope employers must consider in this area, but are not intended to be all inclusive.

a. **Hepatotoxins:** Chemicals which produce liver damage
Signs and symptoms: Jaundice; liver enlargement
Chemicals: Carbon tetrachloride; nitrosamines

b. **Nephrotoxins:** Chemicals which produce kidney damage
Signs and symptoms: Edema, proteinuria
Chemicals: Halogenated hydrocarbons; uranium

c. **Neurotoxins:** Chemicals which produce their primary toxic effects on the nervous system
Signs and symptoms: Narcosis; behavorial changes; decrease in motor functions
Chemicals: Mercury; carbon disulfide

d. **Agents which act on blood or hematopoietic system:** Decrease hemoglobin function; deprive the body tissues of oxygen
Signs and symptoms: Cyanosis; loss of consciousness
Chemicals: Carbon monoxide; cyanides

e. **Agents which damage the lung:** Chemicals which irritate or damage the pulmonary tissue
Signs and symptoms: Cough, tightness in chest; shortness of breath
Chemicals: Silica; asbestos

f. **Reproductive toxins:** Chemicals which effect the reproductive capabilities including chromosomal damage (mutations) and effects on fetuses (teratogenesis)
Signs and symptoms: Birth defects; sterility
Chemicals: Lead; DBCP

g. **Cutaneous hazards:** Chemicals which affect the dermal layer of the body
Signs and symptoms: Defatting of the skin; rashes; irritation
Chemicals: Ketones; chlorinated compounds

h. **Eye hazards:** Chemicals which affect the eye or visual capacity
Signs and symptoms: Conjunctivitis; corneal damage
Chemicals: Organic solvents; acids

REFERENCES

1. Lowry GC, Lowry RC. Right-to-know and emergency planning. Michigan: Lewis, 1988:4.
2. U.S. Department of Labor, Occupational Safety and Health Administration. Hazard communication—final publication. Washington, DC: OSHA, 1987: 52 FR 31852–31886.
3. U.S. Department of Health and Human Services, Public Health Service Centers for Disease Control National Institute for Occupational Safety and Health. NIOSH pocket guide to chemical hazards. Washington, DC: OSHA, 1985:42.
4. Sax NI, Lewis RJ, Sr. Hawley's condensed chemical dictionary. 11th ed. New York: Van Nostrand Reinhold, 1987:725.
5. National Plant and Coatings Association. Hazardous materials identification system's revised raw materials rating manual. Fall. Washington, DC: National Plant and Coatings Association, 1984:RM/8.
6. National Fire Protection Association. Fire protection guide on hazardous materials, NFPA 704, standard system for the identification of the fire hazards of materials. 9th ed. Quincy: National Fire Protection Association, 1986;704.5–704.8.
7. Toxler R. Wegleitung durch die Arbeitssicherheit. Luzer: Eidgenossiche Koordinations Kommission fur Arbeitssicherheit, 1987:303–309.
8. Kuhn R, Birett K. Merkblatter gefahrliche Arbutstoffe, Vol 5. Landsberg/Lech: Ecomed, 1980: Warnsybole, 27.

SUGGESTED READINGS

1. U.S. Department of Labor, Occupational Safety and Health Administration. OSHA 3084—chemical hazard communication. Washington, DC: OSHA, 1989:1–9.
2. U.S. Department of Labor, Occupational Safety and Health Administration. OSHA 3111—hazard communication guidelines for compliance. Washington, DC: OSHA, 1988:1–13.
3. U.S. Department of Labor, Occupational Safety and Health Administration. OSHA instruction CPL2-2.38; inspection procedures for the hazard communication standard, 29 CFR 1910.1250. Washington, DC: OSHA, 1985:1-C-4.

23

Environmental Audits and Property Transfer: Hazardous Material Implications for Real Estate

Gretchen Heins
Steven Pike, M.D.
John B. Sullivan, Jr., M.D.

INTRODUCTION TO PROPERTY TRANSFER AUDITS

The last decade of this century arrives with humankind acutely aware of the detrimental effects careless disposal of waste has had on life and the environment. This waste management problem parallels our growth in population. All biologic systems experiencing exponential growth eventually have their growth retarded either by an inadequate food supply or by the toxic effects of waste products produced by the biologic mass. As our species proliferates, the available space uncontaminated by prior activities becomes more limited, and previously remote deposits of waste are increasingly adjacent to our homes. In some cases, land development for residential and commercial use takes place on previously existing landfills or dump sites. Activities previously considered innocuous are now scrutinized with greater concern, based on recent knowledge of the implications that the application of materials, processes, and residue may have on the health of flora and fauna. Even wastewater treatment, previously considered a beneficial activity, is being reexamined with attention focused on the effects the process and effluent have on the environment.

The cumulative effect of years of unregulated and ignorant production, consumption, and disposal practices becomes more alarming when we examine effects on the quality of life and the detectable concentrations of hazardous materials at locations remote from the site of manufacture, use, or deposition. We now know that hazardous materials migrate off-site and cause contamination of groundwater, surface water, and air. Uptake by aquatic organisms and plants can lead to bioaccumulation and biomagnification of the concentration of hazardous substances in species higher in the food chain. Thus a toxic effect may occur directly by local contact with the hazardous substance, and also indirectly by ingestion of contaminated food.

Most of our knowledge, with respect to biologic systems and human toxicology, was gained during the second half of this century. Sophisticated analytical methods in chemistry, toxicology, physics, and electronics enabled us to detect hazardous materials in environmental and biologic systems and to measure the effects of such substances. The appreciation that low concentrations of chemicals can have profound health effects is relatively new.

This increased awareness of the effects of hazardous materials on health and the environment has been accompanied by the creation of new government agencies that regulate the creation, transportation, use, and disposal of hazardous materials as well as the cleanup of waste deposits inherited from prior practices. Public concern led to a sudden emergence of environmental problems as a leading issue on a national level, manifested dramatically in April 1970 when hundreds of thousands participated in Earth Day events nationwide. That same year Congress passed legislation creating two agencies mandated with protecting the environment and the health of workers, the Environmental Protection Agency and the Occupational Safety and Health Administration.

The Environmental Protection Agency (EPA) is one of the most powerful government agencies in this country. Its regulatory powers were greatly expanded by the late 1980s with the Congressional enactment of the Toxic Substances Control Act (1) (TSCA), the Resource Conservation and Recovery Act (2) (RCRA), the 1980 Comprehensive Environmental Response and Liability Act (3) (CERCLA) also known as the Superfund, and, recently, the Superfund Amendments and Reauthorization Act (4) (SARA) of 1986.

The Occupational Safety and Health Administration (OSHA), also created in 1970, changed the operations of industry by regulating worker exposure to many substances, based on the recommendations of the National Institute for Occupational Safety and Health (NIOSH) created about the same time.

It is against this background that the need for environmental audits has arisen. Under certain provisions in RCRA and SARA the principal responsible parties (PRPs), which may include the present and prior owners of hazardous waste, the present and prior owners of property contaminated by waste, the transporters of waste, and the operators and owners of disposal sites where waste is deposited, may be financially responsible for the costs of any remediation required to clean up contaminated property. The presence of environmental hazards found in real estate and commercial properties is influencing property value and outcome of real estate transactions. While no laws mandate environmental audits except for specific materials in restricted environments, such as polychlorinated biphenyls (PCBs) in transformers and capacitors (5), underground storage tanks (6), and asbestos in schools (7), a 1986 federal district court decision in *United States v. Maryland Bank & Trust Co.* (8) sent shock waves to lenders across the United States and has resulted in the demand for environmental audits being liability driven rather than health or regulatory driven. In the secondary mortgage market, the Federal National Mortgage Association (Fannie Mae) has adopted a policy (9) requiring a phase I audit to ascertain environmental risks on the property and all properties within a 1-mile radius.

Increased public awareness of issues related to environmental contamination has led to much closer scrutiny by both regulatory agencies and public interest groups of the owners and operators of real property. This scrutiny is focused on the possibility that on-site activities, past and present, may lead to increased risk to human health and the environment. Regulations now exist that address site contamination and site cleanup issues. Improper use, storage, or disposal of contaminants on-site can lead to regulatory fines. Real or suspected injury to human health and the environment resulting from site contamination can lead to third party liabilities which can exceed the real value of the property. In this litigous environment, it is prudent for a seller or purchaser of real property to assess the potential for environmentally driven liabilities prior to completion of a property transaction. It is also prudent for an existing property owner or operator to assess whether onsite activities at present are in compliance with both existing environmental regulations and the state of the practice in terms of reducing the potential for future site environmental problems. To address these concerns, two types of site environmental assessments have developed in recent years: the prepurchase or sale property transfer environmental assessment and the existing facility environmental audit. In the United States the potential for hazardous substances on properties and the need for concern about longterm obligations are recognized under the Superfund Amendments and Reauthorization Act of 1986 (SARA). Under this law, the "innocent" purchaser provisions contain "due diligence" language which requires that purchasers of real property have no prior knowledge of, nor any reason to suspect that, a hazardous material has been, or could be, associated with the property. By definition, an "innocent" purchaser must have undertaken, at the time of acquisition, all appropriate inquiry into the previous ownership and uses of the property consistent with good commercial or customary practice in an effort to minimize liability" (SARA, Section 101[f][35B]).

PROPERTY TRANSFER ASSESSMENTS

It is common practice at this time in the United States to conduct property transfer environmental audits prior to property purchase or sale. The requirement for audit can be set by a number of parties to the sale agreement. The assessment can be requested by the buyer, by the loan originator, by the insurance company, and even by the seller. The buyer, the loan originator, and the insurance company are obviously attempting to avoid unseen liabilities that might render the deal financially unattractive or devastating. The desire of a seller to conduct a property assessment may seem less understandable at first glance. It would seem that, by avoiding any mention of environmental issues prior to sale, the seller may be able to transfer hidden liabilities to an unsuspecting buyer, allowing the "caveat emptor" tradition to hold sway. However, the "joint and several liability" provisions of the CERCLA (Superfund) regulations negate this assumption. In addition, the seller may wish to establish the condition of the land at the time of sale to avoid future liability based on the actions of the purchaser. The purchaser might claim that they were not the source of the contamination, or that it occurred prior their purchase of the land. Environmental audits are now common features of business transactions in the transfer of real property ownership.

An environmental audit is designed to identify the presence of hazardous materials on-site as a result of past or present uses of the property and to provide recommendations for further investigations and remediation as required. Environmental audits are broken down into three phases (Fig. 23.1). Phase I audits are restricted to a qualitative determination of contamination by site reconnaissance, records review, and interviews. Phase II audits are a quantitative identification of the contam-

inants and the extent of the contamination determined by surface and subsurface soil and water sampling, air sampling, laboratory analyses, and site visits. This may include assessments of actual and potential risk to biologic species and the public health. Phase III audits involve evaluating actual and potential risks associated with identified contamination and may include a plan for remediation.

In practice, phase I audits are performed initially, with the need for a phase II audit being dictated by the findings of the phase I audit and the needs or desires of the buyer, seller, and lender.

Environmental audits may involve professionals with expertise in occupational medicine, toxicology, industrial hygiene, entomology, aquatic biology, microbiology, hydrology, geology, and civil engineering. While engineering firms may be skilled and experienced in site reconnaissance and soil drilling and sampling, they are limited in their ability to interpret the analytical results and assess the risks to biologic organisms and the public health. Toxicologists, occupational physicians, and industrial hygienists may be able to characterize exposure pathways, evaluate analytical data, and project the impact of detected contamination on the public health but lack the skill and experience of the engineer in understanding what can and cannot be done in the field to sample for contaminants and remediate those found. Understanding groundwater flow, geologic formations, physical properties of contaminants, and meterologic conditions are important factors in determining risk in the same manner as knowledge of the toxic effects, kinetics, metabolism, distribution, target organs, and species differences are with respect to the contaminants.

PROPERTY TRANSFER ASSESSMENT PHASES

In order to allow a potential party in a property transfer to make an appropriate assessment of the liability potential of a parcel without spending prepurchase money needlessly, the concept of phasing of actual site assessment activities has developed. In a phased approach, an environmental site consultant is retained to address the potential for contaminants. The consultant establishes the likelihood of contamination in a step-by-step process, allowing the interested party to decide at any time that enough information has developed to allow a reasoned decision on the real value of the property in the context of potential contamination. As mentioned previously, the three phases of the property transfer audits are (a) phase I, preliminary assessment; (b) phase II, field assessment; (c) phase III, remediation. Utilizing this phased approach allows for termination of the property transaction at several points throughout the assessment if the property becomes undesirable to either the buyer or seller.

PHASE I: PRELIMINARY ASSESSMENT

The elements of a typical phase I assessment include: (a) existing data review, (b) site history, (c) site visit, (d) initial risk assessment. The review of existing data includes assessing existing site maps and surveys, available data on site geology and hydrogeology, available data on nearby sensitive environmental receptors, records within regulatory agency files concerning any permits or violations for the subject property, historical air photos covering the sequence of developments on the subject property, historical documents covering the activities that have occurred on-site during the period of record, and engineering

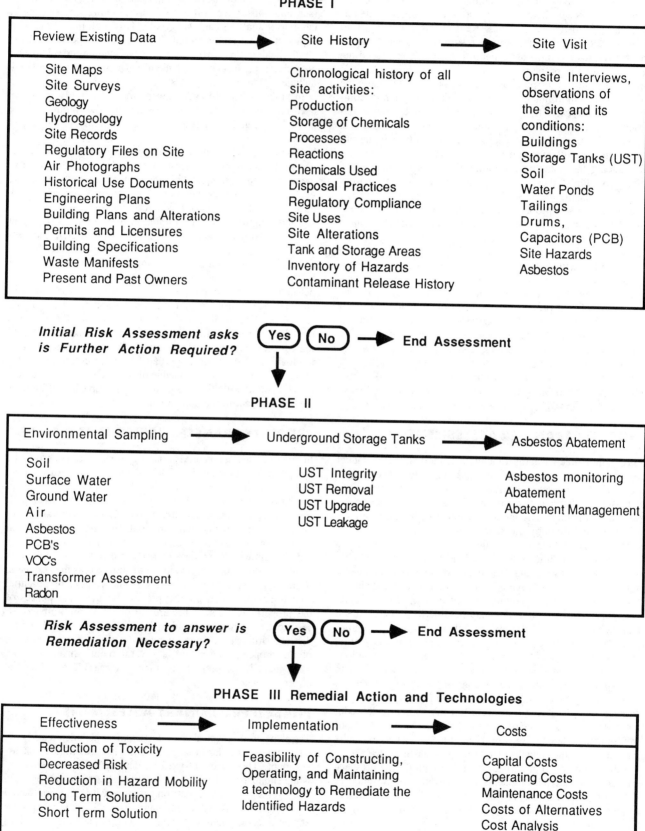

Figure 23.1.   Property transfer audit phases.

plans and drawings covering any on-site improvements. Based on these data, a site history is developed. The site history provides a chronologic listing of site activities that may have included the production, use, storage, and disposal of hazardous substances. Site histories may reveal multiple past uses of property that can reveal types of hazards that could be present. Depending on the type and amount of foundation excavation that occurred on-site during the development of a high rise structure, a potential source of contaminants could still exist on the property. The type of activity that has occurred on-site is used to hypothesize what types of chemical usage may have occurred and what the potential health and environmental impacts of their presence on-site may be.

Questions regarding compliance of the facility with all applicable federal, state, and local regulations must be answered. This is followed by an inventory of hazardous materials and the identification of contaminant sources present. Further inquiry may reveal that contaminant releases to the environment have occurred, and, if so, the extent and distribution of contamination should be ascertained. Contamination of adjacent property of off-site contamination in the area may affect the property under audit even if the subject property is free of past or present contaminant sources. Prior and present working conditions should also be investigated, but may be difficult to ascertain because cooperation is required of the existing operator who may be neither buyer, seller, nor lender. Available records such as site plans, engineering drawings, process flow diagrams, purchasing logs, permits and licenses, waste manifests, and building specifications should be reviewed. Interviewing present and past owners and present and past occupants of the site will often reveal valuable information and leads that would not otherwise be discovered. During the process, it is important to document all sources of information as well as the reliability of the source.

Sources of Historical Information

Specific sources of historical information will vary depending on the property location and current ownership. For example, records regarding federal or state land may be kept in different repositories than are records for privately owned land. Location can be an important factor, because local and provincial agencies may have different responsibilities in different locations. Table 23.1 contains historical information usually researched in a typical property transfer audit.

Public libraries, historical societies, regulatory agencies, and city or regional district offices are good sources of historical information. Historical maps and photographs may be found at the library or at an agency such as the Surveys and Mapping Department of the U.S. Geological Survey.

Records of hazardous material usage on-site are generally available through local and state and regulatory agencies. Local fire departments may also have records on hazardous materials and spills and be good sources of information regarding installation or removal of underground storage tanks. Underground storage tanks (USTs) must be assessed for location, size, use, and leakage. Information on USTs must also include ownership registration papers, permits, and other test data. Interviews with personnel knowledgeable regarding previous site operations are also a good source of information. Retired employees of the company currently operating on-site or employees of companies previously located on-site can be excellent sources of information.

Ideally, the site historical research should be conducted prior to the site visit. Because property transfer assessments are often conducted in a short time frame, this is not always possible. When the historical research must be conducted in conjunction with the site visit, it is important to make any significant historical information available to the site visit personnel as soon as possible. Documentation of the chain of title, business activity on the site, and significant environmental events such as floods and fires requires a review of aerial photographs as far back as they are available.

A review of city and county community planning documents and newspaper articles may reveal valuable information about the past activities on the site. Federal, state, and local agency records should be examined coupled with interviews with the officials responsible for enforcement of regulations or for issuing permits. Sources not to be overlooked include well registrations, sewer and septic tank permits, fire department records, air quality records, business licenses, UST registrations, and designations of properties on state or federal Superfund lists within a 9-mile radius of the subject property.

Research into historical land uses is conducted for several major reasons. One reason is that information gained through the research will help the site visit personnel know what to look for during the walk-through. For example, if historical research reveals that an underground storage tank was installed on the site in the past, the site visit personnel will look for vent pipes or fill pipes that may be associated with that suspected underground tank. Historical information is often useful in evaluating the potential for asbestos-containing materials in a building. If the presence of asbestos-containing materials is determined to be likely, the site visit team can be prepared to collect samples for analysis.

Another reason to conduct careful historical research regarding site uses is that, if the assessment continues into phase II, a more specific sampling and analysis program can be developed. Historical information may help determine the most

Table 23.1. Property Transfer Assessment—Historical Information Concerning Site

Geological/hydrology reports
Geotechnical/soils reports
Well records
Environmental reports
Historical maps
Sanborn maps
Aerial photographs
City directories
Periodical record search (as needed)
Title reports
Building permits
As-built drawings
Permits (environmental)
Fire marshal inspection records
Site maps
Underground storage tanks records
Health department records
Transformer location information
Assessor's office records
Engineering records
Reports of spills and/or releases to soils or water

likely locations for contamination to occur and may help define potential constituents. This can save both money and time during the phase II assessment, as it aids in the design of a logical approach to problem definition.

Finally, sometimes recommendations regarding phase II activities are made based solely on historical information. For example, if historical records indicate that an underground storage tank was installed on the site in the past, but the site visit team could find no evidence of the tank during the walk-through, a recommendation may be that further assessment should be conducted using remote sensing techniques such as metal detection to determine whether a tank is present.

Documentation of File History

Appropriate documentation is a key component of any phase I assessment. Appropriate forms and lists should be used to address specific properties fully. Forms and checklists should be fully completed, dated, and signed by the individual collecting the information. During site visits, photographs should be taken to further document current site conditions. If possible, historical photographs should be obtained to document past site conditions. This information is used to develop the final Phase I report.

Site Visit

Site visits conducted during property transfer assessments consist of two main components, on-site interviews with personnel and the personal observations of the site visit team. The site visit provides an opportunity to interview site occupants regarding current operations and their knowledge of previous operations. The site visit also provides the opportunity to compare documented site history with current site conditions. A site visit questionnaire should be completed during the actual site visit to document observed site conditions.

Visual inspection of a site can reveal important clues about waste management by observing discolored soils, staining of containment vessels or buildings, the presence of drums, capacitor, transformers, surface tanks, wells, impoundment ponds, tailings, railroad easements, and gasoline pumps. The drainage patterns in relationship to these observations should be noted both for surface and groundwater, specific site drainage, and the location of floodplains. The native plant life present should be identified. The density, variety, and health of the flora and fauna will provide valuable hints about the quality of life on site compared with conditions off site. Note should be made of adjacent properties, whether residential or commercial, and activities that may influence conditions on the subject property. The topography of the site should be noted and caution should be exercised where imported mounds of earth preclude accurate assessment of the underlying surface soils.

Site reconnaissance requires actually walking on-site and visually inspecting all buildings, storage facilities, and undeveloped land. Depending on the information obtained from the historical records and review described above, a decision must be made by the project manager regarding the need for a formal health and safety plan as well as the need for personal protective equipment to be worn by the visit team. Some sites may pose significant hazards to the team conducting the environmental audit in the form of dangerous gases, explosives, open pits, and confined spaces. It is highly recommended that each investigator on site complete a 40-hour training course (10) and

Table 23.2.   Potential Site Hazards

Underground storage tanks
Aboveground storage tanks
Waste storage areas
55-gallon drum storage areas
Vehicle or facility maintenance areas
Lead piping in water distribution systems
Effluent discharge areas
Process tankage
Underground process or storage piping
Wells or sumps, active or abandoned
Paint and solvent storage and use areas
Material safety data sheets
Waste piles
Usage of metals in fabrication
Soil staining or order
Special waste generation, storage, and disposal
Solid waste management
Presence of PCB-containing transformers or capacitors
Presence of asbestos
Confined spaces and trenches

be properly equipped to detect organic vapors and other hazards (11). Such potential site hazards must be noted and recorded (Table 23.2). During the site visit, the assessor is looking for evidence of the potential for contamination, direct or indirect. Processes and reactions involving manufacturing can provide clues to the use of certain chemicals.

In addition, the site visit can include a preliminary assessment of the potential for asbestos within insulation, pipe insulation, acoustic panelling, vinyl floor tiling, roofing tars, and other site improvements. Depending on the timing of the property transfer closing, asbestos samples can be collected from readily accessible features suspected of containing asbestos. Asbestos identification is typically accomplished through optical crystallographic techniques, although more sophisticated methodology using transmission microscopy is available and is becoming the standard method for identification. Using the results of phase I task work, the assessment team then determines what the likelihood is that potential contamination may exist on site.

Recommendations are provided for additional phase II tasks which can provide site-specific verification of suspected problem areas.

Occupant Interview

On-site discussions with site occupants often reveal details about the site which would not otherwise be obtainable. During the interview process the tenants are questioned concerning the nature of their operations, length of time on the premises, and knowledge of past operations. They are also asked about the presence, condition, and contents of underground tanks, presence of transformers, knowledge of past spills, utility service to the property, use and management of hazardous materials on the site, and handling of waste materials. The oral record of site activities is as important an indicator of potential site problems as is any actual observation of existing site conditions. Histories of spills or leaks from storage or process tankage on site is often hard to obtain except through discussions with knowledgeable site personnel.

Mortgage Markets and Environmental Audits

The Federal National Mortgage Association requires that the following specific items be addressed in an environmental audit: asbestos, PCBs, radon USTs, waste sites, and additional hazards. Underwriting decisions are based on the findings of the environmental audit. Building construction specifications, a consultant's asbestos report, or actual building inspection data are required for evaluation of the presence of asbestos. Utility transformer records, site surveys of transformers and site soil, or groundwater PCB test results are examples of information sources for the PCB determination. Radon determination in the phase I audit may rely on water utility records, gas utility records, or on-site radon test results. Waste sites and UST determinations require site soil and groundwater test results, EPA Comprehensive Environmental Response, Compensation, and Liability Information System (ECERCLIS) and Hazardous Waste Data Management System (HWDMS) database searches and, for USTs, oil, motor fuel, and waste oil systems reports, UST reports, and site tank surveys. The additional hazards include information such as urea formaldehyde foam insulation survey results, building interior air test results, lead paint surveys, and lead in drinking water test results. The presence of any of the hazards discussed above automatically trigger the need for a phase II audit under current Fannie Mae guidelines.

Phase I Assessment Report

After the completion of the historical research and site walk-through, a Phase I site assessment report is prepared. The report should contain a chronology of the site history and a description of the interviews and observations made during the site visit. The report should also present conclusions regarding the potential risk associated with chemical contamination or asbestos-containing materials on site. It should also present recommendations for further assessment, if appropriate.

Forms documenting historical research, site observations, and interviews should be included as an appendix to the report. Photographs and material safety data sheets, if available, should also be included in an appendix. At a minimum, two figures should be included with the report. The first figure should show the overall location of the site. The second figure should show the layout of the property including all buildings and other items of significance. Additional figures can be added as appropriate.

Phase II: Contaminant Assessment

If the information collected in the phase I assessment suggests that a contamination source may exist on-site, additional work to clarify site environmental conditions is usually necessary. The scope and specific elements of the phase II recommendations may include the following:

1. Define site-specific chemical contaminants and concentration levels.
2. Determine the extent of contamination.
3. Identify contaminant migration pathways (soil, water, and/or air).
4. Assess potential health and natural resources risks related to contaminant type, levels, and volumes present on the property.
5. Identify areas on-site that may require remediation and/or further study.

Table 23.3. Phase II Audit Sampling Strategies

Soil drilling and sampling
Groundwater sampling
Soil vapor probe installation
Surface water sampling
Indoor/outdoor air sampling
Geophysical analysis
Field chemical screening
Laboratory analysis
Asbestos sampling/evaluation
UST leakage and damage
Radon sampling

6. Determine estimated costs for remediation and/or disposal of identified hazardous wastes.
7. Assess the potential liability.

A phase II assessment includes the development and implementation of a site-specific sampling plan, an analytical plan, and a health and safety plan.

The phase II environmental audit attempts to quantitatively identify suspected contaminants reported in this phase I document as well as the extent of the contamination on-site and off-site using a well-designed strategy (Table 23.3). This involves field investigations for underground storage tank leak detection, shallow and deep soil sampling, surface and ground water sampling, air sampling, sampling for asbestos, PCBs, and radon, in addition to other specific chemicals and hazards, and laboratory analyses of each sample. Soil vapor surveys may yield valuable information regarding the presence and identity of volatile organic compounds (VOCs) such as gasoline and organic solvents and can help define contaminant plume boundaries. This activity can be performed by driving vapor probes into the areas of suspected contamination using ''best engineering judgment'' or randomly, based on a sampling grid. This allows for rapid detection of organic vapors in the field which can serve as a guide for further, more accurate, investigations. Shallow soil surface sampling, the use of a split spoon auger for deeper samples, and coring techniques may be needed to obtain the desired information. Attention to the possibility of extraneous contamination by materials such as grease and solvents is critical to preserve sampling accuracy. Quality control of the drilling, sampling, transport, sample preparation, and analyses is imperative.

A sampling strategy is developed prior to conducting a field sampling program in order to efficiently and cost-effectively address the issues. The sampling plan will identify the type and number of samples to be collected (i.e., surface soil, subsurface soil, surface water, groundwater, and/or air) and will be designed to obtain the maximum amount of information using appropriate methodologies. Sample locations will be selected based on areas of concern identified in phase I and other areas as required, to effectively characterize the site. The sampling plan will identify appropriate sample collection methodologies and required drilling or laboratory services.

Sample collection methodologies are selected based on site-specific characteristics, the matrix to be analyzed, types of contaminants, and potential areas of contamination.

Soil Drilling and Sampling

These procedures are used when soil contamination by chemicals is suspected. Locations for sampling are based on historical use patterns, soil staining, or other evidence gathered in the phase I assessment. Where little information on overall contamination sources is available, grid sampling may be useful. Surface and subsurface samples can be collected for subsequent laboratory analysis.

Surface soil samples are collected using stainless steel sample scoops or spoons and placed in clean glass jars provided by the laboratory. If a large area is to be sampled, statistical sampling based on a grid system can be used for collecting discrete and/or composite samples. Sample compositing can be successfully conducted using this approach to provide the necessary information at considerable cost savings.

Subsurface soil sampling can be conducted using test pits and/or soil borings. Test pits would be advanced with backhoe equipment in areas where subsurface contamination is anticipated. If site conditions warrant deeper test pits, however, depths up to 15 feet may be attained. Soil samples are generally collected from test pits using stainless steel scoops or spoons and transferred into clean sample jars provided by the laboratory.

Soil borings are advanced using drill rigs with hollow stem auger, cable tool, and/or air rotary drilling equipment. The choice of drilling method will depend on site geologic conditions and the degree and type of contamination. Soil samples can be collected from soil borings using split spoon samplers and/or Shelby tubes. The soil sample is then transferred (using stainless steel spoons) into clean sample jars provided by the laboratory. Groundwater monitoring wells can be completed in soil boring locations where new or additional groundwater information is required to assess site conditions.

Groundwater Sampling

Groundwater often serves as the "homogenizing agent" for disseminated on-site contamination and is an excellent indicator of the level of site contamination. Groundwater is often the resource that requires highest preservation, particularly in areas of high potable groundwater usage or in areas where groundwater is influent to sensitive surface water receptors. Much lower levels of contamination in groundwater can lead to cleanup requirements than in soil with similar contamination. This is because the water can serve as a direct human and animal ingestion pathway. It is not uncommon for drinking water standards to be applied to the cleanup of potable groundwater supplies. Wells will typically be installed upgradient and downgradient from suspected contamination sources to verify their effect on groundwater quality.

Groundwater samples are collected from wells after the wells have been installed and adequate purged. A minimum of three well casing volumes are purged from wells to allow the collection of representative groundwater samples. Purging is continued until pH and conductivity of the groundwater have stabilized. Purging can be accomplished by using positive displacement lift pumps and/or bailers, depending on the well construction, well depth, purge volume, and well recovery rate. Groundwater samples can be collected using positive displacement lift pumps and/or bailers on the recovery rate and are transferred into clean jars provided by the laboratory.

Soil Vapor Survey

If organic contamination is suspected to be present on site as a result of leaks, spills, or previous disposal practices, soil vapor probe installation may be recommended. The results obtained from these probes can assist in the mapping of the organic plume, thereby further defining the extent of contamination. In addition, the results of a soil vapor survey can be used to select locations for soil borings and groundwater monitoring wells.

Soil vapor surveys are conducted by hand or power-assisted driving of 1-inch slotted steel probes into subsurface soils. Soil vapor is drawn through the probe using a vacuum. The exit port of the vacuum is monitored during purging using an organic vapor analyzer. Sophisticated photoionization detections can detect organic vapor emissions above ground and help direct appropriate soil sampling.

Surface Water Sampling

Runoff or runon from or to the contaminated property can carry both dissolved and particulate contaminants related to the site. Stream or culvert sampling up and downstream of the site can determine whether a contribution from an off-site source may be intercepting the site area. Similar sampling can be done in ponds, lakes, or standing water within or near the site.

Surface water samples are generally in clean jars provided by the laboratory by submerging the sample jar in the source of surface water.

Indoor and Outdoor Air Sampling

Air emissions or dust emissions from a property can often indicate contaminants that are available within a person's breathing zone. Such samples give indications of the potential for human health effects within or near the property. Indoor samples are taken to check for indoor air chemical contaminants. Proper sampling strategy by knowledgeable professionals is crucial to obtaining reliable data on indoor air contaminants. In addition, interpretation of results can be difficult due to the multitude of chemicals that can be present in closed indoor environments.

Geophysical Analysis

For properties with few site improvements but with indications of uncontrolled dumping or of unregistered buried tanks or other fluid receptacles, the consultant may suggest remote methods used to define buried metallic bodies, fluid plumes with varying electrical conductivity, or dimensions of excavation or fill areas. An array of geophysical methods are available for such work, including resistivity, electromagnetic induction coupling, electromagnetic surveying, subsurface interface radar, and other less commonly used methods.

Field Chemical Screening

Depending on the timing of the work and on the actual work being performed, the consultant may recommend some form of on-site field screening for chemical constituents in recovered samples. This may involve the use of such equipment as gas chromatographs and organic vapor analyzers. This approach has the advantage of real-time chemical information which can be used to protect workers from the risk of chemical analysis in the laboratory. Although some techniques can provide concentrations to the parts per billion level, laboratory verification (typically 10% of all samples analyzed) is recommended.

Asbestos Sampling

Asbestos analysis may be required to determine whether asbestos is present in a friable condition on-site. The determination should be made by a qualified asbestos inspector. If asbestos is confirmed on-site in a friable condition, its removal should be accomplished under a plan developed by a certified asbestos abatement specialist, and removal in compliance with the plan should be verified.

Analytical Plan

In most situations, samples of groundwater, surface water, soil, and air collected in the field are submitted to a laboratory for analysis. The requirements for analysis should be determined in conjunction with a chemist familiar with available techniques for identifying contaminants and with the requirements for detection levels based either on health and safety concerns or on existing regulatory standards or protocols. The quality assurance procedures of the selected laboratory should be closely scrutinized. This information should be contained in a detailed analytical plan as well as in the health and safety plan.

The choice of analytical methods utilized during phase II is based on the level of defensibility the project requires. If legal challenge of the results is anticipated, the methods chosen should include only those which provide compound identification confirmation. These methods include gas chromatography-mass spectroscopy (GC-MS) for organic analyses and atomic absorption spectroscopy (AAS) and/or inductively coupled plasma (ICP) spectroscopy for inorganic analyses. These methods are generally more costly than other methods. However, other methods rely on identification by inference and not by direct identification. Therefore, they are not usually defensible if legally challenged.

Oftentimes, in a phase II assessment, screening methods are employed to identify possible contamination in a cost effective manner. Based on the results of these screening analyses, more detailed analytical methods may be used to confirm the presence of the contaminant. Confirmatory analysis by GC-MS can be conducted on a small percentage of those samples identified by the screening methods as containing contaminants of concern. An accredited laboratory with documented quality assurance and quality control procedures should be used to analyze samples. Sample chain of custody and proper sample identification are very important aspects of the analytical plan. Depending on the magnitude of the phase II assessment, the analytical plan may be a part of the sampling plan.

Health and Safety Plan

A health and safety plan for phase II site characterization and/or sample collection is necessary where hazardous material contamination is suspected. The health and safety plan is designed to assess the potential hazards of a site and reduce the potential for illness or injury. The plan is based on available site information, planned site activities, and known or suspected hazards. The health and safety plan functions by prescribing safe work practices, site control measures, personnel protective equipment, personnel training requirements, and emergency procedures and contacts. An individual identified in the plan is designated site safety officer. This individual is responsible for maintaining site control and for ensuring that site personnel have read, have understood, and are in compliance with the procedures outlined in the health and safety plan.

Each firm involved in the site characterization (consultant, driller, excavator) should provide a health and safety plan, personal protective equipment, and monitoring equipment for its operations at the site. Under some circumstances, a single plan may be prepared and used for all operations at the site. The program should include written policy regarding work at hazardous sites, personnel training requirements (40 hours of training specifically designed for work on hazardous waste sites is recommended), and a formal medical monitoring program for employees.

The consultant chosen to oversee work on-site should also be able to provide field monitoring equipment as needed at the site. Examples of monitoring equipment routinely used includes explosimeters, photoionization organic vapor detectors, flame ionization organic vapor analyzers, Geiger counters, oxygen meters, and various colorimetric indicator tubes and pumps.

The phase II environmental audit report should not only present the analytical results but should also interpret and discuss the date, provide some guidance in the form of recommendations for containment, and identify possible exposure pathways for populations at risk. The actual plan for remediation and a quantitative assessment of risk are defined as phase III activities, but the distinction may be blurred in actual practice.

Phase III: Remediation Action

If phase II assessment determines that concentrations and quantities of contaminants are in violation of established regulatory limits or guidelines or that the contaminants pose a threat to human health or the environment, remedial action is usually necessary.

Based on the results of the phase I and II surveys, remediation costs can be estimated. These estimates can then be used to decide whether the costs for remediation can be accommodated within the sale agreement and still allow the transfer to proceed. If so, a decision can be made on who should pay for the remediation, and the remedial activities can be initiated. It is important to realize that the presence of site contaminants need not present a land transfer. If the parties of record understand site conditions and are prepared to responsibly interact to clean them up, the land can still be used for its intended purpose, and the deal can proceed.

The first step in selecting a remedial action is to select and evaluate technology options (Table 23.4). Technologies generally address one component of site problems, such as groundwater contamination. Where multiple media are contaminated, multiple technologies may be combined to form site alternatives. The evaluation of potentially applicable technologies involves four general steps:

1. Develop remedial action objectives specifying the contaminants and media of interest.
2. Identify volumes or areas of media to which objectives might be applied.
3. Identify and screen technologies applicable to each objective to eliminate those that cannot be implemented technically at the site.
4. Assemble the selected representative technologies into alternatives representing a range of treatment and contaminant combinations, as appropriate.

Defined alternatives are evaluated against the short and long-

Table 23.4. Remediation Technologies

Technology Type	Media	Process Options
Capping	Ground water, soil	Clay cap, synthetic cap, multilayer cap
Extraction	Groundwater	Wells, subsurface or leachate collection
Physical treatment	Groundwater	Coagulation, air stripping absorption, neutralization, precipitation, ion exchange
	Soil	Solidification, encapsulation, dewatering
Chemical treatment	Goundwater, soil	Neutralization, precipitation, ion exchange
Biologic treatment	Soil	Cultured microorganisms
Thermal treatment	Soil	Incineration

term aspects of three broad criteria: (a) effectiveness, (b) implementability, and (c) cost.

Effectiveness—Criteria

Each alternative should be evaluated as to the effective protection of human health it will provide as well as the reductions in toxicity, mobility, or volume in the environment that it will achieve. Both short- and longterm components should be evaluated (shortterm referring to the construction and implementation period and longterm referring to the period after the remedial action is complete). Reduction of toxicity, mobility, or volume refers to changes in one or more characteristics of the hazardous substances or contaminated media by the use of treatment that decreases the threats or risks associated with the hazardous material.

Costs—Criteria

Cost estimates for screening alternatives typically will be based on a variety of cost-estimating data. Bases for screening cost estimates may include cost curves, generic unit costs, vendor information, conventional cost-estimating guides, and prior similar estimates as modified by site-specific information.

Both capital and operation and maintenance costs should be considered, where appropriate, during the screening of alternatives. The evaluation should include those operation and maintenance costs that will be incurred for as long as necessary, even after the initial remedial action is complete. Present worth analysis should be used during alternative screening to evaluate expenditures that occur over different time periods. By discounting all costs to a common base year, the costs for different remedial action alternatives can be compared on the basis of a single figure for each alternative.

Implementation—Criteria

Technical feasibility refers to the ability to construct, reliably operate, and meet technology-specific regulations for process options until a remedial action is complete. It also includes operation, maintenance, replacement, and monitoring of technical components of an alternative, if required, into the future after the remedial actions is complete. Administrative feasi-

bility refers to the ability to obtain approvals from other offices and agencies, and the availability of treatment, storage, and disposal service. It also refers to the requirements for and the availability of specific equipment and technical specialists.

After the necessary permits and equipment have been obtained, implementation of the remedial action can begin. During implementation if may be important to conduct site monitoring to assess potential transport of contaminants off-site. It is also important to employ sampling and analysis to verify that the remedial technology is effective.

RISK MANAGEMENT AS A COMPONENT OF ENVIRONMENTAL AUDITS

The term "risk assessment" has been traditionally defined as the quantitative characterization of the probability of a specific injury or disease to a specified target population resulting from exposure to a hazard or combination of hazards over a specific period of time. The exposure must be such that the hazardous substance is able to exert an action at the target organ and generally will require absorption whether percutaneous, gastrointestinal, or respiratory. Exposure does not occur on the basis of a hazard and a susceptible organism existing in the same environment but requires that a pathway exist to enable the hazardous substance to enter the organism. The organism thus exposed incurs a risk for injury or disease. It is important to distinguish "hazard" from "risk" since these terms are often used loosely, causing miscommunication and confusion.

A substance is hazardous if it has the potential to cause injury or disease to an organism. Risk is the measure of the probability of such an injury or disease for a given exposure to the hazard. There can be no risk without both the hazard and the exposure being present. Preventive measures try to eliminate one or both to preclude the development of injury or disease. Remediation techniques attempt to remove the hazard. Personal protective equipment and engineering controls attempt to eliminate the exposure. The degree of effectiveness of either approach affects the risk. The National Research Council defined four stages in the risk assessment process:

1. Hazard identification;
2. Dose response assessment;
3. Exposure assessment;
4. Risk characterization;

Risk assessment as done by regulatory agencies is part of the process for establishing standards for pesticide residue in food, maximum contaminant levels in water (MCLs), and personal exposure limits (PELs). The process generally involves examination of published clinical, epidemiologic, or animal bioassay data. Clinical and epidemiologic data are quite limited and often are severely handicapped by inadequate quantitative exposure data. When animal bioassays are used, the best data are generally the NTP 2-year carcinogenesis bioassays in rodents. These experiments involve dosing groups of animals ($n = 50$ usually), consisting of at least two species and both sexes divided into control groups and exposure groups, at the maximum tolerated dose (MTD), one-half the MTD and one-fourth the MTD. The data on tumor yield and time to tumor are used to construct a dose-response curve. The data are also applied to a mathematical model in an attempt to define the dose-response curve at lower levels, particularly as the dose approaches zero. It is this region of the dose-response curve that is of most interest from a public health point of view, because the magnitude of the effect at low doses may have significant implications for the health of hundreds, thousands, or hundreds of thousands in the population. However, great difficulty exists in the practical application of this process, as the dose-response curves predicted by the various mathematical models can diverge greatly at low doses, producing estimates of risk that can vary by orders of magnitude. The choice of the mathematical model is governed in part by biologic plausibility and theoretical concepts regarding the mechanism of injury or carcinogenesis, which is the usual outcome of concern.

A number of assumptions are made in applying a particular model to the data and in the mathematical derivation of the model itself. One should always be cognizant that the results are dependent on the validity of the assumptions, and, should any one assumption be invalid, the results will vary. An important mathematical assumption that is made to simplify the arithmetical calculations may not necessarily be true. Other assumptions include the existence or lack of existence of a threshold dose, whether the risk is additive to background rates of cancer or multiplies background rates, etc. Much debate exists in the literature and among risk assessors about the direction to take (13). As one would expect from the brief discussion above, the variance in the predicted risk is often at low levels, and the point estimate is often bounded by extremely large values for the 95% confidence limits.

The mathematical models can be divided into two general classes: the tolerance distribution models where dose is a random variable and the mechanistic models where time is a random variable. The Mantel Bryan (14) model is the classic tolerance distribution model and was used by the Food and Drug Administration until the mid-1970s for regulatory purposes. The most commonly discussed mechanistic models are the one hit model, the gamma multihit model, the multistage model, and recently the two stage model (15). Detailed reviews and discussions of these models exist in the literature. There is recently considerable interest by the National Research Council in an approach called physiologically based pharmacokinetics (PBPK) modeling (16).

When the model is fitted to the data, extrapolation of the results to humans, the target species of usual interest, can be performed. To perform the extrapolation, a specific exposure scenario must be defined, and biologic parameters of the target species must be measured or assumed from published values. These parameters include age at first exposure, exposure duration (lifetime, years, weeks per year, days per week, hours per day), route of exposure, life span, body weight, food intake, drinking rate, respiratory rate, etc. Assumptions regarding scaling factors between species and whether to adjust dose on the basis of surface area or weight, adjustments for species differences in life span, respiratory rates, and factors for averaging dose, etc., must also be made. The selected model is then used to extrapolate the animal data to the target species and for the doses of interest. The desired results are estimates of the concentrations that produce a predetermined level of risk (probability of cancer) for the exposure scenario or the derivation of a unit potency factor computed usually for a risk of cancer defined as one in a million [P(Ca) = 10. × E-6] expressed as mg/kg/d, ppm or ppb/d, or mg/m³/d.

The exposure scenario conducted as part of an environmental audit will identify the chemicals posing carcinogenic and noncarcinogenic hazards to workers and the public from those identified as being present in laboratory reports. From these,

a set of indicator chemicals is defined for quantitative risk assessment (QRA). An exposure assessment is then performed which will identify the route of exposure (ingestion, inhalation, or dermal), the exposure pathway (air, surface water, groundwater, food, or soil), and the probable duration of the exposure for the population(s) at risk. Estimates of exposure point concentrations of indicator chemicals using environmental monitoring and appropriate models are compared with applicable or relevant and appropriate requirements (ARARs). If ARARs are lacking for some chemicals, then the risk assessor must estimate human intakes, assess toxicity, and characterize risks using methods described in the Superfund Public Health Evaluation Manual (17).

Where published potency factors are not available, the risk assessor should search the primary scientific literature to identify available toxicity studies conducted by the National Toxicology Program (NTP) and might incorporate the results into a multistage mathematical model (the multistage model is the current standard for quantitative risk assessment used by the EPA for risk assessment. Software developed for the Electric Power Research Institute (EPRI) is available for this purpose.

The same calculation, with relevant parameters changed, is repeated to determine health and environmental risks posed to the environment and humans within 100 yards of each plant due to volatile toxic chemicals emitted by the site. Exposure concentrations and the target populations may vary from site to site.

These data are then reviewed by regulators, policymakers, public health officials, or other interested parties and applied to decision-making for the promulgation of health standards, clean up levels, reentry levels for buildings, residue on foods, etc. The process is recently being applied more to provide lenders with a basis for making financial decisions involving contaminated property.

COSTS OF ENVIRONMENTAL ASSESSMENTS

The range of costs on environmental assessments can be extreme. A decision regarding the appropriate level of expenditure for an assessment relates to the potential benefit of the property transfer as compared with the added expense of the overall environmental audit. Unfortunately, no amount of expenditure provides absolute certainty regarding site contamination issues. It is certainly possible that actual site problems may not be identified despite best efforts of the assessment team that analyzed the property. In the United States, the concept of "due diligence" has been applied to describe how much assessment is enough to allow some statutory protection from joint and several liability under CERCLA. The real questions is how much work is required to make the buyer and/or seller comfortable enough to go forward with a land acquisition. Some level of risk will always be present, so the prudent owner or operator should enter a potential acquisition with an overall risk management strategy, one element of which will be environmental liability. If the strategy is essentially a "zero-risk" strategy, then a large sum of money may be required to reach the required level of environmental security. It is the unknown extent of environmental liability which one may be accepting that makes the decision very difficult indeed. In the case of the risk, a purchaser is willing to accept the realm of earthquake resistance. For instance, there is an existing record of building performance under various types of earthquake loading which can allow some level of rational planning and risk assessment.

engineering community can design in a factor of safety given their knowledge of building performance and the seismic history of the area in which the building exists. No such track record exists for environmental contamination issues. Regulatory and public health standards for various contaminants are constantly reviewed, and most often they are reduced as the reviews proceed. For each property there will be some point at which additional expenditure for environmental characterization will not lead to reduced risk. The challenge of property transfers in the late 1990s will be to find the point of diminishing returns.

REFERENCES

1. Toxic Substances Control Act (TSCA). PL 94-469, 15 USC 2601 et seq., 40 CFR 700-799, 1977.

2. Resource Conservation and Recovery Act (RCRA). PL 94-580, 42 USC 6901 et seq., 40 CFR 240-271, 1976.

3. Comprehensive Environmental Response, Compensation, and Liability Act (CERCLA). PL 96-510, 42 USC 9601 et seq., 40 CFR 300, 1980.

4. Superfund Amendments and Reauthorization Act (SARA). PL 99-499, 1986.

5. Environmental Protection Agency Polychlorinated Biphenyl Regulations. 15 USC 2605 et seq., 40 CFR 761, 1981.

6. Resource Conservation and Recovery Act (RCRA). 42 USC 6991, 6992, and 6996 et seq., 40 CFR 280, 1985.

7. Asbestos Hazard Emergency Response Act (AHERA). PL, 15 USC 2641 et seq., 40 CFR 763, 1986.

8. *United States v. Maryland Bank & Trust Co.*, 632 F. Supp. 573 (D. Md. 1986).

9. Federal National Mortgage Association. Environmental hazards management procedures for the delegated underwriting and servicing product line, Part X.

10. Occupational Safety and Health Standards. 29 USC 655 et seq., 29 CFR 1910.120, 1986.

11. U.S. Department of Health and Human Services, Public Health Service, Centers for Disease Control, National Institute for Occupational Safety and Health. NIOSH/OSHA/USCG/EPA occupational safety and health guidance manual for hazardous waste site activities. DHHS (NIOSH) Publication No. 85-115, Washington, DC: GPO, 1985.

12. National Research Council (NRC). Risk assessment in the federal government: managing the process. Washington, DC: National Academy Press, 1983.

13. Hoel DG, Merrill RA, Perera FP, eds. Banbury report 19: risk quantitation and regulatory policy. Cold Spring Harbor, NY: Cold Spring Harbor Laboratory, 1985.

14. Mantel N, Bryan W. "Safety" testing of carcinogenic agents. Natl Cancer Inst 1961;27:455–470.

15. Krewski D, Van Ryzin J. Current topics in probability and statistics: dose response models for quantal response toxicity data. Amsterdam: North Holland, 1981.

16. National Research Council. Pharmacokinetics in risk assessment. Workshop proceedings, Subcommittee on Pharmacokinetics in Risk Assessment, Safe Drinking Water Committee, Board on Environmental Studies and Toxicology, Commission on Life Sciences. Drinking water and health, Vol. 8. Washington, DC: National Academy Press, 1987.

17. Risk Assessment Guidance for Superfund, Part A, Human Health Evaluation Manual, December 1989, EPA, Washington D.C.

18. Crump KS, Howe RB, Van Landingham C, Clement Associates, K.S. Crump Division. TOX-RISK toxicology risk assessment program. Ruston, Louisiana, for the Electric Power Research Institute, Palo Alto, California, 1988.

24

Personal Protection From Hazardous Materials Exposures

Richard L. Urie, C.I.H.

INTRODUCTION

Protection of employees from hazardous materials consists of three broad areas:

1. Administrative controls;
2. Engineering controls;
3. Personal protective equipment.

Administrative controls consist of managerial efforts to reduce risks of accidents or toxic exposures through planning, training, employee rotation on job sites, changes in processes, and product substitution. These include the development of standard operating procedures along with emergency response plans. The development of environmental and medical surveillance programs may be part of policy and procedures.

Engineering controls are those measures that are planned and constructed for the purpose of reducing accidents and or chemical and physical hazards. Engineering controls may be implemented at the source of the hazard, along the exposure path (such as with a pipeline), or at the operator or receiver of the hazardous substance. Examples include the use of exhaust ventilation, dust suppressants to control fugitive dust emissions, radiation shielding, and the installation of physical protective guards over machinery.

Personal protective equipment (PPE) includes a wide variety of items worn by an individual to prevent injury or exposure. Generally, administrative and engineering controls are used to prevent exposure of personnel to hazardous materials. However, direct personnel response to a hazardous materials site is frequently required in order to conduct environmental sampling, clean up spills, or respond to accidents and injuries. For these instances, protective equipment is required. Such equipment must offer respiratory, ocular, and dermal protection from chemical or physical hazards. Proper protection is important for two reasons:

1. Due to the nature of most hazardous materials incidents and hazardous waste site investigations, the use of personal protective equipment (PPE) is often the only feasible means of preventing or reducing chemically related exposures.
2. The misuse of PPE may directly or indirectly contribute to accidents, chemical or radiologic exposures, dermal injury, burns, heat stress, and related impairments. This chapter will address the fundamental types of respiratory protective equipment and protective garments. Advantages and limitations of the uses of PPE regulations specifications, basic applications for hazardous materials workers, and potential problems associated with misuse will be discussed.

RESPIRATORY PROTECTION (OSHA)

Respiratory protective devices come in a wide variety of configurations, materials, sizes, and intended applications. The selection, use, and maintenance of respirators are complex subjects requiring extensive training and experience. Yet workers are often assigned respirators without consideration given to medical clearance, respirator fit-testing, job-specific selection criteria, or adequate maintenance of the equipment. The large number of Occupational Safety and Health Administration citations issued for inadequate respirator programs attests to this frequent violation. Proper respiratory protection begins with knowledge of the equipment.

Respirators of each class require an apparatus or framework which serves to isolate the wearer from contaminated air. Such apparatus may be provided in the form of a tight-fitting facepiece, a snorkel-like mouthpiece, or a loose-fitting cover such as a hood, suit, hard hat assembly, or blouse.

Examples of tight-fitting facepieces include the quarter-mask which covers the mouth and nose (Fig. 24.1), the half-mask which fits over the nose and under the chin (Fig. 24.2), and the full face mask which covers the face from the hairline to below the chin (Fig. 24.3). These facepieces are generally constructed of neoprene, silicone, or molded rubber. Full face respirators provide limited eye protection against impact and chemical contact.

Mouthpiece respirators are inserted into the mouth in the same fashion as a snorkel (Fig. 24.4). Respirators of this type may include attached nose pinchers to prevent entry of air through the nostrils. Mouthpiece respirators are seldom used for purposes other than emergency escape contingencies.

Loose-fitting respirators typically cover at least the face and a portion of the head and may include full body suits. Some are built into a hard hat/face shield assembly (Fig. 24.5), thereby providing limited protection against impact or chemical contact.

The type of facepiece, cover, or mouthpiece determines the degree of protection provided against barrier breakthrough. Barrier breakthrough is the passage of contaminated air through a breach in the respirator-to-face seal. This level of sealing or barrier protection in conjunction with the efficiency of the air-purifying element or air-supplied system determines the overall protection factor for the protective device.

The National Institute of Occupational Safety and Health (NIOSH) has assigned protection factors to various representative respiratory protection ensembles, as indicated in Tables 24.1 and 24.2. The protection factor is the ratio of the concentration of the contaminant present in the ambient atmosphere to the concentration within the facepiece of the respirator. NIOSH describes the application of the protection factor as follows: "The maximum specified use concentration for a respirator is generally determined by multiplying the exposure limit for the contaminant by the protection factor assigned to a specific class of respirators" (1).

The respirators currently on the market may be broadly classified as the following types:

1. Air-purifying respirator;

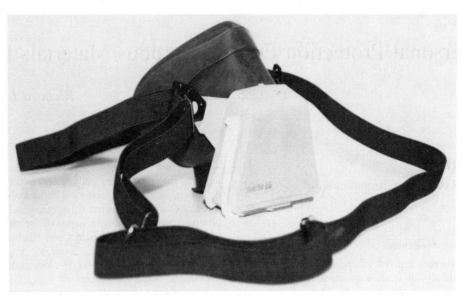

Figure 24.1.   ¼ Mask respirator.

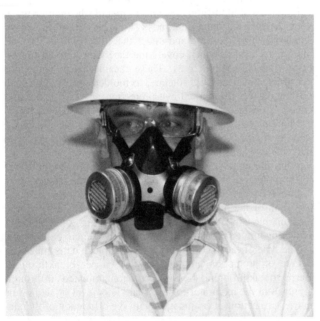

Figure 24.2.   ½ Mask respirator.

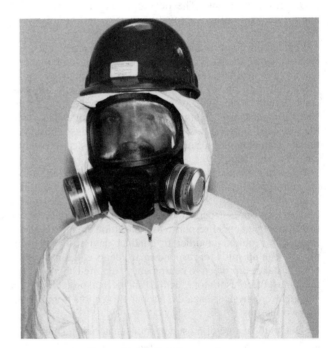

Figure 24.3.   Full face respirator.

2. Supplied air respirator;
3. Self-contained breathing apparatus.

Air-Purifying Respirators

These incorporate any one of the apparatuses previously discussed with a particulate filter(s), gas/vapor removal element(s), or a combination particulate and gas/vapor removal system. Respirators within this class may be powered by a portable battery-driven blower (powered air-purifying respirator), or operated under the negative pressure generated by inhalation (negative pressure air-purifying element).

Particulate filtering respirators use a fibrous material which traps dusts, mists, and/or fumes. Some filters are impregnated with a resin base and are electrostatically charged to enhance the filtration efficiency (2). However, conditions such as high humidity or exposure to oily mists may result in the loss of this electrostatic charge.

Filters can be either standard configuration, offering moderate particulate arresting efficiencies, or approved as high ef-

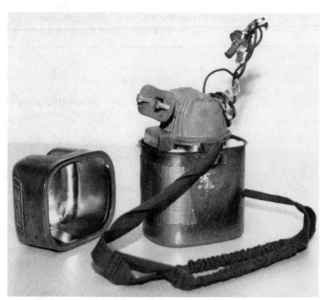

Figure 24.4. Mouthpiece respirator "The Self-Rescuer is a mouth-piece-type respirator."

ficiency particulate air filters (HEPA filters). HEPA filters typically consist of a larger cartridge or canister as opposed to the relatively flat disk-like standard filter element (Fig. 24.6). The standard filter has an approximate efficiency of 80–90% against 0.6-micron particles; the HEPA element has a tested efficiency of 99.9% against 0.3-micron particles. Both classes of filters develop increased efficiency as the particle load within the filter increases with use. Conversely, as the openings within the filter media become smaller, breathing resistance increases. Filters of both types are typically used until such a time as breathing becomes difficult due to this resistance. However the policy of filter reuse should not be followed in situations involving the filtration of radioactive particles which may emit ionizing radiation other than alpha particles.

One piece disposable dust are also available . However, they are seldom used for applications other than those involving nuisance dusts due to poor filtration efficiency and/or inadequate face-sealing properties (Fig. 24.7).

Gas and vapor cartridges or canisters are engineered to collect toxic or irritating gases or chemically convert gases to safe material (Fig. 24.8). The purification device contains a granulated high surface area media referred to as sorbent. Sorbent interacts with the gas molecules through adsorption, absorption, chemisorption, or catalytic chemical reactivity. The most commonly used sorbent media is activated carbon which alone is an effective adsorbent for some organic vapors or gases. Activated carbon may also be impregnated with chemical substances in order to enhance the adsorption action for other specific gases. Examples include iodine-impregnated activated carbon for use against mercury vapor and metallic oxide-impregnated carbon which collects acid gases. Other agents used as adsorbents include silica gel and activated alumina. Absorbents that rely on chemical interactions can include akaline sorbents used to neutralize acid gases. Sorbents can also utilize catalysts to speed up the conversion of toxic gases to relatively nontoxic products. The "self-rescuer" respirators carried by

underground mine workers utilize a catalyst called hopcalite, which converts carbon monoxide to carbon dioxide.

Combination cartridges and canisters are available and consist of multiple elements for various gases or for gases and particulates. Cartridges and canisters are labeled and color coded for their intended use. Table 24.3 depicts the color code system established by American National Standard, K.13.1. All U.S. manufacturers of respirators conform to this color code system, however, cartridges, filters, and canisters are not interchangeable with different brands of respiratory devices, despite the uniform color code.

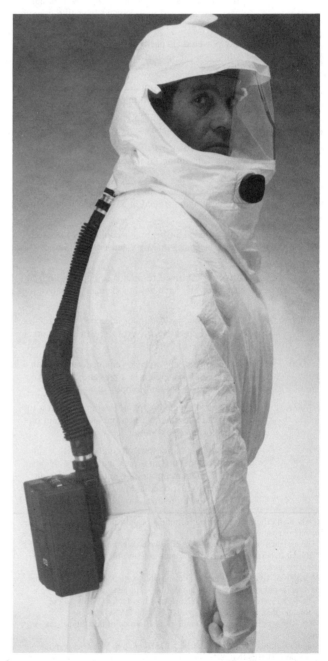

Figure 24.5. MSA PAPR (powered air-purifying respirator) (Total Assembly).

Table 24.1 Assigned Protection Factor Classifications of Respirators for Protection Against Particulate Exposures[a]

Assigned Protection Factor	Type of Respirator
5	Single-use or quarter-mask respirator
10	Any air-purifying half-mask respirator including disposable equipped with any type of particulate filter except single use[b,c]
	Any air-purifying full facepiece respirator equipped with any type of particulate filter[e]
	Any supplied-air respirator equipped with a half-mask and operated in a demand (negative pressure) mode[b]
25	Any powered air-purifying respirator equipped with a hood or helmet and any type of particulate filter[d]
	Any supplied-air respirator equipped with a hood or helmet and operated in a continuous flow mode[d]
50	Any air-purifying full facepiece respirator equipped with a high efficiency filter[b]
	Any powered air-purifying respirator equipped with a tight-fitting facepiece and a high efficiency filter[d]
	Any supplied-air respirator equipped with a full facepiece and operated in a demand (negative pressure) mode[b]
	Any supplied-air respirator equipped with a tight-fitting facepiece and operated in a continuous flow mode[d]
	Any self-contained respirator equipped with a full facepiece and operated in a demand (negative pressure) mode[b]
1000	Any supplied-air respirator equipped with a half-mask and operated in a pressure demand or other positive pressure mode[b]
2000	Any supplied-air respirator equipped with a full facepiece and operated in a pressure demand or other positive pressure mode[b]
10,000	Any self-contained respirator equipped with a full facepiece and operated in a pressure demand or other positive pressure mode[b]
	Any supplied-air respirator equipped with a full facepiece operated in a pressure demand or other positive pressure mode in combination with an auxiliary SCBA operated in a pressure demand or other positive pressure mode[b]

[a]Only high efficiency filters are permitted for protection against particulates having exposure limits less than 0.05 mg/m^3.
[b]The assigned protection factors (APFs) were determined by Los Alamos National Laboratories (LANL) by conducting quantitative fit testing on a panel of human volunteers.
[c]An APF of 10 can be assigned to disposable particulate respirators if they have been properly fitted using a quantitative fit test.
[d]The APFs were based on workplace protection factor (WPF) data or laboratory data more recently reported than the LANL data.
[e]The APF was based on consideration of efficiency of dust, fume, and/or mist filters.
Source: Bollinger NJ, Schultz, RH. NIOSH guide to industrial respiratory protection. DHHS (NIOSH) publication N. 87-116. Washington, DC: GPO, 1987.

Table 24.2. Assigned Protection Factor Classifications of Respirators for Protection Against Gas/Vapor Exposures

Assigned Protection Factor[a]	Type of Respirator
10	Any air-purifying half-mask respirator (including disposable) equipped with appropriate gas/vapor cartridges[b]
	Any supplied air respirator equipped with a half mask and operated in a demand (negative pressure) mode[b]
25	Any powered air-purifying respirator with a loose-fitting hood or helmet[c]
	Any supplied-air respirator equipped with a hood or helmet and operated in a continuous flow mode[c]
50	Any air-purifying full facepiece respirator equipped with appropriate gas/vapor cartridges or gas mask (canister respirator)[b]
	Any powered air-purifying respirator equipped with a tight-fitting facepiece and appropriate gas/vapor cartridges or canisters[c]
	Any supplied-air respirator equipped with a full facepiece and operated in a demand (negative pressure) mode[b]
	Any supplied-air respirator equipped with a tight-fitting facepiece operated in a continuous flow mode[c]
	Any self-contained respirator equipped with a full facepiece and operated in a demand (negative pressure) mode[b]
1000	Any supplied-air respirator equipped with a half-mask and operated in a pressure demand or other positive pressure mode[b]
2000	Any supplied-air respirator equipped with a full facepiece and operated in a pressure demand or other positive pressure mode[b]
10,000	Any self-contained respirator equipped with a full facepiece and operated in a pressure demand or other positive pressure mode[b]
	Any supplied-air respirator equipped with a full facepiece operated in a pressure demand or other positive pressure mode in combination with an auxiliary SCBA operated in a pressure demand or other positive pressure mode[b]

[a]The assigned protection factor (APF) for a given class of air-purifying respirators may be further reduced by considering the maximum use concentrations for each type of gas and vapor air-purifying element.
[b]The APF's were determined by Los Alamos National Laboratories (LANL) by conducting quantitative fit testing on a panel of human volunteers.
[c]The APF's were based on workplace protection factor (WPF) data or laboratory data more recently reported than the LANL data.
Source: Bollinger NJ, Schultz RH. NIOSH guide to industrial respiratory protection. DHHS (NIOSH) publication N. 87-116. Washington, DC: GPO, 1987.

Supplied Air Respirators

Supplied air respirators consist of a source of respirable air which is supplied to the wearer's face or headpiece. They are defined as type A, B, or C (2a).

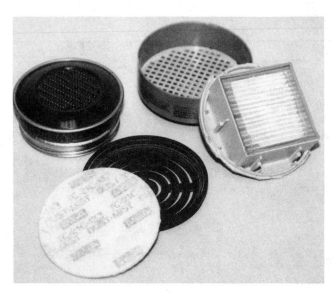

Figure 24.6. Filter pad, HEPA cartridge and canister.

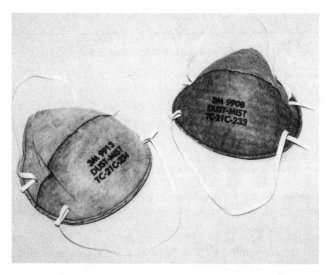

Figure 24.7. Disposable dust respirators.

Type A: Consists of a tight-fitting facepiece attached to a large diameter hose supplied with fresh air from a mechanical blower. The blower may be motor driven or hand operated.

Type B: Respirators also consist of a tight-fitting facepiece attached to a large diameter hose with low breathing resistance. Air is drawn through the hose by the force of inhalation only.

Type C: Respirators consist of a tight- or loose-fitting face or head assembly, a high pressure air line not to exceed 300 feet, couplings, regulators, control valves, and a supply of breathing air typically from compressed air cylinders or an approved compressor (Fig. 24.9).

Breathing air used for any respirator system must meet the requirements for type 1 gaseous air (grade D or higher quality) set forth by the Compressed Gas Association (Table 24.4).

Type C respirators may be further classified with respect to the air flow/pressurization of air in the facepiece. They may be supplied with (a) continuous air flow, (b) air flow which is delivered upon inhalation only (''demand''), or (c) constant pressurization of the mask with additional air flow upon inhalation (''pressure-demand''). The continuous flow system provides constant pressurization of the facepiece but requires a large volume of air. Demand systems conserve the air supply, but do not provide constant positive pressure, thereby potentially allowing contaminants into the mask if the face-to-facepiece seal is broken. Pressure-demand systems provide a constant positive pressure and conservation of air.

Work on hazardous waste sites or chemical incident scenes that warrant supplied air respirator use typically involve the type C pressure-demand system with an auxiliary emergency air supply attached to the wearer.

Self-Contained Breathing Apparatus

Self-contained breathing apparatuses (SCBAs) are individual respirator systems consisting of a portable air or oxygen supply worn by the user (Fig. 24.10). There is no physical link to a stationary air supply as in the case of supplied air respirators. SCBAs may be classified as ''closed circuit'' or ''open circuit'' systems (3). Closed circuit systems, also known as ''rebreathers,'' recycle the user's exhaled breath after removing carbon dioxide and adding oxygen as needed. The gases are recycled within a contained system, except in the event of excess pres-

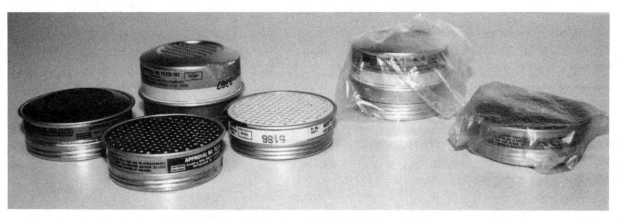

Figure 24.8. Single element and combination cartridges.

Table 24.3.   Atmospheric Contaminants to Be Protected Against

Atmospheric Contaminants to Be Protected Against	Colors Assigned[a]
Acid gases	White
Hydrocyanic acid gas	White with ½-inch green stripe completely around the canister near the bottom
Chlorine gas	White with ½-inch yellow stripe completely around the canister near the bottom
Organic vapors	Black
Ammonia gas	Green
Acid gases and ammonia gas	Green with ½-inch white stripe completely around the canister near the bottom
Carbon monoxide	Blue
Acid gases and organic vapors	Yellow
Hydrocyanic acid gas and chloropicrin vapor	Yellow with ½-inch blue stripe completely around the canister near the bottom
Acid gases, organic vapors, and ammonia gases	Brown
Radioactive materials, excepting tritium and noble gases	Purple (magenta)
Particulates (dusts, fumes, mists, fogs, or smokes) in combination with any of the above gases or vapors	Canister color for contaminant, as designated above, with ½-inch gray strip completely around the canister near the top
All of the above atmospheric contaminants	Red with ½-inch gray stripe completely around the canister near the top

[a]Gray shall not be assigned as the main color for a canister designed to remove acids or vapors.
NOTE: Orange shall be used as a complete body, or stripe color to represent gases not included in this table. The user will need to refer to the canister label to determine the degree of protection the canister will afford.
(Secs. 4(b)(2),6(b) and 8(c), 84 Stat. 1592, 1593, 1596, 29 U.S.C. 653, 655, 657; Secretary of Labor's Order No. 8-76 (41 FR 25059); 29 CFR Part 1911) (39 FR 23502, June 27, 1974, as amended at 43 FR 49748, Oct. 24, 1978)
Source: Pritchard JA. A guide to industrial respiratory protection. Department of Health, Education and Welfare publication N. 760-189. Washington, DC: GPO, 1976 (Reprinted April 1979).

surization, in which case air is vented out the relief valve. Closed circuit SCBAs which provide up to 4 hours of use per charge are available. The two basic types of rebreathers use either a cylinder of compressed oxygen or a solid oxygen generating substance such as potassium superoxide (KO_2). Rebreathers have limited use at hazardous waste sites or chemical spill sites due to the high expense of the units and the danger of flammability associated with oxygen-enriched systems (4).

Open circuit SCBAs exhaust the exhaled air to the atmosphere, rather than recycling it. They typically consist of a 30- or 60-minute supply of compressed grade D air worn on the back of the user and a tight-fitting facepiece (Figure 24.10). As with type C respirators, these SCBAs may use either a demand or pressure-demand regulator system. The complete system typically weighs 30–38 pounds. Open circuit SCBAs are available with an optional valve stem which allows the attachment of an airline from a stationary source of air. (Figure 24.11) This feature allows the option of creating a type C respirator with a 30- or 60-minute escape bottle.

CHEMICAL PROTECTIVE CLOTHING

Chemical protective clothing (CPC) is a broad class of garments worn to protect the wearer against contaminant-related injury or as a means of controlling the spread of the contaminant. The term ''chemical'' protective clothing is somewhat misleading, as it typically includes garments worn in situations involving infectious or radiologic waste as well as chemicals. Hazardous material incidents in which CPC is needed include exposure to any of the following: toxic gases; asphyxiants; corrosive liquids; flammable vapors; solvent vapors; explosives; carcinogens.

Clearly, there is no universal ensemble appropriate to all situations. Such factors as garment flammability, chemical resistance, strength, degree of vapor sealing, heat transfer, cost, and so forth dictate the need for a wide variety of garment materials and designs. A few representative styles and materials are discussed to introduce the reader to some of the most commonly used CPC ensembles.

Fully Encapsulating Suits

These are one-piece garments that provide chemical protection for the entire body (Fig. 24.11). They represent the most extensive degree of PPE skin protection available. The suit also protects the enclosed breathing apparatus from chemical degradation and excessive decontamination requirements. Most resusable encapsulating suits are made of butyl rubber, Viton, or Teflon or a combination of these. The suits may have integral boots and/or gloves made of neoprene, polyvinylchloride (PVC), or other natural or synthetic materials. The face shield may be made of glass or acrylate compounds. Disposable encapsulating suits are also available which are manufactured from a variety

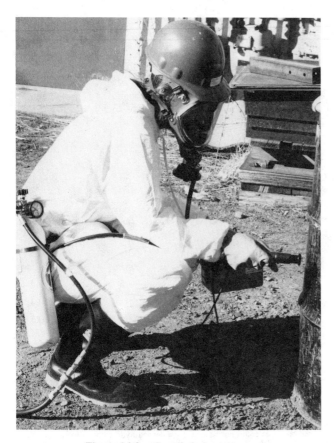

Figure 24.9. Supplied air system.

of polymer-covered fibrous materials. Encapsulating suits are used in conjunction with SCBAs and/or a type C air-line respirator.

Nonencapsulating Suits

Nonencapsulating suits consist of one or two pieces. One-piece hooded coveralls are generally the suit of choice (Fig. 24.12); however, a hooded jacket worn with a pair of pants or bib overalls is also an option. Usually when these suits are worn in the field, seams, gaps, and connection points are tape sealed (5). Nonencapsulating suits are often purchased with the intent of disposing of the garment after a day of field use.

Aprons, Boots, Boot Covers, and Gloves

Aprons are also employed as a means of partial skin protection for such activities as chemical sampling and packaging. Aprons may cover only the chest and abdomen or extend the full length of the chest to the feet and include full sleeves (6).

Boots, boot covers, and gloves are a necessary addition to most ensembles, as the hands and feet are the most likely portion of the body to come in contact with contaminants.

Barrier creams are available which, when applied directly to the skin, offer temporary protection against some chemical products. Barrier creams are more appropriate for use in controlled industrial settings than in hazardous material situations. Such creams may be used to help prevent the dermal absorption of chlorinated solvents.

Specialized Protective Equipment

Specialized protective equipment and accessories are available for applications other than chemical-skin contact and include such items as flame-resistant suits, flotation gear, antiradiation suits, blast fragmentation suits, and cooling accessories.

Flame resistant suits—Consist of aluminized encapsulating suits, fire fighter's bunker coats, or one-piece nonencapsulating suits (Fig. 24.13) such as the Nomex coverall. Garments of this nature are sometimes worn in conjunction with chemical protective clothing which alone offers little protection against a flashback.

Antiradiation suits—Designed to prevent ingestion, inhalation, or spread of radiation-bearing particles. They offer little protection against the effects of electromagnetic radiation exposure (8).

Blast and fragmentation suits—Employed when handling explosive materials. However, there is no gear that will adequately protect against the impact of more than a minute quantity of explosive material at distances less than about 20 feet (9).

Cooling devices—Due to the potential for heat stress associated with chemical protective clothing, cooling accessories are sometimes incorporated into the protective ensemble. These accessories consist of three basic types: (a) evaporation cooling garments involving the circulation of cool, dry air; (b) water/ice jackets utilizing conductive cooling properties (Fig. 24.14); and (c) garments containing battery-powered pumps and tubes which circulate cool liquid across the chest and back. The overall effectiveness of these devices on hazardous waste sites is limited due to the added weight, bulk, and maintenance requirements. Other protective gear commonly used on hazardous waste sites includes hard hats and goggles or face shields.

Levels of Hazardous Material Protection

The Environmental Protection Agency has established distinct combinations of respirators and chemical protective garments for use in certain hazardous materials situations. These classes or "levels of protection" are referred to as A, B, C, and D (10).

Level A: Represents the maximum degree of skin and respiratory protection offered by a combination of a supplied air respirator and an encapsulating suit.
Level B: Consists of a supplied air respirator and a nonencapsulating garment.
Level C: Involves a moderate degree of respiratory protection and skin protection through the use of an air-purifying respirator and a nonencapsulating garment.
Level D: Consists of standard work clothes—no respirator and no chemical protective garment.

The specific EPA ensembles for levels A through D are presented in Table 24.5. Many companies and agencies have adopted the terminology of the EPA.

REGULATIONS AND CERTIFICATIONS IMPACTING ON PPE USE

Respiratory protective devices must be tested and certified by the National Institute for Occupational Safety and Health

Table 24.4. Characteristics of Grade D and Better Breathing Air

Limiting Characteristics	GRADES					
	D	E	F	G	H	I
% O_2 (v/v) Balance predominantly N^2V	atm. 19.5–23.5	atm. 19.5–23.5	atm. 19.5–23.5	atm. 19.5–23.5	atm. 19.5–23.5	atm. 19.5–23.5
Water	b	b	b	b	b	1–10.4°F
Hydrocarbons (condensed) in mg/m³ of gas at NTPᶜ	5	5				
CO	20	10	5	5	5	1
Odor	*	*	*	*	*	*
CO_2	1000	500	500	500	0.5	
Gaseous hydrocarbons (as methane)			25	15	10	0.5
Nitrogen dioxide				2.5	0.5	0.1
Nitrous oxide						0.1
Sulfur dioxide				2.5	1	0.1
Halogenated solvents				10	1	0.1
Acetylene						0.05

*Adapted from Compressed Gas Association, Inc., Air Specification G-7.1.

ᵃThe term "atm" (atmospheric) denotes the normal oxygen content of atmospheric air; numbers indicate oxygen limits for synthesized air.

ᵇThe water content of compressed air required for a particular grade can vary from saturated to dry depending upon the intended use. If a specific water limit is required, it should be specified as a limiting dewpoint (expressed in temperature °F at one atmosphere absolute pressure) or concentration in ppm (v/v).

ᶜNo limits are given for condensed hydrocarbons beyond grade E since gaseous hydrocarbon limits could not be met if condensed hydrocarbons were present.

Source: Pritchard JA. A guide to industrial respiratory protection. Department of Health, Education, and Welfare publication N. 760-189. Washington, DC: GPO, 1976. (Reprinted April 1979).

(NIOSH) and/or the Mine Safety and Health Administration (MSHA). NIOSH and MSHA performance requirements are stipulated in Title 30, Code of Federal Regulations, part II.

Users of respirators must meet a variety of requirements established by the appropriate agency in authority, such as OSHA, the Nuclear Regulatory Commission (NRC), and/or MSHA. The OSHA requirements are representative of other agency requirements. That standard incorporates American National Standards Institute (ANSI) standard Z88.2–1969—"Practices for Respiratory Protection," 49 CFR Part 173—"Shipping of Compressed Gas Cylinders," ANSI standard 248.1–1954—"Marking of Compressed Gas Cylinders," and Compressed Air Standard G-7.1–1966.

The major requirements of the OSHA 29 CFR 1910.134 Respiratory Protection Standard are:

1. Standard operating procedures governing the selection and use of respirators shall be in writing.
2. Respirators shall be selected on the basis of hazards to which the worker is exposed.
3. The user shall be instructed and trained in the proper use of respirators and their limitations.
4. Where practicable, the respirators should be assigned to individual workers for their exclusive use.
5. Respirators shall be regularly cleaned and disinfected. Those issued for the exclusive use of one worker should be cleaned after each day's use, or more often if necessary. Those used by more than one worker shall be thoroughly cleaned and disinfected after each use.
6. Respirators shall be stored in a convenient, clean, and sanitary location.
7. Respirators used routinely shall be inspected during cleaning. Worn or deteriorated parts shall be replaced. Respirators for emergency use, such as self-contained devices, shall be thoroughly inspected at least once a month and after each use.
8. Appropriate surveillance of work area conditions and degree of employee exposure or stress shall be maintained.
9. There shall be regular inspection and evaluation to determine the continued effectiveness of the program.
10. Persons should not be assigned to tasks requiring use of respirators unless it has been determined that they are physically able to perform the work and use the equipment. A physician shall determine what health and physical conditions are pertinent. The respirator user's medical status should be reviewed periodically (for instance, annually).
11. Approved or accepted respirators shall be used when they are available. The respirator furnished shall provide adequate respiratory protection against the particular hazard for which it is designed in accordance with standards established by competent authorities. The U.S. Department of Interior, Bureau of Mines, and the U.S. Department of Agriculture are recognized as such authorities. Although respirators listed by the U.S. Department of Agriculture

Other standards are in effect which define respirator selection and use under specific circumstances. Examples include OSHA standards for asbestos, lead, and arsenic exposure. Due to the complex integration of various agency standards, an organization such as NIOSH should be consulted for clarification.

Unlike respirators, protective garments are not stringently regulated. While there are a variety of recommended tests and manufacturing guidelines available, few have been incorporated into regulatory standards. Many of the more established manufacturers have adopted guidelines from the American Society of Testing and Materials (ASTM), the American National Standards Institute (ANSI), and the National Fire Protection Association (NFPA), regarding permeability/breakthrough testing, sizing, and garment flammability, respectively (13, 14).

Protective accessories including eye and face protection, head protection, and foot protection are well addressed by agencies such as OSHA. OSHA regulations incorporate these standards: ANSI "Occupational and Educational Eye and Face Protection" 287.1-1968, ANSI Safety Requirements for Industrial Head Protection, 289.1-1969, and ANSI Men's Safety-toe Footwear, 241.1-1967.

SELECTION OF PERSONAL PROTECTIVE EQUIPMENT

Much has been written on this complex subject which is too extensive to consolidate in this text. However, detailed decision trees and selection guides are available, including two NIOSH publications:

1. Respirator Decision Logic, publication #87-108
2. Personal Protective Equipment for Hazardous Material Incidents: A Selection Guide, publication #84-114.

Some of the major respirator selection criteria to be evaluated include:

- level of oxygen in the atmosphere;
- toxicity of contaminant, including conditions immediately dangerous to life and health (IDLH values) and permissible exposure limits (PELs);
- sealing efficiency of mask;
- sorption efficiency of cartridge media for the specific contaminant of concern;
- odor or irritant threshold of contaminant;
- concentration of contaminant;
- service life of respirator;
- conditions of use (i.e., fire, humidity, etc.).

The selection of chemical protective clothing is based on a variety of scientific data and judgment. Criteria such as permeation and breakthrough are good indicators of chemical resistance. However, stitching, sizing, dexterity, and general durability must be closely inspected for a given brand. The manufacturing process should also be evaluated. For example, two gloves of the same material and thickness may have different degrees of protection if one is latex-dipped and one is solvent- or cement-dipped, the difference being that solvent dipping involves multiple dipping or layering, whereas latex dipping is a single dip process (7). It has been speculated that the single dip may result in a higher rate of imperfections.

Protective suits, aprons, boots, and gloves are manufactured by different methods and in a wide variety of materials, thick-

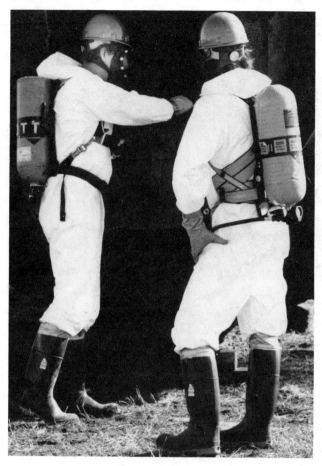

Figure 24.10. SCBA.

continue to be acceptable for protection against specified pesticides, the U.S. Department of the Interior, Bureau of Mines, is the agency now responsible for testing and approving pesticide respirators.

OSHA also prohibits facial hair on respirator users due to data indicating poor respirator-to-face sealing (11). Contact lenses are also prohibited (12). Individuals dependent on the use of corrective lenses will require special respirator spectacle kits.

Respirator filters and cartridges must meet certain test criteria as defined by MSHA in 30 CFR Part II. Particulate filters are tested against silica dust, lead fume, silica mist, and/or dioctylpthalate (DOP). Chemical cartridges are tested with the following agents:

Cartridge	Test Atmosphere
Ammonia	Ammonia
Acid gas	Sulfur dioxide, chlorine, HCL
Methylamine	Methylamine
Organic vapors	Carbon tetrachloride
Pesticides	Silica dust, lead fume, DOP
Carbon monoxide	Carbon monoxide

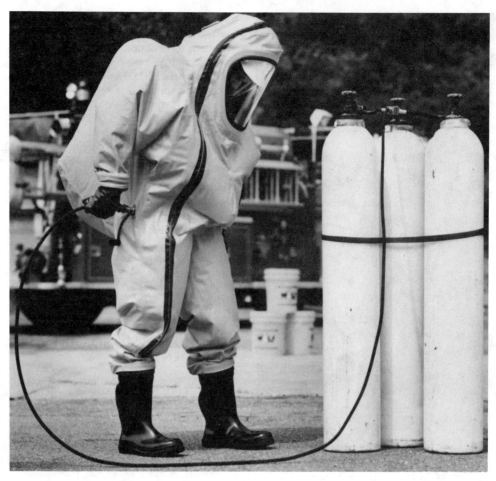

Figure 24.11. Fully encapsulating suit with SCBA in a level A hazardous materials operation. User is changing the SCBA air bottle with air from the stationary bottle.

nesses, and configurations. All of these variables must be considered when selecting a chemical protective garment for a given application. One major set of parameters to be assessed is the breakthrough time and permeation rate of a chemical or group of chemicals for the material used to construct the garments. Breakthrough is defined as the differential time from initial contact of the outside surface of the chemical protective clothing with a chemical to the first detection of the chemical on the inside surface (7). Permeation rate is a numeral expression which indicates the amount of a chemical which passed through a given area of clothing per unit time. It is important to note that these data are based on laboratory conditions. Use in the presence of increased heat will increase the movement of the chemicals through the garment. In addition, the data pertain to the material only; seams, zippers, and face shields, may not offer the same degree of chemical resistance as the material itself. Breakthrough and permeation data for several materials are available from manufacturers of disposable chemical protective garments, e.g., Dupont's Tyvek.

Combining the various criteria for selecting respirators and protective clothing results in some variation of the EPA "Levels of Protection." The basic advantages and limitations of each level are also provided (Table 24.5).

There are many qualifiers to be evaluated before assigning an initial level of protection. However, some general examples are presented based on the experience of the author.

Level A operations: Includes work with concentrated corrosives such as a chlorine cylinder leak or an anhydrous ammonia line repair, handling of highly toxic materials such as military chemical agents or highly infectious microorganisms, and entry into unknown chemical or infectious waste releases.

Level B operations: Includes confined space entry situations where oxygen concentration may be below 19.5% and/or toxic products are present, work involving volatile carcinogens such as hydrazine, and products irritating to the skin which exceed an immediately dangerous to life and health (IDLH) value such as a 200 ppm vapor concentration of hydrofluoric acid.

Level C operations: Includes some low-level uranium tailings cleanup, lead dust exposure, low to moderate asbestos sampling, and low level exposure to solvent vapors.

Level D operations: Operations conducted in the support area, of a hazardous waste operation, equipment mobilization, and noninvasive geophysical surveys.

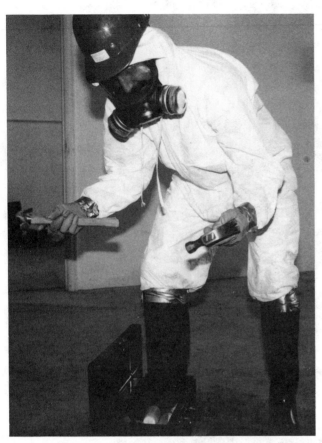

Figure 24.12.   Chemical protective coverall.

PROBLEMS ASSOCIATED WITH PPE USE

While the various forms of eye, skin, and respiratory protection described in this chapter can be critical elements of a safety program, they also present some health concerns related to physical fitness of workers, heat stress, and exposure to multiple chemicals.

Heat stress is a common concern among users of impermeable garments when temperatures exceed 75°F (23.9°C) and/or the physical labor demand is high. The added weight of an SCBA and confinement within a full face mask add to the workload, heat retainment, and loss of evaporative cooling. The end result may be a 35% loss of cooling, an additional 40 pounds of carrying weight, and an environment within the suit equal to 100% humidity. Some suits cannot be worn for more than 15 minutes above 80°F (26.7°C) (15). Therefore, measures must be taken to restrict the wearing time of impermeable garments to temperature-dependent work/rest regimes (16). In addition, workers should be encouraged to replace lost fluids throughout the day, avoid alcoholic beverages, monitor body temperature or heart rate, and schedule heavy work for cooler parts of the day. Workers new to a warm work environment should be acclimated over a week-long period, beginning with a 50% workload which is progressively increased by about 10% each day (17, 18).

Signs and symptoms of heat-related illness and loss of thermoregulatory control should be monitored for and include head-ache, disturbances in gait, tachycardia, dizziness, skin that is warm or hot to the touch with little sweating, rapid respirations, and altered mental status. Supervisors of hazardous materials workers should be aware of these warning signs and intervene immediately if they become apparent. Emergency medical response is required to prevent serious illness or death. Workers in level A protective gear may not be easily observed until they have serious signs and symptoms.

Dermatoses may result from the moisture and abrasion caused by some protective garments. Respirator masks that are disinfected but inadequately rinsed can result in severe skin irritation due to residual chemicals. Suits and masks may be worn for hours at a time before being removed. Any dirt, disinfectant, or moisture trapped within the facepiece seal will remain in contact with the skin under pressure. Workers must be advised of the importance of PPE cleaning, disinfection, and rinsing.

The use of SCBAs and air-line respirators have been related to complaints of headaches and upper airway irritation. Some drying of the mucous membranes can be expected. This is a result of the removal of water vapor from the compressed air, which prevents corrosion within the regulator systems (19). Some symptoms of irritation may be related to the pressure placed on the temples by the respirator straps or the constant flow of cool air across the face and eyes.

The negative pressure requirements, exhalation residence, and dead air space of air-purifying respirators may result in such physiologic changes as increased alveolar carbon dioxide tension, decreased oxygen uptake, and an increased oxygen debt (20). The end result of such reactions may be fatigue, dyspnea, and headache. This may contraindicate the use of negative pressure air-purifying respirators at high altitudes, during heavy exertion, or for workers with significant respiratory impairments.

Restricted vision and reduced dexterity associated with PPE use may increase the possibility of falls, vehicular accidents, and other conventional safety concerns. Workers should be advised to work in pairs (i.e., the buddy system), and take additional time, if needed, to complete field tasks in high risk areas. Mobile equipment operators must be particularly watchful of workers near their operations, as hearing may also be compromised by hoods, shrouds, or masks.

Permeability of Level A garments are typically studied only with single chemicals and not mixtures. NIOSH has stated that the permeation parameters of single chemicals cannot be relied on to determine the permeability of mixtures (18).

SUMMARY

Of the three forms of employee protection, administrative controls, engineering controls, and personal protective equipment, the latter is the least desirable, but often the most applicable to situations involving hazardous materials work. Proper selection of PPE begins with a thorough knowledge of the equipment and the contaminant(s). Users of PPE must be properly trained in its use, fitted, and examined by a physician prior to being qualified for field duty. Some equipment, such as respirators and flotation gear, must meet certain agency approvals. Improper use of PPE may result in a variety of hazardous conditions including chemical or radiologic exposure due to inadequate protection, heat stress, dermatoses, fatigue, and general discomfort.

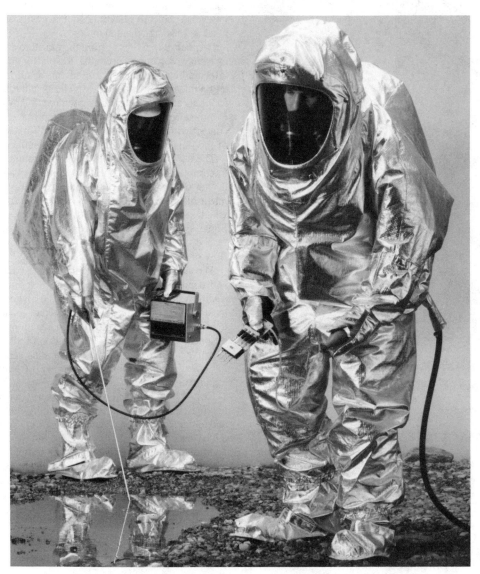

Figure 24.13.   Flame-resistant suits.

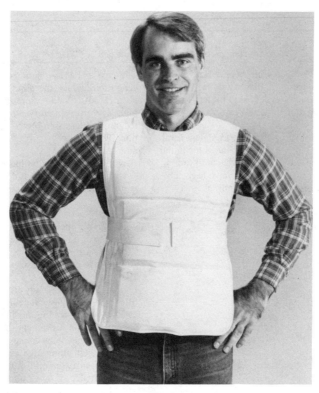

Figure 24.14.   Cooling vest used to prevent heat stress.

Table 24.5.   Sample Protective Ensembles[a]

Level of Protection	Equipment	Protection provided	Should be Used When:	Limiting Criteria
A	Recommended • Pressure-demand, full-face-piece SCBA or pressure-demand supplied air respirator with escape SCBA • Fully encapsulating, chemical-resistant suit • Inner chemical-resistant gloves • Chemical-resistant safety boots/shoes • Two-way radio communications Optional • Cooling unit • Coveralls • Long cotton underwear • Hard hat • Disposable gloves and boot covers	The highest available level of respiratory, skin, and eye protection	• The chemical substance has been identified and requires the highest level of protection for skin, eyes, and the respiratory system based on either: —measured (or potential for) high concentration of atmospheric vapors, gases, or particulates or —site operations and work functions involving a high potential for splash, immersion, or exposure to unexpected vapors, gases, or particulates of materials that are harmful to skin or capable of being absorbed through the intact skin. • Substances with a high degree of hazard to the skin are known or suspected to be present, and skin contact is possible. • Operations must be conducted in confined, poorly ventilated areas until the absence of conditions requiring level A protection is determined.	• Fully encapsulating suit material must be compatible with the substances involved.

Table 24.5.   *Continued*

Level of Protection	Equipment	Protection provided	Should be Used When:	Limiting Criteria
B	Recommended • Pressure-demand, full-face-piece SCBA or pressure-demand supplied-air respirator with escape SCBA • Chemical-resistant clothing (overalls and long-sleeved jacket; hooded, one- or two-piece chemical splash suit; disposable chemical-resistant one-piece suit) • Inner and outer chemical-resistant gloves • Chemical resistant safety boots/shoes • Hard hat • Two-way radio communications Optional • Coveralls • Disposable boot covers • Face shield • Long cotton underwear	The same level of respiratory protection but less skin protection than Level A It is the minimum level recommended for initial site entries until the hazards have been further identified	• The type and atmospheric concentration of substances have been identified and require a high level of respiratory protection, but less skin protection. This involves atmospheres: —with IDLH concentrations of specific substances that do not represent a severe skin hazard; or —that do not meet the criteria for use of air-purifying respirators. • Atmosphere contains less than 19.5% oxygen. • Presence of incompletely identified vapors or gases is indicated by direct-reading organic vapor detection instrument, but vapors and gases are not suspected of containing high levels of chemicals harmful to skin or capable of being absorbed through the intact skin.	• Use only when the vapor or gases present are not suspected of containing high concentrations of chemicals that are harmful to skin or capable of being absorbed through the intact skin. • Use only when it is highly unlikely that the work being done will generate either high concentrations of vapors, gases, or particulates or splashes of material that will affect exposed skin.
C	Recommended • Full-facepiece, air-purifying, canister-equipped respirator • Chemical-resistant clothing (overalls and long-sleeved jacket; hooded, one- or two-piece chemical splash suit; disposable chemical-resistant one-piece suit) • Inner and outer chemical-resistant gloves • Chemical-resistant safety boots/shoes • Hard hat • Two-way radio communications Optional • Coveralls • Disposable boot covers • Face shield • Escape mask • Long cotton underwear	The same level of skin protection as Level B, but a lower level of respiratory protection	• The atmospheric contaminants, liquid splashes, or other direct contact will not adversely affect any exposed skin. • The types of air contaminants have been identified, concentrations measured, and a canister is available that can remove the contaminant. • All criteria for the use of air-purifying respirators are met.	• Atmospheric concentration of chemicals must not exceed IDLH levels. • The atmosphere must contain at least 19.5% oxygen.
D	Recommended • Coveralls • Safety boots/shoes • Safety glasses or chemical splash goggles • Hard hats Optional • Gloves • Escape mask • Face shield	No respiratory protection Minimal skin protection	• The atmosphere contains no known hazard. • Work functions preclude splashes, immersion, or the potential for unexpected inhalation of or contact with hazardous levels of any chemicals.	• This level should not be worn in the Exclusion Zone. • The atmosphere must contain at least 19.5% oxygen.

Source: NIOSH/OSHA/USCG/EPA document: Occupational Safety and Health Guidance Manual for Hazardous Waste Site Activities. Washington, DC: GPO, October 1985.
*Based on EPA protective ensembles.

REFERENCES

1. Bollinger NJ, Schutz RH. National Institute of Occupational Safety and Health guide to industrial respiratory protection. Department of Health and Human Services (NIOSH) publication N. 87–116. Washington, DC: GPO, September 1987.

2. Pritchard JA. A guide to industrial respiratory protection. Department of Health, Education, and Welfare (National Institute of Occupational Safety and Health) publication N. 760-189. Washington, DC: 1976 (Reprinted April 1979).

2a. Code of Federal Regulations. Title 30, Part 2. Washington, DC: GPO, 1984.

3. Code of Federal Regulations. Title 30, Part 2. Washington, DC: GPO, 1984.

4. Ronk R, White MK, Linn H. Personal protective equipment for hazardous materials incidents: a selection guide. Department of Health and Human Services (National Institute of Occupational Safety and Health) publication N. 84-114. Washington, DC: GPO, October 1984.

5. U.S. Environmental Protection Agency. Hazardous materials incident response operations—training manual. Washington, DC: 1982:3–4.

6. U.S. Environmental Protection Agency. Standard operating safety guides. Washington, DC: 1988.

7. Schwope AD, Costas PP, Jackson JO, Weitzman DJ. Guidelines for the selection of chemical protective clothing. Vol. 1: Field guide. Cincinnati, OH: American Conference of Governmental Industrial Hygienists, 1983.

8. U.S. National Bureau of Standards. Safe handling of radioactive materials, Handbook 92. Washington, DC: 1964:33.

9. U.S. Department of the Army: A history of the development of an armor ensemble for mine clearance personnel. Technical Report 71-30-CE. Natick, MA: U.S. Army Natick Laboratories, 1970.

10. National Institute of Occupational Safety and Health, Occupational Safety and Health Administration, United States Coast Guard, Environmental Protection Agency document: Occupational safety and health guidance manual for hazardous waste site activities. Washington, DC: 1985.

11. Stobbe TJ, da Roza RA, Watkins MA: Facial hair and respirator fit: a review of the literature. Am Ind Hyg Assoc J 1988;49(4):199–204.

12. Code of Federal Regulations Title 29, Part 1910.134. Washington, DC: GPO, 1984.

13. North hand protection: permeation resistance guide, publication IH-200. Charleston, SC: Siebe North, 1984.

14. Chempruf II total-encapsulating suit instruction manual, Publication 481127. Pittsburgh, PA: Mine Safety Appliances Company, nd.

15. Raven PB, Dodson A, Davis TO: Stresses involved in wearing PVC supplied air suits: a review. Am Ind Hyg Assoc J 1979;40:592–599.

16. Levine SP, Martin WF: Protecting personnel at hazardous waste sites. Stoneham, MA: Butterworth Publishers, 1985.

17. U.S. Public Health Service, NIOSH recommended standard for occupational exposure to hot environments. Publication no. 757-009/26. Washington, DC: GPO, 1977.

18. Moran, J., Personal protective equipment, Hazmat, Hazwaste, Hazchem and Lady SARA. Appl Ind Hyg 1989;4(2):F7–F9.

19. International Fire Service Training Association. Self-contained breathing apparatus. 1st ed. Oklahoma: Fire Protection Publications, Oklahoma State University, 1982.

20. Raven PB, Dodson AT, Davis TO: The physiological consequences of wearing industrial respirators: a review. Am Ind Hyg Assoc J 1979;40:517–534.

25

Evaluation of Hazardous Environments

John B. Sullivan, Jr., M.D.
Joseph Darcy, Ph.D., C.I.H.
Mark Van Ert, Ph.D., C.I.H.

DEFINING THE HAZARDOUS ENVIRONMENT

A fire, a vapor cloud of a toxic gas such as chlorine, and leaking drums of benzene are easily recognized hazards. However, there are other environmental situations that pose hazards to human health which may not be readily recognized. Toxic hazards may be defined according to the chemical or substance to which a person is exposed, the duration of exposure, the dose, the route of exposure, and the contributing effects of underlying disease states. Exposure to an unknown human carcinogen over a period of years in a work environment is as important to recognize as a potentially explosive concentration of a gas or vapor. Both are health hazards with different potentials to produce serious health effects or death. Thus the importance of defining a hazardous environment can vary from a need to prevent chronic and longterm exposures to prevention of acute toxic injury or death.

Entry into a hazardous environment should not be undertaken before gathering as much data as possible to delineate the risks and hazards present. The presence of chemicals and materials that can produce health effects vary from low level airborne contaminants, to highly toxic vapors and volatile organic chemicals, to explosives, flammable gas, and carcinogens. Knowledge of the type of work performed and chemicals used in an industry or stored at a hazardous waste site is invaluable for determining the risk to entry personnel and for dictating proper personnel protection.

Defining a hazardous environment is based on the specific chemicals present and their physical forms, processes, reactions, and environmental conditions of the site. The overall hazard of an environment is dictated by a variety of conditions:

- site location and terrain;
- chemicals involved and their concentrations;
- presence of radioactive material including ionizing radiation;
- presence of infectious agents and other biohazards;
- physical forms of chemicals (vapor, gases, dusts, liquids);
- processes and reactions involving chemicals;
- presence of explosives, compressed gases, and flammables;
- deficiency of oxygen;
- confined spaces and storage tanks.

The overall health hazard of toxic substances is a function of dose, length of exposure, route of exposure, metabolism to a toxic intermediary substance, target organ susceptibility, and previous health status of the exposed person.

Hazard Evaluation

Recognition of a hazardous material may be as simple as identifying a placard on a transport container or building or a label on a drum. However, hazard recognition can also be difficult,

such as identifying the contents of an unknown or suspected toxic dump site or buried drums of chemicals. In most instances, hazard evaluation will require a systematic approach combining observations, site monitoring, and evaluation. Hazardous materials stored in a building or being transported require certain labeling that identifies the hazard class. These hazardous materials may be identified by use of the United Nations (UN) identification numbers and Department of Transportation (DOT) symbols (See *Recognition of Hazardous Materials*). This general classification system can be useful in determining the presence of a hazard in a transport vehicle or a building (Table 25.1). However, certain sites that have been disposal dumps for years may be storing containers and drums not bearing any label or markings. In addition, the unknown waste site may contain a large inventory of different chemical hazards that have spilled or have been dispersed into the surrounding soil or groundwater without evidence of obvious contamination.

Proper assessment and evaluation of a toxic or a suspected hazardous material site involves a systematic approach utilizing advanced planning to minimize the hazard to personnel and the surrounding community. The overall objective is to identify and define the source, identify and document health effects, protect personnel, and implement controls to eliminate or reduce the hazard to an acceptable level. There are a variety of sites and occupational environments that may require evaluation and characterization to determine whether a chemical pollutant or toxin is actually present or to provide monitoring for known hazards. These areas include but are not limited to the following:

- unknown hazardous waste site;
- known hazardous waste site;
- confined spaces where chemical contamination is known;
- unknown confined space contents;
- indoor environments with low level pollution;
- industrial sites governed by Occupational Safety and Health Administration (OSHA) regulations;
- radioactive contaminated environments;
- medical wastes site;
- pressurized container leaks;
- leaking and spilled containers and drums;
- contaminated water source;
- underground and above ground storage tanks.

Hazardous Waste Standards and Regulation

Hazardous waste regulatory standards have been developed by a variety of governmental agencies including the Environmental Protection Association (EPA), DOT, and OSHA, as well as by individual states. Certain regulatory acts such as the Re-

Table 25.1. United Nations Hazard Classification System

Class 1	Explosives
Class 2	Gases: Flammable, poisonous, or compressed liquefied, or dissolved that are neither flammable nor poisonous
Class 3	Flammable liquids
Class 4.1	Flammable solids
Class 4.2	Flammable solids or substances likely to undergo spontaneous combustion
Class 4.3	Flammable solids or substances that emit flammable gases in contact with water
Class 5.1	Oxidizers
Class 5.2	Organic peroxides
Class 6.1	Toxic substances
Class 6.2	Infectious and medical wastes, biologic hazard
Class 7	Radioactive substances
Class 8	Corrosives
Class 9	Miscellaneous substances

source Conservation and Recovery Act (RCRA) of 1976 and the Comprehensive Environmental Response Liability Act (CERCLA) of 1980 also affect the generation, handling, and disposal of hazardous materials.

RCRA, an amendment to the Solid Waste Disposal Act of 1965, specifically regulates the generation and handling of toxic and hazardous wastes. RCRA was designed to cover areas of solid waste disposal not covered by other federal legislation. RCRA endeavors to regulate the problem of hazardous waste defined as:

A solid waste, or combination of solid waste, which because of its quantity, concentration, or physical, chemical, or infectious characteristics may: (a) Cause, or significantly contribute to an increase in mortality or an increase in serious irreversible, or incapacitating reversible, illness, or (b) Pose a substantial present or potential hazard to human health or the environment when improperly treated, stored, transported, or disposed of, or otherwise managed (1).

Under RCRA the generator of a hazardous material is responsible for the safe disposition and disposal of that material as well as for the proper tracking of the material from generation to disposal. The EPA has reserved the right under the RCRA guidelines to regulate medical wastes as a hazardous waste.

CERCLA, commonly referred to as Superfund, regulates the release and disposal of wastes into the environment by a variety of means such as solid waste dumping into landfills, liquid waste discharge into water sources, transportation of wastes, and incineration of wastes. The liability aspect of CERCLA is limited to reimbursement for waste site cleanup operations and does not include compensation for victims or personal injury from hazardous wastes.

Occupational Safety and Health Standards

Fifty years ago, industrial hygienists employed by governmental agencies formed a group dedicated to the establishment of principles and policy for governing the degree of exposure to which workers could be exposed to airborne chemicals. This group, termed the American Conference of Governmental In-

dustrial Hygienists (ACGIH), composed a list of chemicals which eventually became accepted as threshold Limit Values (TLVs) intended to serve as exposure guidelines for worker protection. The ACGIH has defined three categories of TLVs: (a) time weighted average (TLV-TWA), (b) shortterm exposure limit (TLV-STEL), and (c) the ceiling limit.

THRESHOLD LIMIT VALUES

TLVs are time-weighted average concentrations of airborne chemicals to which nearly all workers may be exposed, day after day, without adverse effect. The American Conference of Governmental Industrial Hygienists (ACGIH) has established these concentrations as guidelines for the control of exposures. The ACGIH further insists that the TLVs are not to be used as fine lines between unsafe and safe levels of exposure. Further, TLVs are not established specifically on health impairment, but may be established on the basis of narcosis, irritation, or other forms of stress.

The TLV-TWA is the airborne concentration of a substance to which workers can be continuously exposed in an occupational setting over an 8-hour period, 40 hours per week, without adverse health effects (2). Known or suspected carcinogens may not be assigned TLVs. The TLV-TWA is calculated as follows:

$$\text{Exposure} = \frac{(C_1T_1) + (C_2T_2) + \ldots \ldots (C_nT_n)}{8 \text{ hours}}$$

C = Concentration (constant level)
T = Time in hours of exposure at concentration, C

PERMISSIBLE EXPOSURE LIMITS

Permissible exposure limits (PELs) are conceptually the same as TLVs but differ in some specific allowable concentrations. The PELs are enforceable standards under OSHA, whereas the TLVs are intended as guidelines. Recently OSHA updated their standards and amended existing air contaminant standards. These revisions were scheduled for implementation on September 1, 1989. Any method of compliance may be used until December 31, 1992, at which time the long established hierarchy of exposure control, i.e., engineering control, administrative control, personal protective equipment, will be reestablished. OSHA has promulgated a list of limitations for certain chemical and physical exposures known as PELs (permissible exposure limits). The PEL for a substance is the 8-hour TWA or ceiling concentration above which workers cannot be exposed (3).

CONDITIONS IMMEDIATELY DANGEROUS TO LIFE OR HEALTH

Immediately dangerous to life or health (IDLH) means an atmospheric concentration of any toxic corrosive or asphyxiant substance that poses an immediate threat to life or would cause irreversible or delayed effects or would interfere with an individual's ability to escape from a dangerous atmosphere. IDLH conditions most generally arise in emergency situations, thus making training essential for situations in which emergencies may arise.

RECOMMENDED EXPOSURE LIMIT

The National Institute for Occupational Safety and Health (NIOSH) develops and periodically revises recommendations for limits of exposure to hazardous substances or conditions in the workplace. These recommended exposure limits (RELs) are published and transmitted to OSHA for use in promulgating legal standards.

With the passage of the Occupational Safety and Health Act in 1970, OSHA was born. Under the authority of the Occupational Safety and Health Act of 1970 (Public Law 91-596), NIOSH continues to develop and periodically revise recommendations for limits of exposure to potentially hazardous substances or conditions in the workplace. This act mandated that OSHA adopt national consensus standards for worker exposure in industry. A list of exposure limits similar to the ones developed by the ACGIH was thus created by OSHA and is now used to regulate human exposure in the work environment. Each year the ACGIH updates and publishes TLVs and biologic exposure indices. These TLVs are to assist in the control of health hazards from chemical as well as biologic and physical agents in the workplace. The TLVs of the ACGIH serve as a guideline and are not legal limitations, whereas those promulgated by OSHA form the basis of legal regulation.

Preventive measures designed to reduce or eliminate health effects of these hazards are also recommended by NIOSH for consideration by OSHA. All known and available scientific information relevant to the potential hazard is evaluated by NIOSH in formulating these recommendations. Exposure limits are based on the best available information from human and animal studies as well as from clinical experience. It should be noted that the PELs established by OSHA are not always in agreement with the TLVs proposed by the ACGIH, due to annual updating by the latter. Traditionally, the ACGIH limits have been more conservative than those established by OSHA.

Exposure recommendations are published yearly and transmitted to OSHA or the Mine Safety and Health Administration (MSHA) of the U.S. Department of Labor for use in promulgating legal standards. These published documents specify NIOSH RELs to a variety of chemical agents. In addition, appropriate preventive measures designed to reduce or eliminate adverse health effects are recommended.

NIOSH is also involved in preparing documents related to special hazard reviews and occupational hazard assessments. These criteria documents provide safety and health assessments of specific chemical hazards along with recommended control and monitoring methods. NIOSH also evaluates new and emerging occupational health hazard data and publishes bulletins on these as necessary. These hazard bulletins provide information on previously unrecognized toxic hazards, report updates on current hazards, or disseminate information on hazard control methods and monitoring.

The Occupational Health Standards promulgated by OSHA require employers to determine employee exposure to contaminants. This regulation obligates employers to "identify and qualify" exposures. For those engaged in hazardous waste operations, this is a very difficult task because of the unknown nature of the mixtures encountered. Presently, identification and quantitation is done only in a few instances. Thus human exposure to a variety of unknown compounds is a possibility.

PRINCIPLES OF ENVIRONMENTAL MONITORING

Environmental monitoring helps determine if the hazard is *real* or *potential*. The purposes of environmental monitoring are many and varied and include the following:

WORKER PROTECTION

Evaluation of worker exposures is accomplished by determining concentration of contaminants within the breathing zone of the employee. These concentrations are then compared with established exposure standards (PELs, RELs, TLVs). If measured concentrations are in excess of standards, engineering controls should be instituted to reduce exposures to within acceptable limits. If these controls are unsuccessful in reducing concentrations, personal protective equipment may be used to control exposures.

PROTECTION OF THE PUBLIC

The primary means by which the general public is exposed to toxic agents is by inhalation of airborne contaminants or by ingestion of waterborne contaminants. Environmental monitoring of both air and water then become essential aspects of a program of protection of the public health. The Environmental Protection Agency (EPA) has responsibility for establishing control of air and water discharges and for enforcing standards established under the Clean Air Act and the Safe Drinking Water Act.

RISK ASSESSMENT

Risk assessment is a means by which the level of risk to human health may be quantified. This risk is usually tied to the carcinogenicity of the compound. Risk assessment may be related to toxicologic evaluation of the compounds and the biologic uptake based on human consumption patterns. For instance, one might consider the contamination level in water and relate it to what is considered the "acceptable daily intake" (ADI).

PROPERTY TRANSFER AUDITS

It is becoming increasingly necessary to determine the degree of contamination on a site, i.e., water, soil, asbestos, and others, because of the potential litigation which may be brought against the seller. Lending institutions are becoming increasingly reluctant to finance (or refinance) projects unless and until environmental audits are conducted.

The presence of a particular toxin or mixture of toxins in an environment does not indicate that human exposure has occurred or that disease exists. The storage of large amounts of chemical solvents in nonleaking containers may constitute a potential hazard to persons and the immediate environment but is not a *toxic* hazard until human or environmental exposure occurs. The exposure must be assessed to determine both risk of toxicity and actual toxicity. Environmental monitoring helps: (a) determine whether the risk of toxic exposure exists, (b) quantify the amount of the toxin, (c) relate the dose to both exposure and response of the organism, (d) prevent disease by maintaining chemical and other hazard exposures below predefined limits in the occupational environment.

Hazard evaluation involves both the toxicity of the chemical or material, and the risk of exposure (2). Therefore, the evaluation must include:

- nature of the chemical or chemicals;
- quantity of material and its physical form;
- route of exposure of the organism;
- potential of multiple exposures;

- exposure-dose-response;
- prior health status of the organism;
- use of medications by the exposed person;
- duration of exposure (acute, chronic, longterm);
- magnitude of the exposure;
- control measures that limit exposure;
- toxicity of the material in biologic systems.

Exposures are generally classified as acute, chronic, or long-term. An acute exposure usually involves a single dose during a rapid time period. Acute exposures can involve multiple chemicals or single chemicals, and the health effects become apparent very quickly. Chronic exposure involves receiving a dose at frequencies over a period of time which may be hours, days, or months. Health effects following chronic exposure are a function of the route of exposure, accumulation and metabolism of the chemical, possible synergism among multiple chemicals, the dose, frequency of the dose, and the inherent toxicity of the chemical or material. Chronic exposures are usually of longer duration and low level in concentration. Long-term exposures are generally considered to be of more than 1 year and are on a continuous basis.

Exposures can be defined on a qualitative and quantitative basis. The most useful information is obtained from quantitative data, since this type of data can best be related to the threshold exposure which may result in a health effect. Threshold is defined as the lowest level of perception for a stimulus (3). In terms of hazardous and toxic materials, a threshold may be defined as the relationship of the lowest detectable level of a biologic or toxic response of the organism to a specific concentration or dose of a toxin below which no toxic effect occurs. It should be noted that the biologic variability in toxic responses among humans as well as among different animals can be tremendous. Some toxins have a small margin of safety, and some have large margins of safety. Exposures may be multiple and erratic in the occupational setting, and the overall biologic response can be influenced by other environmental exposures which may act synergistically.

Physical Classification of Chemical Hazards

It is important to understand the different forms in which chemical hazards can present themselves as well as the terms applied to these physical states (3). The basic forms of chemical hazards are as follows:

Gas: A material that is neither a solid nor liquid. It expands and contracts in response to temperature and pressure and can fill a container of any size completely as it expands. It may change to a liquid or solid state by the effect of increased pressure with the concomitant effect of temperature below the critical temperature of the gas.

Vapor: The gaseous form of a substance which is normally in a liquid or solid state at 25°C and 760 mmHg (standard conditions). When a solid or liquid is heated, it may be converted into a gaseous state which is a vapor.

Dusts: An airborne dispersion of a solid material formed by a mechanical process such as grinding, sanding, or breaking. Dust particles range in size from 0.1–50 microns and larger in diameter. A 50-micron dispersion size can be detected by normal eyesight. Dusts below 10 micron in size are respirable.

Fume: An airborne dispersion of small solid particles such as metals, formed when the solid is heated to the point of volatilization. As the heat is removed, the gaseous phase solid condenses to form small particles of solid material. Fume particles are generally very fine and are smaller than 1.0 micron in diameter, thus being respirable. Usually the solid involved is a metal, and the volatilized material forms an oxide with atmospheric oxygen.

Smoke: An aerosol of carbon or soot less than 1.0 micron. Results from combustion of carbon-containing material.

Fogs and Mists: Dispersed liquids formed by condensation from the gaseous state. A fog is a visible aerosol of a liquid.

Particulates: A composite grouping including dusts, fumes, and smoke which are dispersed solids. Particulates are a concern, due to their size and potential for entering the terminal portion of the respiratory tract. The aerodynamic diameter of particulates is of special interest, since those smaller than 10 micrometers may enter terminal respiratory airways. Particulates are further defined in terms of being respirable (enters terminal respiratory tract) or nonrespirable (trapped in upper airway).

INSTRUMENTS USED IN MONITORING

The purpose of a monitoring program is to detect the presence of toxic and other hazardous environmental threats to personnel and to ensure that concentrations of hazardous substances do not exceed established TLVs or regulatory standards (4, 5). Monitoring helps determine the level of protection required at a hazardous materials site and dictates the types of personal protective equipment required. Two basic approaches are used in monitoring: direct detection (referred to as real-time) and indirect detection. Direct detecting or real-time monitoring instruments can be used on the site to provide instantaneous information concerning ambient air concentrations of certain chemicals, radioactive materials, and IDLH conditions.

Indirect or integrative monitoring is useful for detection of low air concentrations of chemicals over a prolonged period of time to concentrate an occupational environment. Whereas direct-reading instruments are available for only a limited number of specific toxic hazards, indirect analytical techniques can detect numerous, specific chemicals at very low concentrations (Table 25.2). Direct-reading instruments provide real-time assessment of a site's hazards. Indirect reading instruments, due to the fact that collection occurs over a specified period of time and analysis occurs off-site, provides a historical assessment of a site that may have changed since the samples were collected.

The nature of the environment being sampled will help dictate the sampling strategies and kinds of instrumentation to be used. Questions to be answered in any monitoring programs are:

- What is the purpose of the monitoring?
- What is the suspected chemical or contaminant?
- What kind of instrumentation is required?
- Where is the monitoring going to be performed?
- When is it to be performed?
- Over what length of time is the monitoring to occur?
- How many samples are to be collected?

Sampling strategies must include a quality assurance program to account for proper calibration of any instrument used

Table 25.2.   Direct Air Sampling Instruments

Instrument	Detection Method	Chemical	Detection Limits
Compound-specific instruments	Electrochemical cell	Hydrogen cyanide Hydrogen sulfide Oxygen Nitrogen dioxide Carbon monoxide	0–100 ppm 0–100 ppm 0–100% 0.01–50 ppm 0–500 ppm
Portable gas chromatograph	Flame ionization	Organic vapors	0.2 ppm 0–1000 ppm
	Photoionization	Compounds with ionization potential less than or equal to the output energy of the ultraviolet lamp	0.1 ppb
Aerosol monitor	Light scattering	Aerosols	0.001 mg/m^3
Mercury vapor analyzer	Ultraviolet light	Mercury vapor	0–1 mg/m^3
Combustible gas detector	Catalytic combustion	Vapors of combustible gases	0–100% LEL
Portable photoionization detector	Photoionization	Compounds with ionization potential less than or equal to the output energy of the ultraviolet lamp	0.05–2000 ppm
Portable infrared analyzer	Infrared absorption	Infrared absorbing compounds	0–9999 ppm
Portable FID	Flame ionization	Organic vapors	0–1000 ppm
Gamma radiation detector	Scintillation detector	Gamma radiation	Does not detect beat or alpha

before and during sampling procedures, adequate flow and volume, calibration of sensors used, and use of accepted standards and procedures.

Direct (Real-Time) Reading Instruments

The role of direct-reading instruments is very important in evaluating hazardous environments and exposures. However, the user must define the specific role of the instrument. The instrument must be matched with the skill and knowledge of the user. Choice of a particular direct-reading instrument is dependent on the physical and chemical state of the matter to be detected. The kinds of direct-reading instruments that may be used at a hazardous materials site include the following (Table 25.2):

explosimeters and combustible gas indicators;
photoionization detector (UV);
portable gas chromatography;
oxygen meters;
gamma radiation detectors;
portable infrared spectrophotometer.

Direct-reading instruments may be employed as early warning devices in settings where dangerous substances may be present in the air. They are the primary instruments used to initially characterize an unknown hazardous site, since they detect organic vapors being released into the atmosphere, the presence of explosive conditions and flammable gases, lack of oxygen, and the presence of ionizing radiation. Contemporary instruments are very sensitive with detection limits in the parts per million (ppm) and, in some cases, parts per billion (ppb) range such as the photoionization detector. However, due to problems of specificity when multiple chemicals are present, quantitation becomes difficult.

Direct-reading instruments have certain limitations in their capacity to detect hazardous substances. Since they can only

Table 25.3.   Electrochemical Cells for Compound Detection

Simple paraffins
Halogenated paraffins
Aliphatic ring compounds
Nitrogen-containing compounds
Unsaturated acids and esters
Chlorinated aromatics
Chlorinated olefins
Aromatics
Organometallics
Carbon-oxygen compounds
Sulfur-containing compounds
Phosphorous compounds

Adapted from Transducer Research, Inc., 1228 Olympus Drive, Naperville, Illinois

detect or measure certain specific substances or classes of chemicals, it is possible to miss other hazards. Most of these instruments are not designed to detect air concentrations below 1 ppm. False readings can occur due to interference from other chemicals. It is critical that direct-reading instruments be used by highly qualified persons such as certified industrial hygienists who are trained to interpret data provided by these instruments and who are skilled at proper calibration and instrument use.

Real-Time Gas and Vapor Detection Methods

Electrochemical cells, which operate on the principle of membrane electrolysis, are commonly used to detect gases (Table 25.3). The gas passes through a membrane and reacts with an electrolyte. This reaction produces a flow of electrons proportional to the partial pressure of the gas in the air. With the addition of chemical filtration mechanisms preceding the cells, instruments may be made more sensitive and specific for a variety of gases. However, it is uncommon to find direct gas reading instruments that detect more than two gases at a time.

Combustibility or explosivity is generally detected with an instrument that uses catalytic combustion. The gaseous contaminant burns on a heated wire, thus altering resistance to flow of an electric current. The measure of the degree of resistance correlates with percent concentration of the gas. The heat of combustion, a particular physical characteristic of combustible gases, is used for quantitative detection. However, this procedure is nonspecific when mixtures of gases are being analyzed. A gas (or vapor) sample is drawn into the instrument across a heated filament and ignited. The resulting change in electrical resistance of the filament is detected by conventional bridge measurement techniques. The degree of induced electrical resistance is directly proportional to the gas (or vapor) concentration of the gas (or vapor) being drawn into the instrument. Typically, these instruments read in percent of the lower explosive limit and thus are not useful in measuring concentrations in the part per million range. They are not to be used in determining concentrations relative to the PELs.

Monitors with a photoionization detector (PID) represent a nonspecific instrument which employs an ultraviolet lamp. The gas is carried into the ionization chamber and ionized by the ultraviolet beam. The resulting degree of ionization produces an electric signal which is read out on a meter. Some PIDs that are coupled with chromatographic columns can separate gases and identify, as well as quantify gases. Other gas detecting instruments use a flame ionization detector (FID). These instruments are used to detect a volatile hydrocarbon. The hydrocarbon is drawn into the ionization chamber, and a hydrogen flame ignites the compound. The resulting degree of ionization produces an electrical signal which is read out on a meter. The FID is not as sensitive as other detectors and is less sensitive to compounds containing electronegative atoms such as oxygen, sulfur, and chlorine. Instruments with FID's can also separate out and detect multiple gases. The PID and FID are the common direct reading detection instruments employed at unknown hazardous materials sites; however, these instruments do not detect hydrogen sulfide or hydrogen cyanide. Multiple methods of detection are used at such sites to insure safety of personnel.

Other instruments employ infrared absorption as a detection method. The gas is drawn into a chamber through which infrared radiation is projected. The gases are identified by selecting specific wavelengths of infrared light. The measured absorbance is then converted to a parts per million value through appropriate instrument calibration. These instruments allow for the detection of multiple gases such as carbon dioxide, chlorine, hydrogen cyanide, hydrofluoric acid, hydrogen sulfide, hydrogen, sulfur dioxide, ammonia, and nitrogen dioxide.

Elemental mercury, which vaporizes at room temperatures, can be a significant hazard in confined areas. It has no odor, and real-time airborne concentrations can be measured using a gold-film technology mercury vapor detector with a sensitivity of 0.003 mg/m^3 (Jerome Instruments, Arizona).

Gas detector tubes can also be used on the site as direct-reading instruments. These direct-reading colorimetric detector tubes contain a reagent that reacts with a standard volume of air and the gaseous contaminant drawn through it. The reagent changes color in the presence of specific hazardous gases. The concentration of the contaminant in the air is read directly on the calibrated tube in ppm. The length of the color band indicates the quantity of hazardous gas present. Examples of toxic

gases detected include hydrogen sulfide, hydrogen cyanide, carbon monoxide, phosgene, phosphine, arsine, benzene, hydrogen, and general hydrocarbons (Table 25.4).

Real-time monitoring for airborne particulate concentrations with portable instruments has become available in recent years. The principle of operation involves light scattering, piezoelectric effects, or beta attenuation.

Sample Collection Devices

Solid sorbent tubes: Typically, sampling for insoluble gases and vapors is accomplished by drawing contaminant-laden air through a bed of granular sorbent (charcoal, silica gel, etc.). The contaminant is adsorbed onto the granular material from which it is subsequently removed by a desorptive process. The desorbed material is then identified and quantified by laboratory procedures.

Passive diffusional monitors: These sampling devices operate much the same as solid sorbent tubes except that the contaminant is collected by diffusion rather than by actively drawing contaminant-laden air through the collection device. Analysis of the samples is similar to that for solid sorbent tubes.

Bubblers (impingers): Contaminant-laden air is drawn through a liquid media in which the contaminant is soluble. The liquid media contaminant matrix is then chemically prepared for laboratory analysis, e.g., spectrophotometry.

Indirect-Reading Instruments

Indirect-reading instruments, such as charcoal tubes and dosimeters or badges (Table 25.5), are used to detect low concentrations of chemicals that may be present in occupational environments. An important concept in the use of these devices is the selection of the proper sampling media to be employed, which depends on the nature of the substance sampled. The analysis of these samples occurs at a later time in a licensed and/or certified analytical laboratory.

EVALUATING A HAZARDOUS MATERIALS SITE

There are multiple health-related concerns at hazardous materials sites which are a function of the nature and location of the site, the need for personnel protective equipment, and the actual physical or chemical hazards that may be present. Site surveys are conducted to discover situations that potentially pose a threat to human health and safety. Surveys are not useful unless data concerning the use of the site and site activities are available. Familiarity with raw materials and chemicals used, processes and reactions involving chemicals, production steps, and the final product is important for proper assessment of an industrial site.

Every industrial site or plant is required to maintain an inventory of all chemicals used in operations or manufacturing (29 CFR 1910.1200, hazard communication standard). This inventory can serve as a starting point for identifying potential exposure sources. Attention should be directed to the physical forms of the chemicals also.

These health concerns include the following:

1. Chemical and toxic hazards at the site;
2. Potential for explosion and presence of compressed gases;

Table 25.4.   Detector and Indicator Tubes

Chemical	Sensitivity/Range (ppm)	OSHA PEL ppm 1989
Acetone	100–12,000	750
Acetaldehyde	100–1000	100
Acetic acid	5–80	10
Acrylonitrile	0.5–20	
Ammonia	2–30	35 (STEL)[a]
	5–700	35 (STEL)
	25–700	35 (STEL)
Acid compounds (air)	Qualitative	
Aliphatic hydrocarbons	2–23 mg/l	
Aniline	0.5–10	2
Arsenic trioxide	0.2 mg AS/m³	
Arsine	0.05–60	0.05
Organic arsines	Qualitative	
Basic compounds (air)	Qualitative	
Benzene	2–60	1
	0.5–10	1
Bromine	0.2–30	0.1
n-Butane	0.1–0.8%	800
1-Butylene	1–55 mg/l	
Carbon dioxide	1–20 vol %	10,000
	0.5–10 vol %	10,000
Carbon disulfide	3–95	4
Carbon monoxide	10–3000	35
Carbon tetrachloride	1–15	2
Carbonyl chloride	0.05–1.5	
Chlorine	0.2–30	0.5
Chlorobenzene	5–200	75
2-Chloro-1,3-butadiene	5–90	10
1-Chloro-2,3-epoxypropane	5–60	2
Chloroformates	0.2–10	
Chloroprene	5–90	10
Cyanogen chloride	0.25–5.0	0.3 (ceiling)
Chromic acid	0.1–0.5 mg/m³	0.1 (ceiling)
Cyclohexane	100–1500	300
Cyclohexylamine	2–30	10
DDVP[b]	0.05	0.1
Demeton	Qualitative	0.1 mg/m³
Diborane	0.05–3	0.1
p-Dichlorobenzene	2–100	75
Dichlorovos	0.05	
Diethyl ether	100–4000	400
Dimethyl acetamide	10–40	10
Dimethyl formamide	10–40	10
Dimethyl sulfate	0.005–0.05	0.1
Epichlorhydrin	5–50	2
Ethyl mercaptan	0.5–5	0.5
Ethanol	100–3000	1000
Ether	100–4000	
Ethyl acetate	200–3000	400
Ethyl benzene	30–600	100
Ethyl ether	100–4000	400
Ethylene	50–2500	
	0.1–5	
Ethylene glycol	10–180 mg/m³	50 (ceiling)
Ethylene glycol dinitrate	0.25	0.1 mg/m³ (STEL)
Ethylene oxide	1–30	1
Formaldehyde	0.2–5	1
	0.5–10	1
Formic acid	1–15	5
n-Hexane	100–3000	50
Hydrazine	0.2–10	0.1

Table 25.4.   *Continued*

Chemical	Sensitivity/Range (ppm)	OSHA PEL ppm 1989
Hydrocarbons	0.1–0.8	
Hydrochloric acid	0.5–25	
Hydrocyanic acid	2–150	
Hydrogen fluoride	1.5–15	3
Hydrogen peroxide	0.1–3	1
Hydrogen sulfide	1–200	10
Isopropyl alcohol	100–3000	400
Mercaptan	0.5–5	
Mercury vapor	0.1–2 mg/m³	1 mg/m³ (ceiling)
Methacrylonitrile	1–10	1
Methyl acrylate	5–200	10
Methane	Qualitative	
Methanol	50–3000	200
Methyl bromide	3–100	5
Methyl chloroform	50–600	350
Methyl mercaptan	2–100	0.5
Methyl methacrylate	50–50,000	100
Methylene chloride	50–2000	500
Monostyrene	50–400	
Nickel (aerosol)	0.25–1 mg/m³	1 mg/m³
Nickel tetracarbonyl	0.1–1	
Nitric acid	1–50	1 (STEL)
Nitrogen dioxide	0.5–25	1 (STEL)
Nitrous fumes	0.5–10	1 (STEL)
n-Octane	100–2500	300
Oil mist	1–10 mg/m³	5 mg/m³
Olefins (butylene, propylene)	1–55 mg/l	
Organic basic nitrogens	Qualitative	
Oxygen	5–23 vol %	
Ozone	0.05–1.4	0.1
	10–300	0.1
n-Pentane	100–1500	600
Perchloroethylene	5–50	25
Phenol	5	5
Phosgene	0.04–1.5	0.1
Phosphine	0.1–40	0.3
Propane	0.5–1.3 vol %	1000
n-Propanol	100–3000	200
Sulfur dioxide	0.5–25	2
Sulfuric acid	1–5 mg/m³	1 mg/m³
Toluene	5–400	100
Toluene diisocyanate	0.02–0.2	0.005
o-Toluidine	1–30	5
1,1,1-Trichloroethane	50–600	350
Trichloroethylene	2–200	50
Triethylamine	5–60	10
Vinyl chloride	1–50	1
0-Xylene	10–400	100

[a]STEL = shortterm exposure level.

3. Potential for fires;
4. Vapors, fumes, or gases being released;
5. Lack of oxygen;
6. Presence of ionizing radiation;
7. Electrical hazards;
8. Biologic and infectious hazards;
9. Physical hazards such as heat, cold, noise, and confined spaces.

Generally, hazardous materials sites represent the unknown. There is uncertainty as to the kinds of hazards and chemicals that may be found as well as uncertainty as to the correct initial

continues

Table 25.5. Color Badge Detectors

Chemical	Sensitivity/Range (ppm)
Acetic acid	1.3–25
Butadiene	1.3–40
Carbon dioxide	0.13–3.8 vol %
Carbon monoxide	6.3–75
Ethanol	125–3100
Ethyl acetate	63–1250
Hydrochloric acid	1.3–25
Hydrocyanic acid	2.5–25
Hydrogen sulfide	1.3–38
Nitrogen dioxide	1.3–25
Olefin	12.5–250
Sulfur dioxide	0.63–18

From National Draeger, Inc.

identification of those chemicals. Hazardous materials sites that have been characterized have been found to contain a wide variety of toxic chemicals (Table 25.6). Assessment of the actual chemicals present may be impossible in the initial survey of the site. Personnel protective measures are thus selected on the basis of the presence of unknown hazards. A hazardous material site should be approached as if multiple, serious health hazards are present until proven otherwise.

CHARACTERIZING THE WASTE SITE

The following summarizes the general approach to evaluate a real or potential hazardous waste site environment (Table 25.7).

Planning and Organization for Site Evaluation

A team or project leader must be identified who is authorized to direct all activities at the scene or site. The team leader assigns all functions and responsibilities of the various team members. Lines of authority and responsibility need to be clearly delineated to avoid confusion over job task and reporting responsibilities. Planning and organization includes a number of individuals assigned to specific tasks (Fig. 25.1), a work plan, a site safety plan, personnel training, a medical program, technical advisors, and an emergency response plan. Some of these activities and stations may occur off the location of the hazardous material site (6).

Project Management Practices

Worker and public health safety are primary concerns, and commitment to these factors is best defined through the hazardous waste project management practices. A strong public health and worker safety commitment of management must be present and visible before site evaluation commences. Community leaders should be kept informed of the progress of the investigation and work. Prevention and containment of any chemical or hazardous materials release into the environment should be addressed in the plan before work on the site begins. Establishing identifiable lines of communication with the surrounding community is essential. The public must have confidence in the health and safety plan of the team evaluating the hazardous materials site. Identification of community leaders and the establishment of an open communication line with them will prevent rumor and help gain confidence. The following

Table 25.6. Chemicals Commonly Found at Hazardous Materials Sites

Volatiles
Chloromethane
Bromomethane
Vinyl chloride
Chloroethane
Methylene chloride
Acetone
Carbon disulfide
1,1-Dichloroethene
1,1-Dichloroethane
trans-1,2-Dichloroethene
Chloroform
1,2-Dichloroethane
2-Butanone
1,1,1-Trichloroethane
Carbon tetrachloride
Vinyl acetate
Bromodichloromethane
1,1,2,2-Tetrachloroethane
1,2-Dichloropropane
trans-1,3-Dichloropropene
Trichloroethene
Dibromochloromethane
1,1,2-Trichlorolethane
Benzene
cis-1,3-Dichloropropene
2-Chloroethyl vinyl ether
Bromoform
2-Hexanone
4-Methyl-2-pentanone
Tetrachloroethene
Toluene
Chlorobenzene
Ethylbenzene
Styrene
Xylene
4,6-Dinitro-2-methylphenol
N-Nitrosodiphenylamine
4-Bromophenyl phenyl ether
Hexachlorobenzene
Pentachlorophenol
Acenaphthene
2,4-Dinitrophenol
4-Nitrophenol
Dibenzofuran
2,4-Dinitrotoluene
2,6-Dinitrotoluene
Diethyl phthalate
4-Chlorophenyl phenyl ether
Fluorene
4-Nitroaniline
Phenanthrene
Anthracene
Di-n-butyl phthalate
Fluoranthene
Benzidine
Pyrene
Butyl benzyl phthalate
3,3'-Dichlorobenzidine
Benzo(a)anthracene
bis(2-Ethylhexyl)phthalate
Chrysene
Di-n-octyl phthalate
Benzo(b)fluoranthene

continues

Table 25.6. *Continued*

Volatiles (*cont'd*)
Benzo(k)fluoranthene
Benzo(a)pyrene
Indeno(1,2,3-cd)pyrene
Dibenz(a,h)anthracene
Benzo(ghi)perylene

Pesticides, insecticides, and herbicides
delta-HCH
gamma-HCH (Lindane)
Heptachlor
Aldrin
Heptachlor epoxide
alpha-HCH
beta-HCH
Endosulfan I
Dieldrin
4,4'-DDE
Endrin
Endosulfan II
4,4'-DDD
Endrin aldehyde
Endosulfan sulfate
4,4'-DDT
Endrin ketone
Methoxychlor
Chlordane
Toxaphene
Aroclor-1016
Aroclor-1221
Aroclor-1232
Aroclor-1242
Aroclor-1248
Aroclor-1254
Aroclor-1260

Table 25.7.   Steps in the Evaluation of A Hazardous Materials Site

1. Assign a project leader
2. Perform off-site characterization and take site history
3. Collect site data and perform site research
4. Survey perimeter
5. Protect entry personnel
6. Perform initial on-site survey and evaluate for:
   Clues to potential hazards
   Conditions IDLH
   Organic vapors and gases
   Inorganic vapors and gases
   Oxygen deficiency
   Confined space dangers
   Combustible gases
   Explosive conditions
7. Devise sampling strategies for detailed site evaluation
   Soil sampling
   Groundwater sampling
   Surface water sampling
   Air sampling
8. Document
9. Evaluate biota
10. Assess hazard

management practices are recommended to accomplish the overall objective of site evaluation:

A well-designed work plan with clear organizational structure is essential.
Training of workers in hazardous materials site health and safety courses is mandatory.
Administrative and engineering controls of worksite activities should provide for maximum safety of workers and prevent exposure to the public.
Management must be committed to the health and safety of the workers and the public.
There should be close communication with supervisors and employees concerning any issues that affect safety and health.
Communication with responsible community leaders concerning the site planning and activities is a requirement.

Work Plan

The site work plan must be developed before any site activity is undertaken. A comprehensive plan includes reviewing all information available on the site such as site records, photographs, previous soil analysis, any sampling data, waste inventories, generator and transporter records, and state and local environmental agency records, as well as interviews with community members.

Work objectives must be clearly defined in the plan and updated as needed as the work progresses. The work plan must include the following in detail:

- site information;
- work objectives;
- sampling plan;
- inventory of materials found;
- disposal techniques;
- containment plans;
- personnel requirements;
- personnel training requirements and training update;
- equipment requirements;
- safety plan;
- medical surveillance program;
- emergency response plan.

Site Safety Plan

A site safety plan is an important component of the overall work plan that is essential for protecting workers and the community from exposure to hazardous materials originating from site activities (7). The site safety plan must be written so that the initial investigation and survey of the site can safely proceed. The plan is updated as needed depending on materials and conditions at the site. The development of a site safety plan should include input from certified industrial hygienists, health and safety experts, clinical toxicologists, and occupational physicians. Components of the site safety plan include the following:

Risks associated with each operation to be undertaken are well-defined and recognized by management and workers.
Adequate training of personnel in hazardous materials site health and safety as well as in carrying out their assigned tasks is confirmed.
There is a description of personal protective equipment required for the initial site survey as well as for site characterization.

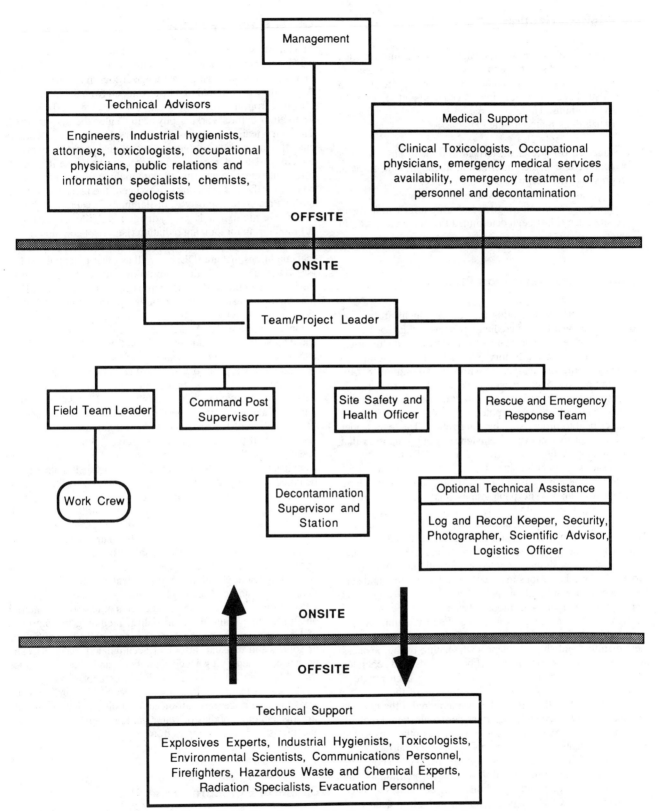

Figure 25.1. Hazardous materials site planning and organization.

Environmental and personnel monitoring procedures are described in terms of air, soil, water, and breathing zone analysis.

Control and containment measures and actions to reduce and eliminate hazards are detailed.

Medical surveillance requirements for workers are described.

Standard operating procedures of the site are detailed.

An emergency response plan should be a major component of the plan.

Site Characterization

The project team leader is responsible for providing detailed information on the site prior to personnel entry. Site characterization provides information necessary to make decisions on potential site hazards, monitoring procedures, and selection of protective clothing. There are three basic phases to characterizing a hazardous materials site (7):

1. Conduct an off-site characterization prior to any entry by personnel, and gather information about the site through records and site perimeter reconnaissance.
2. Conduct an on-site survey with a survey team.
3. Perform proper monitoring for gathering information about the site once it has been determined that the area is safe to enter.

Off-Site Characterization Phase

Prior to any personnel entering the site, as much information about the site must be gathered and evaluated (Fig. 25.2). This information is best gained by records research of the historical use of the site. The site history is actually a very useful tool for managing the risk associated with site exploration (8). Interviewing persons familiar with the site and its activities, examination of records of business activities associated with the site, and types of chemicals potentially stored or used at the site are critical to proper site characterization. The team leader should attempt to identify the existence of any condition that is immediately dangerous to life and health (IDLH).

The exact site location should be noted, and any aerial reconnaissance photographs of the site should be reviewed along with land use maps, site photographs, historical and current site maps, and U.S. Geological Survey topographic maps. Geologic and hydrogeologic data of the site should be reviewed. The populations around the site area should be noted to determine risk factors of exposure. All roads and rail lines to and from the site area should be noted along with any pathway of dispersion for a hazardous material, including ground and surface water and wind patterns.

The presence of any hazardous substances can be researched through interviews with persons living close by, company records and logs, records from state and federal regulatory agencies, manifest and shipping papers, the nature of the business at the site, media reports, fire department records, and generator and transporter records. There may also have been previous survey data available from other investigators of the site.

The perimeter of the site can be reconnoitered if the hazards are unknown. Off-site sampling at the perimeter should include air monitoring for conditions IDLH as well as other suspected airborne pollutants, soil sampling, and ground and surface water monitoring. Visual observations from the perimeter should be performed with the objective of developing a preliminary site map noting terrain, location of buildings, containers, ponds, pits, and wells. Changes in vegetation and the presence of disturbed areas may indicate a toxic waste site. Dead animals and plants should be noted. Any unusual odors or discoloration of water and soil should be noted.

Information obtained from off-site characterization is used to select appropriate protective clothing for the initial on-site survey personnel.

On-Site Survey Phase

The on-site survey is used to verify information obtained from off-site characterization as well as to discover unknown hazards that pose immediate danger to the hazardous materials workers. A site safety plan should first be developed from the information obtained from the site history and off-site characterization investigation before workers physically enter the site area (6). The entry team is composed of four persons. Two workers enter the site in protective equipment while two support workers remain off-site for rescue and emergency response if needed. Initial measures on entering the site include (a) monitoring for conditions IDLH such as lack of oxygen, the presence of combustible material, explosives, or flammable material, or highly toxic chemicals such as hydrogen sulfide or cyanide; (b) monitoring for ionizing radiation (gamma, beta, alpha) with appropriate detectors; (c) observations for signs of potential or real conditions that are IDLH as well as other potential hazards (see IDLH chapter). If there are no immediate health hazards, the survey can proceed. If dangerous conditions are identified, then caution must be exercised before proceeding with further site surveys activity.

Once conditions IDLH are ruled out, the investigation team should note the type, number, and conditions of any containers and/or drums. Chemical hazard storage systems include metal or plastic drums, paper or cardboard containers, glass containers, underground storage tanks, pipelines, compressed cylinders, above-ground tanks, ponds, wells, surface water, debris, pits, and lagoons. Any of these could contain a health hazard. The condition of the waste containers is important. The team should note if the containers are bulging, leaking, or corroded and rusted and if labels are present on these containers. If chemicals or materials are found, their physical state should be noted (gas, liquid, solid, color, foaming, corrosive nature).

Next, the team should note the location and presence of physical barriers such as hills, pits, wells, buildings, potential landfills, and storage tanks. Also noted is the presence of chemical and waste dispersion patterns such as surface water runoff, air and wind direction, soil contamination, and nature of the terrain. The terrain, if unstable, could be a hazard to the investigating team. Observation of physical and/or chemical barriers to entry and exit should be made.

Notation should be made of the effects of any waste material on surrounding plant and animal life, including the presence of dead animals, altered vegetation, surface collection of liquids or solids, and unusual dusts and accumulated materials. The presence of identifying labels, numbers, and chemical names should be recorded. Recordings should be kept in a log book.

The survey team should then collect samples of air, drainage areas, soil (surface and subsurface), pools of liquids, solids, streams and other bodies of water, and groundwater (upstream and downstream), and samples from containers. Sampling should also be performed for biologic and infectious hazards as well as for radioactive hazards as necessary.

Chemical Exposure at the Site

Hazardous materials sites rarely contain only a single type of waste hazard. Multiple chemicals in multiple physical forms can be encountered. These chemicals may be liquid, gases, solids, metals, vapors, radiologic, or biologic (Table 25.6). Main exposure routes for chemicals are dermal and inhalational and can range from acute to chronic. Factors relating to health

☐ Name of Site _____

☐ Property Ownership: _____

☐ Address & Location

☐ Size of Area _____

☐ Historical Use of Property _____

☐ Dates and Duration of Waste Activities _____

☐ **Types of Site Activities & Operations**

☐ Drums & Container Storage   ☐ Waste Water

☐ Mining Operation   ☐ Below Ground Storage Tanks

☐ Mine Tailings   ☐ Above Ground Storage Tanks

☐ Landfill   ☐ Incineration

☐ Terrain Evaluation   ☐ Building Locations

☐ **Composition of Waste Material** _____

☐ Chemicals   ☐ Radioactive   ☐ Medical Waste
☐ Carcinogens   ☐ Flammables   ☐ Explosives

☐ Waste Disposal Methods _____

☐ **Site Incidences** _____

☐ Explosions   ☐ Fires   ☐ Past Injuries

☐ Previous Sampling & Evaluation Information

☐ Records of Prior Response Actions

☐ Previous Site Investigation Records

Figure 25.2. Hazardous waste site survey checklist.

effects of chemical exposure are the type of chemical, dose, route of exposure, duration of exposure, and prior health status. The exposure of personnel to multiple chemicals must be evaluated in a detailed and tailored medical surveillance program. Personnel must be trained according to the standards set forth in OSHA hazardous waste workers training programs and be adept at the use of personal protective equipment.

There are two issues which need to be addressed with respect to the toxic effects of contaminants encountered in hazardous waste operations:

1. Determining the propensity of a contaminant to volatilize from water or soil preferentially to other contaminants may help one to predict which of several contaminants may be airborne before others. This concept is embodied in Henry's law, which relates the degree to which an organic compound is soluble in water and the vapor pressure of the compound. The higher the Henry's law constant, the more likely it will be airborne. If one cannot detect an airborne organic vapor in the molecular boundary layer of air existing above the surface of the water, then it is likely that those compounds of lower Henry's constant are also not airborne.

2. Given the level of contamination of a specific compound in water, what is the worst case scenario for an airborne concentration of that compound? If we know Henry's constant for the compound and the concentration of the contaminant in water, we may determine the vapor pressure of the compound. By application of the gas laws we may estimate the maximum concentration which may exist in the airborne state. This procedure may enable one to reduce (or eliminate) the need for direct reading instruments.

These individual standards mandate such things as medical surveillance, respiratory protection, and action levels at hazardous waste operations. If the route of entry into the body is by inhalation, then instruments for evaluation of airborne contaminants must measure concentrations in the vicinity of the breathing zone. The results of sampling with direct-reading instruments may not be representative of average breathing zone concentrations obtained during investigation of hazardous waste operations. Drilling logs and trenching logs are full of data relating concentrations "downhole" and "in the trench" when the data are intended to be associated with health effects. It may be important to use instruments to determine "hot spots," but they must be reported as such.

Conditions IDLH

Conditions IDLH must be ruled out during the initial site survey (6). Conditions IDLH can be due to the presence of explosive or flammable materials, a deficiency of oxygen such as in a confined space, the presence of a highly toxic compound in high concentration, or the presence of ionizing radiation. Dangerous conditions can also be associated with a variety of processes and reactions involving chemicals as well as physical processes (Table 25.7). Direct-readings instruments are used during this phase of the investigation and should include combustible gas detectors, organic vapor detectors, oxygen meters, radiation monitors, and certain colorimetric indicator tubes. If hazardous atmospheric conditions are present as indicated by monitoring, the entry team must proceed with extreme caution. Also, hazardous conditions may suddenly change at a site.

A confined space is any space having a limited means of egress which is subject to the accumulation of toxic or flammable contaminants or an oxygen-deficient atmosphere. Confined spaces include but are not limited to storage tanks, process vessels, bins, boilers, ventilation or exhaust ducts, sewers, underground utility vaults, tunnels, pipelines, and open top spaces more than 4 feet in depth such as pits, tubes, vaults, and vessels. Hazardous concentrations of gases such as hydrogen sulfide and chlorine or volatile organics can exist in low-lying areas, pits, wells, and any confined space in storage tanks or buildings. Certain chemicals may be lighter than air, such as carbon monoxide, and may accumulate above the ground. Sampling on hill tops, at ceiling levels in buildings, and in other confined high spots may be indicated. Open spaces generally do not concentrate toxic vapors of chemicals due to

dispersion unless there is a large or sudden release. Concentrations in the open air are also influenced by winds.

Personnel entering confined spaces must be protected from structure collapse, exposure to asphyxiants, and exposure to contaminants which may be in excess IDLH levels. In addition, prior to entering a confined space, an evaluation of the environment relative to the potential explosivity of the space must be determined. Entry must be denied if the lower explosive limit (LEL) is exceeded. It is recommended that workers not enter an environment in which 25% of the LEL is exceeded. Prior to and during occupancy, continuous monitoring for toxic and explosive atmospheres must be maintained. Continuous positive ventilation must also be maintained.

Pressurized tanks are those in which contents have reacted releasing a gas (vapor) inside the container. This condition (pressurization) may also occur at elevated temperature or reduced atmosphere pressure. Movement of such containers should be avoided where possible. If movement is necessary, a vehicle with a grappler fitted with some sort of blast shield should be used. If such a container is to be opened, it should be done with an opener operated by remote control.

Leaking drums should be placed in overpack drums before the contents spill. If leaking drums cannot be moved, the contents should be pumped into an intact drum.

The level of protection used during drum-handling operations will be dictated by the condition of the drums and by the content. If the potential for skin absorption is high and respiratory protection is also determined to be necessary, level A protection is necessary [fully encapsulating suit with self-contained breathing apparatus (SCBA)]. If skin protection is unnecessary, then level B (chemical splash suit with SCBA) may be sufficient. If skin protection is of lesser concern and a lower level of respiratory protection is considered adequate, level C may be sufficient. Rarely should level D be used during drum-handling operations.

Oxygen Deficiency at the Site: Normal oxygen content of the air at sea level is 21%. A decrease of O_2 content to 16% can result in mental impairment, difficulty in concentration, and performance impairment. Decreases of the O_2 content of air below 16% can result in unconsciousness and death. Oxygen deficiency is defined as any concentration below 19.5%. Conditions that may result in oxygen deficiency include confined spaces, low-lying areas, pits, and wells that may contain gases or chemical vapors. Monitoring of the O_2 concentration in ambient area is required before entry into an unknown area.

Explosives and Flammables: The potential for an explosion or fire may be present at a site as a result of a chemical reaction, heat, specific chemicals that react violently with water, or ignition of materials in an oxygen rich environment. Explosions or fires can be spontaneous, but they usually occur due to site activity or processes being conducted. Explosive atmospheres and flammable vapors must be monitored with the proper equipment, and personnel must be protected. Ignition sources must be removed and kept apart from these environments. Explosion-proof equipment should be used by workers.

Ionizing Radiation: Radioactive materials may emit alpha particles, and beta and gamma radiation. Alpha particles are stopped by clothing. However, alpha radiation can be harmful if emission materials are inhaled or ingested. Beta radiation can produce burns following intense exposure and is harmful if emission materials are ingested. Proper protective clothing can prevent health effects from both alpha and beta radiation sources of these materials. Gamma radiation passes through clothes and human tissue. Chemical protective clothing does not protect against gamma radiation. Proper monitoring and protective equipment is essential to protect personnel, and site activity should be curtailed if gamma radiation levels are greater than 2 mrem/hour (see chapter on radioactive materials).

Biologic Hazards and Infectious Wastes: Medical waste may contain infectious agents. However, only 15% of medical waste actually contains potential infectious agents (refer to chapter on medical waste). The discovery of medical wastes at a hazardous materials site justifies certain precautions. The risk of infection is related to introducing a pathogenic agent through skin breaks by cuts, needle sticks, and other sharps. Sharp objects should not be directly handled. Instead, a pair of tongs should be used to pick up needles and other sharps (see chapter on medical wastes).

Other Safety and Health Hazards: Hazards can be created by the terrain and the environment of a hazardous materials site as well as by the physical stress produced by protective gear worn at such sites (see chapter on personnel protective equipment). Uneven surfaces, the presence of holes and wells, unstable structures, and the presence of heavy operating equipment all create potential hazards to workers.

Weather can be a factor in the health and safety of personnel at a hazardous materials site. Heat stress is a very real hazard for workers wearing protective clothing and may be more hazardous than the chemicals at the site. Heat stress can result in heat exhaustion, with subsequent loss of fluids and hypovolemia or heat stroke, which can result in seizures, severe hyperthermia, multiple organ damage, and death. Cold environments can result in hypothermia, with subsequent mental and physical impairment or frostbite.

The effect of noise at a site must also be a consideration. Excessive noise from equipment can result in hearing loss, distraction of workers, and interference with worker communication. Administrative and engineering controls for noise reduction must be in place if workers are exposed to a sound level exceeding 90 dBA (decibels on the A-weighted scale) per 8-hour time weighted average (TWA). Workers who are exposed to 85 dBA on an 8-hour TWA must have a hearing conservation program as described in OSHA regulation 29 CFR Part 1910.95.

Sampling and Monitoring Strategies Phase

Sampling strategy is thus a two-stage process: the initial survey followed by a secondary, more specific, characterization of a site. The initial sampling phase is used to establish priorities and identify risks present at a site. Chemicals and other hazardous materials are qualitatively identified in the first phase of sampling and further identified and quantitated in the second phase.

The initial sampling phase allows plans to be developed for safe site entry and dictates the use of proper personal protective equipment. Samples of air, water, and soil are obtained to initially characterize the presence of organic contaminants, dangerous conditions, and the physical forms of hazards present. Air sampling should be conducted with a variety of sampling media to help identify major classes of airborne contaminants as well as their concentrations. Personnel should identify potential sources of generation of hazards and begin sampling

downwind of the suspected source while working in the direct axis of the wind. Sampling should then proceed upwind until reaching the source of highest concentration. Level B personnel protection should be worn during this phase. After the highest concentrations of contaminants are identified, sampling should be conducted at cross-axis with the wind to help determine dispersion patterns. Finally, samples should be obtained upwind from the source.

The second phase of sampling specifies the individual contaminants present, quantitates specific contaminants, allows for collection of samples for more specific studies, and enables the development of control technologies as well as health impact studies (6). Perimeter monitoring at fixed locations around the site where personal protective equipment is not required should also be conducted to determine migration patterns of chemicals. Wind speed and direction should be recorded at these fixed sites. This maneuver helps determine the integrity of the ''clean'' zones.

Periodic monitoring on the site is important to validate the initial data and to protect personnel who engage in work-related activities on the site. Monitoring should be repeated when work activity changes to a new site, when atmospheric conditions change, or when new sources of chemicals are discovered.

The use of personal monitoring for workers who are closest to the source of contamination is recommended. These workers would be exposed to the highest dose of the contaminant. Samples should be collected in the breathing zone areas of workers. If the workers are wearing face masks, then monitoring should be done outside the face mask. Breathing zone monitoring samples the actual inhalational dose of airborne contaminants that is actually occurring. Personal monitoring may require the use of multiple media and the use of constant flow rate pumps to accurately assess exposures. Many samples may be required over a period of days to properly assess the magnitude and variation in exposure. If workers are in teams, a different personal monitor can be attached to each team member at the same site. An alternative measure is to attach the monitoring devices to equipment at the site.

There are two fundamental concepts that describe means by which samples are collected: instantaneous (grab) sampling and integrated sampling. Direct, instantaneous sampling for hazardous conditions is essential to protect personnel and help decide on the types of personnel protective equipment required. Conditions IDLH must first be ruled out using combustible gas detectors, oxygen, sensors, photoionization detectors, flame ionization detectors, and gamma radiation detectors.

At a hazardous materials site where the presence of multiple chemicals is usually the rule, instrument readings should be interpreted conservatively. Also, in these situations, the person actually using the equipment should be fully trained and capable of proper instrument use, such as a certified industrial hygienist. Basic sampling criteria include the following considerations:

Calibration should be performed according to manufacturer's instruction before and after every use.

Chemical response (standard) curves not provided by the manufacturer should be developed by qualified personnel.

A detection reading of ''zero'' should be reported as ''no instrument response,'' since direct-reading instruments will not detect more than one chemical or class of chemicals. Other dangerous substances can be present and not detected by these instruments.

Any positive reading should be reported as a positive response and not a specific concentration unless a single contaminant is known to be present.

Any positive response or needle deflection of an instrument requires repeated sampling with several detection systems. The survey should be repeated with a variety of instruments to minimize the number of chemicals undetected.

Instantaneous Sampling: Instantaneous samples reflect the conditions which exist at the time the sample is collected. The time period may vary from seconds to usually not more than minutes. Any direct-reading instrument may be considered to be an instantaneous sampler. In addition, samples may be collected in some sort of volumetric container (bags, vacuum bottles, etc.) of known volume and transported to a laboratory for analysis.

Indicator tubes used in the analysis of gases and vapors are usually referred to as instantaneous samplers; however, there are other indicator tubes intended to be used over long time periods (hours), in which case they would not be considered to be instantaneous samplers. Many chemical hazards can be detected by detector tubes that are not detected by sophisticated direct-reading instruments.

Many direct-reading instruments may be fitted with an integrator and will thus provide data over virtually any time period selected.

Integrated Sampling: Sampling conducted over an extended period of time (usually hours) such that the results of the analysis represent an average concentration over the time period is referred to as integrated sampling. Integrated sampling is accomplished by use of small sampling pumps drawing contaminant-laden air through sampling media at some known flow rate. The sampling period is timed so that the total volume of air sampled is known. Common sampling media are charcoal tubes and filters. As indicated above, direct-reading instruments may be fitted with an integrator which will provide data indicative of concentrations over virtually any time period.

Area Effects

The effects that toxic materials and waste sites have on the surrounding environment should be assessed. The collection of data on plant, insect, and animal life changes relative to the presence of a site contributes significantly to understanding the hazards of such a site. The concentrations of chemical substances in particularly heavy metals, and in the tissues of plants, animals, and marine life should be determined by appropriate sampling and analysis. Inspection of a site by trained personnel can give clues to the presence or effects of toxic materials.

Soil samples are usually obtained from subsurface locations by placing borings at strategically located positions and sampling the soil extracted from the borings. Groundwater samples are obtained from monitoring wells which have been placed at strategic locations. Generally, monitoring wells are placed to determine the lateral extent of the contaminant plume. Both surface water and soil are collected in carefully decontaminated containers from representative locations throughout the site.

Documentation Issues

Proper documentation practices are important for providing quality control over data collection, providing reasons behind

Table 25.8.   Hazardous Processes, Reactions, and Conditions

Fires and explosions
Flammable liquids
Compressed gases
Confined spaces
Oxygen-deficient areas
Release of chemicals in vapor form
Dust and particulate formation
Fume formation
Release or spill of corrosives
Unknown spilled material
Oxidation reactions
Chemical reactions
Heating chemicals near flashpoints
Release of cryogenic fluids
Sudden release of pressurized gases
Radioactive materials
Thermal reactions
Electrical shock
Loading and unloading processes
Low pressure operations
Handling large quantities of flammable liquids

certain safety practices, tracking results of chemical analysis to their source of origin, ensuring that results of analysis are recognized by proper authorities, and providing for chain of custody in legal matters pertaining to the site. Documentation includes the use of photographs, log books, sample tables, charts and tables, graphics, and chain of custody containers and forms. The task of documentation is assigned to a specific individual to ensure that this important practice is conducted correctly. Written records of sample collection, sample storage and tracking, sample analysis and results, and sample destruction are critical features of expert documentation practices.

Hazard and Exposure Assessment

Following site characterization and documentation of the presence and concentration of substances at a site, the hazards associated with these substances must be established (Table 25.8). There are many variables that have direct influence on the accuracy of toxic hazard assessment and exposure assessment (9). There are usually numerous chemicals at hazardous materials sites, and the hazard assessment must account for the combinations and potential synergism of these multiple substances in their various forms and locations.

Vapor emissions from chemicals can change with atmospheric conditions as well as with work activities. Concentrated pockets of vapors may produce high air concentrations for shortterm intervals until disturbed by worksite exploration. These vapor concentrations will be affected by dispersion and diffusion and can then produce relatively low airborne concentrations over a larger work area.

Changes in temperature will affect vapor pressures of volatile organic solvents. Wind direction and speed will directly influence the concentration of surface chemicals and vapors. These may be further dispersed or concentrated by the wind. Also, the wind may generate respirable contaminated dust particles. Work activities associated with exploration and digging at the site may disturb contaminated areas and alter the airborne concentration of substances. Moisture can affect the sampling of dusts, since very fine dusts of hazardous solids change size

Table 25.9. Newly Regulated Hazardous Substances by OSHA

Acetylsalicylic acid (aspirin)	Diethylene triamine	Methyl isopropyl ketone
Acrylic acid	Diethyl ketone	Methyl parathion
Aluminum pyro powders	Diethyl phthalate	Methyl silicate
Aluminum welding fumes	Dinitolmide (3,5-dinitro-o-toluamide)	Metribuzin
Aluminum soluble salts	Dioxathion (Delnav)	Monocrotophos
Aluminum alkalis	Diphenylamine	Nonane
Amitrole	Dipropyl ketone	Paraffin wax fume
Ammonium chloride fume	Diquat	Phenothiazine
Atrazine	Disulfiram	Phenyl mercaptan
Bismuth telluride, Se-doped	Disulfoton	Phenylphosphine
Borates, anhydrous	2,6-Di-tert-butyl-p-cresol	Phorate
Borates, decahydrate	Diuron	Phosphorus oxychloride
Borates, pentahydrate	Divinyl benzene	m-Phthalodinitrile
Boron tribromide	Endosulfan	Piperazine dihydrochloride
Bromacil	Ethion	Platinum metal
Bromine pentafluoride	Ethylene glycol	Potassium hydroxide
Butane	Ethylidene norbornene	Propargyl alcohol
Butyl acrylate	Fenamiphos	Propionic acid
n-Butyl lactate	Fensulfothion	Propoxur (Baygon)
o-sec-Butylphenol	Fenthion	Propylene glycol dinitrate
Calcium cyanamide	Fonofos	Propylene glycol monomethyl ether
Calcium hydroxide	Formamide	Resorcinol
Caprolactam dust	Gasoline	Rosin core solder pyrolysis products
Caprolactam vapor	Germanium tetrahydride	Silicon tetrahydride
Captafol (Difolatan)	Glutaraldehyde	Sodium azide
Captan	Grain dust (oat, wheat, barley)	Sodium bisulfite
Carbofuran (Furadan)	Hexachlorobutadiene	Sodium metabisulfite
Carbon tetrabromide	Hexachlorocyclopentadiene	Subtilisins (proteolytic enzyme)
Carbonyl fluoride	Hexafluoroacetone	Sulfur tetrafluoride
Catechol (Pyrocatechol)	Hexane isomers	Sulprofos
Cesium hydroxide	Hexylene glycol	Tetrasodium pyrophosphate
Chloroacetyl chloride	Hydrogenated terphenyls	Thioglycolic acid
Chlorodifluoromethane	2-Hydroxypropyl acrylate	Thionyl chloride
Chloropentafluoroethane	Indene	Tin oxide (as Sn)
o-Chlorostyrene	Indium and compounds	p-Toluidine
o-Chlorotoluene	Iodoform	Trichloroacetic acid
Chlorpyrifos	Iron pentacarbonyl	1,2,4-Trichlorobenzene
Cobalt carbonyl	Iron salts	Trimellitic anhydride
Cobalt hydrocarbonyl	Isooctyl alcohol	Trimethylamine
Crufomate	Isophorone diisocyanate	Trimethyl benzene
Cyanamide	2-Isopropoxyethanol	Trimethyl phosphite
Cyanogen	N-Isopropylaniline	Triphenyl amine
Cyanogen chloride	Manganese cyclopenta-dienyltricarbonyl	Tungsten, insoluble compounds
Cyclohexylamine	Manganese tetroxide	Tungsten, soluble compounds
Cyclonite	Methacrylic acid	n-Valeraldehyde
Cyclopentane	Methomyl (Lannate)	Vinyl acetate
Cyhexatin	4-Methoxyphenol	Vinyl bromide
Diazinon	Methylacrylonitrile	Vinyl cyclohexene dioxide
2-N-Dibutylaminoethanol	Methyl 2-cyanoacrylate	Vinylidene chloride (1,1-dichloroethylene)
Dichloroacetylene	Methylcyclopentadienyl manganese tricar-	VM & P Naphtha
1,3-Dichloropropene	bonyl	Welding fumes
2,2-Dichloropropionic acid	Methyl demeton	Wood dust, all soft and hard woods, except western red cedar
Dicrotophos	4,4'-Methylene bis(2-chloroaniline)	m-Xylene α,α'-diamine
Dicyclopentadiene	Methylene bis(4-cyclohexylisocyanate)	
Diethanolamine	Methyl ethyl ketone peroxide	
	Methyl isoamyl ketone	

and weight with changes in moisture content. Water from rainfall can change vapor emissions from a site and effectively reduce air concentrations of volatile contaminants or dilute contaminants in soil.

Once conditions IDLH are ruled out or controlled, the assessment should concentrate on routes of exposure and absorption of the chemicals that are present using the TLVs and PELs as a guide. The site survey should provide the basis for exposure assessment by supplying the following information:

the types and physical forms of the chemicals and hazards present at the site as well as their location;
the media in which these substances are present such as soil, water, air and their dispersion patterns;

the concentrations of substances present;
exposure and effect on the surrounding plant and animal environment.

Additions to OSHA Chemical Listing for PELs

Assessing the potential toxic effects and hazards posed by environmental and occupational exposure to chemicals is a continuing effort on the part of private industry, the government, and consultants to business and the community. As of January 1989, 164 new chemicals have been added to the regulated workplace standards set by OSHA (Table 25.9).

REFERENCES

1. Casto KM. Environmental health law. Chapter 8 in: Blumenthal DS (ed.), Introduction to environmental health. New York: Springer Publishing Co, 1985.

2. Cheremisinoff PN. Evaluating the hazard. Chapter 2 in: Management of hazardous occupational environments. Lancaster, PA: Technomic Publishing Co, Lancaster, PA, 1984.

3. Proctor NH. Setting health standards: toxicologic concepts. Chapter 1 in: Proctor NH, Hughes SP. Chemical hazards of the workplace. Philadelphia: JB Lippincott Co., 1978.

4. U.S. Department of Health and Human Services, Public Health Service, Centers for Disease Control. National Institute for Occupational Safety and Health. Air monitoring. Chapter 7 in: Occupational safety and health guidance manual for hazardous waste site activities. Washington, DC: NIOSH, 1985.

5. Olishifski JB. Air-sampling instruments. Chapter 18 in: Olishifski JB (ed.), Fundamentals of industrial hygiene. Chicago, IL: National Safety Council, 1985.

6. U.S. Department of Health and Human Services, Public Health Service, Centers for Disease Control, National Institute for Occupational Safety and Health. Planning and Organization. Chapter 3 in: Occupational safety and health guidance manual for hazardous waste site activities. Washington, DC: NIOSH, 1985.

7. U.S. Department of Health and Human Services, Public Health Service, Centers for Disease Control, National Institute for Occupational Safety and Health. Site characterization. Chapter 6 in: Occupational safety and health guidance manual for hazardous waste site activities. Washington, DC: NIOSH, 1985.

8. White AL. The site history: a tool for risk management. Hazardous Waste, 1984;1(4):533–543.

9. Important Parameters in Toxicity Assessment. Chapter 4 in: EPA toxicology handbook. Rockville, Maryland: Government Institute Inc., 1988.

26

Situations and Exposures Immediately Dangerous to Life and Health

Clifton D. Crutchfield, Ph.D., C.I.H.
John B. Sullivan, Jr., M.D.

DEFINING EXPOSURES IMMEDIATELY DANGEROUS TO LIFE AND HEALTH

A chemical hazard is a combination of the intrinsic toxicity of the chemical and the quality and quantity of exposure. The environment of the exposure is also a factor that dramatically influences the hazard of a chemical. An example of such an environmental factor is a confined space, which can radically alter the exposure risk.

A variety of situations create conditions which can be immediately dangerous to life and health (IDLH). These include:

1. Confined spaces;
2. Explosive situations and spontaneous combustion;
3. Oxygen deficiency;
4. Acutely toxic concentrations of gases, vapors, or aerosols; and
5. Presence of ionizing radiation.

The term, "immediately dangerous to life or health" (29 CFR 1986), has been defined as "conditions that pose an immediate threat to life or health or conditions that pose an immediate threat of severe exposure to contaminants, such as radioactive materials, which are likely to have adverse cumulative or delayed effects on health" (1). IDLH definitions were originally developed to aid in selection of respiratory protective devices for occupational environments. They identified the concentration of a chemical above which the most protective respiratory device should be used, such as a self-contained breathing apparatus, for a 30-minute exposure period. IDLH values assigned to chemicals are higher than the concentrations found to be toxic in animals (Table 26.1). These IDLH conditions were defined by an exposure time of 10 minutes with severe toxicity being unconsciousness, incapacitation, or intolerable irritation in the animal (2). For all compounds considered, except nickel carbonyl, the IDLH level is higher than the permissible exposure level (PEL) (2). Since IDLH values were developed for occupational exposures, they are not applicable in assessing true health risks of public exposures to acute releases of hazardous substances. Development of IDLH standards was also based on personal awareness of a dangerous condition existing as well as a designated time of escape from the exposure.

The Superfund Amendment and Reauthorization Act of 1986 (SARA) required the U.S. Environmental Protection Agency (EPA) to identify extremely hazardous substances. The EPA subsequently developed a method to evaluate the toxicity of substances for the purpose of community emergency planning. This EPA method initially ranked 92 extremely hazardous substances based on the IDLH values developed by the National Institute for Occupational Safety and Health (NIOSH) (1).

There are problems associated with the original definition of IDLH conditions, as well as the ranking of IDLH values for chemicals: (a) it was designed for the purpose of respirator selection; (b) it ignores the contribution of other environmental factors; (c) it assumes a sudden chemical release scenario; (d) it does not consider preexisting disease or chemical mixtures; and (e) it does not consider carcinogenicity of a chemical or hazard (Table 26.2). In addition, the initial EPA/NIOSH IDLH values were not reviewed for accuracy and reliability in their application to humans, nor have the values been updated since the 1970s (2).

Original IDLH values were based on a 30-minute time of exposure which could produce lethality or toxicity. This 30-minute time frame ignores the health effects that can be produced from sudden exposures, the fact that a person may be quickly impaired or rendered unconscious in much less time than 30 minutes, and the fact that the ability to escape would be impaired due to environmental factors.

IDLH values are also higher in comparison to the Emergency Exposure Guidance Levels (EEGL) developed by the National Academy of Sciences (NAS) (Table 26.3) (2). EEGLs were developed for military personnel to prevent injury and are based on 1-hour exposures compared with the 30-minute exposures of IDLH values (2). For the public, it has been suggested that shortterm Public Emergency Guidance Levels (SPEGL) be created with a 2–10-fold uncertainty safety factor below the EEGL values (2). The term IDLH can, thus, apply to a chemical concentration or a situation of exposure to a hazard. In general, use of the term IDLH should be flexible and can refer to an occupational as well as an environmental exposure that can produce acute health effects or death.

IDLH conditions can also arise from a process in which a hazard is created. Such process hazards include:

1. Handling explosives and flammable materials;
2. Low pressure or high pressure operations;
3. Working with materials close to their flash points or autoignition range;
4. Mixing chemicals;
5. Chain reactions;
6. Radioactive materials and radiation sources;
7. Oxidizing materials;
8. Handling materials that react violently with water;
9. Working with materials that spontaneously polymerize or combust;
10. Working with materials that have properties of explosive decomposition;
11. Presence of high energy electrical sources.

Indications that potential IDLH conditions exist include the presence of underground or above ground storage tanks that

Table 26.1. Comparison of Severe Toxicity Endpoints Resulting from Chemical Exposure to IDLH Values

Compound	IDLH (ppm)	Toxic Concentration (ppm)	Species
Acetaldehyde	10,000	4946	Mouse
Acetic acid	1000	163	Mouse
Acetone	20,000	23,480	Mouse
Acrotein	5	1.68	Mouse
Ammonia	500	303	Mouse
Amyl acetate	4000	1531	Mouse
Arsine	6	13[d]	Mouse
Benzyl chloride	10	17	Mouse
n-Butanol	8000	4784	Mouse
2-Butoxy ethanol	700	2824	Mouse
p-t-Butyl toluene	1000	360	Mouse
Carbon monoxide	1500	1450	Rat
Chlorine	30	9.34	Mouse
Chloroacetophenone	100	0.96	Mouse
Chlorobenzene	2400	1054	Mouse
Chlorobenzylidene malonitrile	0.26	0.52	Mouse
Chloropicrin	4	7.98	Mouse
Crotonaldehyde	400	3.53	Mouse
Cyclohexanone	5000	756	Mouse
o-Dichlorobenzene	1700	182	Mouse
Dimethylamine	2000	511	Mouse
Epichlorohydrin	100	687	Mouse
Ethyl acetate	10,000	614	Mouse
Ethyl acrylate	2000	315	Mouse
Ethyl benzene	2000	4060	Mouse
Fluorine	25	64	Mouse
Formaldehyde	100	3.13	Mouse
Furaldehyde	250	234	Mouse
Hydrogen chloride	100	309	Mouse
Hydrogen cyanide	50	139	Rat
Hydrogen fluoride	20	590	Rat
Hydrogen sulfide	300	125[f]	Rabbit
Isoamyl alcohol	8000	4452	Mouse
Isobutyl alcohol	8000	1818	Mouse
Isophorone	800	27.8	Mouse
Isopropyl alcohol	12,000	17,693	Mouse
Isopropyl benzene	8000	2490	Mouse
Methanol	25,000	41,514	Mouse
Phenol	250	166	Mouse
n-Propanol	4000	12,704	Mouse
Styrene	5000	980	Mouse
Sulfur dioxide	100	117	Mouse
Toluene	2000	5300	Mouse
Toluene diisocyanate	10	0.39	Mouse
Vinyl toluene	5000	16.4	Mouse
o-Xylene	1000	1467	Mouse

[d]Adjusted from a 1-hour exposure.
[f]Adjusted from a 90-minute exposure.
Adapted from: Alexeet GV, Lipsett MJ, Kizer KW. Problems associated with the use of immediately dangerous to life and health (IDLH) values for estimating the hazard of accidental chemical releases. Reprinted with permission by American Industrial Hygiene Association Journal. Vol. 50:598–605 (1989).

Table 26.2. Compounds for Which IDLH Values Are No Longer Listed by NIOSH because of Potential Human Carcinogenicity

Acrylonitrile	Ethylene dibromide
Aldrin	Ethylene dichloride
Arsenic (inorganic)	Ethylene oxide
Arsine	Formaldehyde
Benzene	Hydrazine
Cadmium fume and dust	Lead arsenate
Calcium arsenate	Methyl bromide
Carbon tetrachloride	Methyl chloride
Chlorodiphenyl	Methylene chloride
Chloroform	Methyl iodide
Chloroprene	Monomethyl hydrazine
Coal tar pitch	Nickel carbonyl
Dieldrin	2-Nitropropane
Diglycidyl ether	Phenyl hydrazine
1,1-Dimethylhydrazine	1,1,2,2-Tetrachloroethane
Dinitrotoluene	Tetrachloroethylene
Dioxane	1,1,2-Trichloroethane
Epichlorohydrin	Trichloroethylene

Adapted from: Alexeet GV, Lipsett MJ, Kizer KW. Problems associated with the use of immediately dangerous to life and health (IDLH) values for estimating the hazard of accidental chemical releases. Reprinted with permission by American Industrial Hygiene Association Journal: Vol. 50:598–605(1989).

mon chemicals can produce IDLH situations, especially in confined environments (Table 26.4).

Preventing human exposures to situations or environments that can be classified as IDLH must be a primary concern, from the perspective of both occupational exposures and public exposures. Most human exposures to these situations result from a lack of knowledge or understanding of the conditions that create them.

None of the forms of ionizing radiation can be directly sensed by the body. Many of the simple asphyxiant gases, which have low levels of toxicity apart from their ability to displace oxygen, may not be detected by human senses. Examples of such gases include nitrogen, argon, and carbon dioxide. Other toxic and potentially lethal gases may have characteristic odors, such as hydrogen sulfide. Even when warning properties such as odor or irritation are present, a person may still become desensitized and underestimate the level of danger. Exposure to high vapor concentrations of many of the commonly used commercial and industrial solvents can rapidly produce central nervous system stimulation or depression and impair a worker's ability to rationally assess the level of danger associated with the exposure.

Performance of a worker may also be impaired by prescription medications or the use of illicit drugs. When coupled with certain environmental conditions, such impairment can create a situation that may be dangerous to health and life. Over-the-counter medications containing sedating antihistamines, prescription medications, or drugs of abuse are potential offenders. Many drugs routinely prescribed for hypertension or cardiac disease can produce dizziness, sedation, or syncope. Combined with a particular hazardous environment, a person may become a danger to himself/herself or others. Therefore, knowledge of drugs that a worker is taking is very important to the worker's health and safety, as well as to that of other workers and the public. Management of a company has the responsibility to ensure worker safety. A worker taking medications that can cause impairment must not be assigned to tasks such as driving

require entry by personnel, trenches, low lying spaces, presence of gas cylinders or bulging drums, visible vapor or dust clouds, presence of extremely dangerous chemicals such as cyanide, phosphine, arsine, hydrogen sulfide, phosgene, halogen gases, or ionizing radiation, and presence of an explosive atmosphere. Hazard warning signs may or may not be present. Many com-

Table 26.3.   Comparison of Immediately Dangerous to Life or Health (IDLH)[a] to National Academy of Sciences (NAS)[b] Values

Compound	IDLH (ppm)	EEGL (ppm)
Acetone	20,000	8500
Acrolein	5	0.05
Ammonia	500	100
Arsine	6[c]	1
Benzene	2000[c]	50
Carbon disulfide	500	50
Carbon monoxide	1500	400
Chlorine	30	3
Chlorine trifluoride	20	1
Chloroform	1000[c]	100
Dichlorofluoromethane, FC21	50,000	10,000
Dichlorotetrafluoromethane	50,000	10,000
1,1-Dimethylhydrazine	50[c]	0.24[d]
Ethanolamine	1000	50
Ethylene oxide	800[c]	20
Fluorine	25	7.5
Hydrazine	80[c]	0.12[d]
Hydrogen chloride	100	1[d]
Hydrogen sulfide	300	50[e]
Isopropyl alcohol	12,000	400
Methanol	25,000	200
Methylhydrazine	5[c]	0.24[d]
Nitrogen dioxide	50	1
Ozone	10	1
Phosgene	2	0.2
Sodium hydroxide (mg/m^3)	250	2
Sulfur dioxide	100	10
Sulfuric acid (mg/m^3)	80	1
Toluene	2000	200
Trichlorotrifluoroethane	4500	1500
Xylene	1000	200

[a]The IDLH is a 30-minute value.
[b]Values listed are 60-minute EELs or EEGLs unless specified.
[c]Value not listed in most recent NIOSH publication (3) but replaced by "Ca."
[d]Value listed is a 60-minute SPEGL.
[e]Value listed is a 10-minute EEGL.
Adapted from: Alexeet GV, Lipsett MS, Kizer KW. Problems associated with the use of immediately dangerous to life and health (IDLH) values for estimating the hazard of accidental chemical releases. Reprinted with permission by American Industrial Hygiene Association Journal: Vol. 50:598–605(1989).

or operating dangerous equipment. Company management has a responsibility to ensure that employees taking these medications are not assigned to work in hazardous situations.

Successfully dealing with hazards related to potential IDLH gases and vapors in the environment involves understanding how they create risk and recognizing when and where they may be present. Both the respiratory system and the central nervous system are the primary target organs for most toxic vapors. The lack of a sufficient oxygen supply or the loss of capacity to transport oxygen immediately creates risk. Without sufficient oxygen, the central nervous system is rapidly compromised and the ability to recognize and take steps to correct the dangerous situation quickly diminishes. The body's sensory elements cannot always provide adequate warning of the presence of potential IDLH conditions. Instead, the circumstances under which IDLH conditions are generated must be recognized.

Emergency conditions such as chemical spills, process upsets, tank ruptures, or fires and explosions are obvious potential hazard sources. The airborne composition of the gases and vapors may be the same as the chemicals involved in the release, or they may be composed of reaction or combustion byproducts that have higher toxicities. Since the actual composition and concentration of contaminants in the air at an emergency site are usually unknown, the most prudent procedure is to assume the worst case situation and protect exposed personnel accordingly. The requirement for emergency response personnel to wear self-contained breathing apparatus and full protective clothing when initially approaching an unknown situation is an example of such prudence. The level of required protection can be relaxed only when the actual exposure risks are determined. Limiting emergency response to personnel who are adequately trained and equipped to deal with the situation is one of the best means of preventing overexposure to IDLH environments during emergencies. Preplanning can assist in predicting the levels of response and types of training and equipment that may be needed for specific locations or operations.

Confined Spaces and Chemical Accumulation

A number of seemingly benign situations can also pose IDLH risks. One of the most common of these involves entry of personnel into confined spaces. Examples of typical confined spaces include tanks, vaults, pits, sumps, pipes, and ventilation ducts. Such spaces are typically designed to contain, convey, or process materials, or to isolate high energy sources from the surrounding environment. They are not usually designed for human occupancy. Consequently, a variety of IDLH conditions can be encountered in a confined space (Table 26.5) (3).

Toxic, explosive, or oxygen-deficient atmospheres comprise some of the most immediate hazards that are encountered in confined spaces. The nature of a confined space restricts or prevents the turnover of air in the space. Consequently, extremely high concentrations of flammable or toxic gases and vapors can build up over time. The vapor concentration above a liquid in the space will be primarily determined by the temperature and vapor pressure of the liquid. If the space is essentially airtight, vapor stratification can occur if the molecular weight of the vapor or gas is significantly different from the molecular weight of air.

Two possible sources of toxic or flammable materials must be considered in conjunction with confined spaces. The first source is associated with liquids or gases that are actually stored or contained in a confined space such as a tank or sump. Unless all liquid or gas is drained from the space and its interior surfaces are thoroughly cleaned, high gas or vapor concentrations can occur.

A second, less obvious means of creating flammable or toxic atmospheres in a confined space involves the introduction or seepage of a gas or vapor into the space from an external source. When considering the types of contaminants that may be encountered in a confined space, it is important to look beyond the compounds that are normally stored or used in it. Exhaust emissions from a gasoline engine used on a temporary basis in the vicinity of a tank or vault can transform a normally benign atmosphere into a toxic one.

Volatile organic solvents, such as the chlorinated hydrocarbons trichloroethylene and 1,1,1-trichloroethane, can accumulate in confined spaces and produce dangerous or lethal situations for personnel who enter these spaces. Cases have occurred in which workers who have entered a confined area contaminated with a chlorinated solvent vapor have suffered

Table 26.4.   Chemicals Associated with IDLH Situations

I. Chemical asphyxiants
   Hydrogen cyanide
   Hydrogen sulfide
   Carbon monoxide
   Acetonitrile
II. Hemolytic chemicals
   Arsine
   Phosphine
   Aluminum phosphide (reaction with acid)
   Stibine
   Naphthalene
III. Methemoglobin-forming chemicals
   Aniline and aniline derivatives
   Nitrobenzene
   Dinitrophenol
   O-Toluidine
   Xylidine
   Dinitrotoluene
   Nitrotoluene
   Nitrochlorobenzene
   Monomethylhydrazine
IV. Cholinesterase inhibitors
   Malathion
   Parathion
   Methyl parathion
   Diazinon
   Disyston
   Chlorpyrifos
   Carbamate
   Dichlorvos
V. Physical asphyxiants
   Acetylene
   Argon
   Neon
   Helium
   Ethane
   Hydrogen gas
   Methane
   Propane
   Natural gas
   Liquified petroleum
   Nitrogen
   Carbon dioxide
   Volatile organic hydrocarbons and solvents
VI. Respiratory and sensory irritants
   Acetaldehyde
   Acetic acid
   Formaldehyde
   Furaldehyde
   Toluene diisocyanate
   Methyl isocyanate
   Chlorine
   Phosgene
   Diborane

VI. Respiratory and sensory irritants *continued*
   Dichloroethyl ether
   Ethylene oxide
   Inorganic acid vapors
   Phenol and organic acid vapors
   Ammonia
   Beryllium
   Nitrogen dioxide
   Ethanolamine
   Diethylamine
   Dimethylamine
   Ethylamine
   Fluorine
   Hydrogen fluoride
   Bromine
   Hydrogen bromide
   Butyl mercaptan
   Acrolein
   Chloropicrin
   Chlorine dioxide
   Boron trifluoride
   Ethylene chlorohydrin
   Chlorine trifluoride
   Nickel carbonyl
   Ozone
   Sulfur dioxide
   Lithium hydride
   Halogenated organic solvents
   Methylene chloride
   Trichloroethylene
   1,1,1-Trichloroethane
   Tetrachloroethane
   Carbon tetrachloride
   Chloroform
   1,1-Dichloroethane
   Ethyl ether
   Dichlorodifluoromethane (Freon 12, Halon)
   Dichloromonofluoromethane
   Difluorodibromomethane
   Ethylbromide
   Hexachloroethane
VII. Explosives and flammables
   Hydrogen
   Oxygen
   Organic solvent vapors
   Gasoline
   Sodium
   Potassium
   Ammonium nitrate
   Magnesium
   Trinitrotoluene
   Cyclonite
   Hexogen
   Cyclotrimethylene trinitramine
   Nitrocellulose
   Nitroglycerin

syncope or sustained a cardiac dysrhythmia. Halogenated hydrocarbons are suspected of lowering the threshold of ventricular fibrillation response to circulating epinephrine. An exposed worker observing a coworker in distress or unconscious may attempt a rescue, become excited, and experience a cardiac dysrhythmia due to the synergy of increased blood concentrations of circulating catecholamines and halogenated hydrocar-bons (see Cardiac Toxicology chapter). Thus, the rescuer may actually be the person to die.

Oxygen Deficiency

Oxygen deficiency is another potential killer in confined spaces. The atmosphere normally contains 20.9% oxygen. If the oxy-

Table 26.5. Characteristics of Hazardous Confined Spaces

1. Limited access that could hinder emergency rescue
2. Potentially hazardous atmosphere (e.g., oxygen-deficient, toxic, flammable/explosive)
3. Harmful atmosphere may be inherent to space or introduced during operation in or close to space
4. Presence of one or more energy sources that are controlled at a point external to the space
5. Limited internal operating area that requires workers to remain in close proximity to energy sources
6. Elevated working surfaces with poor or slippery footing
7. Difficulty for external workers to observe or monitor operations inside the space

Adapted from: Firenze RJ. Health and safety in confined workspaces for the construction industry. Division of Training and Manpower Development. Cincinnati, OH: National Institute for Occupational Safety and Health, 1984.

gen content in air falls below 19.5%, it is considered to be oxygen-deficient. A reduction in the oxygen content of air in a confined space can be caused by consumption of the oxygen, displacement of the oxygen by another gas or vapor, or a combination of consumption and displacement. Processes that consume oxygen include combustion, fermentation, and oxidation reactions such as rusting. Inert gases such as nitrogen or argon are often used to blanket materials stored in confined spaces or to purge such spaces or the lines that lead into them. The introduction of an inert gas can displace available oxygen from a confined space and leave an oxygen-deficient atmosphere. Operations such as welding, which must often be conducted in confined spaces, may involve the introduction of flammable and toxic materials, the consumption of oxygen, and the displacement of oxygen by shielding gases.

Control of Confined Spaces

The characteristics listed in Table 26.5 can be used to help identify confined areas that have the potential to contain IDLH atmospheres or conditions. A comprehensive evaluation should be conducted of all areas that have one or more of these characteristics. When a specific confined space is identified, positive steps must be taken to isolate it from routine or unintended entry. The first isolation step involves posting the area with signs that clearly identify it as a controlled confined space. Completion of the isolation procedure may involve limiting access by using barriers, locks, or other personnel/excluding devices. A comprehensive isolation procedure will definitely require a training program that informs all personnel who could possibly gain access to a confined space about the system used to identify and mark such areas, as well as the procedures developed to control entry into them.

One of the most important rules to establish regarding work in and around confined spaces is to prohibit entry into such spaces for all personnel who do not have an absolute need to enter them. A positive entry control program must be established and rigorously maintained. An entry permit procedure is an effective means of establishing positive control over confined space entries. Such a procedure, when rigorously enforced by management, establishes a mechanism to ensure that all persons entering a confined space receive proper training prior to entry.

An essential part of a confined space control program will also prohibit personnel from working alone in such areas. Given the number of things that can go wrong in a confined space,

it is crucial to ensure that continuous, visual communication is established and maintained throughout all operations that involve entries into confined spaces. With an entry permit system, the specialized knowledge required to deal safely with confined spaces can be focused, maintained, and updated in an organization's safety or health function. A number of steps will then become a part of the required permitting process. These steps will generally involve:

1. Review of operations that have previously been conducted in the space;
2. Review of all aspects of the operations that are to be conducted in the space;
3. Review of entry and exit routes that will be utilized during the space entry;
4. Review of the physical layout and energy sources associated with the space, as well as any operation in the nearby area that may affect the space while personnel are in it;
5. Determination of the nature and concentration of contaminants in the space atmosphere, as well as its oxygen content;
6. Review of training level of personnel planning to enter or directly support space entry;
7. Establishment of resource policies and procedures and review of personnel training for rescue efforts.

Review of the historical uses of a space will provide information on residual contaminants that could be left over from previous operations or uses of the space. Any records of previous environmental monitoring conducted in the area may also indicate the possibility of contaminants from outside sources migrating to and concentrating in the confined space. The granting of an entry permit must be predicated on the demonstration of sufficient knowledge of exactly what is to be accomplished in the confined space. If doubt exists about the level of knowledge, work procedures should be practiced and critiqued prior to entry rather than being sorted out once entry is made. The overall objective is to limit exposure time in the confined space as much as possible, and preplanning all aspects of the entry is the most effective way to do so. Personnel positioned outside to support the entry must also be able to demonstrate proficiency with their assigned emergency support role.

Since they are not normally designed for human occupancy, many confined spaces have appreciable physical hazards associated with their entry and egress routes. Storage tanks typically have entry utility holes located on top, where slips and falls are a common hazard, especially when exiting a wet interior. Personnel positioned to visually monitor operations in the tank or to belay lifelines are also placed at increased risk of falling or being less able to effect a rescue if required.

If available, alternate egress routes must be planned and briefed in case the primary route becomes unusable. Such planning should also cover those situations where a confined space is actually located within a surrounding confined space or other potentially IDLH atmosphere. Careful attention must be paid to availability and stability of entry and egress routes during the entry planning phase.

The review of planned operations should cover all aspects of what will take place between entry and egress. All energy sources in or around the space should be reviewed, and those that are not required for the planned entry operation should be deenergized. In addition to monitoring the condition of the space environment at the time of entry, attention must be paid to contaminants that might be generated while working in the space. The potential for oxygen depletion or displacement during the operation must also be assessed.

After the potential hazards of the planned confined space entry have been assessed, an analysis is required to ensure that personnel involved in the entry have sufficient training to accomplish the entry safely. Specific role assignments must be understood and acknowledged by all personnel. Any mismatches between assigned task and physical capacity should be screened out, and training currency for items such as self-contained breathing apparatus (SCBA) should be checked.

Completion of the preplanning steps mentioned above is designed to generate sufficient information to issue a confined space entry permit. The permit should only be issued to a specified crew for a specified period of time. Open-ended permits can easily negate or bypass the controls inherent in the permit system.

With an entry permit issued to trained, knowledgeable personnel, preparations for actual entry into the confined space can begin. Preliminary procedures for entry are covered in American National Standard Institute (ANSI) Z117.1 (4). They generally involve posting or barricading the area so that non-involved personnel do not inadvertently interfere with the operation. Appropriate positive lockout/tagout procedures must be followed to ensure that energy sources that are counted on as being deenergized are actually deenergized. Reliance on an assumed hazard control that is in fact not in place creates a much greater hazard than would exist if the control was not in place and counted on in the first place. In addition to deenergizing nonessential energy sources, hot work, smoking, hot electrical leads, or other potential sources of ignition should be prohibited from the area. All planned draining, cleaning, purging, and/or ventilating of the confined space should also be accomplished.

Entry into Confined Spaces

Immediately prior to entry, all energy states associated with the confined space should be reconfirmed and the atmosphere in the space should be tested. The following questions should be considered when testing the quality of air in the confined space:

1. Is the contaminant in the space heavier or lighter than air?
2. Is there a place for the contaminant to pool?
3. Can a contaminant seep in from external sources?
4. Is the contaminant flammable or explosive?
5. Can static electricity be generated during the operation?
6. Does the atmosphere contain less than 19.5% oxygen?

In the absence of any atmospheric testing, confined space must be treated as IDLH. Testing for toxic concentrations of gases or vapors should be accomplished with real-time instruments such as photoionization detectors, infrared detectors, or organic vapor analyzers. During the testing procedure, it is imperative that the atmosphere throughout the confined space be tested because of the propensity for gases and vapors of different molecular weights to startify in undisturbed air. Fatalities have occurred when only the upper portion of air in a confined space was tested prior to entry. Due to stratification, the oxygen-deficient condition was confined to the lower portion of the space.

Whenever possible, potentially toxic contaminants should be purged from the confined space prior to entry. Purging with fresh air should be used to dilute contaminants to less than one half of their established permissible exposure limit or threshold limit value.

Flammable atmospheres should be purged to less than 10% of their lower explosive limit. When purging a confined space with fresh air, it is important to pay attention to the mixing geometry and effective mixing rate that is achieved during the purging operation so that locally high concentrations of contaminants do not remain when the purge is completed.

The highest level of protection and precaution is required when entries into known or suspected IDLH environments are made. The basic procedure for such an entry will involve the use of SCBA to provide air supply. The nature of contaminants in the space will dictate the other types of protective clothing required. The person making the entry into the IDLH condition must also be attached to a lifeline that is constantly manned by a trained observer positioned outside the space. The observer must also be equipped with an SCBA and must maintain constant visual contact with the worker in the confined space. The trained observer should not be assigned other duties during the course of the entry. Less stringent requirements for respiratory protection and immediate rescue can be established only to the degree that conditions inside a confined space can be tested and absolutely determined to not be IDLH.

SUMMARY

The key to preventing the drastic consequences that can result from toxic exposures from hazardous releases or hazardous environments is recognizing when and where such conditions can exist in occupational settings. Once the potential for IDLH conditions is recognized, programs and procedures can be developed to ensure that only personnel who are thoroughly trained and properly equipped are exposed to the risk. Regarding the public, levels of exposure that are tolerated in occupational and military environments are unacceptably high. The application of shortterm public emergency exposure levels much lower than either IDLH values or EEGL values are needed. Developing and assessing the protective levels of these values is difficult, but necessary to ensure public health and confidence.

REFERENCES

1. National Institute for Occupational Safety and Health and Occupational Safety and Health Administration. NIOSH/OSHA pocket guide to chemical hazards. Publication no. 78-210. Washington, DC: Government Printing Office, 1981:1–191.
2. Alexeet GV, Lipsett MJ, Kizer KW. Problems associated with the use of immediately dangerous to life and health (IDLH) values for estimating the hazard of accidental chemical releases. Am Ind Hyg Assoc J 1989;50:598–605.
3. Firenze RJ. Health and safety in confined workspaces for the construction industry. Cincinnati, OH: Division of Training and Manpower Development, National Institute for Occupational Safety and Health, 1984:33–42.
4. American National Standard Institute. Safety requirements for confined spaces. ANSI Z-117.1. New York: ANSI, 1989.

27

Health Effects from Groundwater Contamination by Volatile Organic Solvents

John A. Lowe, C.I.H.

INTRODUCTION

Public and political concerns associated with clean drinking water have made the study and control of groundwater contamination a high priority in environmental regulation. Several federal environmental protection statutes address the protection of groundwater resources from chemical contamination. The widespread use of groundwater by human populations, the extent of contamination, and the number and types of contaminants present in groundwater suggest that groundwater potentially represents a significant source of exposure to the public. The major reasons to be concerned about contamination of groundwater with toxic substances include the role of groundwater in the water supply, the difficulty of detecting contamination in groundwater, and the difficulty of treating contamination problems once they are detected. The result is that there is substantial uncertainty in regulatory agencies about whether groundwater contamination represents a growing public health concern.

The problem of groundwater contamination by hazardous wastes has become a focal point for marshaling legal, regulatory, and problem-solving resources to reduce exposures and protect public health. On the surface, this concern appears to be highly warranted. Groundwater contamination is the exposure pathway from hazardous waste sites that most commonly results in adverse effects in human populations. However, in pursuit of this goal, insufficient attention is given to the priorities for regulating exposures to groundwater contaminants. For example, of the classes of contaminants present in groundwater (metals, organic compounds, ionic compounds such as nitrates, and microorganisms), a high level of concern is placed on volatile organic compounds, a level of concern that may outweigh the threat to public health presented by these compounds.

The reasons for volatile organic compounds (VOCs) being perceived as a threat to groundwater and public health have to do with a limited number of cases of observed health effects related to high concentrations of VOCs in water, widespread detection of low levels of VOCs in groundwater, the methods used to assess risks associated with low levels of carcinogenic contaminants in groundwater, and risk management policies that place a high priority on controlling cancer risks to extremely low levels. Proper assessment of the risks posed by low level VOC contamination in groundwater is crucial, since mitigation can involve expensive pump-and-treat remediation technologies or the abandonment of contaminated aquifers as water supplies.

Listings of the VOCs detected at disposal sites have been developed largely for sites on the Environmental Protection Agency (EPA)'s National Priority List (NPL) (Table 27.1). A 1983 study performed by Mitre Corporation for EPA indicated that, of the 20 chemicals most commonly detected at NPL sites, 11 of these were VOCs (1). These compounds, in order of frequency and detection, were as follows:

- trichloroethylene;
- toluene;
- benzene;
- chloroform;
- tetrachloroethylene;
- 1,1,1-trichloroethane;
- ethylbenzene;
- trans-1,2-dichloroethane;
- xylene;
- dichloromethane;
- vinyl chloride.

Assessment of the risks from low level VOC contamination in groundwater is based on the following factors:

- The potential for VOCs to migrate through soil into groundwater;
- The difficulty of detecting contamination problems once they are detected;
- The circumstances in which adverse effects from VOC contamination in drinking water have been identified, based on epidemiologic data;
- The conservatism in the underlying assumptions of risk assessment.

ASSESSING EXPOSURES TO VOCs IN GROUNDWATER

VOCs in the soil potentially present in the largest threat of contamination of groundwater. The physical and chemical properties of VOCs facilitate migration through soil. Evaluating the threat of groundwater contamination by VOCs involves consideration of exposure pathways. The exposure pathway provides the framework for evaluating the environmental fate and transport of VOCs in soil and groundwater. An exposure pathway consists of the following elements:

- A source of chemical release to the environment;
- An environmental transport medium (in this case, soil vapor or soil moisture);
- A point of potential human contact with the contaminated medium (also referred to as the receptor); and
- A route of entry into humans, either inhalation, ingestion, or dermal contact with the contaminated soil or water.

Sources of VOC Releases to Soil

VOCs become introduced to the soil by surface disposal to land, spills during handling or transportation, or losses from

Table 27.1. VOCs Commonly Detected in Groundwater at NPL Sites

Chemical	% of Sites Affected	Concentration in Groundwater (ppm) Average	Maximum
Trichloroethylene	34	3.82	790
Chloroform	21	1.46	220
1,1,1-Trichloroethane	16	1.25	618
Methylene chloride	11	11.2	7800
Vinyl chloride	8	0.8	516
Toluene	28	5.18	1100
Benzene	24	5.0	1200
Ethylbenzene	13	0.65	25
Xylene	12	4.07	150

Source: Upton AC, Knerp T, Toniol P. Public health aspects of toxic chemical disposal sites. Annu Rev Pub Health 1989;10:1–25. Based on a survey performed for EPA in 1985 of substances found at hazardous waste sites.

surface or underground storage tanks. The nature of disposal sites, underground tanks, and other sources has been discussed elsewhere (1, 2); however, a brief synopsis of chemical sources for groundwater contamination is presented here. Historically, most chemical wastes were considered unsuitable for most practical purposes, and discharge to land or shallow burial was considered economical disposal practice. Types of practices included disposal of sludges or semisolid materials to the surface or in waste piles, surface disposal or burial of drummed materials, and disposal of liquids in lagoons or impoundments. Early studies of disposal practices indicated that sites could range from secure landfills situated over impermeable soils, with lined impounds and engineered covers, to uncontrolled sites located in permeable soils, over shallow water tables, and near drinking water wells. The number of sites potentially releasing chemicals to groundwater varies from author to author; however, a conservative estimate ranges on the tens of thousands (1).

VOC Transport to Groundwater

The potential for VOCs to contaminate groundwater is based on several factors, including method of containment of the wastes, soil characteristics, depth to groundwater, and chemical properties. The threat to public health from groundwater contamination is related to the proximity and location of groundwater wells to the source of contamination. Transport of VOCs in the unsaturated zone to groundwater occurs largely by transport through soil vapor, with some transport in soil moisture. Soil porosity, variations in rainfall, soil moisture content, and soil organic matter content are some factors influencing VOC transport in the unsaturated zone. VOCs are characterized by relatively high vapor pressures, low-to-moderate solubilities in water, and limited tendency to sorb to soil particulates. Migration will tend to be promoted in porous soils (sands and coarse silts) with low organic matter contents.

Dispersion in groundwater is dependent on numerous factors, including aquifer permeability, local and regional groundwater flow patterns, chemical properties, rate of leaching from the unsaturated zone, and withdrawal rates from surrounding groundwater wells. These factors will influence the resulting shape of the contaminant plume in groundwater. Some plumes may be narrow and of limited extent, while others may be widespread, covering square miles.

Groundwater Receptors for VOC Contamination

The importance of groundwater resources underlies the need for careful assessment of the health risks of groundwater contaminants. Approximately 48% of the total population of the United States relies on groundwater as its drinking water source. The midwest and western regions are more reliant on groundwater, due to the relative lack of permanent lakes, steams, and rivers (2). Roughly one third of the urban population relies on groundwater, while nearly 95% of the rural population uses groundwater sources, supplied largely from individual domestic wells. An additional important use of groundwater is for irrigation purposes.

ASSESSING RISKS ASSOCIATED WITH VOCs IN GROUNDWATER

The adverse effect principally of concern for VOC contamination of groundwater is cancer. Cancer is of concern largely due to the scientific uncertainty over the existence of no-effect threshold for carcinogenic effects, resulting in the conservative assumption of no threshold for carcinogenicity for purposes of regulating VOCs in groundwater. Carcinogens in groundwater are not regulated in terms of concentrations producing no observable adverse effects but in terms of concentrations equivalent to acceptable risk. Public concern over cancer has mandated that regulatory agencies use extremely low acceptable risk levels in setting criteria levels for VOCs in groundwater.

The primary sources of data for evaluating the potential for adverse effects in humans from VOC contamination in groundwater are (a) epidemiologic studies of the cancer incidence associated with trihalomethanes (THMs) due to chlorination of drinking water, (b) epidemiologic studies of groundwater contamination at hazardous waste disposal sites, and (c) chronic exposure studies in laboratory animals.

These categories of data have their own set of advantages and disadvantages in assessing health risks from VOC contamination of groundwater. The THM studies best stimulate the human exposure scenario for VOCs in groundwater, which is longterm exposure to low level contamination, but do not correlate well the relationship between particular concentrations in water and observed effects. Studies of human populations near disposal sites are influenced by lack of information concerning exposure, low power due to the small populations studied, and the ability to draw only limited conclusions, due to various constraints in study design. Longterm animal bioassays potentially can establish a dose-response relationship for numerous compounds but create their own set of uncertainties in the extrapolation of results from animals to humans.

Epidemiologic Studies of Trihalomethanes in Drinking Water

Since the mid-1970s, numerous studies have evaluated cancer rates in populations served by drinking water from surface sources. The putative carcinogens were considered to be THMs (chloroform being a representative member) formed from the chlorination of surface water containing organic matter. A national survey of U.S. drinking water supplies reported the mean trihalomethane concentration was 117 μg/l, with chloroform the major constituent at a mean concentration of 83 μg/l (3). Several studies comparing chlorinated and nonchlorinated water supplies have shown associations, some statistically significant, between chlorinated drinking water and certain gastrointestinal and genitourinary cancers; however, conclusions from these studies are limited because certain confounding variables (such as cigarette smoking) were not considered. Three studies comparing measured THM concentrations with cancer mortality observed increased mortality from cancer of the bladder, large intestine, and rectum with increased THM concentrations in drinking water. In its review of these studies, the National Academy of Sciences (NAS) concluded that the results of these studies did not establish causality and that quantitative estimates of mortality associated with THM concentrations were quite crude (4).

The positive associations observed between cancer and THMs in drinking water are quite small. One example is the regression coefficients developed by Hogan et al. (5) of bladder cancer mortality and chloroform concentrations in drinking water. Assuming the presence of a causal relationship, an increased mortality from bladder cancer of $0.3/10^5$/year for males and $0.2/10^5$/year for females was associated with an increased chloroform concentration of 100 μg/l. This compares with bladder cancer mortality observed in the U.S. National Mortality Rates (1950–1969) of 6.8 (males) and 2.4 (females). The projected increases in mortality have been shown by case-control studies to be explainable by as little as a one- to two-cigarette per day difference in average cigarette consumption and are probably too small to distinguish in the presence of confounding factors (4).

A later review of subsequent studies evaluated the relationship between THMs in drinking water and cancer. The studies evaluated by the NAS provided low risk ratios, typically below 1.5–2. NAS recommended that the Maximum Contaminant Limit for THMs under the Safe Drinking Water Act be reduced from 100 μg/l; however, this was based on the results of a cancer risk assessment, not the epidemiologic evidence (6). Issues surrounding the use of cancer risk assessment for setting acceptable levels in water are discussed below.

Shy (7) has also reviewed the available epidemiologic studies, concluding that some associations found in aggregate risk studies were also observed in a few case-control studies. Exposures based on a crude measure of water quality (surface versus groundwater sources; chlorinated versus nonchlorinated sources) appeared to be associated with a small but statistically significant risk of cancer of the bladder, colon, and rectum. The studies were not consistent in finding a relationship with one or the same set of cancer sites, or in convincingly controlling for potentially confounding factors. Hence, a causal relationship between chlorinated drinking water and cancer has not been firmly established, although the results are sufficiently suggestive to warrant further research (7).

Despite these inconclusive findings, these studies perform an important role in assessing low level VOC contamination in groundwater. The results are not conclusive, but suggestive, and represent concentrations in groundwater at which elevations in cancer risks are barely detectable using epidemiologic methods. Calculating the cancer mortality potentially associated with particular concentrations in water, assuming the presence of an epidemiologic association, can be useful in calibrating cancer risk assessment methods used to develop regulatory standards representing acceptable levels of exposure.

Epidemiologic Studies of Waste Disposal Sites

Relatively few studies have been conducted evaluating the incidence of adverse effects in population living near disposal sites. These studies share many of the limitations common to epidemiologic investigation. Many are cross-sectional studies, better suited for generating hypotheses regarding causes rather than testing hypotheses. Exposure data typically are limited or inadequate; the potential is high for misclassification of exposed individuals, creating errors and uncertainties in study results. More often than not, a study is prompted by community concern over the detection of contaminations, often under considerable political pressure. This leads to examination of a vast array of possible health outcomes, often including self-reported symptoms, without any relation to the types of contaminants and concentrations present, or pathways of exposure (8). Many of the sites studied have played an important role in shaping the public debate concerning VOC contamination in groundwater; however, careful evaluation of these studies often fails to reveal trends between adverse health outcomes and contamination.

It is questionable whether the result of such "fishing expeditions" add to our understanding of the health risks posed from the disposal of hazardous wastes (8). However, a limited number of these studies are useful examples of the extent of VOC contamination in groundwater considered to be associated with adverse health effects. In Hardeman County, Tennessee, following complaints from local residents, high levels of carbon tetrachloride, hexachlorocyclopentadiene, and other chlorinated compounds were detected in samples from local wells near a landfill where 300,000 barrels of wastes from pesticide manufacturing were buried from 1964 to 1972. In 1978, residents were advised to stop consuming well water, and a two-step cross-sectional survey of 49 local residents and 57 unexposed individuals was conducted. The population previously exposed to contaminated well water showed hepatomegaly and abnormally high levels of hepatic enzymes upon initial examination. Levels of hepatic enzymes were significantly reduced during follow-up testing 2 months later. Concentrations of carbon tetrachloride detected in private wells serving the exposed individuals ranged from 61–18,700 μg/l, with a median of 1500 μg/L. The authors concluded that the findings indicated a transitory liver injury probably related to exposure to contaminated groundwater (9).

Animal Bioassays in Evaluating Risks to Humans

Toxicologic data from laboratory animals are more readily available than epidemiologic studies and have the advantage of being able to relate dose and effect. Regulatory agencies have relied heavily on animal studies for evaluating risks; however, there are two problems with this approach. First, the results of animal studies (usually rats or mice) must be extrapolated to humans. Second, doses much higher than those humans are generally exposed to must be used to obtain a dose-response relationship in a small test group of laboratory animals, requiring that effects observed at high doses must be extrapolated to low dose environmental exposures.

In assessing cancer risks to humans from animal data, when there are results from more than one valid and well-conducted bioassay, data are usually selected from the bioassay in which the most sensitive species is used (10, 11). This decision is based on the assumption that, in the absence of data to the contrary, humans should be considered as sensitive as the most sensitive species (12). Some authors have concluded that humans are roughly as sensitive or in some cases more sensitive than experimental animals (11, 13, 14). Allen et al. (15) have compared the carcinogenic potencies estimated from epidemiologic data to those estimated from animal carcinogenesis bioassays. The chemicals were all those for which reasonably strong evidence of carcinogenicity could be found in humans or animals and for which suitable data could be obtained for quantifying carcinogenic potencies in both humans and animals. This study yielded potency estimates from animal bioassays that were highly correlated with potencies estimated from epidemiologic data. The authors concluded that these findings support the general use of animal data to evaluate carcinogenic potential in humans and also for the use of animal data to quantify human risk (15).

Interspecific extrapolation is complicated by the numerous physiologic and metabolic differences that exist between rodents and humans. Physiologic differences between rats and by humans include size, life span, lack of a nonglandular stomach in rats, and differences in the volume of blood flowing to different organs. Metabolic differences include differences in basal metabolic rates, pharmacokinetics, enzyme activity levels, and receptors. These differences between species and their effects on risk assessment have been reviewed by Calabrese (16). Other differences between the animal study and human exposure situation include the route of exposure (i.e., use of gavage in dosing animals) and duration of exposure. Although it may be possible to identify test species with similarities to humans in some respects, it has not been possible to identify the similarities that are most important for comparison of long-term chronic effects, such as carcinogenicity. However, for the near future, chronic animal bioassays are likely to remain the primary source of data for evaluating chronic toxicity and carcinogenicity in humans (12).

Risk Assessment in Developing Water Quality Standards

Risk assessment serves an important function in developing water quality standards and, in large part, is responsible for the direction of federal and state regulation of groundwater contaminants. Risk assessment is defined as the characterization of the potential adverse health effects of human exposures to environmental hazards. A risk assessment results in the presentation of summary judgments on the existence and magnitude of a public health problem (17).

Risk assessments are performed to project future risks that cannot be measured directly from very low levels of chemical exposure. Risk assessments represent only an approximation of actual exposures and health outcomes, resulting in some uncertainty about the risks predicted to be associated with an exposure. Data specifically addressing factors contributing to those risks frequently are not available. These data gaps must then be bridged by using assumptions. The use of health-conservative assumptions is one approach to addressing uncertainty

in the predicted risks. Use of health-conservative methods is unlikely to underestimate chemical exposures or the associated risks.

The types of assumptions made in risk assessments used to develop standards for VOCs in groundwater include the following:

- Chemicals tend to fall into two classes: carcinogens and noncarcinogens; and
- Assessment of exposure is based on the assumptions of (a) lifetime exposure, (b) drinking water consumption of 2 liters per day, and (c) exposure normalized to a body weight of 70 kilograms.

Evidence of carcinogenicity of a chemical comes from two sources: lifetime studies with laboratory animals and human (epidemiologic) studies where excess cancer risk has been associated with exposure to the chemical. Unless evidence exists to the contrary, if a carcinogenic response occurs at exposure levels studied, it is assumed that responses will occur at all lower doses. Exposure to any level of a carcinogen is then considered to have a finite risk of inducing cancer associated with it, i.e., carcinogenic exposure is not considered to have a no-effect threshold.

Since risks at low levels of exposure cannot be measured directly by either animals or epidemiologic studies, mathematical extrapolation models are used to extrapolate from high to low doses. There is no universally acceptable scientific basis for any mathematical extrapolation model that relates exposure to cancer risk as extremely low contaminant concentrations present in the environment. The linearized multistage model procedure for low dose extrapolation is recommended by the U.S. EPA (10). Use of the linearized multistage model leads to a plausible upper limit to the risk which is consistent with some mechanisms of carcinogenesis.

The linearized multistage model incorporates a procedure for estimating the largest possible slope at low extrapolated doses that is consistent with experimental dose-response data (use of a large slope tends to produce a higher estimate of cancer risk). The animal testing data used for the extrapolation are the most sensitive species, based on the assumption that humans is equally as sensitive as the most sensitive animal species. The risk estimates made with this model should be regarded as conservative, representing the most plausible upper limit of risk. That is, the true risk is not likely to be higher than the estimate and is most likely lower.

Numerical estimates of cancer potency are presented as cancer potency slopes (CPSs). Under an assumption of dose-response linearity at low doses, the CPS defines the cancer risk due to continuous constant lifetime exposure of one unit of carcinogen concentration (in units of risk per milligram per kilogram per day).

The U.S. EPA's approach to assessing the risks associated with systemic toxicity is different from its approach to assessing the risks associated with carcinogenicity, because of the different mechanisms of action thought to be involved in the two cases. In the case of carcinogens, the EPA assumes that a small number of molecular events can evoke changes in a single cell that can lead to uncontrolled cellular proliferation. This mechanism for carcinogenesis is referred to as "nonthreshold," since there is theoretically no level of exposure for such a chemical that does not pose a small, but finite, probability of generating a carcinogenic response. In the case of systemic toxicity, however, organic homeostatic, compensating, and adaptive mechanisms exist that must be overcome before a toxic endpoint is manifested. For example, there could be a large number of cells performing the same or similar function whose population must be significantly depleted before the effect is seen.

The measurement used to evaluate health risks potentially associated with exposure to noncarcinogens is the Reference Dose (RfD). The RfD describes the principal approach to and rationale for assessing risk for health effects other than cancer and gene mutations from chronic chemical exposure. The RfD is based on the assumption that thresholds exist for certain toxic effects such as cellular necrosis, but may not exist for other toxic effects such as carcinogenicity. In general, the RfD is an estimate in units of milligrams per killogram per day (with uncertainty spanning perhaps in order of magnitude) of a daily exposure to the human population (including sensitive subgroups) that is likely to be without an appreciable risk of deleterious effects during a lifetime.

RfDs are calculated by dividing a NOEL, NOAEL, or LOAEL dose (units equal milligrams per kilogram per day) by an uncertainty or safety factor that typically ranges from 10–10,000. The acronyms ''NOEL,'' ''NOAEL,'' and ''LOAEL'' are defined as follows (18):

- **NOEL:** No observed effect level. The dose at which there are no statistically or biologically significant increases in the frequency or severity of effects between the exposed population and its appropriate control.
- **NOAEL:** No observed adverse effect level. The dose at which there are no statistically or biologically significant increases in the frequency or severity of adverse effects between the exposed population and its appropriate control. Effects are produced at this dose, but they are not considered adverse.
- **LOAEL:** Lowest observed adverse effect level. The lowest dose of chemical in a study or group of studies that produces statistically or biologically significant increases in the frequency or severity of adverse effects between the exposed population and its appropriate control.

These concepts are important in understanding the development of drinking water standards. Drinking water standards are promulgated under the authority of the Safe Drinking Water Act (SDWA). The primary standards are known as Maximum Contaminant Levels (MCLs) and are federally enforceable. MCLs are derived from Maximum Contaminant Level Goals (MCLGs), which are nonenforceable health goals set at levels at which no known or anticipated adverse effects occur, including an adequate margin of safety. MCLGs are not strictly based on RfDs but are developed from NOAELs and appropriate uncertainty factors. Differences between RfDs and MCLGs are probably due to the fact that different offices within EPA are responsible for development of the different values. MCLGs for carcinogens are set at zero, based on the assumption that the only safe dose of a carcinogen is zero (i.e., there is a finite risk at all non-zero doses). A summary of these values is presented in Table 27.2. With this assumption, estimating acceptable concentrations of carcinogens in water becomes a matter of selecting an acceptable level of excess cancer risk.

MCLs represent a pragmatic though health-conservative approach to establishing acceptable and regulated concentrations of VOCs in water. The EPA is required to set MCLs as close to MCLGs as feasible, with feasibility being based on the

Table 27.2. Risk-Based Concentrations of Selected VOCs in Water

Chemical	RfD[a]	Concentration Equivalent to Health-Based Criteria (μg/l)		
		10^{-6} Risk Level[b]	MCLG[c]	MCL[d]
Benzene		1.0	0	1.0
Chloroform		0.43		
1,2-Dichloroethane		0.4	0	5.0
Methylene chloride	2100	5.0		
Toluene	10,500		2000	2000
1,1,1-Trichloroethane	3150		200	200
Trichloroethylene		3.0	0	5.0
Perchloroethylene	350	0.7	0	5.0
Vinyl chloride		0.02	0	2.0
Xylenes	70,000		10,000	10,000

[a]Reference Dose—calculated for noncarcinogenic, systemic effects, based on a 2-l/day water consumption rate and a body weight of 70 kilograms. RfDs were obtained from the EPA *Health Effects Assessment Summary Tables* (HEAST) (22). Chemicals that do not have RfDs presented are assessed solely on carcinogenic effects.
[b]Concentration in water equivalent to a lifetime cancer risk of 1×10^{-6}, based on a 2-l/day water consumption rate and a body weight of 70 kilograms. Cancer potency slopes used in this calculation were obtained from HEAST (22).
[c]Maximum Contaminant Level Goal (23).
[d]Maximum Contaminant Level (23).

availability of control technologies and analytical detection limits. Selection of an acceptable level of excess cancer risk has proven to be a difficult exercise.

The acceptable cancer risk level of 1×10^{-6} originates from efforts by the Food and Drug Administration (FDA) to use quantitative risk assessment for regulating carcinogens in food additives in light of the zero tolerance provision of the Delany Amendment (19). The associated dose, known as a ''virtually safe dose'' (VSD), has become a natural standard used by many policymakers and the lay public for evaluating cancer risks. However, a recent study of regulatory actions pertaining to carcinogens found that an acceptable risk level can often be determined on a case-by-case basis. This analysis of 132 regulatory decisions, handed down largely during the Reagan administration, found that regulatory action was not taken to control estimated risk below 1×10^{-6} (one in one million), which are called *de minimus* risks. *De minimus* risks are historically considered risks of no regulatory concern. Chemical exposures with risks above 4×10^{-3} (four in ten thousand), called *de manifestis* risks, were consistently regulated. *De manifestis* risks are typically risks of regulatory concern. The risks falling between these two extremes were regulated in some cases, but not in others (20).

The decision to regulate cancer risk is historically a function of population size, as follows:

- Small population risks: as population risk approaches 250 cancer deaths (which could occur only in a population of the United States), the *de manifestis* risk level drops to 3×10^{-4} (three in ten thousand). Below this level, no action had ever been taken to regulate risk.
- For effects resulting from exposures to the entire U.S. population, the level of acceptable risk drops to 1×10^{-6}.

The justification typically given by regulatory agencies for deciding to regulate risks in the region between *de minimus* and *de manifestis* risks is the extent of population exposure and cost-effectiveness. Individual cancer risks above the *de manifestis* level were always regulated, regardless of cost. In the region between *de minimus* and *de manifestis*, substances with risk reduction costs of less than $2 million per life saved were regulated; substances with higher costs were not regulated (20).

SUMMARY AND CONCLUSIONS

The importance of VOC contamination of groundwater in environmental policymaking rests in (a) widespread potential for human exposure, (b) the difficulty in detecting contamination, and (c) the suspected associations between selected hazardous waste disposal sites and adverse health effects. The inability of epidemiology to detect low frequency occurrences in exposed populations, coupled with the desire to regulate contaminants proactively, has led to the use of quantitative risk assessment, particularly for the regulation of carcinogens.

The THM studies potentially represent a baseline for comparison of results obtained from risk assessments and help place VOC contamination in groundwater into a public health perspective. Some authors have raised concerns about the compounding conservatism in risk assessments and the potential for the conservative approach to distort regulation of environmental contaminants (21). The cumulative effects of specific contamination events, regulatory approaches to risk assessment, and uncertainties in assessing adverse effects from exposure to VOCs in groundwater have resulted in great public and regulatory concern and scrutiny. It is likely that health risks associated with VOC contamination are lower than typically are perceived; however, given the current state of knowledge, it is not possible to state how much lower these risks are. Despite these uncertainties, VOC contamination in groundwater will continue to have high priority in environmental regulation and in the public perceptions of environmental problems.

REFERENCES

1. Universities Associated for Research and Education in Pathology. Health aspects of the disposal of waste chemicals. Grisham JW, ed. New York: Pergamon Press, 1986.
2. Patrick R, Ford E, Quarles J. Groundwater contamination in the United States. 2nd ed. Philadelphia: University of Pennsylvania Press, 1987.
3. Williamson SJ. Epidemiologic studies on cancer and organic compounds in U.S. drinking waters. Sci Tot Environ 1981;18:187–203.
4. National Research Council. 1977. Drinking water and health. Vol 3. Washington, DC: National Academy Press, 1980.
5. Hogan MD, Chi P-Y, Mitchell TJ, Hoel DG. Association between chloroform levels in finished drinking water supplies and various site-specific cancer mortality rates. Research Triangle Park, NC: National Institute for Environmental Health Sciences. Unpublished, 21 p.
6. National Research Council. Drinking water and health. Vol. 7. Washington, DC: National Academy Press, 1986.
7. Shy CM. Chemical contamination of water supplies. Environ Health Perspect 1985;62:399–406.
8. Upton AC, Kneip T, Toniolo P. Public health aspects of toxic chemical disposal sites. Annu Rev Public Health 1989;10:1–25.
9. Clark CS, Meyer CR, Gartside PS, Majeti VA, Specker B, Balistreri WF, Elia VJ. An environmental health survey of drinking water contamination from a pesticide waste dump in Hardeman County, Tennessee. Arch Environ Health 1982;37:9–18.
10. U.S. Environmental Protection Agency. Guidelines for carcinogen risk assessment. Fed Reg 51:33992–34003.
11. California Department of Health Services. Guidelines for chemical risk assessments. Berkeley, CA: CDHS. Epidemiologic Studies and Surveillance Section, 1985.
12. National Research Council. Drinking water and health. Vol. 6. Washington, DC: National Academy Press, 1986.
13. Crouch E, Wilson R. Interspecific comparison of carcinogenic potency. J Toxicol Environ Health 1979;5:1095–1118.
14. National Research Council. Drinking water and health. Washington, DC: National Academy Press, 1977.
15. Allen BC, Crump KS, Shipp AM. Correlations between carcinogenic potency of chemicals in animals and humans. Risk Anal 1988;8:531–544.
16. Calabrese EJ. Principles of Animal Extrapolation. New York: John Wiley & Sons, 1983.
17. National Research Council, Committee on the Institutional Means for Assessment of Risks to Public Health. Risk assessment in the federal government: managing the process. Washington, DC: National Academy Press, 1983.
18. Dourson ML, Stara JF. Regulatory history and experimental support of uncertainty (safety) factors. Regul Toxicol Pharmacol 1983;3:224–238.
19. Hutt PB. Use of quantitative risk assessment in regulatory decisionmaking under federal health and safety statutes. In: Hoel DG, Merrill RA, Perera FP, eds. Risk quantitation and regulatory policy. Cold Spring Harbor NY: Cold Spring Harbor Laboratory, 1985.
20. Travis CC, Crouch EAC, Wilson R, Klema ED. Cancer risk management: a review of 132 federal regulatory cases. Environ Sci Technol 1987;21:415–420.
21. Nichols AL, Zeckhauser RJ. The perils of prudence: how conservative risk assessments distort regulation. Regul Toxicol Pharmacol 1988;8:61–75.
22. U.S. Environmental Protection Agency. Health effects assessment summary tables. First/second quarters, FY-1990. Washington, DC: Office of Solid Waste and Emergency Response, 1990.
23. U.S. Environmental Protection Agency. CERCLA compliance with other laws manual. Washington, DC: Office of Solid Waste and Emergency Response. OSWER Directive 9234.1-01. 1988.

28

Toxic Exposure and Medical Causation

John B. Sullivan, Jr., M.D.

INTRODUCTION TO MEDICAL CAUSATION

Organized methods for determining disease causation originated with endeavors to diagnose and treat bacterial infections in the 1800s. Initial investigative methods date from the 1840 concepts of the anatomist Jakob Henle. Henle's pupil, Robert Koch, refined his teacher's concepts regarding infectious diseases between 1884 and 1890 in a series of presentations before the International Congress in Berlin (1). These principles, known as the Henle-Koch postulates, became the foundation for causal thinking in terms of both chronic and acute disease. These postulates were the first systematic approach to defining a cause and effect relationship relating microorganisms to disease, and they stated the following:

The organism must be present in individuals who have acquired the disease spontaneously.

The organism must be able to be isolated from the person with the disease and cultured in the laboratory.

The isolated organism must be able to cause disease in laboratory animals similar to the disease acquired in humans.

The organism must then be able to be isolated from the diseased animal in the laboratory model (2).

The Henle-Koch postulates brought order to the analysis of disease etiology by providing rational methods of investigation and reproducibility of results. However, these postulates fall short of being able to define a causal relationship in toxic exposures: (a) They do not account for individual biologic variability with respect to threshold effects. (b) An exposure-effect relationship can be reproduced in a laboratory model, but extrapolation to human disease is difficult. (c) They defined the relationship between exposure to an agent and production of a disease in a qualitative sense only. (d) They apply in cases of a known, high, acute dose of a single agent which produces easily observable disease. The postulates do not apply to chronic exposures of multiple chemicals in unknown doses (2).

Further difficulties of applying the Henle-Koch postulates to disease were recognized by Dr. Thomas Rivers (1). Viruses could not be grown in lifeless culture media, and many different viruses could be isolated from a person with a specific disease. Association and regularity of occurrence were recognized as conditions necessary to the establishment of disease causation:

A specific virus must be found *associated* with a disease with *regularity*.

The virus must not be an *incidental* finding in the individual with the disease, but must be demonstrated to *cause* the disease (1).

Rivers also introduced the utility of biologic markers as indicators of disease or the presence of infectious agents. It was not obligatory to demonstrate the actual presence of the virus in every case of disease because biologic markers, such as anitibody titers, could be used to link an infectious agent with a disease or carrier state. In addition, Rivers corroborated the concept that asymptomatic carriers of disease could be identified through the use of biologic markers.

Rivers' studies marked the beginnings of the epidemiologic approach to disease causation and biologic monitoring. Pattern recognition and regularity of disease occurrence became important observations in studying causation. The use of epidemiologic data continued to be important in determining disease causation versus association of an agent with disease. These concepts have led to the appreciation that similar clinical disease patterns, or syndromes, can be caused by a variety of different toxic substances.

Epidemiologic concepts of disease causation were refined by Robert J. Hubener in 1957 (1). He examined serum antibody response to infectious disease and added the concepts of disease prevention with antisera and vaccines. Questions concerning the previous health status of the host and the presence of host-modifying factors became considerations in disease causation. Investigators began to focus on the multiple chemical exposure concept in disease causation and examined synergistically acting toxins, prior health status of the person, and biologic variability.

The concepts promulgated by Henle and Koch did not define a quantifiable dose-response relationship between cause and effect. Dose-response relationships of toxins to disease are now standard for chemical and drug toxicity testing. However, most occupational disease states produced by toxins cannot be defined in terms of a dose-response relationship due to the nature of the work environment. Causal thinking at this level failed to address the issue of *exposure-response* relationships where the dose is ill-defined or not known at all (3). The potential of subclinical disease produced by low level exposures over a long period of time was also not considered. Thus, defining the exposure became of paramount importance in terms of identifying toxic causation.

Technologic advances and the development of sophisticated laboratory procedures have improved the ability to define exposures to toxins and other health hazards. Studies in metabolism of chemicals to toxic metabolites further enables scientists to determine the cause of chemically related diseases. The advent of sophisticated methods of environmental monitoring added to the ability to detect exposures in the work environment. Sophistication for detecting disease was provided by the ability to assay toxins and their metabolites in biologic samples. The detection of subclinical disease using biologic markers such as *n*-acetylglucosaminidase, an indicator of renal tubular disease also enhanced early detection. Ancillary medical tests such as computerized tomography, magnetic resonance imaging, nerve conduction studies, electromyography, and pulmonary function tests also contributed to the early diagnosis of disease.

The limitations imposed by the sensitivity and specificity of laboratory measurements greatly affect the ability to detect disease states. Sensitivity is the probability of a test having a positive result in a patient with a specific disease. Multiple testing of patients with the specific disease is necessary in order to derive a sensitive assay. Sensitivity can be expressed as:

$$\frac{\text{True positives}}{\text{True positive + False negative}}$$

Specificity is the probability of having a negative test result in a patient who does not have a specific disease. Testing of patients without the disease is necessary to derive a truly specific test. Specificity is expressed as:

$$\frac{\text{True negative}}{\text{True negative + False positive}}$$

The ability to detect disease is a reflection of the sensitivity and specificity of the assay system being used as well as the patient's biologic response to the exposure.

Investigation of disease causation and work-relatedness of disease relies on the application of a combination of properly conducted epidemiologic studies, environmental monitoring, well-designed toxicologic studies, appropriate clinical evaluation, identification of risk modifiers, and accountability for interfering or contributing factors to disease.

EPIDEMIOLOGIC PRINCIPLES IN TOXIC CAUSATION

Epidemiology is the study of health and disease in populations. The purpose of epidemiology is to discover the cause of disease in order to prevent it by describing determinants of health and disease, including injury. Clinical medicine is individual-oriented; epidemiology is community- and population-oriented. Focusing on rates of morbidity and mortality, epidemiology attempts to discover the environmental and individual causes of disease (4).

Epidemiology cannot determine the cause of disease beyond a doubt. Instead, the use of epidemiologic principles helps determine an *association* between a suspected cause and a disease. Combined with clinical medicine, epidemiology can be a powerful investigative tool in discerning the probability of causation. Epidemiology examines the strength, consistency, and specificity of association between a toxin and a disease.

Such studies can help determine the association between a cause and effect by identifying hazards, testing hypotheses, elucidating dose-response relationships, evaluating measures to prevent disease, and demonstrating that preventive measures eliminate the disease. In studying diseases in populations, epidemiology attempts to discern the presence or the occurrence of a disease. Measures of disease include *incidence* and *prevalence*. Incidence refers to the rate of occurrence of new cases of disease within a defined period of time. Prevalence is the presence of all cases, old and new, expressed as a proportion or percentage of individuals in a population who have the disease at one point in time. Rates of incidence and prevalence of a disease must be adjusted for age differences within populations studied.

Epidemiologic methods can be grouped as : (a) descriptive, (b) analytical, and (c) experimental (4). Descriptive epidemiology is the study of the amount and distribution of a disease within a population: occupation, age, sex, race, social class, geographic location, work environment, exposures, habits, and other possible harmful factors that could be disease-related are

examined. Analytical epidemiology tests hypotheses of disease association using case-control studies (retrospective) or cohort studies (prospective or historical). Experimental epidemiology allows for the alteration of the subject's environment and study of the results of these alterations.

Longterm low level exposure to chemical hazards is difficult to assess in the everyday working environment and is probably the most complex cause of disease. Descriptive epidemiologic techniques are commonly employed to evaluate this problem. A hypothesis of causation is generated from descriptive data gathered, and this hypothesis is tested by analytical studies. Analytical studies commonly used to test hypotheses include (5–8):

1. Cohort studies (prospective or incidence);
2. Case-control studies (retrospective);
3. Noncurrent cohort studies (historical cohort);
4. Cross-sectional studies (prevalence).

Of these methods, cohort and case-control studies are the two most commonly employed methods to investigate the effects of chronic chemical exposure within a population.

Case-Control Studies

Case-control studies are the most commonly employed epidemiologic method used in studying occupationally related disease. Case-control studies provide savings in the expense involved with data collection and analysis. This type of investigation begins by identifying persons with a disease process and comparing them with a control population without the disease. This method appears to proceed from effect to cause. The disease group and nondisease group are then retrospectively studied with respect to exposure, duration of exposure, frequency of exposure, and other related matters. Eventually, an exposure frequency to a chemical or work situation can be established in relation to the specific disease in question as a means to compare the cases and the controls (8). The case-control method, although generally a retrospective comparison of a case group with controls, can also be a prospective study if applied to the discovery of new cases of disease compared to new controls. The case-control method selects individuals with identified disease incidence (cases) and individuals without the disease (controls) and then studies the difference in exposures (5). Case-control studies use small numbers of study subjects and short periods of time, and identify the relative risk of disease from an exposure or a work environment.

Criticisms of case-control studies must be considered. The case-control method is not effective if the exposure is commonly found among the populations, cases, and controls being studied. Arguments also center on issues of bias from the nonrandomized nature of the study (6). The cases being studied are generally selected because of a certain disease process that they have demonstrated, thus introducing a large chance for bias. Another point of criticism concerns the gathering of data on exposures. Exposures are usually obtained from medical clinic registers, job titles, disability claims, and other such "biased" lists. The use of a job title or a job description to indicate an exposure is not always valid. Workers tend to move about, even within the same employment, and job titles do not always indicate exposure duration, frequency, or intensity. The completion of health questionnaires is useful to the investigation but may provide misleading, biased information relating to exposure by the persons with a selected disease in question if not properly designated and administered. Health survey questionnaires that are self-administered should be standardized and contain questions that are unrelated to the disease being studied (8). In order to help compensate for questionnaire bias, it is useful to employ interviewers who are ignorant of the disease being studied and use controls that do not have diseases that can be associated with the exposure in question.

Cohort Studies

Cohort studies are either prospective or historical and have the same basic design (7): (a) identification and enumeration of the population to be studied, (b) identification of a comparison or reference population, (c) determination of the disease incidence through follow-up of the cohort population and, (d) comparison of disease rates between the cohort and the control population. Historical cohort studies are utilized more often than prospective studies.

The cohort study employs a defined group of a population that is exposed, may be exposed, or has been exposed to a defined level of risk from a hazard or chemical and studies the group over a period of time. This study involves large numbers of subjects, is expensive, and takes years to complete. Incidence of disease or death in the studied population is compared with that of groups with different exposures to the hypothesized cause. Cohort studies provide direct measure of risk in the exposed group versus the nonexposed group (7, 9). Relative risk (RR) is the disease rate in the exposed population divided by the disease rate in the unexposed population (5, 7, 9).

	Risk	**Disease**
	Present	Not Present
1. Exposed	a	b
2. Unexposed	c	d

$$\text{Relative risk} = \frac{(a)(d)}{(b)(c)}$$

Cohort studies generate incidence rates. The attributable risk (AR) is a term referring to the health effect produced by a particular exposure factor. The person may be exposed to multiple factors in the environment, but the attributable risk estimates the risk generated by a specific exposure. Attributable risk is calculated as follows:

$$AR = \frac{RR - 1}{RR}$$

Cohort studies may be either retrospective, the most common, or prospective, and require large study populations over lengthy periods of time.

Historical Cohort Study

The historical or retrospective cohort study involves disease and mortality evaluation of a defined population of workers in a similar exposure environment extending longitudinally from the past to the present. Follow-up, retrospective data can be added to this type of study. Conducting either a prospective or retrospective cohort study requires defining the cohort. This process can be difficult since the number of study subjects is crucial. Therefore appropriate sample size must be determined before the study. Latency periods must

be considered, and the time from the initiation of the exposure in question to the end of the study must be long enough to allow for disease development. The exposure must be high enough to sufficiently determine that the population studied was at risk. Contributing factors of multiple exposures will complicate the study. The historical cohort study is derived from records already in existence and relies on the accuracy of such records. These records must define the jobs and tasks of employees as well as their potential exposure. Employees entered into the study are identified by these records. Parameters such as age, race, sex, job description, and length of employment may be restricted.

Defining the level of exposure is crucial to any cohort study, prospective or retrospective. Retrospective studies rely on past records and past data in defining the exposure. Prospective studies rely on industrial hygiene determinations of exposure at the present as well as in the future. Proper environmental monitoring techniques are critical to the success of this study.

Defining the job task and or actual duties of the person being studied can be a complicating factor. People are mobile and jobs frequently change within the same company. Determining which jobs and tasks actually present greater risk of exposure is important to clearly define the population at risk. Excess disease and mortality may not be apparent in a large cohort study if the entire cohort is presumed to be exposed when in actuality only certain job classes were exposed. Thus, a highly exposed, small segment of workers with a high disease incidence can be missed (7, 9, 10). Characteristics such as processes, procedures, and activities of workers may actually be more important than job titles in assessing the exposure of workers. Changes in the chemicals used, introduction of safety features, and alterations of processes of production can influence the historical exposure information. Therefore, restricting the study to one facility or to a single source of data helps maintain consistency. Decisions on which workers are eligible to be included in the cohort are based on the ability to retrieve data from company records or personnel files. However, records may not be available on all workers.

The actual size of the study cohort is critical to statistical analysis of the data. Eliminating chance, that is, a false positive or type I error, in the association of an exposure with a disease is imperative. A second type of error is the false negative. This error is known as a type II error and can be more important, since disease occurrence may be missed if the exposure is felt not to be associated with the disease. Type II errors will result in continued exposure of the workers.

Another source of potential error involves the use of inadequate latency periods in the study. Latency is typically the time from the onset of an exposure to the time of some detectable outcome. In cancer studies, the latency period is typically 15—20 or more years for solid tumors and 5—10 years for hematologic cancers. Insufficient latency periods will underestimate true risks from exposures. The latency period can be affected by a mobile workforce, interchanging jobs within the same company, and insufficient exposure time to a hazard. Workers with short lengths of employment and short lengths of exposure are usually excluded from the cohort study to prevent dilution of the relative risk (7, 9, 10). Shortterm exposures can be important to include if the chemical in question is well-known and its hazard is well-defined. Inclusion of short-term exposures can then help define the true latency period required to develop disease.

Information concerning disease and mortality in cohort studies is gathered from a variety of sources. Traditionally, these sources are company files, death certificates, medical records of the individual workers, employee records, records of environmental monitoring, and local registries of disease. Death certificates, frequently used in mortality studies, may not accurately reflect the actual cause of death, and thus autopsy records and hospital records provide a valuable corroborative resource (7, 9, 10). Using the cause of death as listed on the actual death certificate introduces potential sources of error. Cohort studies should code the death according to the International Classification of Diseases (ICD) as a means of reducing error and standardizing the study (7, 9, 10).

A standardized mortality ratio (SMR) is commonly employed in cohort studies and is calculated as follows:

$$SMR = \frac{\text{Total observed deaths in study population}}{\text{Total expected deaths in study population}} \times 100$$

Age-specific death rates from a standard population are compared with the age-specific death rates in the study population. The total observed deaths in the study population are compared with the expected deaths based on the standard population's death rate. An SMR > 1.0 indicates a possible association between cause and effect. Standard mortality ratios are an indirect method of comparison and assume that the study population is standardized with respect to age, sex, and other conditions and would experience the same mortality rate as the comparison or control population. SMRs are sometimes compared with each other in studies attempting to identify the risks in similar exposures or within the same industry. This comparison can be misleading due to the difference in latency periods of the studies, differences in ages of subjects studied, length of studies, exposure characteristics, and other confounding variables. Thus when SMRs are compared, the factors of age, exposure length, and latency must be considered.

Defining disease risk in cohort studies is generally conducted by comparing a working population to a national standardized population. The standardized population is made up of both healthy and sick individuals whereas the working population is generally healthy. This appearance of the working population as being more healthy than the general population control is known as the "healthy worker effect." This can be controlled to some degree by using other working populations as the standard for comparison.

SMRs greater than 1.0 among different studies of certain industries have been used to implicate a cause and effect relationship. However, the use of SMRs to denote a health effect response or lack of response can be erroneous. In general, SMRs equal to 1.0 denote lack of increased mortality above the control population. However, an SMR equal to 1.0 does not denote lack of cause and effect. Sometimes SMRs must be compared within occupational job descriptions and actual tasks in order to bring out excess mortality that is hidden by a dilution effect of all the workers within one industry. Subgroups of workers within the study may show excess morbidity or mortality, whereas the overall SMR may not reveal any excess. The converse may also exist where an elevated SMR may not imply an association of cause and effect. The results of more than one independent study showing SMRs being greater than 1.0 usually strengthens the argument for a cause and effect relationship. However, one must be alert to the potential probability of a group of SMRs being greater than one by chance

alone (11). This probability is dependent on the total number of studies as well as on the probability that a certain study will show an excess mortality. Demonstrating a significance by chance alone must be considered when using multiple epidemiologic studies with SMRs greater than 1.0 to associate an exposure to an outcome. (11).

Cross-Sectional Studies

Cross-sectional studies examine disease prevalence in a defined population by evaluating the relationship between disease and the variables associated with the environment, such as occupational exposures to chemicals and other important factors. Cross-sectional studies are adversely affected by latency periods in disease processes as well as by the temporal factors associated with exposure preceding the disease. Also, these studies involve only living subjects; they are biased in that those subjects who might have died from the exposure before the study are not included.

PRINCIPLES OF INFERENCE IN CAUSATION

Understanding the basic principles of inference as they apply to logical and analytical decision-making is critical to investigations of toxic causation (12, 13). An example of inferential causation can be seen in the 1964 report by the Surgeon General in his report on smoking and health (14). Since then, causation has become more and more dependent on epidemiologic, inferential, and statistical information, as opposed to clinical and environmental evaluation (15). Toxicology relies on inductive progression of well-organized facts as can be found in the natural sciences. Introduction of uncertainty into the logical progression of cause and effect has clouded the issue of resolving toxic causation.

Five basic tenets of inferential causality must be examined prior to linking an agent with a disease: (a) the strength of the association; (b) the specificity of the association; (c) consistency of disease association with a particular toxin, chemical, or workplace; (d) the coherence of association; and (e) temporal relationship, or time order, of the exposure relative to the disease. The concepts of *time* and *direction* are important in linking disease to causation in persons chronically exposed to multiple chemicals in the workplace.

Strength of Association

The association between a disease and a suspected cause may range from very weak to very strong. The stronger the association, the more likely that the suspected agent is the cause. However, weak associations should not be ignored as lacking sufficient causation. The strength of an association is greatly influenced by the number of subjects in a study. Large numbers of subjects can reveal significant differences that may not appear in studies involving a small number of subjects. Commonly used measures of strength of association are the relative risk, the correlation coefficient, and regression analysis. The correlation coefficient and regression analysis are used to relate data that is quantitative in nature.

Strength of association is better defined in terms of *relative risk*. Relative risk is the incidence of a disease in a population exposed to a chemical source compared with the incidence of the disease in a nonexposed population. Relative risk allows calculation or determination of *attributable risk*, that is, the proportion of a disease associated with a cause. One method to determine disease causation is to remove the exposure and determine whether the disease incidence decreases by a certain proportion that can be attributed to the exposure. This longitudinal study requires control over confounding factors. Assigning attributable risk presents many difficulties: variability in biologic responses of individuals, the confounding factors of multiple chemical exposures, host factors of prior health and disease, and the factors of a mobile workforce.

The strength of association can be affected by a number of important factors related to defining the nature of the exposure and the population exposed. Defining the exposure is critical in determining strength of association. Bias in misclassifying exposures, omitting exposures, or not considering the presence of multiple exposures can create error in determining the strength of association in toxic causation. Timing of the dose is especially important in attempting to associate a chemical with a teratogenic effect (16). Exposures that occur at critical phases of gestation would be more influential in strengthening the degree of association. Thus studying populations exposed only at these critical gestational times will increase the strength of association (16).

Underestimating cofactors or confounding factors associated with the disease can be a major source of error (12). A confounding factor may be associated with the disease or causative of the disease in question. Controlling confounding factors in determining the strength of association is crucial to final outcome. Confounding factors must be studied for their strength of association in relation to their influence over the disease outcome. If a factor thought to be confounding is controlled in the study, and the strength of association is unchanged, then the factor is not influential or confounding (12). If a variable is not tested, then it is potentially confounding. It is less likely that a strong association will be due to a confounding factor. However, a weak association may be influenced by the confounding factor (12). Thus weaker associations require repeated testing before a causal relationship can be determined.

The exposure should thus be defined in terms of the hazard or chemical present, physical forms (vapor, liquid, aerosol, solid, radiation, infectious agent), exposure routes, dose, timing of the dose (in terms of a teratogen), confounding factors, and duration of exposure. Environmental monitoring for conditions at the time of the exposure may not always be possible.

Specificity of Association

Specificity of an association is determined by the relationship that an exposure has with the occurrence of a specific disease. Specificity ultimately refers to the ability to predict with precision that the occurrence of one variable will predict the occurrence of another (12, 13). This occurrence may be a one-to-one relationship, that is, every time the agent is present, the disease occurs. It should be noted that cause and effect observations that approach a one-to-one relationship are frequently artificial and do not absolutely predict a causal relationship.

An example would be the occurrence of peripheral neuropathy following exposure to arsenic. Peripheral neuropathy can also be caused by many other toxins such as solvents and other metals. Arsenic can also produce other disease manifestations besides neuropathies. The disease manifestation may not be specific for the toxin in question; however, the toxin in question can produce the specific disease. Toxins may have multiple effects and thus disease pattern recognition, along with sophisticated monitoring and testing, play important roles in helping to determine specific causes. The individual with peripheral neuropathy can be tested for arsenic exposure, and toxicity and solvents can be quantitated in biologic fluids and in the environment. In addition, specific chelators of arsenic can be used to treat or reverse the pathologic process. Thus specificity of disease causation can be defined in terms of results of clinical evaluation as well as by recognition of disease patterns. Specificity is the consequence of discovering causation.

Specificity of association is subdivided into specificity of *effect* and specificity of *exposure* (12, 13). Specificity of effect is defined as one cause having only one effect, a true one-to-one relationship of cause and effect. As the example above indicates, not all peripheral neuropathies (the effect) are caused by arsenic even though arsenic is a known cause. Thus specificity of effect does not by itself greatly strengthen a causal relationship. Specificity of exposure may add to the strength of causation. There are numerous diseases and disorders associated with certain exposures. For example, pulmonary disease and granulomatous processes are associated with beryllium inhalation. The fact is that similar disease states can be found with exposure to a multiplicity of dissimilar toxins and hazards. Specificity can contribute to defining toxic causation, but the absence of specific effects or specific exposures does not detract from causation.

Specificity of association depends on factors such as defining the exposure through environmental and biologic monitoring and the ability to measure the presence of disease. Thus deficiencies in environmental monitoring and lack of sophistication in detecting disease have a negative impact on specificity of association. The issue of time order of a disease must be addressed with regard to specificity of association. Did the disease precede the exposure and is the exposure now falsely leading one to implicate a causal relationship?

Consistency of Association and Reproducibility

Assigning chemical causation using inferential epidemiology demands that a definable agent or agents be associated with an observable health effect. The toxin or chemical must be available for studies in the laboratory to better define dose-response relationships, as opposed to exposure-response relationships (where the dose is unknown); human population studies over time must demonstrate a relative risk that can be attributed to the toxin or site of exposure; and the findings must be reproducible. Consistency in reproducibility adds great strength to causation. When a disease incidence is reduced to background population occurrence and recurs upon reexposure, the causal nature of the exposure is reproducible. This is a strong argument for disease causation by an exposure. However, this is not always ethically or realistically achievable. Results of studies on the rubber industry indicate that workers in curing areas have higher incidences of respiratory cancer. The actual causative agent has yet to be discovered. It would be unethical to reproduce the disease by altering engineering and industrial hygiene controls to reexpose future populations to confirm the suspected agent.

Consistent replication of results under different study conditions makes the causal association stronger. Therefore, studies confirming the existence of a disorder from multiple sources of investigation using different study designs lend strength to the consistency of association as being causal.

Coherence of Association

Coherence in disease causation refers to the support provided by existing studies and known data. That is, the scientific and medical literature supports causation through scholarly studies. These studies may be clinical, pathologic, animal toxicology studies, dose-response relationships, statistical data, epidemiologic studies, or individual case reports. Coherence of association is strengthened by previous studies indicating that the toxin or industry in question is associated with the disease process. Animal studies are frequently referenced in determining consistency of association. Extrapolation of test results from animal data to humans is difficult. Also, extrapolation of toxin-induced human disease to reproducibility in animal studies with the agent in question may not be possible. Failure to produce similar disease in animals with a suspected toxin, as found in humans, does not rule out a causal connection.

Time Order of Association

To establish the time order of disease is not always easy. The exposure must precede the disease for causation. However, with the addition of multiple confounding factors, along with a mobile worker population and multiple chemical exposures, the time order can be very difficult to establish absolutely in every case. In addition to the proper time order, the toxin or chemical must lead to the disease in question. That is, the chemical exposure must lead to a definable disease state consistent with the exposure. Again, clearly defining the exposure history in terms of onset, duration, and response is critical.

Basis to any epidemiologic principle for determining causation is that the exposure must precede the disease. This determination is influenced by various factors: (a) multiple chemical exposures over a long time, (b) multiple chemical exposures acutely at one time, (c) multiple occupations with unknown multiple exposures, (d) prior health status of the person exposed, (e) dose or lack of dose information, (f) route of exposure, or (g) the presence of cofactors or confounding factors which can give the illusion of a cause and effect relationship when in fact there is none.

TOXIC INJURY AND MEDICAL CAUSATION

Toxicologists rely on a variety of evidentiary practices to help determine causation (15): (a) structure-activity relationships of chemicals to help determine that chemicals with similar structures may have similar metabolites and toxicities; (b) shortterm screening tests for teratogenicity and mutagenicity; (c) animal studies for pathotoxicology, target organ damage, and lethal doses; (d) cohort and case-control studies; (e) clinical case reports and clinical experience; (f) computer modeling for predicting metabolites; (g) in vitro studies for toxicity testing. Toxicology is an inexact science and as such must depend on statistical data and epidemiologic evidence to infer causation. Extrapolating toxicologic studies in animal models to human conditions adds another source of uncertainty. Extrapolation of animal data to the human condition is not always feasible, and animal studies are a poor substitute for well-designed human population studies and clinical experience.

The human response to a toxin can be quite variable and can

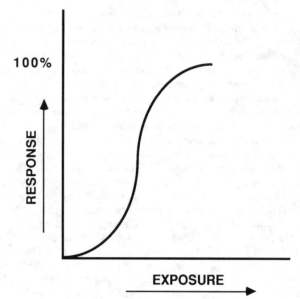

Figure 28.1.   Dose-response relationship curve.

range from nondetectable to subclinical to overt clinical pathology and recognizable disease. The Henle-Koch postulates were starting points for qualitative description of disease. Through the years, the causation concepts were refined an modified as knowledge of disease processes and methods to detect exposure outcome became more sophisticated. However, even with the most modern tools, techniques, and tests, it remains very difficult to determine probable causation in every case of disease associated with an exposure. Toxic causation can be quite apparent in some cases, such as peripheral neuropathy and pancytopenia following exposure to arsenic or pulmonary injury following chlorine gas or beryllium exposure. Causation can also be very difficult to establish, as in the case of cancer, particularly when exposures are chronic or longterm and involve multiple chemicals at low concentrations.

Three difficult aspects involved with proving causation are: (a) defining the exposure, (b) defining a response or health outcome, and (c) accounting for confounding factors or disease effect modifiers.

Defining Exposure, Dose, and Response

The ultimate goal of epidemiologic investigation is to establish a quantitative relationship between the environment, occupation, or exposure and the health effects. This relationship tends to be a curve generated by comparing quantified exposure versus the proportion of individuals with health effects. This curve reflects the variables of individual biologic variability to exposure, the agent, and the environment and expresses relative risk (3). In traditional toxicologic studies, the relationship of exposure and effect is expressed in the classic dose-response curve that compares a particular dose of an agent with a given response of the organism (Fig. 28.1). Occupational and environmental exposures frequently cannot be defined in terms of a traditional dose-response relationship. The response is tempered by a multiplicity of factors that cannot be controlled: the individual variation of the human host, the quality of the exposure, the route of exposure, and the intrinsic toxicity of the agent in question. Defining exposure in occupational environments and determining whether a true association exists between the exposure and the disease can be extremely difficult.

The human environment cannot be controlled as well as the experimental animal environment. Various dimensions of exposure as well as response to toxins may occur given the fact that humans respond differently to different exposures. There is a need to better define the threshold dose of a given toxin in the work environment so that, below a defined level of exposure, no biologic response occurs. However, individual susceptibility to exposures must always be of concern. Traditional dose-response relationships do not account for these susceptibilities (3, 17).

Three questions arise: How is dose defined in human exposure situations? What constitutes toxic exposure? How is the response detected? Dose can be described in terms of concentration of a chemical in the environment, concentration of a chemical in biologic fluids, time and magnitude of exposure, presence of toxic intermediates, and tissue concentrations of chemicals or metabolites at the target organ level. Exposure may be defined in terms of environmental monitoring, concentrations of chemicals or metabolites in biologic fluids, presence of biologic markers, concentrations in breathing zones, routes of exposure, and history. Response to exposure can be a spectrum ranging from none to subclinical target organ stress to observable disease. Response can be described in terms of tissue receptor activity, biologic markers of disease, concentration of chemicals or metabolites in biologic fluids, and pathology.

The sensitivity and specificity of tests are critical to determining the presence of a threshold response following an exposure. However, the human response to exposure can vary tremendously (18). Thresholds are controversial, since they are linked with a measured response once they are reached. However, does a response to an exposure always indicate disease? Certainly, maintaining exposures below response thresholds will help prevent disease in the majority of humans. A response to an exposure is dependent on biologic variability and other host-specific factors such as prior disease status. Due to this biologic variability and interindividual variability in humans, one human's threshold may be lower or higher than another's in terms of response to certain exposures (3, 18). Regulatory agencies assume a factor of 10 in terms of human variation in response to noncarcinogenic toxins (18).

Early detection of health effects is dependent on the ability of clinical evaluation and laboratory tests to detect this first response to stress. Occupational exposure standards and permissible exposure limits are set to prevent injury and disease to the majority of workers. Most clinical tests used in medical surveillance of workers are nonspecific and insensitive to early detection of a response to a toxic exposure. By the time a response is detected, disease has occurred. The use of environmental monitoring and biologic monitoring can help overcome this insensitivity of traditional clinical methods of surveillance. Biologic monitoring can detect exposure below the threshold of response as well as indicate environmental exposure below traditional threshold limit values and permissible exposure limits set by the Occupational Safety and Health Administration (OSHA). The question then arises as to what constitutes adverse health effects as opposed to a biologic response from an exposure.

Attempting to define exposures by job categories can be difficult. Employees may frequently change jobs in one area of an industry, and they may be involved in a variety of processes that can produce multiple exposures associated with a job category. Work areas such as well as job titles can be used to determine whether an exposure has occurred within a certain environment. Observations of actual job duties can help define cumulative exposure. Accompanied by actual industrial hygiene monitoring, these observations can be very important in defining the kinds of chemical hazards present, duration and route of exposure, and cumulative dose.

Confounding Factors and Effect Modifiers

Confounding factors are either direct or indirect factors that occur with the exposure and thus cloud the issue of causation. Confounding factors are separate, alternative causes of a disease; effect modifiers can contribute to a disease. Effect-modifying factors, such as smoking or exposure to other toxins, may contribute to or cause the disease in question separate from the initial exposure. Confounding factors and effect modifiers thus hinder the attempt to make causal connections. Confounding factors also include disease states that are present prior to an exposure. An example would be the confounding effect of a closed head injury in a worker exposed chronically to solvents. Both can produce cerebral atrophy and behavioral changes.

Work-Relatedness of Disease

The relationship of disease to an occupation can be either easily recognized or very nebulous. An easily recognized disease from an occupational toxic exposure may not be a subject for the worker's compensation system, since it is usually not contested. However, worker's compensation systems are replete with examples of cases where lack of clarity in relationships abound, expert's opinions differ, and the legal system must make the final judgment as to the cause of disease. A disease can be judged to be work-related if (a) clinical conditions exist that are compatible with known health effects of an agent or industry in question, (b) there is presently or was previously a sufficient exposure to agents in the work environment that produced health effects, (c) there is sufficient evidence that a preexisting disease was exacerbated by a present or previous exposure in the work environment, (d) the evidence supports an occupational origin.

The first step in defining work-relatedness of a disease involves establishing that a disease or health effect really exists. In many cases of worker compensation hearings, the existence of disease may be a subject of debate, and disagreement may arise in testimonies of medical experts. The second major step after establishing the presence of disease is defining the exposure that could have caused the disease and presenting evidence that the exposure led to the disease.

Evidence of exposure is sought through a combination of clinical evaluation of the worker, biologic sampling, environmental sampling, laboratory testing, and special procedures. All of these may not be possible or required depending on the nature of the case in question. Knowledge of the worker's job, including processes, chemicals used, the nature of the industry, and epidemiologic and industrial hygiene evaluations can be of great benefit in defining the worker's exposure history. The physician should endeavor to obtain a complete description of the worker's activities in the workplace. This includes daily activities, equipment and chemicals used, process and reactions near the worker's station that could potentially be a source of exposure, and exact locations where the individual works. Personal hobbies and other occupations must be explored. The use of an occupational and environmental health questionnaire can be useful in revealing work habits and exposures. The physical form of the agent is important in determining if exposure has occurred or was possible. The physical working conditions can also be important in helping to define exposure history.

Environmental monitoring and surveys can be useful in determining the kinds and qualities of exposures in the workplace. Examination of industrial hygiene monitoring data, if any has been previously performed, may help relate air concentrations to disease. However, all environmental samples must be scrutinized for accuracy and reliability. Confirmation of workplace exposure can be accomplished by environmental monitoring and sampling in the actual work site of the person. It is critical to enlist the expertise of certified industrial hygienists to avoid errors in sampling and to provide the best sampling strategy. True breathing zone samples and monitoring during identical conditions of worker activity are crucial to preventing misleading and erroneous information. Sampling under realistic conditions, appropriate timing and location of sampling devices, the use of certified laboratories to analyze data, and the use of correctly calibrated instruments all affect judgments concerning exposure relationship to health effects.

Exacerbation or aggravation of previously existing disease due to the workplace is considered to be a compensable condition. Determining that a preexisting disease has been exacerbated by an agent or exposure in the workplace can be difficult and is frequently a subject of debate among medical experts, particularly in the worker compensation courts. Clinical and laboratory evaluation may not be sophisticated enough to determine a causal relationship. The initial disease itself must be studied to determine whether its natural course can be separated from the claimed aggravation. Objective evidence may be present in terms of worsening clinical condition. Laboratory evaluation and ancillary studies may support a worsening of the disease process. The working conditions and the agent in question must also be demonstrated to produce or aggravate such disease. Conditions outside the working environment must be examined for possible causes. Drugs and other medications the worker may be taking should be examined for their contribution to the target organ toxicity or potential to cause the disease in question.

A systematic approach must be undertaken to evaluate the work-relatedness of disease and to evaluate the possible cause and effect relationship between exposure and health effects.

A Systematic Approach to Evaluate Toxic Causation

In summary, there are certain crucial steps involved in evaluating a patient with a disease thought to be caused by a chemical exposure. Ruling in or ruling out toxic causation involves detailed investigation using a logical approach combining the various principles of causation (Fig. 28.2).

DEFINE THE EXPOSURE

The exposure history should be documented as completely as possible in terms of time of occurrence, duration of exposure, intensity, and quality. It is imperative that the exposure precede the onset of illness; otherwise, there is no further argument. Determination must be made that the patient was exposed to a chemical, process, or environment that could be causative of

the disease in question. A thorough occupational and personal history must be obtained including a listing of chemicals used in the work and home environment. All potential exposure sources must be identified. A careful history of all past occupations as well as past and present hobbies is essential. The route of exposure is important. The usual routes of exposure are by inhalation, dermal contact, and ingestion. Defining the route can be very important in terms of the clinical toxicity which is manifested by the hazard or agent.

EVALUATE THE EXPOSURE-DOSE-RESPONSE RELATIONSHIP

This may not be present, or it may be difficult to judge. Doses are not always measurable in occupational situations; in such cases, the relationship between exposure and response must be evaluated. Careful questioning should include chemical exposure situations where environmental and/or biologic monitoring may have been performed. This is especially important for those chemicals whose limits of safety have been defined by threshold limit values or permissible exposure limits in the workplace. OSHA publishes such a list. The American Conference of Governmental Industrial Hygienists also has a published list of standards for a large number of toxic and potentially toxic chemicals. It must also be determined whether the dose of the exposure was sufficient to produce the patient's response. Attempts should be made to determine whether the exposure was an acute event versus a chronic or subchronic exposure.

EVALUATE THE TEMPORAL RELATIONSHIP

Does the exposure precede the disease? If not, then causation can be ruled out. Was the disease exacerbated by the exposure? This requires detailed knowledge of the pathotoxicology of the chemical in question as well as sensitive methods to detect toxicity. An example is a mechanic with preexisting liver disease who is exposed to solvents in the workplace. Exacerbation of his liver disease may be blamed on solvents. However, the disease may also be a natural progression. Sophisticated studies including adequate tissue biopsy are required to help determine whether the solvents may have some role. Environmental monitoring for airborne solvent concentrations will help define the exposure.

EVALUATE LATENCY PERIODS

Is there an identifiable temporal relationship from the time of the exposure to disease onset? Is this temporal relationship adequate for causation? Is there an adequate latency period from the time of exposure to clinical disease appearance? In terms of a carcinogenesis, the latency period is more than 15–20 years following a known exposure to a carcinogen. Appearance of cancer within a few years of exposure to a suspected carcinogen source would be highly improbable. The chronicity of the exposure must also be taken into account.

EVALUATE KNOWN ASSOCIATION OF DISEASE BY THE CHEMICAL

Information should be sought that could demonstrate a link between a chemical exposure and a disease. Medical literature research should include known industrial sites and occupations associated with the disease in question. This is particularly

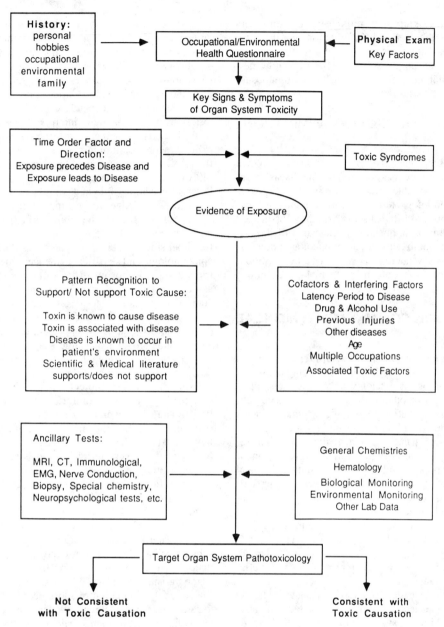

Figure 28.2. Toxic exposure diagnostic strategy.

useful if the etiologic agent is difficult to identify or if multiple chemicals are involved in the exposure. Is the chemical or drug in question known to produce the disease or to be associated with the disease? Do epidemiologic studies support the association or causation? Do animal studies support the association or causation? Have there been other case reports in the literature?

EVALUATE THE PATHOTOXICOLOGY

Is the clinical pathology or pathophysiology consistent with the chemical or drug exposure? An example would be a person exposed to benzene developing acute myelogenous leukemia versus chronic myelogenous leukemia. The pathotoxicology should be defined in terms of signs, symptoms, target organ damage, and immune system lesions. A thorough physical examination along with proper laboratory tests and ancillary spe-

cial tests are important to clearly define pathotoxicology. Toxic syndromes should be noted along with key signs and symptoms indicating organ pathology. In terms of an immune lesion, specialized laboratory investigations can be conducted to evaluate humoral-mediated immunity, cell-mediated immunity, and proper functioning of phagocytes. Medical literature searches may be an important adjunct in helping define the relationship of the lesions to the chemical or drug in question.

CONSIDER CONFOUNDING FACTORS AND RISK MODIFICATION FACTORS

Was only one chemical or drug involved? Was the patient exposed to multiple chemicals which confound the investigation? Workers are exposed to multiple agents and often move between different jobs and job tasks. Other confounding factors include dietary and nutritional status, previous health status, previous infections, family history of cancers and inherited diseases, history of smoking, and multiple occupations with varied exposures. Is there enough information to rule out a modifying or confounding cause of the disease? Secondary immunodeficiencies can be a result of nephrotic syndromes, gut malabsorption, malnutrition, malignancies, or immunosuppressive drugs.

CESSATION OF DISEASE FOLLOWS TERMINATION OF EXPOSURE

When the exposure is terminated, does the disease abate? When the person or population are reexposed, does the disease reappear? This may be impossible to determine in most exposure evaluations. In epidemiologic terms, cessation of chemical exposure to a population with the disease will prevent disease recurrence if the chemical in question is causative of the disease. Reversal of immunotoxicity or pathotoxicology upon cessation of exposure to a xenobiotic is suggestive of causation. Disease recurrence or reexposure helps to make a definitive causation argument.

TOXIC CAUSATION CONTROVERSY: MEDICAL VERSUS LEGAL

Litigation of toxic injury claims reveals differences between medicine and the legal system in decisions regarding cause and effect. Medical toxicology is a science and clinical discipline that deals with poisons or other natural or humanmade substances that cause a harmful effect to biologic or human systems or alters the normal activity of these systems. As such, medical toxicology is involved with the detection, analysis, metabolism, toxicokinetics, health effects, regulation, and prevention of harmful effects from poisons and toxins of any source. Medical toxicology as an applied science relies on epidemiologic studies, statistical analysis of data, environmental data, and analytical laboratory and clinical evaluation of patients to make decisions with respect to cause and effect relationships. The legal system renders decisions based on opinion. Thus an important part of the regulatory process regarding cause and effect stems from courts deciding on which opinion, in an adversarial system, to accept as fact.

The purpose of the legal system is to resolve disputes, whereas the purpose of medical science is to discover the facts of cause and effect involving biologic systems (19). In the civil law of torts, the plaintiff attempts to prove that the defendent caused injury and seeks compensation; the defendant rejects and resists this effort (20). The attorneys for both sides are not coalesced in a cooperative course to discover the true facts of the case, but instead are adversaries seeking to advocate their individual sides as the truth. In this adversarial system, each side attempts to persuade and convince that the preponderance of evidence is in his or her favor. Impediments to objective truth are part of the adversarial system of legal liability.

The law can reach very different conclusions from those established by medical science with respect to causation (21). A cause and effect relationship must be supported by scientific evidence; however, this evidence is not always easy to obtain with absolute certainty. Law suits have become more dependent on the use of statistical and epidemiologic data to support causation. In occupational settings, it is difficult to define exposure in quantitative, dose-response relationships. Instead, toxicologists speak in terms of risk, low level exposures, and subclinical health effects. Much confusion arises over the use of animal experimental data in extrapolating to human disease causation in toxic tort litigation. Animal studies are used for regulatory purposes, yet they cannot be used to validate human causation in toxic exposures without sufficient human clinical and epidemiologic evidence to support a causal relationship.

The legal system depends on expert witnesses to present testimony regarding their interpretations of the case and its facts. Experts must qualify on the basis of their knowledge, skill, experience, training, or experience in toxicology, and their opinions and arguments generally differ as to the probability of cause. Evidence of the experts must meet certain legal criteria to be admissible in a court (19). The legal system takes scientific knowledge of the expert witness and reduces this to opinion (19). Much of the opinion of expert witnesses in toxic tort litigation involves the use of statistical data. The attorneys for either side, as well as the court, may be uncomfortable with epidemiologic and statistical evidence. Indeed, many jurors and triers of fact do not understand that a statistically significant association does not prove a causal relationship. However, courts and juries tend to give validation to numbers and may make decisions regarding cause based on these numbers and opinions of experts. Experts present their opinions in terms of a legal standard of reasonable scientific or medical certainty or probability. Reasonable probability means that there is a 50% plus chance of a causal relationship. This more-probable-than-not standard is imprecise and troubling to a medical or scientific expert more comfortable with narrower confidence limits. The court eventually must decide which expert, when combined with the other facts and attorney arguments, to believe in settling the dispute. Thus, in a court of law, the test for plaintiff recovery in a toxic tort is not scientific certainty, but legal preponderance of the evidence (19).

The difficulty in establishing causation except by varying degrees of uncertainty helps fuel the toxic tort and liability system (23). In effect, the courts provide a regulatory practice with respect to health risks and personal injury involving hazardous materials exposures (24). Courts also tend to regulate substances based on fears of exposure and minimal risk rather than on actual disease resulting from defined exposures. Decisions arising from the legal system may have profound influence in the regulation of substances that have no propensity to cause disease at the levels of exposure claimed or at exposure levels that medical science can demonstrate.

Defining safety and risk in terms of toxic and hazardous exposures is difficult and at the crux of the disagreement between medical science and the legal system in toxic causation issues (25). Legal solutions to managing risk are much different from those proposed by medical science. The legal standard of *de minimis* is applied both by governmental regulatory agencies and by the courts to cases of human exposures to multiple chemicals and other potential hazards (25). The concept of *de minimis* is interpreted to be the smallest amount of a substance that a person (or the public) could be exposed to without fear of health risks. It is virtually a high level of safety based on a low level of risk. However, the interpretation of *de minimis* by many regulatory agencies, including the courts, may be a zero level of exposure. This zero level of exposure is unreasonable, since absolute safety cannot be guaranteed in exposure circumstances, although safety can be maximized and risk reasonably minimized. The Environmental Protection Agency, (EPA) and the Food and Drug Administration (FDA) have adopted the use of the *de minimis* principle in regulating carcinogens in order to prevent exposures to specific substances in a way that limits the health risk to virtually nothing.

The concept of *de minimis* can create individual and/or public fears once an exposure has occurred. These fears have caused governmental agencies and the courts to regulate exposures to substances not because they have proven to be dangerous, but because they create fear of cancer or fear of toxic injury. The regulatory agencies are endeavoring to quantify the level of minimal risk as one in a million over a lifetime. However, this is not an actual risk, as it is sometimes perceived to be by the public and the courts (25). This concept of acceptable risk being one in a million has been employed as a safety standard by the EPA, FDA, and OSHA to indicate a reasonable, acceptable negligible level of risk associated with an exposure. The one in a million number is derived from mathematical modeling based on multiple scientific assumptions (25).

Separating out those substances that do no harm following certain exposures from those that do harm will continue to be a difficult matter for regulatory agencies, physicians, and toxicologists. The courts will continue to apply their standards of judging fault and resolving conflict to this process of risk assessment and health effects compensation. Eventually, all sides may come together in an effort to reform the adversarial approach to deciding causation.

REFERENCES

1. Evans AS. Causation and Disease: the Henle-Koch postulates revisited. Yale J Bio Med 1976; 49:175–195.
2. Hackney JD, Linn WS. Koch's postulates updated: a potentially useful application to laboratory research and policy analysis in environmental toxicology. Am Rev Respir Dis 1979; 119:849–852.
3. Guidotti TL. Exposure to hazard and individual risk: when occupational medicine gets personal. J Occup Med 1988; 30:570–577.
4. Blumenthal DS. A perspective on environmental health. Chapter 1. Introduction to environmental health. In: Blumenthal DS, ed. New York: Springer Publishing Co, 1985:1–22.
5. Karvonen M. Epidemiology in the context of occupational health, Chapter 1. In: Karvonen M, Mikheev MI, eds. Epidemiology of occupational health. Copenhagen: World Health Organization 1986:1–16.
6. Mikheev MI. Evaluation of the long-term effects of harmful occupational factors, Chapter 4, pp. 69–79. In: Karvonen M, Mikheev MI, eds. Epidemiology of occupational health. Copenhagen: World Health Organization, 1986.
7. Pearce N, Checkoway H, Dement J. Design and conduct of occupational epidemiology studies: I. Design aspects of cohort studies. Am J Ind Med 1989; 15:363–373.
8. Pearce N, Checkoway H, Dement J. Design and conduct of occupational epidemiology studies: III. design aspects of case control studies, Am J Ind Med 1989; 15:395–402.
9. Halperin W. The cohort study, Chapter 9, pp. 149–180. In: Karvonen M, Mikheev MI, eds. Epidemiology of occupational health. Copenhagen: World Health Organization, 1986.
10. Axelson O. Case-control studies, with a note on proportional mortality evaluation, Chapter 10. In: Korvonen M, Mikheev MI, eds. Epidemiology of occupational health. Copenhagen: World Health Organization, 1986:181–199.
11. Korelitz JJ, Spivey GH, Schmidt RT. Potential for misleading associations between exposure and disease when reviewing multiple epidemiologic studies. J Occup Med 1988; 30:224–227.
12. Susser M. Rules of inference in epidemiology. Regul Toxicol Pharmacol 1986; 6:116–128.
13. Susser M. Causal thinking in practice: strengths and weaknesses of the clinical vantage point. Pediatrics, 1984; 74:842–849.
14. Surgeon General, Advisory Committee of the U.S. Public Health Service. Smoking and Health, PHS Publication No. 1103. Washington, DC: Superintendent of Documents, 1964.
15. Brennan TA. Untangling causation issues in law and medicine: hazardous substance litigation. Ann Intern Med 1987; 107:741–747.
16. Stein Z., Kline J, Kharrazi M. What is a teratogen? Chapter 2, pp. 23–66. In: Kalter H, ed. Issues and reviews in teratology. New York: Plenum Press, 1984.
17. Hatch TF. Significant dimensions of the dose-response relationship. Arch Environ Health, 1968; 16:571–578.
18. Calabrese EJ. Uncertainty factors and interindividual variation. Regul Toxicol Pharmacol 1985; 5:190–196.
19. Mitchell NR. Legal standards of causation in chemical exposure litigation. Regul Toxicol Pharmacol 1987; 7:206–216.
20. Frankel M. Causation and lawyers' causes. Regul Toxicol Pharmacol 1986; 6:89–94.
21. Harter P. The dilemma of causation in toxic torts. Regul Toxicol Pharmacol 1986; 6:103–107.
22. Gots RE. Medical causation and expert testimony. Regul Toxicol Pharmacol 1986; 6:95–102.
23. Connolly DR. Insurer perspectives on causation and financial compensation. Regul Toxicol Pharmacol 1982; 6:80–88.
24. Huber PW. Little risks and big fears. Regul Toxicol Pharmacol 1987; 7:200–205.
25. Young FE. Risk assessment: the convergence of science and the law. Regul Toxicol Pharmacol 1987; 7:179–184.

29

Legal Causation in Toxic Tort Litigation

William Powers, Jr., J.D.

INTRODUCTION

The law's concept of causation is often a source of consternation and confusion for scientists who encounter toxic tort litigation. Scientists, who usually deal with broad statistical correlations and probabilistic evidence, often complain that the law's seemingly talismanic concern about particularized causal links in individual cases produces naively unscientific and callously unjust results (1). Some lawyers have expressed similar concerns (2).

We should not be surprised that debate about causation is heightened in cases involving longterm exposure to toxic substances. Causation is formally a requirement in all personal injury litigation, but in most cases it is not a source of great controversy. In toxic tort litigation, however, the alleged link between a toxic substance and a plaintiff's injury is often attenuated. Several years or even decades might separate the exposure and the injury's manifestation. Because causation is frequently hotly disputed in toxic tort litigation, the choice among different approaches to causation, which might be inconsequential in most tort litigation, can be critical.

Some of the confusion and consternation about the law's concept of causation is due not to the concept itself; it is due to imprecise thinking about various aspects of causation and their relationship to other elements of a lawsuit. The discussion that follows attempts to clarify the role causation plays in tort litigation generally and in toxic tort litigation specifically.

THE RELATIONSHIP BETWEEN CAUSATION AND OTHER ELEMENTS OF A PERSONAL INJURY LAWSUIT

One source of confusion is a failure to distinguish causation from other elements of a personal injury lawsuit. The details of tort law are extremely complex. All cases, however, present three basic questions: (a) did the defendant engage in tortious (legally wrong) conduct, (b) did the plaintiff suffer a legally cognizable injury, and (c) did a causal link exist between the defendant's tortious conduct and the plaintiff's injury? For a plaintiff to recover damages, the court must answer all three questions affirmatively; causation is a necessary but not sufficient element of the plaintiff's case. A failure to distinguish the question of causation from the other two questions can create a misapprehension about the role causation plays in personal injury litigation. Specifically, a court's failure to impose liability on a defendant should not be understood to be a failure to find causation. It is at least as likely to represent a finding that the defendant did not do anything legally wrong or that the plaintiff did not suffer a type of injury that the law protects.

Tortious or legally wrong conduct comes in a variety of forms. Depending on the circumstances, the plaintiff must prove that the defendant *intentionally* caused the plaintiff's injury, *negligently* caused the plaintiff's injury, or engaged in conduct that is subject to *strict liability*. Accordingly, "tortious conduct" is not always synonymous either with "fault" or with "conduct that caused injury." Legally cognizable injuries also come in a variety of forms, the most common of which are personal injury and property damage. Several types of "real" harm are not protected, especially when the defendant did not intentionally cause the harm. For example, horrified bystanders who watch an airplane crash usually cannot recover for their emotional injury. Nor can a business executive normally recover lost profits because the crash closed the airport and prevented him or her from attending an important meeting. Again, when a court denies recovery on the ground that the defendant did not engage in tortious conduct or on the ground that the plaintiff did not suffer a legally protected injury, its ruling should not be misinterpreted as a conclusion that the defendant's conduct did not "cause" the plaintiff's injury.

Our propensity to confuse causation with other elements of a lawsuit is exacerbated by the fact that we often use "causation" in everyday language as a synonym for "responsibility." When two cars collide we often ask, "Who caused the collision?" as the equivalent of asking, "Who should we hold responsible, and for what?" But according to the law's concept of causation, both motorists "caused" the collision. The issue of responsibility depends on issues other than causation.

THE COMPONENT PARTS OF LEGAL CAUSATION

Even if causation is distinguished from other issues in a lawsuit, a second source of confusion is a failure to separate the multifaceted concept of causation into its component parts. What lawyers call the "causation" issue in personal injury litigation covers two very different inquiries. The plaintiff must prove that the defendant's tortious conduct was both a "cause-in-fact" and a "proximate cause" of his or her (legally cognizable) injuries. Courts sometimes refer to "cause-in-fact" as "actual cause," and they sometimes refer to "proximate cause" as "legal cause." To make matters worse, courts sometimes use the term "proximate cause" (or "legal cause") as an umbrella to cover *both* the "cause-in-fact" and "proximate cause" aspects of the inquiry, and sometimes they use the term to refer only to that part of the inquiry that is separate from "cause-in-fact." Irrespective of the nomenclature, however, all courts divide the overall issue of causation into these two fundamentally different inquiries.

Cause-in-fact is a true causation issue; proximate cause is not. Proximate cause is a policy determination about the scope of the defendant's liability, even when his conduct was tortious and did, in fact, cause the plaintiff's injury. The law of proximate causation is extremely convoluted. The core of proximate causation, however, depends on foreseeability. Unforeseeable results, though in fact caused by the defendant's tortious conduct, are generally beyond the scope of proximate causation. For example, a person who wrongfully places rat poison on a food counter would be liable to someone who ate contaminated food, but he would not be liable for a fire caused by the poison's unexpectedly igniting (3). Poisoning, not fire, is the foreseeable risk that causes us to condemn placing rat poison on a food counter. Courts would reflect this judgment by denying liability through a finding of no proximate causation. Such a policy judgment would not, however, reflect a conclusion that the defendant's conduct was not a cause-in-fact of the fire.

This discussion merely scratches the surface of proximate causation. It is sufficient here to note that proximate causation is not a true causation issue at all. It is a policy judgment concerning an assignment of responsibility in cases where the defendant was, in fact, a cause of the plaintiff's injury. Again, it is wrong to conclude that a denial of liability on the ground of proximate causation has anything to do with what scientists would consider to be a true issue of causation.

CAUSE-IN-FACT

Having clarified the role actual causation plays in tort litigation, we can evaluate the law's concept of actual causation and compare it to the concept of causation used by scientists. Even here, however, it is important to distinguish among three different legal issues: (a) the *concept* of actual causation, (b) *proof* of actual causation, and (c) the *result* that the defendant's conduct must have caused. In fact, most of the controversy over the law's use of actual causation in toxic tort cases focuses on the last two issues, not on the basic *concept* of actual causation.

The Concept of Causation

The basic concept of cause-in-fact is defined by the "but for" or "*sine qua non*" test. Under this test, if a plaintiff's injury would not have occurred in the absence of the defendant's tortious conduct, the defendant's tortious conduct was a cause-in-fact of the injury. This definition is purely operational. It does not, as one commentator has claimed, commit the legal system to a "Newtonian" or "corpuscular"—rather than "probabilistic" or "quantum mechanical"—view of causal mechanisms (4). In fact, the "but for" test does not imply anything about the metaphysics or underlying mechanism of causal links.

As a conceptual definition of actual causation, the "but for" test works well in the overwhelming majority of cases. In one type of case, however, it does not correspond to our intuition. In some cases a result is "overdetermined," meaning that either of two (or any more than two) antecedent conditions would have been sufficient to bring about the result. The most common example in tort literature is two independent fires, both of which approach a house and either of which would be sufficient to burn it down. Neither fire is a "but for" cause of the house's catching fire, because the other fire would still have burned the house. Nevertheless, our intuition tells us that each fire was a cause of the house's burning down. The law accomplishes this result through the "substantial factor" test of causation.

Some courts use the term "substantial factor" as an umbrella term to refer both to the "but for" test and to whatever (unnamed) test tells us causation exists in overdetermined situations. Most courts, however, use the term to refer only to overdetermined situations. The substantial factor test does not, however, mean that a "but for" cause must also be "substantial." All "but for" causes are considered to be actual causes of a result, irrespective of their triviality. Consequently, all results have multiple "but for" causes under the law's concept

of actual causation. The law then uses the requirements of tortious conduct, *proximate* causation, and a legally cognizable injury to determine whether the defendant's conduct should bear the responsibility.

A great deal of philosophical debate has focused on the precise definition of causation that accounts for our intuition in cases of overdetermined results. A common definition formulation is the "NESS" test of actual causation. Under the "NESS" test, an antecedent is an actual cause of a result if it is a *necessary element* of a *sufficient set* of conditions to bring about the result. Even this test leaves some paradoxical cases unresolved, but it is a sufficiently coherent conception of actual causation to handle all but the rarest of legal disputes (5). For our purposes, debate over the law's concept of causation in toxic tort litigation, which centers on the probabilistic nature of epidemiological evidence, does not depend on the philosophical ambiguities of causation in some of these rare cases of overdetermined results.

A more significant issue is whether a *probabilistic* conception of cause-in-fact would be more appropriate than the "but for" test, even in cases not involving overdetermined results. It is important here to distinguish between two different ways probabilities can affect the issue of causation in tort litigation. One way is a *conception* of causation that competes with the "but for" test. Another way is as a method of *proving* that the "but for" test has been satisfied. A failure to distinguish between these different issues has been a source of confusion. Sometimes, a proponent of a probabilistic *conception* of cause-in-fact actually is more concerned with the use of probabilistic evidence to *prove* cause-in-fact. Nevertheless, some courts and scholars have suggested a probabilistic *conception* of causation, which might be attractive to epidemiologists who are comfortable dealing with probabilities.

A case suggesting a probabilistic conception of causation is *Herskovits v. Group Health Co-Op* (6). By negligently failing to diagnose his patient's lung cancer, a physician reduced the patient's chance of survival from 39% to 25%. The patient died, and his estate sued for wrongful death.

Two justices held that the plaintiff's statistical evidence established a causal link between the misdiagnosis and the death, notwithstanding the fact that the patient probably would have died anyway. Had the doctor's misdiagnosis reduced the patient's chances of recovery by 51% or more, these justices could have held that, more likely than not, the patient would not have died "but for" the misdiagnosis. This would have amounted to using probabilistic *proof* of "but for" causation, but it would have been consistent with the "but for" *concept* of causation. But, given the *actual* statistics in the case, the two justices' conclusion was incompatible with the "but for" concept of causation. It could be explained only by a probabilistic concept of causation, whereby any antecedent that (significantly) increases the probability of a result constitutes a cause-in-fact of that result (presumably if the result actually does occur) (7).

A few judges and commentators have urged courts to use the probabilistic concept of causation adopted by the two justices in *Herskovits* (8), but most courts have declined to do so and have continued their adherence to the "but for" test. In fact, the majority of justices in *Herskovits* rejected the two justices' probabilistic concept of causation.

Notwithstanding the probabilistic language of epidemiology, most epidemiologists also seem to rely on a "but for" *concept* of causation. When an epidemiologist cites statistics that exposure to a certain substance increases the risk of disease by 10%, he or she seems to *mean* that "but for" the presence of the toxic substance, the "increased risk" would not have occurred. Similarly, if epidemiological statistics demonstrate that the 10% increase in the risk of disease produces 100,000 additional annual cases of the disease, the statistics seem to *mean* that "but for" the presence of the toxic substance, the 100,000 additional cases would not have occurred.

The Result the Defendant's Tortious Conduct Must Have Caused

Even if epidemiologic statistics show that a toxic substance causes, in the "but for" sense, 100,000 annual cases of a disease, we might still conclude that the disease in any one individual was not, more likely than not, caused by exposure to the toxic substance. These seemingly contrary conclusions do not depend on different *concepts* of causation. Their difference flows from the different *results* to which the "but for" test is being applied. Statistics can justify a belief that *one* result ("increased risk" or "100,000 aggregate cases") was caused, in the "but for" sense, by the toxic substance, but that *other* results (a single case of disease) was not. The result in the individual case is due to the fact that in our legal system, "increased risk" or "aggregate results" normally are not legally cognizable injuries. It is not due to a different *concept* of causation than was used to interpret the aggregate epidemiologic evidence.

The importance of distinguishing between the *concept* of causation and the *result* the defendant's conduct must cause is highlighted by further examination of *Herskovits*. Contrary to the reasoning of the two justices discussed above, three other justices held that the plaintiff had not proved that the defendant's misdiagnosis had caused the decedent's death. But these three Justices also held that the plaintiff could recover for a "lost chance" (14%) of survival. This injury, these justices reasoned, was worth 14% of the value the court would have assigned to the lost life, and it was caused, in the "but for" sense, by the physician's misdiagnosis. These justices were willing to redefine what constituted a legally cognizable injury without altering the basic *concept* of causation under the "but for" test.

A court could use similar reasoning to define an increased risk of a disease as a legally cognizable injury in toxic tort cases. Of course, a court would then have to place a value on *that* injury, which would be less than the value of contracting the disease. Again, the issue here is not primarily the concept of causation, it is the definition of legally cognizable injury.

Proof of Causation

A final area of controversy and confusion is the type of proof courts will accept to prove cause-in-fact. Even if courts agree on the "but for" test as a nonprobabilistic *concept* of causation, they cannot escape the fact that probabilistic evidence is relevant to *prove* causation. Thus, courts have had to grapple with the use of statistics and expert scientific testimony to prove causation. The treatment various courts give to statistical evidence gives the (sometimes accurate) appearance that courts accept evidence scientists would consider dubious and reject evidence scientists would consider sound (9).

The use of statistical evidence is not unique to the issue of causation. Any issue in a lawsuit can raise problems of statistical proof and expert testimony. The use of paid experts on each side of a lawsuit is undoubtedly unseemly to scientists devoted to an unbiased search for truth. Indeed, the practice is not without controversy within the legal community. But it is a problem of the adversary process and of litigation generally, not of the law's specific treatment of causation.

Burden of Proof Understanding the law's treatment of statistical evidence and expert witnesses requires an understanding of the legal concepts of "admissibility" and "burden of proof." In civil cases, the plaintiff must prove his or her case by a preponderance of the evidence. This means that the plaintiff must prove each element "more likely than not." Thus, probabilities are built into the system of legal proof, even if they are not part of the *concept* of causation.

With complicated exceptions, any relevant evidence is generally *admissible*, meaning that it can be put into evidence for the jury's consideration. Of course, jurors are usually not scientists, and they can make naive decisions about statistical evidence or expert testimony. The naiveté of jurors can be a serious problem in any litigation involving technical issues, but it is a general problem, not one unique to the issue of causation.

A separate and more difficult issue is whether statistical evidence is enough, standing alone, to have a case submitted to the jury. This issue depends on the "burden of proof." For every issue in a lawsuit, one party has the burden of coming forward with evidence that can support a jury finding on that issue. The jury can usually choose to disbelieve evidence, and if the record contains conflicting evidence, the jury usually resolves the issue. But the judge determines as a preliminary matter whether the party with the burden of proof has met that burden by coming forward with at least some credible evidence. If the party with the burden of proof does not meet it, the judge is supposed to grant a directed verdict to the opponent. On most issues, the burden of proof is on the plaintiff, though occasionally the burden is on the defendant.

The burden of proof serves an administrative role in civil litigation. "Correct" decisions depend *both* on the decisionmaker making a good decision on the available information *and* on the decisionmaker having an adequate amount of information upon which to base the decision. The burden of proof assigns the responsibility for gathering a minimally acceptable *amount* of information and presenting it to the decisionmaker.

An important question in civil litigation is whether purely statistical evidence is sufficient to satisfy a plaintiff's burden of proof and thereby justify having a case submitted to the jury. Of course, if the statistics themselves do not show a fact existed "more likely than not," the evidence is insufficient. But even if the statistics support an inference "more likely than not," a court might require additional "particularistic" evidence. This seems irrational from the perspective of making the best decision on the available evidence, but courts that require traditional evidence undoubtedly understand this. Their reason is different; it is to encourage the party with the burden of proof to gather more information ad present it to the court.

Courts seem to fall into two camps on the burden of proof (10). Under one view, the plaintiff need only introduce evidence that tends to show more likely than not that the fact alleged existed (here a causal link under the "but for" test). Under this view, often called the "weak view," purely statistical evidence is sufficient to have an issue submitted to the jury, as long as the evidence tends to show the fact "more likely than not.'' Under the second view, often called the ''strong view,'' the plaintiff is *also* required to introduce some further evidence of the alleged fact.

Whether or not the strong view is meritorious, its justification is *not* that probabilities alone cannot create a sound belief (11). It is, instead, that the proponent has not fulfilled his or her obligation under the burden of proof to gather information and present it to the trier of fact.

In fact, a rigid division between the weak view and the strong view is misleading. Courts are increasingly willing to accept purely statistical evidence when the proponent on an issue does not have reasonable access to particularistic evidence. But courts that adhere to the strong view do occasionally keep a case from the jury even when purely statistical evidence would support a finding of the alleged fact.

Expert Witnesses. Statistical evidence is almost always introduced in conjunction with the testimony of an expert witness. The use of expert witnesses is usually governed by the concepts set forth in Rules 702 through 705 of the Federal Rules of Evidence. These Rules apply to federal courts only, but most states have identical or very similar rules. The relevant Rules are as follows:

Rule 702. *Testimony by Experts.*

If scientific, technical, or other specialized knowledge will assist the trier of fact to understand the evidence or to determine a fact in issue, a witness qualified as an expert by knowledge, skill, experience, training, or education may testify thereto in the form of an opinion or otherwise.

Rule 703. *Bases of Opinion Testimony by Experts.*

The facts or data in the particular case upon which an expert bases an opinion or inference may be those perceived by or made known to him at or before the hearing. If of a type reasonably relied upon by experts in the particular field in forming opinions or inferences upon the subject, the facts or data need not be admissible in evidence.

Under these rules, duly qualified experts can testify about a wide range of technical topics, including statistical evidence. They can even give an opinion on an ultimate legal issue, such as causation.

Supposedly, experts help the jury understand technical material that would otherwise be beyond the jury's comprehension. In practice, the adversarial system encourages each side to hire experts in an attempt to persuade the jury toward its own side. Cross-examination by an opposing attorney is a partial safeguard, but juries undoubtedly make mistakes interpreting statistical evidence, even with the 'help'' of experts.

The problem of jurors' lack of sophistication regarding statistical evidence, even with the help of experts, is significant in toxic tort cases involving questions of causation. Lay jurors may not be well-suited to confront the technical nature of causation in toxic tort litigation, and scientists are understandably frustrated to see objective data manipulated in an adversarial process. It is beyond the scope of this survey to analyze possible alternatives to the use of juries to resolve these technical issues. But it is important to understand that *this* problem, as significant as it may be, is a problem of expert testimony and scientific evidence that is not confined to the issue of causation. More specifically, it is certainly not a product of the law's *concept* of causation.

MULTIPLE TORTFEASORS

Divisible and Indivisible Injuries

Special problems involving causation can arise in cases involving multiple tortfeasors. These problems are often acute in toxic tort litigation.

Sometimes a plaintiff sufferers a truly indivisible injury caused jointly by two or more tortfeasors. An example is when one defendant pushes a pedestrian into the street and another defendant then hits the pedestrian with a car. Each defendant in such a case is a ''but for' cause of the entire injury; the injury cannot even theoretically be divided. Under the traditional view of such cases, each defendant is ''jointly and severally'' liable for the injury, meaning that the plaintiff can recover the entire damages from either of them, though the plaintiff cannot recover more than once (12). A joint tortfeasor who pays the plaintiff's entire damages under joint and several liability can then recover ''contribution'' from the other tortfeasor. Joint and several liability normally applies only to indivisible injuries; it does not normally apply to cases in which multiple defendants each cause a portion of a divisible injury.

Sometimes, however, a plaintiff suffers theoretically divisible injuries caused by two or more tortfeasors, but the plaintiff cannot prove which one caused which part of the injury. A common example is where two or more defendants pollute a single body of water (13). Unless the various defendants were acting as a group or were otherwise responsible for each other's conduct (thereby creating ''vicarious liability'') the traditional rule required the plaintiff to prove causation against each defendant independently. If the plaintiff could not prove which defendant caused which part of the injury, the plaintiff could not recover anything.

Most courts now relax or shift the burden of proof to give plaintiffs some relief from the problem. The most common solution is to shift the burden of proof to the defendants to sort out which of them caused which part of the injury (though the plaintiff must still prove that each defendant caused some of the injury) (14). If a defendant cannot sort things out, it is liable for the entire injury, as though it had caused it all. This burden-shifting device effectively treats theoretically divisible but practically indivisible injuries as though they were theoretically indivisible and applies joint and several liability to them.

A less common solution is to relax the plaintiff's burden of proof but not eliminate it entirely. Under this approach the jury is permitted to make its best estimate of the portion of injury each defendant caused. In a pollution case, for example, a jury might divide the damages roughly according to the volume of each defendant's emissions. Failing all else, the jury can divide the damages on a pro rata basis (15). Under this approach, each defendant is *not* jointly and severally liable for the other tortfeasors' shares.

Given the different treatment courts give divisible injuries and indivisible injuries, it is especially important in toxic tort cases to identify carefully the type of causation problem. For example, if two pollutants cause emphysema, one causing some disease and the other causing more disease, the damages are theoretically divisible but practically indivisible. Thus, depending on the jurisdiction, the plaintiff would have to prove either which pollutant caused which portion of the injury or rely on one of the burden-shifting or burden-relaxing devices.

If, on the other hand, the two pollutants work together to cause an injury neither alone would have caused, each would be a "but for" cause of the entire, indivisible injury. Consequently, each defendant would be jointly and severally liable for the entire injury (16). Accordingly, to determine the legal consequences of a toxic exposure, a court must determine not only *whether* a causal link exists, but also the type of causal link.

Market Share Liability

Another problem involving causation in tort litigation generally and in toxic tort litigation specifically is when a plaintiff suffers a single, indivisible injury but cannot prove which of several possible defendants was the actual culprit. A famous example is *Summers v. Tice* (17). Two hunters each negligently shot toward the plaintiff, who was hit by a pellet of shot. The shot clearly came from one of the guns, but the plaintiff could not prove which one. The court gave the plaintiff relief by shifting the burden of proof on causation to the defendants. When neither defendant could prove which gun was the source of the shot, each was held jointly and severally liable.

The most common example of this problem is when a drug causes a side effect and the victim cannot identify the manufacturer of the particular lot. This is an acute problem for drugs whose side effects have a long latency period. Some courts have given the plaintiff relief in this situation, though most courts continue to follow the traditional rule by requiring the plaintiff to prove which manufacturer sold the particular drug. The most common form of relief, for those courts that give relief, is the "market share" theory. Subject to some complicated procedural requirements, under this theory a plaintiff can recover a percentage of his or her damages equal to each manufacturer's share of the relevant market (18). This approach is similar to the "lost chance" cases discussed earlier. The plaintiff can recover from each defendant on the basis of probabilistic evidence less than more likely than not, but the damages are reduced proportionately. Although several courts have adopted the market share theory, several others have reject it (20). It is still too early to tell whether the market share theory will gain wide acceptance.

CONCLUSION

The role of causation in toxic tort litigation is controversial and complex. Most of the controversy focuses on proof of causation, not on the underlying concept of causation. Debate over the role of causation in toxic tort litigation is clarified by distinguishing among (a) the concept of causation, including the difference between cause-in-fact and proximate cause, (b) legally cognizable injuries that are compensable, and (c) problems of proving causation. With these distinctions in mind,

scientists may still object to the law's use of causation in toxic tort litigation and may still disagree with the policies the law seeks to advance. But the source of the disagreement will be more focused, and confusion about the role causation plays in toxic tort litigation can be avoided.

REFERENCES

1. *See e.g.*, Brennan, Untangling causation issues in law and medicine: hazardous substance litigation. Ann Intern Med 1987;107:741.

2. *See* Rosenberg, The causal connection in mass exposure cases: a "public law" vision of the tort system. Harvard Law Rev 1984;97:851.

3. *See* Larrimore v. American National Insurance Co., 184 Okla. 614, 89 P.2d 340 (1939).

A leading case addressing this approach to proximate causation is Overseas Tankship Ltd. v. Morts Dock & Engineering Co., [1961] A.C. 388, [1961] 2 W.L.R. 126, [1961] All E.R. 404 (1961). The defendant's ship negligently spilled bunker fuel into Sydney Harbor. Bunker fuel is designed not to burn when spread on water. Though it was foreseeable that the fuel would pollute the harbor, it was not foreseeable that it would burn. Nevertheless, the fuel ignited and burned the plaintiff's dock. The court held that although the defendant's conduct was a *cause-in-fact* of the fire, it was not a *proximate* cause of the fire. It was a proximate cause only of the pollution.

A small minority of courts do not define proximate causation primarily with reference to foreseeability. *See, e.g.*, Dellwo v. Pearson, 259 Minn. 452, 107 N.W.2d 859 (1961).

4. Brennan T., Untangling causation issues in law and medicine: hazardous substance litigation. Ann Intern Med 1987;107:741.

5. For a brief discussion of "overdetermined result" cases and a claim that no explicit test improves on our intuition in cases not covered by the "but for" test, see Robertson D., Powers W., Anderson D. Cases and materials on torts. West Publishing Co., St. Paul, MN: Stanford Law Rev 1956:9(60);88–90.

6. 99 Wash. 2d 609, 664 P.2d 474 (1983).

7. The other judges who voted for liability used the "but for" concept; they concluded that the diminution of the patient's survival chances (rather than the death itself) was the legally compensable injury in the case.

8. For a survey and criticism of these suggestions, see Wright R., Actual causation vs. probabilistic linkage: The bane of economic analysis. J Legal Stud 1985:14;435.

9. *See, e.g.*, Gots R., Medical and expert testimony. Regul Toxicol Pharmacol 1986:6;95.

10. Rosenberg D. The causal connection in mass exposure cases: a public law vision of the tort system. Harvard Law Rev 1984:97;851.

11. *But see* Wright R., Causation, responsibility, risk, naked statistics, and proof: pruning the bramble bush by clarifying the concepts. Iowa L Rev 1988:73;1001.

12. Joint and several liability also applies to cases in which each of two or more joint tortfeasors constitutes an independently sufficient cause (that is, a "substantial factor" cause) of an indivisible injury.

13. *See, e.g.*, Landers v. East Texas Salt Water Disposal Co., 151 Tex. 251, 248 S.W.2d 731 (1952).

14. *See, e.g.*, Landers v. East Texas Salt Water Disposal Co., 151 Tex. 251, 248 S.W.2d 731 (1952).

15. *See, e.g.*, Loui v. Oakley, 50 Haw. 272, 438 P.2d 393 (1968).

16. If either pollutant alone is sufficient to bring about the injury, each is a "substantial factor" cause of the entire injury. Because the injury again is indivisible, each defendant would be jointly and severally liable.

17. 33 Cal.2d 80, 199 P.2d 1 (1948).

18. *See, e.g.*, Sindell v. Abbott Laboratories, 26 Cal.3d 588, 607 P.2d 924, 163 Cal. Rptr. 132 (1980).

19. *See, e.g.*, Mulcahy v. Eli Lilly & Co., 386 N.W.2d 67 (Iowa 1986). *Mulcahy* ultimately rejects market share liability, but the court's analysis provides a good introduction to the arguments on both sides of the issue.

Emergency Medical Response and Hazardous Materials

30

Toxicologic Disasters: Natural and Technologic

Lee M. Sanderson, Ph.D.

NATURAL DISASTERS WITH TOXIC CONSEQUENCES

Introduction

A natural disaster results from natural environmental hazards which cause widespread damage to the environment and/or its residing population. These disasters usually, but not always, occur suddenly or at least over a relatively short period of time. Natural disasters include phenomena associated with subterranean stress (for example, erupting volcanoes and earthquakes), surface instability (rock slides, mud slides, and avalanches), high winds (hurricanes and tornadoes), and abnormal precipitation or temperature (floods, blizzards, heat waves, and droughts).

The actual documentation of public health impacts from toxic consequences of natural disasters is extremely limited. Based on existing published literature, those disasters presenting the largest risk of actual or potential toxic consequences include erupting volcanoes, floods, and earthquakes.

Volcanoes

Approximately 80% of the 500 active volcanoes around the world are classified as "explosive" (1, 2). Almost 10% of the world's explosive volcanoes are located in the western United States and Alaska (3). This category of volcano erupts suddenly and emits large quantities of ash. "Effusive" volcanoes release large amounts of lava and gas but little ash. "Mixed" volcanoes exhibit both explosive and effusive characteristics. The toxicologic risks of volcanic eruptions are associated with pyroclastic flows, gases, and ashfalls.

Pyroclastic flows consist of a mixture of rocks, pumice, ash, and hot gases. The predominant health effects from exposure to pyroclastic flows include asphyxiation and inhalation injury.

With references to gases, the chief volatile emissions include hydrogen sulfide, sulfur dioxide, carbon dioxide, hydrogen chloride, hydrogen fluoride, hydrogen, helium, and redone. Polynuclear aromatic and halogenated hydrocarbons may also be present (4). Plume analysis of the eruption of Mount St. Helens also identified quantities of carbonyl sulfide, carbon disulfide, and nitrogen dioxide (5). Released gases may be asphyxiants or respiratory irritants. Since the flow of dense, asphyxiant gases is largely determined by gravity, people and animals in valleys or low areas contiguous with the erupting volcano are at greatest risk. Carbon dioxide caused the asphyxiation of 142 people from the eruption of Dieng Plateau, Java, in 1979 (6), 37 people from the underwater eruption of Lake Monoun, Cameroon, in 1984 (7), and 1700 people from the underwater eruption of Lake Nyos in 1986 (8). One of the most important irritant gases is sulfur dioxide, an air pollutant common in many parts of the world. Sulfur dioxide released during volcanic eruptions may result in health effects ranging from subclinical airway constrictions to asthma and bronchitis. Increases in hospitalized pediatric cases of asthma were observed following the 1979 eruption of La Soufriere in St. Vincent (9). Study of the Masaya volcano showed the principal gases of health concern were sulfur dioxide (emission of 1300 metric tons per day), hydrogen chloride (400 tons per day), and hydrogen fluoride (5 tons per day) (10). Populations located downwind may be exposed to sulfur dioxide concentrations (1 parts per million [ppm]) that exceed the World Health Organization (WHO)-recommended maximum level of 0.05 ppm (11). Deaths in Japan from hydrogen sulfide and in Iceland from carbon monoxide have been documented (12, 13).

With respect to ashfalls, ash particles can serve as vehicles for gases and other volatiles, which may then be washed off by rains onto crops and into bodies of water, potential affecting quality of potable water and food. Fine ash particles may have irritation effects on the lungs and eyes. Following the Mount St. Helens eruption, tests for leachable elements (for example, fluoride) were negative. In contrast, following Icelandic eruptions in 1947 and 1970, elevated fluoride levels (9 ppm) were found in streams (14). Fluoride poisoning in animals eating ash-laden vegetation has been described (15).

The only volcano disaster to occur in the contemporary United States was the eruption of Mount St. Helens in 1980 (4). Mount St. Helens is the most active and dangerous volcano in the Cascade range, and prior to 1980 its last active eruptive period was from 1831–1856 (16). The eruption of Mount St. Helens on May 18, 1980, entailed an earthquake-triggered avalanche of the north flank, a laterally directed pyroclastic surge, and a vertical displacement of ash and gas which rose 20 kilometers in less than 10 minutes. This cloud was blown northeastward and deposited ash in eastern Washington, central Idaho, and western Montana. There were 35 known deaths, with necropsy examinations performed on 23 bodies (15). These examinations showed that 18 died from asphyxiation due to ash inhalation, four from burns or associated complications, and one from head injury. Apart from the immediate deaths and injuries, the main potential health problems resulted from the widespread ashfall. Dangerous levels of gas (sulfur dioxide, carbon dioxide, hydrogen sulfide, and hydrogen fluoride) were found only at the crater. More than 90% of the ash particles were within the respirable range. High total suspended particulate (TSP) levels could induce acute respiratory illness in exposed, susceptible persons. Ingestion of ash through contaminated water or vegetables was not a problem for humans or animals. In vitro tests of the ash for mutagenicity were negative. In vitro and in vivo testing showed that the ash might be fibrogenic. In the week following the May 18 eruption, increases in emergency room (ER) visits and hospital admissions for respiratory complaints increased in the areas that had received the heaviest ashfalls and little increase, if any, in rural areas and areas with less ashfall. Record review of patients with respiratory complaints seen at two hospital ERs showed 63 patients with asthma, 91 patients with bronchitis, and 32 patients with chronic obstructive pulmonary disease (15). These two hospital ERs experienced a fourfold increase in the number of asthma patients and twofold increase in bronchitis patients (90% of these ER patients with diagnosed asthma had a history of this disease, while 27% of the bronchitis patients had previously diagnosed asthma). The increased number of ER visits was a direct result of the irritating effects of the elevated TSP levels on the airways (17).

Floods

The occurrence of floods and the damage they cause have been well-documented since the beginning of recorded history. Floods account for approximately 40% of all natural disasters and cause the greatest amount of environmental damage (18). The flood that caused the greatest health impact occurred in 1887 along the Yellow River in China and resulted in the deaths of 900,000 people (18). Floods may indirectly cause toxic exposures when waters encroach upon areas where chemicals are manufactured, stored, or used. Human exposure to released chemicals may result from direct contact with contaminated water, ingestion of such water, inhalation of fumes, or consumption of contaminated vegetables, fish, or animals.

The best documented example of a flood causing the release of chemicals occurred in 1976 along the Teton River in southeastern Idaho (19). On June 5, the Teton Dam broke and released 29.6 billion cubic meters of water. This floodwater damaged three commercial pesticide facilities and many pesticide storehouses on farms. Storage containers at these locations were damaged or broken, and pesticides were dispersed over 200 kilometers of the Snake River. Minimum quantities of chemicals lost included 2000 lbs of Di-Syston (O,O-diethyl S-[-2-(ethylthio)ethyl]phosphorodithioate) and 200 gallons of liquid Furadan (2,3-dihydro-2,2-dimethyl-7-benzofuranyl methylcarbamate). Unknown quantities of other chemicals including dichlorodiphenyltrichloroethane (DDT), polychlorinated biphenyls (PCBs), and malathion were also lost. A pesticide evaluation and recommendation committee was able to recover 1217 containers, less than 60% of all containers lost. Of the recovered containers, 65% were empty. An extensive environmental testing strategy included the collection and analysis of several hundred samples of plants, soil, water, sediments, plankton, fish, and waterfowl. Based on the results of analyzing these samples, no apparent hazard to human health was detected.

Earthquakes

A catastrophic earthquake may be the most destructive type of natural disaster. Earthquakes occur when plates move along fault lines and release sufficient energy. Earthquakes may result in secondary natural hazards which include avalanches, landslides, and tsunamis. Contemporary earthquakes that have resulted in the greatest loss of life include the 1976 China earthquake, which resulted in as many as one million deaths (20), the 1970 Peru earthquake, which resulted in approximately 52,000 deaths (21), and the 1976 Guatemala earthquake, which resulted in approximately 23,000 deaths (22).

The vast majority of deaths and injuries associated with earthquakes results from traumatic injuries resulting from physical (mechanical) energy. However, there are certainly potential risks associated with chemical energy. Primary and secondary hazards associated with a catastrophic earthquake certainly have potential

for causing the release of chemicals and toxic products into the environment. The 1906 San Francisco earthquake resulted in approximately 700 deaths (21), and most of these were due to exposures to the fires (thermal energy and combustion products) that occurred afterwards (23). Contemporary cities around the world contain chemical and petroleum products which could be released during a catastrophic earthquake and cause hazards due to fires and toxic byproducts (21). Horizontal ground displacements around the fault zone may rupture or break pipelines carrying fuel and natural gas (24). Immediately after the 1985 Mexico City earthquake, underground natural gas lines broke and produced geyserlike flames (25), and sulfurous odors from leaking gasoline storage tanks filled the air (26). A catastrophic earthquake could also damage production and storage facilities for other hazardous materials and result in releases of toxic vapors, spills of liquid and solid materials, and contamination of surface water and groundwater (21).

TECHNOLOGIC DISASTERS WITH TOXIC CONSEQUENCES

Introduction

In our contemporary world, the perceived risk of chemical disaster has increased due to numerous factors. The technical sophistication and industrialization of both developed and developing countries have grown. The manufacture, storage, transportation, and utilization of large amounts and varying types of flammable, explosive, or toxic chemicals have increased. Many of these chemicals are either new or result from sophisticated chemical syntheses involving highly reactive and toxic intermediates. A trend toward centralization of industries has increased transportation distances and quantities of chemicals stored. Growing population densities in areas where chemicals are manufactured or transported have increased the numbers of persons potentially exposed. Also, medical knowledge about health effects associated with chemical exposures has increased.

In recent years, public concern about chemical disasters has been fueled by the occurrence of several releases which resulted in public health impacts—the malathion poisoning in Pakistan; the dioxin contamination from an explosion at a trichlorophenol plant in Seveso, Italy; the toxic oil syndrome in Spain; methyl isocyanate release in Bhopal, India; the aldicarb oxime release in Institute, West Virginia; and, the hydrofluoric acid release in Texas. Although these incidents are among the most notable and dramatic examples of how chemicals have the potential to cause disasters, they simply represent the proverbial tip of the iceberg.

Each year, there are thousands of unintentional chemical releases which, had the circumstances of their occurrence been slightly different, could have resulted in significant public health impacts. The United Kingdom chemical industry employs 380,000 people within 4300 facilities. From 1983–1985, there were 362 unintentional chemical releases documented. Approximately two thirds of the incidents occurred during normal operations, while one third occurred during maintenance or cleaning operations. The chemicals most frequently involved included unspecified hydrocarbon materials (52 incidents), sulfuric acid (45), chlorine (35), caustic soda/potash (32), explosives or pyrotechnics (28), vinyl chloride (20), hydrogen chloride (16), hydrochloric acid (14), petrol (13), phosgene (12), xylene/toluene (12), nitrous fumes (11), and hydrogen sulfide (10). Approximately 55% of these releases affected persons in some way (27). The Acute Hazardous Events (AHE) Database characterizes events in the United States which involve the release of acutely toxic substances (28). From 1980–1985, there were 6928 chemical releases, with 7% involving acute health impacts (injury or death) (28). There were a total of 138 deaths and 4717 injuries. Of the releases resulting in health impacts, 25% involved either chlorine, ammonia, hydrochloric acid, or sulfuric acid. Of all releases, 74.8% occurred in plants, and 25.2% occurred during transport.

Bhopal

The release of methyl isocyanate (MIC) at the Union Carbide plant in Bhopal, India, on December 3, 1984, is the worst industrial chemical disaster (29). By 3:00 AM, approximately 2 hours after the release began, all 40 tons of material had escaped from tank 610 (30). The violent reaction causing the release was evident by the large cracks in the concrete foundation on which tank 610 lay. The toxic plume extended as far as 8 kilometers from the plant and covered an area of 40 square kilometers (31). The public siren was not sounded until 1:00 AM and lasted only a few minutes. It was not resumed until 2:00 AM (30). All workers were saved by compliance with an announcement to run in a direction opposite of the wind direction (30).

This release left thousands of local residents dead and hundreds of thousands of others exposed in just a few hours (29). A precise determination of the mortality was not possible due in large part to the fact that over 80% of the deaths occurred before people entered the medical care system. Only 438 deaths were recorded by hospitals on December 3 and 4 (32). In terms of actual and potential morbidity, the most accepted estimates indicate that, of 200,000 persons exposed, 50,000 to 60,000 received substantial exposure (33).

MIC is used for the manufacture of pesticides, including aldicarb, carbaryl, carbofuran, and methomyl (34). It is flammable and highly reactive with water (34). Inhalation of MIC results in severe bronchial spasms, asthmatic breathing, and chemical pneumonia when toxic levels are inhaled (35). MIC exposure causes pulmonary edema by destroying lung tissue, and, depending upon the dose, the victim may die in a matter of minutes. Others exposed to MIC die from anoxia or cardiac arrest (34). Other respiratory problems include difficulties in breathing, coughing, fever, and severe expectoration. Direct contact with eyes, mucous membranes, and skin results in irritation and burns (35). The time-weighted average for 8-hour exposure to MIC is 0.02 ppm as compared with 25.0 for chloroform and 50.0 for carbon monoxide (36).

One study of immediate and delayed effects of acute inhalation exposure to MIC in rats and mice showed necrosis of the epithelial lining of the nasal passages, trachea, and bronchi, fibrosis of the large airways, and focal obstructive lung disease (34). Other target organs were not implicated, and effects on fertility, reproduction, and immune efficiency were not observed.

A study of 978 patients hospitalized as a result of the Bhopal release was conducted (37). Most prominent and common complaints were eye irritation, dyspnea, chest pain, and choking sensation. Many patients had nausea, vomiting, and epigastric discomfort. Cerebral manifestations included apathy, hyper-

somnolence, and coma, while neurologic manifestations included muscle weakness, tremors, paresthesia, and depression. Longterm evaluation of the patients showed residual lung damage, superficial esophagitis and gastritis, and almost complete recovery of neurologic manifestations.

Factors contributing to the Bhopal disaster included weather conditions, location of the plant, disinvestment in the plant by the parent company, failure of engineering controls, lack of adherence to standard operating procedures. A southerly wind and thermal inversion directed and trapped the plume over the most highly populated areas of Bhopal. This population underwent a tremendous increase from 350,000 in 1969 to 800,000 in 1984 (38). Poorer populations gravitated to lands contiguous with the Union Carbide plant. After 1981, the Bhopal plant began losing money, with production never reaching projected levels. The workforce was reduced in size and many skilled employees left for securer positions. Six accidents occurred at the Bhopal plant between 1981 and 1984 (38). Three of these involved the release of MIC or phosgene, with one worker being killed on December 26, 1981 (38). Five different engineering safety systems were designed to prevent such a release and included the refrigeration system, the spare tank, the flare tower, the vent gas scrubber, and the water curtain (33). At the time of the release, the refrigeration system was not working; the spare tank was not used; the vent gas scrubber failed; the flare tower was under maintenance and was inoperative; and the water curtain was unable to reach 35 meters off the ground (the level at which the MIC release occurred).

Example of a Fixed Site Chemical Release in the United States

At approximately 9:25 AM on August 11, 1985, a release of 3850 pounds of chemicals escaped from the aldicarb production unit of the Union Carbide plant in Institute, West Virginia (39, 40). Aldicarb is a cholinesterase-inhibiting pesticide produced from aldicarb oxime, methylene chloride, and MIC. Six employees and 130 community members were treated at local emergency rooms on August 11. Twenty-nine of these patients were hospitalized for one or more days, mostly for observation. Health effects were transient and consistent with exposure to irritating vapors rather than with exposure to MIC or aldicarb. In an effort to ascertain whether other community members who did not seek medical care were potentially exposed and possible symptomatic, a telephone survey of 199 randomly selected households (consisting of 406 persons) was conducted. Most survey respondents reported that they were home when the chemical release occurred. Approximately 27% of the persons perceived themselves as being exposed and reported transient symptoms such as headache, nausea, vomiting, burning eyes, dizziness, coughing, and burning throat. The plant siren alerted only 5% of the surveyed residents to the chemical release. Most people learned of the release by word of mouth, telephone, radio, or television. Approximately 15% of the residents realized there had been a release by seeing an unusual cloud or smelling a peculiar odor. Many persons became exposed from entering the area after the release had occurred. Community members were unnecessarily vulnerable to potential chemical injury because of inadequate warning, lack of an established evacuation plan, and failure to restrict access to the area after the release.

Example of a Transportation-Related Chemical Release in the United States

One representative example of this type of chemical release occurred on Sunday, September 7, 1986. At 11:30 AM, 23 tank cars and three engines from a 46-car train transporting chlorine derailed in a valley four miles north of Collins, Mississippi (41). Two of the tank cars, each containing 20,000 gallons of chlorine, ruptured and released chlorine gas into the environment. Because the release was toxic and could not be controlled, an evacuation was ordered, and approximately 100 families left their homes. Confirmed health impacts were limited to occupational and emergency response-associated exposures. Although formal evacuations for natural disasters (hurricanes) had occurred in the past, a survey to evaluate the evacuation process was conducted, and interviews with 62 families (representing 259 persons) staying in the evacuation center were conducted. Only 52.9% of these families were warned directly by police or other officials. This fact, along with insufficient transportation and preexisting health problems, resulted in delays in evacuating families. Other concerns among the evacuees included nonexplicit directions about where to go, fears of looting, feelings of panic, and questions about how to care for pets. Unnecessary exposure to the chlorine plume may have occurred when members of 39% of the households returned home during the evacuation in order to obtain food or clothing and to care for pets. Evacuation is one strategy for preventing mortality and morbidity from chemical releases. This study showed that, to maximize the preventive nature of evacuations, it is advantageous to educate the public about emergency evacuation plans, make the warning message comprehensive so that it addresses residents' concerns, facilitate departure through availability of augmented transportation, and enforce restricted access to evacuated areas.

PREPAREDNESS AND RESPONSE TO FUTURE CHEMICAL DISASTERS

The Role of Contingency Planning

Disasters resulting from unanticipated and/or uncontrollable releases of chemicals during their production, storage, or usage are not predictable. However, the systematic contingency planning along with appropriate emergency response actions necessary to minimize the associated public health impacts must be well planned. The occurrence of and response to recent chemical disasters have identified the need for better contingency planning because of two major trends: (a) the possibility of another Bhopal disaster and the risk of potential chemical disasters are increasing due to technology transfer from developed to developing countries; and (b) currently governments, corporations, and international agencies are not totally capable of handling large-scale chemical disasters (42). It is therefore important for contingency planning for chemical disasters to delineate through a formal, tested organizational structure a coordination of emergency response activities at all levels. In the United States, the Federal Emergency Management Agency (FEMA) has the lead role for this planning. Plans at any level (local, state, or federal) may become outdated with time, and consequently they need to be constantly evaluated and modified as necessary. Disaster simulations/exercises should be used to evaluate the quality and practical aspects of the

plans. Any actual emergency response should include a component that assesses the effectiveness and weaknesses of the appropriate contingency plan.

The Role of the Epidemiologist

Epidemiology has traditionally been used to identify risk factors and prevention strategies for population-based health impacts from natural and technologic disasters. Consequently, many disaster professionals may regard the epidemiologist as a researcher who is studying the current chemical disaster in order to learn lessons which can be applied to the next chemical disaster.

With reference to phases of chemical disaster preparedness and response (successive continuum of primary prevention, preparedness, emergency relief, rehabilitation, and reconstruction), the role of the epidemiologist should not be limited to primary prevention. The epidemiologist can also provide health-related technical guidance for preparedness and response (emergency relief) activities. Potential preparedness activities that may benefit from epidemiologic input include solicitation of legislative support, augmentation of operational aspects of contingency planning, health and safety training for responders, and education of defined populations at risk. With decentralized response plans (emphasis at the local rather than national level), efforts by the epidemiologist should have similar priority. The epidemiologist should also have input into risk analyses for preparedness planning in terms of assisting with deriving valid and descriptive estimates of associated mortality and morbidity. During emergency response, accurate assessment and prediction of these public health impact estimates are necessary for maximizing efficacy of allocation of finite medical resources.

Rapid Assessment for Chemical Disaster

The primary role of a rapid assessment following chemical disaster is to gain timely, accurate information suitable for directing efficacious action that will minimize all health impacts. The majority of chemical incidents involve fires or spills, are usually small in size, involve little nonoccupational exposure, and have no longterm medical implications. For these events, a responsive rapid assessment may be less sophisticated and easier to conduct. However, when large numbers of people are exposed (e.g., large quantities of toxic substance(s) are blown across populated areas), conducting a comprehensive rapid assessment is essential. A rapid assessment should always be performed; its complexity is relative to the size and characteristics of the release.

Activities of a rapid assessment should focus on information objectives which can be undertaken consecutively and/or concurrently. Examples of such objectives are as follows:

1. Determine the type(s), size, and distribution of the release. The type(s) of releases (e.g., atmospheric dispersion, explosion, fire spill) should be determined. A chemical disaster may involve one or more types of releases. Other characteristics that should be determined include the size of the release (estimated weight/volume of chemicals dispersed) and the distribution (dispersion area) of the release.

2. Identify the specific type(s) of chemicals and their reaction byproducts. Efforts need to focus on ascertaining the identity, quantity, and concentrations of the chemical(s). Emphasis should be placed on both the specific chemical(s) involved and their processes with emphasis on reactivity and physicochemical properties.

3. Identify human exposure pathways. The public health impacts from a chemical disaster are directly determined by the routes and amounts of exposure for humans. During the impact phase (while the release is ongoing) of the disaster, inhalation may be the usual route of chemical exposure. During the postimpact phase, dermal exposure through direct contact with contaminated objects or ingestion of contaminated food or water may be important routes of exposure.

4. Define the population(s) at risk. Information should be ascertained about the number and types of occupational and emergency response workers who are exposed and the types of protection they have during those exposures, the proximity and size of residential neighborhoods, the location and numbers of high-risk people (e.g., nonambulatory individuals with chronic diseases that may be exacerbated, infants), the structure of residential, commercial, and public dwellings, the preparedness response of residents, etc.

5. Conduct toxicologic evaluation and assessment. The identified chemicals may result in many different types of toxicity, depending upon the impact on exposure routes and specific biochemical and physiologic systems. Toxicologic expertise required is usually beyond the capability of the emergency department of the local hospital and, depending upon the specific chemicals involved, may be beyond the capability of state expertise. Efforts should initially identify toxicology expert(s) and possibly clinical epidemiologists and poison information specialists at poison control centers. Current information and recommendations provided by toxicologic databases and poison control centers should be utilized.

6. Describe morbidity and mortality. Characteristics of the chemical disaster may provide or define the need for epidemiologic surveillance to determine the incidence, distribution, location, type, and severity of disaster-related health effects. It is essential to identify as early as possible a case definition that will be universally and consistently applied. Epidemiologic descriptive information is invaluable for assisting with the allocation of medical resources, estimating the need for additional health services, and augmenting efforts to develop rosters of exposed persons or actual censuses of exposed populations.

7. Identify appropriate treatment regimen(s). Based on all relevant toxicologic and epidemiologic information, a consensus of clinical opinions should be used to identify the most appropriate treatment regimen(s) for symptomatic persons. This information should be quickly disseminated to appropriate emergency care and medical care providers.

8. Evaluate emergency medical care and health service capabilities. The role of many public health and medical officials during a chemical disaster may not be that different from routine responsibilities except for exacerbations due to societal disruption, public fear, new operating procedures, amounts of work to be completed, levels of coordination and organization required, etc. The amount of exacerbation is largely determined by and is inversely proportional to the amount of preparedness planning for a chemical disaster. It is very important to evaluate the availability and quantity of appropriate medical care, etc. This evaluation should include a determination of the status of emergency medical care capability, including both medical personnel and facilities with identification of backup capabilities. Once acceptable diagnostic criteria and treatment regimens are established, then the medical care assessment should include evaluation of capability and needs to

diagnose and treat exposed persons. The evaluation should also include consideration of capability for decontamination of patients in order to prevent secondary exposures among medical care providers.

9. Ensure provision of appropriate medical care. Medical treatment protocols should be established and address relevant diagnostic tests, treatment regimens for emergency settings, antidotes, medications, equipment, and medical specialization expertise. This information needs to be disseminated to all appropriate practicing physicians during impact and postimpact phases of the disaster. It is also important to establish procedures to ensure that clinically affected persons enter the medical care system.

10. Identify and evaluate environmental control strategies. As part of the emergency response, environmental control strategies are identified and implemented with the objective of controlling the spread of chemical contaminants in the environment. It is important to minimize additional occupational and nonoccupational exposures.

11. Evaluate evacuation and mass care strategies. As part of the rapid assessment, health input is necessary for evaluating whether population(s) can stay in the affected areas or should temporarily evacuate. Special consideration should be given to high-risk populations. Any recommendation for evacuation should come after thorough review of specific evacuation issues (appropriateness, impediments of effectiveness, feasibility, compliance, health criteria for reoccupation, handling separated family members and pets, etc.) and guidelines (notifying, moving, and providing mass care for the population). If persons are evacuated and placed in mass care shelters, the relevant health and safety guidelines discussed in the rapid assessment for refugees should be followed.

12. Develop criteria for defining comprehensive databases. Actual or potential public health impacts of the chemical disaster may necessitate accurate and comprehensive databases of exposed populations for future socioeconomic assistance, registry development, longterm clinical follow-up, and epidemiologic investigations. Information from prior determinations of case definitions and populations at risk should be used to develop criteria for defining which databases should be developed and what types of information should be included.

REFERENCES

1. Simkin T, Siebert L, McCelland L, et al. Volcanoes of the world. Stroudsburg: Hutchinson Ross, 1981.

2. Francis P. Volcanic hazards. Sydney: Academic Press, 1984.

3. Kerr RA. Volcanoes to keep an eye on. Science 1983;221:634–635.

4. Baxter PJ. Volcanoes. Chapter 5 in Gregg M, ed. The public health consequences of disasters. Centers for Disease Control. Washington, DC: GPO, in press, September 1989.

5. Olsen KB, Fruchter JS. Identification of hazards associated with volcanic emission. Am J Public Health 1986;76:45–52.

6. Le Guern F, Tazieff H, Faiure PR. An example of a health hazard: people killed by gas during a phreatic eruption: Dieng Plateau (Java, Indonesia), February 20, 1979. Bull Volcanol 1982;45:153–156.

7. SEAN Bulletin 1985;10:3–4. Washington: Smithsonian Institute.

8. Kerr RA. Nyos, the killer lake may be coming back. Science 1989;244:1541–1542.

9. Leus X, Kintanar C, Bowman V. Asthmatic bronchitis associated with a volcanic eruption in St. Vincent, West Indies. Disasters 1981;5:67–69.

10. Baxter PJ, Stoiber RE, Williams SN. Volcanic gases and health: Masaya Volcano, Nicaragua. Lancet 1982;2:150–151.

11. World Health Organization. Environment health criteria 8: sulfur dioxide and suspended particulate matter. Geneva: WHO, 1979.

12. Kawari M, Inoue T, Ishida Y. An autopsy case of volcanic hydrogen sulfide intoxication. Kitakanto Med J 1978;28:237–244.

13. Thorarinson S. On the damage caused by volcanic eruptions with special reference to tephra and gases. In: Sheets PD, Grayson DK, eds. Volcanic activity and human ecology. New York: Academic Press, 1979:125–159.

14. Baxter PJ, Bernsein RS, Falk H, et al. Medical aspects of volcanic disasters: an outline of the hazards and emergency response measures. Disasters 1982;6:268–276.

15. Baxter PJ, Ing R, Falk H, et al. Mount St. Helens eruptions, May 18 to June 12, 1980. JAMA 1981;246:2585–2589.

16. Crandell DR, Mullineaux DR. Potential hazards from future eruptions of Mount St. Helens volcano, Washington. Geological Survey Bulletin No. 1383-C. Washington, D.C.: GPO, 1980.

17. Baxter PJ, Ing R, Falk H, Plikaytis B. Mount St Helens eruptions: the acute respiratory effects of volcanic ash in a North American community. Arch Environ Health 1983;38(3):138–143.

18. Frazier, K. The violent face of nature: severe phenomenon and natural disasters. New York: William Morrow and Company, 1979.

19. Perry, JA. Pesticide and PCB residues in the upper Snake River ecosystem, Southeastern Idaho, following the collapse of the Teton Dam 1976. Arch Environ Contam Toxicol 1979;8:139–159.

20. Whittow, J. Disasters—the anatomy of environmental hazards. Athens, GA: The University of Georgia Press, 1979.

21. Stratton J. Earthquakes. Chapter 4 in Gregg, M., ed. The public health consequences of disasters. Centers for Disease Control. Washington, D.C.: GPO, in press, September 1989.

22. Pan American Health Organization (PAHO): Emergency management of environmental health and water supply. Chapter 6. Preparing for earthquakes. Washington, D.C.: PAHO, 1980.

23. Bronson, W. The earth shook, the sky burned. New York: Pocket Books, Simon and Schuster, 1971.

24. Steinbrugge KV, Lagorio HJ, Davis JF, Bennett JH, Borchardt G, Toppozada, TR: Earthquake planning scenario for a magnitude 7.5 earthquake on the Hayward Fault, San Francisco Bay Area. Cal Geol 1986; (Jul):153–157.

25. Disaster in Mexico. Newsweek. September 30, 1985;16–22.

26. Boraiko AA. Earthquake in Mexico. Nat Geographic. May 1986;655–675.

27. Robinson BJ: A three year survey of accidents and dangerous occurrences in the UK Chemical Industry. Proceedings of the World Congress: Chemical Accidents. Edinbergh: CEP Consultants, Ltd, July 1977:33–36.

28. U.S. Environmental Protection Agency, Office of Toxic Substance. Acute Hazardous Events Database, Report No. EPA 560-5-85-029. 1985.

29. Bertazzi PB. Industrial disasters and epidemiology. A review of recent experiences. Scand J Work Environ Health 1989;15:85–100.

30. Khandekar S, Dubey S. City of death. India Today. December 31, 1984;4–24.

31. Bhopal Working Group. The public health implications of the Bhopal disaster. Am J Public Health 1987;77:230–236.

32. The crime continues. Sunday (Calcutta). April 13, 1985;25.

33. Waldoholz M. Bhopal death toll, survivor problems still being debated. Wall Street Journal. March 21, 1985;22.

34. McConnell EE, Bucher JR, Schwetz BA, et al. Toxicity of methyl isocyanate. Environ Sci Technol 1987;21:188–193.

35. Union Carbide Corporation. Methyl Isocyanate, Report F-41443-A-7/76. New York: Union Carbide, 1976.

36. American Conference of Government Hygienists (ACGIH): TLV's: threshold limit values for chemical substances and physical agents in the work environment and biological exposure indices with intended changes for 1984–1985. Cincinnati, OH: ACGIH, 1984.

37. Misra NP, Pathak R, Gaur KJBS, et al. Clinical picture of gas leak victims in acute phase after Bhopal episode. Indian J Med Res 1987;86(suppl):11–19.

38. Bowonder B, Kasperson JX, Kasperson RE. Avoiding future Bhopals. Environment 1985;27(7):6–36.

39. Etzel R, Sanderson L. Chemical release—Institute, West Virginia. Centers for Disease Control. EPI-85-74-2. Atlanta, GA: U.S. Public Health Service, 1986.

40. Baron R, Etzel R, Sanderson L. Surveillance for adverse health effects following a chemical release in West Virginia. Disasters 1988;12:356–365.

41. DuClos P, Sanderson L, Thompson FE, Brackin B, Binder S. Community evacuation following a chlorine release, Mississippi. Disasters 1987;11:286–289.

42. Abraham M: Chemical accidents—a consumer perspective of the tunnel at the end of the light. Proceedings of the World Congress: Chemical Accidents. Edinbergh: CEP Consultants, July 1977:32.

31

Recognition of Hazardous Materials

William V. Gustin

INTRODUCTION

When incidents involving hazardous materials occur, it is usually the "first responder" (the first arriving fire, police, or emergency medical service unit) who must quickly and accurately determine the presence of hazardous materials, identify the specific products involved, and ascertain the degree of hazard inherent in each of them. Often the safe and successful outcome of a hazardous material incident will depend on the action taken in the few minutes following arrival of personnel on the scene.

First responders can use various sources or clues to detect the presence of hazardous materials as well as determining the specific products involved. However, they need to know how to safely approach a hazardous material incident in order to identify materials and determine their hazards while minimizing risk of exposure, contamination, or adding a source of ignition.

The difference between successfully handling a hazardous materials incident or just becoming part of the problem will depend largely on an awareness of the presence of hazardous and toxic materials. Labeling and documentation systems are, at best, tools to assist in product hazard identification. No marking system was designed to identify all hazardous materials before they can do harm to emergency response personnel; they are just one of many possible indicators of the presence of hazards that should be identified, understood, and heeded. Markings and labels are often of no use to the first responder if he/she does not suspect the presence of hazardous materials. Some of the greatest loss of life involving such an incident has occurred when firefighters, who are generally well versed in hazardous identification and procedures, were unaware of their presence and approached an incident as if it were a routine operation. It is incumbent on each emergency responder to know where hazardous materials will most likely be encountered. The next "routine" overturned truck on the highway or patient with chest pain at an industrial site may turn out to be much more than anyone was prepared to handle.

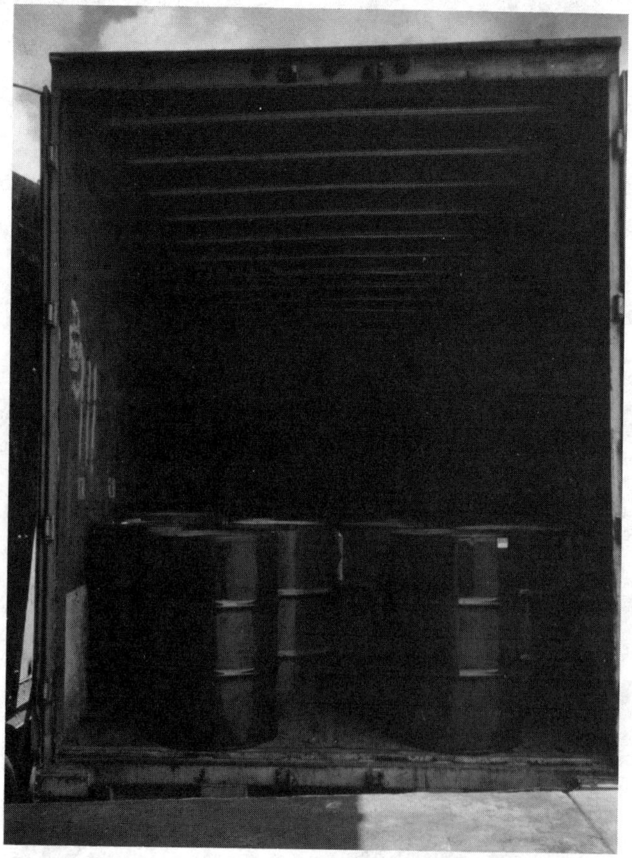

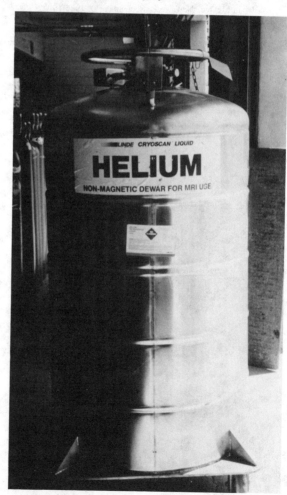

Figure 31.1. 55-Gallon drums unmarked, being transported.

Figure 31.2. Pressurized helium container.

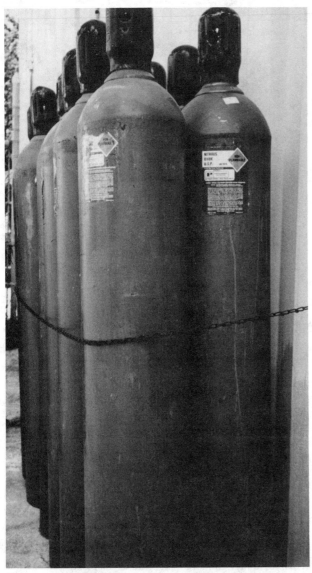

Figure 31.3. Compressed gas cylinders of nitrous oxide.

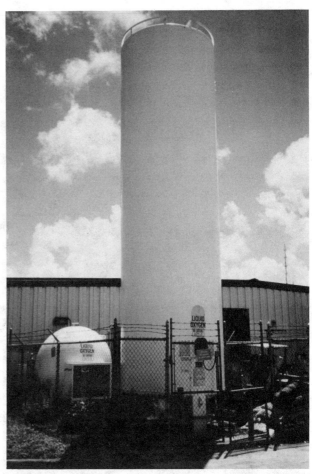

Figure 31.4. Liquid oxygen storage tank typically found near hospitals.

5. Container markings and colors
6. Shape and design of container
7. Other indications (i.e., visual, odors)

Occupancy and/or Location

When the subject of hazardous materials is discussed, many emergency response personnel tend to conjure up thoughts of exotic chemicals with long, multisyllabic names. Actually, the vast majority of hazardous material incidents involve common hydrocarbon gas and liquid fuels, solvents, corrosives, and pesticides. The typical American home contains a variety of chemical hazards: gasoline, solvents, pesticides, fertilizers, chlorine and acids for swimming pools, and propane cylinders. Multiplying the contents of the average home by 10,000 will give some indication of the inventory of potential hazards in stock at a local hardware store or home center.

The degree of danger that emergency response personnel are exposed to is often in inverse proportion to the amount of knowledge they have of the presence of hazardous materials at a particular occupancy. To illustrate this point, consider the clandestine drug laboratory. This operation dangerously and illegally stores, uses, and disposes of toxic, flammable, and corrosive substances, often in the garage or basement of a house in a quiet residential neighborhood. Each "designer drug" requires different chemicals for its production. A typical illegal

IDENTIFYING THE HAZARDOUS AND POTENTIALLY HAZARDOUS SCENE

As previously mentioned, marking and labels are just one of many indicators of the presence of hazardous materials. It would be foolish to determine the initial strategy at a possible hazardous materials incident entirely on the presence or absence of a sign or label. Marking, labeling, and documentation regulations have limitations. The National Fire Academy—Emergency Training Center course materials detail several clues for detecting the presence of hazardous materials which the first responder should apply before intervening in an incident (1):

1. Prior knowledge of an occupancy, processes, reactions, and contents
2. Facility inventory documents Superfund Amendments and Reauthorization Act (SARA Tier I & II) and Material Safety Data Sheets (MSDS)
3. Placards and labels
4. Shipping papers

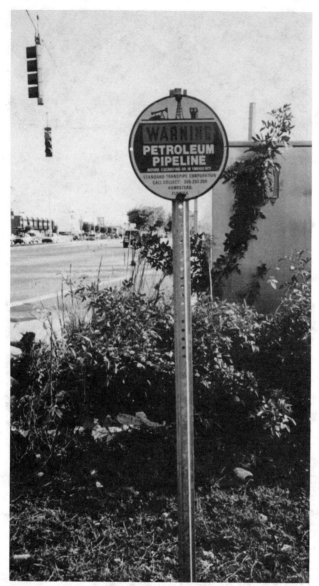

Figure 31.5. High pressure liquid fuel transmission line. Marker posts such as this one will usually be found where the pipeline crosses highways, railways, and waterways.

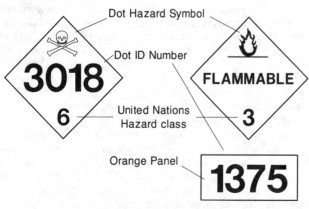

Vehicle Placards

Figure 31.6. Components of a vehicle placard.

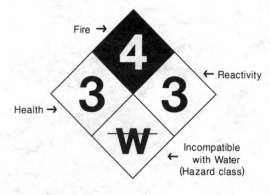

0 = No Hazard   Health = blue   Reactivity = yellow
4 = Extremely Hazardous Fire = red   Hazard class = white

Building Placards

Figure 31.7. Components of a building placard.

laboratory uses large quantities of acetone, ether, and hydrochloric acid in the manufacturing or refining process and often disposes of these volatile materials down the toilet. The unknown presence of hazardous materials poses great risk for emergency responders if they do not anticipate the possibility. If emergency responders are not aware that hazardous materials are present, they cannot protect themselves.

Basically, expect large amounts of hazardous materials and chemicals to be found where they are involved in the following: production, storage, use, and transportation.

PRODUCTION

All industrial manufacturing and processing occupancies are likely sites for hazardous materials. Hazardous materials include ingredients, catalysts, intermediate compounds, by-products or the finished product of almost every manufacturing or industrial process. Relatively safe products, such as plastics or fiberglass boats, require large quantities of toxic, reactive, and flammable ingredients and catalysts in their manufacture.

STORAGE

This category refers to the bulk handling of hazardous materials before and after they are transported to the area of use. Examples of storage facilities include: tank farms of liquid and gaseous hydrocarbon fuels; local chemical distributors (corrosives, oxidizers, solvents, flammable liquids, and gases); bonded warehouses storing liquor (contains alcohol, which is flammable).

Any warehouse can contain large amounts of flammable, corrosive, and/or toxic liquids in the most common, yet potentially, one of the most dangerous containers—the 55-gallon drum. This seemingly innocuous container has earned an ominous safety record over the years. Its familiar presence should not lull emergency responders into a sense of complacency. Fifty-five-gallon drums can be highly dangerous in content (Fig. 31.1):

1. They can be found everywhere, and their presence is hidden behind closed doors.
2. They can easily be punctured, releasing their hazardous

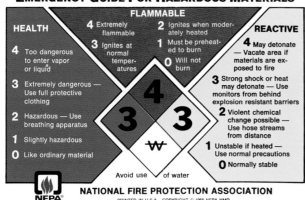

DOMESTIC LABELING

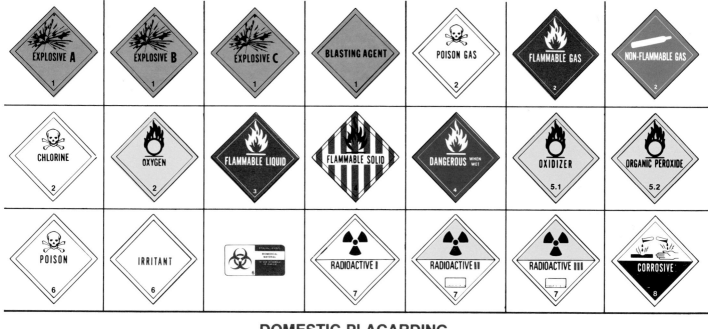

DOMESTIC PLACARDING

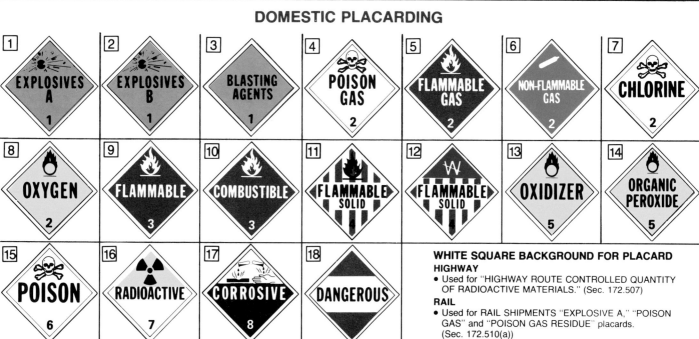

WHITE SQUARE BACKGROUND FOR PLACARD
HIGHWAY
- Used for "HIGHWAY ROUTE CONTROLLED QUANTITY
  OF RADIOACTIVE MATERIALS." (Sec. 172.507)

RAIL
- Used for RAIL SHIPMENTS "EXPLOSIVE A," "POISON
  GAS" and "POISON GAS RESIDUE" placards.
  (Sec. 172.510(a))

Figure 31.8. Placarding system showing shape, color coding, and symbol. Copyright © 1985, National Fire Protection Association, Quincy, MA 02269.

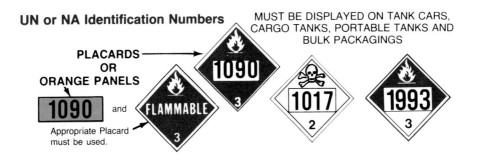

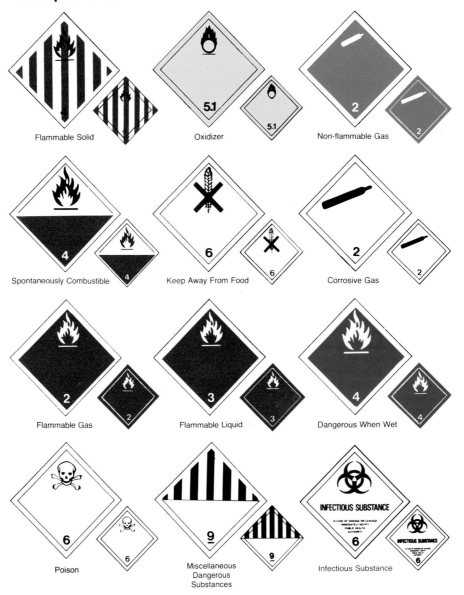

Figure 31.9.   Department of Transportation (DOT) Chart 9. Hazardous materials warning labels and placards, UN and North American (NA) identification numbers, and international labeling.

UN ID Number	DOT Symbol	Hazard Class

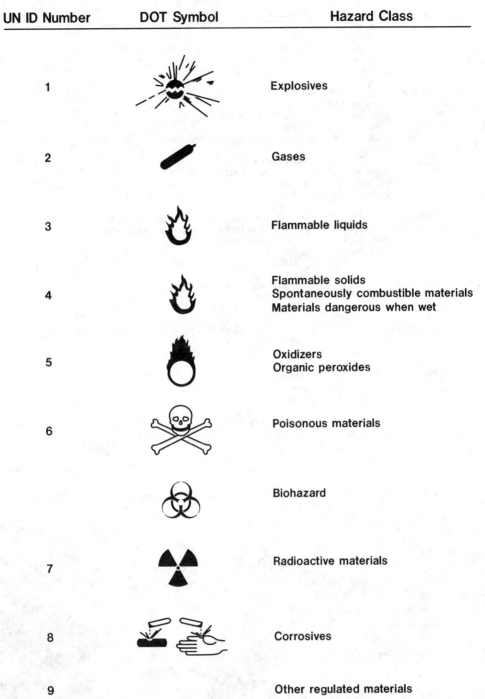

1		Explosives
2		Gases
3		Flammable liquids
4		Flammable solids Spontaneously combustible materials Materials dangerous when wet
5		Oxidizers Organic peroxides
6		Poisonous materials
		Biohazard
7		Radioactive materials
8		Corrosives
9		Other regulated materials

Figure 31.10. Department of Transportation (DOT) hazard symbols describing hazard class in terms of the nature of the hazard and the United Nations (UN) identification number.

contents, by accidental penetration of a forklift fork or by other mechanical damage.

3. They are typically not equipped with pressure relief devices. Rising internal pressures from heat exposure will not be relieved, and there is no reliable indication of impending explosion, a result of rising pressure and container failure.

USE

This grouping refers to handling of hazardous materials on a consumable basis. Examples include facilities using chlorine gas as well as other occupancies using hazardous materials. These include, but certainly are not limited to:

1. Home
2. Office—a blueprint duplication machine leaking anhydrous ammonia can result in a mass-casualty incident.
3. Farm—pesticides, oxidizers, anhydrous ammonia.
4. Schools—high school and college chemistry labs.
5. Health care—radioactive materials, infectious wastes, compressed oxygen, anesthetic gases, and cryogenic liquid oxygen (Figs. 31.2–4).

Class 1		**Explosives**
	Division 1.1	Explosives with a mass explosion hazard
	Division 1.2	Explosives with a projection hazard
	Division 1.3	Explosives with predominantly a fire hazard
	Division 1.4	Explosives with no significant blast hazard
	Division 1.5	Very insensitive explosives
Class 2		**Gases**
	Division 2.1	Flammable gases
	Division 2.2	Nonflammable gases
	Division 2.3	Poison gases
	Division 2.4	Corrosive gases (Canadian)
Class 3		**Flammable liquids**
	Division 3.1	Flashpoint below -18°C (0°F)
	Division 3.2	Flashpoint -18°C and above but less than 23°C (73°F)
	Division 3.3	Flashpoint of 23°C and up to 61°C (141°F)
Class 4		**Flammable solids; Spontaneously combustible materials; and Materials that are dangerous when wet**
	Division 4.1	Flammable solids
	Division 4.2	Spontaneously combustible materials
	Division 4.3	Materials that are dangerous when wet
Class 5		**Oxidizers and Organic peroxides**
	Division 5.1	Oxidizers
	Division 5.2	Organic peroxides
Class 6		**Poisonous and Etiologic (infectious) materials**
	Division 6.1	Poisonous materials
	Division 6.2	Etiologic (infectious) materials
Class 7		**Radioactive materials**
Class 8		**Corrosives**
Class 9		**Miscellaneous hazardous materials**

Figure 31.11. United Nations hazard classification system.

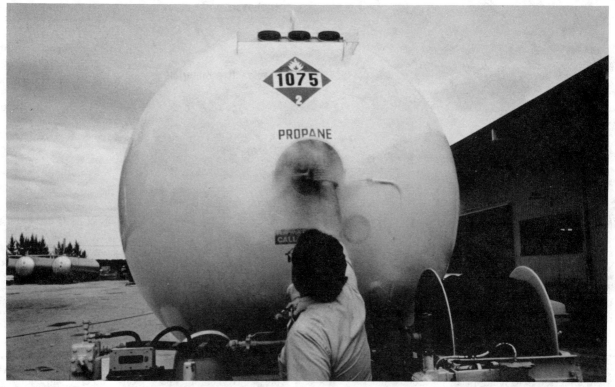

Figure 31.12. Placard on pressurized propane tank has UN/NA identification number, ''1075,'' in the center. Note the DOT symbol for flammable gas at the top.

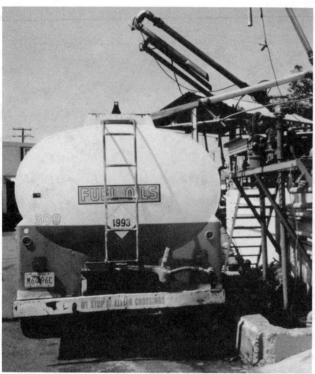

Figure 31.13. Flammable liquid placard with red background bleached by sunlight showing the UN/NA identification number on tanker truck.

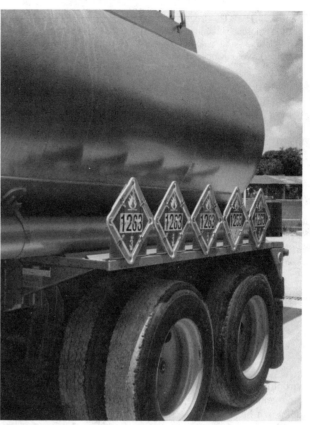

Figure 31.14. A liquid tanker capable of transporting five separate liquids due to compartmentalization. Each liquid requires a separate placard.

The best way to deal with hazardous materials in production, storage, and use is *before* an incident occurs. Progressive fire, rescue, and EMS services prepare themselves for incidents at fixed facilities by:

conducting preplan survey and inspections;

developing preincident plans in cooperation with plant personnel and all responding agencies;

developing a filing system for quick retrieval of material safety data sheets on each occupancy;

requiring by local law, that facilities utilize a marking system for fixed installations and training personnel in its interpretation.

TRANSPORTATION

The nation's industry and economy depends, in part, on the hundreds of thousands of hazardous materials transported each day from the supplier to user and, ultimately, to the waste disposer. All but a very few of these shipments reach their destination safely and without incident. This is due, in part, to the regulations governing the transport of hazardous materials. In the United States, hazardous materials are defined, classified, and regulated by the Department of Transportation (DOT).

The laws for transporting hazardous materials which the DOT administers and enforces are detailed in Title 49 of the Code of Federal Regulations (49 CFR). Forty-nine CFR sections specify the types and quantities of materials that can be transported as well as the type of packaging required to contain specific materials. Additionally there are sections listing requirements for the identification of hazardous materials in transit to assist emergency response personnel in recognizing and understanding their hazard. The regulations are often confusing, difficult to enforce, and in a constant state of revision.

Transportation emergencies are often more dangerous than those at fixed facilities. The materials involved may be unknown, and warning signs may not be visible or may be obscured by rollover, smoke, or debris; the driver may be killed or missing. An understanding of the placarding, labeling, and documentation requirements as outlined in the 49 CFR as well as of the weaknesses of the present system is imperative.

Hazardous materials are transported by five basic modes: (a) roadway; (b) rail; (c) water; (d) air; and (e) pipeline.

Paramedical personnel should be prepared for the possibility of a patient being exposed and contaminated by a hazardous material anytime accidents involve: (a) railroad lines and railyards, (b) trucking and freight terminals, or (c) river and ocean-going vessels, as well as waterfront warehouses.

Pipelines—high pressure gas and liquid interstate transmission lines, as well as local utility distribution systems, may be buried beneath the ground and be located close to residential areas. These lines can be a potential hazard if damaged and leakage occurs (Fig. 31.5).

WHAT IS A HAZARDOUS MATERIAL?

Any study of hazardous material transportation regulations should begin with an understanding of exactly what a hazardous material is. The DOT defines a hazardous material as "a substance or material determined by the Secretary of Transportation to be capable of posing an **unreasonable risk** to health, safety, and property when transported." "Unreasonable risk" obviously covers a very broad spectrum of health, fire, and en-

Figure 31.15. This truck is transporting one-ton chlorine gas containers (UN#1017, Gas Class 2) and calcium hypochlorite (oxidizer). Note incorrect position of placards.

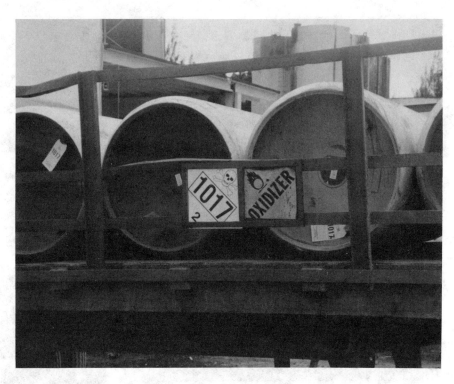

vironmental considerations. Situations can arise when the emergency responder is taken by surprise by a shipment of unknown hazardous materials which pose a risk to his safety but do not meet the criteria of an ''unreasonable risk'' as defined by the Secretary of Transportation.

HAZARD CLASSES

The DOT has placed each hazardous material into one of several hazard classes according to the most significant hazard of the material. The classification system does not give consideration to materials with more than one hazard. For example, a poisonous material may also be flammable. Corrosives are both a toxic hazard from inhalation of their fumes as well as a corrosive hazard if they contact the skin. This is but one of many weaknesses of the system.

PLACARDS

Hazardous material shipments must be placarded according to the requirements applying to its specific hazard class. A placard is a diamond-shaped sign that is displayed on all four sides of a truck, trailer, shipping container, or rail car. Placards indicate the presence of hazardous materials in a number of ways. They are coded according to a number system, a color system, and symbols (2) (Figs 31.6–31.9).

By shape—A distinctive diamond shape, ''square on point,'' measuring 10.75 inches.

Colored background—Knowing which color corresponds with each hazard category is very important. Color will definitely be the first distinguishing characteristic of the placard to be seen. Color may be the only clue to hazard identification if the placard is unable to be read due to distance, damage, smoke, or vapor cloud.

The symbol in the top corner—These symbols graphically describe the hazard class in terms of a poison, explosive, gas,

flammable liquid, flammable solid, oxidizer, biohazard, radioactive material, or corrosive (Fig. 31.10).

United Nations Class Number—The United Nations divides materials into nine hazard classes for shipments throughout the United States and Canada. All placards, except **DANGEROUS** for mixed loads, are grouped into one of eight categories, corresponding to the UN number displayed in the bottom corner of the placard (Figs. 31.6, 31.9, 31.11).

UN/NA IDENTIFICATION NUMBER

UN (United Nations) or NA (North American) identification numbers are found on or beside placards on tank cars, cargo tanks, or portable tanks (Figs. 31.12–31.14). When found on a placard, it will be located in the center where the hazard class name is usually found. If beside the standard placard, as required for POISON GAS, RADIOACTIVE, and EXPLOSIVES, the four-digit identification number will be in an orange rectangle in black digits (Fig. 31.15). This number can be used with the *Department of Transportation Emergency Response Guidebook* (3) to identify the type of product by finding the product or products that correspond to the I.D. number in the yellow section of the book. Each product or products with similar properties have a guide page listing general hazards and initial actions to be taken by first responders (Figs. 31.16, 31.17). Every fire, police, and EMS vehicle should carry the guidebook, and all first responders should know how to use it.

Labels are, in many respects, smaller version placards, which are attached to individual packages when required. They are four-inch diamonds, except for ETIOLOGIC (BIO-HAZARD) which is rectangular, and MAGNETIC HAZARD (air shipments) which is square.

LABELING AND PLACARDING REQUIREMENTS

First responders must not place blind trust on the present DOT placard and labeling system. A study of 49 CFR will indicate

ID No.	Guide No.	Name of Material	ID No.	Guide No.	Name of Material
1040	69	ETHYLENE OXIDE *	1057	17	LIGHTER, for cigars, cigarettes, etc., with flammable gas
1041	17	CARBON DIOXIDE-ETHYLENE OXIDE MIXTURE, with more than 6% ETHYLENE OXIDE	1058	12	LIQUEFIED GAS, nonflammable, charged with nitrogen, carbon dioxide or air
1041	17	ETHYLENE OXIDE-CARBON DIOXIDE MIXTURE, with more than 6% ETHYLENE OXIDE	1058	12	LIQUEFIED NONFLAMMABLE GAS charged with NITROGEN, CARBON DIOXIDE or AIR
1043	16	FERTILIZER AMMONIATING SOLUTION, with more than 35% free ammonia	1060	17	METHYL ACETYLENE and PROPADIENE MIXTURE, stabilized
1044	12	FIRE EXTINGUISHER, with compressed or liquefied gas	1061	19	METHYLAMINE, anhydrous *
1045	20	FLUORINE, compressed	1061	19	MONOMETHYLAMINE, anhydrous *
1046	12	HELIUM, compressed	1062	55	METHYL BROMIDE *
1048	15	HYDROGEN BROMIDE, anhydrous	1063	18	METHYL CHLORIDE *
1049	22	HYDROGEN, compressed	1064	13	METHYL MERCAPTAN *
1050	15	HYDROCHLORIC ACID, anhydrous *	1065	12	NEON, compressed
1050	15	HYDROGEN CHLORIDE, anhydrous *	1066	12	NITROGEN, compressed
1051	13	HYDROCYANIC ACID *	1067	20	NITROGEN DIOXIDE *
1051	13	HYDROGEN CYANIDE, anhydrous, stabilized *	1067	20	NITROGEN PEROXIDE *
1052	15	HYDROFLUORIC ACID, anhydrous *	1067	20	NITROGEN TETROXIDE *
1052	15	HYDROGEN FLUORIDE, anhydrous *	1069	16	NITROSYL CHLORIDE
1053	13	HYDROGEN SULFIDE *	1070	14	NITROUS OXIDE, compressed
1055	22	ISOBUTYLENE	1071	22	OIL GAS
1056	12	KRYPTON, compressed	1072	14	OXYGEN, compressed
1057	17	CIGARETTE LIGHTER, with flammable gas	1073	23	OXYGEN, refrigerated liquid (cryogenic liquid)
1057	17	FLAMMABLE GAS in LIGHTER for cigars, cigarettes, etc.	1075	22	LIQUEFIED PETROLEUM GAS
			1075	22	LPG, liquefied petroleum gas
			1075	22	PETROLEUM GAS, liquefied
			1076	15	CARBONYL CHLORIDE *
			1076	15	PHOSGENE *

* Look for information next to this **NAME** in the TABLE OF EVACUATION DISTANCES in the back of this book. Use this in addition to the Guide Page if there is NO FIRE.

Figure 31.16. Typical page from the *DOT Emergency Response Guidebook*. Note the presence of the UN identification number which corresponds to the guide number. From Department of Transportation.

that not every hazardous material will be placarded or labeled every time, on every container, and in every mode of transport.

There are five classes of materials that require placarding *regardless of any quantity, on any mode of transportation*:

1. Explosive A;
2. Explosive B;
3. Poison A;
4. Radioactive III;
5. Flammable Solids—Use No Water.

All other materials require a placard *only* when 1000 pounds or more are transported by rail or motor carrier. The implications of this regulation are that emergency personnel may approach an overturned or burning truck with no outward indication that it is carrying 999 pounds of flammable, poisonous, corrosive, or oxidizing materials.

MIXED SHIPMENTS

DOT regulations allow for shipments of mixed loads of materials from different hazard classes to be placarded **DANGEROUS** instead of displaying two or more placards for the individual products being shipped. The exception to this regulation is for the five classes of materials that must be placarded at any quantity, and if 5000 pounds or more of one class are loaded at one facility, the specific placard for that class must be displayed. The **DANGEROUS** placard will also be used for shipments of 1000 pounds or more of Class C EXPLOSIVES or IRRITATING MATERIAL. First responders encountering a container displaying the **DANGEROUS** placard should expect a "mixed bag" of goods and should examine shipping papers to determine the exact materials involved.

GUIDE 13

POTENTIAL HAZARDS

HEALTH HAZARDS
Poison; **extremely hazardous.**
May be fatal if inhaled or absorbed through skin.
Vapors non-irritating but may deaden sense of smell.
Runoff from fire control or dilution water may cause pollution.

FIRE OR EXPLOSION
Some of these materials are **extremely flammable.**
May be ignited by heat, sparks or flames.
Vapors may travel to a source of ignition and flash back.
Cylinder may explode in heat of fire.
Vapor explosion and poison hazard indoors, outdoors or in sewers.

EMERGENCY ACTION

Keep unnecessary people away; isolate hazard area and deny entry.
Stay upwind, out of low areas, and ventilate closed spaces before entering.
Self-contained breathing apparatus and chemical protective clothing which is spe-
cifically recommended by the shipper or producer may be worn but they do not
provide thermal protection unless it is stated by the clothing manufacturer.
Structural firefighter's protective clothing is not effective with these materials.
Evacuate the leak or spill area immediately for at least 50 feet in all directions. (See
the Table of Initial Evacuation Distances in the back of this book. If you find the
Name of Material there, call for help to perform the recommended evacuation.)
Isolate for 1/2 mile in all directions if tank car or truck is involved in fire.
CALL CHEMTREC AT 1-800-424-9300 AS SOON AS POSSIBLE, especially if there is
no local hazardous materials team available.

FIRE
Small Fires: Let burn unless leak can be stopped immediately.
Large Fires: Water spray, fog or standard foam is recommended.
Move container from fire area if you can do it without risk.
Stay away from ends of tanks.
Withdraw immediately in case of rising sound from venting safety device or any
discoloration of tank due to fire.
Cool container with water using unmanned device until well after fire is out.
Isolate area until gas has dispersed.

SPILL OR LEAK
Do not touch spilled material; stop leak if you can do it without risk.
Shut off ignition sources; no flares, smoking or flames in hazard area.
Use water spray to reduce vapor. **do not** put water directly on leak or spill area.
Isolate area until gas has dispersed.

FIRST AID
Move victim to fresh air and call emergency medical care; if not breathing, give ar-
tificial respiration; if breathing is difficult, give oxygen.
In case of contact with material, immediately flush skin or eyes with running water
for at least 15 minutes.
Keep victim quiet and maintain normal body temperature.
Effects may be delayed; keep victim under observation.

Figure 31.17.   Typical guide page in the *DOT Emergency Response Guidebook* which refers to the hazardous material section in the front of the book. From Department of Transportation.

"RESIDUE" PLACARD

Rail tank cars, when off-loaded at their destination, are, of course, not completely empty. They contain residual liquid and are usually filled with flammable or toxic vapors. Residues in these tank cars create a dangerous confined space hazard. A **RESIDUE** placard is required to indicate the material last carried by an "empty" tank car (Fig. 31.18).

LIMITATIONS OF PLACARDS AND LABELS AS AN IDENTIFICATION SYSTEM

As mentioned earlier, the present DOT identification system does have its weaknesses. It was, however, never intended to be an all-inclusive system for identifying each and every hazardous material in transit. The following is a summary of the weaknesses and limitations of the placard/label system:

1. Placard and label regulations apply only to materials in transit and may not be present at fixed facilities.

2. Placards and labels indicate only the most significant hazard of a material. For example, a material placarded **CORROSIVE** may also pose a threat as a poison and possibly, an oxidizer. Anhydrous ammonia, placarded **NONFLAMMABLE GAS**, can form a vapor cloud that no one can survive.

3. Materials have to meet narrow criteria to be placed in a specific hazard class. For example, anhydrous ammonia is classified as a nonflammable gas by DOT criteria by virtue of its high upper explosive limit. However, ammonia has fueled some deadly and devastating explosions when allowed to accumulate in a confined space.

4. Most mixed loads qualify for the **DANGEROUS** placard, which provides no outward indication of the hazard(s) of the contents.

5. Shipments of the most hazardous materials (except the five mentioned earlier) do not require placards for less than 1000 pounds. Nine hundred ninety-nine pounds of flammable liquids in a burning truck can be an unrecognized life-threatening hazard for an unsuspecting first responder.

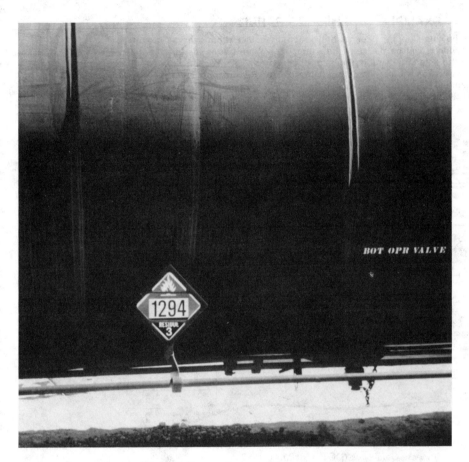

Figure 31.18. Residue placard on off-loaded flammable liquid tank car indicates potential confined space hazard.

Figure 31.19. Placard partially obscured by vapor cloud.

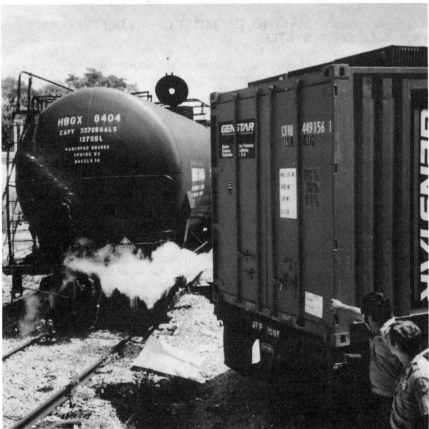

EXAMPLE OF SHIPPING PAPER

The following shipping paper is only illustrative since it may vary in format. However, all descriptions will be basically the same. You should look for this type of entry to determine the shipping name of the hazardous material, its classification, its ID number (ID No.), and a reportable quantity notation (RQ or RQ-number) for use in reporting spill incidents to the National Response Center. With very few exceptions, shipping papers identifying hazardous materials are required when they are being transported:

- To be in the cab of the motor vehicle;
- To be in the possession of a train crew member on a train;
- To be kept in a holder on the bridge of a vessel; or,
- To be in an aircraft pilot's possession.

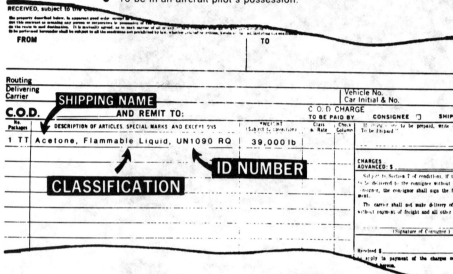

Figure 31.20. Shipping paper example showing location of important information concerning hazardous materials. (From *DOT Emergency Response Guidebook* (DOT p. 5800.4), 1987.

6. Labels are very small, require that the vehicle be opened in order to observe, and are required to be applied to only one side of a package. This makes a label impossible to read if it is in the wrong position or blocked by other packages, as in a loaded semitrailer (Fig. 31.1).

7. Narrow requirements based on container size may allow a substantial amount of flammable liquid to be unlabeled, because it is in small containers (e.g., aerosol cans).

8. Hazardous material shipments are often incorrectly labeled and placarded. Recent surveys reveal that as many as 50% of trucks hauling hazardous materials are either incorrectly placarded or not placarded at all.

9. Placards will deteriorate from weather. Rain, dirt, and snow quickly obliterate cardboard placards. Several weeks of sun will bleach colors out of placards making them difficult to identify from a distance (Fig. 31.13).

10. Placards can be obscured by darkness, rollover, debris, smoke, fire, or vapor cloud (Fig. 31.19).

11. Probably the most significant weakness of labels and placards is that a responder must get dangerously close to the container or vehicle to read them. Often, if emergency personnel are close enough to read a placard, they are too close!

Placards, container markings, and shipping papers cannot give an accurate indication of what will happen when two or more incompatible materials are mixed or come into contact with each other. The result can be the formation of more toxic or more reactive materials, such as the mixture of aluminum phosphide and an acid which releases phosphine gas.

MAKING THE MOST OF AN IMPERFECT SYSTEM

Placards and labels can be a very useful tool for hazard identification if emergency responders follow these guidelines:

1. Memorize the symbols and, more importantly, the colors of all placards and labels.

2. Practice sighting placards on trucks and trains. Look up the four-digit identification number of tank vehicle placards and find the material in the *Department of Transportation Emergency Response Guidebook*.

3. Use binoculars to observe placards at a safe distance.

Shipping Papers

Shipments of hazardous materials must be documented on shipping papers which accompany a shipment to its destination. Due to the present regulation that most shipments of hazardous materials less than 1000 pounds in weight do not require placarding, shipping papers may very well be the first clue to the presence of dangerous materials. The analysis of the limitations of placards in the previous section explain that they, at best, provide only general information of the most significant hazard of a material and usually do not identify specific products. Shipping papers can help to fill the void of information necessary for precise identification of a product, its quantity, and specific hazards (Figs. 31.20, 31.21).

Except for hazardous waste shipments, there is not a specific form required to be used as a shipping paper under DOT reg-

**TRUCK BILL OF LADING
AND DELIVERY RECEIPT**

ORDER TYPE 2	CUSTOMER NO. 309450	LOCATION MIA

BILL OF LADING NO.
▶ 0381-023727-00

CARRIER
ATLANTIC TRUCK LINES

SHIPPING DATE
0/14   1989

SPECIAL INSTRUCTIONS

CONSIGNED TO / DESTINATION
PENTA CHEMICALS
17300 S.W. 87th COURT
FORT LAUDERDALE, FL

CUSTOMER ORDER NO. / CONTRACT NO.
00227-6

SHIPPING POINT (CITY, STATE)
MIAMI

FREIGHT TERMS PREPAID | AREA/DIST. 0381 | SLS. NO. 354

NO OF PKGS OR GROSS GAL ORDERED	PKG TYPE	SHIP POINT	PRODUCT CODE	NET AMOUNT	UOM	H.M.	PRODUCT DESCRIPTION AND FREIGHT CLASSIFICATION
1	DRU	MIA	15030	55	GAL	X	METHYL ALCOHOL, FLAMMABLE LIQUID UN 1230
2	DRU	MIA	15559	724	LBS	X	ISOPROPANOL FLAMMABLE LIQUID UN 1219 / ISOPROPYL ALCOHOL 99%
6	DRU	MIA	15770	2790	LBS	X	MONOETHANOLAMINE / CORROSIVE MATERIAL UN 2491
10	BOX	MIA	16199	1000	LBS		NON-HAZARDOUS / TETRAPOTASSIUM PYROPHOSPHATE
10	CYL	MIA	17236	400	LBS	X	NITROGEN NON-FLAMMABLE GAS UN 1066
10	BAG	MIA	0661	1000	LBS		NON-HAZARDOUS / ABSORBENT MATERIAL - CLAY

IN CASE OF EMERGENCY CALL (800) 424-9300

DATE RECEIVED 04/10/89 | DATE TO SHIP | DELIVERY DATE 04/14/89 | TOTAL PACKAGES DELIVERED 39 | TOTAL GROSS GALLONS POUNDS 6354

If this shipment moves via "for hire" carrier it shall be governed: (a) as to contract carriers by the applicable contract, or (b) as to common or other carriers by the National Motor Freight Classification uniform bill of lading in effect on date of shipment, if applicable, or by such other bill of lading form or conditions as may be prescribed by government authority. If delivery is made by seller's truck or into vehicle of buyer, bill of lading provisions are not applicable and this document will serve as a delivery receipt.

THIS IS TO CERTIFY THAT THE ABOVE NAMED MATERIALS ARE PROPERLY CLASSIFIED, DESCRIBED, PACKAGED, MARKED AND LABELED, AND ARE IN PROPER CONDITION FOR TRANSPORTATION ACCORDING TO THE APPLICABLE REGULATIONS OF THE DEPARTMENT OF TRANSPORTATION

Subject to Section 7 of National Motor Freight Classification (100-H) Rules, if this shipment is to be delivered to the consignee without recourse on the consignor, the consignor shall sign the following statement.

The carrier shall not make delivery of this shipment without payment of freight and all other lawful charges.

Signature of Consignor ▶

LOADER'S SIGNATURE AND DATE | DRIVER'S SIGNATURE AND DATE | RECEIVER'S SIGNATURE AND DATE

SEND FREIGHT BILL TO
CARRIBEAN CHEMICAL COMPANY
3033 N.W. NORTH RIVER DRIVE
MIAMI, FL 33142

FORM C-6F21 (REV. 8-88) PRINTED IN U.S.A.   **ALL UNLOADING DEMURRAGE WILL BE BORNE BY CONSIGNEE**   **1 – TERMINAL**

Figure 31.21. Example of truck transport bill of lading demonstrating information provided on hazardous materials being transported. With permission from National Fire Protection Association.

```
TANK                FLORIDA EAST COAST RAILWAY COMPANY                SHEET   1
TRAIN
                        CONDUCTORS WHEEL REPORT    SEND TO       HIAF2
   TRAIN E675    DEPARTURE TIME 2030    DATE  11/03/88  CONDUCTOR
                AAR  LEFT
  INIT NUMBER   K  CODE   AT CONSIGNEE CONTENT  ORIGIN/PLAN  SHIPPER  FROM DEST

   FEC    675   Z       0366 HELPING   ENGINE                         0007 0366
   FEC    229   Z       0125 IN TOW    ENGINE                         0007 0125
   NAHX  93055  C  C611 0366           MTY       LONESTAR             0007 0366
   SOU  523258  B  B314 0366 JEFSMURFI PULPBD    FERNAND BCONTAINER   0007 0366
   SOU    189   M  R400 0366 GALCUEENT BEER      DOUGHERTYMILBREWIN   0007 0366
   SOU    846   D  A416 0366 GALCUEENT BEER      DOUGHERTYMILBREWIN   0007 0366
   SOU    221   D  A416 0366 GALCUEENT BEER      DOUGHERTYMILBREWIN   0007 0366
   UTLX  81385  T  T389 0125 PETROLAN  CMPGAS    BAYOU SALARCPETRO    0007 0107
        **DANGEROUS***
   UTLX  80836  T  T389 0242 PETROLAN  CMPGAS    BAYOU SALARCPETRO    0007 0242
        **DANGEROUS***
   DUPX  17430  T  T055 0341 TAGTERMIN MTY       HOUSTON PEIDUPONT    0007 0344
   DUPX  17407  T  T055 0341 TAGTERMIN MTY       HOUSTON PEIDUPONT    0007 0344
   DUPX  17402  T  T055 0341 TAGTERMIN MTY       HOUSTON PEIDUPONT    0007 0344
   UTLX  81802  T  T389 0366 PUBGASCO  CMPGAS    BAYOU SALARCPETRO    0007 0366
        **DANGEROUS***
   GATX  49599  T  T104 0366 ALLUNIVE  CRSVMT    BRUNSWICKLCPCHEMI    0007 0366
        **DANGEROUS***
   SOU  585071  M  R400 0366 GALCUEENT BEER      DOUGHERTYMILBREWIN   0007 0366
   PLMX  27111  T  T564 0366 ALLUNIVE  CRSVMT    BRUNSWICKLCPCHEMI    0007 0366
        **DANGEROUS***
   ACFX  77350  T  T564 0366 ALLUNIVER CMPGAS    BECANCOURCIL         0007 0366
        **DANGEROUS***
   SOU    233   D  A416 0366 GALCUEENT BEER      DOUGHERTYMILBREWIN   0007 0366
```

Figure 31.22. Train "consist" report listing contents of each railroad car and its shipment. This form can help locate the presence of a hazardous material. With permission from National Fire Protection Association.

ulations. However, when a hazardous material is listed on a shipping paper along with nonhazardous materials, the hazardous materials must be:

1. Entered first, OR
2. Entered in a color that clearly contrasts with the description of nonhazardous materials, OR
3. Be identified by the entry of an "X" or an "RQ" placed beside the name of the material in the "HM" column.

All shipping papers will provide the following information:

1. Proper shipping name;
2. Hazard class;
3. UN identification number that can be referenced in the *D.O.T. Emergency Response Guidebook*;
4. Number of packages, i.e., drums, boxes, tank load, or car load;
5. Type of packages, i.e., drums, boxes, cylinders, tank load, or car load;
6. Correct weight.

Locating Shipping Papers

Shipping papers should be located and examined as soon as a close approach to an incident can be accomplished safely. A close approach to the scene may be impossible for the first responders due to fire, explosion, toxic fumes, and lack of proper protective equipment.

Truck Transport

The shipping papers, called a "bill of lading" for truck shipment, shall be in the possession of the driver in the cab of the truck (Fig. 31.21). It may be stored in a holder which is mounted to the inside of the door on the driver's side of the vehicle. When attempts to locate the bill of lading beside the driver are unsuccessful, it could possibly be found: (a) attached to packages in the trailer; (b) on the engine cover in the cab; (c) on the dashboard; (d) in the driver's briefcase; or (e) under the mattress in the "sleeper."

Rail Transport

Rail shipping papers must be in the possession of the train crew. If the train has a caboose, they would be in the possession of the conductor at the end of the train. The papers will be found in the engine for trains without cabooses. The train crew should furnish two types of shipping papers. The first is the "train consist" or "wheel report." This computer printout lists all the cars as they appear in the train beginning with the lead engine, a general description of their contents (i.e., merchandise, compressed gas), and if the car is carrying a hazardous material. The consist is valuable in a derailment situation for piecing together cars and their contents when several have left the track (Fig. 31.22). The second document is the "way bill" or bill of lading for individual rail cars (Fig. 31.23). The way bill provides all required information and must also mention the residue of the last hazardous product carried on an "empty" (see Residue Placard) tank car. Content and hazard information can be obtained from the yard master for incidents in a railroad yard.

Air Shipments

Airbills on each piece of the shipment must be in the possession of the pilot in the cockpit and are usually in the pilot's briefcase.

UNIFORM STRAIGHT BILL OF LADING - ORIGINAL - NOT NEGOTIABLE

[redacted] RAILROAD COMPANY

FORM 173 5 RWC
REV 5/78

RECEIVED, subject to the classifications and tariffs in effect on the date of the issue of this Bill of Lading, the property described below, in apparent good order, except as noted (contents and condition of contents of packages unknown), marked, consigned, and destined as indicated below, which said company (the word company being understood throughout this contract as meaning any person or corporation in possession of the property under the contract) agrees to carry to its usual place of delivery at said destination, if on its own road or its own water line, otherwise to deliver to another carrier on the route to said destination. It is mutually agreed, as to each carrier of all or any of said property over all or any portion of said route to destination, and as to each party at any time interested in all or any of said property, that every service to be performed hereunder shall be subject to all the conditions not prohibited by law, whether printed or written, herein contained, including the conditions on back hereof, which are hereby agreed to by the shipper and accepted for himself and his assigns.

TRANSFERRED TO CAR | KIND | WEIGHT IN TONS: GROSS | TARE | NET | LENGTH OF CAR: ORDERED | FURNISHED | MARKED CAPACITY OF CAR: ORDERED | FURNISHED

CAR INITIALS AND NUMBER: GATX 10874
KIND: T9
NET: 64

WAYBILL DATE: APRIL 14, 1989
WAYBILL NUMBER: 74017

T.O.F.C.
TRAILER INITIAL AND NUMBER | LENGTH | PLAN NUMBER
TRAILER INITIAL AND NUMBER | LENGTH | PLAN NUMBER

CONSIGNEE AND ADDRESS AT STOP

STOP THIS CAR
AT
AT
AT

TO | STATION | STATE | ORIGIN ROAD CODE: 712 - SCL (NO. AND INITIALS) | FROM NO. | STATION | STATE

THIS DATA ADDED BY CARRIER

ROUTE (SHOW EACH JUNCTION AND CARRIER IN ROUTE ORDER TO DESTINATION OF WAYBILL)

Show "A" if Agent's Routing or "S" if Shipper's Routing

FROM (SHIPPER) "Bill of Lading number, or Shipper's number, when furnished shall be shown in the shipper's block of the waybill and prefixed by B/L to indicate bill of lading number, or S/N to indicate shipper's number."

AMERICAN PETRO-GAS
HOUSTON, TEXAS

CUSTOMER'S CODE NO: 34991

CONSIGNED TO (MAIL OR STREET ADDRESS OF CONSIGNEE—FOR PURPOSES OF NOTIFICATION ONLY.)

ACME GAS COMPANY
MIAMI, FLORIDA

RWC

BILL OF LADING DATE | BILL OF LADING NO

WEIGHED AT

DESTINATION: MIAMI
STATE OF: FLORIDA
COUNTY OF

ROUTE (FOR SHIPPER'S USE ONLY)

INVOICE NO.

GROSS

TARE

AL'NCE

NET

Subject to Section 7 of Conditions, if the shipment is to be delivered to the consignee without recourse on the consignor, the consignor shall sign the following statement: The carrier shall not make delivery of this shipment without payment of freight and all other lawful charges.

Signature of Consignor

Note—Where the rate is dependent upon value, shippers are required to state specifically in writing the agreed or declared value of the property. The agreed or declared value of the property is hereby specifically stated by the shipper to be not exceeding

PER

*If the shipment moves between two ports by a carrier by water, the law requires that the bill of lading shall state whether it is "carrier's or shipper's weight".

SHIPPER'S SPECIAL INSTRUCTIONS

CAR TRIP LEASED TO CONSIGNEE GROSS GAL. 25427
NET C GAL. 25198 US 30261 TEMP.
65 TARIFF 5.02 GAVITY 503 INSPEC. CAPS
12/6/88 VALVES SAME

IF CHARGES ARE TO BE PREPAID, WRITE OR STAMP HERE "TO BE PREPAID"

PREPAID

NO. PKGS	DESCRIPTION OF ARTICLES, SPECIAL MARKS, AND EXCEPTIONS	COMMODITY CODE NO.	★	WEIGHT	RATE	FREIGHT	ADVANCES	PREPAID
1-T/C	LIQUIFIED PETROLEUM GAS FLAMMABLE GAS UN 1075 PLACARDED: FLAMMABLE GAS			126,494 LBS.	WEIGHTS AND CHARGES TO FOLLOW PREPAID			

SHIPPER

AGENT

PER

PER

AM

PM

PERMANENT POST OFFICE ADDRESS OF SHIPPER

Figure 31.23. Example of shipping paper for railroad shipment of flammable liquid petroleum gas (UN#1075). With permission from National Fire Protection Association.

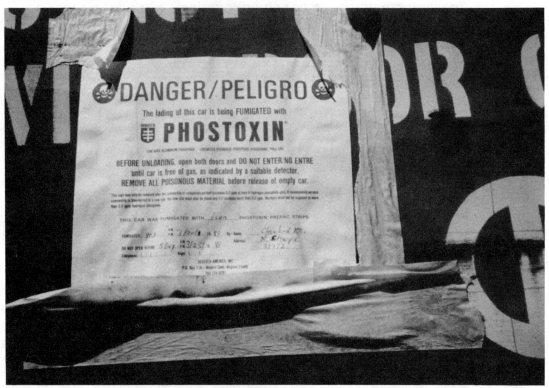

Figure 31.24.   Fumigation notice indicates the potential for a confined space toxic hazard. With permission from National Fire Protection Association.

Water Shipments

A "dangerous cargo manifest" must be on the vessel in a designated holder on the bridge or in the wheelhouse. Barges have a dangerous cargo manifest located in the pilot house of the tug boat. Unmanned barges will keep the manifest in a pipe or cylinder holder near the warning sign indicating hazardous cargo.

Container Markings

Containers used in transport and at fixed facilities will often display the name of the owner or manufacturer as well as the product contained. Obviously, a container bearing the name and logo of Amoco, Texaco, Dow, or Union Carbide would give indication of a possible presence of hazardous materials. A company's name and logo will usually be the largest markings on a container and thus be read from the farthest distance.

Fumigation   Occupancies that store, process, or purvey food, grain, or food products often undergo pesticide fumigation. Rail cars transporting foodstuffs are routinely fumigated with a toxic pesticide such as phostoxin or methyl bromide when they are loaded. Responders to an incident involving such products should look for fumigation notices posted at doors to buildings or transport containers (Fig. 31.24). "Tented" buildings would give immediate indication of a building undergoing fumigation. A light smoke or vapor coming from a restaurant or warehouse after hours should give rise to suspicion of pesticide fumigation.

Rail Cars   Some rail cars are designed or set aside by the owner to transport only one commodity. These cars will generally have the name of the product stenciled on the rail car.

DOT regulations require over 40 hazardous products to have their names stenciled in 4-inch letters on the sides of the rail car. Some of these products are: anhydrous ammonia, chlorine, hydrocyanic acid, liquified hydrogen, liquified petroleum gas, nitric acid, and phosphorous.

National Fire Protection Association 704 SYSTEM

This system, developed by the National Fire Protection Association (NFPA), is for use by fixed storage, buildings, and manufacturing facilities to indicate the presence of hazardous materials as well as their relative degree of hazard. The system uses a diamond which is divided into quadrants of smaller diamonds. Each diamond quadrant addresses a different hazard category (Fig. 31.7).

—The blue diamond in the 9 o'clock position identifies Health Hazard.
—The red diamond in the 12 o'clock position identifies Flammability Hazard.
—The yellow diamond in the 3 o'clock position identifies the reactivity or instability of a material.
—The white diamond in the 6 o'clock position provides information on special hazards of a material. This quadrant may contain a symbol, such as that indicating RADIOACTIVE materials or letters, such as that indicating water-reactive −W or OXY for oxidizer.

The relative hazards of HEALTH, FLAMMABILITY, and REACTIVITY of a product are rated by a number from zero (0), indicating no special hazard, to four (4), indicating severe hazard.

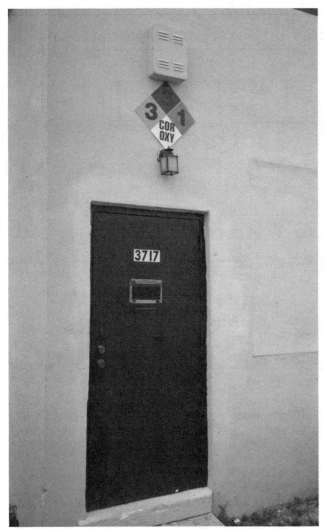

Figure 31.25. The presence of the National Fire Protection Association (NFPA) warning placard above the door indicates the presence of corrosive and oxidizing materials. The placard indicates that the stored material is extremely dangerous to health, ignites at normal temperatures, is unstable if heated, and is not compatible with water.

The 704 system is nationally recognized but is not mandated by federal law. Many industries voluntarily post 704 diamonds at their facilities in cooperation with their local fire department. Many local governments have enacted ordinances requiring the use of the system.

The 704 System provides a simple arrangement of readily recognizable colors, numbers, and symbols which give the first responder an idea of the general hazards of a material at a glance (Fig. 31.8). It does not, however, identify the specific product involved and, unfortunately, is not used in transportation. The presence of such a warning at a building site indicates that hazardous materials are stored (Fig. 31.25).

CONTAINER SHAPE AND DESIGN

Some hazardous materials require specialized containment that have a specific shape, which can give a clue to the identity of its contents. Determining whether a hazardous material is present or not based on container design alone would be dangerously inadequate. New and different container designs are being pro-

duced to meet the needs of changing regulations and technology. A few years ago, pressurized gas rail tanker cars used to be identified by their white color, rounded ends, and dome arrangement. Now DOT regulations require that the cars be retrofitted with thermal insulation that is sprayed on or under a metal jacket. Today, pressurized gas cars may very well be black with squared-off ends. Hazardous materials in small containers up to and including the 55 gallon drums are transported in general cargo trailers and stored in unmarked warehouses—giving no clue to their presence.

All limitations aside, container shape and design can give the first responder a clue to the presence of hazardous materials at a fairly great distance, which can make the task of product identification a lot safer. A complete study of container shape and design is beyond the scope of this chapter. There are many excellent books on hazardous materials which offer an in-depth view of the subject. What follows is a brief overview of container-product relationships.

Trucks

The trucking industry utilizes different types of bulk containers (other than general cargo trailers which are used to ship hazardous cargos in small containers) for shipment of bulk quantities of hazardous materials. These trailers are easily recognized by their shape and may consist of one or more compartments (Figs. 31.26–31.28).

Rail Transport

Railroad tank cars are generally classed as either pressurized or nonpressurized. Pressurized tank cars carry a variety of hazardous liquids and pressurized gases. Some of the most common include chlorine, propane, butane, and anhydrous ammonia. They are recognized by a protective dome on the top of the car, which houses all the valves, gauging fixtures, and relief devices, and by the absence of any valves or piping under the car (Fig. 31.29).

Nonpressurized cars carry flammable, poisonous, and corrosive liquids, as well as a wide variety of nonhazardous products (Fig. 31.30). These cars generally have a variety of valves, pipe outlets, and relief devices along the top of the car and, usually outlets at the bottom. Nonpressurized cars carrying corrosive materials generally can be identified by a black band around the tank at the outlets to protect the tank from spills when loading or off-loading acids or alkalis.

Small Cylinders

The compressed gas industry has a suggested standard for color coding cylinders to indicate their contents. Under the standard, oxygen cylinders are painted green; helium—brown; and nitrous oxide—blue, among others. This color code system is a suggested standard and not required by law. Emergency response personnel should check for the extent of voluntary compliance in their jurisdiction.

Incidents involving liquid propane (LP) gas cylinders are on the rise. As with 55-gallon drums, the hazards of small LP cylinders are taken lightly or ignored because the containers are so common. An exploding 20-pound propane cylinder used to fuel barbecue grills will create a fireball, ground flash, shock wave, and flying metal tank fragments. First responders must anticipate their presence in homes, LP-powered vehicles, and even gas-powered floor scrubbing machines. Their presence may be hidden

4 Basic Designs of Truck Trailers
for Shipment of Bulk Quantities of Hazardous Materials

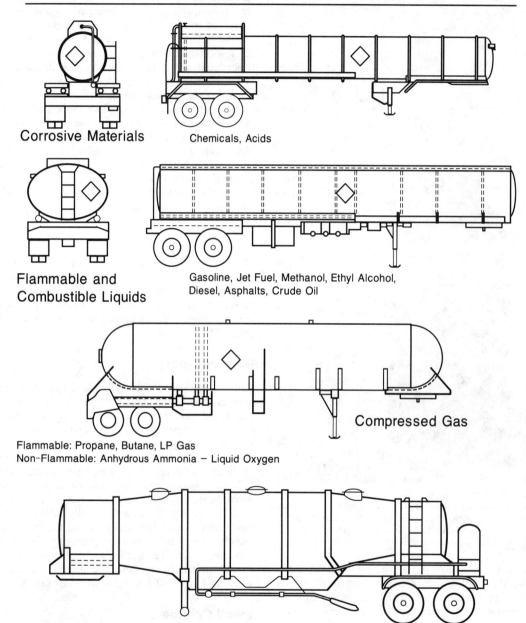

Corrosive Materials — Chemicals, Acids

Flammable and Combustible Liquids — Gasoline, Jet Fuel, Methanol, Ethyl Alcohol, Diesel, Asphalts, Crude Oil

Compressed Gas
Flammable: Propane, Butane, LP Gas
Non-Flammable: Anhydrous Ammonia – Liquid Oxygen

Non-Hazardous Bulk Flowable Commodities – Dry Cement, Lime, Bentonite, Urea Fertilizer, Feed Compounds
Hazardous Bulk Flowable Commodities – Ammonia Nitrate (Oxidizer)

Figure 31.26. Basic shapes of truck trailers that transport hazardous materials.

but must be expected at accidents or fires involving snack trucks, mobile homes, and recreational vehicles (Fig. 31.31).

OTHER INDICATIONS OF HAZARDOUS MATERIALS

Many hazardous materials will behave in ways that can give notice of their presence to first responders. Unfortunately, almost all of this behavior is a result of these materials exiting their containers or being exposed to fire. Therefore, a strange odor, vapor cloud, or noxious fumes are as much a signal to withdraw to a safe distance as they are cause for further investigation.

Emergency personnel should never intentionally expose themselves to odors or close-in views of chemical reactions. They must be observant and respond appropriately to any of the following conditions:

1. Foul, unusual, or noxious odors—some materials, such as hydrogen sulfide (H_2S) will paralyze the olfactory senses after a few whiffs.

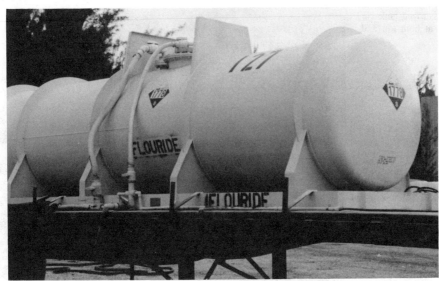

Figure 31.27. Specialized transport container for fluoride. Note reinforcing ribs and protection for valves at the top. This is typical for a tank which contains a corrosive.

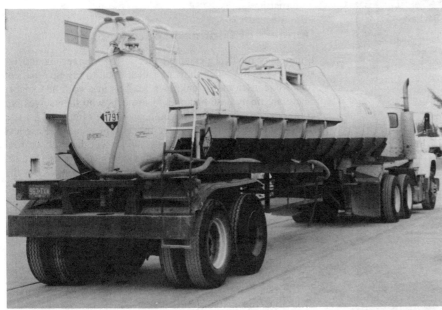

Figure 31.28. Corrosive liquid tanker distinguished by external ribs and relatively small tank container in relation to truck carriage. These features indicate a heavy liquid.

Figure 31.29. Profile of a pressurized tank car carrying chlorine. Note the dome on top which contains all outlets.

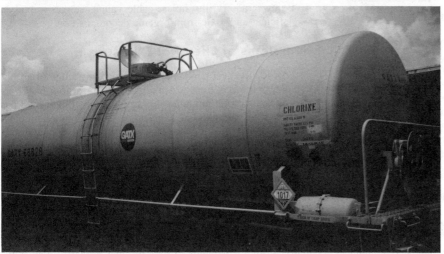

Figure 31.30. Nonpressurized tank car with valves and outlets at both top and bottom of car.

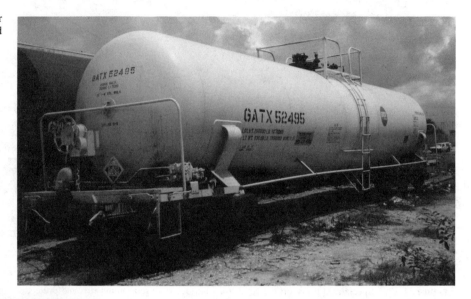

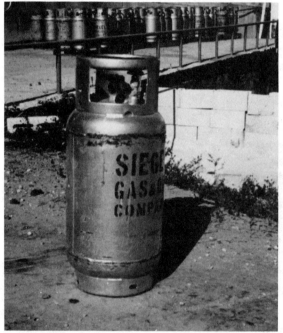

Figure 31.31. Liquid propane gas cylinder.

2. A vapor cloud—a result of the refrigeration effect of a liquified gas, such as propane, or a cryogenic liquid, such as liquid oxygen, boiling into a gas as they leave their containers.
3. Fumes, possibly from a spilled corrosive material—concentrated nitric acid will emit brownish fumes.
4. Irritation to the eyes, nose, and throat—leaking chlorine or anhydrous ammonia can cause slight discomfort one minute and kill the next as the wind direction shifts and blows concentrated fumes towards emergency responders and bystanders.
5. Unusually intense or large fires for the size of the building, vehicle, or container involved.
6. Fires that do not subside, or actually intensify, upon application of water.
7. Loud jet-like noise or jets of flame—indicative of containers

venting and/or relief devices operating to relieve rising internal pressures.

Dangers of Confined Spaces

Emergency medical personnel face a very dangerous and insidious situation when they are called upon to rescue a patient found unconscious for unknown reasons in a confined space. There are many case histories of rescuers who themselves become victims when they succumbed to the effects of a toxic or oxygen-deficient atmosphere in a confined space. Rescuers should suspect oxygen deficiency and protect themselves from toxic and/or flammable gases within confined spaces. The removal of an unconscious or incoherent patient from any of the following confined spaces requires special training, breathing apparatus, and devices to detect and monitor the presence of toxic and or flammable gases:

1. The hold of a ship—contaminated with carbon monoxide, spilled chemicals or leaking refrigerant gases;
2. Cargo trailers and box cars—contaminated with leaking chemicals or fumigated with pesticides;
3. Refrigerated trucks and rail cars—filled with oxygen-excluding refrigerant gases;
4. Below grade: utility holes, cable vaults, sewers—oxygen deficient and toxic from organic decomposition.

Symptoms of Chemical Exposure

Emergency medical personnel with prior knowledge of an occupancy or mode of transport involved with hazardous materials will likely interpret any unusual symptoms exhibited by a patient as signs of possible exposure to hazardous chemicals. Immediate measures must be taken to protect the rescuers from exposure, determine the material involved, and decontaminate the patient prior to his admission to a hospital emergency department (4).

APPROACH AND INITIAL ACTION AT A HAZARDOUS MATERIALS INCIDENT

Emergency responders personnel are conditioned to rapidly intervene in all incidents to save life and property. Naturally,

Figure 31.32. Fire department personnel assessing a hazardous scene with binoculars at a safe distance. Note wind sock showing correct position for personnel to be in (up-wind).

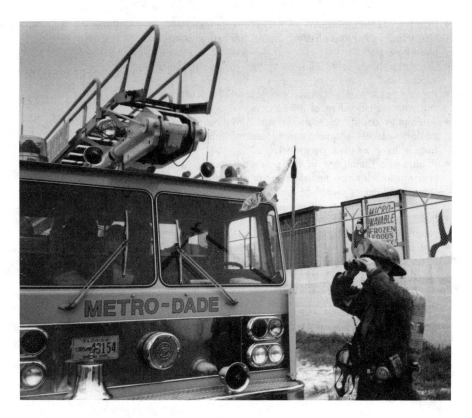

a quick response and rapid fire control or patient stabilization are desirable qualities in any responder. The mindset of emergency responders—to always rush in to save life and property—can cause them to prematurely commit themselves at hazardous material incidents. A known or potential hazardous materials incident requires a much more thorough and cautious assessment of conditions before the scene can be safely approached, victims rescued, and materials identified.

Response Information

An assessment of conditions begins when the emergency call is received. Responding units should obtain as much information as possible from the caller through their dispatcher such as:

1. Exact address and name of occupancy;
2. The name and type of materials involved, spelled out, if possible;
3. Type and number of containers involved;
4. Visible placards, labels, and four-digit UN identification numbers;
5. Whether the placard was being off-loaded, mixed, transferred, etc.?

Responding units should not wait to obtain this information once they are on the scene—conditions may rapidly deteriorate before they arrive.

The wind condition and speed should be ascertained enroute or at least at a great distance from the immediate scene. Wind direction will have a great bearing on the direction of approach and positioning of responding units. Even the slightest breeze can be detected by discharging a small amount of finely divided dry chemical extinguishing agent into the air from a fire extinguisher.

Approaching the Scene

The following guidelines will allow for a safe approach to a known or suspected hazardous materials scene:

- Approach the scene from upwind and uphill.
- Stop at a safe distance and observe conditions (with binoculars, if necessary) before approaching the immediate scene (Fig. 31.32).
- Position the vehicle so that it is heading away from the scene in case sudden retreat is necessary.
- Approach the scene, on foot, with extreme caution. A vehicle's catalytic converter operates at a minimum of 1200°F—a sufficient temperature to ignite all flammables.
- Approach the scene with a minimum number of personnel to conduct the initial assessment—keep the other responding units staged at a safe distance outside the hazard area.
- Use protective equipment. Obviously, units not equipped with protective clothing and self-contained breathing apparatus will not be able to safely intervene in an incident to the extent that a properly protected unit would.

Initial Action

- Isolate the scene and deny entry to bystanders, unprotected responders, and responders who do not have a definite mission in the hazard area.
- Control traffic; but without the use of flares. Don't add an ignition source.
- Eliminate sources of ignition, but do not start vehicles or operate electrical switchgear in the hazard area.
- Post a wind sock and plan for a sudden change in wind direction. A small flag or a piece of police line taped on an antenna or post will do the job.

- Plan for sudden ignition of spilled or leaking materials. Assign standby positions on dry chemical fire extinguishers and foam hose lines.
- Do not walk or drive through spilled material or enter a vapor cloud.
- Perform rescues only at an acceptable level of risk to rescuers and with realistic chances for success.
- Attempt to identify the materials involved through placards, markings, labels, shipping papers, and information received from a driver or plant personnel.
- Realize the limitations of the personnel on the scene. A decision to withdraw and wait for more qualified and protected responders would be based on conditions, level of protective equipment, and collective level of expertise of those on the scene. See chapter on protective clothing and chapter on monitoring devices.
- Understand that the safest and most prudent action for first responders may be to do nothing except to evacuate the area and isolate the scene. Direct involvement in an incident should be preceded by the question: Would the outcome of this incident be any different if we did nothing?

International Placards and Labels

Most international placards and labels are similar to American ones, in terms of colors and symbols (5). Examples of the Canadian system for dangerous goods placarding is presenting is Figure 31.9.

CONCLUSION

It can be very frustrating for emergency personnel who are used to rushing into an incident to do nothing but await the arrival of more qualified responders. The degree of risk to be taken must be commensurate with the amount to be gained by any act on the scene. Detecting the presence of hazardous materials is the goal—but not at the expense of exposure or contamination of personnel.

REFERENCES

1. Hazardous materials incident analysis, student manual. Emmitsburg, MD: National Fire Academy, National Emergency Training Center, Feb. 1, 1985.
2. Official department of transportation hazardous materials placarding and labeling chart. Washington, DC: U.S. Department of Transportation, Research and Special Programs, 1986.
3. Department of Transportation emergency response guidebook (DOT P. 5800.4), September 1987.
4. Bronstein A, Currance P. Emergency care for hazardous materials exposure. St. Louis: C.V. Mosby Co., 1988.
5. Canadian dangerous goods placarding guide. Ontario, Canada: International Compliance Center, Mississauga, nd.

32

Prehospital Organization and Medical Control of Hazardous Materials Incidents

Gerry Bates, C.E.P.
Elizabeth Criss, R.N.
Daniel Spaite, M.D.

In modern civilization, the potential for the accidental release of hazardous chemicals into the environment, with the resultant injury or death to people and destruction of property, is very real. On average, there are 1.6 hazardous materials releases per day in the United States (1). Fortunately, most are small and can usually be handled with a minimum response of emergency personnel and equipment. But whether small or large, these incidents are unlike "normal" responses experienced by emergency medical services (EMS) personnel. By its very nature, a chemical release can continue to affect people and the environment even after containment steps have been taken. A mistake in initial operating procedures can result in injury, death, property damage, and permanent environmental damage.

DEFINITIONS

The U.S. Environmental Protection Agency (EPA) defines extremely hazardous substances as chemicals "that may present severe health hazards to humans following short-term exposure during a chemical accident or other emergency" (2). Perhaps a more useful concept of a hazardous material was developed by Ludwig Benner, Jr., who defines a hazardous material as "any substance which jumps out of its container when something goes wrong and hurts or harms the things it touches" (3). This definition applies to all hazardous materials and punctuates the fact that container problems are part and parcel of hazardous materials issues. A hazardous material incident can thus be defined as the release, or potential release, of a hazardous material from its container into the environment.

PLANNING AND PREPAREDNESS

Safe and effective response to a hazardous materials incident requires special planning and training by all personnel involved. An effective hazardous material incident emergency plan depends on two key elements: hazard analysis and contingency planning (4).

Hazard analysis is the evaluation of the potential risk to and vulnerability of a community in the event of a hazardous chemical release. The purpose of a hazard analysis program is to identify the locations where potential exists for a hazardous incident. In addition, it is designed to evaluate the impact of an incident, in a given location, on a community. It should also assess what resources are available for emergency and cleanup response to an incident.

A hazardous materials contingency plan describes the community's preemergency preparedness. This plan should address the issues of local responsibility and jurisdiction, scene control, medical control, resource availability, and the interrelationship between the hazardous materials emergency activities of each participant in the plan (see chapter 34, Hospital and Community Preparation for Hazardous Material Releases).

The Superfund Amendments and Reauthorization Act of 1986 (SARA), Title III (5), requires state and local governments to establish and maintain emergency preparedness and response systems for chemical incident management.

RESPONSE ORGANIZATION

An effective hazardous materials response system requires coordination and cooperation between the private sector, public emergency response agencies, and health facilities. When developing a community contingency plan, one of the major areas of consideration is how a hazardous materials incident will be managed and controlled. The U.S. Department of Labor requires that any incident involving a hazardous substance be managed by using an incident command system (ICS) (6).

Incident Management

The first and foremost responsibility of responding personnel at any incident is to establish a well-organized command center. The most experienced person on the initial responding unit must assume the role of incident commander. Transfer of command may be considered upon the arrival of a more experienced or senior individual. By placing one individual in command, the responsibility for incident control becomes fixed, and efforts of control are more consistent and efficient. Resources are used more effectively, and a much safer work environment is provided for response personnel.

The site selected by the incident commander for a command (ICS) center should be in a safe location that is highly visible and easily accessible. The command center should provide a good view of the incident and the surrounding area. However, since hazardous chemical releases often spread far beyond their point of origin, this is not always possible. In cases such as this, a position remote from the incident must be established. To maintain the effectiveness of the ICS, all responding personnel must be informed of the command center's location.

Sectoring

The complexity of many hazardous materials incidents becomes nearly indescribable. The tremendous influx of information, the potential for widespread geographic involvement, and the

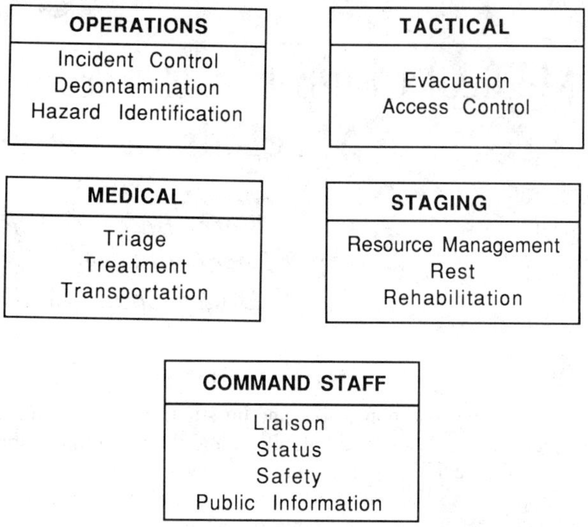

OPERATIONS
Incident Control
Decontamination
Hazard Identification

TACTICAL
Evacuation
Access Control

MEDICAL
Triage
Treatment
Transportation

STAGING
Resource Management
Rest
Rehabilitation

COMMAND STAFF
Liaison
Status
Safety
Public Information

Figure 32.1. Functional Sectors for Effective Scene Management

large volume of responding agencies and personnel can create an overwhelming situation. It is essential that the incident commander develop an organized scene management plan. Effective implementation of this plan is achieved by assigning specific geographic areas and functional activities or sectors to various personnel (Fig. 32.1). Sectoring is a system for dividing an incident management organization into smaller, more manageable units. The incident commander then serves the primary function of providing direction and support to the operating units so that they may achieve their objectives safely and efficiently. An example of sectors that might be required for a hazardous materials incident are included in Fig. 32.1.

Incident Objectives

Every hazardous materials incident response should be directed by a standardized set of priorities. These priorities set a course of action at an incident and provide guidance to the incident commander. This, in turn, increases the effectiveness of the entire management team. The action plan at any incident should be based on four incident priorities:

Life safety: The first responsibility of a hazardous materials incident responder is to provide for the safety of the public and other emergency personnel. This is accomplished by:
a) early recognition and identification of the hazardous material;
b) isolation of the incident from the public and unprotected response personnel;
c) rescuing endangered persons if this can be accomplished without jeopardizing rescuers; and
d) evacuating areas in which a threat to life and/or health exists.
Incident control: these efforts should include:
a) identification of the mechanisms of an uncontrolled release of a hazardous material and
b) developing a course of action to control it, based on a predetermined area-wide management plan.
Environmental concerns: The first issue with this priority is to determine the extent of environmental damage that has occurred. Plans should include identifying:

a) the damaged portion of the environment and
b) methods of securing those resources necessary to restore it to as near normal as possible.
Property conservation: The final incident priority involves:
a) identifying contaminated properties and
b) restoring them to as near a preincident state as possible.

Incident Evaluation

The unique and unpredictable nature of hazardous materials incidents necessitates a thorough evaluation before committing resources to a potentially dangerous situation. An initial approach that is carelessly or naively considered can have dire consequences. Deaths and toxic injury to overzealous responders have been reported from incidents that ultimately required no intervention for neutralization. The incident commander must make a careful evaluation before deciding when and how to commit available resources. The objective of the evaluation is to identify the nature and severity of the immediate problem and gather sufficient information to formulate a valid action plan. A hazardous materials incident requires a more cautious and deliberate evaluation than most other emergency situations (see Chapter 25, Evaluation of Hazardous Environments).

A preestablished set of response guidelines is beneficial in assisting the incident commander in determining whether to intercede or to let an incident run its course. These response guidelines should also include criteria for determining what resources will be needed at the incident. The following is an example of a set of guidelines as established by the Arizona Department of Health Services, Division of Emergency Services (7).

A first responder to a hazardous materials incident should not intervene initially if:

A. Materials are unknown and cannot be readily identified;
B. Atmospheric contaminants, liquid splashes, or other direct contact will adversely affect the responder, and proper equipment is not available to prevent such from occurring;
C. The incident involves a type of material in a quantity that would require placarding by the Department of Transportation (DOT);
D. There is a National Fire Protection Agency 704 M rating of 3 or higher in any category (see Chapter 31, Recognition of Hazardous Materials);
E. There are victims due to exposure to the material, and proper protective equipment is not available to the responder;
F. There will be no adverse environmental impact;
G. The incident occurs in a location where it is unlikely that hazardous vapors or gases will accumulate;
H. Personal protective equipment will not adequately protect personnel.

Initial Radio Report

An important task of the first arriving responder will be to notify dispatch of the conditions upon arrival at the scene. This should include building type and occupancy level, conditions at the scene, actions being taken, special instructions to other incoming personnel, and request for additional units if needed. The primary purpose of this report is to inform both the dispatch center and other responding units about the current status of the incident and whether any special preparation or precautions are required.

Isolation

The major responsibility of emergency responders is to provide for the health and welfare of the public and other emergency personnel at the scene. The first step in meeting this incident priority is to separate the people from the toxic material. To accomplish this priority it is important to identify the affected area and establish a perimeter around the incident. This may be as simple as blocking streets and access to the area, or it may require a massive evacuation effort.

The objective of an isolation procedure is to: (a) limit the number of people exposed to the material, and; (b) rescue endangered persons, if possible, without significant risk of harm to emergency personnel (4). Areas that must be identified during the development of the isolation plan include: all locations endangered by the hazardous product; safe refuge where people can remain clear of the hazard; access points that might allow unauthorized entry into the hazardous area, e.g., doorways, on-ramps, grade crossings, and structures with high hazard potential, e.g., collapse, explosion, entrapment (4).

Generally, hazardous materials incident scenes can be divided into three separate isolation areas: a) exclusion or restricted, b) contamination reduction (decontamination) or limited access, and; c) support or command (Fig. 32.2). The exclusion area or restricted zone is the area immediately surrounding the hazard and poses the greatest danger to responders. Only personnel assigned a specific task and wearing the proper protective clothing are allowed into this area. The contamination reduction or limited access area is a buffer zone between the exclusion area and the support area. If set up properly, personal

protection should not be required. This area must also be restricted to personnel with specific tasks. Decontamination occurs in this area. The support and command area is considered clean and free of contamination. This area is used for staging by all agencies involved in the incident, under the control of the incident commander. Establishment of these isolation areas prevents unnecessary and unprotected people from wandering into the hazard. In addition, incident command is simplified through a clear identification of the controlled access areas and provides an additional margin of safety to all personnel.

Evacuation

Evacuation is the removal of persons from an endangered area. It is usually done as a protective measure and, in residential areas, often results in a prolonged stay away from home. The evacuation zone of a hazardous materials incident is generally very large. All persons not directly involved in incident-related tasks are removed from the evacuation zone.

The size of the evacuation zone depends on the nature and amount of hazardous material and the type of risk it presents to unprotected persons. In some cases, it may be necessary to completely evacuate a large radius around the hazard, e.g., potential explosions. In others, evacuation may only be downwind and/or downhill from the site, e.g., toxic vapors or liquids. An alternative to evacuation for material that dissipates quickly may be to keep people indoors with windows and doors shut.

A comprehensive reference for specific isolation and evac-

Hazardous Materials Accident Site Organization

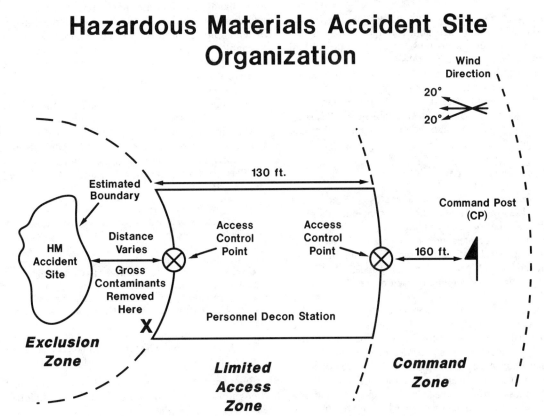

Figure 32.2. Schematic of the recommended isolation areas for a hazardous materials scene. Distances and extent of isolation may vary in relation to the nature and size of the spill. Note that the command zone is upwind of the exclusion zone. (Used with permission of the Tucson Fire Department.)

uation guidelines is the *Emergency Response Guidebook* published by the U.S. Department of Transportation (8).

RECOGNITION AND IDENTIFICATION OF HAZARDOUS MATERIALS

The presence of hazardous materials is often implied by the location of an incident or container, i.e., railroad car, truck, tanker, 55-gallon drum. At other times, the existence of such materials at an incident will be unknown to arriving units as well as to the public. In view of these possible situations and the amount and variety of hazardous chemicals in any community, emergency personnel must develop a high index of suspicion for the existence of toxic hazards even at "routine" calls. Responding units should approach each scene alert to the potential involvement of a chemical hazard. There are several clues that will assist in determining the presence of a hazardous material. These include structure type and location of material, presence of a detectable odor, container type and shape, visible presence of vapors or smoke, and physical complaints of the victims (see Chapter 31, Recognition of Hazardous Materials).

Personnel who are involved in hazardous materials responses should become familiar with several resources and continuously update their knowledge of how to use them. A real incident provides a poor setting for on-the-job training when hazardous materials are involved. Irrevocable harm to the environment and people can result from seemingly trivial mistakes. These incidents are very unforgiving to the poorly trained.

PERSONAL PROTECTION

Entry of toxic materials into the body occurs via four routes: inhalation, skin absorption, ingestion, and injection. At a hazardous materials incident, steps must be taken to prevent all four exposure pathways. Once a toxic situation has been identified and material identified, responders must determine the types of protection required. If the proper equipment is not available, no one should enter the area. In this instance, an isolation zone should be immediately established while personnel await the arrival of units equipped with appropriate protection equipment.

Respiratory Protection

The primary function of a breathing apparatus is to reduce the risk of injury due to inhalation of airborne contaminants. This is accomplished either by removing contaminants from the air or by supplying an alternate source of clean air. The two most common types of basic breathing apparatuses are the filter mask (air purifying) and the self-contained breathing apparatus (SCBA) (Fig. 32.3). A third, less commonly used apparatus is the rebreather.

The air-purifying filter mask removes contaminants by filtering the breathing air through a purifying element. There are a variety of purifying elements for use with the filter mask. Specific purifying agents are designed to protect against certain contaminants. Filter masks are designed to be used in open air and only when the contaminant has been identified (9, 10).

SCBA provides a self-contained supply of clean air and prevents any infiltration of contaminated air through the use of a sealed mask. Positive pressure SCBAs, which provide a constant flow of air to the mask, are required by the Occupational Safety and Health Administration (OSHA) for personnel work-

ing with specific contaminates (see Chapter 24, Personal Protection from Hazardous Materials Exposures). Positive pressure reduces the risk of exposure to contaminated air even in the event of an imperfect seal of the mask or an equipment defect. SCBAs are the safest and most reliable means of respiratory protection. If the nature of the air contaminant is unknown, SCBAs should always be considered.

A rebreather transforms the user's exhaled air through a chemical exchange process and recycles it as a continuous air supply. The exhaled air passes through the chemical chamber, which removes the carbon dioxide; supplemental oxygen is added at a concentration of 21%. Rebreathers allow the responder to work for considerable lengths of time (45–60 minutes) in a contaminated area. Unfortunately, the air becomes extremely hot and dry and therefore increases the fatigue factor for the user.

It is important that all emergency responders be familiar with the use and maintenance of the breathing apparatus. Training should simulate both normal and emergency conditions and should evaluate the individual's fitness for using the equipment which can be heavy and cumbersome.

Protective Clothing

Any and all physical contact with a toxic hazard must be prevented by the equipment utilized by the emergency personnel. The type of protective clothing used is determined by the physical, chemical, and toxic properties of the hazard, the tasks that must be accomplished in the restricted area, and the potential for bodily exposure. Generally, the head, eyes, hands, and feet are most susceptible to exposure, and additional protection should be considered for these areas. When complete protection is necessary, a set of clothing is assembled that includes head protection, face shield and/or safety glasses, chemically resistant boots and gloves, and body protection.

When the hazard has been identified and is known to be minor, minimal protection is needed. As the hazard level increases, so does the level of protection.

The Environmental Protection Agency (EPA) has identified four levels of personnel protection that couple the potential for exposure with the amount of protection provided (see Chapter 24, Personal Protection from Hazardous Materials Exposures) (Fig. 32.4).

Level A. Positive pressure SCBA and a vapor-tight clothing barrier between the wearer and the hostile environment. Level A should be worn when the highest level of respiratory, skin, and eye protection is needed.

Level B. Chemically resistant clothing with positive pressure SCBA. Level B provides protection against splashes and low vapor concentrations but does not afford complete skin and eye protection.

Level C. Respiratory protection and chemical resistant clothing. The main selection criteria for level C are conditions that permit the use of air purifying respirators.

Level D. Minimal clothing protection and no respiratory protection. This level should only be used when no contaminants are present and no potential splash or respiratory hazard exists.

Emergency response personnel should realize that standard firefighting attire, as recommended by the National Fire Protection Association, does not provide adequate protection from the splashes or vapors of many hazardous chemicals. This protective clothing, if combined with respiratory protection, is classified as level C protection.

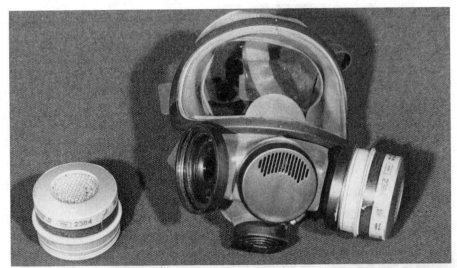

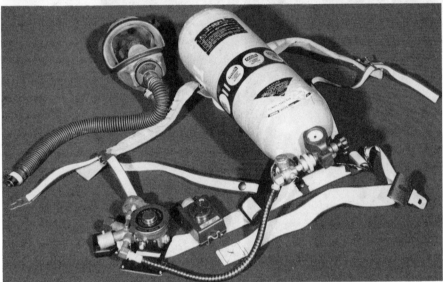

Figure 32.3. A: A standard filter mask. Note the removable filter. Appropriate filters are available to protect against specific contaminants. B: A self-contained breathing apparatus (SCBA). This type of breathing apparatus is required for use with protective clothing levels A and B.

MEDICAL SECTORING

As a general rule, EMS response personnel should not be involved in the direct control or management of a hazardous materials release. Even if there are initially no victims, the risk for injury to the persons handling the incident is so great that the prehospital medical team should be available for potential casualties. In the event of a multiple patient incident, sectoring of the medical priorities is useful to ensure rapid, efficient use of available EMS resources.

Medical Command

The person in charge of the "medical sector" will be directly responsible to the incident commander. The primary responsibilities of the medical sector are twofold: coordination and control of all medical operations at the incident and evaluation of all potential medical problems with communication of this information to the incident commander.

The medical sector can be subdivided into several areas of responsibility. These include patient rescue and/or extrication, patient triage, patient treatment and stabilization, patient transportation and distribution to medical facilities, and medical resources (Fig. 32.5).

Rescue and Extrication

Treatment of patients should not be conducted in the exclusion area. If extrication and/or rescue of a patient from the exclusion area is necessary, it should be performed by the hazardous materials operations team. Attempting impossible rescues should be avoided. Long extrications and rescues should be attempted only if no unnecessary risk to the rescuers exists. To prevent unnecessary exposure and spread of contaminants, anyone involved in the rescue process must be considered contaminated. These personnel should not participate in patient treatment.

Triage

The ultimate goal of the triage process is to provide the best care possible for the greatest number of patients, given the available resources. At a large scale hazardous materials incident, there may be more patients than the medical team can

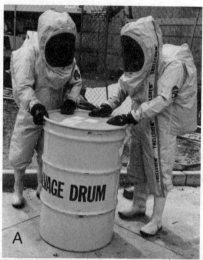

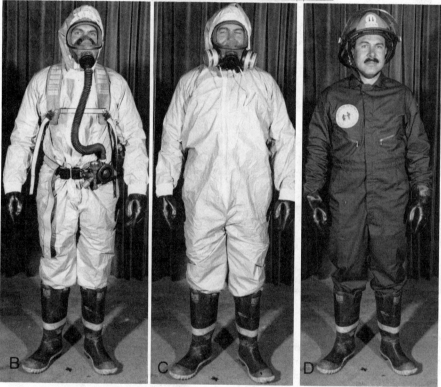

Figure 32.4.   Levels of Personal Protection: A. Workers in level A protective gear handle a disposal barrel. B. Level B protection is characterized by the use of chemical-resistant clothing and positive pressure SCBA. C. Level C protection is characterized by the use of air purifying respirators. D. Minimum clothing protection and no respiratory protection are required for level D protection.

immediately handle. Numerous systems are available that prioritize patients for treatment and transport to a hospital (11). Most use a color and/or numerical coding to categorize patient status and treatment priority (Fig. 32.6). These systems are based on four levels of priority:

Priority I: Critical. Immediate treatment and transport is required.
Priority II: Serious. Emergency transport is required but may be delayed until priority I patients have been removed.
Priority III: No emergency transport is necessary. Evaluation and treatment at the scene in consultation with the base hospital physician is adequate.
Priority IV: Obviously dead or nonviable, given the resources available. No transport required.

Ideally, the most experienced EMS responder should be the triage officer. By its very nature, triage requires the maximum amount of discipline and is potentially the most emotionally demanding. It is important that the triage officer understand his or her responsibility. There is a tendency for medical personnel to treat the first injured person that they encounter. However, if the triage officer falls victim to this tendency, many other potentially more salvageable patients will remain untreated.

Treatment

The treatment zone should be located in an area where patients and medical personnel will be safe from toxic exposure, i.e.,

Hazardous Materials Accident Site
Medical Sectors

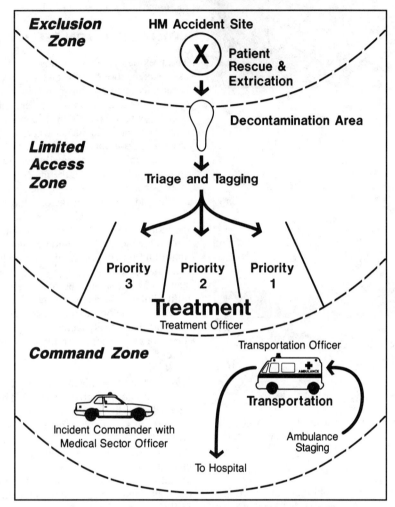

Figure 32.5. Suggested schematic for the medical sectors needed at a hazardous materials site. Size and nature of the hazardous material spill will assist in determining the extent that this plan will be implemented. (Used with permission of the Tucson Fire Department.)

uphill and/or upwind of the incident. The area should also provide good access for transport vehicles. In incidents with large numbers of patients, the treatment area should be divided into three selections, corresponding to the three triage priority levels (Fig. 32.5). This allows categorization of patients requiring differing levels of care into easily identifiable locations and aids in organizing transport priority.

A treatment officer, appointed by medical command, is in charge of all personnel in this area. The treatment officer does not treat individual patients but, rather, conducts secondary patient triage and assigns medical resources to those patients in most need. This person should continually reassess patients and move patients to other treatment priority areas as deterioration occurs.

The initial examination of a chemically contaminated person should determine several things: to what degree the injuries are related to the toxic substance, what body parts have been most severely exposed, the route of entry, and whether the toxic material is continuing to harm the patient.

Chemically contaminated patients should be stripped of *all*

clothing. This should occur prior to entering the treatment section to avoid unnecessary contamination of medical personnel. Simply removing the patient's clothing reduces the potential for contamination of rescue and hospital personnel by as much as 85% (12, 13). All clothing should be properly bagged to ensure safe disposal.

If the patient's condition is life-threatening, advanced cardiac life support (ACLS) and advanced trauma life support (ATLS) protocols will supersede the contamination reduction procedures. If decontamination has not been completed, these procedures should be carried out by properly protected personnel (see Chapter 33, Field Decontamination of Hazardous Materials).

Transportation

The transportation officer is responsible for patient loading, distribution, and transport to area hospitals. This requires coordination with medical command, the treatment officer, and the receiving facilities. Hazardous materials incidents can quickly

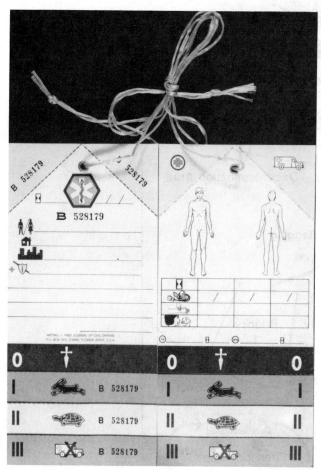

Figure 32.6. Patient triage tags systems assist the personnel at the scene as well as those at the receiving facility in determining the extent of injuries of the incoming patients. (Used with permission of Journal of Civil Defense/Met Tag, Starke, FL.)

overload local medical treatment capabilities; therefore the transportation officer must carefully monitor the status of local medical facilities and their capacity to accept patients. The receiving facilities are given specific information about the number, severity, and estimated time of arrival for incoming patients. The contamination status of incoming patients should be included in the telemetry to the receiving facility. The transportation officer is also responsible for recording the number, condition, and destination of all victims, coordinating traffic flow to and from the scene, and procuring and distributing medical resources at the incident site.

Prior to transport, it may be necessary to prepare transport personnel and their vehicles to protect them from potential contamination. Draping the interior of the vehicle and gurney with a plastic tarp affords some measure of splash and contact protection to the vehicle. Transport personnel should maintain a level of personal protection that is appropriate for the toxic materials involved (see Personal Protection Section). Neoprene or latex gloves, rubber boots, and respiratory protection should be considered.

Leather (shoes, belts, watchbands, etc.) absorbs and retains a host of toxic substances. Decontamination of leather material is not possible following exposure, and these articles must be destroyed. If possible, leather items should be removed from rescuers before contact with the patient. Soft-style contact lenses

should also be removed and replaced with glasses, if possible, before patient contact. If hazardous material becomes trapped behind the lenses, they can act as an occlusive dressing, holding the material to the eye (12, 13).

CONTAMINATION REDUCTION

The previous sections of this chapter have outlined the necessary precautions to be taken to prevent contamination at a hazardous materials incident. However, even with these precautions contamination of rescuers and equipment may occur. A contamination reduction (decontamination) sector should be established at all incidents where the possibility of personnel or equipment contamination exists. The purpose of this sector is to neutralize or physically remove contaminants, thereby preventing the spread of the material beyond the contamination reduction area. The extent of the contamination reduction process depends on several factors, the most important being the type of contaminant. Generally, the more harmful the material the more extensive the contamination reduction process.

Ideally, the contamination reduction site should be located uphill and upwind of the incident. The potential for contaminated water runoff must be considered during the planning stage. The site should be remove from storm drains, sewers, utility holes, and environmentally sensitive areas. It must be located outside of the immediate hazard zone. The area should be isolated and easily identifiable by all personnel. Logistically, it provides for systematic removal of contaminants as the patient or rescuer moves from the ''dirty'' to a ''clean'' area (Fig. 32.7).

All personnel conducting contamination reduction should be in appropriate protective clothing. The process of decontamination begins by removing all the patient's clothing. Plastic garbage cans or similar containers lined with plastic bags can be used to store clothing. If possible, a predecontamination ''swipe'' test should be conducted on the patient's skin. This process involves wiping cloth swabs over contaminated or potentially contaminated areas of the patient's skin. These are then saved in sealed plastic bags for later analysis at the medical facility. This assists in the determination of the patient's initial level of contamination and the effectiveness of the contamination reduction procedures.

The regional poison control center and reference materials can assist in determining whether any special decontamination process is necessary. Ordinarily, scrubbing with a mild soap and water solution using a soft sponge followed by rinsing with copious amounts of water provides a relatively safe and effective means of removing contaminants. Water spray and runoff must be kept to a minimum. Avoid the use of a bristle brush, as this may abrade the skin, allowing contaminants to enter the body.

There will be times when on-scene contamination reduction efforts may not be practical, e.g., extreme cold, high winds, etc. In these cases, life-saving care should be instituted immediately without considering decontamination. If possible, the patient's clothing should be removed while in the transport vehicle. If contaminated clothing cannot be removed safely, the individual should be wrapped in plastic tarps or blankets to decrease the risk of contaminating transport personnel and equipment. Outside garments are then removed and disposed of at the medical facility.

The hazardous materials incident site should remain secure until cleanup procedures are completed. All contaminated ma-

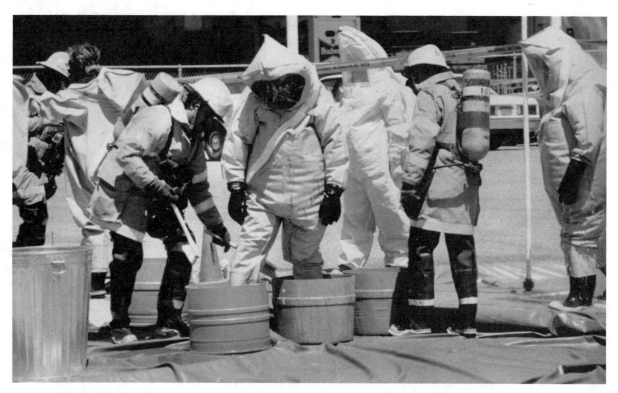

Figure 32.7. Moving from right to left, emergency workers in level A protective garments proceed through a systematic decontamination process. Note the shower in the right corner used to remove gross contamination prior to garment cleaning and removal. (Used with permission of the Tucson Fire Department.)

terials and equipment must be cleaned or disposed of properly. Each piece of equipment must be disassembled, cleaned, and inspected before it is returned to service. Response vehicles must be cleaned and decontaminated. Response personnel must shower and change their clothing. Used clothing should be washed immediately. Items that cannot be decontaminated must be secured in containers for disposal by an authorized agency. Every effort should be made to contain hazardous waste water on the site. Often proper site selection and isolation procedures will aid in reducing the time and energy required for cleanup of waste solutions. These should be secured until they can be removed by an authorized agency.

MEDICAL RECEIVING FACILITIES

Even in the best of circumstances, some patients arriving at the receiving facilities may still be contaminated. If improperly handled, this may result in a second hazardous materials incident at area hospitals. Unfortunately, many medical facilities are poorly prepared to handle the chemically contaminated patient. A well-conceived plan that has been prospectively developed will make provisions for notification of appropriate medical and administrative personnel, a contamination reduction team, and the establishment of an isolated receiving area (see Chapter 34, Hospital and Community Preparation for Hazardous Material Releases). Each hospital must have a well-conceived section in its emergency incident plan that specifically deals with preparation for and management of contaminated patients.

Contamination Reduction Area

As previously stated, many hospitals are not adequately equipped to deal with contaminated patients. It may not seem cost-ef-

fective to allocate funds and space to a designated contamination reduction area when chemically contaminated patients make up such a minute portion of overall patient volume. Despite this, medical facilities should accept this important responsibility to the community.

Basically two options are available for hazardous materials readiness. The first is having a designated zone for receiving and decontaminating patients prior to entry into patient treatment areas. This contamination reduction area is staffed by properly trained and experienced personnel working with appropriate equipment and protective clothing.

If the hospital does not have existing space for such a plan, a second option entails a modified trailer that is a self-contained contamination reduction unit (Fig. 32.8).

MEDICAL CONTROL

The medical control of a hazardous materials incident is extremely important, since it can have such widespread health implications for prehospital and hospital personnel and the community as a whole. The prospective aspect of medical control is probably the most significant with regard to the proper management of patients who have been exposed to toxic materials. An experienced EMS physician should be intimately involved with all of the planning stages of the hazardous materials response. This physician should work with emergency response provider agencies that are well-versed in and experienced at working in the uncontrolled field environment and with the logistics of rescue and decontamination.

On-line medical control during a hazardous materials incident should be established early by EMS responders. In this case the medical control should be a well-trained EMS base

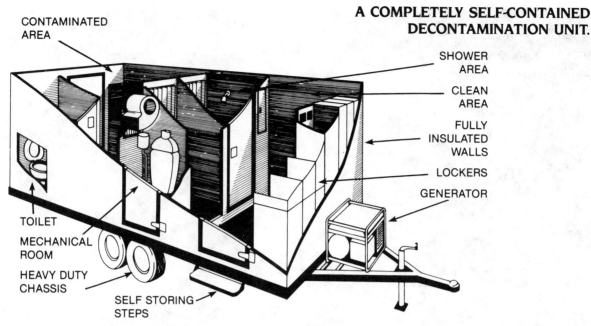

Figure 32.8.   A self-contained contamination reduction unit can be used on site or by hospitals that do not have space to dedicate to contamination reduction. (Used with permission of Evergreen Safety Systems, Inc., Arvada, CO.)

hospital physician who is familiar with the logistics and capabilities of prehospital medical personnel. It will frequently be advantageous for this physician to also be in contact with a toxicologist and/or the regional poison center (see Chapter 35, Role of the Regional Poison Center in Hazardous Materials Accidents).

In some instances, an on-site medical command physician may be requested by personnel at the scene. In large incidents, this provides continuous, ongoing medical control without requiring time-consuming radio contact. If an infield physician is requested, only one who is trained and experienced in the provision of medical care in the field should respond. Other physicians will be likely to have a "tunnel" vision approach which is typical of *any* medical personnel who are thrown into the field environment for the first time. In this kind of setting it is likely that the medical control will be incorrectly prioritized and perhaps even detrimental to the patients as a whole.

Physicians should be aware of the fact that hazardous materials response teams are being developed rapidly throughout the entire country. This is occurring regardless of whether there is significant physician involvement or not. For the health and welfare of the public, it is imperative that physicians uphold their responsibility to supervise all aspects of health care. Recent EMS literature has emphasized the great importance of having intense physician supervision in all aspects of prehospital care. This is to ensure that medical care being practiced by physician extenders in the field is appropriate, timely, efficient, safe, and optimum (14).

REFERENCES

1. Binder S. Deaths, injuries and evacuations from acute hazardous materials releases. Am J Public Health 1989;79:1042–1044.

2. Rules and Regulations. Fed Reg 51:(221) Nov 17, 1986;41573.

3. Benner L, ed. A textbook for use in the study of hazardous materials emergencies. Oakton, VA: Lufred Industries, 1978.

4. Noll G, Hildebrand M, Yvora J, eds. Hazardous materials: managing the incident. Stillwater, OK: Fire Protection Publications, 1988:4, 53–56.

5. Rules and Regulations. Fed Reg 51:(221) Nov 17, 1986;41570.

6. Rules and Regulations. Fed Reg 54:(42) March 6, 1989;9328.

7. Arizona Department of Health Services, Division of Emergency Services. Hazardous materials response training, level one: first on the scene. Instructor guide. Phoenix, AZ: Arizona Department of Health Services, 1985:VII–5,6.

8. U.S. Department of Transportation, Research and Special Programs Administration. Emergency response guidebook. DOT # P-5800.4. Washington, D.C.: DOT, 1987.

9. Arizona Department of Health Services, Division of Emergency Services. Hazardous materials response training, first responder. Phoenix, AZ: Arizona Department of Health Services, 1985:IV–16.

10. U.S. Environmental Protection Agency. Hazardous materials incident response operations. Part 2. Washington, D.C.: U.S. Environmental Protection Agency, 1987:2–1.

11. Isman W, Carlson G. Hazardous materials. Encino, CA: Glencoe Publishing Co., 1980:226–227.

12. Vance M. Hazardous materials training program. Section 1. Phoenix, AZ: Arizona Department of Health Services, 1985.

13. Koleson R. A hazardous materials incident: emergency medicine. (Video). St. Louis, MO: The HazMat Resources, 1985.

14. Peterson JA. The EMS physician and the hazmat team. National Association of Emergency Medical Services Physicians National Conference, 1988.

33

Field Decontamination of Hazardous Materials

Charles E. Stewart, M.D.

INTRODUCTION

The necessity and principles of decontamination are well-known to most medical providers. One form of decontamination, antiseptic technique, is used daily throughout the world. The surgical scrub decontaminates both patient and provider; the scrub clothes, drapes, and sheets provide a "containment vessel," and antiseptics become "neutralizing" solutions. Indeed, the reproductive abilities of viruses and bacteria add a magnitude to biologic decontamination that the radiation physicist or chemical engineer will never know. The release of methyl isocyanate at Bhopal, India, killed 2500 persons, the nuclear accident at Chernobyl contaminated tens of thousands of persons, but smallpox devastated the native population of the Americas and the Sandwich and Polynesian islands (1). The Black Death killed nearly one third of the population of Europe.

Until very recently, emergency providers have not been well trained in hazardous materials management. Physicians who work in emergency departments or who are involved with the emergency medical service (EMS) agencies must understand that an accident involving hazardous materials places the health and possibly the lives of the rescuers, the victims, the surrounding community, and the emergency department staff in jeopardy. When either chemical or radioactive agents are involved, there is the possibility that contamination of both rescuers and victims will occur (2). Emergency providers may not consider the presence of hazards when confronted with an injured patient and an overturned truck unless they are specifically trained in hazardous materials response.

This chapter will present simple guidelines to prevent contamination and explain expedient methods for decontamination of both field casualties and providers. It is not intended to replace specific guidelines for a particular agent, but rather to give an overall approach applicable to all casualties. EMS physicians and providers are reminded that some substances will mandate self-contained protective and airtight overgarments with completely self-contained breathing supplies. Fortunately, these exposures are rare, and shipments of these substances are usually well-controlled.

HAZARD IDENTIFICATION

Vital to all decontamination and containment procedures is the identification of the contaminating material. In many cases, this involves determining what material or chemical a facility or industry is using, storing, or making. In transportation accidents, identification can be accomplished by locating the bill of lading or manifest which may have the contents well-identified or noting the presence of a label or placard. The shipper or the consignee may know the contents of a particular shipment. Usually the manifest and other data are available in the vehicle or with the driver. Problems in identifying hazards occur when these documents are lost, missing, or placarding or labeling is missing or in error.

The Department of Transportation (DOT) controls shipments of hazardous materials by all common carriers and requires the following:

Proper shipping containers;
Acceptable shipping papers;
Shipper certification of content;
Placarding and labeling of container and/or transport vehicle.

DOT has mandated a diamond-shaped placard for hazardous materials, placed on both sides and the rear of the vehicle. This placard contains a 4-digit number keyed into the DOT hazardous materials register. This number can be used to rapidly identify a substance (see chapter on identification of hazardous materials). The placard may also contain a symbol such as a skull and crossbones, flames, or bomb exploding. A single number that refers to the United Nations system for classifying hazards shipped between countries may also appear on the placard (Fig. 33.1). Other hazards may fall under different regulatory agencies such as carcinogens (Fig 33.2) and polychlorinated biphenyls (PCBs) (Fig. 33.3), which are required to have special labeling by the Occupational Safety and Health Administration and the Environmental Protection Agency. Rapid emergency action may be found in the DOT *Emergency Response Guidebook.*

Unfortunately, placards or labels may be missing, incorrect, or destroyed. Placarding is not required when less than 1000 pounds or 300 gallons of hazardous materials are being transported. Military shipments may be unmarked for security reasons. Mixed shipments may not have placards for "small" quantities of substances, and may show only the largest shipment's composition. These rules are somewhat stricter when radioactive materials, biologic agents, or explosives are carried. It is obvious that 1000 pounds of some materials may represent a dangerous or lethal exposure to responding personnel when a spill occurs. In some cases, the substance must be identified by real-time, on-scene environmental monitoring by qualified professionals.

FIELD DECONTAMINATION

Prevention of Contamination

The usual reference books and technical resources available to emergency response personnel will not detail the steps involved in decontaminating either personnel or equipment. Technical data and advice may be conflicting or inadequate. Chemical companies are thought to produce at least 35,000 different dangerous substances. Of these, only 1700 or so have been identified by DOT as hazardous. Most hazardous response teams will refer to the DOT *Emergency Response Guidebook* for advice.

The best method of decontamination is not to become contaminated. This can be done by minimizing contact with po-

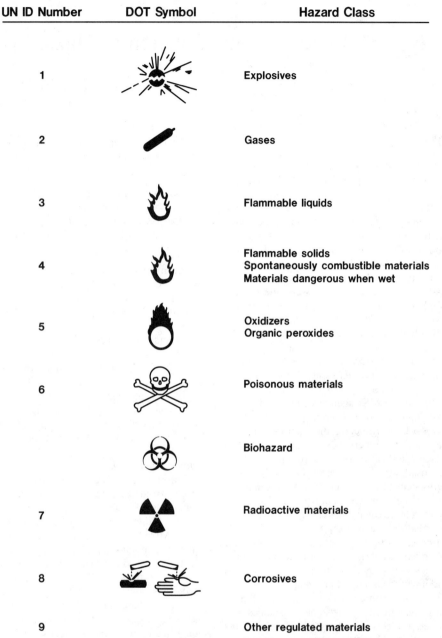

UN ID Number	DOT Symbol	Hazard Class
1		Explosives
2		Gases
3		Flammable liquids
4		Flammable solids Spontaneously combustible materials Materials dangerous when wet
5		Oxidizers Organic peroxides
6		Poisonous materials
		Biohazard
7		Radioactive materials
8		Corrosives
9		Other regulated materials

Figure 33.1.   Department of Transportation Hazard Symbols and Classes with the United Nations identification number.

tentially hazardous substances. When there is a spill of unknown substances at the scene of an accident, ASSUME THAT IT IS DANGEROUS. Medical providers should not walk through areas of obvious contamination and should not touch objects that are potentially contaminated.

The basic principles of field decontamination can be summarized as follows:

1. Containment of the hazard;
2. Prevention of responder exposure and contamination;
3. Decontamination:
   a. Personnel
   b. Victims
   c. Equipment
4. Tracking of contamination and victims;

5. Monitoring victim, personnel, and equipment for contamination;
6. Cleanup of contaminated equipment and personnel.

Disposable outer garments and disposable equipment may prevent spread of contaminants, and should be used when necessary. Monitoring and sampling instruments should be protected by plastic bags or sheaths. Monitor leads should be brought through the neck of the bag and taped. (Sampling ports may be cut in the bags where needed.)

Decontamination Site Selection and Management

Before beginning decontamination, the officer in charge should decide the extent of decontamination necessary and how much

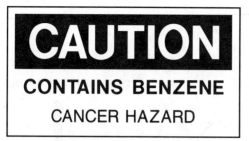

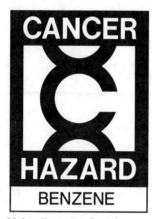

Figure 33.2. Example of carcinogen warning.

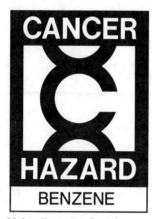

Figure 33.3. Example of PCB warning.

decontamination can be accomplished at the scene of the accident. This depends on the nature of the contaminant, number of victims, location of the victims, the extent of injuries, and the environment. Decontamination at hospitals or fire stations will complicate the problem and will contaminate multiple areas and vehicles and should not be attempted.

The following questions need to be answered regarding the decontamination:

Are existing resources available to decontaminate both personnel and equipment?

If they are not readily available, how long will it take to get them?

Can the decontamination be safely accomplished with the equipment on hand?

Are there environmental factors or factors relating to the particular hazard which alter the decontamination process?

Is the site appropriate?

Dilution is difficult to use as a decontamination technique when the environmental conditions are prohibitive, such as a temperature that is below freezing. Certain radioactive substances should not be diluted, and certain chemicals may not be compatible with water. The toxicity of some agents which contaminate equipment may make equipment unsafe or unusable. Disposal may be the only safe method of handling some agents. Nearby streams and ponds may make sites environmentally unsuitable for certain agents that persist in the environment should runoff occur. Hospitals also generally make poor decontamination sites, due to the added risks to staff and other patients and lack of preparation.

When a suitable decontamination site has been established, a decontamination station is constructed. This decontamination station should be clearly marked and all firefighters, police, rescue workers, and cleanup technicians should be aware of the site. The site decontamination station and the emergency decontamination stations ensure that no contaminated patient is transferred directly into a hospital or emergency department environment. Proper flow of personnel and victims from the zone of contamination through the stations and into the clean areas is essential to containment of the hazard as well as for effective decontamination of victims and personnel (Fig. 33.4).

Decontamination Facilities

These range from portable stretchers to self-contained mobile units (Figs. 33.5 and 33.6). Field decontamination units are portable, easily set up in minutes, and have collection vessels to contain washings. Decontamination stretchers for patients can be easily constructed using saw horses, small plastic swimming pools, and disposable stretchers if necessary. Decontamination of rescue personnel is essential to contain spread of any hazardous material and can be carried out using portable field facilities (Figs. 33.7 and 33.8) as well as the larger self-contained units which are mobile and have the necessary shower stations and changing areas (Figs. 33.5 and 33.9). Decontamination of victims as well as personnel is conducted in the proper zone (Fig. 33.4). Appropriate protective garments must be worn by the responding personnel (Figs. 33.8 and 33.10).

Decontamination Officer

The decontamination officer's responsibilities, duties, and authority should be clearly outlined in disaster plans. An appropriately trained medical triage officer should have joint authority, so that truly life-threatening injuries are not neglected. The decontamination officer and medical triage officer should be responsible to the incident commander.

The decontamination officer, medical triage officer, and incident commander should confer with specialists such as chemical engineers, toxicologists, certified industrial hygienists, nuclear physicians, and radiation physicists as needed to determine which decontamination methods will be used, how much decontamination is required, and how much can be completed at the scene. Patients with life-threatening emergencies

SITE DECONTAMINATION

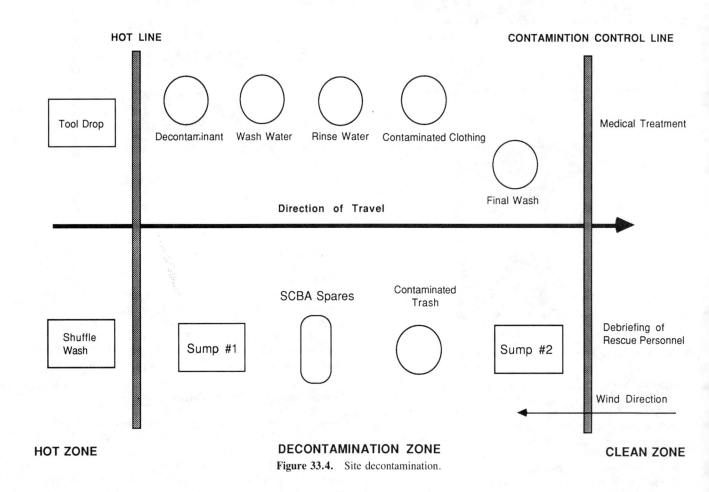

Figure 33.4.   Site decontamination.

Figure 33.5.   Self-contained decontamination facility.

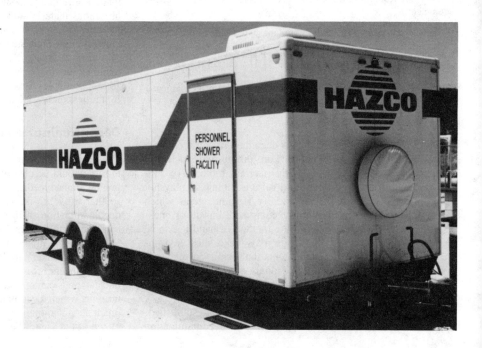

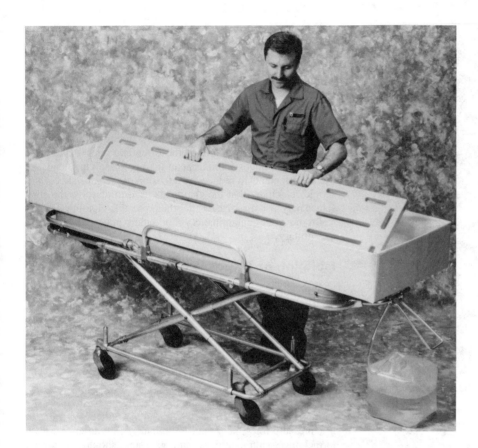

Figure 33.6. Portable field stretcher decontamination unit for patients. Note collection tank. Courtesy RMC, Philadelphia, PA.

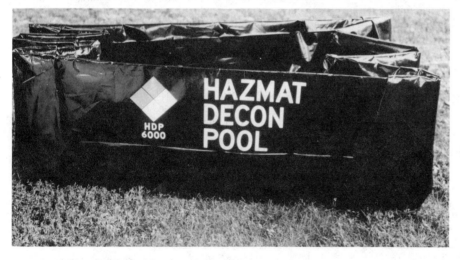

Figure 33.7. Decontamination and containment vessel. Courtesy RMC, Philadelphia, PA.

may have to be treated at the receiving medical facility for contamination. The receiving hospital must be forewarned in this case.

Transport Vehicles

Although ambulances are traditionally used for transport of casualties, this is not ideal for contaminated victims. Ambulances are difficult to decontaminate, are filled with expensive equipment, and can carry very few patients. Multiple radioactive material incidents have proven this point.

Although helicopters can move patients rapidly, they are more expensive than land ambulances and more difficult to decontaminate. A pilot, unaccustomed to protective gear, may not be able to safely pilot the vehicle. An unprotected pilot overcome by contaminants, endangers self, crew, patient, and those on the ground.

Vans and other trucks are far better vehicles to transport the contaminated patient than are ambulances. They have steel beds, carry large numbers of patients, and are relatively easy to decontaminate. In the worst outcome, a pickup truck is far easier to replace than an ambulance in all parts of the United States. Four-wheel-drive trucks provide added mobility in inclement weather and rough terrain. Plain body vans or delivery vans provide acceptable substitutes in cases of inclement weather.

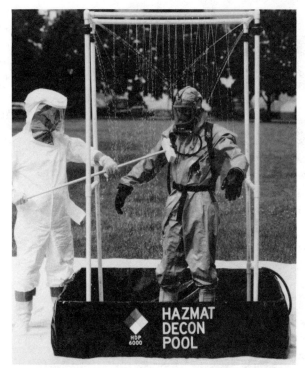

Figure 33.8. Personnel decontamination pool and shower. Courtesy RMC (Radiation Management Consultants), Philadelphia, PA.

TECHNIQUES

Decontamination techniques will depend on the injuries to the victims, the nature of the contaminant, weather, and the tools and equipment available. Likewise, the size and complexity of the decontamination station will depend on the physical and chemical properties of the contaminant, the potential for exposure and location of that exposure for the workers, availability of equipment, and the weather. See Table 33.1 for additional equipment and Table 33.2 for general decontamination procedures.

Physical Removal of Contaminant

The most common technique to get rid of a contaminant is to physically remove it. Physical removal is simple and effective and requires few specialized tools. Physical methods of removal include: brushing, scraping, wiping, diluting, adsorbing, and

vacuuming. In special situations the area may be cleaned by pressurized streams of water, steam, or sand. Some liquids may evaporate or may be vaporized.

Chemical Removal

Chemical removal is the neutralization or dissolution of the substance with another chemical. It is more complex than physical removal, since it requires an understanding of the chemical structure and the reactions of the offending agent. Chemical removal techniques include neutralizing, dissolving, and the use of surfactants to reduce the adhesion of the substance. One should remember that the chemicals used to dissolve the substance may also dissolve or alter the protective clothing. Chemical removal of contaminants is not widely practiced except by the military.

Isolation or Disposal

It may not be possible or practical to decontaminate some equipment or clothing. This is often true with radioactive agents. Special areas for storage of these items will be designated by decontamination officers in conjunction with state and federal officials.

CHEMICAL DECONTAMINATION

Generally, skin exposures should initially be treated by irrigating the contaminated areas with large volumes of water at low pressure for greater than 30 minutes. Only after exposure to metallic sodium, lithium, and potassium should this not be immediately done, since these metals react violently with water. In these cases, the metallic fragments should be expeditiously removed with forceps. Specific "antidotes" for skin exposure do not generally exist, and providers should not waste time looking for these antidotes.

The following guidelines for decontamination solutions may be helpful when medical providers are faced with an unknown hazardous material. The solutions are designed to chemically neutralize agents and not merely remove them. A general understanding of these techniques is useful. The components to formulate these solutions may be prepackaged and stored for long periods of time in an appropriately sized receptacle in dry form. When needed, water can be added to make the appropriate solutions. *In all cases of suspected chemical contaminations, the medical provider should be irrigating with low pressure, high volume water irrigation while awaiting these*

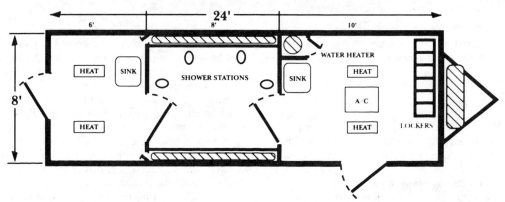

Figure 33.9. Typical layout of field self-contained decontamination unit. Courtesy of HAZCO, Dayton, OH.

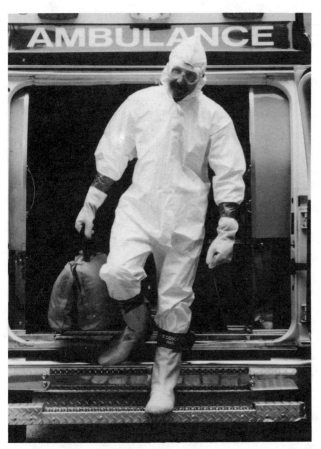

Figure 33.10. Hazardous material protective clothing. Note hood, eyewear, gloves, and boots.

solutions. These solutions are not recommended for routine use but are included for completeness. These solutions are used primarily by the military.

Decontamination Solution A

Decontamination *solution A* contains 5% sodium bicarbonate and 5% trisodium phosphate. These chemicals are available in most hardware stores and chemical supply houses. Four pounds of sodium bicarbonate and four pounds of commercial grade trisodium phosphate should be mixed in 10 gallons of water to obtain the proper concentrations.

Decontamination solution A may be used on intact skin, followed by copious water irrigation. *Solution A is not to be used on open wounds, mucous membranes, or eyes.* Generally these areas are best treated with copious irrigation by large volumes of water at low pressure for long durations.

Decontamination solution A may be used for:

Inorganic acids;
Acidic caustic wastes;
Metal processing wastes;
Solvents and organic compounds (chloroform, trichloroethylene, and toluene);
Plastic wastes and PCBs;
Biologic contamination.

Decontamination Solution B

Decontamination *solution B* is a concentrated solution of bleach (sodium hypochlorite). A 10% solution may be made by mixing 8 pounds of anhydrous calcium hypochlorite powder with 10 gallons of water. Anhydrous calcium hypochlorite powder is commonly known as HTH and is available from swimming pool supply houses. HTH should always be stored in plastic containers. Decontamination solution B may be used on intact skin after it is diluted 50:50 with water to form a 5% solution (similar to household bleach). Regular strength 5% household bleach containing sodium hypochlorite can be substituted for solution B. Use of either solution should be followed with copious irrigation with water. *Solution B is not to be used on open wounds, mucous membranes, or eyes.*

Decontamination solution B may be used for:

Radioactive materials (especially plutonium);
Heavy metals such as lead, mercury, or cadmium;
Pesticides, chlorinated phenols, dioxin, and PCB;
Cyanide;
Ammonia;
Inorganic wastes;
Organic wastes;
Biologic contamination.

Decontamination Solution C (Rinse Solution)

A general purpose rinse solution suitable for use with chemical decontamination solutions A and B is 5% solution of trisodium phosphate. To prepare the rinse solution, 4 pounds of trisodium phosphate should be added to each 10 gallons of water.

Rinse solution is an effective decontaminant for:

Solvents and organic compounds;
Polychlorinated Biphenols (PCB) and Polybrominated Biphenyls (PBB)
Oily wastes not suspected to be contaminated with pesticides.

Following a rinse with *solution C*, the equipment may be rinsed again with water. Decontamination solution C may be used on intact skin and should be flushed off with water. *Solution C is not to be used on open wounds, mucous membranes, or eyes.*

Decontamination Solution D (Alkali Decontamination Solution)

Decontamination solutions listed above are not effective with strong alkali contaminating agents. A dilute solution of hydrochloric acid may be made by mixing one pint of concentrated hydrochloric acid in ten gallons of water. *This solution is used to decontaminate equipment only and should not be used on personnel.*

Decontamination solution D is suitable for:

Inorganic bases;
Alkalies;
Alkali caustic wastes.

All skin, eye, or mucous membrane exposed to any of these alkaline agents should be treated with copious irrigation with water. Irrigation should involve large volumes, low pressures, and long durations.

Table 33.1. General Decontamination Equipment

This equipment list will provide MINIMUM protection to the emergency squad responding to an accident or to the hospital receiving such an accident. It is manifestly not designed or intended to replace specific guidelines for known agents.

Containment Equipment

Decontamination stretchers are available from commercial supply houses (Fig. 33.5–8). These stretchers are portable and lightweight and can be assembled quickly in the field. Military-type litters can be used in place of more expensive commercially available decontamination stretchers. These litters are difficult to decontaminate but can be cheaply disposed of after decontamination is completed.

Larger self-contained decontamination units constructed like trailers are also available. An improvised containment unit can be constructed using a small rigid-sided wading pool to contain contaminated wash water and decontamination solutions.

Plastic tarpaulins may be used to further contain spills and to provide privacy for decontamination operations and may be used as tool or equipment dumps. They may be purchased in a variety of sizes and weights.

Plastic Bags

Bags of all available sizes should be available for preserving samples and disposing of contaminated materials. Small sizes may be used for valuables and specimens, while large sizes may be used for contaminated clothing and equipment. Clear zip-front body bags will minimize contamination to both the transport personnel and the transport vehicle.

Plastic Sheeting

Plastic sheeting may be used to cover nonessential and nonmovable equipment. Ventilation ducts may be sealed with duct tape and plastic sheeting. ''Safe'' corridors may be marked with plastic sheeting.

Tape

Engineer's tape comes in 100-foot rolls of bright colors and may be used to mark out exclusion zones and decontamination stations. Police or special purpose marker tape is somewhat more expensive and serves the same purpose. Marker cones are also useful.

Adsorbent Material

This material is available from commercial supply houses and will allow spills of contaminants to be adsorbed and then cleaned up easily.

Sponges and Soft Brushes

Abundant disposable brushes, cloths, and sponges should be stored. These may be used for cleaning victims or equipment. If possible, access should be arranged to a 55-gallon drum of polyethylene glycol solution (PEG-400).

Disposable Suture Sets

Two or three disposable suture sets should be available for removal of particulate contamination.

Protective Clothing

Multiple types of protective garments are available ranging from nitrile or butyl rubber-hooded suits to charcoal-impregnated military clothing. Proper protective clothing is generally selected for a specific task depending on the type of material from which it is made and the nature of the contaminant (13). Special purpose decontamination squads should have appropriate garments with them or readily available at all times. Decontamination officers should review the available type and compare protection times with the types of agents most commonly found in the community. Remember that no garment is impermeable forever.

Protective Garments

Many types of special purpose protective garments are available. Tyvek garments (DuPont) are relatively inexpensive, easily available, and come in an assortment of sizes. Tyvek suits provide adequate shortterm protection for small quantities of most materials and are disposable. Suits with hoods and attached shoe covers are available. For medical professionals who are not involved in gross decontamination and cleanup, this level of protection will usually suffice (Fig. 33.10).

Nitrile Gloves and Boots

Nitrile materials are chemically resistant and offer superior protection at all temperatures when compared to rubber gloves and boots. They cost only a fraction more than similar rubber products. Since medical providers must often touch casualties before decontamination is complete, they should have this protection. Both short (regular) and gauntlet length gloves should be provided.

Face Protection

Either full-face protection masks (preferred) or eye protection goggles should be available for all medical personnel. These may be built into personal respirators.

Respirators
Self-contained Breathing Apparatus (SCBA)

This is the ideal, but it requires substantial training to use safely. It is also quite expensive both for original purchase and upkeep. Spare cylinders must be stocked in a ratio of about four cylinders for each mask unit in order to ensure a continuous supply in more remote areas. All members of the decontamination squad who enter the exclusion areas should have their own SCBAs.

continues

Table 33.1. *Continued*

Filter Cannister Respirator

For most contaminants, a simple filter respirator will suffice. Particularly with the relatively lower levels of contamination that most medical teams will encounter, these units will suffice. A wide variety of filters is available that protect against special chemicals or combinations of chemicals. Multiple filter sets should be carried that will protect against commonly encountered hazards in the area. Since filters have a finite duration of protection, spare filters of each type selected should be readily available.

Miscellaneous Equipment

There are certain items that are very useful which can be easily stored and provide multiple functions:

Cotton swabs
Blood drawing equipment
Urine collection containers
Sputum collection containers
Triage tags
Labels for patients and bags
Index cards for writing comments to attach to patients
String or rubber bands
Clipboard and paper for keeping track of patients
Logbook for recording
Shoe covers
Protective eyewear with side shields
Vapor barrier masks
Indelible markers for labeling
Masking or gaffer's tape—This tape can be used to secure bags or markers to items. It may also be used to mark containers
Large plastic bags—clear bags as well as red bags (medical waste)
Plastic sheeting for covering floors and walls
Adsorbent materials for small spills
Sponges
Adsorbent gauze
Plastic buckets with lids
Rubber aprons
Rubber and/or latex gloves

Sawhorses

Sawhorses or military litter stands may be used to provide an elevated and level surface to work on patients. Both military litters and backboards can be placed on the stands. Elevation of the litters allows the triage and treatment teams to work with much less fatigue.

Water

This may be more difficult to provide and control than anticipated. Showers and decontamination scrubbings consume large amounts of water rapidly. One should check with the fire department and arrange for water supply prior to an incident. Both hot and cold running water are desirable (and in some climates necessary). Additional supplies of cool potable water are needed for hot climates. Garden hose and a portable shower head may allow the shower to be brought to the patient, rather than moving the patient to the shower. Fifty feet or more of garden hose is recommended. Fire units may charge a small line with a fog nozzle for the same purpose.

RADIOACTIVE DECONTAMINATION

Instruments are available to measure both type and intensity of radioactivity and determine both endpoints and the nature of the contamination. In no other type of contamination is this information so readily obtainable. Monitors are available for gamma, beta, and alpha detection. Equipment for radioactive emergency response is listed in Table 33.3.

Exposure History

It is important to promptly determine the history of the exposure. Exposures should be classified as external contamination, internal contamination, or irradiation. Internal contamination, also termed incorporation, is a medical emergency and occurs following inhalation, wound contamination, or ingestion of radionuclides and other radioactive materials. Emergency providers should realize that operators at "fixed sites," (such as nuclear reactors, medical installations, and industrial radioactive agent production plants) not only have knowledge of the

agents involved but may be able to provide cogent information about the appropriate precautions and treatment for the agent. The patient from such a facility may well be an authority on the treatment or use of this particular radioactive substance. If an accident occurs during transportation of radioactive materials, the exposed patient will probably be less informed or able to cope with the situation.

The exact type of exposure, agent, and route of entry should be determined. Any information sheets available, such as transportation manifests and loading documents, should be secured and transported with the first patient or patients. Remember that *irradiation* accidents need not be decontaminated and represent no danger to providers or staff.

Specific Field Detection Equipment

GEIGER-MULLER SURVEY METER

The Geiger-Muller survey meter will detect both beta- and gamma-emitting radioactive contamination. It will not detect

Table 33.2. Nine-Point Decontamination Plan

Step 1—Entry Point

An entry point allows control of decontaminated personnel. A tool drop will allow any tools which may be needed by other personnel at the accident site to be left in a "dirty" place. This will make the tools available for replacements or for those who only need to decontaminate enough to safely change the SCBA units.

Step 2—Gross Cleaning

In this step as much solid, liquid, or gas as possible is removed from contaminated personnel. When working with high risk agents, everyone who is working at step 2 should be in SCBA and have a level of protection to the person being decontaminated. These step 2 workers will have to be completely decontaminated when their job is done.

Step 3—SCBA/Respirator Service Area

At this point, additional SCBA equipment must be available. For high risk hazardous materials, the entire SCBA must be changed. For lower risk agents, air bottles or filter changes may be appropriate. Clean units are handed from the clean side of the decontamination station, and dirty units are left in the contaminated area for cleaning and resupply.

Step 4—Protective Clothing Removal

Protective clothing should be removed and isolated at step 4. It may be necessary to dispose of protective clothing rather than attempt decontamination. Abundant supplies of protective garments will be needed for replacement workers in these cases.

Step 5—Personal Clothing Removal

In management of extremely hazardous materials, complete removal of personal clothing will be required. This may include undergarments and personal effects such as watches and jewelry.

Step 6—Body Washing

Again, in management of extremely hazardous materials, showers and body washing will be needed. Heated overhead showers are much better than cold water hose lines. Sumps or tubs may be used to control water runoff.

The decontamination officer should ensure that the wash is complete, includes behind and in the ears. Soap and water will usually suffice for these areas.

In extreme cases, hair clipping may be needed. Contact lenses should be removed and the eyes irrigated to remove contaminants.

When materials do not present an extreme hazard, the shower area may be set up at a more controlled site.

Step 7—Dry and Redress

Towels and clean replacement clothes must be provided. Disposable coveralls, surgical scrubs, and disposable slippers are inexpensive and easy to obtain.

Step 8—Medical Evaluation

After decontamination is complete, the decontaminated personnel should be evaluated by medical providers. A log should be maintained of each and every person who was in the "hot" area. Vital signs should be taken on every person.

Any open wounds or skin breaks should be noted by the medical personnel. Even if these are not new injuries, they should be cleansed and properly evaluated for the presence of contaminants. Physicians with advice or training in management of the agent involved should be consulted for direction about these wounds.

Step 9—Observation, Medical Treatment, and Debriefing

Special decontamination for patients with inhalation of agents, wound decontamination, or agents that readily penetrate intact skin may be required. At this point, further observation may be needed for exposure to chemicals with late effects. These personnel should be transported to an emergency department for further medical evaluation and therapy.

All personnel should be debriefed by a recorder who can note duration of exposure, protection used, and any special features of the accident. This information may be quite useful for both medical and administrative investigations about casualties.

neutrons or alpha particles. This instrument can be quite rugged and is suitable for gross detection of most radioactive substances. Spare batteries are necessary.

ALPHA METER

An alpha radiation meter is a sensitive and delicate instrument used for detecting alpha emitter radioactive agents. It is not generally used by field personnel due to its delicate probes. The radiation physicist is most knowledgeable about this instrument. Spare probes should be available.

DOSIMETER

Three different types of dosimeters are available. These include the thermoluminescent dosimeter (TLD), the film badge, and the electrostatic pen dosimeter. Though pen dosimeters are easily read in the field, they are easily damaged. Film dosimeters provide a permanent record, but it can take days to get results. TLDs are easy to read and are relatively rugged but leave no permanent record. Decisions about which dosimeter to use should best be left to the radiation physicist. The decontamination officer should ensure that all members of the decontamination team have at least one dosimeter.

Table 33.3. Radioactive Decontamination Field Equipment

Radiation detection instruments
   Gamma-beta monitor
   Dosimeters or film badges
   Dosimeter charger
   Extra batteries
Body chart survey diagrams for coding contaminated areas
Protective clothing (multiple sets 20–30)
   Surgical scrubs
   Surgical gowns
   Caps and masks
   Shoe covers
   Latex or rubber gloves
   Tape for sleeves
   Protective eye wear with side shields
Neoprene industrial gloves
Tongs and forceps for remote handling
Instruction cards for decontamination
Decontamination stretcher(s) or disposal litters
Large waste containers (44-gallon size) with plastic liners
Clorox and bleach solutions
Abrasive soap
Wipes and sponges
Suture sets for wound debridement
Biologic sampling equipment with vials and swabs
Radiation signs
Yellow rope with stands for demarcating areas
Plastic (polyethylene 8 × 100 feet, 6 mil) floor and wall covering
Plastic (polyethylene 4 × 100 feet, 6 mil) covering for corridors
   and halls
Garden hose and extensions with a variable spray head for low
   pressure washes
Large yellow plastic bags with ties
Two-inch tape
Self-adherent contamination labels
‘‘Radioactive’’ labeled tape
Notebook with pencils
Indelible markers
Filter paper for covering ventilation areas
Towels, sheets, and wash clothes (multiple sets 20–30)
Washbasins
4 × 4 gauze and 2 × 2 gauze
Bandages
Plastic drapes
Kitty litter for adsorbent

Radiation Caution Signs and Labels

The internationally recognized magenta and yellow trefoil will serve to mark hazard areas, sample bags, and equipment or wastes that have been contaminated after radioactive release emergencies. These signs should be carried by all decontamination officers to appropriately mark the contaminated areas.

Decontamination Procedures

UNBROKEN SKIN

Undress the patient. Simply removing the clothing will often eliminate 90% of contaminants. Ensure that the clothing is bagged and tagged with the patient's name. Package wallet and special effects separately from the clothing.

Determine the areas to be decontaminated using the appropriate monitoring equipment. The use of a front and back body chart will help document contaminated areas of the person's body. Priority should be given to areas around breaks in the skin and those areas with the highest levels of contamination. Mark areas with lipstick or felt-tip marker. Hairy areas may be clipped but should not be shaved. Shaving may cause skin damage that allows contaminants to be absorbed.

Isolate areas of contamination with plastic sheets and tape. Self-adherent surgical draping material may be placed on the uncontaminated areas to prevent spread of contamination.

Patients who are awake and medically stable may shower using surgical soap and water. Comatose and severely injured patients should be showered with hoses equipped with mist nozzles. Since this process may take some time, use warm water for patient comfort and to prevent hypothermia. Attendants should be wearing waterproof protective garments. If hairy areas were not originally contaminated, they should be avoided during the shower. After the shower, the patient should be resurveyed.

In patients who are unable to shower, an attendant should wash off contamination with surgical soap and moistened sponges. Ensure that these contaminated sponges are put into a marked waste disposal area. Resurvey the area with the appropriate detection instrument. If contamination remains, gently scrub the area with Schubert's solution. This chelating solution should be used for about 3–5 minutes, taking care not to break the skin.

Schubert's solution consists of the following ingredients:

Citric acid	4.2 g/l
Tartaric acid	3.0 g/l
Disodiumethylene diaminetetraacetic acid (EDTA)	8.0 g/l
Calcium chloride	2.2 g/l

Adjust solution to pH 7.0 with concentrated sodium hydroxide.

After decontaminating again with Shubert's solution, resurvey the area. If contamination persists, repeat the cleansing with Schubert's solution and resurvey. If this fails, scrub the area gently with a concentrated solution of equal parts of soap, detergent, water, and cornmeal (this is often known as decontamination solution E).

Again, ensure that no skin breaks are created to allow incorporation of the radioactive material into the body. If there is a substantial amount of contamination persisting after this scrub, household strength chlorine bleach may be used as a scrub solution. Repeat the scrub until contamination is completely removed, or three scrubs fail to decrease the decontamination appreciably.

At this point, the decontamination officer should consult with both a physician and a radiation physicist to determine the allowable contamination. The patient's current contamination level should be resurveyed, and a joint decision about surgical debridement or more vigorous skin debridement should be made.

BROKEN SKIN AND INCORPORATION

Incorporation of radioactive material via a wound site, inhalation, or ingestion is a medical emergency that must be managed in the pre-hospital environment. Internal tissues can become permanently irradiated. In addition, the material may become incorporated into the normal biochemical processes of the body.

Survey and mark the wounds as noted above. Irrigate wounds and broken skin with copious amounts of water for 5 to 10 minutes. Ensure that no contamination is washed into eyes, mucous membranes, or wounds. Carefully decontaminate intact skin surrounding the wounds as noted above. Do not flush the wound with chelating agents or other decontamination solutions. Resurvey the wound. Continue irrigation with water or saline until the radioactivity is either undetectable or within acceptable limits. If the radioactivity persists, have a health physicist calculate the expected body burden from the residual contamination. This will vary with the nature of the radioactive agent found.

The health physicist and a surgeon or emergency physician jointly should determine the feasibility of sharp debridement of the area. Anesthesia should be given by regional block through uncontaminated skin wherever possible. If possible, tissue dissection is done to preserve tissue margins. The wound should be surveyed after the dissection. The specimen should be treated as radioactive wastes.

Rarely, the wound must be closed and excision performed at a later date. This decision should be made by a senior surgeon, in conjunction with a radiation physicist. The expected absorption of radioactive agent and the potential body burden of radioactive agent should be calculated.

Eyes: In all cases, irrigate the eyes with copious amounts of water or normal saline. Direct the irrigation from the nose to the temples, so that contamination is washed away from the nasal tear drainage. Survey the area frequently. Check nasal washings and swabbings for residual contamination.

Nose and mouth: Ensure that the contamination is truly in the cavity and not the surrounding area. Instruct the patient not to swallow, if possible. Irrigate the mouth and nasal areas with copious amounts of water and gently swab with cotton applicators. Frequent suctioning will help the patient avoid swallowing secretions. Continue irrigation until no further contamination is removed.

Ingested radioactive materials: These should be removed by inducing emesis if at all possible (3, 4). Emesis may be induced by usual doses of ipecac. If the patient is unconscious, then lavage may be necessary. Providers faced with this situation should consult a nuclear medicine physician or radiation medicine specialist. There are no data that activated charcoal is useful for binding radioactive materials. Whole gut lavage can be used to decrease residence time of radioactive materials in the gastrointestinal tract. This solution can be easily monitored for radioactivity. Aluminum-containing antacids can significantly reduce the absorption of radioactive strontium, and a dose of three ounces should be given. Barium sulfate can prevent the absorption of radium and stronium by formation of insoluble sulfates.

PHARMACOLOGIC THERAPY FOR RADIOISOTOPE ABSORPTION

Pharmacologic therapy may be indicated for incorporation of radioisotopes. Certain multivalent radioisotopes, such as the actinide series, uranium, and plutonium, have been effectively chelated using the investigational drug diethylenetriaminepentaacetic acid (DTPA). This treatment must begin within the first few hours of exposure to be effective. Decorporation with chelating agents should be started as soon as possible in patients with contaminated wounds. Patients with residual contamination from skin break or foreign bodies may also benefit from pharmacologic therapy. Treatment depends on the chemical properties of the particular radioisotope involved and should be done in conjunction with advice from a nuclear medicine

physician or radiation medicine specialist (see chapters on radioactive emergencies and pharmacotherapy).

DTPA is available from the Radiation Emergency Assistance Center/Training Site (REAC/TS) in Oak Ridge, Tennessee. Decorporation with chelating agents should be started as soon as possible in patients with contaminated wounds. Patients with residual contamination from skin break or foreign bodies may also benefit from pharmacologic therapy. Treatment depends on the chemical properties of the particular radioisotope involved and should be done in conjunction with advice from a nuclear medicine physician or radiation medicine specialist (see chapters on uranium, radioactive emergencies). DTPA chelates multivalent radionuclides and allows them to be renally excreted. Calcium disodium $CaNa_2EDTA$ (calcium versenate) has also been used as a radioisotope chelator but is not as efficacious as DTPA. Both the calcium and zinc salts of DTPA are approved for human use. CaDTPA is 10 times more effective than ZnDTPA for increasing renal excretion of actinide radionuclides within the first few hours of exposure. ZnDTPA is equally efficacious after the first one or two days of exposure.

In an acute exposure, one gram of CaDTPA diluted in 250 milliliters of dextrose 5% in water should be infused over 60 to 90 minutes. The dose may be repeated daily for 5 days. For immediate field administration, an aerosol inhalation treatment can be accomplished by placing the entire contents of a vial in a nebulizer. ZnDTPA appears to be less toxic then CaDTPA, but due to its lower efficacy it should not be the first drug of choice. CaDPTA should be continued at a once-daily dose of one gram intravenously. During this time blood samples, whole body and chest counts, 24-hour urine collections, and stool samples should be collected and monitored for radioactivity to determine need for further chelation. If further chelation is required beyond 5 days, then ZnDTPA should be substituted for more prolonged therapy. A DTPA administration protocol and consent form is available from REAC/TS (see chapter on radioactive emergencies).

DECONTAMINATION OF BIOHAZARD EXPOSURE

Biologic decontamination has abruptly changed from an issue taught and largely ignored to a ''critical'' step due to the rise of acquired immune deficiency syndrome (AIDS)-related diseases as well as the growing importance of the issue of medical waste disposal. It is interesting to note that the principles taught to medical providers are applicable to every contagious disease. It is equally interesting to note that the hysteria of AIDS has not been supported by an increase in AIDS transmission to medical providers—other than through high risk activities such as illicit drug use. The risk of acquiring an infectious disease from medical waste contact is low if proper precautions are undertaken to reduce exposure and injury (see chapter on medical waste).

PROBLEMS IN DECONTAMINATING INJURED PATIENTS

Vital Signs

It has been well-established that obtaining reliable vital signs is difficult to impossible when either the examiner or the casualty is wearing protective garments (5–7). Adequate monitoring of the patient's condition may require the protective garments to be breached.

Of course, vital signs are easy to obtain and treatment easy to provide when protective garments have been removed. The question is determination of a safe time to remove the garments (8).

It is difficult to detect and monitor the pulse in a normotensive casualty while wearing protective garments, particularly when the examiner is also gloved. Direct contact of the examiner's fingers to the patient's skin will eliminate many of these problems, but at a cost of exposure of both patient and examiner to the noxious agents that prompted the garments in the first place.

Pulses may be remotely measured by piezoelectric crystal plethysmography attached to a finger. An alternative may be the use of infrared light-emitting diodes and receivers such as are used in pulse oximeters. Both of these methods require the exposure of the casualty—at least the finger. If there are only a few people in protective garments, it may be possible to wire the patient with earlobe pulse oximeter probes prior to donning protective garments. This will be an unlikely scenario in most field operations, unfortunately.

Doppler flow devices are quite efficient at detecting flow but require direct contact with gel-coated skin areas. Doppler flow devices will allow very accurate determination of systolic blood pressures.

Oxygenation

The usual field EMT or paramedic has no method for determining oxygenation other than the color of the patient. The respiratory status provides only indirect evidence of oxygenation which can be markedly changed by some chemical agents. Oxygen saturation provides a better guide to the state of tissue perfusion when it is available. Oxygen saturation is easily measured with portable and battery-powered pulse oximeters from a wide variety of manufacturers. These devices will easily provide oxygen saturation and pulse. Probes may be attached to fingers, toes, or earlobes. Probes are simple, relatively inexpensive, and easily applied before the exercise, when they are available.

The respiratory rate can be measured by an attentive observer. If the trained observer has to attend to multiple casualties, this measurement is discontinuous. When the victim is being transported, such observers may be unable to adequately evaluate the patient.

Transthoracic impedance devices, such as used for premature infants, are available and are quite reliable. They are relatively expensive and will require a breach of the protective garments to apply. Diaphoretic patients may rapidly shed the electrodes, necessitating multiple exposures of the patient in order to reapply electrodes.

Problems with Protective Garments

Not only are protective garments annoying, they result in serious decrements of performance. The moment that protective garments are donned, skin irritation and sweating start. These irritations cause distraction. When job performance is critical, distraction may result in an increase in accidental injuries, breaches in protection, and decrements in performance.

As soon as the provider realizes there is a threat, anxiety may cause psychologic casualties. These psychologic casualties may constitute a major problem for the incident scene commander, since the medical services will have to treat casualties not only from the support and evacuation units but from their own ranks. These casualties may not be obvious but may only suffer major decrements in performance.

A major relief to stress is socialization and communication with friends and colleagues. When one is wearing protective gear, normal facial expressions are unreadable even at close distance. Voices are changed and clarity and timbre lost during transmission through masks and facepieces. Eye contact may be lost. Body contact becomes difficult and muffled by the protective garments. This loss of socialization and communication heightens the anxiety.

The process of decontamination itself may cause an increase in anxiety. Unless decontamination is complete, the "clean" areas will rapidly become "dirty." This will produce substantial amounts of distrust and anxiety about the thoroughness of the decontamination. An anxious, hungry, hot, dehydrated, exhausted field worker who is forced to go through the decontamination station "yet another time" is likely to become angry. Obsessive and compulsive decontamination squads must be tempered by leaders with compassion and understanding about the job stress of the field member.

Until one has abundant experience with either a respirator of self-contained breathing apparatus, the increased effort of respirations becomes an annoyance. If the activity requires substantial physical exertion, then the increased work of breathing will cause a decrease in performance. Since difficulty in breathing is an early sign of poisoning by some chemical agents, the increased work of breathing may provoke anxiety about the integrity of protective garments.

High humidity and an occlusive protective garment will increase risk of heat exhaustion and heat stroke. The inability of a person in full protective garments to lose heat by radiation, convection, or evaporation is well-documented (9–11). If a casualty results from this high heat load, it may be impossible to differentiate the early effects of a toxic agent from those of exertional heat stroke. Lesser heat loads may lead to a decrease in attention span and performance, resulting in accidental injuries. The medical team must constantly monitor the team members for such signs of heat stress.

Drinking is possible with only a few of the protective mask designs, and then only from specially designed containers (12). Even when one has all the right equipment, drinking is difficult to accomplish without practice with the assembled equipment. Inadequate amounts of water may be consumed during use of this equipment, especially when one considers the increased water loss due to an increased heat load. Dehydration becomes a distinct possibility. It is well-known that even modest dehydration will produce a marked decrement in both physical and mental abilities.

Damaged or improperly donned protective clothing will allow entry of contaminants with potentially disastrous results. At the very least, decontamination will be more difficult.

Improper protective garments will afford little or no protection. Chemicals may rapidly permeate through and into incompatible garments and respiratory filters.

REFERENCES

1. Lorin HG, Kulling PEJ. The Bhopal tragedy—what has Swedish disaster medicine planning learned from it? J Emerg Med 1986;4:311–316.

2. Heully F, Gruninger M, et al. Collective intoxication caused by the explosion of a mustard gas shell. Ann Med Leg 1956;36:195–204.

3. Milroy WC. Management of irradiated and contaminated casualty victims. Emerg Med Clin North Am 1984;2:667–686.

4. Drum DE. Health implications of nuclear energy (letter). Ann Intern Med 1979;91:127–128.

5. Burgin WW, Gehring LM, Bell TL. A chemical field resuscitation device. Milit Med 1982;147:873–874.

6. Bennion SD. Designing of NBC protective gear to allow for adequate first aid. Milit Med 1982;147:960–962.

7. Hodson PB. Assessment of casualties in a chemical environment. J R Army Med Corps 1985;131:116–117.

8. Gaston B. Casualty decontamination during amphibious assault. Navy Med 1988 Mar–April:8–9.

9. Stephenson LA, Kolka MA, Allan AE, Santee WR. Heat exchange during encapsulation in a chemical warfare agent protective patient wrap in four hot environments. Aviat Space Environ Med 1988;345–351.

10. Nishi Y, Gonzalez RR, Gagge AP. Prediction of equivalent environments by energy exchange and assessments of physiological strain and discomfort. Isr J Med Sci 1976;12:808–61.

11. Stewart C. Heat emergencies. In: Environmental emergencies. Baltimore: Williams & Wilkins, 1989.

12. Cadigan FC. Battleshock—the chemical dimension. J R Army Med Corps. 1982;128:89–92.

13. Wilcher FW. Performance certification of clothing connected to concern for protection. Occup Health Saf 1987;June:39–44.

RESOURCES

The following resources emphasize safety, containment, decontamination, and cleanup. They are weak on medical care. Because of this, the responsibility for care of the patient continues to rest with the treating physician.

CHEMTREK 1-800-424-9300

Chemical Manufacturers Association Chemical Transportation Emergency Center (CHEMTREK) is available for emergency assistance 24 hours per day. This single resource will aid in contacting all other agencies and correlating available data for protection and decontamination hazards. They cannot provide adequate medical help for physicians treating contaminated persons.

OHM-TADS

Oil and Hazardous Materials Technical Assistance Data Service. They will provide help about petroleum and derivatives through physical characteristics. OHM-TADs can be contacted through CHEMTREK listed above.

CHLOREP

Chlorine manufacturers chlorine emergency plan. CHLOREP can be contacted through CHEMTREK, listed above.

Published Resources

Hazardous Materials Incident Response Operations, U.S. Environmental Protection Agency Training Manual, Unit 3, 1981. (Not available for public distribution.)

Radiologic Handbook, U.S. Department of Health, Education and Welfare.

Department of Transportation Hazardous Materials Emergency Response Guidebook (DOT publication 5800.3)

34

Hospital and Community Preparation for Hazardous Material Releases

John B. Sullivan, Jr., M.D.
Mark Van Ert, Ph.D., C.I.H.
Bill Durham

INTRODUCTION

Emergency preparedness for hazardous materials releases is a function of the training and proficiency of fire department and hazardous materials teams, the ability of the community to respond to evacuation and safety procedures, the understanding of the hazards of the involved materials, and adequate preparation of health care facilities to manage victims. In addition, company management has the obligation to provide technical and managerial planning to help prevent releases as well as to respond to releases. The Emergency Planning and Community Right-to-Know Act (EPCRA) was enacted into law to ensure community preparation to properly respond to hazardous materials releases. However, most communities, hospitals, and emergency departments are not prepared to handle releases of materials, disasters involving hazardous materials, or even smaller incidents involving relatively nontoxic material where a few or multiple people are contaminated. Hospital disaster plans may not contain plans for responding to mass exposures to chemical, radioactive, or biologic hazardous materials. Even if the disaster plan does address such emergencies, practice of the plan may be lacking.

Hospitals and emergency departments differ greatly in their ability to respond to spills and releases of hazardous materials. There is no standardization within communities. Improper response to handling of contaminated victims and their clothing can result in contaminant spread into clean areas of a hospital facility as well as in serious injury or death to the victims and response personnel.

The components of a comprehensive, well deliberated contingency plan for hazardous materials releases in a community include: (a) rapid and accurate assessment of the problem, (b) timely response for trained personnel, (c) adequate resources and training for responders, (d) ability to communicate with receiving hospitals before victims arrive, (e) adequate resources and preparation to manage victims at the receiving hospitals, (f) inclusion of the plan as a component of the overall hospital disaster plan that is practiced annually, (g) involvement of local company management which may store or use chemicals and (h) development of company response plans.

A recent review of deaths and injuries from acute hazardous materials spills from three national databases (National Response Center, Department of Transportation Hazardous Materials Information Center, and the Acute Hazardous Materials Events Data Base) in 1986 revealed that 587 chemical releases resulted in 115 deaths, 2254 injuries, and 111 evacuations of areas where spills occurred (1). There was no follow-up of these exposures to determine longterm health effects, and these data represented the minimum number of injuries and deaths.

The data further revealed that a hazardous materials spill or release occurs once every 3 days in the United States due to vehicle accidents or train derailments and that there are 1.6 hazardous material incidents per day in the United States that result in death, injury, or evacuation (1). There is probably gross underreporting and undercollection of hazardous materials incidences by the national databases. The types of materials spilled in these releases demonstrate the typical materials being transported on highways and railways in this country (Table 34.1) (1). Other data from the Department of Transportation in 1983 revealed 4829 highway and 851 railroad hazardous materials incidences costing more than $110,000,000 in damages and resulting in eight deaths and 191 injuries (2).

In addition to rail and truck transport of hazardous materials through many communities, many cities and rural communities are close to manufacturing facilities, businesses, and industries that manufacture, process, or store highly toxic chemicals as well as other hazards. Examples include phosphine, arsine, chlorine, volatile isocyanates, hydrogen cyanide, hydrogen sulfide, corrosives, flammable hydrocarbons, and radioactive materials. Release of a large amount of highly toxic gases into a community can potentially occur and should be considered in emergency planning.

Emergency Planning and Community Right to Know Act

The 1984 release of methyl isocyanates in Bhopal, India, was still a fresh memory when the Superfund Amendments and Reauthorization Act (SARA) became law in 1986. Part of this law, specifically Title III, was a response to the past deficiencies of communities to respond to hazardous materials releases. Title III established requirements for federal, state, and local governments to provide planning for chemical emergencies as well as for informing the public about chemicals stored, used, and released in communities (Appendix 1). This law is known as the Emergency Planning and Community Right to Know Act (EPCRA). The law established structure at both state and local levels of government to assist communities in planning for chemical emergencies. This act requires business and other facilities in the community to provide information to the public on the variety of chemicals stored. Section 313 of the Act requires release of information for over 300 chemicals. Also, businesses are required to report accidental releases and spills of extremely hazardous substances and hazardous substances regulated by the Comprehensive Environmental Response, Compensation, and Liability Act (CERCLA) to state and local response officials. Material Safety Data Sheets (MSDSs) must be available to these officials. Inventories of these chemicals

Table 34.1. Examples of Typical Materials Released in Hazardous Materials Incidents

Chlorine
Toluene diisocyanate
Natural gas
Sulfuric acid
Ammonia
Liquid oxygen
Hydrochloric acid
Corrosives
Phosphoric acid
Polymethylene diisocyanate (PAPI)
Nitric acid
Gasoline
Diesel oil
Sodium hydroxide
Sodium cyanide
Naphtha

Table 34.2. Chemical Categories Listed under the Emergency Planning and Community Right-to-Know Act

Extremely hazardous substances

More than three hundred highly toxic chemicals whose release must be immediately reported. Sections 301-304.

Hazardous substances

Chemicals listed under Superfund cleanup regulations of CERCLA. Includes around 720 chemicals. Releases of these chemicals above a certain amount must be reported immediately. Section 304.

Hazardous chemicals

These chemicals are defined by OSHA as a health hazard. Inventories of these chemicals must be kept along with MSDS and submitted if they are used, stored, or processed in certain amounts. Sections 311-312.

Toxic chemicals

Comprised of more than 320 chemicals or chemical categories selected due to their chronic or longterm toxicity. Estimates of annual releases must be reported and entered into a national database. Section 313.

as well as their location within the building structure must be reported. EPCRA contains the following four main provisions with respect to a community's response and right-to-know concerning hazards:

1. Emergency planning for chemical releases;
2. Emergency notification of chemical accidents and releases;
3. Reporting of hazardous chemical inventories;
4. Toxic chemical release reporting.

In addition, the law deals with trade secrets as well as disclosure of chemical information to the public and health care professionals.

There are four groups of chemicals subject to reporting under EPCRA which are found in the Federal Register (Table 34.2).

Emergency Planning

The emergency planning component of EPCRA involves community preparation for hazardous materials emergencies response. According to the law, every community in the United States must have a plan. Each state must have a State Emergency Response Commission (SERC) appointed by the governor. The SERC may be composed of emergency medical services, environmental services, transportation services, health agencies, and others with an interest in serving the community. Each SERC wil appoint local emergency planning committees (LEPC) around their respective state areas. The LEPC includes owners and operators of industrial plants, representatives of local and state elected officials, health care providers, hospitals, environmental specialists, community and media representatives, law enforcement officials, and fire department officials. The task given to the LEPC is to identify community hazards and develop local plans for their community's response to emergencies involving hazardous materials.

The basic components of a local emergency plan (LEPC) include the following:

1. Use information provided by industries and businesses to identify routes, locations, and facilities where hazardous materials are stored and/or transported in the community.
2. Establish emergency response procedures including an evacuation plan for responding to hazardous materials releases or spills.
3. Set up notification procedures for responders.

4. Establish methods to determine the severity of a hazardous materials release and the areas that will likely be affected by the release.
5. Establish a means to notify the public about a hazardous materials release or spill.
6. Identify the emergency equipment available in the community to respond to hazardous materials releases.
7. Include a program for training local emergency responders and medical workers.
8. Develop methods to test emergency response plans.
9. Designate a community coordinator and facilities coordinator to carry out the plan.

The law requires industries and businesses to notify SERCs and LEPCs if they have certain extremely hazardous substances as defined by the Environmental Protection Agency (EPA) present above threshold quantities on their premises. These businesses then must participate in the emergency planning process. Presently, the EPA has defined 366 "extremely hazardous chemicals," that if present at designated threshold quantities in a business will activate the emergency planning component of EPCRA. The intent of the emergency planning component of EPCRA is for the LEPC to characterize the local community with respect to hazards present and to know the capacities and capabilities of the hospitals and medical facilities in the community. The LEPC must also inform the public about the plan through literature and public meetings. The plan is reviewed and updated annually.

Hazardous Chemical Reporting

Section 313, Title III, of SARA now requires businesses to submit annual reports on the amounts of chemicals stored within their facilities. The purpose of the reporting is to inform the public as well as the government about toxic substances that are present, their location, quantities, and potential health effects. These reports are sent to the SERC, LEPC, and fire department. The EPA is required by law to make this data available to the public via an electronic database.

Businesses and industries must report hazardous chemicals

in two ways: (a) using MSDS, which companies are required to keep on file on their premises for all hazardous materials in the workplace; (b) submitting annual inventories of chemicals to SERC, LEPC, and the fire department.

A separate MSDS is required by the Occupational Safety and Health Administration (OSHA) for each chemical on-site in any business. Under EPCRA, the facility must submit a copy of the MSDS or lists of MSDS chemicals. This MSDS reporting is based on the OSHA definition of chemical hazards and includes over 4.5 million facilities and as many as 500,000 plus products.

The second reporting method required is the submission of annual inventories of hazardous chemicals to SERC, LEPC, and the fire department. A two-tiered approach is required by law. Tier I includes reporting on the amounts and general location of chemicals in a facility if that facility stores 10,000 pounds of materials that can produce health effects. The tier II report includes the same information but names the specific chemical. Unless specified by local community and state law, companies may file only tier I reports. However, companies are always encouraged to file tier II reports since they are more helpful in emergency planning and response.

This information is available to the public by contacting their SERC or LEPC. A listing of locations of chemicals inside the building is not available to the public but is available to emergency responders. Violators of the reporting law are subject to penalties of up to $10,000 per day per violation for failing to submit MSDS information and $25,000 per violation for annual inventory reporting.

Emergency Release Notification

Under EPCRA a business or industry which releases more than the predetermined amount of chemicals included on the EPA extremely hazardous chemical list as well as 700 plus other chemicals must immediately notify the LEPC and the SERC of the release. Superfund requires reporting to the National Response Center (NRC) if any of the chemicals are on the Superfund list. For some chemicals the release of more than one pound must be reported. Reporting quantities range from 10 to 10,000 pounds.

Notification must be immediate and include the following:

Name of chemical;
Location of the release;
If the chemical is on the extremely hazardous EPA list;
How much has been released;
Time and duration of the release;
Whether the chemical was released into the air, water, or soil;
Health risks from the chemicals;
Precautions to be taken including evacuation;
Name of facility contact person.

Follow-up reporting is also required by the facility detailing response taken and health risks update. Failure to notify authorities or to submit a follow-up emergency report is subject to civil penalties of up to $25,000 per day for each day of noncompliance. Repeat offenders can be fined up to $75,000 a day. Criminal penalties may also be imposed.

Toxic Chemical Release Reporting

EPCRA also allows for the community to know if there are releases of chemicals into the environment of the community. Companies who must report are:

1. Those engaged in manufacturing operations who have 10 or more full-time employees.
2. Companies who manufacture, import, process, or use any of the chemicals on the list (appendix) in amounts greater than the threshold quantities listed. Threshold quantities listed are 75,000 pounds during calendar year 1987, 50,000 pounds during 1988, and 25,000 during 1989 and subsequent years.
3. If a company uses any of the listed chemicals without processing them, the threshold quantity for reporting is 10,000 pounds a year.

Beginning in 1989, Section 313 requires suppliers of mixtures and trade name products to notify customers of the presence of any of these chemicals listed in their products beyond certain *de minimis* concentrations (EPA 560/4-88-001, February 1988). *De minimis* concentrations of toxic chemicals in a mixture is defined as a concentration of less than 1% of the mixture or a concentration less than 0.1% of an OSHA defined carcinogen in any mixture. The EPA compiles this information into a Toxic Release Inventory accessible to the public through electronic data bases.

HAZARDOUS MATERIALS RELEASE PLANNING FOR HOSPITALS

Victims of hazardous materials incidences can range from seriously injured and uncontaminated to uninjured and highly contaminated. The degree of injury and contamination must be judged by the prehospital response and triage team and communicated to the medical command in the emergency department receiving the victims. For radioactive contamination, some area hospitals or facilities associated with the use of radioactive materials and radionuclides may be better prepared to receive and decontaminate victims. These facilities should be clearly identified in the hospital disaster plan. The importance of having a hazardous materials plan for chemical, radioactive, and biologic exposures as a component of the facility disaster plan is critical. A limited versus a full emergency disaster response is based on the number of victims as well as on their medical condition. Depending on the contaminant, minimizing its spread is an important consideration. Some chemicals and radioactive materials are very difficult to decontaminate, and expensive emergency department equipment can become contaminated if a proper response plan is not implemented and practiced by the hospital staff.

Upon notification that a hazardous material release has occurred, there are a number of important questions with respect to victims that must be asked by medical command in the hospital:

What is the material?
Is the material radioactive?
If the material is radioactive, what is the route of contamination?
How many victims were exposed?
Are there casualties?
Are the casualties from trauma or the exposure?
What was the degree of exposure?
Is there a physiologic antagonist or antidote for the hazard and, if so, is there enough available in the area hospitals?
Which medical facilities in the community are prepared to respond?

The hospital disaster plan must address the medical, administrative, and technical controls necessary to assure proper response to a community chemical spill or release. The plan should have separate chemical, radioactive, and biologic responses written in easy-to-follow instructions. Many hospital disaster plans contain a response for radioactive substances, but few contain a plan for chemically contaminated victims. Annual drills should be conducted to ensure that the medical staff as well as the administrative staff and technical consultants understand their duties. Drills can concentrate on the types of hazards likely to be encountered in the community. This is especially important if a hospital is located near industries and facilities that use and store hazards. Rural hospitals along major highways in the United States must be prepared to manage spills from transport vehicles that routinely pass through their area.

Hazardous materials response plans are different from the more routine disaster response involving victims from accidents. Triage is different for both prehospital care personnel and hospital personnel. The need to decontaminate will dictate the ability to construct special decontamination zones both in the field and in the hospital. The medical staff will have to become knowledgeable in radiation and chemical safety. In addition, tracking of contaminated clothing and collection of decontamination washings is essential. An improperly conducted response to a real hazardous materials incident can result in improper treatment of patients with increased morbidity and mortality as well as risks to the response team. Staff must be taught the proper use of personal protective garments, how to use radiation detection equipment, how to interact with specialized technical consultants, and how not to spread contamination. The drills should include the construction of the decontamination zones both inside the emergency department and outside the emergency department.

Area surveys and audits of chemicals will help determine the kinds of emergencies likely to be encountered. Proper amounts of physiologic antagonists and specialized treatment protocols should be documented. A health care facility near a plant that stores or uses arsine and phospine must be prepared for the possibility of having to provide numerous blood exchange transfusions as a treatment. Hospitals near agricultural areas or pesticide manufacturing facilities must be sure that enough atropine and pralidoxime are available to manage multiple, severe poisonings from organophosphates. Mining operations may utilize cyanide, and cyanide antidote kits must be stocked and expiration dates routinely checked.

Hospital administrators should be knowledgeable about the need for controlling contaminant spread and the need for specialized patient flow patterns within the hospital. The contamination of a hospital area by an improperly handled chemical will prevent the further use of that area until proper cleanup is accomplished. Therefore, proper storage control and disposal of contaminated clothing and decontamination washings is essential. Administrative controls and planning are essential to contain contamination as well as to prevent contamination of the hospital areas and personnel. Ancillary technical help such as radiology, laboratory technologists, and respiratory therapists must be included in the practice of the plan.

Timely identification of the nature of the problem and the number of victims involved in a hazardous materials release is the duty of the responding emergency services. Identification of the substance is accomplished by a variety of means including hazard warning labels, placards, MSDSs, company records, and information stored by the LEPC (See chapter on recognition of hazardous materials).

Environmental specialists, serving as technical consultants, are usually asked to respond as a component of the disaster plan. Radiation safety specialists should be consulted to help develop the facility's response to radioactive emergencies both external and internal to the hospital. The radiation safety officer is the designated technical control of the radiation decontamination plan. Practice of this response should be yearly and should involve the radiation safety officer or certified health physicist. The chemical response plan should involve consultation with certified industrial hygienists. They have the knowledge and expertise to provide monitoring for chemical contamination of patients as well as for cleanup of the emergency department and hospital. They can help prevent hazardous materials from being disseminated. Industrial hygienists are also knowledgeable about state and federal regulations regarding hazardous materials. Integration of these technical specialists as part of the medical team that responds to a hazardous material release will help ensure the success of the plan.

The regional poison center can be a valuable source of information regarding treatment and decontamination of patients. Physiologic antagonists and special therapies may be necessary, and the poison center can provide expert consultation.

RESPONSE TO CHEMICAL CONTAMINATION

Emergency Department Receiving of Patients

The response of a health care facility to a disaster or release of hazardous chemicals resulting in injured victims and/or victim contamination should consist of the following broad areas:

1. Activation of the appropriate disaster plan;
2. Communication with the prehospital response team;
3. Triage;
4. Decontamination outside the hospital;
5. Medical care and decontamination inside the hospital;
6. Tracking of patients and patient belongings;
7. Cleanup and decontamination of the facility;
8. Appropriate patient follow-up and documentation.

Following the notification of a chemical release involving victims, the response plan should be activated. Depending on the magnitude and the number of victims, secondary help may be required and a call-up list activated. Exposure to a contaminating material can continue if prehospital decontamination procedures are inadequate. In a disaster situation, the first responders may not recognize that an exposure exists, and the initial victims can reach the emergency department without having been decontaminated. Should this occur, the hospital receiving area can be contaminated as well as other areas in the hospital to which the victims are transported. Contaminated victims who have not been seriously injured should be decontaminated outside of the emergency department in an appropriately controlled and demarcated area. Seriously injured and contaminated victims should be triaged to a special resuscitation-decontamination room in the emergency department. This area should be prepared to render both medical care and decontamination as necessary.

Decontamination principles, equipment, and techniques of the field can be applied to the emergency department and hospital. The hospital environment should be easier to control due to advanced planning and preparation. In actual fact, most emergency departments and hospitals are not adequately prepared to manage hazardous material emergencies in their communities. Hospitals in general lack detailed plans for receiving victims of hazardous materials releases, decontamination protocols, movement and tracking mechanisms for patients and their contaminated clothing, and clean-up operations. In addition, formal practice of any plan is frequently absent.

Victim Receiving, Triage, and Decontamination Area

The location of decontamination areas should be part of the overall emergency response plan. Decontamination zones can be outside the hospital or inside the facility. Decontamination of victims outside the emergency department is the ideal, but this is not always practical. Incoming ambulances should be identified as carrying contaminated or decontaminated victims, and a separate entry area to the hospital provided if possible. The receiving triage medical team should meet the victims at the ambulance bay arrival zone and be outfitted with a level of protective clothing that matches the contaminant and level of contamination of the victims. Depending on the substance involved, personnel protection can range from a minimum of surgical gowns and scrubs with shoe covers, masks, caps, gloves, and eye protection to respirators, chemically resistant suits, gloves and boots. If a decontamination area is set up outside the entrance to the hospital, it should be properly demarcated with bright ribbon or rope and signs. Only authorized personnel should enter this area. The decision to have an external decontamination zone is dependent on the temperature outdoors, the nature of the contaminant, the nature of the victim's injuries, and the ability of the personnel to control the contaminant. Portable decontamination stretchers are available which allow for victim decontamination outside or inside the facility (Figs. 34.1

and 34.2). These stretchers have wash containment tanks. For victims that are seriously ill or injured, treatment and decontamination should be conducted inside the emergency department in a specially outfitted room.

Arriving victims should be surveyed for evidence of life-threatening injuries and need for acute medical attention as well as for decontamination need. If the patient is stable, the initial triage should determine whether a residual level of contamination exists to warrant further use of specialized protective garments by medical personnel both in the receiving triage area and in the hospital. Depending on the chemical or substance involved, it is crucial to have proper expertise and monitoring equipment available for both chemical and radioactive contamination to expedite the triage procedure. Patients in need of immediate medical care should be triaged to a separate decontamination-treatment room if the level of contamination is unknown and the patient's injuries are life-threatening. In all cases, simply removing the patient's clothes and washing the skin with water markedly reduces the level of contamination and the burden for other medical staff.

All incoming patients should be regarded as contaminated until proven otherwise. Field decontamination may not have been very thorough or may have been nonexistent. The patients should be scanned for evidence of contamination such as condition of clothing and condition of the skin. The patient should be asked whether he or she received a field wash. One should note whether the odor of a chemical is present. If in doubt, decontaminate before entering the emergency department proper unless the victim has a medical problem or injury requiring immediate attention.

If a patient has bypassed decontamination in the field, this may indicate a life-threatening illness or injury. The difficult question that must be answered by a well-trained medical triage officer both in the field and at the receiving area of the hospital is: Does this patient need treatment or decontamination first? The balance between protection of staff and provision of emer-

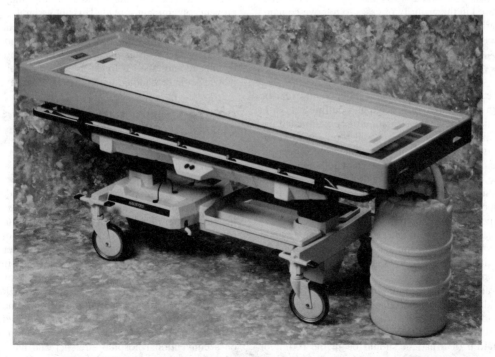

Figure 34.1. Hospital decontamination table. Courtesy RMC, Philadelphia, PA.

Figure 34.2. Hospital decontamination system on stretcher.

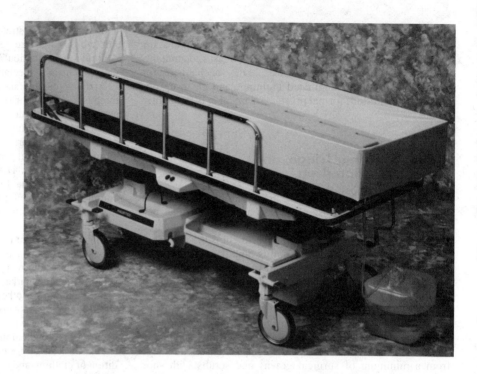

gency medical care requires judgement based on knowledge and practice. Both come with implementation and practicing the hazardous materials disaster plan.

Entry into and out of the decontamination area is restricted to patients and personnel. Protective garments should be worn which can be left in a drop zone in the decontamination area when personnel leave. Following decontamination, patients can then be triaged into the emergency department or other areas of the hospital. Patient belongings and clothes should be left in the plastic bags and placed in a security-controlled area for disposal as necessary. A water wash that includes a mild detergent can be used in the majority of cases to remove contaminating hydrocarbons.

Decontamination and Medical Care in the Emergency Department

Simultaneous decontamination and medical intervention can be accomplished in a specially constructed and outfitted room in the emergency department. Resuscitation of contaminated patients can take place in specially prepared rooms with ventilation ducts obstructed and turned off to prevent chemical seepage into other areas of the hospital. The medical equipment in this room should be considered to be contaminated and remain in this resuscitation room and not removed to other areas until cleared by proper authorities, such as certified industrial hygienists. This special room should be designated in the disaster plan and ideally should have an entrance to the outside with a separate corridor that can be decontaminated. This room would also serve for victims of radioactive accidents and should be isolated from other areas.

The waste drainage from decontamination should be routed to separate holding tanks or containers. Specialized decontamination stretchers are available that allow for this as well as for treatment of victims. Only equipment needed for the active resuscitation of a patient should be in the room, or passed into the room. This equipment remains in this room

until it can be adequately decontaminated or demonstrated to be clean through appropriate monitoring. All articles and equipment that enter the exclusion zones should be considered to be expendable. The use of portable units for suction, plastic disposable equipment, and other such equipment will help to prevent contaminant spread. Portable electrical junction boxes will prevent contamination of wall sockets. An adjacent area should be available for decontamination of medical personnel. This area can also serve as a clothing drop area and a changing area for personnel.

Polyethylene sheeting taped to floors and walls will help prevent contaminant spread. This thick, durable plastic sheeting and tape should be stocked with the disaster equipment. Building and constructing this containment room should be practiced as part of the disaster plan. All contaminated objects should be bagged and labelled for each patient. When possible, these items should be handled with tongs or other remote equipment.

CONTROLLING AND CONTAINING CHEMICAL CONTAMINATION

Decontamination Equipment

Selected equipment properly stored will provide rapid response and protection to the emergency personnel receiving contaminated victims (Table 34.3). Medical personnel should wear protective garments according to the level of protection required. Specialized decontamination stretchers are commercially available for field use as well as for use in the emergency department. These decontamination tables provide easy access to patients for treatment, are reusable, and allow x-rays to be taken. Made of fiberglass materials, they come with their own collection containers (Fig. 34.1). Disposable decontamination units are also available which are easily set up within minutes on a conventional hospital stretcher and have their own collection containers (Fig. 34.2).

Table 34.3.   Equipment for Chemical Decontamination

There are very useful items that can be easily stored and serve multiple functions:

Cotton swabs
Blood-drawing equipment
Urine collection containers
Sputum collection containers
Triage tags
Labels for patients and bags
Index cards for writing comments to attach to patients
String or rubber bands
Clipboard and paper for keeping track of patients
Logbook for recording
Shoe covers
Protective eyewear with side shields
Vapor barrier masks
Indelible markers for labelling
Masking tape can be used to secure bags or markers to items. It may also be used to mark containers.
Large plastic bags—clear bags as well as red bags (medical waste).
Plastic sheeting for covering floors and walls
Adsorbent materials for small spills
Sponges—4 × 4 and large surgical sponges
Gauze
Plastic buckets with lids
Rubber aprons
Latex gloves
Neoprene industrial gloves
Tongs for remote handling

Plastic bags of variable sizes should be available for preserving samples and disposing of contaminated materials. Small sizes may be used for valuables and specimens, while large sizes may be used for contaminated clothing and equipment. Clear zip-front body bags will minimize contamination to both the transport personnel and the transport vehicle. These bags should be labeled with contents and identity of patients.

Polyethylene sheeting may be used to cover nonessential and nonmovable equipment. Ventilation ducts may be sealed with duct tape and plastic sheeting. Corridors of travel may be lined with plastic sheeting.

Rolls of bright colored tape may be used to mark out exclusion zones and decontamination stations. Marker cones are also useful. Self-adhering labels are valuable for tracking clothes, samples, and waste material.

Absorbent Materials

A number of spill control products are available for absorbing inadvertent contamination of surfaces during patient care and decontamination procedures. A variety of these materials is available, and it is best to consult safety supply catalogs for examples of such sorbents and their effectiveness. Dry sorbents used to control solvents, acids (excluding hydrofluoric acid), and caustics contain vermiculite, clay absorbent, corn-cob absorbent, diatomaceous earth, and expanded silicates. Polypropylene microfibers either in sheets or shredded also have excellent chemical resistance and absorptive properties and can be used to control hydrofluoric acid spills. Other absorbents are available for specific applications. Impregnated aluminas function by a process of absorption, adsorption, and chemical oxidation. To further reduce hazards associated with spill cleanup, neutralizer kits for acid and caustic spills are available that include safety glasses, scoops, bags, ties, and labels. Following cleanup, all contaminated materials should be collected in polypropylene bags and properly disposed of in hazardous waste containers.

Protective Garments

Multiple types of personal protective garments are available from safety supply houses. Proper protective clothing is selected for a specific task depending on the type of material from which it is made and the nature of the contaminant. Special purpose decontamination teams should have appropriate garments with them or readily available at all times. Decontamination officers, in consultation with environmental health specialists, should review the types of protective garments used and compare protection times with the types of agents most commonly found in the community. The minimum protective equipment consists of surgical gowns and scrubs with shoe covers, masks, caps, and eye protection. Special disposable coveralls which are tear-resistant as well as chemical-resistant are available from supply houses. These garments come as complete jumpsuits or as coveralls and can be purchased and stored. Aprons made of styrene-butadiene rubber are chemical-resistant and afford protection from caustics as well. Nitrile latex type gloves are chemical-resistant and easy to work with while wearing. Disposable polyethylene shoe covers for short-term use or reusable latex or rubber boots will protect from chemicals and decontamination fluid. Proper training in the use of this equipment for the medial teams is essential. Input into this training by qualified personnel such as certified industrial hygienists and radiation health physicists is crucial.

Nitrile offers superior protection at all temperatures when compared with rubber gloves and boots. They cost only a fraction more than similar rubber products. Since medical providers must often touch casualties before decontamination is complete, they should have this protection. Both short (regular) and gauntlet-length gloves should be available.

Respiratory Protection

For many contaminants encountered in a hospital environment, respirators are not necessary. If needed, a simple organic vapor mask will suffice. If respirator use is anticipated, a respirator training course is required along with proper fit testing for personnel. A wide variety of canister filter respirators is available that protect against special chemicals or combinations of chemicals. Full-face protection respirator masks are rarely, if ever, required. Routine eye protection goggles should be available for all medical personnel.

Decontamination Solution and Water

Decontamination may be more difficult to provide and control than anticipated, particularly if performed outside the facility. Showers and decontamination scrubbings consume large amounts of water rapidly. Additional supplies of water are needed for hot climates. Garden hose and a portable variable pressure shower head may allow one to bring the shower to the patient, rather than move the patient to the shower. Fifty feet or more of garden hose is recommended. In general, a water-detergent solution will suffice in most decontamination scenarios. Portable decontamination showers for outside use are available.

Monitoring of Chemical Cleanup

If decontamination sites are properly constructed and the process of decontamination properly managed, the chance of contamination of a hospital area is minimal. Evaluation of the decontamination area for residual hazards should be performed by a certified industrial hygienist or other professional with similar qualifications. Monitoring techniques are dependent on the nature of the pollutant and require some familiarity with the decontamination procedures conducted. Wipe tests with gauze pads followed by a pH check suffice for acids and alkalis. For suspected organic solvent contamination, photoionization detectors provide a convenient and sensitive approach to monitoring large areas. In other instances where the contaminant has a low vapor pressure, such as polychlorinated biphenyls (PCBs), it may be necessary to evaluate the area with wipes and analyze the samples for the specific contaminant. Many of these techniques can be used to evaluate the effectiveness of patient decontamination procedures.

RESPONSE TO RADIOACTIVE CONTAMINATION

Hospital preplanning for radioactive materials and radionuclide exposures from an accident is crucial to the success of managing these patients as well as to preventing overall contamination of the medical facility and personnel. The 1979 accident at Three Mile Island nuclear plant in Harrisburg, Pennsylvania, revealed the inadequate preparation in the areas of medical response, technical response, and administrative response of hospitals in the community (3). Even worse was the local, regional, and global impact of the Chernobyl reactor accident in 1986. The Chernobyl accident resulted from an uncontrolled power excursion that produced overheating of the reactor and subsequent loss of cooling (4). The initial resulting explosion spewed forth high levels of radioactive emissions and fuel fragments. Several days later, heat from the decaying fission material in the damaged reactor produced tremendous heat, which resulted in distillation of remaining fission products, thus creating highly dangerous radioactive material release for the second time (4). The health effects of the Chernobyl accident are still being tabulated and have included at least 31 acute fatalities, a minimum of 237 cases of acute radiation illness, and an unknown number of persons who have or will develop cancer from the excessive exposure. There were approximately 115,000 persons evacuated from the surrounding area, and estimates are that 122 leukemias will occur in this group over the ensuing 2–12 years (4). The economic losses are difficult to calculate but are estimated at 6.8 billion U.S. dollars direct costs with up to $15 billion in costs to neighboring countries (4). The accident at Chernobyl deposited radioactive material throughout the Northern Hemisphere, increased the longterm risk for cancer in the evacuated population as well as in more distant populations, and resulted in loss of life as well as social costs.

Usually, persons with radioactive contamination are coming from facilities that have very knowledgeable personnel that can aid in the decontamination process. The facility from which the victims will be coming has probably initiated decontamination. Prior planning with such facilities and experts will guarantee greater success with fewer problems for the hospital emergency department personnel. Training in radioactive emergencies cannot be overemphasized. The radiation emergency plan should be an integral component of the overall hospital disaster plan. The plan requires the participation of radiation health experts working in concert with the medical team. The plan should be practiced once a year and involve the emergency medical staff as well as the radiation safety experts. Hospitals near nuclear facilities or isotope production facilities should actively include the professional personnel of those plants in the overall emergency plan and practice the plan with their involvement. Equipment necessary for proper response to a radioactive contamination is listed in Table 34.4.

The need for preplanned and orderly procedures for hospitals to receive, triage, and manage contaminated victims from radiation accidents is well-recognized (5,6). Following notification of an accident and that the hospital will be receiving victims, the radioactive emergency plan must be implemented according to the disaster plan protocol. This includes notification of the health physicists or radiation safety officer and formation of the decontamination medical team. Security and police should be notified to provide traffic control around the area outside the hospital and within the hospital. The radiation safety team headed by the radiation health expert must work closely with the medical command officer. As much information must be obtained as possible and on-site emergency personnel should be in constant contact with the receiving medical facility. The following questions should be answered:

What was the nature of the accident?
What kind of facility is involved?
What type of radionuclide is involved?
Did the accident involve irradiation only?
How many contaminated victims are there?
Is the contamination external or is there a risk of internal contamination from the accident?
What is the extent of contamination?
Has decontamination at the facility been performed?
Are there other injuries that alter the flow and immediate care of the victims being triaged?

Radiation Health and Safety Team

The involvement of a formal radiation health and safety team which supplies direction to the medical team is a requirement. The radiation safety team is responsible for patient and personnel monitoring, monitoring the routes from ambulance entrance to the decontamination room, and decontamination guidance, as well as monitoring of decontamination personnel and cleanup of the facility. Patient care is the medical officer's responsibility. Radiation safety is responsible for collection of personal dosimeters and maintaining control of all specimens from the patients. The radiation health specialist should be notified by the appropriate authority designated in the disaster plan as soon as the plan is implemented.

Preparation to Receive Patients

A restricted area for decontamination and medical management within the emergency department must be designated (5,6). This decontamination area should have the following characteristics: (a) convenience of wash equipment or shower area for ambulatory personnel as well as injured personnel, (b) portable shielding for working with gamma radiation, (c) a generous decontamination floor space area that can hold all personnel as well as more than one victim, (d) adjoining area or room for personnel to be monitored as they go into or leave the area, (e) capacity to hold the necessary equipment, (f) location out

Table 34.4.   Emergency Department Radioactive Decontamination Room Equipment

Two-inch demarcation tape for floor
Four-inch and two-inch-wide tape to secure wall and floor coverings
Plastic (polyethylene, 6 mil, 8 feet × 100 feet) floor and wall covering
Plastic (polyethylene, 6 mil, 4 feet × 100 feet) hall and corridor floor covering
Rolls of adsorbent paper with plastic backing for room and hallway
Ventilation filter paper
Radioactive warning signs
Decontamination stretchers with drainage collection tank
Plastic aprons
Dosimeters and film badges for decontamination team
Direct reading dosimeters plus chargers
Flashlights with extra batteries
Five-gallon wash containers
Cotton sheets and covers
Yellow rope with stands for demarcating zones
Large waste containers with lids (44-gallon drums) with plastic bag liners for waste
Dress-down and decontamination instructions
Sterile suture sets with extra forceps, hemostats, and scissors
Sterile irrigation fluid (several liters)
Sterile dressings
Razors with extra blades
Personal respirators
Surgical gowns, scrub tops and bottoms, shoe covers, caps, masks, and latex gloves, protective eyewear with side shields—for both decontamination team and as extra clothes for victims.
Disposable paper towels
Blankets
Five-gallon plastic buckets with tops
Large barrels for waste disposal
Scrub brushes
Surgical sponges—large
Irrigation syringes
Irrigation basins and bowls
Surgical scrub sponges
Liquid soap—one quart
Neoprene industrial gloves—one or two pairs
Tongs and forceps
Cotton swabs and wipes
Detergent (abrasive soap, detergent-cornmeal)
Clorox solution or other bleach (5% sodium hypochlorite)
3% hydrogen peroxide
Sponge forceps
Cotton-tipped applicators
Tubes with tops to contain cotton-tipped applicator samples
Lead storage containers from nuclear medicine to contain samples
Body chart of front and back for recording contaminated areas
Irrigation bulb syringe
Plastic specimen containers with lids
Hair clippers
Nail clippers
Bandage scissors
Vacutainers, syringes, needles, and blood drawing tubes
Alcohol wipes
Tissue paper
4 × 4 and 2 × 2 gauze pads
Small plastic bags for samples
Large yellow plastic bags (100)
Self-adherent labels and markers
Urine containers (1000-2000 milliliters)
Gamma-beta monitor
Alpha detector
Extra batteries
"Radioactive" tape labels for marking containers
Logbook with pencils
Markers

Table 34.5.   Radioactive Contamination Emergency Department and Staff Preparation

1. Remove all patients and pregnant women out of the area from the arrival zone of the ambulance, the entrance into the emergency department, and the route of all contaminated patients.
2. The route from the ambulance arrival zone to the decontamination room is covered with polyethylene plastic secured to the floor with tape.
3. The arrival route and entry ways for patients are demarcated with rope or radioactive labeled ribbon. Proper "radioactive" signs are in place. This area will remain as such until cleared by radiation safety officers or the health physicists in charge.
4. The decontamination room is marked with proper signs. The floors and walls are covered with polyethylene sheeting secured by tape. A demarcation line of bright, clearly identifiable tape separates "clean" from "unclean" area on entrance to the decontamination room. Ventilation to the room is turned off and ventilation ducts covered with appropriate filters or plastic. The room must be self-contained. Electrical switches and handles of doors and equipment should be covered with tape.
5. A designated radiation safety officer maintains watch at the entrance of the decontamination room to monitor all personnel, equipment, and samples leaving the room.
6. A designated nurse or technical assistant is on standby outside the decontamination room to pass in supplies to the medical team in the room. This person does not enter the decontamination room.
7. All equipment in the room is essential to the care and decontamination of the patient and must remain in the room until cleared by radiation safety.
8. Protective garments are worn by decontamination team. Two pairs of gloves should be worn. The inner gloves are removed as the last pieces of protective equipment as the person exits the room post decontamination. The minimum protection includes surgical scrubwear, pants and shirt, cap, masks, shoe covers, surgical gown with sleeves taped, two pairs of gloves, and eye protection.
9. All personnel entering and leaving the room must be surveyed by radiation safety for contamination. Contaminated items and clothing must remain in the room.

of the way of general traffic and can be entered by a separate corridor not receiving much use. Basic approaches for the emergency department preparation and receiving of patients are presented in Table 34.5.

All pregnant women should be kept away from this area. The route from the ambulance arrival area to the decontamination room should be covered with plastic sheeting secured to the floor by tape. This route should be demarcated as "radioactive," and not used by other personnel until cleared by radiation safety (Fig. 34.3). The floor and walls of the decontamination room should be covered with plastic sheeting and secured. The ventilation duct system and air return vents should be turned off and covered to prevent carrying of contaminant into other areas of the hospital. In some cases, a special filter may be used to cover these air vents. The decontamination room floor and walls should be covered with polyethylene plastic to aid in the cleanup of the room and contain decontamination wash spillage. Clothing should be placed into plastic bags and appropriately labeled with the name, date, time, and nature of the contaminant. A line of demarcation with yellow radioactive tape can be used as a "control" point to separate the clean side of the room from the decontamination side. No

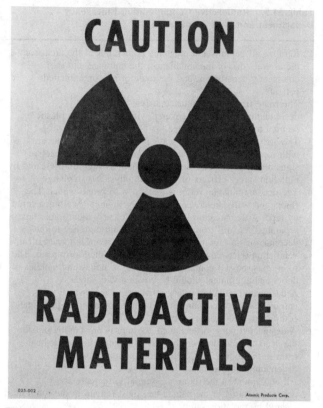

Figure 34.3. Radioactive materials warning signs. Source: Atomic Products Corporation.

Table 34.6. **Identification Tag Information Radioactive Contaminated Patient**

1. Name, employer, company identification number
2. Health physicist name and telephone number
3. Injuries and prehospital treatment
4. Skin contamination
    Type of contaminant (gamma, beta, alpha)
    Location (body chart, front and back)
    Dose rate and/or count measurements
      Before decontamination
      After decontamination
5. Decontamination methods and solutions used
6. Internal contamination
    Name of radionuclide
    Chemical and physical form
    Solubility
    Route of contamination (wound, inhalation, ingestion)
    Nasal swab counts
    Wound counts
    Whole body counts
    Bioassay samples collected
    Prehospital treatment
    Hospital treatment
7. External penetrating radiation
    Location and position of patient, relative to source of exposure
    Time of exposure
    Duration of exposure
    Personal dosimeter collected
    Symptoms
    Treatment

Decontamination of the Patient

Decontamination of a patient must reduce the exposure of the skin to radioactive materials, prevent or reduce systemic absorption, and contain the contaminant (7). The majority of radionuclide contamination will occur to the hands or face; however, the chance of more extensive contamination certainly exists. Hospitals and medical personnel must be prepared to handle the decontamination of small areas of the body as well as larger areas. According to the Joint Commission of Accreditation of Hospitals, each facility must be prepared to properly handle victims of such accidents.

The decontamination team is composed of the physician team leader, nurses, radiation safety experts, and other designated technical assistants. A call-up list of experts should be developed as a component of the disaster plan. No other personnel should be allowed to enter the decontamination zone unless they are part of the team rotating in or out. Personnel should wear surgical scrub suits with masks, caps, two pairs of gloves, and rubber or plastic shoe covers. The team leader should be trained in radiation safety and experienced enough to recognize the need for personal respirators in the event of heavy contamination of the victims by radionuclides. All members of the team should be trained in the use of radiologic monitoring equipment and decontamination procedures. The decontamination team should also wear plastic or rubber aprons during the actual washing of the victims. Excessive splashing of wash solution should be discouraged and eye protection should be worn by the decontamination personnel. Personal dosimeters should be worn by all members of the team (Fig. 34.4). Exposure to radioactive material is monitored by the radiation safety experts, and team members should be rotated as necessary to avoid cumulative doses above 5 rems.

It is imperative to determine whether the victim is contami-

person or equipment should cross this control line unless monitored for contamination. The radiation safety officer controls the flow of personnel and equipment across this line and into and out of the decontamination room. No potentially contaminated personnel or equipment can leave or enter this area unless cleared by the radiation health specialist. All biologic samples which are used to help determine whether internal contamination has occurred (blood, urine, nasal wipes, ears, eyes, skin wipes, nails, and feces) should be placed in appropriate containers, labeled, and placed under the control of the radiation specialty team. Most contamination is spread by the hands of personnel; thus light switches, door handles, and other graspable handles should be covered by polyethylene sheeting to prevent contamination. A decontamination stretcher to properly wash the patients and prevent splashing and spillage of washings should be available in the room.

Heavy duty polyethylene plastic drums with tight fitting lids and plastic liners should be placed in the decontamination room to hold contaminated materials. Identification and warning labels should be applied to these drums and their tops sealed with tape as they are filled. These drums will not be reopened and will be disposed of.

Patient identification tags should contain information relevant to the situation (Table 34.6). This information will usually accompany the patient to the medical facility. However, if the victims have not been tagged, then tagging should be done as part of the triage and decontamination process.

Radiation safety should check hallways and adjacent rooms for tracking of radioactive wastes.

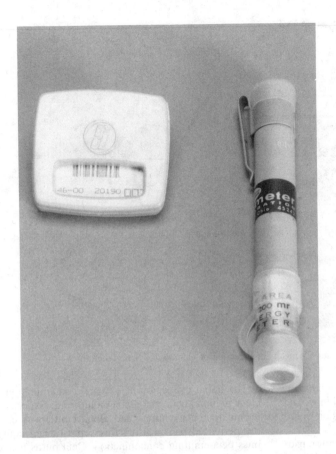

Figure 34.4. Personal dosimeters for radiation decontamination response team.

nated, where the contamination is, and the exact nature of the radioactive material or radionuclide. The decontamination team must address the following in concert with the radiation safety team:

1. Patient triage for serious medical conditions;
2. Management of serious wounds and medical conditions;
3. Evaluation of contamination extent and location;
4. Internal contamination management;
5. External contamination management.

The initial survey of the patient by the triage team occurs in the ambulance arrival zone. This survey will determine the level of contamination as well as whether there are contaminated wounds. Initial triage includes assessment of airway and cardiovascular status. Patients who are critical are triaged immediately to the decontamination-resuscitation room. If the patient is not critical, then clothes are removed in the decontamination zone outside the medical facility and placed in properly marked bags. The radiation safety team then decides the level of contamination and the areas of the skin (back and front) contaminated. These areas are indicated on the triage tags accompanying the patients. Patients without critical illness or injuries can be decontaminated after their clothes are removed. Portable decontamination units with self-attached containment vessels should be available as in chemical decontamination scenarios.

Monitoring a patient for radioactivity requires instruments to detect gamma, beta, and alpha sources. A Geiger-Muller survey meter detects both gamma and beta radioactivity (Fig. 34.5). A special alpha ''window'' is required to detect alpha radioactivity. A radiation health specialist or certified health physicist should be part of the emergency team to monitor for radioactive con-

tamination. It is important to hold the monitoring device the same distance from the site being monitored to determine the extent of contamination. Error in estimating exposures can be made if the instrument is not used properly. These are three basic exposure situations that must be differentiated or determined with regard to medical care of radiation accident victims (6): (a) external or dermal contamination, (b) internal contamination via ingestion or inhalation and (c) irradiation.

Radioactive material contaminating wounds, ingested, or inhaled can result in irradiation of tissues throughout the body as well as in incorporation of the material into biochemical mechanisms, with a resultant permanent radioactivity. Decontamination of any open wound is the first priority. If an open wound is found to be contaminated, decorporation treatment should be started. Decorporation should be instituted for inhaled or ingested radioactive material. Thus identification of the type and nature of the radioactive contaminate is crucial. Copious irrigation of the wounds with normal saline usually removes some of the radioactive material. The most common radioactive materials encountered by medical personnel are beta and gamma emitters. Alpha particle emitters are not as serious and are relatively uncommon. Beta particles are able to penetrate several meters through the air and are emitted from the nucleus of the atom. Beta particles can penetrate a few millimeters of tissue and are a health risk by both external and internal contamination routes. Gamma radiation is electromagnetic waves emitted from the nucleus of an atom which, due to their ability to penetrate both air for several meters and tissue for several centimeters, pose a significant health threat by any route of exposure. Alpha particles, generally isotopes, have a 2^+ charge and can only penetrate air for a few centimeters and

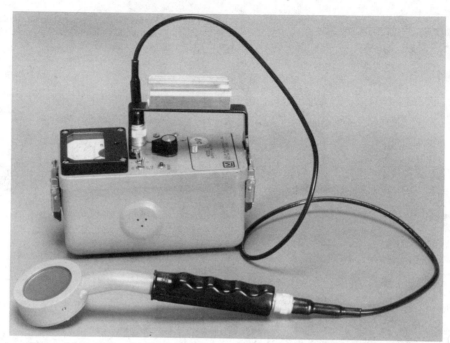

Figure 34.5.   Geiger-Muller survey meter for detection of gamma and beta radiation.

tissue for only a few micrometers. Alpha particles cannot penetrate intact skin. Alpha particles are a health hazard in wound contamination or if inhaled or ingested (see chapters on radioactive and radiation emergencies).

External contamination: This type of contamination usually occurs via a radioactive dust, liquid, or powder. Contamination of clothes, skin, eyes, and hair may occur and can be detected by proper monitoring. External contamination requires decontamination according to an established protocol.

Decontaminating the skin begins with removing the patient's clothes, placing the patient on the decontamination stretcher, bagging the clothes, and thoroughly washing the patient with a detergent-water mix. Washing should be gentle so as not to abrade the skin and cause incorporation. Gentle cleaning with a sponge is recommended. Attention should be paid to the hair, nails, and web spaces of toes and fingers. The wash solution must be collected in a containment vessel and the decontamination team adequately garbed in protective clothing. After the initial decontamination, the patient is then resurveyed for residual radioactivity. For contaminated hair, clipping may be necessary. Alpha radiation will not penetrate the intact skin. The dangers associated with alpha radiation are that of incorporation into the body and subsequent emission of beta or gamma radiation from daughter products (8). One millimeter of tissue will substantially reduce beta radiation effect on the basal cell layer of the epidermis.

Dermal absorption of radionuclides and radioactivity is of primary concern and is a passive process determined by the physical condition of the skin, the extent of contamination, the solubility of the contaminant, and the chemical nature of the radionuclide. The horny layer of the skin is the most important barrier to penetration. Mechanical damage to the skin will substantially increase absorption (8). Injury from acids and alkalis can either facilitate, or in some cases inhibit, percutaneous absorption. Dilute acid burns facilitate the dermal penetration of plutonium (8).

The initial evaluation of external contamination should include gamma, beta, and alpha monitoring. Experience in monitoring for beta emitters and alpha emitters is essential. An inexperienced person using this sophisticated equipment can miss beta-emitting contamination. Beta burns to the skin can occur if this contamination remains in contact too long.

General principles of external decontamination (Table 34.7) involve gently scrubbing the contaminated areas with a water-detergent combination. The use of a soft brush or soft sponge is recommended to prevent abrading the skin. Between decontamination procedures, the skin should be dried and monitored for effectiveness of the decontamination. If contaminant remains, this process should be repeated three more times. Persistence of contamination despite the initial decontamination can be managed by a slightly abrasive method such as a paste of cornmeal and Tide detergent mixed 50:50. The use of 5% sodium hypochlorite (household bleach) solution should be tried prior to a more abrasive measure. A problem with sodium hypochlorite is that a weak acidic solution tends to make plutonium soluble and could increase risk of percutaneous absorption. The use of radionuclide chelating agents in addition to the detergent scrub has been employed. Each method should be followed by monitoring for residual contamination after drying of the skin.

Another aggressive method involves the application of 4% potassium permanganate solution, a staining agent and oxidizer, followed in 2 minutes by rinsing of the skin with 4% sodium bisulfite. This should be undertaken by a person with experience with potassium permanganate since the skin can be damaged (7).

All contaminated hair should be washed and clipped if contaminants remain. All hair samples are saved by radiation safety. Results of decontamination procedures should be checked by monitoring. A detailed decontamination procedure should be a component of the overall hospital radiation disaster plan.

Internal contamination, also termed *incorporation*, results from the inhalation, ingestion, or would contamination of a radioactive material or radionuclide. The radioactive material

Table 34.7. Triage and Decontamination of Patients

1. The physician in charge directs medical care and decontamination of the patients.
2. Radiation safety officer monitors patient front and back on arrival. Contaminated areas are recorded by nurse on patient cards or tags.
3. Patient's clothes are removed and sealed in plastic bag containing proper patient identification.
4. Routine cotton swab samples are obtained of mouth, eye conjunctivae and mucosa, nasal mucosa, and ear canals and placed in sample containers marked with the patient's identification. Other samples are obtained as needed, such as of wound sites and all skin contaminated areas. Samples are given to radiation safety officer for proper storage.
5. Radiation safety officer monitors all decontamination personnel and biologic samples obtained during management and decontamination.
6. Medical assessment identifies medical needs of the patient. Patients with contaminated open wounds have priority.
7. **Contaminated wounds:**
   A. Begin decorporation treatment with DTPA as soon as possible.
   B. Open wounds are washed with normal saline for 3 to 5 minutes and re-monitored for contamination level. This step is repeated if contamination persists.
   C. Persisting contamination of open wounds despite repeated saline washings can be managed with a 3% hydrogen peroxide wash.
   D. Contaminated tissue not successfully removed by repeated washings may require surgical debridement. Surgical debridement may be necessary if the radionuclide is toxic, has a long half-life, and is not removed by appropriate decontamination methods.
   E. Save and label all tissue removed and place in appropriate specimen containers for storage by radiation safety.
   F. Cover all decontaminated wounds with sterile dressing and protect them from other areas of the skin that may be undergoing decontamination.
8. **Contaminated eyes, ears, mouth, nose:**
   A. Irrigate eyes with water or saline. Do not allow cross-contamination to the other eye during irrigation.
   B. Irrigate ears with warm saline or a 50:50 mixture of warm saline with 3% hydrogen peroxide using a bulb syringe. Monitor decontamination process, and repeat irrigation as needed. Do not allow irrigation solution to flow into patient's mouth, eyes, or wounds.
   C. Irrigate nose with saline using a bulb syringe. Have suction available, and do not allow patient to swallow irrigant. Monitor irrigant for radioactivity during the process.
   D. Have patient irrigate mouth without swallowing the water. Insert nasogastric tube into stomach and monitor contents of stomach for radioactivity. If gastrointestinal contents are contaminated, then lavage stomach until clear and begin decorporation with DTPA.
   E. Monitor level of decontamination and repeat irrigations as needed.
9. **External contamination:**
   A. Decontamination of the skin should begin with mild washing and gentle scrubbing using a detergent and water. A soft sponge or soft brush should be used to avoid skin abrasions. Monitor both skin and washing fluid for radioactivity and repeat washing three to four times to remove residual contaminant.

9. **External contamination** *(continued)*:
   B. For residual levels of contamination, use a mixture of 50:50 corn meal and powdered detergent (Tide) mixed in water to form a paste. Gently scrub the skin with this mildly abrasive material using soft sponges.
   C. For contamination persisting beyond the above efforts, a 5% sodium hypochlorite solution (Clorox) can be used either as full strength over most areas or diluted 1:4 with (Clorox:water) over areas like the face and neck.
   D. Citric acid 3% can be applied to the areas and rinsed off with water.
   E. For persistent contamination, and *in extreme cases only*, the application of 4% potassium permanganate followed by a 4% sodium bisulfite rinse may be tried. Potassium permanganate is an oxidizer and will stain the skin as well as remove the outer layer of skin.
   F. All skin areas, front and back, should be decontaminated until radiation safety agrees that the process is successful.
   G. Washings are collected in a containment vessel.
   H. Avoid splashing decontamination fluid, and do not allow washings to contaminate eyes, mouth, other mucous membranes, or wounds of the patient.
   I. Contaminated hair is washed with water and soap, then rinsed and monitored. Repeat as necessary. Hair may have to be cut. Do not shave hair, due to risk of cutting skin.
10. Patients may be removed from the decontamination room after radiation safety indicates that the level of contamination is safe. The patient should be dried. All materials should remain in the decontamination room. Wounds can be closed as needed after decontamination. Monitoring of patients and personnel is performed before anyone is allowed to leave the room.
11. Entire body of patient is monitored by radiation safety before leaving room.
12. All previously sampled areas should be resampled and labeled as "post-decontamination" with time and patient identification.
13. New polyethylene floor covering is laid-out from the patient to the door of the decontamination room and a clean stretcher is brought into the room. The patient is placed on the stretcher by a "clean" team and removed from the room. The process is monitored by radiation safety.
14. **Decontamination team exit:**
   A. The team may be rotated in and out depending on the level of contamination. This will be guided by radiation safety.
   B. An exiting team member will go to the designated "clean" line at the door of the room. All protective clothing will be placed in a predesignated drop zone or placed in a predesignated container. Outer gloves are removed first. Personnel monitors are then given to radiation safety officer. Remove tape from sleeves and trouser cuffs. Remove outer surgical gown then shirt and pants. Shoe covers are removed one at a time. Radiation safety monitors the first shoe and if clean the person can step over the line into the clean area and remove the second shoe cover. The inner gloves are then removed after the person is over the clean line, and they are dropped into the designated area.
   C. The team member then showers and is remonitored by radiation safety officer for any contamination.

thus has the opportunity to become incorporated into the body and irradiate internal tissues. This situation is a serious medical emergency. Some radionuclides can become permanently incorporated into the biological molecules of the body. Methods to decorporate these radioactive materials should be carried out according to a standard protocol.

Prompt and proper handling of contaminated wounds is especially important to prevent further incorporation of radioactive material. Surveying the wound with the radiation detector will indicate if the site is contaminated; sampling of wound tissue, exudate, any foreign bodies, and wound irrigation solution should be accomplished.

Multivalent radioisotopes in the actinide series (transuranic elements plutonium, neptunium, americium) as well as rare earths such as cesium have been effectively chelated using diethylenetriaminepentaacetic acid (DTPA). Although human data on the use of DTPA are limited, its administration is recommended as soon as possible and should be done within the first few hours to be effective. DTPA is available from the Radiation Emergency Assistance Center/Training Site (REAC/TS) in Oak Ridge, Tennessee, telephone number (615)576-1004 (8). Decorporation with chelating agents should be started as soon as possible in patients with contaminated wounds. Patients with residual contamination from skin break or foreign bodies may also benefit from pharmacologic therapy. Treatment depends on the chemical properties of the particular radioisotope involved and should be done in conjunction with advice from a nuclear medicine physician or radiation medicine specialist. DTPA chelates multivalent radionuclides that can then be renally excreted. Calcium disodium ethylenediaminetetraacetic acid ($CaNa_2EDTA$, calcium cersenate) has also been used as a radioisotope chelator but is not as efficacious as DTPA. Both the calcium and zinc salts of DTPA are approved for human use. CaDTPA is 10 times more effective than ZnDTPA for increasing renal excretion of actinide radionuclides within the first few hours of exposure. ZnDTPA is equally efficacious after the first one or two days of exposure.

In an acute exposure, 1 gram of CaDTPA diluted in 250 milliliters of dextrose 5% in water should be infused over 60–90 minutes. The dose may be repeated daily for 5 days. For immediate field administration, an aerosol inhalation treatment can be accomplished by placing the entire contents of a vial in a nebulizer. ZnDTPA appears to be less toxic then CaDTPA, but due to its lower efficacy should not be the first drug of choice. CaDTPA should be continued at a once-daily dose of 1 gram intravenously. During this time blood samples, whole body and chest counts, 24-hour urine collections and stool samples should be collected and monitored for radioactivity to determine the need for further chelation. If further chelation is required beyond 5 days, then ZnDTPA should be substituted for more prolonged therapy. A DTPA administration protocol and consent form is available from REAC/TS.

Irradiation by high energy gamma rays does not result in contamination. Tissue damage occurs immediately at the time of irradiation. The person is free from radioactive contamination unless source material was actually contacted or an explosion has occurred. Irradiation may be localized or it may be total body. It total body irradiation has occurred then the patient may experience the onset of the radiation syndrome. The significance and extent of the irradiation injury can be gauged by the onset of gastrointestinal symptoms (nausea, anorexia, vomiting). If vomiting begins within 1–5 hours, the person has sustained very serious irradiation effects. If vomiting begins within minutes following the exposure, then the person has probably sustained a lethal dose. Vomiting within 1–5 hours indicates a potentially lethal dose. Noting the time of the onset of gastrointestinal symptoms along with vomiting following the exposure is crucial and should be documented on the patient's chart. A complete blood cell count with a differential should be obtained as early as possible to document a baseline and then repeated within 6 hours and again at 24 hours. If the

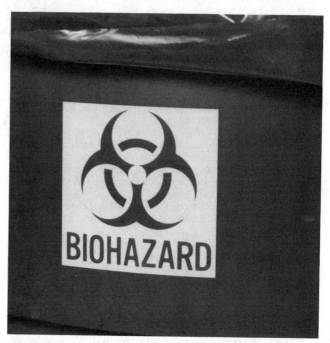

Figure 34.6. Infectious waste and biohazardous materials warning symbol.

absolute lymphocyte count does not fall below $1200/mm^3$ within 24 hours, the patient will probably remain clinically stable. If lymphocytes cannot be detected by the end of 6 hours postexposure, then the dose will be lethal to the patient.

BIOLOGIC AND BIOHAZARDS

The vast majority of medical waste is noninfectious. Most laboratory cultures and culture media are autoclaved prior to disposal. However, there may be occasions when medical waste is spilled or biohazards present a real risk to personnel. In such situations, cleanup and decontamination can follow the basic *CDC Guideline for Infection Control in Hospital Personnel*. Health care facility policies and procedures relating to infection control should be implemented. Some of the basic guidelines are as follows:

1. Physical contact with waste material should be prevented or minimized. Gloves should be worn along with protective eye goggles if blood or fluid is handled. Biohazardous materials should be labeled with the standard warning sign (Fig. 34.6).
2. Sharps, needles, and broken glass should not be directly handled. Remote instrumentation such as tongs can be used to collect such material. Special containers for sharps are available and should be used.
3. A dilute bleach solution (5%) diluted with water (1:10) should be used to clean up body fluids and blood.
4. Hands must be washed immediately if they are potentially contaminated.
5. Personnel familiar with infection control and biologic waste disposal practices should be called on to provide clean-up services.

Any needle stick or sharps injury to personnel must be handled according to infection control policy for such injury. Consultation with an infectious disease expert is highly recommended in these situations.

FOLLOW-UP AND POSTINCIDENT CARE OF HAZARDOUS MATERIALS CONTAMINATION

After patients are stabilized and decontaminated, it is necessary to arrange follow-up for possible health effects as well as provide for cleanup of the facility. There are many important facets of the post-incidence response: (a) decisions of further medical care and clinical monitoring must be made depending on the injuries and nature of the contaminant; (b) facility and equipment decontamination and cleanup must occur before the equipment or rooms can be used for other patients; (c) if the incident involved radioactive material, then radiation safety is responsible for collection of all biologic samples as well as personnel dosimeters worn by the medical decontamination team. Radiation safety must provide an estimate of the exposure to the members of the decontamination team; (d) waste disposal must be properly carried out and all waste must be accounted for by a tracking log; (e) update all logbooks and records concerning the patients; (f) administrative report and critique of the handling of the incident; (g) group meeting with medical team to review the incident; (h) early psychologic debriefing and interviews with patients and personnel can help prevent post-exposure stress syndrome.

Accurate, legible recordkeeping is crucial. Records should document medical care provided, decontamination of patients, difficulties with removing contaminates, wound management, and follow-up instructions. Records regarding technical control and containment of hazards, administrative controls to reduce hazards to patients and staff, tracking of patient's personal belongings and clothes, tracking of wastes and washings, and laboratory reports and biologic samples will provide essential documentation required by risk management and will also help in reviewing and critiquing the incident.

Following a radioactive decontamination scenario, radiation safety should survey all individuals involved for contamination before they leave the restricted area. Dosimeters are collected and wipe surveys must be taken from the instruments used in the room to determine whether they have been contaminated. Wipe surveys of the floor and walls is also necessary. Neither the room nor the equipment can be returned to normal service until it is ascertained that they have been decontaminated to background levels. Disposal of radioactive waste and washings is also a task of radiation safety. All biologic samples must be accounted for and controlled. Records and logs must be updated. Radiation exposure records of the emergency team will be determined and the individuals involved notified of their exposure. The estimated exposure to the patient is calculated and recorded. The responsible nuclear medicine physician will review all information regarding patient and personnel exposure.

Follow-up medical care may be necessary for patients who are not hospitalized, depending on the nature of the contaminating substance. Patients with radioactive contamination should be examined by a nuclear medicine physician. Patients with chemical contamination may require special medical follow-up, again depending on the nature of the contaminant. It is advisable to have one medical resource provide follow-up such as the company's occupational physician or a clinical toxicologist. This allows for continuity of care for all patients involved and provides the patient with a common medical provider knowledgeable in the area of toxic exposures. Clinical toxicologists and the regional poison center can be valuable resources of information regarding health effects and longterm monitoring of patients.

PSYCHOLOGIC EFFECTS OF HAZARDOUS MATERIALS EXPOSURES

Victims of a hazardous material exposure, especially following a disaster where there are multiple victims with injuries and death, may experience a posttraumatic stress disorder. This syndrome consists of anxiety, depression, insomnia, amplification of symptoms, and somatization. Predisposing personality factors are not necessary for this syndrome to occur. The development of such a neuropsychologic disorder has been evident following even mild or low level exposures to unknown agents or agents that are thought to be highly toxic. The situation regarding the exposure, associated injuries, magnitude of the exposure and fears of the unknown all contribute. Early intervention and debriefing with psychologic counseling can be effective in preventing and treating this disorder (see chapter on psychological sequelae). Recognition that a posttraumatic syndrome can develop is essential to longterm management of both victims and rescue personnel.

CONCLUSION

Success in managing patients of chemical or radioactive releases depends on prior adequate preparation of medical staff, administrative staff, and technical staff. Practicing mock scenarios, setting up decontamination zones and constructing decontamination facilities will enable the medical staff to become familiar with the roles of the technical consultants as well as their own roles in decontamination and containment. Practicing with basic equipment will allow the team to become familiar with the use of personal protective equipment, monitoring techniques, and methods to properly handle contaminated patients, as well as proper documentation and patient follow-up. Administrative staff must be trained to respond to the media as well as to provide for an orderly flow of patients, tracking of the contaminant and waste, and proper disposal methods.

A comprehensive disaster policy response inclusive of chemical, biologic, and radiologic victim contamination management is mandated by SARA on a state and local community level. Hospitals, poison centers, and fire departments must be prepared to provide expert response to any of these hazardous material situations.

REFERENCES

1. Binder S. Deaths, injuries, and evacuations from acute hazardous materials releases. Am J Public Health 1989;79:1042–1044.
2. Leonard, RB. Community planning for hazardous materials disasters. Top Emerg Med 1986;7(4):55–64.
3. Maxwell C. Hospital organizational response to the nuclear accident at three mile island—implications for future-oriented disaster planning. Am J Public Health 1982;72:275–279.
4. Anspaugh LR, Catlin RJ, Goldman M. The global impact of the Chernobyl reactor accident. Science 1988;242:1513–1518.
5. Richter LL, Berk HW, Teates CD, et al. A systems approach to the management of radiation accidents. Ann Emerg Med 1980;9:303–309.
6. Leonard RB, Ricks RC. Emergency department radiation accident protocol. Ann Emerg Med 1980;9:462–470.
7. Hubner KF. Decontamination procedures and risks to health personnel. Bull NY Acad Med 1983;59:1119–1128.
8. Management of persons accidentally contaminated with radionuclides. National Council on Radiation Protection and Measurements, NCRP Report No. 65. Bethesda, MD: NCRP, 1979.

Appendix

Title III and Its Enforcement Potential

I. INTRODUCTION—OVERVIEW. TITLE III OF THE SUPERFUND AMENDMENTS AND REAUTHORIZATION ACT OF 1986 (PUB. L. NO. 99–499, TITLE 3, 42 U.S.C. 110001 et seq., effective October 17, 1986).

A. Legislative policy and purpose for enacting Title III was to bring industry, government, and the general public together to prepare for accidental chemical releases in reaction to the Bhopal, India tragedy where a major release of methyl isocyanate killed more than 2000 people and injured thousands more. Title III has two main goals: emergency planning and community right to know.

    1. The emergency planning aspect requires local communities to prepare plans for dealing with emergencies relating to hazardous materials.

    2. The community right-to-know aspect creates new rights for members of the public and local governments to obtain information concerning potential threats in their neighborhoods.

B. Diversity of available information maintained by the State Emergency Response Commission (SERC) is required to be reported by regulated entities, primarily industry, under Sections 302, 311, 312, 313, and 304 may include documentation submitted relating to: specific chemicals present at a facility including quantity and location; health hazards and safety precautions related to particular chemicals at a facility; emergency contacts on-site; and general information concerning a facility, such as name, complete address, Dunn and Bradstreet number, permit information, and operational data.

C. Title III informational use in environmental enforcement and investigation can be very helpful and useful in a variety of ways.

    1. Title III information can aid and assist investigators and enforcement personnel in initial information collection efforts, particularly in gathering basic facts about a specific facility or owner/operator.

    2. Title III information can be utilized in related enforcement actions to demonstrate intent and knowledge on the part of a facility owner/operator concerning hazardous materials.

    3. Title III information can be utilized as supporting evidence and documentation concerning a facility's overall environmental history, including compliance levels and operating patterns.

    4. Title III information can be used independently to determine statutory violations and to initiate enforcement actions pursuant to Title III authority, including criminal, civil, and administrative provisions.

II. INFORMATION AVAILABLE—FIVE SOURCES. CONSISTS OF REGULATED ENTITY REPORTING UNDER SECTIONS 302, 311, 312, 313, AND 304.

A. Section 302. The owner or operator of any facility where extremely hazardous substances (EHSs) are produced, used, or stored in quantities greater than the threshold planning quantity (TPQ) shall report.

    1. Reporting Requirements: Owner or operator shall notify the SERC for the state in which such facility is located that he/she is subject to the requirements of Section 302.

    2. Deadline: May 17, 1987. Thereafter, the owner or operator must notify the SERC and the Local Emergency Planning Committee (LEPC) within 60 days of applicability.

    3. Form: No specific form required. Correspondence on business letterhead outlining responsibilities is acceptable.

    4. Special Considerations: List of Extremely Hazardous Substances, see 40 CFR 355.20 Appendices A and B. Additional changes to this list have been proposed in the Federal Register.

B. Section 311. The owner or operator of any facility which must prepare or have Material Safety Data Sheets (MSDSs) under the OSHA Act of 1970 and regulations promulgated thereunder shall submit either copies of MSDSs or a list of chemicals.

    1. Reporting Requirements: Owner or operator shall submit the MSDSs or list of chemicals to the SERC, LEPC, and the local fire department.

    2. Deadline: October 17, 1987. Thereafter, updates and revisions required within 90 days of new submission to OSHA or of awareness of significant new information.

    3. Form: Material Safety Data Sheet or a list of chemicals subject to OSHA regulation grouped in categories of health and physical hazards.

    4. Special Considerations: Hazard Communication Standard originally applied to SIC Codes 20–39; expansion to nonmanufacturing sector SIC Codes 1–80 became effective June 24, 1988, requiring Title III submissions on September 24, 1988; last expansion to construction industry became effective January 30, 1989, requiring Title III submissions on April 30, 1989. Threshold levels currently are 10,000 pounds for hazardous chemicals and 500 pounds for extremely hazardous chemicals.

C. Section 312. The owner or operator of any facility subject to MSDS requirements for hazardous chemicals under the OSHA Act of 1970 and regulations promulgated thereunder shall prepare and submit an emergency and hazardous chemical inventory form.

    1. Reporting Requirements: Owner or operator shall submit the Tier I inventory form to the SERC, LEPC, and the

local fire department and upon request, shall submit the Tier II form.

2. Deadline: March 1, 1988, and annually thereafter.

3. Form: Tier I and Tier II form.

4. Special Considerations: Factors outlined above as special considerations for Section 311 are applicable here as to regulated SIC Codes and thresholds.

D. Section 313. The owner or operator of a facility that has 10 or more full-time employees and that is in SIC Codes 20–39 and that manufactures, processes or otherwise uses a toxic chemical shall complete a toxic chemical release form.

1. Reporting Requirements: Owner or operator shall submit a toxic chemical release form to the state officials designated. In Illinois, it is the Illinois Environmental Protection Agency.

2. Deadline: July 1, 1988, and annually thereafter.

3. Form: EPA Form R also called Toxic Chemical Release Inventory Reporting Form.

4. Special Considerations: Threshold of 25,000 pounds for a listed chemical that is manufactured or processed and 10,000 pounds for a listed chemical "otherwise used."

E. Section 304. The owner or operator of a facility shall immediately report a release of a CERCLA hazardous substance or a Title III extremely hazardous substance which meets or exceeds the reportable quantity.

1. Reporting Requirements: Owner or operator of a facility shall immediately report to the SERC and the LEPC following a regulated release and provide notice as outlined in Section 304(b)(2) including: chemical name or identity; indication if substance is an EHS; quantity; time and duration; medium or media; health risks; and proper precautions.

2. Deadline: Immediate.

3. Form: None.

4. Special Considerations: Releases reported under Section 304 also require a written follow-up emergency notice as soon as practicable afterwards including: actions taken to respond to or contain the release; known or anticipated acute or chronic health risks; and, where appropriate, advice regarding medical attention. For CERCLA hazardous substances, see 40 CFR 302.4; for Title III extremely hazardous substances, see 40 CFR 355.20 Appendices A and B.

III. TITLE III ENFORCEMENT. STATUTORY AUTHORITY. TITLE III OF SARA AUTHORIZES THE FEDERAL GOVERNMENT, STATE, AND LOCAL GOVERNMENTS, AND CITIZENS TO BRING LEGAL ACTION AGAINST OWNERS OR OPERATORS OF FACILITIES FOR FAILURES TO COMPLY.

A. Subtitle A—Emergency Planning and Notification: Includes for enforcement purposes Sections 302(c), 303(d), and 304.

1. Federal: U.S. EPA Administrator may order owner or operator to comply with 302(c); administrator may order owner or operator to comply with 303(d); and civil and criminal penalties are authorized for 304 violations.

2. State and Local: may initiate civil action for failure of owner or operator to notify SERC for 302(c), venue is United States District Court; SERC or LEPC may start civil action against owner or operator for failure to give information for 303(d); no state or local authority for Section 304.

3. Citizen: no citizen authority for 302(c); no citizen authority for 303(d); may initiate civil action against owner or operator for failure to submit Section 304(c) follow-up report, venue United States District Court.

B. Subtitle B—Reporting Requirements: Includes for enforcement purposes Sections 311, 312(a), and 313.

1. Federal: administrator may assess civil penalty by use of administrative order or United States District Court for failure to prepare or submit MSDS for Section 311; administrator may assess penalty by use of administrative order or United States District Court for failure to submit Tier I form for Section 312; administrator may submit civil penalty by administrative order or United States District Court for failure to submit a toxic chemical release report form for Section 313.

2. State and Local: may initiate civil action for failure of owner or operator to submit MSDS for Section 311, venue is United States District Court; may initiate civil action for failure of owner or operator to submit Tier I form for Section 312, venue is United States District Court; no state or local authority for Section 313.

3. Citizen: may initiate civil action for failure of owner or operator to submit MSDS for Section 311, venue is United States District Court; may initiate civil action for failure of owner or operator to submit Tier I form for Section 312, venue is United States District Court; may initiate civil action for failure of owner or operator to submit a toxic chemical release form for Section 313, venue is United States District Court.

C. Subtitle C—General Provisions: Includes for enforcement purposes Section 322(a)(2), 322(d)(3)(A), 322(d), and 323(b).

1. Federal: administrator may assess civil penalty by use of administrative order or United States District Court for failure to submit information to support trade secret claim for section 322(a)(2); administrator may assess civil penalty by use of administrative order or United States District Court for trade secret claim that is not substantiated or frivolous; administrator may assess civil penalty by use of administrative order or United States District Court for failure of a claimant to provide information to support a trade secret claim; administrator may assess civil penalty by use of administrative order or United States District Court for failure to submit information to a physician who requests for an emergency case for Section 323(b).

2. State and Local: no state or local authority for Subtitle C—General Provisions.

3. Citizen: health professional may initiate action in United States District Court to compel owner or operator to comply.

35

Role of the Regional Poison Center in Hazardous Materials Accidents

Theodore G. Tong, Pharm.D.

Responding to the need for toxicologic information and referral assistance, poison control centers have been established in many communities as an integral part of the emergency medical response effort to deal with hazardous materials incidents. Spills, leaks, fires, and other accidents during the manufacture, transport, use, and storage of hazardous chemicals and toxic substances are occurring throughout communities in the United States with alarming frequency. In many communities where these incidents pose considerable risk, poison control centers have become an important participant in the network of agencies, services, and individuals with designated responsibilities and tasks for managing and giving assistance during these emergencies.

The first poison control center was established in Chicago in 1953. At one time during the late 1960s more than 600 poison centers existed throughout the United States. The range of capability of these centers, most of which were operating on a voluntary basis and in a decentralized manner, were quite variable. Users were often concerned by the lack of skilled medical or toxicologic expertise available from some centers. In some cases several centers could be found in the same area, while in other regions large geographic areas and population bases remained unserved. Medical direction, center organization, staffing, and range of services were not always consistent with the needs of the public and professional communities. During the 1970s, the concept of "regionalization" of poison center activities began to evolve, prompted in large part by the development of regional emergency medical services programs throughout the country (1). In the late 1970s, the American Association of Poison Control Centers (AAPCC) began to establish guidelines and criteria for regional poison control programs. Through the cooperation and collaboration of public, private, and institutional interests and resources, cost-effective and accessible systems of poison information and referral assistance have evolved (2). By the early 1980s, AAPCC efforts with support from organizations such as the American Academy of Clinical Toxicology and the American College of Emergency Physicians to improve the quality of poison control services had largely been successfully accomplished. The development of regional poison centers has occurred under the premise that such centers are capable of providing consistently more comprehensive and proficient services than the traditional center (3). Trained personnel who are either pharmacists or nurses functioning full time as poison information specialists, following established protocols and procedures and supported with skilled medical and clinical toxicologic expertise, are more likely to provide better quality of service than a center depending on staff lacking in formal training in toxicology and whose primary responsibilities and duties do not consist of responding to poison calls. The mission and goals of poison control centers include:

- Respond to inquiries from the public and health professionals for poison information and emergency treatment referral assistance.
- Prevent unnecessary delays in the management of poisonings by early recognition and appropriate assessment of the problem.
- Increase public awareness about poison prevention and what to do when a poisoning occurs.
- Reduce unnecessary emergency room visits and hospital stays for poisonings at considerable cost savings to patients, insurers, and the public
- Provide data collection and research on the incidents and outcomes of poisonings.
- Provide instruction and training on poison management to health professionals.
- Collaborate with local, regional, and state public safety and health agencies to deal with emergencies involving hazardous and toxic materials.

Since acceptance of the concept of regionalization of poison control services has become more widespread, the number of poison centers has declined considerably. As of January 1990, there are 35 AAPCC-certified regional poison centers that have applied for and met the association's regional criteria (Appendix). It has been estimated that approximately 60–70 regional centers are needed to adequately serve the need of the total population estimated to be 245.8 million in the United States (4, 5). During the 1980s, as concerns for environmental and workplace safety became national issues, poison information centers have seen their roles expanded beyond the traditional scope of prevention, education, and treatment of accidental childhood poisonings and acute drug overdoses (2, 6).

Actions taken during a hazardous chemical or toxic substance release are frequently conducted in a confused and inefficient fashion when on-scene responders, in the absence of any coordinated preincident operational plan for response, raise questions concerning what to do and where to obtain help. Response on these occasions typically involves numerous authorities and jurisdictions representing law enforcement, fire, safety, public health, and emergency medical responders. Lack of coordination of warning and notification procedures are further complicated on these occasions by insufficient access to the knowledge and skills needed to identify the materials released and to determine the health problems they may cause. Many poison control centers serving communities where the manufacture, transport, storage, and use of hazardous and toxic materials take place, forced by circumstances, have become a resource for information and referral assistance when these materials have been released into the environment. Poison control centers, during several recent widely publicized hazardous chemical accidents, have found themselves the center of inquiry from on-scene incident responders, the media, and a confused, anxious, and sometimes angry public for information on possible acute health effects, decontamination procedures, and recommendations for treatment (7). The notion that poison control centers have an important responsibility for providing a variety of response activities during hazardous chemical or toxic substances release incidents has been given much recent attention (2, 6, 7). Poison control centers have a vital role to play in minimizing public confusion and anxiety by offering rapidly accessible details on expected health hazards and making appropriate referrals to experts on containment, cleanup, and disposal of hazardous materials. The centers play a critical role by correctly determining the seriousness of the toxic exposure. The experience of centers that have been involved in these circumstances regardless of the chemicals or materials released are quite consistent and similar with regard to the type of information assistance and expertise referral requested. A review of major incidents will show that poison control centers are an excellent resource for notification and coordination of emergency medical personnel efforts to deal with toxic-exposed victims incoming to emergency treatment facilities and the potential medical problems.

Poison control centers have become designated in some local and regional emergency response plans as the focal points for alerting treatment facilities and public safety agencies of possible dangers and appropriate courses of action to take during exposure to hazardous and toxic materials; most centers will not recommend specific testing, containment, decontamination, or disposal procedures but will refer such inquiries to the appropriate local, regional, or state agencies responsible for these activities and services (Table 35.1). Centers engaged in hazardous materials response efforts are expected to have rapid access to computerized information on hazardous materials with listings of their physical and chemical properties and details on their safe handling, containment, and decontamination (10).

Poison control centers that assist in toxic emergency response *must*:

- Have full-time specialists trained and proficient in the retrieval, analysis, and communication of medical, toxicologic, and chemical information.
- Be accessible for information assistance on a 24-hour/day, 7-day/week basis to public safety and medical personnel; they must be similarly available to the public during incidents.
- Have resources organized in such a manner as to permit rapid access to technical and clinical information dealing with hazardous materials.
- Be located in a medical facility with ready access to consultants from various medical, laboratory, industrial, and occupational health-related clinical and scientific specialties.
- Have procedures and capabilities for recordkeeping and review.
- Have interest and capability to provide training to medical and other health specialists on matters related to toxicology and hazardous substances.

As the resource for information on the pathophysiologic effects of many chemicals and toxic substances, a poison control center's immediate goal is to determine: (a) identity and characteristics of the materials released or at risk of being released; (b) real or estimated quantities involved; (c) specific

Table 35.1. Poison Control Center's Role in Hazardous Materials Emergencies

- Participate in a coordinated, community-specific plan with clearly designated responsibilities and defined procedures when a hazardous materials emergency occurs.
- Assist incident responders in identifying and assessing the threat to health and environment.
- Facilitate the linkage between toxicologic expertise and information resources with incident responders and the emergency management system; the goal for such ties is to arrive at appropriate decisions dealing with health and environmental risks.
- Assist in the mobilization of medical resources to provide rescue and emergency care for those injured or ill from exposure to toxic release or spill.
- Provide appropriate medical management information to medical personnel treating victims.
- Be a mechanism by which health effects from exposures can be accurately followed up and documented post incident.
- Be the designated toxicologic focal point for dissemination of accurate, clear, consistent, and appropriate information to the public during toxic incidents.
- Provide technical assistance in efforts to develop emergency contingency and response plans for toxic incidents.
- Offer educational programs and opportunities to public safety and medical personnel on control, management, and response to hazardous chemical incidents.
- Evaluate toxicologic information and data on hazardous materials and become an accessible repository of this information and data.
- Become involved in a surveillance role to help identify and remove undetected environmental toxic hazards from the community.

nature of the release or type of accident; and (d) reactions observed between released materials and the environment or any known casualties or injured. Estimations are then established for the probability of illness, shortterm and longterm toxicity that might be experienced from contact, or exposure to the hazard or hazards. Where the hazardous materials incident is complex and ''major'' in scope, special consultants and expertise are called upon to provide additional support and assistance.

For medical professional inquiries during incidents, physician and toxicologic and hazardous materials specialists are available for consultation. The center often will provide the medical professional access to a range of information and expertise through its consultants—environmental and industrial toxicologists, hazardous wastes and materials management specialists, and occupational health specialists. A poison center should be able to provide information including physical property data, chemical property data, reactivity and toxicity information, and medical management advice. Centers must be prepared to act quickly and correctly during hazardous materials emergencies and accidents. Coordination between poison center, public health and safety agencies, and on-scene incident responders is essential.

The ability of poison control centers to competently and thoroughly assess the health threats of chemical and toxic substance release incidents is a necessity. Several case histories are given here to demonstrate the considerable degree of contribution poison control centers give for accurate risk assessment and advice for immediate action to take in order to minimize the adverse consequences from these threats (7–10).

POISON CONTROL CENTER AND HAZARDOUS MATERIALS INCIDENTS— CASE HISTORIES

November 21, 1979: 3:30 PM, San Francisco, California

A fire was reported to have started and probably ignited by an electric heater at a location in an area of mostly manufacturing and warehousing facilities adjacent to downtown San Francisco. The blaze, fueled by leaking chemicals illegally stored in the structure, had grown to become a four-alarm incident within minutes. As responding firefighters fought the unusually heavy, thick, acrid, and greenish-brown colored smoke, the nearby on-ramps to the San Francisco Bay Bridge were closed, snarling dense rush-hour traffic trying to leave the city on this late November afternoon before Thanksgiving Day.

A number of firefighters at the scene were overcome by smoke and exhaustion. In one instance, a 48-year-old firefighter required transport from the scene to the emergency department at the San Francisco General Hospital for evaluation. On arrival, he was in acute respiratory distress, cyanotic, and lethargic. He was examined and no evidence of myocardial involvement was found. He failed to improve following administration of 40% oxygen. Blood drawn from him for arterial blood gas analysis was an unusual chocolate-brown color.

Specialists in the San Francisco Bay Area Poison Control Center (SFBAPCC), which was situated in the emergency department, were consulted by physicians who were confounded by this dilemma. Methemoglobinemia from a toxic byproduct of combustion was suggested as a possible etiology. Accordingly, on administration of methylene blue, rapid improvement was produced, and the firefighter subsequently recovered.

Early recognition of this firefighter's toxic and life-threatening problem and successful resolution with assistance from the poison center helped to focus attention of the city's fire department, public health department, and media on the importance of a poison center as a resource during emergencies that involve toxic and hazardous materials.

January 13, 1980: 6:55 AM, San Francisco, California

San Francisco firefighters responding to multiple alarms rushed to the scene of a blaze in an area close to the city's downtown. Upon arrival, it was apparent to the incident command that unknown chemicals stored in the structure were involved. The SFBAPCC was called at approximately 7:10 AM by fire and public health department officials urgently requesting the assistance of a poison information specialist at the scene with the assessment and identification of the toxic hazards and threat to health that may arise from this fire. The center responded immediately by dispatching the director to the scene.

The two-story building, which eventually was completely destroyed, was the office and warehouse of the same firm involved in the November 1979, fire. Under the guise of being a pharmaceutical manufacturer, this firm was a leading producer of isobutyl nitrite, a chemical commercially promoted and sold as a perfume or room deodorizer known as "Rush." Vapors of Rush and other butyl nitrite compounds are alleged to enhance sexual performance when inhaled and are purchased solely for this purpose.

This fire took scores of firefighters nearly 6 hours to suppress; it was not until 2 days afterward that workers in surrounding office complexes were able to reenter the area without experiencing respiratory and eye irritation. There were no serious injuries encountered during this episode.

Prompted by the growing number of similar incidents, the

Table 35.2. Findings by San Francisco Ad Hoc Advisory Group on Hazardous Incident Management, 1980

- Fire and police personnel needed technical assistance to effectively and appropriately respond to hazardous materials emergencies.
- A clearinghouse for this technical assistance was needed.
- The poison center is the likely place to serve this function.
- The center did *not* have considerable expertise, experience, or resources dealing with these issues.
- The level of information on hazardous substances could be greatly enhanced for the center by identifying the expertise already present in the region and making it available to the center.
- The emergency response system needed assistance in:
  (a) *identifying* unknown chemical hazards; (b) *assessing* the nature of and toxicity of materials present at any incident;
  (c) *recommending* to the on-scene incident commander appropriate courses of action to take regarding personal protection, containment, identification, removal, and reporting.
- There was a need for training of firefighters in handling hazardous materials.
- There was a need for longterm follow-up for firefighters exposed to toxic materials.

San Francisco Fire Department (SFFD), in late January 1980, convened an ad hoc advisory committee to give guidance in the formulation of a citywide contingency plan in order to respond optimally to the problems of hazardous materials emergencies. This group, composed of designated representatives of the fire department, poison center, city departments of public health, water, public works, the Mayor's Office of Emergency Services, and a number of other experienced individuals with interest in occupational medicine nursing, public health, industrial safety, and emergency planning, met regularly for several months to study the issues. A number of findings were made (Table 35.2) and from them, specific recommendations for implementation were proposed by this group (Table 35.3).

Table 35.3. Suggestions of the Ad Hoc Advisory Group to the San Francisco Fire Department, 1980

- The poison center should be a central communication contact point in any emergency response to hazardous materials incident plan.
- The center should develop standard protocols and references dealing with emergency response.
- A hazardous materials incident response team should be assembled; this team should be comprised of individuals who can be called for technical assistance on toxicology information and can give experienced on-scene help.
- On-scene responders must receive training and/or be experienced in areas of toxicology, industrial hygiene, basic combustion chemistry; have appropriate reference materials; be aware of the department's plan of operation for hazardous emergencies; be familiar with use and limits of personal protective equipment; have skill in the use of essential on-site measurement techniques.
- An emergency response plan should be developed for the city with notification procedures and contingency options clearly outlined.
- A procedure should be developed for medical follow-up care of exposed firefighters.
- Minimal training and personal protective clothing requirements should be established for fire department personnel with responsibilities in hazardous materials response.

These specific action suggestions were then extensively examined and studied by the department with consideration and participation by various city, regional, and state agencies, in addition to hazardous materials management consultants. Nearly 1 year later, a notification plan was developed, adopted, and implemented by the SFFD. The advisory committee was also asked to continue serving the department as a consultant on matters related to the planning and conduct of emergency response to hazardous materials incidents.

August 21, 1981: 1:35 PM, San Francisco, California

A 16-inch natural gas main was punctured by a drill at a site undergoing excavation in San Francisco's financial district. Escaping natural gas blew upward and was carried into nearby businesses and office buildings. There was no ignition; however, the gas did contain oil-containing polychlorinated biphenyls (PCBs). The natural gas escaped into the atmosphere, but the fallout of the PCB oil as a mist contaminated an eight-square block area covering cars, buildings, trees, pedestrians, police, and firefighters. The SFBAPCC received first notification from the fire department of the incident at 3:00 PM, when it became obvious to the incident command that the oil mist may have contained PCB. Approximately 30,000 persons were safely evacuated from the area within 45 minutes. No one was killed or seriously injured, although many persons, automobiles, and buildings were sprayed with the PCB-contaminated mist. It was not until 10:45 PM, nearly 10 hours after the pipe was punctured, that the escaping gas was completely stopped. It was 2 weeks before cleanup and decontamination were completed and clearance was given by health officials, permitting public entry into the area's offices and businesses.

During the first 6 days of this episode, the poison center received inquiries from hundreds of concerned individuals who had been exposed to PCB or were in close proximity to the contaminated area at the time of the incident.

April 3, 1983: 4:15 AM, Denver, Colorado

Just after 4:15 AM on April 3, 1983, a spill of 20,000 gallons of nitric acid occurred in the central Denver railyards. The acid spread over a 300×300-foot area, and an acid cloud began to rise over the city. The rapid spread of fumes ultimately led to an evacuation of 3000 residents. Numerous community agencies were involved in the spill: Police, Fire Department, Office of Emergency Preparedness, the Rocky Mountain Poison and Drug Center, State Highway Patrol, Public Works, Health Department, Emergency Medical Services, Environmental Protection Agency (EPA), Red Cross, and other volunteers.

The poison center was one of the initial agencies involved in the management of the spill. It outlined potential toxic effects of nitric acid fume inhalation and supplied medical treatment information to workers involved in the cleanup of the spill, hospitals and health workers, the media, and the public.

The increased need for information from the poison center resulted in a *200%* increase in the center's average daily call volume with a total of 648 calls received on April 3, 1983 (8).

August 14, 1985: approximately 3:00 PM, New York City

The New York City Poison Control Center was advised by police that a metalworking plant in the Borough of Queens was burning out of control. It was known that the plant contained seventy-four 55-gallon drums of cyanide (exact chemical composition unknown).

An advisory was issued from the center about the hazards of the situation along with instructions about use of protective equipment and on-site first aid. The city's hazardous material emergency unit, several mobile emergency room vehicles, the

Department of Environmental Services, police, fire, and emergency medical services units were all participating as incident responders.

During the first hours of the incident, the poison information specialists contacted all of the emergency departments that would potentially receive patients in order to ensure that they were familiar with the use of the Lilly Cyanide Antidote Kit. In addition, they were reminded of the possibility that any individual brought from the fire site might be poisoned not with cyanide, but with carbon monoxide.

The Poison Control Center became aware that the hospitals likely to receive patients from the scene had very limited supplies of the cyanide antidote kits. The center became the lead agency to coordinate the acquisition of the antidote. A telephone call to Eli Lilly and Company (Indianapolis, Indiana) resulted in an immediate air shipment of 60 cyanide antidote kits into the disaster area within 2 hours (9).

April 24, 1988: 8:45 AM, Tucson, Arizona

Almost 300 pupils and four teachers at a northwest elementary school were rushed to eight area hospitals after the school's evaporative coolers sucked insecticide into classrooms. A 73-year-old neighbor said he had sprayed, with a garden hose sprayer, malathion on four plants at about 8:15 AM in his backyard, which was immediately south of the school. The children described by teachers were "starting to get sick . . . had stomachaches, headaches . . . a lot of them couldn't breathe."

The Arizona Poison Control Center responded to 200 calls by the late afternoon, mostly from worried families; other calls came from triaging medical personnel and the media. The center was an invited participant at a number of postincident meetings to discuss the immediate health concerns with parents, school, and public health and safety officials.

A review of other major and well-publicized hazardous materials incidents where a poison control center played a major role in the emergency response will show that, regardless of the materials or chemicals involved, the type of information and referral assistance needed by public safety, health personnel, media, and the general public are quite consistent and similar. Poison control centers had a key role in minimizing public confusion and anxiety during many of these situations. Equally important, the centers also played a critical role by correctly determining the seriousness of the toxic exposure.

Following the August 25, 1981, incident involving the PCB oil release in San Francisco, a retrospective analysis of the SFBAPCC experience during the incident was initiated; the goal was to characterize and evaluate the utilization of the center on this occasion. The intent of the review was to identify ways that a poison center might anticipate in this preparation and planning in order to more effectively deal with similar toxicologic emergencies in the future (Table 35.4).

All calls to the center were individually entered onto a report form which serves to document and record the caller's name, location, substance involved, history of exposure, assessment, and outcome. All reports involved with the PCB incident entered during the week were reviewed. A total of 510 Reports was retrieved. Of the inquiries, 31% dealt with someone who was symptomatic, probably due to the exposure, e.g., headaches, nausea, and eye and respiratory irritation; 25 persons experienced acute onset of skin irritation with four reporting delayed onset of acneform-type lesions. "Chlorance" characterized by comedones, cysts, pustules, and inflammatory skin changes is a hallmark sign of recent exposure to polychlorinated biphenyl compounds. The largest percentage (50%) of callers

Table 35.4.   Characteristics of Inquiries Received at Poison Center during/after PCB/Gas Leak, San Francisco, California; August 25–26, 1981

Total calls received		510[a]
Reports of symptoms		159[b]
Headache, lightheadedness, nausea, vomiting	79	
Eye and respiratory irritation	56	
Skin irritation and rash	24	
Inquiries regarding decontamination		103
Inquiries regarding reproductive effects		27
Inquiries from medical personnel		28
Inquiries from firefighters		5
Inquiries from cleanup personnel		7
Inquiries from press		8
General information (e.g., cancer risks, reentry to area, information for employees, etc.)		137

[a]Many calls involved several individuals or a large group; more than 50 calls were untallied.
[b]Possible relationship to leak only.

were simply requesting information. Most often these calls dealt with decontamination procedures, cancer risks, and information regarding reentry into the contaminated areas. Risks of PCB-induced teratogenicity were a common concern among callers. There were a number of calls (28) from emergency medical personnel, mostly physicians and nurses, asking for clinical details and specific precautions to take regarding containment and decontamination procedures. The center specialist gave details to medical personnel on decontamination, treatment, and suggestions on what advice to give patients. Members of the local media remained posted with the poison center throughout the critical and uncertain first days of the incident; much interaction between the media and the center staff of specialists concerned corroborating details related to the known health risks from PCB exposure and the proper care of contaminated personal property and persons.

Since multiple chemicals were frequently involved in these release incidents, the symptoms and complaints experienced by individuals in contact or by those who had already been exposed were very often nonspecific in character. Chemical agents usually have multiple organ system effects, and, depending on the route, duration, amount, and concentration of the exposure, the onset and duration of symptoms will frequently vary. Ocular and dermal injury can occur following contact or exposure to materials such as oxidants, corrosives, and vesicants. Chemicals absorbed can produce significant systemic toxicity. Some chemicals can cause both cutaneous damage and systemic toxicity following exposure or contact with them. The majority of toxic injury encountered during hazardous chemical and toxic material incidents is incurred through inhalation (Table 35.5). In any risk analysis process involving toxic substances, there is no substitute for scrupulous collection of details, particularly regarding the physical conditions of anyone exposed and the circumstances that surrounded the incident.

Poison control center evaluation of the toxic exposure will include identifying instances where pharmacotherapy may be of antidotal value. Specific antidotes are indicated for serious poisoning with chemical asphyxiants (i.e., carbon monoxide, cyanide, the methemoglobin formers) and organophosphate and carbamate pesticides (Table 35.6). Consultation with poison con-

Table 35.5.   Special Problems in Hazardous Materials Incidents

Irritant gases
  Chlorine
  Ammonia
  Oxides of nitrogen, sulfur
  Acids
  Phosgene
  Aldehydes
  Isocyanates
Asphyxiants
  Nitrogen
  Halogenated aromatic hydrocarbons
  Methane
  Carbon dioxide
Chemical asphyxiants
  Carbon monoxide
  Nitrites
  Cyanide
  Hydrogen sulfide
Fumes, vapors, smoke
  Heavy metals: zinc, nickel, lead, mercury, arsenic, chromium
  Pesticides: organophosphates, carbamates
Others
  Paraquat
  Polychlorinated biphenyls

trol center medical staff is a policy and procedure whenever advice on specific pharmacotherapy is recommended. Appropriate precautions to avoid contamination of personnel are emphasized on any occasion where the poison control center has determined that a health hazard is present. In the overwhelming majority of cases, casualties from chemical and toxic exposures will only require administration of symptomatic and supportive care.

In summary, the role of many poison control centers has expanded beyond the traditional scope of prevention and treatment of accidental childhood ingestions and acute drug overdoses. Many centers, by circumstance and necessity, have become useful resources of information and referral assistance during chemical release accidents. It should be recognized that, during these toxic crises, a poison center must remain "open" and accessible for people seeking help with other types of poisoning problems far removed from the immediate incident (11). Another issue poison control centers must deal with is: the need to provide off-site interpretive abilities and skills for hazardous materials incidents.

Table 35.6.   Emergency Pharmacotherapy in Hazardous Materials Exposures

Oxygen
Methylene blue
Chelating agents
  Dimercaprol/British AntiLewisite (BAL)
  d-Penicillamine
  Calcium disodium Ethylenediaminetetraacetate (EDTA)
  Dimercaptosuccinic acid (DMSA)
  2,3-Dimercaptopropane-1-sulfonic acid (DMPS)
Pralidoxime
Atropine
Cyanide antidote kit
Calcium gluconate
Bronchodilators
Anticonvulsants
Antidysrhythmics

Legal concerns and liability also need clarification. Additional challenges to poison control centers include satisfying public expectation as the frequency of toxic exposures increases and competition for scarce operational resources grows more intense.

REFERENCES

1. Temple AR, Veltri JC. One year's experience in a regional poison control center: intermountain regional poison control center. Clin Toxicol 1978;12:277–289.

2. Tong TG, Becker CE, Foliart D, et al. A model poison control system. West J Med 1982;137:346–350.

3. McIntire MS, Angle CR. Regional poison-control centers improve patient care. N. Engl J Med 1983;308:219–221.

4. Temple AR. History and present status of American poison control centers. Vet Hum Toxicol 1982;24(Suppl):2–4.

5. Manoguerra AS, Temple AR. Observations on the current status of poison control centers in the United States. Emerg Med Clin North Am 1984;2:185–197.

6. Perrin EV, Micik S. Poison control centers and the toxic environment. Emerg Med 1982;14(17):95–98.

7. Tong TG, Joe G, Morse LH, et al. A poison center experience with environmental emergencies. Vet Hum Toxicol 1983;25(Suppl 1):29–33.

8. Spiller SK, Wruk KM, Montanio CD, et al. Poison center disaster management: a strategic plan. Vet Hum Toxicol 1985;27:301.

9. Weisman RS, Goldfrank L, Bellini R. Chemical disasters (letter). Vet Hum Toxicol 1985;27:439.

10. Mrvos R, Dean BS, Krenzelok EP. A poison center's emergency response plan. Vet Hum Toxicol 1988;30:138–139.

11. Tong TG. Hazardous materials emergencies: how prepared for the next incident. Vet Hum Toxicol 1983;25:295–296.

APPENDIX

American Association of Poison Control Centers
Certified Regional Poison Centers
(January 1990)

ALABAMA

Alabama Poison Center
  809 University Boulevard East
  Tuscaloosa, AL 35401
  Emergency Numbers
    800/462-0800 (Alabama only); 205/345-0600

Children's Hospital of Alabama Regional Poison Control
  Center
  1600 7th Avenue South
  Birmingham, AL 35233
  Emergency Numbers
    205/939-9201 (Alabama only); 800/292-6678; 205/
    933-4050

ARIZONA

Arizona Poison and Drug Information Center
  Health Sciences Center, Room 3204K
  1501 North Campbell
  Tucson, AZ 85724
  Emergency Numbers
    602/626-6016 (Tucson); 800/362-0101 (Arizona
    only)

Samaritan Regional Poison Center
  Good Samaritan Medical Center
  1130 East McDowell, Suite A5
  Phoenix, AZ 85006
  Emergency Number
    602/253-3334

CALIFORNIA

Fresno Regional Poison Control Center
  Fresno Community Hospital and Medical Center
  Fresno and R Streets
  Fresno, CA 93715
  Emergency Numbers
    209/445-1222; 800/346-5922

Los Angeles County Medical Association
  Regional Poison Center
  1925 Wilshire Boulevard
  Los Angeles, CA 90057
  Emergency Numbers
    213/664-2121; 213/484-5151; 800/777-6476

San Diego Regional Poison Center
  UCSD Medical Center
  225 Dickinson Street
  San Diego, CA 92103-1990
  Emergency Numbers
    619/543-6000; 800/876-4766

San Francisco Regional Poison Center
  San Francisco General Hospital
  1001 Potrero Avenue, Room IE86
  San Francisco, CA 94110
  Emergency Numbers
    415/476-6600; 800/523-2222

UC Davis Regional Poison Control Center
  2315 Stockton Boulevard, Room 1511
  Sacramento, CA 95817
  Emergency Numbers
    916/453-3692; 800/342-9293 (Northern California
    only)

COLORADO

Rocky Mountain Poison and Drug Center
  645 Bannock Street
  Denver, CO 80204-4507
  Emergency Number
    303/629-1123 (Colorado)

FLORIDA

Florida Poison Information Center
  The Tampa General Hospital
  Davis Islands
  Post Office Box 1289
  Tampa, FL 33601
  Emergency Numbers
    813/253-4444 (Tampa only); 800/282-3171
    (Florida)

GEORGIA

Georgia Regional Poison Control Center
  80 Butler Street, S.E.
  Atlanta, GA 30335-3801
  Emergency Numbers
    404/589-4400; 800/282-5846 (Georgia only)

KENTUCKY

Kentucky Regional Poison Center of Kosair Children's
  Hospital
  224 East Broadway, Suite 305
  Louisville, KY 40202
  Emergency Numbers
    502/589-8222; 800/722-5725 (Kentucky only)

MARYLAND

Maryland Poison Center
  20 North Pine Street
  Baltimore, MD 21201
  Emergency Numbers
    301/528-7701; 800/492-2414 (Maryland only)

MASSACHUSETTS

Massachusetts Poison Control System
300 Longwood Avenue
Boston, MA 02115
Emergency Numbers
617/232-2120 (Boston area); 800/682-9211
(Massachusetts only)

MICHIGAN

Blodgett Regional Poison Center
1840 Wealthy Street S.E.
Grand Rapids, MI 49506
Emergency Number
800/632-2727 (Michigan only)

Poison Control Center
Children's Hospital of Michigan
3901 Beaubien Boulevard
Detroit, MI 48201
Emergency Numbers
313/745-5711 (Detroit);
800/462-6642 (Michigan only)

MINNESOTA

Hennepin Regional Poison Center
Hennepin County Medical Center
701 Park Avenue South
Minneapolis, MN 55415
Emergency Number
612/347-3141

Minnesota Regional Poison Center
St. Paul-Ramsey Medical Center
640 Jackson Street
St. Paul, MN 55101
Emergency Numbers
612/221-2113; 800/222-1222 (Minnesota only)

MISSOURI

Cardinal Glennon Children's Hospital
Regional Poison Center
1465 South Grand Boulevard
St. Louis, MO 63104
Emergency Numbers
800/392-9111 (Missouri only); 314/772-5200;
800/366-8888

NEW JERSEY

New Jersey Poison Information and Education System
201 Lyons Avenue
Newark, NJ 07112
Emergency Numbers
800/962-1253 (New Jersey only); 201/923-0764
(outside New Jersey)

NEW MEXICO

New Mexico Poison and Drug Information Center
University of New Mexico
Albuquerque, NM 87131
Emergency Numbers
505/843-2551; 800/432-6866 (New Mexico only)

NEW YORK

Long Island Regional Poison Control Center
2201 Hempstead Turnpike
East Meadow, NY 11554
Emergency Number
516/542-2323

New York City Poison Center
455 First Avenue, Room 123
New York, NY 10016
Emergency Numbers
212/340-4494; 212/764-7667

NORTH CAROLINA

Duke Regional Poison Control Center
Duke University Medical Center
Box 3007
Durham, NC 27710
Emergency Number
800/672-1697 (North Carolina only)

OHIO

Central Ohio Poison Center
700 Children's Drive
Columbus, OH 43205
Emergency Numbers
614/228-1323; 800/682-7625

Regional Poison Control System and Cincinnati Drug and
Poison Information Center
231 Bethesda Avenue, M.L., #144
Cincinnati, OH 45267-0144
Emergency Number
513/558-5111

OREGON

Oregon Poison Center
Oregon Health Sciences University
3181 SW Sam Jackson Park Road
Portland, OR 97201
Emergency Numbers
503/279-8968; 800/452-7165 (Oregon only)

PENNSYLVANIA

Delaware Valley Regional Poison Control Center
One Children's Center
34th & Civic Center Boulevard
Philadelphia, PA 19104
Emergency Number
215/386-2100

Pittsburgh Poison Center
One Children's Place
3705 5th Avenue at DeSoto
Pittsburgh, PA 15213
Emergency Number
412/681-6669

RHODE ISLAND

Rhode Island Poison Center
593 Eddy Street
Providence, RI 02903
Emergency Numbers
401/277-5727; 401/277-8062 (TTY)

TEXAS

North Texas Poison Center
5201 Harry Hines Boulevard
Dallas, TX 75235
Emergency Numbers
214/590-5000; 800/441-0040 (Texas only)

Texas State Poison Center
University of Texas Medical Branch
Galveston, TX 77550-2780
Emergency Numbers
409/765-1420 (Galveston); 800/392-8548 (Texas
only); 713/654-1701 (Houston); 512/478-4490
(Austin)

UTAH

Intermountain Regional Poison Control Center
50 North Medical Drive, Building 528
Salt Lake City, UT 84132
Emergency Number
801/581-2151

WASHINGTON, DC

National Capital Poison Center
Georgetown University Hospital
3800 Reservoir Road, N.W.
Washington, DC 20007
Business/Emergency Numbers
202/625-3333; 202/784-4660 (TTY)

WEST VIRGINIA

West Virginia Poison Center
3110 MacCorkle Avenue, S.E.
Charleston, WV 25304
Emergency Numbers
304/348-4211 (local); 800/642-3625 (West
Virginia)

36

Pharmacotherapy of Hazardous Materials Toxicity

Katherine Hurlbut, M.D.
Theodore Tong, Pharm.D.
John B. Sullivan, Jr., M.D.

INTRODUCTION

The medical management of individuals exposed to toxic substances during hazardous material releases may require the administration of specific pharmacotherapy. Pharmacologic intervention is selected on these occasions from a limited number of agents that have antidotal value as antagonists to the harmful effects of these substances. In the overwhelming majority of cases, casualties from chemical and toxic exposures will require only symptomatic and supportive care. Antidotal therapy given to produce physiologic reversal of the systemic effects of a toxin or poison is appropriate only in very specific situations. Antidotes play a life-saving role in the treatment of serious acute intoxication with chemical asphyxiants such as carbon monoxide, cyanide, hydrogen sulfide, methemoglobin formers, and organophosphate and carbamate pesticides; they are also important to consider in some cases of acute and chronic metal poisoning. Used appropriately with attention directed toward establishing realistic therapeutic endpoints, antidotes can reduce the risks of the morbidity and mortality that result from certain toxic exposures. Table 36.1 is a list of commonly used physiologic antagonists and the toxins they antagonize.

ATROPINE

The cholinergic effects of organophosphate and carbamate insecticides are reversed by atropine. Organophosphates and carbamates bind to and inhibit acetylcholinesterase enzymes, thereby allowing acetylcholine to accumulate at receptor sites producing excess cholinergic effects. Signs and symptoms of organophosphate and carbamate toxicity result from the accumulation of acetylcholine at muscarinic and nicotinic receptor sites in the peripheral and central nervous system.

Muscarinic receptors are located at parasympathetic postganglionic sites and anatomically are found in smooth muscle, exocrine glands, and the heart. Accumulation of excess acetylcholine at muscarinic sites produces excessive salivation, urination, lacrimation, diarrhea, bradycardia, pupillary constriction, bronchoconstriction, and increased bronchial secretions. Acetylcholine receptors are widely distributed in the central nervous system also. Excessive stimulation can induce confusion, ataxia, seizures, depression of central respiratory drive and cardiovascular centers, and coma (1). Nicotinic acetylcholine receptors are found at the neuromuscular junction and autonomic ganglia. Excessive stimulation results in muscle fasciculation, weakness and fatigue, diminished respiratory effort, respiratory failure, tachycardia, hypertension, and hyperglycemia.

Atropine antagonizes the central and muscarinic cholinergic

effects of organophosphate and carbamate insecticide poisonings but does not reverse the nicotinic effects. It is important to realize that the doses of atropine required to effectively treat these patients will exceed by severalfold the doses used for other indications. Reluctance to use the doses required will adversely affect patient outcome. Case reports show that amounts required may be as high as 2 grams in 24 hours and 28 grams over the course of hospitalization (2).

The endpoint of atropine therapy is the drying of secretions, particularly pulmonary secretions, and reversal of pulmonary edema. Dry mouth, dry flushed skin, dilated pupils, and tachycardia will also result in most cases of proper atropinization. The initial adult dose varies from 1–2 milligrams intravenously, depending on the severity of symptoms, repeated every 10–15 minutes as needed until atropinization occurs. In severely poisoned patients, atropine will need to be used for at least 24–48 hours, and there have been reports of patients requiring atropine therapy for as long as 24 days (2). In some cases, the use of continuous atropine infusions has been advocated at a rate of 0.02–0.08 mg/kg/hr intravenously titrated to effect (3). Children over the age of 12 years should receive the adult dose of atropine, and those under 12 years should receive an initial dose of 0.05 mg/kg intravenously followed by a maintenance dose of 0.02–0.05 mg/kg every 10–30 minutes until signs of atropinization occur (1).

Since dose and frequency of atropine administration must depend on severity of poisoning, the amount of atropine given should be titrated to whatever is needed to antagonize cholinergic symptoms. An effective endpoint guide to therapy in all serious cases of poisoning is the drying of secretions, which includes reversal of pulmonary edema. Administration of atropine is continued, and the dose only slowly tapered until the organophosphate or carbamate has been completely metabolized and eliminated, which may take several days to achieve. Atropine administration should be stopped if fever, delirium, and other signs of atropine toxicity appear.

A fully atropinized patient may not experience reversal of muscle weakness and respiratory distress which is caused by overstimulation of the nicotinic receptor. In fact, a person may experience respiratory arrest or respiratory depression even if fully atropinized, because atropine does not block the nicotinic receptors at neuromuscular junctions.

Clinical symptomatology of organophosphate poisoning and carbamate poisoning may be limited to muscle weakness only in pediatric patients and in some adult cases. Traditional signs of cholinergic stimulation such as diarrhea, vomiting, and oral secretions may be mild or not evident at all. Neuromuscular weakness, particularly in pediatric patients, may go unrecognized. In such cases, atropine will not be successful in reversing signs and symptoms, and pralidoxime administration will be necessary.

Table 36.1. Common Antidotes for Hazardous Materials

Drug	Toxin Antagonized	Dose	Mechanism
Atropine	Organophosphate and carbamate insecticides	*Adult:* 1–2 mg i.v. starting dose repeated every 10–15 minutes until drying of secretions and atropinization is complete *Pediatric:* 0.05 mg/kg i.v. initial dose. Dose range 0.02–0.05 mg/kg repeated every 10–30 minutes as needed until atropinization is achieved	Blocks muscarinic receptors and antagonizes muscarinic effects
Pralidoxime (2-PAM, Proto-pam)	Organophosphate and carbamate insecticides	*Adult:* 500–1000 mg i.v. over 20–30 minutes; repeat every 4–6 hours as needed to control symptoms Pediatric: 25–50 mg/kg i.v. over 20–30 minutes; repeat every 4–6 hours as needed to control symptoms	Regenerates acetylcholinesterase enzyme and helps reverse both muscarinic and nicotinic effects
DMSA (Chemet)	Lead	30 mg/kg/day (10 mg/kg TID) in 3 divided doses for 5 days, then 10 mg/kg BID for 14 days	Metal chelator
Methylene blue 1% Solution	Methemoglobinemia	0.1–0.2 ml/kg of 1% solution i.v. slowly; repeat once if needed; may have to repeat more often if required up to total dose of 7 mg/kg; endpoint of therapy is methemoglobin <10%	Nonenzymatic catalyst which increases the activity of methemoglobin reductase to reduce methemoglobin to hemoglobin
Calcium gluconate 10%	Hydrofluoric acid	*Topical gel:* 2.5% gel applied locally to area of injury *Injectable:* 5–10% solution injected into injury site. Total injected volume should not exceed 0.5 ml/cm^2; endpoint of therapy is to relieve or reduce pain	Binds fluoride ion and prevents tissue injury
BAL (Dimercaprol)	Lead, Mercury, Arsenic mainly	4–5 mg/kg i.m. every 4 hours for 2–3 days, then every 6 hours for 7 days.	Metal chelator
Cyanide Kit 3% Sodium Nitrite 25% Sodium Thiosulfate	Cyanide, hydrogen sulfide	Administer 10 ml of 3% sodium nitrite (300 mg, 1 vial) i.v. slowly; then administer 50 ml (one vial) of 25% sodium thiosulfate; repeat doses if needed. *Pediatric:* Dose of sodium nitrite must be adjusted for weight and hemoglobin. Sodium nitrite dose of 10 mg/kg i.v. or 0.2 ml/kg not to exceed 300 mg total dose. Sodium nitrite can produce fatal methemoglobinemia if patient receives overdose. The following is a guide to sodium nitrite administration in a child: Hgb 8 g%—0.22 ml/kg Hgb 10 g%—0.27 ml/kg Hgb 12 g%—0.33 ml/kg Hgb 14 g%—0.39 ml/kg Sodium thiosulfate 25% 1.65 ml/kg i.v. should be administered next. Doses can be repeated if necessary.	Sodium nitrite produces met-hemo-globinemia that has high affinity for cyanide, forming cyanmethemoglobin. Thiosulfate converts cyanmethemoglobin to thiocyanate.
Inhalational sodium bicarbonate	Chlorine gas	2 ml of 8.4% sodium bicarbonate mixed with 2 ml of normal saline administered by face mask nebulizer with 6 liters of O_2 per minute; may be used in conjunction with inhaled bronchodilators.	Relieves symptoms of chest burning, throat irritation, and dyspnea secondary to chlorine gas inhalation; combines with hydrochloric and hypochlorous acids.
Oxygen	Carbon monoxide	Hyperbaric or 100% oxygen.	Reduces binding of CO to hemoglobin and other tissues by mass effect; the higher the PaO_2, the faster the decline in COHgb.
D-Penicillamine	Lead, arsenic, mercury	250 mg orally four times per day for 7–10 days.	Metal chelators.

continues

Table 36.1 *Continued*

Drug	Toxin Antagonized	Dose	Mechanism
DTPA ZnDTPA CaDTPA Diethylenetriaminepentaacetic Acid	Radionuclides	Call REAC/TS Oak Ridge Tennessee (615)576–1004. CaDTPA is more effective than Zn DTPA. Administer 1000 mg of CaDTPA diluted in 250 ml of D_5W over 60–90 minutes. May repeat daily for 5 days ***Field treatment:*** Aerosolize contents of one vial in a nebulizer	Chelates radionuclides and allows renal excretion.
CaNa$_2$EDTA	Lead	75 mg/kg/day divided every 12 hours for 5 days or 1000 mg/m^2 divided every 12 hours for 5 days. Same dose is given IV or IM.	Chelator.

PRALIDOXIME (2-PAM, PROTOPAM CHLORIDE)

Pralidoxime (2-PAM) reactivates acetylcholinesterase and is an antidote for organophosphate poisoning. Where the toxic effects from organophosphates are predominantly nicotinic in origin, 2-PAM is particularly beneficial. When administered early in the course of the poisoning, 2-PAM is effective at restoring muscle activity and respiratory effort. It is still beneficial if given as late as 24 or more hours after exposure to the pesticide has occurred. Ineffectiveness of 2-PAM has been described when it is given to symptomatic individuals 36–48 hours after their exposure. However, it should be kept in mind that some patients have responded dramatically to 2-PAM 48 hours or longer after exposure. The "aging" process that results in the formation of a very stable acetylcholinesterase-organophosphate complex resistant to the reactivating effect of 2-PAM is probably responsible for this ineffectiveness. It is sometimes claimed that central effects following organophosphate poisoning do not respond to pralidoxime because of the inability for a quaternary ammonium compound to penetrate the blood-brain barrier. This observation, however, is not universally accepted (4); dramatic central nervous system-originated responses have been noted in pesticide-poisoned children who quickly awakened from a comatose condition when they were given 2-PAM.

A blood sample for red blood cell (RBC) cholinesterase and/or plasma cholinesterase activity should be obtained before the cholinesterase activator is administered; otherwise, the result reported may be spurious. The RBC cholinesterase and plasma cholinesterase values can be useful guides to therapy. Depression of RBC or plasma cholinesterase values can be deceiving, since a range of normal values exists. Depression of enzyme activity in either the RBC or plasma can occur along with symptoms of poisoning, yet the measurable value may still be within the normal limits of the range. Serially following enzyme activity is useful in guiding therapy.

The dose of pralidoxime for a child older than 12 years of age and for an adult are the same, 0.5–1.0 grams administered intravenously over 20–30 minutes. For younger children, 25–50 mg/kg of pralidoxime infused intravenously over 20–30 minutes can be administered. The dose may be repeated following 1–2 hours and then at 12-hour intervals if cholinergic symptoms persist or recur. If these symptoms are severe, the dose may be repeated more frequently at intervals of 4–6 hours as needed.

In healthy adults, the half-life of pralidoxime is about 1.2 hours (5). Animal data suggest that a minimum plasma concentration of 4 μg/ml of pralidoxime is needed for adequate protection against subsequently administered organophosphates (6). Currently recommended dosing schedules would provide levels below 4 μg/ml for most of the dosing interval. Because of this, some authors suggest the use of continuous infusions of pralidoxime (6, 7). The suggested infusion dose is 0.5 g/hr in an adult; however, experience with this regimen is limited, and it must be considered experimental. Close attention should be given to the onset of adverse effects such as muscle weakness, respiratory depression, diplopia, blurry vision, dizziness, headache, nausea, tachycardia, and hypertension. Dosage of pralidoxime should be reduced in patients with renal insufficiency.

Anticholinergic therapy must begin immediately whenever a severe organophosphate poisoning is suspected. Administration of the cholinesterase reactivator should also begin as quickly as possible. Following the reversal of effects from exposure to the cholinesterase-inhibiting pesticides, close observation and monitoring is necessary for as many as several days since the symptoms of organophosphate toxicity may reappear as the effects of atropine and pralidoxime diminish. Cases have occurred in which patients have suffered respiratory arrest and depression days after successful reversal of symptomatology after therapy with both atropine and protopam.

METHYLENE BLUE

Methylene blue is used to reverse the methemoglobinemia caused by nitrates, nitrites, and other nitro compounds. Methemoglobin is the oxidized form of hemoglobin with iron in the ferric state. In this condition, hemoglobin is unavailable for oxygen transport or release to tissues. Methylene blue is a nonenzymatic electron-carrying catalyst for nicotinamide adenine dinucleotide phosphate (NADPH)-dependent methemoglobin reductase activity. Methylene blue, by initially undergoing reduction to form leukomethylene blue in erythrocytes, increases the rate of methemoglobin reduction to hemoglobin. Methemoglobin is then reduced by leukomethylene blue to hemoglobin. As methylene blue is oxidized in the enzymatic process which reduced methemoglobin to hemoglobin, NADPH is required as a cofactor.

Methemoglobinemia in individuals who are deficient in NADPH as a result of a congenital absence of glucose-6-phosphate dehydrogenase (G-6-PD) is not reversed by methylene blue. Individuals with G-6-PD deficiency may develop an acute hemolytic anemia when exposed to methemoglobin-forming oxidant agents. Persons who are deficient or without methemoglobin reductase are also more likely to develop methemoglobinemia following exposure to oxidant agents.

A variety of substances have been associated with the development of methemoglobinemia. A partial list of substances implicated in methemoglobinemia includes organic nitrates (nitrobenzene, nitrophenol) and nitrites, the antipyretics acetanilid and phenacetin, the local anesthetics benzocaine and lidocaine, dapsone, and phenazopyridine (8). Methemoglobinemia has also been reported in infants as part of a syndrome including vomiting, diarrhea, leukocytosis, and acidosis (9). Other causes of methemoglobinemia in infants include formula reconstituted with nitrate-contaminated water, analine ink used to mark diapers, benzocaine, resorcin-containing dermatologic preparations, bismuth subnitrate disinfectants, furniture polish, and silver nitrate treatment for burns (9, 10).

At methemoglobin concentrations of 15–20%, patients are generally asymptomatic, but blood appears "chocolate brown," and clinical cyanosis may be evident. At levels of 20–45%, dyspnea, fatigue, dizziness, lethargy, headache, and syncope appear. The level of consciousness becomes increasingly depressed at levels of 45–55%. With levels between 55% and 70%, major hypoxemia occurs with coma, seizures, circulatory failure, and cardiac arrhythmias. At levels above 70%, the incidence of mortality is high (11). The cyanosis from methemoglobinemia does not respond to oxygen therapy. A quick bedside test for significant methemoglobin level is to place a drop of the patient's blood on a piece of white filter paper. The presence of darker (or resembling chocolate color) than normal control blood should suggest strongly the presence of methemoglobinemia. The treatment of methemoglobinemia is with methylene blue and oxygen. The dose of methylene blue is 0.1–0.2 ml/kg of a 1% solution administered by slow intravenous infusion.

There has been one case reported of the use of continuous infusions of methylene blue as part of the treatment of dapsone intoxication. A 0.05% solution and 0.5% saline were used at a rate of 0.1 mg/kg/hr to achieve a methemoglobin level of 5–10%. The authors recommend stopping methylene blue every 48 hours to reevaluate the need for continued therapy (12).

Side effects of methylene blue therapy include nausea, vomiting, precordial pain, dizziness, headache, diaphoresis, hypotension, and altered mental status. Methylene blue has also been associated with the development of methemoglobinemia by oxidating the ferrous iron of reduced hemoglobin to the nonoxygen carrying ferric state. Usually, this is seen when excessive doses are used. However, it has appeared with doses as low as 5 mg/kg of body weight (13). Excessive doses have also been associated with the development of persistent cyanosis and delayed hemolytic anemia in patients without genetic defects of G-6-PD (14). It should also be noted that the use of methylene blue may interfere with the determination of hemoglobin saturation by pulse oximeter (15). Because of the risks associated with methylene blue, it is generally recommended that the dose be repeated only once if a patient does not respond to the initial infusion and that the total dose not exceed 7 mg/kg. The possibility of G-6-PD deficiency should be considered in any patient with a known exposure to methemoglobin-forming toxins who does not respond to methylene blue therapy.

CALCIUM GLUCONATE

Calcium gluconate is used for the treatment of hydrofluoric acid burns. Hydrofluoric acid poses a greater medical hazard than most common chemically induced burns. It is believed that dermal injury occurs in two stages, the first involving rapidly developing coagulative necrosis on skin contact which is followed by a slower secondary phase, which is the result of hydrofluoric acid penetration into subdermal tissue. It is believed that the fluoride ions resulting in the dissociation of hydrofluoric acid react with tissue calcium ions. This in turn depletes tissue calcium and results in a cellular release of potassium iron from nerve endings, resulting in intense pain. The complex of fluoride ions with tissue calcium is felt to interfere with electrical membrane function and cellular metabolism, ultimately causing cellular death and necrosis (16, 17). The degree of pain and tissue destruction is felt to be related to the concentration of hydrofluoric acid solution. The National Institutes of Health have classified human hydrofluoric acid burns into three categories: Solutions up to 20% may produce pain or redness until as late as 24 hours after exposure, exposure to 20–50% hydrofluoric acid solutions is usually apparent within 8 hours following exposure, and solutions of greater than 50% generally produce immediate intense pain and tissue destruction (18).

Initial therapy for dermal injuries is copious irrigation with water. Various topical treatments for hydrofluoric acid burns hae been proposed, although research in this area is limited. One study suggested that, of various topical treatments tested, only 2.5% calcium gluconate gel significantly reduced burn area. Calcium gluconate is also administered by subcutaneous or interdermal injection into hydrofluoric acid burns. It is generally recommended that 5–10% calcium gluconate be injected into the affected area with a 24–30-gauge needle, using approximately 0.5 ml/cm^2 of surface tissue. It must be remembered that injection into areas containing little soft tissue, such as fingers, can result in significant elevation in tissue pressures, and some authors recommend that palmar fasciotomy be done concomitantly with any injections into the fingertips (18).

With finger burns, often there is involvement of the nailbed requiring partial or complete removal of the nail and either topical application of calcium gluconate gel or injection into the nailbed. While some authors advocate the use of regional anesthesia in calcium gluconate injections, others report that relief of pain rapidly follows adequate calcium injection and suggest that pain relief be used as an endpoint to monitor adequacy of therapy. Again, there have been limited studies to support the use of calcium gluconate injection.

There has been one study which compared the effectiveness of 10% calcium gluconate, 10% magnesium acetate, and 10% magnesium sulfate in interdermal and subcutaneous infiltration for hydrofluoric acid burns in rats. The numbers were small; however, the magnesium-treated groups healed significantly faster and were significantly less severe than the control groups, while the calcium-treated burns were not significantly different than either the control or the magnesium-treated group (19).

Some authors have advocated the use of intraarterial calcium infusion for the treatment of digital hydrofluoric acid burns. While experience with this technique is somewhat limited, it offers the advantage of not requiring injections into injured tissue and obviating the need for nail removal for nailbed burns. The technique used has varied slightly, between investigators but, in general, the arterial supply to the affected areas is identified by arteriogram; a catheter is placed in the appropriate artery in close proximity to the affected area, and a dilute solution of either calcium gluconate or calcium chloride is infused over several hours. This technique allows delivery of higher doses of calcium in a more uniform fashion to affected tissues. Disadvantages of this technique include the fact that it requires an invasive vascular procedure and that attendant risk of arterial spasm or thrombosis. It also requires greater resources and expense, as repeated infusions are often necessary, and hospitalization may be inevitable. Experience with this technique is currently limited to a few centers, and it has not been proven superior to local infiltration. It should probably be limited to severe distal extremity burns and to physicians who are comfortable with its utilization.

Fortunately, hydrofluoric acid burns of the eye are relatively uncommon. While some authors suggest irrigation with 1% calcium gluconate followed by calcium gluconate eye drops, there is little evidence to support this recommendation (20). One study in rabbits suggests that irrigation with water, isotonic saline, or magnesium chloride was the only nontoxic treatment with any therapeutic value. In this study, subconjunctival injection with 10% calcium gluconate caused marked injury in normal eyes, while irrigation with calcium chloride caused significant increase in the frequency of corneal ulceration in eyes burned with hydrofluoric acid (21). At this point, the most effective treatment is believed to be immediate and copious irrigation with water or normal saline. Patients with hydrofluoric acid burn to the eye require careful ophthalmologic follow-up.

Systemic fluoride toxicity has occurred from dermal, inhalation and oral exposures to hydrofluoric acid, and several deaths have been reported. Hypocalcemia should be anticipated in any significant exposure by any route and corrected with intravenous calcium gluconate. Other potential metabolic disturbances include systemic acidosis, hypomagnesemia, hyperkalemia, hyponatremia, and hyperphosphatemia in addition to elevated serum fluoride levels. Cardiac toxicity may be manifested by bradycardia, prolonged QT interval, and malignant ventricular arrhythmias that are not responsive to usual resuscitative maneuvers. Acute pulmonary edema has also been reported with systemic hydrofluoric acid poisoning with apparent inhalation. Serum calcium should be measured in all patients with significant exposure and hypocalcemia corrected and followed. Patients will require general supportive measures to correct hypoxia, acidosis, and renal insufficiency. Occasionally, dialysis may be required to lower serum potassium and fluoride levels. Cardiac arrhythmias may be secondary to electrolyte disturbances, acidosis, or hypoxia and are best treated by identifying and correcting the underlying cause (23). One case report suggests that in severe burns with systemic toxicity and refractory hypocalcemia, immediate excision of the saturated skin may be necessary (24).

HEAVY METAL CHELATORS

Several chelators are available for the treatment of heavy metal intoxication in humans. In 1968, Pearson developed several principles referred to as the hard/soft acid-base theory which allow a qualitative estimation of the chemical affinity between a metal ion and a complexing agent. Using this theory, metal ions are classified as soft, hard, and borderline. Soft metal ions are those with large atomic radii and a high number of electrons in the

outer shell, in contrast, hard ions have smaller atomic radii and smaller numbers of electrons in the outer shell. In forming a metal complex, the metal ion coordinates or accepts free electron pairs supplied by electron donor groups of the ligand molecule. Most therapeutic chelating agents use sulfur, nitrogen, or oxygen as electron donors. Chemically, these groups are also classified as soft, borderline, and hard. According to hard/soft, acid base theory, soft metals, also known as sulfur seekers, form the most stable complexes with soft ligands and hard metals, also called oxygen seekers, form stable complexes with hard ligands. Most therapeutic metal antidotes contain more than one functional group used in chelating the toxic metals (26).

Dimercaprol

Dimercaprol (British anti-Lewisite, BAL) is a dithiol chelating agent which was developed when an antidote to arsenic in the chemical warfare agent Lewisite was needed. The sulfhydryl groups of dimercaprol complex with heavy metals to prevent or reverse the binding of metals to sulfhydryl group containing enzymes. If the affinity of the metal for dimercaprol exceeds that of the enzymes, as with arsenic, mercury, and gold, a water soluble and less toxic mercaptide complex is formed and readily eliminated by the kidney. Dimercaprol not excreted as dimercaprol-metal complex is quickly metabolized by the liver and excreted as an inactive product in the urine. Alkalinization of the urine during dimercaprol therapy may help to prevent the rapid dissociation of the drug-metal complex in an acid medium and may prevent renal toxicity.

Dimercaprol has traditionally been the chelator of choice for arsenic and inorganic mercury poisoning. Dimercaprol is ineffective for the treatment of arsine gas or organic mercury poisoning. Dimercaprol also chelates lead, but there are more useful drugs available today. It comes as an oily liquid, and the usual dose for severe poisoning is 3–5 mg/kg administered by intramuscular injection every 4 hours for 2 days, then every 6 hours for 7 days. In milder cases, the treatment can be limited to 2 days or until another chelating drug is available and able to be administered. In some instances of metal poisoning, dimercaprol is started first and administered until a more tolerable agent is able to be given.

Adverse effects are common but are usually transitory and mild. At the recommended doses, hypertension, tachycardia, fever, nausea, vomiting, headache, seizures, stupor, and rash can occur. These side effects may occur within 30 minutes of drug administration. Systolic and diastolic hypertension can occur within minutes of administration. The hypertension usually returns to normal within 2 hours post injection. However, hypertension may persist with prolonged therapy, necessitating discontinuation of the drug.

Dimercaprol is a nephrotoxin, and the dose administered should be reduced or discontinued in patients with renal failure or if renal compromise occurs during therapy. Since other chelators are now available, prolonged treatment with dimercaprol is usually unnecessary. Approximately 50% of dimercaprol is excreted in the bile, and hepatic dysfunction can interfere with drug elimination.

Penicillamine

Penicillamine is a metabolic breakdown product of penicillin. It exists as two stereoisomers, D- and L-penicillamine. However, the L-isomer is not used therapeutically because of neurologic toxicity. Penicillamine contains three ionizable functional groups: a carboxyl group with a pKa of 1.8, an alpha amino group with a pKa of 7.9, and a beta thiol group with a PKA of 10.5 (26). Penicillamine is rapidly absorbed by the proximal small intestine following oral administration. Biologic availability varies between 40% and 70% of the administered dose (26). Absorption may be decreased significantly if the dose is given with a meal or if taken with antacids containing aluminum and magnesium hydroxides or with ferrous sulfate (26–28). Peak plasma concentrations are achieved 1–3 hours after ingestion and half-life, with oral administration, is between 1.3 and 3.2 hours. Both half-life and time to peak plasma concentration appear to be dose-independent (26).

Some studies of penicillamine elimination have shown a biphasic decrease in plasma concentrations. This byphasic elimination along with a volume of distribution of greater than 50 liters suggests the existence of a deep compartment or a pool of tissue-bound penicillamine which is slowly released (26). Penicillamine is highly protein bound. Radiolabeled penicillamine disappears rapidly from liver and kidneys but only slowly from collagen and elastin tissue such as skin and bone. It does not undergo marked metabolic degradation and is eliminated primarily by the kidneys, mainly as penicillamine disulfides and, to a lesser extent, as unchanged penicillamine or metabolized forms (26).

Penicillamine has the advantage over several other older metal chelators in that it can be administered orally. It has been used primarily for the treatment of mild to moderate lead toxicity. It is generally recommended for use in patients without evidence of lead encephalopathy and with levels below 80 μg/dl. It is generally not used in patients with ongoing lead ingestion, as there is fear that oral penicillamine could lead to increased absorption of lead present in the gastrointestinal (GI) system. It is also used for continuation of therapy after initial treatment with other agents (29–33).

The use of penicillamine has been associated with several adverse reactions, including rash, leukopenia, thrombocytopenia, proteinuria, and abdominal cramping (29–33). More serious toxic reactions such as hemolytic anemia, Stevens-Johnson syndrome, and membranous nephropathy have also been reported (31). Concern has been raised about the safety of administration of penicillamine to individuals with known penicillin allergy, and this has generally been considered a relative contraindication for its use as some cross-reactivity between the two drugs has been documented. One study suggested that while some penicillin-sensitive patients display a positive skin test to D-penicillamine, the actual risk of severe allergic reaction to penicillamine in a penicillin-sensitive patient is actually quite low (34).

The usual adult dose is 15–40 mg/kg/day divided in 2–4 doses with a maximum dose of 2 g/day. Doses in children are generally 25–30 mg/kg/day divided in two or three doses/day (31). Doses as high as 100 mg/kg/day have been used (30). A standard administered dose for an adult is 250 milligrams four times a day for 7–10 days.

Dimercaptosuccinic Acid

Dimercaptosuccinic acid (DMSA, Chemet) is a water-soluble analog of dimercaprol (BAL) which has greater water solubility and limited lipid solubility and is effective orally. DMSA has been studied fairly extensively, both at the basic science and

clinical levels, in China, the Soviet Union, and Japan. Until recently, however, DMSA has received relatively little study in the United States and Europe. Recently, this agent has been rediscovered by clinical investigators in the United States. DMSA has two asymmetric carbon atoms and exists as both the meso form and the DL-form. As the meso form, DMSA is easier to prepare and more available; it is the compound that has been used in most published investigations (35). DMSA has been approved for chelation of lead in the United States for children with blood lead levels greater than 45 μg/dl.

Relatively little is known about the pharmacokinetics of DMSA, primarily because of difficulty encountered in measuring the drug. The drug is absorbed from the GI tract, although it is unclear what percentage is absorbed. In one study, approximately 20% of administered DMSA could be accounted for in the urine. In this study, of the DMSA administered, only 2.5% was excreted as unaltered DMSA, and 18% was excreted as metabolized forms (36). The half-life is 3 hours, but the volume of distribution is unknown (37).

In the United States, DMSA has primarily been used for the treatment of lead poisoning, although much experience has been gained in its use for arsenic and mercury intoxication. Animal studies have demonstrated that DMSA is effective in mobilizing lead from soft tissue with large decrements in blood, brain, and kidney lead concentrations, but no loss from bone and no observable redistribution of lead (38). Several studies on lead intoxication in humans have been performed showing the efficacy of DMSA for the treatment of lead intoxication (39–40). One study in children found that 1050 mg/m²/day of DMSA was significantly more effective than 1000 mg/m²/day of intravenously administered calcium disodium EDTA in reducing blood lead concentrations and restoring erythrocyte amino levulinic acid dehydratase (ALADH) activity (40).

Animal studies have also suggested that DMSA may be useful in the therapy of arsenic poisoning. One study in rats showed DMSA to be as effective as BAL in reducing tissue arsenic concentration in experimentally intoxicated animals (41). There are several case reports of the use of DMSA in treating human arsenic intoxication. However, the results are not as clear (42). DMSA has been shown to be more effective than BAL or D-penicillamine in inducing urinary mercury excretion in rats chronically poisoned with methyl mercury (43). There are limited data available in the treatment of elemental mercury intoxication with DMSA, although several human studies have shown an increase in urinary mercury elimination and a decrease in symptomatology in patients with elemental mercury poisoning treated with DMSA (42–43).

DMSA has the advantage of being an oral agent which appears to be effective against several different heavy metals. Reports of toxicity have been rare and include an increase in urinary and concomitant decrease in plasma zinc concentrations (42) and a transient elevation in serum SGPT (39). Animal studies have also demonstrated an increased urinary excretion in copper, suggesting that the drug might be useful in the treatment of Wilson's disease (41). Recommended dosing for adults and children is 30 mg/kg/day divided into three doses (10 mg/kg TID) for 5 days, then 10 mg/kg/day administered twice daily for 14 days. The strong sulfur odor of any of the thiol chelators makes the medication unpalatable to most patients.

DMPS

2,3-Dimercapto-1-propanesulfonic acid (DMPS), like DMSA, is a water-soluble chemical analog of BAL which is orally effective. DMPS has also been studied fairly extensively in the People's Republic of China, the Soviet Union, and Japan and is now receiving more clinical attention in Western Europe and the United States. DMPS is remarkably stable, especially at acid pH. While it has been prepared both as a racemic mixture and as the dextrorotatory and levorotatory form, most studies involve the racemic mixture.

Relatively little information is available on the pharmacokinetics of DMPS, and most of what little work has been done has been in animals. DMPS is absorbed orally, although there are wide interspecies variations. There is disagreement as to the extent of DMPS binding to plasma proteins. It is also unclear whether DMPS distributes intracellularly. The half-life and volume of distribution in humans is not known at this time (35).

An outbreak of methyl mercury poisoning occurred in rural Iraq in the winter of 1971 and 1972 from the consumption of homemade bread made with wheat treated with a methyl mercury fungicide. This provided an unusual opportunity for testing several therapies for the treatment of methyl mercury poisoning in humans. One study compared the half-life of mercury in patients receiving various forms of therapy. In patients receiving no treatment, the half-life of methyl mercury was about 65 days, while it was 61 days in those receiving placebo, 26 days for those receiving D-penicillamine, 24 days for those receiving N-acetyl penicillamine, 20 days for those receiving a thiolated resin, and 10 days in those receiving DMPS. While all the agents reduced the blood levels of mercury and increased its urinary excretion, DMPS was felt to be the most effective. Unfortunately, no appreciable clinical improvement was noted among the patients who were severely or very severely intoxicated, while those with moderate to mild intoxication improved regardless of therapy (53, 54). In one other human case of methyl mercury poisoning, DMPS did not lower the half-life as effectively (55). Animal studies have demonstrated that DMPS significantly increases urinary excretion and decreases whole body burden of elemental mercury and inorganic mercury in rats (56–57). DMPS has also been shown, in rats, to decrease renal lead concentrations and increase urinary concentrations at relatively low doses, while at higher doses it also removed lead from liver and bone (58). One study in children showed that DMPS significantly lowered blood lead concentrations in intoxicated children without affecting copper or zinc levels, while significantly increasing urinary excretion of lead, copper, and zinc (59).

DMPS has also been shown to prevent lethal effects of many arsenic compounds in animals (35). In rats, DMPS has also been shown to increase the urinary excretion of gold and significantly decrease gold concentrations in kidney and skin. DMPS has also been reported to increase the urinary excretion of copper sulfate in sheep and decrease the lethality of copper sulfate in mice (35).

Toxic effects from DMPS are rare and include nausea, weakness, vertigo, itching skin, mild allergic reactions, and increased urinary excretion of zinc in men. When used intravenously it can cause ulceration at the site of injection (35).

Calcium Disodium Ethylenediaminetetraacetate

Calcium disodium ethylenediaminetetraacetate (CaNa$_2$EDTA) is administered to treat lead and cadmium poisonings. In cases of copper and zinc poisonings, it also finds use. CaNa$_2$EDTA complex is displaced by divalent and trivalent metals to form

a water-soluble complex readily eliminated by the kidneys. The drug is not metabolized, and over 95% is excreted unchanged by the kidneys. CaNa$_2$EDTA has been the treatment of choice for an early treatment of chronic lead poisoning in patients who are symptomatic, have lead encephalopathy, or demonstrate elevated blood lead concentrations. CaNa$_2$EDTA effectively mobilized lead from bone and soft tissue stores. When used alone, CaNa$_2$EDTA may aggravate symptoms of lead toxicity in patients with very high lead levels. In cases with blood levels above 70 µg/dl or with clinical symptoms of lead poisoning, the first dose of BAL should precede the first dosing of CaNa$_2$EDTA by at least 4 hours. CaNa$_2$EDTA may also be used as a provocation test in cases of suspected lead poisoning.

Concomitant adminstration of CaNa$_2$EDTA and dimercaprol (BAL) increases the rate of lead mobilization from tissue depots and probably reduces the incidence of central nervous system toxicity when compared with the single use of CaNa$_2$EDTA. The evaluation of the effectiveness of chelation of lead is conducted by monitoring the blood and urine lead level and the erythrocyte protoporphyrin content. The dose of CaNa$_2$EDTA given in the management of lead poisoning depends on the severity of the intoxication and the patient's response to and tolerance of the drug. CaNa$_2$EDTA is given by slow intravenous infusion or intramuscular injections. Various doses and regimens have been recommended. Dosage of CaNa$_2$EDTA is the same for either intravenous or intramuscular administration. Daily dose of 75 mg/kg/day can be given in two equally divided doses at 12-hour intervals or as a 12–24 infusion. The duration of CaNa$_2$EDTA therapy given in this manner may be for up to 5 days. The usual dose of CaNa$_2$EDTA when given alone in the treatment of symptomatic acute lead poisoning or elevated blood levels (greater than 50 µg/dl) is 1 g/m^2 daily for 3–5 days. Patients with blood level concentrations exceeding 100 µg/dl may be given 1.5 g/m^2 daily for the same period, usually in conjunction with dimercaprol. Children may require several courses of therapy, while advice on adults usually gives no more than two courses of therapy. At least 2–4 days and preferably 2–3 weeks should intervene between courses of treatment with CaNa$_2$EDTA.

For adults with lead neuropathy, the CaNa$_2$EDTA regimen needs to be adjusted according to measures of serum creatinine. At serum creatinine concentrations of 2–3 mg/dl, patients may be given 500 mg every 24 hours for 5 days; and every 48 hours for three doses when creatinine concentrations are in the 3–4 µg/dl range. A simple 500-milligram dose of CaNa$_2$EDTA may be sufficient for a patient with serum creatinine exceeding 4 µg/dl to mobilize lead excretion. The doses and regimens can be repeated at intervals of 1 month until the lead tissue and blood burden has been reduced to an acceptable level.

Acute tubular necrosis is the result of excessive CaNa$_2$EDTA dose. Careful monitoring for signs of renal damage is required. CaNa$_2$EDTA can produce signs that may be confused with lead-caused renal injury, such as proteinuria and microscopic hematuria. Particular attention should be given to establishing urine flow and sufficient hydration before the drug is given. Laboratory determinations to establish level of renal function should be done regularly. Prolonged and continuous chelation may iatrogenically cause zinc, trace metals, and vitamin B6 deficiency, particularly in poorly nourished patients. Too rapid intravenous infusion of CaNa$_2$EDTA may result in intracranial hypertension when used to treat lead encephalopathy.

Anorexia, nausea, vomiting, headache, paresthesia, hypercalcemia, and hypotension have occurred following parenteral

CaNa$_2$EDTA. Sudden chills and fever accompanied by fatigue, malaise, thirst, and asthma-like symptoms have been experienced soon following infusions of the drug. Electrocardiographic changes (i.e., T wave changes) and acute gouty attacks have been other, uncommon, adverse effects reported to follow the CaNa$_2$EDTA therapy. for intravenous infusion, CaNa$_2$EDTA is diluted in 5% dextrose or 0.9% sodium chloride to a 0.2–0.4% concentration (2–4 µg/dl). The manufacturer recommends an infusion rate of over 1 hour for one-half the daily dose determined for asymptomatic patients and at least 2 hours in symptomatic patients. The remaining portion of the daily dose is given 6 or or hours following the first infusion. When administered as an infusion, the daily dose is usually delivered over at least 8 hours.

Intramuscular injection of CaNa$_2$EDTA is quite painful and may necessitate the addition of an anesthetic such as 1% procaine hydrochloride to the chelating solution before administration.

Thrombophlebitis has occurred after intravenous infusions of CaNa$_2$EDTA solutions, particularly when concentrations greater than 0.5% were administered.

Cyanide Antidote

The Cyanide Antidote Kit (E. Lilly) contains amyl nitrite ampule, a 3% sodium nitrite solution, and 25% solution of sodium thiosulfate. The kit is the only treatment for cyanide poisoning available in the United States. Without the sodium thiosulfate solution, the kit can be given to reverse the asphyxiant effects of hydrogen sulfide poisonings.

Nitrite-induced methemoglobinemia frees cytochrome oxidase from cyanide since the cyanide ion has a greater affinity for iron in the ferric state, thus forming a relatively stable cyanomethemoglobin. Sodium thiosulfate serves as a sulfur donor for rhodanese, converting cyanide to the less toxic thiocyanate, which is water-soluble and readily excreted by the kidneys (60, 61).

Amyl nitrite is questionably effective in producing a state of methemoglobinemia; if any such conversion takes place, the level is probably quite low (<5%). Sodium nitrite solution administered intravenously will produce a significant methemoglobinemia. This is followed by infusion of the sodium thiosulfate which has a low toxicity and is well-tolerated.

The adult dose of 3% sodium nitrite is 300 milligrams or 10 milliliters given over 5 minutes. In children, the dose is 10 mg/kg or 0.2 ml/kg adjusted for weight and hemoglobin content. An adult dose of sodium nitrite, if given to a child, can produce a fatal methemoglobinemia. Nitrites infused too rapidly or in excess can produce or aggravate hypotension and hypoxemia; oxygen saturation and level of methemoglobinemia need to be frequently and closely monitored. Should symptoms of hypoxemia recur, more nitrite and thiosulfate solutions can be given at one-half the dose previously administered.

4-Dimethylaminophenol (DMAP) is used in Europe as a methemoglobin-generating agent in the treatment of cyanide intoxication. It was originally hoped that DMAP would be a more effective antidote than sodium nitrite, as DMAP forms methemoglobin much more rapidly. However, it is still unclear whether there is any significant difference in efficacy between the two (62). In using any of the methemoglobin-forming agents, there is always the concern of generating methemoglobin levels which are themselves toxic, as clinically toxic levels can occur even at the recommended doses (63). This is a particular concern in patients whose cyanide intoxication has occurred as a result of fire, as most of these patients already have significant carboxyhemoglobin levels, and induction of methemoglobinemia only compounds the hypoxia. One study demonstrated that the use of sodium nitrite in mice with a simultaneous cyanide and carbon monoxide poisoning significantly increased mortality, although treatment with DMAP did not appear to affect mortality (64).

In part because of these concerns, newer agents for the treatment of cyanide intoxication have been developed. Hydroxycobalamin (vitamin B12A) is widely used in Europe and is currently under an investigational protocol in the United States for the treatment of cyanide poisoning. Hydroxycobalamin detoxifies cyanide by binding a cyanyl group forming cyanocobalamin (vitamin B12), which is then excreted in the urine. Hydroxycobalamin has a greater affinity for cyanide than does cytochrome oxidase. Unfortunately, the reaction requires one molecule of hydroxycobalamin for each molecule of cyanide to be detoxified, and, with the molecular weight approximately 50 times that of cyanide, it requires significant amounts of hydroxycobalamin to detoxify small amounts of absorbed potassium cyanide. Relatively few side effects have been associated with the use of hydroxycobalamin, including transient reddish discoloration of the skin and mucous membranes and urine, urticaria, and rare cases of anaphylaxis (65). Hydroxycobalamin has been shown to be effective in reducing cyanide levels in several animal studies and in humans receiving nitroprusside. In addition, it appears to act synergistically with sodium thiosulfate (65).

Cobalt EDTA has also been proposed for the treatment of cyanide intoxication on the premise that cobalt could combine directly with cyanide, thus reactivating inhibited cytochrome oxidase while the EDTA could chelate any free cobalt, thus decreasing its toxicity. It has been used in Europe, the United Kingdom, and Scandinavian countries. However, it has some associated cardiac toxicity. Of particular concern are reports of ventricular arrhythmias, thus, this appears a less promising new antidote (60).

There are various animal studies suggesting other new antidotes including success with the use of oral activated charcoal in rats subjected to oral potassium cyanide poisoning (66), a single-patient and a dog study showing successful use of hemodialysis in cyanide toxicity (67), and a study in mice showing that pyridoxal 5′-phosphate (vitamin B6) increased the LD$_{50}$ and extended the survival time in cyanide-poisoned animals (68). However, recommendations for clinical use will have to await further studies.

RADIONUCLIDE AND RADIOACTIVE MATERIALS CHELATOR

Internal contamination by radionuclides or a radioactive material can result from the inhalation, ingestion, or wound contamination of a radioactive material or radionuclide. The radioactive material has the opportunity to become incorporated into the body and irradiate internal tissues. This is a medical emergency which must be appropriately treated to remove as much contaminant as possible. Some radionuclides can become permanently incorporated into the biologic molecules of the body. Prompt management of contaminated wounds is important to prevent further incorporation of radioactive material.

Multivalent radioisotopes in the actinide series (transuranic elements plutonium, neptunium, americium) as well as rare earths such as cesium have been effectively chelated using diethylenetriaminepentaacetic acid (DTPA). Although human data on the use of DTPA are limited, its administration is recommended as soon as possible and should be done within the first few hours to be effective. DTPA is available from the Radiation Emergency Assistance Center/Training Site (REAC/TS) in Oak Ridge, Tennessee (telephone number (615)576-1004). Decorporation with chelating agents should be started as soon as possible in patients with contaminated wounds. Patients with residual contamination from skin break or foreign bodies may also benefit from this pharmacologic therapy. Treatment depends upon the chemical properties of the particular radioisotope involved and should be done in conjunction with advice from a nuclear medicine physician specialist.

DTPA chelates multivalent radionuclides that can then be renally excreted. $CaNa_2EDTA$ (calcium versenate) has also been used as a radioisotope chelator but is not as efficacious as DTPA. Both the calcium and zinc salts of DTPA are approved for human use. CaDTPA is 10 times more effective than ZnDTPA for increasing renal excretion of actinide radionuclides within the first few hours of exposure. ZnDTPA is equally efficacious after the first 1 or 2 days of exposure.

In an acute exposure, 1 gram of CaDTPA diluted in 250 ml of dextrose 5% in water should be infused over 60–90 minutes. The dose may be repeated daily for 5 days. For immediate field administration, an aerosol inhalation treatment can be accomplished by placing the entire contents of a vial in a nebulizer. ZnDTPA appears to be less toxic then CaDTPA, but due to its lower efficacy it should not be the drug of first choice. CaDTPA should be continued at a once-daily dose of 1 gram intravenously. During this time blood samples, whole body and chest counts, 24-hour urine collections, and stool samples should be collected and monitored for radioactivity to determine need for further chelation. If further chelation is required beyond 5 days, then ZnDTPA should be substituted for more prolonged therapy. A DTPA administration protocol and consent form is available from REAC/TS.

INHALATIONAL SODIUM BICARBONATE FOR CHLORINE GAS

Chlorine gas inhalation is common and can result in cough, chest pain, dyspnea, chest tightness and burning, ocular irritation, dizziness, headache, throat irritation, and pulmonary edema, depending on the degree of exposure. Chlorine is 2.5 times heavier than air and is stored in pressurized tanks. Signs and symptoms resulting from chlorine gas exposure are dependent on the concentration of the gas, duration of exposure, and water content of the exposed tissues. The odor threshold of chlorine gas is 0.02 ppm, and consequently a person can detect chlorine long before any injury will occur. Nasal irritation can occur at 0.2 ppm. Five to 15 ppm can produce mild upper airway irritation and eye burning; 30 ppm produces dyspnea, chest tightness, and cough. Pulmonary edema can occur following airborne concentrations of 60 ppm. The tissue injury secondary to chlorine gas exposure results from contact with moisture with the formation of hydrochloric and hypochlorous acids. Hypochlorous acid decomposes to hydrochloric acid and liberates nascent oxygen which can damage cells. Serious chlorine gas exposures can result in bronchoconstriction, damage to the pulmonary epithelium, and pulmonary edema.

A series of 14 patients treated (personal data of the author, J.B.S.) with a mixture of 2 milliliters of 8.4% sodium bicarbonate and 2 milliliters of normal saline by face mask nebulizer demonstrated the efficacy of dilute sodium bicarbonate to reverse the symptoms of chlorine gas exposure. This therapy can help relieve the symptoms of chest tightness and burning, throat irritation, and cough. It will not reverse bronchoconstriction, and, if wheezing is present, inhalational treatment with a bronchodilator can be safely performed in addition to the sodium bicarbonate inhalation. Inhalation dilute sodium bicarbonate therapy can be safely and quickly administered in prehospital settings.

REFERENCES

1. Monthesen ML. Management of acute childhood poisonings caused by selected insecticides and herbicides. Pediatr Clin of North Am 1986;33(2):421–445.
2. Golsousidis H, Kokkas V. Letter: Hum Toxicol 1986;4:339–340.
3. Minton NA, Murray VSG. A review of organophosphate poisoning. Med Toxicol 1988;3:350–375.
4. Ellin RI. Anomalies in theory and therapy of intoxication by potent organophosphorus anticholinesterase compounds. Gen Pharmacol 1982;13:457–466.
5. Sidell FR, Groff WA. Intramuscular and intravenous administration of small doses of 2-pyridiniumaldoximethochloride to man. J Pharm Sci 1971;60:1224–1228.
6. Thompson DF, Thompson DG, Greenwood RB, et al. Therapeutic dosing of pralidoxime chloride. Drug Intell Clin Pharm 1987;21:590–593.
7. Thompson DF. Letter: Ann Emerg Med 1987;16:831–832.
8. Smith RP, Olson NV. Drug induced methemoglobinemia. Semin Hematol 1973;10:253–268.
9. Yano SS, et al. Transient methemoglobinemia with acidosis in infants. J Pediatr 1982;100:215–218.
10. Curry S. Methemoglobinemia. Ann Emerg Med 1982;11:214–221.
11. Hall AH, Kulig KW, Rumack BH. Drug and chemical induced methemoglobinemia: clinical features and management. Med Toxicol 1986;1:253–260.
12. Berlin G, Brodin B, Hilder J. et al. Acute dapsone intoxication: a case treated with continuous infusion of methylene blue, forced diuresis and plasma exchange. Clin Toxicol 1985;22:537–548.
13. Whitwan JG, Taylor AR, White JM. Potential hazard of methylene blue. Anesthesiology 1979;34:181–182.
14. Goluboft N, Wheaton R. Methylene blue induced cyanosis and acute hemolytic anemia complicating the treatment of methemoglobinemia. J Pediatr 1961;58:86–89.
15. Kessler MR, Eide T, Humayun B, et al. Spurious pulse oximeter desaturation with methylene blue injection. Anesthesiology 1986;65:435–436.
16. Bracken WM, Cuppage F, McLaury RL, et al. Comparative effectiveness of topical treatment of hydrofluoric acid burns. J Occup Med 1985;27:733–739.
17. Carney, SA, Hall M, Lawrence JC, et al. Rationale of the treatment of hydrofluoric acid burns. Br J Ind Med 1974;31:317–321.
18. Anderson WJ, Anderson JR. Hydrofluoric acid burns of the hand: mechanism of injury and treatment. J Hand Surg 1988;13;1:52–57.
19. Harris JC, Rumack BH, Bregan DT. Comparative efficacy of injectable calcium and magnesium salts in the therapy of hydrofluoric acid burns. Clin Toxicol 1981;18(9):1027–1032.
20. Vance MV, Curry SC, Kunkel DB, et al. Digital hydrofluoric acid burns: treatment with intraarterial calcium infusion. Ann Emerg Med 1986;15:890–896.
21. Trevino MA, Herrmann GH, Sprout WL, et al. Treatment of severe hydrofluoric acid exposures. J Occup Med 1983;25:861–863.
22. McCulley JP, Whiting DW, Petitt MG, et al. Hydrofluoric acid burns of the eye. J Occup Med 1983;25:447–450.
23. Caravati EM. Acute hydrofluoric acid exposure. Am J Emerg Med 1988;6:143–150.
24. Buckingham FM. Surgery: a radical approach to severe hydrofluoric acid burns. J Occup Med 1988;39(11):873–874.
25. Aaseth J. Recent advances in the therapy of metal poisonings with chelating agents. Hum Toxicol 1983;2:257–272.
26. Netter P, Bannwarth B, Péré Petal, et al. Clinical pharmacokinetics of d-penicillamine. Clin Pharmacol 1987;13:317–333.
27. Bergstrom RF, Kay DR, Harkcom TM, et al. Penicillamine kinetics and normal subjects. Clin Pharmacol Ther 1981;30:404–413.
28. Osman MA, Patel RB, Schuma A, et al. Reduction in oral penicillamine

absorption by food, antacid, and ferrous sulfate. Clin Pharmacol Ther 1983;33:465–470.

29. Marcus SM. Experience with d-penicillamine in treating lead poisoning. Vet Hum Toxicol 1982;24:18–20.

30. Bartsocas CS, Grunt JA, Boylen GW, et al. Oral d-penicillamine and intramuscular BAL and EDTA in the treatment of lead accumulation. Acta Paediatr Scand 1971;60:553–558.

31. Shannon M, Graef J, Lovejoy FH. Efficacy and toxicity of d-penicillamine in low level lead poisoning. J Pediatr 1988;112:790–804.

32. Sachs HK, Blanksma LA, Murray EF, et al. Ambulatory treatment of lead poisoning: report of 1155 cases. Pediatrics 1970;46:389–396.

33. Vitale LF, Rosalinas-Bailon A, Folland D, et al. Oral penicillamine therapy for chronic lead poisoning in children. J Pediatr 1973;83:1041–1045.

34. Bell CL, Graziano FM. The safety of administration of penicillamine to penicillin sensitive individuals. Arthritis Rheum 1983;26:801–803.

35. Aposhian HV. DMSA and DMPS–water soluble antidotes for heavy metal poisoning. Annu Rev Pharmacol Toxicol 1983;23:193–215.

36. Aposhian HV, Maiorino RM, Dart RC, Perry DF. Urinary excretion of meso-2,3-dimercaptosuccinic acid in human subjects. Clin Pharmacol Ther 1989;45:520–526.

37. Maiorino RM, Akins JM, Blahak, et al. Determination and metabolism of dithiol chelating agents. J Pharmacol Exp Ther. In press.

38. Cory-Slechta DA. Mobilization of lead over the course of DMSA chelation therapy and long-term efficacy. J Pharmacol Exp Ther 1988;246:84–92.

39. Graziano JH, Siris ES, LoIacono N, et al. 2,3-dimercaptosuccinic acid as an antidote for lead intoxication. Clin Pharmacol Ther 1985;37:431–438.

40. Graziano JH, Lolacono NJ, Meyer P. Dose-response study of oral 2,3-dimercaptosuccinic in children with elevated blood lead concentrations. J Pediatr 1988;113:751–757.

41. Graziano JH, Cuccia D, Friedheim E. The pharmacology of 2,3-dimercaptosuccinic acid and its potential use in arsenic poisoning. J Pharmacol Exp Ther 1978;20:1051–1055.

42. Fournier L, Thomas G, Garnier R, et al. 2,3-dimercaptosuccinic acid treatment of heavy metal poisoning in humans. Med Toxicol 1988;3:499–504.

43. Graziano JH. Role of 2,3-dimercaptosuccinic acid in the treatment of heavy metal poisoning. Med Toxicol 1986;1:155–162.

44. Berlin M, Rylander R. Increased brain uptake of mercury induced by 2,3-dimercaptopropanol (BAL) in mice exposed to phenyl mercuric acetate. J Pharmacol Exp Ther 1964;146:236–240.

45. Magos L. Effect of 2,3-dimercaptoptopanol (BAL) on urinary excretion and brain content of mercury. Br J Ind Med 1968;25:152–154.

46. Glomme J, Gustavson KH. Treatment of experimental acute mercury poisoning by chelating agents BAL and EDTA. Acta Med Scand 1959;164:175–182.

47. Piomelli S, Rosen JF, Chisolm J, et al. Management of childhood lead poisoning. J Pediatr 1984;104:523–532.

48. Chisolm JJ. Treatment of acute lead intoxication, choice of chelating agents and supportive therapeutic measures. Clin Toxicol 1970;34:527–540.

49. Foreman H, Trujillo TT. The metabolism of C-14 labeled ethylenediaminetetraacetic acid in human beings. J Lab Clin Med 1954;43:566–571.

50. Hammond PB, Aronson AL, Olson WC. The mechanism of mobilization of lead by ethylenediaminetetraacetate. J Pharmacol Exp Ther 1967;157:196–206.

51. Hammond PB. The effects of chelating agents on the tissue distribution and excretion of lead. Toxicol Appl Pharmacol 1971;18:296–310.

52. Foreman H, Finnegan C, Lushbaugh CC. Nephrotoxic hazard from uncontrolled edathamil calcium-disodium therapy. JAMA 1956;160:1042–1046.

53. Bakir F, Al-Khalidi A, Clarkson TW, Greenwood R. Clinical observations on treatment of alkyl mercury poisoning in hospital patients. Bull World Health Organ 1976;53(Suppl) 87–92.

54. Clarkson TW, Magos L, Cox C, et al. Tests of efficacy of antidotes for removal of methyl mercury in human poisoning during the Iraq outbreak. J Pharmacol Exp Ther 1981;218:74–83.

55. Lund ME, Banner W, Clarkson TW, Berlin M. Treatment of acute methyl mercury ingestion by hemodialysis with n-acetylcysteine (Mucomyst) infusion and 2,3-dimercaptopropanesulfate. Clin Toxicol 1984;22:31–49.

56. Cikrt M, Lenger V. Distribution and excretion of ^{203}HG^{2+} in rats after spironolactone and polythiol resin treatment. Toxicol Lett 1980;5:51–54.

57. Chrian MG, et al. Estimation of mercury burdens in rats by chelation with dimercaptopropanesulfanate. J Pharmacol Exp Ther 1988;245:479–484.

58. Twarog T, Cherian MG. Chelation of lead by dimercaptopropanesulfanate and a possible diagnostic use. Toxicol Appl Pharmacol 1984;72:550–556.

59. Chisolm JJ, Thomas DJ. Use of 2,3-dimercaptopropane-1-sulfanate in treatment of lead poisoning in children. J Pharmacol Exp Ther 1985;235:665–669.

60. Way JL, et al. Recent perspectives on the toxicodynamic basis of cyanide antagonism. Fundam Appl Toxicol 1984;4:S231–239.

61. Holland MA, Kozlowski LM. Clinical features and management of cyanide poisoning. Clin Pharmacol 1986;5:737–741.

62. Kruszyna R, Kruszyna H, Smith RP. Comparison of hydroxylamine, 4-dimethylaminophenol and nitrite protection against cyanide poisoning in mice. Arch Toxicol 1982;49:191–202.

63. Van Heigst ANP, Douze JMC, Van Kesteren RG. Therapeutic problems in cyanide poisoning. Clin Toxicol 1987;25:383–398.

64. Moore SJ, Norris JC, Walsh DA, Hume AS. Antidotal use of methemoglobin forming cyanide antagonist in concurrent carbon monoxide/cyanide intoxication. J Pharmacol Exp Ther 1987;242:70–73.

65. Hall AH, Rumack BH. Hydroxycobalamin/sodium thiosulfate as a cyanide antidote. J Emerg Med 1987;5:115–121.

66. Lambert RJ, Kindler BL, Schaffer DJ. The efficacy of super activated charcoal in treating rats exposed to lethal oral dose of potassium cyanide. Ann Emerg Med 1988;17:595–598.

67. Wesson DE, et al. Treatment of acute cyanide intoxication with hemodialysis. Am J Nephrol 1985;5:121–126.

68. Keniston RC, Cabellon S, Yarbrough KS. Peridoxal 5-prime-phosphate as an antidote for cyanide, spermine, gentamicin, and dopamine toxicity: An in vivo rat study. Toxicol Appl Pharmacol 1987;88:433–441.

37

Dermal Injuries and Burns from Hazardous Materials

Edward C. Geehr, M.D.
Richard F. Salluzzo, M.D.

BASIC PRINCIPLES AND CONCEPTS OF DERMAL INJURIES FROM HAZARDOUS MATERIALS

Although most thermal burns share common management approaches, chemical burns are distinguished by their broad range of pathophysiologic processes. Unlike thermal sources of burns, chemicals may continue to injure tissue for several days unless neutralized or removed.

The extent of burn caused by chemical agents is a function of several factors, including the quantity and concentration of the agent, the duration of contact, the depth of penetration, the specific agent involved, and the anatomy involved. Some studies have also suggested a possible genetic susceptibility to injury by certain agents. Underlying state of health and age are two other relevant factors.

The use of the term ''burn'' to describe injury by these chemicals is a bit of a misnomer, as tissue destruction by thermal activity is not the primary mechanism of injury. Different classes of agents may destroy tissue proteins by oxidation, reduction, vesicant activity, desiccation, metabolic inhibition, or protoplasmic poisoning, but the final common pathway involves the coagulation of tissue proteins.

Skin is the largest organ of the body, with approximately 15% of the total body weight and a surface area of approximately 9m^2 in the average adult. Given its size and vulnerability, it is not surprising that skin is often injured when patients are exposed to toxic substances. Skin consists of two principal layers, the epidermis and the dermis (Fig. 37.1). The epidermis is approximately 100–200 μg in thickness and composed principally of metabolically active squamous cells which synthesize structural proteins of the outermost stratum corneum. The stratum corneum constitutes the principal anatomic barrier against penetration by exogenous chemicals. For example, the buffering action of lactic acid, amphoteric amines, and weak bases present on this layer affords some protection against alkalies. The remainder of perceptible skin thickness is due to a loose matrix of dermal connective tissue composed of fibrous proteins (collagen, elastin, reticulan) imbedded in a proteinaceous ground substance. By attacking and destroying the various proteins and lipoproteins present in the epidermis and dermis, hazardous chemicals cause local tissue destruction and penetrate into the more vascular tissue layers from which systemic absorption may occur.

Chemical burns may be considered a special form of irritant contact dermatitis in which substantial skin necrosis and inflammation may result from one-time exposure to a chemical substance. For example, exposure to formaldehyde may result in first-degree burns, or a sensitization dermatitis may occur in previously exposed persons. The dermatitis may be characterized by an eczematous vesicular reaction which occurs suddenly with eruptions on the eyelids, feet, neck, scrotum, and arms. Urticaria has been reported as well.

From an occupational standpoint, irritant contact dermatitis is by far the most common dermatosis requiring medical attention. The great majority of cases of irritant contact dermatitis are caused by chemical substances. After contact with a toxic chemical, a series of changes may occur including transudation of serum through the epidermis, desiccation, and erythema, with progression to frank vesicles, blisters, and necrosis. The inflammatory changes induced from skin irritation result from direct local toxic effects on cellular elements in the skin, which in turn lead to release of lysosomal enzymes and insoluble inflammatory mediators. These inflammatory changes may result in eventual tissue destruction and cell death. In some instances, tissue destruction may be extensive and occur after a relatively brief skin exposure to agents such as strong caustics or corrosives.

The majority of cases of irritant contact dermatitis result from repetitive exposures to relatively weak irritants, substances which are not likely to cause visible cutaneous injury following a single exposure. It is important to emphasize that virtually any substance under the proper conditions is capable of causing irritant contact dermatitis, which often results from cumulative exposures rather than from a single injury. A variety of factors predispose to the development of cutaneous injury (Table 37.1).

Clearly, the inherent caustic or corrosive chemical properties of an agent will influence the extent of injury. However, other physical properties such as molecular size, weight, polarity, and ionization will also have an impact on the ability of a substance to penetrate the protective skin barrier and promote injury. In general, larger molecular weight substances, when ionized, are poor penetrants and less likely to cause injury. The concentration of the chemical and the duration and frequency of exposures play an important role in tissue injury. Cutaneous injury is less likely to occur with lower concentrations, shorter exposures, and less frequent contact. Skin becomes more permeable and less of a protective barrier as the temperature rises, which directly increases the irritant potential of toxic substances. If the skin surface is injured or otherwise compromised, chemical irritation is also more likely to develop.

The anatomical skin site influences the extent of injury because of the relative differences in thickness of the protective epidermal layers in different parts of the body. In general, the eyelids, face, and genital skin have the thinnest protective barriers and are therefore the most susceptible to chemical irritation. Finally, there have been several studies to determine the impact of genetics and race on host susceptibility to injury. To date these studies have not demonstrated conclusive evidence that susceptibility is influenced by these factors.

ALKALI DERMAL INJURIES

The inorganic alkalis include sodium, potassium, lithium, barium, and calcium hydroxides, as well as the silicates of these metals. These compounds are used extensively in home and

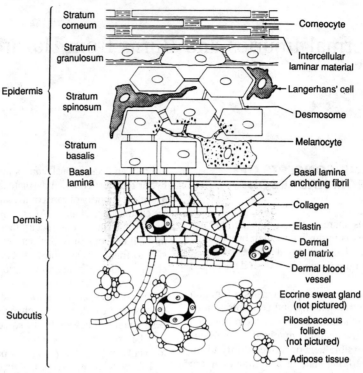

Figure 37.1.   Components of the skin. Source: Rom W. Environmental and occupational disease. Boston: Little, Brown, 1983:302. Reproduced with permission.

Table 37.1.   Factors Predisposing to the Development of Cutaneous Irritation

Potential irritant(s)
  Chemical properties
  Physical properties
Quantitative aspects of exposure
  Concentration
  Duration of exposure
  Frequency and number of exposures
Qualitative aspects of exposure
  Occlusion of substance against skin
  Temperature of substance or skin surface
  Preexisting skin damage to protective skin barrier
  Anatomical skin site
Host susceptibility
  Atopic disease
  Race(?)
  Sex(?)
  Age(?)

industry, in such products as washing powders, drain cleaners, and paint removers. Anhydrous sodium hydroxide may cause severe injury to tissues based upon its ability to saponify lipids, denature proteins and collagen as well as to dehydrate tissues and cells. The alkalis often produce a brown friable gelatinous eschar in the areas of skin contact, referred to as "liquefaction necrosis." The initial injury with alkalis is typically not as fulminant as those caused by acids. Ultimate tissue destruction, however, is often more profound with alkali exposure. As with other chemicals that "burn," the concentration of the alkali and duration of exposure are critical determinants of the degree of tissue injury. Skin biopsies from human subjects having 1 N sodium hydroxide applied to their arms for an average of 80 minutes showed progressive inflammatory changes resulting in the total destruction of the epidermis within 60 minutes.

Management of alkali dermal injury should begin in the prehospital setting with removal of the patient from the source of exposure. All clothing and footwear contaminated with the alkali should be removed and irrigation of the burn areas initiated. Supportive therapy including oxygen and intravenous fluids should be utilized as needed. Upon arrival in the emergency department, irrigation and supportive therapy should continue while a thorough evaluation of dermal injury and systemic toxicity is performed.

In addition to injury from skin contact, alkalis may also cause injury due to ocular exposure, inhalation, and ingestion. Ocular injury may be very severe, including disintegration and sloughing of the conjunctival and corneal epithelium, corneal opacification, and ultimately blindness. Treatment for ocular exposures should begin in the prehospital setting with irrigation utilizing large amounts of water. These patients should be brought immediately to an emergency department where irrigation should continue until corneal pH returns to normal. An urgent referral to an ophthalmologist should be made on all cases with significant exposures.

Inhalation injuries due to alkalies may be life-threatening. Respiratory injury may range from mild irritation of the mucous membranes to significant injuries of respiratory tissues causing pneumonitis and pulmonary edema. Severe tissue hypoxia and shock may occur. Prehospital treatment for inhalation injuries from these agents should include removal from the exposure area, oxygen therapy, and maintenance of airway and blood pressure. Subsequent emergency department care should include continued maintenance of supportive therapy, with specific attention to the degree of systemic injury. Ingestion of these agents may cause extensive injuries to oral, esophageal, and intestinal mucosa. Patients may present with severe oral, chest, and abdominal pain, with hematemesis and bloody diarrhea. Esophageal or intestinal perforation may result in mediastinitis, peritonitis, shock, and subsequent cardiovascular collapse (3). The estimated fatal dose in adults is 5 grams. Gastric lavage or emesis is contraindicated. Initial therapy should involve dilution of the alkali with milk or water as well as airway support and fluid resuscitation where appropriate.

Cement burns represent another common alkali burn seen in emergency departments. Many of the commercial cements in use today are a combination of tri- and dicalcium silicates with varying amounts of alumina, tricalciumaluminate, and iron oxide. When cement becomes wet, sodium, potassium, and calcium hydroxides are formed, and the pH of the cement rises above 12. Wet cement often comes in contact with workers' skin through work clothes or footwear, which provide a partial barrier to these substances. The resultant burn is typically discovered hours after the initial contact. The same principles of management as for alkali burns should be utilized.

CHROMIC ACID BURNS

Chromic acid is commonly used during the electroplating process. Of the three valences of chromium (Cr^{2+}, Cr^{3+}, Cr^{6+}) the hexavalent form is the most toxic due to its ability to freely cross cell membranes. Most tissue damage is caused by the change of valence (from Cr^{6+} to Cr^{3+}) which occurs in the presence of protein. Chromic acid is a strong desiccant, and the readily absorbed hexavalent ionic form causes remote organ injury. Chromic acid is commonly used in combination with sulfuric acid at elevated temperatures in the electroplating process, enhancing its toxicity (4).

Relatively minor exposures of chromic acid cause immediate skin damage, permitting rapid absorption of the toxic chromium ion in the absence of prompt ingestion. If an explosion is part of the injury process, total body exposure may be quite large and include contamination of the mucosa. Full thickness burns covering as little as 1% of the body surface area may lead to irreversible acute tubular necrosis secondary to acute chromium intoxication. The mortality rate is high if the burned area exceeds about 10% of the body surface area.

Presenting complaints of someone exposed to chromic acid include localized pain of the involved skin surfaces, with subsequent diarrhea, gastrointestinal bleeding, hemolysis, hepatic injury, and renal damage. Severe poisoning follows the ingestion of as little as 1–2 grams of compounds containing hexavalent chromium ion. The lethal dose is approximately 6 grams.

Treatment is directed at immediate, copious irrigation of all exposed areas. If irrigation cannot be achieved within seconds to minutes, full thickness burns and cutaneous absorption of the chromium ion will result. A variety of compounds have been recommended for limiting the toxic effects of the hexavalent chromium ion, including dressings of sodium thiosulfate, sodium citrate, or lactate, and sodium metabisulfite. Recommended systemic antidotes include sodium thiosulfate, dimercaptrol, and calcium disodium EDTA.

Some have advocated a prompt, deep, tangential incision of all contaminated tissues in order to present systemic ion penetration. Others have advocated hemodialysis or exchange transfusions in order to reduce the body content of chromium ion. All these approaches must be regarded as experimental,

1. 2R(solid) + 2H$_2$O---2R + 2OH - (aqueous) + H$_2$(gas)

2. 2R + (aqueous) + 2OH - (aqueous) ---2ROH (aqueous)

NET REACTION

2R (solid) + 2H$_2$O---2ROH (aqueous) + H$_2$(gas)

(where R represents either metallic sodium or potassium)

Figure 37.2.   Reaction of water and metallic sodium or potassium.

since most experts agree that once substantial amounts of hexavalent chromium have been absorbed there is no medical or surgical therapy proven to be lifesaving.

ELEMENTAL METALS

The elemental metals, such as sodium and potassium, have several industrial applications including use as coolants in nuclear reactors, as polymerization catalysts in the manufacture of tetraethyl lead, and in the production of photoelectric cells. Injuries caused by the elemental metals may be particularly devastating due to the production of both chemical and thermal burns (5). Upon reaction with water in tissues, these elements form hydroxides, which can cause significant tissue destruction (Fig. 37.2). As a result, the usual therapy of copious water irrigation for chemical burns is not appropriate.

As with other chemicals that "burn," any contaminated clothing or footwear should be rapidly removed, as should any obvious metal particles in tissue. The burn area should be covered with oil (mineral oil or common cooking oils) to prevent further chemical reaction. Any burning metal in tissue should be extinguished by an extinguisher containing sodium chloride, sodium carbonate, or a graphite base.

After the initial therapy in the prehospital setting, the patient should be rapidly transported to an appropriate emergency department where further wound debridement and metal extraction can be performed. Any extracted sodium or potassium particles should be placed for disposal in isopropyl alcohol and terbutyl alcohol, respectively. After excision of all metal particles, treatment is the same as for traditional alkali burns.

WHITE PHOSPHORUS

White phosphorus is an incendiary utilized in modern weaponry as well as in the manufacture of various insecticides, fertilizers, and rodent poisons. It is a translucent, solid substance with a garliclike odor which on exposure to air may fume or flame spontaneously.

White phosphorus is an oxidizing agent which is highly toxic to skin, causing both thermal and chemical burns. Much has been learned about burns caused by this agent from the study of wartime injuries. As a general rule, exposures to this agent cause second- and third-degree burns to the contact area. This substance will continue to oxidize and injure tissue until debrided, completely oxidized, or neutralized by tissue. Particles of this agent are often driven deeply into tissue layers, making neutralization very difficult (6).

Treatment of dermal injuries caused by white phosphorus should begin in the prehospital setting and include copious irrigation, removal of visible particles from the wound, and removal of all garments and footwear contaminated with the substance. Any particles removed from tissue should be placed under water and disposed of to prevent spontaneous combustion with air. In the emergency department setting, more extensive debridement should be performed. Irrigation with copper sulfate solution is often helpful in identifying occult white phosphorus particles in the wound by causing a characteristic black color change. After the identification process is completed, it is very important to fully irrigate the wound to remove all residual copper sulfate to prevent systemic copper toxicity (7). White phosphorus rarely causes systemic toxicity via percutaneous absorption or inhalation. Ingestions of this substance do occur, and a dose of 1 mg/kg is considered potentially lethal (8). Systemic ingestions are associated with fatty degeneration of the liver and with the signs and symptoms of acute liver failure.

ORGANIC ACIDS (PHENOLS, CRESOLS, CHREYSILIC ACIDS)

Organic acids are characterized by the presence of a benzene ring with one or more substituted hydroxyl groups. These compounds are used in the pharmaceutical industry and as deodorant sanitizers and home disinfectants. Organic acids are highly corrosive to skin and mucous membranes and may cause serious systemic effects following percutaneous absorption.

Phenol, also known as monohydroxybenzene, is a white crystalline solid at room temperature. In liquid form, it is known as carbolic acid. Phenol is extremely corrosive to skin surfaces, causing third-degree chemical burns (9). Eye contact may cause severe damage to the cornea, resulting in blindness (10). Phenol is effectively absorbed by inhalation, skin exposure, or ingestions. Systemic toxicity is manifested by tachycardia, tachypnea, muscle pain, cyanosis, convulsion, and, ultimately, coma and death.

Cresol is an organic acid with toxicity similar to phenol. Cresol causes significant dermal injury by its denaturing effect on tissue proteins, leading to inflammation and necrosis of epidermal and dermal tissues. Repeated skin contact with low concentrations may cause tawny discoloration of the skin and chronic inflammatory changes. Cresol may be absorbed systemically after chronic dermal exposure, resulting in some cases in central nervous system, liver, and kidney injury.

Appropriate management of dermal injuries from these agents should begin in the prehospital setting. Removal from the source of the agent is standard, as is removal of all contaminated clothing and footwear. Copious irrigation is performed on all affected areas. Supportive measures such as oxygen therapy and fluid resuscitation are initiated as needed. Emergency department evaluation includes a careful assessment of extent of injury and a careful search for systemic toxicity.

INORGANIC ACIDS

Sulfuric acid, hydrochloric acid, and nitric acid are inorganic acids that are highly corrosive to tissues. These agents injure tissues primarily by dehydration and heat production, resulting in protein denaturation and cellular death.

Sulfuric acid, also known as sodium bisulfate, has a variety of home and industrial uses. Upon contact with skin, a hard eschar forms with deep ulceration into the underlying tissues. Extensive destruction of tissue occurs, and considerable heat is released during this reaction. This process of injury is sometimes referred to as coagulation necrosis. Ingestions from this

substance are rare due to its caustic nature, but may cause shock, glottic and laryngeal injury, asphyxia, and even intestinal perforation.

Injuries caused by hydrochloric and nitric acids are similar to those of sulfuric acid. The burning process is more indolent than that of sulfuric acid, producing deeper, more extensive ulcers.

Therapy for these agents includes removal of all contaminated garments and footwear and copious irrigation with water of all affected areas. If there is any evidence of systemic toxicity, appropriate supportive care is initiated. In the emergency department, appropriate management of burns from these agents often requires debridement and prolonged irrigation to prevent further tissue injury. Due to the highly corrosive nature of these acids, it is critical to quickly neutralize or remove them from tissues. In addition to the danger of injury from oral and skin contact, certain acids, such as nitric acid, are highly toxic if inhaled. Inhalation of the substance may cause severe respiratory irritation with associated burns of the mucous membranes. After severe exposures, pulmonary edema may develop rapidly but generally does so after a latent period of 5–72 hours. Systemic symptoms include dizziness, headache, nausea, weakness, chest tightness, dyspnea, and frothy sputum production. Complete recovery may occur after days to weeks or longer. In severe exposures, death due to anoxia may occur within a few hours of exposure.

Chronic inhalations of lower concentration may lead to erosion of teeth, inflammatory and ulcerative changes in the mouth, chronic bronchial irritation with cough, and chronic dyspnea. Patients exposed to the inorganic acid fumes should be removed from the exposure area immediately and given airway and hemodynamic support as needed. Victims should be brought immediately to an emergency facility for definitive care and evaluation.

HYDROFLUORIC ACID

Hydrofluoric acid is the inorganic acid of elemental fluorine. It is a colorless, fuming liquid or gas with an irritating, pungent odor that has multiple industrial and home uses, including glass etching, rust removal, and cleansing.

The compound is highly corrosive and produces a characteristic injury to skin by two different mechanisms. First, there is tissue destruction through the operation of free hydrogen ions. Second, more extensive injury is caused by penetration of fluoride ions deep into tissues. As with other chemicals that "burn," the extent of injury is dependent on surface area involved, concentration of the acid, and duration of exposure (11).

Hydrofluoric acid burns are characterized by a blanched appearance of the skin with persistent pain, edema, and necrosis (12, 13). When the concentration of acid is less than 20%, pain and erythema may occur after a latent period of up to 24 hours. Concentrations between 20% and 50% cause burns which are often apparent within 1 hour. Burns associated with hydrofluoric acid concentrations above 50% cause immediate tissue damage on contact with resultant severe pain, swelling, and necrosis of tissue (14). With more extensive burns, fluoride ions may penetrate into the deeper tissues, where they can complex with available bivalent cations such as calcium and magnesium to form insoluble fluoride salts. This interaction has several deleterious effects on cellular function including disruption of membrane function and impairment of cellular metabolism which ultimately results in extensive tissue necrosis and cellular death (15, 16).

Patients with hydrofluoric acid burns classically present with pain at the site of contact. The pain is often described as excruciating and may seem out of proportion to the surface area involved. Despite therapy, cellular injury may progress, with vesiculation and eventual necrosis appearing at the contact site. In very serious exposures, fluoride ions may actually penetrate to underlying bone and cause marked demineralization.

Treatment of hydrofluoric acid burns is multifaceted. Initial therapy is aimed at removing the acid from the skin, best accomplished by prolonged and thorough flushing with water or saline. Large volumes of fluid for long periods should be utilized for this purpose. Current therapy also utilizes topical applications and local tissue infiltrates of solutions which will complex with free fluoride ions, the main arbiter of cellular injury. Topical agents include magnesium oxide, calcium gluconate suspension, and the quaternary ammonium salts: benzethonium chloride and benzylkonium chloride (Zephiran) (17). Controlled studies to date have not demonstrated a clear superiority of these agents over water decontamination, perhaps because they are incapable of complexing the fluoride ions in the deeper tissue sites where much of the cellular injury occurs (18).

Over the past 20 years, local injection of calcium gluconate has proved to be superior to topical therapy for significant hydrofluoric acid dermal injuries (19). Many case reports note complete resolution of pain following the injection of calcium gluconate into the dermal tissues and the prevention of serious tissue necrosis. Despite its relative effectiveness, the use of calcium gluconate injections has a number of disadvantages. One drawback of this agent is the degree of pain and mechanical trauma associated with multiple therapeutic injections. Since fingers are a common site of exposure, it is difficult to inject the suggested 0.5 ml/cm^2 of burn due to volume constraints in this area. As a result, injection therapy of the fingers may be inadequate to treat the injury effectively. The problem is compounded in burns that may extend to the nail bed. Some experts recommend nail removal and injection of calcium gluconate directly into the nail bed, but this approach may delay nail regrowth even if burn therapy is effective.

The newest treatment modality for digital burns involves the use of intraarterial calcium gluconate infusion (20, 21). This specific treatment approach has been used extensively in Europe since the late 1970s, and Vance et al. have treated many patients successfully since 1984 in this country. After appropriate arterial catheter placement, a preparation of calcium gluconate (10 milliliters of 10% solution in 50 milliliters of D_5 and water) is infused over 4 hours on a pump apparatus. If after a 4-hour infusion the patient continues to have pain, a second cycle of calcium gluconate intraarterial infusion may be performed. In Vance's series of 10 patients, all had excellent resolution of symptoms within 2 hours. The only complication of this series was one patient with spasm of the radial artery secondary to catheter placement. Intraarterial calcium infusion has several advantages over conventional therapy. First, it eliminates the need for painful local injections. Second, a larger volume of calcium can be delivered to the deep tissues to complex with the fluoride ion which limits tissue injury. The usual calcium gluconate dermal injection of 0.5 ml/cm^2 contains only 4.2 milligrams of calcium, an amount that will neutralize only 0.025 milliliters of a 20% hydrofluoric acid burn solution. In contrast, a 10-milliliter arterial infusion provides 84 milligrams of calcium, enough to neutralize 0.5 milliliter

of a 20% hydrofluoric acid burn. Intraarterial calcium therapy is also effective for burns that extend under the nail into the nail bed. The principal disadvantages to the use of intraarterial therapy relates to its invasive nature. Although several studies have demonstrated its safety, the usual risk from arterial cannulization exists. Hydrofluoric acid may cause systemic toxicity whether absorbed via the skin or through inhalation (22).

ALDEHYDES

Aldehydes are chemical compounds containing the radical −HC=O that is reducible to an alcohol and oxidizable to an acid. A large number of aldehydes are capable of dermal injury and include formaldehyde, acrolein, and glutaraldehyde. These compounds are used in a variety of settings including the production of chemicals, the production of food products, plastics production, the textile industry, and the leather industry. Most aldehydes are highly volatile and tend to cause eye and mucous membrane irritation.

Formaldehyde is well-known as an irritant to eyes and mucous membranes. Skin contact with formaldehyde has a variety of dermal effects including irritation, allergic contact dermatitis, and urticaria. Formaldehyde is a frequent cause of allergic contact dermatitis in the industrial and health care setting. Minor epidemics of allergic contact dermatitis have been described among healthcare workers who handle equipment immersed in formaldehyde solutions. Because of its ubiquity in our environment, humans can come into frequent contact with low concentrations of formaldehyde sufficient to provoke responses in people with allergic contact sensitization (23). These diverse sources include components of plastics, glues, antifungal disinfectants, preservatives, paper, fabrics, leather, coal and wood smoke, fixatives for histology, and photographic materials. Formaldehyde is a skin irritant and a skin sensitizer. The best treatment is to avoid contact by the use of protective wear, including gloves.

Acrolein is a highly volatile aldehyde which in liquid form causes severe skin irritation. Exposure should be treated with copious irrigation; exposures are rarely serious.

Glutaraldehyde is a strong mucous membrane irritant. Occasional contact with skin can cause an allergic response leading to contact dermatitis. Sensitization to glutaraldehyde occurs much less frequently than to formaldehyde, and cross-reactivity with formaldehyde-sensitive individuals does not appear to occur. Exposure should be treated with irrigation, and repeated exposure should be avoided to prevent sensitization (24).

EPOXY RESINS

Epoxy resin systems contain resins, hardeners, and reactive diluents. Other compounds such as tar, glass, dyes, and other plastics are occasionally added to the system. Epoxy resins have a wide range of applications and are increasingly used as a glue for metal, rubber, plastics, and ceramics and for repair work in a variety of areas including concrete, electrical insulation, metals, and floor coverings. Epoxy resin is commonly available as a household glue.

The primary dermal effect of epoxy resin systems is allergic contact dermatitis. More than 90% of those with the contact allergy are sensitized specifically to the resin. The allergic dermatitis is usually evident in localized areas of the hands and forearms, but it occasionally appears on the face and neck (25).

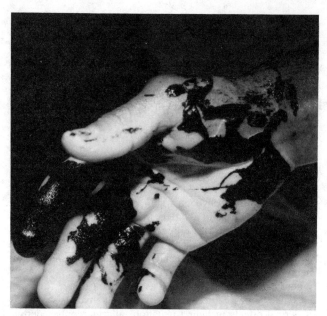

Figure 37.3.   Hot tar burns to the hand.

The treatment of epoxy dermatitis is to avoid ongoing contact. This occasionally necessitates discontinuing of job activity and retraining. Prevention is the best cure.

HOT TAR

Asphalt tar, used in surfacing, is a product of the residues of coal tar. It is heated to about 450°F to maintain its liquid form for application. Upon contact with skin it cools rapidly, but its retained heat is usually sufficient to produce first- and second-degree burns (Fig. 37.3). Burns due to hot tar present a difficult management problem because of the difficulty of removing the hot tar without inflicting further injury to the underlying injured skin (26).

Traditional approaches to tar burn injuries have included cooling of the tar with irrigation or ice pack applications followed by debridement. In recent years, there has been a shift to the use of emulsifying agents which are readily available and can avoid the secondary injury inflicted by debridement procedure. The compound polyoxyethylene sorbitan has been found to have excellent lymphophilic and hydrophilic properties, making it an excellent emulsifier of tar which can be washed off with water (Fig. 37.4). This compound is found in neosporin cream, neosporin ointment, and Tween 80. Liquid Tween 80 is deemed to be preferable to neosporin cream because it is more water soluble and easily washable and emulsification is more rapid (27). However, neosporin is generally more readily available and is perfectly adequate. There are anecdotal reports of the use of mayonnaise as a reportedly highly effective emulsifier.

ORGANIC SOLVENTS

Hydrocarbons are derivatives of petroleum distillation, the major classes of which include straight chain saturated and unsaturated aliphatics, cyclic, and halogenated hydrocarbons. These products are ubiquitous in our environment, and poisoning due to hydrocarbons is a relatively common problem. In 1983, the Association of Poison Controls of America published data from

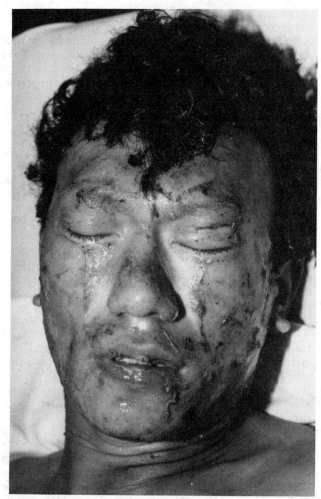

Figure 37.4.   Hot tar burns to the face after removal with polyoxyethelene sorbitan.

16 states in which over 11,000 incidents of hydrocarbon poisoning occurred, resulting in numerous hospitalizations and two deaths.

There are five major clinical syndromes caused by exposure to hydrocarbon products: skin toxicity, gastrointestinal toxicity, pulmonary toxicity, central nervous system toxicity, and generalized systemic toxicity. Acute or chronic exposure to hydrocarbons can result in significant skin injury. Hydrocarbons are directly irritant to the epidermal tissue and as a consequence of their high lipid solubility may cause dissolution of fatty tissues and penetration of cell membranes (28). Varous forms of cutaneous injury may occur including contact dermatitis, eczematoid eruption, burns, and epidermal necrosis. In order of decreasing dermal toxicity are the short-chain aliphatics, aromatics, and chlorinated solvents (Table 37.2). As with other dermal toxins, the depth of injury appears directly related to the duration of exposure and concentration of the specific agent. Prolonged contact with gasoline and other short-chain hydrocarbons has traditionally been felt to cause only partial thickness burns, but recent reports of full thickness injury dispel this notion (29). Significant cutaneous absorption of gasoline and other hydrocarbons is felt to be uncommon. (Table 37.3). Aspiration or inhalation appears to be the major portal of entry for systemic absorption and injury (30).

Table 37.2. Agents Associated with Dermal Injury

Agent	Application	Mechanism of Injury	Therapy
Alkalis	Cement, sugar reagents, drain cleaners, paint removers	Saponify lipids Denature proteins Dehydrate tissues	Water or saline irrigation
Chromic acid	Electroplating Metal cleanser	Oxidizing effects Systemic absorption	Water or saline irrigation, CaNa$_2$ EDTA, dimercaprol for systemic toxicity
Elemental metals	Nuclear coolants Polymerization catalysts	Corrosive Thermal	Wound debridement; excision of all metal particles
White phosphorus	Insecticides Fertilizers Weapons	Corrosive	Water or saline irrigation, copper sulfate irrigation, wound debridement
Phenols Cresols	Pharmaceuticals Deodorants Disinfectants	Corrosive	Water or saline irrigation
Inorganic acid (sulfuric, nitric, hydrochloric)	Glass industry Car batteries Metal cleansing	Corrosive Thermal	Water or saline irrigation
Hydrofluoric acid	Glass etching Rust removal Home cleaner	Corrosive Protoplasmic poison	Water or saline irrigation, subcutaneous or intraarterial calcium
Aldehydes	Plastic, leather, food production	Oxidizers	Water or saline irrigation
Epoxy resins	Floor coverings Glue Electrical insulators	Irritant contact dermatitis	Avoid contact, cortisone ointment
Hot tar	Road surfacing	Thermal	Emulsifying agents (neosporin and Tween 80) then saline or water irrigation
Organic solvents	Solvents Fuels Pharmaceutical	Mild corrosive	Water or saline irrigation
Aliphatic alcohols and glycols	Paint, dye, antifreeze, heat exchangers	Mild corrosive	Water or saline irrigation
Sodium hypochlorite	Bleaches, disinfectants, water purifiers	Corrosive Oxidizer	Water or saline irrigation

At the cellular level, hydrocarbon exposure appears to cause damage to vascular epithelium. In the lungs, for example, lesions may range from small petechiae to large pulmonary hemorrhages. In addition, the hydrocarbons may adversely affect pulmonary surfactant production, which can lead to atelectasis and respiratory distress. The chlorinated aliphatic hydrocarbons such as chloroform, carbon tetrachloride, and trichloroethylene are well-known as hepatic toxins, causing damage to vascular epithelium in the liver. Renal toxicity from these agents is usually associated with more severe systemic exposures and is characterized by glomerular injury as well as by proximal tubular damage present in a patchy distribution (31). Neurologic dysfunction is perhaps the most common sequela from exposure to the hydrocarbon products and ranges from mild euphoria to toxic encephalopathies, including seizures and coma. Benzene and other aromatic hydrocarbons are also known to cause hepatic, renal, and bone marrow toxicity. Ingestion may lead to significant gastrointestinal disturbances including nausea, vomiting, diarrhea, and abdominal pain. Morbidity from oral exposure is primarily due to aspiration because of the otherwise limited absorption across mucus membranes.

Emergency therapy for hydrocarbon dermal injury involves removal from the source of exposure, removal of contaminated clothing and footwear, and copious irrigation with water or saline to the exposed areas. General supportive care should be administered on an individual basis depending on the severity of the exposure and the agent involved.

ALIPHATIC ALCOHOLS AND GLYCOLS

The aliphatic alcohols are hydrocarbon compounds that contain one substituted hydroxyl group. The glycols are alcohols with two substituted hydroxyl groups. Like other hydrocarbons, they are excellent solvents which cause minimal toxicity when associated with routine exposures.

Methyl alcohol, also known as methanol or wood alcohol, is a colorless, volatile liquid utilized as a solvent in the production of paints, dyes, cements, and inks. Toxicity from this agent usually occurs after inhalation, although serious injury and death have occurred from ingestions and percutaneous absorption. Methyl alcohol causes dermal injury similar to other hydrocarbons, the most common being a chronic fissured dermatitis. Systemic toxicity is usually associated with metabolic acidosis and visual disturbances secondary to optic nerve injury. Central nervous system effects include headaches, vertigo, unsteady gait, and inebriation. An ingestion of as little as 15 milliliters has caused death. Recent studies implicate the metabolic products formic acid and formaldehyde as the responsible toxic agents.

Ethylene glycol is employed in hydraulic fluids, antifreeze, and heat exchangers. It causes dermal toxicity similar to other hydrocarbons, and significant percutaneous absorption may occur. Inhalation at room temperature is unlikely due to its low vapor pressure. The estimated lethal dose for adults is 100 milliliters, and in cases of fatal ingestions coma,

Table 37.3. Petroleum Distillates Toxic to Humans

Product	Carbons	Boiling Point Range (°C)	Toxicity[a]		Uses
			Central Nervous System	Lung	
Gas	1–5	40	+	0	Fuel
Benzine	5–6	35–90	+	0	Solvent
Benzene	6	80	+	±	Solvent, degreaser
Gasoline	4–12	40–225	+	±	Fuel
Naphtha	7–10	94–175	+	±	Lighter fluid, lacquer diluent
Mineral spirit	9–12	152–210	+	+	Solvent, degreaser
Kerosene	10–16	175–325	±	+	Lighter fluid, fuel, vehicle
Light gas oil	13–17	230–305	+	+	Diesel, home fuels
Mineral seal oil		260–370	±	+	Furniture polish

[a] + = major; ± = occasional/minor; 0 = generally absent.

respiratory failure, kidney failure, and death may ensue within 72 hours.

Management strategies for dermal injuries secondary to these agents is similar to that outlined for other hydrocarbons.

SODIUM HYPOCHLORITE

This agent is used in disinfectants, bleaches, deodorizers, and water purifiers. As an oxidizing agent, sodium hypochlorite is very corrosive to tissues. The toxicity of sodium hypochlorite is related to available chlorine in solutions containing this substance. Solutions containing less than 6% available chlorine usually cause significant injury to tissues in large volumes only; concentrations of available chlorine greater than 15% can cause significant skin injury in much smaller volumes and after shorter exposures.

The oxidizing potential of sodium hypochlorite is directly related to the concentrations of chlorine present. The more concentrated solutions are associated with greater dermal injury as they are neutralized.

Contact with diluted solutions may cause mild irritation of the skin. However, more concentrated solutions may bleach the skin and cause pain, erythema, blistering, and skin necrosis. Sensitization dermatitis may occur in previously exposed individuals.

Initial treatment for these burns includes removal of contaminated clothing and footwear and irrigation of the affected area with soap or mild detergent and large amounts of water. Patients should be promptly transferred for definitive emergency department care. In addition to its dermal toxicity, sodium hypochlorite may also cause injury from ocular exposure, inhalation, or ingestion. Ocular toxicity is dependent on the concentration of available chlorine, with predictable corneal injury occurring upon exposure to concentrations greater than 15%.

The respiratory effects of sodium hypochlorite are dependent on the concentration, ranging from slight irritation to severe pulmonary compromise. Sore throat, cough, dyspnea, and pulmonary edema have all been reported. Ingestions cause injury to the mucous membranes, with blistering of the mouth, throat, and larynx. Hypotension and shock may ensue secondary to perforation of the esophagus and stomach.

Treatment of such ingestions requires the usual supportive measures including appropriate airway maintenance and fluid therapy. Induction of vomiting and gastric lavage are typically contraindicated. Early endoscopy is recommended to establish the extent of the injury.

PHYSICAL AGENTS CAUSING DERMAL INJURY

High Pressure Injuries

Though the focus of this chapter is clearly on specific chemicals and how they cause dermal injury, consideration must also be given to nonchemical injury associated with the use of these substances. For example, many chemical agents are being utilized in relatively high pressure devices which develop pounds per square inch pressures of 1500 or greater. Injuries from such devices are extremely hazardous for several reasons. As in other chemical burns, there is exposure to a substance that can cause substantial tissue injury. In addition, the chemical may be injected much more deeply into tissues, making removal or neutralization very difficult. Due to the high pressure injection and deep tissue penetration, it is very easy to underestimate the severity of injury. The goal of treatment, as with all chemical burns, is prompt removal of the offending agent by irrigation and debridement. In patients with high pressure injuries, early and adequate exposure of tissue of potentially contaminated tissue should be the main goal of initial therapy. In addition, patients should be carefully observed for evidence of ongoing injury so that further tissue exposure and debridement can be initiated as needed.

Treatment of these injuries is otherwise as outlined in the chapter for the various chemicals involved.

Microwave Injuries

Industrial and home use of microwave energy devices has become very prevalent over the past 15 years. Microwaves are defined as nonionizing high-frequency electromagnetic radiation and are positioned on the high-frequency long wavelength portion of the electromagnetic spectrum (Table 37.4). Though microwave appliances are for the most part quite safe, there are clear hazards associated with their use. The deleterious effects of microwave radiation on the human body are due largely to heat production and subsequent thermal injury. The amount of heat generated is a function of the power output of the microwave device, distance of the tissue from the source, type of tissue involved, and the duration of exposure. Significant dermal injuries secondary to microwave exposure are relatively rare and generally involve the upper extremity. Exposures as brief as 2–3 seconds may cause significant injury, with the occurrence of erythema, pain, blistering, and tissue necrosis. In some instances, the skin may demonstrate only

Table 37.4.   The Electromagnetic Spectrum (Adapted from Tintinalli. Ann Emerg Med, October 1983.)

Frequency (HZ)

10^{16}	10^{15}	10^{14}	10^{13}	10^{12}	10^{11}	10^{10}
Ultraviolet		Vis	Infrared		Radio waves	Microwaves

10^{-8}	10^{-7}	10^{-6}	10^{-5}	10^{-4}	10^{-3}	10^{-2}	10^{-1}

Wavelength (m)

minimal signs of injury, whereas underlying muscle, nerves, and blood vessels may be significantly damaged. Sensory nerves are particularly vulnerable to microwave energy. Cases of persistent neuritis and even compressive neuropathy have been reported following these exposures. Occasionally, burns of the oral mucosa and esophagus have occurred secondary to overheating of food products, particularly by children not familiar with the proper use of these devices.

Much still needs to be learned about injuries resulting from microwave exposure. An emphasis on preventive measures limiting the risk of these devices needs to be an ongoing focus of regulatory and health agencies.

Tissue injury resulting from microwave exposure should be managed by standard wound care techniques. The thermal injury is generally localized to the areas of exposure without propagation along tissue plains or the creation of exit type wounds. Adequate exposure and debridement of injured tissue as well as close observation for potential complications remains the cornerstone of good therapy.

MANAGEMENT SUMMARY

The treatment of dermal injuries from hazardous materials should be approached from the perspective of optimizing local wound care and appropriately evaluating the need for systemic supportive therapy. Emergency treatment is directed at elimination of the offending agent and the accurate diagnosis of extent of injury. Removal of the toxin generally requires dilution, neutralization, and debridement of the burn wound. Additionally, measures to promote systemic detoxification and facilitation of excretion of the offending agent are necessary for certain compounds. Supportive care typically includes adequate fluid resuscitation and ventilatory support.

The rapid removal of contaminated garments and footwear and the initial dilution of the agent should begin in the prehospital setting. The initial irrigation may require gallons of water or saline over a period of several hours. Dilution has many salutary effects including reduction of the concentration of the offending chemical agent and removal of the agent from the contact surface. These effects greatly decrease the rate of chemical reaction and help to restore wound pH levels toward the normal range. It is universally accepted that early intervention is critical in preventing full thickness injury. Thus, it is essential that the irrigation process be started in the prehospital setting.

The neutralization process, whether by water or tissue exposure, usually causes an exothermic reaction which has the potential for further thermal injury. However, this effect may be minimized by continuous irrigation. Certain chemical burns, such as those caused by hydrofluoric acid, may require more specific interventions.

Two issues are of critical importance when confronted with chemical burns and planning a management strategy. First, it is essential not to underestimate the extent of the initial injury. Second, tissue penetration and subsequent injury may continue for several days. Thus, early definitive evaluation and treatment by experienced personnel afford the best chance for minimizing morbidity and mortality.

Dermal injuries from physical agents such as microwaves and high-pressure tissue injectors though uncommon, requires familiarity with their effects for appropriate management of such injuries.

REFERENCES

1. Maibach H. Occupational and industrial dermatology. 2nd ed. Chicago: Year Book Medical Publishers, 1987.
2. Fitzpatrick KT. Emergency care of chemical burns. Postgrad Med 1985;78:189–192.
3. Lecgaard T. Corrosive injuries of the esophagus. J Laryngol Otol 1945;60:389–402.
4. Wang AW, Davis JWL, Sirvant SUU, et al. Chromic acid burns in acute chromium poisoning. Burns 1985;11:181–184.
5. Clare RA. Chemical burns secondary to elemental metal exposure. Am J Emerg Med 1988;6:355–357.
6. Konjoyan TR. White phosphorus burns: case report and literature review. Milit 1983;148:881.
7. Chuttani HK, Gupta PS, Gulati S, et al. Acute copper sulfate poisoning. Am J Med 1965;39:849.
8. Summerlin WT, Adler AI, Moncrief JA. White phosphorus burns and massive hemolysis. J Trauma 1967;7:476.
9. Abraham AJ. A case of carbolic acid gangrene of the thumb. Br J Plast Surg 1972;25:282–284.
10. Freidenwald JS, Hughes WF, Herman H. Acid burns of the eye. Arch Ophthalmol 1946;35:98–104.
11. Derelanko MJ. Acute dermal toxicity of dilute hydrofluoric acid. J Toxicol Cut and Ocular Toxicol 1985;4:73–85.
12. Craig RDP. Hydrofluoric acid burns of the hands. Br J Plast Surg 1964;17:53.
13. Dibbell DG, Iverson RE, Jones W, et al. Hydrofluoric acid burns of the hand. J Bone Joint Surg 1970;52(A):931.
14. Iverson RE, Laub DR, Madison MS. Hydrofluoric acid burns. Plast Reconstr Surg 1971;48:107–112.
15. Burke WJ, Hoegg UR, Phillips RE. Systemic fluoride poisoning resulting from a fluoride skin burn. J Occup Med 1973;15:39–41.
16. Tepperman PB. Fatality due to acute systemic fluoride poisoning following hydrofluoric acid skin burn. J Occup Med 1980;22:691–692.
17. Carney SA, Hall M, Lawrence JC, et al. Rationale of the treatment hydrofluoric acid burns. Br J Ind Med 1974;31:317–321.
18. Bracken WM. Comparative effectiveness of topical treatments for hydrofluoric acid burns. J Occup Med 1985;27:733–740.
19. Blunt CP. Treatment of hydrofluoric acid skin burns by injection with calcium gluconate. Ind Med Surg 1964;33:869.

20. Pegg SP. Intra-arterial infusions in the treatment of hydrofluoric acid burns. Burns 1985;11:440–443.

21. Vance MV. Digital hydrofluoric acid burns. Ann Emerg Med 1986;15:890–896.

22. Mayer L, Guelich J. Hydrogen fluoride (HF) inhalation and burns. Arch Environ Health 1963;7:445–447.

23. Committee on Aldehydes. Formaldehyde and other aldehydes 1981. Washington, DC: National Academy Press.

24. Ballantyne B, Berman B. Dermal sensitizing potential of glutaraldehyde: a review and recent observations. J Toxicol 1984;3:251–262.

25. Fregert S. Contact dermatitis from epoxy resin systems. In: Benneter, HM, Occupational and industrial dermatology. Chicago: Year Book Medical Publishers, 1987.

26. Demling RH, Buerstatte WR, Perea A. Management of hot tar burns. J Trauma 1980;20:242.

27. Bose B, Tredjet T. Treatment of hot tar burns. CMA J 1982;127:21–22.

28. Hunter GA. Chemical burns of the skin after contact with petrol. Br J Plast Surg 1968;21:337–341.

29. Walsh WA, Scarpa FJ, Brown RS, et al. Gasoline immersion burn. N Engl J Med 1974;291:830.

30. Ainsworth RW. Petrol vapour poisoning. Br Med J 1960;5185:1547.

31. Leonard LG, Scheulen JJ, Munster AM. Chemical burns: effect of prompt first aid. J Trauma 1982;22:420–424.

SUGGESTED READINGS

Berkhout PG, Ladd AC, Goldwater LJ. Treatment of skin burns due to alkyl mercury compounds. Arch Environ Health 1961;3:592–593.

Bromberg BE, Song IC, Walden RH. Hydrotherapy of chemical burns. Plast Reconstr Surg 1965;35:85–88.

Bucklow PS, et al. High pressure acid injection. J Trauma 1985;16:552–556.

Cason JS. Report on three extensive industrial chemical burns. Br Med J 1959;1:827–831.

Chan TK, Mak LW, Ng RP. Methemoglobinemia, Heinz bodies and acute massive intravascular hemolysis in Lysol poisoning. Blood 1971;38:739–743.

Ciano M. High frequency electromagnetic imagery to the upper extremity. Ann Plast Surg 1981;7:128–135.

Curreiri PW, Asch MJ, Pruitt BA. The treatment of chemical burns: specialized diagnostic, therapeutic, and prognostic considerations. J Trauma 1970;10:634–642.

Curreri PW. Chemical burns. In: Artz CP, Moncrief JA, Pruitt BA, eds. Burns: a team approach. Philadelphia: WB Saunders Co, 1979.

Flock H. Microwave oven burns. Bull NY Acad Med 1983;59:313–317.

Gruber RP, Laub DR, Vistnes LM. The effect of hydrotherapy on the clinical course and pH of experimental cutaneous chemical burns. Plast Reconstr Surg 1975;65:200–204.

Harris JC, Rumack BH, Peterson RG, et al. Methemoglobinemia resulting from absorption of nitrates. JAMA 1979;242:286–289.

Hodgkinson DJ, Irons GB, Williams TJ. Chemical burns and skin preparation solutions. Surg Gynecol Obstet 1978;147:534–536.

Hunkin F. Contact injuries of the hand. Occup Med 1989;4:473–483.

Hydrofluoric acid chemical safety data sheet SD-25. Washington, DC: Manufacturing Chemists Association, 1968.

Jelenko C. Chemicals that ''burn.'' J Trauma 1974;14:65–72.

Kohnlein HE, Merkle P, Springorum HW. Hydrogen fluoride burns: experiments and treatment. Surg Forum 1973;24:50–51.

Leterman A. Treatment of chemical burns. EMS 1988;36–40.

Lewis BK. Chemical burns. Am J Surg 1959;98:928–931.

Moore PA, Manor RC. Hydrofluoric acid burns. J Prosthet Dent 1982;47:338–342.

Nicholsan CP, et al. Acute microwave injury to the hand. J Hand Surg 1987;12A:446–449.

Rom W. Environmental and occupational medicine. 1st ed. Boston: Little, Brown and Co, 1983.

Shewmake SW, Anderson BG. Hydrofluoric acid burns. Arch Dermatol 1979;115:593–597.

Sinilo ML. Chemical burns and their treatment. Acta Chirurg Plast (Prague) 1961;3:311–317.

Siu V, Kissoon N. Hazards of microwave ovens. Pediatr Emerg Care 1987;3:99–103.

Steinberg UW, Walden RH, Bromberg BE, et al. Hydrotherapy of lye burns. Plast Reconstr Surg 1983;31:481–488.

Stewart DW. Acute poisoning by a barium chloride burn. J Trauma 1984;24:768–770.

Tintinalli JE, Krause G, et al. Microwave radiation injury. Ann Emerg Med 1983;12:645–647.

Trevino MA, Hermann GH, Sprout WL. Treatment of severe hydrofluoric acid exposures. J Occup Med 1983;25:861–863.

Van Rensberg LC. An experimental study of chemical burns. S Afr Med J 1962;36:754–756.

Wilson GA, Sanger RG, Boswick JA. Accidental hydrofluoric acid burns of the hand. JAMA 1979;99:57–60.

38

Acute Pulmonary Injury from Hazardous Materials

John R. Balmes, M.D.

INTRODUCTION

The widespread use in modern society of materials potentially hazardous to the respiratory tract makes inhalational injury a relatively common occurrence. Shortterm exposure to high concentrations of noxious gases, fumes, or mists is generally due to industrial or transportation accidents or fires. The resultant inhalation injury from such high intensity exposures can result in severe impairment or death. Pulmonary insufficiency caused by smoke inhalation probably accounts for more fire-related deaths than any other cause, and the components of smoke most toxic to the lungs are gases produced by the pyrolysis of synthetic materials. Many smoke and toxic inhalation-related deaths occur at the scene, but a large number of patients with inhalation injuries die after hospitalization. Early recognition of inhalation injury in fire and industrial/environmental accident victims could well result in increased survival.

DETERMINANTS OF TOXICITY

The effects of inhalational exposure to toxic materials can range from transient, mild irritation of the mucous membranes of the upper airway to fatal adult respiratory distress syndrome (ARDS). The anatomic site of injury in the respiratory tract depends on what is inhaled. The site of deposition of an inhaled gas is determined primarily by its water solubility, but also by the duration of exposure and the minute ventilation of the victim. Because of the efficient scrubbing mechanism of the moist surfaces of the nose and throat, the concentration of an inhaled water-soluble gas such as formaldehyde is greatly reduced by the time it reaches the trachea. In contrast, a relatively water-insoluble gas such as phosgene is not well-absorbed by the upper airways and thus may penetrate to the alveoli. During vigorous exertion, the oral breathing necessary to meet increased ventilatory demands decreases the contact time between the moist upper airway surfaces and the inhaled gas such that a significant concentration of even a very water-soluble gas may reach the distal lung. Another mechanism by which water-soluble toxic chemicals may penetrate more deeply into the respiratory tract is adsorption onto inhaled particulate matter such as in smoke.

The site of deposition of an aerosol, whether it consists of solid or liquid particles, is determined primarily by particle size. Particles larger than 10 microns in diameter mostly deposit in the nose, oropharynx, and larynx, while particles smaller than 3 microns tend to deposit in terminal lung units. Particles between 0.5 and 10 microns in diameter also will be deposited in the conducting airways. Particle size is not the only determinant of the toxic effect of inhaled particles. For example, acid aerosols are neutralized to some extent by the ammonia generated by oral bacteria, and smaller acid droplets, despite their greater ability to penetrate to the distal lung are more completely neutralized than larger droplets (1).

The toxicity of an inhaled material also is dependent on the varying susceptibility of different populations of respiratory tract cells to the effects of the material. Although ozone is a relatively water-insoluble gas and thus penetrates well into the distal lung, cells of the conducting airways clearly can be injured by inhalation of this gas. The underlying health of the exposed individual can be an important determinant of toxicity. Inhaled sulfur dioxide, which is largely absorbed onto the mucous membrane of the nose and throat because of its water solubility, causes bronchospasm in asthmatic individuals at relatively low concentrations.

MECHANISMS OF TOXICITY

The mechanisms by which inhaled materials can produce toxic effects include the following (Table 38.1): (a) simple asphyxiation due to replacement of atmospheric oxygen by other gases such as methane or nitrogen; (b) tissue asphyxia due to pulmonary absorption of agents capable of interfering with oxygen transport or poisoning cellular respiratory enzymes such as carbon monoxide or cyanide; (c) nonrespiratory effects due to pulmonary absorption of agents such as lead or hydrocarbon solvents; (d) excessive stimulation of physiologic responses by agents inhaled in concentrations below those required to cause morphologic evidence of injury; and (e) direct cellular injury. This chapter will focus only on the emergency medical management of pulmonary injury due to inhaled materials, i.e., toxic effects caused by the last two mechanisms listed above. Toxic effects caused by the first three mechanisms are treated elsewhere in this volume.

Cough, mucus secretion, bronchoconstriction, and perhaps even airway edema are normal physiologic responses to the inhalation of noxious materials. Afferent nerves in the airways which trigger the cough reflex can be stimulated directly by inhaled irritants or indirectly through the release of mediators such as histamine or prostaglandins (2). While the cough re-

Table 38.1. Toxicity from Inhaled Materials

Mechanism	Examples
Simple asphyxia	Nitrogen, methane (replacement of atmospheric oxygen)
Tissue asphyxia	Carbon monoxide, cyanide, hydrogen sulfide
Nonrespiratory effects due to pulmonary absorption	Hydrocarbon solvents, lead
Excessive stimulation of physiological responses	Formaldehyde, sulfur dioxide
Direct cellular injury	Ammonia, chlorine, nitrogen dioxide, phosgene

sponse is generally protective, prolonged or excessive stimulation of this response by inhaled materials can be a cause of significant morbidity in susceptible individuals. Inhalation of concentrations of irritants that cause little effect in most people may induce incapacitating cough in individuals with preexisting airway hyperresponsiveness due to asthma or recent viral upper respiratory infections. Stimulation of mucus secretion from submucosal glands and goblet cells by inhaled materials is another protective response of the airways which also can lead to significant morbidity (3). Hypertrophy of submucosal glands and goblet cell hyperplasia have been demonstrated in both rats and dogs following repeated exposures to sulfur dioxide (4, 5). So-called "benign mucus hypersecretion" or "industrial bronchitis" is common among individuals occupationally exposed to relatively low levels of irritant dusts, gases, fumes, or mists. Whether workers with mucus hypersecretion are at increased risk for the development of chronic airflow obstruction is a matter of current debate, but there are considerable data available to support such a position (6).

Bronchoconstriction is probably a normal response to the inhalation of noxious materials; it serves to protect the pulmonary parenchyma from excessive exposure. While some inhaled materials such as ozone only cause bronchoconstriction at concentrations that also are associated with direct epithelial injury, other materials such as cigarette smoke and sulfur dioxide appear to induce bronchoconstriction at concentrations well below those required to produce morphologic evidence of injury (7).

Airway edema is certainly a feature of direct epithelial injury due to inhaled materials. However, airway edema also may be produced by stimulation of an axonal reflex in airway afferent nerves by exposure to relatively low concentrations of an inhaled irritant (8). Low molecular weight peptides, known as tachykinins, are released from stimulated airway afferent nerves. These peptides cause vasodilation and increased vascular permeability of submucosal vessels (9). Inhaled cigarette smoke, formaldehyde, and toluene diisocyanate (TDI) have been shown to produce tachykinin-mediated airway edema.

Direct injury of the airway mucosa occurs when cytotoxic materials are inhaled at sufficiently high concentrations. Epithelial cell injury and death give rise to a number of effects which impact on a patient's respiratory status. Mucociliary clearance is markedly decreased, the normally tight intercellular junctions become porous (allowing the penetration of foreign material including bacteria), and sloughing of dead epithelial cells may cause mechanical obstruction of airway lumina. In addition, the release of a variety of cytokines and mediators by injured cells of the airway mucosa leads to local inflammation, edema, and constriction of airway smooth muscle. Thus, direct epithelial injury from higher concentrations of an inhaled toxic material amplifies the stimulation of physiologic responses that occurs at lower concentrations.

While much is known about the mechanisms of acute airway injury due to the inhalation of toxic materials, little is known about the possible longterm sequelae of such acute injury. It is clear that most persons who develop acute chemical bronchitis recover completely within a period of weeks, presumably due to the regeneration of a normal airway mucosa. However, a small percentage of persons may develop persistent airway hyperresponsiveness and even clinically significant asthma following a single, high intensity exposure to certain toxic materials. The risk factors for the development of this syndrome, which has been termed "reactive airways dysfunction syndrome" or RADS (10), are unknown, although cigarette smoking is suspected of being one such factor. The observation that many workers who develop TDI-induced occupational asthma have been exposed repeatedly to high concentrations of the material during accidental spills may be relevant to the development of an asthma-like syndrome following single massive exposures to isocyanates and other agents (11).

As described above, inhaled water-insoluble gases and small particles tend to penetrate to terminal lung units where they can cause injury to epithelial cells of the terminal and respiratory bronchioles and of the alveoli, pulmonary capillary endothelial cells, and alveolar macrophages. Also as described above, water-soluble gases can cause such pulmonary parenchymal injury if inhaled in sufficiently high concentrations. Type I alveolar epithelial cells are particularly susceptible to injury presumably due to their high surface area to volume ratio. Pulmonary parenchymal injury is characterized by diffuse bronchiolar obstruction due to edema and infiltration by inflammatory cells of bronchiolar walls and by alveolar flooding (pulmonary edema) due to increased permeability of both layers of the alveolar-capillary membrane. In addition, injury to alveolar macrophages may play a role in the frequent development of superimposed bacterial infection with chemical pneumonitis.

The delayed onset of symptoms and clinical findings that often occurs with chemical pneumonitis may be a result of injury to the alveolar-capillary membrane from inflammatory cells, such as polymorphonuclear leukocytes, recruited to the lungs, rather than from a direct effect of the inhaled material. While most persons appear to recover remarkably well from even severe chemical pneumonitis if they can be adequately supported through the acute phase of their illness, a small percentage will develop progressive inflammation and obliteration of distal airways, i.e., bronchiolitis obliterans, that can be responsible for considerable impairment.

SITE OF INJURY

Upper Airways

The nose, pharynx, and larynx are exposed to the highest concentrations of an inhaled gas and thus frequently bear the brunt of the injury (Table 38.2). In particular, water-soluble gases such as ammonia and chlorine are more likely to cause laryngeal edema and resultant upper airway obstruction than pulmonary parenchymal injury. These gases are capable of producing severe mucous membrane ulceration, hemorrhage, and edema. Although such physical evidence of chemical injury may be present early, it may take several hours for sufficient edema to develop to produce hoarseness and/or stridor. Chemical injury of the face, mouth, and throat may increase upper airway secretions and impair the ability to clear lower airway secretions. Generally, the greater the chemical injury of the upper airways, the greater the likelihood of concomitant chemical injury of the lower airways.

Lower Airways

Breath-holding and laryngospasm in response to irritation of the airways are protective mechanisms that occur in the conscious victim of a toxic inhalation. However, these mechanisms are not operative in the unconscious victim, so that more severe

Table 38.2.   Effects of Irritant Gas Inhalation

Site of Injury	Effects
Mucous membranes of the eyes, nose, and or-opharynx	Erythema Edema Ulcerations/hemorrhage Burns
Upper airways	Mucosal inflammation and/or burns Laryngeal obstruction
Lower airways	Tracheobronchitis Impairment of mucociliary clearance Bronchorrhea Mucosal sloughing Bronchoconstriction Airway edema Atelectasis
Pulmonary parenchyma	Pulmonary edema/ARDS Impaired bacterial clearance/pneumonia
Systemic effects (hydrogen fluoride)	Hypocalcemia, hypomagnesemia Methemoglobinemia (nitrogen dioxide)

injury to the lower airways (and pulmonary parenchyma) is likely to be present in such a setting.

The inhalation of many toxic materials will produce a severe tracheobronchitis (Table 38.2). Cilia become paralyzed, and the clearance of mucus and inhaled particles is reduced (12). Toxic chemicals adsorbed onto the surfaces of inhaled particles will have a greater opportunity to cause airway mucosal injury. Pathologic examination of tissue from fire victims who suffered chiefly from chemical injury to the respiratory tract has shown carbonaceous material (i.e., soot) with adsorbed toxic chemicals to be firmly adherent to the tracheobronchial mucosa (13).

A few hours after a severe chemical inhalation injury, one finds extensive but mild mucosal edema and scattered submucosal hemorrhage without ulceration. The victim may have minimum clinical signs or symptoms at this point. Later (8–48 hours postinhalation), progressive edema develops. A mucopurulent membrane subsequently develops on the mucosal surface. Bronchorrhea also may occur. At 48–72 hours postinhalation, if the injury is severe enough, sloughing of the tracheobronchial mucosa begins, yielding what has been described as a pseudomembranous tracheobronchitis (13). In this stage, expectoration of bronchial casts may be observed.

Even when direct injury to the lower airways is not severe, the stimulation of irritant receptors in the large airways may cause bronchoconstriction. When this effect is coupled with the peribronchial edema that occurs with more severe injury, significant airways obstruction is likely to develop. When sloughing of bronchial mucosa is also present, occlusion of central airways may cause significant atelectasis as well.

Pulmonary Parenchyma

Although less common than injury to the airways, chemical injury at the alveolar level due to the inhalation of toxic materials involves damage to both epithelial and endothelial membranes, resulting in increased permeability-induced edema (Table 38.2). The injury may range from mild interstitial edema to

progressive pulmonary insufficiency. Severe chemical pneumonitis caused by toxic inhalation can be considered a form of ARDS.

Experimental animal evidence confirms that increased pulmonary microvascular permeability to high molecular weight compounds is a feature of chemical pneumonitis (14, 15). While the mechanism(s) by which the increased permeability develops has not been completely defined, it is clear that alveolar flooding may occur even when pulmonary capillary hydrostatic pressure is normal. Because many victims of inhalation injury also have severe cutaneous burns and thus require large volumes of fluid replacement, the management of such patients can be difficult. In addition, there is some evidence that cutaneous burns even in the absence of inhalation injury may induce increased pulmonary capillary permeability (16).

Studies in dogs have demonstrated an immediate reduction in pulmonary surfactant after toxic inhalation (17). This may explain the early development of peripheral atelectasis in many victims of inhalation injury. Loss of surfactant also may play a role in the increased alveolar-capillary membrane permeability that characterizes chemical pneumonitis.

When the pulmonary parenchyma becomes edematous due to toxic inhalation injury, as in the other forms of ARDS, lung compliance decreases, the alveolar-arterial oxygen difference increases (due to shunting of blood away from damaged areas), and pulmonary vascular resistance increases.

The onset of pulmonary edema may be immediate if the injury is severe, although in most cases it is delayed 24–48 hours and may occur as late as one week postinhalation. Several investigators have found little evidence of pulmonary edema in animals who died shortly after smoke inhalation (18–20). Respiratory failure associated with radiographic infiltrates with an onset more than one week postinhalation is likely due to sepsis and/or bacterial pneumonia.

DIAGNOSIS

Due to the delayed onset of many of its clinical features, the early diagnosis of inhalation injury often proves difficult. Certain findings should lead one to suspect the presence of inhalation injury in a fire or environmental accident victim, including facial burns, inflamed nares, sputum production, and wheezing (Table 38.3). Victims of fires or explosions in enclosed spaces, where synthetic materials were burned or where irritating materials were released, should be suspected of having suffered inhalation injury. Because of the likelihood of increased exposure in the unconscious victim, neurologic status at the scene is an important determinant of the severity of lung injury. Firefighters and emergency medical technicians at the scene can often provide information as to how and where the victims were found.

Any fire or explosion victim with actual or suspected altered consciousness should be assumed to have carbon monoxide intoxication. The possibility of cyanide and hydrogen sulfide intoxication should be considered as well. Dizziness, headache, chest pain, nausea, and vomiting should suggest intoxication with a systemic poison capable of causing tissue asphyxia.

Chest radiographic and arterial blood gas values are often normal in the immediate postinhalation period and cannot be relied upon to clear a victim for discharge from an emergency room. A low oxyhemoglobin saturation in the face of a normal PaO_2 should alert one to the likelihood of carbon monoxide intoxication. Simple spirometry or peak expiratory flow rate

Table 38.3.   Action Criteria for Toxic Inhalation Injury

Criteria for transportation to the hospital

    Turned in an enclosed space
    Burning of synthetic material
    Altered mental status
    Facial burns
    Chest pain
    Age greater than 60

Criteria for admission to the hospital

    Altered mental status
    Any respiratory symptoms (i.e., cough, chest tightness, dyspnea)
    Hoarseness, wheezing
    History of ischemic heart disease or chronic obstructive
        pulmonary disease
    Elevated carboxyhemoglobin (greater than 20)

Criteria for admission to intensive care unit

    Depressed consciousness
    Abnormal arterial blood gases
    Abnormal electrocardiogram
    Hoarseness, wheezing
    Decreased peak expiratory flow rates or abnormal spirometry

Criteria for intubation

    Depressed consciousness
    Severe laryngeal obstruction
    Respiratory insufficiency by arterial blood gas measurement

measurements to detect early airway obstruction are often quite useful.

Carboxyhemoglobin saturation should be obtained in all fire or explosion victims. Elevated carboxyhemoglobin levels have been shown to correlate relatively well with the presence of both smoke inhalation injury (21) and concomitant elevated cyanide levels (22). Significant metabolic acidosis should also alert one to the possibility of cyanide or hydrogen sulfide intoxication.

Direct laryngoscopy or fiberoptic bronchoscopy has been advocated by some authors to be performed routinely in the setting of a significant inhalation injury. If laryngeal edema is present, these authors recommend prophylactic endotracheal intubation. However, whole some degree of laryngeal edema is common, most patients improve spontaneously and do not require intubation. Only a small percentage of victims with facial, nasal, and/or oropharyngeal burns (thermal or chemical) go on to develop life-threatening upper airway obstruction, and it is difficult to predict which patients are likely to have such an outcome. This author advocates careful clinical monitoring of fire and toxic inhalation victims, preferably in an intensive care setting, rather than routine laryngoscopy or bronchoscopy. These procedures can be quite uncomfortable when the mucosal surfaces of the nose, throat, and airways are inflamed.

If bronchoscopy is performed, evidence of inhalation injury includes erythema, edema, ulceration, and/or hemorrhage of the airway mucosa (23). If particulate material was inhaled, then its presence on the airway mucosa also may be seen. The presence of endobronchial polyps has been noted on occasion in patients with severe inhalation injury (24). It has been speculated that these polyps are the large airway correlates of the bronchiolitis obliterans which can develop in small airways after inhalation injury.

The results of early ventilation-perfusion lung scanning of victims of toxic inhalation injury have been used to predict subsequent respiratory complications (25). Flow-volume loops have been used both to diagnose upper airway obstruction and as a more sensitive detector of early lower airways obstruction than simple spirometry or peak expiratory flow rates (26, 27). Measurement of diffusing capacity has been suggested as a sensitive indicator of pulmonary parenchymal injury (24). Alveolar epithelial permeability by calculation of lung clearance of inhaled radiolabeled tracers has been used to quantitate the degree of lung injury in patients with ARDS and has been used experimentally in animals to characterize inhalation injury (28). Unfortunately, practical considerations of availability and/or patient ability to perform limit the clinical applicability of these more "sensitive" tests.

TREATMENT

Treatment at the scene of a fire or explosion should assume significant exposure to carbon monoxide and thus high flow (10–15 l/min) oxygen via face mask should be administered to most victims (Table 38.3). Administration of high concentrations of oxygen may cause persons with chronic obstructive pulmonary disease who chronically retain carbon dioxide to stop breathing. Thus, victims must be carefully observed during fire and explosion scene triage and transportation to the hospital. If a victim requires ventilatory support, 100% oxygen should be administered by positive pressure during transportation. Particular attention should be paid to profuse secretions in unconscious victims.

Fire, explosion, or environmental accident victims over the age of 40 years and those with frequent extrasystoles or tachycardia should be monitored via telemetry en route to the hospital. Because seizures may occur as a result of hypoxemia or systemic intoxication with carbon monoxide, cyanide, or hydrogen sulfide, one must be prepared for this complication.

Any victim at the scene observed to have evidence of inhalation injury should be taken to a hospital emergency room for evaluation. At the hospital, the initial history should include a concerted effort to determine the type of materials burned or inhaled and the intensity of exposure. The oral and nasal mucosal membranes should be examined for injury, and concurrent skin burns, even if relatively slight, should not be overlooked. Because of the potential for central nervous system effects from toxic chemical inhalation, a mental status evaluation should always be performed, even in fully ambulatory victims.

All fire or toxic inhalation victims with mental status abnormalities should be hospitalized for at least 24 hours of observation even if they are otherwise without symptoms or signs. Asymptomatic fire victims with a high probability of smoke inhalation injury (i.e., those with facial, nasal, or oral burns; those with significantly elevated carboxyhemoglobulin levels; and those with histories of exposure to toxic fumes or in confined spaces) also should be observed for at least 24 hours. The following parameters should be monitored: vital signs, including respiratory rate; central nervous system status; degree of airway obstruction (serial spirometry or peak expiratory flow rate measurements are better than the stethoscope); arterial blood gases; chest radiograph; and electrocardiogram and cardiac monitoring in patients over 40 years, with chest pain, or with irregular heart rates.

Supportive treatment of victims with evidence of inhalation injury at the time of admission should include: (a) maintenance of an adequate airway; (b) removal of mucus and debris from the tracheobronchial tree; (c) reversal of airflow obstruction; and (d) correction of hypoxemia.

Early intubation may be critical to prevent rapid asphyxia due to upper airway obstruction. A victim of a toxic inhalation with stridor, hoarseness, or severe facial/nasal/oral injuries should be closely monitored with arterial blood gases for respiratory insufficiency, and intubated if necessary. Tracheostomy is rarely required initially and should not be done through burn tissue because of the substantial risk of infection, both in the wound and in the airway.

The severe tracheobronchitis that develops in many patients with inhalation injury requires vigorous bronchial hygiene measures. Adequate hydration, deep inspiratory maneuvers, postural drainage, and chest physical therapy may help promote drainage of mucus plugs and secretions. Frequent suctioning of intubated patients with smoke inhalation injury is a way to debride the airways of the adherent soot that may contain irritant and corrosive chemicals. Some authors have advocated the use of fiberoptic bronchoscopy as a treatment as well as a diagnostic modality in the management of smoke inhalation injury in order to facilitate the removal of adherent soot by lavage (29).

Bronchospasm should be treated with the usual agents as if for acute asthma, except that corticosteroids should be reserved for obstructed patients unresponsive to bronchodilators. Corticosteroids may reduce lung bacterial clearance (30), and sustained use may increase the risk of opportunisitic infection (31).

Hypoxemia can usually be corrected by the administration of oxygen when not complicated by carbon monoxide intoxication. Hypoxemia not corrected by bronchial hygiene measures, bronchodilators, and supplemental oxygen suggests the presence of severe pulmonary parenchymal injury.

Supportive care of patients with severe parenchymal injury which is evolving into ARDS is critical. Mechanical ventilation with positive end-expiratory pressure (PEEP) is usually required to correct hypoxemia with sufficiently low concentrations of supplemental oxygen to avoid oxygen toxicity. Monitoring of pulmonary hemodynamics, cardiac output, and blood gases must supplement the use of formulas in the determination of intravenous fluid replacement in the patient with severe cutaneous burns in order to avoid exacerbation of alveolar flooding.

The use of corticosteroids in the treatment of toxic inhalation injury remains controversial. While some authors have advocated prophylactic corticosteroid therapy to reduce parenchymal inflammation and subsequent fibrosis (32), others have noted increased infectious complications with their use (31, 33). In an animal model of acrolein-induced inhalation injury, the administration of methylprednisone 30 minutes after exposure reduced mortality but was not associated with amelioration of histologic evidence of lung damage (34). The methylprednisone-treated animals had improved survival despite showing more pulmonary vascular congestion than was seen in the control animals. This study confirmed earlier observations and suggests a possible role for steroids in the management of inhalation injury. However, because of the apparent increased risk of pneumonia associated with administration of steroids in patients with inhalation injury, their routine use cannot be recommended.

Pneumonia is the most common late complication in patients with inhalation injury. It can result from either aspiration of microorganisms or hematogenous dissemination from contaminated wounds. Since fever and leukocytosis may be present after inhalation injury in the absence of infection, repeated examination of gram-stained sputum is necessary, and cultures should be obtained if the flora changes. Prophylactic use of antibiotics has not been demonstrated to be of benefit in patients with inhalation injury (31).

PROGNOSIS

The mortality rate from smoke inhalation injury without concomitant severe burns ranges from 5–10%. However, with severe cutaneous burns the mortality rate increases to from 49–80% (18). The cause of this high mortality for combined injury remains unclear. It is likely that the risk of developing ARDS in these patients is determined by the degree of damage to the alveolar epithelium from toxic gas inhalation and to the pulmonary capillary endothelium secondary to complement activation and platelet/leukocyte aggregation (15). As noted above, severely burned patients with inhalation injury often require large volumes of fluid replacement. The inability of their more permeable alveolar-capillary membranes to handle the replaced fluid also may contribute to the high mortality.

Age is a major risk factor for mortality from inhalation injury (35–37). The physiologic stress of inhalation injury is probably less well-tolerated in older persons, who are more likely to have a preexisting cardiopulmonary disorder. An analysis of hospitalized burn patients who were over the age of 60 found that: (a) the cause of death frequently was pneumonia in patients who died but did not have burns over a large surface area; (b) once pneumonia developed, death was almost an invariable outcome; and (c) the mean fluid requirement to maintain adequate vital signs was less for survivors than for those who died (35). An aging cardiovascular system burdened with increased alveolar-capillary permeability due to inhalation injury and/or to severe cutaneous burns is easily pushed into pulmonary edema, which compromises gas exchange and can lead to pneumonia. Patients with inhalation injury are already at increased risk for pneumonia by virtue of their bronchorrhea and impaired respiratory defense mechanisms. Pneumonia is poorly tolerated by elderly patients even in the absence of inhalation injury.

In addition to severity of concomitant cutaneous burns and age, the presence of facial burns (even when the total body surface area burned is small) and elevated carboxyhemoglobin levels (greater than 15% saturation) also have been associated with high rates of inhalation injury and mortality (21, 38).

Because it is difficult to assemble and to study a cohort of patients with inhalation injury that is of sufficient size, there are few data on longterm follow-up of such patients. Anecdotal reports of victims who developed chronic sequelae such as bronchiolitis obliterans and bronchiectasis have existed for some time (39, 40). More recently, persistence of airway hyperresponsiveness and an asthma-like syndrome have been anecdotally reported (10, 41, 42).

One study did systematically characterize the pulmonary function of fire victims immediately after injury and sequentially during treatment and recovery (43). The results of this study confirmed that the incidence of respiratory complications in fire victims is related to the severity of cutaneous burns and the presence or absence of smoke inhalation. Smoke inhalation caused severe airway obstruction in most patients by 9 hours after exposure. Patients with cutaneous burns tended to develop a significant restrictive ventilatory defect over the first several days which correlated with the surface area of the burns, whether or not the chest was burned, the degree of fluid retention, and the reduction in colloid osmotic pressure. As expected, the combination of surface burns and smoke inhalation was associated with the greatest deterioration in pulmonary function. While most parameters of pulmonary function gradually improved over the 5 months following injury, there was still some evidence of mild airways obstruction at this point in those subjects who had sustained smoke inhalation.

The paucity of data regarding follow-up of fire victims leads one to turn to studies of firefighters with repeated occupational inhalation of smoke. It is clear that routine firefighting is associated with acute decrements in pulmonary function (44, 45) and increased airway responsiveness (45, 46). The persistence of these decrements in some firefighters (45, 47) and the apparent increased prevalence of airway hyperresponsiveness among firefighters (48) suggest that inhalation of toxic combustion products may lead to chronic airway inflammation. Of course, the relationship between the effects of recurrent occupational exposure of firefighters and the effects of single massive toxic gas exposures is problematic.

There are data collected in follow-up of victims of massive exposure to chlorine (49, 50) and sulfur dioxide (51) which tend to show a progressive decline in pulmonary function for the first 6 months after exposure. Beyond this point, there usually is either a lack of further deterioration or even a gradual improvement in pulmonary function. However, a persistent restrictive ventilatory impairment and increased airway responsiveness may be present years after inhalation injury in a small minority of patients (50, 51).

SPECIFIC EXAMPLES OF IRRITANT GASES

Ammonia

Ammonia (HN_3) is a highly irritating, highly water-soluble gas which is colorless but with a distinctive odor. It is used extensively as a refrigerant and in the manufacture of plastics, explosives, fertilizers, and pharmaceuticals. Accidental industrial exposure to ammonia usually occurs after rupture of a tank or pipeline (52–54). Transportation accidents have resulted in large scale environmental exposures to ammonia gas (55).

Because ammonia is highly water-soluble, it can cause extensive damage to mucous membranes of the eyes, nose, oropharynx, larynx, and tracheobronchial tree. Ammonia and water combine to form ammonium hydroxide which dissociates to ammonium (NH_4+) and hydroxyl ($OH-$) ions. The latter cause a severe alkaline burn characterized by liquefaction necrosis. In addition, ammonia gas releases heat as it dissolves and is thus capable of causing thermal injury (56).

Exposure to high concentrations of ammonia produces severe burns of the cornea and upper airway. Death may result from acute laryngeal edema (52, 53, 56). Diffuse tracheobronchitis with severe bronchoconstriction and bronchorrhea is a common feature of ammonia inhalation. Mild cases present with inflamed mucous membranes and a normal chest exam. Moderate cases present with wheezing, rhonchi, productive cough, and burns of the cornea, nose, and mouth. Severe cases present in respiratory distress, with blood-tinged sputum, stridor, pulmonary edema, and burns of the upper airway. Severity of inhalation injury relates to both the concentration of the gas and the duration of exposure.

Victims of ammonia exposure require prompt decontamination of eyes and skin, as well as aggressive airway management. Because ammonia tends to cause more airway than parenchymal injury, chest radiographic findings correlate poorly with degree of respiratory distress. Signs of improvement are generally apparent within 48–72 hours of admission, and most patients recover without significant residual impairment. However, anecdotal reports of bronchiectasis and bronchiolitis obliterans exist (54, 55). One case of severe ammonia inhalation injury requiring intubation and mechanical ventilatory support during the acute phase was reported to have been followed by a persistent asthma-like syndrome and airway hyperresponsiveness (57).

Chlorine

Chlorine is an irritant gas which is somewhat less water-soluble than ammonia. It is used widely as a bleaching agent, as a disinfectant, and in the manufacture of many chemicals, plastics, and resins. Chlorine is often transported and stored under pressure in pipes, trucks, or tanks, and exposure occurs during industrial or transportation accidents (49, 58), as a result of mixing chlorine bleach with an acid cleaner (59), or during cylinder changes at swimming pools (60). Chlorine toxicity appears to be mediated both by the evolution of hydrogen chloride upon contact with moist mucous membranes and by the generation of free radicals at the cellular level (61). The oxidant effect of chlorine is thought to be the explanation for the fact that it is approximately 20 times more toxic to the respiratory tract than hydrogen chloride alone.

Because chlorine is less water-soluble than ammonia, inhalation injury due to chlorine is characterized by relatively less upper airway and more parenchymal injury than that due to ammonia. Still, chlorine exposure does cause significant local irritation to mucous membranes. Substernal, burning chest pain and paroxysmal cough are frequent features of chlorine inhalation injury. Headache is also a common complaint. High-intensity exposure can lead to respiratory distress and pulmonary edema. Chest radiographic findings tend to lag somewhat behind the course of the clinical presentation. Pulmonary function tends to be abnormal following chlorine exposure even if pulmonary edema is not clinically evident (49, 58). Typically, both airway obstruction and significant air trapping are found in the immediate postexposure period (49). Over time, pulmonary function tends to improve, although some persons may be left with a residual restrictive ventilatory impairment with increased lung elastic recoil and/or airway hyperresponsiveness (50).

Nitrogen Dioxide

Nitrogen dioxide (NO_2) is a relatively water-insoluble gas that is reddish brown in color. It is encountered in grain storage silos (62), welding (63), combustion of fuels or nitrogen-containing materials (64), production and use of nitrate explosives (63), and handling of rocket fuel oxidizers (65). Because nitrogen dioxide is relatively insoluble in water, there is little absorption by, and irritation of, the mucous membranes of the eyes, nose, and throat. Thus, persons inhaling even high concentrations of nitrogen dioxide may not become immediately aware of their exposure. Again because of its lack of water solubility, inhaled nitrogen dioxide penetrates well to the pulmonary parenchyma where it causes oxidant injury to terminal bronchioles and to both endothelial and epithelial layers of the alveolar-capillary membrane (66–69).

The onset of respiratory symptoms following inhalation of nitrogen dioxide is typically delayed for several hours to up to 30 hours. Cough, dyspnea, fever, and leukocytosis are common clinical features of nitrogen dioxide inhalation injury. As with chlorine, chest radiographs may be normal on clinical presentation but usually progress to show evidence of pulmonary edema. Most victims of nitrogen dioxide inhalation who can be adequately supported throughout the initial acute injury will recover completely, but a few patients go on to develop a late phase of illness 2–6 weeks later. This late phase is characterized by progressive dyspnea, fever, and patchy infiltrates on chest radiographs (70). The mechanism of the late phase of nitrogen dioxide inhalation injury is not understood. Anecdotal reports suggest that treatment with corticosteroids may be beneficial, although no data from controlled clinical trials are available (62, 63, 65, 71, 72). Bronchiolitis obliterans has been described following nitrogen dioxide inhalation injury, but it is not clear that all cases with late phase illness are due to bronchiolitis (73). The likelihood of developing late phase illness does not appear to be related to the severity of the initial illness.

Inhalation of nitrogen dioxide also may lead to the generation of methemoglobin (74, 75), which can complicate hypoxemia due to pulmonary injury by adding an impairment of oxygen transport to extrapulmonary tissues.

SUMMARY

Victims of fires and industrial/environmental accidents may suffer inhalational exposure to a number of agents, including hot air, carbon monoxide, hydrogen cyanide, hydrogen sulfide, and various irritant gases. Victims of fires in enclosed spaces, where synthetic materials were burned or where there was an explosion should be suspected of having sustained inhalation injury. Carbon monoxide intoxication is the most immediate cause of death in fire victims and 100% oxygen should be administered as soon as possible at the scene of the fire. The possibility of cyanide intoxication, especially if plastic materials burned, should be considered as well. Measurement of carboxyhemoglobin is important since a high level increases the likelihood of both pulmonary inhalation injury and cyanide intoxication. The effects of irritant gas exposure depend on the water solubility of the gas inhaled. Water-soluble gases such as ammonia and formaldehyde primarily cause upper airway inflammation, while relatively insoluble compounds such as nitrogen dioxide and phosgene exert their effects primarily on the pulmonary parenchyma. Patients with suspected inhalation injury should be admitted to an intensive care unit for close monitoring of their respiratory status. Intubation may be required early in the clinical course because of life-threatening upper airway obstruction or pulmonary edema. Obstruction of the lower airways should be treated with bronchodilators and efforts to promote clearance of sputum and debris. Careful fluid management is of critical importance in patients with inhalation injury, especially in those who have concomitant extensive skin burns because of the likely presence of increased alveolar-capillary membrane permeability. Treatment with corticosteroids to prevent noncardiogenic pulmonary edema (ARDS) is not supported by data from controlled clinical trials. Patients who develop pulmonary edema will require vigorous respiratory supportive care and invasive hemodynamic monitoring.

REFERENCES

1. Larson TV, Covert DS, Frank R, Charlson RJ. Ammonia in the human airways: neutralization of inspired acid sulfate aerosols. Science 1977;197:161–163.
2. Coleridge HM, Coleridge JCG, Ginzel KN, Baker DG, Banzett RB, Morrison MA. Stimulation of ''irritant'' receptors and afferent C-fibers in the lung by prostaglandins. Nature 1976;264:451–452.
3. Nadel JA. Regulation of bronchial secretions. In: Newball HH, ed. Immunopharmacology of the lung. New York: Marcel Dekker, 1983:109–139.
4. Reid L. An experimental study of hypersecretion of mucus in the bronchial tree. Br J Exp Pathol 1963;44:437–445.
5. Scanlon PD, Seltzer J, Ingram RH, Reid L, Drazen JM. Chronic exposure to sulfur dioxide: physiologic and histologic evaluation of dog exposure to 50 or 15 ppm. Am Rev Respir Dis 1987;135:831–839.
6. Becklake MR. Chronic airflow limitation: its relationship to work in dusty occupations. Chest 1985;88:608–617.
7. Nadel JA, Salem H, Tamplin B, Tokiwa G. Mechanism of bronchoconstriction during inhalation of sulfur dioxide. J Appl Physiol 1965;20:164–167.
8. Lundberg JM, Saria A. Capsaicin-induced desensitization of the airway mucosa to cigarette smoke, mechanical and chemical irritants. Nature 1983;302:251–253.
9. Lundberg JM, Brodin E, Saria A. Effects and distribution of vagal capsaicin sensitive neurons with special reference to the trachea and lungs. Acta Physiol Scand 1983;119:243–252.
10. Brooks SM, Weiss MA, Bernstein IL. Reactive airways dysfunction syndrome (RADS): persistent asthma syndrome after high level irritant exposure. Chest 1985;88:376–384.
11. Moller DR, Brooks SM, McKay RT, Cassedy K, Kopp S, Bernstein IL. Chronic asthma due to toluene diisocyanate. Chest 1986;90:494–499.
12. Loke J, Paul E, Virgulto JA, Smith GJW. Rabbit lung after acute smoke inhalation: cellular response and scanning electron microscopy. Arch Surg 1984;199:956–959.
13. Chu C-S. New concepts of pulmonary burn injury. J Trauma 1981;21:958–961.
14. Rowland RRR, Yamaguchi K, Santibanez AS, Kodama KT, Ness VT, Grubbs DE. Smoke inhalation model for lung permeability studies. J Trauma 1986;26:153–156.
15. Till GO, Johnson KJ, Kunkel R, Ward PA. Intravascular activation of complement and acute lung injury. J Clin Invest 1982;69:1126–1135.
16. Till GO, Beauchalp C, Menapace D, et al. Oxygen radical dependent lung damage following thermal injury on rat skin. J Trauma 1983; 23:269–277.
17. Nieman GF, Clark WR Jr, Wax SD, Webb WR. The effect of smoke inhalation on pulmonary surfactant. Ann Surg 1980;191:171–181.
18. Zawacki BE, Jung RC, Joyce J, Rincon E. Smoke, burns, and the natural history of inhalation injury in fire victims: a correlation of experimental and clinical data. Ann Surg 1977;185:100–110.
19. Stephenson SF, Esrig BC, Polk HC, Fulton RL. The pathophysiology of smoke inhalation injury. Ann Surg 1975;182:652–660.
20. Dressler DP, Skornik WA, Kupersmith S. Corticosteroid treatment of experimental smoke inhalation. Ann Surg 1976;183:46–52.
21. Zikria BA, Budd DC, Floch F, Ferrer JM. What is clinical smoke poisoning. Ann Surg 1975;181:151–156.
22. Clark CJ, Campbell D, Reid WH. Blood carboxyhemoglobin and cyanide levels in fire survivors. Lancet 1981;1:1332–1335.
23. Hunt JL, Agec RN, Pruitt BA Jr. Fiberoptic bronchoscopy in acute inhalation injury. J Trauma 1975;15:641–649.
24. Williams DO, Vanecko RM, Glassroth J. Endobronchial polyposis following smoke inhalation. Chest 1983;84:774–776.
25. Moylan JA, Wilmore DW, Mouton DE, Pruitt BA. Early diagnosis of inhalation injury using 133 xenon lung scan. Ann Surg 1972;176:477–484.
26. Petroff PA, Hander EW, Clayton WH, Pruitt BA. Pulmonary function studies after smoke inhalation. Am J Surg 1976;132:346–351.
27. Haponik EF, Meyers DA, Munster AM, et al. Acute upper airway injury in burn patients: serial changes of flowvolume curves and nasopharyngoscopy. Am Rev Respir Dis 1987;135:360–366.
28. Mason GR, Effros RM, Uszler JM, Mena I. Small solute clearance from the lungs of patients with cardiogenic and noncardiogenic pulmonary edema. Chest 1985;88:327–334.
29. Clark CJ, Reid WH, Telfer ABM, Campbell D. Respiratory injury in the burned patient: the role of flexible bronchoscopy. Anaesthesia 1983;38:35–39.
30. Skornik WA, Dressler DP. The effects of short-term steroid therapy in lung bacterial clearance and survival in rats. Ann Surg 1974;179:415–421.
31. Levine BA, Petroff PA, Slade CL, Pruitt BA. Prospective trials of dexamethasone and aerosolized gentamicin in the treatment of inhalation injury in the burned patient. J Trauma 1978;18:188–193.

32. Welch GW, Lull RJ, Petroff PA, Hander EW, McLeod CG, Clayton WH. The use of steroids in inhalation injury. Surg Gynecol Obstet 1977;145:539–544.

33. Moylan JA, Chan C. Inhalation injury—an increasing problem. Ann Surg 1978;188:34–37.

34. Beeley JM, Crow J, Jones JG, Minty B, Lynch RD, Pryce DP. Mortality and lung histopathology after inhalation lung injury: The effect of corticosteroids. Am Rev Respir Dis 1986;133:191–196.

35. Anous M, Heimbach DM. Causes of death and predictors in burned patients more than 60 years of age. J Trauma 1986;26:135–139.

36. Thompson PB, Herndon DN, Traber DL, et al. Effect on mortality of inhalation injury. J Trauma 1986;26:163–165.

37. Clark CJ, Reid WH, Gilmour WH, Campbell D. Mortality probability in victims of fire trauma: revised equation to include inhalation injury. Br Med J 1986; 1:1303–1305.

38. Wroblewski DA, Bower GC. The significance of facial burns in acute smoke inhalation. Crit Care Med 1979;7:335–338.

39. Donnellan WI, Poticha SM, Hallinger PM. Management and complications of severe pulmonary burn. JAMA 1965;194:1323–1325.

40. Perez-Guerra F, Walsh RE, Sagel SS. Bronchiolitis obliterans and tracheal stenosis: late complications of inhalation burn. JAMA 1971;218:1568–1570.

41. Boulet L-P. Increases in airway responsiveness following acute exposure to respiratory irritants. Chest 1988;94:476–481.

42. Tarlo SM, Broder I. Irritant-induced occupational asthma. Chest 1989;96:297–300.

43. Whitener DR, Whitener LM, Robertson KJ, Baxter CR, Pierce AK. Pulmonary function measurements in patients with thermal injury and smoke inhalation. Am Rev Respir Dis 1980;122:731–739.

44. Musk AW, Smith JT, Peters JM, McLaughlin E. Pulmonary function in firefighters: acute changes in ventilatory capacity and their correlates. Br J Ind Med 1979;36:29–34.

45. Sheppard D, Distefano S, Morse L, Becker CE. Acute effects of routine firefighting on lung function. Am J Ind Med 1986;9:333–340.

46. Sherman CB, Barnhart S, Miller MF, et al. Firefighting acutely increases airway responsiveness. Am Rev Respir Dis 1989;140:185–190.

47. Loke J, Farmer W, Matthay RA, Putnam CE, Smith GJW. Acute and chronic effects of firefighting on pulmonary function. Chest 1980;77:369–373.

48. Niederman MS, Abrams C, Virgulto JA, et al. Increase in bronchial reactivity of firefighters with normal lung function. Am Rev Respir Dis 1981;123:488–491.

49. Charan NB, Lakshinarayan S, Myers CG, Smith DD. Effects of accidental chlorine inhalation on pulmonary function. West J Med 1985;143:333–336.

50. Schwartz DA, Smith DD, Lakshinaryan S. The pulmonary sequelae associated with accidental inhalation of chlorine gas. Chest 1990;97:820–825.

51. Harkonen H, Nordman H, Korhonen O, Winblad I. Long-term effects of exposure to sulfur dioxide. Am Rev Respir Dis 1983;128:890–893.

52. Close LG, Catlin FI, Cohn AM. Acute and chronic effects of ammonia burns of the respiratory tract. Arch Otolaryngol 1980;106:151–158.

53. Walton M. Industrial ammonia gassing. Br J Ind Med 1973;30:78–86.

54. Sobonya R. Fatal anhydrous ammonia inhalation. Hum Pathol 1977;8:293–299.

55. Kass I, Zamal N, Dobry CA, Holzer M. Bronchiectasis following ammonia burns of the respiratory tract. Chest 1972;62:282–285.

56. O'Kane GJ. Inhalation of ammonia vapor. Anaesthesia 1983;38:1208–1213.

57. Flury KE, Dines DE, Rodarte JR, Rodgers R. Airway obstruction due to inhalation of ammonia. Mayo Clin Proc 1983;58:389–393.

58. Weill H, George R, Schwartz M, Ziskind M. Late evaluation of pulmonary function after acute exposure to chlorine gas. Am Rev Respir Dis 1969;99:374–379.

59. Murphy DMF, Fairman RP, Lapp NL, Morgan WKC. Severe airway disease due to inhalation of fumes from cleaning agents. Chest 1976;69:372–376.

60. Decker WJ, Koch HF. Chlorine poisoning at a swimming pool: an overlooked hazard. Clin Toxicol 1978;13:377–381.

61. Adelson L, Kaufman J. Fatal chlorine poisoning: report of two cases with clinicopathologic correlation. Am J Clin Pathol 1971;56:430–442.

62. Lowery T, Shuman LM. Silo fillers disease—a syndrome caused by nitrogen dioxide. JAMA 1956;162:153–160.

63. Jones GR, Proudfoot AT, Hall JI. Pulmonary effects of acute exposure to nitrous fumes. Thorax 1973;28:61–65.

64. Nichols BH. The clinical effects of inhalation of nitrogen dioxide. Am J Roentgenol 1930;23:516–520.

65. Yockey CC, Eden BM, Byrd RB. The McConnell missile accident: clinical spectrum of nitrogen dioxide exposure. JAMA 1980;244:1221–1223.

66. Guidotti TL. Toxic inhalation of nitrogen dioxide: morphologic and functional changes. Exp Mol Pathol 1980;33:90–103.

67. Sherwin RP, Richters V. Lung capillary permeability—nitrogen dioxide exposure and leakage of tritiated serum. Arch Intern Med 1971;128:61–68.

68. Pickrell JA, Hahn FF, Rebar AH, et al. Pulmonary effects of exposure to 20 ppm NO_2. Chest 1981;80:50S–52S.

69. DeNicola DB, Rebar AH, Henderson RF. Early indicators of lung damage: V. Biochemical and cytological response to NO_2 inhalation. Toxicol Appl Pharmacol 1981;60:301–312.

70. Becklake MR, Goldman KI, Boxman AR, Freed C. The longterm effects of exposure to nitrous fumes. Am Rev Tuberc 1957;76:398–409.

71. Horvath EP, do Pico GA, Barbee RA, Dickie HA. Nitrogen dioxide induced pulmonary disease. J Occup Med 1978;20:103–110.

72. Ramirez J, Dowell AR. Silo filler's disease: nitrogen dioxide induced lung injury—longterm follow-up and review of the literature. Ann Intern Med 1971;74:569–576.

73. Milne JEH. Nitrogen dioxide inhalation and bronchiolitis obliterans. J Occup Med 1969;11:538–547.

74. Clutton-Brock J. Two cases of poisoning by contamination of nitrous oxide with higher oxides of nitrogen during anesthesia. Br J Anaesth 1967;39:388–392.

75. Prys-Roberts C. Principles of treatment of poisoning by higher oxides of nitrogen. Br J Anaesth 1967;39:432–438.

39

Acute Ocular Injury from Hazardous Materials

Steven M. Chernow, M.D.

INTRODUCTION

The spectrum of ocular injuries from hazardous materials ranges from minor irritation to binocular blindness. Ocular damage may result from either direct contact with an agent or the effects of systemically absorbed materials (1, 2).

Chemical eye injuries occur both at home and in the workplace. The incidence and epidemiology of these injuries depends on the specific setting (3–5). In a review of cases referred to a regional poison center, 84% occurred at home and 55% of these cases were caused from an alkaline substance. Approximately 10% of all industrial eye injuries involve chemical agents (6). While representing only a small percentage of total industrial eye trauma, chemical burns account for a significant percentage of severe and disabling injuries (7, 8). Despite efforts at prevention, acute chemical ocular injuries continue to occur and require emergent recognition and management.

ANATOMY AND PHYSIOLOGY

The anatomic landmarks of the anterior eye are illustrated in Fig. 39.1. The globe consists of an outer, middle, and inner layer (9). The outer later consists of an opaque, dense sclera which forms the white of the eye. A bulbar conjunctiva covers the lower and upper lids. The remaining element in the outer layer is the transparent cornea. The cornea consists of an epithelial layer, a cellular structure or stroma, and an endothelial layer. The epithelium is 5–6 cells in thickness and protects the anterior stroma of the cornea. Tight junctions of the epithelial cells serve as a barrier to water-soluble compounds and ions. However, lipid-soluble compounds pass readily through the epithelium, because the epithelial cell membranes are composed of lipoproteins. Damaged epithelium allows water-soluble compounds to readily pass. The stroma of the cornea composes 90% of the corneal thickness and is permeable to water-soluble compounds. If destroyed, scarring and irregularities result. The endothelium consists of a single layer of cells and does not regenerate in adults. The cornea and sclera join at the limbus and contain the canal of Schlemm, the drainage system for aqueous fluid.

The middle coat, or uvea, contains the choroid, ciliary bodies, and the iris. The iris rests anterior to the lens and separates the anterior chamber from the posterior chamber. Aqueous humor is secreted by the ciliary process and flows from the posterior chamber through the pupil into the anterior chamber and is drained by the canal of Schlemm. The third coat of the eye is the inner coat and consists of the retina.

PATHOPHYSIOLOGY

The eye is susceptible to damage from contact with many chemicals (1, 10). Splash injuries represent the most common cause of chemical ocular accidents. These may be characterized by the chemical nature of the substance and the resulting ocular injury (Table 39.1). Severe ocular injuries generally result from exposure to alkalis or acids. Hydrocarbons used as solvents frequently cause immediate ocular discomfort with limited corneal damage. While the above agents result in ocular damage based primarily on their physical properties, other chemicals such as formaldehyde and rare earth salts may bind or react chemically with tissue to produce delayed corneal damage. Still other agents act mainly as sensitizing compounds. Many gases and vapors induce a lacrimatory response and may or may not react chemically and lead to ocular damage. Ocular injuries may also occur as a result of particulate matter such as from fibers and dust.

The corneal epithelium and endothelium act as a barrier to water-soluble substances while the corneal stroma inhibits passage of lipid-soluble agents. Chemicals that are both water- and lipid-soluble have the greatest penetration and potential to produce severe tissue injury.

Alkalis

Alkali burns represent some of the most devastating chemical injuries and have received the greatest attention in the medical literature. The severity of the chemical burn is related to the concentration, amount, duration of exposure, cation, and inherent toxicity of the substance (11, 12). Alkaline substances react with cell membranes to cause saponification and lysis, resulting in rapid epithelial destruction and allowing additional alkaline to penetrate and damage the corneal stroma as well as structures of the anterior chamber. The early disruption of the corneal epithelium explains why alkalis rapidly penetrate and involve deeper structures of the eye (13). Differences in penetration rates are also based on the cations involved. Ammonium hydroxide penetrates fastest, followed by sodium hydroxide, potassium hydroxide, and finally calcium hydroxide (Table 39.2) (1).

In a rabbit model, the corneal stroma was resistant to significant damage at pH values as high as 11; however, at pH values of 12 or greater severe corneal stromal injury occurred (14). Ocular alkali burns cause the pH in the anterior chamber to rapidly rise and damage adjacent structures such as the iris, lens, ciliary bodies, and trabecular meshwork (15). Intraocular pressure also acutely rises (16, 17).

Mild burns may result in limited damage isolated to the corneal epithelium whereas more significant burns will result in ischemia and coagulation necrosis. Resulting inflammation may lead to fibrosis and opacification. Secondary glaucoma may also occur if damage to the trabecular meshwork results.

Ammonia is a colorless gas used in fertilization, refrigeration, and the chemical industry (10). It may be liquefied under pressure and readily combines with water to form ammonium hydroxide. Concentrations range from industrial strength of 28% to household solutions of 7%. Aqueous solutions of ammonium hydroxide are highly soluble in both

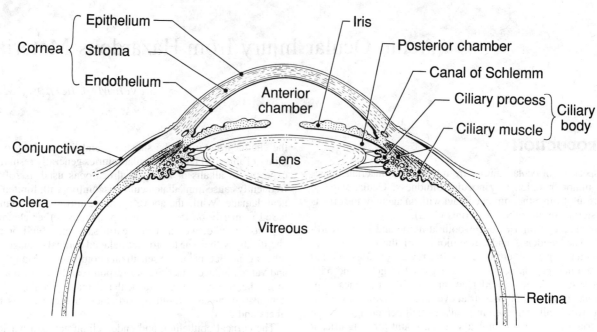

Figure 39.1. Anatomy of the anterior eye.

Table 39.1 Classification of Ocular Toxic Substances

Classification	Mechanism of Injury	Severity of Injury	Prognosis
Caustic			
Alkalis, acids	Physical damage to cornea and anterior chambers	Severe	Guarded
Hydrocarbons			
Inert solvents	Physical damage to corneal epithelium	Mild	Excellent
Organically reactive	Chemical alteration of cellular structures; alkalization	Moderate to severe	Guarded
Metals			
Organically inert	Foreign body reaction	Mild	Good
Organically active	Damage to enzymes and proteins	Severe	Guarded
Nonmetals	Direct corneal damage	Varied	Mixed
Inorganic agents	Damage to enzymes	Varied	Mixed
Sensitizing agents	Autoimmune	Mild	Good

water and lipid. Penetration into the anterior chamber may occur in less than 1 minute (1, 18). The rapid penetration of ammonium hydroxide through the corneal epithelium accounts for the severe ocular tissue damage resulting from contact with this agent.

Sodium hydroxide (lye, caustic soda) is found in many industrial and household cleaning products. Ocular contact results in significant injury (19). The penetration rate in ocular injury resulting from sodium hydroxide is second only to that of ammonium hydroxide. Potassium hydroxide (caustic potash) penetrates the eye slightly slower than sodium hydroxide and produces similar injuries.

Calcium hydroxide (lime) and calcium oxide (quick lime) are used to make plaster, cement, and mortar. Many accidents occur from splash injuries with these substances. Calcium oxide reacts on contact with water to produce calcium hydroxide. Calcium hydroxide penetrates slowly through the epithelium compared with other alkalis. The formation of insoluble calcium soaps with the epithelial cell membrane is believed to explain their relative slow penetration. The particulate matter frequently associated with these injuries has received much attention and is discussed later under the treatment of these injuries.

Organic amines are alkaline compounds that may produce damage to the eye on contact. Certain aliphatic amines cause ocular damage because of their alkaline and fat-soluble properties, while other organic amines act primarily as sensitizing agents (1).

Acids

Acid burns of the eye occur slightly less frequently than alkaline burns. In contrast to alkalis, acids coagulate the protein of the corneal epithelium to form a relative barrier to further penetration of the acid. This explains why acid burns generally produce less severe injuries than alkaline burns (20). The extent of tissue damage depends on the particular acid involved, the concentration, and the time of exposure. With an intact cornea, severe ocular damage does not occur if the pH of the acid is above 2.5 (21). Acids that are more lipid-soluble have greater penetration capability and produce more tissue damage. Sulfurous acid is more lipid-soluble than hydrochloric acid, followed by phosphoric and sulfuric acids (1). The anionic nature of the acid also contributes to its ability to cause severe ocular damage.

Acidic substances may either be organic or inorganic. Many inorganic acids are found in the home and the workplace (Table 39.3). Sulfuric acid is used in the fertilizing, chemical, and metal industry. Ocular injuries have also been associated with accidents resulting from automobile battery explosions (22). Concentrated sulfuric acid releases heat when it reacts with water; therefore, the tissue damage resulting from this agent is generally greater than that explained on the basis of the hydrogen concentration alone.

Hydrochloric acid represents one of the most common acids. Concentrated forms are available at 38% and 32% (muriatic acid). Injuries vary according to the concentration, quantity, and time of exposure; tissue damage ranges from mild irritation to total loss of the eye. Nitric acid is a colorless liquid when pure, and yellow in the commercial form as a result of oxide of nitrogen. Nitric acid burns cause a yellowish opacification of the corneal epithelium. The resulting injuries are otherwise similar to those produced by hydrochloric acid (1).

Hydrogen fluoride occurs in both gaseous and liquid states and produces severe systemic and ocular toxicity. Its indus-

trial use is widespread and includes the semiconductor industry. Ocular injuries are more severe than many other acids as a result of the activity of the fluoride ion (23). Fluoride binds divalent ions such as magnesium and calcium to form insoluble salts. Fortunately, human ocular exposures have been rare. Delayed toxicity has been implicated from an aerosol exposure (24).

Another acid that produces severe ocular burns is sulfurous acid. Sulfurous acid is formed when sulfur dioxide reacts with water. Liquid sulfur dioxide is used in some refrigeration systems. The extensive ocular damage from sulfurous acid is related to its high degree of water and lipid solubility.

Organic acids may destroy the conjunctiva. However, as a rule, they penetrate only slightly into the cornea (25). Commonly occurring organic acids are listed in Table 39.4. Common vinegar is a 4–10% solution of acetic acid and produces only mild irritation, whereas "essence of vinegar" is an 80% solution of acetic acid and may produce severe irreversible tissue damage (20). Phenols and related chemicals can produce corneal hypesthesia and opacification with resulting vision varying from complete recovery to complete loss (1). Acid anhydrides generally produce more ocular damage than their corresponding acids. The ability of the anhydrides to infiltrate through the cornea faster than their acids explains their greater tissue damage (25). Reports of total loss of vision have resulted from acetic anhydride exposure (26, 77). While the reaction for these compounds is acidic, the clinical picture is similar to an alkaline burn (25).

Hydrocarbons

The extent of ocular damage from hydrocarbons depends on their specific physical and chemical properties (Table 39.5). Several references address specific compounds in detail (1, 27, 25). Hydrocarbons such as gasoline and kerosene generally produce a mild conjunctivitis with only minimal or no corneal involvement. Aromatic hydrocarbons such as benzene, toluene, and xylene generally produce mild corneal damage with rapid healing. Halogenated hydrocarbons are used commonly in in-

Table 39.2. Common Alkaline Substances[a]

Chemical Name	Common Name	Industrial Use	Ocular Toxicity
Ammonia (NH_3)		Chemical industry manufacturing fertilizer	Very severe ocular burns
Ammonia hydroxide[b] (NH_4OH)	"Ammonia"	Cleaning agents	Very severe ocular burns
Sodium hydroxide (NaOH)	Lye, caustic soda	Chemical industry manufacturing drain cleaning products	Severe ocular burns
Potassium hydroxide (KOH)	Caustic Potash	Chemical industry	Severe ocular burns
Calcium hydroxide[c] ($Ca(OH)_2$)	Lime, slaked lime	Mortar, plaster, cement	Moderate ocular burn
Calcium oxide (CaO)	Quicklime	Mortar, plaster	Moderate ocular burn
Organic amines	Many	Varied	Ocular burns Sensitizing agents

[a]Arranged in decreasing order of lipid solubility and corneal penetration rates.
[b]Concentrations range from 7–28% for liquid form.
[c]May be removed with EDTA.

Table 39.3. Inorganic Acids

Acid	Industrial Use	Ocular Toxicity
Sulfuric acid (H_2SO_4) (oil of vitriol) (battery acid)	Fertilizer Chemical manufacturing, automobile batteries	Large amount of heat production when combined with water
Hydrochloric acid (HCl) (muriatic acid)	Chemical manufacturing and steel industry	Mild to severe ocular burns
Nitric acid (HNO_3)	Chemical manufacturing	Causes yellow corneal opacifications
Hydrogen fluoride (HF)	Etching agents Semiconductors Cleaning agents	Severe ocular burns Binds divalent ions
Sulfurous acid (H_2SO_3)	Refrigerant Bleach	Very lipid solvent Early ocular anesthesia

Table 39.4. Organic Acids

Acid	Ocular Toxicity
Formic acid (HCOOH)	Conjunctivitis, keratitis
Acetic acid (CH_3COOH)	Low concentration—conjunctivitis, keratitis High concentration—corneal opacification
Trichloroacetic acid (CCl_3COOH)	Similar to acetic acid
Oxalic acid (HOOCCOOH)	Cloudy cornea with eventual healing
Organic anhydrides Acetic anhydride [($CH_3CO)_2O$]	Minor injury to total loss of vision
Maleic anhydride ($C_4H_2O_3$)	Similar to alkali
Succinic anhydride ($C_4H_4O_3$)	Similar to alkali

Table 39.5 Hydrocarbons

Hydrocarbon	Ocular Toxicity
Aliphatic Gasoline Kerosene	Mild conjunctivities with minimal corneal damage
Aromatic Benzene Toluene Xylene	Mild corneal damage
Halogenated hydrocarbons	Minor to severe corneal injuries
Aliphatic alcohols	Mild to severe corneal injuries
Organically active[a] Dichlorodiethylsulfide (mustard gas) Formaldehyde	Severe ocular damage

[a]May have asymptomatic latent period.

dustry and, while systemic absorption may cause major toxicity, direct contact with the eye ranges from minor corneal irritation to severe necrosis. Chloroform, carbon tetrachloride, trichloroethane, and trichloroethylene cause ocular irritation with possible corneal involvement. However, complete spontaneous recovery is the usual course (1).

Aliphatic alcohols mostly cause mild ocular irritation, although some are capable of producing significant corneal damage. Generally dilute alcohols produce mild changes, whereas concentrated liquids cause protein coagulation and cell death.

Other compounds may cause delayed ocular damage. Mustard gas, dichlorodiethylsulfides, reacts as a vesicant, cleaving the epithelial layer of the cornea from the stroma. This occurs after a latent period of up to 6–8 hours (25). Formaldehyde splashed in the eye results in immediate pain and only minimal initial structural damage. However, over the next 12 hours, all layers of the cornea and structures in the anterior chamber may undergo devastating degeneration (1).

Metals

Many metallic salts cause ocular damage upon contact with the eye (28). Dilute concentrations, in the form of dusts and fumes, generally cause mild irritation, whereas concentrated exposures may lead to necrotizing pathology (25). Many of these agents bind to enzymes and proteins to form metallic complexes. The toxicity of these complexes is proportional to their relative solubility; the more soluble complexes penetrate deeper and result in greater ocular destruction (25). Lead is the least soluble, followed by zinc, copper, silver, tin, and finally mercury (Table 39.6). In addition, all heavy metals may form permanent granular deposits in ocular tissue.

Silver occurs in many chemical forms, and several of these cause direct ocular damage. Argyrosis, an ashen-gray discol-

Table 39.6 Metals and Metallic Compounds

Metal	Corneal Solubility	Common Compounds
Mercury (Hg)	High	Mercury chloride Liquid mercury
Tin (Sn)	Moderate	Stannic chloride
Silver (Ag)	Moderate	Silver ammonium Silver nitrate
Copper (Cu)	Moderate	Copper sulfate Copper nitrate
Zinc (Zn)	Low	Zinc salts
Lead (Pb)	Low	Lead acetate

Table 39.7. Nonmetallic Irritants and Corrosives

Agent	Ocular Toxicity
Arsenic (As)	Reacts with sulfhydryl group
Selenium (Se)	Reacts with sulfhydryl group
Phosphorus (PO_4)	Corrosive
Potassium permanganate ($KMnO_4$)	Oxidizing agent
Hydrogen peroxide (H_2O_2)	Oxidizing agent
Silicone organic compounds	Alkylating agent and corrosive
Halogens (Cl, Br, I, F)	Chemically reacts with enzymes

Table 39.8. Summary of Treatment Principles for Chemical Eye Injuries

Immediate

  Copious irrigation at the accident site with the first available
    nontoxic fluid
  Continue irrigation enroute to medical facility

Emergency department

  Instill topical anesthetic and irrigate with 1 liter normal saline
  Evert eyelids and irrigate palpebral conjunctiva
  Double eversion of upper lid and remove any particulate matter
    with moist swab. Use 0.01–0.05 M CaNa$_2$ EDTA to loosen
    calcium hydroxide if necessary
  Check pH of conjunctiva intermittently during and 10 minutes
    after irrigation
  Brief irrigation for neutral and benign agents
  Prolonged (1 hour) irrigation for caustic agents. Insert scleral lens
    with inflow channel (Morgan Therapeutic Lens)
  Document eye exam
  If indicated, instill cycloplegic and antibiotic
  Check tetanus prophylaxis if corneal epithelium is injured
  Consult ophthalmologist for significant injuries

Subsequent care

  Treat secondary glaucoma
  Prevent and treat symblepharon
  Consider further medical and surgical interventions
  Attempt to repair permanent damage

oration of the eye, may occur either by systemic or local absorption of silver. Silver ammonia compounds produce more ocular damage than simple silver salts as a result of strongly alkaline ammonium hydroxide (29). Silver nitrate in a concentration of 0.5% was routinely used for prophylaxis of ophthalmia neonatorum, whereas concentrated solutions have caused necrosis of cell layers and opacification of the corneal stroma (25, 30). Silver precipitates with chloride to form an inactive silver chloride compound, and this may have therapeutic implications for treating ocular accidents. Copper is found in several different forms including copper sulfate and nitrate. Its actions are similar to that of silver (25).

Agents containing mercury include both inorganic and organic compounds. These are primarily toxic when systemically absorbed but may also produce direct corneal damage (1). Liquid mercury (quicksilver) produces little direct epithelial damage to the intact corneal epithelium. Salts of lead and zinc also cause little reaction to an intact epithelium. On the other hand, titanium and tin react similarly to a corrosive acid if concentrated directly on the eye (25). Iron and iron compounds produce little corrosive damage. However, they remain present as an intraocular foreign body. Metallic iron rapidly produces a yellow-brown staining of the surrounding cornea known as a "rust ring."

Nonmetallic and Inorganic Agents

Nonmetallic substances may produce ocular toxicity when in contact with the eye (Table 39.7). Arsenic reacts with sulfhydryl groups of enzyme and structural proteins, the result of which may be devastating. While clinical accidents are rare, complete opacification of the cornea has occurred (25). Selenium is used in the production of pigments, including paints and inks. It is commonly present in the form of selenium dioxide vapor. Chemically it is similar to arsenic in binding with sulfhydryl groups of enzymes and proteins. Both may be treated with British antilewisite agent (BAL).

Phosphorus has two forms: white and gray. The former is highly reactive and ignites at 34°C. The latter is more stable, and is used to produce smoke screens. Case reports are rare; however, ocular damage and chronic conjunctivitis have occurred (25, 31).

Silicon, while inert by itself, may be toxic when combined with organic compounds. Three main classes of such compounds are described: the chlorosilicons (silicons tetrachloride), which are highly corrosive; the organic silicate esters (methoxysilicone), which act as alkylating agents; and the ethoxysilicanes, which are systemically toxic but cause little ocular damage.

The halogens include chlorine, bromine, iodine, and fluorine. These generally cause ocular damage by interfering with vital enzymes. Potassium permanganate and hydrogen peroxide also cause ocular damage as a result of their oxidizing capabilities (25).

TREATMENT

The general principles for treating chemical eye injuries are summarized in Table 39.8. The exact treatment may vary depending on the nature of the inciting agent; more potent agents such as alkali and acids require more intensive treatment. Specific antidotes are rare, and many of these remain controversial.

The most important principle regarding treatment of the chemically injured eye remains copious irrigation of the eye as soon as possible (12, 32, 33). This should occur at the site of the accident with the first available nontoxic fluid. Severe damage may result within seconds after exposure; immediate irrigation may prevent years of corrective therapy or blindness. Adequate eye washes and showers should be standard equipment in the workplace (34, 35). In the home setting any source of water may be utilized, including sinks, hoses, bathtubs, and pools. The eye should be held open during the irrigation. Irrigation fluid should not flow into the unaffected eye from the contaminated eye.

Irrigation should be continued in transport to a medical facility for all significant ocular toxic substances. If the substance is unknown, then it must be assumed to be potentially ocular toxic until proven otherwise. The absence of ocular symptoms cannot be relied upon, as many agents cause loss of ocular sensation. An intravenous solution of normal saline or Ringer's lactate may be utilized for irrigating the eye while transporting the patient. The eye can be flushed using regular intravenous tubing connected to a liter of fluid. Prehospital personnel should

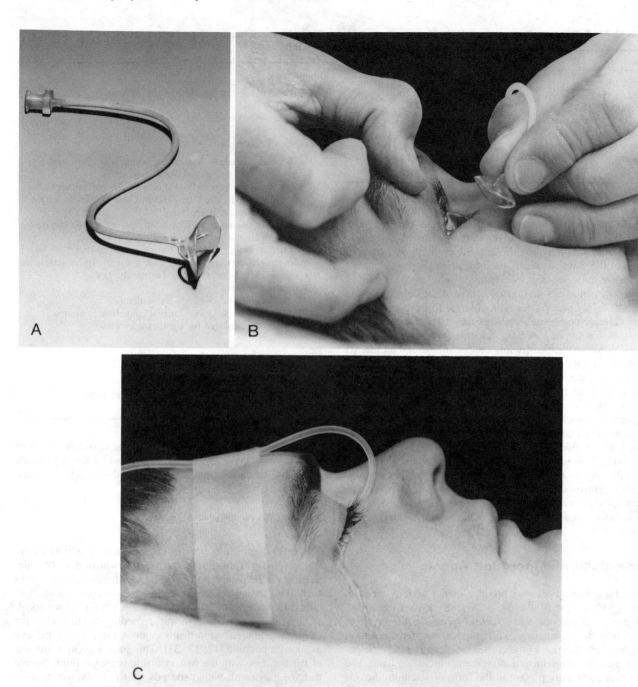

Figure 39.2.   **A**, Scleral lens with an inflow channel (Morgan Therapeutic Lens). **B, C**, Insertion and ocular irrigation utilizing a Morgan Therapeutic Lens.

also obtain the name of the agent involved or bring the container in when feasible.

Treatment in a medical facility differs depending on the nature of the chemical agent. Initially, irrigation is continued with 1 liter of normal saline under medical supervision. Prolonged irrigation is required for caustic agents, whereas brief irrigation is sufficient for less toxic substances. A topical anesthetic, such as proparacaine, may be instilled to facilitate adequate irrigation. The upper and lower lid should be retracted and irrigated. Particulate matter should be removed from the fornices with a sterile moist swab and forceps when necessary.

Alkali and Acids

Alkali ocular injuries mandate the most aggressive treatment protocol. All the general principles apply; however, prolonged irrigation is the standard. Most authors recommend at least 30 minutes, while some advocate 1–2 hours (36). One technique to facilitate prolonged irrigation has been to utilize a scleral lens with an inflow channel (Morgan Therapeutic Lens) (37). This is inserted under the upper and lower lids after instilling topical anesthetic (Fig. 39.2). Alternatively, manual irrigation using intravenous tubing and retracting the lid is also effective (18).

Table 39.9. Prognosis and Grading of Chemical Burns[a]

Grade	Cornea	Conjunctiva	Prognosis
I	Epithelial damage	No ischemia	Good
II	Hazy with iris detail	Ischemia less than 1/3 at limbus	Good
III	Total epithelial loss, stromal haze	Ischemia 1/3 to 1/2 at limbus	Poor
IV	Opaque No view of iris or pupil	Ischemia 1/2 or more at limbus	Very Poor

[a]Adapted from Roper (41).

The pH in the inferior cul-de-sac should be tested with litmus paper intermittently during and 10 minutes after irrigation. Alkaline material may slowly be released from corneal tissue for several hours after irrigation is stopped, especially if particulate matter is present. Irrigation should be continued until a stable pH of 7–8.5 is achieved (1). Double eversion of the upper lid (33) and outward and upward traction of a single everted lid yields excellent exposure of the superior cul-de-sac. Any foreign material should be removed using a moist cotton swab. Calcium hydroxide material such as cement, plaster, and lime may be removed by irrigating the embedded material with 0.01–0.05 M solution of sodium ethylenediaminetetraacetate (EDTA) or using a swab saturated with calcium disodium EDTA (CaNa$_2$ EDTA) (14). Fine forceps may also be necessary.

After prolonged irrigation and removal of all foreign material, a detailed eye examination should be documented. An ophthalmologist should be consulted and the patient admitted for all but the most trivial of injuries. Tetanus prophylaxis should be administered along with topical antibiotics, cycloplegics, and mydriatic agents. If intraocular pressure is elevated or cannot be measured, treatment with acetazolamide and topical timolol maleate should be instituted (18). Topical steroids are generally recommended for the first 7–10 days (18, 38). Collagenase inhibitors have been studied in vitro; however, their in vivo effects are weak (18).

Treatment of acid burns to the eye are similar to alkali burns. Generally these are less severe, require less irrigation, and result in less ocular damage. A notable exception is hydrofluoric acid. However, extrapolating techniques for treating hydrofluoric acid burns of the skin to hydrofluoric acid ocular injuries have not yielded improved results, due to the ocular toxicity of the treatment agents involved (18, 39, 40). An ophthalmologist should be consulted for all significant injuries.

Solvents and Hydrocarbons

Agents that are not chemically reactive such as alcohols, ketones, gasoline, and chlorinated hydrocarbons generally require only brief irrigation to decontaminate the eye. One liter of normal saline is usually sufficient. This is not true if the substance is organically active or very viscous, in which case more prolonged irrigation would be prudent (1). It is safer to err on more prolonged irrigation if the exact nature of the substance is in doubt.

Metallic and Nonmetallic Inorganic Agents

General treatment principles apply to most of the metallic and nonmetallic chemical ocular injuries. Of note, however, is the ability of sodium chloride to bind free silver and form an inert silver chloride (25). Additionally, BAL is effective in binding certain ions such as gold, cadmium, mercury, arsenic, and selenium. Early instillation of a 10–20% solution is required (25). Cocaine is useful to form an insoluble and inactive compound with iodine.

Thermal and Associated Injuries

Thermal burns result from hot and cold vapors and are treated the same way as thermal burns elsewhere in the body. However, exposure to flame rarely involves the cornea and globe, due to the reflex lid closure (33). If there is evidence of a ruptured globe or intraocular foreign body, the eye should be protected, and an ophthalmology consult obtained.

PROGNOSIS AND OUTCOME

Prognosis is related to the degree of tissue damage from caustic agents or structural changes induced from organically active compounds. The speed with which the eye is irrigated at the scene of the accident remains the most critical therapeutic consideration regarding longterm prognosis. Grading of ocular damage from alkali and acid injury may predict the longterm prognosis (Table 39.9) (44). Grade I has epithelial damage only with no ischemia of the conjunctiva. Grade II has a hazy cornea, iris detail preserved, and ischemia limited to one third at the limbus. The longterm prognosis for both is good. Grade III has total epithelial loss with a hazy stroma, loss of iris detail, and ischemia between one third to one half at the limbus. Grade IV has a totally opaque cornea, obscured iris and pupil, and ischemia of more than one half at the limbus. Prognosis is poor to very poor for grades III and IV, respectively (41).

Noncaustic agents such as organic solvents generally cause limited corneal damage with complete recovery, providing they do not react with tissue structures. Initial evaluation of agents that bind chemically and have a delayed onset of action may be misleading. Alklylating agents such as mustard gas and dimethyl sulfate, as well as formaldehyde, arsenic, and some rare earth salts all may exhibit minimal initial pathology but progress to serious ocular damage and blindness.

Factors that also affect longterm prognosis include the development of secondary elevated intraocular pressure, persistent or recurrent corneal ulcers, cataracts, and symblepharon, which are adhesions between the lids and the globe (42, 33). Longterm surgical intervention may be necessary, including corneal transplant, when possible.

MANAGEMENT STRATEGIES AND SUMMARY

Management strategies are outlined in Table 39.8. Immediate irrigation at the scene with the first available nontoxic fluid remains the most critical aspect in the treatment of the chemical eye injuries. Brief irrigation with 1 liter of normal saline or Ringer's lactate is usually sufficient for most benign substances, while prolonged irrigation is necessary for alkali and acids. Commercial eye wash solutions are also available. If any doubt exists as to the nature of the agent, then the injury should be treated as an alkaline burn. The pH should be checked, especially after irrigation, and all foreign material removed. An ophthalmologist should be consulted for all but the most trivial of injuries. Topical cycloplegics and antibiotics should be instilled; elevated intraocular pressure should be assessed and treated. Agents that bind and react chemically frequently have a poor prognosis despite intensive emergent management. Appropriate texts and resources, such as a regional poison center, should be consulted when dealing with unfamiliar specific agents.

REFERENCES

1. Grant WM. Toxicology of the eye. 2nd ed. Springfield: Thomas, 1974.

2. Teir H. Toxicologic effects on the eyes at work. Acta Ophthalmol Suppl 1984;161:60–65.

3. Kersjes MP, Reifler DM, Maurer JR, Trestrall JH, McCoy DJ. A review of chemical eye burns referred to the Blodgett Regional Poison Center. Vet Hum Toxicol 1987;29:453–455.

4. Olson RJ. Occupational eye disorders. In: Rom WN, ed. Environmental and occupational medicine. Boston: Little, Brown, 1983:367–372.

5. Saari KM, Parvi V. Occupational eye injuries in Finland. Acta Ophthalmol Suppl 1984;161:17–28.

6. Pfister RR. Chemical corneal burns. Int Ophthalmol Clin 1984;24:157–168.

7. Morris RE, Witherspoon CD, Helms HA Jr, Feist RM, Byrne JB Jr. Eye injury registry of Alabama (preliminary report). South Med J 1987;80:810–816.

8. Karlson TA, Klein BEK. The incidence of acute hospital-treated eye injuries. Arch Ophthalmol, 1986;104:1473–1486.

9. Newell FW. Ophthalmology: principles and concepts. 6th ed. St. Louis: CV Mosby, 1986.

10. Proctor NH, Hughes JP. Chemical hazards of the workplace. Philadelphia: JB Lippincott, 1978.

11. Hughes WR Jr. Alkali burns of the eye. I. Review of the literature and summary of present knowledge. Arch Ophthalmol 1946;35:423–449.

12. Hughes WF Jr. Alkali burns of the eye. II. Clinical and pathologic course. Arch Ophthalmol 1946;36:189-214.

13. Pfister RR, Koski J. Alkali burns of the eye: pathophysiology and treatment. South Med J 1982;75:417–422.

14. Grant WM, Kern HL. Action of the alkalies on the corneal stroma. Arch Ophthalmol 1955;54:931–939.

15. Paterson CA, Pfister RR, Levinson RA. Aqueous humor pH changes after experimental alkali burns. Am J Ophthalmol 1975;79:414–419.

16. Stein MR, Naidoff MA, Dawson CR. Intraocular pressure response to experimental alkali burns. Am J Ophthalmol 1973;75:99–109.

17. Paterson CA, Pfister RR. Intraocular pressure changes after alkali burns. Arch Ophthalmol 1974;91:211–218.

18. McCulley JP. Chemical injuries. In: Smolin G, Thoft RA, eds. The cornea. 2nd ed. Boston: Little, Brown, 1987:527–542.

19. Stanley JA. Strong alkali burns of the eye. N Engl J Med 1965;273:1264–1266.

20. McCulley JP, Moore TE. Chemical injuries of the eye. In: Leibowitz HM, ed. Corneal disorders. Philadelphia: WB Saunders, 1984:471–498.

21. Friedenwald JS, Hughes WF Jr, Herrmann H. Acid burns of the eye. Arch Ophthalmol 1946;35:98–108.

22. Holekamp TLR, Becker B. Ocular injuries from automobile batteries. Trans Am Acad Ophthalmol Otolaryngol 1977;83:805–810.

23. McCulley JP, Whiting DW, Pettit MG, Lauber SE. Hydrofluoric acid burns of the eye. J Occup Med 1983;25:447–450.

24. Hatai JK, Weber JN, Doizaki K. Hydrofluoric acid burns of the eye: report of possible delayed toxicity. J Toxicol Cut Ocul Toxicol 1986;5:179–184.

25. Duke-Elder S, MacFaul PA. System of ophthalmology. Vol. XIV: Injuries, pt 2. St Louis: CV Mosby, 1972.

26. McLaughlin RS. Chemical burns of the human cornea. Am J Ophthalmol 1946;29:1355–1362.

27. Carpenter CP, Smyth HF Jr. Chemical burns of the rabbit cornea. Am J Ophthalmol 1946;29:1363–1372.

28. Grant WM, Kern HL. Cations and the cornea: Toxicity of metals to the stroma. Am J Ophthalmol 1956;42:167–181.

29. Calvery HO, Lightbody HD, Rones B. Effects of some silver salts on the eye. Arch Ophthalmol 1941;25:839–847.

30. Laughrea PA, Arentsen JJ, Laibson PR. Iatrogenic ocular silver nitrate burn. Cornea 1985–86;4:47–50.

31. Sharir M, Chen V, Blumenthal M. Red phosphorus as a cause of corneal injury: a case report. Ophthalmologica 1987;194:204–206.

32. Brown SI, Tragakis MP, Pearce DB. Treatment of the alkali-burned cornea. Am J Ophthalmol 1972;74:316–320.

33. Paton D, Goldberg MF, Deutsch TA, Feller D. Management of ocular injuries. 2nd ed. Philadelphia: WB Saunders, 1985:93–106.

34. Burns FR, Paterson CA. Prompt irrigation of chemical eye injuries may avert severe damage. Occup Health Saf 1989;Apr:33–36.

35. Weaver LA. Eye washes and showers: ensuring effectiveness. Occup Health Saf 1983;(Aug):13–19.

36. Saari KM, Leinonen J, Aine E. Management of chemical eye injuries with prolonged irrigation. Acta Ophthalmol Suppl 1984;161:52–59.

37. Morgan LB. A new drug delivery system for the eye. Ind Med Surg 1971;40:11–13.

38. Donshik PC, Berman MB, Dohlman CH, Gage J, Rose J. Effects of topical corticosteroids on ulcerations in alkali-burned corneas. Arch Ophthalmol 1978;96:2117–2120.

39. McCulley JP, Pettit M, Lauber S. Treatment of experimental ocular hydrofluoric acid burns. [Abstract]. Invest Ophthalmol Vis Sci 1980;19(ARVO Suppl.):228.

40. McCulley JP, Whitins DW, Pettit MG, Lauber SE. Hydrofluoric acid burns of the eye. J Occup Med 1983;25:447–450.

41. Roper-Hall MJ. Thermal and chemical burns. Trans Ophthalmol Soc UK 1965;85:631–653.

42. Nelson JD, Kopietz LA. Chemical injuries to the eyes. Postgrad Med 1987;81:62–75.

Radiation and Radioactive Emergencies

Peter Pons, M.D.
John B. Sullivan, Jr., M.D.

INTRODUCTION

During the late 1970s and 1980s, major accidents at the Three Mile Island Nuclear Power Plant in Pennsylvania and the Chernobyl Nuclear Power Plant in the Soviet Union, as well as numerous smaller mishaps worldwide, have dramatically demonstrated the hazards associated with radiation and radioactivity. Proximity to a nuclear power generating plant is no longer the only reason for preparation for dealing with radiation emergencies. The widespread use and transport of radioactive materials throughout our communities mandate that every emergency department have a plan in place for responding to an incident involving radiation exposure, and every emergency physician should be familiar with the principles of treatment for these patients. In addition, the common use of radionuclides in a variety of industrial and commercial settings, including hospitals, constitutes another form of risk for which physicians must be prepared.

FUNDAMENTALS OF RADIATION AND RADIOACTIVITY

Generally, the term "radioactivity" refers to the spontaneous release of either particles or energy from a decaying atom. There are numerous sources of radioactivity in the community that may lead to exposure or contamination. These include naturally occurring radioactive substances such as uranium, radionuclides used in medical applications, nuclear reactors, and radiation-producing machines such as x-ray devices or linear accelerators (1). There are many terms and definitions to be familiar with in dealing with radiation and radioactive materials (Table 40.1). Radiation can generally be described as penetrating or nonpenetrating. Penetrating radiation passes into and through tissues and includes gamma rays, x-rays, and fast neutrons. Beta particles can also penetrate tissue to a slight degree. Radiation can be classified as gamma, beta, or alpha.

Alpha particles are heavy particles comprising two protons and two neutrons (thus carrying a plus two charge). These particles have a limited range of only a few centimeters in air when released from a decaying atom and can be stopped by a sheet of paper or epidermis of skin. Therefore, alpha-emitting sources are generally not considered hazardous unless inhaled, ingested, or deposited into open wounds (2–4).

Beta particles are electrons (negatively charged). They may penetrate up to 5 millimeters in human tissue and have a range of several meters of air. Beta particles are hazardous both externally and internally. They can be stopped by a thin sheet of metal (2–4).

Gamma rays are energy waves released from the decaying nucleus and have penetrating characteristics. Gamma rays pose a significant biologic threat. Several centimeters of lead are required to stop gamma rays (2–4).

Neutrons may be released during the process of fission or from the decay of certain isotopes. They may be stopped by a foot (30 centimeters) of water, although they have the ability to penetrate deeply into tissue.

The effect of a dose of radiation is defined in terms of the *rad* (radiation absorbed dose) and refers to the absorption of 100 ergs of energy per gram of tissue. Another term in common use is the *rem* (roentgen equivalent in man). The rem represents the number of rads multiplied by the "relative biologic effectiveness" (RBE) of the type of radiation involved. For example, the RBE of gamma rays is 1, whereas for neutrons it is 2. Therefore, an individual exposed to a particular dose (in rads) of neutrons would have been exposed to the equivalent of twice that number of rads in gamma rays. Exposure to radiation should be kept "as low as reasonably achievable" (ALARA), and current recommendations are for no more than 5 rem/year, whole body exposure.

RADIONUCLIDES

Radioactive forms of elements are termed radionuclides (Table 40.2). Radionuclides are commonly used throughout many industries and medical facilities. The risk of injury to tissues from incorporation of the various radionuclides varies and is a function of the following: (a) specific activity, (b) dose, (c) half-life, (d) biologic elimination, (e) target organ concentration, (f) route of exposure and absorption. The disintegration time (half-life) and the type of radiation emitted vary with the species and are critical features of radionuclide toxicity. The toxicity of a radionuclide to a particular tissue is a function of the type of radiation emitted, the half-life of the radiation, and biologic elimination of the element. Biologic elimination and the actual half-life combine to create an "effective half-life" of elimination. The site of greatest injury from a radionuclide occurs within the tissue (critical organ), which concentrates the radionuclide (Table 40.2). The route of exposure influences toxicity. Inhalation can present a different order of toxicity as compared to ingestion or wound contamination.

RADIATION EXPOSURE AND CONTAMINATION

In determining the appropriate treatment a patient will require and the nature of the precautions taken by those personnel involved in the medical care, the modality of exposure must be considered.

The first situation is irradiation, whereby the patient has been subjected to gamma or x-rays (2–4). In these cases, the patient has been exposed to radiation but is not radioactive and, therefore, poses no risk to medical personnel. The patient has already sustained whatever injury is going to occur, and it will manifest itself over time. Of interest, there is one exception to the rule

Table 40.1. Definitions

Absorbed dose: The amount absorbed per unit mass of irradiated material when ionizing radiation passes through the matter. The unit of measurement of absorbed dose is the rad.

Activity: The number of nuclear transformations occurring in a given quantity of material per unit time.

Alpha particle: A particle with a positive charge made up of two neutrons and two protons emitted by certain radioactive materials. It is the least penetrating of the three types of emitted radiation and can be stopped by a sheet of paper.

Beta particle: An elementary particle emitted from a nucleus during radioactive decay. It has a single electrical charge and a mass 1/1837 of a proton. A negatively charged beta particle is identical to an electron; a positively charged beta particle is a positron.

Curie: The unit of activity of nuclear transformations per unit time. One curie equals 3.7×10^{10} nuclear transformations per second.

Daughter and daughter product: A nuclide formed by radioactive decay of another nuclide the product of which may be stable or unstable.

Effective half-life: Time required for a radionuclide contained in a biologic system to reduce its activity by half as a combined result of radioactive decay and biologic elimination.

Gamma rays: High energy, nuclear in origin, short wave length electromagnetic radiation which are very penetrating.

Ionizing radiation: Any radiation displacing electrons from atoms or molecules, thus producing ions.

Isotopes: One of two or more atoms with the same atomic number but with different atomic weights. The nuclei of isotopes have the same number of protons but different number of neutrons.

Neutron: An uncharged elementary particle with a mass slightly greater than that of a proton. A free neutron is unstable and decays with a half-life of 13 minutes into an electron, proton, and a neutrino.

Physical half-life: The time required for a radioactive substance to lose one-half of its activity by decay.

Proton: An elementary particle with a single positive charge and a mass 1837 times that of an electron.

Rad: The special unit of absorbed dose.

Radionuclide: A radioactive form of an element.

Rem: The special unit of dose equivalent.

X-rays: A penetrating form of electromagnetic radiation which is nonnuclear in origin emitted when the inner orbital electrons of an excited atom return to their normal state or when a metal target is bombarded with high-speed electrons.

that an irradiated victim poses no hazard: the patient who has been exposed to high dose neutron radiation. In these extremely rare cases, the patient may, in fact, become radioactive.

The second situation involves external, surface contamination of the patient (2–4). In these cases decontamination must occur while protecting medical personnel and equipment from exposure. Monitoring of the patient and the decontamination effort must be performed using appropriate radiation detection devices.

Lastly is the case of internal contamination (incorporation) by inhalation, ingestion, or deposition of material into an open wound (2–4). This route of exposure is of particular concern because of the potential for internal irradiation and the permanent incorporation of the radioactive material in the molecules of cells. Usually, the effects of an internal contamination accident such as radionuclide intake manifest themselves over a period of years, except in cases of massive exposure. In these cases, urgent removal is indicated with possible utilization of chelating agents.

DETECTING AND MEASURING EXPOSURE

In order to appropriately determine what steps are needed following a potential exposure, actual contamination is documented by using radiation detection instruments.

The standard device utilized to detect the presence of gamma or beta radiation is the Geiger-Müller Survey Meter (GM meter) (Fig. 40.1) or, as it is more popularly called, the Geiger counter. It is not sensitive enough, however, to detect alpha radiation. This device should be used by qualified individuals knowledgeable in its operation and use. Before a survey is conducted, the machine should be calibrated. Following calibration, the survey is performed by slowly moving the probe over the site of suspected contamination, being certain to avoid touching the probe to the potentially contaminated surface and thus contaminating the device. A written record of the survey results should be kept (a standard burn chart may be used to document contaminated sites on a patient). It is important to hold the monitoring device the same distance from the site being monitored at all times in order to determine the extent of contamination. Error in estimating exposures can be made if the instrument is not used properly.

Differentiation between beta and gamma radiation is accomplished by means of a shield on the probe which will stop beta radiation from being detected. With the shield removed, the GM meter detects total beta and gamma radiation; the difference between the two represents beta radiation. One other important concern is that the GM survey meter may become saturated and subsequently give a false zero reading (1).

The detection of alpha radiation focuses on a different concern. Since alpha radiation has limited penetrating capability and can be stopped by intact skin, the primary hazard is related to actual intake. Therefore, surveys are aimed at detecting contaminated sites that would allow inhalation, ingestion, or absorption via open wounds. Alpha counters are very difficult to use properly and are subject to misinterpretation. Alpha surveys should usually be performed by an experienced health physicist.

Surface swipes are another technique for evaluating the presence of alpha radiation. This method involves wiping the contaminated site with filter paper and then determining alpha activity in a laboratory radiation counter. A variation of this test is the nose swipe, where either a cotton applicator or strip of filter paper wrapped around a swab stick is moistened with distilled water and used to swab each nostril. After drying, the amount of alpha radiation is measured in a gas-flow proportional counter (1).

Different types of personal dosimeters (Fig. 40.2) can be utilized to measure exposure of rescuers and medical personnel to external radiation sources. Film badges can also be utilized as dosimeters and are quite reliable but require careful processing and interpretation (1). A radiation health specialist should be a member of the emergency response team to provide accurate monitoring and interpretation of results.

IRRADIATION AND BIOLOGIC EFFECTS

When radiation passes through cells (irradiation), molecules are bombarded with energy, causing atoms to become excited and bonds to break. This leads to the formation of ions (thus the term ''ionizing radiation'') and charged fragments called radicals which cause further damage and alterations in function when they interact with other cellular components (5–7). The

Table 40.2. Radionuclides

Radionuclide	Radiation Type	Physical $T_{1/2}$	Effective $T_{1/2}$	Organ
Americium-241	Alpha, gamma	458 years	139 years	Bone
Americium-243	Alpha, gamma, daughters	7950 years	195 years	Bone
Arsenic-74	Beta, gamma	18 days	17 days	Total body
Arsenic-77	Beta, gamma, daughters	39 hours	24 hours	Total body
Barium-140	Beta, gamma, daughters	13 days	11 days	Bone
Cadmium-109	Gamma, daughters	453 days	140 days	Liver
Calcium-45	Beta	165 days	162 days	Bone
Calcium-47	Beta, gamma, daughters	4.5 days	4.5 days	Bone
Californium-252	Gamma, alpha, neutron, daughter	2.6 years	2.2 years	Bone
Carbon-14	Beta	5730 years	12 days	Total body
Cerium-141	Beta, gamma, daughters	32 days	30 days	Liver
Cerium-144	Beta, gamma, daughters	284 days	280 days	Bone
Cesium-137	Beta, gamma, daughters	30 years	70 days	Total body
Chromium-51	Gamma	28 days	27 days	Total body
Cobalt-57	Gamma	270 days	9 days	Total body
Cobalt-58	Beta, gamma	71 days	8 days	Total body
Cobalt-60	Beta, gamma	5.3 years	10 days	Total body
Curium-242	Alpha, neutron, gamma	163 days	155 days	Liver
Curium-243	Alpha, gamma	32 years	27.5 days	Liver
Curium-244	Alpha, neutron, gamma	17.6 years	16.7 years	Liver
Europium-152	Beta, gamma, daughters	13 years	3 years	Kidney
Europium-154	Beta, gamma	16 years	3 years	Bone
Europium-155	Beta, gamma	2 years	1.3 years	Kidney
Fluorine-18	Beta, gamma	2 hours	2 hours	Total body
Gallium-72	Beta, gamma	14 hours	12 hours	Liver
Gold-198	Beta, gamma	2.7 days	2.6 days	Total body
Tritium (^{3}H)	Beta	12 years	12 days	Total body
Indium-114m	Beta, gamma, daughters	49 days	27 days	Kidney, spleen
Iodine-125	Beta, gamma	60 days	42 days	Thyroid
Iodine-131	Beta, gamma, daughters	8 days	8 days	Thyroid
Iron-55	Gamma	2.6 years	1 year	Spleen
Iron-59	Beta, gamma	46 days	42 days	Spleen
Lead-210	Beta, gamma, daughters	20 years	1.3 years	Kidney
Mercury-197	Gamma	2.7 days	2.3 days	Kidney
Mercury-203	Beta, gamma	46 days	11 days	Kidney
Molybdenum-99	Beta, gamma, daughters	2.8 days	1.5 days	Kidney
Neptunium-237	Alpha, gamma, daughters	2 million years	200 years	Bone
Neptunium-239	Beta, gamma	2.3 days	2.3 days	G.I. Tract
Phosphorus-32	Beta	14 days	14 days	Bone
Plutonium-238	Alpha, gamma	88 years	63 years	Bone
Plutonium-239	Alpha, gamma	24 thousand years	197 years	Bone
Polonium-210	Alpha	138 days	46 days	Spleen
Potassium-42	Beta, gamma	12 hours	12 hours	Total body
Promethium-147	Beta	2.6 years	1.6 years	Bone
Promethium-149	Beta, gamma	2.2 days	2.2 days	Bone
Radium-224	Alpha, gamma daughters	3.6 days	3.6 days	Bone
Radium-226	Alpha, gamma, daughters	1600 years	44 years	Bone
Rubidium-86	Beta, gamma	19 days	13.2 days	Total body
Ruthenium-106	Beta, daughters	368 days	2.5 days	Kidney
Scandium-46	Beta, gamma	84 days	40 days	Liver
Silver-110m	Beta, gamma, daughters	255 days	5 days	Total body
Sodium-22	Beta, gamma	950 days	11 days	Total body
Sodium-24	Beta, gamma	15 hours	14 hours	Total body
Strontium-85	Gamma	65 days	65 days	Total body
Strontium-90	Beta, daughters	28 years	15 years	Bone
Sulfur-35	Beta	88 days	44 days	Testis
Technetium-99m	Gamma	6 hours	5 hours	Total body
Technetium-99	Beta	200 thousand years	20 days	Kidney
Thorium-230	Alpha, gamma	80 thousand years	200 years	Bone
Thorium-232	Alpha, gamma, daughters	1.4×10^{10} years	200 years	Bone
Thorium (natural)	Alpha, beta, gamma		200 years	Bone
Uranium-235	Alpha, gamma, daughters	7.1×10^8 years	15 days	Kidney
Uranium-238	Alpha, gamma, daughters	4.5×10^9 years	15 days	Kidney
Uranium (natural)	Alpha, beta, gamma	4.5×10^9 years	15 days	Kidney
Yttrium-90	Beta	64 hours	64 hours	Bone
Zinc-65	Beta($+$), gamma	245 days	194 days	Total body
Zirconium-95	Beta, gamma, daughter	66 days	56 days	Total body

Adapted from National Council on Radiation and Protection Measurements, Report No. 65. Management of persons accidently contaminated with radionuclides. Washington, DC: National Council on Radiation and Protection Measurements, 1979.

most radiosensitive tissues are generally those with high cellular turnover, including the hematopoietic, gastrointestinal, and reproductive systems (5–7). The exception to this rule is the lymphocyte, which, although it has a slow turnover rate, is very radiosensitive.

Irradiation by high energy gamma rays produces tissue damage but does not result in contamination. The person is free from radioactive contamination unless source material was actually contacted. Irradiation may be localized or total body. If total body irradiation has occurred then the patient may experience the onset of the radiation syndrome. The significance and extent of the irradiation injury can be determined by the time of onset of gastrointestinal symptoms (nausea, anorexia, vomiting) following exposure. The biologic effects of radiation may become manifest within hours, days, or several weeks, or may take years or even decades to become evident. Those symptoms that occur rapidly are called the acute radiation syndrome, whereas those that occur years later are longterm effects (4).

The acute radiation syndrome is a symptom complex that occurs following whole body exposure (5–7). The severity and nature of the syndrome vary depending on the dose of radiation, dose rate, and individual susceptibility (Table 40.3) (5). Whole body radiation exposure has been characterized as sublethal (<200 rads), potentially lethal (200–1000 rads), or supralethal (>1000 rads). The acute syndrome is divided into four phases: prodrome, latent, manifest illness, and recovery.

Prodrome. This is an initial toxic period characterized by nausea, vomiting, intestinal cramps, diarrhea, salivation, and dehydration (5–7). Fatigue, apathy, fever, and hypotension may also be noted. This phase usually occurs with exposure greater than 100 rads and always with doses greater than 400 rads. Onset of symptoms occurs within 2 hours if doses exceed 600 rads; symptoms may begin in 2–6 hours at doses less than 400 rads. As a general rule, the faster the prodrome occurs, particularly vomiting, the greater the dose received. If vomiting occurs within 1–5 hours, the patient has received a significant dose of radiation; if it starts within 1 hour, the patient has probably received a near-lethal dose; and if vomiting begins within minutes, the patient has likely been exposed to lethal amounts.

Latent Period. This is a period of well-being after the prodrome symptoms resolve, but it is dose-related and may not be present in high level exposure. This period may last days to weeks (5–7).

Manifest Illness. This results from the injury sustained by susceptible organ systems (5–7). The hematopoietic system is exquisitely sensitive, and the result is pancytopenia. The usual sequence of changes is lymphocytopenia, granulocytopenia, thrombocytopenia, and, finally, decreased erythrocytes. Lymphocytes may disappear within 24 hours of exposure. Granulocytes often disappear within several days and platelets in 1–2 weeks. As a result, the patient is at extreme risk for infection or bleeding diathesis. Damage to the gastrointestinal tract may lead to profound electrolyte disturbances and dehydration. Death usually occurs within 2 weeks if the dose of radiation exceeded 1000 rads, and within 2 days if the exposure was greater than 2000 rads.

Longterm effects of radiation may result from a single, acute exposure or from prolonged, chronic exposure. The biologic effects include increased incidence of various types of cancer, shortening of life span, sterility, and cataracts.

CONTAMINATION CONTROL

Every emergency medical services (EMS) system and every emergency department should have in place a comprehensive plan for managing a radiation emergency. The plan should include the following procedures (1, 4, 7):

1. How to assess the extent and type of contamination;

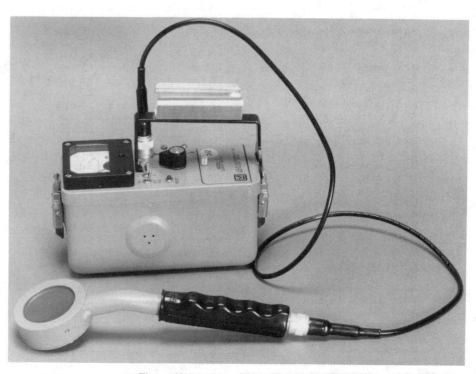

Figure 40.1. Geiger-Müller survey meter.

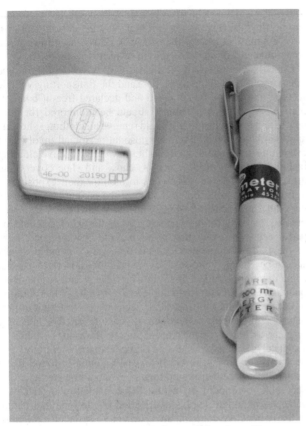

Figure 40.2.   Personal dosimeters worn by staff.

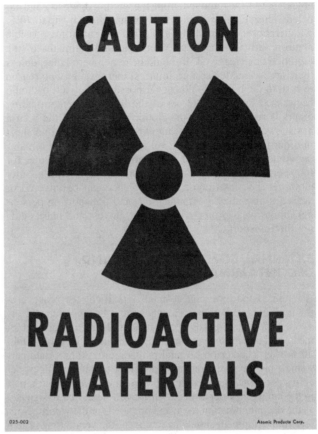

Figure 40.3.   Radioactive hazard warning sign. Source: Atomic Products Corp.

Table 40.3.   Acute Total Body Radiation Exposure Dose-Physiologic Response

Dose in Rads	Medical Effects
20–100	Alterations in number of circulating white blood cells (WBCs) and some chromosomal changes
100–200	Nausea and vomiting along with reduction in circulating WBCs
200–400	Severe reduction in circulating WBCs, nausea and vomiting, hair loss, increased chance of infection, some deaths
600–1000	50% death rate in 30 days, bone marrow suppression, sterility, diarrhea, erythema, and loss of skin cells
1000–2000	Destruction of intestinal mucosa, diarrhea, death in two weeks
2000–3500	Vascular collapse, cerebral anoxia, death within 48 hours

2. How to prevent further contamination;
3. How to decontaminate victims;
4. Who to notify to accomplish steps 1, 2, and 3;
5. A comprehensive list of needed supplies.

At the scene of a radiation accident, a number of tasks must be accomplished rapidly. The site must be secured, a command post set up upwind of the site, and a contamination/decontam-ination perimeter established. The number of personnel inside the contaminated sector should be limited to the minimum necessary to evacuate victims and accomplish necessary tasks. Contaminated clothes and objects should be left inside the control line. The nature of the exposure should be ascertained (irradiation versus radioactive contamination) and a determination of whether the exposure is continuing (2). If, in fact, the exposure is continuing, emergency personnel must ensure their own safety before attempting to rescue any victims. If the radiation source cannot be isolated or shielded, allowable exposure times for rescuers must be calculated before entering the contaminated site.

The immediate priority for any victim of a radiation accident, whether in the prehospital setting or the emergency department, is to address any life threats that may exist, not from radiation, but from concomitant injury. The combination of associated injuries and radioactive contamination requires expert management to prevent incorporation (6, 8). While rescuers and emergency personnel should take appropriate steps to avoid personal contamination, lifesaving interventions should never be delayed. Protective clothing such as shoe covers, gowns, coveralls, masks, and gloves may be donned in order to prevent skin contamination.

As soon as practical, the radiation victim should be moved away from the contaminated site to the control line. Proper signs should be in place to warn of the hazards (Fig. 40.3). At this control site, a survey can be performed using a GM survey meter to determine the extent of contamination. If the meter indicates the presence of radioactivity, all clothing and valuables should be removed from the victim, bagged, and labeled. This step may reduce the contamination by up to 70%. All metal objects should be identified and saved for possible neutron activation analysis which can aid estimates of the radiation dose received. It should be remembered that, unless there are associated serious injuries, there is really no reason to rush to the hospital. Whenever possible, the victim should be washed at the site. Most of the threat of contaminating others is removed when the clothing is gone and the victim has showered. The victim should then be wrapped in a sheet in order to decrease the possibility of spreading any remaining contaminated material and removed to the ambulance for transport. The rescuers should remove the victim's outer clothing. The interior of the ambulance can be covered or draped to minimize contamination, and transporting personnel should wear protective clothing, gloves, and masks during the transport.

EXTERNAL CONTAMINATION AND DECONTAMINATION

As soon as the receiving hospital is notified, the procedures for managing radiation accidents should be implemented (1, 4, 7). Proper emergency department staff preparation, equipment, and patient management are summarized in Table 40.4–40.6. (See chapter on hospital preparation). Appropriate personnel, including the radiation physicist or safety officer, security personnel, and public information officer, should report to the emergency department. One room should be designated as the decontamination room and prepared for the victim. Nonessential equipment should be removed, the ventilation system turned off, and coverings placed on the floor and all door handles, cabinet handles, drawer handles, and light switches. Entry to and exit from the room must be controlled in order to prevent the spread of contamination. Optimally, the room selected should be close to the ambulance entrance to minimize exposure, and the route from the ambulance entrance to the designated room should be covered with paper and sheets. A decontamination table should be available where the victim can

be washed and the effluent collected for disposal. If the effluent can be directly flushed into ordinary drains and diluted with large amounts of water, then there is no risk in allowing the contaminated fluid to be disposed of in this fashion (9).

Once the victim arrives at the hospital, the patient should be transferred to a hospital stretcher, and the transporting vehicle secured until it can be surveyed and declared free of contamination. Ambulance personnel should be monitored for contamination and, if positive, should remove all clothing, shower, and then be checked again. All hospital personnel involved in evaluating and treating victims should wear protective clothing including gowns, gloves, masks, caps, and shoe covers and utilize film badges or dosimeters to monitor their exposure.

Evaluation and decontamination of the patient may proceed once all immediate life-threatening problems have been addressed. A careful, complete survey of the patient should be performed by the radiation physicist, and contaminated areas of the body documented. Nasal, oral, and ear canal swabs should be obtained and sent for analysis. Radioactive material contaminating wounds, ingested, or inhaled can result in irradiation of tissues throughout the body as well as incorporation of the material into biochemical mechanisms, resulting in permanent radioactivity. Treatment of contaminated wounds by surgical debridement may be necessary if wounds cannot be adequately decontaminated (6, 8). Decontamination of any open wound is the first priority. If an open wound is found to be contaminated, decorporation treatment should be started. Also decorporation should be instituted for inhaled or ingested radioactive material. Thus identification of the type and nature of the radioactive contaminate is crucial. Copious irrigation of the wounds with normal saline usually removes some of the radioactive material. If oral contamination is found, ingestion is presumed, and aspiration of stomach contents by nasogastric tube is indicated. If the aspirate is contaminated, gastric lavage follows. The finding of contamination in nasal swabs is considered presumptive proof of inhalation of radioactive material.

Dermal absorption of radionuclides and radioactivity is of primary concern in planning for the management of patients. Absorption is a passive process determined by the nature of

Table 40.4.   Emergency Department and Staff Preparation

1. Remove all patients and pregnant females from the arrival zone of the ambulance, the entrance into the emergency department, and the route of all contaminated patients.
2. The route from the ambulance arrival zone to the decontamination room is covered with polyethylene plastic secured to the floor with tape.
3. The arrival route and entryway for patients are demarcated with rope or radioactive labeled ribbon. Proper ''radioactive'' signs are in place. This area will remain as such until cleared by radiation safety officers or the health physicists in charge.
4. The decontamination room is marked with proper signs. The floors and walls are covered with polyethylene plastic sheeting secured by tape. A demarcation line of bright, clearly identifiable tape separates ''clean'' from ''unclean'' areas on entrance to the decontamination room. Ventilation to the room is turned off and ventilation ducts covered with appropriate filters or plastic. The room must be self-contained. Electrical switches and handles of doors and equipment should be covered with tape.
5. A designated radiation safety officer maintains watch at the entrance of the decontamination room to monitor all personnel, equipment, and samples leaving the room.
6. A designated nurse or technical assistant is on standby outside the decontamination room to pass in supplies to the medical team in the room. This person does not enter the decontamination room.
7. All equipment in the room is essential to the care and decontamination of the patient and must remain in the room until cleared by radiation safety.
8. Protective garments are donned by decontamination team. Two pairs of gloves should be worn. The inner gloves are removed as the last pieces of protective equipment as the person exits the room postdecontamination. The minimum protection includes surgical scrub wear, pants and shirt, cap, masks, shoe covers, surgical gown with sleeves taped, two pairs of gloves, and eye protection.
9. All personnel entering and leaving the room must be surveyed by radiation safety for contamination. Contaminated items and clothing must remain in the room.

Table 40.5. Management and Decontamination of Patients

1. The physician in charge directs medical care and decontamination of the patients.
2. Radiation safety officer monitors patient front and back on arrival. Contaminated areas are recorded by nurse on patient cards or tags.
3. Patient's clothes are removed and sealed in plastic bag containing proper patient identification.
4. Routine cotton swab samples are obtained of mouth, eye conjunctivae and mucosa, nasal mucosa, and ear canals and placed in sample containers marked with the patient's identification. Other samples are obtained as needed, such as of wound sites and all skin contaminated areas. Samples are given to radiation safety officer for proper storage.
5. Radiation safety officer monitors all decontamination personnel and biologic samples obtained during management and decontamination.
6. Medical assessment identifies medical needs of the patient. Patients with contaminated open wounds have priority.
7. Contaminated wounds:
   A. Begin decorporation treatment with DTPA as soon as possible.
   B. Open wounds are washed with normal saline for 3 to 5 minutes and remonitored for contamination level. This step is repeated if contamination persists.
   C. Persisting contamination of open wounds despite repeated saline washings can be managed with a 3% hydrogen peroxide wash.
   D. Contaminated tissue not being successfully removed by repeated washings may require surgical debridement. Surgical debridement may be necessary if the radionuclide is toxic, has a long half-life, and is not removed by appropriate decontamination methods.
   E. Save and label all tissue removed and place in appropriate specimen containers for storage by radiation safety.
   F. Cover all decontaminated wounds with sterile dressing and protect them from other areas of the skin that may be undergoing decontamination.
8. Contaminated eyes, ears, mouth, nose:
   A. Irrigate eyes with water or saline. Do not allow cross-contamination to the other eye during irrigation.
   B. Irrigate ears with warm saline or a 50:50 mixture of warm saline with 3% hydrogen peroxide using a bulb syringe. Monitor decontamination process, and repeat irrigation as needed. Do not allow irrigation solution to flow into patient's mouth, eyes, or wounds.
   C. Irrigate nose with saline using a bulb syringe. Have suction available, and do not allow patient to swallow irrigant. Monitor irrigant for radioactivity during the process.
   D. Have patient irrigate mouth without swallowing the water. Insert nasogastric tube into stomach and monitor contents of stomach for radioactivity. If GI contents are contaminated, then lavage stomach until clear and begin decorporation with DTPA.
   E. Monitor level of decontamination and repeat irrigations as needed.
9. External contamination:
   A. Decontamination of the skin should begin with mild washing and gentle scrubbing using a detergent and water. A soft sponge or soft brush should be used to avoid skin abrasions. Monitor both skin and washing fluid for radioactivity and repeat washing three to four times to remove residual contaminant.
   B. For persisting levels of contamination, use a mixture of 50:50 cornmeal and powdered detergent (Tide) mixed in water to form a paste. Gently scrub the skin with this mildly abrasive material using soft sponges.
   C. For contamination persisting beyond the above efforts, a 5% sodium hypochlorite solution (Clorox) can be used either as full strength over most areas or diluted 1:4 with (Clorox:water) over areas like the face and neck.
   D. Citric acid 3% can be applied to the areas and rinsed off with water.
   E. For persistent contamination, and *in extreme cases only*, the application of 4% potassium permanganate followed by a 4% sodium bisulfite rinse may be tried. Potassium permanganate is an oxidizer and will stain the skin as well as remove the outer layer of skin.
   F. All skin areas, front and back, should be decontaminated until radiation safety agrees that the process is successful.
   G. Washings are collected in a containment vessel.
   H. Avoid splashing decontamination fluid, and do not allow washings to contaminate eyes, mouth, other mucous membranes, or wounds of the patient.
   I. Contaminated hair is washed with water and soap, then rinsed and monitored. Repeat as necessary. Hair may have to be cut. Do not shave hair due to risk of cutting skin.
10. Patients may be removed from the decontamination room after radiation safety indicates that the level of contamination is safe. The patient should be dried. All materials should remain in the decontamination room. Wounds can be closed as needed after decontamination. Monitoring of patients and personnel is performed before anyone is allowed to leave the room.
11. Entire body of patient is monitored by radiation safety before leaving room.
12. All previously sampled areas should be resampled and labeled as "postdecontamination" with time and patient identification.
13. New polyethylene floor covering is laid out from the patient to the door of the decontamination room to the patient, and a clean stretcher is brought into the room. The patient is placed on the stretcher by a "clean" team and removed from the room. The process is monitored by radiation safety.
14. Decontamination team exit:
    A. The team may be rotated in and out depending on the level of contamination. This will be guided by radiation safety.
    B. An exiting team member will go to the designated "clean" line at the door of the room. All protective clothing will be placed in a predesignated drop zone or placed in a predesignated container. Outer gloves are removed first. Personnel monitors are then given to radiation safety officer. Remove tape from sleeves and trouser cuffs. Remove outer surgical gown, then shirt and pants. Shoe covers are removed one at a time. Radiation safety monitors the first shoe and if clean, the person can step over the line into the clean area and remove the second shoe cover. The inner gloves are then removed after the person is over the clean line and dropped into the designated area.
    C. The team member then showers and is remonitored by radiation safety officer for any contamination.

the radionuclide, the physical condition of the skin, the extent of contamination, the solubility of the contaminant, and the chemical nature of the radionuclide. The horny layer of the skin is the most important barrier to penetration. Mechanical damage to the skin will substantially increase absorption. Injury from acids and alkalis can either facilitate or in some cases inhibit percutaneous absorption. Dilute acid burns facilitate the dermal penetration of plutonium (1).

The initial evaluation of external contamination should include gamma, beta, and alpha monitoring. Experience in mon-

Table 40.6. Emergency Department Radioactive Decontamination Room Equipment

Two-inch demarcation tape for floor
Four-inch and two-inch wide tape to secure wall and floor coverings
Plastic (polyethylene, 6 mil, 8 × 100 feet) floor and wall covering
Plastic (polyethylene, 6 mil, 4 × 100 feet) hall and corridor floor
  covering
Rolls of adsorbent paper with plastic backing for room and hallway
Ventilation filter paper
Radioactive warning signs
Decontamination stretchers with drainage collection tank
Plastic aprons
Dosimeters and film badges for decontamination team
Direct reading dosimeters plus chargers
Flashlights with extra batteries
Five-gallon wash containers
Cotton sheets and covers
Yellow rope with stands for demarcating zones
Large waste containers with lids (44-gallon drums) with plastic bag
  liners for waste
Dress down and decontamination instructions
Sterile suture sets with extra forceps, hemostats, and scissors
Sterile irrigation fluid (several liters)
Sterile dressings
Razors with extra blades
Personal respirators
Surgical gowns, scrub tops and bottoms, shoe covers, caps, masks,
  and latex gloves, protective eyewear with side shields—for both
  decontamination team and as extra clothes for victims
Disposable paper towels
Blankets
Five-gallon plastic buckets with tops
Large barrels for waste disposal
Scrub brushes
Surgical sponges—large
Irrigation syringes
Irrigation basins and bowls
Surgical scrub sponges
Liquid soap—one quart
Neoprene industrial gloves—one or two pairs
Tongs and forceps
Cotton swabs and wipes
Detergent (abrasive soap, detergent-cornmeal)
Clorox solution or other bleach (5% sodium hypochlorite)
3% Hydrogen peroxide
Sponge forceps
Cotton-tipped applicators
Tubes with tops to contain cotton-tipped applicator samples
Lead storage containers from nuclear medicine to contain samples
Body chart of front and back for recording contaminated areas
Irrigation bulb syringe
Plastic specimen containers with lids
Hair clippers
Nail clippers
Bandage scissors
Vacutainers, syringes, needles, and blood drawing tubes
Alcohol wipes
Tissue paper
4 × 4 and 2 × 2 gauze pads
Small plastic bags for samples
Large yellow plastic bags (100)
Self-adherent labels and markers
Urine containers (1000–2000 milliliters)
Gamma-beta monitor
Alpha detector
Extra batteries
''Radioactive'' tape labels for marking containers
Log book with pencils
Markers

itoring for beta emitters and alpha emitters is essential. An inexperienced person using this sophisticated equipment can miss beta emitting contamination, and beta burns to the skin can occur if this contamination remains in contact too long.

Decontaminating the skin begins with removing the patient's clothes, placing the patient on the decontamination stretcher, and bagging the clothes. General principles of external decontamination (Table 40.5) involve gently scrubbing the contaminated areas with a water-detergent combination. The use of a soft brush or soft sponge is recommended to prevent abrading the skin. Attention should be paid to the hair, nails, and web spaces of toes and fingers. The wash solution must be collected in a containment vessel, and the decontamination team adequately garbed in protective clothing. Between decontamination procedures, the skin should be dried and monitored for effectiveness of the decontamination. If contaminant remains, this process should be repeated until background levels are demonstrated by monitoring. Persistence of contamination despite the initial decontamination can be managed by a slightly abrasive method such as a paste of cornmeal and Tide detergent mixed 50:50. The use of 5% sodium hypochlorite (household bleach) solution should be tried prior to a more abrasive measure. A problem with sodium hypochlorite is that a weakly acidic solution tends to make plutonium soluble and could increase risk of percutaneous absorption. The use of radionuclide chelating agents in addition to the detergent scrub has been employed. Each method should be followed by monitoring for residual contamination after drying of the skin. An aggressive decontamination method involves the application of 4% potassium permanganate solution, a staining agent and oxidizer, followed in 2 minutes by rinsing of the skin with 4% sodium bisulfite. This should be undertaken by a person with experience with potassium permanganate, since the skin can be damaged (10). Once these procedures are performed, the patient is moved to a clean stretcher and then resurveyed. Hair that cannot be decontaminated should be removed by clipping and saved by radiation safety. Shaving is to be avoided, since small breaks in the skin may be produced.

Following triage and patient assessment, samples of body fluids should be obtained for analysis (2). Blood is sent for a complete blood count, differential, and platelet count. It is essential that samples be drawn as early as possible in order to determine a baseline leukocyte count and to type lymphocytes for possible marrow transplantation later in the patient's course. Absolute lymphocyte count of more than 1500 cell/mm^3 48 hours after exposure indicates minimum exposure, whereas fewer than 1000 lymphocytes at 24 hours or 500 at 48 hours indicates a severe radiation exposure. Serum electrolytes and a chromosome analysis are also performed on blood specimens. Urine and fecal samples are collected daily; however, initial samples that are negative for contamination may be misleading. Several days may be needed before an accurate assessment can be made (1, 2).

INTERNAL CONTAMINATION AND MANAGEMENT

Also termed *incorporation*, internal contamination results from the inhalation, ingestion, or wound contamination of a radioactive material or radionuclide. The radioactive material thus has the opportunity to become incorporated into the body and irradiate internal tissues. This situation is a serious medical emergency. Some radionuclides can become permanently incorporated into the biologic molecules of the body. Methods to decorporate these radioactive materials should be carried out according to a standard protocol (1). Patients who are judged to have high probability of internal contamination should undergo treatment as rapidly as possible in order to minimize incorporation of the radioactive substance (1, 2). Treatment modalities revolve around enhanced elimination or excretion and reduction of absorption; however, specific therapy depends upon identification of the radioactive contaminant involved.

If gastrointestinal contamination is likely, the first procedure utilized is gastric lavage. The stomach is washed with large amounts of water to remove as much material as possible. The aspirate should be tested for contamination and lavage continued until the fluid return is free of radioactivity. Purgatives may be utilized in order to increase the rapidity with which the radioactive material traverses the bowel. In addition, certain cathartics such as magnesium sulfate may produce insoluble salts with some radionuclides and further limit absorption. Barium- and aluminum-containing antacids are used for strontium ingestion and act to decrease uptake by forming insoluble salts. Prussian blue given orally has been utilized experimentally to decrease absorption of some radionuclides (1).

Pulmonary lavage may be used for inhalation of radioactive material that is not soluble. This decontamination technique is performed under general anesthesia and involves the use of a double lumen endotracheal tube so the two lungs can be isolated from each other and lavaged independently to remove deposited material (1).

Blocking agents may be administered to reduce uptake by saturating metabolic pathways with stable or nonradioactive compounds. For example, radioiodine can be competitively blocked by giving potassium iodine. Stable forms of strontium can be used to reduce uptake or radioactive strontium. The same is true for radioactive forms of calcium, zinc, and potassium (1).

Prompt and proper handling of contaminated wounds is especially important to prevent further incorporation of radioactive material. Surveying the wound with the radiation detector will indicate whether the site is contaminated; sampling of wound tissue, exudate, any foreign bodies, and wound irrigation solution should be accomplished. Elimination can be enhanced by the use of chelating agents which bind target compounds and then are excreted by the kidney. Multivalent radioisotopes in the actinide series (transuranic elements plutonium, neptunium, americium) as well as rare earths have been effectively chelated using diethylenetriaminepentaacetic acid (DTPA) (1). Other metal chelators such as calcium disodium ethylenediaminetetraacetic acid (CaNA$_2$EDTA, calcium versenate), dimercaprol (BAL), dimercaptosuccinic acid (DMSA), dimercaptosulfonate (DMPS), penicillamine, and deferoxamine can be used for the appropriate metals (Table 40.7). Calcium disodium EDTA can be used for transuranium metals, but DTPA is much more effective. DMSA and DMPS, analogues of BAL, are newer chelators and are superior to other chelators for removing many metals including cadmium, chromium, mercury, lead, arsenic, and copper (11). The use of combined chelators DTPA and BAL has been successful in removing cadmium in animal models (12).

Although human data on the use of DTPA are limited, its administration is recommended as soon as possible within the first few hours to be effective. DTPA is available from the Radiation Emergency Assistance Center/Training Site (REAC/TS) in Oak Ridge, Tennessee, telephone number (615) 576-

Table 40.7. Chelating Agents for Radioactive Materials

DTPA	Plutonium, americium, curium neptunium, californium, cerium, yttrium, lanthanum, scandium, promethium, niobium, lutetium, zirconium, zinc
CaNa$_2$ EDTA	Lead, zinc, copper, nickel chromium, manganese
Penicillamine	Copper, mercury, lead, gold
Dimercaptosuccinic acid (DMSA)	Mercury, arsenic, lead, copper, cadmium, zinc, nickel, gold
Dimercaprol + DTPA	Cadmium
Dimercaptosulfonate (DMPS)	Cadmium, gold, chromium
Dimercaprol (BAL)	Mercury, arsenic, lead, copper, cadmium, zinc, nickel, gold, bismuth
Deferoxamine	Iron

1004 (1). Decorporation with chelating agents should be started as soon as possible in patients with contaminated wounds. Patients with residual contamination from skin break or foreign bodies may also benefit from pharmacologic therapy. Treatment depends on the chemical properties of the particular radioisotope involved and should be done in conjunction with advice from a nuclear medicine physician or radiation medicine specialist. DTPA chelates multivalent radionuclides that can then be renally excreted. Both the calcium and zinc salts of DTPA are approved for human use. CaDTPA is 10 times more effective than ZnDTPA for increasing renal excretion of actinide radionuclides within the first few hours of exposure. ZnDTPA is equally efficacious after the first 1 or 2 days of exposure.

In an acute exposure, 1 gram of CaDTPA diluted in 250 milliliters of dextrose 5% in water should be infused over 60–90 minutes. The dose may be repeated daily for 5 days. For immediate field administration, an aerosol inhalation treatment can be accomplished by placing the entire contents of a vial in a nebulizer. ZnDTPA appears to be less toxic than CaDTPA, but due to its lower efficacy should not be the first drug of choice. CaDPTA should be continued at a once-daily dose of 1 gram intravenously. During this time blood samples, whole body and chest counts, 24-hour urine collections, and stool samples should be collected and monitored for radioactivity to determine need for further chelation. If further chelation is required beyond 5 days, then ZnDTPA should be substituted for more prolonged therapy. A DTPA administration protocol and consent form is available from REAC/TS.

A nuclear medicine specialist should be consulted as soon as possible in cases of incorporation or if it is suspected to have occurred.

SUMMARY

Although the risk of radioactive contamination to health care providers treating victims of radiation exposure is small, appropriate precautions must always be taken. The type of accident (irradiation, surface contamination, or internal contamination) and the type of radioactivity or radioactive compound involved determines the steps to be taken to treat the patient and prevent further contamination.

REFERENCES

1. NCRP. Management of persons accidentally contaminated with radionuclides. National Council on Radiation Protection and Measurements, Report no. 65. Bethesda, MD: NCRP, 1979.

2. AMA. A guide to the hospital management of injuries arising from exposure to or involving ionizing radiation. Chicago, IL: American Medical Association, 1984.

3. Jacobs LM, Schwartz RJ, Gemmell CH. Radiation injury. Emerg Care Quart 1985;1:41–50.

4. Richter LL, Berk HW, Teates CD, et al. A systems approach to the management of radiation accidents. Ann Emerg Med 1980;9:303–309.

5. Stasiak RS, Stewart CE, Redwine RH. Symptoms and treatment of radiation exposure: an overview for EMS personnel. Emerg Med Serv 1986;15:21–29.

6. Conklin JJ, Walker RI, Hirsch EF. Current concepts in the management of radiation injuries and associated trauma. Surg Gynecol Obstet 1985;156:809–826.

7. Leonard RB, Ricks RC. Emergency department radiation accident protocol. Ann Emerg Med 1980;9:462–470.

8. Eiseman B, Bond V. Surgical care of nuclear casualties. Surg Gynecol Obstet 1978;146:877–883.

9. CDH. Handling the radiation accident victim—a guide for hospital personnel. Colorado Department of Health, Division of Radiation and Hazardous Wastes Control.

10. Hubner, KF. Decontamination procedures and risks to health personnel. Bull NY Acad Med 1983;59:1119–1128.

11. Aposhian HV. DMSA and DMPS-water soluble antidotes for heavy metal poisoning. Annu Rev Pharmacol Toxicol 1983;23:193–215.

12. Cherian M, Rogers K. Chelation of cadmium from metallothionein in vivo and its excretion in rats repeatedly injected with cadmium chloride. Pharmacol Exp Ther 1982;222:699–704.

41

Assessing Community Risk from the Sudden Release of a Toxic Gas

John Lowe, C.I.H.
Gary R. Krieger, M.D., M.P.H.
Steven R. Radis
John B. Sullivan, Jr., M.D.

INTRODUCTION

The risks to health from a sudden release of a toxic gas were demonstrated by the methyl isocyanate disaster in Bhopal, India, in 1984. Since many communities depend economically on the location of plants and facilities that either store, use, or process toxic gases, the ability to model the risk of a toxic gas release to the community is an important aspect of disaster planning. Examples of such toxic gases include arsine, phosphine, phosgene, ammonia, hydrogen sulfide, chlorine, and hydrogen cyanide. Community concern over potential disasters from sudden spills or releases of hazardous materials has led to attempts to predict the risks associated with any such release. Factors that influence the potential health consequences include the volume and duration of gas release, the nature of the toxic gas, the site of release, climate and wind factors, containment technology, proximity of population to the site of release, and emergency medical response. Examining the risk as well as the health concerns requires the use of gas dispersion modeling as a component of the overall risk assessment procedure. This type of model attempts to predict both the concentration of a gas that disperses from a release site into an area as well as the influences of meteorologic factors on these concentrations. This method allows for better community preparation and emergency medical response to any sudden gas release.

Using arsine gas as an example, an estimate of emission and dispersion in air under selected potential sudden release scenarios and evaluation of the possible risks to human health associated with this release will be presented. The air dispersion and risk assessment for potential sudden release scenarios will include:

1. Release of a specific quantity of arsine over a specific duration of time from inside a plant site with the gas being vented into the air from the facility roof.
2. Release of a specific quantity of arsine over a specific duration from compressed gas cylinders damaged during transport and shipping.

To further characterize the airborne concentrations from different release quantities of arsine, the scenarios will include dispersion under varying meteorologic conditions.

Risk assessment for such releases of arsine include:

1. Development of health criteria for shortterm exposure to arsine in the form of an airborne concentration.
2. Exposure assessment and identification of potentially exposed human receptor populations.

3. Modeling dispersion in air of arsine releases under specific conditions of release.
4. Documenting the results of the dispersion modeling and health criteria development.

SITE DESCRIPTION

The facility in which this arsine release occurs will be a four-story semiconductor manufacturing building with 40,000 square feet per floor. The semiconductor industry uses a wide variety of gases as dopants. These materials are used in concentrations ranging from low parts per million (ppm) to 100%. Chemically, dopant gases are hydrides of arsenic, boron, silicon, phosphorus, germanium, and antimony. The corresponding gases are arsine (AsH_3), diborane (B_2H_6), silane (SiH_4), phosphine (PH_3), germane (GeH_4), and stibine (SbH_3). These gases are highly toxic and are flammable or pyrophoric.

DEVELOPING HEALTH RISK CRITERIA

Arsine Gas Toxicity

Acute high dose exposure to arsine is associated with rapid hemolysis of red blood cells and subsequent renal failure. In a variety of industries and exposure situations, over 200 cases of arsine poisoning have been reported, with over 20% of these resulting in fatalities (1). Experimental evidence indicates that the hemolytic activity of arsine is due to its ability to cause a decline in reduced erythrocyte glutathione (GSH) concentrations (2). The hemolysis associated with acute arsine exposure is characterized by a latent period with a length inversely proportional to the extent of exposure. Inhalation of 250 ppm of arsine is instantly lethal; inhalation of 25–50 ppm for 30 minutes is lethal, and 10 ppm is lethal after a longer exposure period (1).

Human exposure data and studies in laboratory animals (rats and mice) illustrate a steep dose-response relationship that results in a sharp threshold between tolerated and lethal doses of arsine. In laboratory animals, exposures to arsine concentrations up to 5 ppm for 28 days were tolerated. However, exposure to 10 ppm for 4 days produced 100% mortality in test populations (1).

These data are consistent with a mechanism of toxicity involving depletion of erythrocyte GSH. GSH is critical for the maintenance of the structural integrity of the erythrocyte membrane (3). If de novo erythrocyte GSH synthesis matches exposure, then significant acute hemolysis is not observed.

However, if arsine doses exceed GSH resynthesis, then acute fulminant hemolysis can be produced. If significant but non-saturating exposure occurs, biochemical evidence of low to moderate hemolysis is produced. A quantitative study of hematologic responses to arsine exposure in mice has been published (2). In this well-designed and -controlled study, hematologic responses were evaluated in mice exposed to 5–26 ppm arsine for 1 hour. The concentrations range from a no-effect level of 5 ppm to a lethal concentration of 26 ppm. This concentration range is extremely narrow and represents less than a 10-fold difference for the 1-hour exposure studied. The lowest hematocrit level was observed 24 hours after exposure, with complete recovery of the surviving mice within 11 days after exposure. Similar results were demonstrated in laboratory animals in a subchronic, low dose study (4). In this study, mice and rats were exposed to arsine for 6 hr/day, 5 days/week at concentrations of 0, 0.025, 0.5, and 2.5 ppm for 90 days. Abnormal hematologic parameters were noted in animals exposed to 2.5 ppm at all time points; hematologic abnormalities were noted after 90 days in those animals exposed to 0.5 ppm. Significantly, after in vitro exposure to arsine gas for 1 hour, GSH levels in rat and mouse erythrocytes were markedly reduced.

These observations confirm a strong inverse correlation between the GSH erythrocyte concentration and the extent of hemolysis in arsine-exposed erythrocytes. Altered erythrocyte osmotic fragility was noted only at the higher dose levels studied (15 and 26 ppm) (2). This observation is consistent with the threshold effect observed in acute lethality studies. Thus, determination of erythrocyte osmotic fragility could represent a biologic exposure index.

In animals, a clear time and dose-dependent threshold exists between subtle hematologic effects and lethality. In humans, the time course for hematologic reaction is similar, although the data are clearly confounded by treatment interventions such as exchange transfusions and hemodialysis. In addition, it is very difficult to document dose and exposure times accurately.

In animal studies, a marked dose-related increase in the activity of δ-aminolevulinic acid dehydratase (ALAD) is observed with exposure to arsine. Furthermore, differential analysis of peripheral blood in rats and mice demonstrate the presence of reticulocytes and Howell-Jolly bodies (1). These findings are consistent with the development of a regenerative anemia. Significantly, the porphyrinuria pattern observed with arsine exposure is different from prolonged oral exposure to arsenate, or acute intratracheal instillation of gallium arsenide. These observations imply that different sites of toxicity and possibly different detoxification mechanisms for arsine compared with other forms of arsenic.

Clinical Toxicology of Arsine

Clinically, the signs and symptoms of poisoning are those consistent with acute and massive hemolysis. Initially, there is painless hemoglobinuria, dizziness, weakness, nausea, vomiting, abdominal cramping, and tenderness. After a dose-dependent latent period, usually 2–24 hours, jaundice accompanied by anuria or oliguria may occur. Evidence of bone marrow depression has also been reported. Individuals with preexisting renal or cardiac disease or with hypersensitivity to hemolytic agents resulting from a congenital deficiency of erythrocyte GSH are potentially highly sensitive to arsine. Treatment of arsine exposure consists of immediate removal of the individual

from the contaminated environment and close clinical evaluation of the subsequent hemolytic crisis. Alkalinization of the urine may help prevent acute renal failure in the event of hemolysis. Exchange transfusion may also be helpful should hemolysis occur. The use of heavy metal chelators does not appear to be efficacious in cases of arsine exposure (1).

Chronic toxicity data are fragmentary, although changes in cardiac performance have been reported. No reports were located concerning neurotoxicity from chronic exposure, although one report details the manifestation of reversible polyneuropathy and a mild psychoorganic syndrome following an acute arsine exposure. In this case, the latency period for the first symptom onset was 1 month. In a separate incident of acute arsine poisoning, the recovered worker demonstrated a peripheral neuropathy for 6 months after exposure (5).

Occupational Exposure Limits of Arsine

Occupational exposure standards are available for arsine. A Threshold Limit Value-Time-Weighted Average (TLV-TWA) for workplace exposure to arsine is 0.05 ppm. This is the concentration to which nearly all workers can be repeatedly exposed, on an 8-hour TWA basis, during a working lifetime without adverse effect. This TLV was adopted by the American Conference of Governmental Industrial Hygienists (ACGIH) in 1977. The Federal Occupational Safety and Health Administration (OSHA) also uses 0.05 ppm as the Permissible Exposure Level (PEL). Notably, the documentation for this value provides little human exposure-response information. There are multiple reasons for this lack of documentation: (a) arsine is colorless, nonirritating, and odorless below 1–2 ppm; (b) at intermediate doses, there is a significant latency period between exposure and hemolytic response. Thus, exposure may be undetected, and airborne concentrations remain undetermined.

The animal database associated with the TLV provides little quantitative dose-response information on the hemolytic effects of arsine exposure. Lethality in mice exposed to arsine concentrations ranging from 8–800 ppm has been evaluated (6). Another older report studied lower airborne concentrations (0.5–2 ppm) but presented few details relevant to exposure conditions or animal responses (6). As discussed previously, a quantitative study of hematologic responses to arsine exposure in mice has been published (2). Hematologic responses were evaluated in mice exposed to 5–26 ppm arsine for 1 hour. The results range from a no-effect level of 5 ppm to a lethal concentration of 26 ppm. This concentration range is extremely narrow and represents less than a 10-fold difference for the 1-hour exposure studied.

Community Exposure Limits/Emergency Planning Guidelines

Several legislative and regulatory efforts have been initiated, both on state and federal levels to regulate toxic gas releases. Since the 1984 Bhopal disaster, the U.S. Environmental Protection Agency (EPA) has established a list of approximately 400 chemicals that are considered extremely hazardous materials (EHMs). EHMs that are gaseous at normal temperature and pressure, or liquids with extremely high vapor pressures are of greatest concern. Arsine is a typical example of an industrial/manufacturing-based EHM.

In California, two pieces of legislation (Assembly Bill (AB) 3777, and Assembly Bill 1021) require facility operators handling EHMs to assess the impact to the community in the event of an accidental discharge. One activity funded under AB 1021 was a study of the use and management of toxic gases. A major aspect of this study was gas dispersion modeling for risk-based evacuation planning (Santa Clara County Fire Chiefs Association, 1987). As part of this emergency response planning exercise, a Community Evacuation Level (CEL) was developed. The CEL was defined as the ''minimum toxic gas concentration level for a single gas at which protection or evacuation of the community is recommended.'' The calculation of a CEL presents a difficult toxicologic and risk management decision. Sherin (1989), at a symposium sponsored by the ACGIH, presented the possible choices for a basis for a CEL (7):

1. The ACGIH Short-Term Exposure Limit (STEL);
2. Two times the TLV-TWA, based on a 60-minute average evacuation time;
3. 1% of the lowest published inhalation lethal concentration (LC$_{50}$) value.

The EPA has also developed a method for evaluating the toxicity of substances for the purpose of emergency planning. This method bases toxicity ranking on the Immediately Dangerous to Life and Health (IDLH) values developed by the National Institute for Occupational Safety and Health.

The IDLH is defined in the Code of Federal Regulations (29 CFR 1986) as, ''. . . conditions that pose an immediate threat of severe exposure to contaminants, such as radioactive materials, which are likely to have adverse cumulative or delayed effects on health.'' Concerns associated with the IDLH concept relative to the calculation of values appropriate for sudden chemical releases have been reviewed (8):

IDLH values were used initially calculated for the purpose of respirator selection.
IDLHs were not intended to be a 30-minute permissible acute exposure standard.
IDLH values were developed for the workplace environment, not for community exposure.
IDLH values emphasized acute noncarcinogenic toxicity, and did not consider possible carcinogenic effects.
One-time exposure to an IDLH concentration may pose a significant cancer risk for some chemicals, when assessed using existing regulatory cancer risk assessment methods.
IDLH values are frequently not consistent with animal-based 30-minute LC$_{50}$ values.
IDLHs are not consistent with the National Academy of Sciences 1-hour emergency exposure guidance levels (EEGLs).

The issue of calculating a cancer risk based on a 30-minute or 1-hour exposure is fraught with potential methodologic problems. Arsine gas has potential carcinogenic effects from the release of elemental arsenic. The carcinogenic potency of inhaled arsenic is derived from epidemiologic studies of miners and smelter workers exposed to inorganic arsenic compounds. Cancer risks are estimated from these data using a linear extrapolation dose-response model that is based on the assumption of continuous inhalation exposure over a lifetime. Attempting to evaluate cancer risks from a one-time shortterm exposure is clearly an inappropriate application of this assessment methodology. Also, there is no toxicologic evidence that supports a conclusion that a 1-hour exposure to arsine presents a significant cancer risk.

Table 41.1 presents a comparison of various values used for arsine emergency response planning. There is a 120-fold var-

Table 41.1.   Arsine Toxicity Values (ppm)

NIOSH (IDLH)	TLV (ACGIH)	PEL (OSHA)	Santa Clara (CEL)	EEGL (NAS)
6	0.05	0.05	0.2	1.0

TLV: Threshold Limit Value
ACGIH: American Conference for Governmental Industrial Hygienist
PEL: Permissible Exposure Limit
CEL: Community Exposure Level (Developed by the Santa Clara County Fire Chiefs Association)
EEGL: Emergency Exposure Guidance Level
NAS: National Academy of Sciences

iation from the TLV/PEL to the IDLH values, and a fivefold difference between the EEGL and the value developed by the Santa Clara County Fire Chiefs Association. It is interesting to compare this range of values with the narrow dose-response relationship that has been demonstrated for arsine.

The determination of the ''true'' health criteria value is critical, because this value is utilized to generate risk-based emergency plans that potentially include community evacuation. The existing, anecdotal human database for arsine exposure is insufficient to calculate a health criteria value; however, the animal database does provide the necessary insight. A 1-hour, no-effect level in laboratory animals was demonstrated at 5 ppm. In developing human health criteria from animal toxicity data, a 10-fold uncertainty factor is considered a conservative factor for extrapolation of results across species. Thus, a health conservative estimate of a no-effect level for 1-hour exposure in humans is then 0.5 ppm. This value is consistent with the National Academy of Sciences 1-hour Emergency Exposure Guidance Levels value of 1 ppm and is consistent with the toxicologic data, which supports a value lower than 5 ppm for a 1-hour exposure. A health criteria of 1 ± 0.5 ppm is an appropriate extrapolation of the database for arsine.

COMMUNITY EXPOSURE SCENARIOS

Two different types of hypothetical arsine gas releases are evaluated in this sudden release model: (a) arsine release from the facility via a roof vent, and (b) arsine release during handling of a cylinder in an outdoor area.

The release from the facility roof vent will be assumed to occur during the use of an arsine cylinder in the semiconductor device manufacturing process. Dopant gases are used in chemical vapor deposition (CVD) processes, which are performed under ventilation control. It is assumed that the arsine-compressed gas cylinder is also under ventilation controls and that any release is exhausted to outside air. The event precipitating the release is assumed to be damage to the cylinder regulator, exposing the cylinder orifice. Arsine is released from the vent as a gas.

Another release will be presumed to have occurred accidentally during handling of a cylinder of compressed arsine gas during transportation and delivery activities. The event precipitating the release is damage to the cylinder regulator, exposing the cylinder orifice. The cylinder is dropped onto the ground and is lodged against an obstruction, which prevents rocketing. The cylinder is assumed to be oriented horizontally, and arsine is released as a denser-than-air aerosol.

EXPOSURE ASSESSMENT

Exposure assessment for such a release of toxic gas into the air must identify zones of vulnerability to the public by incorporating atmospheric dispersion of the gas released with information describing the shortterm health effects of arsine exposure. Assessment must provide the methodology for calculating the arsine release rates and modeling the atmospheric dispersion of these releases. The other prime factor influencing the exposure assessment is the proximity of the community population surrounding the facility.

Characterizing the Surrounding Population

Characterizing the population that surrounds such a facility is critical in assessing the risk. Attention must be paid to the proximity of schools, hospitals, residential areas, and other businesses. Access routes must be identified for their potential use as major exit corridors for the emergency evacuation of the surrounding population.

The facility where the release occurs is located in a small community, furthermore, the land surrounding the building is assumed to be for commercial purposes. The facility property surrounds the building on all other sides at a radius of at least one-quarter mile and extends to the north, east, and west for distances of at least one-half mile. Residential population density in the vicinity of the site is relatively low, with an estimated total residential population of 1500 and a total area of 500 acres.

Arsine Release Rates

The atmospheric dispersion of arsine from the release scenarios is dependent on: (a) the mass release rate and (b) the duration of release. To estimate the release rate, the mode of release must first be selected. These modes could include liquid jets, vapor jets, two-phase jets, and two-phase spills.

Jet releases are applicable when the upstream pressure across a hole or orifice is greater than the downstream pressure. Such releases (gas or liquid) are limited by the sonic or critical velocity (also known as choked flow). Two-phase spills are spills that involve an initial flashing of a cryogenic or pressurized liquid. Two-phase jets involve an initial liquid jet within a duct or long orifice that develop flashing within the duct. The flashing flow is characterized by a turbulent two-phase (vapor and liquid) mixture exiting at a sonic velocity. Vapor releases are low pressure releases, where the momentum of the release is not the dominant factor.

For liquid and vapor jets, there are well-established mathematical correlations that accurately calculate the mass release rates. These correlations depend on the physical thermodynamic properties of arsine at a certain temperature and/or pressure. Two-phase jets are more difficult to predict because of turbulent flashing flow. Recent work in ammonia release studies has helped define the release rate correlation for flashing flow. Two-phase spills depend on atmospheric conditions, the initial properties of the liquid, and the thermodynamic properties of the fluid. The thermodynamic properties are also used in the initial dispersion behavior of the release.

A turbulent two-phase jet flow is assumed to occur through the orifice created by the broken cylinder valve in scenario 2. It is postulated that the 5-pound arsine cylinder is lying horizontal from a fall, thus placing the hole of the broken valve

below the liquid level. Scenario 1 is based on a vapor phase release of arsine gas from the roof vent. Both scenarios consider that the cylinders of arsine are at full capacity, thus producing a constant sonic release flow. Release rates are estimated using the assumption of a flashing flow. Calculation of the release rates for hazard scenario 2 is by the following formula:

$$\text{Arsine amount} = 2.27 \text{ kg (5-pound cylinder)}$$

$$W \text{ (kg/s)} = \frac{F(A \times H_{vap})}{\left[\left(\dfrac{1}{P_v} - \dfrac{1}{P_1}\right)(T_b C_p)^{0.5}\right]}$$

F = frictional loss factor = 0.65 (reference 19)

A = cross-section area of discharge (m²)

  = πr^2 = $\pi (1.524 \times 10^{-4} \text{ m/2})^2$

  = $1.824 \times 10^{-8} \text{ m}^2$

H_{vap} = heat of vaporization (J/kg) = 214,071 J/kg

T_b = boiling point temperature at 1 atm (K°) = 210.7

C_p = specific heat of liquid (J/kg − K°) = 779

P_v = vapor density at pressure = 220 psi (kg/m³)
  = 67.5

P_1 = liquid density at pressure = 220 psi (kg/m³)
  = 1653

W = 4.41×10^{-4} kg/s

$$Release \ duration = \frac{2.27 \text{ kg}}{4.41 \times 10^{-4} \text{ kg/sec}} = 5147 \text{ sec.}$$

Dispersion Modeling of Gas Release

Dispersion models are employed to simulate the airborne concentrations of arsine downwind that could potentially occur following such releases. The objective of dispersion modeling analysis is to provide a conservative estimate of the zone of vulnerability for a given accidental release as a function of a certain meteorologic condition. The zone of vulnerability is determined as the maximum width and distance downwind that a specified level of concern (i.e., an airborne concentration) of arsine may potentially be exceeded. The zone of vulnerability and the distribution of the potentially exposed population are used to rank various releases in terms of significance and to assess the relative merits of any proposed emergency response measures.

The dispersion modeling methodologies applied depend in part on the mode and duration of the release, and hence the nature of the release scenario. The two scenarios under study are:

Scenario 1: A horizontal arsine vapor release resulting from an arsine cylinder valve failure within the facility with emissions occurring through a roof vent.

Scenario 2: A ground-based horizontal arsine aerosol jet release resulting from a 5-pound arsine cylinder valve failure occurring at an outdoor loading area.

The first type of release considered (scenario 1) would produce a near neutral or slightly nonbuoyant vertical arsine vapor jet from the facility roof vent. The second type of release considered (scenario 2) would produce a denser-than-air horizontal aerosol jet of arsine. Observations from field experiments and experience from historical accidents suggest that the majority of releases from pressurized storage vessels produce either a two-phase jet or aerosol cloud (9, 10). The presence of the aerosol and subsequent evaporation produce a cold, denser-than-air plume. While the initial arsine plume would be denser than air, the plume would rapidly mix with ambient air and become a neutrally buoyant vapor plume downwind from the release.

Vapor Dispersion Models (ISCST)

The dispersion modeling techniques applied during the off-site consequence analysis for neutrally buoyant releases of arsine are based on the conventional Gaussian description of an effluent plume. Since the duration of the vapor releases simulated was either longer or shorter than the averaging and expected travel times of concern, the vapor modeling used both continuous and puff release formulations. The Gaussian plume equation forms the basis of the majority of the EPA's suggested dispersion models (11). A screening type of analysis can be performed based on the following conservative assumptions:

No deposition or removal at the surface;
Negligible plume rise and therefore the plume center line remained on the ground throughout the release;
No initial dilution by building wake effects;
Conservative, unfavorable meteorologic conditions that result in relatively higher airborne concentrations.

These conservative assumptions result in prediction concentrations that overstate likely concentrations resulting from simulated accidental releases.

In order to perform the calculations, the EPA's *Industrial Source Complex Short Term* (ISCST) dispersion model can be applied using a range of meteorologic conditions. The techniques employed are similar to the suggestions contained in the EPA's guide for emergency planning for extremely hazardous substances with the exception that more meteorologic conditions are included (12).

The Pasquill-Gifford (P-G) dispersion curves are selected in the ISCST applications due to the mix of rural and moderately developed areas in the vicinity of the facility where release occurs. The Pasquill-Gifford dispersion curves are typically applied to predict concentrations with an averaging time of about 10 minutes. However, since concentration estimates on the order of minutes were required for comparison with short-term health criteria, these dispersion curves are adjusted for averaging times less than 1 hour. Following the suggestions of Hanna et al., the horizontal dispersion parameters were modified for smaller averaging times (13):

Equation 1

$$\sigma_y' = \sigma_y \left[\frac{T_a}{60} \right]^{0.2}$$

σ_y = the Briggs urban horizontal dispersion parameter (m) representing a 60-minute averaging time,

σ_y' = the modified horizontal dispersion parameter (m), and

T_a = the averaging time (minutes).

A conservative estimate for the basis of the P-G curves of 10 minutes is assumed and the 0.2 power law coefficient is recommended. For 1- and 5-hour average concentrations, the application of the relationship results in concentration estimates which were 1.58 and 1.15 times higher than the original ISCST predictions.

The ISCST model can be applied for each release condition, meteorologic case, and averaging time to determine a hazard footprint. The hazard footprint is defined as the crosswind and downwind distances to a given arsine level of concern. Monitoring devices within the hazard footprint would record exposures above the level of concern. In order to define the hazard footprints, monitors can be located at 50-meter intervals in both the downwind and crosswind directions. The downwind distance of the hazard footprint is determined through logarithmic interpolation of the ISCST predictions along the plume centerline. This procedure assumes that the concentration follows a power law with downwind distance, which is a good approximation over short distance intervals.

Once the downwind distance of the hazard footprint is determined, the maximum crosswind distance that exceeds the criteria can be calculated by stepping back in distance and examining the expression:

Equation 2

$$Y_{ref} = \sigma_y' \left[2 \ln \left[\frac{c_{max}}{c_{ref}} \right] \right]^{1/2}$$

c_{ref} = the reference or criteria concentration (ppm) at crosswind distance Y_{ref} (m), and

c_{max} = the plume center line concentration (ppm).

The maximum crosswind width is calculated by applying Equation 2 at each downwind receptor until a maximum is obtained.

Two-Phase and Dense Gas Dispersion Models (SLAB)

The discharge of liquid phase arsine from the cylinder at elevated pressure would likely result in the formation of a denser-than-air aerosol cloud (14). Close to the point of release a volatile two-phase jet would be formed, followed further downwind by a plume dominated by buoyancy-induced spreading, and finally by a well-mixed neutrally buoyant plume. Field experiments examining the release of dense gases have shown that estimates of downwind concentrations were underestimated when the conventional dispersion modeling techniques were employed (15). This is attributed to an overprediction of the vertical dispersion by the Gaussian models which do not consider the stable stratification and reduced vertical mixing of the dense gas cloud.

The physical phenomena influencing the dispersion of such arsine releases either do not occur or are unimportant for simulations of typical vapor emissions. In order to simulate the denser-than-air gas and two-phase releases, such as in scenario 2, the off-site analysis utilizes a modeling system based on the SLAB dispersion model developed by Lawrence Livermore National Laboratory (16). This model has the additional advantages of being: (a) available in the public domain, (b) subjected to scientific peer review, and (c) compared with several other field experiments for validity (17, 18).

The SLAB model was originally intended to simulate steady-state evaporating pools, but has recently been updated to be more robust and include the components required for application to a larger variety of modeling problems (16). The following discussion reproduces several of the pertinent portions of the theoretical description of the SLAB model.

To meet the requirements of denser-than-air situation, the SLAB model is built on a theoretical framework that starts with averaged forms of the conservation equations for mass, momentum, energy, and species. Additional equations are included for the equation of state and the cloud dimensions (plume width in the steady-state mode and puff length and width in the transient puff mode). Turbulent mixing of the cloud with the ambient atmosphere is treated by using the entrainment concept, which specifies the rate of air flow into the cloud. The thermodynamics of liquid droplet formation is modeled by using the local thermodynamic equilibrium approximation. The size of the liquid droplets is assumed to be sufficiently small so that the transport of the vapor droplet mixture can be treated as a single fluid. Consequently, gravitational settling and ground deposition of the droplets are neglected. And finally, ground heating of the cloud when the cloud is cooler than the ground is treated by using the radiation boundary condition and a coefficient of surface heat transfer.

In the steady-state plume mode, the conservation equations are expressed in the steady-state form and are averaged over the crosswind plane of the plume, leaving downwind distance as the single independent variable. In the transient puff mode, the conservation equations are averaged over all three dimensions of the cloud, leaving the downwind travel time of the puff as the single independent variable. The three-dimensional concentration distribution is determined from the average concentration by using similarity profiles that include the calculated cloud dimensions. Concentration can be expressed as both a function of downwind distance and travel time, since these two parameters are related by the calculated downwind cloud velocity. Thus, the SLAB model code is one-dimensional in both modes; however, since the cloud dimensions are also calculated, the model is, in this sense, quasi-three dimensional.

The basic conservation laws, along with the various submodels, form a set of coupled equations that mathematically describe the physics of heavy gas dispersion including: gravity spread which produces a wider and lower cloud; reduced turbulent mixing due to stable density stratification; the thermodynamic effects due to droplet formation and evaporation to ground heating of the cloud; and the indirect effects of temperature change on density stratification and turbulent mixing with the ambient atmosphere. In addition, these equations also include the physical effects due to normal atmospheric advection and turbulent diffusion. The solution of these equations also yields the instantaneous averaged concentration, density, temperature, downwind velocity, and cloud height, width, and length of the released gas plume.

The most important result is the time-averaged concentration as a function of travel time (t) from the source and the three spatial dimensions of downwind distance (x) from the source, the crosswind distance (y) from the cloud centerline, and height (z) above ground level. In the SLAB model, the time-averaged concentration is calculated from the instantaneous ensemble average concentration. The time-averaging calculation uses assumed profiles for the temporal variation in the concentration signal which is a function of the cloud

Table 41.2.   Meteorological Conditions Considered

Wind Speed (m/sec)	Ambient Temperature (K °)	Relative Humidity (%)	Pasquill Stability Class
1.00	291.	62.	A
2.00	291.	62.	A
3.00	291.	62.	A
1.00	291.	62.	B
2.00	291.	62.	B
3.00	291.	62.	B
4.00	291.	62.	B
5.00	291.	62.	B
1.00	291.	62.	C
2.00	291.	62.	C
3.00	291.	62.	C
4.00	291.	62.	C
5.00	291.	62.	C
8.00	291.	62.	C
10.00	291.	62.	C
1.00	287.	69.	D
2.00	287.	69.	D
3.00	287.	69.	D
4.00	287.	69.	D
5.00	287.	69.	D
8.00	287.	69.	D
10.00	287.	69.	D
15.00	287.	69.	D
20.00	287.	69.	D
1.00	283.	83.	E
2.00	283.	83.	E
3.00	283.	83.	E
4.00	283.	83.	E
5.00	283.	83.	E
1.00	283.	83.	F
2.00	283.	83.	F
3.00	283.	83.	F
4.00	283.	83.	F

dimensions, the input spill duration, and concentration averaging time. The effects of plume meander, which increases the effective cloud width as a function of the concentration averaging time, are also included. Thus, the predicted time-average volume concentration takes into account the effects of plume meander, the finite duration of a release, and the length of the averaging time.

SLAB Model Application

The SLAB model can be applied in one mode during the analysis. All scenarios are then treated as continuous horizontal aerosol jets, with the duration of release a function of the amount of arsine in the cylinder. It can be conservatively postulated that the jets were oriented horizontally downwind and were not impeded by obstructions surrounding the release. Finally, the aerosol release is modeled assuming no initial dilution; furthermore, no removal of droplets at the surface was considered for any of the releases.

The initial density and liquid mass fraction of the releases near the source are calculated using the suggestions of Fauske and Epstein (19). The specification of these quantities is important in determining the initial enthalpy of the mixture and hence the energy balance for calculations downstream of the point of release. For an all-liquid discharge, the mass fraction of the vapor component (a) was estimated from:

Table 41.3. Health Effects Criteria for Various Averaging Periods

Criterion[a]	Averaging Period/Concentration (ppm)				
	1-min	5-min	30-min	60-min	120-min
6 ppm	32.9	14.7	6.0	4.2	3.0
1.5 ppm	8.2	3.7	1.5	1.1	0.8
0.6 ppm	3.3	1.5	0.6	0.4	0.3

[a]Criterion levels are based on an exposure period of 30 minutes. Equivalent exposure levels for other averaging periods were estimated based on Haber's law.

Table 41.4. Arsine Release Scenarios 5-Pound Cylinder Accidental Release at Loading Area

Time (minutes)	Arsine (ppm)	Downwind (m)	Crosswind (m)
30	6.0	56	10
	1.5	142	17
	0.6	246	26
60	4.2	69	12
	1.1	167	21
	0.4	282	32
120	3.0	68	12
	0.75	163	21
	0.3	275	33

Equation 3

$$\alpha = \frac{C_{pl}(T_0 - T_{bp})}{h_{vap}}$$

C_{pl} = specific heat of the liquid (J/kg – K°),

α = initial mass fraction of arsine vapor,

T_0 = stagnation temperature (K°),

T_{bp} = boiling point temperature (K°), and

h_{vap} = latent heat of vaporization (J/kg).

For the pressurized arsine storage cylinders considered in the off-site consequence analysis, application of Equation 3 resulted in an initial vapor mass fraction of 0.26 for a stagnation temperature of 238°K (mean annual temperature). This temperature is used as a conservative worst-case assumption.

The initial jet mixture density was determined from:

Equation 4

$$d_{mix} = \frac{1.0}{\dfrac{\alpha}{d_g} + \dfrac{1 - \alpha}{d_l}}$$

where d_{mix}, d_g, and d_l are the respective mixture, gas, and liquid densities (kg/m^3). For the initial mass fractions above and assuming an initial mixture temperature near T_{bp}, the mixture density is estimated to be 17.03 kg/m^3.

Exit velocities for the two-phase jet releases are also calculated using the methods outlined by Fauske and Epstein and the mass discharge rates. Using the principle of conservation of momentum flux, the jet (19), velocity at the end of the zone of depressurization is given by:

Equation 5

$$u_j = u_l + \frac{P(T_0) - P_a}{d_l u_l}$$

u_j = two-phase jet velocity (m/sec),

u = initial liquid discharge velocity (m/sec) determined from the mass discharge rate and the area of the release,

$P(T_0)$ = tank pressure (P_a), and

Pa = atmospheric pressure (P_a).

The initial two-phase jet velocity derived for scenario 2 (5-pound cylinder) based on a 220 psi storage pressure was 73 m/sec. When the source is a two-phase horizontal or vertical jet release, the SLAB model requires the area of the source after it has flashed and formed a liquid droplet-vapor mixture of the pure substance. Given the release characteristics estimated us-

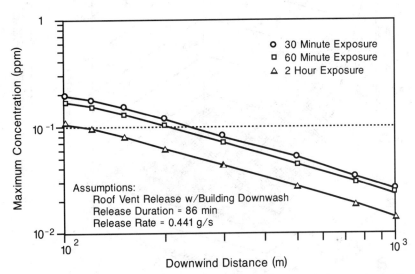

Figure 41.1. ISCST modeling results—Release Scenario 1 Concentration for all meteorologic scenarios roof top vent release scenario.

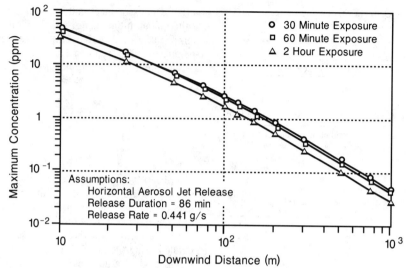

Figure 41.2. SLAB modeling results—highest arsine concentration for all meteorologic scenarios.

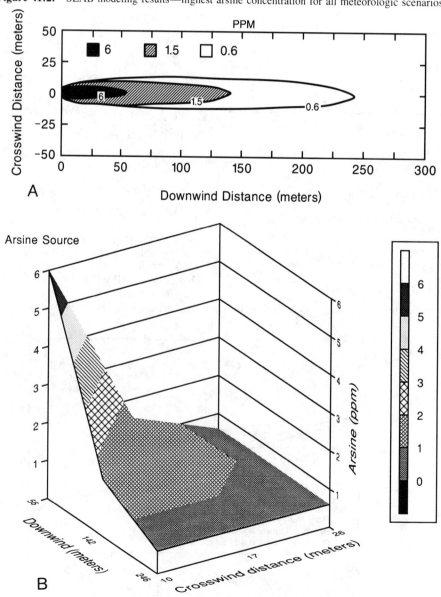

Figure 41.3. **A,** Release scenario 2—30-minute maximum arsine concentration (ppm). **B,** Release scenario 2, 30 minutes, 5-pound arsine cylinder; Note plume dispersion from source in a Gaussian manner decreasing both downward and crosswind.

ing the above equations, the initial area of the release can be calculated as:

Equation 6

$$A_j = \frac{A_b \dfrac{u_l}{d_l}}{U_j d_{mix}}$$

A_j = area of jet at start of entrainment zone (m³),

A_b = area of release (m²).

The area of the jet at the start of the entrainment zone was estimated to be 3.54×10^{-7} m² for scenario 2 based on an initial release area of 1.82×10^{-8} m².

Hazard Footprinting

SLAB model output files are processed to produce tabular and graphical data for off-site consequence analysis. For each meteorologic condition, release scenario, arsine health criteria, and averaging time of concern, a hazard footprint can be determined. The hazard footprint refers to the spatial extent where arsine concentrations exceed a given health criteria. A contour plot is prepared from the composite worst-case concentrations (maximum at each receptor location from all meteorologic conditions) for each release.

The SLAB model does not employ a fixed receptor grid, but indicates plume or puff parameters and concentrations at downwind distances which are dependent on the numerical technique used to solve the model equations. Concentrations along a fixed receptor grid downwind and the downwind extent of the hazard footprints are determined through logarithmic interpolation of the model output files. This procedure assumes that the concentration follows a power law with downwind distance which was found to be a good approximation over short distance intervals based on plots of the model output data.

Crosswind concentrations are determined using the model's crosswind profile function and the shape parameters which were included in the output file. Given the plume centerline concentration, the crosswind concentration was derived from:

Equation 7

$$c(y) = c_{max} \frac{\text{erf}\left[\dfrac{y+b}{\sqrt{2}\beta}\right] - \text{erf}\left[\dfrac{y-b}{\sqrt{2}\beta}\right]}{2(\text{erf})\left[\dfrac{b}{\sqrt{2}\beta}\right]}$$

$c(y)$ = concentration (ppm) at crosswind distance y,

c_{max} = the plume center line concentration (ppm),

erf = error function

b, β = half-width parameters (m). The half width parameters are such that the crosswind profile is uniform when $\beta = 0$ and approaches a Gaussian shape when $\beta >> b$.

Crosswind hazard footprints are determined implicitly from Equation 7 by solving for the crosswind distance y that corresponds to a given level of concern. This calculation can be performed at each downwind distance until a maximum crosswind width of a specified level is determined.

Selection of Meteorologic Scenarios

The SLAB model can be applied for a variety of meteorologic conditions. For the purpose of dispersion modeling the hypothetical meteorologic scenarios considered are indicated in Table 41.2. The range of wind velocities and atmospheric stratifications considered are those recommended by the EPA for screening purposes [20]. Temperature and relative humidities used in the two-phase modeling are based on climatologic averages obtained from the National Oceanic and Atmospheric Administration (NOAA). A surface roughness of 1.5 m was used in the SLAB simulations to accommodate the terrain around the building.

In order to determine how prevalent such wind conditions might be near the site, climatologic average wind conditions can be summarized based on past data.

RISK CHARACTERISTICS

The results of the toxicologic review and health criteria development, along with the results of the exposure assessment, are combined to characterize the possible risks to public health from a sudden release of arsine. A critical part of this analysis is the selection of appropriate Levels of Concern (LOCs). The LOCs were selected after examining a wide range of arsine health effects criteria (Table 41.3). Three criteria were chosen and the analyses and results address each of these criteria. These criteria were identified following consideration of the no-effect levels for arsine exposure and were selected to span the range of airborne concentrations evaluated in the toxicologic review, and provide a range of options for emergency planning. These criteria were as follows:

6.0 ppm for 30-minute exposure;
1.5 ppm 30-minute exposure; and
0.6 ppm 30-minute exposure.

The 6-ppm value represents a conservative estimate of the concentration where rapid evacuation of personnel should occur in the event of a release. Use of respiratory protection by personnel working in areas with this concentration would be advisable, even for short duration activities. As previously discussed, 5-ppm exposure for 1 hour represents a no-effect level in laboratory animals, so that use of the 6-ppm value in this manner is likely to be conservative. The 1.5-ppm value represents an estimate of the concentration presenting a lower level of concern. Emergency response activities in this area would not have to be performed with the same level of rapidity, as compared in areas with the 6-ppm concentration. Note that the 1.5-ppm value is the upper bound of the no-effect level in humans for 1 hour of exposure, based on the toxicology review. The 0.6-ppm value is the EPA's published level of concern, estimated as one tenth of the NIOSH IDLH. Emergency response activities in this area would likely be performed as precautionary measures. Exposure to a concentration of 0.6 ppm for a 30-minute duration is unlikely to result in adverse health effects in humans.

For each of the three criteria, additional averaging periods can be examined to assess shorter term exposure and longer term exposure to arsine concentrations. Exposure times of 60

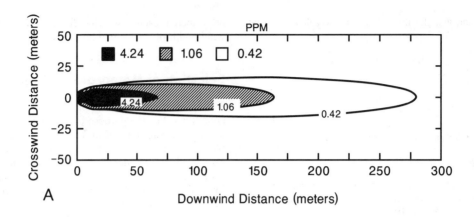

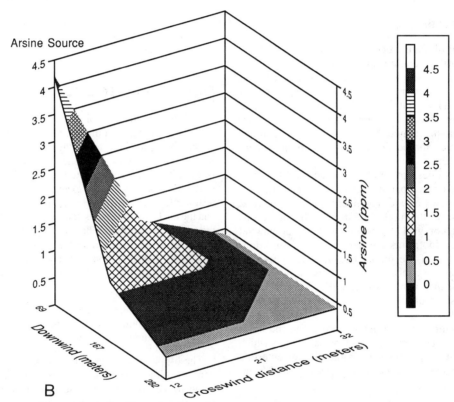

Figure 41.4. **A,** Release scenario 2. 60-minute maximum arsine concentration (ppm). **B,** Release scenario 2, 60 minutes, 5-pound arsine cylinder; Note plume dispersion from source in Gaussian manner decreasing both downwind and crosswind.

and 120 minutes were selected in addition to the 30-minute time. In order to calculate the corresponding arsine concentrations for the three criteria at these averaging periods Haber's law, as expressed, was utilized:

Haber's law:

$$C^n \times t = \text{constant}$$

C is the arsine concentration (ppm);

n is a chemical specific exponent;

t is the averaging time (minutes).

The exponent used in Haber's law is specific to individual chemicals. The United Kingdom Safety and Reliability Directorate has shown the exponent for arsine to be approximately

2. The constant is assumed to stay the same for each criterion, while the time varies. For example, the constant for the 6 ppm level of concern is:

$$(6)^2 (30) = 1080.$$

To obtain a corresponding level of concern for a 5-minute averaging period, the 6-ppm value would be estimated as:

$$(1080/5.0)^{0.5} = 14.7 \text{ ppm}$$

The health effects criteria, or levels of concern (LOC), for each averaging time are presented in Table 41.3.

RISK ANALYSIS RESULTS

The results of the exposure analysis using the two arsine release scenarios, the dispersion modeling techniques, and health cri-

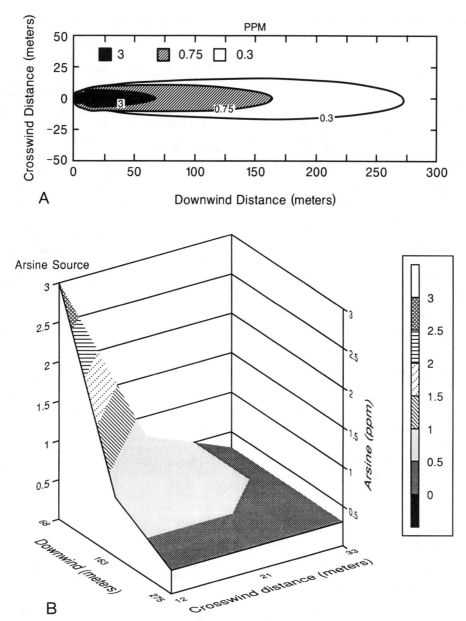

Figure 41.5.   A, Release scenario 2. 120-minute maximum arsine concentration (ppm). **B,** Release scenario 2, 120 minutes, 5-pound arsine cylinder; Note plume dispersion from source in Gaussian manner decreasing both downwind and crosswind.

teria described in the previous discussion were obtained and compared with the chosen arsine health standard. The potential spatial extent of 30-minute arsine concentrations exceeding the levels of concern, and equivalent levels were derived for 60- and 120-minute averaging periods. The zone of vulnerability for each hypothetical accident in terms of the area of potential exposure is then mapped.

The SLAB and ISCST models were applied to predict the resulting downwind arsine concentrations for the two release scenarios under a wide variety of meteorologic conditions. The maximum 30-, 60-, and 120-minute average concentrations predicted for these simulations involving scenario 2 are presented in Table 41.4. For these averaging periods, plots can be used to determine the maximum downwind extent of any given arsine concentration.

Scenario 2 (5-pound arsine cylinder) resulted in the highest

downwind concentrations due to the higher mass emission rate and duration. Estimated concentrations for scenario 1 (roof vent release) were considerably lower than for the outdoor releases as a result of dilution within the laboratory ventilation system, as well as the fact that the release occurred from the roof of the building and not at ground level. Scenario 1 did not result in any dangerous arsine concentrations according to the curves generated by ISCST modeling (Figure 41.1). The highest concentration of arsine achieved in this scenario was 0.2 ppm at the 30-minute release time interval. The concentration-time curves generated in scenario 2 by the SLAB model demonstrate much higher arsine concentrations (Fig. 41.2).

The curves described by Figs. 41.1 and 41.2 appear to be well-represented by power law approximation. In addition, for the near continuous releases the 30-, 60-, and 120-minute concentrations at a given distance were consistent ratios of each other, as averaging time considerations were independent of downwind distance.

Contour plots for scenario 2 were constructed from the output of the SLAB model for each averaging time and release. The plots represent a worst-case composite from all of the meteorologic conditions simulated. In order to show a range of impacts, contours were plotted for the three selected LOCs for arsine. The spatial extent and shape of the areas predicted to potentially exceed these levels are shown in two-dimensional and three-dimensional comparisons in Figs. 41.3–41.5. Note that the downward and crosswind dimensions shown on these plots are in meters.

The shapes of the contours are determined by the release characteristics. Initially, buoyancy-induced spreading of the denser-than-air arsine aerosol cloud produced contours with a wider base close to the point of release, particularly for the low wind speeds. As the arsine vapor cloud moves downwind and mixes with ambient air, the vapor cloud is no longer characterized by a denser-than-air cloud and can be approximated by a Gaussian distribution. Beyond the point at which the arsine aerosol cloud is no longer denser than air, the contours were found to be more elliptical in shape. These contour plots also demonstrate the significantly different areas exposed, depending on the level of concern used. For a majority of the accident scenarios, the distance to the 0.6-ppm level of concern was roughly 3–5 times further downwind than that of the 6-ppm level. Contour plots were not presented for the roof vent release, since none of the LOCs were exceeded for this scenario.

The above modeling results encompass all worst-case meteorologic scenarios. Since deliveries of arsine would likely occur during daylight hours, maximum downwind concentrations under worst-cast meteorologic scenarios were examined. It was still assumed that an accidental release within the laboratory could occur any hour of the day or night.

SUMMARY

The available toxicologic data for arsine supports a no-effect level in humans that is below 5 ppm in air, based on a 1-hour duration of exposure. Extrapolating from the toxicologic data, the no-effect level in humans ranges from 0.5–1.5 ppm in air, based on a 1-hour duration of exposure. Maximum airborne concentrations of arsine from the facility roof vent release ranged from 0.02–0.2 ppm.

Maximum 30-minute (100 meters downwind) airborne concentrations of arsine from an outdoor release of 5 pounds from a cylinder was 3 ppm. The lowest level of concern (0.6 ppm) was predicted to occur at distances up to 250 meters downwind. The highest levels, 6 ppm, occurred within 50 meters of the release.

These maximum airborne concentrations were predicted for worst-case meteorologic conditions at the time of arsine release. The results indicate that, based on the available toxicologic data, available information on the low density of the surrounding community, and the most credible modeling scenarios, adverse effects to the community from arsine exposure are unlikely from the small volume release scenarios evaluated.

Depending on the prevailing wind direction at the time of a release, airborne concentrations above the estimated no-effect level in humans may occur on the premises of the facility. However, in many cases because of its narrow width, the plume could be easily avoided. Potential exposures are likely to be transient because of the limited airborne extent of the plume. Adverse effects that potentially could be associated with a plume with the predicted concentration of airborne arsine should not produce observable symptoms, although some transient, reversible changes in certain blood components and enzyme levels may occur. It is unlikely that exposures at these levels will result in significant or irreversible adverse effects in potentially exposed individuals in the community.

REFERENCES

1. Fowler BA, Weissberg JB. Arsine poisoning. N Engl J Med 1974;29:1171–1174.
2. Peterson EP. BI-ATTACARYYA M-11. Hematological responses to arsine exposure: quantitation and exposure response in mice. Fundam Appl Toxicol 1985;5:499–505.
3. Kosouer NS, et al. Glutathione IV. Intracellular oxidation and membrane injury. Biochim Biophys Acta 1969;192:23–28.
4. Blair PC, et al. Evidence for oxidative damage to erythrocytes in rats and mice induced by arsine gas. Toxicologist 1988;8:19.
5. National Institute for Occupational Safety and Health. Hazard assessment of the electric component manufacturing industry. Bethesda: Department of Health and Human Services, 1985;85–100.
6. Nau CA. The accidental generation of arsine gas in an industry. South Med J 1985;41:341–344.
7. Sherin BJ. Risk assessment and control of toxic gas releases. Arsine: toxicity OATA from acute and short-term inhalation exposure. In: Hazard Assessment and Control Technology in Semiconductor Manufacturing. Cincinnati, OH: American Conference of Governmental Industrial Hygienists: 115–133.
8. Alexeef GV, et al. Problems associated with the use of immediately dangerous to life and health (IDLH) values for estimating the hazard of accidental chemical releases. Am Ind Hyg Assoc J 1989;50:598–605.
9. Wheatley CJ. Discharge of liquid ammonia to moist atmospheres—survey of experimental data and model for estimating initial conditions for dispersion calculations. Safety and Reliability Directorate, Report SRD R410. United Kingdom Atomic Energy Commission, 1987.
10. Kaiser GD, Walker BC. Releases of anhydrous ammonia from pressurized containers—the importance of denser-than-air mixtures. Atmos Environ 1978;12:2289–2300.
11. Environmental Protection Agency. Guideline on air quality models (Revised). EPA-450/2-78-027R. Research Triangle Park, NC: U.S. EPA, Office of Air Quality Planning and Standards.
12. Environmental Protection Agency. Technical guidance for hazards analysis, emergency planning for extremely hazardous substances. Washington, D.C.: U.S. EPA, Federal Emergency Management Agency, U.S. Department of Transportation, December 1987.
13. Hanna SR, Briggs GA, Hosker RP. Handbook on atmospheric diffusion. DOE/TIC-11223. U.S. Department of Energy, Technical Information Center, 1982.
14. Hanna SR, Drivas PJ. Guidelines for the use of vapor cloud dispersion models. New York: Center for Chemical Process Safety, American Institute of Chemical Engineers, 1987.
15. Spicer TO, Havens JA, Key LE. Extension of DEGADIS for modeling aerosol releases. International Conference on Vapor Cloud Modeling, November 2–4, 1987, Cambridge, MA. Sponsored by the Center for Chemical Process Safety, American Institute of Chemical Engineers, New York, 1987.
16. Ermak DL. User's manual for SLAB: an atmospheric dispersion model for denser-than-air releases. Livermore, CA: Lawrence Livermore National Laboratory, Atmospheric and Geophysical Sciences Division, 1989.
17. Ermak DL, Chan ST, Morgan DL, Morris LK. A comparison of dense gas dispersion model simulations with burro series LNG spill test results. J Hazardous Materials 1982;6:129–160.
18. Blewitt DN, Yohn JF, Ermak DL. An evaluation of SLAB and DEGADIS heavy gas dispersion models using HF spill test data. International Conference on Vapor Cloud Modeling, November 2–4, 1987, Cambridge, MA. Sponsored by the Center for Chemical Process Safety, American Institute of Chemical Engineers, New York, 1987.
19. Fauske HF, Epstein M. Source term considerations with chemical accidents and vapor cloud modeling. International Conference on Vapor Cloud Modeling, November 2–4, 1987, Cambridge, MA. Sponsored by the Center for Chemical Process Safety, American Institute of Chemical Engineers, New York, 1987.
20. Environmental Protection Agency. Screening procedures for estimating the air quality impacts of stationary sources. EPA-450/2-4-88-010. North Carolina: U.S. EPA, Office of Air Quality Planning and Standards.

42

Psychologic Sequelae of Chemical and Hazardous Materials Exposures

Richard S. Schottenfeld, M.D.

INTRODUCTION

Neuropsychiatric symptoms, including weakness, fatigue, malaise, anxiety, depressed or irritable mood, difficulty concentrating, distractibility, and memory impairment, are commonly experienced following acute or chronic exposure to a wide range of noxious and toxic substances. These symptoms can result from the direct, toxic effects of exposure on the central nervous system, from psychologic or emotional reactions to exposure, or from a combination of both. Preexisting symptoms may also be mistakenly attributed to exposure. Due to the fact that neuropsychiatric symptoms may lead to considerable disability regardless of etiology, accurate and early diagnosis and institution of appropriate therapeutic interventions are essential (1).

Symptoms following exposure to known or suspected neurotoxins, including heavy metals, pesticides, and organic solvents, often pose a diagnostic challenge. The diagnosis of a toxic syndrome is facilitated when exposures exceed established thresholds for biologic effects and symptoms follow classic patterns for intoxication. Even in situations of definite central nervous system toxicity; however, psychologic and emotional reactions may play a part in the persistence of symptoms and may complicate recovery and exacerbate disability. Conversely, in the absence of definite neurotoxicity or following low level exposure, symptoms can result from psychologic and emotional reactions secondary to the fact that an exposure occurred. They may also result from an increased biologic sensitivity of particular individuals to toxic effects.

The differential diagnosis of neuropsychiatric symptoms includes: (*a*) organic mental disorders; (*b*) psychologic or emotional reactions secondary to exposure and resulting illness; and preexisting or concomitant psychiatric disorders (including psychologic or emotional reactions to life problems or stressors unrelated to exposure and problematic alcohol or other substance use). These diagnoses are not mutually exclusive. Symptoms may reflect a combination of disorders, and complete differentiation of organic from nonorganic disorders is not always possible. Adjustment disorders with anxious or depressed mood following toxic exposures, for example, may be difficult to differentiate from organic affective disorders resulting from direct toxic effects on the central nervous system; both may be present in the same individual. Preexisting psychiatric disorders or coexisting stressors (such as family or economic problems) can also make it difficult to sort out the relative contributions of toxic central nervous system effects and psychologic or emotional reactions to exposure.

Three conditions that merit special attention include the neuropsychiatric syndromes associated with chronic exposure to low levels of solvents and solvent mixtures, multiple chemical sensitivities (MCS), and mass psychogenic illness or "mass hysteria." Recognition that psychologic reactions to exposure,

or a "functional overlay," may complicate recovery following toxic as well as relatively minor or harmless exposures facilitates diagnosis and management of all three conditions.

Accurate diagnosis of neuropsychiatric syndromes associated with exposure will depend on (*a*) a detailed history of exposure and chronology of symptoms; (*b*) knowledge of the possible neurotoxic effects of exposure; (*c*) psychiatric evaluation including a thorough psychosocial history, history of drug and alcohol use, neurologic and mental status examination; and often (*d*) results of special tests, including neuropsychologic testing, electroencephalogram, and diagnostic imaging.

While treatment must be aimed at helping the exposed person and others in his or her environment gain an understanding of the etiology and significance of the neuropsychiatric symptoms. In addition a realistic view of the prognosis for immediate and longterm symptom relief underlies effective preventive interventions and treatments. Cognitive and behavioral treatments are often useful in bringing about symptomatic relief regardless of the specific diagnosis and etiology.

A BIOPSYCHOSOCIAL MODEL OF POSTEXPOSURE ILLNESS

The likelihood that neuropsychiatric symptoms will follow an acute or chronic exposure depends on both environmental and host factors.

Environmental factors are exposure related or psychosocial related. Exposure-related factors include: (*a*) neurotoxicity of the chemical or material, (*b*) dose or concentration of chemical or material, and (*c*) exposure duration (acute, subacute, chronic). Psychosocial-related factors include: (*a*) speed and efficiency of recognition, evaluation, and resolution of problematic exposure, (*b*) shared belief system concerning the danger of the exposure that develops among those exposed; (*c*) shared belief system concerning the danger of the exposure that exists within the community; and (*d*) intensity of preexposure and postexposure social strife and community divisiveness.

Host factors include (*a*) the biologic sensitivity or susceptibility of the exposed person to the toxic effects of exposure and (*b*) the psychologic makeup of the exposed person. The latter includes the tendency of the individual to somatize anxiety; i.e., to interpret the dangers or significance of the exposure (the person's interpretive set), and the individual's coping skills, psychologic defenses, and underlying psychologic vulnerability. These factors will be examined in greater detail.

INCIDENCE OF NEUROPSYCHIATRIC SYMPTOMS FOLLOWING ACUTE AND CHRONIC EXPOSURE

Baseline rates of occurrence of many neuropsychiatric symptoms in the general adult population are quite high, making it difficult to assess whether symptoms resulted from toxic exposure. A National Center for Health Statistics (NCHS) national survey found that 78% of Americans reported being bothered by at least one of 12 common symptoms, such as headache, palpitations, or dizziness (2). Studies of college students show similarly high rates of reported symptoms (3).

Another estimate of population baseline rates of neuropsychiatric symptoms comes from reported prevalence of symptoms in control or referent groups used in studies of the neuropsychiatric effects of exposure. Symptoms of fatigue, for example, were reported by 72% of locomotive engineers and assistants used as case controls in a study of neuropsychiatric symptoms associated with solvent exposure in car painters; 80% of control subjects reported being irritable sometimes or frequently, 70% reported difficulties with concentration and sleep, 44% reported mood lability, and 37% reported being bothered by heart pounding (4). Between one and five chronic neurobehavioral symptoms (including fatigue, sleep disturbances, irritability, lack of concentration, memory problems, instability of mood, headache, decreased libido or potency, and diminished alcohol tolerance) were reported by 56% of papermill workers and urban farm dwellers, used as controls in a study of neurobehavioral changes in shipyard painters exposed to solvents (5).

Despite high baseline rates of neuropsychiatric symptoms in the community, several controlled studies have documented excess rates of neuropsychiatric symptoms following a variety of exposure conditions. Twelve days following exposure to a chemical cloud of malathion, for example, exposed seamen who were compared with seamen on a vessel that was not exposed to the chemical cloud reported significantly more symptoms of headache, dizziness, and fainting (73% versus 24%), visual disturbances (41% versus 10%), nasal or pharyngeal irritation (59% versus 19%), and appetite or taste loss (43% versus 5%). Many of the symptoms reported by exposed seamen were consistent with the acute effects of exposure to malathion, but information about the exposure was limited and did not entirely explain the occurrence of symptoms on the basis of the direct, toxic effects of the chemical. The more knowledgeable workers were about the effects of malathion exposure, the less likely they were to suffer psychologic distress (6). Thirty percent of 20,000 persons evaluated for the effects of ingestion of toxic cooking oil in Spain required psychiatric evaluation because of anxious, depressive, or phobic psychologic reactions. Neuropsychologic testing failed to document evidence of organic brain damage resulting from the toxic effects of the cooking oil. Their psychiatric disorders were classified as adjustment disorders (7). Evaluations of workers involved in the Three Mile Island (TMI) nuclear power plant accident and of workers with longterm occupational exposure to asbestos provide the clearest indication of the incidence of psychiatric symptoms following exposures that are not directly toxic to the central nervous system. Compared with control subjects working at a second nuclear power plant, TMI workers experienced significantly more angry reactions (40% versus 29% among supervisors and 51% versus 31% among nonsupervisors), worry (27% versus 6% and 30% versus 8%), and somatic symptoms (26% versus 12% and 29% versus 17%). Distress levels were in the high normal range, did not appear to interfere significantly with functioning, and declined over the 6 months following the accident (8). Similarly, insulation workers who were at significantly increased risk for asbestosis or lung cancer as a result of high level asbestos exposure also experienced more somatic symptoms, alcohol abuse, and diminished mental health functioning at times of stress compared with postal worker control subjects (9).

ORGANIC MENTAL DISORDERS— NEUROPSYCHIATRIC SYNDROMES ASSOCIATED WITH SPECIFIC NEUROTOXINS

Specific syndromes of neurotoxic and neurobehavioral dysfunction are recognized consequences of toxic exposure to specific chemicals. These exposures can result in pronounced psychiatric manifestations.

Erethism, or the syndrome of organic mental disturbances seen in chronic inorganic mercury poisoning, is characterized by irritability, difficulty concentrating, and insomnia. Affected persons often suffer from overwhelming tiredness, extreme timidity, shyness, embarrassment, discouragement, and apathy. Memory loss and cognitive impairments usually accompany the disorder. Hallucinations and seizures may also occur. Although psychiatric symptoms may be the earliest manifestation of intoxication, gingivitis, dermatitis, and tremor are also characteristic features of inorganic mercury exposure (10).

Although severe intoxication with inorganic lead has long been recognized as a cause of encephalopathy in adults, the more subtle effects of lower level intoxications in adults have been elucidated only in the past decade (11). Severe depression, anxiety, sleep disorders, irritability, fatigue, difficulties in concentration, and memory loss can all be a result of intoxication with inorganic lead. Because not all lead-intoxicated patients with depression or other psychiatric symptoms will suffer from other classic features of intoxication, such as anemia, colic, or peripheral neuropathies, a history of exposure to inorganic lead is the most important clue to the diagnosis. Depressive symptoms may be severe enough to meet criteria for a major depression, but the disorder is best characterized as an organic affective disorder, which places proper emphasis on the etiologic significance of intoxication with inorganic lead (11, 12). Exposure to other metals may also lead to severe neuropsychiatric symptoms. A manic syndrome is associated with manganese intoxication ("manganese madness"); the syndrome is characterized by emotional lability, increased motor activity, auditory hallucinations, irritability, nervousness, and compulsive behavior. The manic syndrome may precede other signs and symptoms of intoxication. A parkinsonian syndrome secondary to manganese toxicity consists of muscular weakness and rigidity, impaired speech and gait, loss of facial expression and usually only appears after the onset of psychiatric symptoms and is irreversible (13). Severe anxiety, fears of dying, and neurasthenia (or severe weakness) caused by intoxication with organic tin compounds are usually accompanied by signs of encephalopathy (severe headache, alterations in consciousness, delirium, and seizures). Chronic intoxication with bromides historically has resulted from medicinal use of bromides but not from environmental or occupational exposure; depression, hallucinosis, and schizophreniform psychosis can be seen in the absence of other signs of intoxication (14).

Intoxication with arsenic, thallium, bismuth, inorganic tin, aluminum, gold, and zinc usually produce widespread systemic signs in addition to central nervous system disturbances, making the diagnosis of an organic mental disorder readily apparent (15–17). Toxic exposure to methyl bromide used as a fumigant can result in psychosis, suicidal ideation, and homicidal thoughts.

PSYCHOLOGIC EFFECTS OF EXPOSURE

Anxiety Reactions and Posttraumatic Stress Disorder

Fear is a feeling of alarm, apprehension, disquiet, or trepidation caused by danger, while anxiety is defined as a similar state of uneasiness, distress, or dread lacking an unambiguous cause or specific threat (18). Both fear and anxiety are commonly accompanied by symptoms of motor tension (trembling, twitching, feeling shaky; muscle tension, aches, soreness; restlessness; easy fatigability), autonomic hyperactivity (shortness of breath; palpitations or tachycardia; sweating or cold, clammy hands; dry mouth; dizziness or lightheadedness; nausea, diarrhea or abdominal distress; flushes or chills; frequent urination; trouble swallowing or ''lump in the throat''), and increased vigilance and scanning (feeling keyed up or on edge; exaggerated startle response; difficulty concentrating or losing train of thought; trouble falling or staying asleep; irritability) (19, 20). The symptoms of fear or anxiety are identical to the chronic neuropsychiatric symptoms that are often experienced following many toxic exposures. No one would doubt that fear could account for the occurrence of these symptoms immediately following a life-threatening event or an acute, frightening toxic exposure. There has been considerable controversy, however, about whether these symptoms could develop in individuals exposed to lesser degrees of trauma or could persist in individuals for prolonged periods following traumatic events in the absence of preexisting personality or anxiety disorders.

Research on posttraumatic stress disorders has provided the most compelling evidence for the widespread persistence of severe anxiety symptoms in persons exposed to traumatic circumstances, regardless of predisposing personality vulnerability. The diagnostic hallmarks of a classic posttraumatic stress disorder (PTSD) include persistent reexperiencing of the traumatic event, avoidance of stimuli associated with the trauma, or generalized numbing of responsiveness, and severe symptoms of anxiety (19). Reexperiencing the traumatic event occurs in the form of recurrent recollections or dreams or reenactments of the trauma. Avoidance is characterized by efforts to avoid thoughts, feelings, activities, or situations associated with the trauma or by psychogenic amnesia regarding aspects of the trauma.

Studies of Vietnam veterans indicate that, even 15 years following the end of the war, 15% of those who served in Vietnam were still suffering from PTSD. Lifetime rates of PTSD approached 50% of Vietnam veterans. Higher rates of PTSD were found in those with the most extensive combat experience, and combat experience opposed to any precombat variables accounted for the greatest amount of variability in development of PTSD (21). Combat veterans of World War II reported similarly high rates of symptoms of depression, anxiety, tension, irritability, startle reactions, impairment of memory, and obsession with thoughts of wartime experiences (22). High rates of PTSD have also been reported in survivors of disasters (e.g., concentration camps or rape).

On the basis of these studies, there can be little doubt that severe traumatic events, including potentially life-threatening toxic exposures, can cause long-lasting and severe psychiatric impairment regardless of preexisting personality vulnerability or underlying psychiatric disorder. There is also evidence suggesting that less severe traumas can also lead to symptoms. Horowitz, for example, conducted an experimental study demonstrating that healthy volunteers experienced greater fear responses after watching a short film depicting bodily injury compared with control subjects watching a neutral film subject, an erotic film, or a film depicting separation. The occurrence of intrusive and repetitive thoughts correlated significantly with exposure to a stressful film (23).

PSYCHOLOGIC EFFECTS MEDIATED BY COGNITIVE APPRAISAL OF DANGER AND COPING ABILITIES

The psychologic consequences of a traumatic experience, including acute or chronic exposure to toxic or noxious substances, depend to a considerable degree on the exposed person's cognitive appraisal of the severity or danger of the experience. Relatively minor or even entirely nontoxic exposures may be interpreted as life-threatening and subsequently may lead to severe psychologic sequelae. Alternatively, extremely dangerous exposures may go unnoticed or unrecognized by those exposed and lead to no psychologic reactions.

Factors affecting the cognitive appraisal of severity of an exposure include (a) the nature and severity of symptoms produced by the exposure; (b) the exposed person's previous experience with similar symptoms and illness; (c) the exposed person's knowledge, expectations, and beliefs about the dangers and potential consequences of exposure; and (d) the type, quality, and credibility of information presented to the person about the exposure (24, 25). Repeated exposures, for example, may become increasingly frightening if they are experienced as unavoidable and believed likely to lead to cumulative effects. Exposures in environments known to contain highly toxic substances will be interpreted differently than identical exposures in environments known to contain nontoxic substances. Based on a combination of these factors, identical symptoms may be interpreted as indicative of entirely benign or extremely malignant conditions. The former interpretive set will evoke little or no anxiety, while the latter may evoke considerable anxiety and a cascade of anxiety-related symptoms that amplify the symptom complex.

The effectiveness of the exposed person's coping skills and psychologic defenses and the adequacy and timeliness of community response also affect the severity of psychologic sequelae to traumatic experiences or toxic exposure. Denial of the significance of exposure can function to ward off what would otherwise be intolerable levels of anxiety. The ability to modulate anxiety by focusing on current activities or future benign outcomes rather than on malignant possibilities may also lessen the severity of adverse psychologic effects. Difficulties coping with emotions that frequently follow traumatic experiences, such as fear, helplessness, anger, guilt, shame, and loss, may complicate the psychologic sequelae. Reassurance in the form of accurate information provided by credible experts, acknowledgment by those responsible for the damage caused, combined with empathic, informed support from family and friends can lessen anxiety following an exposure. Misleading or inaccurate information, refusal by those in charge to accept responsibility, or exaggerated concern of family and friends, however, can exacerbate psychologic reactions.

Depressive Reactions

Although anxiety is the most common psychologic reaction to exposure, significant depression may also result. In addition to depressed mood, depressive states are characterized by diminished interest or pleasure in activities; feelings of hopelessness, helplessness, worthlessness, or guilt; psychomotor agitation or retardation; fatigue; indecisiveness or difficulties concentrating; vegetative symptoms (disturbances of appetite, libido, sleep); and suicidal ideation (19). Depression may result from a loss of bodily functioning or health caused by exposure (depression associated with chronic illness caused by exposure) or from an anticipated or threatened loss of health (depression associated with violation of a person's sense of invulnerability and intactness). Depression may also result from the exposed person's inability or failure to live up to his or her own ideals in response to exposure—for example, becoming frightened or running away from an exposure scene may be experienced as acts of cowardice and lead to loss of self-esteem. Depressive reactions are usually transient but may become persistent if not managed appropriately.

Conversion Reactions

Conversion reactions refer to transformations and attempted resolutions of psychologic conflict into alterations or loss of physical functioning that suggest physical disorder (19, 26, 27). Classical conversion symptoms include paralysis, aphonia, seizures, uncoordination, blindness, tunnel vision, anosmia, anesthesia, and paresthesia. Conversion reactions often develop suddenly during extremely stressful circumstances, such as combat, life-threatening accidents, and environmental or occupational toxic exposures. Symptoms usually achieve some "primary gain" for the exposed person (e.g., paralysis of a limb prevents the person from acting on aggressive and angry feelings) and may also result in "secondary gain" (e.g., the symptom results in evacuation from a dangerous situation or provision of outside support from others).

A case example, altered to disguise the identity of the patient, may be useful to illustrate the often confusing nature of conversion reactions. A 38-year-old, married woman was exposed to vapors containing acetone and methyl ethyl ketone while washing rags that had been soaked in these solvents. She became acutely intoxicated by the vapors, began laughing until she started crying, felt weak and nauseated, and finally began to have some difficulty breathing. Along with several coworkers, she was taken to a local hospital. Although her coworkers recovered rapidly, she developed numbness of her arms, facial grimacing, and dysarthria. Since the exposure, she has felt that her gestures and speech are "retarded." Neurologic examination, neuropsychologic testing, computed tomography (CT) scan, magnetic resonance imaging (MRI) of the brain, and electromyography failed to reveal any consistent abnormality accounting for her persistent neurologic symptoms. Dysarthria, "retarded gestures," and numbness of her arms appeared to resolve her anxiety about how "out of control" she had been while acutely intoxicated, and continued symptoms functioned to keep her from returning to a potentially dangerous job and to express indirectly her anger at her employer for the lack of proper safety precautions and exhaust system.

PREEXISTING OR CONCOMITANT PSYCHIATRIC DISORDERS

The recent Epidemiologic Catchment Area (ECA) survey has documented a high prevalence of anxiety disorders, depression, drug and alcohol use disorders in the general population. ECA documented lifetime prevalence rates of alcohol abuse or dependence in adults of between 11% and 16%; drug abuse and dependence affected between 5% and 6%; major depression was experienced by approximately 5%; panic disorder affected 1.4%; and somatization disorder affected 0.1% (28). Substance use disorders, which are the most common psychiatric disorders experienced by the general adult population, may lead to symptoms or prolonged disability following a toxic exposure that are mistakenly attributed to exposure. A careful history of drug and alcohol use, obtained in a nonjudgmental manner, will often help lead to the diagnosis. Affirmative responses to the questions: Have you tried to cut down on drinking? Have you been annoyed by criticism about your drinking? Have you felt guilty about your alcohol use? or modifications of these questions for other drugs indicate possible alcohol or drug problems (29).

Although somatization disorder is quite rare in the general population, symptoms of the disorder may also be mistakenly attributed to toxic exposure. Somatization disorder is characterized by a history of recurrent and multiple somatic symptoms, of several years duration, for which medical attention has been sought, but that are not due to any physical disorder (19). The disorder usually begins before age 30 and has a chronic, fluctuating course. Predominant symptoms include: gastrointestinal symptoms (vomiting, abdominal pain, nausea, bloating, diarrhea, intolerance of many different foods); pain symptoms; conversion or pseudoneurologic symptoms (amnesia, difficulty swallowing, loss of voice, deafness, double vision, blurred vision, blindness, fainting, seizure, trouble walking, paralysis or muscle weakness, urinary retention); sexual symptoms (burning sensation in sexual organs or rectum, other than during intercourse, sexual indifference, pain during intercourse, impotence); and female reproductive symptoms that occur more frequently or severely than in most women (e.g., painful menstruation). An accurate chronology of symptoms and exposure will usually establish a history of somatization disorder prior to exposure.

Errors in attribution of symptoms to exposure are not usually the result of deliberate falsification. Symptoms of preexisting psychiatric disorders may become more pronounced or noticeable following toxic exposures, and thus come to be associated with the exposure. In addition, there is a natural tendency to search for a specific, discernible cause of symptoms, such as a toxic exposure, rather than to view the symptoms as part of an underlying psychiatric disorder.

SOLVENT SYNDROMES

Although there is an extensive literature describing an association between chronic, relatively low level exposure to organic solvents and solvent mixtures and neuropsychiatric symptoms and disability, there is controversy in the United States about the significance of the deficits reported or the specific etiologic role of repeated exposure to organic solvents.

Spencer and Schaumburg (1985) have recently reviewed the scientific criteria for human neurotoxicity and the evidence suggesting that specific solvents and solvent mixtures are neurotoxic (30). Five solvents meet scientific criteria for proven human neurotoxicity. Central nervous system effects (impaired intellectual functioning and psychomotor deficits) as well as evidence of subclinical peripheral neuropathy have been demonstrated following chronic exposure to *carbon disulfide* at levels previously believed to be safe (10–30 ppm, with brief periods of up to 100 ppm). Deliberate, repeated inhalation of *toluene* for its euphorigenic effect can lead to early emotional and neuropsychologic changes, including anxiety, irritability, mood swings, and forgetfulness. Tremor, nystagmus, slurred speech, hearing impairment, and ataxic gait occur later in the course of repeated exposures. *Hexane* and *ketones* produce primarily peripheral neuropathies in the absence of cognitive or emotional changes. Acute intoxication with *trichloroethylene* and *perchloroethylene* can cause reversible sensory and motor cranial neuropathies, most often of the trigeminal nerve. Chronic, low level exposure to trichloroethylene has also been reported to cause neuropsychologic and emotional changes, but studies have reported contradictory results.

Chronic exposure to other solvents or solvent mixtures has also been reported to result in central nervous system toxicity. After extensively reviewing the literature, Spencer and Schaumberg (1985) concluded that ''while there is cause for concern and a clear need for further research, compelling data are unavailable.''

The neuropsychologic deficits most commonly reported following chronic solvent exposure include shortterm memory deficits, impaired visuomotor performance, and decreased reaction time (4, 5, 31, 32–42). Many of the abnormal findings on neuropsychologic testing are partially explainable on the basis of attention and concentration difficulties and are consistent with an organic affective disorder associated with chronic solvent exposure as well as a primary psychiatric disturbance. Neuropsychologic deficits have been reported to persist for more than 2 years following cessation of exposure, suggesting that the deficits may be irreversible (43).

In many Scandinavian countries, disability is accepted and compensation awarded for neurotoxicity following repeated exposure to paint, lacquers, and solvent mixtures. A uniform nomenclature for solvent-related neuropsychiatric symptoms has been proposed. When cognitive or neurobehavioral deficits are present, a diagnosis of toxic encephalopathy is warranted. In the absence of demonstrable deficits in psychomotor, perceptual, or cognitive function, a mood disturbance associated with chronic solvent exposure characterized by symptoms of depression, irritability, and loss of interest in activities is best considered an organic affective disorder (44).

Three cases of panic disorder have also been reported to have been precipitated by occupational exposure to organic solvents (45). Panic disorder is characterized by the sudden emergence of feelings of intense fear in situations that usually do not cause anxiety. Cognitive, autonomic, and motor symptoms of anxiety are also present during an episode of panic. In all cases, panic attacks were initially experienced only at work following acute exposure to organic solvent mixtures; episodes reoccurred repeatedly at work following subsequent exposures and eventually were experienced spontaneously outside of the work place. One patient had a prior history of panic attacks during adolescence. Two patients experienced panic attacks in response to a diagnostic challenge with sodium lactate. All three patients responded to pharmacologic interventions. The authors suggest that sensitization or a kindling mechanism might account for the disorder.

MULTIPLE CHEMICAL SENSITIVITIES (MCS)

MCS is defined as ''an acquired disorder characterized by recurrent symptoms, referable to multiple organ systems, occurring in response to demonstrable exposure to many chemically unrelated compounds at doses far below those established in the general population to cause harmful effects'' (46). The

disorder often first becomes manifest in association with acute or chronic exposure to toxic or noxious substances. Symptoms that are initially experienced only in response to specific, well-defined exposures are subsequently experienced following exposure to a multitude of odors in environments that are considered benign by the vast majority of the normal population.

There is considerable controversy about the etiology of the disorder. Although clinical ecologists consider the disorder to result from immunologic or allergic reactions, careful and controlled studies have failed to detect consistent immunologic abnormalities (47, 48). Other possible mechanisms to account for the disorder include kindling or sensitization of the central nervous system, sensitization of peripheral tissues, atypical PTSD, and classic learning theory with stimulus generalization (49, 50). None of these mechanisms has been thoroughly investigated in the disorder.

Kindling refers to a process in the genesis of seizures whereby repeated exposure to an epileptogenic stimulus (such as an electrical stimulus or chemical, such as cocaine) leads to seizures at exposure levels that would not initially cause seizure activity (51). Sensitization refers to a modification in nociceptive or pain receptors that results in increased activation of receptors in response to a minimal stimulus (52). The process accounts for the hyperalgesia of skin regions following burn injury and for the severe twinges of pain that are felt following very limited movement during the process of recovery from a sprained ankle. Sensitization may be thought of as the reciprocal of the process of habituation, whereby repeated exposure to the same level of stimulus leads to a diminished response. Kindling mechanisms or sensitization could account for heightened symptom arousal in individuals with MCS following low level exposures.

MCS has also been conceptualized as a variant of posttraumatic stress disorder (53). Rather than reexperience the trauma in words, thoughts, or dreams, persons with MCS reexperience the symptoms associated with the initial exposure (53). Along similar lines, MCS has been conceptualized as a learned behavior. Initial symptoms (the unconditioned response) are evoked by specific exposure (the unconditioned stimulus); subsequent symptoms are conditioned responses evoked by conditioned stimuli (e.g., the odor of the toxic substance). Stimulus generalization would lead to symptoms being experienced following an ever widening array of exposures (53).

Psychologic and emotional reactions to exposure, as discussed above, can exacerbate symptoms of disability of MCS, regardless of etiology. Individuals with MCS are often severely disabled as a result of symptoms. No specific treatment has been demonstrated to be effective for the disorder.

MASS PSYCHOGENIC ILLNESS

Mass psychogenic illness or mass hysteria is defined as ''the collective occurrence of a set of physical symptoms and related beliefs among two or more individuals in the absence of an identifiable pathogen'' (54). Once considered a rare phenomenon, it has been diagnosed with increasing frequency over the past decade in a wide variety of occupational and environmental settings.

The diagnosis of mass psychogenic illness has usually been made by exclusion of causative chemical or biologic agents, leaving open to question the possibility that the investigators have failed to detect an existing pathogen because of a lack of skill or perseverance or the unavailability of adequate detection techniques. Kreiss and Hodgson have proposed that the diagnosis be based on positive criteria as well as negative criteria (the elimination of identifiable chemical or biologic agents) (55). Adequate criteria for a diagnosis of mass psychogenic illness, based on Kreiss and Hodgson's proposal and on published reports of mass psychogenic illness, include: (a) the collective occurrence of symptoms and related beliefs among two or more persons; (b) symptoms occur in the absence of an identifiable pathogen; (c) features or pattern of illness not explained on an organic basis; (d) symptoms are primarily subjective or those associated with anxiety; (e) spread of cases follows a visual or verbal chain of transmission; (f) presence in affected population of factors known to be associated with mass psychogenic illness, such as stressful environmental conditions and characteristic age and gender distribution; (g) preceded by precipitating event, such as exposure to new odor, fumes, or chemicals. The first three criteria are essential for the diagnosis, and the presence of any of the last four criteria increase the certainty of the diagnosis.

Based on a review of 23 cases of mass psychogenic illness, Colligan and Murphy have described characteristic features of the disorder. In the majority of cases, symptoms were largely subjective, nonspecific, and transitory. Symptoms primarily included nausea, dizziness, lightheadedness, sleepiness, headache, and weakness. The onset of symptoms was usually preceded by a triggering event, such as detection of a strange odor or gas or the use of a new chemical or solvent in the environment. Of workers affected by symptoms in the 23 outbreaks, 89% were women, although as noted by the authors, women were also disproportionately represented in the nonaffected population of those in the same environment. Illness outbreaks tended to occur in occupational settings with boring and repetitive work, rigidly paced work, and little opportunity for advancement. Work pressure (including work speed-ups), physical stressors (excessive noise or heat, poor lighting), and psychosocial stressors (labor-management disputes, strife between workers and supervisors, impaired opportunities for interpersonal communication) were all found to be associated with outbreaks of mass psychogenic illness. An outbreak in the Israeli Occupied West Bank also points to the significance of a background of stress and anxiety in the disorder (56). Some ethnic groups with strong superstitions and beliefs in ghosts and spirits (e.g., Malay compared with Chinese workers in Singapore) also appear to be at greater risk for the disorder (57, 58). A history of early childhood loss (divorce of parents or death within the family) was found to be associated with an outbreak of mass psychogenic illness among schoolchildren (59). A relatively large number of reported outbreaks of mass psychogenic illness have occurred in school-aged children or adolescents, suggesting that younger age may also be a risk factor.

Prevention of mass psychogenic illness is directed at reducing environmental and psychosocial stressors. Treatment of an outbreak usually involves removal from the environment of those affected, careful evaluation of the environment for possible biologic or chemical pathogens, and reassurance based on the results of the evaluation that symptoms will resolve over time with no residual harmful effects.

APPROACH TO DIAGNOSIS

Psychiatric disorder or emotional disturbance should be suspected especially in the following circumstances: (a) when recovery appears to be delayed longer than was originally anticipated based on the severity of exposure and resulting impairment; (b) when neuropsychiatric symptoms predomi-

nate, especially in the absence of clear neurologic impairment; and (c) following any severe, life-threatening traumatic situation.

Relatively brief screening instruments can be useful in assessing the likelihood of psychiatric disorder complicating recovery following toxic exposure. The Beck Depression Inventory (BDI) is a 13-item, self-administered questionnaire that can be completed in 5–10 minutes. Scores above 7 on the BDI suggest depression (60). The Hopkins Symptom Checklist (SCL-90) is a 90-item, self-administered questionnaire that can be used to assess general psychiatric severity, anxiety, depression, and somatization (61). Elevated BDI or SCL-90 scores should be followed up with complete psychiatric evaluation.

In the psychiatric evaluation, diagnosis is facilitated by obtaining a complete and accurate history and chronology of symptoms and of the disabling effects of illness. The evaluation needs to include a thorough review of the person's current and past life situation (family relationships and relationships with coworkers, supervisors, or other persons involved in the exposure), prior history of psychiatric disorders, history of somatization, and drug and alcohol use history. The meaning and significance of the exposure to the person, as well as the person's coping skills and characteristic psychologic defenses should also be assessed. A complete mental status examination is also essential.

Neuropsychologic testing can also be useful to assess impairment resulting from exposure, but the interpretation of test results is not always straightforward. Age-adjusted population norms are not available for many of the most commonly used neuropsychologic tests. Preexposure test results are rarely available for comparison, so that the determination of exposure-related neuropsychologic impairment requires estimation of preexposure functioning. School performance or scores on grade school or high school achievement tests often provide the best basis for estimating preexposure functioning. Since considerable variability in cognitive and intellectual functioning in different domains (e.g., verbal abilities, visual-spatial ability) is common in the general population, while intratest scatter on subscales of the WAIS IQ tests, although suggestive of impairment, are not definitive. When there is evidence of overall good preexposure functioning, consistent, recent onset impairment in one area of functioning known to be affected by the toxic substance strongly supports the likelihood of exposure-related central nervous system toxicity.

PREVENTION AND TREATMENT OF POSTEXPOSURE PSYCHIATRIC DISORDERS

The initial response to a toxic exposure of emergency personnel (e.g., firefighters, emergency medical technicians, and emergency physicians) and the subsequent response of work place survivors, employers, and persons with expertise brought in to evaluate the exposure (e.g., toxicologists, industrial hygienists, occupational and environmental physicians) are of critical importance in preventing severe psychologic and emotional sequelae.

During the process of evacuation, reassurance and attempts to maintain some sense of calm are in order. In the days following the discovery of exposure or evacuation, accurate information about dangers of exposure should be presented in a straighforward, clear fashion by knowledgeable persons who are viewed as credible experts by those who have been exposed. Information should be presented accurately and in a way that does not overwhelm a person's defenses—i.e., denial may be quite useful for some people when there's nothing to be done after an exposure to prevent toxic consequences; others will function better only after they have fully reviewed all of the potential sequelae of exposure. Since acute stress may diminish the exposed person's ability to comprehend fully elaborate information, it is important to make sure that those who have been exposed and others in their community develop an accurate understanding of the information presented.

In order to ensure that information is accurately and completely comprehended, presentation of information may need to be repeated, over a period of days or weeks. Distribution of clearly written information, with references to the scientific literature, may also be useful. Persons exposed to toxic or potentially toxic substances, as well as their family members, often need an opportunity to ask questions about the potential dangers of the exposure and to discuss their personal risk of present or future damage with scientific experts. Those responsible for providing information need to take sufficient time to discover what misperceptions, if any, those who were exposed may have and to address these misperceptions. The process is complicated when scientific information about the dangers is limited or nonexistent.

When human error or design problems have led to exposure, psychologic sequelae can be minimized if those in charge of insuring safety (e.g., employers, in the case of occupational exposures) accept responsibility and attempt to rectify problems. Regardless of who is "at fault," an employer's acknowledgment that an exposure has occurred and expression of sincere interest in the recovery of those exposed and in preventing future recurrences can create a climate fostering healing.

Especially following severe, potentially life-threatening exposures, early referral for psychiatric evaluation and assistance may be critical in lessening the psychologic impact of the exposure. Psychotherapy can help exposed persons resolve psychologic conflicts aroused by the exposure. Working through feelings of anger and blame about the exposure, guilt, loss, or vulnerability can ameliorate symptoms associated with emotional disturbance and facilitate recovery. Mistaken attribution of preexisting psychiatric symptoms can be confronted gently in the context of a supportive psychotherapy. Cognitive and behavioral techniques may also be helpful in facilitating successful return to full functioning of traumatized persons. Finally, specific psychotherapeutic or psychopharmacologic treatments may also be useful to treat posttraumatic stress disorders, anxiety disorders, or depression occurring in the aftermath of exposure.

REFERENCES

1. Wells KB, Stewart A, Hays RD, et al. The functioning and well-being of depressed patients. JAMA 1989;262:914–919.
2. National Center for Health Statistics. Selected symptoms of psychological distress. Public Health Services Series 11, Number 37. Washington, DC: U.S. GPO, 1970.
3. Pennebaker J, Skelton J. Psychological parameters of physical symptoms. J Pers Soc Psychol 1978;4:213.
4. Husman K. Symptoms of car painters with long-term exposure to a mixture of organic solvents. Scand J Work Environ Health 1980;6:19–32.
5. Valciukas JA, Lilis R, Singer RM et al. Neurobehavioral changes among shipyard painters exposed to solvents. Arch Environ Health 1985;40:47–52.
6. Markowitz JS, Gutterman EM, Link BG. Self-reported physical and psychological effects following a malathion pesticide incident. J Occup Med 1986;28:377–383.
7. Loper-Ibor JJ, Soria J, Canas F. Psychopathological aspects of the toxic oil syndrome catastrophe. Br J Psychiatry 1985;147:352–365.

8. Kasl SV, Chisholm RF, Eskenazi B. The impact of the accident at Three Mile Island on the behavior and well-being of nuclear workers. Part II: job tension, psychophysiological symptoms, and indices of distress. Am J Public Health 1981;71:484–495.
9. Lebovits AH, Byrne M, Bernstein J, Strain JJ. Chronic occupational exposure to asbestos: more than medical effects? J Occup Med 1988;30:49–54.
10. Kark RAP. Clinical and neurochemical aspects of inorganic mercury intoxication. In: Vinken PJ, Bruyn GW, eds. Handbook of clinical neurology. Amsterdam: North Holland, 1979.
11. Cullen MR, Robins JM, Eskenazi B. Adult inorganic lead intoxication: presentation of 31 new cases and a review of recent advances in the literature. Medicine 1983;62:221–247.
12. Schottenfeld RS, Cullen MR. Organic affective illness associated with lead intoxication. Am J Psychiatry 1984;141:1423–1425.
13. Mena I. Manganese poisoning. In: Vinken PJ, Bruyn GW, eds. Handbook of clinical neurology. Amsterdam: North Holland, 1979.
14. Moses H, Klawans HL. Bromide intoxication. In: Vinken PJ, Bruyn GW, eds. Handbook of clinical neurology. Amsterdam: North Holland, 1979.
15. Foncin JF, Gruner JE. Tin neurotoxicity. In: Vinken PJ, Bruyn GW, eds. Handbook of clinical neurology. Amsterdam: North Holland, 1979.
16. Chhuttani PN. Chopra JS. Arsenic poisoning. In: Vinken PJ, Bruyn GW, eds. Handbook of clinical neurology. Amsterdam: North Holland, 1979.
17. Goetz CG, Klawans HL. Neurologic aspects of other metals. In: Vinken PJ, Bruyn GW, eds. Handbook of clinical neurology. Amsterdam: North Holland, 1979.
18. The American heritage dictionary of the English language. Morris W, ed. Boston: Houghton Mifflin, 1981.
19. American Psychiatric Association. Diagnostic and statistical manual of mental disorders. 3rd ed., revised. Washington, DC: American Psychiatric Association, 1987.
20. Yates FE, Marsh DJ, Moran JW. The adrenal cortex. In: Mountcastle VB, ed. Medical physiology. St. Louis: CV Mosby, 1974.
21. Scrignar CB. Posttraumatic stress disorder: Diagnosis, treatment, and legal issues. New York: Praeger Publishers, 1988.
22. Hocking F. Extreme environmental stress and its significance for psychopathology. Am J Psychother 1970;24:4–26.
23. Horowitz MJ. Stress response syndromes. New York: Jacob Aronsen, 1976.
24. Lazarus RS, Averill JR, Opton EM. The psychology of coping: issues of research and assessment. In: Coelho G, Hamburg DA, Adams JE, eds. Coping and adaptation. New York: Basic Books, 1974:249–315.
25. Schottenfeld RS. Workers with multiple chemical sensitivities: a psychiatric approach to diagnosis and treatment. Occup Med State Art Rev 1987;2:739–753.
26. Laplanche J, Pontalis JB. The language of psychoanalysis. Nicholson-Smith D, trans. New York: WW Norton, 1973.
27. Lazare A. Current concepts in psychiatry: conversion symptoms. N Engl J Med 1981;305:745–748.
28. Robins LN, Helzer JE, Weissman MM, et al. Lifetime prevalence of specific psychiatric disorders in three sites. Arch Gen Psychiatry 1984;41:949–958.
29. Mayfield D, McLeod G, Hall P. The CAGE questionnaire; validation of a new alcoholism screening instrument. Am J Psychiatry 1980;131:1121–1128.
30. Spencer PS, Schaumburg HH. Organic solvent neurotoxicity—facts and research needs. Scand J Work Environ Health 1985;1(Suppl 11)53–60.
31. Orbaek P, Risberg J, Rosen I, et al. Effects of long-term exposure to solvents in the paint industry. Scand J Work Environ Health 1985;11(Suppl 2):1–28.
32. Larsen F, Leira HL. Organic brain syndrome and long-term exposure to toluene: a clinical, psychiatric study of vocationally active printing workers. J Occup Med 1988;30:875–878.
33. Gyntelberg F, Vesterhauge S, Fog P, et al. Acquired intolerance to organic solvents and results of vestibular testing. Am J Ind Med 1986;9:363–370.
34. Lindstrom K. Changes in psychological performances of solvent-poisoned and solvent-exposed workers. Am J Ind Med 1980;1:69–84.
35. Seppalainen AM, Lindstrom K, Martelin T. Neurophysiological and psychological picture of solvent poisoning. Am J Ind Med 1980;1:31–42.
36. Soborg PA, Bruhn P, Gyldensted C, Melgaard B. Chronic painters' syndrome. Acta Neurol Scand 1981;64:259–272.
37. Flodin U, Edling C, Axelson O. Clinical studies of psychoorganic syndromes among workers with exposure to solvents. Am J Ind Med 1984;5:287–295.
38. Elofsson SA, Gamberale F, Hindmarsh T, et al. Exposure to organic solvents. Scand J Work Environ Health 1980;6:239–273.

39. Gregersen P, Angelso B, Nielsen TE, et al. Neurotoxic effects of organic solvents in exposed workers: an occupational, neuropsychological, and neurological investigation. Am J Ind Med 1984;5:201–225.

40. Cherry N, Hutchins H, Pace T, Waldron HA. Neurobehavioural effects of repeated occupational exposure to toluene and paint solvents. Br J Ind Med 1985;42:291–300.

41. Kraut A, Lilis R, Marcus M, et al. Neurotoxic effects of solvent exposure on sewage treatment workers. Arch Environ Health 1988;43:263–268.

42. Oberg RGE, Udesen H, Thomsen AM, et al. Psychogenic behavioral impairments in patients exposed to neurotoxins. Neuropsychological assessment in differential diagnosis. In WHO environmental health series, Document 3: Neurobehavioral methods in occupational and environmental health, Copenhagen: WHO, 1985:130–135.

43. Bruhn P, Arlien-Soborg P, Gyldensted C, Christensen EL. Prognosis in chronic toxic encephalopathy—a two-year follow-up study in 26 house painters with occupational encephalopathy. Acta Neurol Scand 1981;64:259–272.

44. Baker EL. Organic solvent neurotoxicity. Annu Rev Health 1988;9:223–239.

45. Dager SR, Holland JP, Cowley DS, Dunner DL. Panic disorder precipitated by exposure to organic solvents in the work place. Am J Psychiatry 1987;144:1056–1058.

46. Cullen MR. The worker with multiple chemical sensitivities. An overview. Occup Med State Art Rev 1987;2:655–661.

47. Terr A. Environmental illness: a clinical review of 50 cases. Arch Intern Med 1986;146:145–149.

48. American College of Physicians. Position paper: clinical ecology. Ann Intern Med 1989;111:168–178.

49. Schottenfeld RS. Workers with multiple chemical sensitivities: a psychiatric approach to diagnosis and treatment. Occup Med State Art Rev 1987;2:739–753.

50. Shusterman T, Balmee J, Cone J. Behavioral sensitization to irritants/odorants after acute exposure. J Occup Med 1988;30:565–567.

51. Niedermeyer E. The epilepsies: Diagnosis and management. Baltimore: Urban & Schwarzenberg, 1990:22–23.

52. Bonica J. The management of pain, Vol II. 2nd ed. Philadelphia: Lea & Febiger, 1990:95–121.

53. Schottenfeld RS, Cullen MR. Occupation-induced posttraumatic stress disorders. Am J Psychiatry 1985;142:198–202.

54. Colligan MJ, Murphy LR. A review of mass psychogenic illness in work settings. In: Colligan MJ, Pennebaker JW, Murphy LR, eds. Mass psychogenic illness: a social psychological analysis. Hillsdale, NJ: Lawrence Erlbaum Associates, 1982.

55. Kreiss K, Hodgson MJ. Building associated epidemics. In: Walsh PJ, et al., ed. Indoor air quality. Boca Raton, FL: CRC Press, 1983:87–106.

56. Centers for Disease Control. Epidemic of acute illness—West Bank. Morbidity and Mortality Weekly Report. 1983;32:206–208.

57. Chew PK. How to handle hysterical factory workers. Occup Health Saf 1978;47:50–53.

58. Phoon WH. Outbreaks of mass hysteria at workplaces in Singapore: some patterns and modes of presentation. In: Colligan MJ, Pennebaker JW, Murphy LR, eds. Mass psychogenic illness: a social psychological analysis. Hillsdale, NJ: Lawrence Erlbaum Associates, 1982:21–32.

59. Small GW, Nicholi AM. Mass hysteria among school children. Arch Gen Psychiatry 1982;39:721–724.

60. Swiercinsky D. Testing adults: A reference guide for special psychodiagnostic assessments. Kansas City, MO: Test Corporation of America, 1985.

61. DeRogatis LR, Lipman RS, Rickle R. The Hopkins Symptom Checklist (HSA)—a self-report symptom inventory. Behav Sci 1974;19:1–16.

IV

Toxic Hazards of Industries and Sites

43

Semiconductor Manufacturing Hazards

Myron Harrison, M.D., M.P.H.

INTRODUCTION

Electronics is now the world's fourth largest industry, with revenue approaching one trillion dollars annually. By the year 2000, electronics will be the world's largest industry in terms of revenue. Semiconductor integrated circuits, known as "chips," underpin the entire electronics industry. Merchant sales of semiconductors were in excess of $10 billion in the United States in 1987 (1). The United States currently manufactures about 20% of the worldwide volume of semiconductors so that the total world market is probably in the range of $60 billion.

The number of people directly involved in semiconductor manufacture is surprisingly small. Department of Labor figures for 1984 place total employment in the industry in the United States at 270,000 (2). Probably, however, no more than 45,000 people work in "clean rooms" directly handling product. The rest are employed in a variety of engineering, support, sales, and administrative functions. Nevertheless, the relative importance of this small cohort of workers from a health perspective is magnified because of the large number of chemicals used in the processes.

Potential health risks in semiconductor manufacturing occur from the manufacture of substrate through the completed chip. Three broad areas of concern for occupational exposures are:

1. The clean room environment
2. The manufacturing process and tools
3. Selected chemicals used

The complex nature of this highly competitive industry and rapid changes in technology and materials pose obstacles to the delineation of health risks. Knowledge of these processes coupled with an understanding of the inherent toxicology of the materials enables a health professional to make informed assessments of health risks in the semiconductor industry.

THE CLEAN ROOM

Electronic device fabrication occurs in an environment that demands unusual accommodations by workers. Almost all of the health problems currently observable among semiconductor workers are directly attributable to the "clean room" environment rather than to any of the process chemicals. Some of the stressors are relatively easy to identify and to associate with their consequences. Other potential health problems are difficult to characterize because of the ubiquitous epidemiologic problems of long latency, ambiguous case definition, rarity, multifactorial causation, or high background frequencies.

Semiconductor wafers are processed in clean rooms which are designed to minimize deposition of airborne particles onto the product. Federal Standard 209-D defines environmental classes of such rooms with the most frequently used being the maximum number of particles of diameter 0.5 μm or greater per cubic foot of air (0.028 cubic meters). For example, a class 10,000 clean room is defined as having no more than ten thousand 0.5-micron particles per cubic foot of air (0.028 cubic meters). A similar count in normal ambient air would typically exceed 500,000 particles. As circuit geometries shrink, manufacturers concentrate on smaller and smaller particles. Production clean rooms that average much less than one particle equaling or exceeding 0.1 μm diameter per cubic foot are not uncommon.

It is difficult to understand the potential health hazards in clean rooms without understanding the techniques used to create particle-free environments. There are essentially three configurations or generations of semiconductor clean rooms (3):

Mixed-flow rooms usually combined with vertical-laminar-flow work stations
Mixed-flow rooms arranged into aisles and core areas
Vertical-laminar-flow clean rooms

Clean Room Design and Evolution

The original controlled environments in semiconductor manufacturing were relatively air-tight rooms where air was continuously filtered and recirculated in order to remove particles. Filtered air entered through vents in the ceiling and exited through vents placed in side walls near the floor. Air flow in these rooms (often termed "mixed-flow") was random and turbulent, and, therefore, particles remained suspended for long periods of time. Many air changes (one air change is equal to the volume of the air contained in the room) were required before all particles were flushed from the room. Since the point of the design was to minimize airborne particles, makeup air from the outside was often kept at a minimum. Solvent vapors could accumulate to significant concentrations in these primitive clean rooms.

Most often, specially designed clean work stations are used in combination with these mixed-flow clean rooms (Fig. 43.1). These free-standing stations provide a small work space where filtered air flows in parallel lines ("laminar flow"). Laminar flow is extremely efficient at removing particles from the air. The stations also use HEPA (high efficiency particulate air) filters to capture particles. HEPA filters, whether they are in free-standing hoods or in the ceiling of the clean room, effectively remove all particles greater than 0.05 μm in diameter.

Clean room work stations are a decided improvement for the product, but not necessarily for the worker. The appearance of clean room ventilation hoods is initially deceiving. They appear similar to ventilation hoods used in a chemical or biologic laboratory, and it is natural for a health professional to assume that they are pulling air upward and away from the worker. In fact, some air is always being pushed out the front of the hoods toward the worker (Fig. 43.2).

The ventilation technique used in clean room work stations protects the product under the hood from any particles in the room, but can expose the worker to vapors being generated in

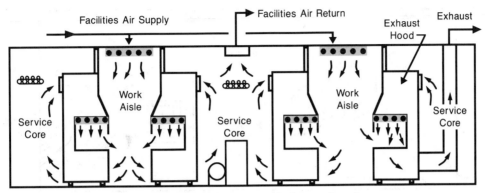

Figure 43.1. Older clean room with clean work stations.

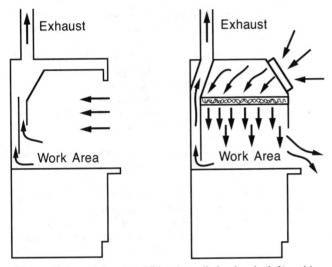

Figure 43.2. Airflow in traditional ventilation hoods (left) and in semiconductor clean room hoods (right).

the work hood. HEPA filters are ineffective at removing gases or vapors. Without the addition of a separate externally vented exhaust system at each work station these stations simply push air contaminants out into the worker's breathing zone.

The next step in the evolution of clean rooms was to arrange work stations adjacent to one another to form aisles. In this arrangement, the rear of the work station faced a service core where all the tool equipment, wet chemicals, and gas distribution facilities were located. Partitions filled the space between the top of the hoods and the ceiling to physically separate the work aisles from the "core" areas (Fig. 43.3).

The work station's hood air intakes are in the core areas. The air is pulled into the back of the work station hood and then goes up to the top of the hood, where a fan pushes it down through a HEPA filter. The air spills over the work surface and out into the work aisle. Approximately 85% of the air flow into the work aisles is coming through these hoods. The remaining air is supplied through HEPA filters in the ceiling of the clean room. The air entering through the ceiling is "conditioned" air whose temperature and humidity have been adjusted within prescribed parameters. Air exits the work aisles through vents in the sidewalls to the core areas. Part of the air in the cores returns via air plenums to the facility ventilation system, but most returns directly to the clean room via the work station hoods.

Airflow remains relatively turbulent in this configuration, although other features yield a significantly cleaner environment for the product. The design focuses all freshly filtered air at the work aisle while return air is channeled through the service core. This results in a high air change rate in the work aisle of 250–300 air changes per hour combining air recirculated through the hoods and facilities ventilation. Consequently, this system is able to achieve airborne particle levels much lower than those found in standard mixed-flow clean rooms. Many of these rooms achieve better than class 100 in the work aisles.

Since the bulk of the air entering the clean room is recirculated from the core areas, workers can be exposed to any contaminants in the core area. Among these contaminants are any gas leaks from lines or cylinders; oil mists from pumps and tools; vapors from wet chemical spills; and air from work aisles that communicate with the same core. Additionally, the equipment in the core areas often generate a large heat load which is circulated directly into the work aisles. This sometimes results in individual aisles that are uncomfortably warm.

Protection of Workers from Airborne Contaminants

Protection of workers needs to be addressed by separate, externally vented exhaust systems at each tool. In the case of "wet stations" which generate mists or vapors, these systems are usually vents around the perimeter of the bench top as well as ventilated subsinks around wet chemical baths. When the perimeter and subsink exhaust systems function as designed, the amount of air escaping out the front of the work station hood toward the worker is minimal. There is a bit of art as well as science in achieving the proper balance between tool exhaust and air flow out of the hood into the work aisle.

Many "dry" processes take place in low pressure closed reactors which are exhausted to a scrubber or other treatment chamber before release to the atmosphere. In the absence of an accident or tool malfunction, operators are not exposed to the gases or exhaust products of these enclosed reactions. Tool maintenance personnel, as will be seen throughout subsequent discussions, have much greater opportunity for exposure.

Air Exchange in Clean Rooms

There is constant loss of air from the clean room circulation through the tool exhausts. These losses are replaced with outside air causing a continual dilution of clean room air. Any makeup

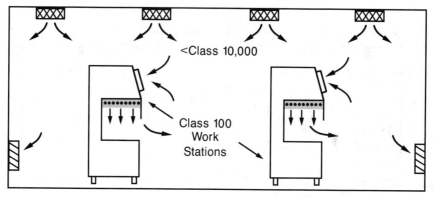

Figure 43.3.   Work aisle/core area type 1 configuration of clean room.

air added to the volume of the clean room adds a new particle load that must be filtered. Facilities engineers would prefer to minimize this burden, but because of losses through tool exhausts, they have no choice but to continually add new air. The volume of makeup air can be considerable. For instance, a single wet station will exhaust approximately 650 cubic feet of air per minute (18.2 cubic meters), and a chemical vapor deposition tool or dry etch reactor between 1500 and 2000 cubic feet per minute (42–56 cubic meters). A good rule of thumb is that 10% of the total clean room volume is being removed (and replaced by outside air) per hour. In the case of a particularly noxious odor or irritating vapor, building engineers can purge the entire clean room volume much more rapidly.

Vertical-Laminar-Flow Ventilation

The state-of-the-art in clean room ventilation is vertical-laminar-flow (VLF) ventilation. Air above the ceiling pressurizes a plenum which is comprised of HEPA filters. The air flows straight down through the room to exit through perforations in a raised floor. Air is captured in a plenum under the floor and is returned through ducts to the ceiling plenum. Straight laminar flow prevents eddying of air currents, and particles are effectively contained within the area where they are generated. Air moves down through the room like a giant piston quickly driving all particles through the floor (Fig. 43.4). In VLF clean rooms the entire volume of air in the room is recirculated and refiltered 9–10 times per minute or approximately every 6 seconds. Better than class 1 environments are easily achieved.

From a health and safety perspective, it is important to realize that airborne chemicals are quickly distributed into the entire volume of the clean room.

Noticeably absent in the VLF environment are the individual work station hoods that are integral to mixed-flow clean rooms. Tool exhaust systems are the same as those in other semiconductor clean rooms. Some VLF facilities isolate the air circulation through the cores. This is done for product protection, but gives additional protection to workers from gas and vapor leaks in the equipment cores.

The VLF clean room is a marked improvement for product yield, and for diminishing worker exposure to chemicals. Even in this environment it must be remembered that low concentrations of vapors are routinely escaping wet tools and entering the clean room circulation. Gas contamination of the clean room environment generally requires a tool failure or other accident. Health professionals faced with specific employee complaints or with more general questions of longterm safety need to take the time to understand the details of any clean room ventilation scheme. Clean rooms are not generic and are no longer exclusive to the semiconductor industry. The aerospace, medical products, ceramics, chemical, biotechnology, and pharmaceutical industries have included clean rooms in many of their processes.

Clean Room Health Problems

Semiconductor clean rooms can be described as hot, dry, and windy. Process optimization requires close control of the tem-

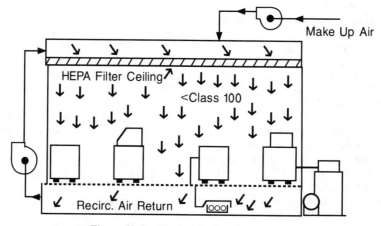

Figure 43.4.   Vertical-laminar-flow room.

perature, which is maintained at about 74°F (23.3°C). Humidity is kept close to 35% to protect wafers from condensation of water droplets. This hot, dry air is moving constantly at about 100 linear feet per minute. These three conditions, especially the extremely low humidity, dehydrate the stratum corneum and can interfere with its ability to protect the underlying epidermis and dermis.

Skin Problems in the Semiconductor Clean Room

Rycroft has written on the importance of "low humidity occupational dermatoses," which can manifest as either pruritis, urticaria, or eczema (4, 5). Recurrent, intractable dermatoses that rarely receive a specific etiologic diagnosis are probably the most frequent cause of medical transfer out of the clean room.

Health professionals faced with dermatits from the clean room too often pursue a chemical irritant or putative allergen when the problem can be easily ameliorated by maintaining hydration of the stratum corneum. Prevention is the best strategy. Some skin problems can be avoided by offering a selection of moisturizing creams or lotions in the change areas. The possibility that the formulation of a specific cream may further aggravate the problem has to be remembered. An added benefit of skin hydration is decreased shedding of dry skin particles into the processing environment.

Sensitization

It is reasonable to speculate that dehydrated, microfissured skin is at increased risk of irritation or sensitization. Unfortunately, health professionals sometimes attempt patch testing to try to rule out the possibility of chemical allergy. However, this diagnostic technique is highly flawed and rarely yields useful information (6, 7). This is especially true when testing with unknown compounds or compounds for which clinical experience is limited.

Upper Respiratory Problems

Other problems beside dermatoses are directly attributable to the hot, dry environment. Recurrent epistaxis, sinusitis, and laryngitis are problems that occur in a very small percentage of workers. All of these upper respiratory problems have caused medical transfer out of the clean room environment.

Asthma

Asthmatics sometimes find that the clean room air worsens their symptoms because of drying of the airways with subsequent formation of mucous plugs. An alternative, but less likely, explanation is that low levels of airborne chemicals are aggravating or precipitating bronchospasm. This problem is not sufficiently predictable to warrant preplacement restrictions for asthmatics, unless the asthma is severe or a specific history of respiratory allergy to chemicals is present.

Eye Problems

The "semi-desert" conditions of the semiconductor clean room can also contribute to eye problems. Some workers complain of constantly irritated eyes, but usually this can be ameliorated by the use of over-the-counter eye drops to moisturize the conjunctivae. Individuals with problems such as a chronic corneal ulcer or chronic or recurring conjunctivitis often fare poorly and may have to be transferred.

Contact lens use is historically not allowed in clean rooms. The reason has been the fear that contact lenses might contribute to a chemical injury of the eye. Prohibition of contact lens use in clean rooms, as in industry as a whole, is an outdated policy that is based on unsubstantiated rumors and fears. The best evidence is that contact lenses serve as protection against either chemical or mechanical insult (8, 9). Obviously, contact lenses by themselves do not serve as adequate protection against either form of injury. Appropriate eye protection must be worn with or without contact lenses.

Contact lenses will be troublesome for some clean room workers, but not because of the intermittent presence of chemicals in the environment. The reason that contact lenses will be aggravating for a portion of workers is the dry, hot air in this environment. Workers requiring visual correction should be allowed to choose between spectacles and contact lenses.

Garments

Clean room garments provide protection of wafers from people. Garments are worn over or in place of street clothes to prevent shedding of contaminant particles from workers. Skin flakes, hair follicles, dust on clothes, cosmetics, and skin bacteria are all frequent sources of contamination. Dressed in ordinary clothes, a person sitting and working sheds from 500,000 to 1,000,000 particles per minute (10). When walking, the number increases to 5,000,000 to 10,000,000 particles per minute. Clean room garments keep most of these particles out of the manufacturing environment.

The suits are designed and woven to minimize fraying and shedding of particles or fibers. Gore-Tex laminate (polytetrafluoroethylene laminate) is sometimes used. Disposable Tyvek (spun-bounded olefin) suits are commonly worn by visitors.

Many garments also incorporate a small percentage of conductive carbon filaments (about 1% by weight) that dissipate static electricity. High density very large scale integrated (VLSI) circuits can be damaged by voltages as low as 20 V—several orders of magnitude less than the charge that can be generated from a clean room worker.

Clean room suits are laundered and repaired at special facilities that maintain a class 100 environment. Workers often attribute skin problems to garment laundering, and occasionally these complaints have been substantiated. One epidemic of contact dermatitis was traced back to high levels of residual tetrachlorethylene used to clean the garments (11). Outgassing of any solvents used to clean these garments is minimal because the garments are sealed in impermeable plastic bags. High levels of tetrachlorethylene were documented inside the sealed bags using organic vapor monitors and subsequently confirmed by gas chromatography. Discontinuation of the use of perchlorethylene and switching to a water-based detergent solved the problem.

Switching to a detergent is not a sure solution. Another clean room was afflicted with an epidemic of dermatitis that was eventually attributed to the alkalinity of residual detergent. This problem was solved when an additional rinse cycle was added to the cleaning procedure.

In a semiconductor facility in Europe, an epidemic (five cases of facial dermatitis) was traced to high residual levels of the laundering chemical—in this case, peroxyacetic acid. Again, the problem was solved with the addition of another rinse cycle.

The possibility of irritation from residual cleaning chemicals trapped in clean room garments is a consideration that should be explored very early in the investigation of dermatitis. Health personnel should be especially suspicious of this possibility if the dermatitis is most noticeable on the skin that is in contact with seams on the garment. These seams are usually areas where the material is folded over and stitched, which makes an efficient trap for residual laundering agents.

Thermal Aspects of Clean Room Garments

Clean rooms garments can also cause thermal discomfort, because they are an additional layer of relatively nonporous clothing in an environment that is already warm. There is no ability to open or shed clothing based on personal comfort. The perception of overheating is not an unusual complaint in areas near furnaces. True hyperthermic syndromes have not been documented.

Fortunately, there is little physical labor required of operators in the semiconductor clean room so that workers are not generating a significant internal heat load. An exception is the maintenance of tools, which can be strenuous.

"Hot flashes" that accompany menopause can be quite intolerable in the clean room garment. Tight, misfitted garments can contribute to overheating in the clean rooms. The need to protect product must be balanced against worker comfort. It is not feasible to create a perfect barrier between the worker and the product.

Headgear

In most instances, headgear is a fabric hood designed to cover the head, mouth, and nose, leaving an exposed area for the eyes. In some situations, goggles have been added to this uniform. A fairly frequent phenomenon with entry into the clean room is the aggravation of facial acne. The problem is usually attributed to irritation from rubbing of the hoods. Work around clean room furnaces can cause sweating and aggravate acne. Acne might seem trivial in an industry replete with potential chemical catastrophes, but it is a genuine cosmetic issue that will demand a solution. Very rarely, the only solution is medical transfer.

Bubble hoods which completely enclose the head and face have been introduced to some fabrication areas. These require a portable powered monitor to draw in air for ventilation of the bubble. Exhausted air passes through a small HEPA filter before exiting into the clean room. Self-contained breathing apparatuses have also been employed in some situations. Any of these initiatives to further enclose the worker will decrease the number who are able to adapt.

Gloves

Polyvinylchloride gloves are usually part of the clean room uniform. Other synthetics such as latex, neoprene, nylon, and polyurethane are sometimes used. Many workers find that their hands perspire. Since the gloves are impermeable to water they can be quite uncomfortable. A small percentage of workers cannot work in clean rooms because of their inability to wear these gloves without developing dermatitis. Occasionally, this inability is due to an allergy to the synthetic, but more fre-

quently it is caused by an occlusive aggravation of a preexisting eczema or other latent dermatitis. Workers with significant histories of eczema, psoriasis, lichen planus of the hands, or with chronic paronychia will not fare well in occlusive gloves. Wearing cotton or nylon liners under the occlusive gloves will sometimes ameliorate a dermatitis.

All the garment items discussed thus far are worn for the protection of product and offer little or no protection from chemicals in the work environment. Additional personal protective equipment must be worn depending on the process.

Illumination

Some employees complain about the yellow or amber light that is one of the hallmarks of any semiconductor manufacturing area. The selective filtration of light is necessary to exclude ultraviolet radiation and the lower end of the visible spectrum as semiconductor photoresists are sensitive in the 300–400 nanometer spectrum. The complaints are nonspecific, but many workers state that they find the lighting depressing. There are presently no documented adverse health effects (physical or psychologic) from exposure to this "unnatural" light. Research into the health effects of light is active (12, 14) and it is possible that clean room illumination will become a health topic in the future.

The perception of heat in the clean rooms can be aggravated by lighting that is unnecessarily bright. Fifty footcandles of illumination (4.6 Lux) is adequate for almost all clean room operations, but higher levels are frequently encountered. Lowering the level of illumination from 80 to 50 (7.4–4.6 Lux) footcandles in one clean room aisle markedly decreased employee complaints of overheating.

Noise

VLF clean rooms can be noisy because of the large ventilation systems and the tool noise. Measurements of 70–75 decibels are common noise levels, but higher readings are occasionally documented. These noise levels pose no potential damage to hearing and are below any threshold for other extra-auditory effects of noise. Nonetheless, visitors will be surprised at the difficulty in carrying on conversation in these environments. The garment hoods covering ears and mouth contribute to this difficulty. Some workers with hearing impairment find the environment very difficult. Completely deaf workers tend to have no problems. Even in the absence of the opportunity to read lips, they usually have developed effective alternative systems of communication.

Ionization of Air

Air filtration removes ions and therefore increases the accumulation of static electricity on surfaces (including wafers). The dryness of the clean room makes control of static electricity all the more difficult. Some semiconductor manufacturers intentionally add ions to the clean room to lessen the possibility of product damage from electrical static discharge (ESD).

Speculation about whether the lack of negative ions in air can cause adverse health effects is a recurring topic. There is no scientific evidence for this proposition. Of more concern is the fact that ionization systems ("static eliminators") used in clean rooms can generate ozone. Health professionals should be aware of this possibility and the possible respiratory effects. Instances have occurred where entire semiconductor fabrication buildings have been evacuated and temporarily closed because of high ozone levels. In one case, six fabrication workers presented simultaneously with symptoms of irritation of eyes and throats, headache, and shortness of breath. Exact ozone levels were not documented but were well in excess of the threshold limit value (TLV) of 0.1 ppm. The building was temporarily closed, the ion generators were eliminated, and the problem did not recur.

Another device used by some manufacturers to lessen ESD are sealed polonium 210 sources which emit alpha particles. These are sometimes placed at every work station. They present a health hazard if the source is broken and workers either inhale or ingest polonium particles.

Problems of Shift Work

Building and equipment overhead contribute a little over 50% to the cost of a completed chip. Chemicals and supplies are about 40% of the cost, and labor is no more than 10%. Semiconductor manufacturers are, therefore, pressured to minimize equipment purchases and operate around the clock. The health effects of unusual shifts are not unique to this industry. Any health professional working in this industry should become knowledgeable about the physiologic and social aspects of this difficult subject. Particularly difficult to solve are work-life issues that often present initially as medical problems.

Psychologic Problems

Clean room environments are notable for emotional sterility and dehumanized surroundings. Walls and furniture are usually gray or white metal. The ambient lighting is a pale yellow or amber color. Windows are rare and usually look out upon equally uninteresting production areas. There is no change in temperature or humidity regardless of time of year. Airflow is even and constant, and the ventilation systems create a persistent mechanical noise. Generally, no music is allowed. Almost the only environmental fluctuation is the intermittent and unpredictable escape of vapors which are rarely dangerous, but often unidentified.

Everyone in the semiconductor clean room is dressed in identical garments which conceal any individual identity. Personal features such as jewelry or makeup are not allowed. Name tags are viewed as a potential source of contamination and are not used. It is difficult to see facial expressions because of the hoods which cover mouths, nose, and forehead. There are no private work spaces or desks nor space that a worker can "own" and individualize.

There are fewer particles generated if human activity is inhibited. Rules or guidelines that discourage assembling in groups, rapid movement, or frequent entry and exit are common. Employees are told to avoid excessive talking and to avoid humming, singing, and laughing since all of these activities release contaminants from the mouth into the clean room. Talking is limited only to that which is necessary for the job. Movements are limited to those which are absolutely essential to the job. Rapid movements such as twitching or gesturing with or clapping hands is avoided. Walking is measured and deliberate.

Unfortunately, many of these rules are unrealistic. It is usual to see small groups of workers talking and laughing while they wait for processes to finish. The benefit upon morale and, ultimately, productivity of this communal behavior probably outweighs the losses incurred from additional particle generation.

The typical work of a semiconductor fabrication worker ("wafer pushers") is inherently repetitive, monotonous, and unchallenging. Basically, the job of many operators is to carry wafers to a tool, load them, and log the job number into a keyboard. The tool is connected to a central computer from which it receives detailed instructions on the parameters of the process. A separate group of process engineers monitors the product and makes all the decisions about changes in the process. Tools are extremely complex, and even routine maintenance is done by a small group of technicians.

With many tasks, the largest part of the job is simply waiting for a tool to finish a process step so that the wafers can be moved to the next tool. It has been estimated that a semiconductor clean room operator typically spends about 10% of the shift actively working and the remainder waiting. Some jobs are exceptions to this generalization. Photoexposure tool work and inspection of wafers with microscopes are two examples where the work is continuous.

Workers have very little sense of ownership of the final product because of the great number of processing steps (often greater than 500). The importance of one's contribution to these microscopic devices is difficult to appreciate. There is little sense of craftsmanship. A striking impression upon talking to many semiconductor fabrication workers is how little they understand about the overall process of semiconductor manufacture.

This type of alienation from one's work is certainly not unique to the semiconductor industry. But from the perspective of a health professional, it can manifest as a host of vague medical complaints that are difficult to diagnose and resolve.

Physical Isolation of the Clean Room

Because of the special garments and, in some cases, the need for multiple clothes changes, clean room ingress and egress are difficult and time-consuming. Other company personnel seldom enter. Management offices are outside the manufacturing floor because of the high cost of clean room space. Clean rooms which are currently under construction offer increased barriers to access—as many as three separate clothes changes before entry.

Psychologic Effects of the Environment

To what extent the unnatural environment, the physical isolation, and the unstimulating work content affect mood, psychology, or motivation is unstudied. Some observers have speculated that the semiconductor clean room operator is more likely to be depressed because of this environment. But there are presently no data to support this idea. Health professionals who work in the industry state that clean room workers as a group seem to be no more afflicted with psychologic problems than other manufacturing groups. In any case, it is important not to forget the unique and alien features of this environment. A few specific syndromes deserve discussion in the context of semiconductor clean rooms.

Phobias

A variety of phobias can be aggravated by the environment and cause a small number of workers to be medically removed from clean rooms. Claustrophobia and chemophobia are the two most common. The former can be precipitated by either the physical environment or the restrictive headgear. Phobias often manifest as classic panic attacks within hours or days of entry into this environment. It is not always easy for health professionals to distinguish between discontent and a true phobia, especially in cases that are slow to manifest. Psychiatric or psychologic referral is important if this diagnosis is entertained. In some cases, desensitization therapy will successfully treat the problem (15–17).

Multiple Chemical Sensitivities

A recently proposed syndrome called "multiple chemical sensitivities" (MCS) is a disorder characterized by recurrent symptoms, referable to multiple organ systems, occurring in response to demonstrable exposure to many chemically unrelated compounds at doses far below those established in the general population to cause harmful effects (18). This case definition will sound very familiar to health professionals experienced with semiconductor clean rooms. Whether these symptoms truly constitute a specific disorder or a group of similar presentations with differing etiologies is not clear.

Other explanations for this constellation of symptoms have been proposed. Several groups conceptualize these reactions as a conditioned stimulus or a conditioned response to a previous overexposure (19, 20). The typical histories of multiple symptoms without objective physical or laboratory findings are also consistent with a diagnosis of somatoform disorder (21).

Whatever the conceptual framework employed, these complaints should be addressed very promptly and very seriously by health professionals. Although it would be naive to think that the complaints are never exaggerated for the purpose of achieving a job transfer or a disability settlement, it is best to avoid such a judgment in any individual case. The large percentage of these patients benefit greatly from psychiatric diagnosis and treatment. Any other approach is likely to steer the patient into the care of clinical ecologists who often inflict serious additional psychologic and financial harm upon these unfortunate people (22).

Mass Psychogenic Illness

Chemical odors are not uncommon in clean room settings. The combination of these odors with work that is often inherently monotonous and the tendency to be isolated from management makes a natural setting for mass psychogenic illness (MPI). The electronics industry has been particularly susceptible to this phenomenon (23, 24).

MPI is suspected when an epidemic of symptoms occur in individual members of a group of people without any objective medical findings and in the absence of any identifiable environmental explanation. MPI is not a clinical diagnosis; it is a sociologic phenomenon describing the collective behavior of a group of people (25).

The current terminology is very unfortunate. The words "psychogenic" and "illness" imply that there is psychopathology in the affected individuals. Quite the opposite, the response, though not conscious, is a natural, healthy coping reaction to a stressful work situation perceived to be unresolvable.

The specific response of the occupational health team and line management to one of these episodes will vary greatly from situation to situation. The best and quickest resolution

will be obtained if qualified occupational health professionals are directing the investigation.

Discussion of MPI is not meant to imply that every unexplained epidemic of symptoms in the clean room falls into this category. MPI should not be automatically proclaimed merely because of the absence of other explanations. There are certain characteristics that make the phenomenon more likely (25). It is also accurate to state that there is much yet to be learned about the health effects of exposure to low levels of chemicals and combinations of chemicals (26). Many episodes of mass symptoms rightfully remain in the "unexplained" category.

PROCESSES AND TOOLS USED IN SEMICONDUCTOR MANUFACTURING

Semiconductor manufacturing can be divided into three groups of processes:

1. Substrate manufacture (making the wafer)
2. Device fabrication (making microelectronic devices such as the transistors in and on the wafer)
3. Device interconnection (wiring together the devices to form a circuit)

In actual production of an integrated circuit, the substrate wafer passes through each process many times.

Substrate Manufacture

Integrated circuits are fashioned onto the surface of thin silicon wafers that vary from 3.25–8 inches in diameter (82.5–200 mm). Silicon is the basic substrate used to make more than 95% of wafers.

Raw silicon dioxide (quartz) is first reduced to silicon by melting in a carbon arc furnace at over 1900°C. This metallurgical grade silicon is ground to a powder, heated, and exposed to high purity hydrogen chloride gas. The product is trichlorosilane ($SiHCl_3$). Trichlorosilane is reduced to very pure silicon by reacting it with hydrogen at high temperature. This "electronic grade" silicon has less than 1 ppb of impurities. The ability to later create microscopic devices by selectively contaminating the silicon depends on starting with a "pure" substrate. As little as one ppm impurity in silicon can profoundly alter its electrical properties.

Crystal Pullers

Almost all crystal growth is done by the Czochralski method. The "crystal puller" tools are large tools in which a "quartzite" (noncrystalline silica) crucible holds molten silicon (1420°C). A starter or seed crystal of silicon is placed onto the end of a rod and dipped into the melt. The rod is pulled out slowly and rotated while the molten silicon crucible is turned in the opposite direction. Silicon atoms attach to the rod and the crystal grows in size.

The melt is usually "doped" with a few grams of boron powder to create silicon with a desired number of electron-deficient areas called "holes." Phosphorus or arsenic is used to dope the melt if an area with a surplus of electrons is desired. The dopant comes in premeasured vials that present little opportunity for exposure.

Crystal growth occurs in an argon atmosphere to prevent oxidation of the silicon crystal and the introduction of impurities from air. Energy to heat the melt is supplied by radio frequency heaters. Magnetic confinement of the melt using large external magnets (1000–5000 gauss, 0.1–0.5 Tesla) is being used experimentally to lessen convective flow in the melt. This results in a structurally more uniform ingot, and is a technique that will eventually be in widespread use. Emerging concerns about electromagnetic field (EMF) exposure will need to be addressed. Finished ingots are usually about 2 feet long (61 centimeters) and weigh approximately 200 pounds (90 kilograms).

The ingot is removed from the reactor employing mechanical hoists, and the crucible is discarded. The graphite susceptor that holds the quartzite crucible needs to be vacuumed and then wiped with methanol or isopropyl alcohol. The debris on the susceptor is primarily silicon dioxide and silicon carbide in large flakes and pieces that pose no inhalation hazard.

Machining Operations

The tools used in milling, grinding, and notching of the ingot, as well as slicing and lapping of the wafers, are standard metal machining tools. The hazards are primarily those of mechanical trauma, machining oils, and noise. Before machining, the ingot is attached to an aluminum or graphite key with an epoxy resin. It is then ground to a uniform diameter cylinder on a lathe. A small notch is machined lengthwise onto the ingot to assist in later positioning of wafers. Wafers are sliced from the ingot at specific angles to ensure the desired crystal orientation on the processing surface. Internal diameter diamond saws are used in this operation. X-ray crystallography is used to position the ingots. Further edge contouring is done to complete the milling operations. Silicon dust from these operations has no special toxicity, but is generally kept well below nuisance standards by using wet processes.

Lapping

Lapping is done to achieve flatness and parallelism on both sides of the wafers. State-of-the-art processing technologies require wafers with 10 angstrom or less variation in the elevations on the surface of the wafer. Most lapping operations use slurries of either alumina or silicon carbide. The machines enclose the wafers, and pressures are adjusted automatically.

Acid Etch

After the machining operations the wafer surface is chemically etched in ''silicon etch,'' a mixture of nitric, acetic, and hydrofluoric acids. This is following by an etch with chromic acid and hydrofluoric acid. Filling the baths and handling the wafers require standard precautions to protect skin and eyes. The ventilation hood over a wet station in these non-clean room settings is a standard hood that pulls air away from the worker. Complaints about acid aerosols are rare to nonexistent at these well-ventilated work stations.

Polishing

Prior to polishing, the wafers are usually ''preannealed'' in furnaces in an atmosphere of nitrogen and hydrogen chloride. To polish wafers, a table holding an abrasive pad rotates while the plates holding the wafers are pressed against it. The wafers are bathed in a slurry of colloidal silica and potassium hydroxide at a pH of about 11. The polishing is accomplished by a chem-

ical-mechanical reaction rather than mechanical friction alone. A celloid of silicon dioxide (SiO_2) and silicon hydroxide (SiOH) forms between the silica particles and the wafer surface and pulls SiO_2 off the wafer. The process is well-enclosed so that exposure to the highly alkaline solution is not a concern while the machines are running. After polishing, class one lasers are used to scribe an identification number on each wafer.

Cleaning

The last step in wafer preparation is removing the silica colloid in a mixture of HCl-H_2O_2 or H_2SO_4-H_2O_2, followed by rinsing in deionized water. These are standard wet station operations with good ventilation. Some manufacturers have substituted less corrosive solutions with which to clean the wafers such as 5% sodium hypochlorite. Some workers develop irritation of eyes and upper airway. There is a tendency in the industry to move away from any chlorine-containing solutions because of contamination problems with chloride ions in later processing. Organic surfactants such as ethoxylated amines are being introduced as substitutes. A final wafer-cleaning step uses ammonium hydroxide solution.

Gallium Arsenide Wafers

While the overwhelming majority of wafers will continue to be silicon for many years, some special applications (generally optoelectronics, military hardware, or very high speed semiconductors) warrant the use of gallium arscnide (GaAs). The primary advantage of GaAs compared with silicon is that electrons move 5–6 times faster in GaAs. Unfortunately, GaAs manufacture is much more hazardous than the manufacture of silicon wafers and therefore requires more stringent industrial hygiene controls than has been customary with silicon.

Polycrystalline GaAs material is formed by reacting elemental arsenic and elemental gallium inside of a sealed tube at high temperatures. Workers are potentially exposed to arsenic when preparing the reaction vessel and removing products. The greatest potential exposure occurs with milling. The polycrystalline GaAs is milled to remove oxides. The ends are sawed off, and the entire chunk is sandblasted. Air levels of arsenic ranging from 540–1500 $\mu g/m^3$ have been measured in these areas (27).

Single crystal GaAs ingots are manufactured from the polycrystalline product by several different methods. The first is a liquid-encapsulated Czochralski technique similar to the crystal pulling of silicon ingots. The main difference is that the surface of the melted GaAs is covered with a layer of molten boron oxide which prevents the loss of vaporized gallium at the high temperatures needed to melt arsenic. The process is enclosed and offers no hazard while in operation. Cleaning a GaAs crystal puller is an extremely hazardous procedure. The graphite susceptor is first vacuumed and the surfaces are wiped with isopropyl alcohol. Personal sampling done by National Institute of Occupational Safety and Health (NIOSH) has documented average exposures in excess of 1000 $\mu g/m^3$ of air during these cleaning operations (27). Self-contained breathing apparatus under positive pressure or an air-supplied respirator must be used to provide adequate protection. Access to the room during cleaning procedures should be highly restricted, and frequent area sampling is necessary to identify potential air contamination.

The other method used to manufacture GaAs ingots is the

horizontal Bridgeman technique. Elemental arsenic is loaded into one end of a horizontal quartz ampule and liquid gallium into a small boat in the other end. A seed crystal of GaAs is placed into the ampule to provide the initial structure for the growth, then heated and cooled. After cooling, the ampule is broken and discarded and the ingot removed. Sampling data has demonstrated that this process is inherently cleaner than the crystal puller method, but the exposures are still well in excess of accepted standards (27).

Subsequent machining operations are similar to those used with silicon ingots, but the GaAs dust must be treated as inorganic arsenic dust. Sampling data in these areas has shown them to be cleaner than some other parts of GaAs processing, but still in excess of the National Institute of Occupational Safety and Health's Recommended Exposure Level (NIOSH REL) of 10 $\mu g/m^3$ (27).

Other III-V Materials

To date, GaAs is the only material that has gained acceptance in the microelectronics industry as a substitute for silicon substrate. Six of the ten elements in columns 3 and 5 of the periodic table lend themselves to electronic device fabrication: aluminum (Al), gallium (Ga), indium (In), phosphorous (P), arsenic (As), and antimony (Sb). The other four are not generally used, because their atomic size precludes easy combination. Boron and nitrogen are too small, and thallium and bismuth are too large. Exotic binary, tertiary, and quarternary combinations of III-V materials are common in research labs and pilot operations. It will not be long before some of these materials enter into widespread production. With them will come more advanced growth techniques, such as molecular beam epitaxy (MBE) and metallo-organic chemical vapor deposition (MOCVD). Unfortunately, investigation of the toxicology of the exotic metallo-organic chemicals used in these processes is in an embryonic stage.

Summary of Wafer Manufacture

The manufacture of substrate wafers, with the exception of gallium arsenide, is relatively safe. Chemical use is less intensive than other parts of semiconductor manufacture, and control engineering is better understood since the processes are not in the clean room environment.

Overview of Device Fabrication

The fabrication of microscopic electronic devices onto the surface of the wafers present tremendous challenges for health and safety professionals. Device fabrication, which is essentially the technology of photolithography, includes the large majority of all the chemical hazards encountered in semiconductor manufacture. Wafers are the basic "parts" that are handled and reprocessed in a photolithography process. Eventually each wafer is cut into a hundred or more individual integrated circuits (chips). Transistors, diodes, resistors, and capacitors are the electronic components fabricated onto each wafer. This is accomplished by creating areas of altered electrical conductivity within the high purity silicon substrate. Unadultered silicon is a poor conductor of electricity, because the four electrons in the outer shell are shared equally with contiguous silicon atoms, creating stable bonds. Addition to the silicon of ma-

terials (such as arsenic and phosphorus) which have an excess of electrons in their outer shell creates an electron rich area. These areas are known as "n" or negative areas. Similarly, addition of materials (most commonly boron) which are deficient in electrons in their outer shell creates an area that is electron poor (a "p" or positive area). The interface between p and n areas is called the "p-n junction." The ability to control the flow of electricity across p-n junctions is the fundamental discovery that is the basis of all microelectronic circuits. Selective contamination or "doping" of microscopic areas of the substrate is achieved through the technology of photolithography.

Lithography

"Lithography" means "writing in stone." In this case, the stone is a layer of silicon dioxide created on the surface of the silicon substrate by oxidation. Patterns can be written into the silicon dioxide by applying a protective layer (a "resist") to selected areas of the silicon dioxide surface and subsequently destroying the unprotected SiO_2 with a chemical etchant such as a strong acid. In essence, the engineers are sculpting a bas-relief impression in the silicon dioxide by means of a chemical attack rather than hammer and chisel. Destroying this protective layer of SiO_2 exposes the underlying silicon substrate to enable implanation with a dopant such as arsenic.

Following the implantation of dopant into the substrate, the resist is stripped away from the remaining silicon dioxide layer. The remaining silicon dioxide can be completely removed or left as a base for a subsequent step in the process. Many processing steps (more than 500 in some complicated logic circuits) are required to manufacture a single microscopic device. Fortunately, many devices (up to 10 billion in memory applications) are created simultaneously on each wafer, and in some steps several hundred wafers are processed simultaneously. Fig. 43.5 is a schematic representation of the basic steps in manufacturing microelectronic devices.

Epitaxy

Epitaxy is often the first production step on the surface of the wafer. Epitaxy is a process of growing a thin elemental crystal layer on top of an identical substrate crystal. The main advantage of epitaxy is that a lightly doped layer of epitaxial silicon can be grown on top of a heavily doped silicon substrate, thus creating a sharp transition of electrical properties between the two layers. This junction can serve as an effective insulating layer between the epilayer and substrate. This prevent currents from flowing via substrate between adjacent devices formed in the epilayer. Silicon upon silicon is the most common epitaxial process. The thickness of the epitaxial layer is usually 5–10 microns. Almost all epitaxial processes are accomplished by chemical vapor deposition (CVD). A general discussion of CVD processes will precede discussion of the specific gases used in silicon epitaxy.

It is important to understand CVD tools in order to appreciate the many potential health and safety hazards (28, 29). Use of these techniques is increasing rapidly, and CVD processes are intensive users of highly toxic gases. CVD is accomplished by using unheated gases to react with heated substrate in a closed chamber. Two configurations of these tools are common, "cold wall" and "hot wall."

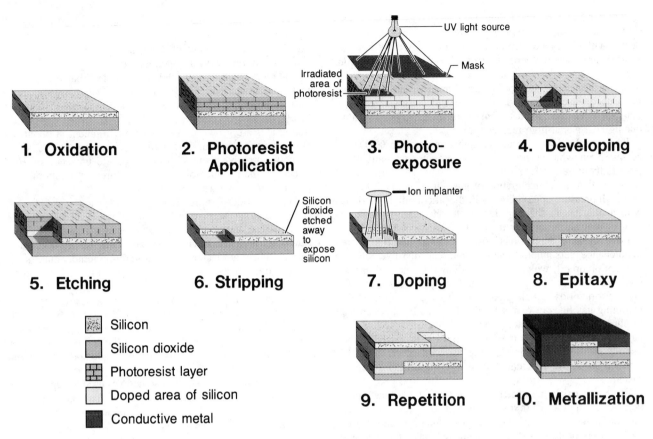

Figure 43.5. Schematic of manufacture of semiconductor devices

1. OXIDATION: The first step is to form a thin layer of chemically-resistant silicon oxide over the surface of the silicon wafer. Sometimes this is preceded by an epitaxial layer of silicon on silicon.

2. PHOTORESIST APPLICATION: The silicon dioxide layer is coated with a thin protective layer called a "photoresist."

3. PHOTO-EXPOSURE: The coated wafer is exposed to UV radiation through a mask that allows light to strike only parts of the photoresist surface. Masks determine the patterns or circuits in the photoresist. With a typical "positive" photoresist the areas struck by light undergo a chemical reaction that will make the photoresist more soluble in an alkaline solution.

4. DEVELOPING: The "developer" is an alkaline solution that will remove the areas of the photoresist that were exposed to UV light. The silicon dioxide under removed areas of photoresist is now protected and can be attacked by etching. The undeveloped or remaining photoresist is hardened by baking to a surface much like the enamel on an automobile.

5. ETCHING: The unprotected silicon dioxide is etched away either by hydrofluoric acid (wet etching) or by ionized gases (dry etching). The photoresist layer protects the silicon dioxide that engineers do not wish to remove.

6. STRIPPING: The remaining photoresist has served its purpose, and is now removed or "stripped" off the wafer surface using highly caustic wet chemicals (wet stripping) or by ionized O_2 (dry stripping or "ashing").

7. DOPING: There are now areas on the wafer where the silicon dioxide layer has been removed to reveal silicon. This silicon can be contaminated or "doped" with atoms such as arsenic to change its electrical conductivity. Altering conductivity in selected areas of the silicon is the essence of creating microelectronic devices such as transistors and diodes. The doping is accomplished by either ion implantation or diffusion.

8. EPITAXY: Another layer of silicon is now applied to the wafer thereby burying the area of silicon that was altered or doped.

9. REPITITION: Subsequent oxidations, resist layers, exposures, etching, doping, etc. create additional areas of either increased or decreased electrical conductivity relative to the substrate silicon.

10. METALLIZATION: The last step is to wire together the devices to create electronic circuits. This is done by depositing patterns of metal by the same photolithographic techniques used to create devices.

In cold wall reactors, 10–50 wafers are held on a metal susceptor which is lowered into a quartz bell jar that is subsequently sealed. The susceptor and wafers are heated to about 1100°C by coupling to a radio frequency energy source. Gases are then introduced into the reaction chamber, and deposit only on high temperature surfaces on the wafers and susceptor. The bell jar—the outside wall of the reactor—is not heated, and no chemical deposition takes place.

Most commonly, cold wall reactions take place at atmospheric pressure, which means that any leak in the chamber can expose workers to reactant gases. Before process gases are introduced into the reaction chamber, pressure checks are done with an inert gas. But manometers occasionally fail, and incidents of leakage have occurred.

Low pressure chemical vapor deposition (LPCVD) at about 50 torr (0.66 ATM) is sometimes used with bell jar type reactors, though more commonly with the hot wall configuration. Low pressure chambers are safer from one perspective in that any leaks will be inward.

Hot wall reactors are essentially typical stack furnaces (described later under "Oxidation"). Quartz boats holding 100–200 vertically standing wafers are slid into furnaces that are heated with electrical resistance. More typically these hot wall reactors are used for deposition of dielectrics or polysilicon, but are sometimes found in epitaxial applications. Since the walls of the reactor are hot in these furnaces, they react with introduced gases just as do the boat and wafers. Deposited material is cleaned from the inside of the chamber by introducing HCl gas at high temperatures.

Increasingly, low pressure vacuums are used in CVD processes. Somewhat surprisingly, low pressure techniques are potentially more dangerous than high pressure depositions. The reason is that the concentration of gases used is much higher. In a high pressure epitaxial growth, the silicon might be doped with arsine gas in the ppm range of concentration. LPCVD epitaxy requires arsine gas in at least 2% concentration.

Low pressure depositions pose additional hazards to tool maintenance personnel. Exhaust gases can dissolve into the vacuum pump oil, which makes handling this material hazardous. (30). Many of the gases used in CVD processes react with air to form solids. Small leaks cause particles to form within incoming gas lines or exhaust lines. Eventually, this can lead to plugged lines and ruptures. Maintenance of these lines can be hazardous, as some of the deposited waste products explode upon exposure to air. Maintenance personnel need to be disciplined about eye protection when working on CVD exhaust systems.

Electric shock is another hazard of CVD tools that require voltages as high as 10,000 volts. In fact, the presence of very high voltages is true of most semiconductor manufacturing tools. Safety professionals in the semiconductor industry often identify the risk of electrocution as their greatest single concern.

Gases Used in Epitaxy

Epitaxial areas use the greatest diversity of potentially very toxic gases of any process in semiconductor manufacture. Typically, in a silicon deposition, HCl gas is used first to etch the wafers. Gases such as silane (SiH_4), dichlorosilane ($SiCl_2H_2$) and trichlorosilane ($SiCl_3H$) are used to deposit silicon. Light doping of the new crystal growth is common and is accomplished by introducing additional gases such as arsine (AsH_3), phosphine (PH_3), or diborane (B_2H_6) to the reactor chamber. Hydrogen is also used in these operations to create a reducing atmosphere and presents a potential explosion hazard.

Generally, operators in epitaxial areas do not have the responsibility of handling or changing gas cylinders. These tasks are done by special "gas teams." State-of-the-art gas delivery systems can greatly minimize the hazard by moving cylinders to a distant gas room.

Many semiconductor workers prefer epitaxy areas because no wet processes are present, and consequently there are no noticeable vapors. Large cylinders of gases such as hydrogen chloride and arsine are typically close by, but usually out of sight and out of mind.

Oxidation

Following epitaxy, a wafer is oxidized to create a thin layer (approximately 300 angstroms) of silicon dioxide. SiO_2 layers are formed repeatedly during the manufacture of semiconductor circuits, mainly as diffusion masks, dielectrics, and passivation layers.

Before oxidation, the wafers are cleaned of all particulate and organic matter in typical wet stations with a solution of H_2O-H_2O_2-HCl at about 80°C. Rinsing with deionized (DI) water and drying with nitrogen gas follows.

The most commonly employed method of oxidation is thermal. Wafers are loaded into quartz boats which are slid into a furnace heated to approximately 1200°C. Thermal oxidation can be divided into dry and wet oxidation. In the dry process thin oxides are grown in a O_2-HCl environment at about one atmosphere of pressure. Dry oxidation processes create extremely corrosive exhaust because of the presence of HCl. Except in the instance of a system failure, operators have no potential for exposure to these gases.

Thicker oxides require higher pressures and the use of steam (wet oxidation). Wet oxidation is accomplished by reacting H_2 with O_2 in the furnace chamber. Hydrogen is used with extreme care because of its potential for explosion. The furnaces must be maintained at or above the autoignition temperature of H_2. Leaks from furnaces are also a concern. Unless the concentration of H_2 in the air is kept below 4%, there is danger of explosion. Area monitors for any H_2 gas leak are very prominent in clean room areas that utilize hydrogen. Because the specific gravity of hydrogen is only 0.07, hydrogen sensors in other industries are typically placed at the ceiling. Clean room ventilation schemes make this strategy inadequate in the semiconductor industry (31).

Chemical vapor deposition is sometimes used to deposit SiO_2. This process is done by reacting silane with oxygen, and gives a better quality oxide. The process temperatures are much lower than those used in typical "wet" and "dry" oxidations.

Furnaces

Furnaces are used not only for oxidation, but also for diffusion, annealing, and some CVD processes. Furnaces are long cylindrical tubes that are typically configured in a "four-stack." Six-to eight-foot-long (1.8–2.4 meters) quartzware "boats" are loaded with wafers and slid into the furnaces. Open-atmosphere furnaces are the usual configuration except for CVD processes. Loading and unloading is usually highly mechanized, though some installations require the workers to push and pull the boats with glass rods. Most commonly, microprocessor-controlled cantilevers handle the quartzware boats. The need to eliminate manual handling of the wafers is driven by process requirements but also lessens human exposure to heat, thermal burns, and exhaust from the furnaces. Heating of the furnace is done with electrical resistance. Most processes occur at either atmospheric pressure or slightly elevated pressures.

Gases are introduced into the reaction chamber from the back of the furnace after the load door is locked. The gas cylinders are stored in well-ventilated gas cabinets. All systems have overrides that purge the furnace with inert gas whenever process conditions exceed preset limits. Both the source and load ends of the furnaces have local exhaust systems.

Worker exposures to toxic exhaust can occur when they open the diffusion furnaces if the furnaces have been inadequately purged or from degassing of the wafers (32, 33).

One persistent problem in furnace areas is that the temperature can be much higher than is typically found in other parts of the semiconductor clean room. Even if the air temperature is not excessive, the infrared radiation from the furnaces can make these areas very uncomfortable for some workers. Facial dermatitis, most commonly acne, can be aggravated by chronic sweating caused by the heat in these areas. Workers in marginal physical condition may also have difficulty in these areas.

Another potential hazard of furnaces is cleaning the quartz-ware tubes that slide into the furnaces. In furnaces used for deposition and diffusion, the glassware is often heavily contaminated with inorganic arsenic. Breakage is not uncommon. The tubes are cleaned by dipping them into large baths of highly concentrated hydrofluoric acid. Workers performing these duties are potentially exposed to inorganic arsenic inhalation, hydrofluoric acid burns, and inhalation of acid aerosols.

Ceramic fiber insulation has replaced asbestos insulation in almost all furnaces. Whenever the operating temperatures are above 1000°C, there is a potential exposure to free silica. Studies have demonstrated that the aluminosilicate fiber divitrifies at about 1100°C to form crystobalite. Release of crystobalite into the air under actual maintenance procedures has been documented (34). Personnel involved in these maintenance operations need to take precautions against inhalation of free silica.

Photoresist Application

Following creation of a silicon dioxide layer the wafer is covered with a photoresist. Although photoresists comprise a very small proportion of the total chemical usage in semiconductor manufacturing, many workers handle these chemicals and are potentially exposed via both inhalation and skin absorption.

Wafer Tracks

The basic tool for application of photoresist is called a wafer track. Unlike most semiconductor manufacturing tools, wafer tracks sit out in the clean room. A cassette of wafers is loaded into one end of these machines by the operator. Individual wafers are moved on air tracks to a photoresist apply station. The entire surface of a wafer is covered with a resist solution by applying a drop of resist to the center of a rapidly spinning wafer. The spinning wafer is contained inside a cup that captures spattered photoresist. The cup is under exhaust ventilation to remove vapors arising from the photoresist solvents.

The wafer is then carried automatically through small ovens or hotplates that bake a wafer at about 80–90°C. This is the "softbake" or "prebake" process, which causes 80–90% of the resist solvent to vaporize. With older or poorly maintained tools, this heating step is a source of high vapor concentrations. In newer tools, the softbake ovens are purged with nitrogen, and exhaust ventilation is adequate to carry away the solvent vapors. Even new, well-designed tools need constant cleaning of the exhaust tubes which become clogged with photoresist polymers. Failure to clean under the tool where resist canisters often spill is a frequent source of solvent vapors.

Environmental sampling at wafer tracks invariably yields results that are under all published exposure standards (32, 35). These data have not been wholly successful in addressing worker preceptions. Workers seem to dislike these tools more than any others in the semiconductor clean room. Odors are common and have the reputation among many workers of being "carcinogenic" and "causing sterility." The latter concern has been generated largely by the presence of glycol ethers in almost all photoresist formulations.

Some manufacturers prime wafers with an application of an adhesive, hexamethyldisilazane (HMDS), prior to photoresist application. Glycol ethers have been a popular solvent in which to carry the HMDS in a liquid application, though most manufacturers have either switched to xylene or substituted an enclosed vapor phase technique.

Wafer track tools are also used to apply materials that are not photoresists. Other polymers such as polysulfone and polyimides are applied as dielectric layers usually in the metallization stage of manufacture. Operators generally make no distinction between photoresists and dielectrics, and anything applied at a wafer track is known as a "resist." The dielectric polymers use different solvents—dichloromethane, n-methyl pyrrolidone, dimethylformamide, and dimethylacetamide are frequent choices.

Photoexposure

Exposure tools, also known as aligners, steppers, or projection tools, use a variety of methods to expose photoresist to ultraviolet (UV) radiation that has passed through a mask. The UV source is an intense mercury arc lamp (about 1500 kilowatts). Although most of the radiation given off by the lamps is greater than 350 nanometers in wavelength, significant amounts are also below 315 nanometers. Leakage of UV radiation during operation or exposure during maintenance can cause serious acute and chronic damage to skin, cornea, and retinae. Photoexposure causes anxiety among operators about the hazards of UV radiation. Frequent monitoring with a UV actinic radiometer is necessary to ensure safety and to reassure the operators.

Another potential exposure of the optical exposure process is to ozone generated by the strong electrical fields surrounding the mercury arc lamps. Levels in excess of published exposure standards have been documented around inadequately ventilated photoexposure tools.

The mercury arc lamps are a potential source of mercury exposure. These lamps eventually fail, burst, and release vaporized mercury (about 2 mg) into the clean room environment. Depending on the volume of the room and the rate of dilution of the air, a significant inhalation exposure could occur. No such overexposures have ever been documented. Routinely changing bulbs after a defined number of hours of operation prevents this possibility.

Photoexposure tools are somewhat unusual in the clean room in that they demand long periods of sitting in static postures. This can generate a variety of musculoskeletal complaints. The work also entails prolonged use of microscopes and/or video display terminals (VDTs) and can be a source of eye strain or fatigue.

Developing

Removal of the exposed photoresist (developing) is accomplished with either a NaOH or KOH bath at a pH of approximately 13. The hazards to skin and eye are easily appreciated, and proper protective equipment is crucial. Alkaline burns are a special hazard to the cornea. Even small splashes into the eye require immediate and copious irrigation followed by prompt referral to an ophthalmologist whether or not symptoms are present.

Developing is but one of many process steps that occur at "wet stations." These tools present the most readily recognized hazards of any tools in semiconductor clean rooms.

Table 43.1. Chemicals Commonly Found at Wet Stations

Alkalis
  Ammonium hydroxide
  Hydrazine monohydrate
  Potassium hydroxide
  Sodium hydroxide

Acids
  Acetic acid
  Hydrochloric acid
  Hydrofluoric acid
  Nitric acid
  Perchloric acid
  Sulfuric acid
  Chromic acid

Other
  Ammonium fluoride
  Hydrogen peroxide
  Methanol
  Isopropyl alcohol
  Sodium peroxide
  Trichloroethylene
  Perchloroethylene
  Freons (many)
  Acetone
  Xylene
  Dimethylacetamide
  N-Methyl pyrrolidone
  Glycol ethers

Wet Stations

Wafers are repeatedly cleaned, developed, etched, and stripped in wet chemical baths. A typical wet station or wet bench consists of a number of process tanks, chemical recirculators and filters, rinse tanks, a wafer dryer, exhaust system, and in some cases automatic chemical dispensing systems. Very often the baths are heated by electric immersion heaters. The use of scrubbing, ultrasonics, megasonics, and acoustics are sometimes added. Robots to handle the wafers have been introduced to some of these operations, especially in vertical laminar flow (VLF) type of clean rooms. Mixed-flow design rooms with individual hoods generally do not have enough space under the hoods to allow robotic tools. Automated handling of cassettes and chemicals is safer than manual techniques, but most accidents at wet stations occur when workers are draining and refilling the baths.

A wide variety of inorganic acids and organic solvents are used at wet stations. Table 43.1 lists some of the chemicals that are found in wet baths in semiconductor manufacturing. Proper personal protective gear must be used, but the hazards are so readily apparent that compliance is generally not an issue.

Possible inhalation hazards at wet stations are more difficult to define. Sporadically and unpredictably, a noticeable amount of chemical vapor is expelled into the worker's breathing zone. This problem is identified primarily at stations where highly irritant chemicals are used. The typical complaints are odors, eye irritation, or throat irritation. Environmental or personal sampling invariably yields numbers that are well within published time-weighted standards. Some of these sampling data have been published (32). As the health profession becomes more knowledgeable about the chronic effects of exposure to low levels of organic vapors or acid aerosols, there may be a reevaluation of these standards.

Wet Station Exhaust Systems

As discussed earlier, perimeter and subsink exhaust systems exist at wet stations in clean rooms to carry away vapors and aerosols. These exhausts must be balanced against positive air flow out of the hood. Ventilation balance is not a static phenomenon. Anytime that an aditional tool is added to an exhaust system, the pull on already established tools is diminished. Likewise, any decrease in air pressure in the clean room will affect the amount of air spilling out of the front of the hoods.

Spills or overflows of acids or solvents into a subsink can be pulled into tool exhaust systems. Nonvolatile chemicals can stay suspended in the exhaust system indefinitely. Eventually, a saturation point will be reached and the chemicals will start to come out of the exhaust system, though not necessarily where they entered. This phenomenon can be an interesting source of odors and exposures in the clean room, and very difficult to investigate.

Fire Hazard at Wet Stations

Fires at wet stations are relatively frequent events. These usually occur when the baths are drained without turning off the heater and are later refilled, igniting the chemicals. In some cases, the electric immersion heater will ignite the bench, which is often constructed of polypropylene. An electric immersion heater will have a surface temperature of approximately 180°F (82°C) in ambient water and 1300°F (704°C) in ambient air. A variety of over-temperature monitors and liquid level controls are available to reduce the chance of accidental ignition. Even when installed, these monitors frequently fail or are ignored by operators. More than half the insurance losses encountered in the semiconductor industry are caused by fire (36). In 1977, an entire semiconductor facility in Scotland was lost to a fire that began at a wet bench.

Fire suppression techniques that are adequate in most industrial settings fail to be effective in the VLF clean room. Laminar flow moves air downward air through the floor while heat-activated sprinklers are naturally placed in the ceiling. In a demonstration study performed in a mock clean room, it was 35 minutes before a conventional fire system detected a wet station fire (36). The current trend in the industry is to install Halon 1301 extinguishing systems at each wet station. New fire codes, specific to the semiconductor industry, state that fire protection systems must be placed directly on the wet station. These codes also address construction of semiconductor fabrication facilities, as well as the handling, storage, and use of the chemicals (37–39).

Hardbake

Following development of the photoresist, a thermal baking process hardens the remaining photoresist to a finish much like the enamel on an automobile. The photoresist is now ready to protect the underlying SiO_2 from an etchant chemical attack. The hardbake process occurs in well-enclosed and well-ventilated ovens.

Etching

SiO_2 that is not protected by resist is removed in the etching process to uncover silicon and enable subsequent doping. Etching is accomplished either by submersion of the wafer in an acid bath or by an enclosed "dry etch," which uses ionized gases.

Acids Used in Wet Etching

Wet etches are most often manual processes, though in some of the most advanced clean rooms, robots move baskets of wafers in and out of the baths. In wet etching, the acids most frequently used are hydrofluoric acid (HF), hydrochloric acid (HCL), sulfuric acid (H_2SO_4), nitric acid (HNO_3), and chromic acid (CrO_3). Dermal hazards are usually very well controlled. Poorly engineered stations can expose workers to significant concentrations of acid aerosols. These are not only irritating, but can damage pulmonary tissue.

HF is the greatest hazard because of its peculiar behavior and the fact that HF burns are frequently undertreated by medical professionals. HF is used in varying concentrations (from 3–50%) for etching silicon.

Dry Etching

Dry etching is supplanting wet etching because of shrinking geometries on the surface of wafers. Wet etching is difficult to control because it etches in all directions.

Dry etching uses ionized gases in closed reactors with most processes carried out at pressures below 1 torr (0.01 ATM). There are at least a dozen different methods of dry etching, but the best known are plasma etching and reactive ion etching (RIE) (40). The only difference between the two is that in RIE the wafers are situated on the anode, while in plasma systems they are on the cathode plate. RIE systems achieve better directional etching action. In either system, activated fluorine-based or chlorine-based etchants are created by exposing a gas to an electrical discharge. The most popular gases are chlorine (Cl_2), trichloroboron (BCl_3), hydrogen chloride (HCl), trifluorocarbon (CHF_3), bromine (Br_2), tetrafluorocarbon (CF_4), tetrachlorocarbon (CCl_4), and trifluoroboron (BF_3), though at least 200 gaseous etchants have been investigated (41, 42). The reactive species etch both physically and chemically. The product of the etching process is usually a halogenated compound of the material being etched. These products are removed continuously by vacuum pumps. There is the remote chance for operators to be exposed to the effluent if an exhaust line leaks or if a tool is opened prematurely. Some of the reactor effluents are highly toxic. They are trapped in either oil or liquid nitrogen, and unless handled appropriately, present a hazard to workers who must maintain the pumps (43).

Dry Etching of GaAs

As gallium arsenide wafers become more widely used, maintenance of dry etching tools will become more hazardous. It has been demonstrated that large amounts of arsenic accumulate in the cartridge filters, nitrogen traps, and pump oil (44).

Radiofrequency Radiation Emissions in Dry Etching

The charged gas plasmas are created with radiofrequency energy, and these tools sometimes leak electric and magnetic energy. In 1983, 23 plasma etching units from four different facilities were monitored by NIOSH for release of radiofrequency (RF) energy. Five of the 23 units emitted electrical field energies above ACGIH standards, and three emitted magnetic fields above ACGIH standards (32). Measurements are done at 10 cms from the units. Since workers generally are not standing near the units when the units are in operation, the actual potential for significant exposure is greatly diminished. Nonetheless, frequent monitoring of the tools for radio frequency emission is warranted. Exposure to less than the current published ACGIH standards will prevent thermal injuries.

Increased Potential for RF Exposure

Crystal pullers, evaporators, and sputterers are among other tools beside etchers and plasma tools that utilize RF energy. The potential for exposure to RF energy is increasing rapidly. Many of the tools used in semiconductor manufacture use wavelengths that are particularly well absorbed by human tissue (13.56 MHz). Careful maintenance and regular monitoring of tools will eliminate the possibility of exposure.

Stripping the Resist

After etching of unprotected silicon dioxide, the resist has served its purpose and must be removed from the protected SiO_2. "Ashing" or "dry stripping" is usually the first step. These tools are essentially the same as dry etch tools. Wafers are placed in a chamber which is pumped down to about 2 torr. Oxygen is introduced and subjected to radio frequency power which creates oxygen radicals. These radicals react with resist to oxidize it to water, carbon monoxide, and carbon dioxide which are pumped away.

The primary reason for the initial introduction of dry stripping was to reduce chemical consumption and disposal problems. At present, process demands require that dry etching replace wet etching. During the dry etch, the top surface of the photoresist mask becomes fluorinated or chlorinated which renders it insoluble to most wet chemistries. Resist that has been exposed to ion implantation is also hardened and difficult to remove with wet processes alone. Therefore an ashing step is used to remove the top layer of the resist, or the "skin" as it is sometimes called. After this top layer of resist is removed, wet or dry processes can be used to strip the remaining resist.

Another approach that has been used to strip resist is to use a combination of UV radiation and ozone at atmospheric pressure (45). This is not a widely employed process at present. Because this process occurs at ambient pressures, rather than in a vacuum, there is increased potential for exposure of workers to the reactant gases.

Wet Stripping

Very corrosive chemicals based on formulations developed in the metal paint industries are used in wet stripping. These processes occur at typical wet stations where cassettes of wafers are dunked into baths. Typically, hot solvent processes (90–120°C) are employed, and ultrasound energy is added to increase the penetration.

The stripper will usually contain a primary solvent, a cosolvent, an activator (penetrant), and a surface wetting agent. Historically, the most popular primary solvent for the diazonaphthoquinone/novolak (DQN) photoresist system has been dichloromethane. The cosolvent used is methanol which prevents the resist from precipitating as oily beads onto the substrate. Added to this mixture is a penetrant, usually phenol. Another popular combination is a mixture of tetrachloroethylene, o-dichlorobenzene, phenol and p-toluene sulfonic acid. Anhydrous hydrazine, H_2O_2-H_2SO_4, Cr_2O_3-H_2SO_4, and an ammonia solution of hydrogen peroxide are other strippers used with DQN.

New Strippers

There is ongoing interest in finding strippers that have less irritating vapors, that are less likely to be chronic health hazards, and that are less expensive to dispose of responsibly. Two chemicals being increasingly used are dimethylacetamide (DMAC) and n-methyl pyrrolidone (NMP). To date, the toxicologic information on these solvents indicates minimal health hazard (46–48). New data may change that assessment. NMP is currently receiving very high focus from the National Toxicology Program (NTP) Chemical Evaluation Committee which is recommending further testing for carcinogenic and reproductive effects (49).

The Future of Wet Stripping Operations

Since wet stripping is considerably more hazardous than dry stripping and is less controllable from a process perspective, it is natural to question why wet stripping is still used. The reason is that photoresist is typically contaminated with metal ions that do not volatilize during the ashing or dry stripping process. These ions are left on the surface of the wafer and will be driven into the wafer during subsequent processing. The metal ions can short microscopic circuits. Wet stripping is much more effective at removing metal ions from the surface of the wafer. Until photoresists are free of metal contamination, wet stripping stations will remain part of the clean room environment.

Doping

Doping of the substrate to create ''n'' and ''p'' regions is achieved either by thermal diffusion or ion implantation. The latter is a more advanced technique that is necessary for smaller geometries. It also has considerably more potential for hazardous exposures than does diffusion.

Diffusion

Diffusion is based on the fact that at 1000°C impurities will diffuse into and through silicon substrate. Since the dopants move much more slowly through SiO_2, a protective layer of that material will allow selective doping.

The first step is called predeposition and coats the wafer with the dopant material. Wafers are placed into quartz tubes which are pushed into a typical stack furnace to heat the wafers. The dopant source is either a gas such as arsine carried in an inert gas, or a powdered form of the desired dopant. Liquid sources can also be used by bubbling an inert carrier gas through a liquid form of the dopant.

The wafers are then put into a second furnace at higher temperatures (about 1300°C) to ''drive in'' the dopant. This step occurs in an oxidizing atmosphere that forms a thin layer of quartz over the freshly doped silicon.

The source cabinets where the dopants are supplied are ventilated to an exhaust system. Scavenger boxes enclose the loading worker end of the furnaces and are also exhausted. All reported sampling data taken while the furnaces are operating have been either undetectable or below published standards (32).

Implantation

Ion implantation is a critical technology in modern semiconductor manufacture. A controllable quantity of almost any element can be mingled with a host material and in this case, it is silicon substrate (50). Ion implantation tools generate a beam of dopant ions by boiling them from a heated filament. The ions are accelerated in electric fields and directed against a gaseous form of the element to be introduced. Arsine, phosphine, and diborane are common dopant gases. Collision with the high velocity electrons strips away the dopants electrons to create a plasma. An electric field pulls the plasma from the chamber. Magnets are used to deflect the ion beam at precise angles causing heavier or lighter ions to be lost from the beam. This results in a highly purified beam of dopant ions that impact the substrate surface. The entire process occurs in a vacuum of 10^{-6} torr (10^{-8} ATM) or less. The vacuums are created by either oil diffusion or cryogenic pumps backed by a mechanical roughing pump.

Operator interaction with the tools is ordinarily limited to loading and unloading a cassette of wafers and entering the job number into a keyboard. Nonetheless, potential health hazards for operators exist. These include catastrophic gas leakage; ionizing radiation; and fumes (such as arsenic trioxide) from newly implanted wafers. Great efforts are taken in the semiconductor industry to ensure against exposure to the toxic gases used in implantation.

All implanters use high voltages to accelerate the charged particles of the ion beam. The energy of accelerated electrons created by this process is high enough to generate x-rays. Much of the ion implanter is lined with lead shielding to protect personnel, but leaks can occur. Film badges are not adequate for identifying exposures from implanters because most emissions are in the form of narrow beams from cracks and holes in the cabinet. It is unlikely that the film badge, whether worn by personnel or placed on the implanter, will be in the line of a leak. X-ray surveys need to be done with a Geiger-Muller counter to ensure that ionizing radiation is not leaking (51). Actual doses can be quantified with an ion chamber.

A study performed by NIOSH in 1985 demonstrated small amounts of inorganic arsenic being emitted from implanted wafers up to 3.5 hours after removel from the tool (33). A survey of ion implantation operations in three semiconductor facilities documented routine worker exposure to levels of airborne dopants below ACGIH or OSHA standards. Area sampling demonstrated the potential for more worrisome exposures (52). A separate study confirmed the presence of low levels of airborne contaminant at these tools (51). The maximum exposure was quite low, 0.04 $\mu g/m^3$. In both studies, surfaces in the implanter areas were contaminated with arsenic, but at very low levels.

Phosphine has also been documented as a gas leaking from wafers implanted with phosphorous even though the source was solid phosphorous.

Workers who maintain or repair the implanters have all the potential exposures described for operators plus additional hazards. Significant levels of arsenic have been documented in pump oils so that maintenance workers are potentially exposed. With the oil acting as an adjuvant, toxic material such as arsenic can easily be absorbed through the skin. Inhalation of toxins contained in the oil mists is a theoretical concern, but of little practical significance. Another hazard of the diffusion pumps is the possibility of thermal burn. These pumps are relatively unprotected and operate at temperatures high enough to boil oil.

Cleaning the tool parts, especially beam line components, is another potential exposure to arsenic for maintenance personnel. A strong odor of garlic (similar to arsine or phosphine) often occurs when beam lines and pumps are opened, and sometimes forces building evacuations. Sampling, even in the presence of the odors, has yet to document the presence of arsine or phosphine. The cause of these odors has not yet been determined. Until proven otherwise, the assumption should be that these odors represent hazardous exposures, and appropriate precautions should be taken.

Bead blasters are used to clean the implanter parts after they have been removed from the tool. Handling of parts and cleaning of the head blasters presents another hazard that requires personal protection. Wet slurry blasters are inherently safer than dry blasters, and have been adopted by some companies.

Several components inside the implanter operate at very high voltages, up to 100,000 volts. Use of grounding hooks prior to any contact with these tools is essential even if the tool is not operating. Ordinarily, it is not possible to get into implanters without turning off the power. But some maintenance and fine tuning requires technicians to adjust these tools with parts charged to high voltage.

Any worker who changes gas cylinders is at risk of a catastrophic accident and should do all gaseous source changes in a self-contained breathing apparatus under positive pressure. Solid sources (usually vaporizers of elemental arsenic) are changed and loaded almost daily for each tool, and present potential for exposure to inorganic arsenic dust. At a minimum, this work should be done under a ventilation hood with appropriate personal protective equipment. Some companies require glove boxes for solid source changes.

Annealing

Implantation damages the surface of the wafer. Slowly heating the wafer returns it to its original condition, as well as incorporating the dopant atoms into the silicon crystal lattice. Annealing is done in stack furnaces at about 800°C.

Occasionally, high energy lasers, electron beams, or flash lamps are used to anneal surfaces because they minimize the diffusion of dopant that occurs with prolonged heating. Rapid thermal annealing (RTA) with lasers can cut the heating time to less than 10^{-7} seconds.

Device Interconnection (Metallization)

Interconnection of completed semiconductor devices is accomplished by depositing patterns of metal ("wiring") onto the surface of the chip. The width of these "wires" varies from 0.5–5 microns in current products. The patterns are created by the use of photolithography as was discussed under device fabrication. Most modern integrated circuits require at least three levels of metallization with each separated by an insulating layer.

Metallization processes are presently less of a health and safety challenge than device formation areas. This is because of the absence of ion implanters and a less frequent use of

chemical vapor deposition tools. Those two types of tools are the heaviest users of hazardous gases. At present, metallization relies on inherently safer physical vapor-depositing methods.

Physical Vapor Deposition of Metals

Deposition of metals has traditionally been accomplished by two physical vapor deposition methods, either evaporation or sputtering. Aluminum is the most commonly used metal for connecting devices. Other commonly deposited metals are chromium, nickel, gold, silver, titanium, tungsten, platinum, and silicon. Combinations such as copper-chrome-gold and lead-tin are frequently employed.

Evaporation

Evaporation uses a two-chambered tool. The wafers are loaded onto a dome and placed into the upper chamber. A solid "slug" of the metal that is to be evaporated and *deposited* is placed in a lower chamber. No reactive gases are used at these tools. The metal is evaporated by *radiofrequency*, thermal, or electron beam heating, and the vapors deposit on wafers in the chamber above. All the reactions occur in a vacuum, and operator exposure to the metals in a vaporized state is not a consideration.

Cleaning of Evaporators

Exposure to metallic dust can occur with cleaning of the tools. Between runs the operator will sometimes vacuum the reaction chamber for any loose flakes or particles of metal. After a certain number of runs the inside of the tool is taken out and cleaned in a bead blaster. Parts of the tool that cannot be removed are mechanically scrubbed with wire pads or brushes. Exposure levels of the metal deposited in the tool are extremely high during these cleaning procedures. For instance, personal sampling on a worker cleaning a lead-tin evaporator documented a 90-minute mean air lead level in excess of 1200 μg per cubic meter (personal communication). Appropriate respirators are one solution to this problem. A preferable solution is to substitute chemical cleaning methods for the mechanical methods.

Sputtering

Sputtering is done by bombarding the target metal with argon ions to release metal ions from the surface of the target. These atoms condense on the substrate to form a film. Sputtering processes are used to deposit semiconductors and dielectrics as well as metals. Sputtering is carried out at relatively high pressures (10^{-2} torr) (10^{-4} ATM). Radiofrequency or direct current power sources are used to create the ionized argon. As with evaporation tools, exposure to metals can occur with cleaning.

Exposure to radiofrequency energy is a possibility at sputterer tools. These emissions are generally the result of incorrect placement of shielding following maintenance procedures.

Chemical Vapor Deposition of Metals

Continued reduction of device and interconnection dimensions is going to cause the current evaporation and sputtering of metals to be obsolete. CVD metal systems allow better contouring as well as better control of composition of binary or tertiary metal systems. Metal silicides are already used in some circuits as first layer metallizations. A typical reaction is to combine tungsten hexafluoride gas with silane to deposit tungsten silicide. Silane is often used in 100% concentrations to ensure the desired composition of the silicide deposition. Metal hydrides, halides, and carbonyls, as well as an infinite variety of organometallics, are also used to accomplish CVD of metals. As these processes become more prevalent in the production environment, they will present a major challenge to health and safety professionals.

Lift-Off

Photoresists are traditionally used in device photolithography to assist in a subtractive or etching process. In metallization processes they are often used to deposit a solid onto the substrate, an additive process. In one technique, the metal is deposited then covered with a patterned resist, and subsequently etched. In another technique the resist is used to "lift-off" deposited metal. This is done by evaporating a metal onto a surface that is partially protected by an already patterned and developed resist. The wafer is then placed in a solvent that causes swelling of the resist. As the resist swells it lifts the overlaid metal away from the surface of the wafer and allows it to be washed away. Metal that was deposited onto the substrate is left behind.

Lift-off stations are much like wet stripping stations in terms of the chemicals employed. The solvent is generally heated which adds to the potential for exposure to vapors. Worker complaints about eye and throat irritation are frequent. Fires are not uncommon.

Silyation

Etching deposited metals requires a more aggressive chemical attack than etching of SiO_2. Consequently, the resists need to be tougher. Silyation is frequently done to harden a photoresist before it is subjected to etching. Silyation is a process of introducing silicon atoms into the surface of the organic resist. The process can be accomplished with either wet or dry procedures. Most commonly, a wet bath using either hexamethyldisilazane (HMDS) or silazone in xylene is used.

Reactive Ion Etching of Metals

As in device formation, dry etching of deposited aluminum is increasingly preferred to wet etching, because smaller geometries can be achieved. The tools and potential means of exposure do not differ from the etching of silicon. Because of the high reactivity of metals with ambient O_2 and H_2O, plasma etching of metals often involves more emphasis on etching oxides of the metal rather than the metal itself. Chlorocarbon and fluorocarbon gases, rather than pure halogens, arc typically used to etch metal films because they are more effective in reducing the metal oxides. Examples of gases used in metal etching are CCl_4 with BCl_3, $SiCl_4$, $C_2Cl_2F_4$, and $CClF_3$.

The exhaust products are a halogenated compound of whatever metal is used for interconnection. Because nitrogen is used as a carrier gas for the reactive halogenated gases, byproducts of the reactions can incorporate nitrogen atoms. Hydrogen cyanide is commonly measured at levels of 1–2 ppm upon opening reactors that are used to dry-etch aluminum; in addition cyanogen chloride has also been detected at excess of the TLV

ceiling (53). These gases have been detected only in aluminum-etch chemistries.

Dielectric Film Deposition

Dielectric layers are electrical insulators used to separate conducting metals or provide protection from the environment. Commonly used layers are polycrystalline silicon, silicon nitride, polyimide, and silicon dioxide. The method of deposition is most commonly physical vapor deposition. Chemical vapor deposition with its attendant use of toxic and flammable gases will be used increasingly as smaller products require more level depositions.

Undoped SiO_2 is used as an insulating layer between multilevel metallizations, and is usually sputtered onto the wafer. Often a tool will be used to do a series of sputter depositions with each followed by an etch cycle in order to try to level or "planarize" the surface of the wafer. The etch cycle is accomplished with a ionized chlorinated hydrocarbon gas.

Passivation

Silicon nitride (Si_3N_4) is often used as a final passivating or protective layer for silicon devices because it is highly impermeable to diffusion of water or sodium from the environment. This CVD process uses two hazardous gases, silane and ammonia. Another final passivating layer that is sometimes deposited is "p-glass." This is a layer of SiO_2 doped with phosphorus to make it more pliant and less likely to crack during the sawing and separation of chips. The source of the phosphorus is phosphine gas. These depositions are two exceptions to the general rule that the use of hazardous gases is not found in metallization processes.

Inspection and Microscopes

Much of the work done in clean rooms is inspection of the wafers through microscopes or, increasingly, by looking at VDTs. Either tends to involve long hours in static postures. Too often, the work stations and tools are not well-fitted to the particular individual. Generalized aches and pains are a frequent complaint as a result of this work. Workers with neck problems seem to have special difficulty. Eye strain and fatigue are also reported with these tools. Complaints associated with microscopic work are among the most frequently reported of all problems in semiconductor clean rooms.

Microscopes pose another interesting hazard, which is the potential for spread of infectious eye disease. Management and health personnel need to be careful that no worker with a conjunctivitis work with microscopes. The most dramatic example of the potential problem occurred in 1987 among microscope users at a microelectronics assembly facility (54). An epidemic of conjunctivitis eventually affected 196 of 350 workers, and caused a 5-day shutdown of the plant. This episode cost the manufacturer more than $600,000. Another epidemic of ocular infections in a class 100 semiconductor facility has been reported (55). The likely pathogen in both epidemics was thought to be an adenovirus. Simple hygiene measures such as handwashing and use of isopropyl alcohol wipes are adequate to prevent transmission of infection. UV lamps are employed in some facilities to sterilize the ocular pieces, but are not entirely effective against viruses. Some workers have solved the problem of dirty oculars by carrying a set of eyepieces in and out of the clean room.

Musculoskeletal Trauma in Semiconductor Manufacture

Aside from the sequelae of inspection work or other tasks requiring prolonged sitting, the semiconductor clean room is remarkably free of musculoskeletal stressors. Heavy physical labor is nearly nonexistent. Repetitive motion tasks, which are often associated with other parts of the microelectronic industry, are absent. OSHA logs from the industry show that sprains and strains are the most frequently reported incidents (56). But, in fact, the actual rate is quite low, and the injuries are largely acute rather than chronic.

Video Display Terminals (VDTs)

As stated above, VDTs are very common in inspection areas. It is not unusual to see a worker using three or four terminals simultaneously at some inspection stations. All the usual ergonomic considerations with VDT use are as important in the clean room as they are elsewhere (57, 58).

One possible outcome of VDT use is especially interesting in the clean room environment. Reports of outbreaks of facial dermatitis among VDT users have been published (59, 60). These rashes usually appear within hours to days after the use of the VDT. Typically, the patient complains of a prickly sensation and eventually develops a facial erythema. It has been proposed that the electrostatic field between the VDT and the operator can cause increased deposition of irritant particles on the face of the user. This is an unproven hypothesis at present, but, given the presence of low concentrations of airborne chemicals and the prevalence of static electricity in semiconductor clean rooms, the hypothesis should be kept in mind. The problem of VDTs and facial dermatitis has usually been solved by raising the ambient humidity, a solution that is not available in the semiconductor environment.

Chip Testing and Separation

Most wafers are put through an automated furnace called a "reflow" oven. This finely controlled warming of the wafers causes the terminal pads, which are usually a lead-tin alloy to soften and reshape into more rounded contours. These are well-ventilated tools that present no hazard to operators except for the use of hydrogen in the ovens to prevent oxidation. The potential for explosion with hydrogen has been discussed previously. Concern has been raised about "reflow" ovens when the substrate is gallium arsenide rather than silicon because of the potential to generate arsine gas.

Testing of the circuits is done by automated tools before the wafers are diced into individual chips. There are almost always a number of defective chips on any wafer.

Diamond wheels are used to dice the wafer into individual integrated circuits. Operators mount wafers onto an adhesive tape that is in a frame. The rest of the procedure is entirely automated including alignment, cutting, cleaning, and selection of good chips. No hazards for operators exist in these operations except for ergonomic stressors of prolonged microscope use. After chip separation, the semiconductor integrated circuit is a finished product. A final visual inspection is done by microscope to identify any gross flaws.

The chips are then packaged individually or into modules by a wide variety of techniques.

Mask Making

Mask making is an integral part of manufacture of semiconductors, and employs many of the same techniques as manufacture of devices. Masks are used in photoexposure tools to determine the patterns of UV light that will be imaged onto a photoresist. Masks are simpler in that only one layer of patterned material is necessary. The process begins with a quartz blank onto which a thin layer of chrome is deposited by an evaporation process. A layer of polymethylmethacylate (PMMA), or a derivative, is deposited over the chrome as a resist. PMMA is a positive, one-component resist. Electron-beam radiation is used to cause scissions of the polymer backbone. The scissioned PMMA polymer is lower molecular weight and more amenable to removal by a ketone solvent developer.

E-beam Tools

An electron beam is used to expose the PMMA resist, which is an example of radiolithography rather than photolithography. Narrow E-beams are used to directly write a pattern of exposure onto the PMMA resist without an intervening mask. The desired pattern is generated from digital data written by circuit engineers and stored electronically. As E-beams cannot exist outside a vacuum, there is no potential for human exposure to this radiation. The beams are focused onto the masks by magnets.

Outgassing of the exposed resist generates a variety of simple hydrocarbons and other organics including CO, CO_2, and aldehydes. These are removed from the vacuum by high speed exhaust so that internal tool surfaces do not become contaminated.

Etching Chrome

Etching of the chrome is done most commonly by wet acid. Newer process requirements are going to force the introduction of more accurate dry etches. One option is plasma etching, which is already widely used in the photolithographic process. Another process called "ion-milling" in which argon is ionized and bombarded against the target is used to etch in some mask-making facilities. No chemical reaction takes place in this process; the argon atoms mechanically sputter against the target.

The plates are cleaned in acid baths and with mechanical brushing. Defects in the chrome pattern on the reticle greater than 1 micron in size can be repaired by depositing additional metal, usually molybdenum. This is accomplished by heating small areas with a laser and then using chemical vapor deposition to deposit metal on the heated areas. Extra metal can be ablated by the same laser tool.

Lasers in Semiconductor Manufacture

Lasers are used widely in semiconductor manufacture. Die separation, trimming, annealing, scribing, mask repair, alignment of wafers, and etching endpoint detection are just a few uses. Visible light lasers offer a hazard, but a well-defined hazard. Rigorous compliance with published American National Standards Institute (ANSI) standards will avoid any injuries. The only fail-safe way to control lasers is to engineer away the possibility of exposure. Experience has shown that a system that depends on personal protection (e.g., goggles) will fail regularly. Incidents of retinal burns are underreported and apparently much more common than generally appreciated (61).

Summary of Semiconductor Manufacturing

The basic processes that need to be understood are crystal growth; machining of wafers; CVD processes including epitaxy; oxidation; photoresist application; exposure; development; wet and dry etching; wet and dry stripping; doping by either diffusion or implantation; and metallization. A reasonable generalization about state-of-the-art facilities is that operators are very seldom exposed to the chemicals they use. Tool maintenance and setup personnel are at greater risk. The specific chemicals and work practices in any particular setting are highly variable, and it is incumbent upon a health professional to take the time to understand each situation before making statements on the presence or absence of health risk. Professionals associated with this industry have invariably commented on the rapid pace of change in tools and materials and on the fact that adequate toxicologic assessment of chemicals almost never proceeds their introduction into manufacturing settings. The pace of change is quickening under the pressure of severe economic competition. As recently as 3–4 years ago a typical schedule of new technology introduction from research through development and pilot lines into full scale manufacturing was typically 6–8 years. The executives who manage microelectronic businesses are now demanding that this schedule be compressed into a 2- or 3-year time-frame. Engineers are not evaluated nor rewarded on their ability to appreciate, understand, new or unusual health hazards. This task is the responsibility of health and safety professionals. Unfortunately, the opportunities for these professionals to be involved before new processes arrive at the manufacturing floor are being diminished by the quickening pace of technologic change.

SELECTED TOXIC HAZARDS

Any large semiconductor facility uses several thousand chemicals. An attempt to review the toxicology of all these materials is doomed to be superficial and of little value. Instead, some issues that are particularly topical in the industry will be discussed:

1. Glycol ethers
2. Gallium arsenide
3. Gases
4. Photoresists
5. Hydrofluoric acid

Glycol Ethers

No health subject is more important to the semiconductor industry than the glycol ethers. These chemicals are used extensively as major components of photoresist solvent systems. A particularly useful characteristic of the glycol ethers is that they are completely miscible with water as well as with most organic solvents, so that they serve as ideal ''coupling'' agents in many solvent systems (62). From a health perspective they have other valuable features. They are nonflammable, noncarcinogenic, and nonmutagenic.

The current OSHA standards were adopted from ACGIH in 1971 and are based on long-recognized effects of glycol ethers upon the kidney, liver, hematopoietic system, and acute central nervous system (CNS) toxicity. Reproductive and developmental hazards that became evident in subsequent animal tests beginning with a report by Nagano in 1979 (63) were not known when the OSHA limits were established.

It is likely that the current OSHA exposure standards will be lowered substantially. Table 43.2 lists current and recommended standards. These inevitable regulatory changes will present a very difficult challenge to the semiconductor industry.

Regulatory History

The following discussion will trace the history of regulatory thinking about the glycol ethers as well as the state of knowledge about their toxicology. Reproductive and developmental effects will be the focus as these outcomes are driving current regulatory thinking.

On May 2, 1983, NIOSH published a Current Intelligence Bulletin on the glycol ethers (64). At that time, NIOSH did not recommend a specific exposure standard. Rather, they stated that 2-methoxyethanol and 2-ethoxyethanol had the potential to cause reproductive effects in male and female workers, and that exposure should be limited as much as possible. NIOSH recommended that standards be reassessed by OSHA.

On January 24, 1984, the EPA published an Advance Notice of Proposed Rulemaking (ANPR) stating its intent to establish stricter standards for the glycol ethers. Recently completed animal studies had been brought to the EPA's attention. On May 20, 1986, the EPA in accordance with the Toxic Substances Control Act referred the responsibility of determining an appropriate standard to OSHA. In the interim the EPA published a risk assessment on the glycol ethers. Their recommended exposure limits are shown in Table 43.2.

ACGIH lowered its TLVs for the four chemicals in 1985, based on animal studies that demonstrated both reproductive and developmental toxicity. Those TLVs have remained unchanged and are shown in Table 43.2. On April 2, 1987, OSHA published an advanced notification to establish health and safety standards for 2-methoxyethanol (2-ME), 2-ethoxyethanol (2-EE), and their respective acetates, 2-methoxyethanol acetate (2-MEA) and 2-ethoxyethanol acetate (2-EEA) (65). A draft of NIOSH's Criteria Document on the Glycol Ethers became available in July 1989. NIOSH proposed exposure limits of 0.1 ppm for 2-ME and 2-MEA, and 0.5 ppm for 2-EE and 2-EEA. These are very close to the EPA recommendations of 1984 (Table 43.2). The NIOSH document also strongly encouraged implementation of biologic monitoring for the metabolites of glycol ethers in recognition of the large contribution of skin absorption.

Animal testing manifested as fetal death or resorptions were observed at inhalation levels as low as 10 ppm in rabbits and 50 ppm in rats (66). The no observed effect level (NOEL) for fetal resorption in these studies was 3 ppm in rabbits and 10 ppm in rats. Other fetal effects such as skeletal and soft tissue lesions were observed at higher levels of exposure.

Testicular damage was observed in rats and rabbits after inhalation exposures of 2-ME (67). The NOEL was 30 ppm. In the rat, inhalation exposures produced similar testicular damage with a NOEL of 100 ppm.

In rabbits, fetal skeletal abnormalities were observed in inhalation studies at 175 ppm (68). Inhalation studies with 2-EE

Table 43.2. Recommended Exposure Standards for Glycol Ethers (in PPM)[a]

Name	Current OSHA Pel (1991)	Current ACGIH TLV (1990-91)	EPA Recommen (1984)	NIOSH Crit Doc (1989)
Methoxyethanol (CH3-O-CH2-CH2-OH)	25	5	0.03	0.1
2-Methoxyethanol acetate (CH3-O-CH2-CH2-COOH)	25	5	0.03	0.1
2-Ethoxyethanol (CH3-CH2-O-CH2-CH2-OH)	200	5	0.5	0.5
2-Ethoxyethanol acetate (CH3-CH2-O-CH2-CH2-COOH)	100	5	0.5	0.5

[a]All standards include a "skin" notation.

in rats also produced skeletal defects as well as decreased birth weight (69). The NOEL in both studies was 50 ppm. 2-EE has been shown to produce similar fetal toxicity in dermal studies (70). Maternal or paternal exposures to 2-EE both result in neurotoxic effects in offspring manifested as impaired neuro-muscular ability (71).

A 2-EEA inhalation study used New Zealand White rabbits and Fischer 344 rats exposed to vapor on gestational days 6 through 18 at concentrations of 0, 50, 100, 200, and 300 ppm for 6 hr/day. Both species showed developmental toxicity and teratogenicity at levels of 100–300 ppm. At 50 ppm both species were free of effect (72). Testicular damage was observed in rabbits after exposure of 2-EE with a NOEL of 100 ppm (73).

Many other bioassays have been reported, but the above are representative of the findings. A complete catalogue of studies can be found in the NIOSH Criteria Document (74). The number of studies and consistency of results is highly persuasive.

EPIDEMIOLOGIC EVIDENCE

The epidemiologic data available on glycol ethers are both meager and poorly controlled. Three studies pertain to male reproduction. A study of men exposed to 2-EE demonstrated a decrease in average sperm count when compared with control subjects. The airborne levels of 2-EE were measured as non-detectable up to 33.8 ppm (75). A study in a glycol ether production facility found decreased testicular size in exposed men, but no decrease in sperm counts or other sperm abnormalities (76).

A study of shipyard painters exposed to 2-ME at a mean concentration of 2.6 mg/m^3 (1.2 ppm) and 2-EE at a mean concentration of 9.9 mg/m^3 (2.6 ppm) had an increased prevalence of oligospermia and azospermia (77). The results, when controlled for smoking, also demonstrated an increased odds ratio for lower sperm count per ejaculation. It is important to note that these exposure levels are well within current OSHA and ACGIH standards. Biologic monitoring for metabolites of 2-ME and 2-EE was positive.

Another study of interest, though not specific to glycol ethers, was published in 1988 (78). This case-control study in a semiconductor clean room facility where glycol ethers are a frequent air contaminant demonstrated a doubling of the odds ratio for spontaneous abortion among clean room-exposed women. The scientific quality of the study is not adequate to allow definitive statements about work in clean rooms, but it presents the hy-

pothesis that clean room work could be associated with adverse reproductive outcomes.

METABOLISM OF ETHYLENE GLYCOL ETHERS

Three general concepts in glycol ether toxicology emerge from pharmacokinetic data (62, 79, 80). The first is the biologic activation of ethylene glycol ethers by liver-dependent alcohol dehydrogenase (ADH) to an alkoxyacetic acid metabolite which is the actual toxin.

Glycol ethers with a secondary alcohol group such as the propylene glycol ethers do not serve as substrates for ADH. Instead, they are metabolized by cytochrome P-450-dependent O-demethylation, and subsequently biotransformed to carbon dioxide. No toxic metabolite is formed.

The second concept is that a mole of a glycol ether is toxicologically equivalent to a mole of its acetate. The glycol ether acetates are rapidly converted to the corresponding glycol ethers by esterases present in the mucosa, liver, kidney, lungs, and blood. Subsequent biotransformation to an alkoxyacetic acid occurs as in Fig. 43.5.

The third important concept is that there is an inverse relationship between the length of the substituted alkyl group and reproductive toxicity. 2-ME is more toxic than 2-EE which is in turn more toxic than 2-butoxyethanol.

MECHANISM OF TOXICITY

The mechanism by which glycol ethers cause reproductive toxicity is not known. Recent studies at CIIT (Chemical Industry Institute of Toxicology) suggest that interference with DNA or RNA synthesis may be involved (81, 82). The current hypothesis is that alkoxyacetic acids interfere with the availability of one-carbon units for incorporation into purine and pyrimidine bases, thereby affecting the formation of nucleic acids. At a time of rapid cellular proliferation such as embryogenesis, a limitation in the availability of these precursors could be highly damaging.

SKIN ABSORPTION

In vitro studies using the skin of beagle dogs demonstrated that 2-EEA is absorbed at a rate of 2.3 mg/cm^2/hr (83). In vitro studies of isolated human skin show absorption rates of 2.8 mg/cm^2/hr for 2-ME and 0.9 mg/cm^2/hr for 2-EE (84). The area of a human hand is approximately 650 cm^2. Therefore, immersion of a hand in 2-ME could result in the absorption of

400 milligrams in 15 minutes. This is equivalent to exposure to 10 ppm in the air for 8 hours. Just 10 seconds of hand immersion would cause absorption of an amount of 2-ME equivalent to 8 hours of exposure at the draft NIOSH recommended exposure level of 0.1 ppm.

BIOLOGIC MONITORING

Since the glycol ethers are rapidly absorbed through the skin, environmental sampling of airborne concentrations is an unsatisfactory assessment of total exposure. Fortunately, analytical techniques exist to determine the levels of alkoxyacetic acid metabolites of 2-ME and 2-EE in the urine (85, 86).

Groeseneken has performed experiments on human volunteers to determine the rate of pulmonary absorption of 2-EE and subsequent excretion of metabolite (87). A steady state was reached almost immediately, and respiratory elimination of unmetabolized 2-EE was only 0.4% of uptake. Ethoxyacetic acid was observed in the urine during exposure and up to 42 hours after exposure. The half-life of absorbed 2-EE in this experiment was 10–12 hours. Ony 23% of inhaled 2-EE is recovered as ethoxyacetic acid. Conjugation of ethoxyacetic acid to glycerine is known to occur in animals, and is assumed to be the reason for this observation in humans. It is possible that a portion of absorbed 2-EE is metabolized to CO_2 and expired. The Groeseneken studies showed that even at exposure levels as low as 10 mg/m³ of air for 4 hours, the metabolite is easily detectable 18 hours after exposure. Since the metabolite is not normally present in human urine, this form of biologic monitoring could serve as a qualitative indicator of exposure.

A field application of this technology studied five women exposed to a combined concentration of 4 ppm of 2-EE and 2-EEA in a silk-screening process (88). All were wearing gloves. The urinary excretion of EEA showed a clear increase over the week, and EEA was still detectable 12 days after exposure ceased. The half-life of EEA excretions was estimated to be 1–2 days. A correlation coefficient of 0.92 was found between average exposure over the week and the EEA excretion at the end of the week.

It is premature to state that a quantitative correlation can be made between the amounts of alkoxyacetic acids found in the urine and absorption of glycol ethers. Most trials have shown great intraindividual variability between the amount of alkoxyacetic acids excreted given the same absorption. The variation was as much as 10-fold in one study (89). Among factors that have been demonstrated to affect the excretion of the toxic metabolite of a glycol ether are metabolic induction by xenobiotics, metabolic inhibition by xenobiotics, and dose-dependent pharmacokinetics. This deficiency in the current data should not discourage the use of biologic monitoring. Although the amount of metabolite in the urine may not be linearly correlated to the absorbed dose of glycol ether, it is likely to be closely correlated to the concentration of toxic metabolite being presented to target organs. Furthermore, as discussed above, the evolving ideas on mechanism of action of the alkoxyacetic acids do not lend themselves to the establishment of a totally safe threshold of exposure.

ENVIRONMENTAL EXPOSURE DATA

There are few published reports of sampling data for glycol ether exposure within the semiconductor industry. The EPA contracted a report on glycol ether exposure data in a variety of industries (65). The data showed that most large industries had exposures below the 0.03 ppm level for 2-ME and below 1 ppm for 2-EE. The exceptions were the trade industries involved in surface coating applications and the use of inks. The former category includes the microelectronics industry. It is important to remember that these data address only exposure via inhalation, and that any skin absorption is additional.

The Semiconductor Industry Association conducted an industry-wide survey of industrial hygiene air sampling data during 1984–85 to describe typical levels of exposure to the ethylene glycol ethers. A total of 227 samples was provided by seven member companies. In 1982, NIOSH had done similar sampling in the semiconductor industry and generated 92 data points. The data from these two studies were published together in 1988 (35). The mean concentration in air of personal samples of 2-EE was 0.55 ppm, just slightly higher than the NIOSH draft REL of 0.5 ppm. A total of 24 area samples was collected, and the arithmetic mean was 0.99 ppm.

The results for 2-EEA were lower with a mean of 0.05 ppm, though the mean of shortterm samples (15 minutes or less) was 2.82 ppm. Area samples were also low at 0.05 ppm.

QUALITATIVE RISK ASSESSMENTS OF GLYCOL ETHERS

The EPA risk assessment of 1984 calculated the margins of safety—defined as the NOEL in the most sensitive species divided by the estimated human exposure level. The NOELs for testicular toxicity were 30 ppm for 2-ME and 100 ppm for 2-EE. For developmental toxicity, the NOELs were 3 ppm for 2-ME and 50 ppm for 2-EE. The NOEL for each acetate was assumed to be the same as its parent compound.

An exposure level with a 100-fold margin of safety is considered unlikely to produce adverse effects in humans. This safety factor is often explained as 10-fold for differences between humans and test species and another 10-fold for protection of hypersusceptible subgroups in the human population. The EPA estimated that between 206,000 and 350,000 workers are exposed to the four ethylene glycol ethers at levels exceeding the 100-fold margin of safety.

The EPA recommended adoption of acceptable exposure levels of 0.03 ppm for 2-ME and 2-MEA and 0.5 ppm for 2-EE and 2-EEA.

Another qualitative risk assessment was published in 1988 (35). This work was done under contract to the Semiconductor Industry Association (SIA). The author chose to use a safety factor of 10 rather than the more traditionally accepted factor of 100. Given the consistency of glycol ether bioassay results among different species, this may be a reasonable decision. The author also chose to reject the Dow Chemical study of 1982 which had demonstrated a NOEL of 3 for developmental effects in rabbits (66). No other study has shown a NOEL this low. The result of these two choices was to conclude that the current ACGIH TLVs of 5 ppm offer adequate margins of safety for reproductive and developmental effects.

QUANTITATIVE RISK ASSESSMENT OF GLYCOL ETHERS

Qualitative risk assessment using a "safety factors" or "uncertainty factors" approach is typical of risk assessment in the area of reproductive toxicology. Quantitative risk assessment, common in the area of carcinogenesis, has rarely been attempted with reproductive or developmental hazards. The EPA has stated that there are not presently any theoretical grounds for adopting mathematical models in these areas (13).

Personnel at OSHA are likewise skeptical that it is possible to do a valid quantitative risk assessment in the areas of reproductive and developmental toxicology. OSHA has, nonetheless, contracted for two separate quantitative risk assessments of the hazards of glycol ether exposure. The practical reason that OSHA has done this is in anticipation of legal challenges to their proposed rule. In the 1980 benzene case the court ruled that OSHA has to make "any reasonable effort" at quantification of risks (90). Other more scientific reasons to seek quantitative models of dose-response are that the reliance on a NOEL places substantial burden on the power of a study to detect low dose effects. Furthermore, a safety factors approach is unable to incorporate any of the pharmacokinetic data that are available on the glycol ethers.

One of the OSHA-contracted quantitative risk assessments on glycol ether reproductive and developmental toxicity has been submitted in the form of three documents: a model of human pharmacokinetics of glycol ethers; a model of increased infertility with male exposure; and a model of developmental toxicity in the fetus with female exposure (62, 91, 92).

In the male study, models were developed to estimate the increase in numbers of infertile couples caused by exposure of men to 2-ME and 2-EE. Exposure data and a "functional intermediate parameter" were based on the Yale-NIOSH study of shipyard painters (77). The "functional intemediate parameter" is a variable assumed to have a strong causal influence on biologic function. The variable used is sperm count. Decreases in sperm count have previously been correlated with increased numbers of couples experiencing delay in achieving pregnancy (93). The results of the model indicate that 1 in 100 additional couples would suffer infertility at 3.3 ppm of 2-EE exposure of 0.76 ppm of 2-ME. Achieving a more stringent goal of limiting excess incidence of infertility to 1 in 400 couples would require that exposures not exceed 0.8 ppm of 2-EE or 0.19 ppm of 2-ME.

The quantitative analysis of developmental effects in women provides models for a variety of outcomes. All of these models extrapolate significant adverse effects at levels of exposure that are much lower than current standards. For example, a 10^{-6} increased frequency of infant mortality is predicted at 0.0085 ppm of 2-ME. For a 10^{-6} increase in miscarriages the best estimate is exposure at 0.067 ppm of 2-ME or 0.53 ppm of 2-EE. Estimates for the same outcome using a more pessimistic assumption about the degree of interindividual variability in susceptibility of the human population yields results of 0.00026 ppm for 2-ME and 0.00056 ppm for 2-EE.

COSTS OF LOWERING GLYCOL ETHER EXPOSURE STANDARDS

OSHA's preliminary evaluation indicated that exposures to glycol ethers could be controlled by a combination of engineering controls, work practices, and personal protective equipment (65). In actuality, the cost of trying to control these exposures to the EPA or NIOSH suggested levels is quite prohibitive and will certainly force substitution of other materials for the glycol ethers in many applications. Indus-

trial Economics Incorporated prepared a draft regulatory impact analysis for EPA (65). They estimated that the cost of instituting all necessary engineering controls and use of personal protective equipment to attain a 0.1 or 0.5 ppm exposure level would be $86.6 million and $42.8 million, respectively. Annual operating costs were more significant—estimated to be about $1.25 billion for either level. EPA assumed that many firms would opt for substitution and therefore estimated the annual costs to industry would be lower at $83 million. Substitution is the route that most industries will be forced to take. The question in the semiconductor industry is whether substitutions can be made without harming the performance of photoresists.

SUBSTITUTES FOR GLYCOL ETHERS IN PHOTORESISTS

Manufacturers and users of photoresists have undertaken efforts to eliminate ethylene glycols from their products and processes. Four commonly explored substitutes are propylene glycol monomethyl ether acetate (PM acetate), ethyl-3-ethoxyproponate, ethyl lactate, and 4-butyrolactone (80). The acute toxicity of the possible substitutes as established by LD_{50} and LC_{50} values is apparently low (80). Furthermore, they seem to be free of chronic toxicity, including reproductive and developmental effects, except at very high exposure levels. As yet unclear is whether they can function as effectively as ethylene glycol ethers in photoresist formulations.

Another solvent that has quickly gained wide use in photoresists is diethylene glycol dimethyl ether, which is commonly known as "diglyme." The industry's use for this material may not be based on a clear understanding of the toxicology of this chemical. Chemists and health professionals stated as early as 1981 that the likely first step in the metabolism of this chemical would be hydrolysis of the ether bond, yielding at least one molecule of 2-ME. Metabolism studies in both rats and mice have demonstrated that diglyme is, as was suspected, biotransformed in part to yield 2-ME and ultimately the toxic metabolite, 2-MAA (94). (Fig. 43.6)

Bioassays demonstrate that all the adverse effects seen with 2-ME occur at similar exposure levels of diglyme (95–98). No exposure standards exist for this chemical; in addition the reproductive toxicity has not been investigated. Diglyme has been substituted widely for 2-ME not only in semiconductor manufacture, but also in other microelectronic uses.

SUMMARY OF THE RISK OF GLYCOL ETHERS

Available animal data on the toxicity of the glycol ethers are unusually consistent and compelling. One would have to be entirely skeptical of the applicability of animal tests to the human species in order to disregard the experimental data. Furthermore, the rapidly evolving data on the possible genotoxic mechanism of the effect of alkoxyacetic acids on nucleic acid formation are difficult to dismiss.

The experimental outcomes—reproductive problems and altered fetal development—are not only very serious, but highly prevalent in our society. Determining the exact contribution of the glycol ethers to these health problems is probably beyond the power of epidemiology. The ability to unequivocably demonstrate the lack of adverse reproductive and developmental hazards from glycol ethers is unrealistic.

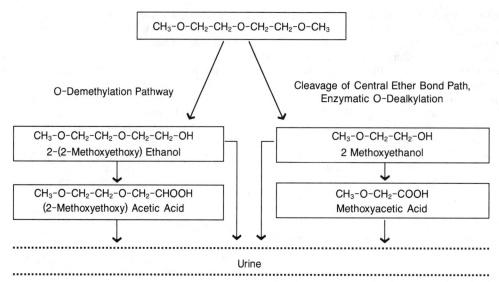

Figure 43.6.   Metabolism of diethylene glycol dimethyl ether.

ADDITIONAL WORKER PROTECTION

There are several areas in which individual employers will have to go beyond the probable OSHA standard in order to fully protect workers from glycol ethers. At present, it seems that the standard will not include biologic monitoring requirements, though the NIOSH Criteria Document on glycol ethers strongly advises that these surveillance tools be adopted. OSHA has stated that they are afraid that employers will ignore engineering controls, environmental monitoring, and personal protection if biologic monitoring results are found acceptable. This philosophy seems to misplace the emphasis on administrative compliance rather than effective prevention. Health professionals should aggressively implement these informative means of monitoring total absorption.

The other weakness of the standard as presently configured is that it will address only the four common ethylene glycol ethers (2-ME, 2-MEA, 2-EEE, and 2-EEA). Other equally toxic glycol ethers may be substituted. The best example, as discussed above, is diglyme (diethylene glycol dimethyl ether), which has already gained widespread use. Many other glycol ethers are used by semiconductor manufacturers, and it is the responsibility of a health professional to learn as much as possible about each of these chemicals encountered in the workplace. The absence of a specific standard is not a certificate of safety.

Gallium Arsenide

In October 1987, NIOSH issued an alert about potential health hazards of gallium arsenide (GaAs) (99). It is important to understand that this alert is based entirely on the known adverse health effects of exposure to inorganic arsenic.

The acute effects of exposure to inorganic arsenic are well characterized (47, 100). Realistically, exposures in the semiconductor industry are very unlikely to be sufficient to cause acute symptoms. Concern about exposure in semiconductor manufacturing is driven by the chronic health effects—primarily cancer, and to a lesser degree, concern about possible effects upon the fetus. Documented chronic health effects in occupationally exposed populations include lung cancer, per-

foration of the nasal septum, laryngitis, pharyngitis, bronchitis, peripheral neuropathy, and encephalopathy. Cutaneous manifestations have been seen in individuals exposed to arsenic in drinking water and drugs, but not in occupationally exposed groups. These clinical findings have included hyperkeratosis of the palms and skin cancer. The possibility of fetal toxicity in humans is not widely discussed, but some animal studies suggest a teratogenic effect (101, 102).

IN VIVO DISSOCIATION OF GaAs

A number of experiments have demonstrated that GaAs dissociates in the lung or gut of mammals to gallium and arsenic with the latter behaving metabolically as any other inorganic arsenic species (103–105). NIOSH has recommended that GaAs be handled in accordance with the 1975 NIOSH recommendation for inorganic arsenic (106). The NIOSH recommendation is that GaAs be controlled to not exceed 2 $\mu g/m^3$ of air as a 15-minute ceiling. OSHA has a less restrictive standard for inorganic arsenic that includes a PEL (TWA-8) of 10 $\mu g/m^3$ of air (107).

THE IMPORTANCE OF BIOLOGIC MONITORING FOR INORGANIC ARSENIC

Dependence on environmental sampling data alone to ensure worker safety can be misleading. Fortunately, biologic monitoring of both total and inorganic arsenic excretion is available to supplement the usual air sampling and wipe samples. Some understanding of the metabolism of arsenic is necessary in order to properly interpret these tests.

Arsenic from dietary sources (primarily seafood) is in the form of either arsenobetaine, arsenocholine, or trimethylarsenic acid. These forms of arsenic are referred to as ''organic'' arsenic and are not associated with any adverse health outcomes.

Exposure to ''inorganic'' arsenic occurs in a variety of environmental and industrial settings. Natural drinking water sources, anthropogenic environmental contamination from minewastes, and seaweed are examples. The latter poses a problem when monitoring Japanese workers, but is generally not a consideration for American workers (108). Inorganic arsenic can be inhaled or ingested in many possible forms. It is excreted in one of three forms—arsenic cations, monomethylarsenic acid or dimethylarsenic acid. Only inorganic arsenic can cause the well-documented acute and chronic adverse health effects of arsenic.

Measurement of total arsenic in urine measures both the organic and inorganic forms. This test is widely available and is what most surveillance programs rely on for evidence of absorption. Workers are generally asked to refrain from seafood for 5 days prior to giving the urine sample. Health practitioners faced with a high result invariably repeat the test after delivering more adamant dietary instructions to the worker. The repeat test is usually normal, and there is a tendency to pursue the problem no further. The abnormal result is written off to "diet," and any investigation of possible workplace exposure may miss subtle exposure. The reality is that a normal repeat urine does not mean that the initial high number was not caused by a workplace exposure. Potentially correctable engineering problems or breaches in safe work practices tend to be overlooked.

There is a solution to this dilemma. It is possible to measure the inorganic component of the total arsenic excreted in urine (109, 110). Until late 1989, this test (often termed "fractionation" or "speciation" of arsenic) was not commercially available, though some companies working with arsenic have been doing the test internally. Measuring inorganic arsenic species in urine is now available from at least one competent commercial laboratory.

Two different strategies for testing urines for arsenic are reasonable. The first is to split spot urine samples and test initially for total arsenic. If the total arsenic exceeds 50 μg/l, the split can be tested for determination of the inorganic arsenic species. Another approach is to simply test for the inorganic arsenic species. Small amounts of inorganic arsenic are absorbed from seafood. For this reason, even if total arsenic is not being determined, it is important to continue to emphasize the usual dietary restrictions prior to routine screening.

Any urine inorganic arsenic levels in excess of 25 μg/l should be pursued very aggressively to find sources of exposure.

One other comment on biologic monitoring for arsenic is warranted. Although some is accumulated in the body—primarily hair, skin, nails, and lungs—most is excreted into the urine quite rapidly (47, 111). Annual samples donated on arbitrary dates such as birthdays are not likely to detect intermittent absorption. Attempts should be made to collect samples soon after potential exposures. Workers should be encouraged to present for monitoring whenever they suspect an exposure may have occurred.

OTHER MEDICAL SURVEILLANCE FOR ARSENIC

In addition to biologic monitoring for inorganic arsenic absorption, few other medical surveillance measures are productive. A good history to try to elicit any symptoms of arsenic exposure or any concerns about the workplace is certainly useful. A good neurologic exam is warranted, as well as a thorough skin examination. The rest of the typical physical exam is unlikely to be worthwhile. No laboratory work except the biologic monitoring discussed above is specific enough to be of value. Of course, if environmental monitoring results exceed the OSHA action level, then a company is legally obligated to conform to the arsenic standard, which unfortunately includes a number of insensitive and nonspecific screening tests (107).

GALLIUM OXIDE TOXICITY

Because experiments to date have shown that gallium is not absorbed from either the lung or the gut, there has been little concern about the systemic effects of gallium. A recent paper raises concerns about local pulmonary toxicity (112). Significant pulmonary pathology in rats was caused by inhalation of gallium oxide particles. The exposure was 4 weeks in duration, at which time alveolar proteinosis was seen. By 6–12 months post exposure, the lesions progressed to fibrosis. The authors stated that the cytotoxic, inflammatory, and fibrotic responses were equal to or greater than that observed with quartz particles. In the future, exposure to gallium may be regulated as more than a nuisance dust. In the meantime, employers should take prudent steps to eliminate inhalation of gallium or its compounds.

GASES

Every semiconductor manufacturer must develop a strategy for the safe handling of gases. These chemicals are not always well understood by the people who work with them, and they possess a potential for catastrophe that is not associated with hazardous solids and liquids. Furthermore, there are four worrisome trends in the use of gases in semiconductor manufacture (46).

1. The total volume of gas usage is increasing.
2. The volume of individual cylinders in increasing.
3. Gases are being used in higher concentrations.
4. More types of gases are being used.

The first step in safe gas handling is to identify every gas used and the potential of each to cause injury or illness. This may be the most important step in the entire sequence of controls. With a clear understanding of the gases and their inherent hazards, it is possible to decide which gases can be brought into work areas by cylinder, which require a more expensive system of gas lines, and which demand substitution as the only rational control.

The International Congress of Building Officials has adopted standards to address the peculiar risks of semiconductor manufacture and its associated chemical storage ("Article 51") (39). Implementation of these standards is far from universal.

SILANE

Silane gas is used extensively in semiconductor manufacture for the deposition of thin dielectric films. Silane presents a significant health hazard because of its potential to detonate. Until the early 1980s the conventional wisdom was that silane, while pyrophoric, could not explode. A series of experiments established that under certain conditions, generally high volume leaks into stagnant air, silane could accumulate and subsequently detonate (113). Manufacturers of monitoring equipment report that 15–20 ppm leaks of silane in semiconductor fabrication areas and around gas cabinets are found routinely (42). One of the major problems of handling silane is that it does not always immediately ignite upon contact with air. Small leaks can produce sizable quantities of silane-air mixtures which have subsequently detonated (114).

As an explosive, 1 pound of silane (0.45 kilograms) is equivalent to 6 pounds (2.7 kilograms) of TNT. A typical 9- by 52-inch (23-132 centimeters) cylinder of silane contains 5000 grams or just over 14 pounds of silane (6.4 kilograms), which is equivalent to 84 pounds (38.2 kilograms) of TNT. An unfortunate demonstration of silane's explosive potential occurred in March 1988. A single cylinder of silane that had been contaminated with nitrous oxide exploded and killed three people. The explosion occurred at an analytical laboratory after the cylinder had been removed from a semiconductor facility because of the contamination problem.

No catastrophic detonations of silane have been reported in the semiconductor industry to date, although in 1988 a silane gas leak at a semiconductor facility in California ignited and caused four injuries and a plant evacuation.

Process demands are increasing both the volumes and concentrations of silane. In the past, a manufacturer could use 2% silane, but today 100% concentrations are increasingly found in production settings. Most manufacturers are responding to this problem by either placing silane cylinders far from populated areas or building explosion-proof concrete bunkers around the cylinders.

ACGIH has a rather curious TLV for silane of 5 ppm (115). This level was adopted in 1983 and replaced a TLV of 0.5 ppm that had been in effect since 1974. The rationale for either concentration is unclear, but is probably a response to the inhalation toxicity of other metallic hydrides. Acute toxicity testing in laboratory animals has shown no toxicity in rats up to 1400 ppm for 6 hours (115). Four-hour inhalation studies established the LC_{50} in rats and mice, respectively, at 4000 and 9600 ppm (116). In any case, the threat of silane is not pulmonary or systemic toxicity via inhalation, but rather the danger of detonation.

Dichlorosilane and trichlorosilane are also used extensively in the semiconductor industry and pose risks similar to silane (117).

ARSINE

At 250 ppm, arsine gas (AsH_3) is instantly lethal to humans. The mechanism of this sudden death is probably a respiratory arrest caused by CNS interruption. At lower concentrations of exposure, the pathologic lesion is hemolysis leading to a severe anemia and hypoxemia. Renal failure also occurs either from direct nephrotoxicty of arsine or from the obstruction of tubules with hemoglobin. Hydration, dialysis, and general support are the mainstays of therapy. Exchange transfusion is always mentioned as a form of treatment for severe hemolysis, but this has probably never been accomplished. Few hospital or medical centers in the United States currently are prepared with an adequate protocol and resources to treat a massive arsine intoxication. The units of blood required to accomplish exchange transfusion would be large and are generally not available. There should be no comforting illusions about the efficacy of health care practitioners in the event of a catastrophic leak of arsine gas. Obviously, an antidote is needed for this toxin.

How likely is such an event in the semiconductor industry? Second-generation ion implanters in some facilities are now using cylinders that contain 40–50 liters of arsine (about two cubic feet). Larger cylinders are found in gas cabinets contiguous to epitaxial areas. To date, arsine has not caused a death in the semiconductor industry, though in 1988 a graduate student who was changing an arsine cylinder in a laboratory on an ion implantation tool was killed by a gas leak (personal communication). Multiple deaths have been caused by arsine in other industries.

Many current processes demand 100% arsine concentrations. A leak of as little as two cubic feet (0.056 cubic meters) of arsine gas could fill a room volume of 8000 cubic feet (224 cubic meters) with gas at the immediately lethal concentration of 250 ppm. A room of 330,000 cubic feet (9240 cubic meters) would be necessary to bring the concentration down to the OSHA IDLH level of 6 ppm. Many facilities have sophisticated gas delivery systems that have been developed to avoid bringing cylinders into work areas. Monitoring systems to detect leakages are also highly sophisticated in most facilities.

SUBSTITUTION FOR ARSINE

The only wholly acceptable solution to the arsine problem is to substitute other sources of arsenic. Several semiconductor manufacturers have been able to completely eliminate arsine from their processes. This is done by using elemental arsenic in implantation tools and alkylated arsine in epitaxy. Elemental arsenic is a solid and is relatively easy to work with safely under a ventilation hood or in a glove box. Alkylated arsines are liquids, so that the potential for catastrophe is minimal. They are also less toxic than the hydride.

GAS DELIVERY SYSTEMS FOR HIGHLY TOXIC GASES

State-of-the-art gas handling systems for highly toxic gases such as arsine isolate all cylinders in remote gas rooms. The gas is delivered to the processing area by coaxial (double-walled) lines. The inside or delivery line containing toxic gas is pressurized to 20–30 psi (1.4–2.0 ATM) while the annular or outside line is pressurized to approximately 100 psi (6.8 ATM) with nitrogen. In the event of a defect in the delivery line, the leak will be inward from the annular space. The pressure in that space is monitored, and a pressure drop of 10% causes a regulator to shut off the source of the toxic gas as well as alarming operators of the gas system.

Unfortunately, gas is not currently piped into ion implanters. These tools use a very high voltage chamber (approximately 100,000 volts). It is, therefore, not possible to safely connect to metal gas lines. Cylinders of gas (typically arsine, phosphine, or diborane) are placed into the tool. The industry is experimenting with sections of glass ceramic delivery line to hopefully allow gas to be delivered from outside lines.

Some highly corrosive etching gases have very low vapor pressure, and therefore must be brought to the tool in cylinders. An example is tungsten hexafluoride, which has a vapor pressure of only 2–3 psi. (0.1–0.2 ATM).

"SAFE" GASES

The highly toxic gases such as arsine or explosive gases such as silane receive the most focus in the semiconductor industry. Inert gases such as argon and nitrogen receive less attention, though these "safe" gases are used in tremendous quantities. Unlike either silane or arsine, inert gases have caused deaths in the industry.

Four cases of oxygen-deficient syncope in 1 year at a single semiconductor facility illustrates the ever-present danger of these gases (personal communication). In two of the cases, workers succumbed after entering rooms with wafer storage cabinets. These cabinets maintain an internal atmosphere of nitrogen at slight positive pressure to protect product from ingress of particles. If a cabinet leaks slightly and is not maintaining positive pressure, the temporary solution is to turn up the flow of gas. This increases flow of nitrogen into the room, and at some point in a small room it will replace enough of the oxygen to present an asphyxiation hazard.

The other two cases occurred in a partially enclosed area at the end of an aisle in a clean room (personal communication). Process engineers introduced a nitrogen drying step to the end of a wet station without installing an exhaust for the nitrogen. It was assumed that the air changes and dilution in the clean room would be adequate to protect workers. The problem was identified when the second of two workers experienced syncope at the tool. The first episode had initially been attributed to the fact that the worker was dieting to lose weight.

In each of these four cases, the worker was a healthy individual, and no permanent harm was suffered. The outcomes might have been disastrous in an individual with coronary artery disease or compromised pulmonary function.

Two lessons may be learned from these incidents. No gas is so safe that engineers can simply depend on environmental dilution to protect workers. The second is that any case of syncope in an industry where gases or vapors are present needs a thorough workplace investigation by health professionals.

Photoresists

There is no reported incident of harm from photoresists as they are used in semiconductor manufacturing. The following discussion is to serve the purpose of introducing health professionals to some areas of reasonable concern. Clearly, the greatest concern about photoresists has been the potential for reproductive and developmental toxicity because of the high content of glycol ether solvents.

CHEMISTRY OF PHOTORESISTS

Photoresists are chemical mixtures which can be altered by exposure to electromagnetic energy such as ultraviolet radiation, electron beams, or x-rays. The radiation is passed through a mask exposing only a desired pattern on the surface of a layer of photoresist. If the photoresist is a "negative" photoresist, the area exposed to light will be hardened and become less soluble. If a "positive" photoresist is used, the exposed area will become weakened and is more easily removed by a solvent during development. The pattern of photoresist left behind after development allows selective exposure of the underlying material to other processes such as etching or ion implantation.

NEGATIVE PHOTORESISTS

Most negative resists become insoluble through some type of radiation induced cross-linking. The first resist used to fabricate solid state devices was a negative resist based on cyclized 1,4-poly(cis-isoprene) that becomes cross-linked upon exposure. Typically, the cyclized rubber matrix was sensitized with a bis(aryl azide) photosensitive cross-linking agent. The use of a negative photoresist in photolithography is severely limited by the fact that the cyclized rubber polymers require organic solvent developers that cause image distortion due to swelling of the photoresist. It is unlikely that a health professional will encounter negative resists in semiconductor manufacture, though they are used to fabricate larger scale components in the electronics industry.

POSITIVE PHOTORESISTS

The mechanism of positive resist action involves either chain-scission or a polarity change in the polymer. Photoresists based on the latter mechanism are the most widely used for semiconductor manufacture because they possess high resolution and excellent resistance to dry etching processes. DQN resists, which will be discussed later, are typically polarity change positive resists.

CHAIN SCISSION RESISTS

The classic "positive" chain-scission resist is poly(methyl methacrylate) (PMMA). It is a widely used electron beam photoresist in some steps of semiconductor manufacture and in mask manufacturing. The acrylic monomer (methyl methacrylate) is a potent sensitizer and causes paresthesias of the fingertips. Sensitization to MMA has occurred in medical professionals who use it to cement a variety of prostheses. No problems have been observed with the use of PMMA in semiconductor manufacturing, probably due to an absence of contamination with the monomer and more easily controlled work practices. The typical developer for PMMA is a combination of methyl isobutyl ketone (MIBK) and isopropyl alcohol (IPA). A great number of substituted methacrylates have been experimented with to try to improve the sensitivity of PMMAs to radiation and its resistance to dry etching.

Another class of positive chain-scission resists is the poly(olefin sulfones). The polymers are alternating copolymers of an olefin and sulfur dioxide. The weak C-S bond is cleaved upon irradiation. These types of resists are typically used in mask making.

DQN PHOTORESISTS

Diazonaphthoquinone-novolak (DQN) resists are typical of the polarity change positive resists. They operate via a dissolution-inhibition mechanism. The major component is an alkali-soluble resin (novolak) that is rendered insoluble in aqueous alkaline solutions through incorporation of a hydrophobic material (a diazonaphthoquinone). Upon irradiation this photoactive hydrophobic material may either be removed or converted to an alkali-soluble species thereby allowing selective removal of the irradiated portion of the resist by an alkaline developer.

The DQN photoresist system is easily the most widely used in semiconductor manufacturing. This system will be discussed in detail to give a sense of potential exposures in photolithography. The overall formulation of a typical DQN resist is shown in Table 43.3.

NOVOLAK RESIN

The resin, polymer, or plastic used to form a protective layer over the wafer is a "novolak" which is a phenol-formaldehyde resin. An important feature of the resin is its insolubility in alkaline solutions. Variations on the solubility of the novolak resin are made by adding other alkyl groups to the aryl ring of the phenol monomer prior to polymerization. A typical resin is formed by the condensation of formaldehyde and a substituted phenol such as meta-cresol.

As a large molecular weight polymer, the novolak resin is without significant health hazard. Small amounts of formaldehyde and substituted phenols contaminate the finished resin

Table 43.3.   Typical Formulation of a DQN Photoresist

Novolak resin	8 grams
Diazonaphthoquinone	2 grams
Glycol ether	20 grams
Butyl acetate	2 grams
Xylene	2 grams
Additives	Trace
Hexamethyldisilazane	
Organic acids	
Phthalic anhydride	
Silanes	
Imidazoles	

and therefore are also present in the final photoresist formulation. It is possible that these monomers are partially vaporized in the softbake process, though the more likely exposure would occur through skin contact with the liquid photoresist (Fig. 43.7).

Formaldehyde presents a concern since it is a sensitizing agent at low air concentrations. Formaldehyde's ability to haptenize human proteins and produce either dermal or respiratory sensitization is a realistic health threat. Experience with phenol-formaldehyde resins in other industries has demonstrated that the possibility of health effects is more than speculative. Contact dermatitis has been the most frequent adverse reaction. Irritant dermatitis has been reported, but most reports document sensitization. Besides formaldehyde, 14 other contact sensitizers have been recognized in resins based on phenol and formaldehyde (118). Para-tertiarybutyl phenol (PTBP) has been the most widely documented. Other contact sensitizers in phenol-formaldehyde resins, and other applications where this problem occurs, including, possibly, semiconductor photolithography will be identified in the future.

DIAZONAPHTHOQUINONE

The sensitizer or photoactive element of the DQN system is diazonaphthoquinone (DQ). Novolak resins are rendered insoluble in alkaline solutions by the addition of 10–20% by weight of DQ. Several hundred variations of DQ have been patented. DQ is often in the form of a diester or triester of sulfonic acid (Fig. 43.8).

TRIHYDROXYBENZOPHENONE

Trihydroxybenzophenone (THBP) is used by many photoresist manufacturers to create diesters and triesters of the diazonaphthoquinones. A small amount of THBP will always contaminate the most fastidiously prepared DQ esters. At least one manufacturer adds THBP to its photoresist formulations in significant amounts to improve the sensitivity of the resist. The interest in this chemical resides in the fact that it was found to

be genotoxic in two tests in vitro. Mutation and chromosomal aberration were observed using Chinese hamster ovary cells (119). Subsequent in vitro tests of THBP were negative. No animal studies have been performed.

The THBP results are not surprising. All photoactivators and sensitizers used in photoresits are, by their nature, expected to be biologically active. Very little testing has been done except for Ames tests and a few in vitro tests for genotoxicity. Surprisingly, when photoactivators or sensitizers are tested they are in their inactivated state. An interesting test that has not been done with these materials would be to paint them onto the skin of animals and then expose the molecules to UV radiation. This would mimic an exposure scenario that may occur to workers when they leave the clean room environment and are exposed to sunlight. Benzophenone is used widely in topical sunscreens to absorb UV-A and UV-C radiation and has shown its ability to cause sensitization.

One can speculate that experience in the printing industry is pertinent to the semiconductor industry. Several recent reports have shown an excess of malignant melanoma among workers in the printing industry (120, 121). This industry uses different specific chemicals than does the semiconductor industry, but uses the same basic process of combining polymers with photosensitive chemicals and exposure to UV radiation to produce an image.

COUPLING OF DQ PHOTOINITIATOR TO THE NOVOLAK POLYMER

Prior to exposure to light the DQ ester acts to inhibit the dissolution of the novolak resin. This inhibition is thought to involve a diazonium-azo coupling reaction promoted by immersion in an alkaline developer (Fig. 43.9).

TOXICITY OF AZO COMPOUNDS

Azo compounds are synthetic compounds not found in nature. They consist of two aromatic rings joined by an azo (-N=N-) bond. They are chromophores and are widely used as dyes. Many have been shown to be carcinogenic in animal studies, though apparently azo dyes with only one azo link are generally not carcinogenic (122). Dyes such as Direct Blue 6, Direct Black 38, and Direct Brown 95 possess multiple azo bonds and are very potent carcinogens (123). Their toxicity is thought to be dependent on biotransformation to benzidine. It is unlikely that the transient azo-coupled diazonium compounds in Figure 43.8 could be similarly metabolized to benzidine.

EXPOSURE OF DQ TO UV RADIATION

After exposure to UV light the DQ inhibitor no longer functions. The exposed DQ is rearranged first to a carbene, then to a ketene, and finally to an indene acid complexed to the

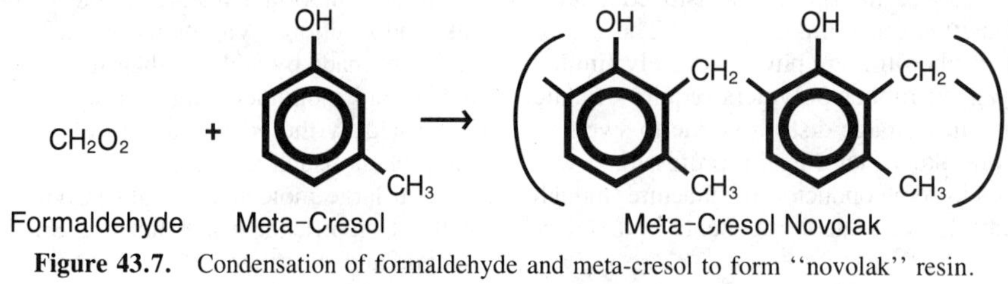

Formaldehyde   Meta-Cresol   Meta-Cresol Novolak

Figure 43.7.   Condensation of formaldehyde and meta-cresol to form "novolak" resin.

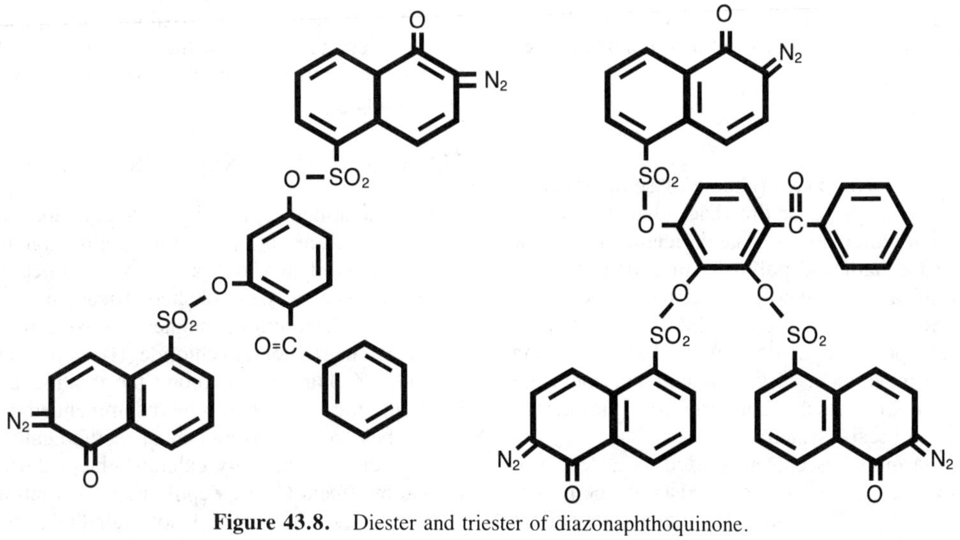

Figure 43.8.   Diester and triester of diazonaphthoquinone.

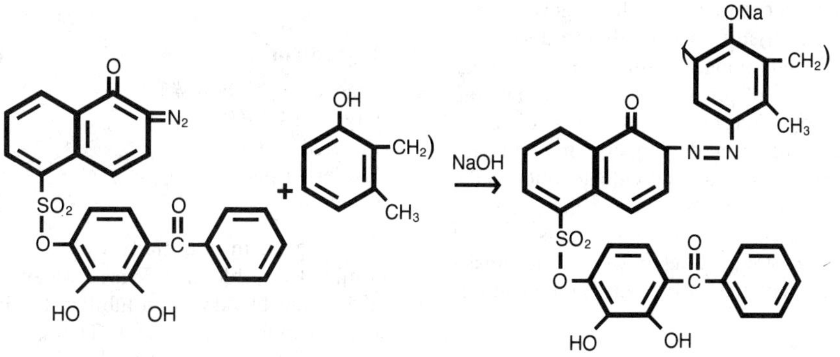

Figure 43.9.   Diazonium-azo coupling reaction.

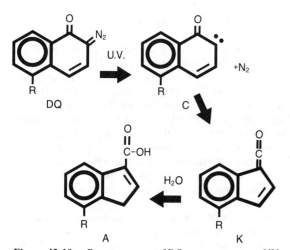

Figure 43.10.   Rearrangement of DQ upon exposure to UV radiation.

novolak resin. This makes the novolak resin more hydrophilic and more soluble (Fig. 43.10)

HEALTH HAZARDS OF DQs

The health hazards of DQs are not known. Their structure is similar to potent antibiotics and cancer chemotherapeutic agents suggesting biologic activity. Some data about similar com-pounds are available. 9,10-Anthraquinone shows evidence of carcinogenic activity when fed to mice and is also a potent skin sensitizer. Hydroquinone is mutagenic, is a well-known skin sensitizer, and has recently been shown to cause respiratory sensitization in humans (124). Its use in the photography industry has shown it to be a skin-bleaching agent (125).

DQN SOLVENTS

A large part of the typical DQN formulation is the solvent carrier combination of *n*-butyl acetate (NBA), xylene, and a glycol ether. The first two are a constant source of troublesome odors in the typical clean room environment. NBA has an odor threshold of less than 1 ppm. The TLV of 150 ppm often becomes a moot point to the workers. Xylene is another chemical with a very low odor threshold and no apparent hazard at levels encountered in the semiconductor industry. Nonetheless, all reasonable engineering controls to reduce these odors should be accomplished. Effective and recurring education about these chemicals is also an important means of addressing perceptions.

The other constituent of the photoresist solvent formulation has typically been an ethylene glycol ether or its acetate. These chemicals continue to pose one of the most worrisome hazards in the semiconductor industry.

ADDITIVES

A variety of additives (listed in Table 43.3) are used in trace amounts to alter the adhesion, speed, and heat resistance of the DQN photoresists. Although they are toxicologically interesting chemicals, there is no significant health hazard given the small amounts.

NEWER RESISTS

The DQN system is the current workhorse of semiconductor photolithography, but has a major drawback that has caused investigators to look for alternatives. That deficiency is the low thermal stability of the hardened polymer. Investigators have experimented with other phenolic polymers to try to find resists that will be stable beyond 120°C. The candidates include poly (p-hydroxystyrene), poly(p-hydroxy-a-methylstyrene), and N-(p-hydroxyphenyl)maleimide. Organosilicon polymers are being used extensively in research laboratories as a photoresist, especially in multilevel resist systems.

Poly(dimethylglutarimide) is currently used as a deep UV resist in production settings. Many new resists are being explored for use with excimer laser radiation, which allows finer resolution than that obtainable with current UV sources. There is a large class of ''inorganic resists'' such as germanium-selenium (Ge-Se) and arsenic trisulfide that will introduce toxic metals into photoresist formulations. Imminent x-ray lithography may require other types of photoresists. Accompanying each new resist polymer are different photoinitiators, different solvent formulations, and different developers. It is the responsibility of a health professional to read with skepticism the material data safety sheets that invariably accompany photoresists. The lack of adverse health effects on these sheets is based on ignorance due to lack of toxicity testing. All photoresist materials should be handled with the most careful and fastidious work practices.

Hydrofluoric Acid

The special dangers of delayed and continuing hydrofluoric acid (HF) burns are widely appreciated in the microelectronics industry. But most burns will be treated by medical personnel outside the industry who understandably are not as sensitized to this topic. HF burns are often undertreated in emergency departments and private physicians' offices. More specifically, calcium gluconate injections should be used to treat almost all HF burns.

INITIAL TREATMENT

The initial treatment of any HF burn is to remove the HF from the skin by irrigation with water for at least 10 minutes. Instead of a gentle stream, the irrigation should be done forcefully enough to accomplish this purpose. Showers or hoses are the ideal methods. A water tap at a sink will suffice for smaller burns. No work area that uses HF should be allowed to operate without these options immediately nearby. Workers should clearly understand the importance of immediate irrigation. Unfortunately, in their haste to transport burned victims to a medical facility, coworkers sometimes forego the crucial initial step of irrigation. Nothing is gained by this delay, which will only allow deeper penetration of fluoride ions into tissue.

Clothes saturated with HF are sometimes a source of continuing exposure. Especially in the instance of a splash, it is best to remove and dispose all clothing. Clothing that has absorbed HF can cause serious burns to anyone who handles it carelessly. Treatment for hydrofluoric acid should proceed immediately if there is any possibility of exposure. The history is often very unclear, and the wise course is to proceed with therapy rather than to agonize over questions that may be unanswerable.

TOPICAL SOLUTIONS, GELS, AND CREAMS

Another treatment option is the application of a topical magnesium, calcium, or quaternary amine salt in order to bind fluoride ions. The wide variety of favorites attest to the fact that none has clearly established efficacy over the others. Magnesium sulfate solution, magnesium oxide paste, calcium gluconate gel, benzethonium chloride (Hyamine), and benzalkonium chloride (Zephiran) are among the treatments that have been used, and they continue to be recommended by many sources.

The best controlled and most methodically sound study to date concluded that only calcium gluconate has efficacy as a topical treatment (126). Zephiran, A&D ointment, magnesium ointment, and aloe gel did not alter the histopathologic progression of the HF burn. Calcium gluconate as a 2.5% gel can be made as follows:

Ingredient	Percent	Weight
Tragacanth ribbon #1	2%	20 g
Glycerin USP	2.5%	25 g
Purified water	68%	680 ml
Liquefied phenol	0.13%	1.3 ml
Calcium gluconate 10%	27.4%	250 ml

The tragacanth is initially weighed, then wet with glycerin and mixed in a blender. Warm water (600 milliliters) is then added to the blender to solubilize the initial mixture. The liquified phenol is added next. This is followed by the calcium gluconate 10% solution, and the concoction is then thoroughly mixed. Afterward it can be stored in tubes for application.

INJECTION OF TISSUE WITH CALCIUM IONS

HF is highly soluble in biologic membranes, and therefore behaves differently from other acids such as HCL and H_2SO_4, whose immediate corrosive and thermal effects are effected immediately and upon the most proximate tissue. HF can absorb deeply and insidiously into tissue before dissociating and releasing highly destructive fluoride ions. The quickest and surest way to bind fluoride ions and halt tissue destruction and symptoms is to inject the afflicted dermal and subcutaneous tissue with calcium ions. This is done with calcium gluconate—most commonly 10% concentration. A rule of thumb is to use 0.5 milliliters for each centimeter squared of burned skin. A 27- or 30-gauge needle is used and multiple injection sites. There is no need to use anesthesia prior to infiltration with calcium gluconate. As with most subcutaneous injections the pain is a function of pressure and tissue distension and can be minimized by injecting slowly.

INDICATIONS FOR CALCIUM GLUCONATE INJECTIONS

There are three clear indications for calcium gluconate injections into the dermal and subcutaneous areas of an HF burn:

1. Any symptom or sign of chemical burn associated with a history of possible HF exposure.
2. A history of a burn with HF of 20% or greater concentration.

If the history of HF burn is clear, but the concentration is unknown then infiltration should be done. With HF concentrations as high as 50%, symptoms may not occur for up to 8 hours. Lesser concentrations may produce symptoms only after 24 hours.

3. A delay in treatment of a clear exposure (such as a splash of HF to the skin). Primarily, this means any delay in appropriate irrigation. HF moves very quickly through intact skin.

The above guidelines leave few circumstances in which calcium gluconate injection is not indicated. The reluctance of physicians to use calcium gluconate injections to treat HF burns is puzzling. When faced with a possible HF burn, the physician is in the fortunate situation where appropriate therapy may be highly efficacious, and in almost no instance will injection be harmful. Granted, injections must be done with reasonable care into small spaces such as digits, but this is not a significant contraindication. Most physicians are comfortable injecting volumes of lidocaine that exceed the volume of calcium gluconate needed to treat HF burns. If 0.5 ml/cm^2 of burn area seems excessive, use less.

Occasionally, the physician is faced with a hard indurated HF burn of a finger into which calcium gluconate injection is neither wise nor possible. This situation may be best treated with intraarterial 10% calcium gluconate infusion. More aggressive use of percutaneous calcium gluconate injections into early HF burns would in many instances prevent progression to induration and tissue destruction.

RISK OF HYPERCALCEMIA FROM INJECTIONS

There is also the remote possibility of causing hypercalcemia with the injections. If large volumes of calcium gluconate are being injected (greater than 10 milliliters of 10% solution), it is prudent to monitor the serum calcium before further injections. In a crisis situation where larger volumes are indicated, a rhythm strip can be monitored for indications of either hypercalcemia of hypocalcemia.

LATE TREATMENT

A late presentation, often after several days, of a probable HF burn is not uncommon. Calcium gluconate injections have caused rapid and dramatic amelioration of both signs and symptoms as late as 5 days after the burn. If there is any reason to think that the tissue is still reacting to fluoride ion, then it is not too late to inject calcium gluconate. Except in the case of fingers or toes, it is always possible to inject around and under the most indurated HF burn. Another situation that arises is the opportunity to repeat the injections. Repeat injections, at an interval of 4–6 hours or a day later, are also perfectly reasonable if clinical signs and symptoms indicate continued tissue destruction.

CALCIUM CHLORIDE CONTRAINDICATED

It is important to mention that calcium chloride cannot be used for dermal or subcutaneous injections. This drug will cause severe irritation and necrosis of tissue. Disastrous incidents have occurred where calcium chloride was mistakenly substituted for calcium gluconate to treat HF burns.

HYDROFLUORIC ACID BURNS OF THE EYE

Splashes of HF into the eye should be irrigated copiously. Introduction of any other chemicals besides water into the eye should be done with caution. Emergency departments may want to take time to research the validity of treatment protocols that seem unusual. The following incident will help illustrate the risk of blindly accepting outside protocols with unusual treatment regimens.

In the early 1980s, some preliminary results were published from experiments done upon the eyes of rabbits that concluded that irrigation of the eyes with Zephiran was the preferred treatment for HF spashes into the eye. One microelectronics company integrated this recommendation into its protocols for HF burns. The protocol was distributed to local emergency departments. The idea of instilling Zephiran into human eyes was quickly discredited, and the microelectronics company changed its protocol within a year.

Unfortunately, several years later when an employee from a different semicondictor company presented with a history of HF splashes into the eye, that outdated protocol was used to treat the patient. The patient was originally asymptomatic. A Morgan lens was placed on the cornea and the eye was irrigated with a solution of Zephiran in water. Almost immediately the patient began complaining of pain. Topical anesthesia was used on the cornea but was only partially successful. The irrigation was completed, the eye was patched, and the patient was discharged. The patient lost her cornea, and the probable cause was an alkali burn caused by Zephiran. Subsequent attempts at corneal transplant met limited success (personal communication).

The best approach at present to an HF splash into the eye is to irrigate with water and refer all these injuries to immediate ophthalmologic consultation.

METABOLIC DISORDERS OF HYDROFLUORIC ACID

Death from systemic fluorosis is a rare, but documented, sequela of topical HF burns (127, 128). One fatality followed an HF burn of only 2.5% of the body surface area (128). All deaths have involved profound hypocalcemia with subsequent arrhythmias and cardiac arrest. The mechanism of this hypocalcemia is probably the removal of free Ca^{++} via the formation of CaF_2.

Patients with significant burns should receive cardiac monitoring and intermittent serum calcium determination for 6–8 hours post exposure. If metabolic problems develop, they will manifest within that period of time. The QT interval is very sensitive to hypocalcemia, and a lengthened QT interval is usually the first sign of hypocalcemia secondary to HF exposure (129). This can occur as quickly as 25–30 minutes post exposure. Classic physical findings such as carpopedal spasm, Chvostek's sign, or Trousseau's sign are often absent even when hypocalcemia, a prolonged QT, and bradycardia are present. Treatment is intravenous injection of calcium and stopping the absorption of fluoride. The latter consists of removal of all clothing, irrigation, topical Ca^{++} treatment, and infiltration of the burn area with Ca^{++}.

SURGICAL EXCISION

Surgical excision of severely HF burned tissue is an option that has been used not only to remove necrotic tissue, but also to remove an ongoing source of fluoride ion. The most dramatic case report describes a worker who suffered a 5% body surface HF burn and who developed a severe hypocalcemia and cardiac arrhythmias. This problem could not be corrected despite large doses of intravenous calcium chloride and appropriate wound therapy, including infiltration of calcium gluconate. The situation was brought under control only when the burned skin on the forearm was surgically removed (129).

INTRAARTERIAL CALCIUM INFUSION

Several articles have been published on the treatment of HF burns with intraarterial calcium infusion (130, 131). This approach has proven to be efficacious in situations where local infiltration was not possible, but logistically it is complicated. This treatment should probably be done only by physicians who can manage any complications. It is not an outpatient procedure.

PREVENTION AND BETTER TREATMENT

The most important strategy for working with HF remains primary prevention, and the semiconductor industry has been quite aggressive in eliminating these burns. Equipment design, increased worker education, better personal protective equipment, and the change to dry etching have all contributed to this progress. Workers at many facilities carry laminated cards in their wallets or purses that instruct private physicians in the treatment of HF burns. Local medical facilities and emergency department personnel may need periodic review of this subject.

REFERENCES

1. Semiconductor Industry Association. Complete semiconductor forecast 1987–1990. Cupertino, CA: Semiconductor Industry Association, 1987.
2. U.S. Department of Labor, Bureau of Labor Statistics. Occupational injuries and illnesses in the United States by industry, 1984. Washington, DC: USDOL Bull. 2259, USDOL.
3. Rapa A. Clean rooms for VLSI Manufacturing, IBM Technical Report (Tr22.2497). East Fishkill: IBM General Technology Division, April, 1983.
4. Rycroft RCG. Low humidity and microtrauma. Am J Ind Med 1985;8:371–373.
5. Rycroft RCG: Low humidity occupational dermatoses. Chapt 1 in: Gardner AW, ed. Current approaches to occupational health. 3rd Ed. Wright, 1987.
6. Fischer T, Maibach HI. Patch testing in allergic contact dermatitis, an update, Chapter 22 in: Maibach, HI, ed. Occupational and industrial dermatology. 2nd ed. Chicago, IL: Year Book Medical Publishers, 1987.
7. Shama SK. Monitoring and updating patch test allergens used in the United States. The Occupational and Environmental Medicine (DEM) Report, 1989, 69–72.
8. Nilsson SEG, Anderson L. The use of contact lenses in environments with organic solvents, acids, or alkalies. Acta Opthalmol 1982;60:599–608.
9. Randolph SA, Zavon MR. Guidelines for contact lens use in industry. J Occup Med 1987;29:237–242.
10. Pogge BH. Metals and semi-metals in the semiconductor device technologies. In Clarkson TW, et al. eds. Biological monitoring of toxic metals. New York, New York: Plenum Press, 1988.
11. Redmond SF, Schappert KR. Occupational dermatitis associated with garments. J Occup Med 1987;29:243–244.
12. Terman M, Terman JS, Quitkin FM, et al. Light therapy for seasonal affective disorder. Neuropsychopharmacology 1989;2(1):1–22.
13. Environmental Protection Agency. Guidelines for the health assessment of suspect developmental toxicants. Washington, DC: (51FR34028) EPA. Sept 24, 1986.
14. Wurtman RJ, Wurtman JJ. Carbohydrates and depression. Sci Am 1989; (Jan) 68–75.
15. Dager SR, Holland JP, Cowley DS, et al. Panic disorder precipitated by exposure to organic solvents in the work place. Am J Psychiatry 1987;144:1056–1058.
16. Klein DF, Zitrin CM, Woerner MG, Ross DC. Treatment of phobias.

II. Behavior therapy and supportive psychotherapy: are there any specific ingredients? Arch Gen Psychiatry 1983;40:139–145.
17. Tearnan BH, Goetsch V, Adms HE. Modification of disease phobia using a multifacted exposure program. J Behav Ther Exp Psychiatry 1985;16:57–61.
18. Cullen MR. Workers with multiple chemical sensitivities. Occup Med State Art Rev 1987;2:655–806.
19. Bolla-Wilson K, Wilson RJ, Bleeker ML. Conditioning of physical symptoms after neurotoxic exposure. J Occup Med 1988;39:684–686.
20. Shusterman D, Balmes J, Cone J. Behavioral sensitization to irritants/odorants after acute overexposure. J Occup Med 1988;30:565–566.
21. Brodsky CM. Allergic to everything: a medical subculture. Psychosomatics 1983;24:731–742.
22. Terr AI. Clinical ecology. Ann Intern Med 1989;111:168–178.
23. Boxer PA. Occupational mass psychogenic illness. J Occup Med 1985;27:867–872.
24. Olkinuora M. Psychogenic epidemics and work. Scand J Work Environ Health 1984;10:501–504.
25. Colligan MJ. Mass psychogenic illness: some clarification and perspectives. J Occup Med 1981;23:635–638.
26. Faust HS, Brilliant LB. Is the diagnosis of "mass hysteria" an excuse for incomplete investigation of low-level environmental contamination? J Occup Med 1981;23:22–26.
27. Lenihan KL, Sheehy JW, Jones JH. Assessment of exposures in gallium arsenide processing: a case study. Chapter 23 in: Hazard assessment control technology in semiconductor manufacturing, ACGIH. Chelsea, MI: Lewis Publishers, 1989.
28. Hammond ML. Safety in chemical vapor deposition. Solid State Technol 1989; (Dec): 104–109.
29. Rhoades BJ, et al. Safety and environmental control systems used in chemical vapor deposition (CVD) reactors at AT&T—microelectronics, Reading, Pennsylvania. Chapter 16 in: Hazard assessment and control technology in semiconductor manufacturing, ACGIH. Chelsea, MI: Lewis Publishers, 1989.
30. Bachmann P, Berges HP. Safety aspects of oil sealed rotary vane vacuum pumps in CVD applications. Solid State Technol 1986; (July): 83–87.
31. Schaeffer J. Hydrogen monitoring throughout the semiconductor manufacturing facility. Semiconductor Safety Assoc J 1988; (Sept).
32. Jones JH. Exposure and control assessment of semiconductor manufacturing. Am Inst Phys Conf Proc (USA) No. 166, 1988:44–53.
33. Ungers LJ, Jones JH, McIntyre AJ, et al. Release of arsenic from semiconductor wafers. Am Ind Hyg Assoc J 1985;46:416–420.
34. Holroyd D, REA MS, Young J, Briggs G. Health related aspects of the devitrification of aluminosilicate refractory fibers during use as a high temperature furnace insulant. Ann Occup Hyg 1988;3:171–178.
35. Paustenbach DJ. Assessment of the developmental risks resulting from occupational exposure to select glycol ethers within the semiconductor industry. J Toxicol Environ Health 1988;23:29–37.
36. Singer PH. Wet bench fire suppression. Semiconductor Int 1987; (Sept):154–157.
37. Uniform building code. Chapt 9, Group H, Division 6, 1988.
38. Uniform fire code. Article 80, 1987. Companion document—The toxic gas model ordinance, 1988.
39. Uniform fire code, Article 51, 1987.
40. Singer PH. Dry etching of SiO_2 and Si_3N_4. Semiconductor Int 1986; (May):98–103.
41. Moreau WM. Semiconductor Lithography. New York: Plenum Press, 1988.
42. Mucha A. The gases of plasma etching: silicon based technology. Solid State Technol 1985; (March):123–127.
43. Ohlson J. Dry etch chemical safety. Solid State Technol 1986; (July):69–73.
44. Ruuskanen J, et al. Gallium arsenide etchers: beware of the pump oil. Semiconductor Int 1988; (June):88–90.
45. Skidmore K. Use the right plasma to strip away resist. Semiconductor Int 1988; (Aug):54–59.
46. Kennedy GL. Biological effects of acetamide, formamide, and their monomethyl and dimethyl derivatives. CRC Crit Rev Toxicol 1988;17:129–182.
47. Fowler BA, ed. Biological and environmental effects of arsenic. Amsterdam: Elsevier, 1983.
48. Becci PJ, Knickerbocker MJ, Reagan EL. Teratogenicity study of N-methylpyrrolidone after dermal application to Sprague-Dawley rats. Fundam Appl Toxicol 1982;2:73–76.
49. Occup Saf Health Rep, (3/22/89): 1780—1781 Bureau of National Affairs.
50. Picraux ST, Percy PS. Ion implantation of surfaces. Sci Am 1985;237:102–113.

51. Baldwin DG, King BW, Scarpace LP. Ion implanters: chemical and radiation safety. Solid State Technol 1988; (Jan):99–105.

52. Ungers LJ, Jones JH. Industrial hygiene and control technology assessment of ion implantation operations. Am Ind Hyg Assoc J 1986;47:607–614.

53. Mueller MR, Kunesh RF: Safety and health implications of dry chemical etching. Chap 15 in: Hazard assessment and control technology in semiconductor manufacturing, ACGIH. Chelsea, MI: Lewis Publishers, 1989.

54. Doyle L, Gallagher K, Heath BS, Patterson WB. An outbreak of infectious conjunctivitis spread by microscopes. J Occup Med 1989;31:758–762.

55. Paul M, Himmelstein J, Weinstein S, et al. Ocular infections and the industrial use of microscopes. J Occup Med 1989;31:763–766.

56. McCurdy SA: Occupational injury and illness in the semiconductor manufacturing industry. Am J Ind Med 1989;15:499–510.

57. Marriott MD, Stuchly MA. Health aspects of work with visual display terminals. J Occup Med 1986;28:833–848.

58. Rose L. Workplace video display terminals and visual fatigue. J Occup Med 1987;29:321–324.

59. Rycroft RJG, Calnan CD. Facial rashes among video display unit operators. In: Pearce BG ed. Health hazards of VDTs. New York: John Wiley & Sons, 1984.

60. Tjonn HH. Report of facial rashes among VDU operators in Norway. In: Pearce BG ed. Health hazards of VDTs. New York: John Wiley & Sons, 1984.

61. Fthenakis VM. Hazards from radiofrequency and laser equipment in the manufacture of a-SI photovoltaic cells. Brookhaven National Laboratory, April 1985:15.

62. Hattis D, Berg R. Pharmacokinetics of ethoxyethanol in humans. MIT Center for Technology, Policy and Industrial Development. Report No. 88–1, February 1988.

63. Nagano K, et al: Embryotoxic effects of ethylene glycol monomethyl ether in mice. Toxicology 1981;20:335.

64. National Institute of Ocuptional Safety and Health. Current Intelligence Bulletin 39. Glycol ethers. Department of Health and Human Services (DHHS) Pub 83–112. May 1983.

65. Occupational Safety & Health Admin. ANPR for Health and Safety Standards. Occupational exposure to 2-methoxyethanol, 2-ethoxyethanol, and their acetates. Fed Reg 1987;52:10585–10593.

66. Hanley TR, Yano BL, Nitschke KD, John JA, et al. Comparison of the teratogenic potential of inhaled ethylene glycol monomethyl ether in rats, mice and rabbits. Toxicol Appl Pharmacol 1984;75:409–422.

67. Miller RR, Ayers JA, Young JT, McKenna MJ, et al. Ethylene glycol monomethyl ether. I. Subchronic vapor inhalation study with rats and rabbits. Fundam Appl Toxicol 1983;3:49–54.

68. Tinson DJ. Ethylene glycol monomethyl ether: inhalation teratogenicity study in rabbits. Submitted to Environmental Protection Agency by ICI Center Toxicology Laboratory, April 21, 1983.

69. Tinson DJ. Ethylene glycol monomethyl ether: Inhalation teratogenicity study in rats. Submitted to Environmental Protection Agency by ICI Center Toxicology Laboratory, April 14, 1983.

70. Niemeier RW, Smith RJ, Hardin ED, et al. Teratogenicity of 2-ethoxyethanol by dermal application. Drug Chem Toxicol 1982;5:277–294.

71. Nelson BK. Ethoxyethanol behavioral teratology in rats. Neurotoxicology 1981;2:231–247.

72. Tyl RW, Pritts IM, France AK, Fisher LC, Tyler TR. Developmental toxicity evaluation of inhaled 2-ethoxyethanol acetate in Fischer 344 rats and New Zealand white rabbits. Fundam Appl Toxicol 1988;10:20–39.

73. Terrill JB. A 13-week inhalation study of ethylene glycol monomethyl ether in the rabbit. Report #82-7589 to the Chemical Manufacturers Association, 1983.

74. National Institute of Occupational Safety and Health draft document: Criteria for a recommended standard . . . occupational exposure to ethylene glycol ethers, May 1989.

75. Ratcliffe JM, Schrader SM, Clapp DE, et al. Semen quality in workers exposed to 2-ethoxyethanol. Br J Ind Med 1989;46:399–406.

76. Cook RR, Bodner KM, Kolesar RC, et al. A cross-sectional study of ethylene glycol monomethyl ether process employees. Arch Environ Health 1982;37:346.

77. Welch LS, Schrader SM, Turner TW, Cullen MR, et al. Effects of exposure to ethylene glycol ethers on shipyard painters: II. Male reproduction. Am J Ind Med 1988;14:509–526.

78. Pastides H, et al. Spontaneous abortion and general illness symptoms among semiconductor manufacturers. J Occup Med 1988;30:543.

79. Andrews LS, Snyder R. Toxic effects of solvents and vapors Chapt 20 in: Casarett and Doull's toxicology. 3rd ed. New York: Macmilnlan, 1986.

80. Boggs A. A comparative risk assessment of casting solvents for positive photoresist. Appl Ind Hyg 1989;4:81–87.

81. Stedman DB, Welch F. Inhibition of DNA synthesis in mouse whole

embryo culture by 2-methoxyacetic acid and attenuation of the effects by sample physiological compounds. Letter: Toxicology 1989;45:111–117.

82. Mebus CA, Welsch F. The possible role of one-carbon moieties in 2-methoxyethanol and 2-methoxyacetic acid-induced developmental toxicity. Toxicol Appl Pharmacol 1989;99:98–109.

83. Guest D, Hamilton ML, Deisinger PJ, Divincenzo GD, et al. Pulmonary and percutaneous absorption of 2-propoxyethyl acetate and 2-ethoxyethyl acetate in beagle dogs. Environ Health Perspect 1984;57:177–183.

84. Dugard PH, Walker M, Mawdsley SJ, Scott RC, et al. Absorption of some glycol ethers through human skin in vitro. Environ Health Perspect 1984;57:193–197.

85. Groeseneken D, VanVelm E, Veulemans H, Masschelein R. Gas chromatographic determinations of methoxyacetic and ethoxyacetic acids in urine. Br J Ind Med 1986;43:62–65.

86. Smallwood AW, Debord KE, Lowry LK. Analyses of ethylene glycol monoalkyl ethers and their proposed metabolites in blood and urine. Environ Health Perspect 57:249–253.

87. Groeseneken D, Veulemans H, Masschelein R. Urinary excretion of ethoxyacetic acid after experimental human exposure to ethylene glycol monoethyl ether. Br J Ind Med 1986;43:615—619.

88. Veulemans H, Groeseneken D, Masschelein R, et al. Field study of the urinary excretion of ethoxyacetic acid during related daily exposure to the ethyl ether of ethylene glycol and ethyl ether of ethylene glycol acetate. Scand J Work Environ Health 1987;13:239–242.

89. Johanson G, Kronborg H, Naslund PH, et al. Toxicokinetics of inhaled 2-butoxyethanol (ethylene glycol monobutyl ether) in man. Scand J Work Environ Health 1986;12:594–602.

90. Industrial Union Department v. American Petroleum Institute, 488 U.S. 622, (1980).

91. Hattis D, et al. Male fertility effects of glycol ethers—a quantitative analysis. MIT Center for Technology, Policy and Industrial Development. Report no. 88-3 1988.

92. Ballew MS, Hattis D. Reproductive effects of glycol ethers in females—a quantitative analysis. MIT Center for Technology, Policy and Industrial Development. Report no. 89-7 1989.

93. Meistrich ML, Brown CC. Estimation of the increased risk of human infertility from alterations in semen characteristics. Fertil Steril 40:220–230.

94. Cheever KL, Richards DE, Weigel WW, et al. Metabolism of bis (2-methoxyethyl) ether in the adult male rat: evaluation of the principal metabolite as a testicular toxicant. Toxicol Appl Pharmacol 1988;94:150–159.

95. DuPont HLR 515-87. Teratogenicity study of diglyme in the rat. Submitted to Environmental Protection Agency under Toxic Substance Control Act.

96. DuPont HLR 129-88. Subchronic inhalation toxicity study with diglyme. Submitted to EPA under Toxic Substance Control Act.

97. DuPont HLR 562-88. Subchronic Inhalation Toxicity Study with diglyme. Submitted to EPA under TSCA.

98. Price CJ, Kimmell CA, George JD, Marr MC. The developmental toxicity of diethylene glycol dimethyl ether in mice. Fundam Appl Toxicol 1987;8:115–126.

99. National Institutes of Occupational Safety and Health alert: request for assistance in reducing the potential risk of developing cancer from exposure to gallium arsenide in the microelectronics industry. DHHS (NIOSH) Publication no. 88-100/October 1987.

100. Finkel AJ. Arsenic. Chapt 3 in: Hamilton and Hardy's industrial toxicology. 4th ed. Littleton, MA: PSG Publishing, 1983.

101. Beaudoin AR. Teratogenicity of sodium arsenate in rats. Teratology 1974;10:153–158.

102. Hood RD, Thacker GT, Patterson BL. Effects in the mouse and rat of prenatal exposure to arsenic. Environ Health Perspect 1977;19:219–222.

103. Rosner MH, Carter DE. Metabolism and excretion of gallium arsenide and arsenic oxides by hamsters following intratracheal instillation. Fundam Appl Toxicol 1987;9:730–737.

104. Webb DR, Wilson SE, Carter DE: Pulmonary clearance and toxicity of respirable gallium arsenide particulates intratracheally instilled in rats. Am Ind Hyg Assoc J 1987;48:660–667.

105. Webb DR, Wilson SE, Carter DE: Comparative pulmonary toxicity of gallium arsenide, gallium oxide, or arsenic oxide intratracheally instilled into rats. Toxicol Appl Pharmacol 1986;82:405–416.

106. National Institutes of Occupational Safety and Health. Criteria for a recommended standard. Occupational exposure to inorganic arsenic, 1975.

107. Occupational Safety and Health Administration. Standard on arsenic (29 CFR1910.1018).

108. Yamauchi H, Takahashi K, Mashiko M, Yamamura Y. Biological monitoring of arsenic exposure of gallium arsenide and inorganic arsenic exposed workers by determination of inorganic arsenic and its metabolites in urine and hair. Am Ind Hyg Assoc J 1989;50:606–612.

109. Foa V, et al. The speciation of the chemical forms of arsenic in the

biological monitoring of exposure to inorganic arsenic. Sci Total Environ 1984;34:241–259.

110. Norin H, Vahter M. A rapid method for the selective analysis of total urinary metabolites of inorganic arsenic. Scand J Work Environ Health 1981;7:38–44.

111. Vahter ME. Arsenic Chapt in: TW Clarkson et al. Biological monitoring of toxic metals. New York, NY: Plenum Press, 1988.

112. Wolff RK, Henderson RF, Edison AF, et al. Toxicity of gallium oxide particles following a 4-week inhalation exposure. Appl Toxicol 1988; 8(3):191–199.

113. Balboni HA, Ziemer EJ. Study of silane self-ignition and explosion-potential. Essex Junction, VT: IBM Gen Tech Div, 1979

114. Ring MA. Silane-O2 explosion, their characteristics and their control. Am Inst Phys Conf Proc (USA) no. 166: 1988, 175–182.

115. American Confederation of Governmental Industrial Hygienists. Documentation of the threshold limit values and biological exposure indices. 5th ed. Cincinnati: American Conference of Governmental Industrial Hygienists, 1986.

116. Stokinger HE. The halogens and the nonmetals boron and silicon. In: Clayton, Clayton, eds. Patty's industrial hygiene and toxicology, 3rd rev. Volume 2B. New York: John Wiley & Sons, 1981.

117. Britton LG. Combustion hazards of silane and its chlorides. Paper 12b, Loss Prevention Symposium, presented at the AIChE Spring National Meeting, Houston, April 6, 1989.

118. Bruze M. Contact dermatitis from phenol-formaldehyde resins. Chapt 40 in: Maibach HI, ed. Occupational and industrial dermatology. 2nd ed. Chicago: Year Book Medical Publishers, 1987.

119. Toxic Substance Control Act TSCA 8e report #HQ-0484-0510.

120. Dubrow R. Malignant melanoma in the printing industry. Am J Ind Med 1986;10:119–126.

121. McGlaughlin JK, et al. Malignant melanoma in the printing industry. Am J Ind Med 1988;13:301–304.

122. Williams GM, Weisburger JH. Chemical Carcinogens. Chapt 5 in: Casaarett and Doull's Toxicology. 3rd ed. NY: Macmillian, 1986.

123. NIOSH Current Intelligence Bulletin #24, Benzidine derived dyes. DHEW Pub. 78–148, April 1987.

124. Choudat D, et al. Allergy and occupational exposure to hydroquinone and to methionine. Br J Ind Med 1988;45:376–380.

125. NIOSH, A recommended standard for occupational exposure to hydroquinone. DHEW Pub. #78-115, Sept. 1978.

126. Bracken W, et al. Comparative effectiveness of topical treatments for hydrofluoric acid burns. J Occup Med 1985;27:733–739.

127. Mullet T, Zoeller T, Bingham H, et al. Fatal hydrofluoric acid cutaneous exposure with refractory ventricular fibrillation. J Burn Care Rehab 1987;8:216–219.

128. Tepperman PB. Fatality due to acute systemic fluoride poisoning following a hydrofluoric acid skin burn. J Occup Med 1980;22:691–692.

129. Buckingham FM. Surgery: a radical approach to severe hydrofluoric acid burns: a case report. J Occup Med 1988;30:873–874.

130. Vance MV, Curry SC, Kunkel DB, et al. Digital hydrofluoric acid burns: treatment with intraarterial calcium infusion. Ann Emerg Med 1986;15:890–896.

131. Velbart J. Arterial perfusion for hydrofluoric acid burns. Hum Toxicol 1983;2:233–238.

44

Toxic Hazards of Plastic Manufacturing

Richard Lewis, M.D., M.P.H.
John B. Sullivan, Jr., M.D.

INTRODUCTION

The emergence of the plastics industry during the past 30 years has had a major impact on many other industries, including manufacturing, construction, and transportation. Articles made from plastics are ubiquitous in industrialized societies, and are found in appliances, automobiles, toys, home furnishings, clothing, insulation, food and beverage containers, and countless other applications. Advances in plastics technology have resulted in the development of materials with properties that equal or exceed those of traditional materials such as metal, wood, and glass. Plastics can be formed into sheets, coatings, or laminates or molded into virtually any shape or size. Plastic materials may have equal strength, durability, and impact resistance compared with some metals but are much lighter, a distinct advantage in the automobile industry. The "synthetic" nature of these materials allows the industry to readily adapt products to current needs. With different combinations of polymers and additives, the production of materials with unique properties and applications is seemingly limitless.

As the plastics industry has grown, the major focus has been on the chemical and mechanical properties of the materials as they relate to specific processes and applications. The presumption has been that high molecular weight polymers are biologically inert. As the industrial and medical experience with these compounds has grown, so has the recognition of a variety of potential health hazards. In the industrial medical setting, health providers need to be familiar with the basic materials and processes of this industry in order to recognize adverse health effects in this ever-expanding and changing industry.

Plastics are synthetic substances which are made by the use of repeating smaller molecular units called monomers. The end product, the plastic, is called a polymer. The intermediate products are termed prepolymers. The intermediate product is termed a synthetic resin. This synthetic resin is the material that is typically shipped in containers to end users or to the producers of plastic substances and urethanes. Generally, the molecules that are the basic building blocks for monomers of plastics have two functional binding sites. When these monomers are made to react with each other, linear macromolecules are formed. By increasing the chain length of these macrocmolecules, the material becomes more solid. There are two basic kinds of plastic with respect to the macromolecules and their reaction to heat: thermoplastic and thermoset.

The term plastic refers to any of a large group of synthetic materials which contain as an essential ingredient a high molecular weight, organic compound produced by polymerization which can be formed into various shapes but is solid in the finished state. A polymer is the essential high molecular weight component of a plastic and is characterized by repeating subunits of simple, low molecular weight molecules, or monomers. An oligomer is a low molecular weight polymer with fewer than 30–40 repeating subunits. When two or more different polymers composed of different monomers are combined they form a copolymer. Health effects related to plastic compounds may be related to biologic interaction with the finished polymer, residual monomer or oligomers, as well as plastic additives.

Plastics are divided into two main classes: (a) thermoplastics, linear or branched polymers, which can be repeatedly softened and reshaped with the application of heat or pressure; these materials are recyclable, although variations in formulations and additives limit the recycling of products after they have reached the consumer; and (b) thermoset plastics, which undergo a chemical reaction during processing that results in permanent cross-linking. The finished materials are resistant to heat and cannot be reformed. Table 44.1 lists the major thermoplastic and thermoset polymers in current use.

Thermoplastics and thermoset plastics are the basic plastic types (1). Thermoplastic compounds have the characteristic that their shape can be altered by heating and then cooling. During heating, the distances between the macromolecules increase with the decrease in Van der Waals forces. During the cooling process, the distances decrease with a subsequent increase in Van der Waals forces. The newly shaped plastic will thus retain the new position. Thermoset plastics cannot be altered by heating because of the fact that the macromolecule basic monomers are linked together. This thermoset linkage usually involves more than two functional chemical groups which are crosslinks between the chains (1).

RESIN MANUFACTURE

Resins are intermediate polymers of monomer subunits which are used to make plastics, foam, and rubber compounds. Resins

Table 44.1. Thermal Degradation Products of Some Plastics

Polymer	Degradation Product(s)	Hazard[a]
Polyethylene	Carbon monoxide	S
Polyvinyl chloride	Vinyl chloride	S, C
	HCl, phosgene	I, R
	Dioxins, furans	C
Polystyrene	Styrene	S
	Benzene	S, C
Fluoropolymers	Carbonyl fluoride	I, R
	Perfluoroisobutylene	I, R
	HF	I, R
Polyurethane	Aldehydes, ammonia	I, R
	Cyanide	S
	Isocyanates	I, R
	Nitrogen dioxide	R
Phenolic	Formaldehyde	I, R, S
	Aldehydes, ammonia	I, R
	Cyanide	S
	Nitrogen dioxide	R

[a]A = asphyxiant; C = carcinogen; I = mucous membrane irritant; R = respiratory irritant; S = systemic toxin.

are the materials mixed with curing agents to form the final product through a polymerization reaction. The raw materials for the production of polymers are derived primarily from crude oil and natural gas, and the growth of the plastics industry is dependent on the availability of these resources. The chemicals that will serve as intermediates or monomers are obtained by crude oil distillation followed by catalytic cracking and reformation. Other chemical reactions, such as the addition of halogens, may take place prior to polymerization (2).

Polymerization reactions occur in closed systems under controlled conditions. Chain reaction polymerization is initiated when a catalyst reacts with a substrate material, forming a free radical from a double bond. Chain growth results when additional monomeric units are added to the growing polymer chain, until either deliberate or spontaneous termination. In step reaction polymerization, two different chemicals react with the elimination of small molecules.

Before polymeric resins are supplied to the manufacturers of plastic products, a variety of additives and fillers may be added in the process of compounding. These include colorants, plasticizers, biocides, antioxidants, flame retardants, and fillers. The intimate mixing of polymer and additives requires heavy machinery including ball mills, high speed propeller mixers, kneading machines, and Banbury mixers or extruders. The compounded polymers may be supplied as sheets or formed into pellets, beads, or powders. In this form, the polymers and intermediates are commonly referred to as resins.

PLASTIC PROCESSING

The plastic processing industry converts a resin into finished products. Granules and powders may be compounded with additives prior to processing, and workers in these operations may have exposures similar to those of the resin manufacturers. Thermoset and partially polymerized materials may be supplied in solid or liquid form, and workers handling these materials may have exposure to unreacted intermediates and catalysts.

Plastic material processing requires that the resin be converted to a soft, malleable state through the application of heat or pressure followed by mechanical constriction to the desired form and cooling. Two of the primary processes used in the manufacture of plastic products are blow molding and injection molding. In blow molding, a hollow tube of heated plastic is formed, usually by extrusion, and placed in a mold with the desired final shape. The tube is filled with air under high pressure which expands the plastic into the mold cavity. The air is exhausted and the finished part ejected. This process can be used to form small bottles or 55-gallon drums. Injection molding uses high pressures to convert thermoplastic materials into articles with complex shapes. Pellets or granules are heated in a barrel, and the melted plastic is injected into a cooled metal mold by a helical screw. The parts are held under pressure until cool, then removed from the mold and trimmed. In compression molding, heat and pressure are applied to resin granules within a mold, forcing the material to conform to the mold shape. In transfer molding, thermoset materials are heated in a cavity and then transferred into a separate mold using a plunger. Extrusion forces a continuous flow of heated plastic through a die of the desired shape and is used for production of piping, tubing, gutters, and sheets. Calendering uses heated rollers to form sheets and coatings. Thermoforming and vacuum forming use pressure or suction, respectively to conform heated sheet plastic to a mold.

Finishing processes include the use of paints, adhesives, and solvents as in many other manufacturing industries. Molded items often need to be trimmed by hand prior to packaging and shipping. Scrap thermoplastic materials are usually recycled after grinding.

HEALTH HAZARDS

Most of the polymerization processes take place in closed systems, and the health hazards of resin manufacture are similar to those of the petrochemical industry (1-4). Workers may have exposure to vapors and dusts containing chemical intermediates, polymers, and additives during loading, mixing, pelletizing, and maintenance operations. Proper storage and handling of chemicals and additives is mandatory. Reactions must be carefully controlled to avoid chemical release or explosion. Dry mixing and pelletizing operations may generate high concentrations of airborne dusts of combustible plastic materials presenting an explosion hazard. The use of heavy machinery requires proper safety measures to avoid worker injury.

The handling of resins, intermediates, and additives may result in worker exposure. Plastic processing equipment operates using high temperatures and pressures and needs to be equipped with proper guards and safety rails to avoid serious burns, amputations, and crush injuries. Plastic grinding may generate polymer dust, resulting in inhalation and a possible combustion hazard. The overheating of plastic materials during processing, cleaning, and maintenance operations may expose workers to the thermal decomposition products of the polymer materials. Finishing operations may expose workers to a variety of other chemical compounds such as solvents and adhesives. In addition, cutting of plastics may result in repetitive motion injuries, such as tendonitis, sprains, and carpal tunnel syndrome.

COMBUSTION PRODUCT HAZARDS

Thermoplastic materials must be heated during processing. The temperatures required to achieve proper fluidity vary with the composition of the polymer and the additives. Overheating of plastics results in thermal decomposition and the release of oligomers, monomers, and other combustion products. The composition of the mixture of gases and vapors which are evolved is complex and is dependent not only on the chemical constituents of the polymer, but also on the temperature. At lower temperatures (300–400°F) combustion is incomplete, releasing larger, more complex molecules, while at higher temperatures (over 1600°F) complete combustion and oxidation produces low molecular weight gases. Workers may be exposed to the thermal decomposition products of plastics through accidental overheating during processing or during clean-out and maintenance operations. In addition, the burning of plastic materials during fires may present a health hazard to firefighters and the public.

The main combustion hazards that have been identified for the major classes of plastic materials are listed in Table 44.1. New thermal degradation products will be identified as research in this area proceeds. It is important to note that, while combustion hazards are primarily respiratory irritants (HCl, aldehydes), significant pulmonary injury from nitrogen oxides and phosgene as well as systemic poisoning from CO and cyanides may occur. The longterm health effects of exposure to combustion products of plastics are unknown.

POLYETHYLENE AND POLYPROPYLENE

High and low density polyethylene resins account for almost one third of the plastics produced in the United States. There are more than 100 different brands of polyethylene available.

Polyethylene is produced by the polymerization of ethylene in either continuous-flow or tubular reactors. Polyethylene is formed from a polymerization reaction of alkenes and conjugated dienes. Ethylene heated under pressure with oxygen produces a high molecular weight compound, polyethylene, made up of many ethylene subunits:

$$nCH_2 = CH_2 \xrightarrow[\text{heat pressure}]{O_2} (-CH_2 - CH_2 -)n$$

This type of polymerization, the end-to-end addition of monomers, is termed *addition polymerization*. The other type of polymerization, in which monomers are combined together, and in the process a molecule is lost, is termed *condensation polymerization*.

Polypropylene is characterized by resistance to heat and chemical corrosion. Propylene polymerization can occur in three different arrangements. All the methyl groups can be on one side of an extended chain (isotactic), methyl groups alternating from side to side (syndiotactic), or methyl groups alternating on each side of the chain randomly (actactic). Isotactic polypropylene is crystalline and forms strong fibers with a high melting point. Atactic polypropylene is a soft, elastic, pliable material. Polymerization of polypropylene generally occurs in a slurry with a hydrocarbon solvent diluent. Production of both plastics uses organometallic catalysts. Solvent vapors are evaporated off during drying and grinding. Liquid polymer is then cooled and formed into pellets.

High density polyethylene is used to form containers ranging from fuel tanks to milk bottles. Low density polyethylene has higher clarity and is used for films. coatings, shrink wrap, and food packaging. Polypropylene is used in containers, including medical syringes, as well as automotive components.

Both ethylene and propylene are asphyxiant gases. Several of the organometallic catalysts used are potent topical irritants. The thermal decomposition products of polyethylene and polypropylene include carbon dioxide as well as formaldehyde and acrolein, both respiratory irritants.

Ethylene and propylene should be stored properly in well-ventilated areas. Workers should not enter reaction vessels without using proper air-supplied respirators. Care should taken to avoid overheating or burning these polymers to prevent the formation of aldehydes and other decomposition products.

POLYVINYL CHLORIDE

Polyvinyl chloride (PVC) is a versatile plastic used widely in diverse applications. This product is produced by polymerization of vinyl chloride monomer, a gas at room temperature:

$$n(CH_2 = CH \xrightarrow{\text{peroxides}} (-CH_2 - CH -)n$$
$$| \qquad\qquad\qquad |$$
$$Cl \qquad\qquad\qquad Cl$$

Polymerization reactions take place in pressure vessels using a process in which vinyl chloride is suspended in water using a colloid with a peroxide catalyst. Residual monomer is removed from the vessels and the slurry is dried, then pelletized.

PVC is used widely in pipe, wire, and cable coatings for its strength and corrosion resistance. Diverse other uses range from floor tile and phonograph records to medical tubing and intravenous solution bags. PVC plastics commonly include plasticizers to increase flexibility. The major class of plasticizers are the phthalate esters, such as di(2-ethylhexyl) phthalate.

From 1927 until 1970, there was extensive exposure to unreacted vinyl chloride monomer in chemical plants producing PVC resin (Fig. 44.1). In the early years of production, air levels of vinyl chloride routinely exceeded 1000 ppm, at times resulting in very high exposure, and workers often became overcome by narcotic concentrations of vinyl chloride (15,000–20,000 ppm).

In the mid-1970s, the toxicity and carcinogenicity of vinyl chloride monomer were recognized after the discovery of several cases of angiosarcoma in workers at a PVC production plant. The marked excess of this rare tumor has subsequently been confirmed in several epidemiologic investigations (5).

At the same time, several other effects related to vinyl chloride exposure were reported. This included a condition termed acroosteolysis, a combination of Raynaud's phenomenon and lytic lesions of the distal phalanges. Subacute liver injury with fibrosis has also occurred with repeated heavy exposure (5).

Over the past 15 years, worker exposure to vinyl chloride has been reduced significantly, from 100–200 ppm in the early 1970s to less than 5 ppm since the promulgation of the Occupational Safety and Health Administration (OSHA) standard in 1974. With this reduction in exposure, the risk of developing acroosteolysis and subacute liver injury appears to be minimal. The risk for developing angiosarcoma, and possibly other malignancies (brain tumors, leukemia), remains uncertain. This is particularly true for workers who were first exposed prior to 1970 (6).

The risk of exposure to unreacted vinyl chloride monomer is much less in the processing of PVC resins into finished products. There has been limited evidence that exposure to PVC dust during grinding and other fabrication operations may result in the development of a pneumoconiosis in some workers accompanied by a slight reduction in pulmonary function. The plasticizer, di(2-ethylhexyl)phthalate, is also hepatotoxic and is an animal carcinogen as well. The thermal decomposition products of PVC include hydrochloric acid and phosgene, both respiratory irritants. Other thermal decomposition products are polychlorodibenzodioxins and polychlorodibenzofurans.

At present, it appears that the marked reduction in exposure to vinyl chloride has been effective in preventing workers from developing the significant health problems of the past. Care should be taken to prevent accidental over-exposure to vinyl chloride during PVC production through the use of proper respiratory protection. Workers should also avoid exposure to polyvinyl chloride dust generated during grinding, drying, or cleaning operations. Medical surveillance under the OSHA standard required annual examinations of workers exposed to vinyl chloride, including liver enzymes. Assessment of lung function is also recommended.

POLYSTYRENE

Styrene-based polymers rank third in production behind polyethylene and polyvinyl chloride. In addition to polystyrene plastics, other styrene polymers are used in the manufacture of synthetic rubber. Polystyrene resins are produced by a bulk polymerization process. A bead polymerization process in sus-

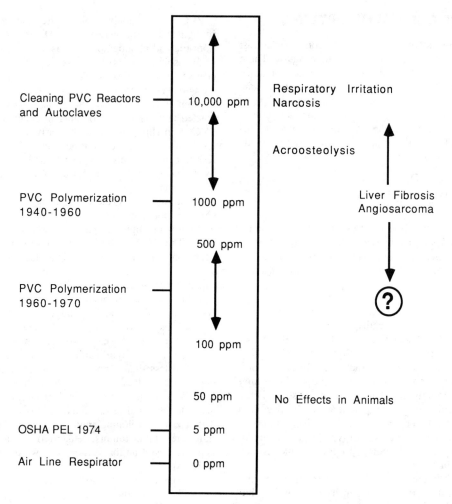

Figure 44.1. Vinyl chloride exposure and health effects at various times and under different conditions.

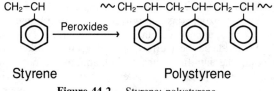

Figure 44.2. Styrene; polystyrene.

pension is used to produce polystyrene foams (Fig. 44.2). Co-polymerization of 1,3-butadiene with styrene produces styrene-butadiene rubber (SBR).

Polystyrene packaging materials are used widely for food products such as egg cartons, plates, cups, and disposable food containers. Copolymers of styrene with acrylonitrile are much more durable and used in machine housings, battery casings, and automotive components.

There is potential exposure to unreacted styrene monomer during resin production, particularly during mixing, loading, and maintenance operations. Styrene monomer may also be released if styrene polymers are heated. Styrene is used as a cross-linking agent in reinforced plastics used in boat building (see Polyesters).

At high concentrations (over 100 ppm), styrene is a respiratory and mucous membrane irritant. Skin contact may result in the development of primary irritant dermatitis. The manifestations of overexposure to styrene include lightheadedness, dizziness, and uncoordination. Limited clinical investigations of workers with longterm exposure to styrene have suggested subtle central and peripheral nervous system injury as well as possible liver damage. Styrene is mutagenic and has been associated with the induction of chromosomal aberrations in humans (7).

Acrylonitrile ($CH_2 = CH - CN$) is an explosive, flammable liquid used in manufacturing acrylic fibers and as an intermediate in pesticide manufacturing. Acrylonitrile (acrylan, vinyl cyanide) vapor is also a potent eye, mucous membrane, and skin irritant and may also cause symptoms of headache, fatigue, and nausea. Acrylonitrile may act as a chemical asphyxiant similar to hydrogen cyanide, and acute poisoning should be managed with amyl nitrate or sodium thiosulfate. Acrylonitrile is also a suspected human carcinogen.

The main measures in protecting the health of workers involved in the production of styrene polymers is control of exposure to styrene and acrylonitrile. Styrene polymers are

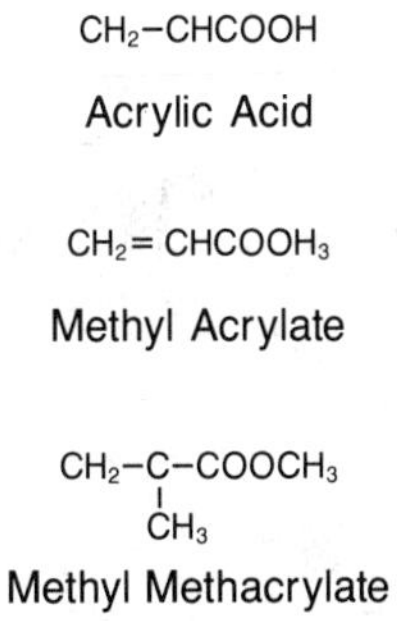

CH$_2$-CHCOOH

Acrylic Acid

CH$_2$= CHCOOH$_3$

Methyl Acrylate

CH$_2$-C-COOCH$_3$
|
CH$_3$

Methyl Methacrylate

Figure 44.3.   Acrylic acid; methyl acrylate; and methyl methacrylate.

generally inert, although free monomers may be released during combustion. Biologic monitoring of worker exposure to styrene involves the measurement of urine metabolites (phenylglyoxylic acid and mandelic acid) or styrene in blood or exhaled air.

ACRYLICS

Acrylic materials are formed from acrylic acid and methyl acrylate (Fig. 44.3). Acrylates have a resilience and clarity that has led to extensive use in coatings, lights, windows, and face shields. Most are polymers of methyl methacrylate, formed through bulk polymerization with peroxide catalysts (Fig. 44.4). Resins are supplied in sheets, pellets, or syrups.

While the methacrylates are upper respiratory and mucous membrane irritants, skin sensitization may occur leading to allergic contact dermatitis. Other symptoms reported after overexposure to methyl methacrylate include headache, fatigue, and irritability.

Prevention of skin sensitization is best achieved through limiting skin contact. Patch testing will confirm the diagnosis. Further work with acrylics should be avoided in sensitive individuals.

FLUOROPOLYMERS AND CHLOROPOLYMERS

Fluoropolymers or chloropolymers comprise a small but growing class of materials that combine resistance with low friction (Fig. 44.5). In addition to nonstick cookware, fluoropolymers are used to form sheaths and coatings for wire and cable. There are a large number of different fluoropolymer resins, most produced using hydrogen fluoride in combination with various aliphatic and chlorinated hydrocarbons. The high viscosity of fluoropolymers requires the use of high pressure and temperature during processing.

During resin production, a variety of fluorinated and chlorinated hydrocarbons may be employed. Many of these are used more commonly as industrial refrigerants and solvents. The main hazard of these materials is the induction of solvent narcosis with overexposure. Hydrogen fluoride is a potent respiratory irritant, potentially causing delayed pulmonary edema (8). Hydrofluoric acid may also be used, an agent notorious for causing extensive necrotic skin burns.

Polymer fume fever is a condition ascribed to the inhalation of the thermal decomposition of polytetrafluoroethylene ($-CF_2 = CF_2 -$)n. After exposure to the overheated polymer, symptoms of fever, chills, cough, and dyspnea develop over several hours, resolving spontaneously in a few days. Smoking cigarettes coated with the polymer has also caused this syndrome. While this has generally been a benign, self-limited condition, there are a few reports of individuals developing chronic pulmonary impairment.

Prevention of illness and injury in fluoropolymer production requires careful recognition of the toxicity of the materials used in production. High temperature processing operations require use of local exhaust ventilation to limit exposure to thermal decomposition products. Respiratory protection must be worn if molds or equipment are heated during cleaning. Good housekeeping practices and restriction of smoking in work areas will prevent inadvertent development of polymer fume fever.

PHENOLIC RESINS

The phenolics are thermoset plastics formed by the reaction of phenol and an aldehyde, usually formaldehyde. Phenolic resins include both resoles and novalacs. Phenol-formaldehyde resins represent a well-known polymer resulting from the reaction of phenol and formaldehyde in the presence of an acid or alkali. Many phenol rings are thus joined together by $- CH^2 -$ groups (Fig. 44.6). The primary use of phenolic resins is in the production of building materials such as plywood and adhesives. Resoles are used in electrical components and laminating. Phenolic resins are also used to coat fabrics, imparting crease resistance.

Most of the components of phenolic resins cause skin irritation, and many are skin sensitizers. Contact dermatitis can result not only from the handling of raw materials or resins but

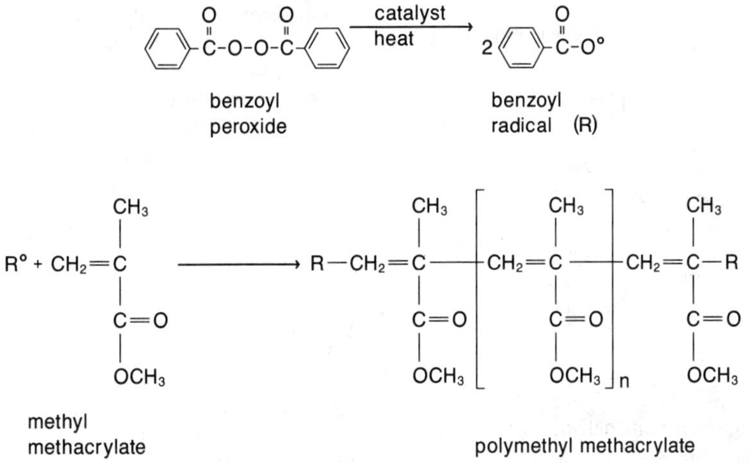

Figure 44.4.

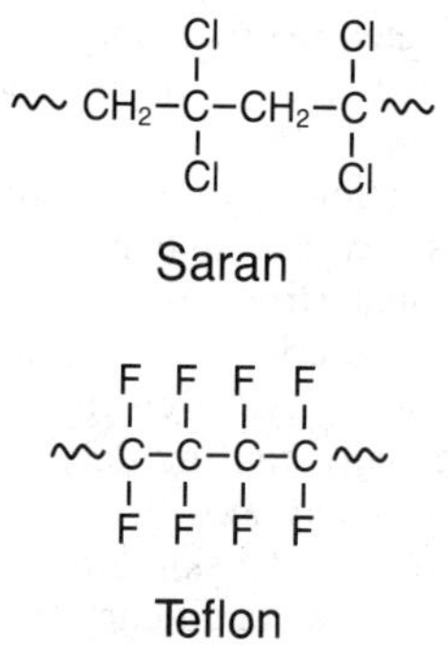

Figure 44.5.   Fluoro and chloro polymers.

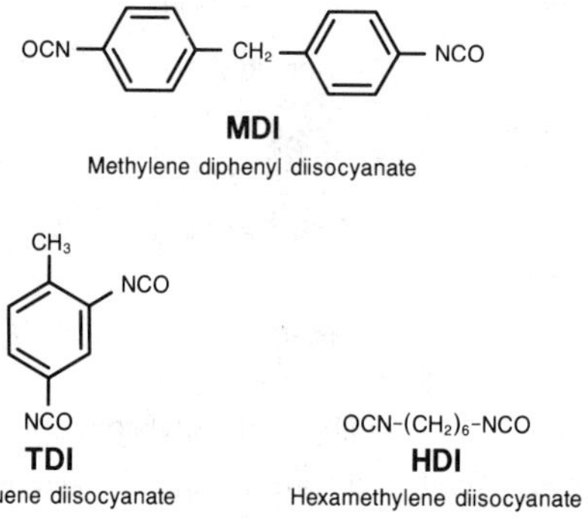

Figure 44.7.

also from the release of uncured resins from finished products. Phenol, formaldehyde, and hexamethylene tetramine are also respiratory and mucous membrane irritants. Phenol may be absorbed through the skin, with overexposure causing fatigue, weight loss, and liver injury. Operations that generate dust such as grinding of phenolic materials have been reported to cause pulmonary impairment and x-ray changes consistent with a penumoconiosis. Thermal decomposition products of phenolic polymers include phenol, formaldehyde, acrolein, and carbon monoxide.

As with acrylics, avoidance of skin contact through proper material handling is essential in the prevention of dermatitis and sensitization. Proper respiratory protection should be worn when handling resin powders and during grinding operations.

POLYURETHANES AND URETHANES

Polyurethanes are used widely in furnishings and construction in the form of flexible and rigid foams. These complex cellular polymers are formed by a reaction of an isocyanate with an alcohol group from a polyol, polyester, or polyether (9). The foams are formed in a one-shot process with the addition of an organometallic catalyst and a blowing agent (water or a chlorofluorocarbon). The liquid polymer is poured on a moving conveyor and heat cured into slabs.

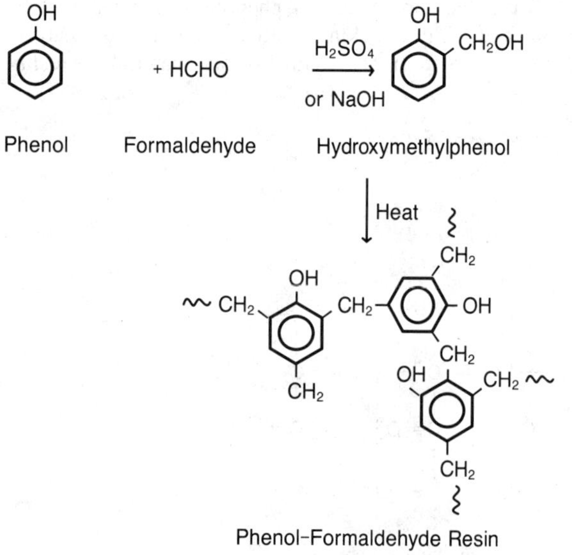

Figure 44.6.   Phenol-formaldehyde resin.

Urethanes are prepared from an isocyanate or polyisocyanate prepolymer. Isocyanates are chemicals that contain the NCO group. Polyisocyanates usually contain three or more NCO groups (10). The basic unit of polyurethane materials is a monomer. Monomers are made to react with each other by an exchange of atoms. A stepwise reaction of monomers is the basis of how diisocyanates are used to make longer chains of polyurethane. The propagation reaction using the monomer-starting material can occur either by the use of radicals or the use of a chemical which transfers a hydrogen atom (1). Usually, a polyol compound is used to transfer the hydrogen atom needed to the isocyanate. This chemical reaction will saturate the double bond between the nitrogen and the carbon in the NCO group. Given the presence of diisocyanate molecules along with hydroxyl groups of a polyol, a repeating exchange of hydrogen atoms occurs which lengthens the repeating molecular structure. This produces a growth in a prepolymer to a large macromolecular end product. Commonly used diisocyanates are toluene diisocyanate (TDI), diphenylmethane diisocyanate (MDI), and hexamethylene diisocyanate (HDI) (Fig. 44.7). These compounds react with the dipolyfunctional hydroxy group such as present on polyol compounds to form polyurethanes (9, 10). Polyurethanes are used as foams and a surface coating as adhesives and sealants. The typical polyol compound is a trihydroxy resin or polyglycol which will react with the diisocyanate to form a prepolymer. The polymerization reaction is an exothermic reaction. The heat that evolves helps cure and set the foam. Because of this exothermic, some diisocyanate may volatilize and escape into the atmosphere of the environment. Other curing agents used in polyurethane manufacturing include amines and esters (Table 44.2).

Diisocyanates are the most commonly recognized isocyanates, with TDI being the most commonly used commercial diisocyanate. Two isomers are available: 2,4-TDI and 2,6-TDI. Other commonly used isocyanates include HDI, naphthalene diisocyanate (NDI), and para-tolyl monoisocyanate (PTI) (11) (Table 44.3). After proper curing, the foams and polyurethanes that have been shaped usually contain no free diisocyanate compounds.

Occupations with the potential of having exposure to isocyanate products include diisocyanate workers, polyurethane manufacturing workers, upholstery workers, spray painters, coating workers, plastic film makers, plastic molders, and rubber workers (11).

Decrement of pulmonary functions and asthma are known consequences of pulmonary exposure to diisocyanate compounds (10–12). Human toxicology from diisocyanates is a result of dermal and inhalation contact with the chemical in a

Table 44.2. Isocyanate Curing Agents

Trihydroxy resin (castor oil)
Polyglycol (dipropylene glycol)
Aromatic amino polyol
Trichlorofluoromethane
Silicone oil
Phosphate esters
Tetramethyl butane diamine
Tetramethyl propane diamine
Diethanolamine
Tetramethylguanidine
Triethylene diamine
Triethylamine
Dimethylethanolamine
Diethylethanolamine
Dichlorobenzidine
Dianisidine
Tolidine
4,4-Methylene-bis(2-chloroamiline)

Table 44.4. Comparison of Physical Features of Certain Isocyanates

	TDI	MDI	PAPI
Molecular weight	174.4	250.3	400
Appearance	Clear to yellow liquid	White solid	Dark amber viscous liquid
Vapor pressures (mmHg)			
50°F (10°C)	0.02	0.00006	0.00024
77°F (25°C)	0.05	0.00014	0.00006
100°F (37.7°C)	0.10	0.00031	0.00016
Relative vapor pressures (mmHg)			
50°F (10°C)	898	1.5	1.0
77°F (25°C)	834	1.5	1.0
100°F (37.7°C)	612	1.5	1.0

liquid or aerosolized form. Dermal contact can be direct or indirect via contact with vapors. Inhalational exposure is via vapor phase of the material or through inhalation of aerosolized material during spraying. Volatility of the isocyanate directly influences toxicity (9–12).

MDI and polyether polyol are frequently used in the formation of urethane foams. The polyol is used to react with the MDI to form a prepolymer, polymethylene polyphenylisocyanate (PAPI) (Fig. 44.8). MDI is manufactured from the condensation of aniline and formaldehyde to form methylene dianiline. This is then reacted with phosgene to form MDI. PAPI is a thick amber gel with little or no volatility and very low toxicity (9).

Exposure hazard of isocyanates is directly related to volatility and molecular weight. Isocyanates with low volatility and larger molecular weight such as MDI and PAPI are much less toxic than highly volatile, low molecular weight isocyanates such as TDI or methyl isocyanate (MIC) (9). The vapor pressures of MDI and PAPI are significantly less in comparison to the vapor pressure of TDI. Since vapor pressure is directly related to

Table 44.3. Common Isocyanates

Toluene diisocyanate (TDI)
Hexamethylene diisocyanate (HDI)
Methylene diphenyl diisocyanate (MDI)
Naphthalene diisocyanate (NDI)
Polymethylene polyphenyl isocyanate (PAPI)
Para-tolyl monoisocyanate (PTI)
Dicyclohexyl methane-4,4-diisocyanate (DMDJ)
Triphenyl methane-4,4',4"-triisocyanate
Isophorone diisocyanate (IPDI)

Diphenyl methane 4,4'-diisocyanate $OCN-\bigcirc-C-\bigcirc-NCO$

Polymethylene polyphenyl isocyanate (PAPI) $OCN-\bigcirc-C-\bigcirc-C-\bigcirc-NCO$
NCO $_{N=0-2}$

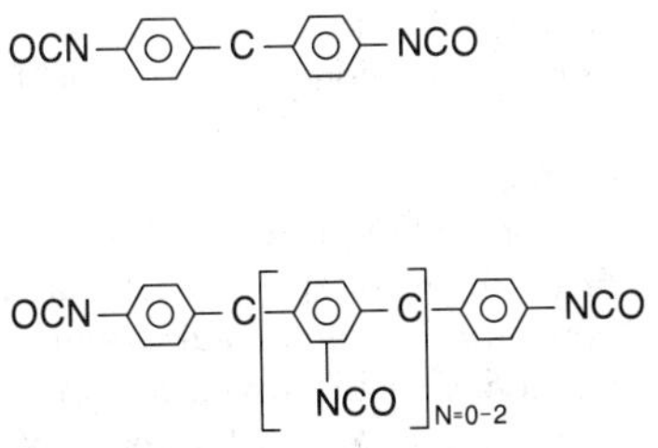

Figure 44.8.

inhalation potential, the pulmonary exposure to PAPI and MDI is less than TDI and would occur only if the material were heated to vaporization or aerosolized (Table 44.4).

Since the isocyanates with higher molecular weight and lower volatility are less toxic, health effects and exposure hazards from polyisocyanates tend to be much less. The low molecular weight and highly volatile MIC and TDI are dermal and pulmonary irritants and can produce severe pulmonary damage in concentrated forms (10–13). The higher molecular weight and less volatile MDI and PAPI are much less toxic than TDI and MIC. The dermal toxicity of MDI and PAPI is limited to mild irritation and requires direct contact.

The respiratory system is the main target organ for isocyanate toxicity and occurs via particle formation or vaporization of the isocyanates. This volatilization can occur with increasing temperatures. Reasonable estimations of the respiratory exposure hazard from isocyanates is based on molecular weight, volatility, ambient temperatures, and the airborne concentration reaching the breathing zone of the individual. If the breathing zone concentration is over 0.5 ppm then pulmonary toxicity is more likely (12). The higher the dose and the longer the exposure, the quicker respiratory symptoms will develop. Usually, with an exposure exceeding 0.5 ppm, symptoms may begin within a few hours (12). Traditionally, these symptoms consist of cough, pleuritis, wheezing, and chest tightness. If concentrations are high enough, pulmonary edema and hemorrhagic alveolitis may occur. This type of exposure results in pulmonary pathology evident within 4–8 hours postexposure. The allergic manifestation of isocyanate exposure in terms of asthma do not occur until reexposure.

Previous human exposures in the medical literature to either TDI or MDI have been in the monomeric form. The main form of MDI used industrially is in the prepolymeric form (polymeric-MDI) or PAPI (Fig. 44.8). This material is a mixture of bifunctional monomers (45–55%) with the remainder being three- and four-ring homologues having three or four NCO groups per molecule. Most of the industrial hygiene work on human exposure standards to isocyanates and diisocyanates has been confined to the monomer form, and not prepolymers. There is ample clinical and experimental evidence that TDI and MDI monomers produce dermal and pulmonary disease in the form of allergic contact dermatitis, pulmonary hypersensitivity, pneumonitis, and asthma (13–17). The medical literature further reflects that MDI monomers and polymers have

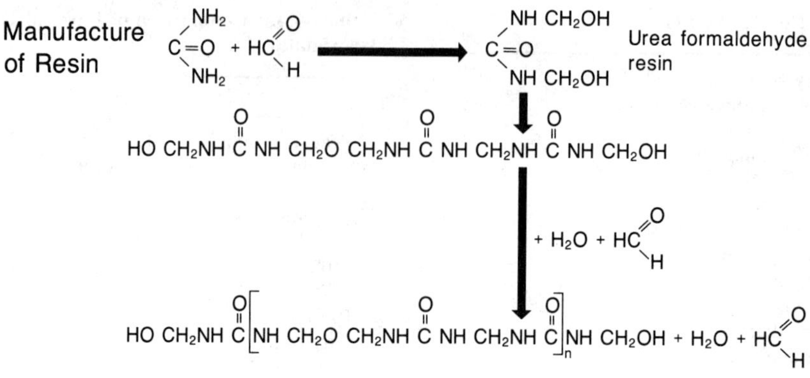

Figure 44.9. Urea-formaldehyde.

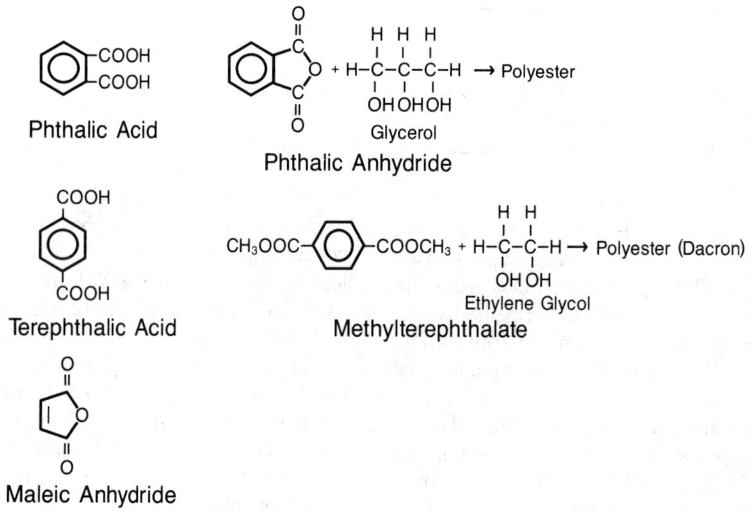

Figure 44.10. Dibasic acids and polyester formation.

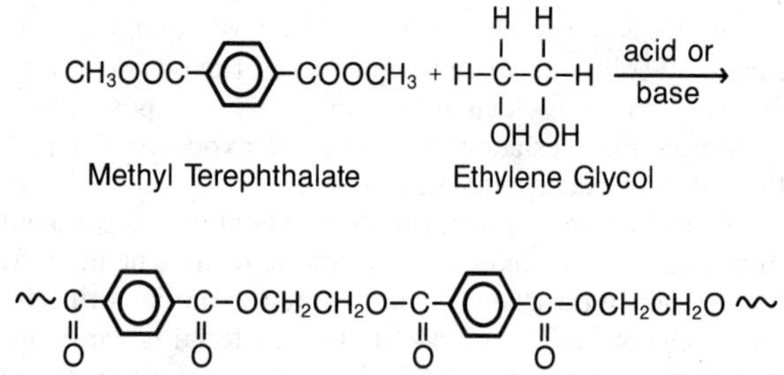

Figure 44.11. Polyester (Dacron).

an impressive safety record in industrial exposures even though direct chronic and longterm exposures are associated with decrements in forced expiratory volume (over 1 second) [FEV_1], forced vital capacity [FVC], and diffusion capacity. However, given adequate safety controls, MDI workers do not demonstrate $FEV_{1.0}$ decrements (18, 19).

OSHA recommends an exposure standard for both TDI and MDI of 0.005 ppm for a time-weighted average (TWA). There

is also a ceiling value of 0.02 ppm recommended for TDI. A ceiling limit cannot be violated at any time. Exposure limits exist only for diisocyanates. Exposure limits for the prepolymeric forms of diisocyanates such as PAPI do not exist, since their volatility is so low and toxicity hazard is minimal (13, 20).

In general, isocyanates are irritants to the skin, cause contact and allergic dermatitis, and are irritants to the mucous membranes. Concentrated forms of the more volatile isocyanates such as TDI and MIC can produce chemical bronchitis and acute asthma at room temperatures in addition to inflammatory changes in the airways. Sensitization to isocyanates in an occupational setting can result in asthma recurring or reexposure to even low concentrations of the same or similar compound (17). The less volatile MDI can produce similar disease on heating.

There is evidence that the exposure level is an important factor in respiratory sensitization and the subsequent development of occupational asthma—thus the importance of prevention. Sensitized workers may develop symptoms of cough, wheezing, and chest tightness even with low levels of exposure upon reexposure. Chronic airway hyperreactivity may persist even after removal from exposure. Other concerns in the pro-

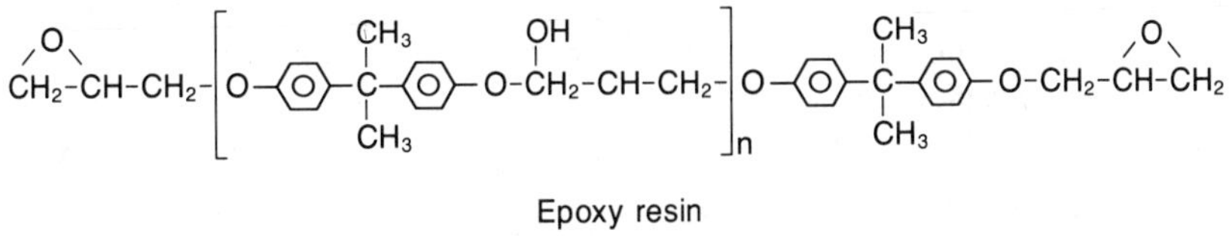

Epoxy resin

when n = 0, molecular weight = 340
n = 1, molecular weight = 624
n = 2, molecular weight = 908
n = 3, molecular weight = 1,192

Figure 44.12. Molecular formula of epoxy resin.

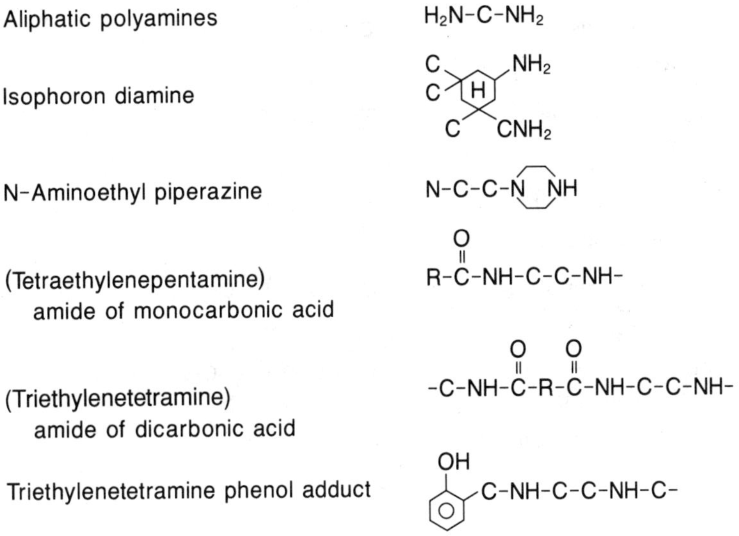

Figure 44.13. Epoxy resin hardeners.

duction and handling of polyurethanes include exposure to chlorinated and fluorinated solvents during batch preparation and curing. Many of the catalysts used are also potent irritants. Thermal decomposition products of polyurethanes, including free isocyanates, hydrogen cyanide, and carbon monoxide, are very hazardous.

Material handling and process ventilation are the key steps in preventing exposures during manufacturing. Proper eye, skin, and respiratory protection are critical in preventing overexposure to isocyanates. Periodic medical surveillance for possible respiratory or skin effects will help ensure the adequacy of these measures in limiting exposure.

AMINO RESINS

The amino resins are thermoset materials used primarily in adhesives, coatings, and insulating materials. These are formed by a reaction of formaldehyde with an amino group from either urea or melamine (Fig. 44.9). The controlled polymerization reaction occurs in the presence of an acid catalyst and heat, with the evolution of water and formaldehyde. Amino resins are supplied as liquids, air-dried solids, or powders.

Exposure to formaldehyde is the main health hazard in the production and use of the amino resins. Formaldehyde is a respiratory and mucous membrane irritant, but may also cause nonspecific symptoms of headache and fatigue. Formaldehyde is also an animal carcinogen and is suspected of being a human carcinogen. The release of formaldehyde from finished products, such as plywood and urea-formaldehyde insulation, may contribute to air quality problems in new buildings (21). Urea-formaldehyde insulation was banned from home use in 1982. Thermal decomposition products include carbon monoxide, formaldehyde, ammonia, and cyanide.

Proper ventilation is important in reducing formaldehyde levels in virtually any use of amino resins. Skin contact should also be avoided to prevent skin irritation or cutaneous sensitization.

POLYESTERS

The basic building components of polyesters are dibasic carboxylic acids (phthalic acids) and anhydrides (Fig. 44.10). Carboxylic acids react with alcohols to form esters. Polyesters are formed when carboxylic acids react with compounds con-

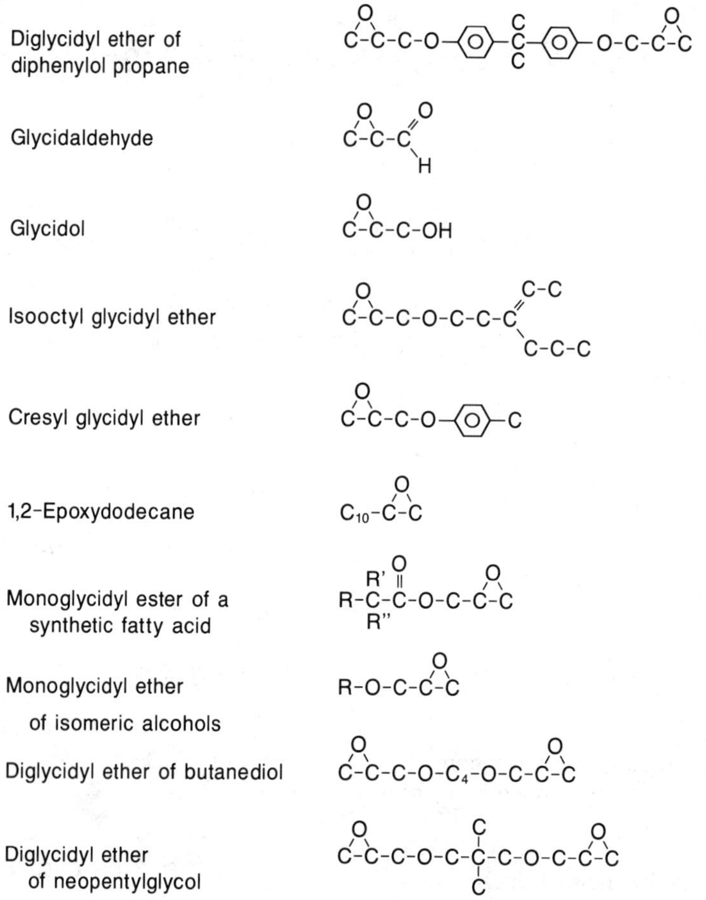

Diglycidyl ether of
diphenylol propane

Glycidaldehyde

Glycidol

Isooctyl glycidyl ether

Cresyl glycidyl ether

1,2-Epoxydodecane

Monoglycidyl ester of a
synthetic fatty acid

Monoglycidyl ether
of isomeric alcohols

Diglycidyl ether of butanediol

Diglycidyl ether
of neopentylglycol

Figure 44.14. Epoxy reactive diluents.

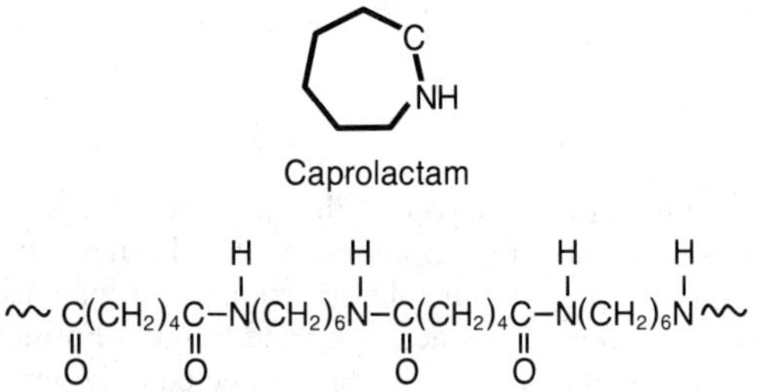

Caprolactam

Figure 44.15. Polyamide (nylon).

taining more than one −OH group. Polyesters include saturated resins, polyethylene terephthalate (PET), and polybutylene terephthalate (PBT) used in containers, coatings, and fabrics. These are formed through a polycondensation reaction of an acid (dimethyl terephthalate, DMT) and an alcohol (ethylene glycol or 1,4-butanediol) (Fig. 44.11).

Unsaturated polyesters are formed from dibasic acids (phthalic or maleic anhydride) and glycol. Styrene is used as a cross-linking agent, and a filler such as fiberglass is also added. The unsaturated polyesters are used in boat hulls, paneling, shower stalls, and automotive bodies. These may be molded or applied by spraying or by hand.

Polyesters do not cause dermatologic or respiratory irritation or sensitization, although their basic building components can. The major hazard in the application of unsaturated polyesters as reinforced plastics is exposure to styrene vapor, particularly during spraying. These operations require the use of proper ventilation and respiratory protection.

EPOXY RESINS

Epoxy resins are formed by the reaction of epichlorhydrin (C_3H_5OCl) and a diglycidyl ether ($C_6H_{10}O_3$) of the bisphenol-A type. Epoxies are used primarily for protective coatings and laminates for metals, woods, and other plastics. Other uses include adhesives and bonding agents, flooring, and reinforced plastics for electrical and tooling applications. The main health hazard of exposure to epoxies is allergic dermal or respiratory sensitization, usually to low molecular weight oligomers of the cured resin (molecular weight = 340) (21). Contact allergies to epoxy resins usually develop following months of exposure. The majority of cases are due to contact with the 340 molecular weight oligomer (Fig. 44.12) (21). The epoxy system consists of a resin, a curing agent (hardener), and a reactive compound. Epoxy resins are used as glues, floor coverings, and paints and coatings. Epoxy resins vary in molecular weight. A low molecular weight resin is below 1000 and is a liquid. High molecular weight resins are greater than 1000 and are typically solids. Resins are made up of oligomers with differing molecular weights. The primary sensitizing oligomer in bisphenol-A resins has a molecular weight of 340 (21). Oligomers of molecular weight 624 are less sensitizing, and those of molecular weight 908 are not sensitizing (21).

Hardeners are curing agents and are usually amines such as aliphatic polyamines (diethylenetetramine, triethylenetetramine, trimethylhexamethylenediamine) are are potent sensitizing agents (Fig. 44.13) (21). Sometimes, cycloaliphatic polyamines are used as curing agents. Hardeners include aliphatic and cycloaliphatic amines, which are strong irritants as well as sensitizers. Amine-curing chemicals are dermal and pulmonary sensitizers. The lower molecular weight aliphatic amines have greater volatility and a much greater chance to contact skin and the airway. Epoxy reactive diluents are also strong sensitizers (Fig. 44.14). Diglycidyl ether is a liquid used as a diluent for epoxy resins and causes ocular, respiratory, and skin irritation. Exposure of the liquid to skin can produce severe damage.

Epichlorhydrin, a curing agent, reacts with nucleic acids and has been shown to induce chromosomal aberrations in lymphocytes of exposed workers. Epichlorhydrin is a liquid and a strong irritant. Dermal contact produces a vesiculated burn and can result in sensitization. Pulmonary exposure to vapor or liquid can result in pneumonitis.

NYLON

Nylon polymers are polyamides formed by either the polymerization of a lactam (caprolactam) (Fig. 44.15) or the reaction of an amine and a dibasic acid. A major use of nylon is in the production of fibers and filaments for textiles and furnishings. Molded compounds are used in automotives, housewares, and appliances. The raw materials are respiratory and skin irritants. Most reductions take place in closed systems. Nylon compounds are a rare cause of allergic sensitization.

CELLULOSICS

Cellulosics are formed by the chemical modification of naturally occurring polymers from wood and cotton. They are used for films, sheeting, tools, and personal items (brushes, pens). Exposure to organic raw wood and cotton fibers may cause allergic respiratory problems. A major hazard with the use of cellulose nitrate films is the formation of high levels of nitrogen oxides with thermal decomposition.

ADDITIVES

Over 500 organic and inorganic compounds are added to plastic materials to alter their physical and chemical properties. There is limited toxicologic information on many of these compounds,

requiring a continuing attention to worker health. Additives include plasticizers, colorants, fillers, foaming agents, asbestos, stabilizers, and flame retardants. Past work practices may also influence worker health, particularly the past use of asbestos and silica as fillers. A detailed assessment of additives used is critical in determining the potential hazard of a specific operation.

REFERENCES

1. Malten KE. Problems in the production and processing of plastics. Chapter 31 in: Maibach H, ed. Occupational & industrial dermatology. 2nd ed. Chicago: Year Book Medical Publishers, 1987.
2. Eckardt RE, Hindin R. The health hazards of plastics. Occup Med 1973;15:808–818.
3. Vainio H, Pfaffli P, Zitting A. Chemical hazards in the plastics industry. J Toxicol Environ Health 1980;6:259–266.
4. Jarvisalo J, Pfaffli P, Vaino H, eds. Industrial hazards of plastics and synthetic elastomers. New York: Alan R. Liss, 1984.
5. Apfeldorf R, Infante PF. Review of epidemiologic study results of vinyl chloride-related compounds. Environ Health Perspect 1981;41:221–235.
6. International Agency for Research on Cancer. IARC monographs on the evaluation of the carcinogenic risk of chemicals to humans. Vol 19. Some monomers, plastics and synthetic elastomers, and acrolein. Lyon: International Agency for Research on Cancer, 1979.
7. Tossavainen A. Styrene use and occupational exposure in the plastics industry. Scand J Work Environ Health 1978;2:7–13.
8. National Institute for Occupational Safety and Health. Criteria for a recommended standard . . . occupational exposure to decomposition products of fluorocarbon polymers. Cincinnati, OH: Department of Health, Education and Welfare (NIOSH), 1977.
9. Woolrich PF, Rye WA. Urethanes: engineering, medical control and toxicologic considerations. J Occup Med 1969;11:184–190.
10. Musk AW, Peters JM, Wegman DH. Isocyanates and respiratory disease: current status. Am J Ind Med 1988;13:331–349.
11. Bernstein IL. Isocyanate-induced pulmonary diseases: a current perspective. J Allergy Clin Immunol 1982;70:24–31.
12. Rye WA. Human responses to isocyanate exposure. J Occup Med 1973;15:306–307.
13. Rando RJ, Abdel-Kader H, Hughes J, Hammad YY. Toluene diisocyanate exposure in the flexible polyurethane foam industry. Am Ind Hyg Assoc J 1987;48:580–585.
14. Malo JL, Zeiss R. Occupational hypersensitivity pneumonitis after exposure to diphenylmethane diisocyanate. Am Rev Respir Dis 1982;125:113–116.
15. Banks DE, Butcher BT, Salvaggio JE. Isocyanate-induced respiratory disease. Ann Allergy 1986;57:389–396.
16. Baur X, Dewair M, Rommelt H. Acute airway obstruction followed by hypersensitivity pneumonitis in an isocyanate (MDI) worker. J Occup Med 1984;26:285–287.
17. Mapp CE, Vecchio LD, Boschetto P, Fabbri LM. Combined asthma and alveolitis due to diphenylmethane diisocyanate (MDI) with demonstration of no crossed respiratory reactivity to toluene diisocyanate (TDI). Ann Allergy 1985;54:424–429.
18. Olsen GW, Shellenberger R, Bodner KM, et al. An epidemiologic investigation of forced expiratory volume at 1 second and respiratory symptoms among employees of a toluene diisocyanate production plant. J Occup Med 1989;31:664–667.
19. Musk AW, Peters JM, Berstein L. Absence of respiratory effects in subjects exposed to low concentrations of TDI and MDI: a reevaluation. J Occup Med 1985;27:917–920.
20. Silk SJ, Hardy JL. Control limits for isocyanates. Ann Occup Hyg 1983;27:333–339.
21. Fregert S. Contact dermatitis from epoxy resin systems, chapter 32 in: Maibach H, ed. Occupational & industrial dermatology. 2nd ed. Chicago: Year Book Medical Publishers, 1987.

45

Chemical Hazards in the Tire and Rubber Manufacturing Industry

John B. Sullivan, Jr., M.D.
Mark Van Ert, Ph.D., C.I.H.
Richard Lewis, M.D., M.P.H.

INTRODUCTION TO RUBBER INDUSTRY HAZARDS

The production of rubber products involves a mixture of complex chemicals to which workers may be exposed. In addition to the multiple chemicals used in rubber production, there are many byproduct chemicals produced by the various processes and reactions.

It was in the early part of the 19th century that the rubber industry began in the United States. The vulcanization process discovered by Charles Goodyear in 1839 (using sulfur and heat to cross-link natural rubber molecules) as well as the use of additives to improve processing led to a demand for rubber products that exceeded supplies. By the end of the 19th century, rubber plants were being exported from Brazil to plantations in southeast Asia, Sri Lanka, Indonesia, Liberia, and Zaire. These countries remain the primary producers of natural rubber today.

The growth of the petrochemical industry and advances in polymer technology, coupled with shortages of natural rubber during World War II, led to the creation of the synthetic rubber industry in the 1940s.

Finished rubber products consist of basic elastomers plus a multitude of chemical additives. The increasing demand for both natural and synthetic rubber has resulted in an increase in the production of processing chemicals. Consumption of rubber is expected to increase by 11% up to 12.1 million metric tons annually before 1993 (1). Today, the demand for synthetic rubber is outpacing the demand for natural rubber. The fastest growing demand will be for ethylene-propylene-diene rubber. Demand for styrene-butadiene synthetic rubber (SBR) was 2.38 million metric tons in 1988 and is expected to reach 2.62 million metric tons by 1993 (1). SBR latex demand will increase to an expected 1.45 million metric tons in 1993.

Four types of synthetic rubbers have become widely used since 1950: (a) styrene-butadiene, (b) butyl rubber, (c) nitrile rubber, and (d) polychloroprene. Other synthetic rubbers are polysulfide, polyurethane, and ethylene-propylene-diene. SBR is used mainly in tire production and is the most commonly used rubber in the world. There were 211 million tires produced in 1988 (1). Approximately $2 billion will be spent on tire manufacturing capacity in 1992 in the United States alone.

In concert with the steady growth in output of the various rubber products, the output of rubber-processing chemicals is expected to be more than 400 million pounds by the end of 1989 (1). These chemicals impart the desirable characteristics for the final rubber product. Tire manufacturing remains the leading consumer of nearly half of all natural and synthetic rubber produced annually. This industry employs over one-half million workers in nearly 400 plants around the world. A single tire may require

the use of several hundred raw materials. Workers' exposures may vary, not only with different jobs within a plant, but with changes in production techniques and material use over time. Many changes have occurred in the industry over the years with regard to the kinds of chemicals used as well as the processes used to manufacture rubber (2).

Natural rubber is obtained from plants, especially the *Hevea braziliensis* tree, native to the Amazon region of South America. Preliminary processing involves filtering to remove dirt and debris and coagulation with formic and acetic acids. The rubber is then rolled into sheets, cut and cured with either smoke or sodium bisulfite bleach, and then formed into bales for shipping (3).

The production of natural rubber shares many of the occupational health hazards of other agricultural industries. These include use of sharp cutting implements, exposure to pesticides (including sodium arsenite), and risk of tropical diseases in endemic areas. The acids and caustics used in processing are potential respiratory and skin irritants. Increasing use of processing equipment requires careful attention to safety practices to prevent worker injuries.

The basic ingredient of synthetic rubber is polymeric material (elastomer) similar to plastic resin. Rubber in its crude state is lacking in strength and resiliency. Cross-linking using sulfur or sulfur donors during the vulcanization process creates a durable, pliable thermoset material.

The manufacturing of synthetic rubber involves the use of large volumes of raw materials. Polymerization of rubber ingredients takes place in enclosed vessels. Leaks from these vessels and maintenance operations, such as the cleaning of reaction vessels and maintenance of distribution pipes have been major sources of exposure in the past, prior to implementation of proper venting and respiratory protection measures.

Cis-1,4-polyisoprene is the basic natural rubber. Styrene-butadiene rubber (SBR), a major synthetic rubber used in tire manufacturing, is produced through an emulsion polymerization reaction of aqueous styrene and gaseous butadiene. Unreacted monomers are recycled. The latex polymer is coagulated with sulfuric acid and dried prior to shipping. Other chemicals may be added, such as carbon black, antioxidants, and curing agents, depending on the intended end use of the product (2).

Overexposure to unreacted styrene monomer can result in central nervous system effects of giddiness, loss of coordination, and possible liver damage. Worker exposure to 1,3-butadiene can result in mucous membrane and respiratory irritation at high concentrations; it is also a suspected human carcinogen.

Neoprene (polychloroprene) combines the mechanical properties of natural rubber with increased resistance to aging, oils, and chemicals. Neoprene is used in belts, hoses, footwear,

Table 45.1. Basic Chemical Groups Used in the Rubber Industry

Elastomers (natural or synthetic)
Fillers
Antidegradents
Vulcanizing agents
Solvents
Acceleraters
Activators
Retarders
Reinforcing agents
Pigments and dyes
Antitack agents
Bonding agents
Miscellaneous chemicals

gloves, and low voltage insulation. Chloroprene (2-chloro-1,3-butadiene) is flammable, and exposure to high concentrations of unreacted monomers as well as partially polymerized intermediates may produce narcosis, respiratory and skin irritation, alopecia, and liver and kidney damage.

Other synthetic rubbers include butyl (isobutylene-isoprene polymers), nitrile (NBR) copolymers of acrylonitrile and butadiene, and polyurethane. Acrylonitrile is a respiratory and mucous membrane irritant, and overexposure can produce cyanide poisoning. Acrylonitrile is a suspected human carcinogen (2).

INDUSTRY PROCESS AND REACTIONS

The rubber industry work environment is quite diverse with respect to physical and chemical exposures. Hundreds of different chemicals are used as rubber additives in the process of manufacturing rubber products (2). These chemicals are grouped into various functional categories (Table 45.1). The major reinforcement and filler materials are carbon black and amorphous silica, although asbestos-containing materials have been used in the past. Vulcanizing agents include sulfur, zinc oxide, stearic acid, and other sulfide and sulfur compounds. Thiurams, thiocarbamates, and various amine and aldehyde compounds are used as accelerators to increase the rate of rubber curing. Additional additives include activators (soaps and fatty acids), extenders (mineral oils), plasticizers (phthalates), antioxidants (amines, quinones), and pigments.

The basic production stages in the manufacturing of rubber tires and tubes are presented in Fig. 45.1 and summarized below. Descriptions for each of these processes are as follows (Table 45.2):

1. Raw material handling, compounding, and mixing;
2. Milling;
3. Extruding and calendering;
4. Component assembly and building;
5. Curing or vulcanizing;
6. Inspection, repair, and finishing;
7. Storage and dispatch.

Raw Materials Handling

The initial step in product fabrication involves weighing and mixing (compounding) various additives with either natural or synthetic rubber. The manual weighing and filling of hoppers results in generation of dust. Additives may be in the form of powders, flakes, or pellets and are supplied in bags or drums.

Carbon black and occasionally zinc oxide arrive in bulk form, either in tankers or metal containers. Antioxidant and other oils are usually received in 55-gallon drums or tank cars. Exposure to dusts or vapors may occur during the handling of these raw materials. Compounding and mixing of materials may be a dusty process, especially when clinical agents stored in open drums and bags are weighed and transferred for mixing in the Banbury units (2).

Raw rubber and other additives are usually fed into a mixer or Banbury unit by conveyor or manual process. These components are mixed together under pressure between the rotors and against the walls of the chamber. The chamber is usually water cooled to reduce heat. However, in some operations, the chamber may be steam heated to reduce the viscosity of the mixture. Retarders, antidegradents, processing oils, reinforcing agents, and fillers are often added to the raw rubber stock at this stage (2).

Milling

The mixer drops its batch of mixed rubber directly onto the rollers of a discharge mill where further mixing takes place. This mixture is then cooled to between 65–80°C and often transferred to other mills for further processing. Local exhaust ventilation is frequently employed to collect fumes and vapors which arise from the process. Workers may be exposed to vapors, aerosols from the hot rubber, and to dust from incompletely mixed additives or other compounding agents added on mix mills.

Rubber comes off the mill in a continuous sheet which is fed by a conveyor to a dip which prevents the rubber from sticking together. Mineral dust (talc and soapstone) slurries are commonly used as antisticking agents. The newly dipped or detackified rubber sheet is dried, folded, and placed on pallets and, in the case of the first stage rubber, it is stored. After this stage rubber is ready for fabrication to the components from which a tire is built.

Rubber stock is heated and remilled to obtain softness and plasticity for further processing. Time and temperature of the milling process governs the chemical reactions within the batch, thus determining the properties of the finished material. As previously described, during the formation of rubber sheets, the uncured rubber is coated with an antitack agent to reduce sticking. In the past, talc (either in a dry or slurry form) was used extensively for this purpose but has now been replaced by the use of amorphous silica and liquid soaps. The rubber stock is cooled in dip tanks generating steam.

All of these operations result in potential exposure to reaction products from heated but unvulcanized rubber stock. In addition, there is potential exposure to dust such as talc or soapstone from the antitack agents.

Extruding and Calendering

The tread and sidewall of a tire are produced by an extrusion process. In the manufacture of tread for tires, the milled rubber sheet is extruded through a die corresponding to specific tread dimensions and weight. It is then cut into specified lengths, and the ends joined manually or automatically with cement at a tire building station.

Rubber sheet may also be formed into plystock by calendering. Steel cord and fabrics (nylon, rayon, polyesters, and fiberglass) may be pretreated using a phenol-formaldehyde solution to improve adhesion.

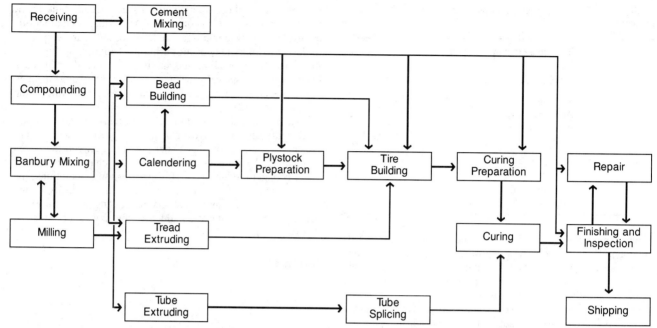

Figure 45.1.   Production stages in manufacturing of tires and tubes. Adapted with permission from Williams T, et al. Worker exposure to chemical agents in the manufacture of rubber tires and tubes: particulates. Am Ind Hyg Assoc J 1980;41:204–211.

The tread and sidewalls of a tire can be manufactured separately or in the same operation. The tread/sidewall extruder laminates the two types of strip to form a tire tread and sidewalls. Strips are bonded by heat and pressure generated by a rotating extruder screw. The tread and sidewall may also be formed separately in similar types of production lines. Extrusion temperatures are in the range of 80°C and may result in volatilization of constituents that are applied earlier in the mixing of the rubber. The extruder operator may also be exposed to volatile organic compounds used at the tread-end cement station or other nearby operations. After extrusion, the tread is sometimes cooled in a water bath and dipped in a solvent bath. Solvents typically used in this phase of the tire building include naphtha, heptane, hexane, isopropanol, and toluene. The continuous rubber tread is then cut into specified lengths and the tread ends tackified. Tackification usually involves applying a cement containing dissolved rubber and solvents (naphtha and toluene) on the tread ends. Local exhaust ventilation may be available to control solvent vapor exposure.

Calendering is the operation that produces plys and belts which form the body of the tire and give it its strength and stability. Plys and belts are composed of rubber reinforcements of fabric, steel wire, or glass fiber. Plys, belts, and liners are made of a calender, a multiple roll mill that produces stock of carefully controlled thickness. A rolled fabric, normally rayon or some other synthetic fiber, is spliced either by adhesive or a high speed sewing machine onto the end of a previously processed roll. This continuous sheet of fabric is then dipped under controlled tension into a tank containing latex. Solutions of formaldehyde, caustic soda, and resorcinol, or other synthetic adhesive combinations may be added to the latex at this point. After dipping, the fabric travels past either rotating meter bars or vacuum suction lines and then through a drying oven to remove excess solvent. The latex-dipped fabric is then passed through a calendering machine which impregnates it with rubber. Temperature during the calendering operation is 70–80°C.

Potential toxins emitted from this process are similar in character to those from milling or extrusion.

Tire Building and Component Assembly

Rubber ties represent combinations of many different rubber components. Tires are assembled on a drum combining ply stock, beads, sidewalls, and other components. The surface of the components may be treated with solvent, primarily naphtha, during the tire-building process. Many rubber products, such as hoses, are already formed into their final shape prior to curing. Tires are sprayed with a mold release agent and placed into steel molds to impart the final shape and surface characteristics during the curing process.

Passenger car tires are built as cylinders on a collapsible rotating drum. First, the inner liner is wrapped around the drum followed by a variable number of rubber impregnated fabric plys. Next, the edges of the fabric and inner liner are wrapped around the bead assemblies. Then, pressure is applied manually or automatically from the tread center out to the bead in order to expel air trapped between the assembled components. Belts made of fabric, steel, or glass fiber are laid onto the cord, and finally the tread and sidewall components are wrapped around the assembled components and are bonded. Organic solvents such as naphtha, heptane, hexane, isopropanol, methanol, and toluene may be used during the building to tackify the rubberized components. Potential sources of human exposure at such stations occur during solvent application and the handling of green (uncured) tire components.

Curing or Vulcanizing

Prior to curing, the assembled unvulcanized part is inspected and repaired if necessary. The tire is then placed in a ventilated booth where it is sprayed on the inside with lubricants and on the outside with release agents, which prevent the tire from

Table 45.2. Summary Description of Major Work Areas (Occupational Title Groups)

1. Shipping and receiving—Receiving unloads and stores all incoming ingredients that go into making the final product, e.g., carbon black, pigments, rubber, etc. Shipping stores and loads the final product (e.g., tires) into trucks or boxcars.
2. Compounding and mixing, cutting and milling: Cement mixing—Raw ingredients (rubber, fillers, oils, pigments) are weighed and mixed together in a Banbury (BB) mixer. Environmental exposure to particulates (e.g., carbon black, accelerators, antioxidants, talc) is high. Cements are solvents such as paraffin HC (e.g., hexane), aromatic hydrocarbons (e.g., toluene, xylene), chlorinated HC (e.g., CCl_4, trichloroethylene), ketones (e.g., methyl ethyl ketone).
3. Mill-mixing: Service to batch preparation—Mill-mixing is a largely superseded mixing process. Service jobs are for the compounding and mixing operations. Environmental exposures are similar to Compounding and Mixing.
4. Milling—Rubber mix from BB is processed further under heat and pressure, till rubber is in a soft, plastic state. This is probably the first work area where there is substantial exposure to reaction products.
5. Calender, plystock handling—The rubber stock from the mill is rolled out into a sheet of controlled thickness, usually covering a fabric. The calender stock (plystock) is then cut and spliced for use in building the ply of the tire. There is some exposure to reaction products and solvents.
6. Tuber (extrusion), Tread Cementing—Rubber stock from a mill is forced through a die forming a tread or tube. The tread is cut in appropriate lengths and cemented with solvents on the cut end so as to be tacky.
7. Tire building, bead building—Beads are rubber-and-fabric-covered wire that in a finished tire rest on the rim of the wheel. The treads, beads, and plystock are used to build the tire. The major exposures are to solvents.
8. Green tire inspection, paint and line—The green (uncured) tire is inspected and repaired, and sprayed with solvents or lined with talc so it will not stick in the curing mold. Solvents and, in some cases, talc are the major environmental exposures.
9. Tube and flap building, valves—The tube from the extruder is cut, valves attached, the inside of the tube coated with talc and then spliced together. The major environmental exposure is to talc. Valve making involves adding a rubber patch to the valve. The rubber is cured, buffed, and sprayed with solvent to make it tacky.
10. Curing—The green uncured product (tire, tube) is cured under heat and pressure. The major environmental exposure is to reaction products, and, in tube curing, to talc.
11. Inspection, finishing, repair—The cured product is inspected (repaired if necessary) and made ready for shipping (finishing). Environmental exposures are in repairing (solvents, rubber dust).
12. Maintenance—This job group includes mechanics, pipefitters, electricians, welders, painters, carpenters.
13. Mechanical and special products—A variety of products and jobs are included in this group, most of them similar to machine shop types of exposures.
14. Reclaim operations—Scrap vulcanized rubber products are shredded, ground up, and "devulcanized." By the application of heat and chemicals, the rubber compound is restored to its original plastic state. Exposures are to particulates and chemicals.
15. Synthetic plant—This is essentially a chemical plant making elastomers that approximate one or more of the properties of natural rubber. SBR is the most important synthetic rubber. Others include neoprene, nitrile, ethylene-propylene-diene, etc. Exposures are to the gases or liquids that are the ingredients for the particular synthetic rubber being made.
16. Janitoring, trucking, power plant, etc.—This is a miscellaneous group with a variety of different jobs and exposures.

Adapted from McMichael AJ, Spirtas R, Gamble JF, Tousey PM. Mortality among rubber workers: relationship to specific jobs. J Occup Med 1976;18:178–185.

sticking to the mold after curing. Either organic-based lubricants or water-based suspensions of silicone solids may be used for outside sprays. Solvent-based lubricants may contain naphtha, hexane, heptane, isopropanol, and toluene. Evaporation of these solvents can contribute to human exposure.

The tire is then molded and vulcanized in a curing press. In this process, the tire is shaped, the tread design created, and chemical cross-linking of the rubber product triggered, allowing the tire to hold its shape. Curing usually takes 20–60 minutes at a temperature of 100–200°C. All freshly molded tires release substantial volumes of curing fumes into the work area and continue to do so as they are transported, usually by conveyor to the finishing and storage areas.

Finishing and Inspection

After vulcanization, tires are inspected for faults and may undergo further processing, such as grinding, trimming, repair, painting, and assembly. Potential occupational health hazards in the refinishing operations involve exposure to rubber dust, particularly from trimming, fumes from grinding, and solvent vapors from cleaning, patching and painting of blemishes.

Storage

Final rubber products can de-gas a variety of chemicals and chemical byproducts during storage, although concentrations are minimal compared to those generated during the cure operation.

CHEMICAL COMPOUNDS USED IN RUBBER COMPOUNDING

Types of Rubber Compounds

A multitude of chemical agents are used to produce the final rubber product. Elastomers, the basic polymers used in rubber manufacturing are divided into three functional classes:

1. General purpose;
2. Solvent resistant;
3. Heat resistant.

General purpose elastomers are the SBR type, butyl, natural rubber, and polybutadiene (Fig. 45.2). Chemical- and solvent-resistant elastomers are nitrile, polyurethanes, and polychloroprene (neoprene). Heat-resistant examples are silicone, polyethylene, and polyacrylates. Today, SBR is the major synthetic rubber produced which comprises about 40% of the world production and is the primary component of tires. Examples of synthetic rubber and their properties are shown in Table 45.3.

Vulcanizing Agents

Vulcanizing agents are necessary to induce cross-linking of rubber elastomers during the process of rubber manufacturing.

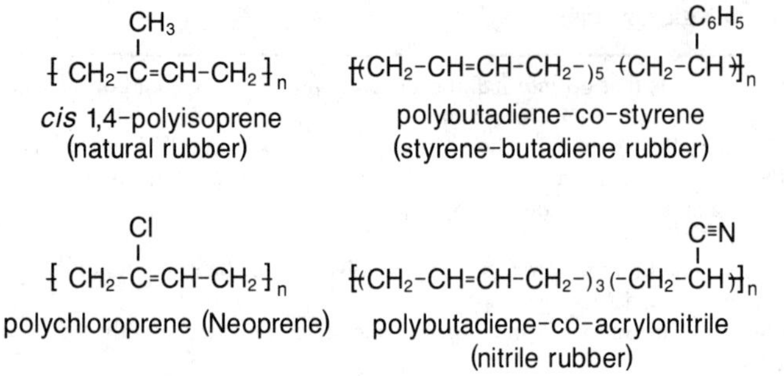

$$\begin{array}{c} CH_3 \\ | \\ \{CH_2\text{-}C\text{=}CH\text{-}CH_2\}_n \end{array}$$

cis 1,4-polyisoprene
(natural rubber)

$$\{CH_2\text{-}CH\text{=}CH\text{-}CH_2\text{-})_5 \; \begin{array}{c} C_6H_5 \\ | \\ \{CH_2\text{-}CH\}_n \end{array}$$

polybutadiene-co-styrene
(styrene-butadiene rubber)

$$\begin{array}{c} Cl \\ | \\ \{CH_2\text{-}C\text{=}CH\text{-}CH_2\}_n \end{array}$$

polychloroprene (Neoprene)

$$\{CH_2\text{-}CH\text{=}CH\text{-}CH_2\text{-})_3 \; \begin{array}{c} C\text{≡}N \\ | \\ (\text{-}CH_2\text{-}CH\}_n \end{array}$$

polybutadiene-co-acrylonitrile
(nitrile rubber)

Figure 45.2. International Agency for Research of Cancer Monograph Vol. 28: The rubber industry. IARC, 1982.

The most common vulcanizing agent in general purpose use is sulfur where both cross-links and cyclic structures are formed (2). Other common sulfur donors used are morpholine, dithiocarbamates, dithiophosphates, and tetraethylthiuram disulfide and tetramethylthiuram disulfide.

Other agents used in the vulcanization process are benzoyl peroxide, dicumyl peroxide, aromatic nitrogen compounds, dioximes, phenols, diisocyanates, and dinitroso compounds (3). Silicone rubber, which is fully saturated, cannot be vulcanized with sulfur. Instead, peroxides are necessary to achieve cross-linking by formation of free radicals on the polymer chain (2).

Accelerators

The reaction between sulfur donors and rubber is very slow, and to speed the process a group of chemicals termed accelerators is used (Table 45.4).

Accelerators function at curing temperatures of 140–200°C. Accelerators can be classified by their chemical structure, their rate of vulcanization, and also by their sulfur demand. Less active accelerators require large amounts of sulfur donors, while more active ones require a smaller quantity.

Slow accelerators are amines and thiourea derivaties. Moderately fast accelerators are sulfenamides, 1,3-diphenylguanidine, and mercaptobenzothiazole (MBT). Very fast accelerators are thiurams, dithiocarbamates, and thiophosphates (Figs. 45.3–45.6).

The variety of chemical structures range from primary, secondary, and tertiary amines, aldehydes, thiophosphates, di-

thiocarbamates, xanthates, sulfenamides, guanidines, thioureas, and benzothiazoles. The need for better accelerators has led to development of a benzothiazole class of chemicals, particularly 2-mercaptobenzothiazole (MBT), which accounts for 90% of the accelerators in use (2, 3). Reacting MBT with amines led to the production of sulfenamide accelerators. Cure rate and scorch safety (scorching devalues a product) are also important factors to consider in the choice of accelerators (2).

Studies have demonstrated that nitrosamines, suspect human carcinogens, are released when compounded rubber is heated as occurs in milling, calendering, and curing operations and are also present as contaminants in accelerator chemicals (Table 45.5; Fig. 45.7). The highest air concentrations of nitrosamines have been measured in curing areas. Changes in rubber formulations have helped to reduce or even eliminate these by-products. Nitrosamines are the result of the use of amines which are nitrosated by nitrogen oxides in the manufacturing process.

Activators

Activators are used to make accelerators more effective and speed the process of vulcanization. Activators are usually inorganic compounds and metal oxides such as zinc oxide, lead oxide, magnesium oxide, and sodium carbamate. Organic acids, such as stearic acid or lauric acid, are used to solubilize the metal oxides in the rubber mixture (2). The most common activator is zinc oxide.

Retarders

Retarders are mainly organic acids, anhydrides, and phthalimides; they delay the action of an accelerator. They are sometimes used to slow the vulcanization process. Also, accelerated rubber may cure prematurely, and retarders slow this process. Commonly used retarders are N-nitrosodiphenylamine, cyclohexylthiophthalimide, and a sulfonamide (2). Cyclohexylthiophthalimide degrades to phthalimide during the vulcanization process (Fig. 45.8) (2).

Antidegradants and Antioxidants

Since rubber deteriorates with aging by oxidation, antidegradants are usually incorporated in the final rubber products to

Table 45.3. Types of Synthetic Rubber

Styrene-butadiene (SBR)—The major synthetic rubber produced. Comprises 40% of the world's production. Weaker than natural rubber but ages more slowly.

Butyl rubber—Low permeability for air and gases. Used for inner tubes.

Nitrile rubber—Abrasion resistant. Resistant to penetration by chemicals, water, and oils.

Polyisoprene—Used mainly as blending component with other rubbers. Synthetic polyisoprene rubber contains a high percentage of cis-isoprene.

Polychloroprene—Known as neoprene. Flame resistant and wears longer than SBR. Possesses resistance to oil, solvent, and water penetration. Used mainly in the transportation industry and for sealants, cables, coatings, and adhesives.

Ethylene-propylene—Possesses resistance to ozone, sunlight, weather, and aging.

Silicone rubber—Resists degradation in temperature extremes. Used in aerospace industry and medical-surgical field.

Polyurethane—Used for coatings, insulation, packaging, and in automotive industry.

Polysulphide—Resistant to solvents and used in sealants in construction and building.

Chlorosulfonated polyethylene rubber—Used in cable covering.

Polyacrylic rubber—Plastic rubber that resists oils and aging. Used as seals and gaskets.

Fluroelastomers—High thermal stability. Used in aerospace industry.

Thermoplastic elastomers—Melt at high temperatures and resolidify on cooling without loss of elastic property.

Adapted with permission from IARC Monographs. Evaluation of the carcinogenic risk of chemicals to humans—the rubber industry. Volume 28. Switzerland: World Health Organization International Agency for Research of Cancer, 1982.

Table 45.4. Common Rubber Accelerators

Thiurams
  Tetramethylthiuram disulfide (TMTD)
  Tetraethlylthiuram disulfide (TETD)
  Dipentamethylenethiuram disulfide (PTD)
  Tetramethylthiuram monosulfide (TMTM)
Mercapto group
  2-Mercaptobenzothiazole (MBT)
  Cyclohexylbenzothiazolesulphenamide (CBS)
  Dibenzothiazoledisulfide (MBTS)
  Morpholinomercaptobenzothiazole (MMBT)
PPD group
  Phenylcyclohexyl-PPD (CPPD)
  Isopropylphenyl-PPD
  Isopropylaminodiphenylamine (IPPD)
  Diphenyl-PPD (DPPD)
  Diaminodiphenylmethane (DDM)
Naphthyl group
  Phenyl-beta-naphthylamine (PBN)
  sym-Di-beta-naphthyl-PPD (DBNPD)
Carbamates
  Zinc diethyldithiocarbamate (ZDC)
  Zinc dibutyldithiocarbamate (ZBC)
Miscellaneous
  1,3 Diphenylguanidine (DPG)
  Dithiodimorpholine (DOD)
  Monobenzyl ether of hydroquinone
  Butyraldehyde-aniline
  Ethylene thiourea

Adapted from Feinman SE. Sensitivity to rubber chemicals, Toxicol Cutan Ocul Toxicol 1987;6(2):117–153.

prevent or to slow oxidation processes. Oxidation can produce cross-linking of butadiene molecules, resulting in stiffness of rubber products. Antioxidants prevent the polymer chain from degrading. Naphthylamine antioxidants, used primarily in the past, were associated with bladder cancer and have been withdrawn from use. Current antioxidants include phenols, thioesters, and amines. Commonly used antioxidants are diphenylamines and dihydroquinolines. P-Phenylenediamine is useful in preventing degradation due to ozone. Antioxidants with phenolic structures fall into five classes: (a) phenols with varying side groups, (b) bisphenols with sidegroups, (c) thiobisphenols, (d) polyphenols, and (e) polyhydroxyphenols (3).

Processing Aids

Processing aids are used to make uncured rubber malleable and more easily mixed, extruded, or calendered. In the early years of rubber manufacturing, pine tars were used for this purpose, but they have been replaced by naphthenic and aromatic mineral oils (2). Aromatic processing oils are widespread in the rubber industry. Many rubber formulations contain as much as 20% or more of aromatic mineral oil with large amounts of polycyclic aromatic hydrocarbons (PAH) present in these oils. Mercaptan derivatives, thiophenols, or mercaptobenzothiazole may also be used to help soften rubber.

Reinforcing Agents

These are very important ingredients in rubber technology and add tensile strength and abrasion resistance to vulcanized rubber (2). The most important reinforcing agents are carbon black and amorphous silicas. Channel black became the carbon black most popular in rubber after 1942. Soon after this, the channel blacks were replaced by furnace blacks. Furnace blacks are manufactured from oil and contain polycyclic aromatic hydrocarbons.

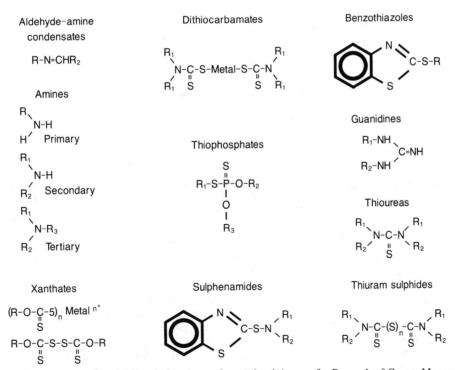

Figure 45.3. Accelerator types classified by chemical structure. International Agency for Research of Cancer Monograph Vol. 28: The rubber industry. IARC, 1982.

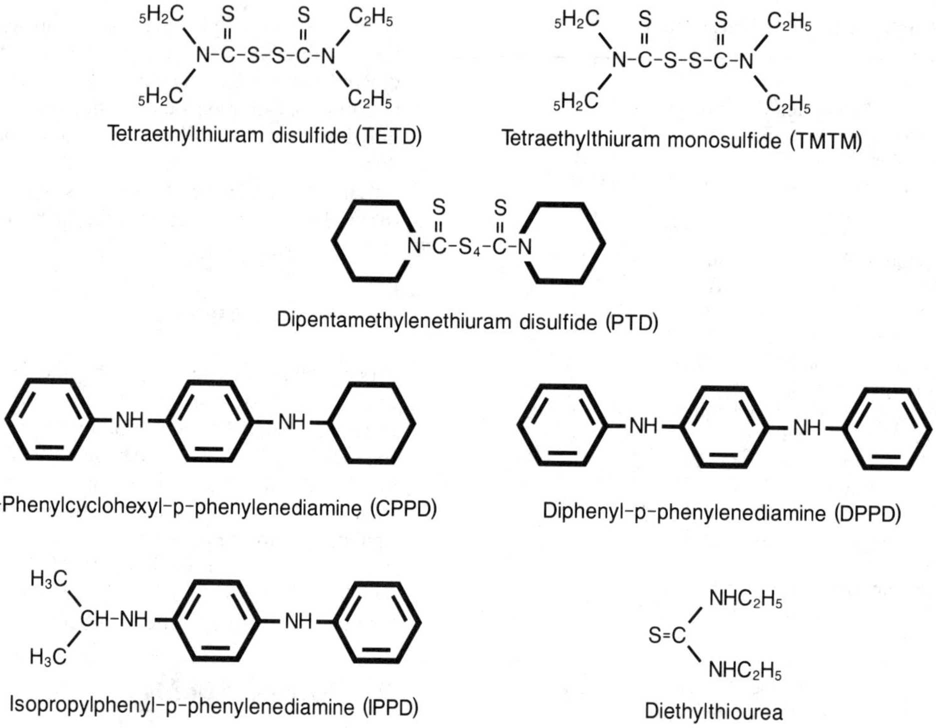

Tetraethylthiuram disulfide (TETD)

Tetraethylthiuram monosulfide (TMTM)

Dipentamethylenethiuram disulfide (PTD)

N-Phenylcyclohexyl-p-phenylenediamine (CPPD)

Diphenyl-p-phenylenediamine (DPPD)

Isopropylphenyl-p-phenylenediamine (IPPD)

Diethylthiourea

Figure 45.4. Thiurams. Adapted from Feinman SE. Sensitivity to rubber chemicals. J Toxicol Cutan Ocul Toxicol 1987;6:117–153.

Dithiocarbamates

Zinc diethyldithiocarbamate
(ZBC; Bis[diethyldithiocarbamato]zinc)

Zinc dibutyldithiocarbamate (ZBC)

Diphenylguanidine

Naphthyl Group Chemicals

Phenyl beta naphthylamine (PBN)

Sym-di-beta-Naphthyl paraphenylenediamine

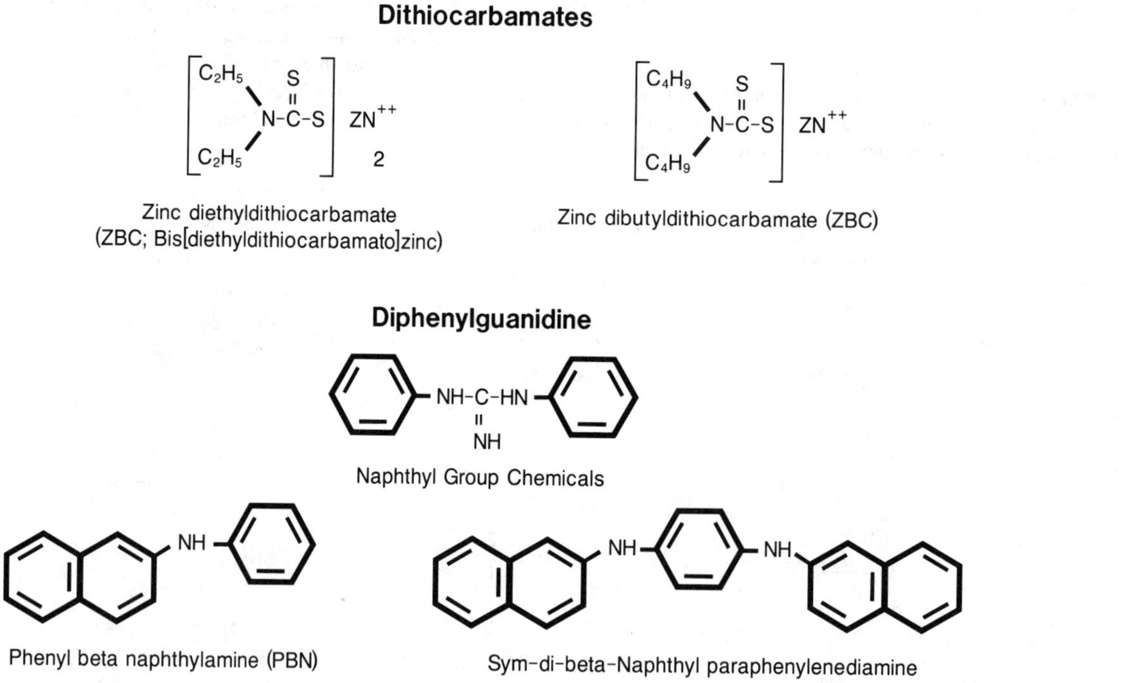

Figure 45.5. Dithiocarbamates and diphenylguanidine. Adapted from Feinman SE. Sensitivity to rubber chemicals. J Toxicol Cutan Ocul Toxicol 1987;6:117–153.

Miscellaneous Agents

A variety of other agents employed in the manufacture of rubber products are silicones, fluorinated hydrocarbons, polyethylene glycols, bonding agents, antitack agents, and a variety of organic solvents including aliphatic hydrocarbons, acetones, 1,1,1-trichloroethane, methyl ethyl ketone, methylene chloride, trichloroethylene, toluene, xylene, tetrahydrofuran, and dimethylformamide. Benzene, employed in the very early history of rubber manufacture, was replaced in the early 1940s with naphtha-type solvents. Flame retardants are added when heat resistance in a required property. These include clay fillers, ammonium phosphates, magnesium hydroxide, aluminum hydroxide, antimony oxide,

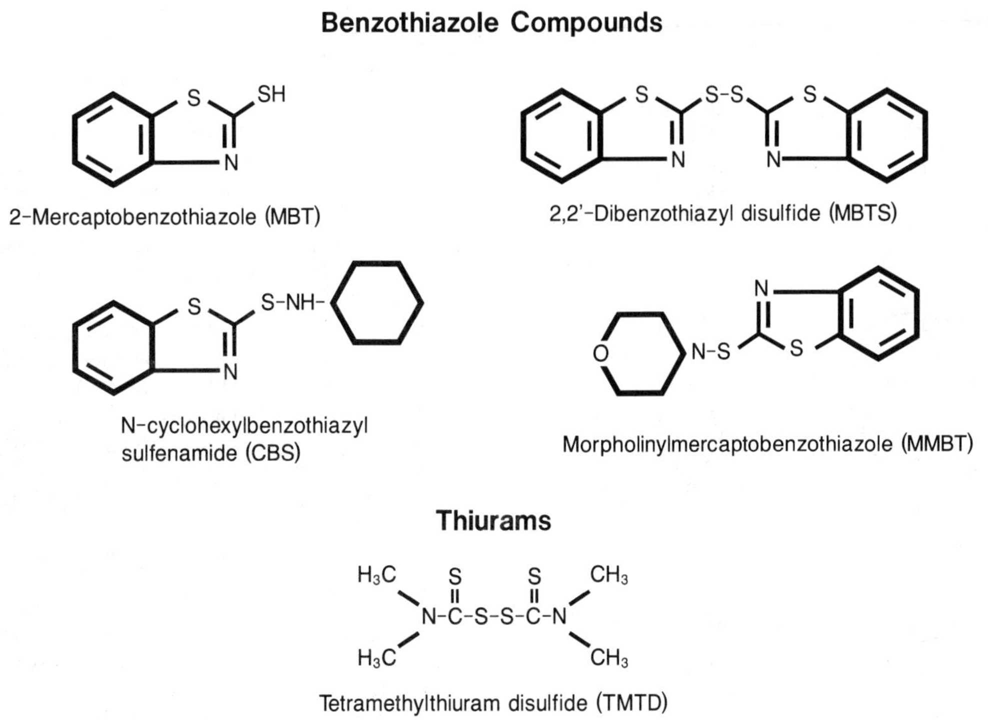

Benzothiazole Compounds

2-Mercaptobenzothiazole (MBT)

2,2'-Dibenzothiazyl disulfide (MBTS)

N-cyclohexylbenzothiazyl sulfenamide (CBS)

Morpholinylmercaptobenzothiazole (MMBT)

Thiurams

Tetramethylthiuram disulfide (TMTD)

Figure 45.6. Benzothiazole compounds and thiurams. Adapted from Feinman SE. Sensitivity to rubber chemicals. J Toxicol Cutan Ocul Toxicol 1987;6:117–153.

Table 45.5. Nitrosamine contamination in Commerical Rubber Chemicals

Accelerator	Nitrosamine Present
N-pentamethylene dithio-carbamate, piperidine salt	N-Nitrosopiperidine
Tetramethylthiuram disul-fide	N-Nitrosodimethylamine
Tetraethylthiuram disulfide	N-Nitrosodiethylamine
Zinc pentamethylene dithio-carbamate	N-Nitrosopiperidine
Zinc dibutyldithiocarbamate	N-Nitrosodibutylamine
Zinc diethyldithiocarbamate	N-Nitrosodiethylamine
Morpholine derivatives	N-Nitrosomorpholine

Adapted from Spiegelhalder B. Carcinogens in the workroom air in the rubber industry. Scand J Work Environ Health, Supplement. 1985;9(2):15–25.

chlorinated paraffins, and brominated aromatics which increase the heat resistance of rubber (3).

Blowing agents are used to produce foam rubber by decomposing at curing temperature to produce gas (Fig. 45.9) (2). Other additive groups are pigments, bonding agents (isocyanates, p-dinitrosobenzene, resorcinol-hexamethylene-tetramine), antitack agents (mica and talc), and mould release agents (silicones, fluorinated hydrocarbons, polyethylene glycols) (2).

GENERAL HEALTH HAZARDS OF THE RUBBER INDUSTRY

As in many other manufacturing industries, noise remains a major concern in the rubber industry. The extensive use of mixing and milling equipment, extruders, calenders, conveyers and hydraulic tools in the tire industry results in noise levels exceeding 85 decibel (dB) throughout most operations. Other physical hazards include risk of thermal and chemical burns and heat stress. Besides trauma, dermal and pulmonary exposures from chemicals are common hazard sources. Health hazards are also peculiar to certain sites and processes in the rubber industry due to the variety of chemicals, processes, and reactions that occur.

Dermatitis

Many rubber additives are capable of producing dermatitis (3). Since natural rubber is not considered a contact allergen, people who develop dermatitis following contact with natural rubber products are reacting to persistent additives (3). Rubber additives can produce dermatitis even from cured products by migrating to the surface of the product over time.

A number of accelerators and other compounds used in the rubber industry, including thiurams, amines, guanidines, disulfides, and certain thiazoles including mercaptobenzothiazole, are skin sensitizers causing both contact and allergic contact dermatitis in rubber workers. Many of the common rubber sensitizers are included in patch test batteries employed by dermatologists and allergists. Cross-reactivity to similar substances may occur, and sensitized individuals generally need to be removed from further exposure to avoid worsening of their condition.

Irritant dermatitis may be precipitated or aggravated by contact with solvents, caustics, and acids. Treatment with topical steroids and emollients is usually effective. Minimizing skin contact with these substances is the best means of prevention. Phenols and hydroquinones can cause focal hypopigmentation (leukoderma).

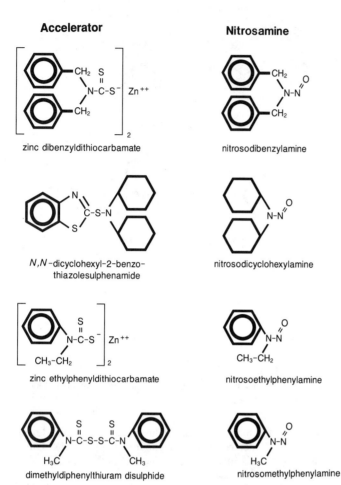

Accelerator

zinc dibenzyldithiocarbamate

N,N-dicyclohexyl-2-benzo-
thiazolesulphenamide

zinc ethylphenyldithiocarbamate

dimethyldiphenylthiuram disulphide

Nitrosamine

nitrosodibenzylamine

nitrosodicyclohexylamine

nitrosoethylphenylamine

nitrosomethylphenylamine

Figure 45.7. Accelerators and corresponding non-volatile nitrosamines. International Agency for Research of Cancer Monograph Vol. 28: The rubber industry. IARC, 1982. Adapted with permission from International Agency for Research of Cancer.

Respiratory Disease

Several studies have demonstrated an excess of respiratory symptoms and pulmonary function abnormalities in rubber workers. Studies have documented that asthma, chronic lung changes, respiratory problems, and bronchitis have been prevalent in the rubber industry, particularly in dusty areas such as compounding and mixing (4). Findings consistent with mucous hypersecretion and mild airways obstruction have been reported in workers exposed to carbon black, additives, talc, and curing fumes (4). Symptoms reported by these workers have included cough and sputum production, frequent upper respiratory infections, and episodes of bronchitis. Spirometry has shown decrements in flow rates with preservation of lung volumes.

In general, the effects of smoking and workplace exposures appear to be additive.

The longterm impact of exposures in the rubber industry on respiratory status is uncertain. Radiographic evidence of pulmonary fibrosis has been reported only rarely in rubber workers and has been related to specific materials and work practices. Mortality studies have not shown excess mortality from these respiratory diseases. If the primary pulmonary insult is the inhalation of particulates and mild irritants, then improved ventilation, material substitution, and better work practices should lessen these effects.

Silicosis and talcosis have also resulted from the substitution of talc for other powder. Talc dust may be of respirable size and contain crystalline silica and fibrous tremalite.

Workers exposed to curing fumes may have a higher prevalence of chronic bronchitis. Respiratory morbidity is related to the intensity and length of exposure to these fumes (4, 5). Other studies have shown that employment in the curing departments is associated with shortness of breath, chest tightness, wheezing, and changes in respiratory function tests (4–6).

Chronic lung diseases such as pneumoconiosis, pulmonary fibrosis, bronchitis, and emphysema can occur in workers overexposed chemically to carbon black as well as to dusts and particulates (7).

Due to the multitude of chemicals that are either used or formed in the manufacture of rubber products, and the observation that workers are frequently exposed to mixtures of chemical agents, it is often difficult to pinpoint a specific chemical in the etiology of disease. General mortality patterns among rubber industry workers have been investigated in relation to the overall industry as well as to the specific jobs or tasks (8, 9).

MEDICAL SURVEILLANCE AND PREVENTION

Health surveillance programs for rubber workers should include periodic audiometry and spirometry. If possible, the information should be standardized to allow assessment of the effectiveness of controls in high risk areas. Physical examinations should focus on the respiratory system as well as the skin. Despite the many uncertainties regarding the true cancer risks in the rubber industry, screening for gastrointestinal cancer should be considered. This is relatively common in the general population, and early detection can markedly improve outcome, particularly for cancer of the colon.

Reduction in the release of air contaminants into the work environment through the use of proper ventilation and substitution of less toxic materials presents a continuing challenge for the rubber industry. Given the potential risks of respiratory disease and cancer in this industry and that smoking tends to potentiate the effects of some chemicals, workplace smoking

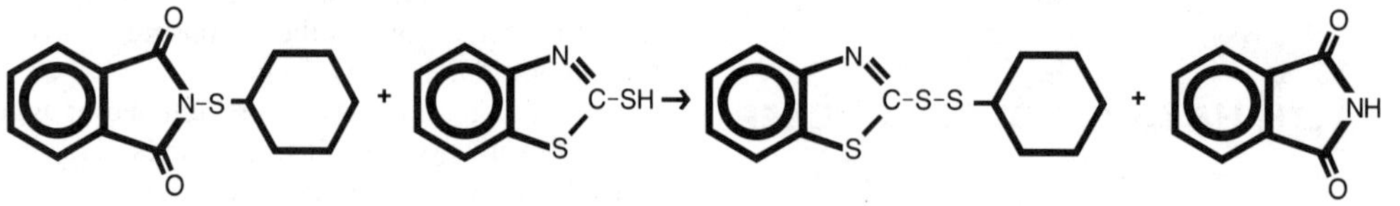

N-cyclohexylthiophthalimide   mercaptobenzothiazole   2-cyclohexylthiobenzothiazole   phthalimide

Figure 45.8. Decomposition of the retarder N-cyclohexylthiophthalimide during vulcanization. International Agency for Research of Cancer Monograph Vol. 28: The rubber industry. IARC, 1982. Adapted with permission from International Agency for Research of Cancer.

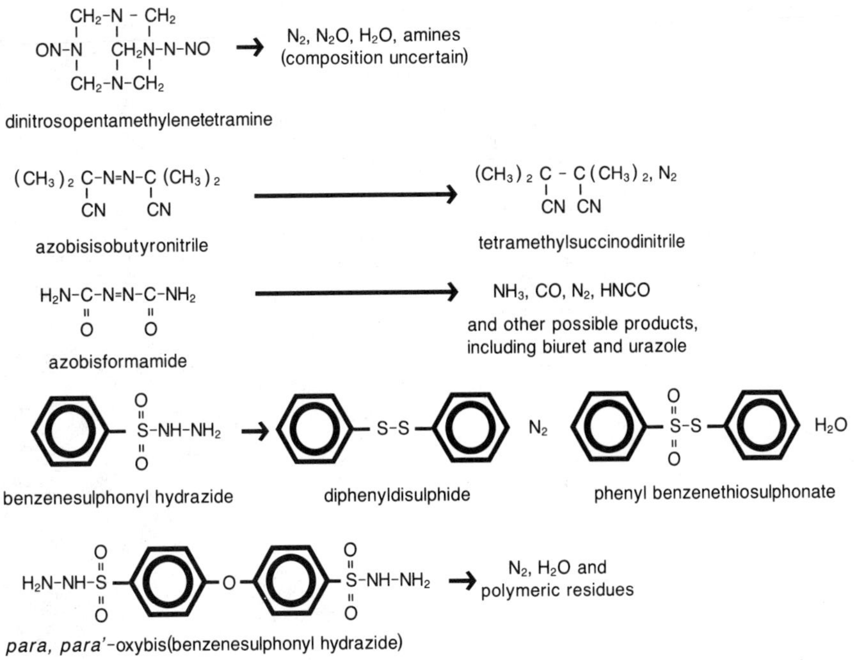

Figure 45.9. Blowing agents and their routes of decomposition. International Agency for Research of Cancer Monograph Vol. 28: The rubber industry. IARC, 1982. Adapted with permission from International Agency for Research of Cancer.

restriction policies and smoking cessation programs may be extremely beneficial for rubber workers.

HEALTH HAZARDS BY AREAS

Raw Material Handling, Weighing, and Mixing Areas

Raw material handling, weighing, and mixing exposes the worker to particulate matter (7). In some rubber manufacturing plants, the majority of particulate exposure consists of carbon black, whereas in others, talc and compounding agents may be significant. Cross-contamination of other areas may also occur due to ventilation patterns, although the magnitude of such exposures is relatively much less (7).

Mill operators can also be exposed to incompletely mixed compounds from the Banbury mixers and from compounding materials added during mix milling. Talc exposures were common in the past due to the use of this compound as a detackifier for stored rubber sheets (2, 7).

In cement mixing, workers may be exposed to solvents employed to prepare "cements" for use in extrusion, calendering, tire building, repair, and other operations. These solvent mixtures, which often include the addition of dissolved rubber solids, are prepared in the cement house.

Component Assembly and Tire Building

Various organic solvents, including petroleum naphthas, often are employed in specific tire manufacturing operations (2, 8). These include tuber or tread-end cementing, bead building, tire building, and spray booth (doper) operations for green (uncured) tires.

Although petroleum naphtha is a common component of many of the solvents applied to green tire components, other solvents including toluene (tread-end cementing) and N-hexane (bead building) are also employed (8). Since petroleum naphthas may contain small amounts of aromatics such as toluene, benzene, and xylene, proper evaluation of worker exposure should include monitoring for these chemicals as well.

Repair of cured tires sometimes requires the use of solvents to preclean flawed areas of the tire prior to application of solvent-rich rubber repair material. Mixtures of toluene and naphtha and other petroleum solvents may be employed in such preparations.

Curing or Vulcanization

Prior to curing, rubber products, including green tires, are frequently sprayed with a solvent-based lubricant in a spray booth (doping) operations. This process generates solvent vapors. The subsequent cure cycle generates condensed volatiles, vapors, gases, and reaction products (2, 9, 10). The curing fume itself consists of a complex array of organic compounds including nitrosamines which arise from the actual cure of the tires (2, 6, 9, 11). Nitrosamines which have been found in curing as well as milling, extrusion, and calendering include N-nitrosodibutylamine (NDBA), N-nitrosodimethylamine (NDMA), N-nitrosodiphenylamine (NDPhA), N-nitrosomorpholine (NMOR), N-nitrosopiperidine (NPI) T, and N-nitrosopyrrolidine (NPYR) (Table 45.6) (11–13).

Final Inspection/Repair and Finishing Area

Inspection may involve the handling of hot cured rubber products. As a result, workers other than those in curing may be exposed to condensed volatiles, vapors, and gases although in

Table 45.6. Exposure Situation for N-Nitrosamines in the Rubber Industry

Job Description	Concentration in the Air ($\mu g/m^3$)
Raw material handling, weighing mixing	
Nitrosodimethylamine	0.2–0.9
Nitrosomorpholine	0.1–2
Milling, extruding, calendering	
Nitrosodimethylamine	0.1–2
Nitrosomorpholine	0.1–9
Assembly and building	
Nitrosodimethylamine	0.1–1
Nitrosomorpholine	0.5–3
Curing or vulcanizing	
Nitrosodimethylamine	0.1–2
Nitrosodimethylamine	15–130
Nitrosodimethylamine	1–4.5
Nitrosomorpholine	0.1–17
Nitrosodimethylamine	1–40
Nitrosodiethylamine	0.1–5
Nitrosomorpholine	0.1–3
Nitrosodimethylamine	40–90
Nitrosomorpholine	120–380
Nitrosodimethylamine	500–1,060
Nitrosomorpholine	200–4,700
Nitrosodimethylamine	1
Nitrosodiethylamine	5
Nitrosopiperidine	0.3
Nitrosomorpholine	0.1
Nitrosodimethylamine	1–3.5
Nitrosomorpholine	3–9
Nitrosodimethylamine	0.2–3.5
Nitrosodimethylamine	1
Nitrosodiethylamine	3
Inspection and finishing	
Nitrosodimethylamine	0.1–1.5
Nitrosomorpholine	0.1–20
Nitrosodimethylamine	1–10
Storage and dispatch	
Nitrosodimethylamine	0.2–10
Nitrosodimethylamine	1–19
Nitrosomorpholine	0.3–17
Nitrosodimethylamine	0.2–1

Adapted from Spiegelhalder B. Carcinogens in the workroom air in the rubber industry. Scand J Work Environ Health, Supplement. 1983;9(2):15–25.

Table 45.7. Summary of Vapor in Air Concentrations of Solvent Components from Selected Work Areas

Work Area Component	Range (ppm)
Cement mixing	
Pentane	0.91–61.2
Hexane	0.83–98.5
Heptane	0.39–90.7
Octane	0.16–7.64
Benzene	0.18–16.5
Toluene	0.37–19.3
Xylene	0.02–1.50
Isopropanol	0.01–28.5
Tire building	
Pentane	0.29–5.45
Hexane	0.30–135.
Heptane	0.06–12.2
Octane	0.19–1.79
Benzene	0.09–1.52
Toluene	0.13–3.29
Xylene	0.01–1.38
Isopropanol	0.07–6.83
Final inspection	
Pentane	0.04–0.82
Hexane	0.59–6.40
Heptane	0.09–0.81
Octane	0.02–0.27
Benzene	0.01–0.19
Toluene	0.03–0.64
Xylene	0.02–0.54
Isopropanol	0.08–0.44
Warehouse	
Pentane	0.03–0.56
Hexane	0.02–0.45
Heptane	0.07–0.19
Octane	0.02–0.21
Benzene	0.01–0.48
Toluene	0.01–0.37
Xylene	0.03–0.51
Isopropanol	

Adapted from Van Ert M, et al. Worker exposures to chemical agents in the manufacture of rubber tires. Solvent vapor studies. Am Ind Hyg Assoc J 1980;41:212–219.

much lower levels. In final inspection, repair activities may require the use of solvent-based rubber products leading to employee exposure to these vapors (Table 45.7) (8).

Storage and Dispatch Area

Stored rubber products release or degas low concentrations of solvent vapors which were employed in the manufacturing process as well as other less volatile products (Table 45.7) (8).

CARCINOGENIC AND MUTAGENIC PROPERTIES OF CHEMICALS

Commonly used accelerators and curing agents (thiuram compounds including tetramethylthiuram disulfide, tetraethyl-thiuram disulfide, and tetramethylthiuram monosulfide) have been demonstrated to be carcinogenic in animal studies (2).

Solvents used in the rubber industry include petroleum naphthas, toluene, hexane, isopropyl alcohol, trichloroethylene, 1,1,1-trichloroethane, and methylene chloride. Occupational studies suggest some evidence of increased carcinogenesis secondary to solvent exposure (14).

Small amounts of monomers such as acrylonitrile, butadiene, chloroprene, ethylene, propylene, styrene, vinyl acetate, vinyl chloride, and vinylidene chloride remain in solid rubber polymer and could be released into the work environment, but probably at concentrations below existing standards. Most of these monomers have not been known to bind directly with cellular macromolecules, but their metabolites might do so (2, 10). There is sufficient evidence to implicate acrylonitrile as a suspected human carcinogen based on animal studies (2, 10). Vinyl chloride is a confirmed human carcinogen (2). There is limited animal evidence of the carcinogenicity of styrene (2, 10).

Epichlorhydrin is also used in the manufacture of elastomers.

Table 45.8. Polycyclic Aromatic Hydrocarbons (PAH) in Rubber Factory Atmospheres

Fluoranthene
Pyrene
Benzo(a)fluorene
Benz(a)anthracene
Chrysene
Benzo(b)fluoranthene
Benzo(a)pyrene
Dibenz(a,j)anthracene
Dibenz(a,h)anthracene
Indenopyrene
Benzo(ghi)perylene
Anthanthrene
Perylene

It can react directly with macromolecules and serum proteins. It is a mutagenic chemical and is also carcinogenic in mice and rats (2, 10). No adequate epidemiologic observations are in the literature as to its carcinogenicity in humans.

Talc, widely used as an antitacking agent, is mainly associated with respiratory disease. However, some talcs may contain asbestos fibers and fibrous tremalite.

Carbon blacks contain variable amounts of compounds, some of which have not been identified. The most probable carcinogenic hazard of carbon black is associated with benzene-extractable chemicals consisting mainly of aromatic hydrocarbons and sulfur compounds (15–17). Among these chemicals are benz(a)anthracene, benzo(a)pyrene, and indenopyrene, which are known carcinogens (Table 45.8). Crysene has been described as a tumor-initiating agent, and nitro derivatives of polycyclic hydrocarbons have also been found in extracts of commercial carbon black (15–17). Data indicate that the known carcinogens present in carbon blacks are strongly absorbed but can be eluted by biologic fluids (15–17). A 1962 study reported that the polycyclic hydrocarbons, including benozopyrene, present in the furnance and channel blacks were not eluted by human blood, plasma, or gastric juice (16). Cancer of the bladder has long been recognized as a problem within the rubber industry and has been associated with specific aromatic hydrocarbons. The cause was probably an organic antioxidant added to the rubber mixture, beta-naphthylamine, although subsequent concern has focused on alpha-naphthylamine, benzidine, and 4-aminobiphenyl (xenylamine). Bladder cancer has been associated with three occupational title groups (OTGs) in the rubber industry including Receiving and Shipping, Compounding and Mixing, and Milling, although the number of bladder cases is small. Reactive metabolic intermediates from aromatic amines and their interaction with cellular macromolecules has been extensively reviewed (2, 10, 18, 19). The carcinogenic or genotoxic activity of aromatic amines and amides is dependent on metabolic activation or N-hydroxylation to hydroxyl-amines. Naphthylamine-acetaldehyde was introduced as an antioxidant in the rubber industry in 1928. It was associated with an increase in incidence of bladder cancer. 4-aminobiphenyl, benzidene, and beta- or 2-naphthylamine are known to be carcinogenic for humans. Their use was discontinued in the early years of the industry. Phenyl beta-naphthylamine (PBNA) was employed, even more recently, as an antioxidant. Research indicated that PBNA is metabolized by the body to beta-naphthylamine. There is sufficient evidence for the carcinogenicity of simpler amines, 2,4-diaminotoluene and 2-chloroaniline, in experimental animals.

Phthalate Esters

Phthalate esters are plasticizers used in numerous "plastic" products including rubber tires. Consequently, they are widely distributed. The two most common plasticizers are diethylhexylphthalate (DEHP) and di-n-butylphthalate (DBP). Phthalate esters are not known to be acutely toxic. They contaminate soil and water in wide-ranging areas of the United States. DEHP and DBP are considered weak animal carcinogens.

Curing Fumes and Other Curing Emissions

During the vulcanization process fumes and vapors are emitted into the air due to volatilization of rubber ingredients. There are no experimental data available concerning the longterm toxicity of curing fumes. Curing fumes from the tire vulcanization process contain a number of chemicals and chemical byproducts (2, 5, 6, 9, 10). These products are dependent on the temperature and the type or composition of the rubber and the presence of absence of oxygen. Increased incidence of lung cancer in workers who are in the curing area has been demonstrated in various epidemiologic studies (9, 20–21). Many airborne nitrosamines are formed during rubber processing and are found in the work atmosphere (2, 11–13, 22). As yet, there is no direct evidence that nitrosamines cause cancer in humans.

Polycyclic Aromatic Hydrocarbons (PAHs)

PAHs are fused benzene ring compounds present in crude oil as well as generated by burning organic materials. PAHs are found in aromatic oils, which are extensively used in the rubber industry as plasticizers and softeners. A tire may contain up to 20% aromatic and paraffinic oils (2). These aromatic oils may contain large amounts of PAHs, some of which contain concentrations of carcinogens. Benzo(a)pyrene is a well-known PAH carcinogen (Table 45.8) (2, 15–17).

PAHs are potent skin carcinogens in animal models. Normally, in the rubber industry, humans do not frequently come into direct contact with these aromatic oils. However, uncured rubber, with which workers have much contact, contains large amounts of these oils. Thus, PAH transfer to the skin may be facilitated. Carbon black also contains PAHs. Fortunately, only small amounts of PAHs are released into biologic fluids by carbon black due to its high absorption feature. Solvent extract of carbon black is carcinogenic, but carbon black itself is not.

PAHs are undoubtedly released during the heating of rubber, yet studies have not demonstrated this to be a significant problem in the industry in relation to existing airborne concentrations.

PAHs are metabolized by the P-450 mixed oxidase enzyme system in the liver to carcinogenic compounds. DNA binding studies have shown that several benzo(a)pyrene metabolites bind covalently to DNA.

Mineral oils such as coal tar oils, petroleum, and other tar products are widely used in the rubber industry as extenders. The use of mineral oils has increased considerably over the years since they are cheap and impart desirable properties to the finished rubber. These oils contain relatively large quantities of PAHs. PAHs also may be formed when the tars and mineral oils are heated. These mineral oils and tar products vary in composition. They all, however, may induce carcinogenic effects in mammals, including humans. This carcinogenic effect may be due to the presence of the PAHs.

Nitroso Compounds and Nitrosamines

Very little information is available on the health effects of chemical byproducts generated during rubber processing. During vulcanization, air is excluded and the mold contains a reducing atmosphere. Products that can be formed during vulcanization and released from the surface of the rubber include amines and organic sulfides derived from accelerators (Fig. 45.10). There are many reports of these chemicals breaking down during curing temperatures. Because the maximum temperature of the vulcanization or curing of rubber is approximately 240°C, pyrolysis does not normally occur (2). Upon removal from the mold, the rubber can undergo oxidating reactions in which peroxy substituted amines and acids can be formed such as N-nitrosomorpholine (NMOR), N-nitrosodimethylamine (NDMA), and N-nitrosopyrrolidine (Table 45.6) (2, 18, 22). These compounds, demonstrated to be carcinogenic in a number of animal models, have been identified in the extrusion, milling, calendering, curing, and cooling (postcuring) areas of tire factories (9, 11–13). The discovery of such compounds in the air of specific areas of tire plants has led to control measures such as improved ventilation and compound substitutions to reduce or eliminate these agents from the workplace environment.

N-Nitroso compounds are produced by acid-catalyzed reactions of nitrites with certain nitrogen-containing amine compounds (18). Nitroso compounds are divided into nitrosamines and nitrosamides. Most of these have been demonstrated to be potent carcinogens. The antidegradant process and curing process involves amines, nitrosamines, and quinolines which are suspected carcinogens. Possibly, these compounds are precarcinogens which require metabolic activation by the body to carcinogens (18).

N-Nitrosomorpholine (NMOR), a known animal carcinogen, has been quantitated in rubber industry factory air sampling (11). Also, small amounts of another carcinogen, N-nitrosodimethylamine (NDMA), have been identified. NDMA was found as an indoor air pollutant at concentrations ranging from 0.07–0.14 $\mu g/m^3$. NMOR was also found in the rubber factory

as an impurity in morpholine and in the cross-linking accelerator bismorpholinecarbamylsulfenamide (BMCS). NMOR was found at all sites sampled in the rubber industries surveyed including milling, extrusion, calendering, and curing. The lowest level was in the finishing area and the highest levels in the extruding areas (11).

Chemicals containing nitro or nitroso groups can serve as nitrosating agents (12). These chemicals can thermally decompose in hot processes to form nitrogen oxide and directly nitrosate amines contained in rubber (Fig. 45.11) (12). Nitrogen oxides can also be formed as byproducts of internal combustion processes secondary to machine use.

Nitrosamines have been reported in numerous worksite air samples in both the United States and Germany in breathing zone samples (12). These nitrosamines included N-nitrosodimethylamine, N-nitrosomorpholine, N-nitrosodiethylamine, N-nitrosobutylamine, N-nitrosopiperidine, and N-nitrosopyrrolidine. The nitrosatable precursor of each of these compounds is used in the rubber industry with the exception of N-nitrosopyrrolidine.

In addition to the nitrosation of secondary amines, reactions involving tertiary amines or amine derivatives occur in aqueous systems and solid systems, as well as in the gaseous phase. The following two nitrosation reactions are possible: (a) Nitrosatable compounds dissolved or dispersed in latex solution can be nitrosated during the production of latex articles. Nitrogen oxide from the air has been proposed as the nitrosating agents in this case. Atmospheric levels of nitrogen oxides that can be complemented by other combustion processes such as open flames and other pollutant sources (11, 12, 18). (b) Chemicals that contain nitro or nitroso groups are potential nitrostating agents as some of these chemicals may decompose thermally during processing of the rubber to form nitrogen oxides. Direct nitrosation of specific compounds contained in solid rubber is therefore possible. Animal studies have demonstrated that airborne concentrations of nitrosamines, similar to those found in the rubber industry, can induce cancers of the lung, kidney, and liver (12).

The rubber industry as a whole has several hundred different chemicals involved in the manufacture of various rubber products. The choice of chemicals employed in different stages of the processing of the rubber varies from company to company, and even within the different departments and factories within the same company.

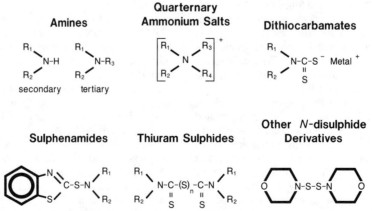

Figure 45.10. Groups of chemicals that can be converted to N-nitrosamines. Adapted with permission from Spiegelhalder B. Carcinogens in the workroom air in the rubber industry. Scand J Work Environ Health, Supplement 1983;9(2):15–25.

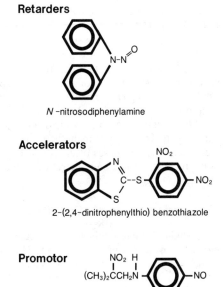

Retarders

N -nitrosodiphenylamine

Accelerators

2-(2,4-dinitrophenylthio) benzothiazole

Promotor

$(CH_3)_2CCH_2N$ — NO

N -(2-methyl-2-nitropropyl)-
4-nitrosoaniline

poly- *N* -nitroso-2,2,4-trimethyl-
1,2-dihydroquinoline

$(CH_3)_2N$ — NO

N,N -dimethyl-*para* -nitrosoaniline

Blowing Agent

dinitrosopenta-
methylenetetramine

Figure 45.11. Nitro and nitroso compounds used in the rubber industry that can act as precursors of nitrogen oxides. Adapted with permission from Spiegelhalder B. Carcinogens in the workroom air in the rubber industry. Scand J Work Environ Health, Supplement. 1983;9(2):15–25.

RUBBER INDUSTRY AND CANCER

Studies of rubber workers in the United States and other countries have demonstrated that the death rate due to all cancers appears lower than in the general population. Yet, a detailed review of the mortality experience of these cohorts has shown excesses for specific causes of death (20–34). Among U.S. rubber workers, excess malignancies of the lung, lymphatic, and hematopoetic systems, particularly lymphatic leukemia, have been associated with certain jobs in the rubber industry (20–34). Stomach cancers have been associated with jobs in the production line including compounding and mixing, milling, and extrusion. Lung cancer has been associated with curing jobs in certain rubber industries (20–34). Establishing causation of these health outcomes with many of the materials and chemicals that occur in the work atmosphere in the rubber industry has been difficult because of the diverse and changing nature of exposures within the rubber industry, the multiple exposures experienced by many workers due to job mobility over a working lifetime, and the lack of historical industrial hygiene data. Most epidemiologic studies of cancer and other diseases in rubber workers have not always been exposure specific, or they have used job descriptions as a substitute for exposure estimates. Consequently, there is sometimes considerable difficulty in identifying etiologic factors in cancer and other disease causation (23). This process is confounded by the need to estimate exposures that occurred several decades ago in relation to cancer occurring in more recent times. Evidence of human carcinogenicity to either a single chemical or a complex mixture of chemicals in the rubber industry has been derived from the following types of studies (23):

1. Reports on individual cancer patients who have a history of exposure to the suspected carcinogen;
2. Descriptive epidemiologic studies in which the incidence of cancer in human populations is found to vary with exposure to the agent or agents in question;
3. Analytical epidemiologic evidence such as case control or cohort studies in which individual exposure to the agents is found to be associated with an increased risk of cancer.

The first two study types provide only suggestive evidence of causation. The third one, an analytical epidemiologic study, provides better insight if there is no identified bias, error in the design of the study, or confounding factors.

The rubber industry has gone through many evolutionary changes involved with technology and chemicals. To try to define a typical rubber manufacturing operation is difficult in terms of either the process or the end product or environmental controls. There are multiple processes in the rubber industry that can be associated with different exposure hazards. The variables that arise include variations in production and control technology, variations in process requirements, and variations in work practice (2, 9, 23).

Assessing exposures of rubber workers is also rather difficult for the following reasons (2, 23):

1. An individual experiences a large variety of exposures from the multiple chemicals used in a given job and cross-contamination from adjacent work areas.
2. Several hundred chemicals, including some complex solvent mixtures, are used in the rubber industry.
3. Few workers in the industry remain in the same job during the entire period of their employment, although job mobility for these workers may be minimal. However, they may work at many different jobs over the course of their employment, making it very difficult to track their exposure history.
4. Cancer excesses that occur in the industry may have resulted from chemical exposures that occurred within or outside the industry many years prior to the clinical diagnosis of the disease.

5. Industrial processes can result in the formation of new materials as byproducts of those processes.

Excess mortality from various cancers has been reported in rubber workers, and the International Agency for Research on Cancer has classified specific exposures in the rubber industry as potentially carcinogenic in humans (2). In spite of changes in manufacturing materials, operations, and work conditions, and worker mobility over the past 60 years, epidemiologic investigations have identified excesses of several different cancers in rubber workers depending on the study population and time frame of interest. While in some instances specific causes have been suggested, specific factors contributing to cancer excess in rubber workers remain uncertain.

The first cancer identified in rubber workers was an excess in bladder cancer in Great Britain. The cancer excess in workers studied was ultimately attributed to the use of aromatic amines, primarily beta-naphthylamine, as an accelerator. The use of this chemical was discontinued by 1950, and excess bladder cancer has not been identified in subsequent studies.

Studies have also shown certain rubber workers to be at an increased risk for developing leukemia (33). Excess has been found in other studies, including a risk of lymphocytic leukemia with exposure to solvents other than benzene (20–34). Limited studies of workers producing synthetic rubber (SBR) have also suggested an excess of leukemia risk (33).

While rubber workers overall have not been found to be at an increased risk for developing lung cancer, excess lung cancer has been identified in a variety of rubber worker subpopulations. Lung cancer has been associated with exposure to compounding, mixing and milling, and curing fume exposure, but these studies are inconsistent (20–33). Smoking, interactions of smoking with other exposures in the industry, and chance clustering (given the extensive investigation of this industry) all remain possible explanations for the findings related to lung cancer to date.

Most epidemiologic studies of the rubber industry are retrospective follow-up studies of cohorts of rubber workers or case control studies of people with cancer. Typically, the rate of occurrence and/or death from cancer is compared with the rates in a control population. This control may be the general population.

Frequently, in follow-up studies, the rate of death in the study population is less than that in the general population. This difference is termed the "healthy worker effect." This selection bias occurs because only relatively healthy people enter the employment force, but it usually applies less to cancer than to other causes of death.

In occupational cohort studies, the standardized mortality ratio (SMR) is commonly used. The SMR is the number of deaths observed in a group divided by the number expected in the same group. The quotient is multiplied by 100. The expected numbers, which are customarily based on the mortality experience of the general population, are usually standardized for age and calendar time. In case-control studies, disease rates are not computed because of the small size of the population studied.

The main studies of the rubber industry in the United States consist of those from the Harvard School of Public Health and the University of North Carolina (2, 20). Data in the Harvard study included 13,571 white male production workers (20). These people were working at a plant on or after January 1, 1940, and worked at least 5 years at the plant between that

time and June 1971. They were followed from January 1940, through June 1974. During that period, 980 deaths from cancer were observed; 1046 were expected. In the second phase of the study, cancer morbidity between 1964 and 1974 was examined by a review of the area tumor registry. The rates of cancer were measured among workers in specific areas of the rubber plant. Lung cancer excesses were noted in the tire-curing area in people who had worked there for at least 5 years, tire-moulding people who had worked there for at least 5 years, and in the fuel cell de-icer manufacturing area. In the tire curing area, there were 31 cases of cancer with 14.1 cases expected; in the fuel cell de-icer area, there were 46 cases of cancer with 29.1 expected (20).

University of North Carolina Studies

In the studies from the University of North Carolina (UNC), 6678 production workers were studied, and 351 cancer deaths occurred during a 9-year follow-up; 336.90 deaths were expected, based on the U.S. male, age, race-specific rate (2, 22, 23).

McMichael et al., in 1976, detailed job histories of seven specific cancer case groups in this industry (9, 34). Their findings were as follows: respiratory cancer excess was found in the receiving and shipping area, compounding and mixing, milling, extrusion, tubing, and reclaim areas.

Excess mortality from lung cancer was found in one United Kingdom study; an excess of lung cancer was found among workers in many occupations in the tire industry and non-tire sectors. Excess cases of lung cancer in U.S. studies were associated with work in compounding and mixing, extrusion, tire curing, and rubber reclaim (2, 9, 20, 26, 27, 34).

Two populations were defined in the UNC study. The first population consisted of 6678 men who were alive on January 1, 1964, and had worked for at least 10 years in a large Akron, Ohio, tire plant (34). This population was followed for 9 years, from 1964. Overall results of the study demonstrated cancers of other organ systems without excess lung cancer. A parallel study of 1339 men in a second tire factory in Akron showed essentially the same, with no evidence of increased lung cancer rates (9, 34). A case-control study conducted on 61 cases of lung cancer and 61 matched control subjects did demonstrate a strong correlation between the rubber curing process and lung cancer. Twenty-five percent of the cases were exposed to curing agents versus 15% of control subjects (9, 34).

The second UNC study was conducted on 8418 white male production workers from 1964–1973. Again, lung cancer was not a prominent disease among the cancers observed.

Harvard School of Public Health Studies

This study defined a population of 13,570 white male workers employed in an Akron plant from 1940–1971 (2, 20). All members of the study had worked for at least 5 years. The number of overall cancer deaths was less than the general population. Bladder cancer appeared in excess. A subsequent cancer study was carried out in this particular plant showing correlations between type of job and excess cancers. The results of this study demonstrated an excess of lung cancer in the curing, moulding, and fuel cell area of the plant (36). The mortality of 13,571 white, male rubber employees was studied from 1940 through 1974 as part of the Harvard study. An excess of lung cancer in the tire curing area (observed = 20, expected = 12.4) was identified. In addition, the curing workers had a higher incidence of chronic bronchitis. Of the curing workers with at least 10 years experience or greater, 25% had chronic obstructive lung disease (COPD). Smoking did not account for the difference between the curing versus the control group in terms of increased respiratory disease.

Results of a 5-year analysis from 1967–1971 of 40,807 British rubber workers demonstrated an overall 19% increase in the incidence of cancer (28). There was also excess lung cancer in the tire manufacturing area (28).

Smoking habits were not accounted for in this large study; however, the SMR for other smoking and urban-related disease was approximately the same in all sectors. This suggests that smoking is not a primary cause for the excess lung cancer seen in this study (28).

The risk of neoplasms in general were higher for the tire industry as compared with the cablemaking industry. No evidence was found to suggest this excess might be due to smoking habits. The death rates for smoking-related causes, in particular for COPD and bronchitis, in the tire industry is approximately the same for the cablemaking industry (28). The first prospective study to report on excess lung cancer deaths in the rubber industry was by Mancuso (23).

BRMA/Birmingham University Study

The British Rubber Manufacturer Association (BRMA) initiated a retrospective study that covered 33,815 men who worked in the rubber industry from 1946–1960. Thirteen factories were included, eight tire and five general rubber products. The study population worked for a minimum of 1 year and was divided into three cohorts (22):

Cohort 1, January 1946 to December 1950
Cohort 2, January 1951 to December 1955
Cohort 3, January 1956 to December 1960

The study looked at all causes of death and not just cancer and was extended until 1975. The final report focused only on cancer cases in the industry.

The initial study analyzed deaths from cancer by studying only members of the population who survived for a minimum for 10 years past beginning employment. This removed all cases of cancer deaths that occurred close to the point of entry into employment. Using this refined 10-year latency technique, an excess of cancer was observed (22).

The lung cancer mortality was analyzed in terms of occupational groups in the rubber industry. The results of this analysis suggested that certain occupations in the rubber industry were associated with higher than expected mortality rates for respiratory cancer (22).

Excess lung cancer has been associated with work in the curing, inspection, and mixing areas of the rubber industry in general, as demonstrated by a number of studies. In the BRMA study, the individual environmental exposure of workers was considered to be important in delineation of carcinogenesis. These work environments were identified by obtaining detailed occupational histories as well as job descriptions from workers. For each chemical exposure, the fraction of the subgroup reported to have some exposure to that chemical was recorded and generated data that indicated excess lung cancer with exposure to curing vapors.

A case-control study was conducted with four control subjects being chosen for each case of lung cancer. These control subjects were matched for age, factory, cohort, and duration of service. No single environmental area stands out as a cause of lung cancer; however, curing vapors (vulcanizing) were highlighted.

Extended BRMA Study

Reported in 1982, the extended BRMA study followed the original study population through December 31, 1975, allowing another 5 years of analysis. This study excluded all those workers who died in the 10 years following the beginning of their employment. This restraint reduced the study population from 36,695 participants to 33,815 and removed the "healthy worker effect" influence (22). The overall results for cancer deaths in the population showed increased SMRs for all cancer types, excess lung cancer, excess leukemia, and excess stomach cancer (22). Lung cancer excess seen in the previous study was reconfirmed by this extended study data. The extended study also confirmed suspected information regarding occupational site and the excess lung cancer cases. In addition, the results were worse for general rubber goods than for tire industries alone.

Both the general rubber goods and the tire manufacturing rubber industries show excess lung cancer rates in the curing, tire-building, and inspection and finishing areas of the workplace.

CONCLUSION

The rubber industry employs hundreds of chemicals in a variety of processes and reactions. Hazardous exposures can occur in multiple environments. Decomposition products from chemical reactions may account for many unknown exposures to potential carcinogens at various sites. Control of exposures is an important preventive health issue. The rubber industry is associated with an excess of cancer in workers. In particular, an excess of lung cancer, leukemia, and lymphomas has been described.

REFERENCES

1. Greek BF. Rubber chemicals face more demanding market. Chem Eng News 1989;25–54.

2. International Agency for Research on Cancer. Monographs on the evaluation of carcinogenic risk of chemicals to humans. Vol. 28: The rubber industry. Lyon: IARC, 1982.

3. Feinman SE. Sensitivity to rubber chemicals. J Toxicol Cutan Ocul Toxicol 1987;6:117–153.

4. Weeks JL, Peters JM, Monson RR. Screening for occupational health hazards in the rubber industry. Part 1. Am J Ind Med 1981;2:125–141.

5. Weeks JL, Peters JM, Monson RR. Screening for occupational health hazards in the rubber industry. Part II: Health hazards in the curing department. An J Ind Med 1981;2:143–151.

6. Fraser DA, Rappaport S. Health aspects of the curing of synthetic rubbers. Environ Health Prospect 1976;17:45–53.

7. Williams TM, Harris RL, Arp EW, Symons MJ, Van Ert MD. Worker exposure to chemical agents in the manufacture of rubber tires and tubes: particulates. Am Ind Hyg Assoc J 1980;41:204–211.

8. Delzell E, Monson RR. Mortality among rubber workers: IV. General mortality patterns. J Occup Med 1981;23:850–856.

9. McMichael AJ, Spirtas R, Gamble JF, Tousey PM. Mortality among rubber workers: relationship to specific jobs. J Occup Med 1976;18:178–185.

10. Fishbein L. Core problems in chemical industries: additives used in the plastics, polymer, and rubber industries. In: Stich HF, ed. Carcinogens and mutagens in the environment. Boca Raton, FL: CRC Press, 1982.

11. Fajen JM, Carson GA, Rounbehler DP, et al. N-Nitrosamines in the rubber and tire industry. Science 1979;205:1262–1264.

12. Spiegelhalder B. Carcinogens in the workroom air in the rubber industry. Scand J Work Environ Health 1983;9:15–25.

13. Nutt A. Rubber work and cancer: past, present and perspectives. Cancer Mortal Morbid 1983;9:49–57.

14. Wilcosky TC, Checkoway H, Marshall EG, Tyroler HA. Cancer mortality and solvent exposures in the rubber industry. Am Ind Hyg Assoc J 1984;45:809–811.

15. Nutt A. Measurement of some potentially hazardous materials in the atmosphere of rubber factories. Environ Health Perspect 1976;17:117–123.

16. Neal J, Thornton M, Nau CA. Polycyclic hydrocarbon elution from carbon black or rubber products. Arch Environ Health 1962;4:46–54.

17. Locati G, Fantuzzi A, Consonni G, Li Gotti I, Bonomi G. Identification of polycyclic aromatic hydrocarbons in carbon black with reference to cancerogenic risk in tire production. Am Ind Hyg Assoc J 1979;40:644–652.

18. Mirvish SS. Formation of N-nitroso compounds: chemistry, kinetics and in vivo occurrence. Toxicol Appl Pharmacol 1975;31:325–351.

19. Dipple A, Michejda CJ, Weisburger EK. Metabolism of chemical carcinogens. Pharmacol Ther 1985;27:265–296.

20. Monson RR, Fine LJ. Cancer mortality and morbidity among rubber workers. J Natl Cancer Inst 1978;61:1047–1053.

21. McMichael AJ, Andjelkovic DA, Tyroler HA. Cancer mortality among rubber workers: an epidemiologic study. Ann NY Acad Sci 1976;271:125–137.

22. Parkes HG, Veys CA, Waterhouse JAH, Peters A. Cancer mortality in the British rubber industry. Br J Ind Med 1982;39:209–220.

23. Mancuso TF. Problems and perspective in epidemiological study of occupational health hazards in the rubber industry. Environ Health Perspect 1976;17:21–30.

24. Delzell E, Manson R. Mortality among rubber workers: III. Cause-specific mortality, 1940–1978. J Occup Med 1981;23:677–684.

25. Delzell E, Monson RR. Mortality among rubber workers: VII. Aerospace workers. Am J Ind Med 1984;6:265–271.

26. Delzell E, Monson RR. Mortality among rubber workers: X. Reclaim workers. Am J Ind Med 1985;7:307–313.

27. Delzell E, Louik C, Lewis J, Monson RR. Mortality and cancer morbidity among workers in the rubber tire industry. Am J Ind Med 1981;2:209–216.

28. Fox AJ, Lindars DC, Owen R. A survey of occupational cancer in the rubber and cablemaking industries: results of five-year analysis, 1967–1971. Br J Ind Med 1974;31:140–151.

29. Kilpikari I. Mortality among male rubber workers in Finland. Arch Environ Health 1982;37:295–298.

30. Delzell E, Andjelkovich D, Tyroler HA. A case-control study of employment experience and lung cancer among rubber workers. Am J Ind Med 1982;3:393–404.

31. Norseth T, Andersen A, Giltvedt J. Cancer incidence in the rubber industry in Norway. Scand J Work Environ Health 1983;9:69–71.

32. Meinhardt TJ, Lemen RA, Crandall MS, Young RJ. Environmental epidemiologic investigation of the styrene-butadine rubber industry. Scand J Work Environ Health 1982;8:250–259.

33. Matanoski GM, Santos-Burgoa C, Schwartz L. Mortality of a cohort of workers in the styrene-butadiene polymer manufacturing industry (1943–1982). Environ Health Perspect 1990;86:107–117.

34. McMichael AJ, Spirtas R, Kupper LC. An epidemiologic study of mortality within a cohort of rubber workers, 1964–1972. J Occup Med 1976;18:178–185.

46

Automobile Airbag Industry Toxic Exposures

J. Michael Hitt, M.D., M.S.

INTRODUCTION

The automobile airbag industry in the 1990s will grow from an infant industry, relegated to the periphery of the automotive industrial complex, to an important component of automotive manufacturing. Federally mandated driver's airbag requirements on 1990 and later model-year vehicles will transform a little-ordered new car option into a standard equipment item. The technology needed to mass produce this product has been developed for the past 15 years. Eight companies worldwide are involved, or will be involved, in airbag production. Two are in Japan, four are in the United States, and two are in Germany. There are an estimated 4000 employees directly involved in its manufacture.

The toxic product of this small product industry, however, will eventually be in the possession of 80% of adults and Americans. Any toxic effects of the product will therefore have major implications on American and world health. The deployment of the airbag requires a controlled rapid generation of gas within centimeters of the driver's face. This results in the release of the products of combustion and creates a unique and potentially hazardous situation within the confines of the passenger compartment. Previously, reactions of this nature have been isolated to the engine compartment and, in the case of the internal combustion engine, are shielded by massive metal blocks. The airbag, however, is designed so that the driver is the target of the deployment, shielded only by the cloth bag, fiber screens, and metal inflator body.

THE AUTOMOBILE AIRBAG MODULE

Fig. 46.1 demonstrates the major components of a driver's side automobile airbag module. This system operates by placing the module in the center of the steering wheel. The back side of the inflator is attached to the steering wheel and the opposite side, facing the driver, contains the airbag, housed within a plastic container and cover. The module is connected to crash sensors at the front and front sides of the vehicle. The sensor will signal at extremely rapid deceleration (Fig. 46.2) causing an electrical current to activate the inflator.

The inflator is the heart of the system consisting of a lightweight, stainless steel or aluminum housing, which contains a stack of gas-generating discs or pellets (Fig. 46.3). The disks are stacked to form an explosive core. This core is housed within a combustion chamber, which occupies the space between the core and the walls of the inflator. The inflator walls are permeated by windows, which allow gas to escape. The windows are screened by a final filter, which serves to cool the gases and protect the airbag itself from particles that might burn or rupture. The entire inflator sits within the circular opening of the airbag. The bag is woven of soft, porous fabric, allowing rapid inflation and deflation.

Combustion occurs when an electronically active squib ignites the enhancer (booster) charge, which ignites the main charge placed within the core of the gas-generating disks. This process is assigned by ignition enhancer chemicals that surround the auto ignition materials.

Chemical Constituents

The following chemicals and agents are used in air bags (Table 46.1): sodium azide, ceramic fibers, 2,4-dinitrotoluene, boron potassium nitrate, nitrocellulose, and cupric oxide.

The principal chemical component of the entire system, and certainly the major potential toxin, is sodium azide, which makes up the bulk of the gas-generating disks. Sodium azide has caused at least seven fatalities following ingestion (1). It is a common preservative for laboratory reagents and is widely used in the explosive industry. Sodium azide is a white crystal. The pK_a of sodium azide is 4.8, so in acidic fluids such as gastric juice a large amount of hydrazoic acid HN_3 will be present (5).

In the industrial setting, low levels of exposure over long periods of time are likely to produce diarrhea and a mild lowering of blood pressure. Sodium azide has been studied as an antihypertensive drug in human clinical trials. It appears to be an effective pharmaceutical agent with no adverse effects noted in 25 years of study, when dosages were kept below 0.75 mg/day. This dose is significant because it represents the approximate daily dose of an industrial worker working one shift at the ceiling exposure limit of 0.3 mg/m^3 (3). For this reason, mild depression of blood pressure may be expected in sodium azide workers. Anecdotal reports cite a greater hypotensive effect in hypertensive workers as compared with normotensive workers. There have been no reports of rebound hypertension on weekends or vacations.

Diarrhea appears to be a common complaint of sodium azide workers. Nausea, vomiting, and abdominal pain have also been noted (3).

Sodium azide is not listed as a carcinogen, although it is a known plant mutagen. Some conflicting animal studies have been performed with no clear evidence of animal mutagenicity (14). There are no known teratogenic or reproductive effects (3).

Toxicity can occur from inhalation of azide gas (hydrazoic acid), which is released through hydrolysis in aqueous solutions of the azide salt or from ingestion of the sodium azide salt. Clinical toxicity mainly targets the cardiovascular system, blood, neurologic, and pulmonary system. Cardiovascular toxicity consists of arteriolar vasodilation, hypotension, syncope, angina, and tachycardia. Neurologic symptoms can include syncope, headache, muscular weakness, decreased reflexes, seizures, and coma. Respiratory toxicity can involve respiratory failure and pulmonary edema. Methemoglobinemia can occur due to oxidation of hemoglobin similar to nitrites. Clinical signs and symptoms of toxicity are dose dependent. Ingestions of 40 milligrams and less (1) have produced headache. Doses of up to 60 milligrams have resulted in syncope and hypotension (1). Doses of 80–150 milligrams (1) have resulted in angina, dysp-

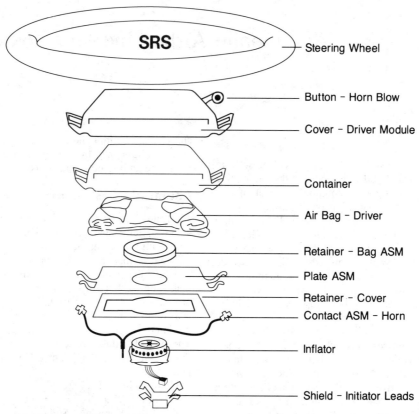

Figure 46.1.   Major components of a driver's side supplemental restraint system (SRS), automobile airbag module.

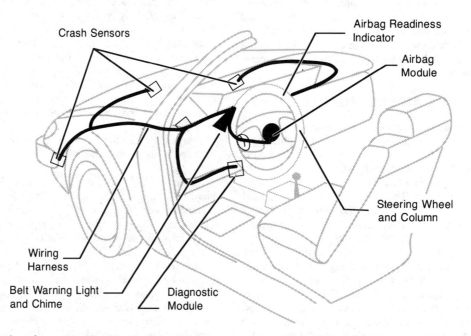

Figure 46.2.   Operation of an automobile airbag module. At extremely rapid deceleration the sensor will signal, causing an electrical current to activate the inflator.

nea, tachycardia, nausea, vomiting, diarrhea, and headache. Ingestion of larger amounts can cause more severe symptoms and even death. Cases of fatal sodium azide poisoning have clinically been associated with severe hypotension, metabolic acidosis, pulmonary edema, cardiac dysrhythmias, bradycar-

dia, and asystole (1). Death has occurred in as short a time as 40 minutes and as long as 30 hours postingestion (1). High-dose inhalations can also produce cardiovascular and pulmonary effects. Pulmonary edema is a common autopsy finding in both humans and laboratory animals. A fatal ingestion can

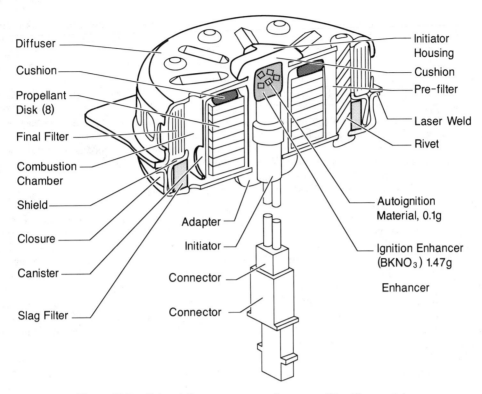

Figure 46.3. Driver inflator component of an automobile airbag module.

Table 46.1. Chemical Hazards of Air Bag Industry

Agent	Use	Exposure	Hazard
Sodium azide salt	Propellant and source of detonation	Ingestion of salt or inhalation of hydrazoic acid	May affect cardiovascular, neurologic, pulmonary, and blood. Blocks cytochrome oxidase and mitochondrial phosphorylation. Can cause hypotension, syncope, headache, muscular weakness, seizures, metabolic acidosis, pulmonary edema, methemoglobinemia, angina, cardiac dysrhythmias, cyanosis
2,4-Dinitrotoluene	Explosive, used in enhancer assembly	Dermal absorption Inhalation Ingestion	Mucous membrane irritant, methemoglobinemia, weakness, dyspnea, cyanosis, nausea, headache, syncope
Ceramic fibers	Filter assembly	Inhalation Dermal Ingestion	Irritant to skin and mucous membrane, nausea, vomiting, and diarrhea may occur following fiber ingestion
Boron	Boron in enhancer present as boron potassium nitrate	Dermal Inhalational of boron as the oxide after ignition	Irritant to eyes and mucous membranes in aerosolized form
Potassium nitrate	Enhancer assembly	Dermal Ingestion	Dermatitis, methemoglobinemia, vasodilator, hypotension, syncope, angina
Cupric oxide	Inflator and module component	Inhalational Dermal Ingestion	Irritant to mucous membrane, chronic exposure may cause nasal septum necrosis, dermatitis
Nitrocellulose	Enhancer assembly	Inhalational Dermal Ingestion	None

be as little as 1–2 grams (2). Demyelination of nerves can occur in chronic large doses. Azides can produce methemoglobinemia and block cytochrome oxidase enzymes as well as mitochondrial phosphorylation. A clinical picture similar to cyanide intoxication may occur in large doses with metabolic acidosis, severe hypotension unresponsive to fluids and vasoconstrictors, and seizures. In unknown ingestions, sodium azide poisoning may be mistaken for cyanide poisoning.

Risk to the public from sodium azide poisoning from airbags is minimal because thermal degradation yields principally nitrogen gas with traces of sodium metal and carbon from scrapping of cars containing airbags (4, 5). Reassuringly, azides are quickly detoxified by bacteria and fungi, and in fact are commonly used in the agriculture industry and in fungicides, herbicides, and nematodecides. More concern is present for rapid release of gas during scrapping operations, tampering, and repair. Azide toxicity, however, should not be a problem in these circumstances.

A second potential hazard utilized in the manufacture of automobile airbags is ceramic fiber. The ceramic fiber used in the process consists of vitreous luminosilicate fibers. These fibers are used as components of the filter assemblies. There are no known chronic health effects in humans from longterm exposure to ceramic fibers. Ceramic fibers have been injected into the peritoneal cavity of laboratory animals as well as into the pleural cavity, and tumors have been produced. This is not a unique effect, and similar results have been detected in various fibrous materials. Several studies have suggested a low order of potential of inducing pulmonary tumors in animals while others have contraindicated this. The International Agency of Research on Cancer (IARC) recently classified fibrous glass wool, mineral wool, and ceramic fiber as Group 2B carcinogens. Group 2B agents are possibly carcinogenic to humans (6).

Ceramic fibers also are irritating to skin and mucosal membranes. Ingestion may cause gastrointestinal disturbances such as irritation, nausea, vomiting, and diarrhea.

The enhancer assembly contains powdered ignition and enhancer material commonly consisting of boron potassium nitrate, nitrocellulose, and 2,4-dinitrotoluene.

Boron potassium nitrate has toxic properties similar to any nitrate and also is mildly irritating to mucous membranes. Environmental monitoring in the enhancer assembly operation has demonstrated that exposure to all propellant dusts and particles is well below Occupational Safety and Health Administration (OSHA) standards. Heavy exposures to processes involving potassium nitrates can cause dermatitis and dermal burns, and chronic exposure to low levels can cause chronic coronary vessel dilation. This coronary artery dilation can be a problem during worker furlough, weekends, and holidays, since the possibility of reflex constriction or spasm or the coronary vessels may occur. However, this only happens in longterm, heavy exposures. Ingested nitrates can be converted by enzymatic activity to nitrites, which can cause methemoglobinemia. Nitrites can also be converted by the body into nitrosamines. Several members of this class of compounds have been identified as carcinogens or potential carcinogens. Boron itself is relatively nontoxic and is a mild irritant.

2,4-Dinitrotoluene is toxic by inhalation and ingestion. It is a mucous membrane irritant and may cause methemoglobinemia. In animals, central nervous system, reproductive, and bone marrow abnormalities have been noted. 2,4-Dinitrotoluene is an animal carcinogen. Tests for mutagenic activity of this compound are ambiguous.

In industry, the principal effects are mucous membrane and skin irritation, but in large exposures cyanosis, weakness, and shortness of breath are common findings. Workers will occasionally have nonspecific complaints such as nausea, headache, confusion, uncoordination, loss of consciousness, cough, and joint pain. Interestingly, the compound appears to permeate the skin to a significant extent. Workers with preexisting central or peripheral nervous system, lung, or reproductive disorders

may have increased susceptibility to 2,4-dinitrotoluene exposure. The IARC, OSHA, and National Toxicology Program (NTP) have not rated 2,4-dinitrotoluene as a carcinogen. Nitrocellulose is not known to have harmful toxic effects in humans (7).

Cupric oxide is also a component of the airbag inflator/module. This chemical has a low inherent toxicity, but some studies demonstrate that exposure to copper-containing material may cause ulceration and perforation of the nasal septum over time. Sensitization to copper does rarely occur in the rarely reported cases of dermatitis associated with copper.

Worker Protection

Clearly the most hazardous component of the airbag manufacturing industry is that of fire or explosion. Automobile airbags are much more than explosive devices attached to cloth bags. They represent a vast amount of engineering effort, stress analysis, and finite element analysis. Despite the superb engineering utilized by this industry, the potential for explosion throughout the manufacturing process is inevitably present. Raw materials must be ground to appropriate size, mixed with other chemical constituents, pressed into appropriate form, and packaged with other components. All of these parts of the process have some inherent risk associated with them. Workers need to be isolated from the most hazardous parts of the process. These components (principally grinding, pressing, and blending) can be done by automated equipment behind reinforced concrete walls and monitored by closed circuit television.

The dust generated from the grinding and pressing process is a potential health hazard, both from inhalation and skin exposure. Workers cleaning and servicing equipment as well as working around the grinding process should have dermal protection with appropriate garments. The use of appropriate respiratory protective devices is also required. Worker protection is required until the disk is sealed into the cannister.

Employees who cut or manipulate the ceramic fiber may be exposed to airborne fiber components and should wear respiratory protection or perform such work in appropriate hooded work stations. Air flows should be adjusted so that the fiber products are not released into the environment at levels exceeding the threshold limit value.

Care should be taken to electrically ground the entire manufacturing process from start to finish. This precaution, however, may not be totally necessary as the sodium azide propellant is not very static sensitive. Ignition of sodium azide requires 250 times the Department of Defense standard for electrostatic discharge sensitivity. To date, no fire or explosive accident involving sodium azide-based propellant has been clearly linked to electrostatic discharge. Nonetheless, all explosives and propellants should be treated as electrostatically sensitive simply as a matter of prudence.

Medical Monitoring

Not all workers in the manufacture of airbags need to be medically monitored. Only those employees whose jobs require the use of respirators, that is, those directly involved in the manufacture, grinding, pressing, and to a lesser extent the packaging of the explosive components require monitoring. The only additional job classification personnel that would require such monitoring would be those working around ceramic fiber. All of these need to have periodic respirator physicals. The

American National Standard for Respiratory Protection—Respirator Use, specifies that any employee who is required to wear a respirator in the course of his or her duties must be appropriately medically monitored. Industrial hygienists and safety engineers must establish the type of respirator indicated for the particular components being utilized. The position then shall classify each employee as class I, II, or III. Class I individuals have no restrictions in respirator use. Class II individuals have some restrictions. Class III individuals are restricted from respirator use. The physician must perform a medical evaluation, stressing cardiac, pulmonary, auditory, and psychologic factors. The employee must be examined for facial deformities, adequate hearing, adequate respiratory and cardiovascular function, endocrine disorders, neurologic disorders, and psychologic conditions; assessment is necessary of any medications that the employee may be taking, including legal and illegal drugs and alcohol. Generally, the physician will want to perform spirometry and may occasionally require an exercise stress test, depending on the type of respirator used and the conditions under which the use occurs, as well as the employee's physical condition. These examinations may be repeated as often as the physician feels necessary, but generally this type of examination is not required any more frequently than every 5 years below age 35, with exams every 2 years up to age 45, and annually thereafter. Examination on termination is usually advisable, as well as on return from prolonged absences or disability (8).

Workers who have potential skin or inhalation exposure to sodium azide should have periodic blood pressure screening. Hypertensive individuals should be identified and their blood pressure should be monitored weekly. Other individuals not found to be hypertensive initially should be monitored weekly for 4 weeks until a baseline is obtained, then every 2–4 weeks thereafter. Monitoring is for the purpose of identifying hypotension, which may or may not be symptomatic in individuals exposed to sodium azide.

Individuals with heart disease or at high risk for heart disease should be restricted from working with sodium azide and potassium nitrate. Both of these chemicals potentially could exacerbate preexisting cardiac conditions.

Preplacement physicals should be performed on all workers in these areas to identify cardiac, pulmonary, dermatologic, neurologic, and any other medical conditions that might place a worker at increased risk in this environment.

As with any plant environment, periodic audiograms should be performed in any areas identified as noisy or borderline noisy. Noise level monitoring in a work environment should be routinely performed as good industrial hygiene and safety practice dictates.

Cumulative Trauma Disorders

In this era of prevalence and concern for cumulative trauma disorders, no discussion of any manufacturing process would be complete without some mention of this problem. The automobile airbag industry, like most industries, involves some jobs that have repetitive use of the upper extremities. Most of the positions within the automobile airbag industry are auto-

mated, so that repetitive use of the hands and wrists is minimal in most areas. One area of concern, however, is the very traditional function—that of sewing. The airbags themselves are hand sewn by workers sitting or standing at an industrial sewing machine. This work usually involves repeated ulnar and radial deviation of the hands throughout an 8-hour day. There is also some flexion and prolonged gripping in this process. Individuals with histories of carpal tunnel syndrome, tendonitis, neck, shoulder, and elbow problems should be restricted from duty in this area. Individuals who become symptomatic with any of these problems while working in the sewing area should be taken off work or transferred, at least temporarily, to a different function within the plant. The module assembly operation also has ergonomic implications, considering the repetitive use of the hands and arms.

Hazards to Occupants of an Automobile

Potential hazards to automobile occupants can be encountered following activation or deflation of an airbag. Similar hazards may be encountered by paramedical personnel responding to an accident. Exposure to irritating gas on deflation of an airbag can occur. The airbag is inflated with nitrogen, which is produced when about 80 grams total of sodium azide is detonated. Byproducts of detonation of sodium azide include sodium hydroxide and nitrogen. Powder residue can produce ocular and nasal irritation. Upon detonation of the sodium azide, nitrogen gas explodes the bag. Nitrogen gas is also vented to the sides of the steering column toward the driver's feet. The nitrogen gas is warmed by the explosion, and an alkaline powder will be present around the driver's compartment.

SUMMARY

The automobile airbag industry is a uniquely new manufacturing process utilizing several potentially hazardous chemicals (Table 46.1). As the deployment of airbags progresses under federal mandate, this industry will grow and new work-related medical conditions will most probably be identified. Now in its infancy, the industry appears to be relatively safe. Only longterm observation and experience will determine other areas for future concern.

REFERENCES

1. Klein-Schwartz W, et al. Three fatal sodium azide poisonings. Med Toxicol Adverse Drug Exp 1989;4:219–227.
2. Lott AL. Material safety data sheet—airbag inflators/module. In: TRW safety systems. Mesa, AZ: 1989.
3. Material safety data sheets. Sodium azide: EXP 0064/88D. 1989.
4. Pietz JF. Problem considerations of using sodium azide in the air cushion restraint system. In: Talley Industries of Arizona. Report #11988. 1978.
5. Abrams A, El-Mallakh JL, Meyer R. Suicidal sodium azide ingestion. Ann Emerg Med 1987;16:1378–1380.
6. Material safety data sheets. Fiberfax. The Carborundum Company—Fibers Division. MSDS #AVP/B07-2, 1980.
7. Material safety data sheets. Single base smokeless powder. Exbro Chemical Products Company, 1988.
8. American National Standards Institute. American National Standard for Respiratory Protection—Respirator Use—Physical Qualifications for Personnel. ANSI, 1984.

47

Aerospace Industry Exposure Hazards

Bradley Y. Dennis, M.D.

POTENTIAL HAZARD EXPOSURES IN AEROSPACE FABRICATION, MAINTENANCE, AND REPAIR

Aerospace manufacturing and repair include numerous potential hazardous exposures. There is a lack of knowledge among many workers and employers concerning these health risks.

This chapter deals primarily with advanced composites and solvents but will also cover other common chemical hazards found in the aerospace industry. While specific health and safety information will be provided concerning several chemicals, it is important to consider some basic health and safety issues. Hazardous exposure may be by oral ingestion, dermal contact, or inhalation. Because the industrial setting does not lend itself to frequent oral ingestion, data from skin contact and inhalation studies are much more relevant than the readily available information on the oral toxicity of a compound.

Regardless of a substance's hazard or toxicity, careful steps should be taken to minimize individual exposure when handling any chemical. If chemicals are handled correctly, even the most toxic substance will pose little hazard to the worker.

While supplier material safety data sheets are helpful, control measures are available to ensure a safe work environment on an individual basis. For instance, administrative controls are provisions made by a company's management to control hazards. They include material handling, training, isolation of operations (lunch areas separate from work areas), personal protective equipment, personal hygiene (hand washing before eating, drinking, and smoking), warning labels, housekeeping, work practices for chemical storage and transportation, and emergency instructions. Engineering controls such as closed-system processing and effective ventilation should provide, as nearly as possible, complete containment of dusts, fumes, and vapors from hazardous materials. When general ventilation is not sufficient to control airborne exposures, engineering controls such as local exhaust ventilation at the emission source should be provided and supplemented by personal protective equipment when necessary.

Workers should not be exposed to airborne contaminants in excess of the Threshold Limit Values as set by the American Conference of Governmental Industrial Hygienists (ACGIH) or the Occupational Safety and Health Administration (OSHA) Permissible Exposure Limits (PEL). Personal breathing zone air monitoring should be considered to establish baseline exposure levels with periodic assessments conducted where toxic chemicals are processed or when unusual odors exist, or heavier than normal visible contamination appears.

ADVANCED COMPOSITES

The definition of a composite is a material made from several components. An early example of a composite is reinforced concrete, in which a reinforcement is embedded in a type of matrix. A composite is expected to have mechanical properties superior to those of its components. The 1950s saw the modern era of composite materials begin with the introduction of metal alloys, fiberglass, and plastics. However, lightweight materials with increased strength, stiffness, and resistance to high temperatures were not introduced until the more recent development of carbon and graphite fiber composites. Since the early 1980s, there has been a significant increase in the use of carbon/graphite composites in sports equipment, industrial machinery, medical prostheses, and especially in the aerospace industry.

Advanced composites consist of carbon or graphite fibers bound in a resin matrix, which provides the insulation and physical resistance properties of composites. The resin matrix that binds the fibers may consist of several different substances, such as epoxy, polyester, polyacetal, polyethylene, and polystyrene. The most commonly used resin is epoxy, which is usually derived from diglycidyl ether of bisphenol A (DGBA) or from a nonbisphenol A epoxy such as 4-glycidiloxy-N,N-diglycidilaniline (GDOGDA). Epoxy resins are reacted with curing agents to solidify the epoxy and convert it to a thermoset plastic.

The primary concerns in the production, machining, and maintenance of advanced composites involve the release of low molecular weight and high vapor pressure compounds. These compounds include solvents, reactive diluents, epoxies, and hardeners released during preimpregnation or evaporation from the stored prepreg material; in addition, the inhalation of carbon fibers and dust can occur during grinding and cutting. Dermal exposure with potential skin sensitization/contact dermatitis, and local eye and skin irritation are possible.

TOXICOLOGIC PROPERTIES OF COMPOSITES

Epoxy Resins

Propylene and chlorine react to form epichlorohydrin, which is mixed with bisphenol A, a backbone chemical formed from acetone and phenol. Epichlorohydrin and bisphenol A form a glycidyl group, which is reacted with hardeners/curing agents (normally amines) to produce epoxy resin for preimpregnating fibers (Fig. 47.1). The term epoxy is applied to compounds containing one or more oxirane rings. The term prepreg defines sheets of pyrolized carbon fibers impregnated with a liquid binder, such as epoxy resin, and then reacted with a curing agent to solidify the epoxy and convert it to a thermoset plastic, molded into a desired shape. Approximately 30–45% of prepreg is resin, and 1–10% is solvent.

Almost all bisphenol A-based epoxy resins contain less than 1 ppm residual epichlorohydrin. The Chemical Abstract Service notes a Threshold Limit Value/Permissible Exposure Limit-Time Weighted Average (TLV/PEL-TWA) of 2 ppm and carries a "skin" notation. However, care should be taken with any resin containing epichlorohydrin, as the International Agency for Research on Cancer (IARC) has classified

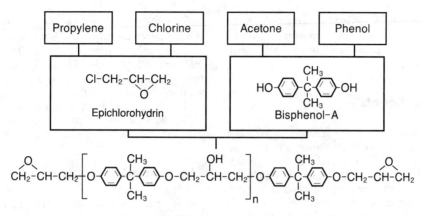

Figure 47.1. Manufacturing process for bis A-based epoxy resins.

epichlorohydrin as a probable human carcinogen (Group 2A) based on animal data (1), and the National Toxicology Program (NTP) has classified it as a substance anticipated to be carcinogenic (2). The IARC has decided that there are insufficient data to classify Bisphenol-A epoxy resin (DGBA) as a potential carcinogen (3).

Epoxy resins formed from bisphenol A and epichlorohydrin have a low order of acute toxicity and cause only slight to moderate skin irritation. Rare individuals may develop a skin sensitivity. Chronic dermal application of DGBA on mice did not cause skin cancer, nor did it cause any hematologic or clinical chemistry changes (4, 5). Bisphenol F epoxy resins cause minor skin and eye irritation and are felt to be toxicologically similar to bisphenol A resins.

Cycloaliphatic epoxy resins have an irritant effect on the skin and mucous membranes, but most are not considered mutagenic. Neither NTP, IARC, nor OSHA considers them carcinogenic. However, there are animal studies indicating a possible carcinogenic effect for certain members of this group, and, therefore, precautionary measures should be followed carefully when handling these products. Cycloaliphatic glycidyl ethers and esters irritate the skin and mucous membranes and may have a sensitizing effect. Neopentylglycol diglycidyl ether has been reported to cause skin tumors with chronic exposure to shaved mice skin (6).

Polyurethane Resins

Polyurethane resins consist of isocyanates and polyols. Most commercial isocyanates are highly toxic from either skin absorption with systemic toxicity or to skin and lung sensitization. Proper ventilation is a necessity because of the high inhalation toxicity. Respiratory sensitization has also been described for some isocyanate exposure.

Toluene diisocyanate (TDI) has a TLV-TWA of 0.005 ppm and TLV-STEL (Shortterm Exposure Limit) of 0.02 ppm. PELs are set at the same levels. Because TDI has no odor warning characteristics, it is hazardous in vapor or liquid forms and causes skin and respiratory sensitization. Some cross-reactivity may occur with other isocyanates. Once sensitization occurs, even a few hundredths of a part per million will cause recurrent allergic reaction. TDI is a strong skin and eye irritant, and prolonged contact with skin will cause burns. Exposure to high vapor concentrations may cause pulmonary edema.

TDI has been classified as possibly carcinogenic by IARC, Group 2B, based on animal, but no human data (10). This classification has been criticized for its poorly conducted oral intubation route of administration, high test doses used, and lack of characterization of the test substance in the body. A study utilizing an inhalation administration did not confirm the earlier NTP study findings (11).

Polyols include polyether and polyester and are used for cross-linking isocyanate compounds. They provide no health hazard other than the occasional presence of unreacted ethylene oxide in some polyols used in poorly ventilated work areas.

Phenolic and Amino Resins

Phenol-, urea-, and melamine-formaldehyde resins have a low toxicity potential. However, contact with the phenol-formaldehyde resin in the uncured state should be avoided because of potential phenol absorption through the skin. Also, small amounts of formaldehyde and phenol may be given off during the curing process, thus requiring good ventilation.

The current TLV-TWA for formaldehyde is 1 ppm, with a STEL of 2 ppm. The PEL-TWA for formaldehyde is a 1 ppm, with a STEL of 2 ppm. Formaldehyde is a strong skin sensitizer and an eye, skin, and respiratory irritant (12). Formaldehyde is an animal carcinogen but study results are inconclusive in humans.

Bismaleimide Resins

Bismaleimide resins (polyimides) have not been studied extensively. Prolonged or repeated skin contact has been reported to cause irritation or sensitization, and dust may cause eye, nose, and throat irritation.

Thermoplastics

Other than the styrene group of thermoplastics (polystyrene), these compounds are not considered harmful to humans. Most cause no toxic effects by ingestion, skin contact, or inhalation. The *styrene* monomer is of concern because its vapors can cause eye irritation, and liquid exposure causes eye, skin, and mucous membrane irritation. Central nervous system (CNS), liver, and kidney effects have also been reported (8). "Styrene sickness," a syndrome characterized by drowsiness, dizziness, nausea, and headache, has been reported in workers exposed to 200 to 700 ppm styrene (8). The styrene monomer has been labeled ''possibly carcinogenic to humans'' by the IARC based on limited animal studies (25).

Hardeners/Curing Agents

Aromatic amine hardeners are slightly irritating to skin and mucous membranes. Inhalation has been shown to cause damage to internal organs such as the liver and may form methemoglobin to decrease the blood's oxygen transporting ability. *Methylene dianiline*—4,4-methylene dianiline has a TLV-TWA of 0.1 ppm with a recommended PEL of 0.01 ppm. Chronic exposure is capable of causing liver damage in humans following oral or dermal exposure (7, 8). NTP has recently classified MDA to be a carcinogen; however, there have been no confirmed reports of MDA-related cancer in humans.

The manufacturer's prepregging and ''B-staging'' operations will usually markedly decrease any free MDA which may be present in an amine-cured epoxy resin system. Although no free MDA is likely to be detected in cured laminates, it is recommended that a high efficiency particulate air (HEPA) filtered ventilated hand tool be considered for cutting and trimming MDA-containing prepregs instead of stripping and peeling by hand. *4,4'-Sulfonyl dianiline* (Dapsone, DDS) has no established workplace standards, and there is no history or evidence of human carcinogenicity with this substance (9).

Aliphatic and cycloaliphatic amine hardeners are strong bases and should be considered severe irritants or corrosives, and some are sensitizers. Polyaminoamide hardeners have a slightly irritating effect on skin but may cause sensitization. Amide hardeners are only slight irritants. Anhydride curing agents are severe eye irritants and strong skin irritants. Good ventilation is necessary for work areas where these curing agents are used.

Solvents

Solvents are utilized at numerous stages in the preparation of composite materials, such as manufacture of the basic resin and fibers, impregnating reinforcements, and in tool and work area cleanup. Skin contact with most organic solvents results in drying, defatting, and dermatitis. Because some solvents are absorbed directly through the skin, there is an additional potential hazard when other materials are dissolved and carried through the skin along with the solvent. For instance, although it should never be allowed, solvents are occasionally used to remove sticky epoxy resins from the skin, which may facilitate the penetration of epoxy resin into the body (12, 13).

Inhalation of solvent vapors may cause delayed pulmonary edema, respiratory irritation, and CNS depression with narcosis, uncoordination, dizziness, unconsciousness, and even death.

Ketone Solvents

Acetone has a TLV and PEL-TWA of 750 ppm and a TLV and PEL-STEL of 1000 ppm. Inhalation may cause mucous membrane irritation, nausea, and headache. Skin contact can cause defatting and dermatitis. Systemic injury probably does not occur with skin absorption, but, repeated exposure to high levels of acetone may cause CNS depression.

Methyl ethyl ketone (MEK) has TLV- and PEL-TWAs of 200 ppm and TLV and PEL-STELs of 300 ppm. MEK causes nose, throat, and eye irritation above 200 ppm (8). A recognizable odor is noted at the TLV for MEK, but very few serious health effects have been reported at this level (8). Minor embryo- and fetotoxic effects have been observed in female rats exposed to MEK levels greater than 1000 ppm (14).

Chlorinated Solvents

Exposure to very high concentrations of halogenated hydrocarbon solvents have been reported to cause CNS depression and cardiac muscle sensitization. Animal studies have demonstrated liver and kidney changes with chronic exposure. Two separate case-control studies have suggested a possible association of chlorinated organic solvents, used in de-icer and fuel cell manufacturing, with excess lung cancer (15, 16).

Methylene chloride (dichloromethane) has a TLV-TWA of 50 ppm, and OSHA has established a PEL of 500 ppm with an acceptable ceiling concentration of 1000 ppm. Exposure to methylene chloride vapors well above the TLV may cause CNS depression, but, use at or below the TLV has caused no adverse health effects (8). Liquid methylene chloride may cause eye and skin irritation, and high concentrations of vapors may cause respiratory irritation. Methylene chloride is metabolized to carbon monoxide, which forms carboxyhemoglobin, thus decreasing the body's ability to carry oxygen to the tissues. Several chronic studies have shown that methylene chloride causes cancer in animals, and the NTP concluded that methylene chloride was carcinogenic in rodents based on inhalation studies (17). Methylene chloride appears to be a genotoxic carcinogen, exerting its effect through the direct chemical interaction of itself or one of its metabolic products with genetic structures of the cell (18).

New toxicokinetic studies, which reduce reliance on animal experiments and provide a more systematic approach to hazard evaluation, have found that the conventional research approach overestimates the human risk from methylene chloride by a factor of 100. Because of the discrepancy between the toxicokinetic approach and conventional risk assessment, the U.S. Environmental Protection Agency (EPA) has reconsidered its rule-making for methylene chloride.

1,1,1-Trichloroethane (methylchloroform) has TLV- and PEL-TWAs of 350 ppm. The TLV and PEL-STELs are 450 ppm. Trichloroethane is generally less toxic than methylene chloride, and exposure of humans to 500 ppm for seven hours per day for five days showed no evidence of abnormal clinical findings (8). Severe overexposure can cause CNS depression, which may lead to respiratory arrest, but rapid and complete recovery usually follows if the victim is alive when removed from exposure (19). Overexposure is also reported to cause fat deposits and necrosis in the liver and occasional kidney damage (20). Alcohol should be avoided before, during, and after trichloroethane exposure because both are metabolized by the liver. This solvent is not teratogenic, and carcinogenicity/mutagenicity testing has proven inconclusive (21).

Other solvents include *dimethylformamide* (DMF) and *N-methylpyrrolidone* (NMP). DMF has a TLV- and PEL-TWA of 10 ppm-skin. It is irritating to the eyes, skin, and mucous

Table 47.1. Controlled Chemicals

Chemical	Prop. 65	Rule 1401*	Typical use
Acetaldehyde	X	X	Solvent-structural adhesives
Acrylamide		X	Adhesives
Acrylonitrile	X	X	Acrylic and elastomers
* Allyl chloride		X	Resin for varnish/plastic/adhesive
* Benzene	X	X	Solvent-phenol prepregs
* Benzidene	X	X	Stiffening agent-rubber
* 1,3-Butadiene	X	X	Synthetic elastomers
Cadmium	X	X	CD plating-ceramics
* Chlorobenzene		X	Solvent-methylene diisocyanate
Chloroform	X	X	Laboratory solvent
* Chromium (hexavalent)	X	X	Paints-plating
* Dichlorobenzidene		X	Cure agent-urethanes
Diethanolamine		X	Cutting oils-detergent for emulsion paints
* Dioxane		X	Lacquers/paints/strippers
* Methylene chloride	X	X	Solvent-paints
* Epichlorohydrin	X	X	Epoxy prepregs-resins
Ethylene dichloride		X	Paint strippers
* Formaldehyde	X	X	Phenol prepregs
* Lead	X	X	Paints
Maleic anhydride		X	Polyester resins
* 4-4'-Methylene dianiline	X		Polymide prepregs
* Nickel		X	Plating-paints
* Phenol		X	Phenolic prepregs
* Propylene oxide		X	Polyols for urethane foams
* Titanium oxide		X	White pigment in paints
* Toluene		X	Solvent-paints
Trichloroethylene		X	Solvent-paints
* Xylene		X	Solvent-paints
* Urethane	X		Elastomers-paints

* (Proposed) new source review of known and suspected carcinogenic air contaminants.
Source: South Coast Air Quality Management District in Los Angeles.

membranes. Overexposure may cause nausea, abdominal pain, loss of appetite, and possible liver damage (8). The IARC has classified DMF as possibly carcinogenic to humans, Group 2B, based on controversial studies linking DMF to the development of testicular cancer (22, 23). NMP has a TWA of 100 ppm (vapor) suggested by the manufacturer. It can cause dermatitis with blistering, edema, and erythema with prolonged or repeated contact. It is not a skin sensitizer. Vapor contact may cause eye irritation (24). No teratogenicity has been noted in animal studies.

REINFORCING MATERIALS

Reinforcement materials are added to the resin matrix of advanced composites to provide strength to the cured material. Once the composite is produced, exposure is limited to that encountered during drilling, grinding, and sanding operations.

Dusts generated during such operations should be controlled by "nuisance dust" standards. Based on chemical and morphologic studies showing high chemical stability of composites, and the fact that most secondary products from machining composites are particulate rather than fibrous, it is more important to consider the size and shape of the particles than the resin chemical or fabric composition (26).

The difference between "total" and "respirable" dust should be considered. Only particles less than 3.5 micrometers can reach the deep lung without being trapped in the nasal hairs or deposited on bronchial walls. Particles greater than 7 micrometers in diameter cannot reach the deep lung tissues. These particles are not considered "respirable." Dusts with a mean aerodynamic diameter of 3.5 micrometers or less are considered respirable (27).

Carbon and Graphite Fibers

Carbon fibers can be made from any carbonaceous, fibrous raw material that pyrolyzes to a char and leaves a high carbon residue. Early carbon fibers were made from rayon but are now made from polyacrylonitrile (PAN) or petroleum pitch. The precursor is heated to 1200°C to produce a carbon fiber and 2200–2700°C to produce a graphite fiber. These carbon-based fibers provide the strength of composites, as graphite fibers are 1.5–2 times stronger than steel.

The TLV-TWA for synthetic forms of *graphite* has been established at 10 mg/m^3. Natural graphite is to be controlled to 2.5 mg/m^3 (respirable dust), but proposals are being considered to specify 10 mg/m^3 for all forms of graphite, natural and synthetic. There are no established limits for carbon fibers, although the U.S. Navy has established a limit of three carbon fibers/cm^3. As a minimum, the OSHA nuisance dust standard of 10 mg/m^3 total dust, 5 mg/m^3 respirable fraction, should not be exceeded. The size of carbon fibers produced by machining of composites is considered too large to be damaging to the respiratory system, but it does cause mechanical abrasion and irritation of the skin and eyes (28). Allergic or sensitizing reactions are not reported to occur when handling unsized carbon or graphite fibers (29, 30).

Animal studies found no tumors or scar tissue in the lungs of guinea pigs after significant exposure to carbon fibers (31). The Health and Environmental Review Division, Office of Toxic Substances at EPA felt there were insufficient data to classify the carcinogenic potential of carbon fibers (32).

Aramid fiber (Kevlar) is another type of reinforcing material. DuPont has established an acceptable exposure limit of five respirable fibers/cm^3. Aramid fiber is not a sensitizer and shows only occasional mild irritation of skin. There is little evidence of lung damage in animal inhalation studies. The EPA has classified aramid fibers as "possible human carcinogen," utilizing especially weak evidence (33).

Fiberglass is a type of humanmade fiber which is supplied in two basic forms: textile (continuous filament) fibers and wool-type fibers used in insulation. The TLV-TWA for fiberglass dust is 10 mg/m^3. OSHA has not established a PEL, but a TWA of 15 mg/m^3 of total dust and 5 mg/m^3 of respirable fraction is presently used. NIOSH is pursuing a standard level of 3 fibers/cm^3.

The continuous filament fibers used in composite reinforcement differs from the wool-type, in that all textile fibers are greater than 6 microns in diameter and thus are nonrespirable (34). The glass fibers may break into shorter lengths, but their diameter will not permit them into the deep lung areas. Fiberglass itself causes only mechanical irritation of the eyes, nose, and throat, but skin sensitization may occur from the uncured resins and hardeners used to manufacture the reinforced laminate (35). Human and animal studies have failed to demonstrate a cancer risk, and the IARC has categorized continuous filament fiberglass as not classifiable for human carcinogenicity. Fiberglass wool was classified as a possible human carcinogen by IARC, based on animal studies utilizing nonnatural routes of exposure, such as injection or implantation (34).

Ceramic fibers are another reinforcement material with no specific TLV or OSHA PEL. A manufacturer has recommended using the airborne concentrations established for fiberglass. Ceramic fibers may cause temporary local skin or respiratory irritation. There are no studies available on the health effects from exposure to ceramic fibers in humans.

Composite Hazard Controls

Proper ventilation systems are most important in controlling potential composite hazards. Dilution ventilation, such as open hangars, are probably inadequate. Paint booths are often inadequate because the filters become saturated quickly by the dust concentration generated; in addition, makeup air volumes are often too small. Aerospace manufacturers traditionally have a metallic background, and older facilities have ventilation systems designed for metallic rather than chemical use.

Composite machining should be performed, when possible, in shops dedicated to this operation. A two room format should be considered with lay-up operations performed in a room ventilated for solvents. A separate room should be utilized for machining of composites where skin protection is provided by full body coveralls (preferably disposable), side shield safety glasses, and gloves.

Local exhaust ventilation should be utilized to remove composite particulates. An exhaust hood designed for air flow to be drawn from under a sanding operation is preferable. A direct tool attachment with high velocity low volume exhaust, or plastic bags designed to fit around or near the tool in use are also acceptable.

Dust masks are adequate respiratory protection for most operations. The NIOSH respirator selection guide should be consulted for airborne concentrations above acceptable exposure levels. When very small composite particulates in the 0.5–1.0-micron range are generated, the use of HEPA filters should be considered. A high efficiency vacuum system is a very helpful general housekeeping tool for eliminating significant proportions of dust and fibers. Compressed air should not be used to blow dust off workers. Hand washing should be mandated, and hands, arms, and face should be thoroughly washed prior to eating.

Repair Material Toxicity

Composite repair materials include polymers such as adhesives and prepregs, as well as aerosol coatings. Repairs may take place in the manufacturing facility, in depots, or in the field. The potential routes of exposure are the same as those for composite fabrication and include skin contact, inhalation, and ingestion.

Polymers

Polymeric materials may be staged into three categories. The *A stage* is an early stage in the preparation of thermosetting resins in which the material is still soluble in certain liquids and fusible. Monomeric reactants are present, and health concern is highest in this stage, especially for two-part room temperature adhesives. The *B stage* is an intermediate stage in the reaction of thermoset resins in which the material swells and softens in contact with liquids and softens when heated but may not dissolve or fuse. B stage materials are partially polymerized into long chain molecules and are less chemically reactive. Health concern is moderate in this stage, which includes epoxy and condensation polyimide prepregs and most film and foam adhesives. The *C stage* is the final, fully cured state of composites and adhesives. There is no chemical reactivity, and the health concern is for dust from machining and sanding.

More than 90% of polymeric materials used are epoxy. The characteristics of epoxy prepregs and film/foam adhesives are the same as those discussed earlier under composite fabrication. They include a glycidyl ether family, mild pulmonary, and eye irritation from dusts and vapors, and potential for sensitization with exposure to uncured resin. Epoxy paste adhesive is 100% resin and has a similar chemistry to the epoxy prepregs and adhesives. It is important to keep in mind that mixing paste adhesives in batches greater than one pound may result in an exothermic reaction in the container, thus releasing toxic gases.

Polyimide polymer materials also include prepregs, film adhesives, and paste adhesives. These materials are also occasionally used in high tech, advanced composites repair work. The condensation polyimide prepreg has a low toxicity in B stage, but mild irritation and dark staining of the skin may occur. Polyimide film adhesive (B stage) may cause moderate skin and eye irritation. The presence of xylene may act as a pulmonary irritant, and silica may cause lung injury. Polyimide paste adhesive (A stage) contains MDA (Methylene dianiline), which may cause liver damage. Silica and xylene are also found in the paste adhesive, as well as ethanol, which acts as a CNS depressant.

The skin route of entry for the polymeric repair materials is of concern only in the A and B stages. It is prevented by using nonpermeable gloves and shop coats which can be cleaned frequently or of Tyvek disposable material. Protective clothing is especially important during the lay-up of prepregs or adhesive mixing operations. Inhalation occurs with the low volatility of B stage polymers and the higher volatility of A stage products as well as C stage dust from machining and sanding operations. Proper ventilation or outdoor work will help prevent inhalation toxicity. Manufacturing and depot areas must have ventilation systems suited to chemical, not metal, operations. All polymers should be cured under vacuum bags with a carbon filter on the exhaust hose. Respirators should be worn to prevent dust inhalation. Ingestion has a very low probability of occurring.

Coating Repairs

Coatings are applied as respirable aerosols, usually within paint booths or paint hangars. They are more toxic than polymer materials because they contain lead in topcoats, chromium VI in primers and topcoats, methylene chloride in solvents, diisocyanates in urethane topcoats, and MDA in a few topcoats. Coatings may enter the body more easily than polymer materials and protective clothing is less effective.

Plating—Surface Preparation Operations

Potential exposures in plating include cadmium, chromium, and nickel. Plasma spraying can cause a potential exposure to chromium. There is a high risk of ground water contamination from repeated spills in plating operations. Risk assessment may be required for cadmium and chromium.

Paint Strippers

Paint strippers are potentially exposed to several solvents such as dioxane, methylene chloride, ethylene dichloride, phenol, toluene, xylene, and trichloroethylene. All depainting operations should be performed in paint booths, utilizing catch basins to eliminate potential for sewer runoff. Exposure to methylene chloride may require a risk assessment performance.

Controlled Chemicals

States such as California are beginning to develop strict laws to control certain chemical exposures. California has already adopted Proposition 65, the Safe Drinking Water and Toxic Enforcement Act of 1986, and has proposed Rule 1401, which controls known or suspected carcinogenic air contaminants. Because so many aerospace manufacturers are located in California, a list of controlled chemicals and their typical use is provided (37) (see Table 47.1).

Administrative controls to ensure employee education in proper maintenance and cleanup methods and correct use of personal protective equipment and respirators are very important. Material Safety Data Sheets (MSDS) should be made available to personnel.

CONCLUSION

The potential hazards encountered in the aerospace industry can be controlled with a better understanding of advanced composites and other potentially toxic substances. Proper handling procedures must be established and enforced to ensure workers' safety.

REFERENCES

1. IARC. Epichlorohydrin. In: International Agency for Research on Cancer monographs on the evaluation of carcinogenic risk to humans. Supplement 7: Overall evaluations of carcinogenicity: an updating of IARC monographs volumes 1 to 42. Lyon, France: WHO, IARC, 1987.

2. National Toxicology Program. Fourth annual report on carcinogens, summary. NTP 85-002. U.S. Department of Health and Human Services, Public Health Service, 1985.

3. IARC. Vol. 47. Organic solvents, some resin monomers, some pigments, and occupational exposures in the painting trades. Lyon, France: WHO, International Agency for Research on Cancer, 1989.

4. Holland JM, et al. Chronic dermal toxicity of epoxy resins. I. Skin carcinogenic potency and general toxicity. ORNL 5762 Special. Oak Ridge National Laboratory, 1981. Holland JM, et al. Test of carcinogenicity in mouse skin: methylenedianiline, gamma-glycidyloxytrimethyloxysilane, gamma-aminopropyltriethoxysilane and a mixture of m-phenylenediamine, methylenedi-

aniline and diglycidylether of bisphenol-A. ORNL/TM-10472. Oak Ridge National Laboratory, 1987.

5. Zakova N, et al. Evaluation of skin carcinogenicity of technical 2,2′-bis-(p-glycidyloxyphenyl)-propane in CF1 mice. Food Chem Toxicol 1985;23:1081–1089.

6. Environmental Protection Agency 8EHQ-0481-0397 and 8EHQ-0481-0397S In: Preliminatry evaluations of initial TSCA section 8(e) substantial risk notifications; February 1, 1980 to December 31, 1982. EPA 560/2-83-001. Environmental Protection Agency, 1983.

7. Kopelman H, et al. The Epping jaundice. Br Med J 1966;1:514–516.

8. American Conference of Governmental Industrial Hygienists. Documentation of the threshold limit values and biological exposure indices. 5th ed. Cincinnati, OH: American Conference of Governmental Industrial Hygienists, 1988.

9. Mandell GL, Sande MA. Antimicrobial agents (continued): drugs used in the chemotherapy of tuberculosis and leprosy. In: Gilman AG, Goodman LS, Gilman A, eds. Goodman and Gilman's The pharmacological basis of therapeutics. 8th ed. New York: Macmillan, 1990.

10. IARC Toluene diisocyanate. In: IARC monographs on the evaluation of carcinogenic risk to humans. Vol 39: Some chemicals used in plastics and elastomers. Lyon, France: WHO, International Agency for Research on Cancer, 1986.

11. Loeser E. Long-term toxicity and carcinogenicity studies with 2,4/2,6-toluene diisocyanate (80/20) in rats and mice. Toxcol Lett 15:71–81, 1983.

12. Greenblatt M. Formaldehyde toxicology: a review of recent developments. Proc Int Cong Role Formaldehyde Biol Syst 2nd. 1987, 53–59.

13. Clayton GD, Clayton FE. Patti's industrial hygiene and toxicology. 3rd revised ed. New York: John Wiley & Sons, 1981, 2141–2159, 2217–2232.

14. Deacon MM, et al. Embryo- and fetotoxicity of inhaled methyl ethyl ketone in rats. Toxicol Appl Pharmacol 1981;59:620–622.

15. Delzell E, et al. A case control study of employment experience and lung cancer among rubber workers. Am J Ind Med 1982;3:393–404.

16. Manson RR, Fine LJ. Cancer mortality and mobidity among rubber workers. J Natl Cancer Inst. 1978;61:1047–1053.

17. National Toxicology Program. Toxicology and carcinogenesis studies of dichloromethane (methylene chloride) (CAS No. 75–09–2) in F344/N rats and B6C3F1 mice (inhalationstudies). NTP Technical Report 306, 1986.

18. Clewell HJ, et al. Toxicokinetics: an analytical tool for assessing chemical hazards to man. Aviat Space Environ Med 1988; A125–A131.

19. Gosselin RE, Smith RP, Hodge HC, Braddock JE. Clinical toxicology of commercial products. 5th ed. Williams & Wilkins, 1984.

20. Prendergast, JA, et al. Effects on experimental animals of long-term inhalation of trichloroethylene, carbon tetrachloride, 1,1,1-trichloroethane, dichlorodifluoromethane, and 1,1-dichloroethylene. Toxicol Appl Pharmacol 1967;10:270–289.

21. Environmental Protection Agency Draft criteria document for 1,1,1-trichloroethane. NTIS Doc. No. PB84-199520. 1984.

22. Chen JL, Kennedy GL. Dimethylformamide and testicular cancer. Lancet 1988;8575-6:55.

23. Levin SM, et al. Testicular cancer in leather tanners exposed to dimethylformamide. Lancet 1987;8568:1153.

24. GAF Material Safety Data Sheet; M-pyrol. Wayne, NJ: Gaf Chemicals Corporation, 1986.

25. IARC. Styrene. IARC Monographs on the evaluation of carcinogenic risk to humans. Supplement 7. Overall evaluations of carcinogenicity: an updating of IARC monographs volumes 1 to 42. Lyon, France: WHO, International Agency for Research on Cancer, 1987.

26. Boatman ES, et al. Physical morphological and chemical studies of dusts derived from the machining of composite-epoxy materials. Environ Res 1988;45:242–255.

27. ACGIH. TLVs. Threshold limit values and biological exposure indices for 1990–1991. Cincinnati, OH; American Conference of Governmental Industrial Hygienists, 1990–91.

28. Kowalska M. Carbon fiber reinforced epoxy prepregs and composites—health risks aspects. SAMPE Quarterly 1982;(Jan):13–19.

29. Schwartz CS, et al. SACMA Task Force: Monograph on safe handling of advanced composite materials components: Health Information. SAMPE, 1989; April.

30. Zumwalde RD, et al. Carbon/graphite fibers: environmental exposures and potential health implications. Cincinnati, OH:NIOSH Div of Surveillance, Hazard Evaluation and Field Studies 1980; Dec.

31. Holt PF, Horne M. Dust from carbon fibre. Environ Res 1978;17:276–283.

32. Vu V. Health hazard assessment of nonasbestos fibers, final draft. Washington, DC: EPA Health and Environmental Review Division, Office of Toxic Substances, 1988.

33. Zahr GE. DuPont comments: Health hazard assessment of nonasbestos fibers (final draft). OPTS 62036E (Appended to letter from Zahr to SACMA, August 19, 1988).

34. IARC. IARC Monographs on the evaluation of carcinogenic risks to humans-man-made mineral fibres and radon. Vol. 43. Lyon, France: WHO, International Agency for Research on Cancer, 1988.

35. Dahlquist I, Fregert S, Trulsson I. Allergic contact dermatitis from epoxy resin finished glass fiber. Contact Dermatitis 1979;5:190.

36. Zustra M. Evaluation of the potential health hazards associated with the machining of carbon fiber composites. Chapel Hill, NC: University of North Carolina, Masters Thesis, 1987.

37. Morris VL. Repair material toxicity. A presentation to workshop on composites—Northrop Corp., B-2 Division-Materials and Processes, Los Angeles, California, March 23, 1989.

38. Morris VL. Aerospace polymer materials. A presentation to composites workshop, Northrop Corp., B-2 Division, January 18, 1989.

48

Toxic Hazards of Firefighters

Linda H. Morse, M.D., M.P.H.
Gary Pasternak, M.D., M.P.H.
Gary Fujimoto, M.D.

INTRODUCTION

Firefighting has always been considered hazardous work because it is performed in an uncontrollable environment. Fire, heat, and risk of explosion and/or structure collapse are dangers not amenable to an industrial safety specialist's careful quantification and control mechanisms. While there are dozens of studies of exposures and methods of control in stationary hazardous environments such as oil refineries and auto body painting operations, there are very few actual studies of the environment that firefighters face during a "working fire," the dose of toxins that enter the body from that environment, or the effects of the chemicals. Firefighter exposure to toxic chemicals occurs in four situations:

1. The traditional exposure to combustion products in the course of firefighting;
2. The more recent job duty of response to hazardous chemical releases;
3. The even more recent assignment of providing "backup" to law enforcement agencies during arrest of drug dealers and illegal "designer drug" laboratories;
4. Through exposure at the fire station to diesel exhaust, cigarette smoke, cleaning supplies, and other commonly used chemicals.

TOXICOLOGY OF FIRES AND COMBUSTION

Prior to the 1940s, active duty firefighting involved primarily exposure to chemical combustion (burning) and pyrolysis (melting) products from natural materials such as wood and wood products (e.g., paper), cotton, silk, other natural fibers, and grass, trees, and bushes in wildland fires (1). Combustion of any of these products always produces massive quantities of carbon dioxide (CO_2) and carbon monoxide (CO), consuming available oxygen in the process. Oxygen deficiency through either simple asphyxia (from CO_2 displacement of O_2) or chemical asphyxia (from CO interference with O_2 transport) are, therefore, the first toxic hazards of concern in firefighting.

Similarly, all fires, including natural material fires, produce irritants such as ammonia (from silk and wool), aldehydes, and acroleins from wood and wood products.

Finally, all fires, including natural materials fires, produce polyaromatic hydrocarbons (PAH), which contain both irritants and carcinogens. Early studies in the carcinogenicity of these materials include Sir Percival Pott's research into the elevated incidence of scrotal cancer in chimney sweeps from soot exposure. Hundreds of PAHs have now been identified, with 11 now recognized as proven carcinogens in animals (2).

From the 1940s through the present, there have been an increasing number of synthetic products used in our society.

The introduction of these materials into widespread use has greatly increased the toxic exposures of firefighters (1). Combustion and pyrolysis of synthetic materials produce carbon dioxide, carbon monoxide, and irritant hazards similar to those seen in combustion of natural products. In addition, however, there is release of additional irritants such as hydrogen chloride from polyvinyl chloride plastics; hydrogen bromide from flame retardant on children's clothes; isocyanates from urethane foam used in upholstery cushions, and nitrogen oxides (2). Unexpected effects have included methemoglobinemia in firefighters exposed to combustion of nitrates or nitrites, cyanide poisoning from the combustion of urethane foam cushions in homes and offices, and production of increasing numbers of carcinogens and suspect carcinogens (such as benzene emissions from both combustion and pyrolysis of the ubiquitous plastic polyvinyl chloride).

Because of the unstable and unpredictable nature of the fire environment and the massive technical difficulties involved, very few studies have examined chemical exposures in the firefighters' environment, and those have been limited to a few common combustion products: CO_2, CO, HCN, HCl, NO_2 aldehydes, particulates, and halogenated solvents (1, 2). The most exhaustive study utilized a portable vacuum cleaner that drew air through a variety of collection tubes inserted in the sides of the machine, that hung from the waist of firefighters. Successful samples were obtained in 24 fires. All fires had one or more samples for the following classes of chemicals: acids, acid gases, gases, aromatic hydrocarbons, particulates, aldehydes, oxyhydrocarbons, furans, nitrohydrocarbons, metals, and halogenated hydrocarbons (Table 48.1). Of these, six known carcinogens were found: acrylonitrile, arsenic, benzene, benzopyrene, chromium, and vinyl chloride.

Multiple toxins are produced by fires, and the generation of these by-products of combustion is directly influenced by factors such as closed space versus open space, the nature of the solid or liquid materials being pyrolized, and thermal factors. Most deaths from fires are caused by hypoxia, either from carbon monoxide or smoke inhalation. In order to burn, solids must volatize to form gases. Studies involving fires and toxic gas production confirm that carbon monoxide is the main toxic gas produced (1). There appears to be no correlation between the materials being burned and the types of gases produced. However, correlations do exist relating to thermal factors and gases produced. Further studies of controlled low energy fires demonstrated the formation of free radicals as a toxic by-product of combustion (1–3). It is now believed that morbidity and mortality secondary to a fire are not only due to carbon monoxide causing hypoxia and asphyxia, but also incapacitation of the victim secondary to intense sensory and respiratory irritation.

Table 48.1. Common Chemical and Environmental Exposures of Firefighters

Carbon monoxide
Carbon dioxide
Ammonia
Acrolein
Acetaldehyde
Formaldehyde
Hydrogen chloride
Hydrogen bromide
Hydrofluoric acid
Polyaromatic hydrocarbons
Sulfur dioxide
Nitrogen dioxide and nitrogen oxides
Hydrogen cyanide
Volatile isocyanates
Particulates
Metals
Chlorine
Volatile nitrates and nitrites
Halogenated hydrocarbons
Aliphatic hydrocarbons
Aromatic hydrocarbons
Oxyhydrocarbons

The toxic products of combustion can be divided into the following functional categories, and their production is dependent on the oxygen content of the burning environment as well as on the products present and the temperature of the fire:

a) **Asphyxiants:** This includes both physical and chemical asphyxiants. The physical asphyxiants in a fire are gases such as nitrogen and carbon dioxide, as well as a low oxygen atmosphere such as could occur in an enclosed space. Chemical asphyxiants include carbon monoxide, hydrogen cyanide, hydrogen sulfide, and methemoglobin-producing chemicals such as nitrates and nitrites.

b) **Pulmonary irritants:** Numerous by-products of combustion are respiratory irritants. These include both particulate matter and gases produced by fires. Smoke, one of the main by-products of fires, is an aerosol of carbon and soot which is less than 1 μm in diameter and is a by-product of burning carbon-containing material. Particulate matter comes in a variety of sizes and includes dust, fumes, and smoke that can penetrate to various portions of the airwave, depending on size of particulate matter. Particles between 1 and 3 μm can penetrate to lower airways, and those less than 1 μm can reach the alveoli. Smoke is a combination of vapor phase and particulate phase. Respiratory irritants which are present in smoke include a number of chemicals such as acrolein and a variety of acids such as hydrochloric acid, ammonia, nitrogen oxides, sulfur dioxide, phosgene, chlorine, and formaldehyde (Table 48.1).

Free Radicals

The formation of free radicals during fires has been investigated as a source of pulmonary damage and incapacitating factors to humans. Free radicals generated during fires may react with lung surfactant and reduce oxygen uptake, thus producing hypoxia (1–3). Animal studies have confirmed that free radicals produce pulmonary toxicity by a mechanism of altering the pulmonary surfactant (dipalmitoyl phosphatidylcholine). Free radicals produced in combustion environments can range from

very stable compounds, such as chlorine, to more explosive species that are unstable at room temperatures. Free radical formations require dissociations of the high energy bonds that bind carbon to carbon, carbon to hydrogen, or carbon to oxygen. The energy required to dissociate such bonds thermally requires temperatures ranging from 840 to 1200°F (450 to 650°C) (3). Free radicals are produced by the pyrolysis of a variety of plastic products, and their production depends upon the temperature of the pyrolysis process. Free radicals that are produced are contained in the smoke of fires. The mechanisms of toxicity of free radicals is the peroxidation of unsaturated lipids within the pulmonary surfactant system. This alters the surface tension of the lungs and reduces oxygen uptake. Incapacitation results from this rapid decline in oxygen uptake by victims. Once incapacitated, a victim is exposed to the other toxic products of smoke, such as carbon monoxide. Lipid peroxidation is the oxidative deterioration of unsaturated lipids. It involves the reaction of oxygen with unsaturated lipids to form free radicals and unstable hydroperoxides (3).

COMBUSTION PROCESS AND THERMAL DECOMPOSITION

Combustion is propagated by the reaction of oxygen in the air with the gases produced by the thermal decomposition of a solid material (4). Typical irritant products of a fire are listed in Table 48.2. Propagation of the fires occurs if heat is transferred back to the material to continue the production of combustible gases. The nature of the toxic by-products of combustion is dependent on the amount of oxygen available, and thermal energy is transferred back to the burning material. Synthetic polymers have been studied with respect to their thermal decomposition and have been shown to release smoke that is different than that found in the thermal decomposition of natural polymers such as wood, cotton, and others (5). Some of these synthetic polymers release larger amounts of carbon monoxide. Synthetic polymers have higher nitrogen content and, depending upon the fire conditions, may release large amounts of hydrogen cyanide. Also due to the chlorine content, large amounts of hydrogen chloride and chlorine gas may be released. Fluoropolymers release toxic gases consisting of fluorinated hydrocarbons. Gases such as hydrogen chloride, hydrogen fluoride, and hydrogen bromide may be produced in such synthetic polymer combustion. These gases are intense irritants of the mucous membranes, eyes, and respiratory tract. Smoke is very irritating to the nose and face, breathing through the mouth, exposes upper airways to highly irritant particulate matter and highly irritant gases.

PULMONARY INJURY AND RESPIRATORY ABNORMALITIES

The inhalation of products of combustion can produce a range of injuries to the airway including irritation of the upper airway, laryngospasm, brochospasm, and alveolar injury with pulmonary edema. Smoke contains sensory irritants in both the vapor phase and the particulate phase. Toxic gases such as chlorine, hydrochloric acid, hydrofluoric acid, and acrolein can be easily inhaled by victims in fires. In addition, pulmonary insufficiency can be produced by the inhalation of particulate matter and soot that have toxic chemicals adhering on their surfaces (6, 7). Individuals who are in a closed environment are at high risk for inhalation of these products of combustion. Symptoms

Table 48.2. Incapacitating and Irritant Toxic By-Products of Fires

Toxin	Sources	Toxic Effects
Hydrogen cyanide (HCN)	From combustion of wool, silk, polyacrylonitrile, nylon, polyurethane, and paper	Binds to cytochrome oxidase and interferes with cellular respiration
Nitrogen dioxide (NO_2) and other oxides of nitrogen	Produced in small quantities from fabrics and in larger quantities cellulose nitrate and celluloid	Pulmonary irritant capable of causing immediate death as well as delayed injury to lungs
Hydrogen chloride (HCl)	From combustion of polyvinyl chloride (PVC) and some fire-retardant treated materials	Respiratory irritant; potential toxicity of HCl coated on particulate may be greater than for an equivalent amount of gaseous HCl
Other halogen acid gases (HF and HBr)	From combustion of fluorinated resins or films and some fire-retardant materials containing bromine	Respiratory irritants
Sulfur dioxide (SO_2)	From materials containing sulfur	An irritant, intolerable well below lethal concentrations
Isocyanates	From polyurethanes and polymers	Potent respiratory irritants and sensitizers are believed to be the major irritants in smoke produced by isocyanate-based urethanes
Acrolein	From pyrolysis of polyolefins, cellulose and wood containing materials at temperatures around 400°C	Strong respiratory irritant

and signs of smoke inhalation include: tachypnea, cough, stridor, shortness of breath, bronchial spasm, rales, chest pain, and chest tightness, as well as central nervous system signs of headache, confusion, dizziness, and coma. Individuals who inhale smoke may also show signs of singed nasal hairs or carbonaceous soot sputum or soot in the oropharynx. Burns of the face may also be present, as well as edema of the upper airway above the epiglottis. Victims of fire and inhalational injury from by-products of combustion should be evaluated with arterial blood gases, methemoglobin concentrations, chest x-rays, electrocardiogram, spirometry, and if necessary, bronchoscopy. Upper airway damage can result from thermal injury or edema from toxic gases and other by-products of combustion. Injury to the lower airways is not from heat but is secondary to toxic gases, free radicals and small particles that can penetrate to lower airways and alveolar surfaces carrying toxic byproducts of combustion. Symptoms of lower respiratory tract injury include shortness of breath and bronchospasm, manifested by hypoxemia seen in arterial blood gases.

Early pulmonary responses can be demonstrated in victims of a fire environment due to decrements in the FEV_1 and the FVC (6, 7). Unconscious victims found in a fire environment have a greater chance of having a lower airway injury because they have lost their protective mechanism of breath holding and laryngospasm. The presence of facial burns or soot in the upper airway are not indicators of lower airway injury. Superheated air is rapidly cooled before reaching the lower respiratory tract due to the efficient heat-exchanging mechanism of the oropharynx and the nasopharynx (7). An exception to this is the inhalation of hot steam that contains 4000 times the heat capacity of superheated air and can produce heat injury to the lower lungs (7). Smoke, as well as heat, can cause upper airway injury and tracheobronchitis, which can lead to upper airway obstruction.

Radiographic manifestations of smoke inhalation may not be apparent on the first chest x-ray. Radiologic findings are generally nonspecific, and most of the findings appear within the first 24 hours after the injury. The admission chest x-ray may be normal because pathology may require hours to develop. Pulmonary infiltrates may require several hours to be recognizable on a chest x-ray. The abnormalities seen on the chest x-ray may include alveolar edema and perivascular and peribronchial infiltrates, as well as interstitial edema (8). The acute effects of firefighting on pulmonary function have been studied and have shown significant changes in spirometry after exposure to smoke (9, 10). Routine firefighting has been shown to cause acute decrements and FEV_1 and FVC, as well as being associated with an increase in airway responsiveness (9).

Hazardous Materials Incidents

Toxic chemical spills and leaks are familiar to almost every professional fire department in the United States. Indeed, the past decade has witnessed the development of a distinct new suboccupation, "hazardous materials teams," with attendant training materials routinely incorporated into new firefighter education and marketed for experienced firefighter review.

Currently, there are more than 100,000 chemicals used in United States industrial operations daily, with almost 2000 new ones added each year. Occupational Safety and Health Administration (OSHA) safety standards for work week exposure exist for approximately 500 substances. Standards for toxicity testing in new chemicals have only been in place since 1976. The vast majority of the chemicals used in industrial operations were put into use prior to passage of that law. While a number of the larger chemical companies have gone back and tested particularly suspect chemicals, rigorous analysis has still been applied to few chemicals used in industrial operations. Increasing use and transport has led to a rapid rise in the number of hazardous materials spills and leaks. The fire service has always been responsible for handling these incidents, although only recently has appropriate training and protective equipment been available.

Drug Labs

The newest and very hazardous task of the fire department is provision of "backup" to Drug Enforcement Agency (DEA) and local police agencies during the capture and arrest of criminals producing designer drugs. The growth of the industrial chemical industry has been matched by a similar spurt, particularly in the 1980s in "designer drug" production. Drugs such as heroin, marijuana, and cocaine are produced from natural plants, although the production operation (particularly cocaine) may require the use of toxic chemicals. However, since the days of lysergic acid diethylamide (LSD) in the 1960s, production of illegal synthetic drugs has grown dramatically. Most frequently, these require a small amount of space (motel room, rented apartment), minimal equipment, and some chemical knowledge. Firefighters are frequently exposed, because inadequate knowledge or carelessness on the producer's part leads to a fire, explosion, or toxic chemical leak. Chemicals can be left behind after production operation is over, and the fire department may be called to identify and remove them. For example, a recent designer drug, "ICE" or U4EA," was found to be produced from cyanogen bromide (cyanide and bromine) and an over-the-counter decongestant.

Awareness of the danger of these drug laboratories led in late 1989, to law enforcement agencies requesting that a fire department hazardous materials team be standing by during the dramatic (and often violent) forced entry and arrest action. In these situations firefighters have been required to help handle chemical "booby traps" in addition to other tasks.

Fire Stations

Traditionally, fire stations have received little health and safety attention. Recent understanding of the hazards of passive cigarette smoke has led to a ban on smoking in many (but by no means all) fire stations. Research into the effects of diesel exhaust has resulted in attempts (again, by no means universal) to capture the diesel exhaust from the firefighting apparatus and vent it outdoors instead of into living quarters of the firefighters. Washing machines for turnout gear are being demanded so that turnout gear can be decontaminated immediately after service.

PERSONAL PROTECTIVE GEAR

Standard personal protective equipment or "turnout gear" consists of 65 pounds of boots, pants, jacket, helmet, gloves, and selfcontained breathing apparatus (SCBA). Wearing this equipment increases body heat, respiratory rate and depth, and heart rate, which can significantly affect intake and transport of chemicals. Until about 1980, firefighters were not encouraged and, in fact, were frequently discouraged from wearing their SCBAs during any but the worst fires. Most departments did not even supply SCBAs to all members until the mid-1970s. Currently, SCBAs are frequently not worn during the "take down" or "overhaul" period after the active fire has been extinguished. "Wet bandanas" are the standard respiratory protective equipment provided to wildlands firefighters. First responders to chemical incidents are most frequently the closest station, equipped with only standard gear, which may provide little protection to chemicals that can damage or penetrate the skin. Hazardous materials team members are now better equipped with complete occlusive suits and SCBA, but the suits add significant heat stress to the body.

MEDICAL APPROACH

Primary care physicians, emergency physicians, and occupational physicians need a practical approach to the complicated occupation of firefighting. The initial evaluation should ascertain whether the exposure was significant. Risk factors and signs suggestive of inhalation injury include enclosed space fires, burning synthetic materials, steam exposure, altered mental status, chest pain, age greater than 40, and loss of consciousness. Firefighters should be asked whether a self-contained breathing apparatus was used, for how long, and whether there were any episodes of equipment failure such as running out of air. Was there a prolonged period of overhaul (the cleanup period following the "knock down" phase of fire extinguishing) when protective equipment was not being used? Did the firefighter require supplemental oxygen at the scene because of "minor" symptoms of fatigue or smoke inhalation? If the firefighter is unconscious or unable to provide a coherent history, other firefighters should be asked about how and where the injured worker was found.

Firefighters with mental status abnormalities, even in the absence of other signs and symptoms of significant smoke inhalation injury, should be hospitalized for observation. Asymptomatic patients with high risk exposures (i.e., facial or nasal burns, confined space exposure, elevated carboxyhemoglobin, increased age, chest pain) should also be observed for at least 24 hours.

In the setting of acute toxic exposures, the evaluating clinician must deliberate carefully before returning a firefighter to duty. Residual mild CO poisoning effects (headache, etc.), which might be well-tolerated by an otherwise healthy individual returning home, could pose a serious danger to the firefighter and to others (coworkers and the public) if the firefighter was called out to handle another incident. The best approach is the conservative one.

Chronic Problems

Because of the uncontrolled occupational environment and the varying nature of exposures, there are only a few studies of firefighters that examined morbidity or mortality. Moreover, many of the existing studies are flawed due to changes in the work environment during the study period or because of comparison of firefighters to the general population (i.e., the "super healthy worker effect"). Another flaw occurs when state or local workers' compensation statistics are used in areas where "presumptions" exist. In California, for example, "heart trouble" is presumed under state workers' compensation statute to be work-related in law enforcement and firefighting positions because of occupational stress. The same is true for cancer and pulmonary problems for firefighters. All studies utilizing workers' compensation data show a high rate of cardiac and pulmonary disease and cancer in firefighters as a result.

The best designed studies utilize police (another super healthy worker group) as a control. In these studes an elevated rate of chronic respiratory disease mortality has been identified. Studies on the acute effects of firefighting on the lungs show significant abnormalities of pulmonary function and methacholine challenge test results after exposure, persisting beyond the temporal period expected for an acute irritant airway reaction (9, 10). These results are biologically plausible given the highly irritating nature of many of the chemicals in a fire environment and/or hazardous material release incidence.

Studies have identified elevated rates of different cancers such as hematopoetic, brain, and gastrointestinal. There has been great controversy over the issue of whether these cancers are occupationally induced, because in the few studies that have been performed, chemical exposures concentrations were often below those thought to be hazardous. The mechanism of carcinogenesis postulates an initiation, promotion, and progression model. The classic initiator chemical in carcinogenesis research is benzopyrene, a combustion product found in 100% of fires studied. Promoter chemicals may or may not be carcinogens themselves, and exposure to them in the presence of an initiator need not be large. Progression involves multiple factors including host defenses and other environmental insults. The elevated rates of hematopoetic cancers fit this model, where there is recurrent exposure to initiators and promoters.

Epidemiologically, there has been a population rise in the rate of glioblastoma brain cancers mirroring the rise in chemical production in the United States. Similarly, this is now reported as a cancer occurring with increased frequency in firefighters. The types of cancers reported in firefighters will be better characterized over the next decade as more attention is paid to identifying medical risks in this occupation.

Surveillance

Because of the limited number of biologic monitoring tests available and the huge number of possible occupational chemical exposures in firefighting, medical surveillance should be oriented toward potential target organs as well as fitness for duty issues.

Pre-Placement and/or Baseline Examinations

Examinations are now recommended by the National Fire Protection Association and mandated for hazardous materials team members by the OSHA 1910:120 hazardous waste regulation.

The *baseline* evaluation should include the following:

1. *Complete* medical history, including past and current problems, allergies, immunizations, review of systems.
2. *Complete* occupational history, including all jobs since high school, hobbies, *and* moonlighting or secondary jobs. (Firefighters quite frequently have secondary jobs with significant chemical exposures such as house painting, construction work, and chimney cleaning.)
3. *Personal exposure record* (PER) and significant past exposures should be documented. (Actual copies of the PER or incident report should be photocopied for the chart.)
4. *Complete physical examination* including careful musculoskeletal and neurologic evaluation.
5. *Screening pulmonary function tests* (PFT)—$FEV_{1.0}$, FVC, $FEV_{1.0}$/FVC and a curve with a peak expiratory flow rate (PEFR) should be documented on a *calibrated* spirometer by a qualified technician from a pulmonary function facility or one holding National Institute of Occupational Safety and Health (NIOSH) certification. These baseline records are critical to the individual and department for workers' compensation and epidemiologic purposes.
6. *Screening audiometry*—studies show a high rate of noise-induced hearing loss among firefighters. Documentation of

hearing ability and risk factors (past or present) for hearing loss is important.
7. *Chest x-ray* for baseline and comparison later if hospitalized or needing treatment.
8. *ECG* for baseline, and comparison later if hospitalized or needing treatment.
9. *Laboratory tests:*
   Urinalysis
   Stool occult blood—Occult blood tests should be part of routine evaluation.
   Complete blood count with differential—firefighters are frequently in low oxygen situations where anemia would pose a hazard. Also, firefighting is associated with an elevated rate of hematopoietic cancers.
   Chemistry panel—baseline for kidney and liver function (which may be damaged by toxic exposures) and "lifestyle" issues (liver function tests for alcohol, cholesterol, and triglycerides for fats and cholesterol intake).
   Red blood cell cholinesterase—in any department responding to pesticide spills, a baseline is necessary. Two of the seven classes of pesticides inhibit cholinesterase. Since the range of normal is wide, a significant decline may be misread as still within normal limits unless there is a baseline value for comparison.
   Fitness testing—some form of strength, agility, and endurance evaluation is usually required by the department prior to hire and, with increasing frequency, on a periodic basis. A fitness physiology laboratory is best equipped to provide the range of services. Alternatively, an exercise pulmonary test plus strength and limberness testing through a hospital or physical therapy group can suffice. Cardiac treadmill tests are not indicated, since there is a high rate of false positives in healthy asymptomatic adults.

Periodic Medical Surveillance Evaluations

NFPA 1500 mandates periodic surveillance examinations; OSHA requires yearly evaluation for hazardous materials team members.

Periodic surveillance include the following (every year for hazardous material if the firefighter is over age 40, every 2 years if under age 40).

1. Update of medical history (review of systems, new problems, new medications)
2. Update of occupational health history (past year)
3. Updated exposure records
4. Complete physical exam
5. Spirometry
6. Audiometry
7. Stool occult blood
8. Lipid panel alternating with general chemistry
9. Repeat strength endurance and agility testing

Records from these evaluations should be available 24 hours a day in case the firefighter is injured and baseline data are needed. A copy of pertinent information should also be given to the firefighter at the time of each exam.

Prior to retirement or leaving the department, a repeated or updated complete evaluation should be performed. Records of all prior evaluations and this exit evaluation must be saved for 30 years *after* the last visit, as all firefighters are exposed to carcinogens.

All contact with the firefighter must remain confidential except for those incidents involving workers' compensation. Personal lifestyle and job hazards overlap so much in the profession that the clinician must win the trust of the firefighter in order to practice good medicine. (This is also in accordance with the American College of Occupational Medicine Code of Ethics and civil court rulings in the past 15 years.)

Health Promotion

Explanation of good personal lifestyle and occupational health habits should prove the most rewarding part of a clinician's interaction with firefighters. The same drive and competitive edge which led him or her into the fire service will prove useful in health promotion. Initiation of cholesterol testing can lead to a competition among the firefighters as to whose level is lowest.

SUMMARY

Clinician involvement with the fire service includes not only provision of acute and chronic injury/disease care but also involvement with other issues related to firefighter health and safety. Better studies are needed regarding the effects of multiple chemical exposures on morbidity and mortality, fitness and cardiopulmonary response. The fire service needs medical advice and support in its efforts to identify better protective equipment and to raise funds from sorely pressed municipal budget for things such as washing machines for decontamination. Firefighters are on the front line in our community defense against hazardous materials incidents and fires and deserve the medical community's vigorous involvement and support.

REFERENCES

1. Lowery WT, Juarez L, Petty CS, Roberts B. Studies of toxic gas production during actual structural fires in the Dallas area. J Forensic Sci (JFSCA) 1985;30(1):59–72.
2. Decker WJ, Garcia-Cantu A. Toxicology of fires: an emerging clinical concern. Vet Hum Toxicol 1986;28(5):431–433.
3. Lowery WR, Peterson J, Petty CS, Badgett JL. Free radical production from controlled low-energy fires: toxicity considers. J Forensic Sci (JFSCA) 1985;30(1):73–85.
4. Hartzell GE, Packham SC, Switzer WG. Toxic products from fires. Am Ind Hyg Assoc J 1983;44(4):248–255.
5. Alarie Y. The toxicity of smoke from polymeric materials during thermal decomposition. Annu Rev Pharmacol Tox 1985;25:325–47.
6. Cohen MA, Guzzardi LJ. Inhalation of products of combustion. Ann Emerg Med 1983;12:628–632.
7. Cahalane M, Demling RH. Early respiratory abnormalities from smoke inhalation. JAMA 1984;251(6):771–773.
8. Texidor HS, Rubin E, Novick GS, Alonso DR. Smoke inhalation: radiologic manifestations. Radiology 1983;149:383–387.
9. Sheppard D, Distenfano S, Morse L, Becker C. Acute effects of routine firefighting on lung function. Am J Ind Med 1986;9:333–340.
10. Large AA, Owens GR, Hoffman, LA. The short-term effects of smoke exposure on the pulmonary function of firefighters. Chest 1990;97:806–809.

49

Toxicology Laboratory Hazards

William M. Snellings, Ph.D.

INTRODUCTION

Safety awareness programs, along with well-thought out workplace policies and procedures on accident prevention, are key to a safe workplace environment. Sometimes, unfortunately, it takes an actual injury to provide the necessary impetus to develop more effective safety programs. The observation of adverse effects in animals from exposure to toxic chemicals may be partly responsible for causing toxicology laboratories to improve their safety programs. Compared with other chemical industries, the toxicology industry works with a wider range of toxic to nontoxic chemicals, although the daily quantities of chemicals that are handled are considerably less. Hence the overall level of risk may be less in a toxicology laboratory.

Safe handling and storage practices involving chemicals are essential in the toxicology laboratory environment. Exposures to personnel can range from acute to chronic due to accidental spills or from low level prolonged exposure.

DESCRIPTION OF THE BUSINESS

One of the main objectives in many toxicology studies is to study the effects or mechanisms of action of chemicals in a laboratory animal. The ultimate goal in this type of work is to better define the effects of these agents on humans and their environment. Usually, in mechanistic or threshold determination studies, one of the dosage levels is high enough to cause an adverse reaction in the test species. The concern, then, is that the potential for the same toxic reaction exists for the researcher, although the response will probably be less intense. However, it should be pointed out that, as long as proper safeguards are maintained, the presence of a toxic agent does not necessarily imply that the work environment is unsafe.

Toxicology laboratories are usually sponsored either by chemical or pharmaceutical industries; by private industry that contracts out its services; by government, such as the National Institute for Occupational Safety and Health; or by universities or colleges. In an unpublished questionnaire of several major chemical and contract laboratories, it was found that considerable emphasis is placed on programs associated with safety awareness and safety procedures. However, the means to obtain these goals varied considerably.

Toxicology testing laboratories may specialize in only a few toxicity evaluation tests or perform a complete battery of tests ranging from one-time (acute) exposure to lifetime (chronic) exposure. In general, methods of containment of test chemicals for acute studies can be accomplished more easily than those for the chronic studies. This is because the smaller number of animals used in acute studies allows much of the work to be conducted in exhaust hoods, whereas this is not practical for studies with a larger number of animals, as in chronic studies. However, in acute testing, usually much higher concentrations of the test chemical are used than in chronic studies. Also, and perhaps most importantly, far less safety information—in some cases, no information—is available when the acute tests are performed. Consequently, one small change in safety procedures could result in a hazardous situation.

The major routes of animal exposure for toxicology studies are oral, dermal, and inhalation; each administration route is associated with a different set of hazards.

Oral

When a test compound is administered orally, it is usually administered by gavage or mixed in the animal feed or drinking water. Several factors will usually influence the decision regarding the appropriate means of oral administration: the palatability of the test material; its potential to evaporate from or react with water or powdered feed; and the overall design of the study, which may be to assimilate actual exposure conditions or to deliver a calculated dose based on body weight.

If the test material is a solid, it may be ground before it can be mixed with powdered feed in order to make a homogeneous mixture. Exposure to the test material as a dust could occur during the milling and mixing operations. Other tasks associated with the handling of the powdered test diets that could result in worker exposure are the transfer of the test diet from mixing equipment to storage containers or the dumping of the unused test diet from the animal feed cup.

When the test material is volatile or cannot be mixed with the diet, gavage and encapsulation are two possible techniques. A problem that can occur when the test material is administered by gavage is that the incidence of animal bites increases as the irritability of the test material increases. Encapsulation of the test material and the subsequent mixing with the powdered diet is a technique that may result in a much lower potential for worker exposure to the test material.

Dermal

For dermal application of test materials that are volatile or that are a powder, special precautions should to be taken to contain the applied materials. For test liquids that dry and leave a residue on the skin, Darlow et al. (1) described expected hazards from experimental skin-painting studies. This work was based on dissemination of fungal spores that were applied to a clipped-hair area on the backs of mice. They found that reclipping of the hair, changing the animal bedding, and sweeping the animal room floor increased the spread of spores that had been applied on the mice.

Another hazard associated with dermal applications is the potential increased incidence of animal bites during the restraint of the animal and the application of an irritating test material. Increased animal movement during the application also may put the laboratory technician at increased risk of accidental chemical exposure.

Inhalation

A test atmosphere for an inhalation study can be generated as a vapor or as an aerosol. Depending on the test material and the exposure concentration, both generation procedures may have certain hazards associated with the physical characteristics of the test material.

One of the more important safety concerns in a vapor study is the potential for a fire or explosion, especially if elevated temperatures (i.e., above the autoignition temperature) or high vapor concentrations (i.e., above the lower explosion limit) are necessary. Other unwanted reactions can occur depending on the reactivity of the test material. Certain chemicals, for example pyrophoric agents, must be diluted with nitrogen before they can be safely mixed with air, or a fire can occur. Electrostatically charged particles in an aerosol study can also cause an explosion.

Another concern in an inhalation study is the potential risk of exposure to the test material, which may occur during the removal of the animals from the inhalation chamber following the termination of the test atmosphere generation. Even with procedures in place to increase the inhalation chamber ventilation rate by the addition of clean air, certain chemicals will linger on the animal fur or will adhere to the inside walls of the inhalation chamber and animal cages. This is especially true for dust inhalation studies. For certain test materials, wearing an appropriate respirator and/or protective clothing may be necessary.

POTENTIALLY HAZARDOUS WORK FUNCTIONS FOUND IN MOST TOXICOLOGY LABORATORIES

There are physical and toxicologic hazards associated with improper storage of flammable, toxic, or unstable (highly reactive) test and reagent chemicals. The procedures for prevention of accidents were well addressed in a symposium sponsored by the American Chemical Society (2). Other discussions on this subject can be found in other parts of this textbook.

There are no available published reports on the type and frequency of injuries in a toxicology laboratory, but it is expected that animal bites and scratches may be one of the most prevalent. Other areas of concern include injuries or illnesses associated with allergic reaction to animals, diseases that can be passed from animals to humans, needle-stick accidents, exposure to anesthetizing or tissue-preserving agents, and the washing of animal caging equipment.

Animal Bites and Scratches

Handling animals has one of the highest potentials for causing an injury in a toxicology laboratory involved in animal testing. Injuries include bites and scratches that can result in an inflammatory or allergic reaction or in a zoonotic disease. For these potential injuries, there are procedures and protective equipment that will decrease the frequency of the injuries. However, for some operations, particularly when handling a large number of animals, the potential for an injury increases (refer to section in this chapter on gloves).

Another possible concern from animal bites or scratches is the reaction of the worker to the introduction of a small amount of test chemical into the wound from the treated animal. However, no significant problems have been noted in the literature from this type of occurrence. The most likely problem from a bite or scratch is a local irritation or an allergic reaction to an animal protein.

Allergic Reactions to Animals

For certain individuals, an allergic response can occur from working in an animal room or with equipment or materials that have been in a room with animals. It has been reported that between 11 and 30% of laboratory personnel who are in close contact with laboratory animals have developed an allergic reaction to these animals (3). The response has most often been characterized by a spectrum of acute respiratory disorders and has been called laboratory animal allergy (LAA). It is believed that certain antigens of animal origin, e.g., urinary proteins, dander, hair, or ectoparasites, may stimulate specific antibody production in susceptible individuals that results in an immediate type of allergic hypersensitivity. The causes and control methods for this condition have been discussed in detail by Newman-Taylor (4) and Lincoln et al. (5).

Some of the clinical signs associated with this condition are asthma, rhinitis, conjunctivitis, sneezing, and skin reactions. Lutsky et al. (6) have reported on the results of a survey from 155 animal facilities, including academic, government, and commercial laboratories. Causes of LAA were reported in 70% of the facilities. The rat and rabbit were reported to be the species that most frequently evoked the hypersensitivity signs of LAA. Sensitivities to mice, guinea pigs, cats, hamsters, and primates were also reported.

Zoonoses

An additional concern when handling laboratory animals is the transmission from the animal to the handler of a virus, bacteria, or parasite through general contact, through an animal bite, or through the respiratory tract by inhalation of aerosols from animal waste.

Toxicology laboratories that conduct research with large mammals have more concerns about zoonoses because the supply sources of these animals are sometimes not as well-controlled for the prevention of diseases as are the rodent sources. Examples of diseases, some fatal, in laboratory workers associated with large animal research are Q fever from sheep (7); listeriosis from sheep, goats, and cattle; toxoplasmosis from cats (8); monkey virus B (9) and tuberculosis (7) from primates.

Eradication programs have greatly reduced the occurrence of zoonotic diseases. Most toxicology laboratories use only specific pathogen-free rodents from vendors with an active quality control program. Therefore, viral infections associated with rodents that have been reported in laboratory animal handlers, e.g., Prospect Hill (10) and Hantaan virus (11), should not be a concern, if the proper quality control exams are performed on incoming animal shipments. In addition, stringent procedures and practices should be in place to prevent the entry of feral rodents and the immediate safe removal of these animals from the laboratory if entry should occur. For example, Fox (12) reported on an outbreak of dermatitis in laboratory personnel which was due to a mite that gained access to the animal facility from wild rodents.

Additional information concerning factors affecting the diagnosis, prevention, and control of zoonoses can be found in a thorough report published by the World Health Organization (13).

Injecting Chemicals into Animals

As indicated in a 25-year review of accidents in a United States Department of Agriculture (USDA) animal research facility, self-injection of infectious agents can be an area of major safety importance (14). In a toxicology laboratory, self-injection of a chemical probably results most often in a local irritation; however, the potential for significant health effects from certain highly toxic agents is possible. The highest potential for needle-stick injuries may be while preparing the syringe or needle for disposal (15). During intravenous or subcutaneous injections of test material, the researcher should be aware of the potential for piercing through the vein or skin of the test animal and accidentally injecting his/her own finger. For example, injections into the ear vein of rabbits may be riskier than most injection procedures because the thinness of the ear necessitates the technician's placing his/her fingers very close to the injection site.

Preparing Tissues for Pathologic Evaluation

Histology technicians prepare sections of animal tissues for pathologic evaluation. Tissues that are fixed in solutions containing formaldehyde or other aldehyde fixatives are then trimmed, dehydrated in a series of alcohol mixtures, and infiltrated and embedded in paraffin. Slices from the paraffin block are mounted on slides, cleared with xylene or toluene, and then stained with a dye.

Formaldehyde has been shown to be carcinogenic in laboratory animals (16). In addition, the acute effects of formaldehyde in humans include dermatitis and irritation of the eyes, nose, and throat (17). The current Occupational Safety and Health Act (OSHA) Permissible Exposure Limit (PEL) for formaldehyde is a 1 ppm (TWA 8-hour) with a Short-Term Exposure Limit (STEL) of 2 ppm.

Neither xylene nor toluene is carcinogenic, but they can cause gastrointestinal and neurologic disturbances (18). The current PEL for both xylene and toluene is 100 ppm (TWA 8-hour) with a STEL of 150 ppm. Kilburn et al. (19) reported on the results of area sampling for these three chemicals in 10 histology laboratories performing tissue and slide preparations. Formaldehyde levels in tissue specimen preparation areas ranged from 0.2–1.9 ppm. In rooms where tissues or slides were processed, xylene ranged from 3.2–102 ppm, and toluene ranged from 8.9–12.6 ppm. The date of their investigation was not given (prior to 1985), and the wide variations in levels were explained by the diversity of activities and by large differences in ventilation rates among the laboratories.

There are a variety of dyes for tissue staining that can be used with a wide range of potential toxic responses from overexposure, including cancer. Because these dyes are not very volatile, the hazards associated with these dyes are minimal if appropriate safeguards are used.

Anesthetizing Animals

When anesthetizing animals, workers may be exposed to volatile anesthetic gases. Milligan and Sablan (20) have reported on the exposure levels of veterinary personnel to halothane. While teratogenic effects of halothane have been shown in rats

(21), the effects of exposure to anesthetics on women in the veterinary and human medical professions are unclear, because there are specific recognition and reporting problems in reproductive epidemiology studies. Several studies have reported an increased risk of spontaneous abortions (22–25); however, the validity of these studies is questionable, since they were carried out using subjective information on spontaneous abortion, and a relatively low response rate was observed. In addition, Baltzar et al. (26) have reported that there were no increases in congenital malformations in medical personnel working with anesthetics. This area, waste anesthetic gas exposure, requires further investigation.

Washing Animal Caging Equipment

Laboratory personnel who are responsible for animal cage cleaning are involved with tasks in which their hands are simultaneously exposed to several potential harmful situations (i.e., chemicals, mechanical friction, high temperature, and physical trauma). In addition, high pressure water is used to remove the waste from certain equipment, and can result in potentially contaminated aerosols. Workers who do not wear protective equipment and clothing (for example, the correct respirator and appropriate gloves, clothing, and eye protection) may be at a higher risk of exposure to chemicals or potential pathogens.

POTENTIALLY HAZARDOUS WORK AREAS FOUND IN A LIMITED NUMBER OF TOXICOLOGY LABORATORIES

Microbiology Laboratory

Only a few toxicology laboratories have developed in vivo immune response testing, called host resistance assays, by challenging the chemically treated test animal with a virus, e.g., influenza, or bacterium, e.g., listeria. Without the proper safeguards, these agents could infect exposed workers. Precautionary safety measures include totally isolated areas for animal quarters and also isolated areas for cage washing and destruction of waste materials.

Work Areas with Special Physical Hazards

Ionizing radiation, microwaves, and laser beams are a concern in the toxicology laboratory. However, because of the current control and licensing placed on facilities, the risk associated with their normal use is not great. There are a number of special uses associated with these types of radiations. For example, radiotracer techniques are used in metabolism and pharmacokinetics, as well as for quantification of certain biologic samples in radioimmunoassays. Also, microwaves are used to immediately denature certain proteins, while lasers are used for aerosol particle sizing.

PROTECTIVE PERSONNEL EQUIPMENT THAT CAN BE ASSOCIATED WITH HAZARDOUS CONDITIONS

Lab Coats

Lab coats that become contaminated with a chemical must be removed and discarded appropriately as soon as the contamination is recognized. Chemical burns have occurred because the contaminated clothing was not discarded, and an unaware employee, while putting on the clothing, came in contact with the caustic chemical.

The type of material and design of the lab coat should be considered in order to make an appropriate selection for particular laboratory activities. Lab coats that button down the front may not protect the worker as well as the wraparound type, because there may be gaps between the buttons.

Gloves

The hands of technicians in a toxicology laboratory can be exposed to chemical hazards from spills or splashes of a test chemical, or physical and biologic hazards from an animal bite or scratch. However, the disadvantages connected with the use of protective gloves, as discussed by Estander (27), should also be taken into consideration. That is, skin irritation and allergy have been associated with glove materials, such as colorants, additives (like thiuram accelerators), some plasticizers and stabilizers, glove powders, and barrier creams, which may even promote the retention of harmful chemicals on the skin. In addition, once a chemical permeates a glove, harmful effects of the chemical are often enhanced by the increased moisture of the skin. Finally, if wearing a particular type of glove impairs the needed hand dexterity, this could result in a different type of safety hazard.

Since small quantities of chemicals are usually used in toxicology testing, the immersion of the gloved hand in the test chemical is not necessary. The appropriate glove material must be selected to protect from spills or splashes of the test chemical. The problems in selection are usually associated with the lack of information concerning what glove material affords the best protection. Unfortunately, there is no universal material suitable for protection from all possible chemicals.

Because of their excellent tactile quality and lower cost, latex disposable gloves are used for many laboratory functions in which contact with a test chemical is not expected. These functions include handling animals and equipment containing test materials. However, care should be taken in the use of this type of glove because of the false sense of security that one may have when wearing "protective" gloves. Latex disposable gloves afford little or no protection from animal bites or from contact with chemicals that readily penetrate the glove material or pass through defects in the glove.

If it is decided in presafety evaluation discussions that latex disposable gloves are appropriate for a short exposure to the test material, then a good practice is to wear two pairs of gloves. If any test material comes in contact with the glove, one or both should be immediately removed and discarded appropriately. It is interesting to note that Smith and Grant (28) reported an approximately six times lower puncture rate for the inner glove when two pairs of latex gloves were worn while performing surgery.

For handling primates and other large animals, leather gloves afford good protection from bites and scratches; however, performing a function such as i.v. injection or palpation is impossible because of the lack of sufficient dexterity or sensitive tactile response. In this case, technicians wearing a more protective type of glove can restrain the animals while technicians wearing a minimum protective type of glove can perform the necessary job task. This same procedure could be followed for

the smaller animals, but due to the large number of animals, the increased labor cost could be prohibitive.

Other problems associated with glove use in animal rooms include handling sticky tape or labels and finding a manufacturer that can supply small glove sizes. As with other safety protective equipment, if it is not easy or comfortable, the worker will avoid its use.

Respirators

In toxicology testing laboratories, there is a tendency to depend on cartridge-type respirators rather than developing improved procedures or mechanical ventilation. Yet, when working in laboratories on tasks such as inhalation testing or diet preparation, dependence on this type of respirator may not fully protect the worker and is not a substitute for the appropriate review of potential safety issues and the establishment of safe operating procedures. In addition, OSHA rules require a formal respiratory protection program for respirator use. The following points are briefly presented to substantiate the stated concern that dependence on cartridge respirators without appropriate review of the safety issues or potential problems could result in a false sense of security and increased risks to the worker.

1. Unacceptable risk to the worker could occur if the following is unknown: the odor characteristics of the test material, including level of detection for odor, taste, or irritation; the breakthrough times for the respirator cartridges; and health status of the workers.

2. Prediction of the time to cartridge exhaustion can be based on theoretical models; however, Nelson et al. (29) and Hall et al. (30) have demonstrated under field use that the effects from competitive adsorption of water vapor or other organic vapors can result in overestimating (>75%) the breakthrough times. In addition, caution should be taken in depending on certain types of respirators to completely remove particles and fibers. Ortiz et al. (31) have evaluated asbestos penetration for several commercially available respirator filters. The data indicated that each of the filter models tested, except for the high efficiency filter (HEPA), was affected adversely to some degree (up to 18% penetration) by one or more of the simulated field/environmental conditions, which included storage at high humidity and preexposure to water mist.

3. An improperly fitted mask could result in an increased exposure to the test material. The effect of facial hair on seal leakage of the respirator continues to be a controversial subject. Stobbe et al. (32) have reviewed the literature and have reported that two of 14 studies found no significant leakage differences, but the rest of the studies reported an increase in leakage from 20–1000 times due to facial hair.

4. Improper selection of the best respirator cartridge for a particular job could result in a false sense of security. As an example, respirators for the removal of dusts can be used effectively by those who have developed an allergy to animal allergens. Sakaguchi et al. (3) have measured three allergens in an animal room and determined that commercially available respirators, claiming to exclude 97% of the particles larger than 0.5 microns, did eliminate a significant amount of the allergens that were in the room air. Allergens were reduced to undetectable levels (<1 ppb) or by as much as 98%. However, these authors pointed out that one respirator for laboratory animal practices had an efficiency as low as 65%.

There are other concerns that contribute to the problems of respirator use. One is that certain individuals are allergic to the mask material that is in contact with the face. Facial dermatitis has been discussed by Fowler and Callen (33). Second, it has been reported that temperature and humidity conditions within the respirator influence the acceptability of respirator use. At respirator air temperatures above 33°C or at dewpoint temperatures above 20°C, the worker may be bothered with breathing difficulties (34). This may result in less adherence to suggested or required respirator use. Finally, with increased dependence on the use of respirators, the technician may decide to take more risk in other areas of the laboratory, rather than following a more laborious, but proven safe, procedure that does not require the use of a respirator.

REFERENCES

1. Darlow HM, Simmons DJC, Roe JC. Hazards from experimental skin painting of carcinogens. Arch Environ Health 1969;18:883–893.

2. Pipitone DA, ed. Safe storage of laboratory chemicals. New York: John Wiley & Sons, 1984.

3. Sakaguchi M, Inouye S, Miyazawa H, Kamimura H, Kimura M, Yamazaki S. Evaluation of dust respirators for elimination of mouse aeroallergens. Am Assoc Lab Anim Sci 1989;39:63–66.

4. Newman-Taylor AJ. Laboratory animal allergy. Eur J Respir Dis 1982;63(suppl. 123):60–64.

5. Lincoln TA, Bolton NE, Garrett AS. Occupational allergy to animal dander and sera. J Occup Med 1974;16(7).

6. Lutsky II, Kalbfleisch JH, Fink JN. Occupational allergy to laboratory animals: employer practices. J Occup Med 1983;25:372–376.

7. Lennette, EH. Potential hazards posed by nonviral agents. In: Hellman A, Oxman MN, Pollack R, eds. Biohazards in biological research. Cold Spring Harbor, NY: Cold Spring Harbor Laboratory, 1973:3–40.

8. Milligan JE, Sarvaideo RJ, Thalken CE. Carcinogens, teratogens and mutagens: their impact on occupational health, particularly for women in veterinary medicine. J Environ Health 1983;46:19–245.

9. Hull RN. Biohazards associated with simian viruses. In: Hellman A, Oxman MN, Polack R, eds. Biohazards in biological research. Cold Spring Harbor, NY: Cold Spring Harbor Laboratory, 1973:3–40.

10. Yangihara R, Gajdusek DC, Gibbs CJ, Traub R. Prospect Hill virus: serologic evidence for infection in mammalogist. N Engl J Med 1984;310:1325–1326.

11. Tsai TF. Hemorrhagic fever with renal syndrome: mode of transmission in humans. Lab Anim Sci 1987;37:428–430.

12. Fox JG. Outbreak of tropical rat mite dermatitis in laboratory personnel. Arch Dermatol 1982;118(Sept).

13. Acha PN, Szyfres B. Zoonoses and communicable diseases common to man and animals. Scientific Publication No. 354. Washington, DC: World Health Organization, 1980.

14. Miller CD, Songer JR, Sullivan JF. A twenty-five year review of laboratory-acquired human infections at the national animal disease center. Am Ind Hyg Assoc 1987;48:271–275.

15. Jagger J, Hunt EH, Brand-Elnaggar J, Pearson RD. Rates of needle-stick injury caused by various services in a university hospital. N Engl J Med 1988;319:284–288.

16. European Chemical Industry Ecology and Toxicology Centre. The mutagenic and carcinogenic potential of formaldehyde. Technical report 1981:2.

17. National Research Council. Formaldehyde—An assessment of its health effects. Prepared for the Consumer Product Safety Commission, National Academy of Sciences, Washington, DC, 1980:1–38.

18. ACGIH. Documentation of TLV, 1989. 5th ed. Cincinnati, OH. American Conference of Governmental Industrial Hygienists, 1989.

19. Kilburn KH, Seidman BC, Warshaw R. Neurobehavioral and respiratory symptoms of formaldehyde and xylene exposure in histology technicians. Arch Environ Health 1985;40:229–233.

20. Milligan JE, Sablan JL, Croy JF. Trace substances in environmental health—XIV. Columbia: University of Missouri, 1980:436–443.

21. Basford AB, Fink BR. The teratogenicity of halothane in the rat. Anesthesiology 1968;29:1167–1173.

22. Cohen EN, Bellville JW, Brown BW. Anesthesia pregnancy and miscarriage. Anesthesiology 1971;35:343–347.

23. Spence AA, Knill-Jones RP. Is there a health hazard in anaesthetic practice? Br J Anaesth 1978;50:713–719.

24. Vessey MP, Nunn JF. Occupational hazard of anesthesia. Br Med J 1980;281:696–698.

25. Edling C. Anesthetic gases as an occupational hazard—a review. Scand J Work Environ Health 1980;6:85–93.

26. Baltzar B, Ericson A, Kallen B. Pregnancy outcome among women working in Swedish hospitals. N Engl J Med 1979;300:627–628.

27. Estander T, Jolanki R. How to protect the hands. Dermatol Clin 1988;6(1):105–114.

28. Smith JR, Grant JM. Does wearing two pairs of gloves protect against skin contamination? Br Med J 1988;297:1193.

29. Nelson G. Correia AN, Harder CA. Respirator cartridge efficiency studies: VII. Effect of relative humidity and temperature. Am Ind Hyg Assoc J 1976;37:280–288.

30. Hall T, Breysse P, Corn M, Jonas LA. Effects of adsorbed water vapor on the adsorption rate constant and the kinetic adsorption capacity of the Wheeler Kinetic Model. Am Ind Hyg Assoc J 1988;49:461–465.

31. Ortiz LW, Soderholm SC, Valdez FO. Penetration of respirator filters by an asbestos aerosol. Am Ind Hyg Assoc J 1988;49:451–460.

32. Stobbe TJ, daRoza RA, Watkins MA. Facial hair and respirator fit: a review of the literature. Am Ind Hyg Assoc J 1988;49:199–204.

33. Fowler JF, Callen JP. Facial dermatitis from a neoprene rubber mask. Contact Dermatitis 1988;18:310–311.

34. Gwosdow AR, Nielsen R, Berglund LG, DuBois AB. Terminal PG. Effect of thermal conditions on the acceptability of respiratory protective devices on humans at rest. Am Ind Hyg Assoc J 1989;50:188–195.

50

Worker Hazards in the Biotechnology Industry

Alan M. Ducatman, M.D., M.Sc.
Daniel F. Liberman, Ph.D.

INTRODUCTION

Historians of science may argue that "biotechnology" is not a new industry. Biotechnology began when humans first fermented honey and grapes for wine, or improved cultivated crops, or began breeding programs to select desirable traits in domesticated animals. This historical perspective is unassailable and unimportant. The public has a clear perception of "biotechnology." It involves specialized research leading to products produced through molecular biology techniques. These use recombinant DNA and protein engineering processes that markedly increase the precision and shorten the time period required for genetic experimentation.

Health and safety professionals will also recognize that this "new" industry is part of a long continuum of human endeavor. As with other "high tech" industries that are now well-established, biotechnology research and production may create risks for occupational illness. A significant challenge will be to anticipate the hazards of this work and prevent the illnesses as new processes and products are introduced.

It is because of health and safety concerns that research facilities for these activities are heavily engineered and rather expensive. Any operation that may generate a workplace aerosol or inadvertently release an organism to the environment is a candidate for *containment*. Containment is achieved through local barriers, building barriers, and personnel practices and procedures.

Local barriers in biotechnology laboratories may include any or all of the items listed in Table 50.1 (1). Biologic safety cabinets may be open-fronted (Class I and Class II). Workers are protected by the air curtain formed when laminar air flow meets the air stream drawn into the front face opening. Gases and aerosols generated in the cabinet are carried into the air stream to the exhaust filter or the recirculation air filter. Class III cabinets, or "glove boxes," have closed fronts and afford an additional level of protection. Work with dangerous agents is performed in Class III cabinets, which have glove ports for access. All equipment necessary for work with dangerous organisms, including incubators, autoclaves, centrifuges, and even animal storage cages, may be contained within a series of contiguous Class III cabinets (2). Routine maintenance and testing programs are critical for biologic safety cabinets of all

classes, as malfunctioning equipment may actually *increase* the risk of infection (3).

Laboratory hoods work by the same general ventilation principle as the Class I biosafety cabinets. A hood should be able to maintain a constant inward velocity at the sash face, in order to move noxious chemicals away from biologists during operations. In addition, the movable sash should be positioned to provide barrier protection against chemical explosions, fires, and splashes. As with biologic safety cabinets, laboratory hoods require balancing, routine testing, and maintenance.

At present, laboratory facilities are frequently laid out to meet the particular needs of a specific investigator or research and development enterprise. Siting concerns include conforming usage (zoning), transportation access, and compatibility of abutters and neighbors, as well as availability and constraints upon utilities (4) (notably waste disposal). The presence of local regulations, especially those constraining the use or application of certain technologies, will be an important citing consideration for biotechnologists, although this concern is unrelated to the health and safety considerations described above. Laboratories are an obvious part of the facility, but insufficient attention may be paid to health and safety support spaces listed in Table 50.2.

CHEMICALS COMMON TO THE BIOTECHNOLOGY INDUSTRY

Common operations of biotechnology include gel electrophoresis, high performance liquid chromatography (HPLC), and

Table 50.1. Local Barriers in Biotechnology Laboratories

Biological safety cabinets (Classes I, II, and III)
Chemical fume hoods
Glove bags
Enclosed centrifuges
Enclosure for sonicators
Safety blenders
Enclosed fermentation equipment

Table 50.2. Laboratory Support Spaces with Health and Safety Implications for Biotechnology

Glasswashing and autoclaving room
Bulk chemical and supply storage area
Laboratory washroom
Low level radiation waste handling area
Radiation counting room and support area[a]
Equipment rooms
Waste storage rooms
Biologic waste incinerator[b]
Wastewater treatment systems
Animal facilities[c]
Interstitial spaces for ventilation
Dedicated access hallways for waste disposal and other maintenance tasks

[a]Smaller facilities often contract this activity to an outside vendor, who offers scintillation equipment and other radiation support facilities at a remote site.
[b]On site incineration is economically desirable for large operations. A variety of clean air standards, which may change over time, have to be met.
[c]At large research institutions, animal housing facilities are often remote from research facilities. There is usually some need for temporary housing and handling on site as well.

protein and nucleic acid engineering. Table 50.3 lists the chemicals frequently used by biotechnologists for HPLC. Although health-related incidents have not been the norm, those that have occurred commonly involved exposure to acetonitrile.

Acetonitrile (CH_3CN) is a common solvent and extractant. It is toxic by any route of exposure, and massive exposures have been reported to cause death by cyanide asphyxiation after inhalation in workplaces. Intoxication and death following inhalation (5) or accidental ingestion (6) are delayed, sometimes for hours. The course is distinctly different than for inorganic cyanides. Unmetabolized acetonitrile is not lethally toxic (7). Cyanide is only one of the toxicants liberated by acetonitrile metabolism, but it is probably the most important one. Thiocyanate production may also contribute to reported fatal outcomes. Survivors of acute exposures have suffered from a variety of reversible symptoms and findings affecting the central nervous system, blood, and possibly the kidneys (5).

Such dramatic outcomes have not been reported for exposed biotechnologists. Yet biologists and support staff, including custodial personnel, do not always have the training to recognize the dangers of their chemicals. The absence of life-threatening exposures to acetonitrile is likely due to relatively small quantities used so far by biotechnologists rather than to universally adequate training or workplace hygiene. There have been a number of less dramatic overexposures to laboratory personnel, characterized by malaise, nausea, and headache, followed in at least two cases by subjective dyspnea. Blood gases were normal, save for evidence of hyperventilation, in two cases where they were obtained. To our knowledge, neither cyanide nor thiocyanate levels have been obtained for exposures in a biotechnology setting. Blood cyanide and thiocyanate measurements are not considered to be well-correlated with dose at lower levels of exposure, in any case (8). One exposure was to a custodian who was inappropriately involved in the cleanup of a broken storage bottle. It is likely that the shortterm exposure limit of 60 ppm was exceeded. This worker experienced delayed, prolonged, and temporarily incapacitating anxiety, once the toxic potential of acetonitrile was recognized. Epi-

sodes such as this one illustrate the importance of training personnel in spill control protocols and restricting "cleanup" to trained personnel.

Other chemicals used in HPLC have toxic properties not always recognized by laboratory personnel. Methylene chloride (dichloromethane) is a multipurpose solvent, used commonly as a degressor or paint remover, which is recognized as an animal (9) and possible human carcinogen (10, 11). An often mentioned additional hazard is metabolic conversion to carbon monoxide (12, 13); this is probably an important hazard at higher doses more characteristic of exposures to paint strippers than to research laboratory workers. Skin absorption is an important mode of exposure (14).

Of the common HPLC chemicals listed in Table 50.3, the following toxins are absorbed through skin: methanol (which is said to have caused deaths by skin absorption) (15), acetonitrile, methylene chloride, dimethylformamide, pyridines, and fluoroacetic acid. Trifluoroacetic acids are less toxic than the highly hazardous monofluoracetates (16, 17) but are still capable of being absorbed through skin. Bipolar compounds such as dimethylformamide are particularly interesting in this regard, as they may enhance the entry of other toxic agents through their "universal solvent" activity as well as by altering the natural barrier mechanisms of the skin. Skin permeability is particularly important to biotechnologists, who may appropriately use chemical hoods or other ventilation mechanisms of protection yet still expose their hands to a variety of chemicals.

Table 50.4 lists some of the chemicals that might be encountered in laboratory reagent preparations. Amyl alcohol is not infrequently responsible for "odor calls," when neighboring laboratory and office inhabitants become concerned by the presence of a fruity but distinctly chemical smell. Unstable compounds such as dimethyl sulfate (18) and hydrazine (19) are capable of causing spectacularly destructive incidents. Fortunately, biotechnologists generally use small quantities of these chemicals. Chronic diseases related to exposure have not been seen in this population so far. Skin splashes, with accompanying burns or local irritation, have occurred. An ongoing

Table 50.3. Chemicals Used by Biotechnologists for HPLC (Ranked by Approximate Usage)

Chemical	Primary Toxicity
Methanol	Metabolic acidosis, optic neuropathy, CNS[a] depression
Ammonium hydroxide	Strong irritant
Acetonitrile[b]	Cyanide-like
Methylene chloride	CNS, animal carcinogen
n-Hexane	Central and peripheral neurotoxicity
Dimethylformamide	Liver
N-Methylpyrrolidinone	Animal teratogen; heat decomposition to NOx
Ethyl acetate	Relatively low toxicity, dermatitis
Trifluoroacetic acid	Strong irritant
Tetrahydrofuran	Irritant
Triethylamine	Irritant and sensitizer, CNS
Ethanolamine	Irritant and sensitizer, CNS
Acetic anhydride	Strong irritant
Dimethylaminopyridine	Irritant, heat decomposition to toxic fumes

[a]CNS, central nervous system.
[b]Most common chemical causing health-related incidents to date in biotechnology research.

Table 50.4. Reagents Used in Biotechnology Laboratories, Ranked by Approximate Usage

Chemical	Primary Toxicity
Glacial acetic acid	Irritant
Hydrochloric acid	Severe irritant
Trichloroacetic acid	Irritant
Isoamyl alcohol	Low toxicity, irritant
Phosphoric acid	Irritant
Formaldehyde	Irritant, sensitizer, animal carcinogen
Glutaraldehyde	Irritant, sensitizer
Dimethyl sulfate	Severe irritant, animal carcinogen
Dimethyl sulfoxide	Central nervous depressant, gastrointestinal
Sulfuric acid	Severe irritant
Hydrazine	Severe irritant; liver, blood, nervous system, and kidney toxicity
Cyanogen bromide	Metabolic asphyxiant, pulmonary toxicity
Hydrofluoric acid	Severe irritant

Table 50.5. Gel Electrophoresis Chemicals

Acrylamide
N,N'-Methylene-bisacrylamide
Ammonium persulfate
Ethidium bromide
N',N',N',N'-Tetramethylethylenediamine
Tris-acetate-EDTA

challenge in research laboratory environments is to inculcate good personal hygiene and work practices, so that buffers are mixed in hoods—with the sash down to prevent eye splashes—and so that personnel are not found with sandals, shorts, or without lab coats and safety glasses.

As biotechnology moves from lab bench to production, the quantities of chemicals including acetonitrile will increase from subliter volumes to 20 or more liters at a time. Spill control and potential exposure will become important planning challenges as scale increases.

Gel electrophoresis is used to examine DNA fragments. Chemicals used in the preparation and staining of polyacrylamide gel electrophoresis are listed in Table 50.5. Three deserve special comment. Tetramethylethylenediamine (TEMED) is a severe eye irritant as well as a potential sensitizer. Ethidium bromide is used, in a combination with ultraviolet light, to visualize DNA bands by fluorescent staining. Biotechnologists have been sufficiently concerned by the mutagenic properties [20] of ethidium bromide that it is one of the first toxins to undergo partial characterization of DNA damage pattern [21]. Another potential source of exposure comes during large scale preparation of closed circular plasmid DNA, when ethidium bromide is added to cesium chloride gradients.

Acrylamide is a white, crystalline powder used to make polyacrylamide gel. Researchers have commonly made up their own gels from acrylamide powder, with potential for dust exposure during weighing, transferring, and mixing operations. It is common to see waste acrylamide powder around balances during visits to molecular biology laboratories. Acrylamide may be the second most common potential source of toxic exposure for biotechnology researchers, including skin contact with powder and with gel preparations. Recently, it has been available in gel form, which should reduce the hazard.

At high doses, acrylamide is an important human neurotoxin whose likely portal of entry is through the skin. A characteristic contact dermatitis of the palms often precedes the neurologic syndrome. Nonspecific central nervous system signs such as fatigue and malaise also precede the classical progressive, symmetric, distal peripheral neuropathy [22, 23]. Neither the dermatitis nor the neurologic syndrome have so far been reported from molecular biology workplaces. The cumulative nature of acrylamide neuropathy [23, 24] nevertheless dictates that skin exposure not be permitted. Furthermore, acrylamide has other, less appreciated toxic properties. It crosses the placenta and causes both experimental reproductive loss and neurotoxic effects in neonates at doses insufficient to cause overt maternal toxicity [25]. Acrylamide also causes direct testicular degeneration in exposed rodents [26], and is recognized as a genotoxin whose primary mechanisms are heritable translocations [26] and spermatic chromoclastogenesis [27]. It is unequivocally an animal carcinogen at several sites [25], although there are inadequate data for deciding if this applies also to humans [28].

Given these toxic properties, it is distressing that biologists endure routine, voluntary dermal exposures. The most likely explanation for this behavior is inadequate education. Suggested standard policies for reducing acrylamide exposure are listed in Table 50.6.

An important procedure in current cell research uses gene markers in selection techniques. Methotrexate is a folic acid antagonist, which will kill cells unable to express the gene product dihydrofolate reductase. Researchers can "link" a second gene of interest, such as insulin or growth hormone, to the gene for dihydrofolate reductase. Then cells surviving antimetabolite treatment will inherit *both* the selected gene and the additional gene linked to it. This process is called "selection for the linked gene."

Although any number of antimetabolites could have been used for linked gene selection, the initial work was carried out with methotrexate. Biologists have taken a generally benign view of methotrexate toxicity, perhaps because the product solutions contain only micromolar quantities.

Methotrexate has been used in pharmacologic treatment of leukemia, several other neoplasms, nonmetastatic trophoblastic diseases, and psoriasis. Toxicity of folic acid antagonists such

Table 50.6. Policies for Reducing Acrylamide Dermal Exposure

Policy	Advantage
1. Source reduction. Purchase in smallest container	A. Economic—saves on waste disposal B. Mixing can be accomplished without weighing
2. Weight out in tared closable containers, kept in fume hood	A. Reduces exposure of weighing
3. Purchase in solution form	A. Reduces exposure of weighing B. Reduces skin exposure
4. Use ventilated glove box or hood with dedicated balance	A. The bottle of powder is open only under local exhaust B. Reduces skin exposure
5. Require gloves for any skin exposure	A. Reduces skin exposure

as methotrexate is correspondingly impressive. At therapeutic doses, it is a proven teratogen, affects male and female reproductive capability, and causes bone marrow aplasia, severe stomatitis, and other gastrointestinal symptoms which may be fatal. In addition, methotrexate is responsible for hepatotoxicity, nephrotoxicity, and immunosuppression (29). Work-related exposures should obviously be controlled vigorously for a known human reproductive hazard. Skin exposure is unacceptable under industrial conditions. Waste liquor from cell growth media may be regarded as hazardous for regulatory purposes if it contains methotrexate.

While occupational professionals would clearly prefer that some other, less human cytotoxic, chemical be used for selective resistance, it is most unlikely that important research, development, or production activities will use any other selective approach. The U.S. Food and Drug Administration regards methotrexate selection as a standard technique. Neither pharmaceutical companies nor independent researchers have incentives to find replacement methodologies. It is essential that potential exposure activities, such as weighing, mixing, and waste handling, be carried out with sufficient planning and attention to occupational and environmental safety to prevent exposure.

Chilled water is used to meet the precise temperature and humidity conditions required for cell line production. Chemical hazards of chilled water unit maintenance include exposure to a variety of corrosive or sensitizing chemicals including strong alkaline and acid chemicals, amines, and hepatotoxic solvents such as dimethylformamide. This problem is not unique to the biotechnology industry. Workers in power plants, industries, and office buildings also work with chilled water units. Personnel will have to control the chemical and biologic hazards associated with servicing chilled water systems. It is of obvious importance to install personal protective gear and a training program for chilled water maintenance workers; manufacturers of chilled water treatment chemicals are sometimes willing to collaborate in this process. Recirculating chilled water units also pose a potential nuisance odor hazard. Such units often contain antifreeze additives such as ethylene glycol. Foul-smelling bacteria, such as *Clostridia glycoliticum*, may metabolize the antifreeze within standing chilled water during intervals between operation. Any break in the chilled water pipes will release the odorous metabolites. It is difficult and possibly unrealistic to persuade building inhabitants that the odor is not hazardous to health. Odors may finally be controlled when walls are scrubbed, furniture cleaned or repainted, and rugs replaced.

Recirculating chilled water is also a source of *Legionella pneumophilia*, the organism responsible for Legionnaire's disease (30). Prevention of this work-related illness requires frequent biocidal treatments and routine microbiologic sampling of treated water.

A frequently ignored chemical hazard common to research and production microbiology is cleanup. Scientists, technologists, and support staff such as glass washers are exposed to a variety of soaps and detergents. Some of these are phenolic-based, some quaternary amines, and most can be sensitizing after longterm use.

PHYSICAL HAZARDS OF PRODUCTION SCALE-UP

Biotechnology is a dynamic industry. There is no standard set of procedures or products. New products create new market niches. Competition is frequently on the basis of new patents rather than cost control or marketing. Under these circumstances, manufacturers rush new discoveries from the laboratory to consumers, without exploring other technologies that might facilitate production engineering. Most often, biotechnology production is a "scaled up" version of laboratory methods.

Biologists may not appreciate that there are important physical hazards associated with scale-up activities, listed in Table 50.7. Laboratory scientists may fail to recognize that laboratory grade materials will not support production technology. The lesson is learned when laboratory grade tubing ruptures and an employee is burned. Steam burns are a fairly common problem. It is to be hoped that maturation of the industry will encourage more innovative use of production and industrial hygiene engineering, with reassessment of production technology. Other physical hazards include large glass bottles, which are heavy to lift and dangerous when dropped. A variety of heavy materials invite improved ergonomic approaches.

Shift work is required in biotechnology because microbial production and harvest do not follow human timetables. As a result, support workers work 12-hour days in some cyclic pattern such as 2 days on, 3 off, 3 on, and 2 off. The problems of shift work are well known and include an effect on virtually every organ system (31). Shift work is commonly thought to play a contributing role in industrial accidents. While a typical biotechnology schedule appears more humane than shift work schedules commonly cited for other industries (32), the obligate round-the-clock nature of the work schedule may provide safety concerns in typically small, sparsely staffed enterprises.

BIOLOGIC HAZARDS OF BIOTECHNOLOGY

Biotechnologists may work with virtually any organism studied by conventional biologists. To date, remarkably few infectious diseases have been reported. The risk of work with engineered

Table 50.7. Physical Hazards of Production Activities

Type	Source
Burn	Pressurized steam. liquid nitrogen/acetone/dry ice
Hypothermia	Cold room (up to 12 hours continuously)
Electrical	Heavy equipment, electrophoresis units
Cuts	20-liter glass bottles, glass bioreactors
Anoxic	CO_2 and N_2 lines
Ergonomic	Drums, large bottles, media preparation and other "scaled up" equipment
Repetitive trauma	Computer modeling
Shift work	Round-the-clock microbial support (monitoring) of large scale production; product isolation and purification

organism may be less than work with nonengineered organisms, because typical engineered organisms have been selected for properties unrelated to infectivity.

There are no limits to the organisms selected for engineering. Some of the more important activities now under way involve the large scale production of epidemic organisms such as the human immunodeficiency virus, hepatitis B, and hepatitis delta. These are used for applied (vaccine) research and basic understanding of their biologic properties. Table 50.8 lists a cross-section of organisms used in industrial applications. Of these, the vaccinia virus may be of considerable concern to immunosuppressed researchers, to their families and friends who may be immunosuppressed, and to exposed individuals with skin disorders. In addition, there is a recent tendency toward host work with specific genes from dangerous organisms. As biotechnologists attempt to develop vaccines and other treatment strategies for serious diseases, researchers must grow these organisms before they can isolate specific genes. The National Institutes of Health *Guidelines for Research Recombinant DNA Molecules* is an important resource for information about control of biohazards (33).

An interesting problem for biotechnologists is how to dispose of research organisms that have been radiolabeled. Strong public interest in biologic waste and evolving infectious waste regulations (34, 35) require that some acceptable form of biologic decontamination be found. Chemical decontamination or usual modes of heat sterilization, such as incineration, are undesirable in this circumstance because they will only further disperse any radioactivity used to label research materials. A possible solution is the judicious use of filters within autoclave bag systems (36), so that steam sterilization can be accomplished without release of radioactivity. Waste disposal is but

one of the safety and regulatory considerations for recombinant biologists who use radiolabeled materials. This broad topic is treated elsewhere for human immunodeficiency virus laboratories (37) and for microbiologic laboratories in general (38).

EPIDEMIOLOGY OF BIOTECHNOLOGY EXPOSURE

There are no peer review data concerning population outcomes in biotechnology. The science is too new, the populations at individual sites too small, the movement of trained personnel from employer to employer too rapid, and the enthusiasm of scientist-entrepreneurs for nonproduct research too small to have encouraged any systematic looks at health outcomes among biotechnologists.

Epidemiologic studies are definitely needed. Perceived soft tissue cancer miniepidemics have been reported among scientists using recombinant technology at Pasteur Institute in Paris and the Agricultural Research Institute of Ireland (39–41). Cancer prevalence miniepidemics may indicate an underlying occupational health problem, or they may be simply the result of chance. Designed population studies are needed to decide whether there is an increased incidence of cancer, or any other chronic disease outcome, among biotechnologists. Studies showing the absence of excess disease would also be extremely important to the industry. Chemical and biologic exposures of recombinant DNA work may vary greatly depending on the type of research or production activity. This is an impediment to epidemiologic research because it may prove difficult to identify sizable populations with similar exposures for study, even if the research question is excess cancer.

Infectious diseases have not yet proved an especially im-

Table 50.8. Common Host and Vector Organisms

Host	Vector
Escherichia coli k12	Plasmids, phage, shuttle vectors[a]
Bacillus sp. (asporogenic strains)	Plasmids
Saccharomyces cerevisiae	Plasmids, shuttle vectors[a]
Corynebacteria glutamicum	With and without plasmids
Streptomyces sp.	With and without plasmids
Mammalian tissue culture cells	*Vaccinia virus, Herpes virus, Murine retrovirus, Papilloma virus*
Insect tissue culture cells	*Bacculovirus*

[a]These vectors can be grown in more than one host; for example, yeast and bacteria or bacteria and tissue culture cells, etc.

portant epidemiologic problem for recombinant biologists. The introduction of more dangerous research organisms is likely to change this pattern, however. Recombinant vaccine research with retroviruses or mycobacteria provides examples of evident infectious hazards. Even research with noninfectious genome may incur the risk of misleading seroconversion. False seroconversions are already a concern of human immunodeficiency virus researchers who work with noninfectious pieces of genome material.

To date, chemical and physical hazard exposures have resulted in acute rather than chronic or permanent problems. Informal reports indicate that transient malaise from acetonitrile overexposure, acid burns, and steam burns from ruptured lines are the most common problems. Support personnel may also have problems from shiftwork.

ENVIRONMENTAL CONTROLS AND PREVENTION OF EXPOSURE

Tables 50.1 and 50.2, discussed in the introduction, review some of the facility requirements of the biotechnology industry. While the information presented in these tables relates to worker health and safety, it turns out that a considerable portion of the biotechnology facility investment relates to protecting the larger community rather than workers. The public has reacted strongly to the conscious manipulation of genetic material at the molecular level, as opposed to the chance changes of natural selection in the environment or the conscious but less precise changes of traditional breeding programs. In the context of public fear, it may seem to health care professionals that workers bear the brunt of real risks but receive few of the resources intended for environmental health. Even Level III biosafety designations relate more to protecting the public from laboratory releases than to protecting workers within laboratories.

The role of health and safety professionals in improving this ironic situation involves education and engineering. Workers, from custodial personnel to Nobel scientists, require information about hazards and how to mitigate them. The present cavalier attitude toward acetonitrile and acrylamide can best be reversed with strong educational programs. Even highly goal-oriented scientists can be convinced to protect their hands from a potent skin absorbable toxin. Availability of protection plays a role in this process. Gloves adequate to prevent penetration, lab coats, and safety goggles are as important to biologists as they are to chemists. Preengineered laboratory hoods, adequately vented biologic cabinets, specially designed centrifuges, and frequent preventive maintenance of ventilation facilities are essential to the protection process. Industrial hygiene and biohazard monitoring should be continuous, in order to discover unexpected breaks from containment.

Uncontained aerosols and skin exposures are major issues in chemical and biologic safety. Each process and procedure can be designed to prevent them, providing personnel have adequate education. Interestingly enough, this prudent safety measure is also critical to preventing contamination at production facilities, so that commerical needs will dictate some critical safety measures at large scale facilities.

REFERENCES

1. Liberman DF. Identification and control of human health hazards associated with current and emerging technology. In: Draggen SS, Cohrssen JJ, Morrison RE, eds. Environmental impacts on human health: the agenda for long-term research and development. New York: Praeger, 1987:193–219.

2. National Institute of Health. Laboratory Safety Monograph. Bethesda: National Institute of Health, 1979.

3. Clark RP, et al. Microbiological safety cabinets and laboratory acquired infection (Letters). Lancet 1988;2:844–845.

4. Wolfe MI. Facility considerations. In: Liberman DF, Gordon J, eds. Biohazards management handbook. New York: Marcel Dekker, 1989:1–45.

5. Amdur ML. Accidental group exposure to acetonitrile. J Occup Med 1959;1:627–33.

6. Caravati EM, Litovitz TL. Pediatric cyanide intoxication and death from an acetonitrile-containing cosmetic. JAMA 1988;260:3470–73.

7. Tanii H, Hashimato K. Studies on the mechanisms of acute toxicity of nitriles in mice. Arch Toxicol 1984;55:47–54.

8. Pozzani VC, Carpenter PC, Palm PE. An investigation of the toxicity of acetonitrile. J Occup Med 1959;1:634–42.

9. National Toxicology Program, National Institute of Health. NTP technical report on the toxicology and carcinogenesis studies of dichloromethane in F344/N rats and B6C3F$_1$ mice (inhalation studies). NIH no. 86-2562, NTP-TR 306, 1986.

10. Hearne FT, Grose F, Pifer JW, et al. Methylene chloride mortality study: dose response characterization and animal model comparison. J Occup Med 1987;29:217–228.

11. Mirer FE, Silverstein M, Park R. Methylene chloride and cancer of the pancreas (Letter). J Occup Med 1988; 30:475–478.

12. Stewart RD, Fisher TN, Hosko MJ, et al. Experimental human exposure to methylene chloride. Arch Environ Health 1972;25:342–48.

13. Stewart RD, Hake CL. Paint-remover hazard. JAMA 1976;235:398–401.

14. Proctor NH, Hughes JP, Fischman ML, eds. Chemical hazards of the workplace. Philadelphia: JB Lippincott, 1988.

15. Henson EV. The toxicology of some alphatic alcohols—Part II. J Occup Med 1960;2:497–502.

16. Parmagianni L, ed. Encyclopedia of occupational health and safety. Geneva: International Labor Office. 1983.

17. Peters RA, Spencer H, Bidstrup PL. Subacute fluoroacetate poisoning. J Occup Med 1981;23:112–113.

18. Ip M, Wong KL, Wong KF, So SY. Lung injury in dimethylsulfate poisoning. J Occup Med 1989;31:141–143.

19. Sotaniemi E. Hirvonen J, Isomaki H, et al. Hydrazine toxicity in the human: report of a fatal case. Ann Clin Res 1971;3:30–33.

20. McCann J, Choi E, Yamusaki E, Ames BN. Detection of carcinogens as mutagens in the Salmonella/microsome test. Proc Natl Acad Sci USA 1975;72:5135–39.

21. Cariello NF, Keohavong P, Sanderson BJS, Thilly WG. DNA damage produced by ethidium bromide staining and exposure to ultraviolet light. Nucleic Acids Res 1988;16:4157.

22. Garland TO, Patterson M. Six cases of acrylamide poisoning. Br Med J 1967;4:134–138.

23. Spencer PS, Schaumberg HH. A review of acrylamide neurotoxicity. I: properties, uses, and human exposure. Can J Noon Sci 1974;1:143–50.

24. Takahashi M, Ohara T, Hashimoto K. Electrophysiological study of nerve injuries in workers handling acrylamide. Int Arch Arbeitsmed 1971;28:1–11.

25. Dearfield KL, Abernathy CO, Ottley MS, et al. Acrylamide: its metabolism, developmental and reproductive effects, genotoxicity, and carcinogenicity. Mutat Res 1988;195:44–77.

26. Hashimoto K, Sakamoto J, Tanii H. Neurotoxicity of acrylamide and related compounds and their effects on male gonads in mice. Arch Toxicol 1981;41:179–189.

27. Shiraishi Y. Chromosome aberrations induced by monomeric acrylamide in bone marrow and germ cells of mice. Mutat Res 1978;57:313–324.

28. Sobel W, Bond TW, Parsons TW, Brenner FE. Acrylamide cohort mortality study. Br J Ind Med 1986;43:785–788.

29. Klassen CD, Amdur MD, Doull J, eds. Casarett and Doull's Toxicology: the basic science of poisons. New York: Macmillan, 1986.

30. Muraca PW, Stout JE, Yu VL, Yee YC. Legionnaire's disease in the work environment: implications for environmental health. Am Ind Hyg Assoc 1988;49:584–590.

31. Rutenfranz J, Knouth P. Shift work. In: Zenz C, ed. Occupational medicine: principle and practical applications. Chicago: Year Book, 1988. 1087–1095.

32. Krieger GR. Shift work studies provide clues to industrial accidents. Occup Health Saf 1987;(Jan):21–34.

33. DHHS/NIH. Guidelines for research regarding recombinant DNA molecules. Fed Reg May 7, 1986:(16) 958–985.

34. Environmental Protection Agency. EPA guide for infectious waste management. US Dept Commerce/NTIS PB86–199130, EPA/530–SW–86–014, 1986.

35. Environmental Protection Agency. Standards for the tracking and management of medical waste; interim final rule and request for comments. 40 CFR Parts 22 and 259. March 24, 1989;54:12326–12395.

36. Stinson MC, Galanek MS, Ducatman AM, Masse FX. Inactivation and disposal of human immunodeficiency virus and radioactive waste in a P3 facility. Appl Environ Microbiol 1990;56:264–268.

37. Stinson MC, Kuritzkes DR, Masse FX. Guidelines for an effective radiation safety program in a human immunodeficiency virus laboratory. Submitted for publication.

38. Staiger JW. Techniques for safe handling of radioactive material. In: Miller B, et al. eds. Laboratory safety: principles and practices. Washington, DC: American Society for Microbiology, 1986:242–260.

39. Inquiry into lab's bone cancers. Nature 1986;321:649.

40. Cancer deaths probed at Pasteur Institute. Science 1986;237:1597.

41. Pasteur Institute invites worldwide help to track r-DNA-lab cancer risk. McGraw-Hill's Biotechnology Newswatch 1986;6:1–2.

51

Medical Waste

John B. Sullivan, Jr., M.D.
Linda Micale, M.S.

MEDICAL WASTE GENERATION

Infectious waste is defined as that waste which is capable of producing infection or characterized by a pathogen that can produce human disease. Infectious waste, generally categorized as a biohazard, possesses the risk or potential risk to humans of producing disease. Such wastes can include highly infectious pathogens including hepatitis, human immunodeficiency viruses (HIV), pathogenic fungi, and other unusual biologic materials. Difficulties in defining infectious waste hazards are due to the variety of material found in waste containers, the nature of the pathogen, the large variety of waste sources, the types of wastes and disposables, and the many different clinical as well as laboratory areas that generate the waste. Many of the components of medical wastes are not themselves infectious, but may be contaminated by biologic fluids or blood that is infectious. Medical waste is an emotional issue as well as a health hazard. Recent events involving public contact with medical wastes has resulted in governmental action to reduce risks of public exposure. It is the individual health care worker, though, who has the highest risk of infectivity and injury (1).

The familiar "red bags" and biohazard-labeled containers are common features of health care environments (Figs. 51.1–51.3). The contents of these waste containers vary tremendously. In addition to the common sharps and needles, the addition of plastic disposables, latex products, and paper contribute greatly to the medical waste load that must be properly disposed. The health care industry is the primary generator of medical waste. The wide variety of hospitals, clinics, laboratories, and extended care facilities provide a varied source of wastes. Medical waste is not always infectious. Estimations are that only 15% of hospital-generated waste is infectious, with the remaining 85% being a combination of disposable, gloves, plastics, paper, needles, syringes, and other medical disposable items (2, 3). Estimations of waste generation in the United States varies from 4–8 kg/bed/day (8–14 pounds/bed/day), with a high end estimate being close to 6000 tons/day nationwide for 1985 alone (2). Other recent surveys indicate that large hospitals generate on the average 4.18 killograms of waste per bed per day (6063 tons/day based on 1.267 million hospital beds that existed in 1987 in the United States) (3). The U.S. Environmental Protection Agency (EPA) currently recognizes six broad categories of infectious waste:

1. Isolation wastes
2. Cultures, biologics, stocks of infectious agents
3. Human blood and blood products
4. Pathologic wastes
5. Contaminated sharps
6. Contaminated animal carcasses, body parts, and bedding

Waste byproducts can be categorized as isolation wastes, cultures, blood and blood products, dialysis unit wastes, used hypodermic needles and syringes, pathology and autopsy wastes, discarded biologics, remains of surgical procedures, laboratory waste, contaminated disposables, animal bedding and animal body parts (Table 51.1). Other components of medical wastes may include antineoplastic agents, radiopharmaceuticals, and the myriad plastics and papers that end up in the "red" containers.

The Centers for Disease Control (CDC), differing slightly from the EPA recognize five categories of infectious medical waste (3): (a) microbiologic, (b) sharps, (c) blood, (d) pathologic, and (e) contaminated animal carcasses. The CDC and the EPA also differ with respect to an optional waste category which the EPA identifies as surgical and autopsy wastes, contaminated wastes from laboratories and dialysis units, and contaminated equipment.

The vast majority of medical waste generated is noninfectious. The fact that many noninfectious materials are disposed of in medical waste containers attests to the uncertainty and

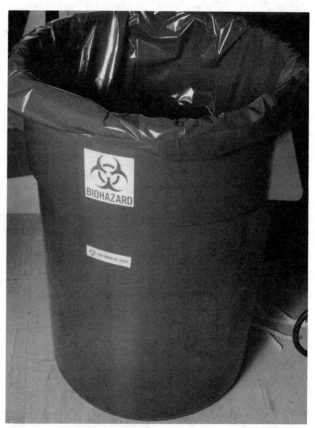

Figure 51.1. Typical biohazardous waste container showing the biohazard symbol.

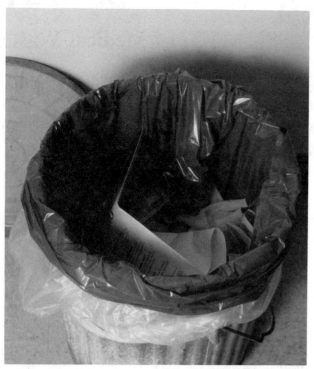

Figure 51.2. Red bag medical waste container.

anxieties surrounding the issue and the definitions of infectious waste versus medical waste. How these types of wastes are defined will directly influence the cost of management and disposal. Hospitals have found that large monetary savings can be realized by adopting the CDC guidelines and definitions as opposed to EPA guidelines (3). However, if EPA guidelines bcome the final regulatory basis for medical waste management, many hospitals would have to spend millions of dollars

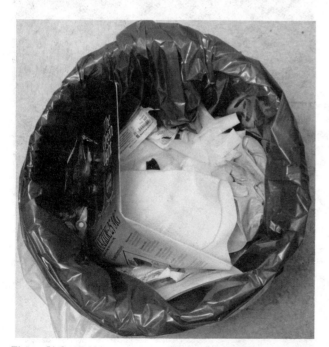

Figure 51.3. Red bag waste container showing variety of noninfectious items as content.

Table 51.1.   Categorization of Medical Wastes

Isolation Wastes

This involves materials that come into contact with blood, secretions, excretions, feces, and other biologic fluids of patients with communicable diseases. This includes a variety of wastes such as needles, disposal plastic items, gowns, masks, paper products, bandages, rubber drains, suture material, and tubing.

Cultures and Stocks of Infectious Agents

These have high concentrations of pathogens which is an important factor in risk management and are usually associated with pathology laboratories. Included are blood cultures, agar plates, and cultures of a variety of biologic fluids which can serve as a medium of infectivity. Also included is a wide variety of pathogens. Culture media are usually sterilized before being discarded.

Blood and Blood Products

Blood should always be considered infectious. Common infectious problems include hepatitis, HIV, malaria, rubella, measles, and others.

Autopsy and Surgery Wastes

These wastes are generated in hospital emergency departments, surgery, pathology departments, and autopsy areas. Included are body parts, tissues, biologic fluids, organs, and secretions from infected or potentially infected patients. Such wastes may also contain plastic, metal, or cardboard. All surgical dressings from patients should be regarded as contaminated and sources of infection. In addition to gauze dressings and bandages of many varieties, these wastes include some biopsy and tissue specimens, cast materials, drapes, silastic tubing, needles, pads, biologic fluids, metal instruments, and latex gloves.

Laboratory Wastes

Includes all culture plates (glass and plastic), transfer devices, plastic tops, agar, paper, plastics used in automated chemical processes, autopsy wastes, blood and blood products, urine and blood containers, and glass tubes.

Sharps

This includes needles and other sharp objects, syringes, needles of all sizes, scalpel blades, pipettes, and broken glass. This category of waste materials has the highest risk of causing injury and transmission of disease.

Dialysis Unit Wastes

Includes sheets, towels, gloves, aprons, bandages, tubing, gloves, filters, and dialysis membranes. These wastes carry a high incidence of hepatitis.

Animal Body Parts

Carcasses and parts of dead animals. Usually confined to research facility or university setting. Parts may be infectious and contain experimental biologic agents as well as experimental pharmaceuticals including antineoplastic drugs, carcinogens, and potent immunosuppressants.

Discarded Biologics

Includes vaccines and drugs that are either outdated or used in animals and humans with infectious diseases. Also included could be antineoplastic drugs and discarded serum from multiple sources (human and animal).

Contaminated Equipment

Includes equipment and equipment parts that come into contact with infectious agents. Patient care equipment, filters, metals, plastics, rubber, cloth, and fabrics.

yearly to be in compliance (3). An overall cost savings in the millions would be realized if the hospitals currently following EPA guidelines switched to CDC guidelines.

Sources of medical and infectious wastes have traditionally been hospitals. However, given that there are over 180,000 private physician offices, over 98,000 dental offices, 16,400 nursing homes, 2900 ambulatory healthcare centers, 650 ambulatory surgical centers, 860 dialysis units, and 225 blood banks, it is clear that the volume of wastes generated will continue to increase (3). Also, as greater efficiencies in health care are necessary, the increase in ambulatory-generated waste may alter the overall nature of the waste streams (3). United States hospitals alone are said to generate 900 tons of medical wastes per day (3). Many states do not regulate private dental and physician offices regarding generation and disposal of medical wastes.

Even the use of the terms *medical waste* and *infectious waste* have been debated regarding a determination of the correct label to apply in order to best categorize both the hazard and nature of the waste streams. However, the Medical Waste Tracking Act of 1988 adopted the term *medical waste* in order to broadly encompass the remote possibility of infection transmission.

SAFETY AND DISPOSAL PRACTICES

The EPA and the CDC have published guidelines which differ on the designation and the disposal of medical wastes. The CDC and the EPA agree on the definition of medical wastes as infectious waste in five categories but disagree on the one category of isolation wastes as being communicable. The EPA also has an optional medical waste which may be derived from sources such as surgical procedures, dialysis wastes, contaminated equipment, and autopsies. The EPA allows local responsible hospital or clinic authorities to decide whether these wastes should be managed as though they were infectious (3).

Disposal practices among large medical facilities such as hospitals and large outpatient clinics are fairly uniform. Policies for managing biohazards and medical waste as well as disease prevention and infection control are required by accrediting agencies. Safe practices regarding disposal of needles and sharps, bagging and labeling of medical waste, storage of waste, and disposal are components of the overall quality assurance program. It is wise to have an individual such as an infection control nurse oversee this program. This individual can ensure proper training of staff who handle infectious waste and ensure compliance with the institution's policies and procedures.

A sharps injury and/or biologic fluids exposure program is another important component of the overall safety and disposal program. These types of injuries and exposures are the most common reason for employees to seek medical care in the handling of such waste. A well-designed and comprehensive program is necessary. Included in these are steps to be taken following a needle stick by personnel from a known or unknown source.

HEALTH RISK ISSUES

The salient risk management issues regarding medical waste generation and disposal involve needlesticks, mucous membrane exposures of workers, handling, storage, and transport. These items include initial disposal practices in clinical areas, storage in clinical areas, tracking of wastes, storage in depository areas, handling at the site of origin by employees of the

facility as well as the transport company, transportation, and handling at the incineration facility.

The Occupational Safety and Health Administration (OSHA) on May 30, 1989, issued a proposed standard relating to the regulation of occupational exposure to hepatitis B virus, HIV, and other blood and biologic fluid-transmitted pathogens (CFR 54, 23042). The standard applies to all occupational exposures to blood and/or other potentially infectious materials. The *definition* of occupational exposure is a reasonably anticipated skin, eye, mucous membrane, or parenteral contact with potentially infectious material that may result from the performance of an employee's duties. This standard requires employers with such employees to identify and document tasks where an occupational exposure may occur. The employer is also required to have a written infection control plan. The OSHA standard establishes four compliance methods:

1. **General compliance:** OSHA has adopted the universal precautions recommended by the CDC.
2. **Engineering and work practice:** Serves to reduce exposures in the workplace by eliminating and/or controlling the hazard.
3. **Personal protective equipment:** Requires employers to provide and employees to use appropriate protective devices and garb such as eye shields, gowns, gloves, head and foot coverings, as well as proper resuscitation devices to prevent exposure.
4. **Housekeeping:** Requires cleaning and disinfection of contaminated areas and items that contact potentially infectious media.

The OSHA standard will also require employers to develop an appropriate employee health program and offer hepatitis B vaccine to all employees who are exposed to potential sources one or more times per month. The health program must also provide post-exposure evaluation and medical follow-up of exposed employees. This evaluation includes HIV as well as hepatitis B exposure evaluation. Postexposure evaluation must offer collection and testing of the source's blood (if permission is granted) and review of the source's medical records for risk factors. The employee's blood must also be tested and the employee offered counseling as well as appropriate prophylaxis if available.

Further, the OSHA standard requires appropriate labeling of containers of infectious waste and refrigerators containing blood and blood products, and containers used to transport and store potentially infectious materials. Training of employees who will have occupational exposure is also mandated. This training must include modes of transmission, safe practices to reduce exposures, personal protection, and the use of personal protective devices, and explanation on how to handle an exposure and the medical evaluation, along with vaccines, available. Medical record documentation of exposures is also necessary, and these must be kept confidential. Documentation of employee training is also included in the standard.

Infection Risks

Health care workers who come into contact with biologic secretions, blood and blood products, and excretions of patients with communicable diseases are at risk with respect to medical waste and infectious hazards. Accidents at this stage are usually due to injury from needles and syringes or contamination of open wound sites or mucous membranes with biologic fluids

Table 51.2.   Human Risks from Medical Waste

Bacteria

Bordetella pertussis
Mycobacterium tuberculosis
Treponema pallidum
Staphylococcus aureus
Streptococcus pyogenes
Neisseria meningococcus

Viruses

Human immunodeficiency virus (HIV)
Hepatitis B
Hepatitis A
Non-A, non-B hepatitis
Cytomegalovirus
Herpes simplex
Measles
Mumps
Rubella
Respiratory syncytial virus

from an infectious source. A variety of infectious agents are recognized as etiologic sources for which health care workers are at risk (Table 51.2). Currently, transmission of hepatitis B and HIV are the primary concerns of health care personnel. Prevention of the disease is the most important risk management issue. The factors that can result in disease production must be controlled. Necessary factors to produce disease are as follows:

1. Presence of a pathogen;
2. Presence of a host;
3. Route of exposure for transmission;
4. Exposure to the pathogen;
5. Exposure to infective dose.

Prevention of disease is part of risk management, and practices of health care facilities to prevent disease from infectious hazardous materials must be part of risk management strategy. Isolation of infectious waste with specialized precautions are a component of hospital and clinic policy and procedures. Overall, the risk of acquiring an infection from medical waste is very remote. Solid municipal waste is said to be manyfold more microbially contaminated than medical waste (3).

Antineoplastic Drug Hazards

These pharmaceuticals are handled routinely by pharmacists and nurses in caring for patients with cancer. The risk from exposure to these personnel is due to the chronicity of low level exposure during preparation and administration to patients. Exposure occurs via skin contact, inhalation, and ingestion of minute amounts of these drugs (4). Personal protective equipment such as gowns, gloves, and properly ventilated mixing hood areas are vital to minimize any potential exposures. Accidental spills are also a source of exposure. Antineoplastic drugs are potent poisons and are recognized teratogens, mutagens, and carcinogens. Another important issue of relative risk involves the handling and disposal of antineoplastic drugs. Epidemiologic studies have revealed that nurses handling antineoplastic drugs have a 2.3 times higher incidence of spontaneous abortion as compared with other nurses (4). A variety of health complaints have been documented in workers mixing and preparing these drugs (4).

Antineoplastic drugs have an irritant effect on the skin, eyes, and mucous membranes. Toxicity of these types of drugs includes mutagenic, teratogenic, and carcinogenic health effects (4). Local allergic reactions can also occur, such as urticarial rashes. These health effects can be prevented using proper safe handling practices. Health care workers, exposed in preparing and handling neoplastic drugs have reported headache, alopecia, rashes, dizziness, facial flushing, abdominal pain, nausea, vomiting, malaise, nasal irritation and sores, neurologic complaints, and skin changes (4). Biologic monitoring of these employees has demonstrated an increase in mutagenic activity in the urine that abates with proper venting and protective equipment (4).

Guidelines for handling and storing antineoplastics have been developed including the use of vertical laminar flow hoods for mixing antineoplastic drugs. A summary of antineoplastic drug precautions for health care workers includes the following (4):

Protective clothing and disposable gloves must be used during preparation and administration of drugs.
Drugs must be prepared in a vertical laminar flow hood.
Proper antiseptic and personal hygiene techniques must be used by employees who handle these drugs.
Waste products must be properly labeled as a hazardous material and disposed of as such.
Biologic fluids of patients who receive these drugs must be handled and disposed of as potentially hazardous.
Health care workers and pharmacists must be properly trained in handling and preparing antineoplastic drugs.
Written instructions discussing proper use of these drugs and precautions must be available to all potentially exposed personnel.
Spills must be properly contained and cleaned up with appropriate protective equipment used.

STORAGE AND TRANSPORTATION OF WASTE

Other risk management issues involve the handling, storage, and transportation of medical wastes. Medical waste is collected in either red bags or plastic sharps containers (Figure 51.4). These smaller plastic collection containers are placed in large, 40-gallon plastic drums for transport and disposal, usually by incineration. These red 40-gallon drums are clearly marked with a biohazard symbol (Figure 51.5). The transporting truck may not always be marked with any symbol or placard to indicate its contents. An accident involving such a transport truck could result in spills of medical wastes that would be a health hazard to responding fire and paramedical personnel. The transport vehicle is large enough to carry multiple drums stacked on top of each other.

FEDERAL REGULATION OF MEDICAL WASTES

The EPA is charged with implementing the federal solid and hazardous waste management program under the Resource Conservation and Recovery Act of 1976 (RCRA; (5). RCRA amended the 1965 Solid Waste Disposal Act. Under RCRA, the EPA was mandated by the U.S. Congress to develop criteria for identifying and listing ''hazardous waste.'' EPA regulations encompass medical or infectious waste as a solid waste although the agency does not recognize the potential health risks of these wastes. Years after the passage of RCRA, the federal government is now reevaluating its position on medical waste.

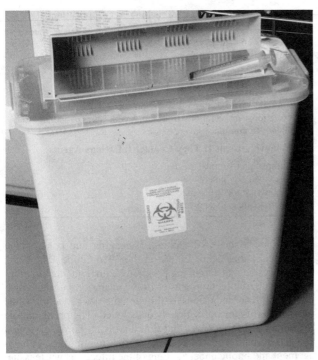

Figure 51.4.   Sharps container.

In December 1978, the EPA proposed regulations that would have placed infectious medical wastes under the category of hazardous waste and therefore under regulatory control by the

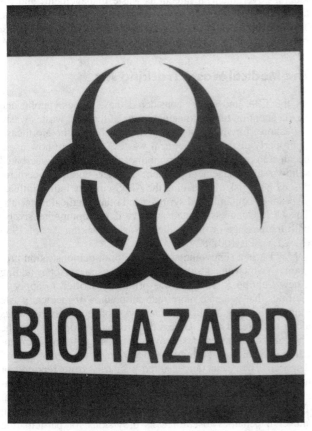

Figure 51.5.   Biohazard symbol.

Resource Conservation and Recovery Act (RCRA). Following public comment, medical waste was not included in the 1980 RCRA regulations. In 1982 and 1986, the EPA published guidelines concerning medical waste handling and disposal. EPA has been in the process of gathering data with regard to medical waste incineration in general. This data gathering is expected to result in performance and operating standards for incineration of medical wastes. Also, OSHA has issued an advanced notice of proposed rulemaking to solicit comment on worker protection requirements for the prevention of infectious disease.

The CDC also have issued guidelines on medical waste handling. The EPA and CDC definitions of hazardous infectious waste differ in that the EPA considers communicable disease isolation wastes as hazardous. The CDC recommend that such waste be managed according to individual hospital policy.

Categorizing Infectious Wastes

In RCRA Section 1004, the Congress defined hazardous wastes as a "solid waste or combination of solid wastes, which because of its quantity, concentration, or physical, chemical, or infectious characteristics may (a) cause or significantly contribute to an increase in mortality or an increase in serious irreversible, or incapacitating reversible, illness; or (b) pose a substantial present or potential hazard to human health or the environment when improperly treated, stored, transported, or disposed of, or otherwise managed" (5). Solid wastes may be solid, semisolid, liquid, or contained gaseous material which is discarded or has fulfilled its intended use, with some exceptions noted in the law (6).

In response to their congressional mandate to identify and list hazardous wastes, the EPA proposed regulations in December 1978 which would have placed certain "infectious" wastes under the hazardous waste provisions of RCRA, Subtitle C. *The Federal Register* (10, p. 20141) described these as "infectious waste[s] generated by certain departments in health care facilities and veterinary hospitals, by laboratories handling etiologic agents, and by sewage treatment facilities, unless these wastes were sterilized or incinerated in accordance with specified methods." The EPA's proposal was based on the rationale that improper management of these infectious wastes could result in a substantial risk to human health and environment. Such a risk was considered at variance with the objectives of RCRA.

Nevertheless, the EPA received about 60 comments on the 1978 proposal expressing concerns about the listing of these infectious wastes. Reportedly, there was insufficient information to establish that exposure to infectious wastes causes harm to human health (7, 9). On the basis of these comments, the EPA postponed its rulemaking on infectious wastes and deleted the proposal in the final rules issued on May 19, 1980. The EPA decided instead to collect technical information and evaluate problems related to infectious waste management. In 1982 and 1986, the EPA published draft and final guidelines, respectively, concerning proper infectious waste handling and disposal rather than develop enforceable standards. In 1987, the EPA met with health care experts to further consider problems associated with infectious waste management.

Guidelines for Infectious Waste Management

The 1986 Guide for Infections Waste Management (Guide) provides recommendations aimed at reducing risks from managing these wastes. The Guide addresses problems associated directly with their infectious characteristics and identifies the six broad categories of infectious wastes discussed earlier in this chapter. The Guide cautioned that other characteristics that may render certain infectious wastes "hazardous" may also subject them to RCRA Subtitle C regulations.

The recommendations contained in this document generally follow accepted practices for safe waste management. The EPA suggested that generators develop a comprehensive system to handle wastes. To reduce health risks, these wastes should be segregated during handling and treatment and packaged in containers appropriate for and compatible with the waste type. Additional packaging or rigid containment may be necessary to reduce risks during storage and transport, and care should be taken to prevent its impairment. Storage areas should be specially designated, and access should be restricted. Wastes should be treated prior to disposal to alleviate their infectious characteristics. Treatment may involve steam sterilization, chemical disinfection, and incineration. Compaction of the wastes should be avoided prior to treatment to ensure the integrity of the packaging; further, the agency noted that compaction may inhibit effective treatment. Although the EPA appeared to favor incineration, it did not preclude the use of other current or future treatment alternatives. Disposal alternatives correspond to the treatment method selected by the generator and include discharge of treated liquids or ground-up solids to sewage systems, and land disposal of treated solids and incinerator ash.

The EPA did not intend for the Guide to hinder states from passing laws and developing regulations to manage infectious wastes (10). Since the enactment of RCRA, many states passed hazardous waste legislation that includes controls for infectious wastes. The EPA noted, however, that most requirements were general, involving facility licensing and treatment or disposal methods. Specific standards for risk management were not typically identified as of the 1986 document. The EPA invited states to use the Guide as a reference source to assist development of their regulatory programs.

The CDC has issued guidelines on medical waste handling. The EPA and CDC definitions of infectious waste differ. The EPA Guide identifies communicable disease isolation wastes as one of the six categories recommended for across-the-board controls. The CDC recommends that such waste be managed according to individual hospital policy. In addition, the CDC does not recognize the optional infectious wastes identified by the Guide, including dialysis unit wastes and miscellaneous laboratory wastes. The difference reflects the persistent difficulty that EPA and other entities have experienced when trying to quantify the potential for an infectious waste to transmit disease (8).

On November 12, 1987, the EPA met with health care experts to evaluate whether the agency should develop regulatory measures to handle infectious wastes (8). The panel agreed that contaminated needles, laboratory wastes, and bulk blood had the greatest potential for transmission of disease, although laboratory wastes and blood may be treated on-site to minimize risks. The potential for exposures of all types increased in occupational settings. Public exposures were expected primarily from improper disposal practices. Given this belief, employers should institute a suitable waste management program and properly train health care workers and infectious waste handlers. The EPA should consider working with OSHA to develop standards for these workers. Small quantity generators of infectious wastes should be evaluated in addition to tradi-

Table 51.3. Medical Waste Tracking Act Application

1. Cultures and stocks of infectious agents, vaccines
2. Human tissues and organs
3. Blood and blood products
4. Needles, sharps, syringes, glass, blades
5. Wastes that contact blood of dialysis patients
6. Biologic waste or discarded equipment that contacts blood or excretions, or secretions from humans or animals isolated secondary to communicable disease

The Following Items If They Contact Infectious Agents

7. Autopsy and surgical waste
8. Discarded equipment
9. Laboratory waste
10. Animal carcasses and bedding

tional sources such as hospitals. Packaging and containment recommendations echoed those in the 1986 Guide. The panel also suggested that a tracking program be implemented to monitor the path of infectious wastes from generation through transport, treatment, and disposal, although the risk reduction value of such a program was seriously questioned. The principal role recommended for EPA at that time involved the development and dissemination of educational materials to improve risk management and public understanding of the infectious waste issue.

In June 1988, the EPA provided information on available literature, including the Guide and a hospital combustion study (10). The *Federal Register* entry also contained a request for comment on the adequacy of the EPA's current definition of infectious wastes, potential risks from exposure, the role of the federal government in infectious waste management, and the appropriateness of exemptions for small quantity generators. The infectious waste tracking system was noted as a means to reduce the potential of improper disposal of these wastes.

The Medical Waste Tracking Act

As the EPA and others considered these issues, public and media attention turned to news stories of medical wastes washing ashore, forcing closure of some beaches in the Northeast. Improperly disposed "chemical wastes," the term now used, became an effective visual symbol of the nation's exacerbated solid waste management problem. Further, public concern focused on the risk of spreading the AIDS virus by indiscriminate disposal of contaminated syringes and other medical materials. The U.S. Congress reacted swiftly, if not comprehensively, with the passage of the Medical Waste Tracking Act of 1988 (MWTA), PL 100-582 (11).

MWTA is a semivoluntary, 2-year pilot demonstration program (6) which amends the Solid Waste Disposal Act by adding a new Subtitle J. The Act was originally written to apply to facilities that generate more than 50 pounds of medical waste monthly in New York, New Jersey, Connecticut, and states along the Great Lakes. Unless they formally "opt out" of the program, these states must provide written, uniform documentation in a chain-of-custody manner to track waste storage and disposal. Their selection resulted primarily from reported or high potential for disposal problems. Other states may be included in the program on petition of the governor of the state. This act provides compliance orders and substantial criminal and civil penalties to enforce its provisions for participating states (Table 51.3).

MWTA, Section 3, defines medical waste as "solid wastes generated in the diagnosis, treatment, or immunization of human beings or animals, in research pertaining thereto, or in the production or testing of biologicals" (11). Like previous EPA guidance, the act does not include hazardous wastes identified or listed under Subtitle C. The act also excludes household wastes, typically commercially available products, as defined under Subtitle C (12). Ten types of medical wastes covered under the program are listed in Table 51.3. Medical wastes are estimated to comprise 2–3% of the nation's total solid waste stream (7).

EPA regulations implementing MWTA are published in the *Federal Registers* of March 24, June 2, and August 24, 1989 (10, 13, 14). While the March 24th entry describes the demonstration program, the latter entries note changes in states covered by MWTA. Each of the Great Lakes states formally opted out of the program. The governor of Louisiana and the mayor of Washington, DC, petitioned for inclusion, but later requested deletion. The state of Louisiana had prepared its own regulations; the mayor reevaluated the ability of the capitol city to implement the program before the second year of demonstration. Authorities in Rhode Island and Puerto Rico petitioned for and were granted inclusion in the program.

At the conclusion of the demonstration program in 1990, Section 11008 of MWTA requires the EPA to make a final report to Congress on a range of topics including: types and sizes of generators, potential risks, costs associated with proper and improper waste management, changes in practices attributable to the program, effectiveness of treatment methods, existing controls and the potential for waste reduction, and the appropriateness of penalties for noncompliance.

The MWTA represents a first federal legislative effort to control infectious/medical wastes. Health care experts, legislators, and regulators are likely to agree that a serious waste management problem is necessary on some level. Speakers at a hearing before the U.S. House of Representatives on July 25, 1989, testified of the need for a national, longterm solution to the problem of medical wastes. The usefulness of the demonstration program was severely questioned (7). Some speakers called for federal regulations, while others recommended a federal requirement for states to adopt permitting programs based on a federal model. It was reported that 22 states were already upgrading or enacting new programs to control medical wastes.

OSHA has also become interested in the opportunity to reduce risks from occupational exposure to medical wastes. This agency has issued an advanced notice of proposed rulemaking to solicit comment on worker protection requirements for the prevention of infectious disease.

The U.S. General Accounting Office (GAO) is preparing a report discussing findings of a medical waste study conducted in a number of states (7). The GAO report is expected to confirm that states are taking a stronger role in medical/infectious waste management. Extensive problems were observed at federal facilities during the study. The study also found that hospital incinerators, often outdated and inefficient, may be unable to comply when EPA's regulations for these treatment/disposal units become effective. GAO is expected to call for more studies on the health effects of handling, and incinerating medical wastes will be emphasized. The GAO's effort did not report on the extent of the public health problem posed by infectious wastes.

In May 1990, the EPA released its first interim report to Congress, "Medical Waste Management in the United States" (15). The report was generated as part of the requirements of MWTA. EPA estimates that ½ million tons of "regulated medical wastes" are generated by 375,000 facilities. Most of these wastes (77%) are generated by hospitals. The EPA also characterized the wastes by types and described the range of management practices observed. The EPA could not readily define the impact of medical waste handling and disposal on public health and the environment. Instead, the EPA proposed a detailed assessment coordinated with the Agency for Toxic Substances and Disease Registry. Such a study would be required, according to the EPA, prior to identifying the scope of a nationwide regulatory program to track medical waste generation and disposal. Nevertheless, the scope of nationwide regulations is likely to include certain uniform labeling requirements, according to the report.

Finally, entities seeking to control medical wastes will eventually face the clouded line between RCRA-regulated hazardous wastes, MWTA medical wastes, and other environmental regulations. First, health care facilities have traditionally generated small quantities of hazardous wastes (between 100 and 1000 kg/month (5). Hazardous wastes generated include waste solvents like xylenes and acetones, and metal-containing wastes like mercury and silver solutions. Waste streams listed in RCRA regulations or which exhibit one of four hazardous waste characteristics must be stored, treated, disposed, or recycled in accordance with RCRA standards regardless of their medical waste status (6).

MEDICAL WASTE DISPOSAL

Medical waste is disposed of by landfilling or by incineration. Incineration is the current method of disposal. However, incinerators with inadequate controls may produce emissions subject to air quality control laws (16). Generators may also be constrained in their treatment, storage, or disposal methods as a result of EPA's plans to increase controls over disposal of treated medical wastes in sanitary landfills (17). Costs of waste management are expected to increase with decreasing landfill capacity, and generators may find the need to develop waste reduction programs patterned after RCRA models (18).

Medical waste generators must know enough about their waste streams to segregate solid, medical, toxic, and hazardous components and handle them in accordance with all of the rules that may apply. Although rules controlling medical wastes may be fragmented and weak at the present time, public and legislative interest in the future of medical waste management is likely to ensure that increased federal controls will be instituted in the next decade.

Medical Waste Incineration

Special concerns regarding medical waste incineration revolve around the nature of the plastics, the amount of paper products, moisture content, and metal content. While some facilities segregate radioactive waste from standard medical waste, some facilities may not. Since incineration reduces waste volume approximately 90%, predicting and eventually documenting emissions from incineration sites is a major feature of human risk assessment. Incineration also produces ash as a byproduct. For 1000 pounds of medical waste incinerated, 200 pounds of ash would be produced (19).

Previous characterization of hospital medical waste from

California in 1987 revealed the following approximate composition (20).

Product	% by Weight
Paper	65
Plastics	30
Moisture	10
Other	5

The plastic content of medical waste is an important variable relating to the chlorinated chemical emissions from incineration processes. Previous estimates of the plastic content of medical wastes have only been as high as 30% (21). The plastic composition of medical waste has definitely increased and now is a major component of waste.

Plastics most commonly found in medical waste include the following:

polyethylene
polystyrene
latex
polyurethane
polypropylene
polyvinylchloride

These plastics contain varying amounts of nitrogen, sulfur, and chlorine in addition to carbon, hydrogen, and oxygen.

Analysis of Common Medical Waste Plastics (Wt %)

	Polyethylene	Polyvinylchloride	Polyurethane
Nitrogen	0.06	0.08	5.98
Sulfur	0.03	0.14	0.02
Chlorine	Trace	45.32	2.42

Other special concerns of medical wastes which must be addressed are radioactive wastes not segregated from bulk medical wastes, the presence of cytotoxic drugs, mercury from dental offices, and other heavy metals as well as the butadiene-styrene content of rubber and latex products. These special concerns are not currently regulated by RCRA and could conceivably be present in incinerator emissions as well as providing an extra risk factor for transport and handling of wastes.

TOXIC BYPRODUCTS OF MEDICAL WASTE INCINERATION

Typical pollutants produced by hospital waste incineration can be characterized according to the size, efficiency, and temperature of the incinerator. Data available for large air-controlled incinerators in the United States and Canada reveal the following emission contaminants: (Table 51.4)

trace metals
polycyclic organics
low molecular weight organics
acidic gases
particulates
carbon monoxide
pathogens

Byproducts of incineration are related to the efficiency of the combustion process as well as the chemical nature of the medical wastes being incinerated. Time, temperature, turbulence, and dwell time are critical variables for proper incineration. The EPA currently recommends a 2-second dwell time

Table 51.4 The Individual Contaminants That Can Be Expected To Be Present In Medical Waste Incineration Emissions

Trace Metals	Polycyclic Organics	
Arsenic	Dioxins	
Cadmium	Furans	
Chromium		
Iron		
Manganese		
Lead		
Nickel		
Mercury		
Zinc		
Vanadium		
Selenium		
Molybdenum		

Low Molecular Weight Organics		
Ethane	Trichlorotrifluoroethane	Propylene
Ethylene	Trichloroethylene	
Propane	Tetrachloroethylene	

Acidic Gases	Others
Sulfur dioxide	Particulates
Hydrochloric acid	Carbon monoxide
Nitrogen oxides	Pathogens
Hydrofluoric acid	Low level radioactive

for biomedical waste. Most available incinerator emission data come from larger hospital-controlled air incinerators. Most hospital incinerators have a 1-second dwell time and cannot meet the requirement. Incineration temperatures must be between 1000–1200°C (1800–2400°F) to destroy dioxins, furans, and antineoplastic agents.

INCINERATION BYPRODUCT FORMATION AND SOURCES

Acid Gases

These consist mainly of hydrochloric acid, sulfur dioxide, and nitrogen dioxides. Chlorine is present in plastics found in syringes and other disposable products commonly used in medical environments. Reacting with hydrogen during the combustion process, hydrochloric acid will be formed. Hydrogen sources in medical waste include paper, plastics, rubber and latex products, as well as any biologic fluids and moisture. The high hydrogen content of medical wastes, along with the ready availability of chlorine from plastics, will make the generation of hydrochloric acid from incineration processes the predominant acid gas. Studies have reported that up to 65% of chlorine in medical waste will be converted to HCl during combustion.

Sulfur present in medical waste will be oxidized to SO_2 during incineration. The rate of production is proportional to the sulfur content. Due to the presence of high HCl content in emissions and the fact that HCl is a stronger acid, most alkaline compounds will bind first with HCl, thus allowing for SO_2 to remain as an emission contaminant.

Nitrogen oxides formed during incineration of medical waste predominantly consist of NO. Oxidation of NO to NO_2 is limited in the combustion process. Most of the nitrogen oxides are formed in the combustion air via reaction of molecular nitrogen with oxygen.

Trace Metals

Trace metal emission quantity is directly proportional to the amount of metal introduced into the incineration process. Sources include needles, surgical instruments, and other sharp objects. Plastics made of polyvinyl chloride contain cadmium. Inks on paper and wrappers contain lead, chromium, and cadmium. Metals may be deposited on particulates emitted from the incineration process. This is termed "fine particle enrichment." Metals have been found predominantly in the respirable particulate fraction of incineration processes. Less particulate enrichment occurs at higher incineration temperatures. Other metals found in emissions are arsenic, manganese, nickel, mercury, antimony, selenium, tin, zinc, molybdenum, and vanadium. Controlling temperature and particulate size will reduce metal enrichment of particulates that can be inhaled.

Particulates

Produced by the incomplete combustion of wastes and entrapment of noncombustible items in emission gases. Sources of particulates include inorganic compounds, ash, and organometallics. Particulate emissions are largely inorganic compounds and are inorganic salts of metals and oxides. Up to 50% of these compounds are soluble in water. Water-soluble particulates are mainly sulfate salts of sodium, phosphorus, calcium, zinc, and ammonium. Insoluble particulates consist mainly of oxides, silica, and phosphate salts of aluminum, silica, calcium, lead, zinc, and iron. The fuel used in the incineration process itself can contribute to the particulate matter emitted. Large organic molecules can be formed in pyrolysis that contain an inorganic nucleus. As the residence time in the incineration process increases along with the temperature, particulate size decreases along with the volume of particulates emitted.

Organics

Sources include the medical waste as well as the incinerator fuel used in the pyrolysis process. Waste emits both water and organics as it is being heated during combustion. Volatile organic compounds escaping from the waste mass will be pyrolyzed above the mass in the process. An efficient thermal process will result in a high degree of CO_2 and water from the combustion of medical waste organics.

Dioxins and Furans

Data indicate that the formation of polychlorodibenzodioxins and polychlorodibenzofurans is related to the efficiency of the combustion process as well as to the chlorine content of plastics being incinerated. Increased temperature and increased efficiency reduce the production of these compounds. The source of these polychlorinated organic compounds is largely the plastics found in medical wastes. Since the predominant content of medical waste appears to be plastics, these contaminants become a major byproduct of incineration and must be specifically addressed in risk management. A low chlorine content in medical plastics will help significantly reduce the dioxin and furan content of incinerator emissions. If the health facilities were to use plastics composed of polyethylene and polystyrene in place of polyvinyl chloride, the dioxin and furan pyrolysis byproducts would be greatly reduced.

Dioxin and furan emissions can thus be controlled and reduced by creating optimal incineration conditions, controlling the oxidizing environment of incineration, and controlling the chlorine content of plastics incinerated.

Other Organics

Intermediate Organic Compounds: Products formed in the combustion of medical wastes include chlorobenzenes and chlorophenols. These byproducts are most likely intermediates in the production of polychlorinated biphenyls.

Low Molecular Weight Organics: Products of an incomplete combustion. Emissions of these compounds can be controlled by time, temperature, and turbulence factors in the incineration process.

Carbon Monoxide

A product of incomplete combustion, carbon monoxide emissions are regulated by both state and federal standards.

Radioactives

Medical waste may contain some low level radioactive contamination. Not all facilities in the survey segregate radioactive waste from other medical waste. This issue can best be addressed and risk minimized by requiring separation of radioactive waste from other waste at the site of origin.

SUMMARY AND CONCLUSION

The future of medical waste management is more federal regulation. The final establishment of federal guidelines will have economic impact on generators of such waste. Health care facilities must comply with the EPA's RCRA regulations regarding medical waste. Also, hospitals must comply with the standards set by accrediting bodies regarding biohazards, infection control, and infectious waste management. Ambulatory health care facilities and smaller generators must also comply with RCRA regulations; however, it is only recently that ambulatory care facilities have begun being accredited by recognized accrediting agencies. This accreditation procedure will force these health care facilities to adopt proper policies and procedures regarding medical waste from generation to disposal. Included in these standards are protection of personnel, visitors, and patients, establishment of policy and procedures for waste management, personnel training, and review and evaluation of policy. Accreditation standards for hospitals and ambulatory care facilities force them to be in compliance with applicable laws and regulations.

The nature and volume of medical waste is directly influenced by the types of plastics used, the nature of infectious diseases, and the use of disposable products. Public concern with medical waste revolves around disease transmission, disposal practices, and toxic byproducts of incineration. Federal guidelines will influence costs related to management and disposal of these wastes. Given the current volume of medical waste generated and the public's response to AIDS and other infectious disease transmission, it is anticipated that the volume of disposable products will continue to rise. Steps that may reduce the volume of medical waste as well as control incineration products include the use of plastics that contain no chlorine, using biodegradable plastics, increase the use of recyclable products, and segregate noninfectious waste from potentially infectious waste at the points of origin. Another reduction feature might be accomplished by the transfer of more health care from the hospital inpatient environment to the ambulatory environment that can operate more efficiently and with greater cost-effectiveness.

REFERENCES

1. Fleming D. Hazard control for infectious agents. Occup Med: State Art Rev 1987;2:499–511.
2. Coucil on Scientific Affairs. Infectious medical wastes. JAMA 1989;262:1669–1671.
3. Rutala W. Management of infectious waste by U. S. hospitals. JAMA 1989;262:1635–1640.
4. Rogers B. Health hazards to personnel handling antineoplastic agents. Occup Med: State Art Rev 1987;2:513–524.
5. U. S. Congress. Resource Conservation and Recovery Act of 1976, PL 94-580, 1976.
6. Code of Federal Regulations. Title 40, Parts 261 through 265. Washington, DC:GPO.
7. Bureau of National Affairs, Inc. Call for long-term national solution to medical waste made at house hearing. Environ Rep: Cur Dev 1989;20(13).
8. Slavik N. Report on the proceedings of the EPA infectious management meeting. Washington, DC: EPA Headquarters, 1987.
9. U. S. Environmental Protection Agency. Guide for infectious waste management. PB86-199130. Washington, DC: National Technical Information Service, 1986.
10. U. S. Environmental Protection Agency. Hazardous waste management system; identification and listing of hazardous waste; infectious waste management. Fed Reg 1988;53(106).
11. U. S. Congress. Medical Waste Tracking Act of 1988, PL 100-582, 1988.
12. Raupp J. Health care institutions. The Resource Conservation and Recovery Act (RCRA): the teenage years. Scottsdale, AZ: Arizona Bar Association, 1989.
13. U. S. Environmental Protection Agency. Standards for the tracking and management of medical waste. 54 Fed Reg (12326) 1989.
14. U. S. Environmental Protection Agency. Standards for the tracking and management of medical waste. 54 Fed Reg (35189) 1989.
15. U. S. Environmental Protection Agency, Office of Solid Waste. Medical waste management in the United States. First Interim Report to Congress, May 1990.
16. McCoy and Associates, Inc. Municipal incinerator ash studied. Haz Waste Consult 1988;6(2).
17. Bureau of National Affairs, Inc. House staff member predicts little action on RCRA this session, no house bill this year. Environ Rep: Curr Dev 1989;20(5).
18. McCoy and Associates, Inc. Minimizing hazardous wastes from medical facilities. Haz Waste Consult 1987;5(2).
19. Brunner C, Brown C. Hospital waste disposal by incineration. JAPCA 1988;38:1297–1309.
20. Jenkins A. Evaluation test on a hospital refuse incinerator at St. Agnes Medical Center, Fresno, California. California Air Resource Board, Stationary Source Division, 1987.
21. Murnyak G, Gazenich D. Chlorine emissions from a medical waste incinerator. J Environ Health 1982.
22. Kaiser E, Carotti A. Municipal incineration of refuse with two percent and four percent additions of four plastics: polyethylene, polyurethane, polystyrene, and polyvinyl chloride. Proceedings of the 1972 National Incinerator Conference, June 1972, 230–245. California Air Resources Board. Air Pollution Control at Resource Recovery Facilities, May 24, 1984.

52

Hazards and Exposures in Dentistry

Jacqueline Messite, M.D.
Harriet S. Goldman, D.D.S., M.P.H.
Ana Taras, M.P.H.

INTRODUCTION

Dentists and dental health professionals comprise a sizeable group at risk for multiple occupational exposures. Approximately 320,000 dental professionals are employed in dental offices, laboratories, nursing homes, hospitals, outpatient care facilities, and an additional 71,000 are self-employed dentists (*Federal Register*, 1989). Well over 93% of dentists employ at least one auxiliary person, with about 33% employing four or more auxiliaries including hygienists, chairside assistants, laboratory technicians, secretarial, and clerical personnel (1).

While dental professionals are exposed to chemical, physical, and biologic agents, the degree of exposure commonly is within limits set by the Occupational Safety and Health Administration (OSHA) (2). However, unacceptable hazards and exposures—including excessive amounts of mercury and waste anesthetic gases in the environment—have been found in a number of dental offices and clinics. In addition, several offices and clinics have been cited by the Occupational Safety and Health Administration (OSHA) for not following proper infection control guidelines and for exposing office personnel to dangerous pathogens (3).

Dental practice is generally not considered to be a high risk occupation and the degree of exposure to chemical agents is not life-threatening. However, depending on the type of toxic agent and the degree of exposure, the potential for increased morbidity does exist. This chapter will review the major occupational exposures in the dental workplace and discuss recommended preventive measures.

CHEMICAL AGENTS

During the routine practice of dentistry, dentists and dental personnel are at risk for multiple exposures to chemical agents. Though considered benign at the levels of exposure experienced by most dental patients, prolonged or repeated exposure to many of these chemicals can result in adverse health effects to the dental staff. Acute exposures resulting from chemical releases in the workplace are also cause for concern. Well-documented are the effects of exposure to mercury, a key ingredient in dental amalgam. Dental personnel can inadvertently inhale waste anesthetic gases, the longterm exposure to which has been associated with a variety of deleterious health effects. Operations involving dental alloys containing metals such as nickel and beryllium may also expose dental staff to potential health risks. Finally, a number of adverse health consequences may result following exposure to certain disinfectants, sterilants, and photographic materials.

Fortunately, mitigating the inherent risks associated with the practice of dentistry can be accomplished by simply creating a healthy workplace environment and encouraging safe work habits. By keeping abreast of up-to-date chemical and health hazard information, the dental team can take steps to minimize their exposure during various procedures. To this end, there are a variety of resources to utilize. Among the most important sources of information are the material safety data sheets (MSDSs), which present summarized information about the health hazards of the chemical substances in the workplace. Provided by the manufacturer, the MSDS contains information about the product's hazard ingredients and physical/chemical characteristics. Fire and explosion hazard data, reactivity data, health hazard data, precautions for safe handling and use, and control measures are also included. Another important resource for dental staff is the product label. These references provide information on safe work practices, protective equipment, and procedures to follow in case of an emergency. State and local health departments and the National Institute for Occupational Safety and Health (NIOSH) also provide fact sheets about hazardous substances and the effects of exposures. The dental team should note that the 1988 OSHA hazard communication regulation requires employers to implement a written hazard communication program. This program mandates the labeling of hazardous materials as well as the updating of MSDSs.

In maintaining safe chemical exposure levels, dentists and dental personnel are bound by federal standards set by OSHA. Certain states, including New York and New Jersey, may set additional legal standards. NIOSH and the American Conference of Governmental Industrial Hygienists (ACGIH) also develop recommended standards. All legal and recommended standards, however, should be considered as guides. In order to avoid any possible health effects, dental personnel must always attempt to keep their exposure to potentially hazardous chemicals as low as possible. Table 52.1 is a quick reference chart of some of the most common and/or potentially dangerous chemical hazards in the dental workplace.

Waste Anesthetic Gases

The administration of inhalation anesthesia in dental operatories has resulted in considerable exposure of dental personnel to waste anesthetic agents. Although anesthetic gases have long been used in medicine and dentistry, deleterious effects on those occupationally exposed were not reported until the 1960s. Subsequently, effects of exposure to these gases have received a great deal of attention from scientific and medical communities. Reported effects in humans include decrements in motor, perceptual, and cognitive skills; liver disease; cancer; spontaneous abortion; and birth defects in offspring.

NIOSH estimates that more than 100,000 dentists and dental assistants in the United States are directly exposed to trace concentrations of inhalation anesthetics every year. These gases

Table 52.1. Most Common and/or Potentially Dangerous Chemical Hazards in the Dental Workplace

Name	Sources of Exposure	Health Effects	OSHA (PEL)[a] TWA	OSHA (PEL)[a] STEL	NIOSH (REL)[b]	ACGIH (TLV)[c] TWA	ACGIH (TLV)[c] STEL	Preventive Measures
Acetic Acid	Photographic solutions	Eye, nose, throat, and skin irritation; bronchitis; skin and eye burns	10 ppm 25 mg/m³	— —	— —	10 ppm 25 mg/m³	15 ppm 37 mg/m³	1. Use proper protective gloves and eyewear. 2. Allow adequate ventilation. 3. Wash any skin or eye contact immediately with running water for 5 to 10 minutes. Seek medical assistance. 4. In the event of a spill, keep neutralizing agents such as soda lime or commercial acid spill cleanup kit available. 5. Handle solutions carefully. Avoid splashing. Always add water to acid when mixing. 6. Properly label and store all acid-containing solutions. 7. Use forceps to handle any object being treated in acids.
Acetone	Solvents	Eye, nose, throat, mucous membrane and skin irritation; dermatitis	750 ppm 1800 mg/m³	1000 ppm 2400 mg/m³	— —	750 ppm 1780 mg/m³	1000 ppm 2380 mg/m³	Proper protective eyewear and gloves.
Asbestos	Lining material for casting binders in periodontal dressings	Pulmonary fibrosis; lung cancer; mesothelioma. Identified by NIOSH as a potential human carcinogen and by ACGIH as a confirmed human carcinogen.	200,000 fibers/m³ TWA*; Action level of 100,000 fibers/m³ TWA*		100,000 fibers/m³ TWA in a 400 liter sample	Amosite Chrysotile Crocidolite Other forms	0.5 fibers/cc* 2 fibers/cc* 0.2 fibers/cc* 2 fibers/cc*	Proper protective eyewear, gloves, and NIOSH-approved mask.

*Fibers >5 μm long

Note: The ADA's Council on Dental Therapeutics has eliminated asbestos from its program of accepted therapeutics.

Substance	Use	Health effects						Protective measures
Beryllium	Casting alloys	Dermatitis; eye irritation; pulmonary edema; pneumonitis; pulmonary granulomatosis (delayed onset). Identified by NIOSH as a potential human carcinogen and by ACGIH as a confirmed human carcinogen.	.002 ppm	.005 ppm (30 min) .025 ppm (C)	Do not exceed 0.5 µg Be/m³	.002 mg/m³	—	Proper protective eyewear, gloves, and NIOSH-approved mask. Use power suction methods to remove dust.
Calcium Carbonate	Polishing agents	Eye, nose, throat, and respiratory irritation	15 mg/m³ (total dust) 5 mg/m³ (respirable fraction)	—	—	10 mg/m³	—	Proper protective eyewear, gloves, and NIOSH-approved mask.
Chlorine	Disinfectants	Eye, nose, throat, mucous membrane, and skin irritation; bronchitis; dermatitis; dental erosion	0.5 ppm 1.5 mg/m³	1 ppm 3 mg/m³	0.5 ppm (C) 1.45 mg/m³ (C)	0.5 ppm 1.5 mg/m³	1 ppm 3 mg/m³	Proper protective eyewear and gloves.
Chromium (metal)	Casting alloys	Dermatitis; histologic fibrosis of the lung	1 mg/m³	—	—	0.5 mg/m³	—	Proper protective eyewear, gloves, and NIOSH-approved mask.
Cobalt (metal)	Casting alloys	Eye, nose, throat, and skin irritation; dermatitis; respiratory hypersensitivity	.05 mg/m³	—	—	0.05 mg/m³	—	Proper protective eyewear, gloves, and NIOSH-approved mask.
Ethylene oxide	Sterilizing agents	Skin, respiratory, and eye irritation; skin sensitization; peritoneal cancer; leukemia; adverse reproductive effects. Identified by NIOSH as a potential human carcinogen; by ACGIH as a suspected human carcinogen.	1 ppm 1.8 mg/m³ (5 ppm excursion limit)	5 ppm (10 min/day C) 9 mg/m³ (10 min/day C) <0.1 ppm (0.18 mg/m³) TWA	—	1 ppm 1.8 mg/m³	1 ppm 1.8 mg/m³	1. Direct exhaust from sterilizers to a safe outdoor location. 2. Purge sterilizers with a sufficient amount of air before opening. 3. Ensure use of interlocks to prevent opening of sterilizers while they are being operated. 4. Check equipment for leakage or malfunctioning parts.

continues

Table 52.1. *Continued*

Name	Sources of Exposure	Health Effects	OSHA (PEL)[a] TWA	OSHA (PEL)[a] STEL	NIOSH (REL)[b]	ACGIH (TLV)[c] TWA	ACGIH (TLV)[c] STEL	Preventive Measures
								5. Use protective gloves and forceps to remove items from sterilizers. 6. Store in adequately ventilated areas where sources of ignition are strictly controlled.
Glutaraldehyde	Sterilizing agents	Eye, nose, and throat irritation; dermatitis; contact with eye may cause severe burns	0.2 ppm (C) 0.8 mg/m³ (C)	— —	— —	0.2 ppm (C) 0.7 mg/m³ (C)	— —	Proper protective gloves.
Hydrogen fluoride	Etching agents for porcelain	Nose, throat, and respiratory irritation; bronchitis; burns	3 ppm	6 ppm	3 ppm 10 hr-TWA 2.5 mg/m³ 10 hr-TWA 6 ppm (C)	3 ppm (C) 2.6 mg/m³ (C)	— —	Proper protective eyewear and gloves.
Hydroquinone	Methacrylate and denture base resins; photographic solutions	Eye and skin irritation, conjunctivitis, and keratitis	2 mg/m³	—	0.44 ppm (C) 2 mg/m³ (C)	2 mg/m³	—	Proper protective eyewear and gloves.
Isopropyl alcohol	Solvents, wiping agents	Eye, nose, throat, and skin irritation; dermatitis	400 ppm 980 mg/m³	500 ppm 1225 mg/m³	— —	400 ppm 985 mg/m³	500 ppm 1230 mg/m³	Proper protective gloves.
Mercury	Amalgam	Loss of appetite, nausea, diarrhea, speech disorders, ulceration of mucosa, gingivitis, central nervous system disorders, nephritis, thrombocytopenia, aplastic anemia	.05 mg/m³	—	.05 mg/m³ TWA	.05 mg/m³	—	1. Adequate ventilation. 2. Office monitoring for mercury vapor at least once a year, more if contamination is suspected. 3. Personal monitoring. 4. Biologic evaluation of all dental personnel at least once a year. 5. Work area with continuous, seamless sheet flooring that extends up the

Material	Source/Use	Health Effects	Exposure Limits					Recommendations
								walls for one foot. Tiled or carpeted floors should be avoided. 6. Nonporous cabinet tops with protective edging or a border to confine spills to the area. 7. Proper amalgam handling, using a no-touch technique. 8. Proper mercury storage away from heat sources in unbreakable, tightly sealed well-labelled containers. 9. Cleaning-up spills immediately. DO NOT USE A VACUUM CLEANER. A wash bottle trap or a syringe can recover all visible droplets. Adhesive tape to clean up small spills can be used. Area should be decontaminated with sulfur-containing compounds. 10. Avoidance of skin contamination. 11. Use face mask to avoid breathing amalgam dust.
Methyl Alcohol	Denatured alcohol	Dermatitis, erythema, scaling, optic neuropathy, metabolic acidosis	200 ppm 260 mg/m³ SKIN	200 ppm 10-hr TWA 262 mg/m³ 10-hr TWA 800 ppm (C) 1048 mg/m³ (C)	250 ppm 310 mg/m³	200 ppm 262 ppm SKIN	250 mg/m³ 328 mg/m³	Proper protective eyewear and gloves.
Methyl Methacrylate	Denture base resins	Eye, mucous membrane, respiratory, and skin irritation; dermatitis	100 ppm 410 mg/m³	— —	100 ppm 410 mg/m³	100 ppm 410 mg/m³	— —	Proper protective eyewear and gloves.

continues

Table 52.1. *Continued*

Name	Sources of Exposure	Health Effects	OSHA (PEL)[a] TWA	OSHA (PEL)[a] STEL	NIOSH (REL)[b]	ACGIH (TLV)[c] TWA	ACGIH (TLV)[c] STEL	Preventive Measures
Nickel (metal)	Casting alloys	Eye, mucous membrane, and respiratory irritation; allergic responses; dermatitis. Identified by NIOSH as a potential human carcinogen.	1 mg/m³	—	—	1 mg/m³	—	Proper protective eyewear, gloves, and NIOSH-approved mask.
Nitric acid	Pickling solutions	Nasal and lung irritation, skin and eye burns from splashes; dental erosion	2 ppm 5 mg/m³	4 ppm 10 mg/m³	2 ppm 10-hr TWA 5 mg/m³ 10-hr TWA	2 ppm 5.2 mg/m³	4 ppm 10 mg/m³	1. Use proper protective gloves and eyewear. 2. Allow adequate ventilation. 3. Wash any skin or eye contact immediately with running water for 5 to 10 minutes. Seek medical assistance. 4. In the event of a spill, keep neutralizing agents such as soda lime or commercial acid spill cleanup kit available. 5. Handle solutions carefully. Avoid splashing. Always add water to acid when mixing. 6. Properly label and store all acid-containing solutions. 7. Use forceps to handle any object being treated in acids.
Nitrous oxide	Nitrous oxide	Decrements in motor, perceptual, and cognitive skills; liver disease; cancer; spontaneous	—	—	25 ppm TWA	50 ppm 90 mg/m³	— —	1. Use effective scavenging equipment and monitoring devices. 2. Regularly inspect anesthetic adminis-

Substance	Use	Potential Health Effects						Precautions
		abortion; and birth defects in offspring						...tration equipment for leaks. 3. Direct waste gas away from windows, ventilators, air conditioning inlets, or other areas that might allow gases back into the office. 5. Maintain adequate ventilation. 6. Minimize conversation with patients. 7. Check for snug fit of face mask. 8. Maintain and service equipment regularly.
Phenol	Disinfectants	Mouth, nose, throat, and skin irritation; liver and kidney damage; severe skin burns from contact	5 ppm 19 mg/m³ *SKIN*	— —	5.2 ppm 10-hr TWA 20 mg/m³ 10-hr TWA 15.6 ppm (C) 60 mg/m³ (C)	5 ppm 19 mg/m³ *SKIN*	— —	Proper protective gloves. If potential for high exposures present, wear NIOSH-approved mask.
Phosphoric acid	Etching agents, phosphate cements	Nose, throat, and lung irritation; bronchitis; dermatitis; skin and eye burns from splashing	1 mg/m³	3 mg/m³	—	1 mg/m³	3 mg/m³	1. Use proper protective gloves and eyewear. 2. Allow adequate ventilation. 3. Wash any skin or eye contact immediately with running water for 5 to 10 minutes. Seek medical assistance. 4. In the event of a spill, keep neutralizing agents such as soda lime or commercial acid spill cleanup kit available. 5. Handle solutions carefully. Avoid splashing. Always add water to acid when mixing. 6. Properly label and store all acid-containing solutions. 7. Use forceps to handle any object being treated in acids.

continues

Table 52.1. *Continued*

			Standards					Preventive Measures
			OSHA (PEL)[a]		NIOSH (REL)[b]	ACGIH (TLV)[c]		
Name	Sources of Exposure	Health Effects	TWA	STEL		TWA	STEL	
Picric acid	Pickling agents	Eye, nose, and throat irritation; dermatitis; yellow-stained hair and skin	0.1 mg/m³ *SKIN*	0.1 mg/m³	—	0.1 mg/m³ *SKIN*	0.3 mg/m³	1. Use proper protective gloves and eyewear. 2. Allow adequate ventilation. 3. Wash any skin or eye contact immediately with running water for 5 to 10 minutes. Seek medical assistance. 4. In the event of a spill, keep neutralizing agents such as soda lime or commercial acid spill cleanup kit available. 5. Handle solutions carefully. Avoid splashing. Always add water to acid when mixing. 6. Properly label and store all acid-containing solutions. 7. Use forceps to handle any object being treated in acids.

Silver (metal)	Amalgam and casting alloys	0.01 mg/m³	Eye, nose, throat, and skin irritation; dermatitis	—	—	0.1 mg/m³	Proper protective eyewear, gloves, and NIOSH-approved mask.
Sulfur dioxide	Tanks containing photographic mixers	2 ppm 5 mg/m³	Eye, nose, mucous membrane, and throat irritation; eye and skin burns	5 ppm 10 mg/m³	0.5 ppm 10-hr TWA 1.3 mg/m³ 10-hr TWA	2 ppm 5.2 mg/m³	5 ppm 13 mg/m³ Proper protective eyewear and gloves.

[a]From Air Contaminants—Permissible Exposure Limits (Title 29 Code of Federal Regulations Part 1910.1000) 1989.
[b]From NIOSH Recommendations for Occupational Safety and Health Standards, vol. 37, 1988.
[c]From Threshold Limit Values and Biological Exposure Indices for 1990–1991. American Conference of Governmental Hygienists.

Action Level—exposure concentration at which employers must initiate certain provisions of the recommended standard
ACGIH—American Conference of Governmental Industrial Hygienists
C—denotes ceiling limit
cc—cubic centimeters
mg/m³—milligrams per cubic meter
NIOSH—National Institute for Occupational Safety and Health
OSHA—Occupational Safety and Health Administration
PEL—permissible exposure limit
ppm—parts per million
REL—recommended exposure limit
SKIN—denotes skin designation
STEL—short-term exposure limit, calculated for a 15 minute period unless otherwise noted
TLV—threshold limit value
TWA—time-weighted average, calculated for an 8-hour work day unless otherwise noted
μg/m³—micrograms per cubic meter
μm—micrometer

include nitrous oxide, halothane, enflurane, and others. Studies (4) in dental operatories in the late 1970s indicated a mean concentration of 900 ppm of nitrous oxide in the breathing zone of the dentist, far in excess of the 50 ppm indicated by NIOSH as achievable during analgesic anesthesia. In 1986, Middendorf et al. found ambient concentrations of nitrous oxide ranging from 132–880 ppm in the breathing zone of surveyed dentists (5). Scavenging equipment was used in only 17 of the 27 dental operatories, and the major sources of exposure were identified as leaks around the mask and exhaled air from the patient's mouth. Nitrous oxide levels ranging from 3–239 ppm were found in 18 scavenged offices surveyed by Kugel et al. (6). The authors underscored the importance of using an *adequate* scavenging system that should be checked periodically.

Perceptual, cognitive, and motor skills were studied in 40 male medical and dental students exposed on two occasions of 4 hours each by inhalation to either air or 500 ppm nitrous oxide with 5 ppm halothane (7). Compared with responses after breathing air, responses after exposure to nitrous oxide and halothane showed statistically significant decrements in the performance of tasks in which attention was divided between auditory and visual signals, a visual tachistoscopic test, and memory test involving digit span and recall of word pairs. After nitrous oxide alone, there was significant decrement in responses on digit test span only. Measurable decrements in performance of volunteers during testing at concentrations as low as 50 ppm nitrous oxide with 1 ppm halothane were noted in subsequent studies. Similar effects were not seen with 25 ppm nitrous oxide and 0.5 ppm halothane (8).

Both maternal and paternal exposure to waste anesthetic gases have resulted in statistically significant increases in spontaneous abortion. A large-scale epidemiologic survey (30,650 dentists and 30,547 chairside assistants) grouped subjects according to occupational exposure to inhalation anesthetics (9). The results showed a statistically significant 1.5-fold increase in the rate of spontaneous abortion among the wives of the exposed dentists. Exposed female assistants experienced a 1.7- to 2.3-fold increase in the rate of spontaneous abortions compared with the unexposed female dental assistants (9).

Exposure to waste anesthetic gases occurs primarily from leakage of gases from the anesthetic system, poor fit of the masks on patients, and improper work practices. In addition, cleansing (blowing out) the system after use can release considerable residual gas from the tubing into the environment, which contributes to staff exposure. In order to provide a safer workplace for those at risk for exposure to waste anesthetic gases, the following preventive measures should be implemented:

1. Use effective scavenging equipment and monitoring devices.
2. Regularly inspect anesthetic administration equipment for leaks.
3. Direct waste gas away from windows, ventilators, air conditioning inlets, or other areas that might allow gases back into the office.
4. Maintain adequate ventilation.
5. Minimize conversation with patients.
6. Check for snug fit of face mask.
7. Maintain and service equipment regularly.

Mineral Dusts (Airborne Particulates)

Clinical dental procedures such as high-speed grinding of silica-containing composite restoratives, the contouring of fused por-celain, and the polishing of metals and plastics with silica- or metallic oxide-containing materials are routine in the dental work environment. Though the effects of these agents are not well characterized, the compositional and physical properties of some of the commonly employed dust-producing minerals closely resemble the features of minerals such as asbestos and silica that have been identified as causative agents in dust diseases of the lungs (pneumoconioses).

Asbestos has been used chiefly as a binder in periodontal dressings and as a lining material for casting rings and crucibles. Airborne asbestos is known to cause pulmonary fibrosis (asbestosis), lung cancer, and mesothelioma of the pleura and peritoneum. Studies of airborne fibers of asbestos during preparation of gingivectomy packs have shown asbestos fibers in the atmosphere at inhalation levels of 3 feet (91 cm) above the height of the table (10). Concern for the potential danger to dental personnel from asbestos exposure has led the Council on Dental Therapeutics of the American Dental Association to eliminate this material from its program of *Accepted Dental Therapeutics*. Dentists should be aware of the occupational hazards surrounding asbestos and use packs that do not contain this material. Additionally, dentists should avoid sanding or drilling on countertops which may contain asbestos.

METALS

Beryllium

Exposure to beryllium, a highly toxic metal, can occur during the melting, grinding, buffing, and general lathing operations of beryllium-containing alloys in the preparation of prosthetic devices. Acute exposure to high concentrations of beryllium compounds can cause marked irritation of the eyes and respiratory tract, including the lung. Rom reported three cases of acute chemical pneumonitis in dental laboratory technicians analogous to acute berylliosis as described by Denardi in the 1940s (11). The technicians were overexposed from the grinding and melting of a nonprecious alloy containing 2% beryllium. All three presented with dyspnea and reticulonodular infiltrates in their chest radiographs. Biopsies in these cases showed acute pneumonitis in one, interstitial fibrosis in another, and granulomas in the third. In addition, Rom reported finding two of seven personal samples for beryllium analysis taken on dental laboratory workers in Utah as being in excess of the OSHA permissible exposure limit.

Chronic exposure to beryllium can produce delayed-onset pulmonary granulomatosis and damage the liver, kidney, and circulatory system. Skin exposure can cause dermatitis, and beryllium metal or compounds implanted in lacerations may result in skin ulcers or granulomas.

Proper protective gloves, eye protection and NIOSH-approved masks should be worn when casting, polishing, or grinding beryllium containing alloys. Power suction methods rather than air hoses are recommended to clean machinery and remove dust from clothing. Wastes and contaminated clothing should be disposed of properly.

Mercury

The dental profession uses more than 100 tons of mercury each year (approximately 2–3 pounds of mercury per dentist office) in dental restorations (12). Dental personnel are exposed to this metal through the contact or handling of mercury and mercury-containing compounds and/or inhalation of mercuric vapors and respirable dusts. The greatest single source of mercury vapor contamination is accidental spillage.

The literature on mercury contamination in the dental office is vast, and observations regarding safety range from reports of low risk to those of alarming danger. Several cases of mercury toxicity in dentists has been documented in the literature (13–16). Reported symptoms of chronic mercurialism include: loss of appetite, nausea, diarrhea, speech disorders, ulceration of oral mucosa, gingivitis, central nervous system disturbances, nephritis, possible thrombocytopenia, and aplastic anemia.

At least 10% of all dental offices in the United States may have ambient mercury vapor levels above the NIOSH recommended threshold limit value (TLV) of 0.05 mg/m³ (17). Dentists, with average mercury blood levels from 5–10 ng/ml, have higher blood mercury levels than those of the general population (18, 19). One comprehensive assessment of the magnitude of mercury exposure among dentists in the United States which measured urinary mercury concentrations in 4272 dentists found a mean urinary mercury concentration of 14.2 μg/l (range 0 to 556 μg/l) (12). Over 90% of the dentists surveyed had urinary concentrations between 0 and 35 μg/l and almost 5% had levels greater than 100 μg/l. Mean mercury concentrations in urine increased as the number of hours in practice each week increased, and those dentists who prepared their own silver amalgam mixture had a statistically significant higher mercury urine level than those who did not. Dentists using preportioned capsules had mean mercury levels that were significantly lower than those of dentists who used all other capsule types. In general, dental offices associated with higher exposure risk were related to increased urinary mercury levels.

In a study by Ship and Shapiro (20), body mercury concentrations of a group of 300 practicing dentists were measured for both longterm and shortterm accumulation. Those dentists with high mercury accumulation, evidenced by x-ray fluorescence of the head and wrist (over 40 μg/g), had neurologic and neuropsychologic problems as well as deterioration in their visual graphic performance (20). The authors concluded that ''the results of the study indicate that the current standards of mercury hygiene in dentistry are not consistent with safety in the dental office.''

In order to investigate whether infants of mothers occupationally exposed to low levels of elemental mercury had increased mercury level, Wannay and Skjaerasen studied a group of 19 female dentists, dental assistants, and dental technicians and compared them with a group of 26 nonexposed women (21). No measure of their workplace exposure was made, but it was inferred from other studies that the exposure was around the recommended threshold limit value of 0.05 mg/m³ or lower. Tissue analysis indicated that the mercury content of the placenta in the exposed group (24.5 ng/g) was twice that of the unexposed and that both the chorion and the amnion membrane showed corresponding differences between the exposed and the nonexposed group (21 and 11.5 ng/g for the chorion and 14.6 and 5.3 ng/g for the amnion membrane, respectively) (21). The placentas for both groups and the chorion in the exposed group contained more mercury than the corresponding erythrocytes and plasma; the amount of mercury in the blood of the mothers and infants in both groups at the time of delivery was similar (21).

The key to prevention of mercury contamination is in reducing the risk of mercury escaping into the environment. Precautions to take in working with mercury should include:

1. Adequate ventilation.

2. Office monitoring for mercury vapor at least once a year, more if contamination is suspected.
3. Personal monitoring.
4. Biologic evaluation of all dental personnel at least once a year.
5. Work area with continuous, seamless sheet flooring that extends up the walls for one foot. Tiled or carpeted floors should be avoided.
6. Nonporous cabinet tops with protective edging or a border to confine spills to the area.
7. Proper amalgam handling using a no-touch technique.
8. Proper mercury storage away from heat sources in unbreakable, tightly sealed, well-labeled containers.
9. Cleaning up spills immediately. DO NOT USE A VACUUM CLEANER. A wash bottle top or a syringe can recover all visible droplets. Adhesive tape to clean up small spills can be used. Area should be decontaminated with sulfur-containing compounds.
10. Avoidance of skin contamination.
11. Use of face mask to avoid breathing amalgam dust.

Nickel

The wider application of nickel-containing base metal alloys has sparked concern over the safety of this material in the dental environment. Nickel is used in the production of prosthetic devices, where nickel content of the base alloy can range up to 81%. Exposure to nickel has been associated with lung and nasal cancer in certain nondental industrial settings, and NIOSH has designated the metal as a potential carcinogen. Nickel is also a powerful allergen, since approximately 10% of women and almost 1% of men are sensitive to this agent (22).

Sources of exposure to dental personnel include the inhalation or ingestion of the dust produced during the grinding of this material or the vapor produced by overheating during the casting procedure. Acute exposure to the dust and fumes can result in irritation to the eyes, mucous membranes, and respiratory system. Proper protective gloves, protective eyewear, and NIOSH-approved masks should be worn when fabricating or grinding nickel-containing alloys. The use of high-velocity evacuation systems is recommended. Though exposure to nickel can be minimized by adequate controls, the risk of allergic response may remain (23).

DISINFECTANTS AND STERILANTS

Dental personnel use a variety of agents to sterilize and disinfect instruments and equipment in the workplace. If not used properly, these chemicals can produce toxic reactions. The following disinfectants and sterilants may be found in the dental workplace.

Chlorine Solutions

Diluted chlorine solutions such as sodium hypochlorite are used in the dental work environment to disinfect surface areas such as countertops, trays, and mirrors. Chlorine can be a severe irritant to the eyes, nose, throat, mucous membranes, and skin. Contact with eyes or skin may also cause severe burns. Chronic exposure to this chemical can lead to lung irritation, bronchitis, and dental erosion. Chlorine should only be used in well-ventilated areas, and proper protective gear should be worn.

Ethylene Oxide

Ethylene oxide (EtO), an alkylating agent, is used as a sterilant in dental offices. Exposure to dental personnel can occur when excessive quantities of EtO are released during routine use of sterilizers. NIOSH recommends that EtO in the workplace be regarded as a potential occupational carcinogen. This recommendation is based on results of animal studies demonstrating EtO to be associated with increased rates of leukemia, stomach and brain cancer. Evidence of mutagenicity in at least 13 biologic species, and epidemiologic investigations at work sites suggested an excess risk of cancer mortality among the EtO-exposed workers (2). In addition, EtO can cause skin, respiratory and eye irritation, skin-sensitization, cutaneous burns, nausea, vomiting, diarrhea, and nervous system effects. Ethylene oxide also is a potential hazard to both male and female reproduction (24). Dental staff performing sterilization operations with EtO should be informed of its potential toxicity, and exposure to this agent should be minimized. The following controls should be implemented when working with EtO (25):

1. Direct exhaust from sterilizers to a safe outdoor location.
2. Purge sterilizers with a sufficient amount of air before opening.
3. Ensure use of interlocks to prevent opening of sterilizers while they are being operated.
4. Check equipment for leakage or malfunctioning parts.
5. Use protective gloves and forceps to remove items from sterilizers.
6. Store in adequately ventilated areas where sources of ignition are strictly controlled.

It is important to emphasize that, when control is not assured, alternate means for sterilization should be considered.

Glutaraldehyde Solutions

Glutaraldehyde is used in solutions for sterilization of non-heat-resistant instruments and for disinfection of handpieces. This chemical can cause severe irritation to the eyes, nose, and throat at very low concentrations in the air. Contact with glutaraldehyde solutions can severely burn the eyes and may cause permanent damage. According to the *Right to Know Handbook for Dental Clinical Staff*, produced by the City of New York Mayor's Office of Operations, Citywide Office of Occupational Safety and Health, and District Council 37 Education Fund, a 5% glutaraldehyde solution, at first use, can cause dermatitis at much lower concentrations on repeated exposures. Glutaraldehyde should be used in well-ventilated areas, and heavy duty rubber gloves should be worn. Chemical residues of glutaraldehyde on instruments should be wiped clean with alcohol. OSHA has recently published a ceiling concentration of glutaraldehyde of 0.2 ppm (29 CFR 1910, January 9, 1989). Cold sterilization procedures use solutions of glutaraldehyde ranging from 0.13% up to 2%. A 2% glutaraldehyde solution left uncovered can generate airborne breathing zone concentrations in excess of this 0.2 ppm ceiling limit set by OSHA. Proper ventilation and use of butyl rubber gloves instead of latex gloves are necessary to protect workers.

Phenols and Phenolic Compounds

Phenols and phenolic compounds are toxic substances that should only be used in the dental work environment for emergencies.

Skin irritation can occur on contact with 0.5% phenol solution. Skin contact with stronger solutions of phenol or phenol compounds is not immediately painful, but deep damage and even local gangrene can result. Extensive skin absorption can affect both the central nervous system and the circulatory system, subsequently causing difficulty in breathing, ringing in the ears, tremors, and convulsions. Vapors can cause irritation of the nose and throat, nausea and vomiting. Repeated exposure may damage the liver and kidney. Strict precautions must be instituted if work with this substance is necessary. Adequate ventilation must be present and protection given to the skin, eyes, and face.

ORGANIC CHEMICALS

Methyl Methacrylate

Methyl methacrylate is used in the production of prosthetic devices. The monomer component of methyl methacrylate is an irritant to the eyes, mucous membranes, skin, and respiratory system. The material can be absorbed through the skin and produce neurologic effects such as finger and palmar paresthesia, pain, and whitening of fingers in cold (26). Contact with methyl methacrylate may cause dermatitis and eye irritation and inhalation of the vapor causes salivation and respiratory irritation. Exposure to high concentrations can cause unconsciousness and death, but the agent's powerful odor should alert most dental workers to its presence.

Pregnant rats exposed to methacrylate esters demonstrated embryo/fetal toxicity and teratogenic effects (27). Exposure of a human to methacrylate vapors has resulted in a prompt decrease in gastric motor activity that lasts for 20–30 minutes after cessation of exposure (28).

When using this material, dental personnel should wear safety glasses and gloves and work in a well-ventilated area or use a supplied air respirator to avoid breathing the vapor. Any spills should be cleaned up promptly, and any areas of skin contact washed thoroughly.

Alcohols

Most alcohols are of relatively low toxicity but can be hazardous without proper precautions. Solutions of isopropyl alcohol can cause skin irritation and dryness with direct contact. Vapors from this agent can also cause eye, nose, and throat irritation. At very high levels, isopropyl alcohol is considered a narcotic. Alcohols should be used only to remove chemical residues and not to disinfect or sterilize equipment or surfaces.

PHOTOGRAPHIC DEVELOPERS AND FIXERS

Dental personnel who come into contact with photographic developers and fixers can be exposed to a variety of chemicals. Staff who work with these agents should be aware of their potential hazards.

Hydroquinone, used in developers can severely irritate the skin and burn the eye. Repeated exposure can stain and discolor the mucous membranes covering the eyes, possibly leading to permanent damage. Limited evidence shows that chronic exposure to hydroquinone may lead to adverse reproductive effects (29).

Sulfur dioxide can build up in tanks containing photographic fixers. At low levels, vapors can cause eye, nose, and throat irritation. Exposure to high levels may result in dyspnea, coughing, and choking. Repeated exposure can lead to nosebleeds and irritation of the throat and lungs.

Control measures in working with photographic chemicals should include use of protective eyewear and heavy duty rubber gloves. Contact lenses should be avoided as they may absorb vapors. Adequate ventilation is imperative, and spilled chemicals should be cleaned up immediately. Exposure to dry powder during solution preparation should be minimized, and skin that comes in contact with these chemicals should be washed off immediately with a pH-balanced soap.

ACIDS

Acids are used in dentistry in pickling solutions and in acid etch solutions and gels. Skin contact with these corrosive chemicals can cause serious injury. Eye contact may lead to permanent eye damage and blindness. Inhalation of vapors can cause nose, throat, and lung irritation. Exposure to high concentrations of these substances may result in unconsciousness and even death. Phosphoric acid and sulfuric acids are commonly used in acid etch solutions. Hydrochloric acid, nitric acid, picric acid, and sulfuric acids are used in pickling solutions. Acetic acid is found in photographic solutions.

Dental personnel who work with acids should take the following precautions:

1. Use proper protective gloves and eyewear.
2. Allow adequate ventilation.
3. Wash any skin or eye contact immediately with running water for 5 to 10 minutes. Seek medical assistance.
4. In the event of a spill, keep neutralizing agents such as a soda lime or commercial acid spill cleanup kit available.
5. Handle solutions carefully. Avoid splashes. Always add water to acid when mixing.
6. Properly label and store all acid-containing solutions.
7. Use forceps to handle any object being treated in acids.

SOAPS AND DETERGENTS

On average, dental personnel wash their hands over 15 times a day (30). Such frequent contact with soaps and detergents is the most common cause of contact dermatitis among dental workers. The most likely reason for these dermatoses is destruction of the protective layers of the epidermis. Consequently, hand cleaners should be used that do not contain abrasives, defat the skin, cause allergic sensitization, and break down with storage.

PHYSICAL AGENTS

Ionizing Radiation

There is a considerable benefit from the judicious use of radiographic examinations in dental practice to evaluate such clinical situations as caries, peridontal disease, cysts and tumors of the jaws. However, dental personnel should be familiar with the adverse effects of such exposure and the measures needed to reduce the potential hazards for themselves as well as for their patients. Over the last few decades, with the development of more sensitive fast speed films, and better techniques, equipment, and monitoring devices, the exposure of dental personnel and patients has been reduced considerably. Such effects as

leukemia and shortened life span, etc., noted in the early dental literature no longer represent a significant risk for dental personnel. Nevertheless, there can be no apathy in the concern for unnecessary radiation exposure. Constant vigilance is required to assure that all measures are being taken to reduce the exposure to as low as possible. The Center for Devices and Radiologic Health of the United States Public Health Service has published guidelines on when, what type of radiographs, and at what intervals dental radiographs should be taken (31).

Nonionizing Radiation

Ultraviolet radiation exposure in dental practice may occur from such sources as devices for curing resins and sealants, plaque lights, and molten metal used in casting. Clinical effects of such exposure include eye irritation, redness of skin and/or mucous membranes, and malignant changes in cells.

Visible light exposure can occur in curing resins. Animal studies have noted retinal damage as a result of continuous eye exposure to such light.

For both ultraviolet and visible light, sources for such exposure should be properly maintained, located, and shielded so that eye exposure and skin contact are minimized. Protective glasses are available.

INFECTIOUS AGENTS

The dental office is a site for transmission of infectious diseases. These infectious diseases are transmitted by airborn organisms (as a result of high speed drilling) as well as bloodborne ones. Airborne illnesses consist of upper respiratory infections including tuberculosis and pneumonia. Bloodborne diseases include hepatitis B, herpes, and acquired immune deficiency syndrome (AIDS). Table 52.2 is a chart on the transmission of the most common infectious diseases in the dental office.

Herpes simplex infections are of great practical importance to dentists because lesions of the eyes and fingers will produce temporary inability to practice (32). Repeated recurrences of ocular herpes can lead to blindness and permanent inability to practice (33). The disease, which is caused by two viruses—type 1 and type 2—is spread predominantly by direct contact. The virus is found in gingival saliva and throat swabs. Clinically, the disease appears initially as vesicles which then break down to form ulcers. They heal without scarring in 14–21 days. The disease orally affects all mucous membranes and the lips (''cold sore'' or ''fever blister'') and recurs throughout a person's lifetime.

It is estimated that anywhere from 30–80% of adults in the general population have been exposed to the virus, depending on socioeconomic status (34). In the dental population, the prevalence of herpes virus increases with age, and therefore the young dentist, because he or she has probably had less exposure to the virus, is most susceptible to infection. Although eye and lip lesions occur more often in the general population, finger infection occur twice as frequently in practicing dentists (32).

Hepatitis B can be devastating to the dental professional. Transmission of the virus in dental personnel is primarily by direct contact through contaminated blood or saliva through a break in the skin of the hands or possibly through the mucous membranes of the eyes, mouth, or nose. The organism can survive for days on countertops, switches, and other environmental surfaces. The incubation period is long, usually between

Table 52.2. Serious Infectious Diseases Found in Dentistry

Disease	Agent	Route of Transmission	Incubation Period	Potential Complications
Acquired immune deficiency syndrome (AIDS)	Virus	Contact from blood, other body fluids	Lifetime(?)	Death
Chicken pox	Virus	Saliva, blood, droplets	10–21 days	Conjunctivitis, shingles Encephalitis
Common cold	Virus	Saliva, blood, droplets	48–72 hours	Temporary disability
Cytomegalovirus	Virus	Oral	2–8 weeks	Birth defects, death
Gonorrhea	Bacteria	Mucous membrane contact	1–7 days	Arthritis, female sterility, infant blindness
Hepatitis A	Virus	Oral, fecal	2–7 weeks	Disability
Hepatitis B	Virus	Saliva, blood, droplets	6 weeks–6 months	Chronic disability, carrier mode death
Hepatitis (non-A, non-B)	Virus	Saliva, blood, droplets	6 weeks–5 months	Chronic disability, death
Hepatitis delta	"Piggyback" virus	Blood, other routes under investigation	Not known	Death, chronic carrier
Hepetic conjunctivitis	Virus	Saliva, blood, droplets	6–10 weeks	Potential blindness
Herpes simplex II	Virus	Mucous membrane contact, possible saliva, blood	Up to 2 weeks Also latent	Painful lesions, disability, death in children
Herpetic whitlow	Virus	Saliva, blood, droplets	2–12 days Also latent	Extreme pain, disability
Infectious mononucleosis	Virus	Saliva, blood, droplets	4–7 weeks	Temporary disability
Influenza	Virus	Saliva, droplets	1–3 days	Death
Legionellosis	Bacteria	Respiratory	2–10 days	Death
Measles (German)	Virus	Saliva, nasal, droplets	9–11 days	Congenital defects, infant death
Measles (rubeola)	Virus	Saliva, nasal, droplets	9–11 days	Temporary disability, encephalitis
Mumps (men)	Virus	Respiratory	14–25 days	Temporary disability, sterility
Pneumonia	Bacteria, Virus	Respiratory, blood blood	Varies with organism	Death
Staphyloccus infections	Bacteria	Saliva, droplets, nosocomial	4–10 days	Skin lesions, osteomyelitis, death
Streptococcus infections	Bacteria	Saliva, blood, droplets	1–3 days	Rheumatic heart, kidney problems, death
Syphilis	Bacteria	Mucous membrane contact, congenital	2–12 weeks	Central nervous damage, death
Tetanus	Bacteria	Open wound	7–10 days	Disability, death
Tuberculosis	Bacteria	Saliva, droplets	Up to 6 months Also latent	Disability, death

Courtesy: Infection Control in the Former Wet Finger Environment. Runnells R. (I.C. Publications, No. Salt Lake, UT) 1984.

6 weeks and 6 months. Early symptoms include extreme fatigue, headaches, malaise, joint pain, fever, and finally jaundice. Work may be impossible for as long as 6 months (34). OSHA estimates that each year in the health care environment there are from 6000 to 7000 new hepatitis B infections. Between 1500 and 1900 persons develop acute symptoms, 300 to 400 persons are hospitalized, and between 130 and 165 persons die each year (35).

The dental profession has a risk of acquiring hepatitis B that is four times that of the general population (34). The prevalence among dentists is 28% with an illness rate of 6% (36, 37). It is estimated that there are about 3000 asymptomatic carriers among dentists. This is not surprising since an office seeing 20 patients/day will treat one active hepatitis carrier patient in seven working days (36, 37).

Acquired immunodeficiency syndrome (AIDS), a disease with a 100% mortality rate, is transmitted by a virus through direct contact with body fluids, specifically blood and semen. A devastating disease marked by a decrease in the immune response, AIDS leaves an individual susceptible to life-threatening opportunistic infections as well as to various cancers (38).

Over 100,000 deaths from AIDS have been reported to the Centers for Disease Control (CDC) from 1981 to 1990, and approximately one million individuals are estimated to be infected with the HIV virus (39, 40). As of December 1990, 40 documented cases of health care workers who seroconverted to HIV after being occupationally exposed have been reported to the CDC (41). Studies of more than 2300 dental workers, many of whom cared for AIDS or high risk patients, have shown only one dentist with no other risk factors who had antibodies to HIV (42).

Of further interest is a report from CDC that states that at least three patients have been infected in the course of treatment by an HIV-infected dentist (43). CDC investigation of the dental practice in which this occurred found serious deficiencies in infection control practices. There was no written policy or training course on infection control practices provided for staff by the dentist, and no office protocol existed for reporting injuries such as needlesticks. Barrier precautions were used, but the dental practice did not have written protocol or a consistent pattern for operatory cleanup and instrument reprocessing.

Tuberculosis is a leading cause of death related to infectious diseases worldwide (44, 45). Predominantly an airborne disease, the contaminated droplets are discharged into the air by

Figure 52.1

DENTAL WORKPLACE CHECKLIST
Some General Practice Guidelines

CHEMICAL AGENTS:

For each of the chemical processes or products used, the following should be considered:

1. Do you know the generic name and potential toxic effects of each ingredient?
2. Have you obtained material safety data sheets from the manufacturer?
3. Are all employees aware of proper handling practices, precautions, and cleanup instructions for spills?
4. Are all hazardous substances properly labeled and stored?
5. Is proper protective equipment available and used as indicated?
6. Are in-service training sessions carried out at least annually?
7. Are you and your employees aware of signs and symptoms of accidental exposures?
8. Are records kept of the dates, quantities, and names of all chemicals used?
9. Is the office adequately ventilated?
10. Is eating, drinking, and smoking prohibited in the work area?
11. Do you and your employees always try to use the least toxic substance for any operation or procedure?
12. Is an eye wash fountain present in case of emergencies?
13. Is hazardous waste disposed of properly?

PHYSICAL AGENTS

Ionizing radiation

1. Are you and your staff aware of the latest techniques and requirements for the safe use of radiation?
2. Does you equipment meet the state and federal requirements in regard to the x-ray beam diameter and filtration, and do you minimize the time and amperage needed to obtain satisfactory results?
3. Is your examination room set up to permit adequate distance (at least 6 feet or 2 meters) for x-ray operator to stand when the equipment is functioning?
4. Do you have an adequately screened and shielded area for your workload?
5. Do you use x-ray holders or other devices to hold film in place?
6. Do you provide patients with a lead apron?
7. Do you only use high speed film?
8. Do you have a quality control program for developing and fixing solutions to assure consistent film quality?
9. Do you have your office inspected periodically by qualified persons to ensure that all equipment and shielding are properly maintained?
10. Have you considered personnel dosimeter measurements for you and your staff to assure control?

Nonionizing radiation

1. Are the sources of this radiation properly maintained and serviced?
2. Are the operators properly shielded from the exposure?

INFECTIOUS DISEASES

Prevention of transmission include the following:

1. Are all employees as well as the dentist properly vaccinated?
2. Do you take a thorough medical history on all patients?
3. Are proper barrier techniques being utilized? These include gloves, masks, glasses, gowns, and protection of environmental surfaces.
4. Are sharps being disposed of properly?
5. Are proper sterilization and disinfection modalities being utilized?
6. Is infectious waste being disposed of properly?

a person with active disease. These droplets can remain suspended in the air for a period of time, ready to be inhaled by a susceptible individual, even after the infected person leaves the immediate area. It is caused by the *Mycobacterium tuberculosis* bacillus. If the initial lung lesions do not heal, active disease will occur later on. Symptoms include fatigue, cough, weight loss, fever, chills, night sweats, malaise, and loss of appetite (34). About 15 million persons have been infected, 90% of whom are asymptomatic and will not develop active tuberculosis (33). For many years, tuberculosis has been declining, but the disease is again on the increase among specific groups: immigrants from areas in the world where there is a high incidence of this disease and where many have received no or inadequate therapy, HIV-positive individuals, migrant farm workers, and Native Americans.

With all these infectious diseases, the possibility for trans-

mission in the dental profession is significant. Unfortunately, the actual number of cases is difficult to determine because specific morbidity is lacking (46). It should be stressed, however, that all dental personnel should be familiar with infectious control procedures specified by Centers for Disease Control and the American Dental Association, and that these procedures be rigorously enforced (47, 48).

DENTAL WORKPLACE CHECKLIST

The key to maintaining safety in the workplace is knowledge and prevention. If potential for exposure to harmful agents is minimized, then dental personnel will reduce their risk for adverse health effects. Appropriate infection control mechanisms must be in place to assure prevention of infectious diseases. Figure 52.1 consists of a checklist that can serve as general practice guidelines in surveying a dental workplace.

REFERENCES

1. American Dental Association, Bureau of Economic Research and Statistics. The 1977 Survey of Dental Practice. Chicago, IL: American Dental Association, 1978.

2. Messite J. Occupational safety and health in the dental workplace. In: Goldman HS, Messite J, eds. Occupational hazards in dentistry. Chicago: Year Book Medical Publishers, 1984.

3. Jakush J. OSHA pays dentists visit; dentists pay sometime later. American Dental Association News. April 17, 1989.

4. Whitcher CE, Zimmerman DC, Piziali RL. Control of occupational exposure to N$_2$O in the dental operatory. Publication 77-171. U.S. Department of Health, Education, and Welfare, National Institute on Occupational Safety and Health, 1977.

5. Middendorf PJ, Jacobs DE, Smith KA, Mastro DM. Occupational exposures to nitrous oxide in dental operatories. Anesth Prog 1986;33:91–97.

6. Kugel G, Norris L, Zive M. Nitrous oxide and occupational exposure: it's time to stop laughing. Anesth Prog 1989.

7. Bruce DL, Bach MJ, Arbit J. Trace anesthetic effects on perceptual, cognitive, and motor skills. Anesthesiology 1974;40:453–458.

8. Bruce DL, Bach MJ. Trace effects of anesthetics gases on behavioral performance of operating personnel. Publication 76-169. Cincinnati, OH: U.S. Department of Health and Human Services, Public Health Service, National Institute of Occupational Safety and Health, 1976.

9. Cohen EN, et al. Occupational disease in dentistry and chronic exposure to trace anesthetic gases. J Am Dent Assoc 1980;101:21–31.

10. Dyer MR. The possible adverse effects of asbestos in gingivectomy packs. Br Dent J 1967;122:507.

11. Rom W. Personal communication, Salt Lake City, Utah, 1983–1984.

12. Naleway C, et al. Urinary mercury levels in U.S. dentists, 1975–1983: review of health assessment program. J Am Dent Assoc 1985;111:37–42.

13. Cook TA, Yates PO. Fatal mercury intoxication in a dental surgery assistant. Br Dent J 1969;127:553.

14. Merfield DP, et al. Mercury intoxication in a dental surgery following unreported spillage. Br Dent J 1976;141:179–186.

15. Symmington IS, Cross JD, Dale IM. Mercury poisoning in dentists. J Soc Occup Med 1980;30:37–39.

16. Shapiro IM, et al. Neurophysiological and neuropsychological function in mercury exposed dentists. Lancet 1982;2:1147–1150.

17. Mantyla DG, et al. Mercury toxicity in the dental office: a neglected problem. J Am Dent Assoc 1976;92:1189.

18. Battistone GC, Hefferren JJ, Miller RA, Cutright DE. Mercury: its relation to the dentist's health and dental practice characteristics. J Am Dent Assoc 1976;92:1182–1188.

19. Goldman HS. Mercury: problems and control. In: Goldman HS, Hartman KS, Messite J, eds. Occupational hazards in dentistry. Chicago: Year Book Medical Publishers, 1984.

20. Shipp II, Shapiro IM. Mercury poisoning in dental practice. Compendium of Continuing Education on General Dentistry. 1983;4:107–110.

21. Wannay A, Skjaersen J. Mercury accumulation in placenta and foetal membranes: a study of dental workers and their babies. Environ Phys Biochem 1975;5:348–352.

22. National Institute of Dental Research. Workshop: biocompatibility of metals in dentistry. J Am Dent Assoc 1984;109:469–471.

23. Newman SM. The relationship of metals to the general health of the patient, the dentist and office staff. Int Dent J 1986;36:35–40.

24. Dixon RL. Toxic responses of the reproductive system. In: Klaassen CD, Amdur MO, Doull J, eds. Casarett and Doull's toxicology. New York: MacMillan Publishing Company, 1986.

25. Cooley RL. Physical, chemical and thermal injuries. In: Goldman HS, Hartman KS, Messite J, eds. Occupational hazards in dentistry. Chicago: Year Book Medical Publishers, 1984.

26. Rajaniemi R, Tola S. Subjective symptoms among dental technicians exposed to the monomer methyl methacrylate. Scand J Work Environ Health 1985;11:281–286.

27. Singh AR, Lawrence WH, Autian J. Embryonic-fetal toxicity and teratogenic effects of a group of methacrylate esters in rats. Appl Pharmacol 1972;22:314–315.

28. Tansy MF, Benhoyem S, Probst S. The effects of methyl methacrylate vapor on gastric motor function. J Am Dent Assoc 1974;89:372–376.

29. New Jersey State Department of Health. Hazardous substance fact sheet—hydroquinone. NJSDH, September 1985.

30. Caruso RJ. Dermatitis: a dentist's occupational hazard. NY State Dent J 1981;47:543–545.

31. US Department of Health and Human Services, Public Health Service, FDA. The selection of patients for x-ray examinations, dental radiographs examinations. HSS/PHS/FDA 1987;88-8273:10–21.

32. Rowe NH, Neine CS, Kowalski CJ. Herpetic whitlow: an occupational disease of practicing dentists. J Am Dent Assoc 1982;105:471–473.

33. Hartman KS. Infectious and communicable diseases. In: Goldman HS, Hartman KS, Messite J, eds. Occupational hazards in dentistry. Chicago: Year Book Medical Publishers, 1984.

34. Burket LW. Oral medicine, diagnosis and treatment. Philadelphia: JP Lippincott, 1984.

35. Proceedings of the National Symposium on Hepatitis B and the Dental Profession. J Am Dent Assoc 1985;110:613–650.

36. Siew C, et al. Screening dentists for HIV and hepatitis B. N Engl J Med 1988;318:1400–1401.

37. Siew C, et al. Survey of hepatitis B exposure and vaccination in volunteer dentists. J Am Dent Assoc 1987;114:457–459.

38. Robertson P, Greenspan D. Perspectives on oral manifestations of AIDS. Littleton, MA: PSG Publishing Co, 1988.

39. Centers for Disease Control. Mortality attributable to HIV Infection/AIDS—United States, 1981–1990. MMWR 1991;40:41–44.

40. Centers for Disease Control. HIV prevalence estimates and AIDS case projections for the United States: report based on a workshop. MMWR 1990;39:1–30.

41. Fallis C. Personal communication, Office of Public Affairs, Centers for Disease Control, March 1991.

42. Klein RS, et al. Low occupational risk of human immunodeficiency virus infection among dental professionals. N Engl J Med 1988;318:86–90.

43. Centers for Disease Control. Update: transmission of HIV infection during an invasive dental procedure—Florida. MMWR 1991;40:21–27.

44. Centers for Disease Control. Tuberculosis—United States, 1984. MMWR 1985;34:229.

45. Woodruff G. Tuberculosis and the dentist. Aust Dent 1957;2:7–12.

46. Zwemer J, Williams J. Dentists' health status and risks. J Am Coll Dent 1987;54:7–12.

47. Centers for Disease Control. Recommended infection control practices for dentistry. MMWR 1986;35:237–42.

48. American Dental Association. Infection control recommendations for the dental office and the dental laboratory. J Am Dent Assoc 1988;116:241–8.

Jacek Dutkiewicz, Ph.D.

DEFINITION AND CLASSIFICATION

Definition

Biohazards are micro- and macroorganisms or substances derived from these organisms which can exert deleterious effects on exposed individuals. This term and definition are mostly utilized in occupational situations (1).

Classification

The total number of biohazards is very large and difficult to estimate. They comprise a broad spectrum of various biologic agents from simple viruses through bacteria and agents associated with vertebrate animals (1). At least 193 of them must be considered as significant, due to high pathogenicity and wide distribution in the working environment (1). This group of important agents includes 27 species of viruses, 38 species of bacteria, 28 species of fungi, 4 species of lower plants other than fungi, and 23 allergenic agents associated with vertebrate animals (1).

The biohazards may act as infectious, allergenic, toxic, or carcinogenic agents in humans.

INFECTIOUS BIOHAZARDS

The infectious agents can be divided into three major subgroups: (1) human origin, (2) animal origin, and (3) others.

Infectious Agents of Human Origin Presenting a Risk for Health Care and Laboratory Workers

These agents have been extensively studied and are identified with the term ''biohazards.'' Data concerning epidemiology and prevention of infections in health care providers have been extensively reviewed (2–6). The hepatitis B virus is the most serious risk factor in health care settings (in particular for workers having frequent contact with blood), and vaccination of the at risk personnel is the most effective prevention measure (4, 6). Other important agents include rubella virus, respiratory syncytial (RS) virus, herpes simplex virus, influenza viruses, slow viruses, *Mycobacerium tuberculosis*, *Salmonella*, and *Staphylococcus aureus* (4, 6). Although the incidence of the occupational infections caused by the human immunodeficiency virus (HIV, AIDS virus) seems to be low, standard universal precautions to prevent transmission of the virus should be taken by all health care and laboratory workers exposed to blood or body fluids (7).

Infectious Agents of Animal Origin Causing Zoonoses

This group comprises about 30 agents indigenous to domestic and wild mammals and birds can cause occupational zoo-noses in farmers, animal breeders, laboratory workers, veterinarians, forestry workers, and in workers processing animal carcasses and products (meat, skins, hair, feathers). They include viruses (Orf virus, foot-and-mouth disease virus, vesicular stomatitis virus, Newcastle disease virus, rabies virus, and others), bacteria (*Coxiella burnetii, Chlamydia psittaci, Leptospira interrogans, Brucella abortus, B. suis, B. melitensis, Francisella tularensis, Bacillus anthracis, Listeria monocytogenes, Erysipelothrix rhusiopathiae, Mycobacterium bovis*, and others), fungi (*Trichophyton verrucosum, T. mentagrophytes*), and protozoans (*Toxoplasma gondii*) (1, 8–10). Occupational zoonoses present a serious problem in developing countries (9). However, outbreaks of some zoonoses (brucellosis, leptospirosis) still occur among workers in North America and Europe (11, 12). In addition some new modes of transmission of the agents are observed, by aerosols generated during industrial processes (10, 11, 13).

Another group of zoonotic agents are those transmitted by invertebrate animals of which the most important are liver flukes of the genus *Schistosoma* transmitted by water snails (causing schistosomiasis), and the nematode *Onchocerca volvulus* transmitted by flies of the genus *Simulium* in central Africa (causing river blindness). These parasitic worms are a great threat for agricultural workers and fishermen in warm climate zones, in particular *Schistosoma*, which affects several hundred million people in Africa and Asia (14).

Other Infectious Agents

This group includes viruses, bacteria, and protozoa present in sewage, water (15), and geophilic fungi (16). One of the most important agents is the gram-negative bacterium *Legionella pneumophila*, which grows in water at the temperature range of 20–50°C and may cause legionellosis in the workers maintaining water systems at power plants, oil drilling platforms, and other such settings (17–19).

The yeast-like geophilic fungi (*Coccidioides immitis, Histoplasma capsulatum, Sporothrix schenckii*, and *Blastomyces dermatitidis*) present in soil, decayed wood, and other vegetable matter and may cause deep mycoses in agricultural workers, gardners, woodworkers, miners, construction workers, and archeologists (16, 20).

Noninfectious Biohazards

These agents are typically allergens. Some of them (aflatoxin and wood dust) have been identified as carcinogens. Most of the agents in this group are associated with organic dusts in agricultural working environments. These include endotoxins from gram negative bacteria.

TOXIC AND/OR ALLERGENIC BIOHAZARDS

General Types of Biohazards

Three basic types of biohazards can be distinguished:

Microbial Factors. These include a vast number of toxin-producing and/or allergenic bacteria and fungi that grow on plant and animal surfaces as well as on different organic and inorganic materials. In the course of various industrial processes, these microbial products can be inhaled together with dusts or droplet aerosols and cause inflammatory reactions of the respiratory tract.

Plant Factors. These include a variety of plant toxins (alkaloids, glycosides), volatile oils, aeroallergens (pollen), and allergenic and/or toxic dusts that are released during processing of plant materials (tea dust, wood dust, buckwheat dust, cotton dust).

Animal Factors. These include toxin- and venom-producing animals (mites, ticks, spiders, stingrays, snakes) or allergens of animal origin (mite and insect particles, feather, epithel, hair, urine, feces, powdered enzymes) that may cause respiratory symptoms, conjunctivitis, and/or dermatitis.

Exposed Occupational Groups

The population at risk from toxic and/or allergenic biohazards is at least several hundred million belonging mostly to the following occupational groups (1).

Farmers and Workers of Agricultural Industry—These individuals are at highest exposure risk, in particular to organic dusts, which may contain high amounts of allergenic and bacteria, fungi, allergenic or toxic substances of plant origin (toxalbumins, lectins), and animal allergens (epithel, hair, feather, excreta) (21, 22). The other adverse agents are allergenic and/or biting insects, mites, and ticks (23, 24).

Gardeners and Orchard Workers—These persons are exposed to contact allergens and toxins of plant origin, pollen, and mites.

Foresters and Wood Processing Workers—These workers are exposed to allergenic fungi, contact allergens of lichens and liverworts, allergens and toxins of trees (pollen, terpen oils, resins), allergenic and toxinogenic caterpillars feeding on trees, and respirable wood dust having allergenic and carcinogenic properties (24–26).

Fishermen and Producers of Seafood—These individuals are exposed to venomous sponges, coelenterates, fish, and snakes (13, 27), and to airborne allergens of sea-squirts, crustaceans, and fish meal (28–31).

Cooks and Salespersons in Food Stores—may be exposed to contact allergens of plant and animal origin.

Laboratory and Health Care Workers—are threatened by a variety of agents, of which the most important are protein allergens of laboratory animals (32, 33) and powdered enzymes used as drugs or reagents (34).

Pharmaceutical Workers and Pharmacists—may be exposed to powders of plant and animal origin containing allergens (mainly enzymes) and toxins (alkaloids, glycosides) (35, 36).

Personal Care Workers (Cosmeticians, Hairdressers, Chiropodists)—are exposed to respiratory allergens in human hair, dander, nail dust, and to allergens of dermatophytic fungi (*Trichophyton rubrum*, *Trichophyton mentagrophytes*) (37).

Biotechnology Workers—could be endangered by bacterial endotoxin during processing of the cultures of gram-negative bacteria (38, 39) and by proteolytic enzymes of *Bacillus subtilis* when producing biologic detergents (40). Processing of fungal cell mass seems to be safe (41). The rapid development of biotechnology (including recombinant deoxyribonucleic acid techniques) must be accompanied by awareness of possible new biohazards, although experience to date does not indicate a great risk for the workers (42, 43).

Workers in the Textile Industry—may be exposed to respirable endotoxin produced by gram-negative bacteria on plant fibers (cotton, flax, hemp) (44, 46), to immunotoxic substances in cotton itself, as tannin (47), and to allergens of the silkworm (48).

Printers and Workers in Other Plants Where Air Must Be Humidified—are under risk to endotoxin-producing gram-negative bacteria (*Pseudomonas spp.*, *Cytophaga allerginae*) and, to allergenic micro-organisms (thermophilic actinomycetes, amoebae of the species *Naegleria gruberi*) which develop in humidifiers and are dispersed into air causing "humidifier fever," asthma, or allergic alveolitis in exposed people (49–52).

Sewage and Compost Workers—are exposed to endotoxin of gram-negative bacteria and to allergenic fungi (*Aspergillus fumigatus*) (15, 53).

Miners—may be endangered by mycotoxin-producing or allergenic fungi developing in mine shafts (54).

Librarians, Archivists, and Art Renovators—may be exposed to allergenic and/or toxinogenic fungi and bacteria growing on moist books, paintings, sculptures, and other objects (55–57).

Solderers—may be exposed to fumes of colophony (rosin, product of pine resin) which may be a cause of asthma (58).

Machine Operators—workers in metallurgical industry may have exposure to oil mist polluted with the toxins produced by bacteria and fungi developing in cutting oil emulsions (59). This hazard, could be prevented by the application of safe and effective biocides to the oil emulsions.

Range of Exposure

Tables 53.1–53.4 show that various toxic and/or allergenic biohazards may attain high levels in organic dusts and in the air of various occupational environments, thus increasing a risk of respiratory disease in exposed workers. In many cases they exceed the safe colony-forming unit (CFU) levels suggested for gram-negative bacteria (1×10^3 to 25×10^4 CFU/m^3), endotoxin (0.1–0.2 mg/m^3) and fungi (5×10^4 to 1×10^7 CFU/m^3) (98–100). There are no comparable reference levels for mycotoxins and for protein allergens of animal origin. For better protection of the workers in at risk professions, there is an urgent need for establishment of recommendations for exposure limits to different respirable biohazards.

Effects on Humans

Respiratory disorders, often associated with fever, are common among agricultural workers doing certain jobs (silo unloading, haymaking, handling of grain, work in animal confinement buildings) associated with the exposure to high concentrations of organic dusts (over 10 mg/m^3), endotoxin (over 1.0 mg/m^3) and microorganisms (over 10^5 CFU/m^3). The incidence of work-related symptoms (dyspnea, cough, chest tightness, fever) in the people performing such jobs has been estimated to be as high as 40–75% of the total working population (1, 101–103).

Table 53.1.   Concentrations of Dust-Borne Microorganisms in the Air of Different Working Environments (CFU/m^3)**

Environment	Total Microorganisms	Gram-negative Bacteria	Fungi
Farming			
Handling of hay	8.4×10^4–1.4×10^7 (60)	*	8.0×10^4–1.6×10^6 (60)
Handling of corn	*	*	9.3×10^5–1.2×10^8 (61)
Silo opening	1.5×10^5–4.4×10^9 (62)	*	1.0×10^4–1.2×10^7 (62)
Cattle farms	5.2×10^4–2.0×10^5 (63, 64)	9.4×10^3 (63)	1.3×10^4 (63)
Swine farms	1.7×10^4–1.4×10^6 (64–66)	8.4×10^3–7.5×10^4 (65, 66)	2.0×10^2–3.0×10^4 (65, 66)
Poultry farms	1.7×10^5–1.8×10^7 (63–65)	6.3×10^3–4.5×10^5 (63, 65)	5.0×10^2–9.1×10^4 (63, 65)
Industry			
Grain stores	1.3×10^5–1.3×10^6 (63)	5.9×10^4–5.5×10^5 (63)	7.4×10^3–4.5×10^4 (63)
Grain mills	2.2×10^4–1.9×10^5 (63, 67)	7.8×10^3–1.2×10^5 (63, 67)	2.6×10^3–1.2×10^4 (63, 67)
Malt-house	5.4×10^5 (63)	1.4×10^5 (63)	1.8×10^4 (63)
Herb processing	9.4×10^4–6.3×10^5 (67)	5.0×10^3–5.8×10^4 (67)	1.7×10^4–1.1×10^5 (67)
Citrus fruit store	*	*	3.3×10^4–7.7×10^8 (68)
Poultry processing	3.0×10^4–1.3×10^6 (63, 69, 70)	1.0×10^3–9.1×10^4 (63, 69, 70)	3.0×10^2–2.0×10^4 (63, 70)
Tobacco processing	1.5×10^3–1.1×10^4 (71)	*	1.4×10^3–1.0×10^4 (71)
Sawmills, furniture	3.1×10^3–6.5×10^5 (72–74)	1.0×10^2–2.2×10^4 (74)	1.7×10^2–6.5×10^5 (72–74)
Wood chip processing	2.7×10^2–3.8×10^5 (74–76)	3.7×10^3–7.0×10^3 (74)	2.7×10^2–3.8×10^5 (74–76)
Cotton mills	1.3×10^5–1.4×10^6 (77)	5.0×10^3–1.1×10^5 (78)	1.8×10^4–8.1×10^4 (77)
Waste processing			
Sewage treatment	*	1.0×10^1–1.0×10^5 (79)	*
Compost plants	*	7.0×10^1–9.6×10^4 (53)	1.0×10^2–1.5×10^6 (53)

CFU = colony forming units; * = no data available; references are given in parentheses.
**Courtesy of Dr. Barbane Ochalska, Krakow, Poland.

It was found that farmers showing symptoms of "organic dust toxic syndrome" or hypersensitivity pneumonitis have been exposed during work to significantly higher amounts of airborne microorganisms than asymptomatic ones (60, 82). The prevalence of respiratory symptoms may be also high in industry workers processing certain plant and animal materials (21, 30, 31, 34, 36, 46) and in laboratory animal care workers (32, 33). The airborne allergenic and/or toxic biohazards may be a cause of the following diseases: hypersensitivity pneumonitis (allergic alveolitis), allergic rhinitis, asthma, byssinosis, organic dust toxic syndrome (toxin fever, grain fever, silo unloader's syndrome), and chronic bronchitis (21, 36, 104–108). According to Rylander (104, 105), most of the disease symptoms are caused by reactions of lung cells to inhaled biologic agents. The process usually begins with the activation of alveolar macrophages which release biologically active substances, as endogenous pyrogen (interleukin-1), and chemotoxins attracting neutrophils and platelets which in turn secrete other inflammatory mediators. Other pathogenic pathways include activation of complement and reactions with specific antibody, as immunoglobulin E in asthma (108).

Effects on skin, appear as atopic allergic reactions to factors in organic dusts (urticaria), as contact allergic dermatitis, and as local inflammatory reactions caused by contact with toxic plants (dermatitis phytogenes) or by bites of insects, mites, and ticks (24, 35, 109–111).

Other irritant effects such as conjunctivitis are due to organic dusts (110, 111). Systemic reactions can be caused by stings or bites of venomous animals such as spiders, ray fishes and snakes (13, 27).

Review of Important Hazards

GRAM-NEGATIVE BACTERIA

Numerous gram-negative bacteria of plant origin represent potential respiratory hazards as a source of endotoxin and allergens.

The most well-known among them is the epiphytic species *Erwinia herbicola* (synonym: *Enterobacter agglomerans*) (44, 46, 112). Bacteria belonging to this species are yellow-chromogenic, facultatively anaerobic, fermentative rods with peritrichous flagella (Fig 53.1). They occur on a variety of plants and plant products and are very common on grain and on cotton (113), in grain and cotton dusts (44, 63, 84), and in the air of grain stores (63) and cotton mill cardrooms (78). *Erwinia herbicola* produces endotoxin which has been determined as a main cause of the acute byssinosis symptoms (46, 114) and allergens that may be a cause of allergic alveolitis or asthma (112, 115, 116).

The other gram-negative species that occur commonly in organic dusts and represent a potential risk for exposed persons belong to the following organisms: *Pseudomonas, Klebsiella, Alcaligenes, Acinetobacter, Citrobacter,* and *Enterobacter* (45, 78, 112, 117). Droplet aerosol from humidifiers and sewage may contain toxins of *Cytophaga allerginae, Pseudomonas, Flavobacterium,* and *Aeromonas nydrophila* (49, 50, 79).

ENDOTOXINS

Endotoxins are high molecular weight, heat-stable lipopolysaccharides (LPSs), consisting of a characteristic lipid component, the lipid A, covalently bound to a heteropolysaccharide. They are present in the outer membrane of gram-negative bacteria as heteropolymers with proteins and phospholipids, and could be easily released to the surrounding dusty environment in the form of the membrane disks measuring 30–50 nm (118). The inhaled particulate endotoxin activates alveolar macrophages and induces the release of inflammatory mediators causing fever (interleukin-1), bronchoconstriction (leukotriene C4, prostaglandin F2, thromboxane A2, platelet-activating factor), and influx of neutrophils and platelets to the lung (46, 114, 119). The effects of the endotoxin inhalation include endothelial alterations and increased pulmonary capillary permeability (114). The concentration of endotoxin in various organic dusts

Figure 53.1. *Erwinia herbicola* (synonym: *Enterobacter agglomerans*), × 30,000, (reproduced with permission from Dr. B. Ochalska, Laboratory of Electron Microscopy, School of Medicine, Cracow, Poland).

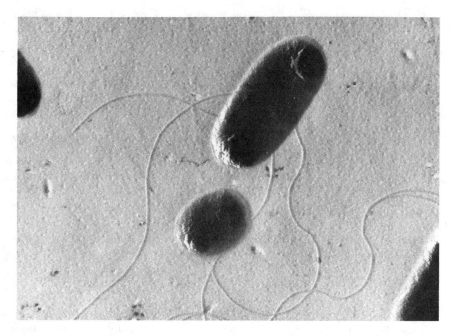

Table 53.2. Concentrations of Bacterial Endotoxins in Organic Dusts and in the Air of Different Working Environments

Environment	Concentration in Dust (μg/g) parts per million	Concentration in Air (μg/m³)
Farming		
Grain harvesting	*	0.01–102.4 (80)
Silo opening	87.2 (81)	0.16–8.85 (62)
Cattle-hay farms	440.0–980.0 (65)	18.0–34.0 (82)
Swine farms	5.0–100.0 (65, 66)	0.12–1.2 (45, 65, 66)
Poultry farms	10.9–120.0 (65, 81)	0.13–1.42 (65, 83)
Industry		
Grain stores and mills	22.5–500.0 (67, 84)	54.9 (67)
Rice production	21.2 (85)	0.49 (84)
Peanut shelling	22.6 (81)	*
Herb processing	200.0–400.0 (67)	4.0–756.8 (67)
Poultry processing	186.8 (81)	0.63–0.92 (86)
Sawmills	*	0.24–4.0 (74)
Furniture factories	*	0.0012–0.35 (72)
Wood chip processing	*	1.23–40.0 (74)
Cotton mills	40.3–780.0 (65, 81)	0.001–0.6 (45)
Cotton gin	*	0.20–2.0 (45)
Waste processing		
Sewage treatment	195.0 (79)	0.10–0.78 (79)
Compost plants	7.0–870.0 (53)	0.001–0.042 (53)

References are given in parentheses; *no data available.

and in the air polluted with the dusts could be high and exceeds levels considered safe (Table 53.2). A significant correlation has been found between the concentration of endotoxin in the airborne cotton dust and decrease of lung function values (expressed as forced expiratory volume in one second) in exposed persons (120). Similar effects of endotoxins were observed in poultry farmers (83).

Respiratory exposure to endotoxin contained in aerosolized dusts can result in an acute pulmonary response. Endotoxins on respirable particulate matter can penetrate deeply into areas such as bronchioles and alveoli. Endotoxin produces an inflammatory response once it comes into contact with pulmonary epithelium. Endotoxin activity is via an indirect inflammatory response by the pulmonary macrophages, and by itself it has no direct toxic activity. Mediators of inflammation are released by macrophages and neutrophils that have direct effect on the distal pulmonary tract. Clinically, exposure to endotoxin can produce acute fever, cough, dyspnea, and wheezing. Chronic exposure may result in hyperactive airway dysfunction.

THERMOPHILIC ACTINOMYCETES

Hazardous Species. The actinomycete *Micropolyspora faeni* (synonym: *Faenia rectivirgula*) was identified by Pepys et al.

(121) as a main source of the allergen causing farmer's lung disease, the best known form of hypersensitivity pneumonitis. The organisms grow in form of branching filaments (Fig. 53.2) bearing short chains of small sperical spores (0.7–1.3 μm in diameter). They develop in damp self-heating plant materials like hay. During handling of moldy hay, large amounts of spores are released into the air, and after inhalation by an individual, the spores may initiate cell-mediated or precipitin-mediated allergic reaction in the lung (21, 107, 122).

Thermoactinomyces vulgaris and *Thermoactinomyces candidus* are other thermophilic species involved in the etiology of farmer's lung disease (21, 122, 123). The spores are formed singly, directly on filaments. Biology of these organisms is similar to *M. faeni*. The relative species *Thermoactinomyces sacchari* has been identified as a cause of bagassosis, the form of hypersensitivity pneumonitis due to inhalation of dust from bagass (extracted sugar cane) (21).

Active substances.   It is assumed that inflammatory reaction in the lung is evoked by the glycopeptide and protein allergens released from actinomycetal spores (122, 124). Some authors also suggest that extracellular proteinases produced by *M faeni* and *Th. candidus* play a significant role in pathogenesis of the disease (22, 123, 125).

MOLD FUNGI

Hazard species.   Many species of molds that develop on various vegetable materials (grain, silage, tobacco, peanuts, fruits, wood, compost) produce allergens and/or toxins causing respiratory disease in the people inhaling dust from these materials contaminated with fungal products. The majority of the hazardous species belong to the genera: *Aspergillus, Penicillum, Absidia, Alternaria, Cladosporium, Cryptostroma, Fusarium, Mucor,* and *Stachybotrys* (16, 126, 127). The greatest risk are posed by the strains of *Aspergillus* and *Penicillium*.

Most of the pathogenic effects of molds on the respiratory system are due to allergenic response mediated through specific antibodies or sensitized cells (21, 107, 126, 127). Some dis-

eases may be caused by the inhalation of mycotoxins, but this problem is still not fully known. There are also suggestions that the symptoms of the organic dust toxic syndrome (ODTS) observed after inhaling of dust containing large amounts of mold spores may be due to nonspecific stimulation of the human immune system by some other substances produced by fungi (enzymes, glucans) (128, 129).

The best known pathogen is *Aspergillus fumigatus*, a common grey-greenish mold that occurs in large numbers on different materials (compost, silage, wood, tobacco) and in air polluted with organic dusts (53, 71, 117, 130). Spherical spores measuring 2.0–3.5 μm are formed on columnar conidial heads (Fig 53.3). Inhalation of the dust massively laden with spores may cause hypersensitivity pneumonitis (16, 71, 130), asthma (21, 122, 126), pulmonary mycosis (aspergillosis) (131), and organic dust toxic syndrome (117). The fungus also produces tumorigenic mycotoxins that pose a risk for sawmill workers (132).

Other species of the genus *Aspergillus* have been described as causative agents of hypersensitivity pneumonitis: *Aspergillus clavatus* has been identified as an agent of malt worker's disease, whereas *A. versicolor, A. flavus, A terreus* and *A. umbrosus* (species predominant in Scandinavia) have been implicated in the etiology of farmer's lung disease (21, 133). *Aspergillus flavus*, a known producer of aflatoxins, occurs commonly on corn and peanuts and in airborne dust from these products (61, 88).

Genus *Penicillium* comprises over 150 species of blue or green molds forming characteristic, brushlike conidiophore heads. They are widely distributed on decomposing organic matter and in air polluted with organic dusts. Penicillia have been described as causative agents of asthma (126) and of various forms of hypersensitivity pneumonitis: suberosis due to exposure to moldy cork, cheese worker's disease, disease due to exposure to moldy fuel chips, and disease of wood cutters (21, 134, 135).

Other allergenic molds include: *Cryptostroma corticale* described as an agent of the maple bark disease (136) and species

Figure 53.2.   *Micropolyspora faeni*, × 1500.

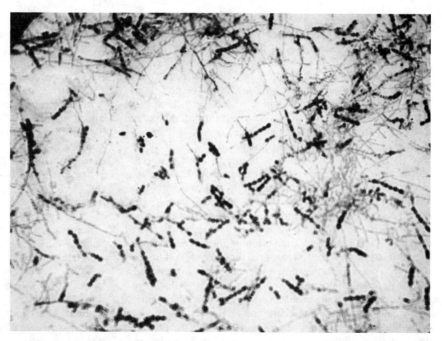

Figure 53.3. *Asperigillus fumigatus* × 1500.

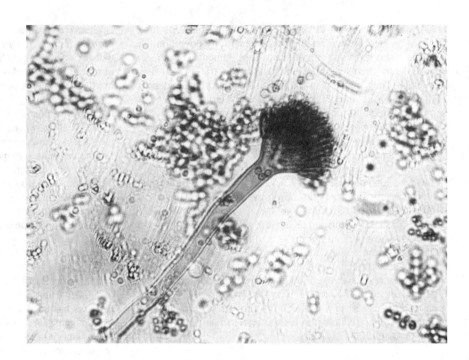

of the genera *Cladosporium* and *Alternaria* considered as a frequent causes of allergic rhinitis and asthma (126, 127).

Effects of Mycotoxins. Mycotoxins are low molecular weight, cyclic metabolites produced by different species of fungi, e.g. those belonging to the genera *Aspergillus*, *Penicillium*, *Fusarium* and *Stachybotrys*. The best known mycotoxins are aflatoxins B_1, B_2, G_1 and G_2 which are produced by *Aspergillus flavus* and *A. parasiticus*. The other important mycotoxins include: ochratoxins (produced by *Aspergillus* and *Penicillium* species), trichothecene toxins (produced by *Fusarium* species and *Stachybotrys atra*), zearalenone (produced by *Fusarium* species), patulin (produced by *Aspergillus* and *Penicillium* species), and cyclopiazonic acid (produced by *Penicillium cyclopium*).

Alimentary effects of mycotoxins on humans and animals may be toxic, carcinogenic, teratogenic, and mutagenic. Much less is known about their effects by inhalation route. The hypotheses relevant to their significant role as a cause of respiratory diseases via inhalation of organic dusts (102, 123) have now been confirmed. Usually only low levels of mycotoxins are found in organic dusts (Table 53.3). Nevertheless, there are strong indications that the levels of airborne aflatoxins and some other mycotoxins (secalonic acid D) may be relatively high in some occupational dust-polluted areas, such as processing peanuts and corn (89, 94). In these areas, a possibility of toxic and carcinogenic effects of mycotoxins must be considered (128, 137) as mycotoxins were found to be in association with fine, respirable fractions of vegetable dusts (91).

Van Nieuwenhuize et al. (87) and Hayes et al. (88) reported a high mortality for cancer in a group of aflatoxin-exposed workers of a plant that extracted oil from linseeds and peanuts. The cases of lung cancer and cancer of the colon were described in people occupationally exposed to contaminated peanut meal and to purified aflatoxin (137). Kusak et al. (54) had a hypothesis that the occupational bronchogenic carcinoma in uranium mines workers (Schneeberg and Jachymov disease) was caused by the inhalation of spores of *Aspergillus flavus* which grow in mine shafts. According to the authors, pathogenic

effects of the spores are due both to aflatoxins and to radioactive substances which are absorbed by molds.

Carcinogenic effects of mycotoxins may be due, at least in part, to the experimentally proven deleterious effects of these substances on alveolar macrophages (138, 139). Impairment of this anticancer defense line may enable fast growth of neoplastic cells.

BASIDIOMYCETOUS FUNGI

Parasites of wheat. Spores of rust (*Puccinia graminis*) and of smuts (*Ustilago*, *Tilletia*) are considered as important aeroallergens which may be a cause of rhinitis, asthma, and conjunctivitis in farmers, millers, workers of granaries, and other exposed persons (21, 126, 127, 140).

Edible mushrooms. There is growing evidence that spores of the commonly cultivated oyster mushroom (*Pleurotus ostreatus*) are highly allergenic and may be a cause of hypersensitivity pneumonitis and asthma in exposed persons (21, 141, 142). It was recently shown that this fungus produces two cytolytic proteinaceous toxins that may contribute to its pathogenic effects (143). Symptoms of respiratory allergy were described also in mushroom growers and processors of dried mushroom soups exposed to spores and mycelium of other mushroom species (*Agaricus bisporus*, *Lentinus edodus*, *Boletus edulis*, *Psalliata hortensis*) (141, 144).

LICHENS AND LIVERWORTS

Allergens produced by lichens (*Parmelia*) and liverworts (*Frullania*, *Radula*) that grow on trees may be a cause of contact dermatitis in wood cutters and sawmill workers (25).

HIGHER PLANTS

Pollen. The flower pollens of grasses, weeds, and trees are well known aeroallergens that may cause allergic rhinitis (pollinosis), asthma, and airborne dermatitis in sensitive persons.

Table 53.3. Concentrations of Mycotoxins in Organic Dusts and in the Air at Different Working Environments

Mycotoxin, Environment	Concentration in Dust (μg/g) parts per million	Concentration in Air (μg/m^3)
Aflatoxins		
Peanut processing	0.25–0.41 (87, 88)	0.0004–0.072 (87, 89)
Handling of corn	0.013–0.19 (90, 91)	*
Grain stores	0–0.0005 (92, 93)	*
Zearalenone		
Grain stores	0.02–0.1 (92, 93)	up to 0.15 (92)
Silo opening	0 (62)	*
Secalonic acid D (SAD)		
Grain stores	0.0005–0.02 (93)	*
Handling of corn	0.3–4.5 (94)	*
Deoxynivalenol		
Grain stores	0.0005–0.02 (93)	*
Silo opening	0.1–0.2 (62)	*

References are given in parentheses; *no data available.

Symptoms of pollinosis are observed during flowering season in a wide range of urban and rural populations, but it is assumed that people of certain professions (farmers, orchardmen, gardeners, greenhouse workers) are under greater risk of disease (22, 109, 145). The concentration of pollen in the air is greatly influenced by weather conditions. Values over 20 grains of grass pollen per one cubic meter of air are considered as hazardous for the sensitive person (146).

Plant Toxins and Allergens. A number of cultivated and wild growing plants produce toxins (alkaloids, glycosides, toxalbumins, photosensitizing substances, volatile oils, resins) and allergens. These may affect gardeners, farmers, herb processors, pharmacists, cooks, and salespersons by direct skin contact or by air, causing dermatitis phytogenes (urticaria, erythema, vesicles) and/or respiratory symptoms. The best known allergenic plants include: different vegetables (bean, celery, capsicum, carrot, and others), different decorative plants (tulips, hyacinth, chrysanthemum, buttercups, *Scilla*, *Euphorbia*, *Dieffenbachia*, *Laportea*, and others), common rue (*Ruta graveolens*), cator bean (*Ricinum communis*), soapwart (*Saponaria officinalis*), vanilla, and poison ivy (*Toxicodendron radicans*) (35, 109, 147). Colophony (rosin), a solid substance obtained by distillation of pine resin and used as a solder flux or as an additive to glues and other products, can cause occupational asthma in electronics workers exposed to soldering fumes and can cause contact dermatitis in other workers (58).

Vegetable dusts. The pathogenic effects of the dusts released from crushed or pulverized plant materials may be due to the associated microbial antigens, and to specific allergens of plant origin. Various allergic disorders (asthma, rhinitis, conjunctivitis, urticaria) were observed in the workers exposed to the dusts from tea, coffee, rice, herbs, buckwheat, ''Maiko'' dust from tuberous root of devil's tongue (*Amorphophalus konjac*) cultivated in Japan, and to powdered plant proteases (papain, bromelain) (13, 36, 48, 110, 111, 147). More recently, the possible role of the tannin component of cotton in evoking respiratory symptoms due to exposure to cotton dust has been suggested (47).

Wood dust. Wood dust exposure appears to be linked to the occurrence of adenocarcinoma of the nasal sinuses. The incidence of this disease is about 1000-fold greater in wood-workers than in other people (26, 149). Exposure to dust from certain woods may cause dermatitis, rhinitis, conjunctivitis, and asthma (13, 26, 150). The greatest risk for asthma is posed by exotic woods (13, 150) and western red cedar (*Thuja plicata*) which contains plicatic acid, a low molecular weight allergen (36). Other allergenic woods include walnuts, locusts, and pines (13, 150).

ARTHROPODS

Crustaceans. Allergenic particles of the processed prawn (*Nephrops norvegicus*) and snow crab (*Chionecetes opilio*) may cause hypersensitivity lung disease in exposed workers producing sea food (29, 30).

Arachnids. Ticks (*Ixodidae*, *Argasidae*) and certain species of spiders (*Latrodectus*) and mites (*Dermanyssum gallinae*, *Ornithonyssus bacoti*, *Pyemotes ventricosus*, *Neotrombicula autumnalis*) may actively attack persons (farmers, foresters) causing local inflammatory reaction (151). Allergens of acarid mites (*Acarus siro*, *Tyrophagus putrescentiae*, *Leipdoglyphus destructor*, *Glycyphagus domesticus*) feeding on stored products (hay, grain) may cause respiratory and nasal symptoms in exposed farmworkers (23, 152). Two species of pyroglyphid mites living in homes and feed on human dander (*Dermatophagoides pteronyssinus* and *Dermatophagoides farinae*) are known causative agents of allergy to house dust (153).

Insects. Contact with allergenic particles of insect origin (poisonous hairs, body fragments, excreta, feces) may cause asthma, rhinitis, conjunctivitis, and dermatitis in the exposed laboratory workers (mainly entomologists), foresters, silk producers, granary workers, and farmers (24). Gypsy moth (*Lymantria dispar*), Douglas fir tussock moth (*Orgyia pseudotsugata*), silkworm (*Bombyx mori*), locust (*Locusta migratoria*), cockroaches (*Periplaneta*, *Blattella*), and grain weevil (*Sitophilus granarius*) are strong sensitizers (21, 24, 48, 140, 154). Bee keepers are at risk of allergy to bee venom and hive particles (155).

OTHER INVERTEBRATE ANIMALS

Contact with poisonous sponges, coelenterates, and bryozoans may cause skin inflammation or systematic reaction in fishers,

Table 53.4. Concentrations of the Animal Protein Allergens in the Air of Occupational Settings

Place, Allergen	Concentration ($\mu g/m^3$)
Egg processing plant	
Egg white components	
Ovalbumin	50.0 (95)
Ovomucoid	10.7 (95)
Lysozyme	2.0 (95)
Cowsheds	
Bovine epithelial antigen	0.04–9.5 (96)
Laboratory animal facilities	
Urinary allergins:	
Different animal species	0.054–50.6 (33)
Rat urinary allergen	0–50.0 (97)
Rat epithelial allergen	0–40.0 (97)

Determinations were made with chemical and immunochemical methods (ELISA inhibition test, RAST inhibition assay). References are given in parentheses.

sailors, divers, and swimmers (13). The respiratory disease of oyster breeders in Japan called "Hoya asthma" is caused by allergens of sea-squirts (*Ascidiacea*) growing on oysters that become airborne during the process of opening of shells (28). People inhaling the airborne dust from pearl-oyster shells during manufacturing of ornaments may develop fever reaction and hypersensitivity pneumonitis (156).

VERTEBRATE ANIMALS

Fishes, amphibians, and reptiles. Contact with antigens and/or venoms present in slime of fishes and frogs may cause allergy in exposed persons (fishermen, cooks, laboratory workers) (109, 157). Sailors, fishers, divers, and swimmers are threatened by the sting of poisonous fish and the bite of the poisonous sea snakes (*Hydrophiidae*), while agricultural workers in tropical regions and zoologists are endangered by the bite of the terrestrial poisonous snakes (13, 27). Inhalation exposure to fish meal may cause asthma and hypersensitivity pneumonitis in factory workers (31).

Birds. Inhalation of the allergenic particles of bird origin (droppings, feather, epithel) may cause respiratory disorders in bird breeders and in workers of poultry processing plants (21, 31, 158). The well-known form of hypersensitivity pneumonitis called "bird fancier's lung" is most common among breeders of pigeons and budgerigars, but also occurs in people that have contact with hens, ducks, turkeys, and pheasants (122, 159). The incidence of this disease among poultry breeders in many countries is between 2–6% (158, 159). The workers of egg-processing plants that produce whole egg powder, egg yolk powder and liquid egg white can develop asthma due to exposure to high concentrations of the airborne egg allergens (Table 53.4) (95, 160).

Mammals. Farmers that breed domestic animals (cows, pigs) and owners of pets (dogs, cats) may develop allergic symptoms due to contact with the airborne particles of animal epithel, hair, urine, feces, milk, and saliva (22, 96, 161). A particular risk exists with laboratory animals (rats, mice, guinea pigs, rabbits) that produce strong protein allergens. These allergens can occur in high concentrations in the air of animal facilities (Table 53.4) (33, 97). It is estimated that 11–30% of

all laboratory animal care workers have a syndrome called laboratory animal allergy (LAA) characterized by rhinitis, asthma, conjunctivitis, and dermatitis (32, 97). At risk of allergy from animal protein are pharmaceutical and laboratory workers exposed via inhalation to powdered enzymes (pepsin, trypsin) (34). Furriers, tanners, and wool processors are also exposed to antigens in animal hair (162). A skin allergy due to contact with meat and cheese ("protein dermatitis") has been observed in butchers, in workers of meat and dairy package plants, and in cooks. Allergic dermatitis after contact with amniotic fluid has been described in veterinarians (109).

ACKNOWLEDGMENTS

This work was in progress while the author held the National Research Council Associateship at the National Institute for Occupational Safety and Health (NIOSH) in Morgantown, West Virginia.

REFERENCES

1. Dutkiewicz J, Jabionski L, Olenchock SA. Occupational biohazards: a review. Am J Ind Med 1988;14:605–623.

2. Pike RM. Laboratory-associated infections: incidence, fatalities, causes and prevention. Annu Rev Microbiol 1979;33:41–66.

3. Collins CH. Laboratory-acquired infections. London: Butterworths, 1983.

4. Patterson WB, Craven DE, Schwartz DA, Nardell EA, Kasmer J, Noble J. Occupational hazards to hospital personnel. Ann Intern Med 1985;102:658–680.

5. Miller BM, Groschel DHM, Richardson JH, Vesley D, Songer JR, Housewright RD, Barkley WE, eds. Laboratory safety: principles and practices. Washington, DC: American Society for Microbiology, 1986.

6. Gestal JJ. Occupational hazards in hospitals: risk of infection. Br J Ind Med 1987;44:435–442.

7. Centers for Disease Control. Recommendations for prevention of HIV transmission in health-care settings. MMWR 1987;36(suppl 2S):3S–18S.

8. Hubbert WT, McCulloch WF, Schnurrenberger PR, eds. Diseases transmitted from animals to man. 6th ed. Springfield, IL: Charles C Thomas, 1975.

9. Steele JH. Zoonoses as occupational diseases in agriculture and animal related industries. Chicago: American Medical Association, 1977.

10. Collins JD. Abattoir associated zoonoses. J Soc Occup Med 1983;33:24–27.

11. Kaufmann AF, Fox MD, Boyce JM, Anderson DC, Potter ME, Martone WJ, Patton CM. Airborne spread of brucellosis. Ann NY Acad Sci 1980;353:105–114.

12. Waitkins SA. Update on leptospirosis. Br Med J. 1985;290:1502–1503.

13. International Labour Office. Encyclopaedia of occupational health and safety. 3rd ed. Lyoun, 1983.

14. Garfield E. Schistosomiasis: the scourge of the Third World. Part 1. Etiology. Cur Con 1986;(29)9:3–7.

15. Clark CS. Potential and actual biological related health risks of wastewater industry employment. J Water Poll Con Fed 1987;59:999–1008.

16. DiSalvo AF, ed. Occupational mycoses. Philadelphia: Lea & Febiger, 1983.

17. Fraser DW, Deubner DC, Hill DI, Gilliam DK. Nonpneumonic, short-incubation-period legionellosis (Pontiac fever) in men who cleaned a steam turbine condenser. Science 1979;205:690–691.

18. Castellani PM, Greco D, Cacciottolo JM, Vassalo A, Grech A, Bartlett CLR. Legionnaires disease on an oil drilling platform in the Mediterranean: a case report. Br J Ind Med 1987;44:645–646.

19. Sykes JM, Brazier AM. Assessment and control of risks from Legionnaires' disease. Ann Occup Hyg 1988;32:63–67.

20. Howard DH. The epidemiology and ecology of blastomycosis, coccidioidomycosis and histoplasmosis. Zbl Bakt Hyg A 1984;219–227.

21. Lacey J. Occupational and environmental factors in allergy. In: Ganderton MA, Frankland AW, eds. Allergy 74. London: Pitmans Medical Press, 1974:303–318.

22. Donham KJ. Hazardous agents in agricultural dust and methods of evaluation. Am J Ind Med 1986;10:205–220.

23. Cuthbert OD, Brostoff J, Wraith DG, Brighton WP. "Barn allergy": asthma and rhinitis due to storage mites. Clin Allergy 1979;9:229–236.

24. Wirtz RA. Allergic and toxic reactions to nonstinging arthropods. Annu Rev Entomol 1984;29:47–70.

25. Catilina P. Work with wood. Professional risk and prevention. Arch Ma Prof 1981;42:253–285 (in French).

26. Whitehead LW. Health effects of wood dust—relevance for an occupational standard. Am Ind Hyg Assoc J 1982;43:674–678.

27. Kizer KW. Marine envenomations. J Toxicol Clin Toxicol 1984;21:527–555.

28. Jyo T, Komoto K, Tsubai S, Katsutani T, Otsoka T, Oka S. Sea squirt asthma—occupational asthma induced by inhalation of antigenic substances contained in sea squirt body fluid. Allerg Immunol (Paris) 1974;20/21:435–448.

29. Gaddie J, Legge JS, Friend JAR, Reid TMS. Pulmonary hypersensitivity in prawn workers. Lancet 1980;2:1350–1353.

30. Cartier A, Malo JL, Forest F, LaFrance M, Pineau L, St-Aubin JJ, Dubois JV. Occupational asthma in snow crab processing workers. J Allergy Clin Immunol 1984;74:261–269.

31. Avila R. Extrinsic allergic alveolitis in workers exposed to fish meal and poultry. Clin Allergy 1971;1:343–350.

32. Beeson ME, Dewdney JM, Edwards RG, Lee D, Orr RG. Prevalence and diagnosis of laboratory animal allergy. Clin Allergy 1983;13:433–443.

33. Edwards RG, Beeson ME, Dewdney JM. Laboratory animal allergy: the measurements of airborne urinary allergens and the effects of different environmental conditions. Lab Anim 1983;17:235–239.

34. Cartier A, Malo JL, Pineau L, Dolovich J. Occupational asthma due to pepsin. J Allergy Clin Immunol 1984;73:574–577.

35. Lewis WH, Elvin-Lewis PF. Medical botany. Plants affecting man's health. New York: John Wiley, 1977.

36. Pepys J. Occupational asthma—an overview. J Occup Med 1982;24:534–538.

37. Davies RR, Ganderton MA, Savage MA. Human nail dust and precipitating antibodies to *Trichophyton rubrum* in chiropodists. Clin Allergy 1983;13:309–316.

38. Ekenvall L, Dolling B, Goethe CJ, Ebbinghaus L, Von Stedingk LV, Wasserman J. Single cell protein as an occupational hazard. Br J Ind Med 1983;40:212–215.

39. Olenchock SA. Quantitation of airborne endotoxin levels in various occupational environments. Scand J Work Environ Health 1988;14(suppl 1):72–73.

40. Flindt MLH. Pulmonary disease due to inhalation of derivatives of *Bacillus subtilis* containing proteolytic enzyme. Lancet 1969;1:1177–1181.

41. Seeliger HPR, Hof H. Annotation to the pathogenicity and toxicity of yeasts as used in production of single cell proteins. Mykosen 1981;24:381–388.

42. Walgate R. How safe will biobusiness be? Nature 1980;283:126–127.

43. Landrigan PJ, Harrington JM, Elliott LJ. The biotechnology industry. In: Harrington JM, ed. Recent advances in occupational health, no. 2. Edinburgh: Churchill Livingstone, 1984:3–13.

44. Rylander R, Lundholm M. Bacterial contamination of cotton and cotton dust and effects on the lung. Br J Ind Med 1978;35:204–207.

45. Rylander R, Vesterlund J. Airborne endotoxins in various occupational environments. In: Watson SW, Levin J, Novitsky TJ, eds. Endotoxins and their detection with Limulus Amebocyte Lysate test. New York: Alan R. Liss, 1982:399–409.

46. Rylander R. The role of endotoxin for reactions after exposure to cotton dust. Am J Ind Med 1987;12:687–697.

47. Specks U, Kreofsky TV, Rohrbach MS. Tannin mediates secretion of neutrophil chemotactic factor (NCF) from alveolar macrophages (AMo) in rabbits and humans. In: Jacobs RR, Wakelyn PJ, eds. Cotton dust: Proceedings of the 13th Cotton Dust Research Conference. Memphis, TN: National Cotton Council, 1989.

48. Kobayashi S. Different aspects of occupational asthma in Japan. In: Frazier CA, ed. Occupational asthma. New York: Van Nostrand, 1980:229–244.

49. Rylander R, Haglind P. Airborne endotoxins and humidifier disease. Clin Allergy 1984;14:109–112.

50. Liebert CA, Hood MA, Deck FH, Bishop K, Flaherty DA. Isolation and characterization of a new *Cytophaga* species implicated in work-related lung disease. Appl Environ Microbiol 1984;48:936–943.

51. Burge PS, Finnegan M, Horsfield N, Emery D, Austwick P, Davies PS, Pickering CAC. Occupational asthma in a factory with a contaminated humidifier. Thorax 1985;40:248–254.

52. Edwards JH, Griffiths AJ, Mullins J. Protozoa as a source of antigen in humidifier fever. Nature 1976;264:438–439.

53. Clark CS, Rylander R, Larson L. Levels of Gram-negative bacteria, *Aspergillus fumigatus*, dust and endotoxin at compost plants. Appl Environ Microbiol 1983;45:1501–1505.

54. Kusak V, Jelinek S, Ula J. Possible role of *Aspergillus flavus* in the pathogenesis of Schneeberg and Jachymov disease. Neoplasma 1970;17:441–449.

55. Kowalik R. Microbiodeterioration of library materials: microbiodecomposition of basic organic library materials. Restaurator 1980;4:135–219.

56. Kowalik R. Microbiodeterioration of library materials: Microbiodecomposition of auxiliary materials. Restaurator 1984;6:61–115.

57. Strzelczyk AB. Paintings and sculptures. In: Rose AH, ed. Microbial deterioration, vol. 6. London: Academic Press, 1981:203–234.

58. Burge PS. Occupational asthma due to soft soldering fluxes containing colophony (rosin, pine resin). Eur J Respir Dis 1982;63(suppl 123):65–77.

59. Hill EC. Microbial aspects of health hazards from water-based metal working fluids. Tribology Int 1983;16:136–140.

60. Kotimaa MH, Terho EO, Husman K. Airborne moulds and actinomycetes in the work environment of farmers. Eur J Respir Dis 1987;(suppl 152):91–100.

61. Hill RA, Wilson DM, Burg WR, Shotwell OL. Viable fungi in corn dust. Appl Environ Microbiol 1984;47:84–87.

62. May JJ, Pratt DS, Stallones L, Morey PR, Olenchock SA, Deep IW, Bennett GA. A study of dust generated during silo opening and its physiologic effects on workers. In: Dosman JA, Cockroft DW, eds. Health and safety in agriculture. Boca Raton, FL: CRC Press, 1989.

63. Dutkiewicz J. Exposure to dust-borne bacteria in agriculture. I. Environmental studies. Arch Environ Health 1978;33:250–259.

64. Lehnigk K, Thiele E. Review of the data on exposure of the workers of animal farms to airborne microorganisms. Z ges Hyg 1978;24:331–335 (In German).

65. Clark CS, Rylander R, Larsson L. Airborne bacteria, endotoxin and fungi in dust in poultry and swine confinement buildings. Am Ind Hyg Assoc J 1983;44:537–541.

66. Donham KJ, Popendorf W, Palmgrem U, Larsson L. Characterization of dusts collected from swine confinement buildings. Am J Ind Med 1986;10:294–297.

67. Dutkiewicz J. Microbial hazards in plants processing grain and herb. Am J Ind Med 1986;10:300–302.

68. Strom G, Blomquist G. Airborne spores from mouldy citrus fruit—a potential occupational health hazard. Ann Occup Hyg 1986;30:455–460.

69. Lenhart SW, Olenchock SA, Cole EC. Viable sampling for airborne bacteria in a poultry processing plant. J Toxicol Environ Health 1982;10:613–619.

70. Dutkiewicz J, Smerdel-Skorska C, Krysinska-Traczyk E, Molocznik A, Uminski J, Roman J, Buchawska M, Lebiocki W, Gorny J. Air pollution with microorganisms and dust in modern poultry processing plants. Med Wiejska 1982;17:65–74 (In Polish).

71. Huuskonen MS, Husman K, Jarvisalo J, Korhonen O, Kotimaa M, Kuuseia T, Nordman H, Zitting A, Mantyjarvi R. Extrinsic allergic alveolitis in the tobacco industry. Br J Ind Med 1984;41:77–83.

72. Wilhelmsson B, Jernudd Y, Ripe E, Holmberg K. Nasal hypersensitivity in wood furniture workers. Allergy 1984;39:586–595.

73. Terho EO, Husman K, Kotimaa M, Sjoblom T. Extrinsic allergic alveolitis in a sawmill worker. A case report. Scand J Work Environ Health 1980;6:153–157.

74. Dutkiewicz J. Bacteria, fungi and endotoxin in stored timber logs and airborne sawdust in Poland. In: Ilewellyn GC, O'Rear CE, eds. Biodeterioration research II. Washington, DC: Plenum Press, 1989.

75. Halweg H, Krakowka P, Podisadlo B, Owczarek J, Ponahajba A, Pawlicka L. Studies on the pollution of air with fungal spores on selected working posts in a paper mill. Pneum Pol 1978;46:577–585 (In Polish).

76. Jappinen P, Haahtela T, Liira J. Chip pile workers and mould exposure. Allergy 1987;42:545–548.

77. Tuffnell P. The relationship of byssinosis to the bacteria and fungi in the air of textile mills. Br J Ind Med 1960;17:304–306.

78. Haglind P, Lundholm M, Rylander R. Prevalence of byssinosis in Swedish cotton mills. Br J Ind Med 1981;38:138–143.

79. Rylander R, Lundholm M, Clark CS. Exposure to aerosols of microorganisms and toxins during handling of sewage sludge. In: International Conference on Biohazards of Sludge Disposal in Cold Climates. Calgary, 1982:69–78.

80. Lundholm M, Palmgren U, Malmberg P. Exposure to endotoxin in the farm environment. Am J Ind Med 1986;10:314–315.

81. Olenchock SA. Endotoxins in agricultural dusts. In: Barry S, Houghton DR, Llewellyn GC, O'Rear CE, eds. Biodeterioration 6. London: C.A.B. International, 1986;312–315.

82. Malmberg P, Rask-Anderson A. Natural and adaptive immune reactions to inhaled microoganisms in the lungs of farmers. Scand J Work Environ Health 1988;14(suppl 1):68–71.

83. Thelin A, Tegler O, Rylander R. Lung reactions during poultry handling related to dust and bacterial endotoxins levels. Eur J Respir Dis 1984;65:266–271.

84. DeLucca AJ II, Godshall MA, Palmgren MS. Gram-negative bacterial endotoxins in grain elevator dusts. Am Ind Hyg Assoc J 1984;45:336–339.

85. Olenchock SA, Christiani DC, Mull JC, Shen Yi-e, Lu Peillian. Airborne endotoxins in a rice production commune in the People's Republic of China. J Toxicol Environ Health 1984;13:545–551.

86. Olenchock SA, Lenhart SW, Mull JC. Occupational exposure to airborne endotoxins during poultry processing. J Toxicol Environ Health 1982;9:339–349.

87. Van Nieuwenhuize JP, Herber RFM, DeBruin A, Meyer PB, Duba WC. Epidemiological study on the carcinogenicity of prolonged exposure to low levels of aflatoxins among factory workers. Tijd Soc Geneesks 1973;51:754–760 (In Dutch).

88. Hayes RB, Van Nieuwenhuize JP, Raatgever JW, Ten Kate FJW. Aflatoxin exposures in the industrial setting: An epidemiological study of mortality. Fd Chem Toxic 1984;22:39–43.

89. Sorenson WG, Jones W, Simpson J, Davidson JI. Aflatoxin in respirable airborne peanut dust. J Toxicol Environ Health 1984;14:525–533.

90. Burg WR, Shotwell OL. Aflatoxin levels in airborne dust generated from contaminated corn during harvest and at an elevator in 1980. J Assoc Off Anal Chem 1984;67:309–311.

91. Sorenson WG, Peach MJ, Simpson JP, Olenchock SA, Taylor G. Size range of viable fungi particles from aflatoxin-contaminated corn aerosols. In: Dosma JA, Cotton DJ, eds. Focus on grain dust and disease. New York: Academic Press, 1980:527–536.

92. Palmgren MS, Lee LS, DeLucca AJ II, Ciegler A. Preliminary study of mycoflora and mycotoxins in grain dust from New Orleans area grain elevators. Am Ind Hyg Assoc J 1983;44:485–488.

93. Ehrlich KC, Lee LS. Mycotoxins in grain dust: method for analysis of aflatoxins, ochratoxin A, zearalenone, vomitoxin, and secalonic acid D. J Assoc Off Anal Chem 1984;67:963–967.

94. Ehrlich KC, Lee LS, Ciegler A, Palmgren MS. Secalonic acid D: natural contaminant of corn dust. Appl Environ Microbiol 1982;44:1007–1008.

95. Halverson PC, Swanson MC, Reed CE. Occupational asthma in egg crackers is associated wit hextraordinarily high airborne egg allergen concentration (Abstract). J Allergy Clin Immunol 1988;81:321.

96. Virtanen T, Vilhunen P, Husman K, Happonen P, Mantyjaravi R. Level of airborne bovine epithelial antigen in Finnish cowsheds. Int Arch Occup Environ Health 1988;60:355–360.

97. Lewis DM, Bledsoe TA, Dement JM. Laboratory animal allergies. Use of the radioallergosorbent test inhibition essay to monitor airborne allergen levels. Scand J Work Environ Health 1988;14(suppl 1):74–76.

98. Popendorf W. Workgroup report on agents. Am J Ind Med 1986;10:251–259.

99. Clark CS. Workgroup report on prevention and control. Am J Ind Med 1986;10:267–273.

100. Dutkiewicz J. Recommendations of the threshold limits for exposure to microorganisms in agricultural working environments (unpublished).

101. Kovats F, Bugyi B. Occupational mycotic diseases of the lung. Budapest: Academiai Kiado, 1968.

102. Warren CPW, Manfreda J. Respiratory systems in Manitoba farmers: Association with grain and hay handling. Can Med Assoc J 1980;122:1259–1264.

103. Donham KG, Haglind P, Peterson Y, Rylander R. Environmental and health studies in swine confinement buildings. Am J Ind Med 1986;10:289–293.

104. Rylander R. Lung diseases caused by organic dusts in the farm environment. Am J Ind Med 1986;10:221–227.

105. Rylander R. Organic dusts and lung reactions—exposure characteristics and mechanisms for disease. Scand J Work Environ Health 1985;11:199–206.

106. DoPico GA. Workgroup report on diseases. Am J Ind Med 1986;10:261–265.

107. Richerson HB. Hypersensitivity pneumonitis—pathology and pathogenesis. Clin Rev Allergy 1983;1:469–486.

108. Burrell R, Rylander R. A critical review of the role of precipitins in hypersensitivity pneumonitis. Eur J Respir Dis 1981;62:332–343.

109. Rudzki E. Occupational dermatoses. Warszawa: PZWL (in Polish).

110. Uragoda CG. Tea maker's asthma. Br J Ind Med 1970;27:181–182.

111. Gothe CJ, Wieslander G, Ancker K, Forsbeck M. Buckwheat allergy: health food, an inhalation health risk. Allergy 1983;38:155–159.

112. Dutkiewicz J. Bacteria in farming environment. Eur J Respir Dis 1984;71(suppl 154):71–88.

113. Morey P, Fischer J, Rylander R. Gram-negative bacteria on cotton with particular reference to climatic conditions. Am Ind Hyg Assoc J 1983;44:100–104.

114. Burrell R. Lantz RC, Hinton DE. Mediators of pulmonary injury induced by inhalation of bacterial endotoxin. Am Rev Respir Dis 1988;137:100–105.

115. Kus L. Clinical and experimental studies on allergic alveolitis due to exposure to antigens present in grain dust. Med Wiejska 1980;15:73–80 (in Polish).

116. Dutkiewicz J, Kus L, Dutkiewicz E, Warren CPW. Hypersensitivity pneumonitis in grain farmers due to sensitization to *Erwinia nerbicola*. Ann Allergy 1985;54:65–68.

117. Dutkiewicz J, Olenchock SA, Sorenson WG, Gerencser VF, May JJ, Pratt DS, Robinson VA. Levels of bacteria, fungi and endotoxin in bulk and aerosolized corn silage. Appl Environ Microbiol 1989;55:1093–1099.

118. Dutkiewicz J, Tucker J, Woodfork K, Burrell R. The identification of extracellular endotoxin molecules by immunoelectron microscopy. In: Jacobs RR, Wakelyn PJ, eds. Cotton dust: Proceedings of the 13th Cotton Dust Research Conference. Memphis, TN: National Cotton Council, 1989.

119. Holt PG. Current trends in research on the etiology and pathogenesis of byssinosis. Am J Ind Med 1987;12:711–716.

120. Castellan RM, Olenchock SA, Kinsley KB, Hankinson JL. Inhaled endotoxin and decreased spirometric values. An exposure-response relation for cotton dust. N Engl J Med 1987;317:605–610.

121. Pepys J, Jenkins PA, Festenstein GN, Gregory PH, Lacey ME, Skinner FA. Farmer's lung: thermophilic actinomycetes as a source of "farmer's lung hay" antigen. Lancet 1963;2:607–611.

122. Pepys J. Hypersensitivity diseases of the lungs due to fungi and organic dusts. Basel: S. Karger, 1969.

123. Emanuel DA, Marx J Jr, Ault B, Treuhaft M, Roberts R, Kryda M. Pulmonary mycotoxicosis revisited. Am J Ind Med 1986;10:305–306.

124. Edwards JH. The isolation of antigens associated with farmer's lung. Clin Exp Immunol 1972;11:341–355.

125. Nicolet J, Bannerman EN. Extracellular enzymes of *Micropolyspora faeni* found in moldy hay. Infect Immun 1975;12:7–12.

126. Lacey J, Pepys J, Cross T. Actinomycete and fungus spores in air as respiratory allergens. In: Shapton DA, Board RG, eds. Safety in microbiology. London: Academic Press, 1972:151–184.

127. Austwick PKC. Fungi and actinomycetes. In: Scadding JG, Cumming G, Thurlbeck WM, eds. Scientific foundations of respiratory medicine. London: W. Heinemann, 1981;396–413.

128. Sorenson WG. Health impact of mycotoxins in the home and workplace: an overview. In: Llewellyn GC, O'Rear CE, eds. Biodeterioration research II. Washington, DC: Plenum Press, 1989.

129. Rylander R. Fogelmark B, Goto H. Acute pulmonary inflammation induced by glucans. In: Jacobs RR, Wakelyn PJ, eds. Cotton dust: Proceedings of the 13th Cotton Dust Research Conference. Memphis, TN: National Cotton Council, 1989.

130. Minarik L, Mayer M, Votrubova V, Uregeova N, Dutkiewicz J. Allergic alveolitis due to antigens present in mouldy beech chips—description of two cases. Studia Pneumol Phtiseol Cechoslov 1983;43:38–45 (in Slovak).

131. Minarik L, Skalsky T, Heyna A, Steklacova E. Occupational aspergillosis of the lung. Rozhl Tuberk 1969;29:169–173 (in Slovak).

132. Land CJ, Hult K, Fuchs R, Hagelberg S, Lundstrom H. Tremorgenic mycotoxins from *Aspergillus fumigatus* as a possible occupational health problem in sawmills. Appl Environ Microbiol 1987;53:787–790.

133. Terho EO, Lacey J. Microbiological and serological studies of farmer's lung in Finland. Clin Allergy 1979;9:43–52.

134. Van Assendelft AHW, Raitio M, Turkia V. Fuel chip induced hypersensitivity pneumonitis caused by *Penicillium species*. Chest 1985;87:394–396.

135. Dykewicz MS, Laufer P, Patterson R, Roberts M, Sommers HM. Woodman's disease: hypersensitivity pneumonitis from cutting live trees. J Allergy Clin Immunol 1988;81:455–460.

136. Emanuel DA, Wenzel FJ, Lawton BR. Pneumonitis due to *Cryptostroma corticale* (maple bark disease). N Engl J Med 1966;274:1413–1418.

137. Jesenska Z. Current problems of fungi and mycotoxins in working environments. Pracov Lek 1985;37:133–138 (in Slovak).

138. Sorenson WG, Gerberick GF, Lewis DM, Castranova V. Toxicity of mycotoxins for the rat pulmonary macrophage in vitro. Environ Health Perspect 1986;66:45–53.

139. Sorenson WG, Simpson J. Toxicity of penicillic acid for rat alveolar macrophages in vitro. Environ Res 1986;41:505–513.

140. Jimenez-Diag C, Lahoz C, Canto G. The allergens of mill dust (asthma in millers, farmers and others). Ann Allergy 1947;5:519–525.

141. Lopez M, Salvaggio J, Butcher B. Allergenicity and immunogenicity of basidiomycetes. J Allergy Clin Immunol 1976;57:480–488.

142. Cox A, Folgering HTM, Van Griensven LJLD. Extrinsic allergic alveolitis caused by spores of the oyster mushroom *Pleurotus ostreatus*. Eur Respir J 1988;1:466–468.

143. Anderson J, Trivedi A, Toogood JH. Cytolytic toxins extracted from *Pleurotus ostreatus* (PO) spores (Abstract). J Allergy Clin Immunol 1988;81:274.

144. Symington IS, Kerr JW, McLean DA. Type I allergy in mushroom soup processors. Clin Allergy 1981;11:43–47.

145. Saweda Y. Epidemiological study of apple pollinosis among apple farmers. Jpn J Allergy 1980;29:293–297.

146. Solomon WR. Aerobiology of pollinosis. J Allergy Clin Immunol 1984;74:449–461.

147. Hennebreg M, Skrzydlewska E, eds. Intoxications due to higher plants and fungi. Warszawa: PZWL, 1984 (in Polish).

148. Cartier A, Malo JL, Dolovich J. Occupational asthma in nurses handling psyllium. Clin Allergy 1987;17:1–6.

149. Wills JH. Nasal carcinoma in woodworkers: A review. J Occup Med 1982;24:526–530.

150. Woods B, Calnan CD. Toxic woods. Br J Dermatol 1976;94(suppl 13):1–97.

151. Zoltowski Z, ed. Medical arachnoentomology. Warszawa: PZWL, 1976 (in Polish).

152. Blainey AD, Topping MD, Ollier S, Davies RJ. Respiratory symptoms in arable farmworkers: role of storage mites. Thorax 1988;43:697–702.

153. Voorhorst R, Spieksma FTM, Varekamp H, Leupen MJ, Lyklema AW. The house dust mite (*Dermatophagoides pteronyssinus*) and the allergens it produces. J Allergy 1967;39:325–339.

154. Etkind PH, O'Dell TM, Canada AT, Shama SK, Finn AM, Tuthill RW. The gypsy moth caterpillar: a significant new occupational and public health problem. J Occup Med 1982;24:659–662.

155. Bousquet I, Menardo JL, Michel FB. Allergy in beekeepers. Allergol Immunopathol (Madr) 1982;10:395–398.

156. Weiss W, Baur X. Antigens of powdered pearl-oyster shell causing hypersensitivity pneumonitis. Chest 1987;91:146–148.

157. Armentia A, Martin-Santos J, Subiza J, Pola J, Zapata C, Valdivieso R, Losada E. Occupational asthma due to frogs. Ann Allergy 1988;60:209–210.

158. Petro W, Bergmann KC, Heinze R, Muller E, Wuthe H, Vogel J. Long-term occupational inhalation of organic dust—effect on pulmonary function. Int Arch Occup Environ Health 1978;42:119–127.

159. Molina C, Brun J, Tourreau A, Godefroid JM, Aiache JM. Respiratory disorders in poultry breeders. Rev Franc Malad Resp 1974;2:849–866 (in French).

160. Centers for Disease Control. Occupational asthma from inhaled egg protein—Iowa. JAMA 1987;257:904.

161. Harries MG, Cromwell O. Occupational asthma caused by allergy to pigs' urine. Br Med J 1982;284:867.

162. Pimentel JC. Furrier's lung. Thorax 1970;25:387–398.

54

Toxic Hazards of Sewers and Wastewater Facilities

Allen G. Kraut, M.D.

WORK PROCESS

Sewage is a mixture of liquids and solids of domestic and industrial origin which varies in composition from sewer to sewer and from hour to hour (1). Sewage collects through a system of sewer pipes ranging between 20 centimeters and 3.5 meters in diameter which terminate in wastewater facilities (2). Initial treatment involves passage of sewage through screens to remove large debris. Wastewater is then diverted to large tanks, where heavier wastes settle to the bottom. Materials lighter than water float to the top and are skimmed off. Partially purified sewage flows over the edge of the tank for further processing. Settled sludge is collected for concentration and disposal.

Colloidal particles such as proteins and oily emulsions which do not naturally separate from sewage are coagulated by the addition of inorganic compounds such as aluminum sulfate. Under appropriate pH conditions, the positive metal ions in the coagulant materials neutralize the negative charge of the colloid, promoting coagulation. Particles greater than 0.4 micrometers in diameter precipitate from solution (3).

Secondary sewage treatment refers to the biodegradation of sewage by aerobic or anaerobic bacteria. Aerobic processes are divided into those that do and those that do not actively provide oxygen to the microorganisms. Activated aerobic processes accelerate sewage metabolism by providing additional oxygen to the bacteria. Under appropriate conditions this process has a purification efficiency of greater than 95% (2). When oxygen is not actively added to the system, sewage remains in stabilization ponds, usually 3–4 meters deep, for between 10 and 60 days. This process is used when sufficient space is available and the underlying soil can retain toxic effluents, preventing ground water contamination.

Anaerobic sewage treatment takes place in closed steel digesters and is temperature-dependent. It is less efficient than the aerobic processes but can provide methane as an energy source for the plant. This method is used to treat activated sludge or effluents from industries such as sugar processing, where the amount of oxygen necessary to degrade sewage makes aerobic processes impractical (3).

In both aerobic and anaerobic treatments, sewage must be examined by trained individuals to ensure that conditions are appropriate for waste degradation. The presence of adequate amounts of nitrogen, phosphorus, and trace elements, the absence of toxic metals, and optimal temperature and pH are all important considerations.

The majority of domestic sewage is released into natural bodies of water after secondary treatment. In some instances, when sewage has not been purified sufficiently, it is chlorinated prior to release.

Tertiary sewage treatment is reserved for industrial sewage containing a higher percentage of nonbiodegradable contaminants. A variety of chemical and physical reactions, most commonly precipitation, oxidation, and absorption, are used for additional purification. The precise mechanisms and compounds used are dependent on the pollutant in question: lime is used in the precipitation of fluorides and phosphates in the fertilizer industry, cyanides are oxidized by adding sodium hypochlorite, and dyes may be adsorbed by using activated charcoal powder. Remaining pathogens are killed by chlorination or oxygenation, allowing the purified water to be released or recycled (3).

Accumulated sludge from sewage treatment is dewatered by sedimentation, centrifugal separation, or filtration to reduce bulk prior to deposition. Sludge volume may also be reduced chemically, most commonly with ferric chloride, or by bacterial digestion. Metal-containing sludge can be detoxified by treatment with sodium silicate, producing insoluble metal silicates. Sludge is disposed of in a number of ways, including incineration, ocean dumping, placement in a landfill, or use as fertilizer (3).

POTENTIAL TOXICOLOGIC HAZARDS

Sewage treatment workers perform a large number of tasks in a variety of conditions, ranging from monitoring electronic equipment in office-like settings to fixing pumps in potentially toxic confined spaces. Workers processing sewage and maintaining sewage systems are exposed to a variety of biologic and toxicologic hazards. An increased risk of self-limited diarrheal diseases has been seen in sewage treatment workers employed in various jurisdictions (4, 5). Listeriosis is also a well-known occupational disease of sewer workers (1).

Although no large scale epidemiologic studies have been performed addressing overall mortality and morbidity in sewage treatment workers, many case reports and case series attest to the potential toxicologic hazards of this work (6–8).

Chemical exposures occur through three major mechanisms in wastewater facilities: exposure to compounds necessary to process sewage, exposure to those produced by sewage decay, and exposure to toxic wastes disposed of in the sewage.

Hazards Related to Chemicals Used in the Treatment Process

Preliminary results from the National Occupational Exposure Survey reveal that sewage system workers use over 90 different chemical compounds in their work (9). Compounds routinely used include alkaline cleaners, organic solvents, disinfectants, chemicals for sewage treatment, laboratory reagents, paints, lubricants, hydraulic fluids, and pesticides (10).

Various organic solvent-based materials used in adhesives, cements, and cleaners can routinely cause skin and mucosal irritation and neurologic symptoms such as headache, lightheadedness, and fatigue. In addition certain of these compounds also have specific organ toxicities, e.g., hepatotoxicity secondary to chlorinated hydrocarbon exposures.

A number of disinfectants including alcohols, ammonia, liquid chlorine, and iodine are used in cleaning wastewater facilities. Workers must be warned that ammonia and chlorine should not be mixed, as pulmonary edema may result from inhalation of the resulting chloramines.

Aluminum sulfate and ferric chloride are chemicals commonly used in sewage treatment. Aluminum sulfate, a sewage coagulant, is irritating to the skin and mucous membranes and can produce sulfuric acid when mixed with water. Ferric chloride, a sludge dewatering agent, decomposes to hydrochloric acid in the presence of moisture or light. When either of these compounds is used, workers must wear protective equipment to avoid exposure to breakdown products.

A vast variety of laboratory chemicals including potassium iodide, potassium dichromate, and various acidic and basic buffers are used to assess the efficiency of sewage processing. As the majority of persons performing laboratory testing have little or no formal training in chemistry, appropriate safety practices should be included in any testing instructions.

The largest classes of chemical compounds found in some sewage treatment plants are lubricants and hydraulic fluids (10). Used to service plant equipment, these compounds can cause dermatitis and folliculitis. Other potential hazardous exposures in treatment plants include pesticides used to control flies and rodents, mercury used in gauges and switches, and asbestos insulation materials.

Chlorine is used in wastewater treatment facilities for a wide variety of purposes including disinfection, odor control, grease and scum removal, and chemical neutralization. Approximately 6% of the United States chlorine production is used to chlorinate drinking water and sewage (11).

Workers potentially exposed to chlorine should be informed of its extreme toxicity and of the proper ways to handle this compound. Due to the risk of explosion, chlorine should not be added to sewage containing ammonia, sulfur, or gasoline (12).

Full face respirators are the minimal level of protection necessary for workers changing chlorine cylinders or tank car connections; impermeable gloves and protective clothing must be worn when working with liquid chlorine (13). Emergency eye wash facilities should be located in areas where chlorine is used or stored.

The odor threshold for chlorine is 0.02 ppm (14). Gaseous chlorine exposures cause nasal irritation at concentration of 0.2 ppm, and severe eye and nose irritation at concentrations between 1 and 3 ppm (15). Further symptoms include irritation of the throat, cough which may be productive of whitish or blood-tinged sputum, chest pain, and chest tightness. Systemic symptoms including nausea, vomiting, dizziness, and stupor may develop depending upon the degree of exposure (16, 17). Death due to pulmonary edema has occurred in overexposed individuals (18, 19).

Both acute restrictive (20) and obstructive (18, 21) pulmonary function decrements have been reported in individuals surviving initial exposures. Most survivors, including those hospitalized, do not develop persistent pulmonary function abnormalities (17, 22).

Studies quantifying symptoms following low level chlorine exposures have lacked objective exposure measurements. One study of current employees (23), failed to show dose-response relationships between chlorine exposures of 0.006–1.42 ppm and symptoms, radiographic abnormalities, and pulmonary function results.

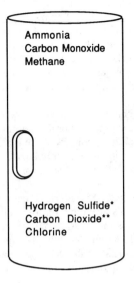

*May rise in hot or humid conditions

** May rise if heated

Figure 54.1. Location of highest concentrations of gases in a confined space such as a container.

Clinical assessments of workers overexposed to chlorine gas should be performed as soon as possible, and workers should be admitted to hospital for observation and supportive treatment if necessary. Precautions should be taken against the possibility that workers may develop pulmonary toxicity a number of hours after the exposure has ended. Although steroids have been used and are thought by some to be helpful (24), controlled clinical trials have not been performed to show whether they are efficacious. Prophylactic antibiotics have not been proven to be efficacious in the management of chlorine toxicity.

Hazards Related to Products of Sewage Decay

A number of sewage and sludge gases are produced during sewage treatment. Depending on their density, they may be located at the top or bottom of an enclosed space (Fig. 54.1).

Hydrogen sulfide (H_2S) is a dense gas, which usually concentrates at the bottom of enclosed spaces. Although its characteristic "rotten egg" odor is easily detectable at low levels, olfactory paralysis may occur at higher concentrations (25). H_2S is a potent irritant and a toxic asphyxiant. Eye irritation may occur after several hours of exposure at the 10–20 ppm range. Higher levels of exposure produce keratoconjunctivitis or "gas eye." Pulmonary edema may result from acute overexposures (26). H_2S reversibly inhibits the cytochrome oxidase system blocking aerobic metabolism. At high concentrations it directly produces toxic inhibition of the respiratory center, causing death from respiratory arrest (27). Treatment should be supportive; nitrite induction of methemoglobinemia has been used to block the inhibition of the cytochrome oxidase system (27).

Carbon monoxide (CO) may be introduced into sewer systems from fires or faulty equipment. Carbon monoxide's strong affinity for hemoglobin and its ability to shift the oxygen dissociation curve to the left make it a toxic asphyxiant gas. Carboxyhemoglobin (HbCO) concentrations of 10% can cause headache, while collapse and coma may occur at HbCO concentrations of 35–45%. Higher levels may lead to death.

Ammonia, a natural breakdown product of sewage, can be very irritating to the eyes and respiratory system. Due to its high solubility, ammonia first affects the upper airway. Respiratory distress follows exposures to levels greater than 100 ppm.

Methane, a highly flammable colorless, odorless gas, is produced by anaerobic digestion or the natural breakdown of sewage. Lighter than air, it collects at the top of enclosed spaces. A simple asphyxiant gas, it is only hazardous due to displacement of oxygen. Methane can spark or flame at air concentrations of 5%.

Carbon dioxide (CO_2) is colorless, odorless, and nonflammable. It concentrates at the bottom of enclosed spaces, and at high concentrations may lead to oxygen deficiency. CO_2 narcosis may ensue following breathing air containing 7–10% CO_2 for a few minutes (28). Table 54.1 summarizes the characteristics of gases commonly encountered in the wastewater industry.

Workers may be exposed to mixtures of these gases when maintaining sludge digesters. Digester gas produced during anaerobic sludge digestion is composed primarily of methane (65–70%) and carbon dioxide (25–30%); small amounts of nitrogen, hydrogen, oxygen, and hydrogen sulfide can also be present (13).

Sewage systems contain many confined spaces which, due to inadequate ventilation, develop hazardous atmospheres. The three major hazards associated with working in confined spaces are oxygen deficiency, explosions, and the toxicities of any gases present. An oxygen concentration of 19.5% has been

recommended as the lower limit below which workers must use supplied air (29).

Gases are combustible throughout a range of air mixtures, starting at the LEL (lower explosive limit), where the minimal concentration of gas required to support combustion is available, and ending at the UEL (upper explosive limit), above which the concentration of oxygen will no longer support combustion. Both the LEL and UEL are expressed in percent by volume in air at sea level (29).

Confined spaces have been classified based on their explosivity, oxygen level, and toxicity into three classes; class A confined spaces are immediately dangerous to life; class B are dangerous but not immediately life threatening; and class C, although potentially hazardous, do not require modifications of work procedures. Classification is determined by the most hazardous existing condition (Table 54.2).

Work procedures for confined spaces having A or B classifications require that, prior to the initiation of work, trained individuals with fully charged self-contained breathing apparatus be present in case of emergency. Backup personnel should not enter confined spaces until adequate assistance has arrived (29).

Hazards Related to Industrial Wastes Present in Sewage

In recent years a growing number of reports have identified toxic exposures to sewage workers following disposal of industrial wastes in sewage systems.

Hexachlorocyclopentadiene (HCCPD) was found to cause eye and throat irritation and headache in heavily exposed sew-

Table 54.1.   Characteristics of Common Wastewater Gases[a]

Gas and Chemical Formula	Explosive Limits		Limits for Trans. PEL (ppm)	Air Contaminants Final[c]		Common Properties	Most Common Sources of Exposure	Preferred Method of Testing
	LEL	UEL		TWA (ppm)	STEL (ppm)			
Chlorine Cl_2	Non-flammable		1 Ceiling	0.5	1	Yellow, green color; pungent odor	Chlorine cylinders and feed line leaks	Chlorine detector
Hydrogen sulfide H_2S	4.3	46	20 Ceiling	10	15	Colorless, characteristic rotten egg odor at low levels	Sewer and sludge gas; petroleum coal gas	H_2S detector Lead acetate paper and ampules
Ammonia NH_3	16	25	50	25	35	Colorless, pungent	Sewer gas	Oxygen deficiency indicator, odor
Carbon monoxide CO	12.5	74.2	50	35	200 Ceiling	Colorless, tasteless, odorless, nonirritating	Product of combustion	CO monitor
Carbon dioxide CO_2	Non-flammable		5,000	5,000	30,000	Colorless, odorless, acid taste at high levels	Sludge, sewer gas, combustion products	Oxygen deficiency indicator
Methane CH_4	5	15	No limits providing sufficient oxygen available			Colorless, odorless, tasteless	Digestion of sludge	Combustible gas indicator Oxygen deficiency indicator
Nitrogen N_2	Non-flammable					Colorless, odorless, tasteless	Sewer and sludge gas	Oxygen deficiency indicator

[a]Table 54.1 Adapted from reference 13.
[b]Transitional OSHA provisions, 29 CFR 1910.1000 Permissible exposure limits through December 30, 1992. All values are 8-hour, time-weighted averages unless otherwise noted.
[c]Final OSHA provisions, 29 CRF 1910.1000 Permissible exposure limits after December 30, 1992. TWA are 8-hour time-weighted averages. STEL are 15-minute weighted averages unless otherwise noted.

Table 54.2. Types of Confined Spaces[a]

Parameter	Class A	Class B	Class C
Characteristics	Immediately dangerous to life	Dangerous, but not immediately life-threatening	Potential hazard
Rescue procedures	At least two individuals fully equipped with life support equipment. Maintenance of communication requires an additional person stationed within the confined space.	One individual fully equipped with life support equipment; indirect visual or auditory communication with workers	Standard procedures. Direct communication with workers outside the confined space.
Oxygen	≤16 or ≥25%	16.1–19.4% 21.5–24.9%	19.5–21.4%
Explosivity	≥20% LEL	10–19% LEL	≤10% LEL
Toxicity	IDLH[b]	Greater than contamination level referenced in OSHA regulations	Less than contamination level referenced in OSHA regulations

[a]Adapted from reference 29.
[b]Immediately Dangerous to Life or Health as referenced in NIOSH Registry of Toxic and Chemical Substances or other recognized sources.

age treatment workers in Louisville, Kentucky (30). A mixture of waste compounds, consisting mostly of Stoddard's solvent and hydrochloric acid, caused a group of sewer repairmen to develop nausea, vomiting, dizziness, and eye and throat irritation (31).

Chronic effects of exposure to industrial compounds are less well documented in sewage treatment workers. Morgan described increased risk of spontaneous abortion in the spouses of sewage treatment workers (32). HCCPD was detected in urine of sewage treatment workers chronically exposed to sewage from a pesticide plant (33). Elevated levels of urinary mutagens have been reported in sewage treatment workers (34).

A medical survey of primary sewage treatment workers exposed to industrial sewage containing benzene, toluene, and other organic solvents revealed that 14 of 19 workers complained of acute central nervous system (CNS) symptoms (lightheadedness, fatigue, increased sleep requirement, and headache) consistent with solvent exposure. The majority of these symptoms resolved with transfer from the plant. Individuals working less than 1 year at this plant were more likely to complain of two or more CNS symptoms than individuals working there longer than 1 year. Objective abnormalities in neurobehavioral testing were found in all four individuals working longer than 9 years at this plant, but in only five of 15 employed there for a shorter period. Exposure to organic solvents present in sewage could have caused these acute and chronic effects (8).

Protective Measures

Proper education and training is the most important aspect of any occupational safety and health program for sewage treatment workers, as it will enable them to identify and limit potentially toxic exposures. A number of excellent resources are available to unions and management for worker education (10, 12, 13).

Continuous air monitoring is used throughout wastewater facilities to warn of potential hazards. Stationary devices alarm at high levels of hydrogen sulfide and combustible gases and signal oxygen deficiency. Portable explosivity indicators used by workers prior to entering and during work in confined spaces measure relative combustibility compared to a suitable standard (35). Odor, particularly in sewage treatment plants, should not

be relied upon to detect toxic chemicals, as the smell of these materials may be masked by the presence of other compounds.

Individuals implementing occupational safety and health programs in sewage treatment plants should utilize the "hierarchy of protection" used for other chemical exposures. Initial approaches to controlling exposures should include replacement of toxic compounds with less dangerous ones and engineering measures to lower exposures. Adequate sources of fresh air should be ensured wherever possible.

Due to the vast array of both anticipated and unanticipated chemical exposures that can occur in treatment plants, workers must have access to and be trained in the use of respiratory protective equipment.

A large number of compounds used in sewage treatment plants are irritating to or absorbed through the skin. Protection from such exposure should be provided by chemical resistant latex, neoprene, or rubber gloves. Shower and eyewash facilities should also be available in cases of emergency (12).

REFERENCES

1. Hunter D. Occupational diseases due to infections. In: The diseases of occupations. Boston: Little Brown, 1969.
2. Bell J. Sewers. In: Parmeggiani L, ed. Encyclopedia of occupational safety and health. Geneva: International Labour Office, 1983.
3. Agamennome M. Waste water treatment and disposal. In: Parmeggiani L, ed. Encyclopedia of occupational safety and health. Geneva, International Labour Office, 1983.
4. Clark CS, Cleary EJ, Schiff GM, Linneman CC, Phair JP, Briggs JM. Disease risk of occupational exposure to sewage. J Environ Engin Div 1976;102:375–388.
5. McCunney RJ. Health effects of work at waste water treatment plants: a review of the literature with guidelines for medical surveillance. Am J Ind Med 1986;9:271–279.
6. Uragoda CG. A case of chlorine poisoning of occupational origin. Ceylon Med J 1970;15:223–224.
7. Adelson L, Sunshine I. Fatal hydrogen sulfide intoxication. Report of three cases occuring in a sewer. Arch Pathol 1966;81:375–380.
8. Kraut A, Lilis R, Marcus M, Valciukas J, Wolff M, Landrigan P. Neurotoxic effects of solvent exposure in sewage treatment workers. Arch Environ Health 1988;43:263–268.
9. National Occupational Exposure Survey. Cincinnati, OH: National Institute for Occupational Safety and Health. Submitted for publication.
10. Caravanos J. Right to know handbook for sewage treatment workers. New York, 1987.
11. Stokinger HE. The halogens and the nonmetals boron and silicon in Patty's industrial hygiene and toxicology Vol 2B. 3rd ed. Clayton GD, Clayton FE, eds. New York: John Wiley and Sons, 1981.

12. Risky Business: an AFSCME health and safety guide for sewer and sewage treatment plant workers. American Federation of State County and Municipal Employees. n.d.

13. Safety and health in wastewater systems—manual of practice. VA: Water Pollution Control Federation Alexandria, 1983.

14. NIOSH criteria for a recommended standard . . . chlorine. Publication no. 76-170. DHEW (National Institute for Occupational Safety and Health).

15. Conradi Fernandez L, Inclan Cuesta M. Chlorine and inorganic compounds. In: Parmeggiani L, ed. Encyclopedia of occupational safety and health. Geneva: International Labour Office, 1983.

16. Chlorine Poisoning. Lancet 1984;1:321–322.

17. Weill H, George R, Schwatz M, Ziskind M. Late evaluation of pulmonary function after acute exposure to chlorine gas. Am Rev Respir Dis 1969;99:374–379.

18. Kaufman J, Burkons D. Clinical, roentgenologic, and physiologic effects of acute chlorine exposure. Arch Environ Health 1971;23:29–34.

19. Adelson L, Kaufman J. Fatal chlorine poisoning: report of two cases with clinicopathologic correlation. Am J Clin Pathol 1971;56:430–442.

20. Polysongsang Y, Beach BC, DiLisio RE. Pulmonary function changes after acute inhalation of chlorine gas. South Med J 1982;75:23–26.

21. Hasan FM, Gehshan A, Fuleihan FJD. Resolution of pulmonary dysfunction following acute chlorine exposure. Arch Environ Health 1983;38(2):76–80.

22. Barret L, Faure J. Chlorine poisoning. Lancet 1984;1:561–562.

23. Patil LRS, Smith RG, Vorwald AJ, Mooney TF. The health of diaphragm cell workers exposed to chlorine. Amer Ind Hyg Assoc J 1970;31:678–686.

24. Chester EH, Kaimal PJ, Payne CB, Kohn PM. Pulmonary injury following exposure to chlorine gas. Possible beneficial effects of steroid treatment. Chest 1972;72:247–250.

25. Milby TH. Hydrogen sulfide intoxication. Review of the literature and report of unusual accident resulting in two cases of nonfatal poisoning. J Occup Med 1962;4:431–437.

26. Hydrogen sulfide environmental health criteria: Number 19. Geneva: World Health Organization, 1981.

27. Stine RJ, Slosberg B, Beacham BE. Hydrogen sulfide intoxication: a case report and discussion of treatment. Ann Intern Med 1976;85:756–758.

28. Courville CB. Forensic neuropathology: the asphyxiant gases. J Forensic Sci 1964;9:19–46.

29. NIOSH criteria for a recommended standard . . . working in confined spaces. Publication No. 80-106. DHEW (National Institute for Occupational Safety and Health).

30. Morse DL, Kominssky JR, Wisseman CL, Landrigan PJ. Occupational exposure to hexachlorocyclopentadiene: how safe is sewage? JAMA 1979;241:217–279.

31. Sewer collapse and toxic illness in sewer repairmen-Ohio. MMWR 1981;30:89–90.

32. Morgan RW, Kheifets L, Obrinsky DL, Whorton MD, Foliant DE. Fetal loss and work at a waste water treatment plant. Am J Public Health 1984;74:499–501.

33. Elia VJ, Clark CS, Majeti VA, et al. Hazardous chemical exposure at a municipal wastewater treatment plant. Environ Res 1983;32:360–371.

34. Scarlett-Kranz JM, Babish JG, Stickland D, Goodrich RM, Lisk DJ. Urinary mutagens in municipal sewage workers and water treatment workers. Am J Epidemiol 1986;124:884–892.

35. National Safety Council Atmospheres in Sub-surface structures and sewers. Data sheet i-550-Rev.85. Chicago: NSC, 1985.

55

Toxic Hazards of the Pulp and Paper Industry

Melanie A. Marty, Ph.D.
Dennis J. Shusterman, M.D., M.P.H.

The pulp industry in the United States annually produces about 54 million metric tons of cellulose material for the subsequent manufacture of paper, cardboard, and fiberboard, or almost one-quarter ton per capita (1). The process of transforming a corresponding volume of wood chips into pulp requires large scale industrial facilities with major economic, environmental, and aesthetic impacts upon adjoining communities. A long-standing public awareness of the nuisance quality of odorous air emissions from pulp mills has been joined in recent years by concerns regarding compounds of potential toxicologic significance in the mills' air and water effluent. In addition, intensive use of a variety of hazardous materials raises inevitable questions regarding worker health and safety.

PROCESS DESCRIPTION

Pulp mills function to extract and process cellulose fibers from wood, simultaneously removing unwanted constituents, such as lignin (wood's intercellular "glue"). The majority of pulp mills operating in the United States use the sulfate or "kraft" method. This method relies heavily on chemical digestion. Perhaps 20% of domestic pulp production involves nonkraft processes, including the groundwood, semichemical, and sulfite techniques (1). Because of the small fraction of production represented by each of these methods, our detailed consideration of production processes will be limited to kraft mills.

Figure 55.1 is a simplified process diagram for a kraft mill. Included in this representation are input (raw materials), output (product and by-products), and closed-loop (recycled) processes. The principal raw materials for the kraft process are wood chips, water, fuel, and bleaching agents (most commonly, chlorine and chlorine dioxide). Sodium sulfide (used in the digestion of the pulp) is recycled through operation of the recovery furnace, evaporators, and lime kiln; however, the escape of even a small fraction of the recirculating sulfur (as hydrogen sulfide, organic sulfides, and various mercaptans) gives pulp mill air emissions their characteristic odor.

The operation of a kraft pulp mill can be summarized as follows. Wood chips are broken down by a combination of sodium sulfide (in basic solution) and heat. The resulting pulp is washed and bleached with a combination of molecular chlorine and chlorine dioxide or hypochlorite. The washed pulp is rolled and dried, and the dried pulp cut and baled for shipment. Wastewater from the bleaching process is typically discharged directly, or with minimal treatment (e.g., an aerated stabilization basin), into a nearby body of water. Spent digester fluid is concentrated in evaporators and fed into the recovery furnace, which recycles solid sodium sulfide and combusts the dissolved lignin as a source of energy. A lime kiln recovers calcium oxide for regeneration of the caustic component of the digester fluid (2–4).

AIRBORNE EMISSIONS FROM KRAFT PULP MILLS

Irritant and Odorant Chemicals

Reduced sulfur compounds are remarkable for their odorant potency; the odor threshold of ethyl mercaptan, for example, has been measured as low as 0.01 ppb (5). The U.S. Environmental Protection Agency (EPA), which has regulated pulp mill emissions since 1978, has formulated an aggregate measure of reduced sulfur gas emissions from pulp mills, known as total reduced sulfur (TRS). Principal sources of TRS emissions in pulp mills include the lime kiln and main recovery furnace (as stack gases) and various "rooftop" sources (e.g., offgasing from the digester). Operational upsets (e.g., breached seals on the digester) can produce significant transients in TRS emissions.

The single most prominent fraction of pulp mill TRS is hydrogen sulfide (H_2S). Published odor thresholds for H_2S range from 0.5–20 ppb, with a geometric mean of 8.1 ppb (5, 6). Upper respiratory irritation does not occur below about 10 ppm. Objective signs of H_2S upper respiratory irritation occur between 50 and 100 ppm. Concentrations in the range of 100–200 ppm produce olfactory fatigue, while 250–500 ppm exposures have been associated with pulmonary edema. Exposures in the 500–1000 ppm range are associated with systemic toxicity including confusion, dysequilibrium, convulsions, respiratory paralysis, and death (7). Systemic toxicity occurs via inhibition of the cytochrome oxidase system, in a manner analogous to cyanide (8).

Controversy exists concerning whether H_2S exposures produce subacute or chronic effects. The vast majority of case reports of severe H_2S intoxication (those involving loss of consciousness with or without convulsions) report either a fatal outcome or recovery without permanent sequelae (9, 10). The World Health Agency defines chronic, "low-level" H_2S exposures as those occurring between 50 and 100 ppm, and associates these with ". . . lingering, largely subjective manifestations of illness" (11). In experimental systems, mice exposed to 100 ppm H_2S by inhalation for 2 hours/day over 4 days showed progressive inhibition of cerebral cytochrome oxidase activity (12), while guinea pigs exposed to 20 ppm of H_2S for 1 hour/day over 11 days showed significant lowering of phospholipid concentrations in the cerebral hemispheres and brainstem, but not in the cerebellum (13). The human health significance of these animal observations is unclear.

The other reduced sulfur gases of concern in pulp mill air emissions—methyl mercaptan, dimethyl sulfide, and dimethyl disulfide—have been less extensively studied than has hydrogen sulfide, but appear to exhibit the same general toxicologic properties (14, 15). Reported odor thresholds for methyl mercaptan range from 0.02–42 ppb, with a geometric mean of 1.6 ppb; for dimethyl sulfide the range is 1–20 ppb, with a mean

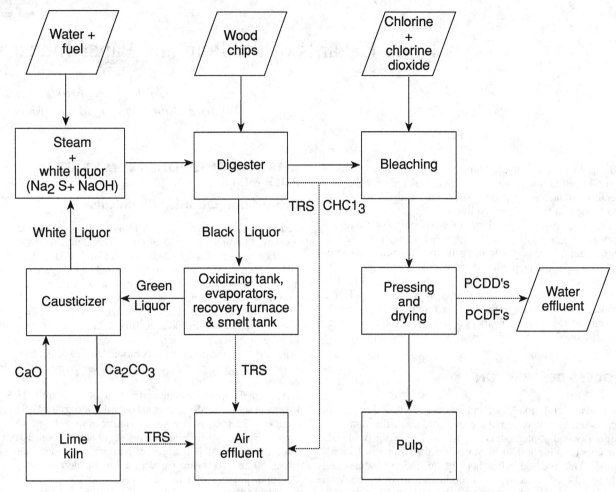

Figure 55.1.   Kraft pulping process.

value of 11 ppb, and for dimethyl disulfide the corresponding values are 0.3, 90, and 41 ppb (5, 6). The relative odorant potencies of these compounds exceed their irritant and systemic toxicity by an even greater factor than is the case for hydrogen sulfide, making it difficult for irritant or toxic exposures to occur except in situations of impaired escape.

In contrast to the reduced sulfur gases, sulfur dioxide (SO_2), an odorant above about 0.5 ppm and respiratory irritant over 2 ppm (5), has relatively poor warning properties. Some asthmatics may be sensitive to SO_2 concentrations as low as 0.25–0.3 ppm, particularly when exercising (16, 17). Community monitoring for SO_2 is required under the Federal Clean Air Act, but given the dilution factor from stack to community, the compound is more likely to pose a hazard to pulp mill workers than to the general public (18). For example, acute SO_2 overexposures among pulp mill workers have resulted both in immediate fatalities and in the development of chronic, irreversible airflow obstruction, with or without bronchiolitis obliterans (19, 20). Similarly, pulp mill workers who report having been exposed to leaks of chlorine or chlorine dioxide, two other irritant gases, appear to be at risk for developing subsequent obstructive pulmonary symptoms and spirometric abnormalities (21).

Table 55.1 summarizes the toxicology and occupational exposure standards for irritant and/or odorant chemicals used in (or emitted from) kraft pulp mills, including digester chemicals,

bleaching agents, reduced sulfur gases, and sulfur dioxide. The occupational standard for hydrogen sulfide exposure, for example, has been set by the Occupational Safety and Health Administration (OSHA) at 10 ppm (8-hour, time-weighted average) and 15 ppm (15-minute, short-term exposure limit), based on the compound's irritancy (22). The State of California treats H_2S as an ambient criteria pollutant, with a 1-hour ambient standard of 30 ppb; this level was set at a multiple of the odor threshold calculated to produce an annoyance reaction in the public (23). Sulfur dioxide is regulated at the federal level as a criteria pollutant, with an annual average limit of 0.03 ppm and a 24-hour standard of 0.14 ppm. California has a lower (0.05 ppm) 24-hour SO_2 standard, as well as a 0.25 ppm 1-hour limit.

Industrial hygiene surveys of kraft pulp mills have documented peak H_2S levels within work areas up to 20 ppm (with mean levels between 0.05 and 2.0 ppm) and peak methyl mercaptan levels up to 15 ppm (mean levels between 0.07 and 3.7 ppm). Specific locations with high exposure potential include the chip chute and evaporation vacuum pumps. Sulfur dioxide tends to be more of a problem in sulfite mills, with peak levels up to 23 ppm (mean levels ranging from 0.05–5.7 ppm) (18). Because of the oxidizing environment of the recovery furnace and lime kiln, most H_2S entering these combustion devices is converted to sulfur dioxide. Given the further dilution of stack and fugitive emissions as they disperse offsite, community ex-

Table 55.1. Irritant and Odorant Chemicals in the Kraft Pulp Process

Source	Chemical	Toxicity	ACGIH TLV-TWA	OSHA PEL-TWA
PROCESSING				
Digestion	Sodium sulfide	Caustic; skin, eye, and upper respiratory irritant	10 ppm (H_2S)	10 ppm (H_2S)
	Sodium hydroxide	Caustic; skin, eye, and upper respiratory irritant	2 mg/m*	2 mg/m*
	Anthraquinone	Phototoxic dermatitis		
Bleaching	Chlorine gas	Upper + lower respiratory irritant	0.5 ppm	0.5 ppm
	Chlorine dioxide	Upper + lower respiratory irritant	0.1 ppm	0.1 ppm
EFFLUENT				
Air	Hydrogen sulfide	Odorant; upper + lower respiratory irritant; cellular poison	10 ppm	10 ppm
	Methyl mercaptan	"	0.5 ppm	0.5 ppm
	Dimethyl sulfide	"	—	—
	Dimethyl disulfide	"	—	—
	Sulfur dioxide	Upper + lower respiratory irritant; bronchoconstrictor	2 ppm	2 ppm

ABBREVIATIONS:
TLV-TWA = ''Threshold Limit Value — [8-hour] Time-Weighted Average'' (Recommended standard of the American Conference of Governmental Industrial Hygienists)
PEL-TWA = ''Permissible Exposure Limit — [8-hour] Time-Weighted Average'' (Enforceable standard of the Occupational Safety and Health Administration) •
     * = ''Ceiling'' Standard (not to be exceeded at any time)

REFERENCES:
American Conference of Governmental Industrial Hygienists: Threshold Limit Values and Biological Exposure Indices for 1990–1991. Cincinnati, ACGIH, 1990.
U.S. Department of Labor, Occupational Safety and Health Administration: Air Contaminants — Permissible Exposure Limits. Washington, D.C., USGPO, 1989.

posures to reduced sulfur gases are generally in the low ppb range, above the odor threshold but below levels known to produce objective irritant effects.

Chlorinated Compounds

The major chlorinated hydrocarbon emitted into ambient air from bleached kraft pulp mills is chloroform. The U.S. EPA estimates that approximately 3340 metric tons chloroform per year is emitted from the pulp and paper industry, accounting for 40% of all chloroform air emissions in the U.S. (24). Chloroform is produced during the pulp bleaching process by the reaction of chlorine or chlorine compounds and lignins in the pulp suspension, followed by degradation of chlorinated lignins in the alkaline extraction stage. The chloroform subsequently evaporates into the air from the wastewater stream. Use of hypochlorite for bleaching pulp results in the greatest production of chloroform. Substitution of chlorine dioxide for hypochlorite salts has been suggested as a control measure for chloroform that would result in a 92% reduction in chloroform emissions from pulp mills (24).

Chloroform is acutely toxic at high concentrations (e.g., anesthetic concentrations of 5000 ppm), producing adverse effects in the liver and kidney, the cardiovascular system, and the central nervous system. At concentrations in ambient air, one would not expect acute or chronic noncancer health effects to occur (25). The major concern in terms of public health is a potential increased risk of cancer from inhalation of chlo-

roform in ambient air. Chloroform carcinogenic potency and classification are summarized in Table 55.2.

Other halogenated volatile organics that may become airborne as a result of evaporation from wastewater include methylene chloride, trichloroethylene, tetrachloroethylene, carbon tetrachloride, bromodichloromethane, and chlorodibromomethane. All of these compounds are mutagenic, and the first four have tested positive in animal carcinogenicity bioassays. As is the case for chloroform, the major public health concern would be a potential increase in the risk of cancer from inhalation of these compounds in ambient air.

No studies have adequately documented concentrations of volatile halogenated organics in ambient air near pulp mills. However, measurements of chloroform in many locations in California (not near pump mills) indicate that chloroform is a ubiquitous contaminant of ambient air, with concentrations ranging from 0.13–1.8 μg chloroform per m^3 of air. The excess cancer risk could range up to about 5 in a million from inhalation of chloroform in ambient air (25). The risk in a community surrounding a major source of chloroform, such as a pulp mill, could conceivably be higher.

The concentrations of 2,3,7,8-tetrachlorodibenzo-p-dioxin (2,3,7,8-TCDD) toxic equivalents in the stack gases of three kraft mill recovery furnaces were <0.01, 0.01, and 0.12 ng/dscm at 3% O_2 (26). These data indicate that recovery furnaces are not as important a source of environmental polychlorinated dibenzo-p-dioxin (PCDD) and dibenzofuran (PCDF) as other combustion sources.

Table 55.2.   Some Carcinogens Present in Bleached Kraft Mill Effluent

Compound	Class[a]	Cancer Potency[b]	Level of Evidence[c] Human	Animal
Benzene	A	2.9×10^{-2}	S	S
Carbon tetrachloride	B2	1.3×10^{-1}	I	S
Chloroform	B2	8.1×10^{-2}	I	S
1,2-Dichloroethane	B2	9.1×10^{-2}	I	S
Hexachlorobenzene	B2	1.7	I	S
Hexachlorodibenzodioxin	B2	$6.2 \times 10^{+3}$	I	S
Methylene chloride	B2	1.4×10^{-2}	I	S
2,3,7,8-Tetrachlorodibenzo-p-dioxin	B2	$1.6 \times 10^{+5}$	I	S
Tetrachloroethylene	B2	5.1×10^{-2}	I	S
Trichloroethylene	B2	1.1×10^{-2}	I	S
2,4,6-Trichlorophenol	B2	2.0×10^{-2}	I	S

[a]Classification of carcinogen under the U.S. EPA. A = sufficient evidence of carcinogenicity in humans and animals. B2 = inadequate evidence of carcinogenicity in humans, and sufficient evidence of carcinogenicity in animals.

[b]These cancer potency values, expressed in units of inverse dose, (mg/kg-day)$^{-1}$, were derived by the U.S. EPA. When multiplied by lifetime dose, the product is the theoretical lifetime risk of contracting cancer when exposed to the chemical at the given dose level.

[c]The level of evidence refers to the basis for classification into EPA's class of carcinogen. I = inadequate; S = sufficient.

Particulate Emissions

Particulate emission sources at a pulp mill include the kraft recovery furnaces, lime kilns, smelt dissolving tanks, and power boilers, which are frequently wood-fired (27). The typical kraft recovery furnace equipped with an electrostatic precipitator emits about 0.2 g particulate per m^3, mainly as sodium salts and black ash, with mass mean diameters on the order of 1.5 μm. Average emissions from existing lime kilns controlled with venturi scrubbers are about 0.15–0.3 g particulate per m^3. Particulates from the lime kilns consist of relatively large (>10μm) particles of lime dust, and small (mass mean diameter < 1μm) particles of sodium sulfate and sodium carbonate. Smelt-dissolving tanks emit primarily sodium sulfate and sodium carbonate particles less than 1 μm in mass mean particle diameter, at rates of about 0.1 g particulate per m^3.

U.S. EPA estimates the production of particulate from the recovery furnace at 0.5–12 kg/kkg (kilokilograms) of product. Estimates for other units include: 0.01–0.5 kg/kkg from the smelt dissolving tanks; 0.15–2.5 kg/kkg from lime kilns; and 0.012–0.4 kg/kkg from power boilers (28).

The major health impact of particulate emissions is dependent on the chemical composition of the particulate matter, the particle size distribution, and air dispersion and dilution. Little data exist that quantify particulate matter in the ambient air surrounding pulp mills. However, the potential exists for adverse respiratory health effects under appropriate meteorologic conditions, particularly from small particles (e.g., respirable particles 1–10 μm in diameter) of lime and sulfates that escape from the lime kilns and smelt tanks.

WATERBORNE EMISSIONS FROM KRAFT PULP MILLS

The kraft pulping process results in production of a large amount of contaminated water, which is discharged with little treatment into a receiving body of water. The processes of wood digestion and subsequent bleaching produce an enormous number of chemicals, many of them chlorinated. Hundreds of these chemicals have been identified (29, 30) and associated with a particular process or bleaching stage within the kraft mill (31–

35). The compounds formed vary with the type of wood being processed, as well as the process itself. Among the compounds identified in bleached kraft pulp mill effluents are resin acids, organic acids and their chlorinated derivatives, and small chain volatile chlorinated organics, as well as chlorinated phenols, guaiacols, benzenes, aldehydes, ketones, thiophenes, terpenes, and large polycyclic compounds including PCDDs and PCDFs. It has been estimated that a kraft mill with production of 1000 tons of pulp per day using conventional chlorine bleaching produces 50–65 tons of chlorinated organic substances per day and discharges 30–40 million gallons (120–160 million liters) effluent/day (36, 37). Estimation of the concentrations of some of these compounds in treated and raw effluent is found in Table 55.3.

Recently, concern has been building over the production of PCDDs and PCDFs in the pulp mill bleaching processes, and the resulting environmental contamination with these highly toxic compounds. The U.S. EPA analyzed samples of fish from many bodies of water in the United States and noticed a correlation between levels of 2,3,7,8-tetrachlorodibenzo-p-dioxin (2,3,7,8-TCDD) in fish tissue and the frequency of pulp and paper manufacturing plants in the watershed of contaminated fish (38). The U.S. EPA and the paper industry are currently conducting a joint study to document the extent of dioxins discharged by the industry. The study will sample effluent, sludges, and pulp at each of 104 pulp mills in the United States that bleach with chlorine. Preliminary results of effluent analyses for 72 mills show an average concentration of 58 parts per trillion (ppt) 2,3,7,8-TCDD and 415 ppt 2,3,7,8-tetrachlorodibenzofuran (2,3,7,8-TCDF) (39). Applying the March 1989 U.S. EPA toxicity equivalents scheme, the mean concentration expressed as 2,3,7,8-TCDD equivalents is 100 ppt.

Keuhl and colleagues found that samples of sludge from seven pulp and paper mill plants contained 2,3,7,8-TCDD ranging from nondetectable at 1 pg/g to 414 pg/g (40). The variability is probably the result of different process parameters at the different mills. Sludge from one mill was characterized further; this sample contained 1860 pg octaCDD per g, 800 pg 2,3,7,8-TCDF per g, 640 pg other TCDF per g, and 150 pg 2,3,7,8-TCDD per g. The finding of PCDDs and PCDFs in pulp mill sludge has raised concern about the practice of using

Table 55.3.   Common Contaminants of Bleached Kraft Pulp Mill Effluents Before and After Biologic Treatment. Adapted from U.S. EPA (1984).

Chemical	Pulp Mill[a]	Concentration (μg/l)		%R[b]
		Untreated Average	Treated Average	
Benzene	M	1	2	0
1,1,1-Trichloroethane	F	24	0	100
2,4,6-Trichlorophenol	M	11	5	55
	B	8	1	88
Chloroform	D	647	67	90
	M	1,405	12	99
	B	1,550	16	99
2,4-Dichlorophenol	M	4	4	0
	B	2	1	50
Dichlorobromomethane	D	1	0	100
	F	15	0	100
Pentachlorophenol	B	19	19	0
	F	8	1	88
Tetrachloroethylene	B	3	0	100
	F	1	0	100
Trichloroethylene	B	2	0	100
Abietic acid	D	11,800	1,467	88
	M	178	767	0
	B	1,043	119	89
	F	470	3	99
Dehydroabietic acid	D	3,500	520	99
	M	232	431	86
	B	861	123	86
	F	273	5	98
Isopimaric acid	D	887	380	57
	M	115	407	0
	B	107	21	80
	F	74	98	
Pimaric acid	D	1,357	710	48
	M	157	430	0
	B	115	22	81
	F	63	0	100
Epoxystearic acid	D	817	0	100
Chlorodehydroabietic acid	D	1,433	473	67
	M	50	42	16
	B	78	11	86
	F	44	0	100
Dichlorodehydroabietic acid	M	57	39	32
	B	3	1	67
	F	6	0	100
Trichloroguaiacol	M	18	0	100
	B	1	0	100
	F	4	1	75
Tetrachloroguaiacol	M	11	0	100
	B	8	1	88
	F	7	3	57

[a]Data were obtained for various subcategories of bleached kraft pulp mills. B = bleached kraft pulp mills producing pulp for coarse paper uses, such as paperboard, tissue. D = bleached kraft pulp mills producing dissolving pulp, a highly refined pulp containing virtually no lignin used in the manufacture of rayon, cellophane, and cellulose acetate and nitrate. F = bleached kraft pulp mill producing fine pulp for use in printing and writing paper. M = bleached kraft pulp mill producing market pulp from wood not destined for a particular use, and sold on the open market.

[b]%R = approximate percent reduction in concentration by biologic treatment. These are only approximations as they are taken from averages of a number of mills with variations in treatment. However, one can see that certain chemicals are biodegraded or volatilized more readily than others. Note the large variability in amount of chemical produced with the type of pulp produced.

pulp mill sludge as a soil amendment with concomitant contamination of the environment, particularly with respect to contamination of the agricultural food chain (41).

The pulp, filtrate, and fines from an 850 ton/day bleached softwood kraft pulp mill contained about 90–100 pg 2,3,7,8-TCDF per g, and about 10 pg 2,3,7,8-TCDD per g after the first chlorination stage (35). Gas chromatography/mass spectrometry chromatograms revealed that the predominant isomers were 1,2,7,8- and 2,3,7,8-TCDF and 2,3,7,8-TCDD. Recent studies have documented the presence of ppt levels of PCDDs and PCDFs in finished paper products including newsprint, coffee filters, cosmetic tissue, and recycled scrap paper (42).

Several studies have shown that the pulp bleaching processes substantially influence the amount of PCDDs/PCDFs formed (35, 39, 40, 43–45). Substitution of chlorine dioxide for chlorine, a reduction in the ratio of chlorine to lignin, and use of oxygen delignification result in significant drops in the production of PCDDs and PCDFs.

The toxicity of kraft pulp mill effluents to fish has been extensively studied and is summarized below. There are a limited amount of published toxicologic data for a handful of the compounds present in pulp mill effluent. Mutagenicity and carcinogenicity of some important constituents of pulp mill effluent are reviewed below. The review by Soklow describes other toxicologic endpoints of some constituents of bleached kraft mill effluent (28).

Aquatic Toxicity

The constituents of bleached kraft mill effluent (BKME) considered to be most toxic to fish are resin acids, chlorinated phenolics, and low molecular weight chlorinated neutral compounds (46, 47). 2,6-Dichlorohydroquinone and some polychlorodihydroxybenzenes have also been implicated as acute toxicants present in first chlorination stage effluents (33, 48).

Neutralized BKME (without further treatment) commonly have 96-hour LC50 values ranging from 15–50% (v/v) (48). Exposures to various concentrations of BKME resulted in a number of adverse physiologic and biochemical changes in a variety of fish species (48–54). Adverse effects in fish have been noted both in the laboratory and in the field in fish caught near effluent outflows. Such changes included decreased swimming speed and stamina, changes in respiration and arterial tension, changes in blood cell count, aberrant carbohydrate metabolism, elevated hepatic cytochrome P-450-dependent monooxygenase activities, impaired ion homeostasis, and pathologic changes. Reproductive toxicity observed following exposure to bleached kraft mill effluent (BKME) includes: decreased egg hatchability, decreased egg survival, developmental abnormalities, retarded growth and development, increased mortality, reduced sperm motility, and inhibited fertilization (55–61).

Mutagenicity of Chemicals in Bleached Kraft Pulp Mill Effluent

Several investigators have reported that chlorination-stage effluent from bleaching of kraft pulp produced positive dose-related mutagenic responses in the Ames-Salmonella assay (46, 62–64). The response was reduced upon addition of rat liver S9 mix or following passage of the effluent through XAD-2 resin. Virtually all of the mutagenic activity was recovered in

the neutral fraction, which contained compounds of moderate polarity. Several chloroacetones and aldehydes were found to induce dose-related increases in mutation frequency in *Salmonella* (Table 55.4) (62, 64). Douglas and colleagues state that chloroacetones appear to be major contributors to mutagenic activity of chlorination stage effluents and that mutagenicity of a mixture of chloroacetones was greater than additive. However, levels of chloroacetones in chlorination stage effluents vary considerably. In addition, chloroacetones are labile in alkaline solution (62), and the contribution to mutagenicity of total pulp mill effluent may be pH-dependent.

Other compounds present in BKME identified as mutagenic in the Ames/Salmonella assay are presented in Table 55.3 and include resin acids and chlorinated propenes, methanes, ethanes, and a furanone (64–69). 2,3,7,8-TCDD has been tested in the Ames/Salmonella test system and is generally regarded as non-mutagenic in bacteria (70–72).

Chlorination-stage effluent concentrate was found to induce gene conversion, mitotic recombination, and aberrant colony formation in *Saccharomyces cerevisiae* strain D7 (63). Several constituents of pulp mill effluent, including chlorinated catechols, guaiacols, acetones, aldehydes, and propenes, are mutagenic in strains of *S. cerevisiae* (Tale 55.3), inducing reversions in strain XV185-14C in the absence of exogenous metabolic activating system (73, 75). Several chlorinated acetones and ethanes, 2,3,7,8-TCDD, dibromochloromethane and dichlorobromomethane produced gene conversion in *S. cerevisiae* strain D7 (74–76). Addition of S9 as an exogenous metabolic activating system increased the activity of 1,1,3-trichloroacetone and trichloroacetaldehyde but not the other test compounds.

Priha and Talka found that certain fractions of BKME induced threefold increases in sister chromatid exchange (SCE) in Chinese hamster ovary cells without metabolic activation (46). Several constituents of BKME induced increases in SCE, chromosomal aberrations, micronuclei formation, cell transformation, and mutation frequency, as well as changes in mitotic index in mammalian cell lines and vertebrates in vivo (Table 55.4) (67, 69, 77–79).

Carcinogenicity of Constituents of Bleached Kraft Mill Effluent

Several compounds identified in BKME are considered to be carcinogens by the U.S. EPA and the International Agency for Research on Cancer, including the volatile organic compounds chloroform, trichloroethylene, methylene chloride, ethylene dichloride, tetrachloroethylene, and benzene (80). These chemicals are volatilized into the air during effluent treatment and discharge. As such, some of the volatile organic compounds may be more important in terms of air contaminants than as water pollutants; however, the concentrations of chloroform, for example, are quite high in the effluent prior to dilution in receiving waters (see Table 55.2).

Other less volatile chlorinated carcinogens present in BKME include 2,4,6-trichlorophenol, pentachlorophenol, hexachlorobenzene, 2,3,7,8-tetrachlorodibenzodioxin and hexachlorodibenzodioxins. The known carcinogens and their classification and approximate potencies are listed in Table 55.2. Of these carcinogens, the most potent are the PCDDs.

Other toxic effects of a number of BKME constituents are reviewed in U.S. EPA (28).

Table 55.4.   Some Mutagenic Constituents of Bleached Kraft Mill Effluent

Compound	Test[a]	Strain/Cell[b]	Concentration[c]	Reference
Neoabietic acid	Ames/Salm	TA1535, TA100, TA1538, TA98	250–1000 µg/plt	Nestmann et al. (66)
	Reversion Trp +	S. cerevisiae XV 185-14C	100–1000 µg/ml	Nestmann and Lee (73)
1,1,2,3-Tetrachloro-2-propene	Ames/Salm	TA1535, TA100, TA98	10 µg/plt	Nestmann et al. (66)
	Fluctuation	S. typhimurium TA1535	0.2 µM	Ellenton et al. (67)
	Fluctuation	E. coli WP2	0.1 mM	Ellenton et al. (67)
	Reversion	S. cerevisiae	0.1–0.4 µl/ml	Nestmann and Lee (73)
	SCE	CHO	0.1 mM	Ellenton et al. (67)
	Chrom. Aber.	CHO	5.0 mM	Ellenton et al. (67)
	Chrom. Aber.	CHO	1.0 mM	Ellenton et al. (67)
1,1,2,3,3-Pentachloropropene	Ames/Salm	TA1535, TA100	10 µg/plt	Nestmann et al. (66)
	Reversion Trp +, Hom +	S. cerevisiae XV185-14C	0.1–0.2 µl/ml	Nestmann and Lee (73)
1,2-Dichloroethane	Ames/Salm dessicator	TA1535, TA100	3–9 mg/plt	Nestmann et al. (66)
	Conversion Trp +	S. cerevisiae D7	0.001–0.1 µl/ml	Nestmann and Lee (75)
1,3-Dichloroacetone	Ames/Salm	TA1535	4.5 µg/plt[d]	Kringstad et al. (64)
	Conversion Trp +	S. cerevisiae D7	0.0001–0.01 µg/ml	Nestmann and Lee (75)
2-Chloropropenal	Ames/Salm	TA1535	0.1 µg/plt[e]	Kringstad et al. (64)
Trichloroethylene	Ames/Salm	TA1535	0.1 mg/plt	Kringstad et al. (64)
Monochloroacetaldehyde	Ames/Salm	TA1535	45 µg/plt	Kringstad et al. (64)
Trichloroacetaldehyde	Reversion Trp +	S. cerevisiae XV185-14C	50–1000 µg/ml	Nestmann and Lee (75)
XF[f]	Ames/Salm	TA100	4.5 µg/plt	Holmbom (68)
	Chrom. Aber.	CHO	4.0 µg/ml	U.S. EPA (69)
	Mitotic Index	CHO	8.5 µg/ml	U.S. EPA (69)
Acetovanillone	Reversion Trp +, Hom +	S. cerevisiae XV185-14C	200–800 µg/ml	Nestmann and Lee (73)
3-Chloro-cis-muconic acid	Reversion Trp +, Hom +	S. cerevisiae XV185-14C	10–250 µg/ml	Nestmann and Lee (73)
4,5-Dichlorocatechol	Reversion Trp +, Hom +	S. cerevisiae XV185-14C	25–100 µg/ml	Nestmann and Lee (73)
4,5-Dichloroguaiacol	Reversion Trp +, Hom +	S. cerevisiae XV185-14C	25–75 µg/ml	Nestmann and Lee (73)
Dichloromethane	Ames/Salm dessicator	TA1535, TA100	0.5 ml/dess	Nestmann et al. (66)
Dibromochloromethane	Conversion Trp +	S. cerevisiae D7	0.001–0.5 µl/ml	Nestmann and Lee (75)
1,1,1-Trichloroethane	Ames/Salm dessicator	TA1535, TA100	0.1–1.0 ml/dess	Nestmann et al. (66)
1,1,3-Trichloroacetone	Ames/Salm	TA100	0.01–0.05 µl/plt	Douglas et al. (62)
	Conversion Trp +	S. cerevisiae D7	0.001–0.1 µl/ml	Nestmann and Lee (75)

continues

Table 55.4. *Continued*

Compound	Test[a]	Strain/Cell[b]	Concentration[c]	Reference
1,1,1-Trichloroacetone	Conversion Trp +	*S. cerevisiae* D7	0.001–0.1 μl/ml	Nestmann and Lee (75)
1,1,1,3-Tetrachloroacetone	Reversion His +	*S. cerevisiae* XV185-14C	0.0005–0.005 μl/ml	Nestmann and Lee (75)
1,1,3,3-Tetrachloroacetone	Ames/Salm	TA100	0.01–0.05 μl/plt	Douglas et al. (62)
	Conversion Trp +	*S. cerevisiae* D7	0.0001–0.01 μl/ml	Nestmann and Lee (75)
Pentachloroacetone	Ames/Salm	TA100	0.01–0.2 μl/plt	Douglas et al. (62)
	Conversion Trp +	*S. cerevisiae* D7	0.001–0.1 μl/ml	Nestmann and Lee (75)
Hexachloroacetone	Ames/Salm	TA100	0.1–0.5 μl/plt	Douglas et al. (62)
	Ames/Salm	TA1535	1.0 mg/plt	Kringstad et al. (64)
7-Oxodehydroabietic acid	Reversion Trp +	*S. cerevisiae* XV185-14C	100–1000 μg/ml	Nestmann and Lee (73)
2,3,7,8-Tetrachlorodibenzo-p-dioxin	Conversion	*S. cerevisiae*	?	Bronzetti et al. (76)
	Cell transf.	BHK	0.025–0.25 μg/ml	Hay et al. (79)
	Mouse lymph. mutat. freq.	L5178Y	0.05–0.5 μg/ml	Rogers et al. (78)

[a]genotoxicity assay; Ames/Salm = the Ames assay using *Salmonella typhimurium* in a plate incorporation system; Reversion = gene reversion assay using the yeast *Saccharomyces cerevisiae*; Conversion = gene conversion assay using *S. cerevisiae*. Loci which the reversion and conversion test systems examine are indicated in this column; Cell transf. = cell transformation assay; SCE = sister chromatid exchange; chrom. aber. = chromosomal aberrations.
[b]The strain of *S. typhimurium* and *S. cerevisiae* are indicated in this column. Mammalian cell types used in SCE and cell transformation assays are as follows: CHO = Chinese hamster ovary cells; BHK = baby hamster kidney cells.
[c]Unless otherwise noted, the lowest concentration tested that produced at least a doubling in the mutation frequency, or, concentration range over which a positive dose-response was observed. μg/plt = micrograms/plate; ml/dess = milliliters per dessicator, referring to the assays for volatile compounds conducted by placing the compound in a dessicator containing plates of bacterial tester strains.
[d]This concentration of 1,3-dichloroacetone induced a 13-fold increase in mutation frequency relative to controls.
[e]This concentration of 2-chloropropenal induced a 20-fold increase in mutation frequency relative to controls.
[f]XF = 3-chloro-4-(dichloromethyl)-5-hydroxy-2(5H)-furanone

Human Exposure

BIOACCUMULATION IN FISH

Some of the compounds in BKME may reach the human food chain through bioaccumulation in fish. Rainbow trout bioconcentrated 2,4,6-trichlorophenol, trichloroguaiacol, and tetrachloroguaiacol in liver and muscle tissue (81). 2,4,6-Trichlorophenol, 2,3,4,6-tetrachlorophenol, 4,5,6-trichloroguaiacol, 3,4,5,6-tetrachloroguaiacol, and pentachlorophenol were found at concentrations greater than 1 mg/ml in the bile of fish living 1 kilometer from a pulp mill outflow (49, 82). Resin acids (pimaric, isopimaric, abietic, and dehydroabietic acids) were also found in the bile at concentrations of about 1 mg/l. Resin acids and chlorophenolics were measurable in the bile of perch *Perra fluviatilis* and roach *Rutilis rutilis* 15 kilometers downstream from the effluent outflow (82). These compounds were not detected in fish upstream of the effluent outflow.

Concentrations of 2,4,6-trichlorophenol, 2,3,4,6-tetrachlorophenol, and pentachlorophenol in the plasma of lake trout exposed to simulated BKME were, respectively, 50, 150, and 275 times higher than in the water (49). Bile concentrations of these compounds ranged up to 32,000 times (pentachlorophenol) higher than in the water.

Bioconcentration factors (BCFs) for a number of compounds including chlorinated guaiacols, chlorinated aliphatics, and chlorinated benzenes are tabulated in Suntio et al. (29). BCFs for several carcinogenic constituents of BKME are listed in this review including those for benzene, chloroform, carbon tetrachloride, dichloromethane, and hexachlorobenzene. Pentachlorobenzene and hexachlorobenzene have the highest bioconcentration factor (log of the BCF in rainbow trout ranges up to 5.37). Other toxic compounds with notable BCFs listed in Suntio et al. (29) include monochlorobenzene, dichloro-, trichloro-, and tetrachlorobenzenes. Lindstrom and Osterberg (31) state that about 10–15% of total organically bound chlorine in the bleach plant effluent is lipophilic and may pose a hazard through bioaccumulation.

PCDDs and PCDFs are lipophilic compounds and are readily bioaccumulated in aquatic organisms. BCFs have been measured for 2,3,7,8-TCDD by a number of investigators and range from about 1000 to upwards of 86,000 (83–86). Variability in measured BCFs can be attributed to fat content, species, presence of humic material and sediment, and a host of other factors. Preliminary results of the U.S. EPA National Bioaccumulation Study revealed that PCDD/PCDF concentrations in fish sampled near pulp mill outflows were in the 10–200 ppt range (39). In addition to cancer risk from PCDDs and PCDFs, bioaccumulation of these compounds may present a risk of other toxic effects including immunotoxicity, reproductive toxicity, and endocrine abnormalities (87–95). Cancer risks to humans from consumption of carcinogen-contaminated fish may be significant and would depend on a number of factors including extent of recreational or commercial fishing of contaminated fish, per capita fish consumption, extent of contamination, and validity of extrapolation of results from animal cancer bioassays to humans.

DRINKING WATER

Swedish investigators observed longrange transport of chlorinated organics originating from a 200,000 ton/year kraft pulp mill through a river basin with ultimate contamination of a public drinking water supply (96). In the finished drinking water, pulp mill effluent constituents accounted for more than 50% of the chlorinated organics, while chlorination of the finished drinking water accounted for the rest. However, the chlorinated drinking water was more mutagenic in the Ames assay than diluted biotreated pulp mill effluent. Gas chromatography/mass spectrometry indicated that as many as 15–20% of the peaks in the drinking water intake seemed to originate from the pulp mill. Retention times of some peaks corresponded to sesquiterpenes and trichlorobenzene previously identified in kraft pulp mill effluent. Further study to characterize potential health impacts of BKME contamination of drinking water supplies is needed.

KRAFT PULP MILLS—COMMUNITY EPIDEMIOLOGY

Numerous studies, both in the United States and in Scandinavia, have examined the health status of communities near kraft pulp mills. Health endpoints examined have included acute and chronic respiratory diseases and a variety of annoyance symptoms (including headaches, nausea, and eye and throat irritation). These studies implicate odorous pulp mill air emissions in the genesis of community annoyance reactions, but do not suggest that significant respiratory irritation is occurring offsite.

Jonsson et al. (97) conducted a community odor annoyance study in Eureka, California, downwind from two pulp mills. Odor annoyance was found to be positively related to odor exposure zone, as validated by olfactometry. A follow-up community symptom survey found that self-reported headache, sputum production (females only), and odor annoyance were related to residential proximity to pulp mills, but this relationship did not hold for a variety of other respiratory, gastrointestinal, or neurologic symptoms. Some respiratory and ocular symptoms actually showed an inverse relationship to odor exposure (i.e., were more prevalent at greater distance from the mills) (98).

Deprez et al. (99) examined respiratory disease hospital admission rates in 66 Maine towns located between 0 and 15 miles from kraft pulp mills. Age- and sex-adjusted respiratory admission rates were positively related to both unemployment rates and to the proportion of the town's workforce employed at the local pulp mill, but distance between the mill and the geographic center of the town (regardless of the wind direction) did not explain variations in admission rates. Mikaelsson et al. (100) conducted an interview and clinical screening study in a sulfite (nonkraft) pulp mill community in northern Sweden; the principal air pollutants identified in the community were sulfur dioxide and chlorine. They found no communitywide excess prevalence of either asthma or chronic bronchitis compared to other regions in the country. On a case by case basis, however, both smoking and employment in the pulp mill were strong

risk factors for chronic bronchitis. Stjernberg et al. (101, 102) extended this study to include not only additional subjects, but also measures of community air quality. They again found no communitywide increase in asthma or bronchitis prevalence, with mean annual ambient levels of SO_2 averaging between 0.008–0.013 ppm (levels below the U.S. annual average standard of 0.03 ppm or the 24-hour standard of 0.14 ppm).

KRAFT PULP MILLS—OCCUPATIONAL EPIDEMIOLOGY

The occupational health status of pulp mill workers has been studied for a variety of endpoints, including cancer, pulmonary function, skin diseases, and hearing impairment. For some health endpoints, findings have varied sufficiently across studies that there remains significant controversy regarding their interpretation. This is particularly true for cancer and respiratory effects.

The effects of pulp mill work on pulmonary function are controversial. Community studies of chronic respiratory disease (in particular, bronchitis) near pulp mills have typically shown excesses in relationship to both smoking and mill employment, but not to residence proximity to mills per se (99–102). On the other hand, the significance of pulp mill employment has been variable in those cross-sectional and longitudinal respiratory health studies that have been carried out among mill workers themselves. Combined survey and clinical studies conducted in New Hampshire (103) and British Columbia (104) have failed to show a higher prevalence of chronic pulmonary disease in pulp mill workers than in the community at large. Another Canadian study highlighted two specific kraft mill work activities—bleaching and maintenance—as possible risk factors for obstructive lung disease (105). The above studies and others (106, 107) all emphasize the importance of smoking as a risk factor for respiratory disease within the pulp mill workforce.

Chip pile workers at pulp mills have been shown to be exposed to high concentrations of airborne mould spores. Although few cases of hypersensitivity pneumonitis could be found in the Finnish occupational disease registries, a limited study there found a tendency toward subclinical pulmonary impairment among chip pile workers who were precipitin positive for *Aspergillus fumigatus* (108). Attention to biologic agents in the process water of paper mills has also led to studies of microbial aerosolization and respiratory tract colonization. One such study confirmed increased rates of nasal colonization by *Klebsiella pneumoniae* among workers so exposed, but no concomitant increase in respiratory symptoms or illnesses (109).

Cancer mortality patterns among pulp mill workers have been examined in a number of cohort studies, yielding both proportional mortality ratios (PMRs) and standardized mortality ratios (SMRs), and in case-control studies and tumor registry-based standardized incidence ratio (SIR) studies. A variety of methodologic limitations, including potential ascertainment bias, the "healthy worker effect," and spurious correlations due to "multiple statistical comparisons," exist. Accordingly, caution is indicated in the interpretation of individual study results.

Table 55.5 summarizes the results of four PMR, two SMR, three SIR, and four case-control studies of pulp or paper mill workers (110–122). In no case was the same malignancy found to be significantly elevated in more than one study. However, for two sites—gastric cancer and lymphosarcoma—there was

Table 55.5. Studies of Cancer Incidence and Mortality in Pulp Mill Workers

Reference Number →	110	111	112	113	114	115	116	117	118	119	120	121	122
Study Type →	PMR	PMR	PMR	PMR	SMR	SMR	SIR	SIR	SIR		Case-Control		
Malignancies													
Lymphopoietic		*											
Leukemias			**								(−)		
Hodgkin's lymphoma	*												
Lymphosarcoma	*			**	*								
Reticulosarcoma					*								
Genitourinary													
Bladder	*												
Gastrointestinal													
Pharyngeal			**										
Gastric	*		**		*								
Pancreatic	*						*						(−)
Colorectal		*	**										
Respiratory													
Sinonasal										**	(−)		
Laryngeal			**										
Lung		**							**				
Mesothelioma								*					

Key to Symbols: * = Nonsignificant excesses
                ** = Significant excesses
                (−) = No association (Case-control studies)

Notes:
Reference 111 examined "pulp, paper, and paperboard mill workers."
Reference 114 found an excess of gastric cancers in sulfite mill workers.
Reference 115 examined "paper workers."
Reference 119 examined "paper and wood industries."

one study each with significant excesses and two studies each with nonsignificant excesses. (One of the studies showing nonsignificant excess of gastric cancer was among workers in sulfite, but not sulfate pulp mills.) To our knowledge, there have been no published attempts to ascertain the comparability of these studies for purposes of performing pooled tests of statistical significance (i.e., meta-analysis).

Finally, a variety of cutaneous hazards also exists in pulp mills, including "wet work" and botanical allergens (123), phototoxic chemicals (e.g., anthraquinone) used in delignification (124), and cutaneous irritants used in "slimicides" (including methylene-bis-thiocyanate, bis-1,4-bromoacetyoxy-2-butene, and 2,3-dichloro-4-bromotetrahydrothiophene-1,1-dioxide) (125–126).

REFERENCES

1. American Paper Institute. U.S. wood pulp data. New York: API, 1988.

2. Britt KW, ed. Handbook of pulp and paper technology. New York: Reinhold, 1964.

3. Minor J. Pulp. In: Grayson M (ed.). Kirk-Othmer encyclopedia of chemical technology. Vol 19. New York: Wiley, 1983:379–419.

4. Ross CR. Paper and paper pulp industry. In: Encyclopedia of occupational health and safety. Vol 2. Geneva: ILO Press, 1983:1588–1591.

5. Ruth JH. Odor thresholds and irritation levels of several chemical substances: a review. Am Ind Hyg Assoc J 1986;47:A142–151.

6. Amoore JE, Hautala E. Odor as an aid to chemical safety: odor thresholds compared with threshold limit values and volatilities for 214 industrial chemicals in air and water dilution. J Appl Toxicol 1983;3:272–290.

7. Beauchamp RO, Bus JS, Popp JA, Craig JB, Andjelkovich DA. A critical review of the literature on hydrogen sulfide. CRC Crit Rev Toxicol 1984;13:25–97.

8. Ellenhorn MJ, Barceloux DG. Medical toxicology. New York: Elsevier 1988:836–840.

9. Burnett WW, King EG, Grace M, Hall WF: Hydrogen sulfide poisoning: review of five years' experience. Can Med Assoc J 1977;117:1277–1280.

10. Deng J-F, Chang S-C. Hydrogen sulfide poisonings in hot-spring reservoir cleaning: two case reports. Am J Ind Med 1987;11:447–451.

11. World Health Organization (WHO). Hydrogen sulfide. Environmental Health Criteria. Vol 19. Geneva: WHO Press, 1981.

12. Savolainen H, Tenhunen R, Elovaara E, Tossavainen A. Cumulative biochemical effects of repeated subclinical hydrogen sulfide intoxication in mouse brain. Int Arch Occup Environ Health 1980;46:87–92.

13. Haider SS, Hasan M, Islan F. Effect of air pollutant hydrogen sulfide on the levels of total lipids, phospholipids and cholesterol in different regions of the guinea pig brain. Indian J Exp Biol 1980;18:418–420.

14. Sandmeyer EE. Organic sulfur compounds. In: Clayton GD, Clayton FE, eds. Patty's industrial hygiene and toxicology. 3rd ed. New York: Wiley, 1981:2061–2111.

15. Rose VE. Thiols. In: International labor association. Encyclopedia of occupational health and safety. Vol 2. Geneva, ILO Press, 1983:2172–2173.

16. Bethel R, Sheppard D, Geffroy B, Tam E, Nadel J, Boushey H. Effect of 0.25 ppm sulfur dioxide on airway resistance in freely breathing, heavily exercising, asthmatic subjects. Am Rev Respir Dis 1985;131:659–661.

17. Horstman D, Roger LJ, Kehrl H, Hazucha M. Airway sensitivity of asthmatics to sulfur dioxide. Toxicol Ind Health 1986;2:289–298.

18. Kangas J, Jappinen P, Savolainen H. Exposure to hydrogen sulfide, mercaptans and sulfur dioxide in pulp industry. Am Ind Hyg Assoc J 1984;45:787–790.

19. Charan N, Myers C, Lakshminarayan S, Spencer T. Pulmonary injuries associated with acute sulfur dioxide inhalation. Am Rev Respir Dis 1979;119:555–560.

20. Woodford D, Coutu R, Gaensler E. Obstructive lung disease from acute sulfur dioxide exposure. Respiration 1979;38:238–245.

21. Kennedy S, Enarson D, Janssen R, Chan-Yeung M. Lung health consequences of reported accidental chlorine gas exposures among pulpmill workers. Am Rev Respir Dis 1991;143:74–79.

22. U.S. Department of Labor, Occupational Safety and Health Administration (OSHA). Air contaminants—permissible exposure limits. Washington, D.C.: USGPO, 1989.

23. Amoore JE. The perception of hydrogen sulfide odor in relation to setting an ambient standard. Sacramento, CA: California Air Resources Board, Contract A4-046-33, 1985.

24. U.S. Environmental Protection Agency. Survey of chloroform emission sources. EPA-450/3-85-026. Research Triangle Park, NC: Office of Air Quality Planning and Standards, EPA, 1985.

25. California Department of Health Services. Health effects of chloroform. Berkeley, CA: Air Toxics Unit, CDHS, March 1989.

26. U.S. Environmental Protection Agency. National dioxin study tier 4-combustion sources. EPA-450/4-84-014h. Research Triangle Park, NC: Office of Air Quality Planning and Standards, EPA, September 1987.

27. Pinkerton JE, Blosser RO. Characterization of kraft pulp mill particulate emissions—a summary of existing measurements and observations. Atmos Environ 1981;15:2071–2078.

28. U.S. Environmental Protection Agency. Paper production and processing — occupational exposure and environmental release study. EPA Report No. EPA-600/2-84-120. PB84-215730. Cincinnati, OH: Industrial Environmental Research Laboratory, Office of Research and Development, EPA, 1984.

29. Suntio LR, Shiu WY, Mackay D. A review of the nature and properties of chemicals present in pulp mill effluents. Chemosphere 1988;18:1249–1290.

30. Kringstad KP, Lindstrom K. Spent liquors from pulp bleaching. Environ Sci Technol 1984;15:236A–248A.

31. Lindstrom K, Osterberg F. Chlorinated carboxylic acids in softwood kraft pulp spent bleach liquors. Environ Sci Technol 1986;20:133–145.

32. Knuutinen J. Analysis of chlorinated guaiacols in spent bleach liquor from a pulp mill. J Chromatogr 1982;248:289–295.

33. McKague AB. Some toxic constituents of chlorination-stage effluents from bleached kraft pulp mills. Can J Fish Aquat Sci 1981;38:739–743.

34. McKague AB. Phenolic constituents in pulp mill process streams. J Chromatogr 1981;208:287–293.

35. Swanson SE, Rappe C, Malmstrom J, Kringstad KP. Emissions of PCDDs and PCDFs from the pulp industry. Chemosphere 1988;17:681–691.

36. Bonsor N, McCubbin N, Sprague JB. Kraft mill effluents in Ontario. Municipal-industrial strategy for abatement. Canada: Environment Ontario, 1989.

37. Graves WC, Burton DT, Richardson LB. Effect of 20–30-day continuous exposure of treated bleach kraft mill effluent on selected freshwater species. Bull Environ Contam Toxicol 1980;25:651–657.

38. U.S. Environmental Protection Agency. The national dioxin study: tier 3,5,6,7. Washington, DC: Office of Water Regulations and Standards, 1986.

39. Bodien DG. Statement of Danforth G. Bodien (U.S. Environmental Protection Agency, Seattle WA) before the California Regional Water Quality Control Board, Central Valley Region, Redding, CA, 27 April 1989.

40. Kuehl DW, Butterworth BC, De Vita WM, Sauer CP. Environmental contamination by polychlorinated dibenzo-p-dioxins and dibenzofurans associated with pulp and paper mill discharge. Biomed Environ Mass Spectrom 1987;14:443–447.

41. Olson LJ, Anderson HA, Jones VB. Landspreading dioxin-contaminated papermill sludges: a complex problem. Arch Environ Health 1988;43:186–189.

42. Beck H, Eckart K, Mathar W, Wittkowski R. Occurrence of PCDD and PCDF in different kinds of paper. Chemosphere 1988;17:51–57.

43. Axegard P, Renberg L. The influence of bleaching chemicals and lignin content on the formation of polychlorinated dioxins and dibenzofurans. Chemosphere 1989;1–6:661–668.

44. de Sousa F, Kolar M-C, Kringstad KP. Influence of chlorine ratio and oxygen bleaching on the formation of PCDFs and PCDDs in pulp bleaching. Part 1: a laboratory study. Tappi 1989;72:147–153.

45. Heimburger SA, Blevins DS, Bostwick JH, Donnini GP. Kraft mill bleach plant effluents: recent developments aimed at decreasing their environmental impacts, Part 1. Tech Assoc Pulp Pap Ind J 1988;71:51–60.

46. Priha MH, Talka ET. Biological activity of bleached kraft mill effluent (BKME) fractions and process streams. Pulp Pap Can 1986;87:143–147.

47. Leach JM, Thakore AN. Isolation and identification of constituents toxic to juvenile rainbow trout (*Salmo gairdneri*) in caustic extraction effluents from kraft pulpmill bleach plants. J Fish Res Board Can 1975;32:1249–1257.

48. Walden CC, Howard TE. Toxicity of pulp and paper mill effluents—a review. Pulp Pap Can 1981;82:115–124.

49. Oikari A, Lindstrom-Seppa P. Kukkonen J. Subchronic metabolic effects and toxicity of a simulated pulp mill effluent on juvenile lake trout, *Salmo trutta m. lacustris*. Ecotoxicol Environ Safety 1988;16:202–218.

50. Andersson T, Bengtsson B-E, Forlin L, Hardig J, Larsson A. Long-term effects of bleached kraft mill effluents on carbohydrate metabolism and hepatic xenobiotic biotransformation enzymes in fish. Ecotoxicol Environ Safety 1987;13:53–60.

51. Hardig J, Andersson T, Bengtsson B-E, Forlin L, Larsson A. Long-term effects of bleached kraft mill effluents on red and white blood cell status, ion balance, and vertebral structure in fish. Ecotoxicol Environ Safety 1988;15:96–106.

52. Woelke CE. Measurement of water quality with the Pacific oyster embryo bioassay. In: Water quality criteria, ASTM STP 416. Philadelphia: American Society for Testing Materials, 1967.

53. Thakore AN, Howard TE. Site of action of chemicals from pulp mill effluent that are toxic to fish. Ottawa, Ontario: Canadian Forestry Service 1976. CPAR Project No. 488.

54. Couillard CM, Berman RA, Panisset JC. Histopathology of rainbow trout exposed to a bleached kraft pulp mill effluent. Arch Environ Contam Toxicol 1988;17:319–323.

55. Kovacs T. Effects of bleached kraft mill effluent on freshwater fish: a canadian perspective. Water Poll Res J Can 1986;21:91–118.

56. Graves WC, Burton DT, Richardson LB, Margrey SL. The interaction of treated bleached kraft mill effluent and dissolved oxygen concentration on the survival of the developmental stages of the Sheepshead minnow (*Cyprinodon variegatus*). Water Res 1981;15:1005–1011.

57. Vourinen M, Vourinen PJ. Effects of bleached kraft mill effluent on early life stages of brown trout (*Salmo trutta* L.). Ecotoxicol Environ Safety 1987;14:117–128.

58. National Council on Air and Stream Improvement. Effects of biologically stabilized bleached kraft mill effluent on cold water stream productivity as determined in experimental streams—first progress report. Technical Bulletin No. 368. New York, NY: NEASI, 1982.

59. Tana J, Nikunen E. Impact of pulp and paper mill effluent on egg hatchability of pike (*Esox lucius* L.). Bull Environ Contam Toxicol 1986;36:738–743.

60. Burton DT, Hall WL, Klauda RJ, Margrey SL. Effects of treated bleached kraft mill effluent on eggs and prolarvae of striped bass (*Morone saxatalis*). Water Res Bull 1983;19:869–879.

61. Cherr GN, Shenker JM, Lundmark C, Turner KO. Toxic effects of selected bleached kraft mill effluent constituents on the sea urchin sperm cell. Environ Toxicol Chem 1987;6:561–569.

62. Douglas GR, Nestmann ER, McKague AB, et al. Mutagenicity of pulp and paper mill effluent: a comprehensive study of complex mixtures. Environ Sci Res 1983;27:431–459.

63. Kamra OP, Nestmann ER, Douglas GR, Kowbel DJ, Harrington TR. Genotoxic activity of pulp mill effluent in Salmonella and *Saccharomyces cerevisiae* assays. Mutat Res 1983;118:269–276.

64. Kringstad KP, Ljungquist PO, de Sousa F, Stromberg LM. Identification and mutagenic properties of some chlorinated aliphatic compounds in the spent liquor from kraft pulp chlorination. Environ Sci Tech 1981;15:562–566.

65. Nestmann ER, Lee EG-H, Mueller JC, Douglas GR. Mutagenicity of resin acids identified in pulp and paper mill effluents using the Salmonella/mammalian microsome assay. Environ Mutagen 1979;1:361–369.

66. Nestmann ER, Lee EG-H, Matula TI, Douglas GR, Mueller JC. Mutagenicity of constituents identified in pulp and paper mill effluents using the Salmonella/mammalian-microsome assay. Mutat Res 1980;79:203–212.

67. Ellenton JA, Douglas GR, Nestmann ER. Mutagenic evaluation of 1,1,2,3-tetrachloro-2-propene, a contaminant in pulp mill effluents, using a battery of *in vitro* mammalian and microbial tests. Can J Genet Cytol 1981;23:17–25.

68. Holmbom BR. Isolation and identification of an Ames-mutagenic compound present in kraft chlorination effluents. Tappi 1981;64:172–174.

69. U.S. Environmental Protection Agency. Biological and chemical studies on 3-chloro-4-(dichloromethyl)-5-hydroxy-2(5H)-furanone: a potent mutagen in kraft pulp chlorination effluent and chlorinated drinking water. Research Triangle Park, NC: Health Effects Research Laboratory, EPA, August 1988.

70. Geiger LE, Neal RA. Mutagenicity testing of 2,3,7,8-tetrachlorodibenzo-p-dioxin in histidine auxotrophs of *Salmonella typhimurium*. Toxicol Appl Pharmacol 1981;59:125–129.

71. Gilbert P, Saint-Ruf G, Poncelet E, et al. Genetic effects of chlorinated anilines and azobenzenes on *Salmonella typhimurium*. Arch Environ Contam Toxicol 1980;9:533–541.

72. Mortelmans K, Haworth S, Speck W, et al. Mutagenicity testing of agent orange components and related chemicals. Toxicol Appl Pharmacol 1984;75:137–146.

73. Nestmann ER, Lee EG-H. Mutagenicity of constituents of pulp and paper mill effluent in growing cells of *Saccharomyces cerevisiae*. Mutat Res 1983;119:273–280.

74. Callen DF, Wolf CR, Philpot RM. Cytochrome P-450 mediated genetic activity and cytotoxicity of seven halogenated aliphatic hydrocarbons in *Saccharomyces cerevisiae*. Mutat Res 1980;77:55–63.

75. Nestmann ER, Lee EG-H. Genetic activity in *Saccharomyces cerevisiae* of compounds found in effluents of pulp and paper mills. Mutat Res 1985;155:53–60.

76. Bronzetti G, Zeiger E, Lee I, et al. Genetic effects of 2,3,7,8-tetrachlorodibenzo-p-dioxin (TCDD) in yeast *in vitro* and *in vivo*. In: Hutzinger O, Frei RW, Aerian E, Pocchiari F, eds. Chlorinated dioxins and related compounds, impact on the environment. Proceedings of a workshop held at the

Instituto Superiore di Sanita, Rome, Italy, 22–24 October, 1980. New York: Pergamon Press, 1982:429–436.

77. Das RK, Nanda NK. Induction of micronuclei in peripheral erythrocytes of fish *Heteropneustes fossilis* by mitomycin C and paper mill effluent. Mutat Res 1986;175:67–71.

78. Rogers AM, Anderson ME, Back KC. Mutagenicity of 2,3,7,8-tetrachlorodibenzo-p-dioxin and perfluoro-n-decanoic acid in L517BY mouse lymphoma cells. Mutat Res 1982, 105:445–449.

79. Hay A, Ashby J, Styles JA, et al. The mutagenic properties of 2,3,7,8-tetrachlorodibenzo-p-dioxin. Am Chem Soc J, Div Environ Chem 1983;3:14–22.

80. International Agency for Research on Cancer. IARC monographs on the evaluation of carcinogenic risk to humans. Overall evaluations of carcinogenicity: an updating of IARC Monographs Volumes 1 to 42. IARC Monographs:Suppl 7. Lyon, France: World Health Organization, 1987.

81. Landner L, Lindstrom K, Karlsson M, Nordin J, Sorenson L. Bioaccumulation in fish of chlorinated phenols from kraft pulp mill bleachery effluents. Bull Environ Contam Toxicol 1977;18:663–673.

82. Oikari AOJ. Metabolites of xenobiotics in the bile of fish in waterways polluted by pulp mill effluents. Bull Environ Contam Toxicol 1986;36:429–436.

83. Corbet RL, Muir DCG, Webster GRB. Fate of 1,3,6,8-TCDD in an outdoor aquatic environment. Chemosphere 1983;12:523–527.

84. Isensee AR, Jones GE. Absorption and translocation of root and foliage applied 2,4-dichlorophenol, 2,7-dichlorodibenzo-p-dioxin, and 2,3,7,8-tetrachlorodibenzo-p-dioxin. J Agr Food Chem 1971;19:1210–1214.

85. Yockim RS, Isensee AR, Jones GE. Distribution and toxicity of TCDD and 2,4,5-T in an aquatic model ecosystem. Chemosphere 1978;3:215–220.

86. Petty JD, Smith LM, Peterman PH, Mehrle PM, Buckler DR, Stalling DL. Bioconcentration of TCDD and TCDF by rainbow trout in a flow-through exposure. Presented at Society of Environmental Toxicology and Chemistry Seventh Annual Meeting, Alexandria, VA, November 2–5, 1986.

87. Courtney KD, Moore JA. Teratology studies with 2,4,5-T and 2,3,7,8-TCDD. Toxicol Appl Pharmacol 1971;20:396–403.

88. Neubert D, Dillman I. Embryotoxic effects in mice treated with 2,4,5-trichlorophenoxyacetic acid and 2,3,7,8-tetrachlorodibenzo-p-dioxin. Arch Pharmacol 1972;272:243–264.

89. Sparschu GL, Dunn FL, Rowe VK. Study of the teratogenicity of 2,3,7,8-tetrachlorodibenzo-p-dioxin in the rat. Food Cosmet Toxicol 1971;9:405–412.

90. Murray FJ, Smith FA, Nitschke KD, Humiston CG, Kociba RJ, Schwetz BA. Three-generation reproduction study of rats given 2,3,7,8-tetrachlorodibenzo-p-dioxin (TCDD) in the diet. Toxicol Appl Pharmacol 1979;50:241–252.

91. Schantz SL, Barsotti DA, Allen JR. Toxicological effects produced in nonhuman primates chronically exposed to fifty parts per trillion 2,3,7,8-tetrachlorodibenzo-p-dioxin (TCDD). Toxicol Appl Pharmacol 1979;48:A180.

92. Kociba RJ, Keyes DG, Beyer JE, et al. Results of a two-year chronic toxicity and oncogenicity study of 2,3,7,8-tetrachlorodibenzo-p-dioxin in rats. Toxicol Appl Pharmacol 1978;46:279–303.

93. Gorski JR, Muzi G, Weber LWD, et al. Some endocrine and morphological aspects of the acute toxicity of 2,3,7,8-tetrachlorodibenzo-p-dioxin (TCDD). Toxicol Pathol 1988;16:313–320.

94. Jones MK, Weisenburger WP, Sipes IG, Russell DH. Circadian alterations in prolactin, corticosterone, and thyroid hormone levels and down-regulation of prolactin receptor activity by 2,3,7,8-tetrachlorodibenzo-p-dioxin. Toxicol Appl Pharmacol 1987;87:337–350.

95. Kociba RJ, Cabey O. Comparative toxicity and biologic activity of chlorinated dibenzo-p-dioxins and furans relative to 2,3,7,8-tetrachlorodibenzo-p-dioxin (TCDD). Chemosphere 1985;14:649–660.

96. Wigilius B, Boren H, Grimvall A, Carlberg GE, Hagen I, Brogger A. Impact of bleached kraft mill effluents on drinking water quality. Sci Total Environ 1988;74:75–96.

97. Jonsson E, Deane M, Sanders G. Community reactions to odors from pulp mills: a pilot study in Eureka, California. Environ Res 1975;10:249–270.

98. Deane M, Sanders G. Health effects of exposure to community odors from pulp mills, Eureka, 1971. Environ Res 1977;14:164–181.

99. Deprez RD, Oliver C, Halteman W. Variations in respiratory disease morbidity among pulp and paper mill town residents. J Occup Med 1986;28:486–491.

100. Mikaelsson B, Stjernberg N, Wiman L-G. The prevalence of bronchial asthma and chronic bronchitis in an industrialized community in northern Sweden. Scand J Soc Med 1982;10:11–16.

101. Stjernberg N, Eklund A, Nystrom L, Rosenhall L, Emmelin A, Stromqvist L-H. Prevalence of bronchial asthma and chronic bronchitis in a community in northern Sweden: relation to environmental and occupational exposure to sulfur dioxide. Eur J Respir Dis 1985;67:41–49.

102. Stjernberg N, Rosenhall L, Eklund A, Nystrom L. Chronic bronchitis in a community in northern Sweden: relation to environmental and occupational exposure to sulphur dioxide. Eur J Respir Dis 1986;69:153–159.

103. Ferris BG Jr, Burgess WA, Worcester J. Prevalence of chronic respiratory disease in a pulp mill and a paper mill in the United States. Br J Ind Med 1967;24:26–37.

104. Chan-Yeung M, Wong R, MacLean L, Tan F, Dorken E, Schulzer M, et al. Respiratory survey of workers in a pulp and paper mill in Powell River, British Columbia. Am Rev Respir Dis 1980 Aug;122:249–257.

105. Enarson DA, Johnson A, Block G, Maclean L, Dybuncio A, Schragg K, et al. Respiratory health at a pulpmill in British Columbia. Arch Environ Health 1984 Sep–Oct;39:325–30.

106. Poukkula A, Huhti E, Makarainen M. Chronic respiratory disease among workers in a pulp mill: a ten-year follow-up study. Chest 1982;81(Mar):285–289.

107. Huhti E, Ryhänen P, Vuopala U, Takkunen J. Chronic respiratory disease among pulp mill workers in an arctic area in Northern Finland. Acta Med Scand 1970;187:433–444.

108. Jappinen P, Haahtela T, Liira J. Chip pile workers and mould exposure. A preliminary clinical and hygienic survey. Allergy 1987;42:545–548.

109. Niemela SI, Vaatanen P, Mentu J, Jokinen A, Jappinen P, Sillanpaa P. Microbial incidence in upper respiratory tracts of workers in the paper industry. Appl Environ Microbiol 1985;50:163–168.

110. Milham S Jr, Demers RY. Mortality among pulp and paper workers. J Occup Med 1984;26:844–846.

111. Solet D, Zoloth SR, Sullivan C, Jewett J, Michaels DM. Patterns of mortality in pulp and paper workers. J Occup Med 1989;31:627–630.

112. Schwartz E. A proportionate mortality ratio analysis of pulp and paper mill workers in New Hampshire. Br J Ind Med 1988;45:234–238.

113. Svirchev LM, Gallagher RP, Band PR, Threlfall WJ, Spinelli JJ. Gastric cancer and lymphosarcoma among wood and pulp workers. J Occup Med 1986;28:264–265.

114. Robinson CF, Waxweiler RJ, Fowler DP. Mortality among production workers in pulp and paper mills. Scand J Work Environ Health 1986;12:552–560.

115. Ferris BG, Puleo S, Chen HY. Mortality and morbidity in a pulp and a paper mill in the United States: a ten-year follow-up. Br J Ind Med 1979;36:127–134.

116. Malker HS, McLaughlin JK, Malker BK, Stone BJ, Weiner JA, Ericsson JL, et al. Biliary tract cancer and occupation in Sweden. Br J Ind Med 1986;43:257–262.

117. Malker HSR, McLaughlin JK, Malker BK, Stone BJ, Weiner JA, Erickson JLE, et al. Occupational risks for fleural mesothelioma in Sweden, 1961–79. J Natl Cancer Inst 1985;74:61–66.

118. Jappinen P, Hakulinen T, Pukkala E, Tola S, Kurppa K. Cancer incidence of workers in the Finnish pulp and paper industry. Scand J Work Environ Health 1987;13:197–202.

119. Hayes RB, Gerin M, Raatgever JW, De Bruyn A. Wood-related occupations, wood dust exposure and sinonasal cancer. Am J Epidemiol 1986;124:569–577.

120. Fukuda K, Motomura M, Yamakawa M. Relationship of occupation with cancer of the maxillary sinuses in Hokkaido, Japan. Natl Cancer Inst Monogr 1985;69:169–173.

121. Morton W, Marjanovic D. Leukemia incidence by occupation in the Portland-Vancouver metropolitan area. Am J Ind Med 1984;6:185–205.

122. Norell S, Ahlbom A, Olin R, Erwald R, Jacobson G, Lindberg-Navier I, et al. Occupational factors and pancreatic cancer. Br J Ind Med 1986;43:775–778.

123. Storrs FJ. Dermatitis in the forest products industry. In: Maibach HI, Gellin GA, eds. Occupational and industrial dermatology. Chicago: Year Book, 1982:323–328.

124. Menezes Brandao F, Valente A. Photodermatitis from anthraquinone. Contact Dermatitis 1988;18:171–172.

125. Jappinen P, Eskelinen A. Patch tests with methylene-bis-thiocyanate in paper mill workers. Contact Dermatitis 1987;16:233.

126. Rycroft RJ, Calnan CD. Dermatitis from slimicides in a paper mill. Contact Dermatitis 1980;6:435–439.

56

Hazardous Materials Incinerators and Waste Sites

John A. Lowe, C.I.H.

INTRODUCTION

On the surface, hazardous waste sites and hazardous materials incinerators appear to be very disparate aspects of hazardous waste management. However, the unifying feature of waste sites and incineration is that they are both associated with the introduction and distribution of toxic substances into the environment. These releases to the environment potentially result in chemical exposures that raise concerns about increased risks to human health. These concerns about increased health risks fall into three broad categories of adverse health effects: carcinogenicity; noncancer systemic effects, including teratogenicity and developmental toxicity; and immunotoxicity. Several well-publicized cases of reported symptoms and adverse health effects associated with some sites (for example, Love Canal, New York, and Times Beach, Missouri) cast suspicions over all sites where chemical wastes are treated, stored, and disposed. However, assessment of the health risks associated with specific sites must account for the nature of the site (such as the local geology and hydrology), characteristics of the wastes disposed there, and characteristics of the surrounding populations and resources. The pathways of exposure to the surrounding populations greatly influence whether adverse effects will be associated with a specific site.

Public Health Concerns

Carcinogens pose a special problem in hazardous waste management. Carcinogenic chemicals are treated as a special class of toxicant. This class is not considered to have a threshold of exposure defining no adverse effect; hence, any level of exposure above zero is associated with a finite risk of developing cancer. Assessing whether waste site contaminants are associated with increased risks of cancer involves linear extrapolation of the cancer incidence observed with highly elevated exposure levels (from epidemiologic studies or animal bioassays) to much lower levels of exposure. The health significance of carcinogens in hazardous wastes or incinerator emissions is assessed by invoking an acceptable risk level that is specified by regulatory agencies and that reflects societal norms. These risk levels often are much lower than the cancer risks posed from exposures to toxicants originating from natural or background sources, or they represent concentrations in soil, water, or air that fall below the limits of detection in chemical analyses. Some of the outcomes of controlling carcinogens in this manner are: (a) specifying clean-up standards for hazardous waste sites well in excess of what is needed to protect public health; (b) slowing the development of waste treatment technologies such as incineration; and (c) giving an arbitrarily high priority to the control of trace levels of environmental carcinogens over other public health problems.

Noncarcinogenic chemicals, or those giving rise to adverse effects other than cancer, are assessed using more traditional toxicologic concepts of dose-response relationships and assuming the presence of no-effect thresholds. Because no-effect thresholds are assumed to be present, levels of exposure to noncarcinogenic chemicals in hazardous wastes or incinerator emissions that protect public health typically are several orders of magnitude greater than acceptable risk for carcinogenic exposures. Hence, site clean-ups are more often driven by the presence of carcinogens rather than noncarcinogens. However, some noncarcinogens are of greater concern, such as kidney toxicity from cadmium exposures or neurobehavioral effects from lead exposure, where appreciable background exposures may be present.

Immunotoxicity has been of growing concern because of its role in protection against adverse effects associated with exposures to toxic substances, particularly to carcinogens. Due to its complexity, the immune system is prone to interference by chemical exposure as well as biologic factors including age and health, nutrition, and disease status. Due to its host defense nature and its intimate association with the circulatory and lymphatic systems, the immune system is broadly exposed to chemicals. Some toxicants specifically affect cell-mediated immunity, while others affect both cell- and humoral-mediated immune mechanisms. Furthermore, since immune response is modulated by T-cells, chemical exposure may decrease immunity by affecting various aspects of T-cell functions. Several studies have documented immunosuppression in both animals and humans from chemical exposure, potentially increasing susceptibility to adverse effects from chemicals and pathogens. Immunotoxicity remains an unknown quantity in assessing health effects associated with chemicals released from hazardous waste sites or in incinerator emissions. Regulatory agencies currently do not provide any guidance for evaluating immunotoxic effects or their interactions with carcinogenic or other systemic adverse effects.

Responses to Hazardous Wastes Problems

The importance of hazardous waste sites as a perceived threat to public health is exemplified by the passage (and amendment) of the Comprehensive Environmental Response, Compensation and Liability act (CERCLA), which has authorized over $10 billion to study and clean up sites. This is in addition to funding and regulatory efforts allocated at the state and local levels for site investigation and enforcement activities, and for activities at land disposal facilities under the Resource Conservation and Recovery Act (RCRA). RCRA also serves an all-encompassing role in the management of hazardous wastes and permitting of waste treatment, storage, and disposal facilities.

CERCLA was amended in 1986 by the Superfund Amendments and Reauthorization Act (SARA). A principal change in CERCLA as amended by SARA is a statutory preference for permanent remedies that protect public health, with cost-effectiveness of the remedies being a secondary consideration. (Formerly under CERCLA, protection of public health and cost-effectiveness were weighted equally in selecting remedies). Numerous sites have been investigated and characterized, and are now moving into the process of remediation, through the RI/FS process. (RI/FS means **R**emedial **I**nvestigation/**F**easibility **S**tudy, which is the primary tool for implementing CERCLA. RI is the mechanism for collecting data needed to select a remedy for the site. FS is the mechanism for development and evaluation of the remedial action.) However, the costs for eventually cleaning up the thousands of identified sites, as well as sites as yet unidentified, potentially represents a significant social and financial cost to the public for the forseeable future. Nonetheless, the public's intent to clean up hazardous waste sites is clear, as expressed by the passage and amendment of legislation such as CERCLA and RCRA.

Increasingly, concern has focused on minimizing degradation of soil and water resources by preventing disposal of hazardous wastes in land facilities. As a result of this concern, there is greater reliance on "terminal" treatment technologies, including thermal treatment, or incineration. While incinerators can destroy numerous types of hazardous chemicals, these projects have encountered significant public opposition, due in part to concerns over the health risks associated with emissions to the air and disposal of residues.

With the close attention from the media and policymakers, and the extensive regulatory and legal attention, concern is raised about the continuing lack of focus on public health in the controversy over managing hazardous waste sites. There is a need to more carefully define the problems and issues associated with hazardous waste sites and treatment technologies. A better understanding of the problems and a health-related perspective (rather than a policy-related one) could lead to a more efficient use of the resources for controlling the public health hazards associated with existing hazardous waste sites and the management of ever-increasing amounts of generated waste. The health considerations can be expressed in more detail, as follows:

- The need for remediation or restoration of a hazardous waste site must be judged against the health hazards, threats to resources (such as ground water) and future uses of the site.
- Potential pathways of exposure from sites must be carefully identified and evaluated for proper decision-making concerning site remediation.
- Risk assessment methods, particularly health conservative methods, greatly influence the perceived risks associated with hazardous waste sites. Risk assessment is then an important determinant in the level of remediation required at a site.
- Existing clinical and epidemiologic studies of populations near hazardous waste sites are of limited value in drawing a baseline useful for evaluating potential health effects from low level exposures.

The significance of potential exposures of the public from hazardous waste sites, when considered from the epidemiologic perspective, has two parts: first, epidemiologic observation of disease trends associated with waste sites is clouded by uncertain estimation of exposures, presence of multiple contaminants, and small exposed populations, which reduces the power of studies to detect the increased incidence of disease; second, epidemiologic observation seldom provides the quantitative relationship between the potential for increases in adverse health effects (or "health risks") and chemical exposure, which is provided by risk assessment. Risk assessment readily provides this quantitative determination of health risks, including risks that could not be detected by epidemiology; hence, risk assessment has become the primary tool for making decisions in the investigation and remediation of hazardous waste sites. The distinctions between epidemiologic investigation and risk assessment in managing hazardous waste sites can be drawn as such:

- Epidemiologists and clinicians measure and evaluate health effects that can be clinically detected. This provides a scientifically defensible assessment of conditions under which a hazardous waste site may affect the health of a community; however, these studies may not quantitatively identify public health goals needed to develop remedial action plans for hazardous waste sites.
- Risk analysts, in using risk assessment, provide an approach for quantitatively expressing public health goals. This allows public health considerations to be factored into the selection of remedial action alternatives for hazardous waste sites, along with considerations of costs and technical feasibility. However, many of the underlying assumptions used in quantitating health risks are the focus of considerable scientific controversy, creating uncertainty about the extent of remedial action needed to protect public health.

Making rational decisions concerning how to spend our dollars on environmental protection involves developing a perspective about the magnitude of health hazards presented by hazardous waste sites and cultivating the ability to rank these hazards with other public health problems.

HAZARDOUS WASTE SITES

Humans can potentially become exposed to substances disposed in hazardous waste sites through the air, soil, water, and food. An exposure pathway consists of the following elements (1):

- A source of chemical release to the environment;
- An environmental transport medium (e.g., air, groundwater, soil);
- A point of potential human contact with the contaminated medium (also referred to as an exposure point); and
- A route of entry into humans, either via inhalation, ingestion, or dermal contact with the contaminated soil or water.

It is of value to first consider the possible pathways of exposure from the public health and epidemiologic perspective, as a comparison to perspective of risk assessment and remedial action. The pathways of human exposure from a hazardous waste site include:

- Emissions into the air of volatile organic compounds or fugitive dusts from surface soils;
- Migration of contaminants to ground water used for drinking water;
- Runoff of contaminants into surface waters used for fishing or for drinking water;
- Contamination of food sources (gardens, agricultural fields, or feedlots) from deposition of contaminated dusts onto foliage and irrigating crops or watering livestock with contaminated water; and
- Direct contact (dermal and ingestion exposures) to contaminants in surface soils.

These pathways are presented in Figure 56.1. Example of sources of chemical releases through these exposure pathways are pre-

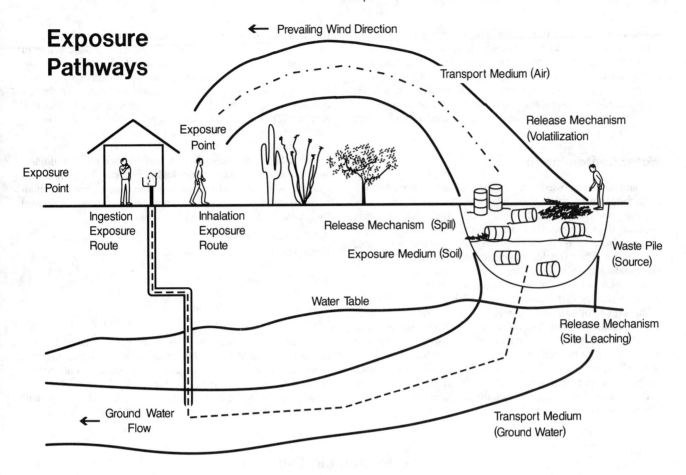

Figure 56.1.

Table 56.1. Common Chemical Release Sources at Hazardous Waste Sites

Receiving Medium	Release Mechanism	Release Source
Air	Volatilization	Surface wastes (lagoons, ponds, pits, spills)
		Contaminated surface water
		Contaminated surface soil
		Contaminated wetlands
		Leaking drums
	Dust resuspension	Contaminated surface soil
		Waste piles
Surface water	Surface runoff	contaminated surface soil
	Episodic overland flow	Lagoon overflow
		Spills, leaking containers
	Groundwater seepage	Contaminated ground water
Groundwater	Leaching	Surface of buried wastes
		Contaminated soil
Soil	Leaching	Surface or buried wastes
	Surface runoff	Contaminated surface soil
	Episodic overland flow	Lagoon overflow
		Spills, leaking containers
	Dust resuspension/deposition	Contaminated surface soil
		Waste piles
	Tracking	Contaminated surface soil
Biota (including humans)	Uptake (direct contact, ingestion, inhalation, bioaccumulation)	Contaminated soil, surface water, sediment, groundwater, or air
		Other biota (crops, livestock, prey organisms)

Source: EPA, 1989.

sented in Table 56.1. Information characterizing the extent of exposure and threat to public health from the foodchain pathways (fish consumption and agricultural production) from hazardous waste sites is too limited for evaluation of the potential for exposure. However, concentrations of contaminants in air near hazardous waste sites, exposure through soil ingestion, and exposure through ingestion of contaminated drinking water have been evaluated.

Water Contamination

Contaminants from waste sites can reach water sources through a combination of the actions involving the hydrologic cycle and the geologic cycle (Figs. 56.2 and 56.3) (2). The geologic cycle involves movement of rock, sediment, and soil. Geologic characteristics of rock can play a role in contaminant spread or retention. The hydrologic cycle involves water evaporation, precipitation, groundwater flow, water runoff, and aquifers.

The sources of pollution and contamination can be either point sources or distributive sources (Tables 56.2 and 56.3). Point sources of contamination can be geometrically defined, are mappable, and are discernible in size, shape, and location (2). Distributed sources of contamination are spread throughout a large area with boundaries which are difficult to define. Point sources include hazardous waste sites, chemical spills, mining operation wastes, and sewage areas. Distributed sources are widespread and may receive contaminate input from a variety of sources. These sources include hazardous waste sites, ag-

ricultural activities involving pesticide and chemical application to soil and crops, sewage disposal practices, and spreading of contaminants by rain, soil erosion, wind, flooding, and other natural elements (2). Through a complex interplay of both hydrologic and geologic cycles, a combination termed the hydrogeopollution cycle (Fig. 56.4), contaminate and pollution spread can be enhanced from either point sources or distributive sources. Groundwater is repleted by water passing through soil, sand, and rock.

Groundwater may contain a variety of trace metal pollutants such as mercury, lead, arsenic, cadmium, iron, barium, boron, cyanide, selenium, chromium, uranium, sulfur, nitrates, manganese, and aluminium (2). Contaminants can be introduced by a variety of activities such as:

Solid waste dumping
Hazardous materials disposal
Sewage disposal
Radioactive waste disposal
Agriculture chemical use
Mining activities and waste disposal
Industrial waste disposal and underground storage tank leakage

Biologic contamination of groundwater is caused by discharge of human and animal sewage into or near water supplies. Most pathogenic microbial organism contamination of groundwater is from a fecal source (Table 56.4). Coliform bacteria, normally found in the gastrointestinal tract, are commonly monitored for in water supplies as measures of fecal contamination.

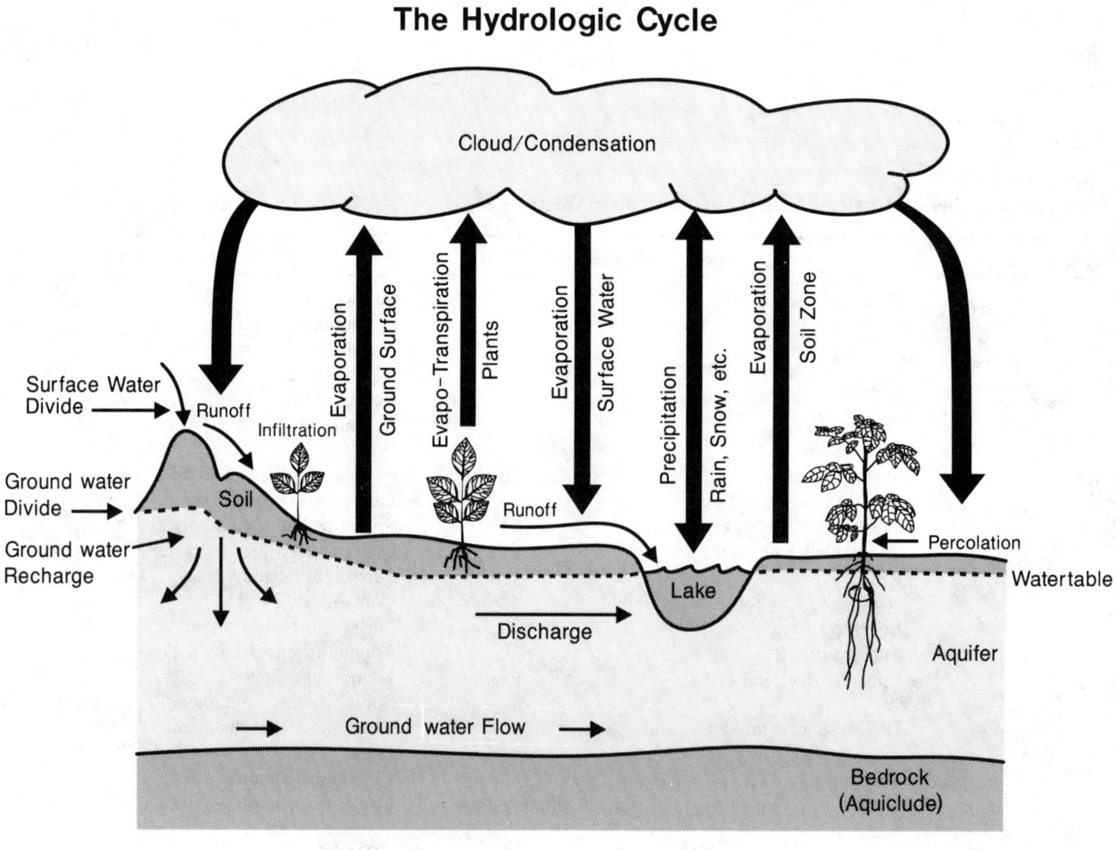

Figure 56.2. From Egboka B, Nwankwor G, Orajaka I, Ejiofor A. Principles and problems of environmental pollution of groundwater resources with case examples from developing countries. Environ Health Perspect 1989;83:39–68.

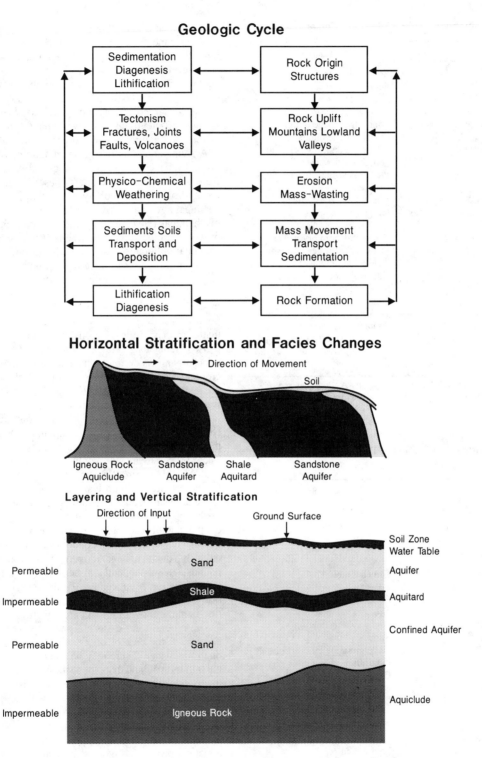

Figure 56.3.   From Egboka B, Nwankwor G, Orajaka I, Ejiofor A. Principles and problems of environmental pollution of groundwater resources with case examples from developing countries. Environ Health Perspect 1989;83:39–68.

These bacteria include the gram-negative bacilli *Escherichia coli*, *Citrobacter*, *Klebsiella*, and *Enterobacter* species (2). Nonpathogenic organisms may also pollute ground water. Chief among these nonpathogens are sulfur and iron bacteria (2). Sulfur bacteria include sulfate reducers which produce elemental sulfur from sulfates. Iron bacteria oxidize ferrous or manganous iron. Both pathogenic and nonpathogenic bacteria occur as contaminants in either oxidizing or reducing environments. These organisms break down organic and inorganic material, releasing byproducts.

Drinking Water Pathways

The pathway of exposure typically of greatest concern has been ingestion of drinking water, particularly from ground water

Table 56.2. Point Sources of Pollution and Contamination[a]

Pollution	Examples
Sewage disposal systems	Sewage lagoons
	Septic systems
	Cesspools
	Barnyards/feed lots
Surface waste disposal sites	Landfills/garbage dumps
	Surface waste dumps
Underground waste disposal sites	Storage tanks (low, medium, high level wastes)
	Pit latrines, tunnels, trenches, caves
	Waste subsurface injections
Spills, washings, and intrusions	Oil/gas/waste spills
	Auto workshop washings
	Research/laboratory washings
	Seawater/saltwater intrusions
Mining	Acid mine drainages
	Gas explosions/seepages
	Mine dumps and gangue deposits
	Tunnels/excavations outflows
Natural mineral/ore deposits	Saline ponds/lakes
	Hot springs/mineralized waters
	Anhydrite/pyrite deposits/evaporites

[a]From Egboka B, Nwankwor G, Orajaka I, Ejiofor A. Principles and problems of environmental pollution of groundwater resources with case examples from developing countries. Environ Health Perspect 1989;83:39–68.

Table 56.3. Distributed Sources of Pollution and Contamination[a]

Source	Examples
Agriculture	Cropland
	Pasture and rangeland
	Irrigated land
	Wood land
	Feed lots
Forestry	Growing stock
	Logging
	Road building
Construction	Urban development
	Highway construction
Mining	Surface
	Underground
Terrestrial	Landfills
	Dumps
Utility maintenance	Highways and streets
	Deicing
Urban runoff	Floods and snowmelt
Precipitation	Rainfall and snowfall
Background sources	Native forests
	Prairie land

[a]From Egboka B, Nwankwor G, Orajaka I, Ejiofor A. Principles and problems of environmental pollution of groundwater resources with case examples from developing countries. Environ Health Perspect 1989;83:39–68.

sources. Several sites located near communities reporting adverse effects in health surveys also have a ground water exposure pathway. In their review of epidemiologic studies of hazardous waste sites, Buffler et al. (1985) state that ingestion was the most frequently reported route of exposure in episodes of environmental contamination (3). Several studies have reported associations between contaminated water supplies and adverse effects in humans (3–6). Many of these studies are ecologic in nature, and do not explicitly trace pathways of exposure from sites to nearby populations, or are able to associate observed effects with levels of exposure. Thus, they are not sufficiently quantitative in nature to determine the level of remedial actions needed to protect public health.

Arriving at a quantitative understanding of the magnitude of groundwater contamination associated with chemical releases from a hazardous waste site is based on an understanding of the hydrology and geology of the site, properties governing chemical fate and mobility in soil, and the nature of the source of chemical release (Fig. 56.2). Figure 56.5 depicts the fate processes in the soil environment. The major fate processes of chemical pollutants in soil are adsorption, dispersion, and diffusion (i.e., chemical movement through the soil moisture and gas in soil pores), volatilization, and degradation. Conditions favoring chemical migration through soil include high solubility in water, porous, sandy soil, and high rainfall rates, or water ponded over the site. Conversely, soils that are high in organic matter or clay are less porous and tend to strongly sorb chemicals. Chemicals in soil are also degraded or transformed by microorganisms or abiotic mechanisms such as hydrolysis. Microbial or abiotic processes can reduce the concentration of a chemical in soil (hence reducing the concentration in ground water and risk to public health); however, these processes can result in more toxic transformation products. For example, chlorinated volatile organic compounds (VOCs) are degraded in the soil both by abiotic fate processes and biodegradation. These processes are slow, with half-lives for several chlorinated VOCs ranging from 0.5–2.5 years. The mechanisms of transformation include hydrolysis, dehydrohalogenation (in the absence of electron donors), and reductive dehalogenation. Under methanogenic conditions (i.e., anaerobic (1,1-DCA) and reducing conditions), 1,1,1-trichloroethane is transformed sequentially to 1,1-dichloroethylene (1,1-DCA), then vinyl chloride, or to 1,1-DCA, then to chloroethane. These compounds are subsequently mineralized to carbon dioxide. The transformation products 1,1-dichloroethylene and vinyl chloride are more toxic than the parent compound, with vinyl chloride being a known human carcinogen.

The groundwater exposure pathway is also of high concern because of the lack of observable effect of chemical disposal on groundwater. There may be a lag time of several years from the initiation of land disposal to the occurrence of contamination in groundwater. There may be exposure for several years before contamination in groundwater is detected and alternate water supplies are obtained for the affected communities. Exposures can potentially occur in communities that are distant from the source of contamination. There are numerous technical and logistical problems involved in evaluating this pathway, such as the installation of monitoring wells and laboratory analysis of groundwater samples.

Evaluating the magnitude and extent of a groundwater contamination problem involves an extensive hydrogeologic study that sometimes requires years to complete. Assessing longterm exposure to contaminants in groundwater is a particularly significant problem in evaluating the potential for health effects, since sampling and analysis provide only a snapshot of contaminant levels in water at a specific time. Groundwater mod-

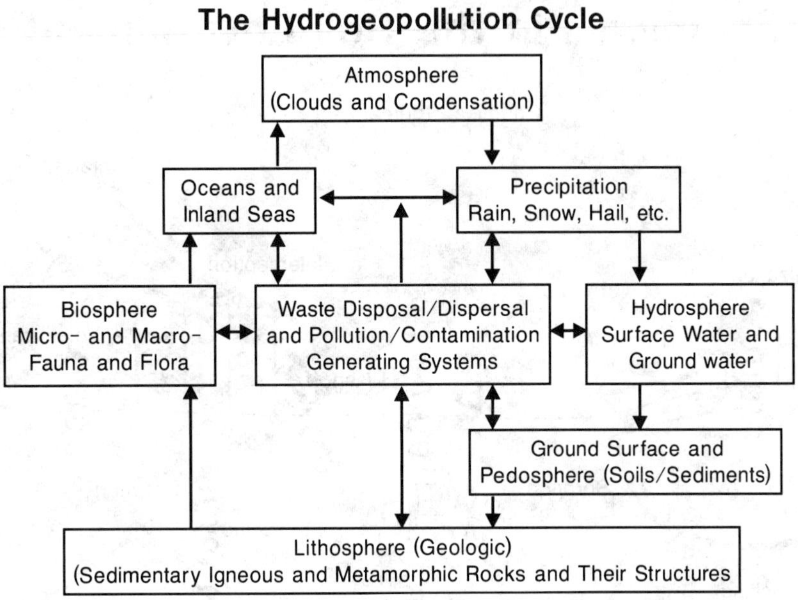

The Hydrogeopollution Cycle

Figure 56.4.   From Egboka B, Nwankwor G, Orajaka I, Ejiofor A. Principles and problems of environmental pollution of groundwater resources with case examples from developing countries. Environ Health Perspect 1989;83:39–68.

Table 56.4.   Pathogens Associated with Water Supplies[a]

Pathogens	Diseases Caused
Bacterial	
Salmonella typhis	Typhoid fever
Salmonella paratyphi A and B	Paratyphoid fever
Salmonella typhimurium	Salmonellosis
Shigella sonnei	
Shigella dysenteriae	Bacillary dysentery
Shigella flexneri	
Hycobacterium tuberculosis	Tuberculosis
Vibrio cholerae	Cholera
Francisella tularensis	Tularemia
Enteropathogenic Escherichia coli	Enteritis
Leptospira icterohaemorrhagia	Leptospirosis
Viral	
Hepatitis A virus	Viral hepatitis type A
Enteroviruses (polio, Coxsackie A and B and echo)	Respiratory tract infection, nonbacterial enteritis
Adenoviruses	
Parvoviruses	
Reoviruses	
Protozoan and metazoan	
Enteamoeba histolytica	Amoebic dysentery
Acanthamoeba spp.	Amoebic meningoencephalitis
Naegleria spp.	Amoebic meningoencephalitis
Giardia lamblia	Giardiasis
Ascaris lumbricoides	Helminthiasis
Trichuris trichura	
Taenia spp.	

[a]Adapted from Egboka B, Nwankwor G, Orajaka I, Ejiofor A. Principles and problems of environmental pollution of groundwater resources with case examples from developing countries. Environ Health Perspect 1989;83:39–68.

eling can allow longterm evaluation of exposures from this pathway; however, collection of the required data for developing and calibrating a model can be expensive and time-consuming.

Soil Ingestion

Soil ingestion as a pathway of exposure from hazardous waste sites has been of concern primarily due to adverse effects associated with childhood exposure to lead in the urban environment, and potential exposures to dioxins at Times Beach, Missouri.

The concern over dioxin (specifically 2,3,7,8-TCDD) in soil initially was based on incidents in the early 1970s where a waste oil dealer disposed of 2,3,7,8-TCDD-containing wastes by mixing it with salvage oil and spraying it on dirt roads and riding arenas for dust control (7). TCDD contamination was also detected in soils in residential areas, necessitating a determination of the levels representing unacceptable risks to those populations. The Centers for Disease Control, U.S. Department of Health and Human services, concluded that ingestion of soil containing greater than 1 ppb (part per billion) TCDD represented a public health concern (8).

The 1-ppb level of concern was based on the assumption that most soil ingestion occurs before the age of 5 years, with consumption of 10 g/day occurring from the ages of 1.5–3.5 years. These data were reportedly based on studies of childhood lead exposure (8). However, further evaluation of these data suggest that the soil ingestion estimates were unduly conservative, and probably considered the presence of pica, an abnormal condition. Soil ingestion of 50–100 mg/day was reported to be a reasonable estimate of soil ingestion rates, based on childhood lead exposure studies (9).

Exposure to lead in the urban environment has been the subject of numerous clinical investigations, with several recent studies demonstrating a relationship between lead levels in soil and increased blood lead levels in children. These studies represent the best available scientific basis for concerns about

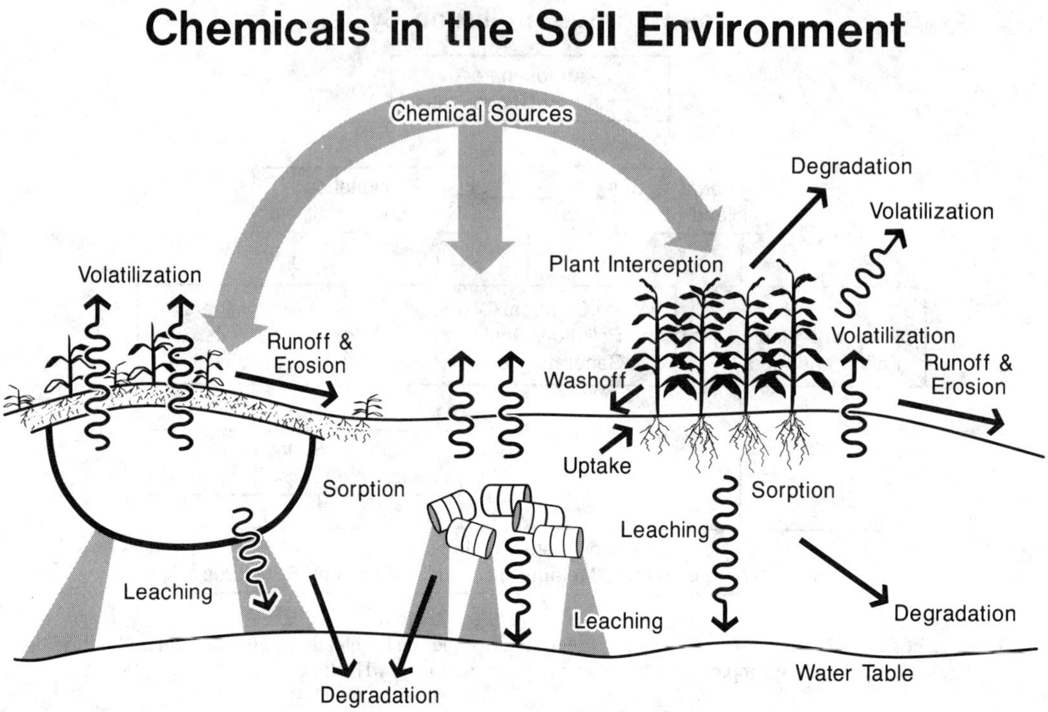

Chemicals in the Soil Environment

Figure 56.5. From Egboka B, Nwankwor G, Orajaka I, Ejiofor A. Principles and problems of environmental pollution of groundwater resources with case examples from developing countries. Environ Health Perspect 1989;83:39–68.

adverse effects from direct contact with soil (10–12). Young children are at a greater health risk from lead exposure, because they absorb proportionally more lead from ingestion exposure, and because normal childhood behavior facilitates contact with a lead-contaminated environment.

Based on these findings, investigators have attempted to quantify the amounts of soil ingested by young children. A few investigators have also addressed soil ingestion rates of older children and adults. These, and other studies based on similar approaches suggested that reasonable estimates of childhood soil ingestion rates were below 250 mg/day. Tracer studies using elements in soil that are poorly absorbed in the gastrointestinal tract (such as aluminum or silicon) have also been used to estimate soil ingestion rates in children. These studies involved analyzing for these elements in stool samples and estimating the tracer contribution from dietary sources. Daily soil ingestion based on these studies is probably between 50 and 100 mg/day (13, 14). Soil ingestion rates have not been estimated for age groups other than children; however, some authors have attempted to make assumptions about types of activities bringing individuals into contact with soil and the frequency of contact in order to estimate ingestion rates for purposes of risk assessment (15–17).

Reported incidents of adverse effects associated with soil ingestion of toxic substances are not common in the literature, outside of childhood exposures to lead. Inhalation, ingestion of drinking water or food, and dermal contact are more commonly reported as exposure pathways in the literature. However, experience with risk assessment has shown that the soil ingestion pathway often provides a significant contribution to estimated risks and can often determine the cleanup level mandated for a site.

Inhalation Exposure

Inhalation exposures and emissions to the air from hazardous waste sites, have been reportedly associated with adverse effects in communities near hazardous waste sites (3, 5). However, the air pathway has received relatively less study than exposures from contaminated groundwater. Shen (1985) states that volatilization is a major loss mechanism for organic compounds disposed to land, and that the public health risk (related to air quality) from hazardous waste landfills and lagoons is greater than from hazardous waste incinerators, due to the presence of pollution controls on incinerators (18). Despite this, there is a relative lack of information on the ambient concentrations associated with emissions from hazardous waste sites.

In one study, air monitoring was performed at a hazardous waste remedial action site to measure inhalation exposure at a drum repackaging process. Area samples were collected from the perimeter of the site and were analyzed for organic amines, polychlorinated biphenyls (PCBs), polynuclear aromatic hydrocarbons, chlorinated hydrocarbon pesticides, and volatile organic compounds (VOCs). VOCs were the only compounds detected, with the highest concentrations being toluene, 1200 $\mu g/m^3$ on site, and 220 $\mu g/m^3$ downwind. Numerous other VOCs were detected downwind, all in the range of $\mu g/m^3$ in air (19). Vinyl chloride emissions from the BKK landfill in California were monitored for the purpose of evaluating the performance of atmospheric dispersion models. The average vinyl chloride concentration over 5 days of monitoring was 6.5 ppb (16.7 $\mu g/m^3$), with a range of <2–12 ppb (<5–30.9 $\mu g/m^3$) (20). Over a 3-year period, the National Institute for Occupational Safety and Health (NIOSH) had collected 500 air samples at hazardous waste sites, including a remedial action where drum handling was performed, a municipal landfill where hazardous wastes were codisposed, and a hazardous waste treatment, storage, and disposal facility. The substances analyzed included organic vapors, heavy metals, pesticides, PCBs, and cyanides. Of these 500 samples, no contaminant exceeded 10% of the OSHA 8-hour time-weighted average permissible exposure limit. For example, toluene concentrations ranged from 900–14,800 $\mu g/m^3$, whereas the OSHA standard is 750,000 μ/m^3. At one site, there is some evidence that particulate-bound polynuclear aromatics were responsible for eye and respiratory irritation among workers and within the nearby community (21).

While the air pathway remains a concern for hazardous waste sites (due primarily to the lack of information concerning the magnitude of exposure), the most definitive studies on human exposure to air pollutants have implicated sources other than waste disposal as significant sources of exposure to airborne toxic substances. For example, the EPA Total Exposure Assessment Methodology (TEAM) study has identified environmental tobacco smoke, gasoline emissions while fueling vehicles, dry cleaning solvent emissions from clothes, moth balls, and indoor air sources as significant sources of exposure to volatile organic compounds (22).

EXPOSURE PATHWAYS AND RISK ASSESSMENT

Risk assessment provides an analytical tool for evaluating the potential for exposure and health risks associated with contaminants at a hazardous waste site. Risk assessment is a systematic study of the possible relationships between exposure to toxic substances in the environment and the occurrence of adverse health effects, based on available scientific evidence. Risk assessments are conducted to project future risks that cannot be measured directly, from very low levels of chemical exposure. Health Risk Assessments (HRAs) represent an approximation of actual exposures, resulting in some uncertainty about the risks predicted to be associated with an activity. Data specifically addressing factors contributing to those risks frequently are not available. These data gaps must then be bridged by using assumptions. The use of health-conservative assumptions is one new approach that addresses uncertainty in the predicted risks. Use of health conservative methods results in estimated levels of health risk that are greater than would actually be experienced as a result of exposure to chemical constituents at the site. Health conservative methods are unlikely to underestimate the exposures or risks from site constituents.

The steps involved in a risk assessment, adapted from the Nuclear Regulatory Commission (NRC, 1983), are as follows:

- Hazard identification, or selection of indicator chemicals, which are the chemicals of greatest health concern (i.e., are the most toxic, mobile, or prevalent of those detected) from among the entire set of chemicals associated with the site;
- Toxicity assessment, which involves estimating no-adverse-effects levels and health criteria;
- Exposure assessment, which involves the identification of potentially exposed populations, sources, and pathways of potential exposure, and estimation of exposures through those pathways; and
- Risk characterization, which combines the results of the exposure and toxicity assessments to provide numerical estimates of health risks.

Hazard Identification

Hazard identification is the process of assessing whether exposure to a substance can be associated with an increase in the incidence of an adverse health effect. Current EPA guidelines have greatly simplified the hazard identification process by recommending that the risk assessment must consider those chemicals detected in soil and groundwater at a hazardous waste site that present 99% of the health risk associated with that site, and must consider all of the carcinogenic compounds detected (1).

Toxicity Assessment

The toxicity assessment derives the numerical criteria used for evaluating the potential for systemic, or noncarcinogenic, effects and cancer risks associated with exposure to contaminants. A reference dose (RfD) is a health-based criterion often used in evaluating noncarcinogenic effects. RfD levels are developed by the U.S. EPA's Environmental Criteria Assessment Office (ECAO). The RfD is based on the assumption that thresholds exist for certain toxic effects such as cellular necrosis but may not exist for other toxic effects such as carcinogenicity. In general, the RfD is an estimate (with uncertainty spanning perhaps an order of magnitude) of a daily exposure to the human population (including sensitive subgroups) that is likely to be without an appreciable risk of deleterious effects during a lifetime. Numerical estimates of cancer potency are presented as slope factors (SFs). Under the assumption of dose-response linearity at low doses, the SF defines the cancer risk due to continuous constant lifetime exposure of one unit of carcinogen concentration, expressed in units of risk per mg/kg/day or $(mg/kg/day)^{-1}$. Individual cancer risk (a unitless number) is calculated as the product of pollutant intake (in mg/kg/day) and the SF for that pollutant, in $(mg/kg/day)^{-1}$. For both carcinogens and noncarcinogens, effects from exposures to multiple chemicals are assumed to be additive (23–24); however, noncarcinogens are additive only for similar end-target organs. This appears to be a reasonable approach to addressing effects from exposures to mixture.

Exposure Assessment

The exposure assessment component of a risk assessment provides the most direct comparison between the historical and epidemiologic information evaluating the significance of certain exposure pathways. Exposure assessment is the estimation of the magnitude, frequency, duration, and routes of exposure to humans. The exposure is typically evaluated by estimating the amount of a chemical which could come into contact with the lungs, gastrointestinal tract, or skin during a specific time. The exposure assessment for this site is based on scenarios that define the potentially exposed populations, frequencies and duration of potential exposures, the possible exposure pathways, and the concentrations in air, food, or soil that potentially contact these populations through the pathways delineated in the exposure scenarios (23, 24).

Exposure assumptions for risk assessments performed for CERCLA (Superfund) sites are based on a reasonable maximum exposure (RME) scenario. The RME scenario is defined as the highest exposure that is reasonably expected to occur at a site. The intent of the RME scenario is to develop an estimate of exposure well above an average exposure level that is still within the range of possible exposures. The assumptions used in estimating the RME and the rationale for those assumptions are those that provide a 95% upper confidence limit (UCL) of the average level of exposure associated with chemicals at a site. Such methods have been developed by the U.S. Environmental Protection Agency because they are not likely to underestimate the exposures or risks from site contaminants in actuality (1). Typical assumptions include:

- Exposure for a lifetime or near-lifetime duration (ranging from 30–70 years, in the absence of other data indicating a different exposure duration);
- Daily exposure, typically for 365 days/year (in the absence of other data indicating a different frequency of exposure);
- Specified contact rates with contaminated media (100 mg/day soil ingestion rate, 2 l/day drinking water ingestion rate);
- Concentrations in environmental media do not degrade or transform over time.

It is difficult to evaluate these assumptions in light of the historical or epidemiologic experience with exposure pathways other than to note that it is likely that these assumptions substantially overestimate health risks. For example, experience with these methods indicates that they predict the soil ingestion exposure pathway as providing as significant a contribution to total exposure (hence total estimated risk) as ingestion of contaminated groundwater; however, available epidemiologic evidence has not indicated increased rates of adverse effects associated with soil ingestion, with the exception of childhood lead exposures. Use of these exposure assumptions address the EPA's mandate under SARA to have remedial actions that primarily protect public health (with cost and feasibility considerations being secondary); however, use of such methods could drastically overestimate health risks, as is discussed below.

Risk Characterization

Risk characterization provides a quantitative description concerning the existence and magnitude of potential public health concerns related to contamination detected at the site. Risk characterization involves combining the results of the exposure and toxicity assessments, providing numerical estimates of health risk, and characterizing the magnitude of uncertainty associated with the risk estimates. A risk assessment for arsenic presents an example of this approach and illustrates the magnitude of conservatism associated with arsenic risks estimated through risk assessment.

Certain areas of Taiwan have high background concentrations of arsenic in groundwater, which have been correlated with rates of hyperpigmentation, skin cancer, and black foot disease (a peripheral vascular disease). Concentrations in water range from 0.01–1.8 ppm; lowest concentrations associated with adverse effects ranged from 0.4–0.6 ppm, and a dose-response relationship has been demonstrated for these adverse effects (25). Similar studies in the United States have not reproduced these results; however, the concentrations in groundwater were approximately 10-fold lower (26). The EPA, using the Taiwan data in a linear extrapolation model, has predicted a cancer risk of 5×10^{-5} associated with lifetime ingestion of 1 µg/l arsenic in drinking water at 2 l/day. Using a 70-kg body weight, this value can be recalculated to a slope factor of 1.75 $(\text{mg/kg/day})^{-1}$ which can be used to characterize risks associated with other exposure pathways, such as soil ingestion of arsenic by a child.

Childhood exposures to arsenic in soil are estimated using the following calculation (1):

Intake (mg/kg-day)
$$= \frac{CS \times IRSOIL \times CF \times FISOIL \times EF \times ED}{BW \times AT}$$

Where:

CS = chemical concentration in soil (mg/kg)
$IRSOIL$ = ingestion rate (mg soil per day)
CF = conversion factor (10^{-6} kg/mg)
$FISOIL$ = fraction ingested from contaminated source (unitless)
EF = exposure frequency (days/year)
ED = exposure duration (years)
BW = body weight (kg)
AT = averaging time (period over which exposure is averaged—days)

Variable Values:

CS: Site-specific measured values
$IRSOIL$: 200 mg/day (children, 1 through 6 years old)
CF: 10^{-6} kg/mg
$FISOIL$: Pathway-specific value (should consider contaminant location and population activity patterns)
EF: 365 days/year
ED: 6 years, assumed exposure duration for a child
BW: 16 kg (children 1 through 6 years old, 50th percentile)
AT: Pathway-specific period of exposure for carcinogenic effects (i.e., 70 years $\times$ 365 days/year).

The default input parameters recommended by EPA for estimating childhood exposure from soil ingestion are summarized in Table 56.5. The cancer risk associated with childhood exposure to arsenic through soil ingestion is then estimated as:

$$RISK = INTAKE \times SF$$

where

$RISK$ = potential cancer risk adjusted for lifetime exposure (unitless)
SF = oral slope factor for arsenic, 1.5 $(\text{mg/kg/day})^{-1}$
$INTAKE$ = chemical intake (mg/kg/day)

The nationwide geometric mean concentration of arsenic in surface soil (i.e., the arsenic background in soil) is estimated to be 5.2 mg/kg (27). With the risk assessment methodology described previously, the lifetime risk associated with childhood exposure to this concentration of arsenic in soil is 1×10^{-5}, based on a lifetime average exposure rate of 0.0000056 mg/kg/day. Risk levels from 1×10^{-4} to 1×10^{-6} are specified as the range of acceptable risk for remedial actions for hazardous waste sites in the RI/FS process, with the extent of population exposure determining the level of risk to be selected for a site. With this consideration, it is possible that background levels of arsenic in soil could present unacceptable levels of cancer risk at certain hazardous waste sites, using this risk assessment methodology. It is reasonable to conclude that the assumptions used in the EPA risk assessment guidance overestimate potential exposures; however, in the absence of data further characterizing the parameters used to express the magnitude, frequency, and duration of exposure, it is likely that

Table 56.5.   Exposure Parameters Used in Soil Ingestion Risk Assessment

Pathway	Parameter	Abbreviation	Units	Parameter Value		Comments	Citation
				Carcinogen	Noncarcinogen		
General parameters	Body weight	BW	kg	16	16	Child body weight recommended by EPA	EPA, 1989
	Exposure frequency	EF	days/year	365	365	Highest possible exposure frequency	
	Exposure duration	ED	years	6	6	Exposure duration recommended by EPA	EPA, 1989
	Averaging time	AT	days	25,500 (70 years × 365 days/year)	2,190 (6 years × 365 days/year)		EPA, 1989
Soil ingestion	Ingestion rate	IRSOIL	kg/day	0.0002	0.0002	Reasonable maximum exposure values recommended by EPA	EPA, 1989
	Fraction of soil ingested from the site	FISOIL	—	1.0 (conservative default value)		Maximum exposure value	

these methods will continue to be employed for estimating health risks.

HEALTH RISKS ASSOCIATED WITH HAZARDOUS MATERIAL INCINERATOR EMISSIONS

Most of the considerations in epidemiology and risk assessment for hazardous waste sites discussed previously also are applicable to hazardous materials incinerators. Incinerator emissions provide environmental concentrations well below those levels at which adverse effects would be detectable by epidemiologic methods. Incineration is an engineered process that employs thermal oxidation at high temperatures (usually 900°C or greater) to destroy the organic fraction of waste and reduce waste volume. Of all of the "terminal" treatment technologies, incineration has the capability for the highest degree of destruction and control of the broadest range of hazardous waste streams. Incineration has been employed for the disposal of hazardous waste for little more than 20 years, although municipal solid waste incineration has been performed for over a century and may offer substantial advantages over other hazardous waste treatment technologies (28). However, with concerns about increased health risks associated with incinerator emissions, significant public opposition has grown against the permitting and operation of new incinerators.

Evaluating health risks associated with hazardous waste incineration involves consideration of several factors, including incineration technologies, operating conditions, types of waste streams, air pollution control devices, meteorologic conditions, and locations of populations and sensitive receptors (such as agricultural areas, livestock, hospitals, schools, and surface water supplies). Identification of the hazards associated with incinerator emissions beings with an overview of incineration processes.

Incineration Processes

Hazardous waste incinerators are found in a variety of designs but share these major components:

- Waste preparation and feeding;
- Combustion chamber(s);
- Air pollution control devices; and
- Residue/ash handling.

The four most common incinerator designs (in order of use) are liquid injection, rotary kiln, fixed hearth, and fluidized bed incinerators (28). Rotary kiln incinerators are more versatile than other designs in the sense that they can incinerate solid wastes, slurries, and containerized wastes as well as liquids. The rotary kiln incinerator, shown in Figure 56.6, is most widely used in commercial incinerators and is presented here as an example of the incineration process.

The rotary kiln is a cylindrical refractory-lined shell that is mounted on a slight incline. The shell rotates to move the waste through the kiln and improve mixing of the waste. The kiln converts solid and liquid wastes to gases, which are then released into an afterburner to complete the combustion. Following incineration of hazardous wastes, the combustion gases are further treated in air pollution control devices before being emitted from a stack. The gases may be scrubbed to remove hydrogen chloride and other acid gases. Ash in the waste is not destroyed in the combustion process. Depending on its composition, the ash will either exit as fly ash (i.e., suspended in the combustion gas stream) or as bottom ash. Fly ash particles are removed from the gas stream using a particle collection device. Bottom ash is removed from the incinerator and disposed of in a landfill.

Hazard Identification

Ideally, the primary products of combustion are carbon dioxide, water vapor, and inert ash. While combustion and incineration devices are designed to optimize destruction of wastes, they never completely attain this ideal. Rather, small quantities of byproducts can be formed. These products along with the potentially uncombusted waste components form the emissions from the incinerator. Each of the major components influences the type and magnitude of chemicals emissions from an incinerator.

Typical Rotary Kiln/Afterburner Combustion Chamber

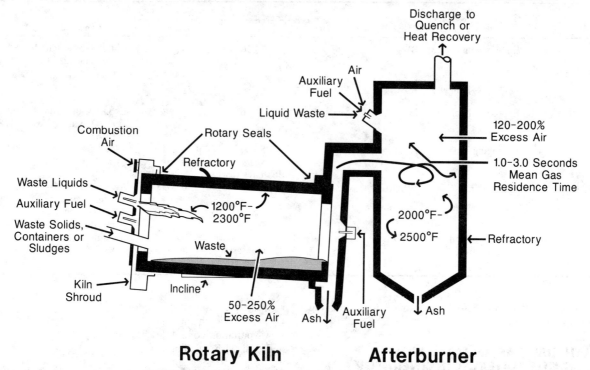

Figure 56.6. From Oppelt ET. Incineration of hazardous wastes: a critical review. J Air Pollut Control Assoc 1987;37:558–586. Reprinted with permission.

Table 56.6. Overview of Incinerator Emissions

Incinerator Component	Emission
Waste preparation and feeding	Fugitive emissions from tanks, values, and fittings
Combustion chambers	Stack emissions of organic compounds and combustion byproducts
Air pollution control devices	Stack emissions of particulate matter (fly ash) and acid gases
Residue/ash handling	Particulate emissions during ash handling and disposal

The major public health concerns with incineration have been associated with emissions to the air and the disposal of incinerator ash (Table 56.6). Emissions to the air from an incinerator may take two forms: stack emissions and fugitive emissions. Stack emissions, consisting of the combustion gas containing traces of fly ash, organic combustion byproducts, and acid gases, may comprise several classes of chemicals, including volatile and semivolatile organic compounds, trace metals, polycyclic aromatic hydrocarbons (PAHs), polychlorinated dibenzodioxins and polychlorinated dibenzofurans (PCDD/PCDFs), and "traditional" air pollutants such as sulfur dioxide, nitrogen dioxides, ozone precursors, and particulate matter. Fugitive emissions consist largely of volatile organic compounds (VOCs) that escape from tanks, valves, and fittings. If the incinerator is associated with a landfill, then incinerator emissions may include resuspension of dust during ash handling and disposal.

METALS

Metals, including arsenic, beryllium, chromium, cadmium, lead, mercury, nickel, and zinc, are not destroyed by incineration. The total metals input to an incinerator emerges associated with either with the fly ash or bottom ash. Most of the metals input emerging from the combustion zone is associated with the bottom ash. However, some of the more volatile metals (i.e., metals with lower boiling points), such as arsenic, lead, cadmium, and mercury may emerge in a vapor state. These volatile metals will condense onto fly ash particulates being emitted from the stack. These metals will exhibit enrichment onto fine particulate matter (i.e., higher concentrations relative to the concentrations on larger particles). Fine particulate enrichment of metals is of public health concern because air pollution control devices provide less control for fine particulate emissions, and fine particulates are more readily inhaled and deposited in the lung. Metals are also of concern in incinerator emissions because, once dispersed into the air, they can deposit onto the soil and provide exposure through the foodchain. Several metals are carcinogenic based epidemiological studies of high exposure levels in workers, including arsenic, beryllium, chromium, cadmium, and nickel. Other metals have been shown to produce adverse effects in humans, including lead and mercury.

COMBUSTION BYPRODUCTS

Even with good combustion conditions, incomplete combustion byproducts may be emitted from an incinerator. Testing of combustion byproducts has focused largely on Principal Or-

Table 56.7. Most Frequent Combustion Byproducts from Incinerators

Volatile Organic Compounds	Semivolatile Organic Compounds
Benzene	Naphthalene
Toluene	Phenol
Carbon tetrachloride	Bis(2-ethylhexyl)phthalate
Chloroform	Diethylphthalate
Methylene chloride	Butylbenzylphthalate
Trichloroethylene	Dibutylphthalate
Tetrachloroethylene	
1,1,1-Trichloroethane	
Chlorobenzene	

Source: Oppelt ET. Incineration of hazardous wastes: a critical review. J Air Pollut Control Assoc 1987;37:558–586.

ganic Hazardous Constituents (POHCs), those compounds identified as hazardous under Appendix VIII of RCRA. Appendix VIII is a list of approximately 400 organic and inorganic hazardous chemicals, first published in 1980 in 40 CFR 261. The list is updated semiannually. Appendix VII compounds that are present in highest concentrations in the waste feed and are the most difficult to destroy are typically selected as POHCs.

RCRA specifies that an incinerator must attain at least 99.99% destruction and removal efficiency (DRE) for each POHC. This means that the quantities of each POHC emitted from an incinerator must be less than 0.01% of the quantity fed to the incinerator. EPA source tests data from existing incinerators. However, even with good combustion conditions, combustion byproducts may be emitted from an incinerator. Comparison of total hydrocarbon emissions with the total quantities of specific organic compounds identified in incinerator emissions during testing has revealed that only a percentage of the total hydrocarbon emitted has been characterized. Testing of combustion byproducts has focused largely on POHCs, and currently a complete database on combustion byproducts is not yet available (28). Combustion byproducts are of concern because of the uncertainty of their identities. Studies of combustion byproducts show that they include the following:

- POHCs not destroyed in incineration (0.01% of quantity fed to the incinerator);
- Products of the incomplete combustion from auxiliary fuel;
- Formation of "new" compounds (compounds not initially in the waste feed) from chemical reactions in the combustion zone of the incinerator;
- Byproducts from other sources (such as air pollutants in combustion air or trihalomethanes in scrubber water).

EPA-sponsored tests of incinerators identified nine volatile organic compounds and six semivolatile organic compounds that were observed most frequently and at highest concentrations in combustion byproducts (Table 56.7) (28–30). The volatile compounds tended to be detected more often and at higher concentrations in stack gases than the semivolatile compounds. These incineration tests also compared emissions of organic compounds from facilities incinerating hazardous waste and those same facilities burning only fossil fuel. The data from these tests indicated that there is little inherent difference between waste and fuel combustion emissions of organic compounds (28, 30).

The principal health concerns with combustion byproducts is the lack of information identifying the chemicals present in the emissions. Risk assessments performed by EPA indicate that the health risks associated with combustion byproducts are two to three orders of magnitude lower than the risks associated with metals emissions. However, considering the uncertainties about the chemical constituents, EPA has recently proposed an alternate approach in assessing and minimizing health risks associated with combustion byproducts. EPA states that operating incinerators at a high combustion efficiency reduces combustion byproducts (31).

DIOXINS AND FURANS

Polychlorinated dibenzodioxins (PCDDs) and polychlorinated dibrenzofurans (PCDFs) are of concern because of carcinogenicity and other toxic effects reported in studies with laboratory animals. There are over 75 possible PCDD isomers and 135 possible PCDF isomers, with the 2,3,7,8-tetrachlorodibenzo-p-dioxin isomer (2,3,7,8-TCDD) receiving the most extensive study. However, emissions testing of incinerators typically has been limited to quantitating total PCDD/PCDFs and the 2,3,7,8-TCDD isomer. The available emissions testing data for hazardous waste incinerators indicate that PCDD/PCDFs are typically not detected in the emissions. Of 17 facilities that have been tested, only five detected levles of PCDD/PCDFs in the emissions. 2,3,7,8-TCDD, the most toxic member of this class of compounds, was not detected in emissions from any of the tested incinerators. The highest PCDD levels were detected in an incinerator using creosote and pentachlorophenol sludges as a fuel, where PCDDs were detected in the waste feed (28, 30). Oppelt (1987) has also noted that emissions measured from hazardous waste incinerators are approximately 1000-fold lower than emissions from municipal solid waste incinerators.

Emissions of PCDD/PCDFs are influenced by the type of waste feed and combustion temperature. Waste feeds containing PCDDs/PCDFs or precursor compounds have a greater tendency of producing PCDD/PCDF emissions. Precursor compounds for PCDD/PCDFs include PCBs, chlorinated phenols, and chlorinated benzenes.

Exposure Pathways and Risk Assessment

The extent to which exposure occurs from emissions to the air differs between stack and fugitive emissions, and between particulate and volatile emissions. Fugitive emissions occur largely at ambient temperatures from low-lying sources. Because of the low temperature and elevation, they do not disperse very far and tend to produce relatively higher concentrations close to the point of emission. Stack emissions occur at higher temperatures and from more elevated sources, which tend to provide greater loft to the plume, and produce dispersion over greater distances. The significance of these different dispersion processes is that fugitive emissions (consisting of VOCs) potentially are associated with inhalation exposures of individuals located close to the incinerator, while stack emissions are potentially associated with both inhalation exposure and ingestion exposure from particle deposition and pollutant transport through the food chain; impacts from stack emissions also fall over a more widespread area compared with fugitive emissions. Figure 56.7 presents the exposure pathways associated with incinerator emissions.

Risk assessment of emissions from hazardous materials in-

Environmental Exposure Pathways

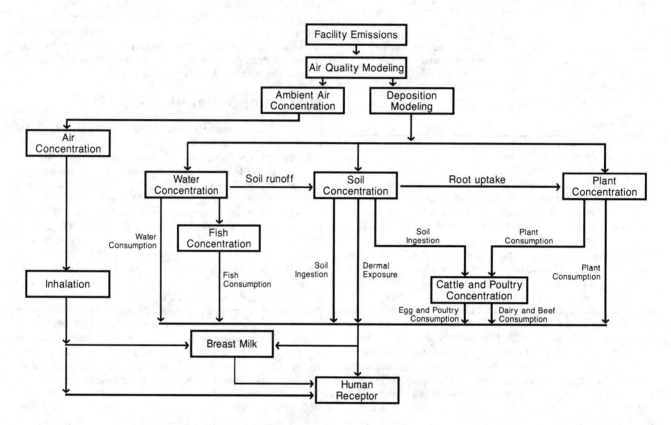

Figure 56.7.   From Lowe JA, et al. Health effects of municipal waste incineration. Boca Raton, FL: CRC Press, 1991. Reprinted with permission.

cinerators involves the use of air dispersion and particle deposition modeling. Gaussian plume-based dispersion models typically are used to estimate ambient concentrations associated with incinerator emissions. Figure 56.8 presents a schematic of Gaussian plume dispersion characteristics. Dispersion modeling estimates concentrations in air taking into consideration meteorological conditions (windspeed, wind direction, and vertical stability), source characteristics (stack height, and temperature and velocity of the gases existing the stack), and locations of human populations relative to the incinerator. Guidelines for the use of dispersion models are provided by the EPA (29). Pollutant concentrations in air are used to estimate inhalation exposures to incinerator emissions. evaluating secondary exposure pathways (soil ingestion, crop ingestion, meat and milk ingestion, and dermal contact with soil) requires calculation of the particle deposition flux to the soil. Deposition flux is influenced by particle deposition velocity, which in turn is a function of particle diameter, density, and meterologic conditions near the ground surface.

Risk assessments for municipal solid waste incinerators, which have similar exposure pathways to hazardous materials incinerators typically show that food chain exposure pathways provide the major contribution to estimated exposures (32). However, this is probably due to overestimation inherent in deposition modeling methodologies. Deposition algorithms in EPA "guideline" models such as the Industrial Source Complex

(ISC) model are not mass conservative and, under certain conditions, the quantity of pollutant deposited could exceed the quantity emitted. Deposition algorithms in guideline dispersion models also neglect plume depletion (i.e., reduction in the concentration in air as deposition occurs), also contributing to overestimation of both inhalation and ingestion exposures (33).

Studies of human exposure to VOCs have identified more likely sources than hazardous materials incinerators for this class of compounds. For example, the EPA's Total Exposure Assessment Methodology (TEAM) study provided the first large scale, direct measurement of personal exposures to chemical pollutants, outside of the workplace (22). This study involved over 600 individuals who each carried a personal air monitor for two consecutive 12-hour periods and who maintained a diary of their activities during the monitoring period. Compounds monitored in this study were VOCs, including benzene, tetrachloroethylene, and 1,1,1-trichloroethane. Study areas were selected to identify contrasts in exposures between heavily industrialized areas and lightly industrialized areas. Although fixed-area outdoor air samples could distinguish a difference in airborne concentrations between heavily and lightly industrialized areas, personal air monitoring results did not distinguish between these areas, indicating that the greatest level of exposure occurs indoors. It is likely that the sources of most of these exposures are common activities: benzene from sidestream smoke from cigarettes, tetrachloroethylene from

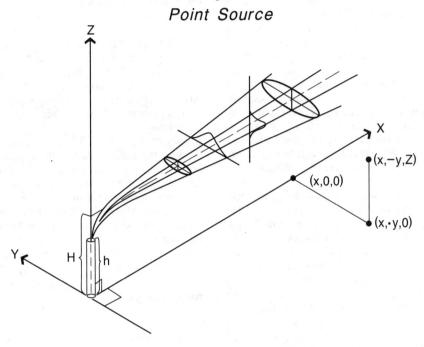

Gaussian Dispersion Model
Point Source

Figure 56.8. From EPA. Guidelines on air quality models. Rev ed. Publ. No. EPA-450/2-78-027R. Research Triangle Park, NC: Office of Air Quality Planning and Standards, 1986.

wearing and home storage of clothes that have been dry cleaned, and the use of p-dichlorobenzene in moth balls and air fresheners.

Health risks from dioxin and furan emissions from both municipal solid waste and hazardous materials incinerators typically have been of great concern by the public. However, environmental monitoring studies of these compounds have shown similarities in isomers, levels detected in the environment, isomeric patterns and congereric profiles in samples collected from several industrialized nations. A notable finding was the similarity of dioxin data between Sweden, which has 25–40 municipal solid waste incinerators, and Yugoslavia, which has no incinerators. This comparison suggests that sources other than incineration might contribute significantly to background levels of dioxins and furans in the environment. These sources could include automobile exhaust and forest fires (34). One hypothesis suggests that dioxins and furans are ubiquitous by-products of any combustion process (35).

PERSPECTIVES ON PUBLIC EXPOSURES TO CHEMICALS

Both hazardous waste sites and hazardous waste incinerators are perceived as significant sources of exposure to chemical substances, and as health risks, by the general public. Given the nature of the study of adverse effects from low level exposure to toxic substances, it is problematic to answer the question of whether hazardous waste and its management is a risk. However, for certain pollutants, it has been possible to draw some conclusions pertaining to exposure sources.

Despite years of effort, relatively few studies conducted

to evaluate the potential human health effects from hazardous waste sites have been sufficiently well-designed or well-conducted to yield meaningful results (36). Studies are frequently unable to estimate exposure or proximity to the site. Often the potentially exposed populations are small, limiting the power of an epidemiologic study to detect adverse effects. Risk assessments provide the opportunity to evaluate risks that cannot be evaluated using epidemiologic methods, and they provide a method for ranking risks associated with different sites and establishing priorities for site remediation. Predicting the occurrence of adverse effects from low levels of exposure requires consideration of natural processes that cannot be directly studied or measured scientifically. The health risk assessment process necessarily invokes numerous assumptions about the behavior of chemicals in the environment and the potential for adverse health effects based on the best available scientific evidence. Since risk assessments are based largely upon assumptions, there is uncertainty about whether the results accurately reflect the actual risks associated with environmental pollutants. One approach to addressing this uncertainty is to use health-conservative assumptions that deliberately overstate the magnitude of the health risks. However, the results of a health-conservative risk assessment must be used judiciously in making decisions about how much remediation a hazardous waste site requires or whether or not to construct an incinerator. Risk assessments overstate health risks, potentially resulting in selection of options for managing hazardous waste that are both costly and overly protective of public health.

While the health-conservative approach is qualitatively correct, its application in a quantitative risk assessment is problematic. If each assumption or parameter in a risk assessment, where uncertainty was present, were selected as a 95% upper confidence level (i.e., only one of 20 values would be more conservative), the resulting risk (probability of cancer occurring in the exposed individual) would have a minute chance of occurring; it could occur only if all of the unlikely assumptions had occurred. For example, if there were two such uncertain assumptions used, the probability of the joint conservative event occurring would be one in 400. If there were four such assumptions, the probability of the joint conservative event would be 1 in 160,000 (i.e., there would be a 160,000-fold overestimate of the risk of cancer associated with a specific exposure situation). Thus, quantitatively, the risk estimate from a health-conservative assessment becomes a remote event of little value in managing risk (37).

An important element in making informed decisions about how to clean up a hazardous waste site or where to build incinerators (if at all) is communicating the nature of the decision-making process. Successfully communicating the results of risk assessment requires an understanding of how different groups perceive health risks from environmental pollutants. Different institutional settings (i.e., proponents of incinerator projects, parties responsible for investigating and cleaning up waste sites, members of potentially affected communities, agency officials or environmental activists) view health risk issues differently due to different cultural biases (38). Laypersons tend to view the acceptability of risks in terms of familiarity, control over decision-making, controlability of the risk, catastrophic potential, voluntariness of the risk-producing activity, familiarity with the risk-producing activity, and uncertainty over the level of risk (39). An expert's view of risk consists of the probability of an adverse event and the magnitude of its consequences. However, "common sense" definitions of risk frequently do not consider the probability of occurrence, but rest entirely upon the magnitude of the consequence (38). Hence, a health-conservative, worst case scenario in a risk assessment is not viewed by the public in terms of how unlikely its occurrence may be, but in terms of the severity of its consequences, should it occur. Additionally, activists may assert that health risks imposed by one group (such as project proponents or responsible parties) fall unevenly on another group (affected communities). The activist viewpoint is that a risk that threaten's an individual's health cannot be spread equitably, and under such circumstances any risk to an exposed population is unacceptable (38).

These represent the concerns that must be addressed when communicating to the public the risks associated with contaminants at hazardous waste sites or incinerator emissions. Information addressing public concerns about low level chemical exposure can include expressions of the credibility of a risk assessment (through external peer review or "blue ribbon" panels), accessibility of the risk assessment process to public comment, and certification of the risk assessment results through agency review. In the case of hazardous materials incinerators, discussions of administrative and engineering controls for the facility may address public concerns about the level of control over potential risks.

CONCLUSIONS

Predicting or inferring the occurrence of adverse health effects from exposures to low levels of chemicals, either released from hazardous waste sites or emitted from hazardous materials in-

cinerators, often cannot be addressed with any certainty by observational methods such as epidemiologic studies. These potential occurrences are then addressed through the process of risk assessment. Risk assessment involves numerous assumptions about the behavior of chemicals in the environment and the potential for adverse effects at low levels of exposure. Since assumptions are used in risk assessment, there is uncertainty about whether the results reflect the potential for adverse effects associated with a particular exposure situation. These uncertainties often cannot be resolved through observational means, due to an extremely low potential frequency of occurrence. The uncertainty is typically addressed through the use of health-conservative methods that deliberately overstate the magnitude of health risks. However, the use of conservative assumptions must be considered carefully, or else the resulting risk assessment presents an extremely unrealistic depiction of the risks associated with a particular exposure situation and hence is of little use in decision-making. Communicating the results of a risk assessment requires consideration of the perceptions and cultural biases of the members of the public.

REFERENCES

1. EPA. Risk assessment guidance for superfund. Vol I. Human health evaluation manual (Part A). Interim Final. EPA/540/1-89/002. Washington, DC: Office of Emergency and Remedial Response, 1989.
2. Egboka B, Nwankwor G, Orajaka I, Ejiofor A. Principles and problems of environmental pollution of groundwater resources with case examples from developing countries. Environ Health Perspect 83:39–68, 1989.
3. Buffler PA, Crane M, Key MM. Possibilities of detecting health effects by studies of populations exposed to chemicals from waste disposal sites. Environ Health Perspect 1985;62:423–456.
4. Shy CM. Chemical contamination of water supplies. Environ Health Perspect 1985;62:399–406.
5. Levine R, Chitwood DD. Public health investigations of hazardous organic chemical disposal in the United States. Environ Health Perspect 1985;62:415–422.
6. Griffith J, Duncan RC, Riggan WB, Pellum AC. Cancer mortality in U.S. counties with hazardous waste sites and groundwater pollution. Arch Environ Health 1989;44:69–74.
7. Carter CD, Kimbrough RD, Liddle JA, Cline RF, Zack MM, Barthel WF, Koehler RE, Phillips PE. Tetrachlorodibenzodioxin: an accidental poisoning episode in horse arenas. Science 1975;188:738–740.
8. Kimbrough RD, Falk H, Stehr P, Fries G. Health implications of 2,3,7,8-tetrachlorodibenzodioxin (TCDD) in residential soil. J Toxicol Environ Health 1984;14:47–93.
9. Paustenbach DJ, Murray FJ. A critical examination of assessments of the health risks associated with 2,3,7,8-TCDD in soil. Chemosphere 1986;15:1867–1874.
10. Sayre JW, Charney E, Vostal J, Pless BI. House and hand dust as a potential source of childhood lead exposure. Am J Dis Child 1974;127:167–170.
11. Needleman HL, Landrigan PJ. The health effects of low level exposure to lead. Annu Rev Public Health 1981;1:277–298.
12. Bander LK, Pirkle JL, Makuc D, Neese NW, Bayse DD, Kovar MG. Dietary lead intake of preschool children. Am J Public Health 1983;73:789–793.
13. Binder S, Sokal D, Maughan D. Estimating soil ingestion: the use of tracer elements in estimating the amount of soil ingested by young children. Arch Environ Health 1986;41:341–345.
14. Clausing P, Brunerkreef B, Van Wijnen JH. A method for estimating soil ingestion by children. Int Arch Occup Environ Health 1987;59:73–82.
15. Hawley JK. Assessment of health risks from exposure to contaminated soil. Risk Anal 1985;5:289–302.
16. LaGoy PK. Estimated soil ingestion rates for use in risk assessment. Risk Anal 1987;7:355–359.
17. Calabrese EJ, Strand EJ, Barnes RM. Preliminary adult soil ingestion estimates: results of a pilot study. Regul Toxicol Pharmacol 1990;12:88–95.
18. Shen TT. Air pollution assessment of toxic emissions from hazardous waste lagoons and landfills. Environ Int 1985;11:71–76.

19. Levine SP, Costello RJ, Geraci CL, Conlin KA. Air monitoring at the drum bulking process of a hazardous waste remedial action site. Am Ind Hyg Assoc J 1985;46:192–196.

20. Baker LW, Mackay KP. Screening models for estimating toxic air pollution near a hazardous waste landfill. J Air Pollut Control Assoc 1985;35:1190–1195.

21. Costello RJ. NIOSH air monitoring at hazardous waste sites. In: Levine, SP, Martin WF, eds. Protecting personnel at hazardous waste sites. Boston: Butterworth Publishers, 99–128.

22. EPA. The total exposure assessment methodology (TEAM) study: summary and analysis. Vol I. Publ. No. EPA/600/6-87/002a. Washington, DC: Office of Acid Deposition, Environmental Monitoring and Quality Assurance, 1987.

23. EPA. Guidelines for exposure assessment. Fed Reg 1986;51:34042–34054.

24. EPA. Guidelines for carcinogen risk assessment. Fed Reg 1986;51:33992–34003.

25. Tseng WP. Effect and dose-response relationships of skin cancer and black foot disease with arsenic. Environ Health Perspect 1977;19:109–119.

26. Morton W, Starr G, Pohl O, Stoner J, Wagner S, Weswig P. Skin cancer and water arsenic in Lane County, Oregon. Cancer 1976;37:2523–2532.

27. Shacklette HT, Boerngen JG. Element concentrations in soils and other surficial materials of the conterminous United States. U.S. Geological Survey Professional Paper No. 1270. Washington, DC: USGPO, 1984.

28. Oppelt ET. Incineration of hazardous wastes: a critical review. J Air Pollut Control Assoc 1987;37:558–586.

29. EPA. Guidelines on air quality models, Rev ed. Publ. No. EPA-450/2-78-027R. Research Triangle Park, NC: Office of Air Quality Planning and Standards, 1986.

30. EPA. Dioxin emissions from industrial boilers burning hazardous materials. EPA 600/2-85-118. Cincinnati, OH: Hazardous Waste Engineering Research Laboratory, 1986.

31. EPA. 40 CFR Parts 260, 261, 264, and 270. Standards for owners and operators of hazardous waste incinerators and burning of hazardous wastes in boilers and industrial furnaces; proposed and supplemental proposed rule, technical corrections and request for comments. Fed Reg 1990;55:17862–17921.

32. Levin A, Fratt DB, Leonard A, Bruins RJF, Fradkin L. Comparative analysis of health risk assessments for municipal waste combustors. J Air Waste Management 1991;41:20–31.

33. Tesche TW, Kapahi R, Honrath R, Dietrich W. Improved dry deposition estimates for air toxics risk assessments. Paper No. 87-73B.1, presented at the 80th Annual Meeting of the Air Pollution Control Association, New York, June 21–26, 1987.

34. Rappe C, Andersson R, Bergqvist P-A, et al. Overview on environmental fate of chlorinated dioxins and dibenzofurans. Sources, levels and isomeric patterns in various matrices. Chemosphere 1987;16:1603–1618.

35. Crummett WB, Townsend DI. The trace chemistries of fire hypothesis: review and update. Chemosphere 1984;13:777–788.

36. Upton AC, Kneip T, Toniolo P. Public health aspects of toxic chemical disposal sites. Annu Rev Publ Health 1989;10:1–25.

37. Lave LB. Methods of risk assessment. In: Lave, LB, ed. Quantitative risk assessment in regulation. Washington, DC: Brookings Institution, 1982.

38. Raynor S, Cantor R. How fair is safe enough? The cultural approach to societal technology choice. Risk Anal 1987;7:3–9.

39. Slovic P, Fischoff B, Lichtenstein S. Why study risk perception? Risk Anal 1982;2:83–93.

57

Health Hazards of Shipbuilding and Ship Repairing

Katherine L. Hunting, Ph.D., M.P.H.
Laura S. Welch, M.D.

INTRODUCTION

Shipyard work involves construction and repair of merchant vessels, Navy and Coast Guard ships and submarines, non-self-propelled vessels such as barges, off-shore drilling rigs, and platforms. The U.S. shipbuilding and ship repair industry employs approximately 128,000 production workers, equally divided between Naval and private shipyards. This employment figure does not include supervisory, administrative, and professional workers such as engineers (1).

The construction of a ship is a complex task, involving many trades and skills and the use of many hazardous substances. Much of the ship is constructed in a berth or a building dock; preliminary work is also done in offices and ancillary shops which are an integral part of the shipyard. In the shops, conditions are similar to those in engineering or manufacturing facilities, whereas work aboard ship is similar to construction conditions.

The basic construction of a ship's hull is accomplished by measuring, cutting, assembling, and welding steel plates. In the shop, the plate is cut to size, usually with flame cutting, formed to shape by cutting or rolling, and fabricated into subassemblies by welding. Subassemblies are then transferred to the building dock by cranes or vehicles; assembled by welding; finished with pneumatic chisels, gouging, or grinding; and sandblasted and painted. The ship is finished with the installation of plumbing, ventilation, machinery, flooring, berths, decking, and electronic equipment. Each of these tasks is performed by a different trade or set of trades, each with a unique set of hazards. Table 57.1 lists the primary shipyard trades and the proportion of shipyard workers represented in each occupational group.

DESCRIPTION OF SHIPYARD TRADES AND EXPOSURES

Since many readers may not be familiar with shipyard work, this section will describe the work done by the most important shipyard trades. Exposures typically experienced by each trade will also be discussed. It should be noted that the following descriptions are generalized; even among workers in the same trade, tasks and exposures vary considerably. The most important distinction, for most trades, is whether individuals work in the shop, aboard the ship (exterior or interior), or, as in some cases, in shipyard facilities (''maintenance'' trade workers).

Welders

Welders join metals by heating them to high temperatures. These processes result in emissions of toxic fumes, dusts, gases, and vapors. The principal components of welding fumes from carbon steel are oxides of nitrogen and vaporized iron, which condenses to a fine dust (2). In addition, fumes from welding or cutting may contain ozone, carbon monoxide, zinc, fluorides, silica, lead, chromium IV, nickel, aluminum, beryllium, cobalt, copper, manganese, magnesium, vanadium, arsenic, or other metals (3, 4). The composition of welding fumes varies depending on the type of metal being welded, the presence of a coating on the metal, the welding technique, and the type of electrode and filler wire used (3). Ship hulls are typically constructed of carbon steel; alloys may, however, be used to construct the ship's superstructure (5) and for numerous specialty applications. Many different welding or cutting techniques, including gas metal arc, low hydrogen, submerged arc, gas tungsten, plasma arc, gas welding, gas/flame cutting, and arc air gouging are employed in shipyard work (6). Hand welding and machine welding, in which joints are welded without manual manipulation of the welding electrode or torch, are both employed in shipyard work (1).

Nonfume chemical exposures experienced by welders include decomposition products (most notably phosgene) of organic solvents used to degrease metals prior to welding. Fuel gases such as propane, acetylene, and hydrogen may also be released. Physical hazards of welding work include electricity, heat, noise, vibration, ionizing radiation, and ultraviolet (UV), visible, and infrared (IR) radiation (3).

Prior to the mid 1970s, shipyard welders were frequently exposed to asbestos. The highest exposures occurred when welders worked around delagging operations (removal of asbestos insulation) or in areas where asbestos was being sprayed.

Table 57.1. Major Occupational Groups, Shipbuilding and Ship Repairing (Production Workers Only)[a]

Occupational Group	%[b]
Welders	10.6
Machinists and machine tool operators	6.8
Pipefitters and insulators	6.8
Shipfitters	6.6
Electricians	5.9
Painters	5.1
Material movement and service workers	3.7
Sheet-metal workers	3.5
Shipwrights, carpenters, and loftworkers	3.3
Marine trade helpers	3.0
Riggers	2.1
Electronics technicians and mechanics	1.6
Other tradeworkers	41.0
Total	100.0

[a]Source: United States Department of Labor. Bureau of Labor Statistics.
[b]These data are from a 1986 survey of private U.S. shipyards, which estimated 65,309 production workers in the private sector of the industry. Naval shipyards were not included in the survey; however, the distribution of trades is expected to be similar to private yards.

Welders occasionally removed asbestos insulation themselves in order to weld fixtures into place. Also, welders typically used asbestos blankets for protection from sparks and hot metal slag (7).

Machinists

A machinist fabricates metal parts, mechanisms, or machines and may install ship machinery as well (1). Turners, planer operators, drillers, grinders, milling machine operators, press machine operators, and tool makers are classified as machinists (8). Exposures include use of antioxidants, synthetic cutting fluids, cutting oils, chromates, greases, lubricants, rust inhibitors, and solvents.

Cutting oils vary in their content of polycyclic aromatic hydrocarbons, some of which are thought to be carcinogenic in humans (9). Machinists have a high risk of occupational dermatitis, on both an irritant and an allergic basis, and may develop acne from cutting oils. Allergy may develop to additives and antimicrobial agents in the oils or synthetic fluids (10). Due to working in close proximity to other crafts during ship construction, shipyard machinists also have significant exposure to products used by other trades, including asbestos.

Pipefitters and Insulators

The marine pipefitter lays out, installs, and maintains a ship's piping systems, which include steam heat, power, hot water, hydraulic, air pressure, and oil supply pipes. This job includes laying out pipe sections, cutting and boring holes, operating shop machines for cutting and threading pipe fittings, and bolting or welding pipes together. A pipefitter's work involves both installation and insulation of pipes. An insulator covers boilers, pipes, tanks, and refrigeration units with insulating materials. These materials include asbestos, manmade mineral fibers (MMMFs), cork, plastic, and magnesium; their purpose is to reduce loss or absorption of heat, prevent moisture condensation, and deaden sound (1). The most significant hazard for insulators and pipefitters in shipyards has been to asbestos; 70% of pipefitters surveyed in 1975 had x-ray changes secondary to asbestos (11). Asbestos is now present during ship repair, but not during new construction. As MMMFs have replaced asbestos for shipyard applications, these exposures are of increasing concern to pipefitters and insulators, as well as to those who work near them in dusty environments.

Shipfitters

A shipfitter lays out and fabricates plates, bulkheads, frames, and other metal structural parts and braces them in position within the hull of the ship for riveting or welding (1). The most significant exposure to a shipfitter is to fumes from welding and cutting. These exposures may occur in the shop during fabrication; during hull construction, as structural parts are tack welded prior to permanent welding; or indirectly, from work near welders. Platers, a subgroup of shipfitters who mark and position steel plates ready for welding, often work in close proximity to welders (4). Like most other shipyard trades, shipfitters may have indirect asbestos exposure.

Electricians

A marine electrician installs and repairs wiring, fixtures, and equipment for shipboard electrical systems. The counterpart to this position is the maintenance electrician, who installs, maintains, and repairs equipment for the generation, distribution, or utilization of electric energy in the shipyard (1). Exposures of concern are solvents (formerly including benzene), metal fumes, fluxes, chlorinated biphenyls, epoxy resins, chlorinated naphthalenes, and electrical current (12). Electricians often must remove or replace insulation material and may also work in the vicinity of insulators (4). Electricians, particularly those who work aboard ship or in shipyard power plants, can have considerable exposure to asbestos. Many studies of shipyard workers, which have included electricians, have found an increased lung cancer risk. Electricians have also been found to have an increased risk chest of x-ray changes (7, 13), and mesothelioma (14, 15). Shipyard electricians have also been found to have increased rates of leukemia (12).

Painters

A painter applies paint, varnish, lacquer, or other finishes to the surfaces of the ship, primarily using brushes or spray guns. Maintenance painters perform similar work in the shipyard facilities (1). Prior to application of coatings, painters also prepare ship surfaces, removing scale, rust, and old paint. Surface preparation is done by abrasive blasting or by wiping surfaces with solvents (16, 17). Shipyard painters are exposed to a wide variety of organic solvents, including aliphatic hydrocarbons, alcohols, ketones, glycol ethers, chlorinated hydrocarbons, and aromatic hydrocarbons. Benzene is present now only as a very low level contaminant, but significant exposures were present prior to 1977. Painters are also potentially exposed to numerous metals and metal oxides, including lead, chromium, cadmium, nickel, and organotins, which are used in coatings as antifouling agents (18). Metal exposures may occur as a result of paint removal operations; painters must be protected from exposure to lead dust when preparing red lead painted surfaces (17–19). Painters may be exposed to silica if they sandblast or work in the vicinity of sandblasting operations. Work in confined spaces adds another hazardous element to painting work.

Painters working aboard ships, like workers in most other shipyard trades, are potentially exposed to asbestos and have been shown to be at risk of mesothelioma (14) and other asbestos-related diseases. Organic solvents impair nervous system function; solvent-exposed shipyard painters have been found to have increased acute neurologic symptoms (20, 21), neurobehavioral performance decrements (21), and increased vibratory perception thresholds indicative of peripheral polyneuropathy (22). Other organ system effects have also been found in association with shipyard painting exposures. For example, epoxy resin systems contain irritant, and often sensitizing, compounds. Recent studies by Welch et al. (18, 23) showed increased hematologic and sperm abnormalities among shipyard painters exposed to ethylene glycol ethers.

Material Movement and Service Workers

This category of workers includes several different occupational groups whose exposures may vary depending on their work location. Crane operators run various types of cranes to hoist, move, and place materials, machines, and products within a shipyard. Guards, janitors, truck drivers, and forklift operators are also classified with material movement and service workers (1).

Sheet-Metal Workers

A sheet-metal worker fabricates, assembles, installs, and repairs sheet-metal products and equipment (1). Welding exposures, which are particularly likely to occur among shop workers, are of concern. Sheet-metal workers are also exposed to asbestos and manmade mineral fibers during shipboard installation or repair of ducts or other products. Since many ducts are fabricated with MMMF liners, exposure to MMMF dust also occurs during in-shop fabrication or during on-ship installation.

Shipwrights, Maintenance Carpenters, and Loftworkers

All of these trades involve wood carpentry work. The shipyard carpenter constructs and maintains woodwork and equipment such as docks, structures to support ships in dry dock, bins, cribs, counters, partitions, framing, doors, floors, stairs, casings, and trim. Carpentry work is done in the shop and aboard the ships by shipwrights and in the shipyard facilities by the maintenance carpenter (1). Shipyard carpenters have had significant exposures to asbestos, and are also exposed to wood dust, glues, and solvents. At the Portsmouth Naval Shipyard, for example, the solvents with which carpenters worked included xylene, toluene, acetone, methylene chloride, tetrachloroethane, methyl ethyl ketone, and (formerly) benzene (12). Loftworkers lay out full scale models of the ship and construct templates and molds to be used as patterns and guides for layout and fabrication of various structural parts of ships (1). Loftworkers work in a separate shop area, the "mold loft." As such, these workers are exposed to wood dust, glues, and solvents, but not generally to asbestos.

Riggers

A rigger's job involves movement of machinery, equipment, structural parts, and other heavy loads aboard ships. The job includes installation and repair of rigging and weight-handling gear on ships, and attaching necessary hoists and pulling gear to rigging in order to lift, move, and position heavy loads (1). As with other material movement workers, riggers' chemical exposures will vary depending on work occurring in their vicinity.

Electronics Technicians and Mechanics

Electronics workers install, maintain, repair, overhaul, construct, and test electronic equipment and related devices (1). This work is carried out both in the shop and aboard ship (where asbestos exposure may occur). Hazardous exposures include solvents used in cleaning components, electrical current, and electromagnetic radiation.

HEALTH EFFECTS OF SHIPYARD EXPOSURES

The major classes of shipyard hazards are summarized in Table 57.2. The many trades involved in building and repairing ships have differing exposures. There are exposures to asbestos, radiation, and heat, that are widespread in the shipyard and common to many trades. This complex exposure picture makes it difficult to assess the health hazards to shipyard workers. Table 57.3 lists some of the most important occupational diseases that occur in shipyards. While some of what we know about

Table 57.2. Major Classes of Shipyard Hazards

Physical hazards
  Extremes of temperature
  Oxygen deficiency in closed spaces
  Ergonomic stress of work in confined spaces
  Noise
  Vibration
  Ionizing radiation
  Electricity
  Airborne particles

Chemical hazards
  Diesel exhaust and other combustion products
  Fumes and gases from welding and burning
  Dusts from asbestos and other insulation, sandblasting
  Vapors from paints, thinners, resins
  Lead
  Organic tins
  Oils
  Epoxy resins systems

Table 57.3. Occupational Diseases of Particular Interest in Shipyards[a]

Conjunctivitis or keratitis from welding arcs
Deafness due to pneumatic hammers, chippers, arc air gouging
Vibration white finger
Acute lung irritation from zinc, oxides of nitrogen, and ozone from welding and burning
Siderosis from welding
Silicosis from sandblasting
Solvent narcosis
Occupational asthma from epoxies and isocyanates
Asbestosis and asbestos-related cancers
Cataracts from lasers and ionizing radiation
Irritant contact dermatitis

[a]Modified from Bridges VG, Campbell J, Howe W. Shipbuilding. In: Parmeggiani L, ed. Encyclopedia of Occupational Health and Safety. 3rd ed. Geneva: International Labour Organization, 1983:2027–2032.

shipyard-related occupational diseases comes from shipyard worker health studies, much of what is known comes from health studies carried out among relevant trades in other industries.

A number of mortality studies have been carried out among shipyard worker populations. A limitation of these studies is that exposures have been evaluated by using job title as a general indicator of exposure. For instance, cancer studies of welders may presume that increased risks are attributable to welding fume exposure, without doing an assessment of the degree of asbestos or radiation exposure. Results of such studies should therefore be interpreted with caution regarding causal exposures.

Welding

Welding work takes place in shops, during hull assembly, during interior construction, and in finishing phases. Trades that weld include welders, caulker/burners, boilermakers, platers, shipfitters, and sheet-metal workers (4). Welders and boilermakers have the highest exposure to welding fumes. Caulker/burners and platers are also exposed, generally to a lesser degree. Workers in other trades are also exposed to welding fumes, as they often work in the vicinity of welding. In addition to fume proximity, factors such as work location (e.g., shop, open air, confined space), provision of exhaust ventilation, and use of personal protective equipment modify exposure.

Health effects of welding exposures are specifically covered in a variety of sources (3, 24, 25) (see Chapter 90).

Exposure to welding fumes, while working in confined or other poorly ventilated areas, can cause metal fume fever. This acute condition often resembles an upper respiratory infection, acute bronchitis, pneumonia, or upper gastrointestinal infections (3) and is relatively common. It has been estimated that nearly 40% of welders over age 30 have experienced metal fume fever (24). Pneumonitis has been less commonly reported in association with welding work; it may result from acute high concentration exposures to nitrogen dioxide, ozone, and a number of metal fumes (3).

Chronic respiratory disease also occurs among welders. Siderosis, or "welders lung," is a benign condition resulting from the accumulation of iron oxides in the lung. Fibrosis may also develop in response to many other welding exposures (2, 3, 24).

Numerous studies have reported an increased risk of chronic bronchitis among both smoking and nonsmoking welders compared with nonwelders (24). The risk is more pronounced among smokers (2, 3). Shipyard welders appear to be at risk of developing obstructive chronic bronchitis; in other industries welding has not been associated with obstructive changes. Sjögren (24) suggests that inhalation of air contaminants is higher for shipyard welders than for other welders due to their work in semiconfined or confined spaces.

Welding fumes may contain a variety of metals, such as chromium (VI) or nickel, which are either known or suspected carcinogens. Epidemiologic studies carried out in many occupational settings have found welding to be associated with a moderately increased risk of lung cancer (3, 24). Several studies have specifically addressed the risk attributable to shipyard welding exposures and have found an excess risk of lung cancer among welders or other workers with welding exposures (4, 8, 26, 27). The studies by Tola et al. and Schoenberg et al. controlled for smoking; the other studies had no data on smoking. Many shipyard welders have had substantial asbestos exposures, and it is not known how much of their observed excess risk of lung cancer is attributable to this versus welding exposures or to other possible carcinogens such as ionizing radiation. Shipyard welders (7, 28) as well as other welders (24) have an increased risk of mesothelioma.

Epidemiologic evidence is equivocal for the relationship between welding and cancers at sites other than the lung (3, 24). Cancers of concern include laryngeal, nasal, sinonasal, kidney, and other urinary tract organs. Stern et al. (12) noted an increased risk of leukemia among shipyard welders. Limited epidemiologic evidence (3) indicates that welders may have increased cardiovascular disease death rates, as well as increased risk of reproductive disorders.

Asbestos

Asbestos materials are now infrequently used in new ship construction, but were extensively used in vessels constructed before 1975. As a consequence, there will be asbestos-related disease appearing in current workers from past exposures and the potential for exposure in the repair of vessels constructed before 1975. Present-day exposure to asbestos is carefully reg-

ulated and exposures are expected to be quite low when the work is carried out according to regulations.

Crocidiolite, amosite, and chrysotile have been used extensively in shipyards since the beginning of the century. In shipyards in the United States, amosite was added to chrysotile just before and during World War II (11). Asbestos was used as insulation for pipes, boilers, and steam lines and in welders' blankets. Carpenters used asbestos board in constructing fireproof doors. Because of the confined spaces in ships and the overlapping of jobs and processes between trades, one must assume that all production workers who worked on the ship have had some exposure to asbestos. In addition, many shop workers have had asbestos exposure.

Dust concentrations were not measured to any degree in the 1940s and 1950s, but the mobile nature of the work resulted in dust concentrations that varied from day to day and from one part of a ship to another. In general, the process of removing insulation generates higher fiber counts than the application, and the highest fiber levels were present in the confined spaces of boiler and engine rooms. Samples taken during the removal of lagging had mean values of 171 fibers/ml in boiler rooms and 88 fibers/ml in engine rooms in one shipyard in England (28). Nicholson (29) conducted an integrated analysis of monitoring data in shipyards in the 1960s and estimated an overall time-weighted average (TWA) for shipyard work at between 4 and 12 fibers/ml for fibers longer than 5 microns.

The well-recognized health hazards of asbestos exposure in shipyards and elsewhere include asbestosis, pleural fibrosis, lung cancer, and mesothelioma; increased rates of colon cancer, laryngeal cancer, and other cancers have been reported as well.

A survey of chest x-ray abnormalities in a large shipyard during the 1970s found that 46% of 1000 shipyard production workers (most with more than 20 years of employment) had pleural or parenchymal changes compatible with asbestos disease (11). The prevalence of abnormalities ranged from 36% in carpenters and 40% in painters to 74% in pipefitters. The rates of abnormalities were even higher in workers engaged exclusively in ship repair in the same period; 86% of repair workers with 20 years or more of experience had pleural or parenchymal abnormalities (30).

Sandén et al. (31) found an increased odds ratio (OR) for lung cancer (OR = 2.3) and gastric cancer (OR = 1.4) among Swedish shipyard workers. Fletcher (32) found an incidence of lung cancer 2.5 times expected in British shipyard workers. Edge (33) found a twofold increased risk of lung cancer among men with pleural plaques in a British shipyard. Putoni and coworkers (34) found a standardized mortality ratio (SMR) for lung cancer of 2.2 in shipyard workers in Genoa. In a population-based case-control study of lung cancer, Blot et al. (35) found an odds ratio of 1.4 for shipyard work. Most of these studies attributed the increased risk to heavy asbestos exposure in shipyards; none included a detailed exposure assessment.

Shipyard workers suffer from excess mortality due to mesothelioma. Selikoff et al. (11) found that 10% of deaths among 440 shipyard workers were from pleural or peritoneal mesothelioma. Kolonel et al. (15) reported eight cases of mesothelioma among 7000 men followed prospectively after work in the Pearl Harbor Naval Shipyard. As discussed under "Welding," studies of shipyard welders have found excess mortality from mesothelioma (7). Shipbuilding was also found to convey an increased risk of mesothelioma in a study using the Swedish Cancer Registry (28). Cases of mesothelioma were reported in nine different shipyard trades: laggers, painters, boilermakers, shipwrights, welders, electricians, fitters, plumbers, and joiners. Many of these trades do not work directly with asbestos, but rather, work in proximity to workers using asbestos products. Since most cases of mesothelioma are attributable to asbestos exposure (36), we can conclude that all these trades, and by analogy other trades without daily use of asbestos products, have had significant asbestos exposure in shipyards.

Manmade Mineral Fibers

Manmade mineral fibers (MMMFs) are used in ship construction as an insulating material and have been the primary substitute for asbestos in that application. Valić and coworkers (37) measured fiber counts during insulation work in shipbuilding and found that respirable fiber counts ranged from 2.6–35 fibers/ml in the engine room and 27.7–23.9 fibers/ml in the auxiliary engine rooms.

MMMFs have long been recognized as acute irritants to the skin and the respiratory tree. More recently, several studies have investigated the chronic health effects of exposure to MMMFs. Cohort studies of disease incidence and mortality have been conducted in populations exposed to MMMFs. Bayliss et al. (38) studied the causes of death for a cohort of 14,000 men working in fibrous glass production and found an excess of deaths due to nonmalignant respiratory disease. A case-control study within this cohort found an association between nonmalignant respiratory disease and exposure to small diameter glass fibers. Enterline et al. (39) also found an excess of nonmalignant respiratory deaths in a cohort of 15,000 fibrous glass production workers. A nested case-control study of the Enterline cohort suggested the excess was attributable to smoking. Robinson et al. (40) also found an excess of deaths from nonmalignant respiratory disease. None of these cohort analyses found a dose-response relationship, and other mortality studies have not found such an excess of nonmalignant respiratory disease (41, 42).

Two studies have found an increased prevalence of small opacities on chest x-rays in men exposed to MMMFs in fibrous glass production (43, 44); Weill et al. demonstrated a dose-response relationship. Others have not observed this effect (45).

Several cross-sectional studies have investigated the prevalance of respiratory symptoms or pulmonary function abnormalities in workers exposed to MMMF. Sixt (46) found an increase in elastic recoil in sheet metal workers exposed to fibrous glass. Hill et al. (47) found an increase in spirometric abnormalities in a group exposed to fibrous glass, but without a dose-response relationship. A large study by Engholm and associates (48) found an increased rate of chronic bronchitis in 135,000 Swedish construction workers exposed to fibrous glass. Several other cross-sectional studies, many in smaller populations, found no effect of MMMF exposure on either respiratory symptoms or pulmonary function.

MMMFs are classified as a IIB carcinogen by the International Agency for Research on Cancer (49). Animal studies have demonstrated that MMMFs introduced into the pleural or peritoneal space can cause cancer, if their size and shape characteristics are similar to asbestos fibers. Stanton and coworkers (50) have described the characteristics of fibers that carry the most carcinogenic potential; most MMMF products have some proportion of fibers with these size characteristics. Two large epidemiologic studies, one in the United States (51) and one in Europe (52, 53), have not shown a definite increase in lung or other cancers, overall. In the European study, however, the

subpopulation working with rock/slag wool did have an excess of lung cancer, while the U.S. study found an excess of lung cancer at one MMMF plant and not at others.

These studies as a whole suggest that there is an effect of MMMFs, and of fibrous glass in particular, on respiratory tract, but no consistent pattern is present in the existing data. It is worth noting that the cohort studies were conducted in MMMF manufacturing facilities, where fiber counts are significantly lower than in secondary uses such as insulation applications or sheet metal fabrication shops (54).

A few studies have specifically looked at the health effects of MMMF in shipyards. Valić et al. (37) found that insulators without prior exposure to asbestos who worked with MMMFs had an increased frequency of nonspecific respiratory complaints and decreased values for midexpiratory flow, MEF_{50} and MEF_{75}, compared with normal values. Smoking was not specifically controlled for in either analysis. Sandén and Järvholm (55) compared the frequency of respiratory symptoms and ventilatory function in 1682 shipyard workers, with and without exposure to MMMFs. They found an increased frequency of chronic cough and phlegm among the men with MMMF exposure, but no difference in lung function. The men with MMMF exposure had a higher prevalence of pleural plaques; whether this was due to MMMFs or to prior asbestos exposure could not be determined.

Physical Hazards

VIBRATION

Shipbuilding entails a great deal of metal working. One of the tools used for cutting metal is a chipping gun. This tool has caused many cases of vibration white finger disease (VWF) in shipyard chipper-grinders. Since around 1970 much of the cutting of metal is performed with lasers, so the risk of VWF has decreased for recently employed workers. A good deal of ship construction is outside work and may entail exposure to cold environments; working in the cold may contribute to the development of VWF and certainly contributes to the degree of symptoms a worker experiences. In one study, 20% of shipyard workers using pneumatic chipping and grinding tools had VWF (56).

Vibration white finger is occupationally induced Raynaud's phenomenon and usually results from the longterm use of hand-held vibrating tools. The disease worsens with continued exposure to vibration but does not remit with cessation of exposure; this makes prevention and early diagnosis very important. Several investigators have suggested methods for early detection; changes in tool design have also been recommended to reduce the extent of VWF in many industries. Appropriate changes in a shipyard include introduction of dampers, addition of vibration-absorbing handles to tools, and tool redesign (17).

NOISE

Pneumatic hammers, gouging tools, and chipping machines are sources of significant noise exposure in shipyards. Noise-induced hearing loss from such exposures has been well described (57).

TEMPERATURE

Since much ship construction is outside work, shipbuilding and repair entails exposure to extremes of both hot and cold. In addition, work in confined spaces, such as ballast tanks, is common; these spaces can become extremely hot in summer.

Excessive heat exposure decreases workplace productivity and can also cause serious adverse health effects and even death. These adverse effects include (58–60):

1. **Heat cramps:** When prolonged exposure to heat causes sweating that is not adequately replaced by fluid intake, muscle cramps may occur, even among trained athletes. The appropriate treatment is *rest*, with fluid replacement.
2. **Heat exhaustion:** Weakness, headache, nausea, and fainting may occur. Rest, removal to a cool area, and replacement of fluids with frequent small sips of liquids treat the condition or intravenous dehydration.
3. **Heat stroke:** Dizziness, headache, irritability, nausea, and confusion are accompanied by *hot, dry skin*. Collapse, coma, renal failure, and death may occur. First aid must be immediate with rapid cooling of the affected person.

Other adverse effects include prickly heat, diminished work capacity, and perhaps decreased sperm quality (61). Sustained body temperature elevation is also known to adversely affect both sperm production and pregnancy outcome.

Heat may contribute to safety hazards as well, due to decreased alertness. In addition, increased sweating may create slippery surfaces, fog safety eyewear, and otherwise make personal protective equipment difficult to wear.

Contributing factors to heat stress include ambient temperature, humidity, and the use of protective clothing. Protective gear, required for a number of jobs, including asbestos removal, welding, and work in confined spaces, may substantially increase the heat hazard both by decreasing convective, evaporative, and radiant heat loss and by increasing work load. Working generates metabolic heat, ranging from 60–120 kcal/hr with light work (typing, desk work) to 240–300 kcal/hr with heavy levels of work (painting) or >360 kcal/hr with extremely heavy work (climbing ladders, lifting 20 kg cases 10 times/minute) (60).

The adverse health effects of heat can be decreased by monitoring the response to heat stress and adapting work loads by increasing the number of workers performing a given task, increasing rest breaks, and providing cool areas and liquids. Accurate assessment of workloads and heat exposure should include industrial hygiene monitoring of wet bulb globe temperature and assessment of work site and of work practices (59).

CONFINED AND ENCLOSED SPACES

Confined spaces are areas that are difficult to get into and get out of. Toxic or explosive gases can build up in confined spaces; they are not designed for continuous worker presence. Such spaces include ballast tanks, bilge tanks, missile tubes, tunnels, pipelines, and open-top spaces more than 4 feet (1.2 m) in depth. Enclosed areas are easier to get into or out of and include spaces such as pump stations. Three main dangers exist in confined spaces and enclosed areas; (1) toxic and corrosive vapors and fumes, (2), explosive gases and flammable substances, and (3) lack of oxygen.

A prime hazard of confined spaces is oxygen deficiency. The normal percentage of oxygen in air is 21%, but the chemical decomposition process plus heat and humidity often decrease oxygen in a confined space. Other gases such as nitrogen and carbon dioxide displace oxygen in the air. Workers should not enter any confined space where the oxygen percentage is below 19.5% unless equipped with a supplied air respirator.

The effects of oxygen deficiency are often difficult to identify because one of the first signs is a feeling of well-being. As the level falls to around 14–16%, a person will begin to feel tired, weak, and light-headed. When levels drop to 6–10% a worker will rapidly lose consciousness and can die in minutes.

One toxic substance that accumulates in poorly ventilated areas is carbon monoxide, a colorless, odorless gas. At lower levels it causes headaches and dizziness; loss of consciousness occurs at higher levels. National Institute for Occupational Safety and Health recommends a limit for carbon monoxide of 35 ppm averaged over 10 hours; levels higher than 200 ppm should never be exceeded.

There are certain procedures and controls that must be followed before workers enter any confined space or unventilated area. Strict written procedures must be established for entering confined spaces or enclosed areas where gases can accumulate, and poorly ventilated areas must be routinely monitored for dangerous gas levels.

IONIZING RADIATION

Shipyard workers engaged in the construction and repair of nuclear-powered vessels may be exposed to ionizing radiation in addition to other shipyard hazards. The primary source of ionizing radiation is exposure to corrosion products in the primary coolant system of the nuclear reactor; these corrosion products are neutron-activated by the reactor. Water in the reactor circulates through a closed piping system to transfer heat away from the reactor core to a heat exchange system; steam generated in the process of cooling the core is used as a power source for propulsion. Trace amounts of corrosion and wear products from the interior surface of the primary coolant system become radiation-contaminated; anyone handing the coolant water or the piping may be exposed. The coolant water contains several short-lived and longer-lived radionuclide. The most significant radiation source is cobalt-60, which has a half-life of 5.3 years (62).

Radiation exposure of shipyard workers occurs after reactor shutdown for repair and in shops where contaminated components of the ship's materials are repaired. The shipyard workers are not directly exposed to uranium, and internal ingestion of radionuclides is not thought to be a significant factor. The first exposure to these radiation sources began in 1957 in the Groton shipyard, with the overhaul of a nuclear-powered submarine (62), and subsequently in other yards. At eight naval and private shipyards studied by Matanoski (62), there were 35,000 nuclear shipyard workers with more than 0.5 rems of cumulative radiation exposure, out of over 106,000 total nuclear workers.

Ionizing radiation is well-known to cause acute radiation sickness, cataracts, and cancer at a variety of sites. The question with shipyards work in general is whether the radiation exposure has been sufficient to cause disease at the generally low level exposures encountered in routine work. Specific shipyard studies have concentrated primarily on cancer.

Najarian and Colton (63) reported that shipyard workers in the Portsmouth Naval Shipyard in Kittery, Maine, had a fivefold increase in deaths from leukemia and a twofold increase in deaths from all cancers, using a PMR (proportionate mortality rate) analysis. This report prompted further and more extensive studies. Rinsky (26, 64) and Stern (12) and their associates have reported the results of several studies of cancer in the same shipyard. A cohort study (64) did not find excess mortality for any cause in shipyard workers exposed to radiation; the authors attributed the difference in results between the PMR and SMR analyses to exposure misclassification. The SMR for leukemia was raised to 1.6 in the group with a lifetime exposure of at least 1 rem at least 15 years before death, but the confidence interval was 0.51–3.86. The SMR for lung cancer in the same group was 1.98. To further investigate these two findings, two case-control studies were conducted. One, investigating leukemia deaths (12), did not find an association with exposure either to solvents or radiation, but did find that both electricians and welders had an excess risk. The other investigated lung cancer deaths (26) and found that radiation workers were more heavily exposed to asbestos and/or welding fumes; controlling for these exposures to the extent possible reduced the risk from radiation. It was not possible to completely separate the effects from asbestos and radiation in this study.

Matanoski (62) studied the mortality of nuclear workers in eight shipyards and compared three groups: nonnuclear workers, nuclear workers with a cumulative dose of greater than 0.5 rem, and nuclear workers with a cumulative dose of less than 0.5 rem. No significant mortality differences were found between the groups for all causes, leukemia, lymphoma, or lung cancer.

These epidemiologic studies, taken together, do not provide clear information to determine whether exposure to ionizing radiation in shipyards elevates cancer risk to workers.

CONCLUSIONS

This chapter has summarized the toxic exposures encountered by workers building and repairing ships, and the disease risks faced by these workers. Because of the variety of shipyard trades, exposures, and health risks, a work history will be of the utmost importance to anyone providing clinical services to shipyard workers. Similarly, researchers in this field will also want to obtain detailed information on the jobs performed by the individuals studied.

Clearly, the shipyard industry is hazardous, with numerous exposures to physical agents and chemical substances. The most important hazard in a historical sense has been asbestos; the most significant hazards in a prospective sense will be determined by existing and new construction technologies and by the degree of attention to control of exposures.

REFERENCES

1. United States Department of Labor, Bureau of Labor Statistics. Industry wage survey: shipbuilding and repairing. October 1986 (Bulletin 2295). Washington DC: GPO, 1988.

2. Cotes JE. Occupational health today and tomorrow: a view from two shipyards. J R Coll Phys Lond 1988;22:232–236.

3. National Institute for Occupational Safety and Health. Criteria for a recommended standard: welding, brazing, and thermal cutting (Publication No. 88-110). Washington DC: U.S. DHHS (NIOSH), 1988.

4. Newhouse ML, Oakes D, Woolley AJ. Mortality of welders and other craftsmen at a shipyard in NE England. Br J Ind Med 1985;42:406–410.

5. Bridges VG, Campbell J, Howe W. Shipbuilding. In: Permeggiani L, ed. Encyclopedia of occupational health and safety. 3rd ed. Geneva: International Labour Organization, 1983:2027–2032.

6. Burgess WA. Potential exposures in industry: their recognition and control. In: Clayton GD, Clayton FE, eds. Patty's industrial hygiene and toxicology. Vol 1. 3rd ed. New York: John Wiley & Sons, 1978:1149–1221.

7. McMillan GHG. The health of welders in naval dockyards: the risk of asbestos-related diseases occurring in welders. J Occup Med 1983;25:727–730.

8. Tola S, Källiomaki PL, Pukkala E, Asp S, Korkala ML. Incidence of cancer among welders, platers, machinists, and pipe fitters in shipyards and machine shops. Br J Ind Med 1988;45:209–218.

9. International Agency for Research on Cancer. Polynuclear aromatic hydrocarbons, part II. Carbon blacks, mineral oils (lubricant base oils and derived products) and some nitroarenes. IARC monographs on the evaluation of carcinogenic risk of chemicals in man. Vol 33. Lyon: International Agency for Research on Cancer, 1984:87–168.

10. Rycroft RJG. Cutting fluids, oils, and lubricants. In: Maibach HI, Gellin GA, eds. Occupational and industrial dematology. Chicago: Year Book Medical Publishers, 1982:233–236.

11. Selikoff IJ, Lilis R, Nicholson WJ. Asbestos disease in United States shipyards. Ann NY Acad Sci 1979;330:295–312.

12. Stern FB, Waxweiler RA, Beaumont JJ, et al. A case-control study of leukemia at a naval nuclear shipyard. Am J Epidemiol 1986;123:980–982.

13. Anton-Culver H, Culver BD, Kurosaki T. An epidemiologic study of asbestos-related chest x-ray changes to identify work areas of high risk in a shipyard population. Appl Ind Hyg 1989;4:110–118.

14. Malker HSR, Mclaughlin JK, Malker BK, et al. Occupational risks for pleural mesothelioma in Sweden. J Natl Cancer Inst 1985;74:61–66.

15. Kolonel LN, Yoshizawa CN, Hirohata T, Myers BC. Cancer occurrence in shipyard workers exposed to asbestos in Hawaii. Cancer Res 1985;45:3924–3928.

16. Sparer J, Welch LS, McManus K, Cullen MR. Effects of exposure to ethylene glycol ethers on shipyard painters: I. Evaluation of exposure. Am J Ind Med 1988;14:497–507.

17. Kovshilo VE. Environmental hygiene in shipbuilding and ship repairing. In: International Symposium on Safety and Health in Shipbuilding and Ship Repairing, ed. Safety and health in shipbuilding and ship repairing: proceedings of a symposium organized by the government of Finland [and others], held in Helsinki, 30 August–2 September, 1971. Geneva: International Labour Office, 1972:63–75.

18. Welch LS, Cullen MR. Effect of exposure to ethylene glycol ethers on shipyard painters: III. Hematologic effects. Am J Ind Med 1988;14:527–536.

19. Georgiev L. Exposure to dust and harmful chemicals in shipbuilding and ship repairing. In: International Symposium on Safety and Health in Shipbuilding and Ship Repairing, ed. Safety and health in shipbuilding and ship repairing: proceedings of a symposium organized by the government of Finland [and others], held in Helsinki, 30 August–2 September, 1971. Geneva: International Labour Office, 1972:103–105.

20. Cherry N, Hutchins H, Pace T, Waldron HA. Neurobehavioural effects of repeated occupational exposure to toluene and paint solvents. Br J Ind Med 1985;42:291–300.

21. Valciukas JA, Lilis R, Singer RM, Glickman L, Nicholson WJ. Neurobehavioral changes among shipyard painters exposed to solvents. Arch Environ Health 1985;40:47–52.

22. Halonen P, Halonen JP, Lang HA, Karskela V. Vibratory perception thresholds in shipyard workers exposed to solvents. Acta Neurol Scand 1986;73:561–565.

23. Welch LS, Schrader SM, Turner TW, Cullen MR. Effects of exposure to ethylene glycol ethers on shipyard painters: II. Male reproduction. Am J Ind Med 1988;14:509–526.

24. Sjögren B. Effects of gases and particles in welding and soldering. In: Zenz C, ed. Occupational medicine: principles and practical applications. 2nd ed. Chicago: Year Book Medical Publishers, 1988:1053–1060.

25. Zenz C. Occupational medicine: principles and practical applications. 2nd ed. Chicago: Year Book Medical Publishers, 1988.

26. Rinsky RA, Melius JM, Hornung RW, et al. Case-control study of lung cancer in civilian employees at the Portsmouth Naval Shipyard, Kittery, Maine. Am J Epidemiol 1988;127:55–64.

27. Schoenberg JB, Stemhagen A, Mason TJ, Patterson J, Bill J, Altman R. Occupation and lung cancer risk among New Jersey white males. J Natl Cancer Inst 1987;79:13–21.

28. Sheers G, Coles RM. Mesothelioma risks in a naval dockyard. Arch Environ Health 1980;35:276–282.

29. Nicholson WJ. Case study: asbestos—the TLV approach. Ann NY Acad Sci 1976;271:152–169.

30. Selikoff IJ, Nicholson WJ, Lilis R. Radiological evidence of asbestos disease among ship repair workers. Am J Ind Med 1980;1:9–22.

31. Sandén A, Näslund PE, Järvholm B. Mortality in lung and gastrointestinal cancer among shipyard workers. Int Arch Occup Environ Health 1985;55:277–283.

32. Fletcher DE. A mortality study of shipyard workers with pleural plaques. Br J Ind Med 1972;29:142–145.

33. Edge JR. Incidence of bronchial carcinoma in shipyard workers with pleural plaques. Ann NY Acad Sci 1979;330:289–294.

34. Putoni R, Vercelli M, Franco M, Valerio F, Santi L. Mortality among shipyard workers in Genoa, Italy. Ann NY Acad Sci 19799;330:353–377.

35. Blot WJ, Morris LE, Stroube R, Tagnon I, Fraumeni JF Jr. Lung and laryngeal cancers in relation to shipyard employment in coastal Virginia. J Natl Cancer Inst 1980;65:571–575.

36. Mossman BT, Gee JBL. Asbestos-related diseases. N Engl J Med 1989;320:1721–1730.

37. Valić F, Beritić-Stahuljak D, Skurić Z, Cigula M. Exposure to man-made mineral fibers and respiratory effects in users industry: shipbuilding. Acta Med Iugosl 1986;40:21–29.

38. Bayliss DL, Dement JM, Wagoner JK, Blejer HP. Mortality patterns among fibrous glass production workers. Ann NY Acad Sci 1976;271:324–335.

39. Enterline PE, Marsh GM. The health of workers in the MMMF industry. In: Biological effects of man-made mineral fibers. Vol 1. Proceedings of a WHO/IARC Conference, Copenhagen, Denmark, 20–22 April 1982. Copenhagen: World Health Organizational Regional Office for Europe, 1982:311–339.

40. Robinson CF, Dement JM, Ness GO, Waxweiler RJ. Mortality patterns of rock and slag mineral wool production workers: an epidemiological and environmental study. Br J Ind Med 1982;39:45–53.

41. Shannon HS, Hayes M, Julian JA, Muir DCF. Mortality experience of glass fibre workers. Br J Ind Med 1984;41:35–38.

42. Saracci R, Simonato L. Man-made vitreous fibers and workers' health. Scand J Work Environ Health 1982;8:234–242.

43. Weill H, Hughes JM, Hammad YY, Glindmeyer HW, Sharon G, Jones RN. Respiratory health in workers exposed to man-made vitreous fibers. Am Rev Respir Dis 1983;128:104–112.

44. Nasr ANM, Ditchek T, Scholtens PA. The prevalence of radiographic abnormalities in the chests of fiber glass workers. J Occup Med 1971;13:371–376.

45. Wright GW. Airborne fibrous glass particles: chest roentgenograms of persons with prolonged exposure. Arch Environ Health 1968;16:175–181.

46. Sixt R. Lung function of sheet metal workers exposed to fiber glass. Scand J Work Environ Health 1983;9:9–14.

47. Hill JW, Rossiter CE, Foden DW. A pilot respiratory morbidity study of workers in a MMMF plant in the United Kingdom. In: Biological effects of man-made mineral fibres. Vol 1. Proceedings of a WHO/IARC Conference, Copenhagen, Denmark, 20–22 April 1982. Copenhagen: World Health Organization, 1982:413–426.

48. Engholm G, Von Schmalensee G. Bronchitis and exposure to man-made mineral fibres in non-smoking construction workers. Eur J Respir Dis 1982;63 (suppl 118):73–78.

49. International Agency for Research on Cancer. Man-made mineral fibres and radon. IARC monographs on the evaluation of the carcinogenic risks to humans. Vol 43. Lyon: International Agency for Research on Cancer, 1988: 152.

50. Stanton MF, Layard M, Tegeris A, et al. Relation of particle dimension to carcinogenicity in amphibole asbestoses and other fibrous minerals. J Natl Cancer Inst 1981;67:965–975.

51. Enterline PE, Marsh GM, Henderson V, Callahan C. Mortality update of a cohort of US man-made mineral fibre workers. Ann Occup Hyg 1987;31:625–656.

52. Saracci R, Simonato L, Acheson ED, et al. Mortality and incidence of cancer of workers in the man made vitreous fibres producing industry: an international investigation at 13 European plants. Br J Ind Med 1984;41:425–436.

53. Simonato L, Fletcher AC, Cherrie J, et al. The International Agency for Research on Cancer historical cohort study of MMMF production workers in seven European countries: extension of the follow-up. Ann Occup Hyg 1987;31:603–623.

54. Esmen NA, Sheehan MJ, Corn M, Engel M, Kotsko N. Exposure of employees to man-made vitreous fibers: installation of insulation materials. Environ Res 1982;28:386–398.

55. Sandén A, Järvholm B. Pleural plaques, respiratory symptoms and respiratory function in shipyard workers exposed to man-made mineral fibres. J Soc Occup Med 1986;36:86–89.

56. National Institute for Occupational Safety and Health. Vibration white finger disease in U.S. workers using pneumatic chipping and grinding hand tools. I: Epidemiology. Cincinnati, OH: U.S. DHHS (NIOSH), 1982.

57. Olishifski JB. Occupational hearing loss, noise, and hearing conservation. In: Zenz C, ed. Occupational medicine: principles and practical applications. 2nd ed. Chicago: Year Book Medical Publishers, 1988:274–323.

58. Keilblock AJ, Schutte PC. Physical work and heat stress. In: Zenz C, ed. Occupational medicine: principles and practical applications. Chicago: Year Book Medical Publishers, 1988:334–356.

59. National Institute for Occupational Safety and Health. Proceedings of a NIOSH Workshop on Recommended Heat Stress Standards (Publication No. 81-108). Washington DC: U.S. DHHS (NIOSH), 1981.

60. Eastman Kodak Company/Human Factors Section/Health Safety and Human Factors Laboratory. Ergonomic design for people at work. Vol 1. New York: Van Nostrand Reinhold, 1983:241–281.

61. Levine RJ, Bordson BL, Matthew RM. Deterioration of semen quality during summer in New Orleans. Fertil Steril 1988;49:900–907.

62. Matanoski GM. Health effects of low-level radiation in shipyard workers, final report (Dept. of Energy Contract Number DE-AC02-79EV10095). Baltimore: The Johns Hopkins University, 1989.

63. Najarian T, Colton T. Mortality from leukemia and cancer in shipyard nuclear workers. Lancet 1978;1:1018–1020.

64. Rinsky RA, Zumwalde RD, Waxweiler RJ, et al. Cancer mortality at a naval nuclear shipyard. Lancet 1981;1:231–235.

58

Health-Related Hazards of Agriculture

John B. Sullivan, Jr., M.D.
Melissa Gonzales, M.S.
Gary R. Krieger, M.D., M.P.H.
C. Ford Runge, Ph.D.

INTRODUCTION AND OVERVIEW

Farming has the allure of a healthy lifestyle. Farmers usually live far from congested and polluted urban areas and are generally healthier than their urban counterparts. Farmers have lower mortality rates from ischemic heart disease and cancer as compared with other occupations on the basis of age and sex (1). Despite this seemingly idyllic lifestyle, there are health risks associated with farming that underscore the serious nature of the labor endured by those in agribusiness. Estimates from the United States Department of Agriculture (USDA) indicate that 3.7 million people are employed in farming in the United States (2). The Office of Migrant Health, of the Department of Health and Human Services, estimates that between 2.7 and 5 million hired employees in agribusiness are seasonal and migrant workers, with approximately 30% being migrant (2). Farming remains dependent on seasonal and migrant work forces in most areas of the country.

Prominent health and safety issues in agriculture involve exposure to a variety of chemicals and pesticides, trauma, respiratory disease, and cancer. Agricultural production is one of the most accident-prone occupations in the United States (1). Farmers have higher incidences of certain types of cancer as well as higher incidences of morbidity and mortality from respiratory disease (1). As contrasted with other industries, there has been a paucity of organized occupational safety and health programs dedicated to disease prevention, health promotion, and medical care of the farm worker. In addition to the injuries and illnesses sustained by farm workers, broader public health issues have also come to attention in the form of the spread of pesticide and chemical residues from the farm land into groundwater, air, and soil. The contamination of rural groundwater with pesticides and other chemicals is just being recognized as a potential health problem.

In developing countries, more than 50% of the population is involved in agriculture and farming, whereas in industrialized nations less than 5% of the population is involved in agricultural business (3). Since food must be provided to the world's population of 5 billion, agriculture remains an important contributor to the world economy. Despite this economic importance, farming as a business and way of life has faced financial and political hardships (4). American farmers produce enough food to feed the population of the United States and export $40 billion in produce annually (5). Despite the fact that the family farm is the single most common unit for the production of the agriculture economy, the family members who work on farms are not protected by state or federal labor regulations (5). All age groups work on farms and thus injuries and illnesses are common to those under 18 as well as those over 65 years of age.

Overall mortality for common diseases in farmers appears to be less than the general population; however, injuries and illness related to farming continues to rank as high as the mining and construction industries. Strategies to improve the delivery of occupational and environmental health services to farming communities are needed (6). Such health programs must focus on critical areas with regard to the business of farming:

1. Injury prevention;
2. Prevention of respiratory disease;
3. Medical surveillance for health effects from exposure to pesticides;
4. The increasing incidence of certain forms of cancer in farm workers;
5. Prevention of toxic effects from chemicals;
6. Environmental chemical pollution of soil and water;
7. Exposure of the public to pesticides;
8. Education and health surveillance programs.

Rural health care has always been a difficult service to deliver, and occupational health care delivery to farming communities is no better. There continues to be a decline in the availability of health care to rural populations. Rural hospitals continue to close at a rate higher than urban hospitals. Physicians have little incentive to practice in these underserved areas, and if they do, they are usually not trained in occupational and environmental health. During the 1980–1987 period, 161 rural hospitals located mainly in farming states (Minnesota, Wisconsin, Illinois, Texas, Oklahoma, and Louisiana) closed (5). These closures followed the implementation of Medicare's Prospective Payment System, which pays rural hospitals 36% less than urban counterparts for the same service (5). Physician-to-population ratios in rural areas continues to be less than in urban areas. Recruitment of physicians is hampered by attractive urban reimbursement standards and lifestyle (7).

Research into novel health care delivery programs to farming communities is occuring in some states, but more is needed (7). State and federal regulations to protect farmers and farm workers are also needed. The National Association of Community Health Centers and the National Rural Health Association have pointed out that the United States spends 42% less on funding of rural health care versus urban health care despite the fact that rural populations have higher rates of chronic disease.

EPIDEMIOLOGY OF INJURIES AND ILLNESS

The National Safety Council ranks agriculture as one of the nation's most dangerous industries, with high annual work death rates (Table 58.1, Figs. 58.1 and 58.2) (8). Tractor-related

Table 58.1. National Safety Council's Work Accidents Per 100,000—1989

	Workers	Deaths	Death Rates	Disabling Injuries
Agriculture	3200	1300	40	120,000
Mining, quarrying	700	300	43	30,000
Construction	6500	2100	32	190,000
Manufacturing	19,500	1100	6	340,000
Transportation, public utilities	5900	1400	24	140,000
Services	36,200	1500	4	300,000
Government	17,300	1600	9	240,000
Trade	27,400	1100	4	340,000

Source: With permission from National Safety Council. Accident Facts. Chicago, IL: NSC, 1990.

accidents are the leading cause of fatal injuries (4, 8). Machinery, animals, and trucks are the leading causes of nonfatal injuries (4, 8). These figures may actually be underestimates, since agricultural facilities with fewer than 11 employees are exempt from the Occupational Safety and Health Administration's (OSHA) legal injury and illness reporting requirements, and more than 95% of farms have less than this number of employees (9). Estimations of work-related deaths and serious injuries are based on multiple sources such as the National Safety Council, Department of Labor, and the Centers for Disease Control. Data on accidents and injuries are frequently difficult to collect (8, 9).

To help correct the problems associated with multiple federal agencies collecting data on mortality statistics from accidents and injuries, the National Institute of Occupational Safety and Health recently created the National Traumatic Occupational Fatalities database (NTOF), which provides a uniform approach of work-related health surveillance for trauma-linked mortality (10). In addition, the NTOF includes agriculture in its surveillance program. However, the NTOF only uses information from death certificates and can overlook fatalities.

The accident surveillance program of OSHA covers less than 11% of farming business due to the small number of employees per business in the farming industry (10). In contrast, NTOF has no exclusions for certain worker groups. The NTOF database shows that the overall agribusiness, which included production, services, forestry, and fishing, had an annual mean mortality rate of 20.7 deaths per 100,000 workers from 1980–1985 compared with a mean of 7.9 deaths per 100,000 workers in the general work force (10). If agriculture production is separated out from services, and forestry and fishing are excluded, the producing agribusiness has a mortality per 100,000 three times that of general industry (Fig. 58.3). Age-specific mortality rates are highest in the 55–64-year-old group (Fig. 58.4).

National Safety Council statistics from 1989 show that there were 40 deaths per 100,000 population in the agriculture industry compared with 9 per 100,000 in all other industries (8). Mining in 1989 had 43 deaths per 100,000 (Table 58.1). However, these statistics do not include anyone under the age of 14. Some states have data on children under the age of 14: Indiana, 14% of fatal farm injuries involved children under 15 years; Wisconsin, 24%; and Pennsylvania, 19% (8, 9).

Despite the difficulty in obtaining accurate health surveillance data, a pattern of disease and injury linked to farming as an occupation has been identified (4). Most fatalities in farming are due to trauma secondary to machinery and tractors (Figs.

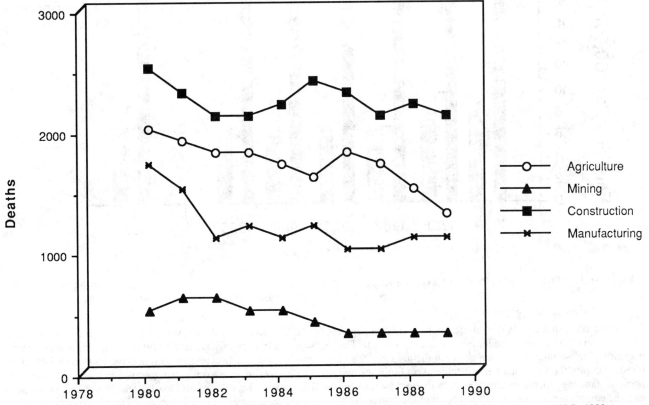

Figure 58.1. Work deaths by industry division, 1980–1989. National Safety Council. Accident facts. Chicago: NSC, 1990.

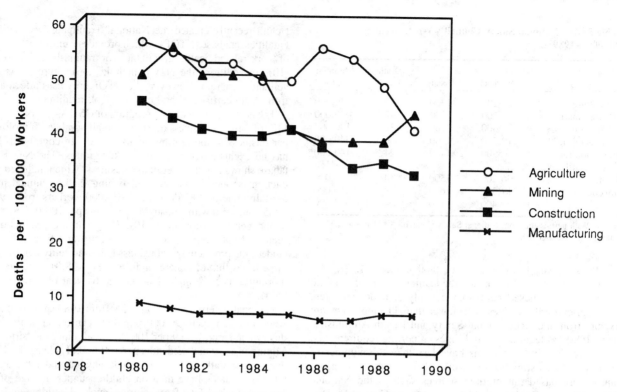

Figure 58.2. Death rate by industry division, 1980–1989. National Safety Council. Accident facts. Chicago: NSC, 1990.

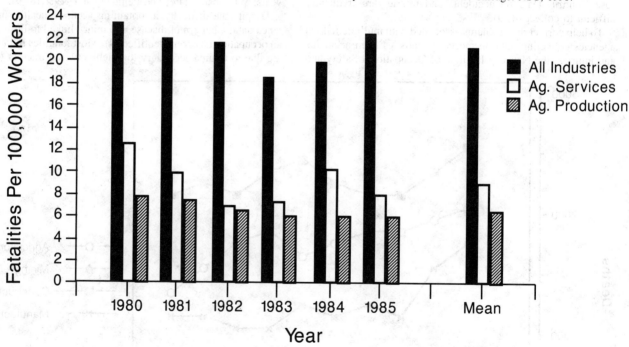

Figure 58.3. Fatality rates per 100,000 workers for all industries, agricultural services, and agricultural production, 1980–1985. Source: Centers for Disease Control, 1980–85.

58.5A and B). Other causes of fatalities include animals, electricity, drowning, trauma, and toxic exposures (4, 8). The majority of those injured are men between the ages of 20 and 60 (4). Despite the large number of accidents and injuries that occur in farming, there continues to be a distinct lack of organized comprehensive health and safety programs that address the problems unique to this business.

The type of labor involved in farming gives rise to other sorts of injuries that are more chronic, such as muscle, joint, and bone injuries secondary to repetitive motion or vibration. The effects of noise on hearing constitutes another problem. The type of farm labor and associated illness and injury also varies depending on the developing status of a country. Physical activity and manual labor are characteristics of Third World

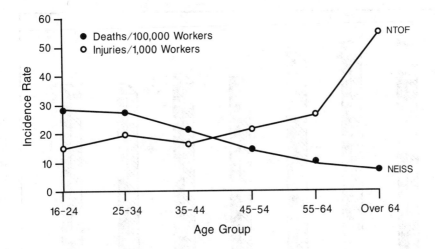

Figure 58.4. Mortality and injury rates for the agricultural industry. Centers for Disease Centrol, 1980–85; US Consumer Products Safety Commission, May 1981–April 1987.

agribusiness. Developed countries use more mechanized approaches to labor. Exposures to toxic chemicals are more common among laborers in developing countries.

Fatal agriculture-related accidents far exceed the number of work-related deaths in other industries. Workers are potentially exposed to a tremendous variety and quantity of synthetic chemicals used as fertilizers, pesticides, and fumigants. These chemicals pose both acute and chronic health hazards. Exposure to organic materials and microorganisms from plant and animal origin have also been shown to have detrimental effects on the respiratory system. Organic dust toxic syndrome (ODTS) and farmer's lung disease, an allergic alveolitis, are well-known agricultural occupational diseases. Farmers have also been shown to have increased incidence of lymphatic and hemopoietic, stomach, brain, prostate, lip, skin, and connective tissue cancers than to do other occupational groups. An excess mortality rate due to respiratory disorders is attributed to exposure to dust and molds from grain and hay. Skin disease in the form of mechanical trauma, overexposure to sunlight and chemicals, and dermatitis are commonly seen occupational hazards of the industry.

The aggressive use of chemicals, pesticides, fumigants, and fertilizers has resulted in a variety of health concerns to both the individual laborer as well as to the public. The use of pesticides is both an emotional and a political issue as well as an economic concern. Aerial spraying and crop dusting can expose both workers and members of the public. In addition, the widespread contamination of groundwater and soil beyond the point of pesticide and chemical application raises concerns of larger environmental pollution and public exposure to low levels of pesticides, nitrates, and other chemicals.

Health problems of farming can be ordered in nine general categories:

1. Trauma and injury—acute and chronic;
2. Respiratory disease;
3. Toxic exposures to chemicals;
4. Cancer;
5. Skin disease;
6. Infections;
7. Hearing loss;
8. Neurologic disorders;
9. Muscle and joint disorders.

The extent to which occupationally related exposures are associated with various health disorders is difficult to assess accurately. Unlike other industries which have access to specialized occupational medicine programs and physicians, the agriculture industry has traditionally lacked the dedicated and organized health and safety approach common to other industries. This is especially true in Third World countries or in the case of migrant farm workers. The lack of uniformity in diagnosis, testing, and evaluation of occupational factors makes it difficult to perform effective epidemiologic evaluations. Worker compensation data are also inconsistent due to various exclusions, exemptions, and loopholes in state laws.

Agriculture is a unique industry because people of all ages are at risk. Farms are often both work sites and homes, so that even nonworkers can be exposed to hazards. Thus, it cannot be assumed that the majority of farm injuries and illnesses occur with full-time farmers, since hired workers, spouses, young children, retired and part-time farmers are also at risk. The diversity of the workers differs from one area of the country to the other, and within each area agriculture workers differ from the work force in other industries (11). For example, each year more than 300,000 agricultural laborers work in the state of California. These workers differ from the rest of the work force in the state in the nature of their work, ethnic and cultural makeup, and in their socioeconomic and employment relationships. A significant portion are Mexican nationals who work transiently, moving to a new location as work becomes available (11). The great diversity of crops cultivated in California creates a multitude of job tasks, each of which may entail its own particular risk. Workers in southwestern states share these characteristics. The work forces in the southeastern states differ in ethnic makeup and sociologic factors. Workers are often informally recruited by labor contractors and have no idea in whose field they are working. These factors combine to make it difficult to obtain valid data to ascertain the extent to which occupational health problems exist among migrant agricultural workers.

Agricultural workers in other regions have their own set of occupational exposures varying with crop selection and type of animal production. In the midwestern and north central United

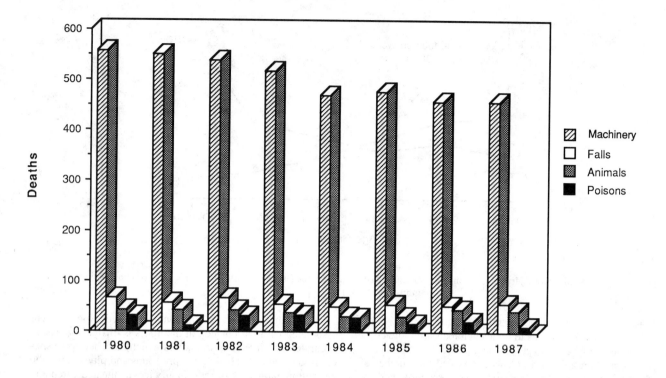

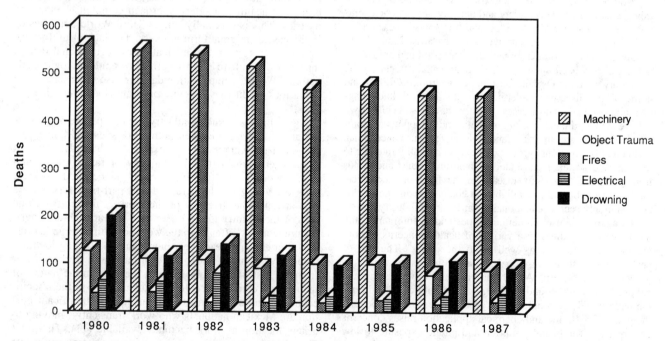

Figure 58.5. **Top,** Deaths from farm accidents, 1980–1987. Source: National Safety Council. Accident facts. Chicago: NSC, 1990. **Bottom,** Deaths from farm accidents, 1980–1987. Source: National Safety Council. Accident facts. Chicago: NSC, 1990.

States, where crops and harvesting practices differ, automated farm equipment is extensively used in the harvest of grains and cereals. Animal confinement systems, grain silos, and hay storage each have characteristic hazards and associated health effects.

Comparisons of respiratory disease rates for farmers and farm laborers show regional differences between Iowa and California; California showed an elevated rate relative to Iowa. Although the reason for this difference is not fully understood,

the differences in the mobility and the socioeconomic and ethnic backgrounds of the worker populations and difference between crops and work practices are cited as potential explanations (12). For example, pesticide usage is high in both areas; however, the crop mix is substantially different between the two states. Iowa has greater acreage of corn, while California has substantial commercial vegetable acreage. Thus while California requires intensive applications of halocarbon fumigants for controlling nematodes, in Iowa this problem is typically con-rolled by granule-formulated organophosphates. Fumigant gases may be widely used in warehouses containing perishable crops; elemental sulfur dusts are used as miticides and fungicides, and large quantities of organophosphate and carbamates are applied to orchards, vineyards, and row crops.

COMPREHENSIVE OCCUPATIONAL AND ENVIRONMENTAL HEALTH PROGRAMS FOR THE FARMING BUSINESS

Recognition of the unique problems related to occupational and environmental health of the farmer and farm workers has led to the call for improved medical surveillance and health services in the United States and other developed nations. Policies and strategies for future disease prevention have been the focus of conferences at the university and government level (6). Despite the fact that farming is one of the top three hazardous occupations ranked with mining and construction, there is no industry-specific comprehensive occupational health and safety service established in the United States. Whereas mining and the construction industry are regulated by the Mining Safety and Health Administration (MSHA) and OSHA, respectively, and served by existing occupational health and safety programs, farming has not enjoyed this integrative medical and technical approach. Industrial hygienists, safety specialists, engineers, and specialized health care providers have not been available to meet the needs of the agribusiness in an organized and comprehensive fashion.

Model farmer health and safety programs have been functioning in Sweden and Finland (3, 13, 14). Many of these programs may serve as models for future program development by other countries. Sweden provides occupational health services to farmers in all regions of the country through 33 specialized occupational health centers (15). Comprehensive health services are provided by a team of physicians, occupational health nurses, safety engineers, and other related health and safety specialists. This provides a dual medical-technical approach that can address farming issues ranging from clinical treatment and prevention services to medical surveillance and industrial hygiene (15). At the governmental level, there is a regional director for each of six regions in Sweden which coordinates the activities of the local health centers in that region. A central office in Stockholm administers these six regions.

In the United States, Iowa has implemented a model community-based health and safety program which targets the family farm and small agribusiness using local community health care facilities to deliver services while the University of Iowa acts as an overall management center (14). Eighty percent of the economy of Iowa is dependent either directly or indirectly on agriculture; thus illness and injury in the farming community can have tremendous impact (14). The Iowa Agricultural Health and Safety Service Program was a 2-year study funded by the state legislature in 1987 in an effort to develop a model program for disease prevention. It used existing health services within communities to deliver sophisticated occupational health and safety programs. Its organizational structure (Fig. 58.6) is dependent on the University of Iowa College of Medicine to manage the project, train physicians and staff, develop educational programs, provide medical consultation, serve as a tertiary care referral resource, and provide consultation in industrial hygiene and environmental health. The community hospital in conjunction with local clinics provides the direct services. A multidisciplinary approach is used at the clinic level by a staff of specially trained physicians and nurses. Safety specialists and industrial hygienists are available from the University. Telephone consultation and basic educational programs are provided free or at low costs to all farmers. On-site industrial hygiene consultation is also available if an accident or injury occurs.

Colorado has had successful experience with an agriculture safety and health program since the late 1970s (16). Based and managed from Colorado State University, the program was funded by a W. K. Kellogg Foundation grant and initially provided workplace health and safety consultation to small business throughout the state and the Rocky Mountain region, including farmers. The success of this venture led to further funding of the program now named the Colorado Occupational Safety and Health Consultation Program. However, it was recognized that direct consultative services were not utilized as much by the small farmers as they were by other nonagriculture-based businesses. A redirection of this effort created the Workplace Health in Agriculture Program (WHIAP), which sought to educate farmers and ranchers with respect to the relationship of health hazards to the agribusiness, using a variety of educational media and techniques. An essential feature of the project was the addition of expertise in toxicology and occupational health that could address issues of chemicals and pesticides. In addition to educating the individual farmer, educational forums were held for the medical community to make physicians and other health care providers aware of the unique work-related accidents, illnesses, and injuries associated with the agribusiness (16).

Another unique health care delivery network was initiated in Wisconsin by the Marshfield Clinic in 1979 (5). This system utilized existing rural medical facilities and practitioners and linked them to the Marshfield Clinic via telecommunications and transport systems. Primary care was provided locally, and the clinic served as a resource center for consultation, diagnostic services, tertiary care referral, and continuing medical education.

Overall, health care delivery to farming communities has initiated new policies and strategies in a variety of countries and states. The needs of agricultural workers can be met when innovative policies and approaches are adopted.

RESPIRATORY HEALTH HAZARDS IN AGRIBUSINESS

Farmers are subject to develop a variety of pulmonary diseases identified as occupational hazards: chronic bronchitis, abnormal pulmonary functions with limited airflow, emphysema, allergic alveolitis, asthma, farmer's lung disease, silo filler's disease, and ODTS. The increase in respiratory disease in farmers is of concern, and prevention can play a role in decreasing morbidity and mortality (1).

Chronic Bronchitis and Respiratory Disorders

Farmers have a high incidence of pulmonary symptoms which are attributed to exposure to dusty environments. The ambient air in and around various agricultural production, storage, and transportation facilities is laden with a variety of gases, dusts, suspended particles, and bioaerosols which pose a risk to the respiratory system. These include organic antigens such as pollen, fungal spores, animal danders, grain dust, and mites; synthetic chemicals such as fertilizers, insecticides, and herbicides;

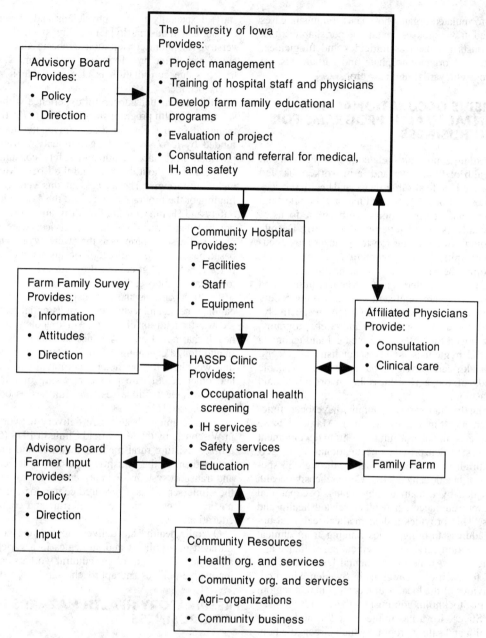

Figure 58.6. Agricultural health services. Reprinted from Gay J, Donham K., Leonard S.: Iowa Agricultural Health and Safety Service Project (HASSP). Am J Ind Med 1990;18:385–389.

and toxic gases released from decomposing plant or animal material. It has long been noted that farm workers are at risk of developing respiratory health disorders; however, limited information is available on the prevalence and specific causes of lung dysfunction in this segment of the work force. Although the reason for excess mortality from respiratory disease is not known, it is suspected that exposure to organic dusts, endotoxins, and thermophilic fungi are primary factors in the production of pulmonary diseases.

Studies have shown that organic dust and tobacco smoke are independent and additive causes of chronic bronchitis (17). Only 6% of nonsmoking farmers, compared with 10–14% of smoking farmers, have chronic bronchitis (17). Table 58.2 outlines the

physiologic responses to commonly encountered causative agents characteristic to particular respiratory disorders.

Agricultural lung diseases can be divided into immunologic and nonimmunologic (18):

Immunologic Type I: Acute or chronic asthma
Immunologic Types III–IV: Acute, chronic, subacute
  Hypersensitivity pneumonitis
  Allergic alveolitis
Nonimmunologic: Acute, chronic, subacute
  Irritant pulmonary response
  Reactive airway dysfunction
  Pulmonary fibrosis

Table 58.2. Respiratory Health Risks

ASTHMA/BRONCHOSPASM

A) Immunoglobin E-mediated

Causative agents:
Pollen from cereal grains
Dander from livestock
Fungal antigens in grain dust and on crops
Dust mites

B) Nonimmunologic Asthma

Causative agents:
Organic dusts

Insecticides, and pesticides, irritant dust, fumes, gases, vapors

HYPERSENSITIVITY PNEUMONITIS (extrinsic allergic alveolitis)

Causative agents:
Fungal spores of thermophilic actinomycetes released from moldy hay or grain

Aspergillus and *Micropolyspora* fungal spores

Antigens of less than 5 μm in diameter

Penicillium fungal spores of proteins in bird droppings

PULMONARY MYCOTOXICOSIS

Causative agents:
Toxins released from fungal spores

Moldy grain or hay

Health effects:
Early asthmatic response within 10–20 minutes after exposure caused by or associated with allergen-induced nonspecific bronchial reactivity. May also have a late asthmatic response 3–8 hours after exposure with recurrent nocturnal asthma several days postexposure

Health effects:
"Grain Dust Asthma" cough, chest tightness, fever, immediate onset to 4 hr onset, airway obstruction, stimulates release of histamine from mast cells

Bronchospasm with preexisting nonspecific bronchial hyperreactivity

Health effects:
Local formation of immune complex mediated immunity
IgE precipitation of antibodies, specific lymphocyte stimulation
"Farmer's lung": cough, dyspnea, fever with onset 3–4 hours postexposure.
Cellular infiltration of alveolar and bronchiolar walls with formations of granulomas and giant cells; progressive interstitial pulmonary fibrosis.
"Bird fancier's lung"

Health effects:
Acute febrile pulmonary illness lasting several days or weeks.
Chest radiograph: interstitial or alveolar infiltrate pattern or both
"Grain fever": fibrosis of the lung, rhinitis, conjunctivitis, or allergic alveolitis

OTHER INFECTIONS

Brucellosis	Staphylococcal and streptococcal infection
Leptospirosis	Echinococcosis
Toxoplasmosis	Salmonellosis
Rabies	Rocky Mountain spotted fever
Psittacosis	Tularemia
Tetanus	Sporotrichosis
Anthrax	Ascariasis
Erysipelas	Plague (*Yersinia pestis*)
Q-fever	Balantidiasis
Histoplasmosis	Listerosis
Blastomycosis	Valley fever (coccidioidomycosis)
Tuberculosis	

GASES AND CHEMICALS

Causative agents:
Gases from decomposing materials and manure:
ammonia, hydrogen sulfide, carbon dioxide, carbon monoxide, methane

Gases and other chemical agents:
phosgene, chlorine, sulfur dioxide, ozone, paraquat (herbicide), anhydrous ammonia (fertilizer), chlorine

Nitrogen dioxide released from decaying fodder in silos

Other oxides of nitrogen

Health effects:
Acute pulmonary inflammation from inhalation of H_2S, acute asthma-like illness, bronchitis, delayed pneumonitis

Immediate irritation of the mucous membranes of the eyes, nose, mouth, larynx, trachea, and bronchi
Delayed pulmonary edema (12–24 hrs) caused by damage to alveolar capillary membrane

"Silo filler's disease," cough, dyspnea, delayed pulmonary edema

Acute respiratory distress, delayed febrile respiratory illness leading to adult respiratory distress syndrome fibrosing bronchiolitis and/or interstitial pulmonary fibrosis

Adapted from: Cockcroft DW, Dosman JA. Respiratory health risks in farmers. Ann Intern Med 1981; 95(3):380–382. Lowry T, Schuman LM. "Silo-filler's disease—a syndrome caused by nitrogen dioxide. JAMA 1956; 162:153–160. Madsen D, Klock LE, Wenzel FJ, et al. The prevalence of farmer's lung in an agricultural population. Am Rev Respir Dis, 1976; 113:171–174. Warren CPW. Lung disease in Farmers. CMA Journal. 1977; 116:391–394.

Granulomatous disease
Chronic bronchitis

Immunologic or hypersensitivity pneumonitis is best represented by a condition termed farmers lung disease (FLD), and the nonimmunologic condition is best represented by ODTS.

Farmer's Lung Disease

Inhalation of material from moldy forage containing thermophilic spores is most commonly associated with a syndrome known as "farmer's lung disease (FLD)." After handling moldy crops, workers may experience symptoms such as cough, dyspnea, and fever. In acute cases, symptoms are manifested 3–4 hours after exposure and may resemble viral or bacterial pneumonitis. Fatigue, fever, weight loss, malaise, and a nonproductive cough may be the major complaints. However, the disease may develop gradually, producing permanent dyspnea and pulmonary impairment (19). The chest x-ray may show bilateral reticular patterns. Recurrence of symptoms when the worker returns to the job and to exposure to moldy hay or grain would indicate the possibility of farmer's lung disease. Pulmonary function tests may show a loss of FVC and $FEV_{1.0}$ as well as ventilation-perfusion imbalance which may produce hypoxemia.

In the United States, case reports of farmer's lung have centered in the Wisconsin area where climatic conditions are conducive to the development of mold (20). The prevalence of the disease is directly related to the rainfall in the area. Medical surveillance programs for farmers conducted at the Marshfield Clinic have monitored pulmonary problems of the agricultural work force in the Wisconsin area since 1963 (21). Serologic monitoring for farmer's lung disease in more than 1000 blood samples per year at the Clinic have shown that 8–10% of farmers are serologically positive for antigens thought to produce the disease. The clinic has not been able to establish any causative relationship between seropositivity and the subsequent development of the disease; however, seropositivity for antigens does correlate with pulmonary symptoms (21). An increase in chronic cough, bronchitis, and decreased pulmonary functions has been seen in workers serologically positive to farmer's lung disease antigens. The most common seropositive response in one study group was to *Micropolyspora faeni* (18). Chronic pulmonary symptoms have been positively correlated with the presence of positive antibody serology (18).

Cases of FLD in rural cattle and dairy communities in Maryland and Wyoming have also been reported. The prevalence of farmer's lung in epidemiologic studies of farming and dairy production workers in Wisconsin was 3% and 9% in Wyoming. Prevalence rates in Scotland have been reported at 2–9%, and 12% in England and Wales (19).

Organic Dust Toxic Syndrome

Exposure to respirable organic dust can occur in removing layers of silage and in other dusty processes. Exposure to farm dusts is associated with a pulmonary syndrome known as organic dust toxic syndrome (18, 22). The syndrome is noninfectious and presents with fever, chills, malaise, cough, myalgias, headache, and dyspnea soon after heavy exposure to dust (22). ODTS is thought to be nonimmunologic in origin and due to a direct inflammatory response of the lungs to respirable particles of organic material. Agricultural dust is composed of a wide variety of organic materials in addition to inorganic materials (Table

Table 58.3. Contents of Organic Dusts

Plant debris
Starch granules
Molds
Endotoxins
Mycotoxins
Spores
Fungi
Gram-negative bacteria
Enzymes
Grain extracts
Allergans
Insect parts
Silica
Soil particles
Chemical residues

58.3). This wide variety of dust components is implicated in the etiology of ODTS. The composition of the dust depends on the type of operation or farm environment in which the dust is produced. High concentrations of gram-negative bacteria, endotoxin, and mold such as actinomycetes occur in operations involving moldy grains and silage (18). Cotton dusts have a higher concentration of endotoxin-containing gram-negative bacteria (18).

Exposure to 90–100 mg/m^3 of respirable grain dust for 1–2 hours provoked the syndrome in 2 of 6 control subjects (1). Symptoms include productive cough, facial warmth, headache, throat irritation, chest tightness, burning chest pain, and dyspnea (1). These symptoms may be followed several hours later by myalgias, fever, chills, and elevated white blood cell counts (1). Organic dusts containing endotoxin, mold, spores, and bacteria can produce an acute pulmonary inflammatory response with a predominance of polymorphonuclear leukocytes in the lungs. The disease is usually self-limited without permanent sequelae. Therapy is symptomatic and supportive.

It is now thought that exposure to organic dusts causes a cascading effect (Fig. 58.7) involving pulmonary macrophages (21). The activated pulmonary macrophages trigger phagocytic responses in the lungs with an infiltration of polymorphonuclear leukocytes. In addition, complement activity may be triggered, T-cells activated to respond to these antigens, and inflammatory mediators released (21).

Despite the different pathogenesis between OTDS and FLD, it is difficult to separate these two syndromes by clinical symptoms and physical examination on all occasions (Table 58.4). Both FLD and ODTS can present with cough, leukocytosis, fever, dyspnea, chills, malaise, myalgia, and pulmonary function decrements (21). ODTS is characterized by a history of high level dust exposure with negative serology for FLD antigens. The cause of ODTS is an acute inflammatory pulmonary response to inhaled dusts; there are usually no longterm sequelae (21). FLD has a higher incidence in late winter and early spring. ODTS has a higher incidence in late summer and early fall (21). The prevalence rate for FLD has been calculated to be 4.2/1000 (21). The incidence of ODTS versus FLD is difficult to ascertain given the common symptoms of both diseases. The incidence of ODTS is estimated to vary from 10–190 per 10,000 population at risk (22).

Animal Confinement Areas

Animal confinement areas represent a distinct pulmonary health hazard. This method of production, where a large number of

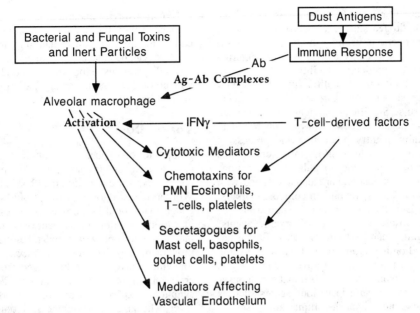

Figure 58.7.   Inflammatory cascade induced by organic dusts containing microbial contaminants. Reprinted from Holt PG. Inflammation in organic dust-induced lung disease: new approaches for research into underlying mechanisms. Am J Ind Med 1990;17:47–54.

Table 58.4.   Comparison of Agriculture-Related Lung Disease

Organic Dust Toxic Syndrome	Farmer's Lung Disease
Onset in 4–12 hours	Onset 4–8 hours
Fever, chills, dyspnea, myalgias, headache, nonproductive cough, malaise	Fever, chills, malaise nonproductive cough, dyspnea
Duration of 12–24 hours, may last up to 5–7 days	Duration 12–36 hours and disease may progress with permanent damage
Rales on examination	Rales on examination
Leukocytosis with predominance of neutrophils	Leukocytosis with lymphocytosis and eosinophils
Mild hypoxemia with alveolar-arterial gradient	Mild to severe hypoxemia with an increased gradient
Negative serology to antigens	Positive antigen serology
Lung lavage cells are PMNs	Lung lavage cells are lymphocytes
Chest x-ray is normal or shows only mild interstitial infiltrate	Chest x-ray may show more dense infiltrates
Biopsy shows acute inflammation	Biopsy shows mononuclear cells or granulomas
Pulmonary function tests demonstrate mild restriction and decreased diffusion of CO (DLCO)	Pulmonary function tests show severe restriction, obstruction, and decreased DLCO
Nonimmunologic etiology	Immunologic etiology

Adapted from Von Essen S, Robbins R, Thompson A, Rennard S. Organic toxic dust syndrome: an acute febrile reaction to organic dust exposure distinct from hypersensitivity pneumonitis. J Toxicol Clin Toxicol 1990;28:389–420; Marx J, et al. Am J Industrial Med 1990;18:263–268.

animals are raised in an enclosed structure with a limited amount of area provided per animal, has brought about a tremendous increase in productivity. The increased use of confinement systems has been associated with an increase in physical, chemical, and biologic health hazards to the agriculture worker. An estimated 500,000 workers are employed in swine confinement operations, and an additional 500,000 work in poultry, veal, beef, or dairy confinement operations.

Exposed production workers show a high prevalence of respiratory symptoms including cough, excess sputum and phlegm production, and wheezing and irritation to the nose and throat. Feeds and particulates of animal origin are the greatest contributors to the total dust load, which reaches excessively high levels during feeding (23). Human antibodies found specific for feed dusts suggest an immunologic basis for the respiratory symptoms observed. Biologic materials also contribute adversely to the effects on the respiratory tract. Since a single antigen has not been identified as the primary source of sensitization, in order to test for sensitization it would be necessary to use a large antigen panel to assess the many types of dust present in barns and confinement systems.

Symptoms in swine confinement workers can be grouped to include the following (24): (a) upper and lower airway irritation and inflammation, (b) chronic bronchitis, (c) rhinitis and sinusitis, and (d) hyperactive airway. A summary of the symptoms reported by swine confinement workers includes cough with sputum production, chest tightness, dyspnea, wheezing, malaise, fever, dizziness, myalgias and arthralgia, fatigue, and throat irritation (23). Pulmonary function studies have shown decrements in flow volumes as well as the parameters of FEV_1 and $FEV_{1.0}/FVC$ (24).

The incentive for energy production from methane released by anaerobic decomposition of wastes from animal confinement units has made liquid manure storage a common component of confinement systems. The uncontrolled activity of anaerobic and facultative microbes in stored manure produces metabolic byproducts including as many as 150 different gases, many of which are known to be toxic (25). Ambient concentrations of methane, ammonia, carbon dioxide, and hydrogen sulfide can easily exceed chronic and shortterm exposure limits if proper controls are not practiced and maintained. In addition to respiratory symptoms, workers are also subject to the central nervous system depressant effects of carbon dioxide and the metabolic effects of hydrogen sulfide and carbon monoxide. Displacement of atmospheric oxygen by the mixture of gases has lead to asphyxiation, especially among workers entering confined spaces within the production facility.

The development of allergic alveolitis (hypersensitivity pneumonitis) has been shown to be a risk from exposure to airborne microorganisms. Significant amounts of suspended endotoxins from gram-negative bacteria have been found in swine confinement units, poultry production and processing facilities, and in airborne grain dusts (26). Similar endotoxins have been thought to be responsible for pulmonary reactions in persons exposed to cotton dust and are also associated with headache, diarrhea, and other symptoms in compost workers.

An immunoglobin E-mediated asthmatic response can be precipitated by the exposure to a variety of organic agents. Pollen from cereal grains, dander from livestock, fungal antigens in grain dust and on live crops, or dust mites in organic dusts are among the most common causative agents for this type of response (27). Nonimmunologic asthmatic responses can also be elicited from exposure to various agents such as organic dust, pesticides, and irritant dust fumes and gases.

Grain Dust

Grain dust is a product of the handling of grain. There are several processes in which workers are exposed, ranging from grain elevators to transporting, milling, and baking (28). Grain elevators are sources of high particulate pollutants, both inside the elevator and outside. Dust levels vary, depending on ventilator effectiveness, between 5 and 50 mg/m^3. Air particulates as high as 1000 mg/m^3 have been recorded (28). Particles less than 10 micrometers are considered respirable, and up to 10% of grain dust would fit this size (28). The components of grain dust will vary with the grain and location. Common constituents of grain dusts are (28):

grain kernel pieces
pieces of seeds
trichome particles
insect parts
allergans
silica
mite parts
bacteria
mold and fungi
residues of pesticides, fungicides, and herbicide

Clinical symptoms following exposure may vary depending on the composition of the grain dusts inhaled. Skin irritation and pruritis are common complaints following exposure to oat and barley dusts due to the trichome particles that penetrate the skin (28). A syndrome known as a "grain itch" is caused by a mite (28). Irritation of the eyes, nose, and upper airway are common complaints following grain dust exposure.

Respiratory diseases following exposure to grain dusts vary from hypersensitivity pneumonitis to asthma and grain fever. Chronic exposure results in airflow limitations evident on pulmonary function testing. Grain fever is an acute febrile illness occurring after exposure to dusts and is reported to occur in up to 30% of farmers (28). Symptoms of grain fever include malaise, cough, dyspnea, chills, and fever. Grain fever is actually classified as an organic dust disease and is probably nonimmunologic (28). Symptoms may last from hours to days.

Hypersensitivity pneumonitis (allergic alveolitis or FLD) is associated with the handling of moldy materials. This is not commonly associated with handling dry grain (28). Asthmatic reactions can be induced by both allergic and nonallergic causes. Overall, grain dust exposure can produce symptoms associated with chronic bronchitis, asthma, allergic alveolitis, and chronic airflow limitations.

Cotton Dust

Symptoms of exposure to cotton dusts are similar to those caused by other organic dusts. Pulmonary disease caused by chronic exposure to cotton dust has been known as *byssinosis*. Workers exposed to cotton dust would slowly develop a chronic cough that would be particularly worse on returning to work on Monday, with improvement over the weekend. Over time, the cough became worse and relenting with no weekend improvement (29). The term *byssinosis* traditionally is reserved for symptoms related to chest discomfort experienced by workers returning to work on Monday (29). Overall, respiratory symptoms experienced by cotton workers include low grade fever, wheezing, chest tightness, initially a dry cough followed by productive cough with longer exposure, and asthma (29).

The pathophysiology of cotton dust exposure is an inflammatory response in the lungs due to responses of pulmonary macrophages and the release of mediators of inflammation. The causative agents in cotton dust are thought to be products of the plant as well as endotoxin, molds, and gram-negative bacteria. Plant products include: histamine, phenols, epoxides, terpenoids, tannin, and lacinilene C7-methyl ether (29).

Mycotoxicosis and Silo Filler's Disease

Pulmonary mycotoxicosis can be caused by exotoxins of fungal spores in moldy grain or hay. This condition is more commonly known to grain handlers as "grain fever," an acute febrile pulmonary illness that may develop into fibrosis of the lung (27). This condition is not to be confused with "silo filler's disease" a condition that results from nitrogen dioxide release from decaying fodder in silos (20, 30, 31). The nitrogen dioxide is released as a product of the oxidation of nitrate groups in silage and nitrogen-rich soils. As the fodder decays in this manner, the silos in which it is stored begin to fill with the gas. Sufficient concentrations can produce respiratory irritation. Higher concentrations can precipitate acute pulmonary edema. If the worker survives this event, the condition may relapse within a few weeks. Survival after relapse is less likely. Without relapse, complete recovery can be expected (31). Gases released from decomposing fodder and other chemical agents used in agricultural practice pose a significant hazard to pulmonary function. Chlorine, sulfur dioxide, ozone, phosgene, herbicides such as paraquat, and fertilizers such as anhydrous ammonia produce immediate irritation of the mucous membranes of the upper respiratory track. If the exposure is great enough, delayed pulmonary edema may develop.

Endotoxin Exposure

Gram-negative bacteria and endotoxin are found in many farming environments (32). Endotoxin is a heat-stable, lipopolysaccharide-protein complex derived from the cell wall of gram-negative bacteria (32). Endotoxin-contaminated dusts are encountered in harvesting, transport, processing, and storage of agriculture products as well as in livestock production areas (32). The target organ for endotoxin-induced injury is the lung, and in particular, the pulmonary macrophage, which is very sensitive to inhaled endotoxin. Dusty farming operations are a prime source of endotoxin pulmonary exposure, and calculated levels can exceed the airborne threshold of 90 endotoxin units per cubic meter (90 EU/m^3). This threshold is set for a zero mean $FEV_{1.0}$ response following exposure to endotoxin-containing dusts of a respirable size. Some environments have recorded endotoxin air concentrations as high as 13,210 EU/m^3 in respirable dust (32). Other studies have confirmed these airborne concentrations of endotoxins well beyond the 90 EU/m^3 threshold limit and that these high concentrations can vary in different locations of a processing area (32).

Green Tobacco Sickness

Green tobacco sickness is an occupational illness occuring among workers who crop or harvest tobacco leaves which are damp from rain or dew. The incidence of the illness is regularly noted in the tobacco fields of North Carolina where workers complain of headache, pallor, nausea, vomiting, and prostration after handling wet tobacco leaves. Symptoms resemble nicotine poisoning but may simulate organophosphate poisoning and heat exhaustion and thus may be treated inappropriately. The moisture on the tobacco leaves probably acts as a solvent for the nicotine, facilitating dermal absorption, especially as work clothing becomes wet (33). Sufficient urinary excretion of nicotine and its major metabolite, cotinine, have been observed in conjunction with the symptoms of green tobacco sickness. Workers who smoke rarely experience symptoms. This is probably due to the fact that smokers are more tolerant to the amount of nicotine they absorb while working on the harvest (34).

CLINICAL EVALUATION OF RESPIRATORY DISEASES

Distinguishing among the various respiratory disorders that occur in farm workers can be difficult because the symptoms of each disease process are quite similar. Also, the combination of smoking and agricultural exposure can be additive. The duration and amount of exposure to certain dusts and environmental contaminants is also important to consider in evaluating symptoms (35). In evaluating exposure to dusts, the dose, length of exposure, type of dusts, dust components, and size are all factors that contribute in different ways to produce different disease processes.

Clinical symptoms of cough, fever, fatigue, dyspnea, and $FEV_{1.0}$ declines can occur with both acute as well as chronic exposures. Thus, symptoms alone, without a historical time course of the exposure and an understanding of the true nature of the exposure, may not be helpful in disease differentiation. Immediate pulmonary responses may or may not be predictable of the development of chronic or future pulmonary disease (35).

Disease process and syndromes that require differentiation include pulmonary hypersensitivity, organic dust toxic syndrome, mucous membrane irritation, chronic bronchitis, byssinosis, and occupational asthma. Clinical evaluation should focus on smoking history, allergies, personal protection methods, previous work and exposures, and prior cardiac and pulmonary disease (36). A useful guide to the clinical evaluation of some of the more common pulmonary diseases of farmers is presented in Table 58.5 (36).

Table 58.5. Clinical Evaluations of Respiratory Disorders in Agricultural Workers

Chronic Bronchitis

History: Consider exposure history, amount of sputum produced, duration of symptoms, time of day that cough is worse and sputum production is the most. Any symptom change away from work should be noted. Inquire about night sweats, fatigue, and other vague symptoms.

Physical Examination: Auscultation of lungs for diminished breath sounds, presence of ronchi or rales, and quality of breath sounds. Respiratory effort and respiratory rate should be noted. General condition and level of physical activity should be noted. Note temperature patterns during day and night.

Ancillary Testing: Chest x-ray with a PA and lateral view should be obtained. Look for absence of hilar adenopathy or other lesions. Pulmonary function testing should include $FEV_{1.0}$, FVC, and $FEV_{1.0}$/FVC ratio. Sputum should be examined for types of inflammatory cells and can be cultured if necessary. A complete blood count (CBC) with differential should be obtained. Appropriate skin test can be applied, and serology may be considered for common fungal infections such as coccidioidomycosis and histoplasmosis.

Assessment: Exclude asthma, bronchiectasis, infections, neoplasms, and other causes of chronic cough.

Occupational Asthma

History: Occupational history and exposures are important. Asthma can be caused by a wide variety of exposures, chemical as well as biologic. Asthmatic-like syndromes can be allergic or nonallergic in nature. Evaluate hereditary predisposition. Seek presence of work-related wheezing. Define the times of onset and the activity engaged in at the time of onset.

Physical Examination: Pulmonary auscultation may reveal inspiratory as well as expiratory wheezes. Note respiratory rate and effort. Note temperature. Look for use of accessory muscles.

Ancillary Testing: Chest x-ray, PA and lateral, should be obtained. Chest x-ray may reveal signs of hyperinflation. Pulmonary function testing should include $FEV_{1.0}$, FVC, and $FEV_{1.0}$/FVC ratio. Reversible airway obstruction with β-adrenergic agonists. Peak flow recordings during the week may indicate times of airway obstruction.

Assessment: Exclude reactive airway disease process. Bronchodilators are usually helpful. Referral to a pulmonary specialist.

Hypersensitivity Pneumonitis

History: Explore symptom onset in relation to certain types of exposures. Define the exposure in terms of location and nature. Inquire about cough, sputum production, myalgias, fever, chills, malaise, dyspnea.

Physical Examination: May reveal rales and ronchi. May note increased respiratory effort and rate.

Ancillary Testing: Chest x-ray, PA and lateral, may reveal reticulonodular pattern bilaterally. Absence of hilar adenopathy. Pulmonary function testing should include $FEV_{1.0}$, FVC, and $FEV_{1.0}$/FVC ratio looking for restrictive airway defects. Positive serology for fungal antigens. CBC with differential may reveal a leukocytosis with increased lymphocytes.

Assessment: Referral to pulmonary specialist if suspected.

Organic Dust Toxic Syndrome

History: Symptoms usually occur a few hours after a high level dust exposure. Consider the nature of the dust. Symptoms include cough, fever, chills, myalgias, and dyspnea and are usually self-limited to hours or days.

Physical Examination: Auscultation of the chest is usually normal. Note respiratory effort and rate. Note temperature.

continues

Table 58.5. *Continued*

Ancillary Testing: Chest x-ray with Pa and lateral is usually normal. Pulmonary function testing should include $FEV_{1.0}$, FVC, and $FEV_{1.0}$/FVC ratio. These are usually normal. CBC with differential may reveal a leukocytosis. Examine sputum for microorganisms and cell types.

Assessment: Refer to pulmonary specialists if no improvement in 7 days. Rule out pneumonias and other causes.

Adapted from: doPico G. Am J Ind Med 1990; 17:132–135.

AGRICULTURAL CHEMICAL EXPOSURES

The use of chemicals, particularly fertilizers, pesticides, fumigants, and herbicides, is pervasive in agriculture. This results in agricultural use of approximately 65% of the registered pesticides in the United States. The primary use of these and other insecticides is for the control of insect vectors and to reduce crop loss. Insecticides have helped reduce disease in our environment through control of insects as well as improving living conditions by increasing the amount of available food. Pesticides include organophosphates, carbamates, rodenticides, herbicides, and fungicides. Additional agents found to be useful include food preservatives and seed dressings. Human exposure to insecticides and pesticides is widespread in developing countries as well as in more industrialized nations. Agricultural workers represent approximately 52% of the occupational labor force in developing countries (37). In 1984, insecticides made up 32% of the world's market of pesticide sales (37). There are more than 900 different pesticides registered for use by the Environmental Protection Agency (EPA) in the United States, and these compose more than 25,000 brand names of agrochemicals and pest control agents (37).

The use of pesticides in agriculture has produced an improvement in the financial investment of the farmer (38). To improve crop production, losses to insects and pests must be minimized. Third World countries, especially, have a need to improve agriculture production. This poses health problems, since these countries make extensive use of pesticides and workers in developing nations are generally unaware of safety aspects in the distribution and application of pesticides.

Insecticides can be classified into four main chemical groups (37):

1. Synthetic organic chemicals: organochlorines, organophosphates, carbamates
2. Inorganic chemicals: metals (arsenic, thallium, cyanide)
3. Biologics: pheromones, bacteria, viruses
4. Botanicals: pyrethrins

A more extensive classification of pesticides is presented in Table 58.6.

There are two categories of workers who are occupationally exposed to pesticides. The first group consists of those workers described as mixers, loaders, and applicators of pesticide formulations. A high rate of occupational injury in these workers is due to their acute exposure to high concentrations of pesticides at full strength. Illnesses usually evolve from accidental spills. The second category consists of a much larger number of field workers who are exposed to pesticide residues on the foliage of crops and in soils of the treated fields in which they harvest or otherwise do work. The exposure of this group differs from that of the mixer-loader, applicator group in that it is a

Table 58.6. Partial Listing of Pesticides

Inorganic and organometal pesticides
  Barium carbonate
  Sodium dichromate
  Copper sulfate
  Zinc chloride
  Zinc phosphide
  Cadmium chloride
  Elemental mercury
  Mercuric chloride
  Thallium sulfate
  Lead arsenate
  Methylmercury
  Ethyltin and related organotins
  Bismuth subcarbonate
  Bismuth subsalicylate
  Antimony potassium tartrate
  Arsenical pesticides
  Phosphorus
  Elemental sulfur
  Sodium selenate
  Sodium fluoride
  Sulfuryl fluoride
  Zinc hexafluorosilicate
  Sodium chlorate
  Boric acid

Pyrethrins, Pyrethroids, and Plant-Derived Pesticides
  Pyrethrins
  Phenothrin
  Decamethrin
  Cypermethrin
  Cyfluthrin
  Deltamethrin
  Cyhalothrin
  Fenvalerate
  Cyfluthrinate
  Fluvalinate
  Tralomethrin
  Tralocythrin
  Permethrin
  Resmethrin
  Rotenone
  Nicotine
  Anabasine
  Sabadilla and related compounds
  Strychnine
  Ricin
  Blasticidin-S

Propellants, solvents, and oil insecticides
  Dichlorodifluoromethane
  Kerosene
  Tetralin
  Xylene

Fumigants and nematocides
  Hydrogen cyanide and the cyanide salts
  Acrylonitrile
  Isobornyl thiocyanoacetate
  Carbon disulfide
  Aluminum phosphide and phosphine
  Naphthalene
  Epoxyethane
  Methyl bromide
  Dichloromethane
  Chloropicrin
  Boron trifluoride
  Carbon tetrachloride
  1,2-Dibromoethane
  1,2-Dichloroethane
  1,1,1-Trichloroethane

continues

Table 58.6. *Continued*

Trichloroethylene
Tetrachloroethylene
1,1-Dichloro-1-nitroethane
Dibromochloropropane
1,3-Dichloropropene
1,2-Dichloropropane
p-Dichlorobenzene

Chlorinated hydrocarbon insecticides

DDT
TDE
Ethylan
Methoxychlor
γ-Hexachlorocyclohexane (lindane)
Chlordane
Heptachlor
Aldrin
Dieldrin
Endrin
Isobenzan
Endosulfan
Mirex
Chlordecone
Toxaphene
Kelthane

Organophosphate pesticides

Mipafox	Mevinphos
Dimefox	Azinphos-methyl
DFP	Bromophos
Malathion	Dicapthon
Parathion-methyl	Monocrotophos
Demeton-methyl	Dicrotophos
Oxydemeton-methyl	Dimethoate
Dichlorvos	Endothion
Trichlorfon	Fenitrothion
Naled	Fenthion
Jodfenfos	Formothion
Methidathion	Parathion
Phenthoate	Diazinon
Phosphamidon	Demeton
Pirimiphos-methyl	Phorate
Temephos	TEPP
Thiometon	Carbophenothion
Schradan	Chlorfenvinphos
Merphos	Chlorphoxim
Leptophos	Chlorpyrifos
Carejin	Dialifos
Edifenphos	Dichlofenthion
Fonofos	Dioxathion
	Fensulfothion
	Phosalone
	Phoxim

Carbamate pesticides

Carbaryl
Aldocarb
Propoxur
3-Isopropylphenyl-N-methylcarbamate
4-Benziothielyn-N-methylcarbamate
Bufencarb
Carbofuran
Dioxacarb
Isolan
Landrin
Methomyl

Table 58.6. *Continued*

Carbamate pesticides (cont.)

Mexacarbate
Oxamyl
Phencyclocarb
Promecarb
Bendiocarb

Nitro compounds and related phenolic pesticides

2,4-Dinitrophenol
Binapacryl
Dinocap
Dinoseb
Pentachlorophenol
TCDD

Synthetic organic rodenticides

Sodium fluoroacetate
Fluoroacetamide
Fluoroethanol
Gliftor
MNFA
Pyriminil
ANTU
Warfarin
Difenacoum
Brodifiacoum
Diphacinone
Chloralose
Norbormide

Herbicides

2,4-D-Dichlorophenoxyacetic acid	Diuron
2,3,5-Trichlorophenoxyacetic acid	Dichlobenil
MCPA	Ioxynil
Silvex	Paraquat
Dicamba	Diquat
TCA	Atrazine
Propanil	Propazine
Phenmedipham	Simazine
Cycloate	Amitrole
Molinate	Pyrazon

Fungicides and biocides

Captan	Thiram
Captafol	Ziram
Tetrachlorophthalide	Maneb
Dichloran	Zineb
Quinotozene	Benomyl
1-Chlorodinitrobenzene	Thiabendazole
Diphenyl	Thiophanate-methyl
	Organotins (tributyltin)

Miscellaneous pesticides

Chlorfenxon	Busulfan
Propargite	Chlorambucil
Azoxybenzene	Thiotepa
Chlordimeform	Hexamethylmelamine
Metaldehyde	5-Fluorouracil
DEET	Methotrexate
	Porfirmycin

Adapted from Hayes W: Pesticides Studied in Man, Williams & Wilkins, Baltimore.

more chronic, low dose exposure, primarily involving dermal absorption (39–41).

The pesticides most frequently implicated in acute field exposures have been the organophosphates and carbamates. These pesticides exert their primary and acute toxic effects by inhibiting acetylcholinesterase by phosphorylation of the enzyme.

continues

A 60% depression in cholinesterase activity can produce relatively mild nonspecific symptoms such as nausea, headaches, malaise, constriction of pupils, and an asthma-like tightness of the chest. Greater depressions of cholinesterase activity may produce pulmonary edema, unconsciousness, respiratory failure, and even death. Cholinesterase depressions resulting from carbamate exposures are usually reversed more rapidly than those resulting from organophosphate exposure. Depression in plasma cholinesterase can also occur from pregnancy and birth control pills, which can make interpretation difficult if there are no symptoms associated with exposure.

Symptoms of organophosphate and/or carbamate poisoning can range from mild to severe. The degree of symptoms is dependent on the nature of the pesticide and its toxicity, absorbed dose, and prior level of cholinesterase activity. Weakness, abdominal pain, nausea, diarrhea, vomiting, and visual changes are associated with mild toxicity. Workers who are chronically exposed to organophosphate and carbamate insecticides without proper protection can deplete their cholinesterase activity to seriously low levels and be at an increased risk for developing poisoning even following a mild exposure that would normally not be serious. These individuals are at an increased risk for other work-related accidents and injuries also. Workers can be poisoned from crop residues as well as from direct contact during application (41–45). The rationale behind the legal reentry intervals has been to prohibit entry into treated fields to allow sufficient decay of the pesticide such that potential health risks should be mitigated.

Pesticide-related illness in agricultural production workers is an occupational hazard. A study of Nebraska farmers and pesticide applicators discovered that 30% of these individuals had significant reductions in serum cholinesterase activity, and 22% had pesticide poisoning symptoms (46). These types of exposures could certainly be an important variable contributing to the high incidence of accidents in this population. One example occurred when a field crew began harvesting in a mevinphos (Phosdrin)-treated field 2 hours after the pesticide was applied. Members of the crew sought medical treatment for a variety of symptoms ranging from nausea and visual disturbances to chest pain and shortness of breath. Plasma cholinesterase levels were depressed 15%, and red blood cell cholinesterase depressed almost 6%. Symptoms persisted for up to 10 weeks after exposure, which was longer than the 14 days it took for cholinesterase levels to normalize (42).

In response to serious illnesses and deaths among agricultural pesticide applicators, the state of California introduced a medical surveillance requirement in 1974 (47). The primary goal of medical surveillance is to prevent the development of profound cholinesterase depression and pesticide toxicity. California employers are required to provide wash and change facilities, clean work clothing, and the use of closed mixing and loading systems for the most toxic pesticides. Medical surveillance is also required for all agricultural pesticide applicators whose exposure to cholinesterase-inhibiting pesticides in toxicity category I or II (Table 58.7) is expected to reach 30 hours in any 30-day period. Mixer and loaders exclusively using closed systems are exempt from this requirement. Workers are referred to a physician medical supervisor for baseline red blood cell and plasma cholinesterase determination not less than 30 days after the last exposure to a cholinesterase-inhibiting pesticide. Workers are retested during their exposure period to detect any probable pesticide overexposure. If red blood cell cholinesterase activity is depressed to 60% or below baseline

Table 58.7.   U.S. EPA's Toxicity Categories for Pesticides

Category	LD$_{50}$[a]
I	≤50 mg/kg
II	51–500 mg/kg
III	>500 mg/kg

[a]Animal, oral, and dermal median lethal dose

or plasma cholinesterase to 50% or below, the worker must be removed from all exposure to organophosphate or carbamate pesticides. Removed workers may not resume handling cholinesterase-inhibiting pesticides until their cholinesterase activity levels have returned to at least 80% of baseline values. However, although the regulations also require enclosed mixing and loading systems or enclosed cabs and industrial hygiene measures in conjunction with medical supervision, surveys of workers demonstrate that cholinesterase depression exceeding the state's requirements for removal still exist (43). This suggests that the present regulatory mechanism is inadequate to control occupational pesticide exposures, and reevaluation of the individual components of the system is necessary to determine where improvements can be made.

The Federal Food, Drug, and Cosmetic Act originally established harvest intervals restricting the time between pesticide application and harvest, based on pesticide residue levels on foodstuffs, for the purpose of consumer protection. Today, it is the EPA that lists tolerance levels of residues on food under the Toxic Substances Control Act (TOSCA). The intervals themselves, however, are established by the individual states (48). Reentry intervals for the purpose of worker safety did not become a regulatory issue until the passage of the Occupational Safety and Health Act of 1970 creating the Occupational Safety and Health Administration (OSHA), and the passage of the 1972 amendments to the Federal Insecticide, Fungicide, and Rodenticide Act (FIFRA). OSHA became the first federal agency to propose pesticide reentry standards to protect the health of field workers. The first standards included 21 organophosphorous insecticides and five crops (citrus, peaches, grapes, tobacco, and apples). After protest from several agricultural groups, these standards were replaced within 6 weeks with less stringent standards covering only nine organophosphates with intervals ranging from 1–3 days for wet areas and 14 days for dry areas (based on average rainfall greater of less than 25 inches) (49). In 1973 the federal court gave jurisdiction to set and administer reentry standards to the EPA. Final EPA reentry standards, published in the Federal Register in 1974, required 48-hour reentry intervals for 11 organophosphate pesticides, endrin, and endosulfan (50).

States were given the responsibility and authority to set additional restrictions to address local problems. California has been the only state to establish its own reentry standards, which require longer intervals of between 5–30 days (51). Even with these longer intervals, there have still been numerous cases of illnesses among field worker crews that were induced by contact with residues on leaf surfaces (41, 42, 52).

The extent to which field workers are adversely affected by contact exposure to pesticide residues is a controversial subject. Many factors or a combination of factors may be necessary to produce an actual episode of poisoning by residues. Also, the dose-response mechanisms are difficult to assess because of the great variation in the types of pesticides used, work rate, quantity of pesticide contacted, and individual metabolism. The use of biologic markers such as pesticide metabolites has been attempted as a means of determining absorption. However, biologic monitoring is costly and, as noted earlier, the agriculture work force does not lend itself well to any longterm surveillance. In an effort to overcome this obstacle, exposure assessment models have been attempted for individual types of crops which involve similar maintenance and harvest so as to have similar exposure patterns. These models correlate the dislodgeable foliar residues (DFR) available for contact with daily dermal dose rates of an average harvester. The result is an empirical transfer factor expressed in terms of quantity of residue per unit of body surface area (40, 41). Thus far, transfer factors for tree fruits such as citrus and peaches are in the range of 4000–30,000 cm^2/hour. A substantial amount of data needs to be amassed under varying climatic conditions in order for the transfer factor to be an effective method of quantifying exposure without the use of biologic monitoring.

The number of officially reported cases of residue-related illness is estimated to be only 1–2% of the actual number. Epidemiologic evidence backs this up. Considerable indirect evidence suggests that farm workers are adversely affected by pesticide residues, but the true magnitude of the problem is uncertain because cases are largely undetected and grossly underreported. There are important socioeconomic and cultural factors that must be understood and carefully evaluated in any attempt to study this problem.

Pesticide-Related Dermatitis

Other pesticide-related exposure health problems include contact and allergic dermatitis. Chlorinated compounds, organophosphates, sulfur compounds, fumigants, herbicides, and fungicides may cause dermatitis in exposed individuals. Some pesticides are skin sensitizers. These include dithiocarbamates, pyrethrins, thioates, thiurams, parathion, and malathion (53, 54). Contact dermatitis is also common following exposures to animal hair and some plants. Contact dermatitis may also be related to the solvent used to dilute certain pesticides for application.

Cancer Risk, Pesticide Exposure, and Agriculture

Overall incidence of cancer in agricultural workers is lower than in the general population. However, there is concern over the widespread exposure and longterm exposure of farm workers to the myriad pesticides and other agricultural chemicals. Agricultural workers tend to have a decreased risk for cancers of the lung, colon, bladder, nose, rectum, and liver (55, 56). There is an increased risk for hematologic malignancies and for cancers of the brain, lip, stomach, and prostate (55). Mortality from multiple myeloma, leukemia, non-Hodgkin's lymphoma, brain cancer, and connective tissue cancer has been increasing in the farming communities more than in the general population over the period from 1950–1980 (55). The question is whether chemical exposure is associated with this increased cancer risk. Groundwater and soil contamination with pesticides, nitrates, and nitrosamines is increasing in rural communities from the extensive use of chemicals. In Nebraska farming areas alone there were an estimated 30 million pounds of pesticides and 2 million tons of fertilizer used in 1982 (46). Mortality studies published in 1985 looked at the years 1950–1979 and revealed an excess mortality for lymphoma and leu-

kemia in Nebraska (46). Case-control studies from Iowa farming communities in the 1980s do not indicate that the occupation of farming itself is a risk for increased lymphocytic leukemia; however, this study does point toward pesticide use as a risk factor in multiple myeloma (57).

Investigations into the possible etiologies or associated risks have focused on chemicals and animal viruses (57). An elevated risk for lymphosarcoma, reticulosarcoma, and other lymphomas in areas with heavy insecticide, herbicide, and fertilizer use has been noted (58). These cancers may, however, also be related to dietary factors, sun exposure, the handling of synthetic chemicals, or inhalation of mycotoxins (59). An identifiable risk pattern in association with chemical exposure has not yet been established.

To evaluate the potential carcinogenic risk of pesticides the National Cancer Institute developed a large scale routine bioassay in 1960 as a preliminary means of testing pesticides and other chemicals (56). This program is now being conducted by the National Toxicology Program. Criteria were established to ensure the validity of animal tests as a qualitative predictor of human effects. For example, a test using the maximum tolerated dose of a pesticide would require that it induce cancer in at least 7–10% of the animals being tested to be a statistically significant risk. Various federal and state agencies use this data in their regulatory decision-making process. In addition to the EPA, The U.S. Department of Agriculture, the Food and Drug Administration, and the Consumer Product Safety Commission are also authorized to exercise specific controls for limiting human exposure (56).

Arsenic exposure is associated with human lung cancer and hematologic malignancies (55). Exposure of Egyptian farmers to organophosphates, vinyl chloride, and arsenical pesticides has been noted to be associated with a higher incidence of hepatic angiosarcoma (56). Arsenic compounds are used still as wood preservatives, but the use of arsenical compounds as pesticides has greatly declined.

Many studies have examined the suspected link between cancers and pesticide exposure in farmers. Using death certificates for Nebraska farmers from 1957–1974, one study found a statistically significant increase in chronic myelogenous leukemia (59).

Many pesticides have demonstrated carcinogenic and genotoxic properties in animals (Table 58.8). Only a few of these have been human carcinogens (arsenic and vinyl chloride). The organochlorine pesticides such as chlordane, heptochlor, dieldrin, aldrin, lindane, and DDT have been scrutinized as potential causes of increased risk of cancer. However, reviews of most of the significant studies performed through the years show inconclusive evidence for carcinogenicity of the organochlorine pesticides (55, 56).

Certain cancers have been found to be in an excess in agricultural workers, especially for hematologic malignancies (55). Similar cancer patterns have been observed in other countries in farm workers. The reasons for this increased risk of cancer remain unknown. Studies have been focusing on the exposures to pesticides and to animal viruses (55). Multiple epidemiologic studies examining the relationship of chemical exposures and cancers in agricultural workers have been performed. As would be expected, acute and chronic exposures to multiple chemicals occur.

Difficulties are encountered in trying to assess the exposure to pesticides and determine any increases in relative cancer risks. Phenoxy herbicides such as 2,4,5-trichlorophenoxyacetic

Table 58.8.   Evidence for Carcinogenicity of Pesticides

Compound	Animal	Human	In Vitro	IARC[a]	EPA[b]
Aldrin	Limited	Inadequate	Inadequate	3	C
Amitrole	Sufficient	Inadequate	Inadequate	2B	B2
a-Naphthylthiourea	Inadequate	Inadequate		3	C
Aramite	Sufficient				
Arsenicals	Inadequate	Sufficient	Limited	1	A
Benzal chloride	Limited	Inadequate	Limited	3	C
Benzotrichloride	Sufficient	Inadequate	Limited	2B	B2
Benzoyl chloride	Inadequate	Inadequate	Inadequate	3	C
Benzyl chloride	Limited	Inadequate	Sufficient	3	C
Captan	Limited	Insufficient			
Carbon tetrachloride	Sufficient	Inadequate	Inadequate	2B	B2
Chlordane	Limited	Inadequate	Inadequate	3	C
Chlordimeform (metabolite)	No data	Insufficient			
Chlorobenzilate	Limited	Insufficient			
Chlorophenols		Limited		2B	B2
Chlorothalonil	Limited	Insufficient			
Diallate	Limited	Insufficient			
1,2-Dibromochloropropane	Sufficient				
p-Dichlorobenzene	Sufficient	No data		2B	B2
2,4-Dichlorophenoxyacetic acid esters	Inadequate	Inadequate	Inadequate	3	C
p,p'-Dichlorodiphenyltrichloroethane	Sufficient	Inadequate	Inadequate	2B	B2
Dicofol (Kelthane)	Limited	Insufficient			
Dieldrin	Limited	Inadequate	Inadequate	3	C
Ethylene dibromide	Sufficient	Inadequate	Sufficient	2B	B2
Ethylene oxide	Limited	Inadequate	Sufficient	2B	B2
Ethylene thiourea	Sufficient	Inadequate	Limited	2B	B2
Fluomenturon	Inadequate	No evaluation			
Formaldehyde	Sufficient	Inadequate	Sufficient	2B	B2
Heptachlor	Limited	Inadequate	Inadequate	3	C
Hexachlorobenzene	Sufficient				
Kepone (chlordecone)	Sufficient				
Lindane (γ-hexachlorocyclohexane)	Limited	Inadequate	Inadequate	3	C
Malathion	No evidence	No data			
4-Chloro-2-methylphenoxy acetic acid	Inadequate	Inadequate		3	C
Methyl parathion	No evidence	No evidence		3	C
Mirex	Sufficient				
Nitrofen	Sufficient	No data			
Parathion	Inadequate	Insufficient			
Pentachlorophenol	Inadequate	Inadequate	Inadequate	3	C
Phenoxy acids		Limited		2B	B2
o-Phenylphenol	Limited	Insufficient			
Piperonyl butoxide	No evidence	No evidence			
Sulfallate	Sufficient	No data			
2,3,4,8-Tetrachlorodibenzo-p-dioxin	Sufficient	Inadequate	Inadequate	2B	B2
Tetrachlorovinphos	Limited	Insufficient			
Thiourea	Sufficient				
Toxaphene	Sufficient				
Trichlorofon	Inadequate	Insufficient			
2,4,5-Trichlorophenol	Inadequate	Inadequate	No data	3	C
2,4,6-Trichlorophenol	Sufficient	Inadequate	No data	2B	B2
2,4,5-Trichlorophenoxyacetic acid	Inadequate	Inadequate	Inadequate	3	C
Vinyl chloride	Sufficient	Sufficient	Sufficient	1	A

Reprinted with permission from Council of Scientific Affairs. Cancer Risks of Pesticides in Agricultural Workers. J Am Med Assoc 1988;260:959–966.

[a]IARC indicates: International Agency for Research on Cancer. Evidence is divided into the following categories: 1, evidence is sufficient to establish a causal relationship between the agent and human cancer; 2, agent or process is probably carcinogenic to humans; 2A, limited, almost sufficient evidence for carcinogenicity in humans; 2B, combination of sufficient evidence in animals and inadequate human data; and 3, cannot be classified according to carcinogenicity in humans.

[b]EPA indicates: Environmental Protection Agency. Evidence is divided into the following groups: A, carcinogenic to humans (epidemiologic evidence supports a causal relationship); B, probably carcinogenic to humans (B1, epidemiologic evidence is limited or the weight of evidence from animal studies is sufficient or B2, evidence is sufficient from animal studies but epidemologic studies provide inadequate evidence or no data); and C, possibly carcinogenic to humans (limited evidence from animal studies and no human data).

acid (2,4,5-T) and 2,4-dichlorophenoxyacetic acid (2,4-D) have been extensively studied with respect to potential carcinogenesis (55). These herbicides had been contaminated with 2,3,7,8-terachlorodibenzo-*p*-dioxins (TCDD), a known animal carcinogen.

Multiple case-control and cohort studies of phenoxy herbicide-exposed agricultural workers have been published since 1979 (59–68). The major case-control studies performed in Sweden, New Zealand, and the United States can be questioned with respect to the reliability of data collection and exposure assessment (60). These studies, published between 1979 and 1988, demonstrated widely ranging relative risks (55).

Swedish case-control studies published in 1979 and 1981 indicated an increase in soft tissue sarcoma and lymphoma in exposed workers (55, 61–64). Studies in New Zealand and the United States published between 1986 and 1988 as well as a newer Swedish study in 1988 and 1989 have demonstrated varying relative risks (55, 65–69). Swedish case-control studies of 1979 and 1981 showed a five- to sixfold relative risk for soft tissue sarcomas in workers exposed to these herbicides (55, 61–64), whereas more recent Swedish studies (1988) showed only a 3.3-fold relative risk for sarcoma (55). A twofold relative risk for soft tissue sarcoma was found in Italian rice field workers in a 1987 study (55, 66). However, U.S. studies published in 1986 and 1987 along with New Zealand studies in 1984 and 1986 demonstrated a relative risk of only 1.0 (55, 65–67). Swedish cohort studies differed from case-control studies and found a relative risk of only 0.9 for soft tissue sarcomas, compared with the five- to sixfold relative risk in earlier Swedish studies involving herbicide exposure (55).

Case-control studies in 1981 showed an increased relative risk of six for non-Hodgkin's lymphomas in phenoxy herbicide-exposed workers, but a 1989 Swedish study found a relative risk of only 1.6 (55, 62). A Kansas study in 1986 found a risk of 2.0, which increased to sevenfold if workers had used the herbicides for more than 20 days (55). Other studies from New Zealand in 1987 and from Washington in 1987 failed to show an increased risk for lymphomas in persons exposed to phenoxy herbicides (55, 65, 67).

Definite conclusions from all of these cohort and case-control studies cannot be reached. All of these studies suffer from lack of variables control: methods of herbicide application, dose absorbed, length of exposure, route of exposure, cofactors such as presence of other chemicals or potential carcinogens, and genetic background. The increase in certain cancers in agricultural workers appears real; however, the etiology remain unknown.

REGULATION OF PESTICIDES

The primary federal statute for the regulation of manufacturing, use, and distribution of pesticides is the Federal Insecticide, Fungicide, and Rodenticide Act (FIFRA) which was enacted in 1947. Since then, FIFRA has been amended in 1972, 1975, and in 1978. The EPA has had the responsibility to regulate pesticide use since 1970. Pesticide regulation first occurred under the Insecticide Act of 1910, which was a consumer protection measure against mislabeling and distribution of ineffective pesticides. FIFRA replaced this act. Pesticides are also regulated by the EPA under the following acts:

1. Federal Envrionmental Pesticide Control Act
2. Resource Conservation Recovery Act of 1972 (RCRA)

3. Comprehensive Environmental Response, Compensation, and Liability Act (Superfund)
4. Toxic Substances Control Act (TSCA)
5. Clean Water Act
6. Safe Drinking Water Act

A pesticide is defined under FIFRA as "any substance or mixture of substances intended for preventing, destroying, repelling, or mitigating any pest, and . . . any substance of mixture of substances intended for use as a plant regulator, defoliant, or dessicant" (70). Pesticides thus include insecticides, fungicides, herbicides, rodenticides, dessicants, disinfectants, defoliants, and nematocides (70). FIFRA requires all pesticides sold or distributed to be registered with the EPA. Once registered, FIFRA classifies the pesticide as general or restricted in use. The application and use of pesticides is tightly controlled by the EPA under FIFRA.

FIFRA prohibits the sale of unregistered pesticides, the production of pesticides by unregistered manufacturers, the use of adulterated pesticides, and the use of a pesticide in a manner inconsistent with its labeling. The EPA has the authority to enforce FIFRA by legal sanctions, including civil penalties, criminal fines, injunctions, product seizure, termination of product sales, or recalls (70). When evidence indicates that a particular pesticide may be a significant health hazard, the appropriate regulatory agency or agencies can take any of the following actions (56):

1. Issue permissible exposure limits for the workplace;
2. Cancel registration and order withdrawal of the product from the market;
3. Place restrictions on use or application of the compound;
4. Set tolerance limits for pesticide residues on foodstuffs;
5. Cancel registration;
6. Establish maximum permissible contamination levels for the pesticides in drinking water.

In addition to the regulation of pesticide use and application, FIFRA requires the pesticide manufacturer to be registered with the EPA. The EPA, under agreement with the Food and Drug Administration, establishes pesticide tolerance for raw foods and produce (70). Pesticides that might be considered food additives are controlled by the EPA under the Food, Drug, and Cosmetic Act (70). It is of interest that once a pesticide is discarded, it becomes a hazardous waste and is then under regulation by RCRA and not FIFRA.

The 1978 amendment to FIFRA allows manufacturers of pesticides to have a waiver on submission of data demonstrating efficacy of their product, except where the product has a direct relation to or effect on public health. In addition, the 1978 amendment allows for public disclosure of the safety and health data regarding pesticide regulation (70). The 1978 amendment also transfers to states the responsibility to enforce pesticide use regulations if they can demonstrate that they possess the means to do so. The EPA reserves the right to revoke any state's responsibility for pesticide regulation if that state is unable or unwilling to enforce the regulations (70).

Regulation of a pesticide suspected to be a carcinogen is not uniformly applied by all federal agencies (56). However, these agencies have been consistent in regulating a substance when it is expected to cause an increase of more than four cases of cancer per 1000 persons (56). If the expected increase in cancer is less than one in a million, then regulation is unlikely (56). Cost-effectiveness of regulation is also considered, if the cost of regulation is anticipated to be less than $2 million per life saved (56).

ENVIRONMENTAL CONCERNS REGARDING CHEMICALS AND PESTICIDES

Soil, Air, and Groundwater Contamination

There are approximately 1 billion pounds of pesticides applied to crops in the United States annually (71). The main route of application is spraying, and it is estimated that only 1–3% of these pesticides reach their point of action (71). Application via spraying covers wide agricultural areas as well as potentially exposing workers and the public.

Since World War II, the widespread and intensive use of pesticides has been associated with persistent and broad spectrum agents such as DDT. DDT and its related chlorinated compounds have been associated with residues throughout the environment, including accumulation in both the food chain and living systems. Although DDT was banned in the United States in 1972, it continues to be used widely outside North America. However, new nonresidual chemicals and agents that can be specifically targeted to certain pests have been developed in response to environmental concerns. These newer chemical agents, despite substantial improvements, still generate concern because of their potential impacts on soil fertility and their long term effects on ground and surface water (Figure 58.8).

Chemical pesticides reach the soil by direct application and from aerial and ground sprays. Overall, there are three main processes which affect the efficiency and ultimate fate of pesticides in soil:

1. Absorption-desorption;
2. Transformation via biologic and chemical degradation;
3. Transport into the soil, atmosphere, surface water, and groundwater.

Investigations have demonstrated the groundwater can suffer contamination attributable to the widespread application of agricultural chemicals. Specific chemicals, such as atrazine, can now be measured in aquafers and wells. The problem is to determine the origin of these chemicals, which have been widely applied over periods of decades.

This non-point source problem involves both time sequence and location. Recent work by the Tennessee Valley Authority involving stereoscopic infrared color aerial photography has begun to demonstrate that source and time sequence problems may no longer be insurmountable (72). Computer databases can be constructed that include land use category, site number, surface area and topography, and hydrogeologic codes for both aquafer and stream systems. As this technology becomes more sophisticated, the quality and specificity of the database will improve such that the term "agricultural non-point source pollution" may become an anachronism.

Contamination of groundwater, well water, and soil by farm chemicals occurs due to water runoff, drainage, seepage, and spraying. Environmental contamination by nitrates, pesticides, halogenated hydrocarbons, and other toxic chemicals is now recognized as a health risk.

Nitrate contamination of well water and groundwater in rural areas has been a source of methemaglobinemia in infants and children and in some occasions, even adults (73). Nitrates from fertilizer and livestock excrement are the main sources of this type of water contamination. Water contamination with nitrates and nitrites is common, and illness and death secondary to methemoglobinemia was recognized as early as 1947 and as late as 1987 from ingestion of contaminated water sources (74, 75). Well water surveys in South Dakota revealed that up to 39% of dug or bored wells contained nitrates at unsafe concentrations (73).

The EPA defines the acceptable limit of nitrates (NO_3-N) as 10 mg/l of water (10 ppm). Most cases of methemoglobinemia involve water concentrations above 100 mg/l (73). It should

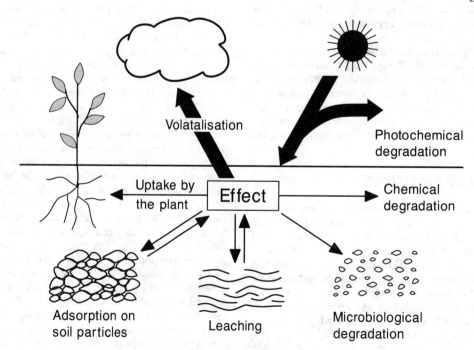

Figure 58.8. Scheme of pesticide degradation. Reprinted from Buchel KH. Political, economic and philosophical aspects of pesticide use for human welfare. Regul Toxicol Pharmacol 1984;4:174–191.

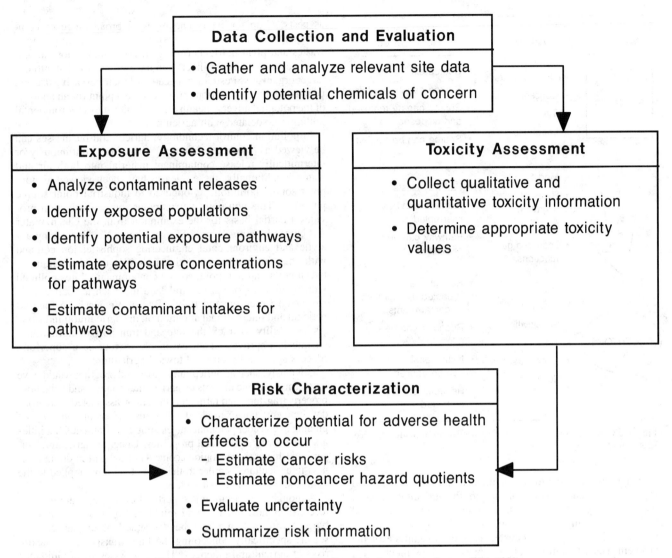

Figure 58.9.   Specific tasks of a Baseline Risk Assessment. Source: EPA 1989.

be noted that the production of methemoglobinemia is not always associated with symptoms. Illness is associated with the amount of hemoglobin available as well as the percent oxidized to methemoglobin. Rural children and adults who have relatively lower levels of hemoglobin will tend to manifest illness more easily.

An additional potential health concern involves the conversion of nitro-containing compounds to potentially carcinogenic nitrosamines that can be consumed. Aldicarb, atrazine, carbaryl, simazine, and carbofuran can react with nitrites at acidic pHs to form nitro compounds (73). Aldicarb, a highly toxic carbamate has been detected in groundwater samples (76). The degradation and persistence of aldicarb in soil and water are influenced by the type of soil, pH, plant application, and moisture (76).

Volatilization of pesticides into the air is determined by the vapor pressure of the active ingredient (71). Pesticide loss into the air occurs during application of vapors, aerosols, and dusts as well as from retained crop residues. The transport of pesticides beyond the sites of application into nearby homes, public roadways, water, and nonagricultural land is a realistic concern.

The legal, economic, regulatory, political, and social forces directed at the agriculture business are growing. Practices that reduce pesticide loss from point of application are being explored: (a) efforts to increase effectiveness and reduce the amount required per application; (b) new formulations that result in improved biodegradability; and (c) improved application methods (77, 78). Innovative changes include improving chemical formulations to prevent release into the atmosphere as well as reducing soil and groundwater release and the use of recombinant DNA biotechnology to provide viruses and bacteria as biologic pesticides (78).

An Agricultural Superfund

The agricultural sector as a whole is increasingly under fire as a source of pollution. Extending the "polluter pays" principle to agriculture and to individual farmers, based on an agricultural "superfund" is a novel idea with technical, health and public policy implications. The superfund concept arises from P.L. 94-580, which effectively spreads the costs of industrial pollution by imposing fees on industry, the proceeds of which are available to pay for hazardous waste cleanup at "superfund sites" (79).

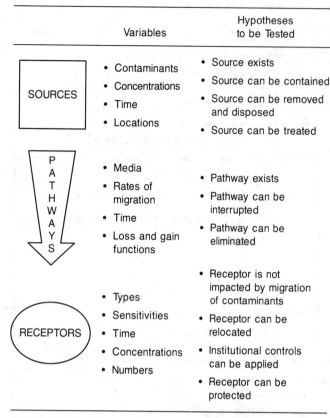

	Variables	Hypotheses to be Tested
SOURCES	• Contaminants • Concentrations • Time • Locations	• Source exists • Source can be contained • Source can be removed and disposed • Source can be treated
PATHWAYS	• Media • Rates of migration • Time • Loss and gain functions	• Pathway exists • Pathway can be interrupted • Pathway can be eliminated
RECEPTORS	• Types • Sensitivities • Time • Concentrations • Numbers	• Receptor is not impacted by migration of contaminants • Receptor can be relocated • Institutional controls can be applied • Receptor can be protected

Figure 58.10. Elements of a conceptual evaluation model. Source: EPA, 1989.

If agriculture were to be included in the superfund, or a separate such fund were established for the agricultural sector, the costs of agricultural pollution would effectively be spread to all those paying into the fund. Who will pay, of course, is an issue likely to prompt debate, as is the magnitude of the problem itself. Regardless of who pays and how much, such cost spreading may be preferable to allowing full liability to be borne in agriculture by a few companies producing chemicals found to have adverse effects or by farmers found to have used these chemicals over time.

Based on methods currently in use in connection with the superfund, the type of information that would be demanded in characterizing the risks associated with agricultural pollution can be explored. These risks are at present largely unknown. If the public increasingly demands information on the human health impacts of agricultural pollution, the framework developed under superfund legislation in the nonagricultural sector can be useful in agriculture as well. After considering this information, what would be the implications of public policy issues involved in implementing an agricultural superfund?

Chemicals and fertilizers used in crop production have, until recently, been regarded as less significant causes of pollution than more localized hazards resulting from landfills, industrial disposal, and other "point sources." Yet recent evidence implicates agricultural contributions over wide areas as significant "non-point sources" of pollution, which despite the lack of a single source, are nonetheless identifiable. Broadly speaking, the two main sources are pesticides and fertilizers.

Pesticides are generally synthetic organic chemicals used to kill or inhibit the growth and reproduction of species viewed as pests. Crop fertilizers encompass a broad range of commercially available and indigenous sources, including animal wastes and plant nutrients (nitrogen, potassium, phosphorus). Both pesticides and fertilizers can have effects on distant nontarget organisms. Pesticides, because of their pervasive use and negative public perception, provide a focal point for an analysis of the potential adverse health effects induced by environmental pollution associated with agriculture.

In pollution control technology, agricultural businesses can be viewed as "source generators" that either continuously or intermittently release contaminant material into both air and water. Traditionally, these releases have been viewed as non-point source pollution, as opposed to industrial point source pollution. This non-point versus point source distinction provides a partial basis for the exemption from the Clean Water Act currently enjoyed by U.S. agriculture. Yet, increasing analytic and environmental engineering sophistication coupled with changing public perception may blur the distinction between point and non-point source contaminants. Sites polluted with byproducts of agricultural land use such as California's Kesterson Reservoir and Italy's Bay of Venice have focused national and international attention on the agricultural industry. As the ability to track the fate and transport of agricultural chemicals improves, it is reasonable to foresee a superfund process specifically directed toward agriculture.

Obviously, such an agricultural superfund program would have longterm economic impacts on agricultural policy, land valuation, property transfers, and farmland conversion associated with urban development. For example, lending institutions are already beginning to consider potential and existing environmental liabilities associated with agricultural properties. Under an agricultural superfund, this practice would become a normal part of doing business in agriculture, similar to the current scrutiny applied to the industrial and commercial sectors.

Although no agricultural superfund exists, it is appropriate to consider how such a fund might be constructed and what type of information might be demanded of the agricultural sector, specifically concerning the fate, transport, and health risks of agricultural practices. The Risk Assessment Guidance for Superfund process provides a framework for developing the risk information necessary to assist in this process (80). There are four primary objectives of this assessment:

1. To provide an analysis of baseline risks;
2. To generate data that provide a basis for determining what levels of chemicals are environmentally acceptable;
3. To provide a basis for comparing potential health impacts of various remediation strategies;
4. To provide a consistent process for evaluating and documenting public health threats associated with a given pollution source.

The analysis of agricultural use of pesticides fits well into this overall framework. Typically, the baseline risk assessment of potentially widespread contamination utilizes a four-part approach:

1. Historical overview, data collection, and evaluation;
2. Exposure assessment;
3. Toxicity assessment;
4. Risk characterization.

Each of these categories is further subdivided into specific tasks (Fig. 58.9) which will produce an overall conceptual

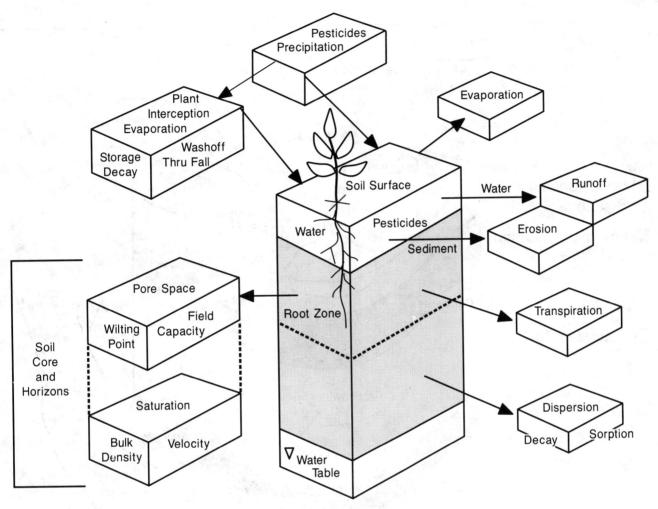

Figure 58.11.   Pesticide root zone model. Source: EPA, 1984.

evaluation model (Fig. 58.10). Pesticides can be considered in terms of this four-part process.

Exposure Assessment

Exposure assessment is the determination or estimation of the magnitude, frequency, duration, and route of exposure of a particular chemical pollutant. These estimations can be based on long duration real-time measurement or a variety of mathematical models. Typically, these "fate and transport" models provide conservative estimates of the amount of chemical available at the human exchange boundaries (lungs, gastrointestinal tract, skin) during a specified time period. There are several specific instances in which real-time monitoring data are not adequate and fate-transport models must be utilized. These include:

1. Cases in which potential exposure points are spatially separate from the monitoring point. Examples of this situation include groundwater transport and air dispersion of chemicals.
2. Cases in which time-series data are lacking. Longterm site-specific data are generally unavailable; therefore, even though there may be situations in which it is reasonable to assume constant conditions, it is necessary to predict future exposure employing a model.
3. Cases in which monitoring data are difficult to quantify.

Examples are the case of a groundwater plume discharging into a river or other surface water body. The dilution in the river water can result in concentration of the chemical below limits of detection, despite the fact that the chemical can bioaccumulate and ultimately raise health concerns.

Fortunately, while much could be done to improve our knowledge of agricultural chemical use, a reasonably large and well-documented database exists for the determination of the environmental fate and transport of pesticides in soil. Soils poses a large and physiochemically active surface area. This surface area provides a site for multiple surface reactions and a reservoir for the retention of pesticides; in addition, the chemical character of pesticides affects the extent and nature of pesticide absorption by soils. The overall distribution of pesticides in soil phases is influenced not only by intrinsic soil properties, but also by external factors, including climatic conditions and agricultural practices (81).

Fate-transport models have been devised to incorporate both these external factors and various physiochemical factors to address the following fundamental questions:

1. What are the principal mechanisms for change or removal in each soil type and horizon?
2. How does the chemical degrade or accumulate in air, water, soil, and other biologic material?

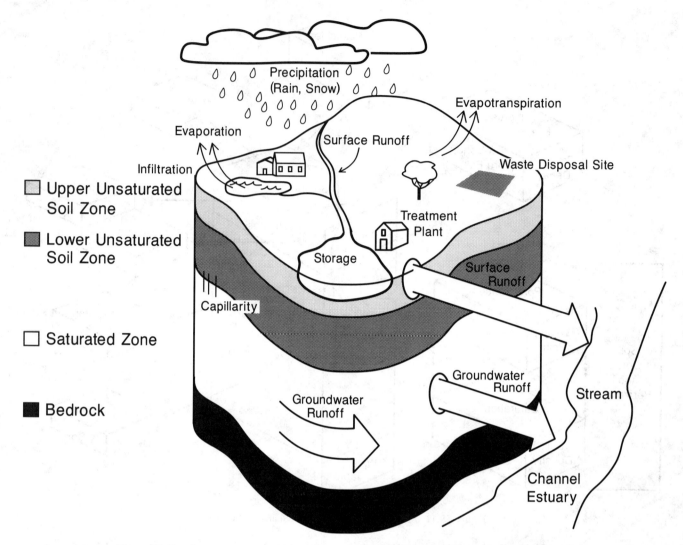

Figure 58.12. Seasonal soil compartment model. Source: Environmental Protection Agency, 1987.

3. Does the agent react with other compounds in the soil environment?
4. Is there transfer from the soil surface to ground water, and, if so, what are the mechanisms, rates, and reactions of this process?
5. What is the longterm (air, water, soil) environmental persistence of each chemical?
6. Are potentially toxic byproducts produced, and, if so, how are they to be analyzed?
7. Is a steady-state concentration distribution achieved?

Each of these questions is applicable to the general transport of chemicals in ground and surface water, air, soil, and the food chain.

The Superfund Exposure Assessment Manual provides specific guidance for the selection of contaminant release and fate analysis models; in addition, there is a large selection of situation-specific models (82). Two particularly well-documented models relevant to pesticide fate and transport are the Pesticide Root Zone Model (PRZM, Fig. 58.11) and the Seasonal Soil Compartment Model (*SeSoil*) (Fig. 58.12) (83, 84).

PRZM simulates the vertical movement of pesticides in the unsaturated soil and within and below the plant root zone. Simulations can also be extended to the water table where groundwater models can be utilized. The PRZM model analyzes runoff, erosion, plant uptake, leaching, decay, foliar washoff/volatilization, vertical movement, dispersion, and retardation (Fig. 58.11). Predictions can be made daily, monthly, or annually. The cumulative frequency distribution wave of a given pesticide leaving the root zone is illustrated in Fig. 58.13. Extensive documentation, including modeling specifics and limitations, are available for PRZM and other pesticide models from the EPA (82).

SeSoil is a general water and sediment transport model that allows specific analysis of pesticide and sediment transport on water sheds (Fig. 58.12). This model has particular utility because it merges with preexisting longterm climate files, and it is integrated into the Graphical Exposure Modeling System (GEMS) family of air and water models. GEMS is user friendly and allows the complete fate and transport analysis of most chemicals. There are, of course, many limitations to these models; however, they are constantly improving and provide an initial screening tool with wide applicability to pesticide use in agriculture.

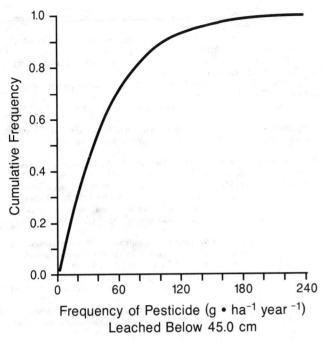

Figure 58.13. Cumulative frequency distribution of pesticide leaving root zone. Source: EPA, 1984.

Toxicity Assessment

The primary hazard of pesticide exposure is the development of acute toxic effects associated with dermal contact or inhalation. The medical literature is replete with studies of pesticide-related illness (52). The health effects of low level or prolonged pesticide exposures via drinking water are less clear. Controlled epidemiologic studies of longterm exposure to pesticides has generally been focused on farmers and pesticide production workers. Qualitative and quantitative risk assessment suggests the possibility of incremental increased cancer risk, although human epidemiologic data are less clear. Specific health-based recommendations for acceptable pesticide levels in ground water have been formulated. The ability to recommend no adverse effects levels for pesticides in groundwater is controversial, although the limit-setting process and methodology are well established by the EPA. Risk-based toxicity assessments for pesticides are common despite the lack of strong evidence to support or negate a causal relationship between low level exposure and disease. This scientific uncertainty does not effect the increasing public pressure to monitor and regulate low doses of pesticide exposure in food and water.

Risk Characterization

Risk characterization combines toxicity and exposure assessments into quantitative and qualitative expressions of risk. Risks are estimated as projected excess rates of cancer for chronic disease associated with a set of chemical exposures. Risk characterization also provides key information for policy makers. Pesticide risk methodology involves the same assumptions and calculations as for other chemical exposures. Those are (a) standard intake assumptions; (b) EPA potency factors (carcinogenic risk) and reference doses (noncarcinogenic); (c) risks combined across exposure pathways; (d) carcinogenic risk assessed and analyzed; (e) noncancer hazard quotients calculated;

and (6) sensitivity and uncertainty analysis of all assumptions performed. The current risk assessment guidance manual for Superfund (80) provides further detail and documentation of the entire process.

Implications for Policy

Overall, traditional non-point source pollution problems such as agriculture, in fact appear highly amenable to a superfund risk evaluation process. As the distinction between point and non-point source pollution becomes harder to sustain, non-point source pollution in agriculture may well become subject to regulations under existing superfund laws, or through creation of a separate agricultural superfund. An agricultural superfund would, no doubt, be controversial, since it would involve major shifts in liability assignment for farmers and suppliers of farm chemicals. Yet, members of the U.S. Committee on Irrigation and Drainage have suggested that some members of industry might be happy to see the focus and costs for cleanup of contaminated water shifted in part to an additional sector of the economy that has heretofore escaped responsibility (79). As the technology of chemical detection and fate-transport improves, agriculture may well become exposed and vulnerable to the increasing regulatory and financial pressure associated with environmental contamination.

REFERENCES

1. Malmberg P. Health effects of organic dust exposure in dairy farmers. Am J Ind Med 1990;17:7–15.
2. Schenker MB, McCurdy SA. Occupational health among migrant and seasonal farmworkers: the specific case of dermatitis. Am J Ind Med 1990;18:345–351.
3. Hoglund S. Farmers' occupational health care—worldwide. Am J Ind Med 1990;18:365–370.
4. May JJ. Issues in agricultural health and safety. Am J Ind Med 1990;18:121–131.
5. Emanuel DA, Draves DL, Nycz GR. Occupational health services for farmers. Am J Ind Med 1990;18:149–162.
6. Donham KJ. Prologue: agricultural occupational and environmental health: policy strategies for the future. Am J Ind Med 1990;18:107–119.
7. Hartye J. Physicians as the weak link in agricultural health services—defining the agenda for action. Am J Ind Med 1990;18:421–425.
8. NSC. Accident Facts. Chicago: National Safety Council, 1990.
9. Purschwitz MA, Field WE. Scope and magnitude of injuries in the agricultural workplace. Am J Ind Med 1990;18:179–192.
10. Myers JR. National surveillance of occupational fatalities in agriculture. Am J Ind Med 1990;18:163–168.
11. US Department of Commerce, 1982 census of agriculture. Vol. 1. Geographic area series, part 51. US Publication AC82-A-51. Washington, DC: Bureau of Census, 1982.
12. Burmeister LF, Morgan DP. Mortality in Iowa farmers and farm laborers, 1971–1987. J Occup Med 1982;24:898–900.
13. Husman K, Notkola V, et al. Farmers' occupational health program in Finland, 1979–1988: from research to practice. Am J Ind Med 1990;18:379–384.
14. Gay J, Donham KJ, Leonard S. Iowa agricultural health and safety service project. Am J Ind Med 1990;18:385–389.
15. Hoglund S. Farmers' health and safety programs in Sweden. Am J Ind Med 1990;18:371–378.
16. Sandfort D. Reaching the difficult audience: an experiment to provide occupational health services to farmers and ranchers in Colorado, USA. Am J Ind Med 1990;18:395–403.
17. Chan-Yeung M, Enarsm D, Gryzbowski S. Grain dust and respiratory health. Can Med Assoc J 1985;133:969–973.
18. Marx JJ, Guernsey J, Emanuel DA, et al. Cohort studies of immunologic lung disease among Wisconsin dairy farmers. Am J Ind Med 1990;18:263–268.
19. Warren CPW. Respiratory disorders in Manitoba cattle farmers. Can Med Assoc J 1981;125:41–46.
20. Madsen D, Klock LE, Wenzed FJ, et al. The prevalence of farmer's lung in an agricultural population. Am Rev Respir Dis 1976;113:171–174.

21. Holt PG. Inflammation in organic dust-induced lung disease: new approaches for research into underlying mechanisms. Am J Ind Med 1990;17:47–54.

22. Von Essen S, Robbins RA, Thompson AB, Rennard SI. Organic dust toxic syndrome: an acute febrile reaction to organic dust exposure distinct from hypersensitivity pneumonitis. Clin Toxicol 1990;28:389–420.

23. Katlia ML, Mantyjarvi RA, Ojanen TH. Sensitization against environmental antigens and respiratory symptoms in swine workers. Br J Ind Med 1981;38:344–348.

24. Donham KJ. Health effects from work in swine confinement buildings. Am J Ind Med 1990;17:17–25.

25. Donham KJ, Knapp LW, Monson R, Gustafson K. Acute toxic exposure to gases from liquid manure. J Occup Med 1982;24:142–145.

26. Clark S, Rylander R, Larson L. Airborne bacteria endotoxin and fungi in dust in poultry and swine confinement buildings. Am J Ind Hyg Assoc J 1983;44:537–541.

27. Cockcroft DW, Dosman JA. Respiratory health risks in farmers. Ann Intern Med 1981;95:380–382.

28. Hurst JS, Dosman JA. Characterization of health effects of grain dust exposures. Am J Ind Med 1990;17:27–32.

29. Rylander R. Health effects of cotton dust exposures. Am J Ind Med 1990;17:39–45.

30. Lowry T, Schuman LM. Silo-filler's disease: a syndrome caused by nitrogen dioxide. JAMA 1956;162:153–160.

31. Moskowitz RL, Lyons HA, Cottle HR. Silo-filler's disease: clinical, physiological and pathological study of a patient. Am J Med 1964;36:457.

32. Olenchock SA, May JJ, Pratt DS, et al. Presence of endotoxins in different agricultural environments. Am J Ind Med 1990;18:279–284.

33. Gehlbach SH, Williams WA, Perry LD, Woodall JS. Green tobacco sickness: an illness of tobacco harvesters. JAMA 1974;229:1880–1883.

34. Ghosh SK, Parikh JR, Govani VN, Roa MN, Kashyap SK, Chatterjee SK. Studies on occupational health problems in agricultural tobacco workers. J Occup Med 1980;29:113–117.

35. Thelin A. Workgroup report: exposure pattern in relation to symptoms—clinical findings. Am J Ind Med 1990;17:129.

36. doPico G. Workgroup report: guidelines for evaluation of clinical cases. Am J Ind Med 1990;17:132–135.

37. Minton NA, Murray VSG. A review of organophosphate poisoning. Med Toxicol 1988;3:350–375.

38. Buchel KH. Political, economic and philosophical aspects of pesticide use for human welfare. Regul Toxicol Pharmacol 1984;4:174–191.

39. Gunther F, Westlake W, Barkley J. Establishing dislodgeable pesticide residues on lead surfaces. Bull Environ Contam Toxicol 1973;9:243–249.

40. Knaak JB, Yutaka I, Maddy KT. The worker hazard posed by re-entry into pesticide-treated foliage: development of safe re-entry times with emphasis on chlorthiophos and carbosulfan. In: Paustenbach DJ, ed. The risk assessment of environmental and human health hazards: a textbook of case studies. New York: John Wiley & Sons, 1989.

41. Popendorf WJ, Leffingwell JT. Regulating OP residues for farmworker protection. Residue Rev 1982;82:125–201.

42. Coye MJ, Barnett PG, Midtline JE, Valesco AR, et al. Clinical confirmation of organophosphate poisoning of agricultural workers. Am J Ind Med 1986;10:399–409.

43. Brown SK, Ames RG, Mengle DC, et al. Cholinesterase activity depression among California agricultural pesticide applicators. Am J Ind Med 1989;15:143–150.

44. Spear RC, Poppendorf WJ, Spencer WF, Milby TH. Worker poisonings due to paroxone residues. J Occup Med 1977;19:411–414.

45. Brown SK, Ames RG, Mengle CD. Occupational illnesses from cholinesterase-inhibiting pesticides among agricultural applicators in California 1982–1985. Environ Health 1989;44:34–39.

46. Weisenburger DD. Environmental epidemiology of non-Hodgkin's lymphoma in Eastern Nebraska. Am J Ind Med 1990;18:303–305.

47. State of California Department of Food and Agriculture. Title 3, Code of Regulations, Chapter 6, Section 6728, Medical Supervision, 1989.

48. US Environmental Protection Agency. Harvest Intervals, EPA Code of Federal Regulations, Title 40, 1989.

49. US Department of Labor, Occupational Safety and Health Administration. Emergency temporary standard for exposure to organophosphorous pesticides. Fed Reg 1973;38:10715.

50. US Environmental Protection Agency. Farm workers dealing with pesticides. Proposed health-safety standards. Fed Reg 1974;39:9457.

51. State of California Department of Food and Agriculture. Title 3, Code of Regulations, Chapter 6, Section 6772, Re-entry Intervals, 1989.

52. Kahn E. Pesticide related illness in California farm workers. J Occup Med 1976;18:693–696.

53. Maibach H, Rycroft R. Contact dermatitis from organophosphorus pesticides. Br J Dermatol 1977;97:693–695.

54. Nater J, Goosken V. Occupational dermatosis due to a soil fumigant. Contact Dermatitis 1979;2:227–229.

55. Pearce N, Reif JS. Epidemiologic studies of cancer in agricultural workers. Am J Ind Med 1990;18:133–148.

56. JAMA Council of Scientific Affairs. Cancer risks of pesticides in agricultural workers. JAMA 1988;260:959–966.

57. Burmeister LF. Cancer in Iowa farmers: recent results. Am J Ind Med 1990;18:295–301.

58. Staftlas AF, Blair A, Cantor KP, Hanrahan L, Anderson HA. Cancer and other causes of death among Wisconsin Farmers. Am J Ind Med 1987;11:119–129.

59. Blair A, Malker H, Cantor KP, Burmeister L, Wiklund K. Cancer among farmers: a review. Scand J Work Environ Health 1985;11:397–407.

60. Blair A, Zahm SH. Methodologic issues in exposure assessment for case-control studies of cancer and herbicides. Am J Ind Med 1990;18:285–293.

61. Hardell L, Sandstrom A. Case-control study: soft-tissue sarcomas and exposure to phenoxyacetic acids or chlorophenols. Br J Cancer 1979;39:711–717.

62. Hardell L, Eriksson M, Lenner P, Lundgren E. Malignant lymphoma and exposure to chemicals, especialy organic solvents, chlorophenols and phenoxy acids: a case-control study. Br J Cancer 1981;43:169–176.

63. Eriksson M, Hardell L, Berg NO, Moller T, Axelson O. Soft-tissue sarcomas and exposure to chemical substances: a case-referent study. Br J Ind Med 1981;38:27–33.

64. Hardell L. Relation of soft-tissue sarcoma, malignant lymphoma and colon cancer to phenoxy acids, chlorophenols and other agents. Scand J Work Environ Health 1981;7:119–130.

65. Smith AH, Pearce NE, Fisher DO, Giles HJ, Teague CA, Howard JK. Soft tissue sarcoma and exposure to phenoxyherbicides and chlorophenols in New Zealand. J Natl Cancer Inst 1981;73:1111–1117.

66. Vineis P, Terracini B, Ciccone G, et al. Phenoxy herbicides and soft-tissue sarcomas in female rice weeders. Scand J Work Environ Health 1986;13:9–17.

67. Woods JS, Polissar L, Severson RK, Heuser LS, Kulander BG. Soft-tissue sarcoma and non-Hodgkin's lymphoma in relation to phenoxyherbicide and chlorinated phenol exposure in Western Washington. J Natl Cancer Inst 1987;78:899–910.

68. Wiklund K, Dich J, Holm LE. Risk of malignant lymphoma in Swedish pesticide appliers. Br J Cancer 1987;56:505–508.

69. Wiklund K, Lindefors BM, Holm LE. Risk of malignant lymphoma in Swedish agricultural and forestry workers. Br J Ind Med 1988;45:19–24.

70. Casto KM. Environmental Health Law. Chapt 8 in: Blumenthal DS, ed. Introduction to environmental health. New York, NY: Springer Publishing Company, 1989:215–247.

71. Plimmer JR. Pesticide loss to the atmosphere. Am J Ind Med 1990;18:461–466.

72. Perchalski FR, Higgins JM. Pinpointing non-point pollution. Civil Engineering, February 1988:62–63.

73. Johnson CJ, Kross BC. Continuing importance of nitrate contamination of groundwater and wells in rural areas. Am J Ind Med 1990;18:449–456.

74. Comly H. Cyanosis in infants caused by nitrates in well water. JAMA 1945;129:112.

75. Johnson C, Bonrud P, Dosch T, Kilness A, Senger K, Meyer M. Fatal outcomes of methemoglobinemia in an infant. JAMA 1987;257:2796–2797.

76. Zaki MH, et al. Pesticides in ground water: the aldicarb story in Suffolk County, NY. Am J Public Health 1982;72:1391–1395.

77. Bode LE. Agricultural chemical application practices to reduce environmental contamination. Am J Ind Med 1990;18:485–489.

78. Menn JJ. Current trends and new directions in crop protection. Am J Ind Med 1990;18:499–504.

79. Fairweather V. Future shock for farmers. Civil Engineering, February 1988:78–79.

80. Environmental Protection Agency (EPA). Risk Assessment Guidance for Superfund, Vol 1. Human health evaluation manual: Part A. Interim final EPA/540/1-89-002 OERR, December 1989.

81. Saltzman S, Yaron B, eds. Pesticides in soil. New York: Van Nos Travel Reinhold Company, 1986.

82. Environmental Protection Agency (EPA). Superfund exposure assessment manual. EPA/540/1-88/001. Environmental Protection Agency, 1988.

83. Environmental Protection Agency (EPA). Pesticide root zone model. EPA/600/3-84/109. Environmental Protection Agency, 1984.

84. Environmental Protection Agency (EPA). SeSoil, A seasonal soil compartment model. EPA/68-01-6271. Environmental Protection Agency, 1987.

59

Indoor Air Quality and Human Health

John B. Sullivan, Jr., M.D.
Mark Van Ert, Ph.D., C.I.H.
Gary R. Krieger, M.D., M.P.H.

INTRODUCTION

Health effects associated with poor indoor air quality (IAQ) have increasingly become a public concern. Changing energy use strategies in the 1970s resulted in construction of buildings with improved energy efficiencies and tighter sealing to prevent energy loss. As a consequence, health complaints relating to indoor environments began to increase, and the term "tight building" or "sick building syndrome" was adopted to describe this problem (1–3). Complaints relating to the environment had previously been attributed to either poor working conditions or physical factors. It soon became apparent, however, that health complaints could also be attributed to poor ventilation, lack of fresh air exchange, or inadequate dilution of indoor contaminants. The seriousness of building-related illness became apparent in the evaluation of 182 cases of illness in members of the American Legion attending a convention in 1976 in Philadelphia where *Legionella pneumonia* resulted in 29 fatalities (3, 4). The dissemination of this bacteria from contaminated ventilation systems emphasized one role of ventilation in producing illness.

Epidemiologic studies have indicated that vague complaints relating to mucous membrane irritation and headache occurred more commonly in office environments (1, 3). It is now recognized that the sources and causes of indoor air-related health effects can be multiple as well as difficult to identify. Also, the syndrome itself is usually vague and not easily substantiated by clinical findings or clinical laboratory testing. Multiple chemical contaminants have been identified in indoor air environments but at concentrations well below regulatory action. Typically, symptoms relating to indoor air quality occur in new building environments, newly remodeled office areas, and even in home environments.

Air quality in home environments is becoming recognized as a new source of illness. Consistent with the workplace, the home has multiple sources of contamination: pesticides, environmental tobacco smoke, cleaning agents, furnishings, building products, and contamination of ventilation systems with mold or fungi. As a result, the home may not offer significant improvement in air quality.

The general sources of poor indoor air quality may be grouped into several broad categories:

1. Exposure to low concentrations of one or multiple chemicals over a prolonged period of time.
2. Exposure to one or more chemicals at a high concentration over a short or prolonged period of time.
3. Exposure to biologic agents such as molds, spores, fungi, and endotoxins.
4. Exposures to infectious agents (bacteria, viruses, rickettsial organisms, and other microbes).
5. Exposure to physical agents such as dusts and particulates.
6. Low fresh air intake (<5%) coupled with poor ventilation distribution parameters.

Diseases related to indoor air pollution include asthma, hypersensitivity reactions, pneumonitis, infections, reactive airway dysfunction, and rashes. Health problems consist of a variety of subjective complaints including headache, nausea, fatigue, mucous membrane and eye irritation, shortness of breath, and musculoskeletal pains. The relationship of the heating, air conditioning, and ventilation system (HVAC) to indoor air quality can be significant. Increases in respiratory symptoms have been traced to ventilation systems. Also, mold and fungus are well-known contaminants of ventilation systems, particularly coolers.

Despite the numerous studies performed over the last decade in relation to indoor air quality and illness arising from indoor environments, the diagnosis of building-related illness remains one of exclusion. Thus it is critical to eliminate objective sources and diseases before establishing a diagnosis of building-related illness.

EPIDEMIOLOGY OF INDOOR AIR QUALITY-RELATED HEALTH EFFECTS

Studies indicate that, depending on age, up to 90% of human activity is spent indoors, with most of this time spent in the home environment versus the work environment (1, 3, 5). Consequently, health effects due to poor indoor air quality are difficult to study. Due to the simultaneous increase in building efficiency and decrease in energy costs, reduced amounts of fresh air are introduced into HVAC systems. Consequently, indoor air receives less fresh air for dilution of indoor air contaminants, which tend to concentrate over time.

Studies of volatile organic hydrocarbons in indoor air environments indicate that they are very low in concentration, usually in parts per billion, but may become more concentrated than in a typical outdoor environment. Characterization of the quantity and types of indoor air chemical contaminants has been undertaken using gas chromatography-mass spectrometry in an effort to better understand the kinds of chemicals to which humans are clinically exposed. Emission sources of these pollutants include interior furnishings such as carpets and fabrics, renovations, building materials, and human sources. Another source of pollution is from the external environment such as pollen, mold, dust, chemical odors, and vapors which may be transferred indoors.

Thermal comfort, temperature, humidity, and air movement factors play a large role in health and perceptions of health in work and home environments. The majority of subjective health complaints associated with poor IAQ have been attributed to

Table 59.1. Symptoms Commonly Expressed in Building-Related Illness

Irritation
   Ocular, nose and throat irritation
   Drying of mucous membranes
   Drying of skin
   Rashes
   Sinus congestion
Respiratory symptoms
   Cough
   Wheezing
   Hoarseness
   Difficult breathing
   Chest tightness
Other symptoms
   Fatigue
   Nausea
   Abdominal pain
   Dizziness
   Myalgia
   Headache
   Lethargy
   Difficulty concentrating
Odors—The identification of certain odors adds to the psychogenic
   factors for investigation and remediation of indoor air pollution

temperature, humidity, fresh air, and air flow factors. This observation may explain the relatively high prevalence of perceived problems associated with IAQ. Studies consistently show that between 20% and 35% of office workers perceive indoor air quality problems in their work environment (1, 3, 5).

Decline in worker productivity can occur as a result of poor air quality. Savings of energy and operation of buildings in terms of cost have to be balanced by loss of worker productivity in terms of the individuals who experience adverse health effects (6). Future developments relating to indoor air quality can be predicted (7):

1. Energy is going to be more costly.
2. Buildings will have increased numbers of occupants.
3. Building materials will be manufactured from synthetic materials rather than natural materials.
4. The time spent in mechanically ventilated buildings will continue to increase.
5. There will be diminishing individual control of personal microenvironments in the workplace.

Given the fact that the individuals will continue to breathe higher volumes of air from the indoor rather than the outdoor environment, the presence of indoor air pollutants may constitute an important longterm chemical exposure risk. Comprehensive assessments of health effects from chemicals in the environment have been investigated using a total exposure assessment methodology (TEAM) (7). This methodology has been undertaken in particular reference to benzene and leukemia occurrence in the United States (7). Due to the fact that the total dose of benzene inhaled is much greater indoors than outdoors over the period of a person's life, the TEAM study attempted to calculate the attributable incidence of leukemia resulting from this longterm exposure. This and other similar studies indicate that the respirable concentration of chemicals in the indoor environment can be excessive over the lifetime of a person.

Symptoms typically associated with indoor air pollution (Table 59.1) are found with a 10–20% background rate in any

population of people (7, 8). This underscores the difficulty in attempting to attribute vague feelings of illness to specific indoor environments. Typically, the symptoms of building-related illness occur within the work environment, abate upon leaving that office environment, and return upon re-entry to the environment. It is also very unusual to find one particular chemical or pollutant that would be causative of these symptoms. In multiple investigations, the National Institute for Occupational Safety and Health (NIOSH) found that inadequate ventilation was the most common cause identified for indoor air pollution (7, 9). Alteration of ventilation with the introduction of more fresh air alleviated symptoms in many of these cases. This observation suggests that chemical pollutants, which may have become concentrated, are then diluted beyond irritant levels by introduction of fresh air. An inadequate supply of fresh air alone, as well as poor air distribution within a building environment, may be sufficient to induce symptomatology. Since occupants in most modern buildings with centralized air conditioning have no direct control over the ventilation and fresh air content, changing ventilation to suit individual needs is difficult, if not impossible.

In contrast to the industrial or occupational environment, residential environments allow significant personal control of thermal comfort factors as well as ventilation. This sense of personal empowerment may be an important psychologic factor that explains the observation of workplace symptom exacerbation followed by home environment improvement. Revisions of the American Society of Heating, Refrigeration, and Air Conditioning Engineers (ASHRAE) ventilation standard 82–1989 are an attempt to deal with current and future needs of building designers, architects, engineers, and building owners and operators with regard to thermal and ventilation comfort and general indoor air quality in the environment (10).

PRIVATE DWELLINGS AND INDOOR AIR QUALITY

Since people spend most of their time at home, the quality of home indoor air is as important as the work environment (11). The spraying of pesticides, smoking, the use of fabricated materials containing a variety of volatile hydrocarbons such as formaldehyde, benzene, toluene, and xylene, and the use of many plastics and foams within the home can all contribute to a low-level chemical environment in which we dwell for most of our lives. Since the 1980s, houses and individual dwellings have become more energy efficient (11). Estimations are that 85% of the new homes built annually, of which there are more than 1.5 million, have better insulation, better vapor barriers, and less air exchange than older homes (11). Health issues include the use of mercurical-containing fungicides in latex paint, the presence of radon, asbestos lining and insulation of furnaces and pipes prior to 1980, the use of various pesticides as termiticides, the general application of indoor and outdoor pesticides, and the use of urea formaldehyde foam insulation. All have played a role in producing health concerns in home environments.

In 1985, public concern over radon gas emissions into homes began to peak (12). Radon gas is a naturally occurring indoor air pollutant, and unsafe air concentrations can occur in houses built over naturally occurring uranium deposits. The association of home air contamination with radon has been blamed for excess lung cancer and has resulted in litigation (12).

The home environment is not regulated by any governmental body, and large numbers of hazardous chemicals are used yearly

Table 59.2. Organic Compounds Found in Indoor Home Environments

Paradichlorobenzene
1,1,1-Trichloroethane
Chloroform
Trichloroethylene
Tetrachloroethylene
Formaldehyde
Carbon tetrachloride
Benzene
Styrene
Methylene chloride
Xylene
Chlordane
Toluene

Adapted with permission from Spengler JD. Shelter for the twenty-first century. Environ Health Perspect 1990;86:281–284.

and disposed of from the home. These chemicals include pesticides, solvents, oils, gasoline, cleaning chemicals, and plastics as well as other solid and liquid wastes. Calculated cancer risks for airborne chemicals have been demonstrated to be higher for indoor home environments than for many hazardous waste sites (11). Multiple chemicals have been identified in indoor air of the home environment (Table 59.2) (11, 13). Individuals and families are thus chronically exposed to these types of chemicals in low concentrations.

Sources of indoor air pollutants in the home that emit hydrocarbon vapors include deodorizers, pesticide sprays, adhesive materials, cosmetics, insulation, fabrics, pressed wood, paints, paint removers, cleaners, cigarette smoke, and other sources of combustion, gasoline, plastics, carpets, furniture, and a variety of other chemical products (11, 13). Tobacco smoke, a common indoor pollutant, contains multiple chemicals that can concentrate in and contaminate the home environment. Environmental tobacco smoke contributes high concentrations of carbon monoxide, formaldehyde, acrolein, benzene, and other potentially harmful chemicals to the indoor arena (Table 59.3).

Residential waste water has been shown to have contaminants of similar chemicals discharged from the home environment (11). It is an established fact that the use of many compounds that are considered hazardous are released from the home environment into waste water (Table 59.4) (11). One survey result showed that improper waste disposal from homes was common (14). Four percent of hazardous waste generated in the state of Massachusetts come from home environments (14). Commonly disposed of chemicals in this survey were motor oils (8.8 million quarts annually), pesticides, paints, radiator fluids (ethylene glycol and methanol), batteries, asphalt, herbicides, solvents, and gasoline (14). These wastes were disposed of in the ground, sewers, or landfills. Due to absence of regulations and the inability to enforce regulations for such small generators, the disposal of home hazardous wastes will continue to contaminate groundwater and soil and be a major contributor to environmental pollution.

EVALUATING IAQ-RELATED HEALTH PROBLEMS

Background Information

The evaluation of indoor air quality-related illness should proceed in a systematic fashion. The objectives of the investigation

are to gather information about the building, identify signs and symptoms, locate and identify causes, audit the building site, determine work-relatedness of any illness, and remediate the cause, if possible (Table 59.5). Ideally, the investigating team should consist of individuals with expertise in industrial hygiene, occupational and environmental health, toxicology, epidemiology, ventilation engineering, construction, and building maintenance. The consulting team should have one identified leader who interfaces with the management and employees. It is essential that clear communication channels be established early to avoid rumor and mixed messages among the triad of management, employees, and investigators. In the event that the business being investigated is located in a rental space, the building owners should also be involved in all phases of the investigation. An organized approach to investigating indoor air quality-related illness is essential to avoid errors of both omission and commission (8, 15, 16). Anxiety and fears of building occupants can actually be exacerbated by the investigation; thus, a proper approach should begin by informing employees in an objective and sensitive manner that an investigation will occur. The employees should be informed that they will participate in this investigation by helping supply data to the investigators. Employees should be informed about the investigation team, that health questionnaires or interviews will be included, and that a building inspection will occur. The anxieties and fears that arise from unknown health risks can be ameliorated to some degree by the initial approach or can be heightened. The sophistication and ability of the investigators to interact with employees will help establish the credibility required to successfully carry out the investigation. Depending on the nature of the company and the sophistication of the workers, the IAQ investigation can be positively or negatively facilitated. Problems with indoor air quality can occasionally create tension and opposition between management and employees. The consultants must be aware that investigations can be interpreted differently by employees.

Schools can be particularly difficult to investigate due to certain unique features. The consultants must effectively interface with administration, teachers, and students, as well as addressing concerns of the family. IAQ problems can create anxieties and fears of longterm health consequences.

Interviews should be conducted privately in all cases in order to establish employee views on the problems and causes. No matter what type of business is involved, it is critical that the investigating consultants maintain objectivity, establish rapport with workers, maintain confidentiality regarding health issues, and be credible to all involved.

Health Audit

Since symptoms associated with indoor air quality problems are vague, identifying the cause of the problem can be difficult. A questionnaire is useful in determining the health status of employees and can help identify individuals who are manifesting symptoms associated with poor indoor quality. The questionnaire should include location of the employee in the worksite, dates the employee experienced illness, whether or not smoking is allowed, presence or absence of allergic conditions, and location where employees experience symptoms. The questionnaire should also help discern psychogenic illness from real illness in the workplace. After employees complete the questionnaire, symptoms can be tabulated so the actual incidence and prevalence of illness can be determined and the

Table 59.3. Major Constituents of the Vapor Phase of the Mainstream Smoke of Nonfilter Cigarettes

Compound	Concentration/cigarette
Nitrogen	280–320 mg (56–64%)
Oxygen	50–70 mg (11–14%)
Carbon dioxide	45–65 mg (9–13%)
Carbon monoxide	14–23 mg (2.8–4.6%)
Water	7–12 mg (1.4–2.4%)
Argon	5 mg (1.0%)
Hydrogen	0.5–1.0 mg
Ammonia	10–130 μg
Nitrogen oxides (NO)	100–600 μg
Hydrogen cyanide	400–500 μg
Hydrogen sulfide	20–90 μg
Methane	1.0–2.0 mg
Volatile alkanes	1.0–1.6 mg
Volatile alkenes	0.4–0.5 mg
Isoprene	0.2–0.4 mg
Butadiene	25–40 μg
Acetylene	20–35 μg
Benzene	12–50 μg
Toluene	20–60 μg
Styrene	10 μg
Volatile aromatic hydrocarbons	15–30 μg
Formic acid	200–600 μg
Acetic acid	100–1700 μg
Propionic acid	100–300 μg
Methyl formate	20–30 μg
Volatile acids	5–10 μg
Formaldehyde	20–100 μg
Acetaldehyde	400–1400 μg
Acrolein	60–140 μg
Volatile aldehydes	80–140 μg
Acetone	100–650 μg
Volatile ketones	50–100 μg
Methanol	80–180 μg
Volatile alcohols	10–30 μg
Acetonitrile	100–150 μg
Volatile nitriles	50–80 μg
Furan	20–40 μg
Volatile furans	45–125 μg
Pyridine	20–200 μg
Picolines	15–80 μg
3-Vinylpyridine	10–30 μg
Volatile pyridines	20–50 μg
Pyrrole	0.1–10 μg
Pyrrolidine	10–18 μg
N-Methylpyrrolidine	2.0–3.0 μg
Volatile pyrazines	3.0–8.0 μg
Methylamine	4–10 μg
Aliphatic amines	3–10 μg
Nicotine	1000–3000 μg
Nornicotine	40–150 μg
Anatabine	5–15 μg
Anabasine	5–12 μg
Tobacco alkaloids	NA
Bipyridyls	10–30 μg
n-Hentriacontane (n-$C_{31}H_{64}$)	100 μg
Total nonvolatile hydrocarbons	300–400 μg
Naphthalenes	3–6 μg
Phenanthrenes	0.2–0.4 μg
Anthracenes	0.05–0.1 μg
Fluorenes	0.6–1.0 μg
Pyrenes	0.3–0.5 μg
Fluoranthenes	0.3–0.45 μg

continues

Table 59.3. *Continued*

Compound	Concentration/cigarette (μg)
Carcinogenic polynuclear aromatic hydrocarbons	0.1–0.25
Phenol	80–160
Other phenols	60–180
Catechol	200–400
Other catechols	100–200
Other dihydroxybenzenes	200–400
Scopoletin	15–30
Other polyphenols	NA
Cyclotenes	40–70
Quinones	0.5
Solanesol	600–1000
Neophytadienes	200–350
Limonene	30–60
Other terpenes (200–250)	
Palmitic acid	100–150
Stearic acid	50–75
Oleic acid	40–110
Linoleic acid	60–150
Linolenic acid	150–250
Lactic acid	60–80
Indole	10–15
Skatole	12–16
Other indoles	
Quinolines	2–4
Other N-heterocyclic hydrocarbons	NA
Benzofurans	200–300
Other O-heterocyclic hydrocarbons	NA
Stigmasterol	40–70
Sitosterol	30–40
Campesterol	20–30
Cholesterol	10–20
Aniline	0.36
Toluidines	0.23
Other aromatic amines	0.25
Tobacco-specific N-nitrosamines	0.34–2.7
Glycerol	120

Reprinted from: US Dept. HHS. Reducing the health consequences of smoking. Rockville, MD: Centers for Disease Control, 1989.

location associated with symptoms identified. An example of a general health questionnaire is presented in Appendix A.

Symptoms of building-related illnesses include complaints of headache, fatigue and drowsiness, sore throat, nasal or sinus

Table 59.4. Common Organic Compounds Found in Residential Waste Water

Phenol
Naphthalene
Diethylphthalate
Di-N-butylphthalate
Butyl benzyl phthalate
Methylene chloride
Chloroform
Trichloroethylene
Tetrachloroethylene
Benzene
Ethyl benzene
Toluene

Adapted with permission from Spengler JD. Shelter for the twenty-first century. Environ Health Perspect 1990;86:281–284.

Table 59.5. Indoor Air Quality Evaluation Checklist

I. Building survey and environmental audit
1. Building design and age
2. Building location
3. Building materials: exterior, mortar, flooring, ceilings, interior walls
4. Interior furnishings: furniture, carpets, drapes, fabrics
5. Interior finishing, paints, coatings, plastics
6. HVAC: Location of intake and exhaust vents, coolers, last cleaning date, filters
7. Recent renovations and changes to building
8. Windows: Can they be opened and are they opened? Location of windows
9. Movement of air mass when windows are opened

II. Interviews and health questionnaire
1. Health survey and identification of ill workers
2. Location of ill workers
3. Location of workers relative to building alterations
4. Identification of asthmatics and allergic individuals
5. Description of syndrome
6. Occurrence of syndrome relative to season
7. Occurrence of syndrome relative to HVAC

III. Pollution source identification
1. Chemicals
2. Volatiles, vapors, and semivolatile chemicals
3. Cleaning agents
4. Particulates, metals, dusts
5. Biologics: mold, endotoxin, bacteria
6. Inorganics
7. Processes and reactions that produce pollutants
8. CO and CO_2
9. Tobacco use
10. Physical sources and thermal comfort factors (lighting, air flow, noise, humidity, temperature)
11. Outside environmental sources (dust, odors, molds)
12. Appropriate environmental monitoring

IV. Medical evaluation of employees
1. Health evaluation
2. Evaluation of signs and symptoms related to organ system
3. Pulmonary functions if indicated
4. Other studies as indicated

V. Remediation
1. HVAC alterations and cleaning
2. Engineering and technical controls
3. Decontamination
4. Removal of source
5. Alteration of work habits
6. Moving workers
7. Control external sources
8. Control psychogenesis

congestion, nausea, dizziness, sneezing, eye irritation, and chest tightness (8, 15, 16). Identifying the prevalence rate of affected employees in the workplace can help determine whether there is an excessive number of complaints related to a possible indoor air pollution cause. If more than 20% of a workforce have health complaints or discomfort from IAQ, then an investigation is necessary to attempt to establish a cause and take corrective action (16). However, since many individuals at a variety of times manifest a number of these vague complaints, it can be difficult to derive a true prevalence rate for indoor air pollution-related illness.

Building Inspection and Site Visit

In conjunction with the background work, interviews, and health questionnaire evaluations, the investigators should perform a site survey of the building. This site audit may lead to more in-depth environmental and evaluation of the building and medical evaluation of affected workers. The building survey should be conducted by a qualified environmental specialist such as an industrial hygienist, with other members of the investigation team, management, and an employee representative involved (16).

Indoor air, either in a work environment or individual home environment, has been shown to contain air contaminants up to 20 or more times higher than that of outdoor air. Investigations have demonstrated an increased number of complaints in air-conditioned sites versus naturally ventilated sites. Identifying the source, or sources, of poor air quality can require extensive investigation including environmental monitoring for pollutants. In general, the following should be included in the evaluation of air quality problems in the site visit and initial building inspection:

1. Building materials and age of building.
2. Location of building with respect to surrounding sources of contamination.
3. Activities in the building.
4. Heating, ventilation, and air conditioning systems functioning, operation, filters, maintenance, and condition.
5. Adequacy of fresh air supply.
6. Number of occupants in affected areas.
7. Building maintenance and cleaning.
8. Interior fabrics, drapes, carpets, and other items.
9. Presence of environmental tobacco smoke.
10. Characterization and inspection of HVAC system including humidification, location of ventilation ducts (exhaust and intake), movement of air, and air exchange.
11. Window locations and window openings.
12. Outdoor environmental sources of pollution near ventilation intakes.
13. Stagnant air and poor areas of air movement.
14. Physical factors such as thermal comfort, lighting, noise, and humidity.
15. Dust and dirt on floors, desks, and in ventilation system.
16. Microbial and dust contamination of ventilation system coolers and/or ducts.
17. Chemicals used in the environment.
18. Location of copying machines and other equipment.
19. Renovations and building changes.
20. Changes to the immediate outdoor environment.
21. Location of outdoor air intake vents.

Upon concluding the building inspection, the investigators should provide a preliminary assessment of their findings, recommendations for changes, and recommendations for any further evaluations and monitoring. Easily identified causes of health complaints should be addressed immediately.

Known Causes of Building-Related Illness

Some diseases and health problems can be directly traced to indoor sources or directly attributable to certain indoor environments. Most of these illnesses are related to microbiologic sources or to known chemical contaminants:

1. **Commonly recognized chemical sources** — There are several chemical sources that have been identified as causes of IAQ-related health effects. The use of tobacco indoors or other combustion is a source of carbon monoxide, acrolein, formaldehyde, and many other chemicals and particulates.

Carbon monoxide can produce headaches, fatigue, nausea, and vomiting. Carbon monoxide can also arise from other combustion sources outdoors and be brought inside through a ventilation intake system. Formaldehyde is another common chemical contaminant that occurs in the air of both residential environments as well as work environments. Formaldehyde is a component of tobacco smoke as well as wood composites and insulation. The latest Occupational Safety and Health Administration (OSHA) TWA (time-weighted average) standard regulating airborne concentrations of formaldehyde has been decreased to 1 ppm. However, investigations suggest that health-related complaints are associated with formaldehyde concentrations much less than 1 ppm. Acrolein, an aldehyde that arises as a product of incomplete combustion, is a strong eye, skin, and mucous irritant. The use of carbonless copy paper has been associated with mucous membrane irritation and dermatitis, as well as contact urticaria. Detergents, alkaline solutions, or acidic solutions and cleansing agents can leave residues in carpets as well as on large surfaces that may result in irritation to eyes, airway, and skin. Over time, these residues can accumulate in the environment and produce symptoms. Sealants on floors can also be mucous membrane irritants. The application of pesticides in home environments as well as in commercial environments may contribute to symptoms. The solvent diluent of the pesticide may be the main agent contributing to such illness, not the pesticide itself.

2. **Hypersensitivity diseases and aeroallergens** — Hypersensitivity pneumonitis is a known entity consisting of fever, cough, chest tightness, fatigue, and pulmonary infiltrates (8, 17, 18). Hypersensitivity pneumonitis may occur after inhalation of a variety of organic materials such as thermophilic actinomycetes. Most cases of hypersensitivity pneumonitis result from frequent exposures to organic dust, endotoxins, or to aerosols from cooling or heating systems that are contaminated with microorganisms (8, 17, 18). A variety of microbiologic organisms and aeroallergens can be isolated from air cooling and other ventilation systems in buildings or home environments (Table 59.6) (18–20). Evaporative coolers, commonly used in hot and dry climates, can be a source of airborne fungi such as *Alternaria, Aspergillus, Cladisporium, Fusarium*, and *Penicillium* (19) (Table 59.7). Specific microbial sources implicating a single source for hypersensitivity pneumonitis may be impossible to identify. Another disease entity, termed humidifier fever (4), is characterized by fever, chills, myalgias, and malaise with absence of pulmonary symptoms (3, 8). Symptoms arise within 4–8 hours following exposure and generally abate within 24 hours.

Asthma or wheezing related to a building environment is also not uncommon. Also, other symptoms and signs of allergic manifestation such as rhinorrhea, sneezing, and ocular irritation can be associated with contaminated building environments. The majority of hypersensitivity diseases can be related to individual susceptibility to allergens in the environment. Following sensitization, an allergic reaction to extremely low concentrations of the antigenic material can recur (3, 8, 18, 19). The vast majority of allergens which produce hypersensitivity diseases within indoor environments are biologic in origin such as mold, fungi, endotoxins, and bacteria. Pulmonary function tests of individuals susceptible to such allergens may not be abnormal. Disease and symptoms may abate once the individual has left the

Table 59.6. Volatile Organic Compounds Found Indoors

Aliphatics	Halogenated hydrocarbons
Cyclohexane	Chloroform
Decane	Dichlorobenzenes
Dodecane	Dichloromethane
2,4-Dimethylhexane	Tetrachloroethylene
1,3-Dimethylcyclopentane	1,1,1-Trichloroethane
Eicosane	Trichloroethylene
Heptane	Trichlorofluoromethane
Hexane	
Methylcyclohexane	Alcohols
4-Methyldecane	2-Butyloctanol
2-Methylheptane	1-Dodecanol
2-Methylhexane	2-Ethyl-1-hexanol
3-Methylhexane	1-Hexanol
3-Methylnonane	Phenol
2-Methylpentane	
Nonane	Esters and Ketones
Octane	Ethyl acetate
Pentadecane	1-Hexyl butanoate
Pentane	Acetone
Tetradecane	Methylethyl ketone
Undecane	3-Methyl-3-butanone
1-Octane	4-Methyl-2-pentanone
1-Decene	
4-Phenylcyclohexene	Terpenes
	Pinene
Aldehydes	Limonene
Decanal	Carene
Nonanal	
Formaldehyde	Miscellaneous
Acetaldehyde	Acetic acid
N-Pentanol	Dimethylphenols
N-Hexanol	
Aromatic hydrocarbons	
Benzene	
Diethylbenzene	
Dimethylethylbenzene	
Ethylbenzene	
Ethylmethylbenzene	
Methylnaphthalene	
1-Propylbenzene	
Naphthalene	
Propylmethylbenzene	
Styrene	
Toluene	
Trimethylbenzenes	
Xylenes	
Chlorobenzene	

environment. One study identified 16 genera of fungi, of which 80% were of respirable size (20). The fungi, *Cladosporium* and *Aspergillus*, made up 75% of respirable particulates of fungi found in this study (20).

3. **Infections** — Infections secondary to building sites became recognized with the advent of Legionnaire's disease in 1976. This disease was traced to aerosolization of bacteria from cooling towers, humidifiers, and evaporative condensers within buildings. The incubation period for *Legionella pneumonia* is 5–6 days (3, 8, 21). The Legionella organism is present in soils, and its dissemination from ventilation and cooling systems can be controlled by using a biocide in the cooling system. Another disease associated with the Legionella bacterium is Pontiac fever. This disease was described in an epidemic of 144 cases in Michigan in 1968

Table 59.7. Mold Commonly Found in Ventilation Systems and Indoor Environments

Cladosporium
Penicillium species
Nonsporulating mycelia
Alternaria
Streptomyces
Epicoccum
Aspergillus species
Aureobasidium
Helminthosporium
Cephalosporium
Acremonium
Fusarium
Botrytis
Aspergillus niger
Rhizopus
Rhodotorula
Beauvera
Chaetomium
Scopulariopsis
Mucor
Curvularia
Rhinocladiella
Verticillllium
Plenozythia
Pithomyces
Zygosporium
Paecilomyces
Stachybotrys
Aspergillus fumigatus
Nigrospora
Stysanus
Leptosphaerulina
Botryosporium
Trichoderma
Chrysosporium
Phoma
Sporobolomyces
Trichothecium
Ulocladium
Yeast
Geotrichum

Adapted with permission from Kozak PP, Gallup J, Cummins LH, Gillman SA. Currently available methods for time mold surveys. II. Examples of problem homes surveyed. Ann Allergy 1980;45:167–176.

(3, 8, 17, 21). Other agents of infection which can be transmitted within indoor air environments include a variety of viruses, bacteria, fungi, and rickettsial organisms (21). The rickettsia *Coxiella burnetii*, which causes Q fever, has been discovered in ventilation systems in proximity to where infected sheep, goats, or other animals are housed. Q fever can be manifested as fever, chills, headache, myalgias, pneumonia, hepatitis, and occasionally endocarditis (21). A variety of other febrile and coryzal-related illnesses can be associated with recirculation of stale air or contaminated air. Outbreaks of febrile illness related to indoor environments have been documented in a variety of studies. An outbreak of febrile illness in Knoxville, Tennessee, in 1981 involved 40% of 325 office workers in a seven-story building (17). The individuals manifested headaches, myalgias, fever, chills, cough, or wheezing. A temporal relationship was observed between starting the HVAC system and the onset of the symptoms in these individuals. Another illness in 1982 was identified in Washington, DC, in the occupants

of a large office building (17). Twelve of 41 employees manifested headache, myalgia, chest tightness, fever, chills, or nausea occurring within the work environment, with relief on weekends (17). Numerous microorganisms were isolated from the HVAC system. Hypersensitivity pneumonitis, humidifier fever, and other allergic manifestations of disease which have included symptoms of fever, chills, myalgias, and headache have been identified since the 1970s. Most of these outbreaks have been attributed to thermophilic actinomycetes, a variety of fungi, and endotoxins. Sources of the microbial contamination were mainly contaminated ventilation systems and air-handling units.

4. **Thermal factors and physical factors** — Physical factors in the environment can have a great impact on illness and perceptions of illness.

   Temperature: Thermal comfort has a profound impact on the perception of health. A temperature range of 68–79°F (20–26°C) is thought to be an acceptable thermal comfort range, depending on activity, clothing, and relative humidity. Temperatures that exceed this range may help to increase the outgassing of volatile organic compounds from building materials and furnishings present in the environment. Attempts should be made to keep temperatures in the lower portion of the temperature range. Reduction in mental performance has been observed at temperatures that exceed these. *Humidity*: There is no agreement on the ideal range of relative humidity. Relative humidity values exceeding 70% are often associated with microbial growth and contamination of ventilation systems. In environments in which the relative humidity is below 20%, individuals will experience drying of mucous membranes and skin. Dermatitis has been associated with warm, dry environments. The Environmental Protection Agency (EPA) currently suggests a humidity range of 45–50%. American Society of Heating, Refrigeration, Air Conditioning Engineers (ASHRAE) recommends that relative humidity be kept below 60%. *Artificial lighting*: Visual stress such as inappropriate levels of lighting, inadequate contrast, and excessive glare all contribute to the development of eye irritation and headaches in the environment. Adjustment of ventilation rates as well as ultraviolet illumination has been reported to reduce ocular symptoms in people experiencing eye irritation. *Vibration and noise*: Health effects or physical complaints can also be related to vibration and noise in the environment. Not only the level of the noise, but the nature of the noise itself is important in producing some physical symptoms. Infrasound (0.1–20 Hz) has been known to cause dizziness and nausea, but usually only in levels above 120 decibels. It is probable that low frequency noise between 20 and 100 Hz which is commonly found in buildings containing industrial, heating, ventilation, and air conditioning equipment can also produce physical problems.

Ventilation and IAQ

Between 1971 and 1988, NIOSH conducted 529 investigations of indoor air quality problems. The overwhelming majority of these evaluations were conducted in response to worker symptoms or illnesses which were thought to be related to the building environment in which the people were working.

A summary of the type of problems and their approximate frequency observed in these investigations is as follows:

1. Inadequate ventilation (52%)

2. Inside contamination (17%)
3. Outside contamination (11%)
4. Microbiologic contamination (5%)
5. Building fabric (3%)
6. Unknown (12%)

Significantly, since 1983 and through 1986, the relative percentages associated with each problem have not substantially changed. Thus, in situations in which there is widespread reporting of nonspecific symptoms, no documented specific sources of external environmental contamination, and extremely low concentrations found with specific environmental monitoring, investigations have usually concluded that inadequate building ventilation is the cause of the employee's complaints. Insufficient information on the health effects of low level pollutants, however, may lead to conclusions that ventilation rather than chemical agents themselves are responsible for reported problems. Improved ventilation, nonetheless, dilutes such contaminants and often alleviates symptoms.

Since 1979, for energy conservation reasons, the amount of fresh air being introduced into the office environment has been limited. The amount of fresh air introduced into the office environment can be quite variable; seasonal cooling or heating requirements often lead to intermittent reduction of fresh air through the building ventilation system. Design modifications to the office environment made after construction may interfere with fresh air distribution and can generate microenvironments of inadequate air flow.

Separately, investigators from NIOSH and the U.S. Center for Disease Control (CDC)—Center for Environmental Health (CEH) have pointed out three interlocking areas of problems associated with building investigations:

1. Inadequacy of initial HVAC assessment methods.
2. Inadequacy of variability or epidemiological and medical studies.
3. Inadequacy of follow-up measures after changes are made in the HVAC system.

It has been repeatedly noted that symptoms can be generated by the buildup of low concentrations of multiple "natural" building contaminants, including off-gasing from building materials, emissions from office machinery, and solvents and other chemicals used in the office work and building maintenance. This synergy of low level multiple pollutants is accentuated by the suboptimally performing HVAC system.

Ventilation systems have traditionally been designed to provide odor control and thermal comfort under the assumption that the air in a building is perfectly mixed. Increasing experience demonstrates that nonuniform mixing is common and that the task of predicting pollution transport produced by the ventilation systems is not simple. Currently, in the United States building ventilation adequacy is measured and compared with ASHRAE guidelines. These guidelines (ASHRAE 62–1981, 55–1981) recommend a minimum of 5 cubic feet per minute (cfm) (0.14 M^3/min) of outdoor air per person in an office area to prevent excessive buildup of CO_2 (22). The recommended minimum was increased to 20 cfm (0.56 m^3/min) if smoking was permitted in the office. More recent ASHRAE guidelines (62–1989) have employed a 20-cfm figure for the general office environment. Carbon dioxide concentrations should remain below 0.5% to prevent headaches and loss of judgment, although the industrial standard for nuclear submarines is 1%. The 5 cfm/person should maintain CO_2 level sat 0.25% when outside

CO_2 levels are about 0.03% (22). If indoor CO_2 concentrations are more than 1000 ppm (3–4 times the outside level), however, there is probably a problem of inadequate ventilation, and complaints such as headache, fatigue, and eye and throat irritation are frequently prevalent. There are also standards set for a few specific pollutants to some extent, based on industrial standards. Unfortunately, there is no specific pollutant standard and no satisfactory measurement for cigarette smoke, the major office pollutant. Considering off-gassing from new plastics, paneling, particle board, and floor glues, new buildings should probably be ventilated at the smoking-permitted rate for the first 2 years.

The anticipated CO_2 levels in a building at various ventilation rates and various outside CO_2 levels can be calculated by the following equation:

$$CO_2 \text{ (inspired)} = [CO_2 \text{ (outdoor)} + (N \times 100)/cfm \times 60)]$$

Where N = generation of CO_2 = 0.63 cu ft/hr/person, this formula rearranges to (22):

$$cfm = \frac{1.05}{CO_2 \text{ (inspired)} - CO_2 \text{ (outdoor)}}$$

This calculation assumes sufficient time for the building to reach a steady state. The rate of CO_2 production is dependent on the number of people present rather than the size of the room, and the ventilation standard is also stated in terms of the number of people present. The room size will not affect CO_2 levels present in the steady state, only the length of time it takes to reach the steady state (22).

Using this formula, a ventilation rate of 5 cfm/person should allow the CO_2 in the building to rise to 0.21 volume % above outside CO_2 levels. A ventilation rate of 20 cfm/person will only allow the CO_2 levels to rise about 0.05 volume % (22).

One cannot directly relate CO_2 levels to ventilation rate in cfm. In evaluating a building, it may be easier to determine air changes per hour (ach) with outside air than to determine the volume of outside air being introduced into the system. Actual occupancy figures and volume figures can be used in determining air changes per hour necessary to meet the standard. When the actual occupancy is not known, ASHRAE suggests using seven occupants per 1000 square feet (93 m^2) for the occupancy figure. Assuming the office ceilings are about 10 feet (3 m) (a fairly standard figure), this amounts to seven persons per 10,000 cubic feet (280 m^3) of office space (10 feet × 1000 square feet). If smoking is permitted, for seven occupants there should be 8400 cu ft/hr of outdoor air (7 × 20 cfm × 60 min/hr). This amounts to 0.84 air changes per hour (ach) (8400/10,000 cubic feet). The corresponding figures if there is no smoking are: for seven occupants, 2100 cu ft/hr (59 m^3) of outdoor air (7 × 5 cfm × 60 min/hr); and 0.21 ach (2,100/10,000 cubic feet) (22).

Since problems related to ventilation are responsible for 50–60% of IAQ problems, altering and adjustments in ventilation can result in improvement or resolution of symptoms. The volume of fresh air should be increased if possible. Sometimes decreasing the occupancy numbers will be helpful. Smoking should be eliminated totally. Local exhaust ventilation may also serve to reduce a pollutant source.

Inadequate outside air intake can be assessed by measuring the rise in carbon dioxide (CO_2) levels in the building over the day and subsequent fall in the evening with the building unoccupied but the ventilating system running at daytime levels. Low range detector tubes are available which can give a reading for outside air to use as a baseline. It is assumed that, if the outside air intake is sufficient to adequately manage CO_2, other contaminants will be managed also. If windows are opened routinely or the rooms served by the ventilation system are usually unoccupied, this method of monitoring will not work. Also, it is important to remember that people can tolerate CO_2 levels nearly 10 times the concentration typically found in a building (22). If it appears appropriate, CO_2 can also be monitored using low range detector tubes to help assess the effect of combustion in the building, or other combustion or traffic sources close to air intakes (22).

Temperature and humidity should also be checked, and, if necessary, air flow at vents and return air grills. Although wet bulb, dry bulb thermometers can be used, that degree of accuracy is generally unnecessary (22). A desk thermometer and relative humidity meter should be adequate. Measurements for air flow assure that a vent is functioning and indicate if the airflow is directed in a suitable direction (22). In general, exact measurements of these parameters are less critical except in special circumstances (22).

These guidelines are based on whole building analysis rather than an analysis of the spatial distribution of the building's ventilation. Pollutant transport depends, in general, upon building geometry, pollutant source characteristics, and thermo/fluid boundary conditions such as flow rate, thermal stratification, duct location, and diffuser type (22). If the air in the room is well-mixed, then the concentration can be predicted based on knowledge of the room ventilation rate, the pollutant source strength, and the concentration in the supply air. In situations where the well-mixed assumption does not apply, knowledge of local concentration distributions is required to determine average ventilation system performance. Even if an acceptable average room concentration can be achieved at a given ventilation rate, the sensitivity of concentration to flow nonuniformities can produce localized areas with acceptably high concentration levels. As a result, a detailed knowledge of source strengths and local ventilation system performance is required to ensure that the ventilation system provides pollutant control at reasonable ventilation rates (22).

To properly evaluate indoor air problems, it is necessary to have some basic knowledge of ventilation. Since buildings are not constructed to contain air pressures significantly different from outside pressures, to move air into a building it is necessary to move air out of the building, and vice versa. If there is a system imbalance in a building it may be noticeable when outside doors or windows are opened, resulting in a rush of air either into (excessive exhaust or insufficient intake) or out of (insufficient exhaust or excessive intake) the building. However, with the slight pressure difference between inside and outside, only as much air will enter the building as is able to leave the building (22).

Volatile Organic Chemicals (VOC) and IAQ

One of the more interesting aspects of indoor air contamination has been the discovery of large numbers of volatile organic chemicals in indoor environments (Table 59.6) (23–27). The source of these chemicals can be attributed to building materials, plastics, carpet, adhesives, wallpaper, insulating materials, sealants, and cleaning materials. These organic chemicals have been identified in indoor air at very low concentrations using gas chromatography-mass spectrometry (GCMS).

Whether these chemicals are the cause of building-related illness must be determined by proper investigation, since they are usually present in concentrations in the low parts per million or parts per billion range. The concentration of these and other chemicals can be much higher in new or refurbished buildings or residences. Buildings with new carpeting and new furnishings will present fingerprints of volatile organic chemicals (VOCs) at much higher concentrations than older buildings without new pollutant sources. However, the concentration of volatile organic compounds found in such indoor environments are usually well below any OSHA standards established for the work environment (23–27).

Chemicals profiled in such studies can produce symptoms typical of these associated with other building-related illnesses. Interestingly, there are often no health problems prior to the renovation activity. Volatile organic chemicals commonly found outgassing in indoor environments can be grouped as follows (23):

1. Alkanes
2. Alkenes
3. Aromatics
4. Aldehydes
5. Ketones
6. Esters
7. Alcohols
8. Chlorinated aliphatics
9. Chlorinated aromatics
10. Terpenes
11. Organic acids

Investigations of building-related illness more frequently include a sophisticated approach termed ''fingerprinting,'' employing GCMS to characterize the chemicals in indoor air. Chemical comparison of different indoor sites can be accomplished using this fingerprinting technique. Such GCMS fingerprinting techniques have been used to positively identify a certain chemical contaminant, its source, and the effectiveness of remediation activities. The GCMS profile of chemicals present in the indoor air of a school classroom where no health complaints were occurring is shown in Figure 59.1 (A–C). Collection of air samples over an extended period of time using charcoal tube sampling techniques allows for the concentration of low level pollutants for analysis. Low level chemicals such as alpha-pinene, carene, and methylhexane can be detected in indoor air using such techniques (Fig 59.1C).

A further example of indoor air pollution investigation using this technique compared two new buildings located at different sites, but constructed with the same materials and occupied at the same time (Figs. 59.2 and 59.3). Buildings A and B were shown to have a similar chemical indoor air profile of volatile organics. However, the occupants of building B had no health complaints, whereas the occupants of building A did. Figures 59.2 and 59.3 compare the GCMS fingerprint of the respective administrative areas of these buildings. Employees in the administrative area of building A complained of odors, eye irritation, chest tightness, nausea, headache, and sore throat, whereas occupants of building B expressed no health complaints. This observation suggests that volatile organics alone cannot always be implicated as the cause of building-related illness. One should also consider that the method of collection and analysis may preclude the detection of other chemical agents of significance.

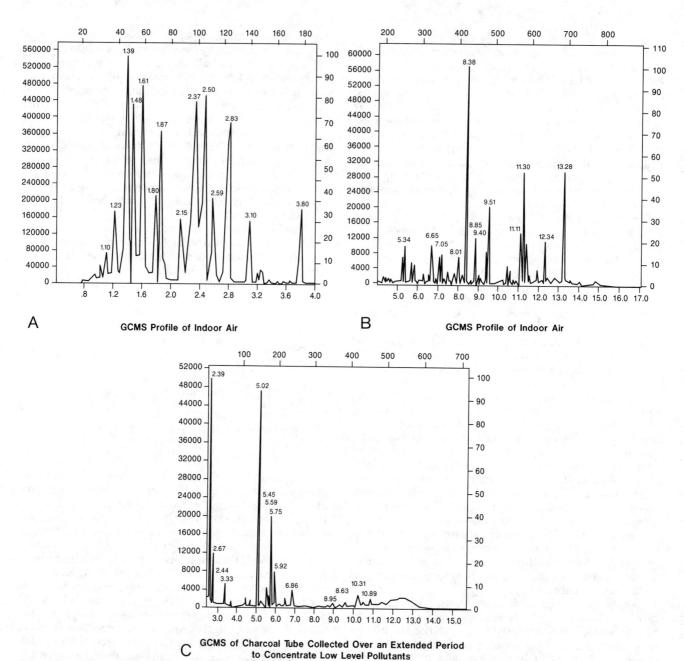

A   GCMS Profile of Indoor Air

B   GCMS Profile of Indoor Air

C   GCMS of Charcoal Tube Collected Over an Extended Period
to Concentrate Low Level Pollutants

Figure 59.1. **A–C,** GCMS profile of chemicals present in the indoor air of a building where occupants had no health complaints. **C,** Charcoal tube collection of hydrocarbons in administrative area.

Sample Volume	**Contaminant Concentration**
957 liters	Alpha pinene 0.08 $\mu g/m^3$
	Carene 0.03 $\mu g/m^3$
	Methylhexane 0.11 $\mu g/m^3$

However, as volatile organic chemicals become concentrated within an indoor environment, certain individuals may be more prone to have sensitivities to these low concentrations.

GCMS fingerprinting can also be used to determine whether removal of a chemical source is associated with abatement of health effects. An example of this approach is shown by a case involving the presence of a solvent diluent of a pesticide, which was injected along the perimeter of one area of a home. Indoor air samples collected in stainless steel cannisters revealed a GCMS fingerprint pattern similar to that of the solvent carrier. The presence of this petroleum solvent (Fig. 59.4A and B) was associated with irritant symptoms in the occupants. Attempts at remediation resulted in reduction of indoor air concentrations of the solvent after removal of exterior wall dirt where the pesticide was sprayed (Fig. 59.4C). Finally, cleaning the contaminated air return of the ventilation system resulted in almost total elimination of the airborne solvent as well as relief of health effects (Fig. 59.4D).

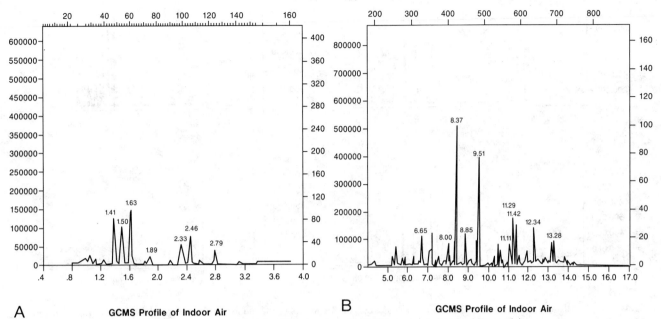

A   GCMS Profile of Indoor Air

B   GCMS Profile of Indoor Air

Figure 59.2.   Building A—Administrative Area in which occupants had health complaints.

C5–C7 Aliphatic hydrocarbons 5 ppb
Benzene 0.6 ppb
Toluene 0.4 ppb
Trichloroethylene 0.1 ppb

Trace amounts of the following chemicals were found in both building A and B: Xylene, benzaldehyde, octanal, nonanal, decanal, acetophone, naphthalene, cyclopentasilone, C11–C14 aliphatic hydrocarbons.

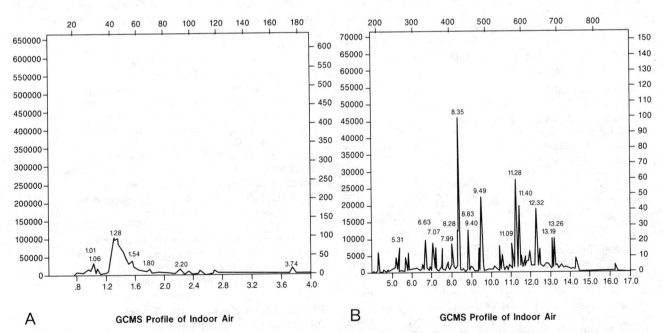

A   GCMS Profile of Indoor Air

B   GCMS Profile of Indoor Air

Figure 59.3.   Building B—Administrative Area in which occupants had no health complaints.

C5–C7 Aliphatic hydrocarbons 23 ppb
Toluene 0.5 ppb
Methylcyclohexane 0.7 ppb
1,2-Dichloroethylene 0.8 ppb
1,1,1-Trichloroethane 0.6 ppb

Trace amounts of the following chemicals were found in both building A and B: Xylene, benzaldehyde, octanal, nonanal, decanal, acetophone, naphthalene, cyclopentasilone, C11–C14 aliphatic hydrocarbons.

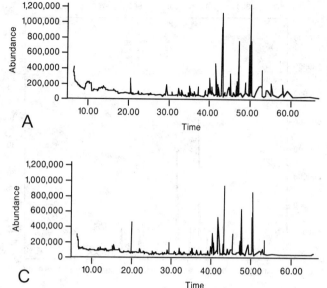

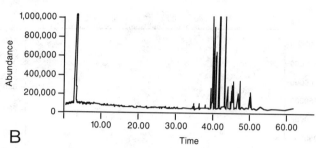

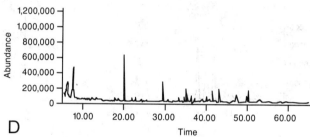

Figure 59.4A. Identification of solvent in indoor air by GCMS. Air samples were collected in stainless steel canisters. A pesticide with a solvent-based carrier had been applied outside the home next to an exterior wall, and the occupants were experiencing irritant symptoms. **B.** GCMS fingerprint of the solvent used with the pesticide confirms similar pattern to the samples collected indoors. **C.** Repeat sampling results of the indoor air following removal of exterior wall soil contaminated with the pesticide and solvent. Results show failure to remediate contamination of the indoor air. **D.** GCMS pattern demonstrates that cleaning of ventilation air duct returns in addition to removal of the exterior wall soil resulted in effective elimination of the air contaminant.

VOCs occur as emissions from a variety of building materials, furnishings, and interior finishes. Most outgassing of VOCs occurs when the building is new and slowly declines over time with a variety of half-lives, depending on the chemical, environmental factors, and the material (13, 24, 27). In addition, there are many odors associated with VOCs in a closed environment and these odors can be associated with health complaints in some instances. Common sources of indoor chemical contaminants include:

—building materials
—furnishings
—plastics, wood products, paints, sealants
—cleaning products
—combustion processes
—carpets and fabrics
—environmental tobacco smoke
—occupants
—outside sources brought indoors
—cements and mortar

Building material such as self-leveling mortar containing casein has been shown to release trace amounts of 2-ethyl-1-hexanol, ammonia, isopropylamine, ethylamine, triethylamine, dimethylamine, trimethylamine, and dimethyl sulfide. Amines have been found in the 0.003–.013 ppm range in indoor air following use of such mortar (28). In addition to the irritant effects from the chemical emissions, an objectionable odor occurs due to the casein content of the mortar and possibly texturing materials for ceilings and outgassing of sulfhydryl compounds into the indoor environment (28).

The vapor emissions for building materials can vary from days to months and even up to years for formaldehyde emissions from particle board and pressed wood products (13, 24, 27). Sources of formaldehyde emissions are sealants, mortar, caulk-

ing compounds, paints, woods, plastics, vinyl products, foams, paper products, and insulation material.

Cleaning products are also responsible for a variety of odors as well as volatile irritants in indoor environments. Most of these products contain amines, ammonia, acids, hypochlorites, phenols, alcohols, and caustics. Accumulation of these chemicals can occur with residual buildup over time. Substituting these cleaning agents for less irritating agents can be helpful in eliminating indoor pollution sources.

Human exposure to volatile chlorinated organic chemicals may result in low plasma concentrations according to studies in humans (29). Blood concentrations of volatile halogenated compounds among residents of Turin City, Italy, were higher in winter months, when residents spent most of their time indoors (29). These halogenated hydrocarbons included 1,1,1-trichloroethane, tetrachloroethylene, trichloroethylene, chloroform, and carbon tetrachloride in atmospheric samples (29). The mean blood concentration in this study during the winter was 1.33 and 0.46 μg/l during the summer (29). Interpreting blood concentrations of organic chemicals is difficult. The presence of such hydrocarbons in low concentrations may be indicative of lifelong or chronic exposure from a wide variety of sources or environments. The presence of such chemicals certainly does not constitute the existence of a disease process.

New Carpet and Health Effects: New Carpet Syndrome

Recognition that carpet vapors can be a cause of human illness and discomfort is relatively new. There are a variety of chemicals which may volatilize from new carpets and glues used to attach carpet. The distinctive new carpet odor has been traced to a new chemical, 4-phenylcyclohexene (4-PC), which has previously been implicated as a potential cause of illness in the Environmental Protection Agency building complex in Wash-

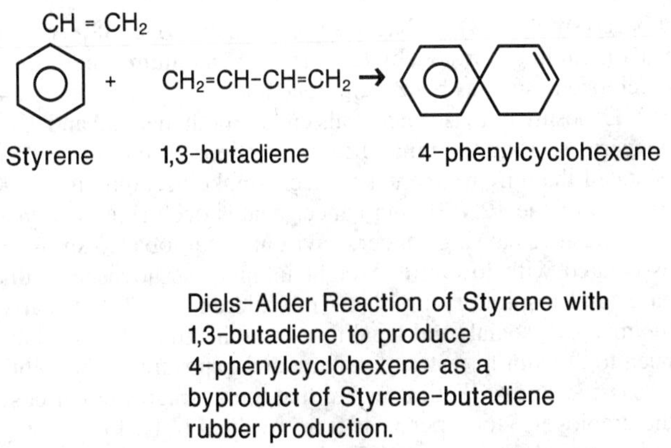

Diels-Alder Reaction of Styrene with
1,3-butadiene to produce
4-phenylcyclohexene as a
byproduct of Styrene-butadiene
rubber production.

Figure 59.5. Diels-Alder reaction of styrene with 1,3-butadiene to produce 4-phenylcyclohexene as a byproduct of styrene-butadiene rubber production.

Table 59.8. Signs and Symptoms in 21 of 34 Workers with 1.9 ppb of 4-phenylcyclohexene and other VOCs in the environment

Headache (14) 67%
Throat soreness (11) 52%
Fatigue and lethargy (10) 48%
Upper airway irritation (7) 48%
Nausea (10) 48%
Ocular irritation (8) 38%
Dizziness (6) 29%
Chest tightness (6) 29%
Skin irritation (5) 24%
Visual disturbance (5) 24%
Unusual taste (4) 19%
Myalgias (4) 19%
Shortness of breath (3) 14%

ington, DC. The source of 4-PC appears to be styrene-butadiene rubber (SBR) latex used to bind the backings of new carpet (30). Professionals involved in the evaluation of carpet-related health episodes should consider other sources of VOCs which may have been simultaneously introduced into the affected environment. Such sources include adhesives employed to adhere commercial carpets, tile and covering to floor or wall surfaces, and other materials employed in construction or finishing such as particle board shelving, synthetic paneling, wallpaper, paint, and even new furnishings.

Knowledge of the health effects and toxicology of 4-PC is limited. Acute and subacute exposure to low parts per billion may be responsible for a syndrome consisting of moderate to severe headaches, lethargy, and skin and mucous membrane irritation (31). The limited human and animal toxicology data from chronic exposure make this an important chemical to study due to the large numbers of people potentially exposed to new carpet vapors.

Using headspace analysis and GCMS, it has been demonstrated that 4-PC is released from new carpet. Analysis of carpet pieces had demonstrated that 4-PC was the common contaminant in several environments reported to cause health effects after new carpet had been installed (30). Further investigation demonstrated that the source of 4-PC was the styrene-butadiene rubber latex backing of the carpet samples. Production of styrene-butadiene rubber latex could result in the formation of 4-PC as a chemical contaminant by the Diels-Alder reaction (Fig. 59.5) (30, 32). When isolated, 4-PC is a clear, oily liquid, possessing the distinctive new carpet odor.

Air monitoring in office and home environments for 4-PC has revealed concentrations ranging from 0.3–40 ppb (33). Data suggest that 4-PC air concentrations decay over several months from a high of 30 ppb to 1–2 ppb after carpet installation. Airborne concentrations of 5 ppb are very odiferous. 4-PC concentrations below 1 ppb have not been associated with illness following installation of new carpet in homes and work environments.

An investigation of an office space in which 21 of 34 workers complained of health effects showed 4-PC present as an air contaminant at 1.9 ppb as well as a variety of VOCs from the adhesive employed to glue the carpet to the floor (31). Formaldehyde, detected at 0.03 ppm, was not considered to be a source of worker illness. New carpet had been installed in this work area one week prior to employees moving into the site.

No other source of indoor air pollution was found. Chemical odors were noted by the majority of workers occupying the site almost immediately. Within a few weeks of occupancy, health complaints were registered by the majority of the employees. The first indication of a health problem occurred when one of the workers presented to an emergency department with severe headache, vomiting, and upper airway irritation. The patient reported that headaches and nausea began within 3 weeks of moving into the new building. The patient also complained of ocular and skin irritation. These symptoms lessened during off-work hours. Surveys revealed 21 of the 34 workers (62%) occupying the building site had adverse health effects. The syndrome experienced by workers is summarized in Table 59.8 (31).

Of the 21 patients with symptoms, 10 described some form of past allergic condition such as hay fever or seasonal rhinitis. The other 11 had no previous allergic manifestations. Smoking was not allowed in the worksite, and six of the 21 affected workers were smokers. The building was a one-story modular type with a large opened area partitioned into smaller cubicles. The area housed clerical staff using video display terminals previously used in the old work area. The entire work area was open except for two administrative offices.

The illness experienced by these employees is similar to that seen in other tight building syndromes with the exception of more pronounced headaches and lethargy. Headaches (67%) and lethargy (48%) may be due to central nervous system effects of 4-PC at low air concentrations. Prominent mucous membrane irritant effects was also apparent; sore throat (52%), eye irritation (38%), chest tightness (29%), upper airway irritation (48%), cough (24%), and skin irritation (24%) accounted for a large number of complaints, indicating the irritant nature of the mixed chemical exposure.

New carpet and other volatile organics are chemicals that appear to produce noticeable health effects at low parts per billion air concentrations. Indeed, emissions from new carpets and adhesives employed in commercial applications of carpets could very well explain some of the elusive causes of illness in new buildings in the past. None of the 21 patients appeared to be seriously ill, and all symptoms resolved following steam cleaning of the carpets and improvement in fresh air ventilation.

It is evident that 4-PC may be a significant chemical which may pose health effects for workers and home owners exposed to new carpet emissions. The extent of these health effects is not entirely known, but appears to be similar to other indoor air pollutants except that clinical symptomatology occurs in the low parts per billion range. 4-PC decays over several weeks to months in the indoor environment and even after 3–6 months may be detected in the 1–2 ppb range. The level of this compound can be reduced in the indoor environment by steam cleaning carpet and simultaneously improving ventilation. Explanation to workers of the expected health effects along with assurance that this and other chemicals can be removed from the environment should be part of the management plan.

The magnitude of illness from 4-PC is unknown despite the fact that new carpet installation in both the home and work environment could expose millions of people. Animal studies indicate that direct contact with liquid 4-PC is cytotoxic to lung tissue and may produce alterations of lymphoid tissue. Due to the ability of 4-PC to produce human health effects at very low air concentrations in addition to the large numbers of exposed persons, and the relatively unknown toxic properties of the chemical, further epidemiologic, clinical, and immunologic investigations of this compound are needed.

ENVIRONMENTAL TOBACCO SMOKE AND IAQ

Smoking, either at work or at home, is probably the most common source of indoor pollutants. Forty percent of all homes in the United States are subject to environmental tobacco smoke on a regular basis (23). Given the conclusions from research regarding adverse health effects due to smoking as well as from exposure to passive smoke, environmental tobacco smoke is now recognized as a serious source of poor indoor air quality and illness. There are numerous chemical as well as particulate pollutants from indoor smoking which can accumulate in the environment and contribute to IAQ complaints (Table 59.3) (23, 34). Odor and irritant complaints are common in work areas where smoking is allowed. Studies have documented that there are increased ventilation requirements in areas where smoking occurs (34). Irritation secondary to smoking-generated pollutants are due to both the vapor phase chemicals and the particulates. In poorly ventilated areas, the ambient carbon monoxide concentration can exceed 9 ppm, and the particulate concentration can exceed 1 mg/m^3, both in violation of ambient air quality.

Tobacco smoke is a combination of vapor phase and particulate aerosol phase. The aerosol of a common puff of mainstream tobacco smoke contains particles ranging in size from 0.1–1 micrometer. The particulate phase contains around 3500 different compounds, and the vapor phase contains 300–500 compounds. The major components of the vapor and particulate phases (Table 59.3) contribute significantly to the overall indoor air pollution chemical environment. Common volatile organic chemicals such as toluene, benzene, styrene, formaldehyde, acetone, methanol, acetic acid, and acetylene are produced by smoking indoors and contribute significantly to human exposure.

Health effects related to passive environmental tobacco smoke are now documented (34, 35). Cardiovascular disease, cancer, respiratory diseases, and asthma have been directly associated with passive smoke (34, 35). The current ventilation standard established by ASHRAE in environments where smoking is allowed is inadequate to protect the health of passively exposed individuals. The current ASHRAE standard calls for 20 cfm of fresh air per occupant where smoking is allowed. However, this standard is probably not adequate in controlling the odors, irritation, and other health effects generated by environmental

tobacco smoke (34). Tobacco smoke contains over 3800 chemicals including formaldehyde, acrolein, cadmium, and known carcinogens such as benzo(a)pyrene and nitrosamines (23, 24, 36). Exposure to these chemicals creates both medical and legal concerns relating to human health of indoor air quality (37). It is stated that environmental tobacco smoke accounts for 2500 to 8700 of the 12,700 lung cancer deaths occurring each year (37). Besides causing cancer, environmental tobacco smoke is associated with low birth weight infants, cardiovascular disease, and respiratory problems in children (34–36). Clearly, the medical, social, and legal thrusts in the United States have been to attempt to restrict smoking and exposure of the public to passive smoke. Estimates are that the average smoker costs the employer $4600 per year from medical bills, lost productivity, and cleaning costs (37).

NEW APPROACHES FOR ASSESSING VENTILATION

As previously discussed, half of IAQ health complaints are related to inadequate ventilation. While ventilation systems are designed primarily to provide control over thermal comfort, it has been assumed that air flow is evenly mixed by the ventilation system. However, this assumption is not always true. Uniform distribution of fresh air via the ventilation systems for maximum dilution of indoor pollutants is not always a reality, and microenvironments of ventilation-distribution mismatches can occur. These mismatches can result in areas of poor air quality or "dead zones," where the air may be stale.

Recent work at the Solar Energy Research Institute (SERI) located in Golden, Colorado, has been directed toward the development of control volume techniques that provide measures of ventilation rates and pollutant removal rates (38). These measures can be used to diagnose specific performance problems:

1. Flow recirculation—pockets of air remain unmixed within a room because of blockage by partitions, furniture, or other large objects.
2. Flow short-circuiting—part of the air supply bypasses a room because of poor system design.
3. Duct leakage.

The SERI system employs an image analysis system similar to those in remote-sensing applications to study the performance of a building's ventilation system (Fig. 59.6) (38). The SERI system is a significant improvement over traditionally used point measurement systems which sample air at only a few points in the occupied zone. The SERI analysis system expands this capability by producing a digitized image of tinted fluid in a simulation of air movement through the occupied zone. This digitized image provides more than 367,000 points at which optical density can be measured to determine pollutant concentration. The system's greater spatial resolution allows highly accurate local measurement of air movement and pollutant distribution so that a realistic assessment of the human exposure to room contaminants can be accomplished (Figs. 59.7 and 59.8). Therefore, remedial corrective actions are possible, and retesting can confirm that positive change has occurred.

An additional benefit of the SERI system is that a real time video of the digitized results are produced and can be used in employee information sessions. Furthermore, the detailed spatial analysis can be correlated with health surveys of the build-

Image Processing for Pollutant Measurements

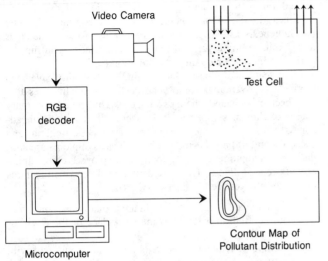

Figure 59.6. Solar Energy Research Institute (SERI) Building Energy Technology Program method to evaluate effectiveness of ventilation using a simulated model of air flow designed to reproduce patterns of air movement and indoor air pollutant distribution.

ing's occupants. Thus, localized ventilation problems can be correlated with the presence or absence of employee health symptom complaints.

With the advent of a strong emphasis on energy conservation, there has been a tendency to limit outdoor air intake during adverse temperature conditions as much as possible to avoid having to heat or cool incoming air. In modern buildings of tight construction which depend entirely on their ventilation system(s) for outside air, this is relatively easy to accomplish. However, the persons designing the ventilating system are seldom the persons trying to reduce energy use and so, after adjustments, it is not uncommon for the amount of outside air being introduced into the system to be considerably below what is necessary to maintain a comfortable indoor environment. Similar problems can occur if inadequate provisions have been made for exhausting air from the building or if the exhaust is blocked. In addition, occasionally the outside exhaust vent faces the fresh air intake portal. Thus the HVAC perpetually recycles contaminated air. Careful sequential review and analysis of the HVAC system is always a critical and rewarding exercise. Therefore, a multidisciplinary approach involving health professionals, industrial hygienists, and mechanical engineers is required.

Radon and IAQ

Radon (radon-222) is a naturally occurring radioactive gas that is present in outside and indoor air resulting from decay of trace amounts of uranium in soil. The decay process of radon releases alpha particles. Radon eventually decays through a number of intermediates to lead-206, a stable end product (39, 40). Concentrations of radon gas can be higher in many indoor air environments compared to outdoors.

The EPA has been studying both the airborne concentrations of radon and the health risks associated with longterm human exposure. Soil and rock naturally contain uranium in the range of 1–4 ppm (40). As a gas, radon can diffuse through soil and rock and enter home environments. Soil contains approximately 1 picocurie (pci) of radium per gram, which provides an emission of 0.5 pci of radon per meter^2 per second (40). Outdoor radon concentrations average 200 pci/m^3, and indoor air concentrations can be up to four times higher (40). Measurements of radon exposure are expressed in terms of working levels (WL) or working levels per month (WLM), an accumulation measurement. In general, 1 pci of radon per liter is equivalent to 0.005 WL (40, 41). The WLM assumes 170 hours per month of exposure (40). Occupational exposure to radon in the United States was reduced from 12 WLM/year to 4 WLM/year in 1971 (41). The level for remediation activity in the home environ-

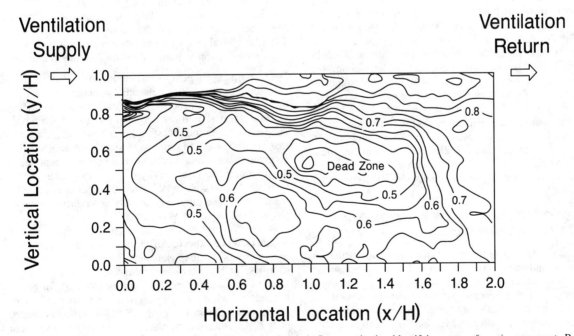

Figure 59.7. Two-dimensional mapping of the results of simulated air flow monitoring identifying areas of no air movement. Reprinted from Anderson R: Determination of ventilation efficiency based upon short-term tests, USDOE, Solar Research Energy Institute, 1988.

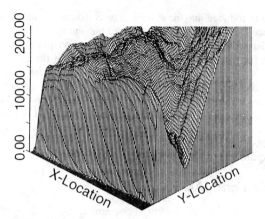

Figure 59.8. Three-dimensional model showing "dead" space areas representing little or no effective air movement as areas of depression. Reprinted from Anderson R: Determination of ventilation efficiency based upon short-term tests, USDOE, Solar Research Institute, 1988.

ment is considered to be 2 WLM/year (41). As of 1989, EPA monitoring has shown radon concentrations to be less than 4 pci/l in 74% of homes across the United States (40). Health concerns are due to the fact that radon decay products (termed "daughters") are chemically active and can thus attach to particles, surfaces, and human tissue (39–41). Thus, inhaled radon contributes to the risk of lung cancer (40, 41). The EPA recommends that home concentrations not exceed 0.02 working levels of radon which is about 4 pci/l of air (40).

The airborne radon concentration in a home is a factor of the earth surrounding the home, ventilation, air changes per hour in the home, amount of radon in water and in natural gas, and construction of the home (40). Radon can diffuse through cracks in foundations and walls, openings for plumbing, and cinder block (40). Radon does not pass easily through solid concrete foundations. The World Health Organization has set limits of radon at 0.11 WL for existing buildings (40).

Health effects from excessive radon exposure relate mainly to an increased risk of lung cancer. Most studies of the relationship of lung cancer and radon exposure are from uranium miners. Studies indicate that all forms of lung cancer are increased by radon exposure (41). Also, the contribution of smoking to lung cancer is a confounding factor in determining the exact etiology. Radon exposure and smoking are thought to increase the risk of lung cancer 10-fold over nonsmokers (41). Over the lifetime of an individual, exposure to 1 WLM/year is thought to increase the number of deaths from lung cancer by a factor of 1.5 over the current rate in men and women (42). The National Council on Radiation Protection and Measurements (NCRP) has published guidelines on remediation and control of radon in indoor environments (NCRP Report No. 77, 1984).

PSYCHOLOGIC ASPECTS OF INDOOR AIR QUALITY IN HUMAN ILLNESS

The presence of illness in the workplace can be unsettling to employees, stimulate anxieties about possible toxic exposures, and accentuate worker anxiety with exacerbation of symptoms. IAQ investigation can generate strong emotional responses, especially if negative results are found by environmental investigation. The overall effect leaves building occupants discouraged, suspicious, and unconvinced that the problem has been discovered and a proper solution proposed.

It is important for the investigator to discern psychogenic-related illness from other physical and chemical-related sources of illness in the environment. It is not uncommon that the psychogenesis aspect can be overwhelming for the manager and dominate employee and management relations during the period of indoor air quality investigation.

Many features of illness relating to indoor air quality have been ascribed to psychologic or psychosocial aspects. In cases that have been investigated where psychogenesis has been the primary source of illness, symptoms of headache, dizziness, lightheadedness, nausea, drowsiness, weakness, numbness, tingling, and chest discomfort have been described. These symptoms are similar to the symptoms typically found in employees complaining of work-related illness. There are certain well-described features that suggest psychogenic illness (43, 44):

1. An incidence of the problem in areas that is not consistent with ventilation patterns in the workplace or the environment.
2. A temporal sequence of events that is not consistent with ventilation flow patterns and ventilation flow rates or chemical sources.
3. An absence of medical findings compatible with exposures.
4. Outbreak of illness consistent with person-to-person transmission rather than transmission from a source.
5. Severe symptoms of sudden onset among a number of people, particulary if the symptoms begin after leaving the source of exposure or do not resolve upon leaving the worksite.
6. Moderate to severe symptoms that are unrelated to the nature of a contaminant found.
7. A diversity of symptoms without collaborating objective findings.
8. The discovery of individuals who are affected, not because they are near the source of the exposure, but rather become affected after learning of the exposure or learning that someone else is exhibiting signs of illness.
9. Pattern of the illness following a classic epidemic curve where conversation is the vector of spread.
10. Managerial or supervisory change or changes in work flow or production volume including deadline requirements.

The term psychogenesis has emotional connotations and can contribute to difficulties between management and workers in the investigation of indoor air-related illness (43). Physicians and managers should refrain from the use of the word "psychogenic" while the investigation is proceeding. Also, factors that create anxiety in employees should be avoided. It should be noted that psychogenic illness can be as disruptive, or more disruptive, to the productivity of the worker as an actual identified chemical or physical source. Sources of conflict between management and employee usually arise once the idea of employee psychogenesis is raised.

Anxiety disorders can also occur following suspected exposure or actual exposure of employees to hazardous chemicals. Symptoms of postexposure anxiety include rapid heart rate, shortness of breath, dizziness, nausea, diarrhea, fatigue, difficulty concentrating, and irritability (45, 46). In general, organizations whose employees have a propensity to develop psychogenic illness are generally rigid and authoritarian with poor communication between workers and management (44). Workers may not feel that management is serious about the problem, and the worker feels an inability to control environmental conditions. Multiple stresses can affect a worker's ability to relate to the environment. These stresses may be fear of loss of job, external forces, and the thought of environmental contamination (46). The perception of risk can also play an important part in the psychogenesis phenomena in the work environment related to indoor air quality (44). Risk of exposure to toxins can add to anxiety. The public is repeatedly exposed to the news media and their presentation of hazardous materials sites, toxic waste dumps, and chemical exposures. Workers may become alarmed if they feel that a chemical contamination in an environment may cause them longterm health consequences. Also, heightened concern will occur if the source of the potential problem, such as an odor, cannot be established or identified and remediated. Odors in the environment can create anxieties and psychogenesis that are very difficult to control. The psychologic responses to indoor air quality problems may relate more to an odor of a chemical than to its toxic effects. Odors such as sulfur odors, odors of rotten eggs, or odors of chemicals or hydrocarbons can be very distressing to workers. Poor air quality is a source of stress in the work environment (46). Authors have summarized psychosocial factors involved in these psychogenic outbreaks (45). These factors are:

1. The environment itself
2. Boredom associated with the job
3. Pressure to produce
4. Physical stresses such as noise, lighting, thermal factors, odors
5. The relationship between labor and management
6. Lack of communication and social support within the work environment

There is also key evidence that there are certain characteristics or personality traits of persons who trigger these psychogenic outbreaks (45). Psychogenic epidemics usually begin suddenly with dramatic symptoms. A thorough investigation can aid in assuring workers that the environment is safe; however, since the symptoms of a psychogenic illness resemble the symptoms commonly found in physical disease, it is often very difficult to allay the fears of these individuals (45). Many times, one individual or a group will serve to accentuate symptoms of others.

There are a variety of strategies that management can use in order to prevent the generation of psychogenic source illness in the indoor environment. The number of outside consultants involved should be limited (44). The more consultants involved, the more likelihood for numerous and conflicting opinions. This conflict of opinions can magnify concern of workers and contribute to the problem (44). Management should have one consultant or one consultant team in charge of both the investigation and dissemination of information to management and employees. Also, there should be only one manager designated to oversee the investigation and implement recommendations. Having different managers involved is distracting and often results in miscommunication to workers and consultants. The sensitivity of managers and consultants is also very important to help resolve a psychogenic-related indoor air quality problem. Insensitive comments and comments that can be taken out of context should not occur. The relationship of management and employee can be greatly tested during these times.

Workers affected by indoor air quality problems generally do not need to be seen in an emergency department or hospital. However, workers may be sent to an emergency department

or hospital, which further serves to intensify the anxiety of the other workers (44). The use of a knowledgeable, single source physician can also help alleviate distortion of facts and decrease rumors. Closing the workplace is not recommended unless there is a serious and significant threat to the health of the workers. Once a workplace has been closed, it is very difficult to reopen again.

Workers should have involvement in the investigation, but their participation should be subject to guidance by the principal consultant. Multiple, independent investigations by citizens or worker groups will be disruptive and create mistrust. Communication should be open and should be timely. Since rumor is the most common source of information, rumors should be controlled by having frequent meetings with employees and open discussions regarding the investigation. Communication with the media may be important in some situations where there is a public health concern. The media, if not properly educated, can help foster sensationalism and rumor. Regular press releases can be important to help neutralize rumors. A single spokesperson who responds to the media should be available.

Due to the nature of indoor air quality-related health problems, a primary source may not be found. Workers may then be told that their problem was psychogenic or related to stress (44). Management should be prepared to deal with this factor and remediate the stressors in the environment that can contribute to illness.

WORK-RELATEDNESS OF IAQ PROBLEMS

The work-relatedness of a disease is important to establish for worker compensation reasons. A disease can be stated to be work-related if the following criteria are met (47):

1. Medical conditions exist that are compatible with known health effects of exposure to a chemical, industrial site, or agents in question.
2. There was previously or is presently a sufficient exposure to agents or chemicals in the work environment to produce health effects or disease.
3. A preexisting disease is exacerbated by a previous or present worksite exposure.
4. Evidence supports an occupational etiology.

Health effects related to poor IAQ, whatever the source, are typically vague and subjective. In addition, environmental monitoring and investigations may not produce evidence of a single objective source, and since most chemicals found in indoor environments are very low in concentrations, there is rarely a demonstrable violation of OSHA regulatory standards. Thus the environmental evaluation may not identify a source of illness, despite persistent health complaints.

Cases of work-related illness secondary to poor IAQ are now reaching worker compensation courts. Producing objective evidence of a disease process in these individuals can be difficult since no clinical or laboratory abnormalities confirm the objective existence of a disease process. Given the lack of objective clinical evidence and lack of existing regulatory standards regarding low level pollutants and their relationship to illness, proving the work-relatedness of IAQ problems will continue to be difficult.

CONCLUSION

Problems associated with IAQ are clearly at an early stage of investigation and analysis. There is a clear disparity between the number and intensity of complaints and the investigative ability to pinpoint specific sources. Health professionals should expect to see a steady increase in the number of health problems attributed to the indoor air quality environment.

A systematic, nonjudgmental, and scientific approach is indicated. Such an approach requires the assistance of industrial hygienists and mechanical engineers and medical professionals. This multidisciplinary team has become essential for most building investigations. Research is being directed toward improving HVAC system performance and the analysis of health effects associated with low concentrations of multiple contaminants in the environment.

The problems associated with IAQ will continue to increase during the 1990s, and the health professional team will play a prominent role.

Appendix A
Indoor Air Quality

(Employee Health and Building Survey)

Company: _____ Type of Business _____

Date built: _____ Address: _____

Date occupied: _____

1. Name _____ Age _____ Male/Female _____

2. Medical illness for which you are being treated: _____

   _____

   Allergies: _____

   Medications you are taking: _____

   _____

3. Do you smoke? Yes _____ No _____ How many packs per day _____

   For how many years _____

4. Date symptoms first noticed: _____

5. Describe how fast the symptoms came on: _____
   (Over what period of time: minutes, hours, days)

   _____

6. Location at worksite when symptoms first began: _____

   Time of day or shift: _____

7. Do your symptoms improve when you leave work? Yes _____ No _____

   Please explain if no: _____

   _____

8. Is there a particular place in the building where your symptoms are worse? Yes _____ No _____

   If yes, explain where: _____

   _____

9. Is there a particular time of the day when symptoms are worse? Yes _____ No _____

   Explain _____

   _____

10. Ventilation type: Central air conditioning _____
                        Open windows _____
                        Humidification _____
                        Coolers _____

11. Please check the symptoms that you have:

    _____ Headache
    _____ Fatigue/drowsiness
    _____ Noticeable odors
    _____ Sore throat
    _____ Nasal/sinus congestion
    _____ Nausea
    _____ Dizziness
    _____ Sneezing
    _____ Eye irritation
    _____ Chest tightness

——— Backpain
——— Trouble sleeping
——— Unusual taste
——— Disorientation
——— Contact lens irritation or inability to wear contact lenses
——— Chest congestion
——— Aching joints
——— Rapid heartbeat
——— Skin irritation/itching
——— Chest pains
——— Unusual vaginal discharge
——— Contact lens problems
——— Tongue/lip numbness
——— Bladder infections/dysuria
——— Nosebleed
——— Cough
——— Shortness of breath
——— Visual disturbances
——— Blurred vision
——— Irritability
——— Loss of smell
——— Loss of taste
——— Abdominal pain
——— Rashes
——— Skin irritation
——— Extremity tingling/numbness

12. Is there a specific location where symptoms most frequently occur?

13. Did a fellow employee describe their illness to you before you became ill?   Yes ——— No ———

14. Do you notice any strange odors in the workplace?   Yes ——— No ———

    If yes, detail the characteristic of the odor:

    ——— Bitter
    ——— Sweet
    ——— Perfume
    ——— Burning substance
    ——— Hydrocarbon or solvent
    ——— Tobacco smoke
    ——— Other (describe) ——————————————————————

15. If you notice any strange workplace odor, where is it located? ——————————————————

    What time of day do you first notice it? ——————————————————————

    Does it disappear during the workday?   Yes ——— No ———

16. Is there tobacco smoke in your work environment?   Yes ——— No ———

17. Do you work next to a smoker?   Yes ——— No ———

18. Description of building and work environment (check all that apply)

    Age of building: New ——— 1–5 years ——— >5 years ———

    ——— Office space in new building
    ——— Office space in old building
    ——— Detached single building
    ——— Multiple rooms
    ——— Highrise
    ——— More than one level but not highrise
    ——— Single level
    ——— Single level attached to other buildings
    ——— Building additions
    ——— Space renovations
    ——— New machines
    ——— New carpet

_____ New insulation
_____ Presence of attached garage
_____ Windows that open
_____ Windows that do not open
_____ High humidity
_____ Open-space worksite
_____ Multiple offices, doors closed
_____ Multiple offices, doors open
_____ Smoking allowed at worksite
_____ Storage of chemicals
_____ Storage of solvents
_____ Central air conditioner
_____ No air conditioning
_____ Recent carpet cleansing
_____ Window air conditioner unit
_____ Recent pesticide spraying
_____ Presence of copier machines
_____ Humidifier

Other descriptive features of work environment: _____
_____
_____

19. List general furnishings and contents of your environment:
_____
_____
_____
_____

Draw a sketch of your work area and location of ventilation ducts, doors, and windows.

Source: Sullivan, Krieger, and Van Ert.

(Adapted from Thoburn T. Presentation at Annual U.S.P.H.S. Professional Association Meeting. NIOSH. April 12, 1985.)

Outside air intake: Brings fresh air into building and will often have adjustable louvers so the amount of outside air admitted can be varied. Louvers do not seal out all outside air when they are closed. Open louvers do not mean 100% outside air is being delivered inside. A normally functioning system often delivers 10–15% outside air.

Filters: Filters keep out dust and other particulate matter. They will not remove gasses and vapors. They are not designed to remove very fine particulates. Dirt on the filter will increase its efficiency, but further dirt buildup can lead to excessive pressure drops across the filter, thus reducing the air flow. Filters can be a source of contamination in the ventilating system. Filter changes can be prompted by visual inspection, monitoring the pressure drop across the filter, or simply on a routine basis.

Fans: Fans move air through the system. The main fans are usually located just after the filters. Other fans may be located for localized exhaust or for returning air. Fans can move large quantities of air but can only work against a small pressure gradient. Obstructions in the ventilating system can reduce air flow in the obstructed ducts even if the fan is working properly.

Cooling and/or dehumidifying coils: Air is passed over cooling coils. If the air temperature is cooled below the dew point, water will condense out on the coils. If the water is not adequately drained away and the coils are not kept clean, molds can grow in the moisture and become a source of contamination. Although the air leaving these coils will have a high relative humidity, as the air warms the relative humidity will drop.

Heating devices: These depend on combustion devices, and the combustion chamber is separate from the ventilation. The products of combustion are vented to the outside. In a new building, the air for combustion is also drawn from the outside. Other sources of heat might be electric heating coils or coils that are heated by a circulating fluid which is heated somewhere outside of the ventilated area. This could be a furnace, a heat pump, or even the cooling coils of a dehumidifier. Heated surfaces will remain dry and should only cause problems if they collect dust or if they leak. In some tight new buildings, heat is primarily supplied around the outer walls to balance heat loss. The remainder of the building receives heat from the occupants and the office machines and lights which generate heat as a byproduct. In these situations, the main ventilation system is primarily called upon for cooling.

Humidifier and/or evaporative cooler: In cold climates, heating outside air to comfortable temperatures greatly reduces its relative humidity. Moisture can be added to the air by introducing steam into the air stream, spraying water into the air stream, or passing the air over or through moist plates or mats. Evaporative coolers pass warm dry air through moist mats. As the water evaporates it cools and humidifies the air. As with cooling coils, the moist surfaces can support mold growth and may require cleaning. If there is no water runoff from steam humidifiers, these would be less likely to cause problems than systems in which there is liquid present.

Distribution ductwork: The conditioned air is distributed from the central air handling unit to the various office areas by a series of multiple branching ducts. As the number of ducts increases, the rate of air flow in each decreases. The air enters the office area through diffusers which hopefully keep the occupied areas from feeling drafty while mixing the air. The amount of air passing through any particular duct can usually be controlled by dampers, usually set to respond to a thermostat. Unless the system is set to deliver at least a minimum of air, some individual offices may get no air exchange during times when the thermostat does not call for temperature modification. Air blowing from the end of a duct can travel as a stream from an appreciable distance without mixing uniformly in a room.

Air return: Either in the individual rooms or in the corridors there will be grill work which allows air to move into return air ducts or plenums. Even if there is a fan to aid this movement, there will be measurable air flow in the room only very close to the vent. It is quite common to use the space above the drop ceiling as the return air plenum.

Outside exhaust: In older buildings, sufficient air would usually leak out through cracks to make a general exhaust to the outside unnecessary. In tight buildings, exhausts are necessary. It will probably have louvers to allow control. Again, 100% closed will probably not completely seal the vent, nor will 100% open mean that all air is being exhausted. In addition to an exhaust on the main system, there will be some local exhaust systems which take air from a problem area (a rest room or a particular machine) and exhaust it to the outside. Most building codes will require the rest rooms and kitchens to have such exhaust ventilation.

Recirculation: Because heating or cooling a building takes energy, and because draft-free temperature control requires that air entering the offices be of only a slightly different temperature than room air, it is the usual practice to circulate greater volumes of air than those needing to be drawn from the outside. Thus there will be ducts which allow much of the air returning from the offices to mix with outside air and go through the filters and back into the system. There will probably be dampers to help control this. Some systems are set so that there will be no recirculation when outside temperatures will allow the use of outside air with virtually no heating or cooling. A very common ventilating unit in new buildings is the roof-mounted integrated unit which contains the intake, exhaust, and recirculating vents and controls. In other arrangements, it is possible that exhaust venting has been neglected. Where quite a few local exhaust vents are needed, it is not uncommon that adequate makeup air has been neglected, particularly in manufacturing settings. Another common practice to save energy is to only run the ventilating system when the building is in use and for a limited period before and/or after hours. This may be automatically or manually controlled. Even if the recirculating system is running, the outside air intake may be shut down at a set time.

REFERENCES

1. Kreiss K. The sick building syndrome: where is the epidemiologic basis? (editorial). Am J Public Health 1990;80:1172–1173.

2. Bardana EJ, Montanaro A. Tight building syndrome. Immunol Allergy Pract 1986;8:17–31.

3. Kreiss K. The epidemiology of building-related complaints and illness. In: Cone JE, Hodgson MJ, eds. Occupational medicine: state of the art reviews. Vol 4. Philadelphia: Hanley & Belfus, October–December 1989:575–592.

4. Feeley JC. Impact of indoor air pathogens on human health. In: Gammage RB, Kaye SV, eds. Indoor air and human health. Chelsea, MI: Lewis Publishers, 1987:183–187.

5. EPA. The exposures factor handbook. Environmental Protection Agency, Office of Health and Environmental Assessment. EPA/600/8-89-1 043. Washington, DC: GPO, 1989.

6. Woods JE. Cost avoidance and productivity in owning and operating buildings. In: Cone JE, Hodgson MJ, eds. Occupational medicine: state of the art reviews. Vol 4. Philadelphia: Hanley & Belfus, October–December 1989:753–770.

7. Stolwijk JA. Shelter and indoor air. Environ Health Perspect 1990;86:271–274.

8. Hodgson MJ. Clinical diagnosis and management of building related illness and the sick building syndrome. In: Cone JE, Hodgson MJ, eds. Occupational medicine: state of the art reviews. Vol 4. Philadelphia: Hanley & Belfus, October–December 1989:593–606.

9. Melius J, Wallingford K, Keenlyside R, Carpenter J. Indoor air quality—the NIOSH experience. Ann Am Conf Gov Ind Hyg, 1984;10:3–7.

10. Morey PR, Shattuck DE. Role of ventilation in the causation of building-associated illnesses. In: Cone JE, Hodgson MJ, eds. Occupational medicine: state of the art reviews. Vol 4. Philadelphia: Hanley & Belfus, October–December 1989:625–642.

11. Spengler JD. Shelter for the twenty-first century. Environ Health Perspect 1990;86:281–284.

12. Radon Gas. Contractor liability for an indoor health hazard. Am J Law Med 1986;12:241–272.

13. Ozkaynak H, Ryan PB, Wallace LA, Nelson WC, Behar JV. Sources and emission rates of organic chemical vapors in homes and buildings. In: Seifert B, Esdorn H, Fischer M, Ruden H, Wegner J, eds. Indoor air '87: proceedings of the 4th International Conference on Indoor Air Quality. Berlin: Institute for Water, Soil and Air Hygiene, 1987:3–7.

14. Stanek EJ, Tuthill RW, Willis C, Moore GS. Household hazardous waste in Massachusetts. Arch Environ Health 1987;42:83–91.

15. Whorton DM, Larson SR, Gordon NJ, Morgan RW. Investigation and work-up of tight building syndrome. J Occup Med 1987;29:142–147.

16. Quinlan P, Macher JM, Alevantis LE, Cone JE. Protocol for the comprehensive evaluation of building associated illness. In: Cone JE, Hodgson MJ, eds. Occupational medicine: state of the art reviews. Vol 4. Philadelphia: Hanley & Belfus, October–December 1989:771–797.

17. Morbidity and Mortality Weekly Report (Vol 33, 1984) Centers for Disease Control, Atlanta, Georgia. Leads from MMWR. JAMA 1984;252:1843–1844.

18. Arnow PM, Fink JN, Schlueter DP, Barboriak JJ, et al. Early detection of hypersensitivity pneumonitis in office workers. Am J Med 1978;64:236–242.

19. Sneller MR, Pinnas JL. Comparison of airborne fungi in evaporative cooled and air conditioned homes. Ann Allergy 1987;59:317–320.

20. Kodama AM, McGee RI. Airborne microbial contaminants in indoor environments. Naturally ventilated and air-conditioned homes. Arch Environ Health 1986;41:306–311.

21. Burge HA. Indoor air and infectious disease. In: Cone JE, Hodgson MJ,

eds. Occupational medicine: state of the art reviews. Vol 4. Philadelphia: Hanley & Belfus, October–December 1989:713–721.

22. Thoburn T. Presentation at Annual U.S.P.H.S. Professional Association Meeting. NIOSH. April 12, 1985.

23. Lewtas J. Toxicology of complex mixtures of indoor air pollutants. Annu Rev Pharmacol Toxicol 1989;29:415–439.

24. Girman JR. Volatile organic compounds and building bake-out. In: Cone JE, Hodgson MJ, eds. Occupational medicine: state of the art reviews. Vol 4. Philadelphia: Hanley & Belfus, October–December 1989:695–712.

25. Sheldon LS, Sparacino CM, Pellizzari ED. Review of analytical methods for volatile organic compounds in the indoor environment. In: Gammage RB, Kaye SV, eds. Indoor air and human health. Chelsea, MI: Lewis Publishers, 1987:335–349.

26. Wallace LA, Pellizzari ED, Gordon SM. Organic chemicals in indoor air: a review of human exposure studies and indoor air quality studies. In: Gammage RB, Kaye SV, eds. Indoor air and human health. Chelsea, MI: Lewis Publishers, Inc, 1987:361–378.

27. Ember LR. Survey finds high indoor levels of volatile organic chemicals. Chemical Eng. News; December 5, 1988:23–25.

28. Lundholm M, Larrell G, Mathiasson L. Self-leveling mortar as a possible cause of symptoms associated with ''sick building syndrome.'' Arch Environ Health 1990;45:135–140.

29. Gilli G, Bono R, Scursatone E. Volatile halogenated hydrocarbons in urban atmosphere and in human blood. Arch Environ Health 1990;45:101–106.

30. Van Ert MD, Clayton JW, Crabb CL, Walsh DW. Identification and characterization of r-phenylcyclohexene—an emission product of new carpeting. Presented at the Am Ind Hyg conference in San Francisco, May 1988.

31. Van Ert MD, Sullivan JB. Personal data. University of Arizona, Tucson.

32. Morrison R, Boyd R. Organic chemistry. Chapt 32, 2nd ed. Boston, MA: Allyn & Bacon, 1966.

33. Vogelman I, Clayton JW, Crutchfield CD, Van Ert MD. Evaluation of 4-phenylcyclohexene concentrations in home and chamber environments. Presented at the Am Ind Hyg conference in San Francisco, CA, May 1988.

34. Hodgson MJ. Environmental tobacco smoke and the sick building syndrome. In: Cone JE, Hodgson MJ, eds. Occupational medicine: state of the art reviews. Vol. 4. Philadelphia: Hanley & Belfus, October–December 1989:735–740.

35. Humble C, Croft J, Gerber A, Casper M, Hames C, Tyroler H. Passive smoking and 20-year cardiovascular disease mortality among non-smoking wives, Evans County, Georgia. Am J Public Health 1990;80:599–601.

36. Godish T. Formaldehyde exposure from tobacco smoke—a review. Am J Public Health 1989;79:1044–1045.

37. Uzych L. Passive smoking and the law. Arch Environ Health 1990;45:72–73.

38. Anderson R: Determination of Ventilation Efficiency Based Upon Short-term Tests, USDOE, Solar Energy Research Institute, 1988.

39. Nero AV. Indoor concentrations of radon-222 and its daughters: sources, range, and environmental influences. In: Gammage RB, Kaye SV, eds. Indoor air and human health. Chelsea, MI: Lewis Publishers, Inc, 1987:43–67.

40. Council on Scientific Affairs. Radon in homes. JAMA 1987;258:668–672.

41. Harley N, Samet JM, Cross FT, Hess T, Muller J, Thomas D. Contribution of radon and radon daughters to respiratory cancer. Environ Health Perspect 1990;70:17–21.

42. Fabrikault J. Shelter and indoor air in the twenty-first century—radon, smoking, and lung cancer risks. Environ Health Perspect 1990;89:275–280.

43. Guidotti T, Alexander R, Fedoruk M: Epidemiologic features that may distinguish between building-associated illness outbreaks due to chemical exposure or psychogenic origin. Brief Communication from Building-Associated Outbreaks. J Occup Med 1987;29:148–150.

44. Boxer PA. Indoor air quality: a psychosocial perspective. J Occup Med 1990;32:425–443.

45. Olkinuora M. Psychogenic epidemics and work. Scand J Work Environ Health 1984;10:501–504.

46. Colligan MJ. The psychological effects of indoor air pollution. Bull NY Acad Med 1981;57:1014–1026.

47. DHEW. A guide to work-relatedness of disease. DHEW (NIOSH), Publication No. 79-216, 1979.

60

Art and Artists

Steven Pike, M.D., M.Sc.

Art has been a human endeavor since prehistoric times, and artists have been experimenting with new techniques, materials, and processes since that time. Artists, in their quest for expressing their emotions, use materials that are found in use in almost every commercial undertaking. These materials used in industry are regulated to protect the health of workers, but the artist often is exposed to much greater concentrations and for longer durations than the average worker. This occurs because artists are intimately involved with their work and the effect they are trying to achieve, while they are often uninformed and unaware of the chemical and physical properties of the materials and their attendant affects on human physiology. Artistic endeavors are also usually solitary or limited to few participants over prolonged periods of time and practiced in homes, studios, lofts, or other locations that are not subject to regulatory compliance.

Since art and crafts work is associated with recreation and pleasure, a limited amount of study has been done on the effects that a lifetime of such work has on the human. There is now an increasing interest by health professionals and professional artists in understanding the materials, the health hazards they pose, and ways of working and handling the materials safely. One of the first to recognize the relationship between occupation as artist and diseases associated with artistic activities and the materials used was the Italian physician and acknowledged father of occupational medicine, Bernardino Ramazzini. Ramazzini, in his 1713 classic *De Morbis Artificum*, describes the diseases of many workers and portrays vividly the appearance and health of painters, potters, gilders, weavers, and woodworkers. Excerpts from his description of potters and painters are of historical interest, and serve as a fitting introduction even 278 years later:

. . . In almost all cities there are other workers who habitually incur serious maladies from the deadly fumes of metals. Among these are the potters . . . Now when they need roasted or calcined lead for glazing their pots, they grind the lead in marble vessels, and in order to do this they hang a wooden pole from the roof, fasten a square stone to its end, and then turn it round and round. During this process or again when they use tongs to daub the pots with molten lead before putting then into the furnace, their mouths, nostrils, and the whole body take in the lead poison that has been melted and dissolved in water; hence they are soon attacked by grievous maladies. First their hands become palsied, then they become paralytic, splenetic, lethargic, cachectic, and toothless, so that one rarely sees a potter whose face is not cadaverous and the color of lead. . . .

. . . Painters too are attacked by various ailments such as palsy of the limbs, cachexy, blackened teeth, unhealthy complexions, melancholia, and loss of sense of smell. It very seldom happens that painters look florid or healthy, though they usually paint the portraits of other people to look handsomer and more florid than they really are. I have observed that nearly all the painters whom I know, both in this and other cities, are sickly; and if one reads the lives of painters it will be seen that they are by no means long-lived, especially those who were the most distinguished . . . But for their liability to disease there is a more immediate cause, I mean the materials of the colors that they handle

and smell constantly, such as red lead, cinnabar, white lead, varnish, nut-oil and linseed oil with they use for mixing colors; and the numerous pigments made of various mineral substances. The odors of varnish and the above-mentioned oils make their workrooms smell like a latrine; this is very bad for the head and perhaps accounts for the loss of the sense of smell. Moreover, painters when at work wear dirty clothes smeared with paint, so that their mouths and noses inevitably breathe tainted air; this penetrates to the seat of the animal spirits, enters by the breathing passages the abode of the blood, disturbs the economy of the natural functions, and excites the disorders mentioned above. . . .

Although the materials may be different, and artists need not grind their own pigments because of the wide commercial availability of paints and oils, Ramazzini's description of the manner in which artists create their works and the clothes that they wear is applicable even today.

Today much of the manufacture of artistic products, i.e., pottery, glass, furniture, and prints, is commercialized and many of the hazards from the materials used in the commercial production of these products are controlled by automation and quality control processes. However, a cottage industry of artists exists that is not well-organized and includes artists working alone or in small groups, crafts workers, and hobbyists. These artists may have studios or workshops in their homes or garages. This discussion applies primarily to this group of artists and to students in art schools and departments in colleges, universities, and high schools and in private settings, where students and instructors continue to be exposed to many hazardous components of art materials. The exposure in schools may be greater than is commonly appreciated because of the number of students that are using solvents, paints, and thinners, coupled with inexperience, lack of knowledge, poor ventilation, and confined spaces.

The hazards to which artists are exposed are myriad and include dusts, metals, solvents, heat, noise, and radiation. These hazards are countered as raw components in the materials used, released, or generated by the processes required for creation of the artwork, or as hazards of the devices and tools used in fabrication, molding, curing, glazing, or otherwise finishing a work of art.

HAZARDS OF SPECIFIC CREATIVE ENDEAVORS

Painting

Painters are exposed to an extensive variety of hazardous substances. Solvents, pigments, preservatives (some of which may contain mercury), varnishes, and oils are representative of the types of materials that may pose a health hazard. Painters who point the tips of their brushes with their lips or who eat in their studio with paint on their hands or food are at increased risk of chronic toxicity due to ingestion of the heavy metals contained in the pigments. Many of these metals are toxic to en-

Table 60.1.   Hazardous Materials Used in Arts and Crafts

I. Metals	
Arsenic	Arsenic is a gray metal present as an impurity in many metal ores. It is used in the production of pigments, glass, enamels, and in textile printing, and thus the artist may be exposed. It is corrosive to the skin and mucous membranes, and in an acute intoxication can cause massive destruction of the gastrointestinal mucosa, resulting in severe fluid and blood loss, which may produce shock and death. It is also toxic to the peripheral nervous system, and chronic intoxication may result in numbness of the hands and feet, in addition to weight loss, diarrhea, eczema, and possibly skin or lung cancer.
Cadmium	Cadmium is a bluish-white metal used as a pigment in cadmium red, cadmium yellow, and naples yellow; as a component of glazes; and in glassmaking and photography. It is irritating to the nose and throat, and may cause respiratory failure in acute high exposures. Cadium is poorly absorbed by ingestion but very well-absorbed by inhalation. It is found in cigarette smoke and chronic exposure may cause kidney damage, anemia, and emphysema. Fumes are formed at kiln firing of ceramic glazes.
Chromium	Chromium is a metal which is used as a colorant in ceramic glazes; in the pigments chrome yellow, chrome green, barium yellow, lemon yellow, molybdate orange, strontium yellow, and zinc yellow; and as a chromate salt and acid use in the photographic and lithographic processes. Chromates may cause skin and respiratory allergies, ulcers of the skin and nasal septum with possible perforation, nasal cancer, and lung cancer, and may be mutagenic and teratogenic. Acute exposures may cause coughing, headache, fever, wheezing, conjunctivities, and epistaxis.
Cobalt	Cobalt is a relatively rare silver-gray metal. Compounds of cobalt are used as pigments in enamels, glazes, and paints, and in glassmaking, pottery, and photography. Cobalt dust is irritating to the mucosa of the eyes and mouth, and may cause skin allergies, coughing, wheezing, and dyspnea. Severe exposure by inhalation may cause pulmonary fibrosis. Ingestion may cause vomiting, diarrhea, and a sensation of warmth.
Copper	Copper is a metal used as an alloy in brass and bronze, as a component in some solders, in pigments such as emerald green, and as a salt in the lithographic process. The salts are irritating to the skin, eyes, and mucous membranes. The inhalation of the metal fumes produced at high temperature, such as from welding, may cause metal fume fever, nasal ulcers, and respiratory irritation. Ingestion of copper salts may cause vomiting, diarrhea, hemorrhagic gastritis, and excessive salivation. The chronic accumulation of copper in the body is rare and occurs in the progressive and sometimes fatal autosomal recessive condition called Wilson's disease (hepatolenticular degeneration).
Lead	Lead is a soft blue-gray metal with a low melting point, used by artists as an ingredient in solder, in the creation of leaded glass, and as a component in pigments, ceramic glazes, enameling, and glassblowing. it serves no useful purpose in the body and is a hemotoxin as well as being toxic to nerves, kidneys, and gastrointestinal tract. At low concentrations symptoms of lassitude and sleep disturbance develop, which later progress to abdominal pain, mental confusion, anemia, paralysis, renal failure, convulsions, coma, and death as concentrations increase.
Manganese	Manganese is a soft gray metal used in the manufacture of some paints, varnishes, dyes, and inks, and is a component of coloring agents used in the manufacture of some glass and ceramics. It is mildly irritating to mucous membranes in the dust or fume state. Chronic exposure by inhalation may lead to nervous system toxicity manifested as confusion, aggression, hallucinations, speech disorders, and gait disturbance, progressing to a condition which may be indistinguishable from Parkinson's disease.
Mercury	Inorganic mercury is a silver liquid at room temperature. It is used in gold, silver, and bronze plating, photography, paints, and pigments. Chronic inhalation of the vapor may cause psychosis, muscle tremors, and weight loss. Acute exposure may cause respiratory tract inflammation. Ingestion of organic mercury or mercury salts may cause similar symptoms plus blindness, deafness, gait disturbance, renal toxicity, and brain damage to children whose mothers were exposed during pregnancy.
Nickel	Nickel is a hard silver metal often alloyed with copper, aluminum, and iron. It is a component of some enamels, ceramics, and glass. It may cause skin allergies and the probability of the salts causing nasal and lung cancer has been mentioned.
Silver	Silver is a soft metal used to make jewelry and is a component of some solders, photographic film, inks, dyes, pigments, and ceramics. The dust of silver salts is an irritant to skin and mucous membranes. Permanent pigmentation may result in tattoos from imbedded particles in the skin, or diffusely, from chronic ingestion, producing the condition argyria.
Tin	Tin is a soft metal used to make alloys of many metals, and in the production of ceramics and pigments. Tin compounds may burn the skin and some organic compounds are very toxic to the nervous system causing headache, vomiting, weakness, and paralysis.
Titanium	Titanium is a dark gray metal used to produce white pigments used in ceramics, paints, and varnishes. Titanium compounds are practically nontoxic to humans except for the tetrachloride, which is quite an irritant to skin and mucous membranes.

continues

Table 60.1.   *Continued*

I. Metals	
Zinc	Zinc oxide is used to produce a white pigment for paints, ceramics, lacquers, and varnishes. It may cause skin irritation and the fumes may cause metal fume fever if inhaled, although high temperatures are required for fume formation.

II. Woods	
Cedar, Western Red (*Thuja plicata*)	Western red cedar may cause skin allergies, asthma, mucosal irritation (manifested as rhinitis and conjunctivitis), and gastrointestinal symptoms.
Cocobolo (*Dalbergia retusa*)	Cocobolo may cause a contact dermatitis from finished products such as musical instruments. It is also a skin and mucous membrane irritant and may cause allergies.
Ebony (*Diospyros*) Mahogany (*Kaya ivorensis, Swietenia macrophylla*) Rosewood (*Dalbergia nigra* and *latifolia*) Teak (*Tectona grandis*)	These woods may all cause skin allergies, irritation, and sometimes asthma, especially when exposure to fine sawdust occurs.
Satinwood (*Fagara flava, Chloroxylon swietenia*) Boxwood (*Gonioma kamassi*) Ipe (*Tabebuia ipe*)	These woods are actually toxic when absorbed by ingestion or inhalation and may cause headaches, vomiting, dyspnea, and bradycardia. The active principles are generally alkaloids. Papular eruptions and weeping with crusting may occur after a few hours of skin contact with ipe sawdust.

III. Dusts	
Agate, granite, jasper, marble, pumice, soapstone, silica flour	These minerals contain silica. Large amounts of free silica dust may cause silicosis, a progressive pulmonary disease. This disease causes pulmonary destruction, fibrosis, and dyspnea, and may cause death with exposure to high concentrations or for prolonged periods.
Greenstone, serpentine, soapstone	These minerals may contain asbestos fibers which may cause lung cancer, gastrointestinal cancer, or mesothelioma, particularly if exposure is complicated by heavy cigarette smoking.

IV. Chemicals	
Acids and alkali	All acids and alkali are caustic to skin and mucous membranes, and can cause severe burns upon exposure. Many of these chemicals are used in photography and lithography. Hydrofluoric acid is used to etch glass and deserves special comment because its toxic effect to tissue may not be manifest for several hours after skin contact. This acid can penetrate quite deeply into tissue with little or no apparent surface injury, only to result later in severe necrosis of tissue and bone. Washing the exposed skin surface with copious amounts of water may not be sufficient, and all cases of hydrofluoric acid burns should be treated by a knowledgeable physician.
Plastics	Toxicity to plastics may result from inhalation or ingestion of the monomer precursors or toxic additives released during the process of polymerization, or from vapors liberated during shaping and molding by the application of heat. Heat application may cause chemical decomposition and complex chemical reactions, producing toxic gases such as hydrogen cyanide, phosgene, formaldehyde, carbon monoxide, and isocyanates.
Acrylics	Acrylics decompose at 750°F, producing the highly toxic monomer, methylmethacrylate. Chlorinated acrylics may yield phosgene, hydrochloric acid, and carbon monoxide at high temperatures. Acrylic paints owe most of their toxicity to the pigments and solvents that they contain and under normal use are no more toxic than oil based paints.
Epoxides	Epoxides are very reactive cyclic ethers used as plasticizers. Many epoxides are mutagenic and carcinogenic. Acute exposures may cause blisters, burns, dermatitis, vomiting, bronchitis, and pulmonary edema.
Epoxy	Epoxy is used to bond materials together and usually at the time of use the resin is mixed with a hardener. The epoxy solvents may cause dermatitis, and the resins may contain plasticizers, such as dibutylphthalate and tricresyl phosphate, which are strong skin irritants. Curing agents, such as the highly alkaline polyamines (e.g., metaphenylene-diamine), and phthalic anhydride, are the most frequent causes of asthma and dermatitis. Aromatic amines, such as pyridine and piperidine, may cause liver and kidney damage.
Foams	Plastic foams may be produced or molded by artists. The foams are often polymers of diisocyanate, either toluene (TDI), or diphenylmethane (MDI). Both are skin irritants and TDI can cause asthma. Artists using heat to mold, cut, or sculpt rigid urethane foams may be exposed to toxic byproducts including hydrogen cyanide.
Peroxide	Peroxides are often used as catalysts to initiate polymerization. Sculptors who may be making their own polymers should regard them as unstable explosives if they are used in relatively concentrated formulations. They may cause blisters, bleaching, and burning of the skin. Inhalation may result in bronchitis or pulmonary edema.
Styrene	Styrene is a colorless oily liquid that polymerizes to form a plastic, polystyrene. Styrene vapors are strong skin irritants and acute exposure to high concentrations may cause narcosis, cramps, and respiratory paralysis resulting in death.

continues

Table 60.1. *Continued*

IV. Chemicals

Vinyls	The monomers used to produce polyvinyl chloride (PVC) esters, alcohols, and ethers, are strong irritants. Vinyl chloride causes hepatic angiosarcoma, and destruction of bone at the distal phalanges, acroosteolysis. As with all plastics containing chlorine, exposure to high temperature may produce hydrochloric acid and phosgene. Phosgene is a gas capable of penetrating into the alveoli without causing any immediately noticeable discomfort. It decomposes to hydrochloric acid and carbon dioxide in the presence of water, causing pulmonary inflammation and edema, which may not be symptomatic until hours after the exposure.
Benzene (C_6H_6)	Benzene (benzol) has been linked to leukemia in humans and should not be used by artists in any concentration. Acute exposure may cause headaches, confusions, coma, and death. Chronic exposure may cause aplastic anemia and chromosomal aberrations. Artists should read labels carefully, as benzene may be a component of a mixture of organic solvents.
Turpentine	Turpentine is a colorless, volatile liquid formed by distillation of the resin from pine trees. The vapors are irritating to the mucosa of the respiratory tract. It is also irritating to the eyes, and may cause corneal burns if splashed. Skin allergies may develop. Inhalation may result in headache, excitement, confusion, convulsions, coma, and death. Chronic exposure may lead to kidney damage, bladder damage, and a susceptibility to pneumonia.
Methanol (CH_3OH)	Methanol, or wood alcohol, should not be used by artists in poorly ventilated spaces. It is rapidly absorbed by inhalation and by skin exposure. It may be an ingredient of paint and varnish removers, wood stains, dyes, and enamels. It may cause blindness and acidosis from acute exposure, particularly if ingested.
Carbon tetrachloride (CCl_4)	Carbon tetrachloride was formerly used as a solvent for dry cleaning, but is found in some solvents for oils, lacquers, and varnishes. It is quite volatile and can be absorbed by inhalation and skin exposure. It is a potent liver and kidney toxin. Absorption may cause drowsiness, headache, gastrointestinal disturbances, and abdominal pain, besides the organ toxicity mentioned above.
Methyl butyl ketone ($CH_3COCH_2CH_2CH_2CH_3$)	Methyl butyl ketone may be found as a component in a solvent mixture used in photo processes. Besides causing a scaly, fissured dermatitis, exposure to high concentrations may result in narcosis, headache, nausea, loss of consciousness, and peripheral neuropathy.
Methyl cellosolve acetate ($CH_3OCH_2CH_2OOCH_3$)	Methyl cellosolve acetate is used as a solvent for resins, lacquers, varnishes, dyes, and inks. The vapors may cause blurred vision due to corneal clouding, and acute absorption can cause narcosis, pulmonary edema, kidney damage, and liver damage. A toxic encephalitis can develop which may be difficult to distinguish from viral or other infectious causes.
Methylene chloride (CH_2Cl_2)	Methylene chloride is used as a paint stripper. Besides the usual toxicity that solvents have on the nervous system, methylene chloride produces additional toxicity because it is metabolized by the body to yield carbon monoxide. Thus, acute exposure may precipitate symptoms of chest pain and may cause myocardial infarction in individuals with atherosclerotic heart disease.

V. Physical hazards

Ultraviolet radiation	Ultraviolet radiation is produced during arc welding and can react with oxygen to produce ozone. Ozone is irritating to the respiratory passages. The radiation can physically damage the epithelial surface of the cornea to produce a painful condition, "welder's flash." Prolonged exposure to ultraviolet radiation may cause skin burns.
Infrared radiation	Infrared radiation is emitted by all matter and is sensed by humans as heat. The lens of the eye is susceptible to cataract formation from chronic exposure to infrared radiation at wavelengths below 1400 nm. This is sometimes called glassblower's or furnaceman's cataract because of the high prevalence of this finding among persons in those occupations. The cataract formation requires approximately 10–15 years of exposure.
Noise	We are surrounded by sound constantly. Noise has been described as any unwanted sound. What we hear is due to rapid oscillations of atmospheric pressure between the frequencies of 50 Hz and 20,000 Hz. The intensity of the pressure changes, or sound pressure level, is damaging to the human ear above 85 dB. Chronic exposure to noise at or above that level results in hearing loss to frequencies generally between 4000 and 8000 Hz. Artists operating machinery such as grinders, drills, and saws should protect their ears from high level sound pressure.

zymes and interfere with normal metabolism because of their reactivity in the ionized state and their ability to combine with protein anions. Metals such as chromium, arsenic, and nickel have been associated with lung and skin cancers. These and other metals and their salts may cause skin sensitization and allergies. Heavy metals are generally nephrotoxic and neurotoxic.

Toxicity of the metals in pigments is generally of a chronic type among artists. Pigments are present in pastels and acrylics

also, so similar risks may be present with these materials. Artists are exposed at low levels and the accumulation of metals over the course of 20–30 years may finally manifest itself as irritability, renal damage, neuropathy, cancer, gastrointestinal problems, reproductive problems, and sleep disturbance. Some metals such as lead and mercury may pose reproductive hazards with the potential to cause birth defects and retardation. These hazards are of great concern where the artist's studio is in the home and children have free access to the studio. The airborne dusts and vapors produced in the studio can be transferred to the other rooms in the home via the heating or cooling system to expose other members of the family. With the advent of energy-efficient construction, little to no outside makeup air can result in significant 24-hour exposures.

Large quantities of solvents are used by artists, who often use them in open containers such as cups, jars, cans. This results in evaporative losses, which can create significant air concentrations that are hazardous, particularly in confined, poorly ventilated spaces. Inhalation of solvent vapors is the most likely type of exposure that may cause adverse health effects to painters. This is of more concern if the artist is using solvents containing benzene or hexane. Inhalation is the most common route of entry of solvents, although skin absorption may be significant when cleaning brushes. Ingestion of solvents occurs to a lesser extent but is likely to occur if the artist eats in the studio or has the habit of pointing the tips of the brushes with his lips. Solvents are often not used in pure forms, but as components in mixtures.

The use of alcohol may potentiate the toxic effects of solvents, and nearly all solvents are flammable. Most solvents share common effects on the nervous system because of their lipid solubility and sequestration in the brain and other fatty tissues. Some owe their major toxicity to metabolites that are formed in the body rather than to their parent forms. Examples are methanol and methylene chloride, which are metabolized to formaldehyde and formic acid, and carbon monoxide, respectively. An atmosphere that is saturated with solvent vapors may acutely cause headache, narcosis, dizziness, euphoria, and nausea. Memory loss and peripheral neuropathy may occur if exposure becomes chronic.

Solvent exposure is probably the single most hazardous feature of arts and crafts work. Efforts to improve ventilation and minimize exposure to solvents will provide the greatest benefit for optimizing the health of artists.

Increased death rates due to cancer of all sites combined and arteriosclerotic heart disease have been reported to be significantly elevated among painters in a proportional mortality study by Miller et al. (1986) of artists listed in the obituaries in *Who's Who in American Art*, published between 1940 and 1969. Miller et al. report an excess proportion of deaths due to cancer of the rectum, lung, and breast among women artists. Leukemia, prostate, bladder, kidney, brain, and colon cancer excesses were observed among artists when compared with the expected proportions based on rates for the general U.S. population. A greater than twofold excess for bladder cancer mortality and for leukemia was observed among painters. A case-comparison study adjusted for smoking revealed a relative risk of 2.5, and there was a significant increase in risk with increasing duration of employment as a painter. Details of exposure were not available, so this study is not conclusive but indicates a need for more detailed and controlled research concerning this group. Claude et al. (1988) reported similar odds ratios for bladder cancer associated with occupation as artists.

Sculpture, Ceramics, and Pottery Making

Sculptors working with stone face three major risks; the risk of silicosis due to inhalation of free silica contained in stones, e.g., granite and slate; the risk of asbestos-caused disease, e.g., mesothelioma, lung, and gastrointestinal cancer, from asbestos fibers in serpentine stone, e.g., soapstone; and the risk of vascular disease of the extremities, e.g., Raynaud's phenomenon,

due to segmental vibration from the use of hand power tools, e.g., pneumatic drills.

Silica dust may be produced during grinding and polishing stone or pottery. The dust settles in the alveoli, where it may be consumed by macrophages. The macrophages are destroyed, releasing proteolytic enzymes and other biologically active products that incite an inflammatory response and the migration of more macrophages. The macrophages phagocytose the free silica and the cycle repeats itself. This process eventually causes tissue destruction, deposition of collagen, and impedance of gas transport across the alveolar membranes. The disease, silicosis, is progressive, resulting in fibrosis, dyspnea, and possibly death. Most studios are dusty and there is a great danger of silicosis from inhalation of fine dusts generated from feldspar- and flint-containing glazes and silica flour. Silicosis has been termed ''potter's rot'' due to the high prevalence of the disease among potters in years past.

Asbestos dust may arise from frayed gloves or aprons, insulation around kilns, French chalk used to dust lithographic plates, talc, instant papier mâché, welding curtains, vermiculite dust, and serpentine stones such as soapstone and African wonderstone. Asbestos dust also penetrates deep into the lungs, where it causes destruction of macrophages trying to engulf fibers that are physically too large for the cell. High concentrations of dust can cause a fibrotic disease, asbestosis.

Asbestosis is not likely to be a disease of artists because their exposure is at a low level. However, the asbestos fibers contribute to the development of lung cancer, gastrointestinal cancer, and mesothelioma. The mechanism is not understood but there is some speculation that the fibers may carry carcinogenic contaminants or act as promoters. The risk of lung cancer is increased 80-fold if asbestos exposure is accompanied by cigarette smoking. Asbestos-related disease has occurred in members of the families of asbestos workers who took dust-contaminated clothing home. As little as 1–3 months of exposure may be sufficient to produce mesothelioma, although there is insufficient evidence to support this claim unequivocally.

Sculptors working with wood may be at increased risk of nasal adenocarcinoma due to chronic inhalation of fine wood dust. No specific wood can be incriminated, but the epidemiologic evidence indicates a greater risk from hardwoods. Nasal carcinoma among woodworkers has been reported from France, Sweden, Austria, the United States, Canada, Germany, and several other countries.

Some woods containing alkaloids may cause systemic symptoms of nausea, vomiting, headache, and dyspnea. Many woods are irritants that cause skin allergies and asthma. The dusts produced from sawing and sanding woods may be composed of respirable particles capable of penetrating deep into the lungs. The particles may be contaminated by chemicals which have been applied to woods such as pesticides and preservatives. In addition, woods may contain biologically active chemicals such as resins, alkaloids, oils, aldehydes, quinones, and proteins. Many of the proteins may be derived from fungi in the form of spores or hyphae. These proteins may cause pulmonary disease manifested by chills, fever, cough, headache, dermatitis, and increasing dyspnea. Systemic effects due to the active chemicals may cause irritation and sensitization of the skin, asthma, vomiting, headaches, dyspnea, and bradycardia.

Sculptors working with metal may be exposed to heavy metal fumes containing lead, cadmium, or copper, if the source of their metal is scrap iron or steel that has been painted to prevent corrosion. The pigments of corrosion-resistant paints often contain heavy metals. The metal fumes are released during arc welding or cutting with a torch. Welding creates its own specific hazards of ultraviolet radiation and the production of ozone and nitrogen oxides.

Potters are exposed to many heavy metals that are components of the pigments or glazes that they use. Lead toxicity is a particular problem as it is a component of lead frits. Other metals that may pose a hazard to potters include chromium, manganese, and cadmium. The toxicity of each has been described above. The use of kilns may release gases such as carbon monoxide, sulfur dioxide, chlorine, and metal fumes.

Glassblowing, Stained Glass, and Enameling

The glassblower's most frequent hazard is heat. It is not unusual to find glassblowers with scars on their arms and hands from burns. They often use asbestos gloves or aprons and this may pose a significant hazard if the fibers are frayed, become airborne, and are inhaled. The infrared radiation emitted from the furnace may contribute to cataract formation. If grinding operations are performed, there may be a risk of silicosis or heavy metal toxicity due to inhalation of the dust. Hydrofluoric acid burns may result if the glass is also etched.

Stained glass work presents a hazard of lead poisoning due to inhalation of lead dust from cutting or sanding the lead strips, or from vaporized lead released during soldering. The acid flux used in the soldering process may contain zinc chloride, which is a strong irritant capable of causing pulmonary edema if the fumes are inhaled when heated. Organic fluxes release decomposition products, such as formaldehyde. Besides the irritant effect of formaldehyde, sensitization may develop, resulting in allergic reactions to the many consumer products containing formaldehyde. Such products include formica countertops, furniture made from particle board, and sizing in permanent press clothing.

The enamels contain metals such as lead, antimony, and zirconium in the first coat. The colors may have pigments based on nickel, chromium, and heavy metals.

Lithography, Photography, and Printmaking

A multitude of reactive chemicals pose hazards for this group of artists. It is the reactivity of the chemicals that allows these artists to produce the effects desired in their works. The pigments used in lithography and printmaking are relatively concentrated forms. It is a messy job requiring the frequent use of solvents with all their attendant hazards. Some solvents contain benzene, e.g., Red Devil Paint and Varnish Remover (50% benzene), and the ingredients may not be listed on the container. Thus, artists should buy generic products or request a material safety data sheet (MSDS) or a list of ingredients when purchasing solvents, aerosols, inks, dyes, or other chemicals.

Acids are used in lithography, and photography, e.g., phosphoric acid and nitric acid, and may cause the release of noxious vapors or gases when mixed with other chemicals, e.g., bleaches. Hydrochloric acid releases chlorine gas when Dutch Mordant is first made. Brown nitrogen oxide vapors are released from the nitric acid used for etching. When dusting plates the talc and French chalk may contain and release up to 40% asbestos fibers.

The intensifiers used in the photographic processes may contain corrosive chromates or mercury compounds. Chemical reducers may release cyanide or chlorine gas; the hardeners and stabilizers contain formaldehyde, and the negative cleaners are often chlorinated hydrocarbons.

The greatest hazard occurs during the pouring and preparation of the various baths needed for photographic processing, with part of the hazard being the fact that they are contained in wide, shallow containers. These containers present a large surface area for evaporative losses. Since great efforts are made to control unwanted light, these processes are generally done in small, unventilated, dark rooms. The reduced lighting, or sometimes no lighting, creates an opportunity for accidental immersion of hands in caustic baths or sensitizing baths, e.g., paraphenylenediamine-containing baths. Absorption of chemicals takes place by inhalation and percutaneous absorption. Rubber gloves should always be used, combined with carefully designed exhaust ventilation.

EVALUATING POTENTIAL HEALTH HAZARDS

The American Conference of Governmental Industrial Hygienists (ACGIH) publishes Threshold Limit Values (TLVs) for materials used in the workplace. The TLVs are defined as either ceiling limits (C) or time-weighted averages (TWAs). They are concentrations of the material in air that should not be exceeded at anytime (C) or an average concentration that should not be exceeded over a specific period of time, usually 8 hours (TWA). They are intended to serve as guidelines, and theoretically a worker with an exposure within the limits would suffer no adverse effects from such an exposure 40 hours weekly over the course of a lifetime. Over the years the TLVs have been reduced as more information regarding the toxic effects of low level exposure has been documented.

The Occupational Safety and Health Administration (OSHA) adopted a number of the TLVs in the early 1970s as Permissible Exposure Levels (PELs). For a number of substances, standards have been written into law, whereby the PEL must not be exceeded. The National Institute of Occupational Safety and Health (NIOSH) periodically reviews existing PELs and materials for which PELs are lacking and recommends to OSHA revised standards that should be set. The process is lengthy and controversial. Opposition to new standards usually comes from industry, while support for standards generally comes from organized labor. The decision regarding what a standard should be is influenced by scientific evidence and opinion, economic impact, legal opinion, and politics.

The artist at work in the studio should strive to reduce exposure to below the published TLVs and PELs. The industrial hygienist can be of great help in this regard by collecting air samples and measuring the ambient concentrations in the air by analytical techniques in the laboratory.

To monitor for dusts or fumes, e.g., asbestos and silica, the industrial hygienist will collect his samples through a special filter using an open face cassette. Total dusts can be quantified by weight, chemical analysis, light microscopy, and electron microscopy. Respirable dusts can be collected through a cyclone assembly, which simulates the deposition of particles in the lung. Particles above a certain size and weight are removed by centrifugal force, allowing only respirable size particles to be collected and quantified.

To monitor for gases and vapors released from solvents, paints, or welding, spot checks can be made using color indicator tubes. These tubes are not very accurate and give only a crude estimation of concentration and identity (some chemicals may give false readings or interfere with the test). A more accurate, but more expensive, means of monitoring is by the continuous sampling of the atmosphere using charcoal tubes, impingers or bubblers, gas badges, or direct reading monitors. The material is adsorbed onto the charcoal, trapped within the solvent in the impinger, or adsorbed in the gas badge. In the laboratory, the material is desorbed and analyzed using sophisticated analytical techniques, i.e., gas or liquid chromatography, mass spectroscopy, atomic absorption, or emission spectroscopy.

In the event of acute exposure causing immediate symptoms, the patient should seek out a well-ventilated area, e.g., outdoors, and should contact the poison control center. Splashes should be diluted thoroughly with copious amounts of water. There should be a strict refrain from eating or drinking in the studio or other location where hazardous materials are in use.

PREVENTION AND CONTROL OF POTENTIAL HEALTH HAZARDS

The first step toward preventing health hazard risks from causing damage is for the artist to become informed about the materials used in the arts and crafts. An inventory of the materials should be maintained along with a description of the adverse effects of their components and the means that should be taken to use the materials safely.

Specifically, the artist should know the chemical or generic name of the materials, the appearance and odor, the permissible exposure level (PEL), and the routes of absorption and toxicity, e.g., ingestion, percutaneous absorption, inhalation. The physical and mental effects that may be produced from excessive exposure should be known.

Solvents should be used in well-ventilated rooms, and containers should not be left open to the atmosphere when not in use.

Simple exhaust ventilation can be installed by running a swamp cooler in reverse. Ventilation should draw fresh air down past the breathing zone before contacting solvent or gas sources and then exit the exhaust system. Vapors, gases, and fumes should not be drawn into the breathing zone on the way out the exhaust system.

Personal protective devices should be used when necessary, but only when work practices and engineering controls have been tried first. Rubber gloves and respirators are examples. Respirators must be chosen properly to ensure that they are designed to protect users from the materials they may be exposed to. A dust respirator is of no use for a chemical exposure. Respirators also must be properly fitted to the user's face. Generally speaking, they do not offer protection over beards.

The artist should substitute less toxic materials whenever possible. The physician can serve as a valuable resource and influence for the artist by alerting the artist patient to potential hazards and providing guidelines for prevention. The treating physician should always inquire about occupation and hobbies, and when arts and crafts are mentioned, the possibility that presenting symptoms may be related to some of the potential hazards mentioned here should be explored.

SUGGESTED READINGS

Bird TS, Wallace DM, Labbe RF. The porphyria, plumbism, pottery puzzle. JAMA 1982;247:813–814.

Braun SR, Tsiatis A. Pulmonary abnormalities in art glassblowers. J Occup Med 1979;21:487–489.

Claude JC, Frentzel-Beyme RR, Kunze E. Occupation and risk of cancer of the lower urinary tract among men. A case control study. Int J Cancer 1988;41:371–379.

Conklin BR. Environmental hazards to elderly artists [Letter]. JAMA 1984;252:3130.

Eckardt RE, Hindin R. The health hazards of plastics. J Occup Med 1973;15:808–819.

Finkel AJ, Hamilton A, Hardy HL. Hamilton and Hardy's Industrial Toxicology. 4th ed. Littleton, MA: John Wright, 1983.

Fischbein A, Wallace J, Anderson KE, Sassa S, Kon S, Rohl AN, Kappas A. Lead poisoning in an art conservator. JAMA 1982;247:2007–2009.

Glasbrenner K. Maladies may be linked to artists' materials [Editorial]. JAMA 1984;251:1391–1395.

Hart C. Art hazards: an overview for sanitarians and hygienists. J Environ Health 1987;49:282–287.

Key MM, Henschel AF, Butler J, Ligo RN, Tabershaw IR, Ede L. Occupational diseases: a guide to their recognition. DHEW (NIOSH) Publication No. 77-181. U.S. Department of Health, Education, and Welfare. Public Health Service. Washington, DC: GPO, 1977.

Lee TC. Van Gogh's vision: digitalis intoxication? JAMA 1981;245:727–729.

Mattison DR, ed. Reproductive toxicology. (Progress in clinical and biological research; vol 117). New York: Alan R. Liss, 1983.

McCann M. The impact of hazards in art on female workers. Prev Med 1978;7:338–348.

McCann, M. Artist beware. New York: Watson-Guptill Publications, 1969.

McCunney RJ, Russo PK, Doyle JR. Occupational illness in the arts. Am Fam Phys 1987;36:145–153.

Miller BA, Silverman DT, Hoover RN, Blair A. Cancer risk among artistic painters. Am J Ind Med 1986;9:281–287.

Morgan WKC, Seaton A. Occupational Lung Diseases. 2nd ed. Philadelphia: WB Saunders, 1984.

Pedersen LM, Permin H. Rheumatic disease, heavy-metal pigments, and the great masters. Lancet 1988;1:1267–1269.

Proctor NH, Hughes JP. Chemical Hazards of the Workplace. Philadelphia: JB Lippincott, 1978.

Ramazzini B. Diseases of workers. New York: Hafner Publishing Company, 1964.

Siedlecki, JT. Potential health hazards of materials used by artists and sculptors. JAMA 1968;204:1176–1180.

U.S. Congress, Office of Technology Assessment. Reproductive health hazards in the workplace. Washington, DC: U.S. Government Printing Office, OTA-BA-266, 1985.

Waller JA, Whitehead L, Donnelly K, Gallagher J, ed. Health hazards in the arts: Proceedings of 1977 Vermont workshops. Burlington: University of Vermont, 1977.

Wills JH. Nasal carcinoma in woodworkers: a review. J Occup Med 1982;24:526–530.

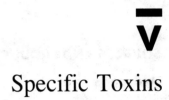

Specific Toxins

61

Hydrogen Cyanide and Inorganic Cyanide Salts

Steven C. Curry, M.D.

SOURCES AND PRODUCTION

Hydrogen Cyanide

Hydrogen cyanide (HCN) has a boiling point of 27.7°C, allowing it to be found as a gas or liquid in the workplace (Table 61.1). As a gas, it is explosive, colorless, and has a faint odor that is variously described as bitter almonds, sweet, pungent, or metallic. Liquid HCN is a colorless or a bluish-white solution that has a similar odor due to the release of HCN gas into surrounding air. While most persons are able to smell HCN, the minority identify it as being similar to bitter almonds. Furthermore, wide individual variations in odor threshold and rapid olfactory fatigue make it very possible for an entire group of persons to be exposed to toxic concentrations of HCN without anyone noticing any abnormal odor (1–3).

The main method used in manufacturing HCN in the United States involves reacting ammonia and methane in controlled conditions. HCN is also manufactured by reacting sodium carbonate with coke-oven gas, by reacting cyanide salts with mineral acids, by reacting ammonia with air and natural gas, and from the decomposition of formamide (4).

HCN is sold as a gas, is available as technical grade liquids in concentrations of 5%, 10%, and 96–99.5%, or is sold as a 2% USP grade solution. It is sold or transported in bottles, drums, cylinders, and tanks. Almost all grades of HCN contain a stabilizer such as phosphoric acid to prevent decomposition and explosion. Impure or unstabilized HCN can undergo spontaneous exothermic polymerization with explosive violence (4).

Table 61.1. Chemical and Physical Properties of Hydrogen Cyanide

Molecular formula	HCN
Atomic weight	27.03
Physical form	Liquid or gas
Boiling point	27.7°C for a 96% solution
Freezing point	−16.8° for a 96% solution
Color	Colorless to tint of blue
Odor	Variously described as bitter almond, metallic, sweet; not detectable by many persons, with wide variation in odor threshold
Water solubility	Very miscible in water
Density	0.7 g/ml for a 96% solution
Vapor density	0.93 (air = 1)
Vapor pressure	807 mm Hg
Flashpoint	−17.8°C (closed cup)
Lower explosive limit	6% by volume in air
Upper explosive limit	41% by volume in air
pKa	9.3 at 25°C
1 mg HCN/m^3	0.906 ppm
1 ppm HCN	1.14 mg/m^3 as HCN, or 1.06 mg/m^3 as CN

Inorganic Cyanide Salts

A number of inorganic cyanide salts are commercially available, and the more commonly used ones are summarized in Table 61.2. Sodium, potassium, and calcium cyanide account for the majority of industrial consumption (4) and are described below in more detail.

Sodium and potassium cyanide are crystalline, white solids at room temperature. The three main methods of commercial production are reacting sodium or potassium carbonate with carbon and ammonia, reacting HCN with sodium or potassium hydroxide, or using a process involving coke-oven gas (4, 5).

Both NaCN and KCN are sold as powders, flakes, granules, pillow-shaped 1-ounce (28 grams) blocks, or pellets or as 30% aqueous solutions. On the commercial scale, solid NaCN and KCN are packed in steel or fiber drums before shipping. Aqueous solutions are shipped in tanks by truck or rail (4).

Calcium cyanide [$Ca(CN)_2$] is manufactured by heating calcium cyanamide with a source of carbon in electric furnaces at temperatures greater than 1000°C. Countries accounting for the majority of $Ca(CN)_2$ production include South Africa, Germany, and Canada. $Ca(CN)_2$ is sold on the commercial scale as flakes or blocks (4, 5).

SITES, INDUSTRIES, AND BUSINESSES ASSOCIATED WITH EXPOSURES

Hydrogen cyanide and inorganic cyanide salts are used in a wide variety of commercial processes. The National Institute of Occupational Safety and Health (NIOSH) estimates that 20,000 workers are exposed daily to NaCN alone (4). When one considers the plethora of cyanogenic compounds found in industry, tens of thousands of workers potentially come in contact with cyanide every working day.

HCN Formation from Cyanide Salts

The release of excessive amounts of HCN gas into the breathing zone of workers can result in collapse and death within seconds to minutes. While workers frequently are aware of the potential danger when using liquid or gaseous HCN, they typically are unaware of the great potential for formation of lethal quantities of HCN from processes utilizing cyanide salts.

When most inorganic cyanide salts come in contact with mineral acids, large quantities of HCN are formed and are released into the atmosphere. Using NaCN and hydrochloric acid as an example:

$$NaCN + HCl \longrightarrow HCN + NaCl$$

Two common scenarios for generation of HCN include the accidental mixing of acid and cyanide solutions in electroplating baths and the accidental pouring of cyanide waste solutions into acid waste containers or into other waste solutions with pHs below 10.5–11.

Table 61.2. Chemical and Physical Properties of Selected Cyanide Salts

Compound	Molecular Formula	CAS #	Atomic Weight	RTECS #	Synonyms	Comments
Ammonium cyanide	NH_4CN	12211-52-8	44.1			Very soluble in cold H_2O; decomposes at 36°C to form HCN and NH_3
Barium cyanide	$Ba(CN)_2$	542-62-1	189.4	CQ8785000	Barium dicyanide; UN 1565 (DOT)	Very soluble in H_2O
Cadmium cyanide	$Cd(CN)_2$	542-83-6	164.5			Solubility in H_2O 1.7 g/100 ml at 15°C
Calcium cyanide	$Ca(CN)_2$	592-01-8	92.1	EW0700000	Calccyanide; UN1575 (DOT)	Releases HCN in H_2O or humid air
Copper(I) cyanide	CuCN	544-92-3	89.6	GL7150000	Cuprous cyanide	Almost insoluble in H_2O; decomposed by H_2NO_3
Copper(II) cyanide	$Cu(CN)_2$	14763-77-0	115.6	GL7175000	Cupric cyanide; copper cyanamide; UN 1587 (DOT)	Insoluble in H_2O
Gold(I) cyanide	AuCN	506-65-0	223		Aurous cyanide; gold monocyanide	Insoluble in H_2O or dilute acids; releases HCN when heated in HCl; dissolved by aqua regia; ignition causes formation of metallic gold and CN
Gold(II) cyanide	$Au(CN)_2$	535-37-5	275.05		Auric cyanide; gold tricyanide	Usually found as trihydrate $Au(CN)_2(H_2O)_3$ with a molecular weight of 329.1; very soluble in H_2O; decomposes at 50°C
Lead cyanide	$Pb(CN)_2$	592-05-2	259.2	OG0175000	C.I. pigment yellow 48; UN 1620 (DOT)	Slightly soluble in cold H_2O; soluble in hot H_2O
Mercury(II) cyanide	$Hg(CN)_2$	592-04-1	252.6	OW1515000	Mercuric cyanide; cianurina; UN 1636 (DOT)	Solubility in cold H_2O of 9.3 g/100 ml
Potassium cyanide	KCN	151-50-8	65.1	TS8750000	Cyanide of potassium; UN 1680 (DOT)	Solubility in cold H_2O of 50 g/100 ml; yields HCN on contact with H_2O or acids
Potassium cyanoaurite	$K[Au(CN)_2]$	13967-50-5	288.1		Gold potassium cyanide; potassium aurocyanide; potassium dicyanoaurate (I); aurate (1-), bis(cyano-C-), potassium	Less HCN liberated from aqueous or weakly acidic solutions than with other water-soluble salts
Silver cyanide	AgCN	506-64-9	133.9	VW3850000	UN1684 (DOT)	Almost insoluble in H_2O and dilute acid, *but* dilute HCl will cause formation of HCN and $AgCl_2$
Sodium cyanide	NaCN	143-33-9	49.0	VZ7525000	Cyanide of sodium	Solubility in cold H_2O of 48 g/100 ml; yields HCN on contact with water or dilute acids
Sodium cyanoaurite	$Na[Au(CN)_2]$	15280-09-8	272.0		Gold sodium cyanide; sodium dicyanoaurate (I); aurate(1-), bis(cyano-C)-, sodium	Less HCN liberated from aqueous and weakly acidic solutions than with other salts
Zinc cyanide	$Zn(CN)_2$	557-21-1	117.4	ZH1575000	Zinc dicyanide	Insoluble in H_2O; readily releases HCN on contact with mineral acids

What is even less recognized by workers is the potential for generation of large quantities of HCN simply from mixing water-soluble cyanide salts with water. For example, NaCN dissolves in water according to the following equilibrium:

$$NaCN <\text{----}> Na^+ + CN^-$$

Sodium cyanide is relatively soluble in water, and large quantities of free CN^- ions are formed. However, the pK_a of HCN is relatively high at 9.3. Therefore, CN^- splits water to form HCN according to the following reaction:

$$CN^- + H_2O <\text{----}> HCN + OH^-$$

In the case of NaCN, the entire reaction becomes:

$$NaCN + H_2O <\text{----}> HCN + NaOH$$

The percentage of cyanide converted to HCN in aqueous solutions of cyanide salts is dependent on the pH of the solution as illustrated in Figure 61.1. Hydrogen cyanide's pK_a of 9.3 makes it necessary for pHs to be well above 10.5–11 to prevent formation and release of significant quantities of HCN.

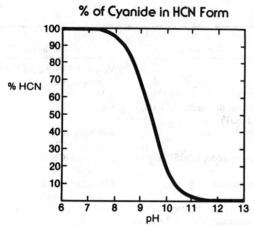

% of Cyanide in HCN Form

Figure 61.1.   Percentage of cyanide present as HCN in an aqueous solution of a cyanide salt is dependent on the pH of the solution. The pK_a of HCN is 9.3.

An employee who does nothing but add a cyanide salt to pure water (pH 7) or to tap water (pH 5–7) can initially cause the generation of lethal quantities of HCN before enough hydroxide (e.g., NaOH) is formed to raise pH and limit HCN formation. Simply using a stream of water to clean up a spill of cyanide salts (e.g., rinsing them into a drain or mopping the floor) can result in serious poisonings and fatalities. Poisonings and deaths from the inhalation or dermal absorption of HCN have occurred when workers contaminated with powdered inorganic cyanide salts have decontaminated themselves in water showers, but continued to wear wet clothing rather than undress (6).

Metal Extraction and Recovery

Aqueous solutions of cyanide are able to complex with gold and silver to form compounds that remain soluble in alkaline solutions of cyanide salts. On the smallest scale, a person may reclaim gold and silver in his or her home by placing old jewelry in small jars of alkaline cyanide solutions. On the largest scale, copper mines maintain lakes and ponds containing hundreds of thousands of gallons of aqueous alkaline cyanide salts for extracting gold, silver, and other metals from impure ore. Operations of intermediate scale involve crushing waste products containing precious metals (e.g., circuit boards, transistors, used x-ray film) and then agitating them in rotary drums containing alkaline cyanide solutions.

Once the desired metal has moved into solution by complexing with cyanide, the metal is extracted back out of solution by various methodologies, including electroplating the metal out of solution onto a cathode.

The most commonly used cyanide salts in metal leeching operations are NaCN, KCN, and Ca(CN)₂ (4). Because cyanide is converted to HCN in aqueous solutions of these salts at pHs near and below the pK_a of HCN, solutions are kept very alkaline, with typical pHs ranging from 10.5–12. This often involves the addition of sodium or potassium hydroxide.

In metal reclaiming operations there are several sources of exposure to cyanide salts. Skin contact with granular cyanide salts can occur during the preparation of leeching solutions. Improper techniques may allow for skin contact with alkaline cyanide solutions (7, 8) during the leeching process from splashing of the solution out of the mixing container, from reaching into the solution to retrieve work pieces or to agitate

the mixture, or from mists created above tanks of metal-cyanide solution during the electroplating phase. Contamination of air with significant amounts of granular cyanide salts (9) or with fine mists of cyanide solutions (10, 11) may also result in inhalation and mucous membrane contact (mouth, throat, nose, large airways) with cyanide.

Electroplating

In electroplating operations, a metal-cyanide salt is dissolved in an electroplating bath containing pieces that are to be plated serving as cathodes. As current flows through the bath, the metal is reduced and deposited on the desired substrate. Many different metals can be plated in this manner, including gold, silver, copper, cadmium, zinc, tin, and indium.

Scenarios for employee contact with cyanide in electroplating operations are the same as those from metal reclaiming operations. Most electroplating baths contain NaCN or KCN in addition to the metal-cyanide, making it mandatory that plating solutions be kept at very alkaline pHs. However, some gold electroplating operations can be performed at neutral or mildly acid pHs if sodium or potassium cyanoaurite (Na[Au(CN)₂] or K[Au(CN)₂] is used as the source of gold in the bath. During normal electroplating operations, sodium and potassium cyanoaurite do not release large quantities of HCN when dissolved in water or weak acids, *although adequate ventilation is required to prevent accumulation of HCN*. It has been suggested that death following suicidal ingestion of Na[Au(CN)₂] does not appear to be from cyanide poisoning (12). However, if significant quantities of sodium or potassium cyanoaurite mix with strong mineral acids, large amounts of HCN can be quickly formed.

Pesticides

Cyanide compounds are used in agricultural and horticultural pest control. Cyanide fumigation powders containing NaCN or Ca(CN)₂ are sprinkled on floors or down rodent burrows. In the presence of water, HCN is released and reaches lethal concentrations in air. In the case of Ca(CN)₂, moisture in the air is enough to allow for significant HCN formation by the following formulas:

$$Ca(CN)_2 + H_2O \longrightarrow Ca(OH)CN + HCN$$

$$Ca(OH)CN + H_2O \longrightarrow Ca(OH)_2 + HCN$$

Earlier this century death from hydrogen cyanide exposure during fumigation was not rare. For example, five sailors died after dropping cyanide "eggs" into vats of acid while fumigating a ship (13). In 1935, Cousineau and Legg reported that one human death occurred for every 2000 cyanide fumigations in Detroit (14).

Metal Hardening

The penetration of a metal's surface by nascent carbon and/or nitrogen results in a hardened, weather-resistant exterior. One method to achieve this end is called cyaniding, and involves heating the metal in a liquid solution such as NaCN, NaCl, and Na₂CO₃ in the presence of atmospheric oxygen (4, 5).

At temperatures above 50°C, NaCN decomposes to formate and ammonia:

$$NaCN + 2H_2O \longrightarrow NH_3 + HCOONa$$

Table 61.3. Occupations or Manufacturing Process Associated with Cyanide Exposure

Dyeing	Metal hardening
Printing	Paper production
Soldering	Cement stabilizer
Metallurgy	Chemical synthesis
Fumigators	Rubber manufacturing
Firefighting	Leather manufacturing
Photography	Plastics manufacturing
Electroplating	Synthetic fiber production
Metal polishing	Precious metal extraction
Mirror making	Pesticide workers and manufacturing

The presence of NaCl in the cyanide solution retards NaCN's decomposition to ammonia and formate. However, NaCl enhances the hydrolysis of NaCN to HCN at temperatures below 80°C.

Skin contact with hot solutions can result in burns, allowing for enhanced absorption of cyanide through injured skin. Splashes or mists of cyanide solution allow for mucous membrane, inhalational, and skin exposure to cyanide. Of course, if the pH of the solution falls, HCN can be released in large quantities, especially in the presence of heat and NaCl.

Miscellaneous Uses of Cyanide

Table 61.3 lists various commercial applications for cyanide. Calcium cyanide is used as a cement stabilizer. Cyanides are essential for the synthesis of various inorganic and organic chemicals, including plastics and rubbers. Various ferrous and ferric cyanides serve as blue pigments in the dyeing and printing industry. Significant quantities of cyanide are not released after ingestion or inhalation of these ferrocyanide or ferricyanide dyes (15, 16).

Many metal polishes contain NaCN or KCN. Poisonings were reported in the early 1900s when workers would rub tarnished silver with chunks of cyanide salts or would remove silver stains from their hands by vigorously rubbing skin with pieces of KCN (17). Of course, the ingestion of a cyanide-containing metal polish can result in severe poisoning and death (18).

HCN is commonly found in smoke (19–21), including that from cigarettes. The burning of most any organic compound containing carbon and nitrogen can generate HCN under the correct conditions (22). Firefighters are commonly exposed to atmospheres containing significant quantities of HCN, and cyanide poisoning may be a major factor in death from smoke inhalation, especially in fires involving plastics.

CLINICAL TOXICOLOGY OF EXPOSURE

Route of Exposure

The main routes of exposure to cyanide in the industrial setting are from skin contact and inhalation (4). Exposure to air containing cyanide dust or mists of aqueous cyanide salts may also allow for significant mucous membrane contact. The placing of contaminated hands into the mouth or the inhalation of dusts or mists may also allow for swallowing and gastrointestinal absorption of cyanide compounds.

Because cyanide salts are rapidly absorbed from mucous membranes, symptoms following acute inhalation of or mucous

membrane contact with toxic concentrations of cyanide salts may begin within seconds to a few minutes after exposure (7, 9). A worker who accidently receives a mouthful of aqueous or powdered cyanide may quickly collapse. However, the absorption of cyanide from the gastrointestinal tract is slower, allowing for delayed toxicity if cyanide compounds are swallowed, assuming survival after initial mucous membrane contact with the poison.

Hydrogen cyanide is extremely well-absorbed by inhalation and can produce death within seconds to minutes (1, 23–25). Because it is unionized and of low molecular weight, significant absorption of HCN can occur through skin if high enough concentrations are present (26, 27).

While brief contact between small areas of skin and dry, powdered NaCN, KCN, or Ca(CN)$_2$ would be unlikely to produce toxicity, short exposures of large areas of skin to solid cyanide salts or their aqueous solutions can result in dermal absorption of lethal quantities of cyanide. The rate of absorption of cyanide across skin increases as the pH of the cyanide solution decreases due to more of the cyanide being present as unionized HCN at lower pHs (6).

Prolonged skin contact with smaller skin areas can still produce toxicity (17). Damaged skin from abrasions (28) or from burns due to alkaline cyanide solutions allows for increased dermal absorption of cyanide. In contrast to the rapid onset of symptoms from the inhalation of HCN, the onset of symptoms following large acute dermal exposures sometimes may be delayed for as long as 30 minutes if decontamination has not been effective, especially if the worker continues to wear wet, contaminated clothing (6).

In many instances, several routes of exposure to cyanide may exist. A 19-year-old man who collapsed after a bag of powdered KCN burst in his face probably suffered inhalational, dermal, and mucosal contact with the powder (9). One man died and two men were found comatose after working in a truck that threw Ca(CN)$_2$ powder 24 feet (7.3 meters) at a height of 6 feet (1.8 meters) onto grapevines (29). Probable exposures included inhalational, mucosal, and dermal contact with the powder as well as inhalation of HCN formed when Ca(CN)$_2$ reacted with water vapor.

Metabolism

Humans detoxify cyanide by transferring sulfane sulfur [R–S$_{(x)}$–SH] to cyanide, thus converting it to thiocyanate (SCN). Thiocyanate is excreted in the urine with an elimination half-life of about 2.5 days in those with normal renal function (30).

There are two main enzymes thought to be capable of converting cyanide to thiocyanate (31, 32). The first is rhodanese (thiosulfate sulfurtransferase, EC 2.8.1.1), an enzyme restricted to mitochondria. Rhodanese is found in various tissues, especially liver, kidney, and skeletal muscle. The most commonly described reaction catalyzed by rhodanese involves the transfer of a sulfur atom from thiosulfate (S$_2$O$_3^{2-}$), a source of sulfane sulfur, to cyanide:

$$CN^- + S_2O_3^{2-} \longrightarrow SCN^- + SO_3^{2-}$$

The second enzyme capable of forming thiocyanate transfers sulfur from mercaptopyruvate to cyanide and is named β-mercaptopyruvate-cyanide sulfurtransferase (EC 2.8.1.2).

$$HSCH_2COCOO^- + CN^- \longrightarrow SCN^- + CH_3COCOO^-$$

In addition to being found in liver and kidneys, this latter enzyme is also found within erythrocytes (32).

While rhodanese has traditionally been credited with cyanide's detoxication, current data indicate that this may not in fact be true. Thiosulfate, a substrate for rhodanese, is thought to be unable to penetrate the inner mitochondrial membrane where rhodanese is located (33, 34). Ballantyne and others (32, 33, 35) suggest an overall scheme whereby numerous sulfur sources are acted upon by various sulfurtransferases, including rhodanese and mercaptopyruvate sulfurtransferase, to form sulfane sulfur, which then complexes with albumin in blood. A nonenzymatic reaction of the sulfane-albumin complex with cyanide may actually account for thiocyanate formation. This hypothesis is in keeping with kinetic studies suggesting that cyanide detoxication takes place in a volume of distribution similar to blood volume (36).

However, other data clearly demonstrate that the albumin-sulfane complex appears to play a minor role in the in vivo detoxication of cyanide. In bloodless rats in which blood is replaced by a fluorocarbon emulsion, sodium thiosulfate still efficiently antagonizes cyanide (37). In the absence of blood or circulating albumin, cyanide's detoxication can only be attributed to sulfurtransferase reactions occurring in tissue sites other than blood.

Out of these disparate data, investigators generally do agree that sulfane sulfur such as thiosulfate is required for and greatly accelerates detoxication of cyanide by converting cyanide to thiocyanate regardless of mechanism.

Cyanide is rapidly taken up and sequestered by red blood cells (38, 39). Such action does not appear to enhance the metabolism of cyanide, but might act to partially lessen toxicity by preventing the diffusion of cyanide out of blood into tissues.

Cyanide's affinity for the cobalt ion (Co^{2+}) causes it to combine with hydroxycobalamin to form cyanocobalamin, which is then excreted in the urine and bile. This route of detoxication normally plays a very minor role in acute cyanide poisoning. However, the administration of large amounts of hydroxycobalamin is used as antidotal therapy in some countries (40). Hydroxycobalamin is not available in suitable form for this purpose in the United States.

Pathophysiology

The major immediate energy source for living cells is adenosine triphosphate (ATP). ATP is mainly produced either in the cytoplasm via glycolysis or through oxidative phosphorylation in the mitochondrium (Fig. 61.2).

In glycolysis two moles of ATP are generated from the metabolism of each mole of glucose to pyruvate. Glycolysis can proceed in the absence of oxygen as long as pyruvate is converted to lactate, regenerating nicotinamide adenine dinucleotide (NAD^+). Unfortunately, the minimal amount of ATP produced in glycolysis will not support life except in selected tissues (e.g., erythrocytes).

In the mitochondrium, pyruvate from glycolysis is decarboxylated before combining with oxaloacetate to form citrate, the first step in the tricarboxylic acid cycle (Krebs' cycle). Citrate then undergoes a series of reactions that generate CO_2, H_2O, GTP, and reduced nicotinamide and flavin adenine dinucleotides (NADH and FADH, respectively).

The major route of ATP production is by oxidative phosphorylation in mitochondria. In the inner mitochondrial membrane, electrons are transferred from NADH and FADH to various cytochromes before finally combining with oxygen to form H_2O. As electrons are transferred among cytochromes, energy is released and used to generate ATP and H_2O from adenosine diphosphate (ADP) and inorganic phosphate (HPO_4^{2-}). Oxygen's role in life, then, is to serve as the final electron acceptor in the cytochrome system.

With the addition of oxidative phosphorylation to glycolysis, a total of 36–38 moles of ATP can be generated from each mole of glucose. ATP production via oxidative phosphorylation can only take place when oxygen is present and when electrons are allowed to proceed down the cytochrome system in a normal fashion.

Cyanide combines with and inhibits a number of mammalian enzymes (33, 41) (Table 61.4). However, it is cyanide's great affinity for ferric iron in cytochrome oxidase, the last enzyme of the cytochrome system, that appears to account for the majority of its toxicity. At physiologic pH, most cyanide in the body is present as HCN. By combining with cytochrome oxidase, HCN prevents electron transport in the cytochrome system, bringing oxidative phosphorylation and the majority of the cell's ATP production to a halt (Fig. 61.2) (36). Cyanide's ability to inhibit glutamate decarboxylase may result in a fall in brain γ-aminobutyric acid (GABA) concentrations and contribute toward convulsions (42).

A metabolic acidosis and fall in oxygen consumption always accompany serious cyanide poisoning. The metabolic acidosis deserves particular discussion since most authors have incorrectly attributed acidosis to elevated circulating lactate concentrations resulting from glycolytic conversion of glucose to lactate. Unquestionably, as ATP production via oxidative phosphorylation is impaired, the conversion of glucose to lactate via glycolysis is accelerated and becomes an important source of ATP, resulting in elevated lactate concentrations. However, ATP production via the conversion of glucose to lactate is not acidifying; it does not produce a net increase in the number of hydrogen ions (43–45). For example, Gevers (46) illustrated glycolysis at pH 8.2:

$$\text{glucose} + 2\,ADP^{3-} + 2\,HPO_4^{2-} + 10\,H^+ \longrightarrow$$
$$2\,\text{lactate}^- + 2\,ATP^{4-} + 2\,H_2O + 10\,H^+.$$

The amounts of ATP and lactate generated in glycolysis certainly vary according to cellular pH and concentrations of available substrates (44). However, the fact that glycolytic production of lactic acid and ATP is not acidifying holds true regardless of pH (44, 47, 48).

An understanding of the generation of ATP in oxidative phosphorylation and of ATP's hydrolysis in metabolic processes explains the metabolic acidosis accompanying cyanide poisoning. Viable cells utilize ATP as an energy source by hydrolyzing ATP to ADP and phosphate. The hydrolysis of ATP results in the net production of hydrogen ions (44). Again, both pH and concentrations of available substrates influence dissociation of hydrogen ions from ATP, ADP, and phosphate. A net increase in hydrogen ion concentration will always occur from the hydrolysis of ATP.

$$ATP^{4-} + 4\,H^+ + H_2O \longrightarrow ADP^{3-} + HPO_4^{2-} + 5\,H^+$$

In oxidative phosphorylation via the cytochrome system, hydrogen ions are consumed in the opposite reaction as ATP and water are generated from ADP and phosphate:

GLYCOLYSIS

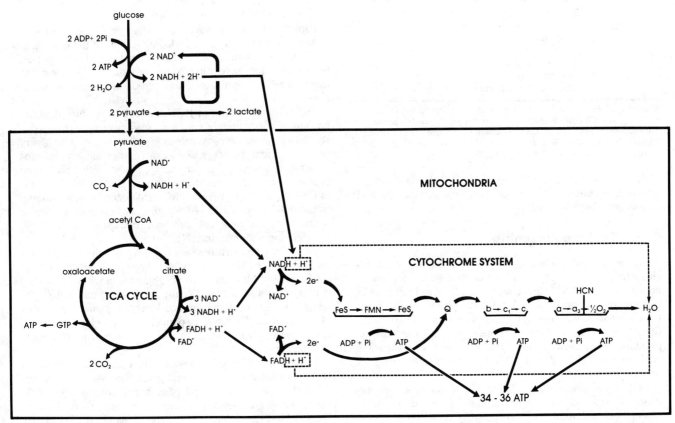

Figure 61.2. Simplified, schematic diagram of cellular ATP production. ATP, adenosine triphosphate; ADP, adenosine diphosphate; Pi, inorganic phosphate; NAD^+ oxidized nicotinamide adenine dinucleotide; NADH, reduced nicotinamide adenine dinucleotide; acetyl CoA, acetyl coenzyme A; GTP, guanosine triphosphate; FAD^+, oxidized flavin adenine dinucleotide; FADH, reduced flavin adenine dinucleotide; FeS, iron-sulfur protein; FMN, flavin mononucleotide; Q, coenzyme Q; b, cytochrome b; c_1, cytochrome c_1; c, cytochrome c; a, cytochrome a; a_3, cytochrome a_3; TCA cycle, tricarboxylic acid cycle (Krebs' cycle).

The conversion of 1 mole glucose to 2 moles pyruvate via glycolysis produces a net 2 moles ATP. Normally, pyruvate enters the mitochondrium where it is metabolized in the tricarboxylic acid cycle (TCA cycle or Krebs' cycle) to produce NADH and FADH. Electrons donated by NADH and FADH are transported down the cytochrome

system and eventually onto oxygen. Energy released during electron transport is harnessed to generate the great majority of the cell's ATP (oxidative phosphorylation). Depending on the mechanism by which NADH from glycolysis is shuttled into the mitochondrium, a total of 36–38 moles ATP (including the indirect synthesis of ATP from GTP in the TCA cycle and ATP generated in glycolysis) can be generated from each mole of glucose.

Cytochrome oxidase comprises cytochrome a and cytochrome a_3. HCN combines with cytochrome a_3 of cytochrome oxidase and interrupts electron transport, causing a decline in both oxygen consumption and oxidative phosphorylation. ATP production in glycolysis (glucose to lactate) becomes an increasingly important pathway for ATP synthesis as oxidative phosphorylation is impaired. Although lactate concentrations rise in cyanide poisoning, they are not responsible for metabolic acidosis (see text).

$$ADP^{3-} + HPO_4^{2-} + 5\,H^+ \longrightarrow ATP^{4-} + H_2O + 4\,H^+$$

With regard to oxidative phosphorylation, when normal homeostatic mechanisms are operating, a normal pH is maintained because ATP is being used throughout the body at the same rate it is being produced in mitochondria. In other words, hydrogen ion production via the cellular hydrolysis of ATP is balanced by the ability of the cytochrome system to utilize hydrogen ions in aerobic generation of ATP (47). When electron transport in the cytochrome system is impaired and oxidative phosphorylation slows or stops, hydrogen ions created by the cellular hydrolysis of ATP are no longer buffered by aerobic ATP production (44). As the hydrogen ion concentration rises, the pH falls.

Thus, in cyanide poisoning, the binding of cyanide to cyto-

chrome oxidase stops electron transport. This impairment of the cytochrome system results in a fall in oxygen consumption and ATP production. Cells must then rely on anaerobic ATP production via glycolysis with the conversion of glucose to lactate. The lack of utilization of NADH in the cytochrome system also results in elevation of the NADH:NAD ratio, a factor that serves to enhance conversion of pyruvate to lactate (44). While cellular and circulating lactate concentrations rise, the elevated lactate levels are not responsible for acidosis. Rather, they serve as a marker for anaerobic ATP production in glycolysis. The acidosis of cyanide poisoning occurs because cells hydrolyze ATP generated in glycolysis, producing H^+, while, at the same time, the ability to buffer hydrogen ions via oxidative phosphorylation is impaired. In fact, any metabolic or physiologic imbalance resulting in a greater hydrolysis of ATP than synthesis of ATP in

Table 61.4.   Partial List of Enzymes Inhibited by Cyanide

Xanthine oxidase
Carbonic anhydrase
Nitrite reductase
2-Keto-4-hydroglutarate aldolase
Acetoacetate decarboxylase
Cytochrome oxidase
Succinate dehydrogenase

Adapted from: Ballantyne B. Toxicology of cyanides. In: Ballantyne B, Marrs TC, eds. Clinical and experimental toxicology of cyanides. Bristol: IOP Publishing, 1987:41–126 and Solomonson LP. Cyanide as a metabolic inhibitor. In: Vennesland B, Conn E, Knowles CJ, et al., eds. Cyanide in biology. London: Academic Press, 1981:11–28.

oxidative phosphorylation can result in metabolic acidosis, whether it be from impaired oxidative phosphorylation or excessive ATP consumption by tissue (44, 47).

Acute Cyanide Poisoning

There are several reasons why cyanide poisoning is mainly characterized by dysfunction of the cardiovascular and central nervous system (CNS). In the face of acidosis and falling ATP concentrations from impaired oxidative phosphorylation, organs most sensitive to energy deprivation (brain, heart) suffer first. Cytochrome oxidase in the heart is also more sensitive to inhibition by cyanide (49). Finally, cyanide concentrations are higher in brain and myocardium than in other organs at the time of death (33).

CNS abnormalities range from agitation and anxiety to confusion, lethargy, coma, convulsions, and cerebral death. Initial stimulation of carotid body receptors by relatively low concentrations of cyanide results in tachypnea. However, lethal concentrations of cyanide rapidly produce apnea.

Cardiovascular toxicity early in cyanide poisoning results in tachycardia and, at times, hypertension. In more serious or lethal poisonings, hypotension, bradyarrhythmias, heart blocks, ventricular arrhythmias, and asystole develop. Wexler and colleagues (50) recorded electrocardiographic changes in 16 men who received intravenous injections of up to 0.2 mg cyanide per kg body weight (one subject suffered a ''momentary dim-out''). Respiratory stimulation was immediately preceded by sinus arrests lasting from 0.88–4.2 seconds that were thought to be vagally mediated. Immediately following sinus arrests there were irregularities in sinus rhythms with slowing of heart rates for periods of a few seconds to as long as 2 minutes. This was then followed by gradual accelerations of heart rates to levels higher than control values. These investigators also reported on electrocardiographic changes in four men executed by inhalation of HCN. Among various arrhythmias reported, a progressive shortening of the ST segment was noted until, terminally, the T wave originated on the R wave. This ''T on R'' phenomenon has since been noted in other cases of severe cyanide poisoning (51).

Nonspecific findings accompanying many cases of cyanide poisoning include diaphoresis, weakness, nausea, and vomiting (25). Other abnormalities resulting from impaired ATP production include rhabdomyolysis, renal failure, hepatic necrosis, and adult respiratory distress syndrome (ARDS) (33, 52, 53).

Because of their alkaline nature, solid or aqueous solutions of cyanide salts can produce corrosive injury when coming in contact with moist mucosal surfaces. This author witnessed massive upper gastrointestinal bleeding with hematemesis in a

physician who died within 20 minutes after ingesting KCN powder. Severe skin burns can also occur after acute dermal contact with alkaline cyanide solutions (8).

Patients who survive severe poisoning may be left with permanent neurologic deficits, including lesions in the basal ganglia (54, 55). Lesions in the striatum are not specific for cyanide, but are seen after severe hypoxemia or following poisoning by many metabolic toxins, including carbon monoxide and methanol.

The minimal amount of HCN required to produce death in humans is not definitely known as most acute poisonings are secondary to massive overdoses. Fatal doses of HCN vary among different species, making exact extrapolation to humans difficult. In general, these animal data indicate that prolonged exposures to HCN concentrations above 90 ppm (95.7 mg/m^3 as CN) are incompatible with life, and concentrations ranging from 10–45 ppm (10.63–47.8 mg/m^3 as CN) may produce a plethora of symptoms with thresholds in each species difficult to determine with certainty (4).

Commonly reported dose-response relationships in humans for inhalation of HCN usually have been referenced to a 1931 publication by Flury and Zernik (56), or to other authors who, in turn, reference Flury and Zernik. However, Flury and Zernik referred to data by Lehmann and Hess that cannot be located (4). McNamara (57) has since pointed out that Lehmann worked almost entirely with rabbits, a species more sensitive to HCN than humans.

From cases of human exposures where air concentrations of HCN have been reported, several generalizations can be made. Headache, metallic taste, and other minor symptoms certainly may develop after several minutes of exposure to 10–30 ppm HCN (10.6–31.9 mg/m^3 as CN) in breathing air (4). Death may occur within 1 hour when breathing 100 ppm HCN (106 mg/m^3 as CN) (4, 33), and fatalities have been reported after exposure to greater than 300 ppm (319 mg/m^3 as CN) for a few minutes. Survival has been reported after a 90-second exposure to HCN at an estimated concentration of 500–615 mg/m^3 (453–557 ppm) and after 3 minutes exposure to 500 ppm HCN (531 mg/m^3 as CN) (23, 24). Ballantyne has suggested an inhalational 5-minute LC$_{50}$ of 680 ppm (723 mg/m^3 as CN), and a 30-minute LC$_{50}$ of 200 ppm (213 mg/m^3 as CN) (33).

The lethal oral dose of HCN is estimated to be about 50 milligrams in an adult. Oral ingestion of 5 milliliters of 20% hydrocyanic acid has been fatal. Lethal oral doses of KCN or NaCN are estimated to be 200–300 milligrams. However, survival has been reported after much larger ingestions with intensive supportive care (51, 52, 58).

Chronic Exposures

Skin contact with aqueous solutions of cyanide salts can be very irritating due to the alkaline pH of such liquids (59, 60). Prolonged contact with alkaline cyanide solutions may result in severe corrosive burns (8). In the author's experience, deep burns from cyanide-containing electroplating solutions may require several weeks to heal, possibly from metals also present in the bath. Topical contact with HCN may produce a blotchy rash of the face (4). Dermatitis associated with gold cyanide electroplating has also been attributed to hydrazine present in plating solutions (61). Some authors believe that allergic reactions to metals in the solutions or to cyanide itself may contribute to dermatitis (62).

Cyanide salts are also irritating to the upper respiratory tract.

Chronic nasal mucosal irritation and ulceration of the nasal septum have been noted in electroplaters (63, 64). Caution must be taken before attributing such changes to cyanide, however, since many metals used in electroplating operations (e.g., chromium, nickel) can cause identical findings. Cohen reported no irritating effects in electroplaters exposed to breathing air cyanide concentrations of 0.006 mg/m³ (0.0056 ppm) (65).

Several authors have discussed the possibility of chronic systemic cyanide poisoning resulting from industrial exposure to cyanide (66–69). Suggested disorders resulting from longterm, low level cyanide exposure have included headache, weakness, dysgusia, vomiting, abdominal pain, chest pain, and nervousness. After an extensive review of the world's literature, NIOSH concluded that convincing evidence for chronic cyanide poisoning from regular exposures to air cyanide concentrations below 10 ppm (10.6 mg/m³ as CN) is lacking (4). Almost all such symptoms are subjective (e.g., headache, nausea, nervousness) and can be produced by a multitude of stress factors in any working environment. In most reports describing chronic cyanide poisoning, cyanide levels in air were not reported or were reported as area measurements that may not have reflected cyanide concentrations in the breathing zone near plating baths or other cyanide solutions. In some reports describing electroplating operations, articles suggest such poor housekeeping that dermal contact with cyanide solutions seemed likely. Most importantly, reports utilizing control groups of workers with which to compare symptoms are the exception.

There is no doubt that some workers may suffer recurrent signs and symptoms of mild cyanide poisoning (e.g., headache, lightheadedness, nausea, metallic or bitter almond taste) each time they work for significant amounts of time in air containing cyanide concentrations greater than 10–20 ppm (10.6–21.3 mg/m³ as CN). Furthermore, repeated episodes of acute, *severe* cyanide poisoning may be accompanied by serious neurotoxicity and result in permanent neurologic deficits (25). While there are no convincing data to suggest permanent effects from working in air containing 10 ppm (10.6 mg/m³) cyanide, NIOSH recognized that some workers did develop a constellation of subjective symptoms such as those noted above when working in air with *average* cyanide concentrations between about 7 and 10 ppm (between 7.4 and 10.6 mg/m³). Partly because transient exposures to air cyanide concentrations far above 10 ppm can occur when 8-hour TWA concentrations are 5 ppm, NIOSH recommended that the 8-hour TWA PEL for all cyanide be changed to a 10-minute ceiling limit of 5 mg/m³ (4.7 ppm), as cyanide in 1976 (4).

Thiocyanate competes with iodine for thyroidal uptake, potentially producing hypothyroidism (70, 71) Because of thiocyanate's long elimination half-life, concern has been raised that accumulation of thiocyanate in those chronically exposed to cyanide may result in goiters (72, 73). El Ghawabi reported "mild to moderate" thyroid enlargement in 36 electroplaters exposed to cyanide for many years (73). Air concentrations of cyanide averaged between 6.4 and 10.4 ppm (between 6.8 and 11 mg/m³). Nevertheless, Hartung (74) notes that the occurrence of thyroid abnormalities after longterm cyanide exposures has been only rarely reported. In fact, rats sensitive to goitrogenic agents that were fed food containing up to 300 ppm HCN did not develop changes in the thyroid, even though tissue levels of thiocyanate were elevated (75). Finally, others have suggested that smoking (a source of cyanide) has more of an influence on urinary thiocyanate levels than occupational exposure to cyanide at concentrations below 8 ppm (8.5 mg/m³)

(76). This implies that occupational exposures to cyanide below 8 ppm are no more likely to produce thyroid disease than smoking.

Several debilitating neurologic disorders have been described in developing countries in which plants rich in cyanide glycosides (e.g., cassava) serve as the main diet. These disorders are probably variants of the same disease and have been called tropical ataxic neuropathy, tropical ataxia, subacute spastic paresis, West Indian neuropathy, and mantekassa, as well as other names. Whether cyanide has any role in these diseases has been debated for years (77, 78). Some investigators have hypothesized that depletion of vitamin B12 occurs in these patients from the conversion of hydroxycobalamin to cyanocobalamin, which is more easily excreted from the body. However, recent reports present convincing evidence that the majority of these disorders actually result from infection by human T cell lymphotropic virus type 1 (HTLV-I) (79, 80).

No data could be located to suggest that occupational exposure to cyanide is carcinogenic or mutagenic.

The continuous subcutaneous infusion of NaCN into gravid Golden Syrian hamsters was embryofetotoxic during organogenesis, especially with regard to neural tube development (81). However, even at the lowest cyanide dose, some maternal toxicity was evident. No data could be located suggesting that maternal exposures to cyanide concentrations that do not produce maternal toxicity are embryofetotoxic. However, studies in this area are notably lacking.

DIAGNOSIS

In blood, most cyanide is concentrated within red blood cells, making red cell cyanide concentrations two to three times higher than those in plasma (38, 39). Plasma cyanide is thought to be in equilibrium with tissue cyanide and may be a more reliable indicator of tissue cyanide levels (39, 82). In part because higher levels of cyanide are more easily measured in red cells than in plasma, however, red cell or whole blood cyanide levels are generally used to confirm the diagnosis of cyanide poisoning when such is suspected.

Normal whole blood cyanide concentrations vary in the adult population. Smokers have higher concentrations than nonsmokers (83–85). In general, whole blood cyanide concentrations are less than 50 μg/l (1.9 μmol/l), although some authors have reported normal mean values up to 180 μ/l (6.9 μmol/l) (86).

There are also tremendous variations in what have been reported to be lethal or near-lethal whole blood cyanide concentrations. This is due, in part, to differences in plasma cyanide concentrations in patients with similar whole blood levels, the time after the onset of poisoning that blood samples were obtained, whether any antidotes for cyanide were administered, and the instability of cyanide in stored blood or in postmortem tissue (1, 84, 87). The medical literature indicates that the lowest whole blood cyanide concentrations compatible with death from cyanide are probably on the order of 1–2 mg/l (38.5–76.9 μmol/l) (84).

Unfortunately, when confronted with a patient who is suspected of suffering from cyanide poisoning, physicians must make decisions regarding therapy before results of cyanide levels are available. Other physical and laboratory data must be examined for clues to the diagnosis of cyanide poisoning.

An anion gap metabolic acidosis is invariably present in serious cyanide poisoning. While the arterial lactate concentrations may be elevated, the lactate concentration frequently does not account for the entire anion gap or base deficit since lactate is not actually responsible for acidosis (discussed earlier).

The fall in oxygen consumption accompanying cyanide poisoning can allow for increased oxygen content of peripheral and mixed venous blood (87–89). The presence of bright red venous blood or retinal veins, then, suggests the possibility of cyanide poisoning (90). However, many persons suffering from cyanide poisoning are cyanotic (55, 91, 92). While arterial PO_2 can be normal in cyanide poisoning, low cardiac output and intrapulmonary shunting in any patient with severe shock can cause arterial hypoxemia, including those suffering from cyanide poisoning.

Cardiovascular and metabolic parameters obtained from invasive monitoring with systemic and pulmonary artery catheters may reveal changes compatible with either sepsis or cyanide poisoning. Both conditions can cause a metabolic acidosis, hypotension, a fall in oxygen consumption, a rise in mixed venous oxygen content, and a fall in the arterial-venous oxygen content difference.

The toxicologic differential diagnosis of cyanide poisoning includes methemoglobinemia (when cyanosis is present), asphyxia (e.g., inert gases, methane), and poisonings by sulfide, azide, arsine, phosphine, phenol, methyl halides, and carbon monoxide. Unfortunately, any intoxication characterized by the sudden onset of seizures may be accompanied by hypotension, hypoxemia, and a metabolic acidosis, making the differential diagnosis large (e.g., monomethylhydrazine, cicutoxin, isoniazid, strychnine). However, sudden unexpected collapse into unconsciousness or convulsions accompanied by metabolic acidosis and decreased oxygen consumption in spite of adequate oxygen delivery makes one lean toward the diagnosis of cyanide or sulfide poisoning.

MANAGEMENT OF ACUTE TOXICITY

Antidotal Strategy

In the United States, the two main antidotal strategies for treating cyanide poisoning are the induction of methemoglobinemia with amyl nitrite or sodium nitrite, and the enhancement of conversion of cyanide to thiocyanate by the administration of sodium thiosulfate.

Cyanide binds to cytochrome oxidase because of its attraction to its ferric iron (Fe^{3+}). Normal hemoglobin contains ferrous iron (Fe^{2+}), explaining why cyanide does not significantly bind to this pigment. When iron of reduced hemoglobin is oxidized to the ferric state, methemoglobin is formed. Because methemoglobin cannot carry oxygen and shifts the hemoglobin-oxygen dissociation curve to the left, the body has extensive mechanisms for maintaining methemoglobin levels within erythrocytes below 1–2% (i.e., <1–2% of all heme pigments are in the met form). In the absence of anemia, methemoglobin fractions of 20–30% are tolerated without life-threatening symptoms in the healthy person (93).

Sodium nitrite and amyl nitrite overwhelm the erythrocyte with oxidant stress, raising methemoglobin concentrations. This source of circulating ferric iron then competes with cytochrome oxidase for binding by cyanide, causing cyanide to dissociate from cytochrome oxidase in tissue and to move into blood,

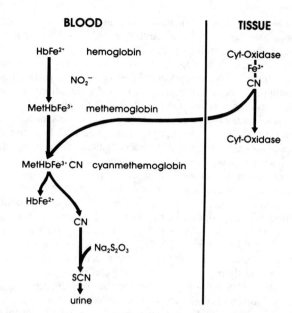

Figure 61.3   Antidotal strategy for cyanide poisoning. Cyanide binds to ferric iron on cytochrome oxidase in tissue, producing cyanide poisoning. Nitrite (NO_2) converts a fraction of circulating ferrous hemoglobin to ferric methemoglobin. Because cyanide's binding to cytochrome oxidase and methemoglobin is reversible, ferric iron of methemoglobin competes with cytochrome oxidase for binding by cyanide. Cyanide moves out of tissue and into erythrocytes as it binds with methemoglobin to form cyanmethemoglobin. Conversion of cyanide released from cyanmethemoglobin to thiocyanate (SCN) is markedly enhanced by the administration of sodium thiosulfate ($Na_2S_2O_3$).

where it combines with methemoglobin in erythrocytes to form cyanmethemoglobin (36) (Fig. 61.3).

The historically suggested dose of sodium nitrite for adults without anemia is 10 milliliters of a 3% solution (300 milligrams) over several minutes. This dose has remained unchanged from that originally suggested and reiterated by Chen (94). While circulating methemoglobin fractions of 25–40% (assuming no anemia) have been advocated to be most effective (95–97), these recommended levels of methemoglobinemia are based mainly on simply producing the highest fraction of methemoglobin that can be achieved in the nonanemic patient without seriously compromising oxygen delivery. This degree of methemoglobinemia is rarely achieved with currently recommended doses of sodium nitrite (94, 95). For example, Moser reported peak methemoglobin fractions in humans of only 10.1% after intravenous administration of 400 milligrams sodium nitrite and of 17.5% after 600 milligrams of sodium nitrite (99). Kiese and Weger reported that methemoglobin fractions rose to a mean of 7% in six volunteers receiving sodium nitrite 4 mg/kg (95). A single volunteer who received sodium nitrite 12 mg/kg developed a methemoglobin fraction of 30%.

Sodium nitrite is also a relatively slow methemoglobin-producing agent. Thirty minutes may be required to raise methemoglobin fractions to 7% after sodium nitrite 4 mg/kg and 60 minutes may be required to reach 30% after sodium nitrite 12 mg/kg (95). Despite the slow onset of relatively low grade methemoglobinemia following the administration of 300 mg sodium nitrite, the combination of sodium nitrite and sodium thiosulfate remains superior to more rapid methemoglobin-forming agents (34), possibly because of a more sustained methemoglobinemia produced by nitrite (34). Furthermore, the fact that dramatic improvements in symptoms have occurred well before methemoglobin levels have peaked (88, 100) also suggests that mechanisms other than methemoglobin production may be important in nitrite's antidotal action (34, 101).

Sodium thiosulfate is a source of sulfane sulfur that enhances the conversion of cyanide to thiocyanate. Thiosulfate generally is not given alone in the treatment of symptomatic cyanide poisoning because of what has been believed to be a slow action as compared with sodium nitrite (animal data concerning the speed with which thiocyanate reverses cyanide poisoning are conflicting) (102, 103). Furthermore, while induction of nonlethal methemoglobinemia can rapidly reverse serious cyanide poisoning, cyanide eventually will be released from cyanmethemoglobin, at least partly by reduction of cyanmethemoglobin to normal hemoglobin (104). Therefore, coadministration of sodium thiosulfate with sodium nitrite ensures cyanide's rapid conversion to thiocyanate as it is released from cyanmethemoglobin (Fig. 61.3). The combination of sodium nitrite and sodium thiosulfate increases the required lethal dose for cyanide up to 13 times in some animal models as compared to increases of 3–4-fold when each agent is given alone (105).

The main adverse effect from sodium or amyl nitrite is vasodilation and hypotension (96). Nitrite-induced hypotension, in part, has caused physicians in other countries to switch to other antidotes in the treatment of cyanide poisoning. These include other methemoglobin-producing agents such as 4-dimethylaminophenol (106) (DMAP) or cyanide-chelating agents such as cobalt edetate (107) (CoEDTA) and hydroxycobalamin (40).

However, there are data suggesting that vasodilation actually may be beneficial in cyanide poisoning. Vasodilators that do not produce methemoglobinemia (e.g., phenoxybenzamine, chlorpromazine) are only slightly protective against cyanide when given alone. However, these vasodilators significantly enhance the antidotal effect of thiosulfate in animal models (108, 109). Other data indicate that vasodilation plays a relatively unimportant role as compared with methemoglobin induction in explaining the antidotal effect of nitrite. The injection of erythrocytes exposed to nitrite in vitro and then washed free of excess nitrite provides a degree of protection equivalent to that produced by nitrite directly injected into animals poisoned with cyanide (104).

The administration of 100% oxygen along with nitrite and thiosulfate to poisoned animals enhances survival over animals breathing room air. Animal studies reveal no advantage of hyperbaric oxygen therapy over the administration of 100% oxygen at one atmosphere (110).

"Solutions A and B" is an antidotal strategy mentioned only to be condemned. Solution A is 15.8% ferrous sulfate in 3% citric acid. Solution B is 6% sodium carbonate. Extensive research has been unsuccessful in determining the origin of this antidotal strategy (111). However, it has been recommended that two solutions be mixed together in equal parts and drunk immediately following the oral ingestion of cyanide. Ferrous iron liberated from the reaction of solution A with solution B is supposed to combine with cyanide in the gut to form relatively harmless ferrocyanide, preventing serious cyanide toxicity. Unfortunately, there are no animal or human data to justify its use. Unpublished data in small groups of rats indicate that the antidote is effective if given *within 60 seconds* of the instillation of cyanide into the stomach by a plastic tube. The administration of the antidote after 60 seconds has no effect (111). Furthermore, a human being drinking cyanide would

Table 61.5   Initial Pediatric Dosage of Sodium Nitrite Based on Hemoglobin Concentration

Hemoglobin Concentration (g/100 ml)	3% Sodium Nitrite Solution (ml/kg)
7.0	0.19
8.0	0.22
9.0	0.25
10.0	0.27
11.0	0.30
12.0	0.33
13.0	0.36
14.0	0.39

Adapted from: Berlin CM. The treatment of cyanide poisoning in children. Pediatrics 1970;46:793–796.

absorb significant, if not lethal quantities from mucous membranes of the mouth and throat. Callaghan and Halton (111) concluded: ". . . the preparation and administration of the *unproved* A and B remedy would delay the institution of measures with proved antidotal value. Therefore, we discourage the use of solutions A and B since the origin, theoretical basis and efficacy of this remedy reside primarily in folklore myth, not in proved antidotal action."

Lilly Cyanide Antidote Kit

The Lilly Cyanide Antidote Kit (Eli Lilly and Company, Indianapolis, IN) contains breakable amyl nitrite pearls for induction of methemoglobinemia by inhalation as well as injectable solutions of sodium nitrite and sodium thiosulfate.

The inhalation of amyl nitrite is meant to be a temporizing measure until sodium nitrite can be given intravenously. A crushed pearl is held in front of the patient's nose and mouth, or in front of an intake valve of a ventilation bag for 30 seconds of every minute. Amyl nitrite pearls are rather ineffective at producing methemoglobinemia as compared with intravenous sodium nitrite (94), and it is far more important to adequately ventilate and oxygenate the patient than to administer amyl nitrite by inhalation.

Sodium nitrite should be given as soon as intravenous access is established. The adult dose is 10 milliliters of a 3% solution (300 milligrams). The administration of an entire ampule (10 milliliters) of 3% sodium nitrite to a child can produce overwhelming, lethal methemoglobinemia (97). The same is true for an adult suffering from significant anemia. Children without anemia can receive 0.33 milliliters of 3% sodium nitrite per kilogram body weight, up to 10 milliliters. If a child's hemoglobin concentration is known, Table 61.5 can be consulted for more specific doses.

After the administration of intravenous sodium nitrite, 50 milliliters of 25% sodium thiosulfate should be administered intravenously to adults over several minutes. The pediatric dose is 1.65 milliliters of 25% sodium thiosulfate per kilogram body weight (97).

If signs of cyanide poisoning persist for 30 minutes or recur after an initial response to the antidote kit, sodium nitrite and sodium thiosulfate doses may be repeated. While some authorities suggest that half the initial dose be used, this author's experience is that two doses of 300 milligrams sodium nitrite given as close as 10 minutes apart do no not produce methemoglobin fractions greater than 20% in otherwise healthy nonanemic adults. Nevertheless, it is highly recommended that total hemoglobin and methemoglobin concentrations be rapidly measured, when possible, before repeating a dose of sodium nitrite to be sure that dangerous methemoglobinemia will not occur, especially in children.

Medical Management

When it is suspected that a worker is unconscious from exposure to cyanide, the most important task for those not yet affected is to protect themselves and immediately leave the area. Rescue of an incapacitated victim should only be performed by personnel equipped with protective clothing or suits, respirators, and devices that can quickly measure cyanide concentrations in air (e.g., Draeger Tubes). Rescue personnel should not enter areas containing greater than 200 ppm HCN unless they are wearing gas-tight suits (4). After the victim has been moved to a safe environment, an airway should be established and adequate ventilation assured, preferably with 100% oxygen. Direct mouth-to-mouth resuscitation should not be performed if it is thought that cyanide was orally ingested. Rather, bag-mask-valve ventilation or endotracheal intubation and bag ventilation should be used. Cardiopulmonary resuscitation should be initiated in those without a pulse. The Lilly Cyanide Antidote Kit should be administered as described above and the patient transported to a health care facility after dermal decontamination (see below). Other than administration of cyanide antidotes and oxygen, treatment of cyanide poisoning is one of supportive care. For instance, severe acidosis may require correction with sodium bicarbonate. ARDS may require positive pressure ventilation and continuous positive airway pressure.

During the rescue and resuscitation of a victim, personnel must be careful not to contaminate themselves with cyanide by coming in direct contact with the victim's contaminated clothing or with spilled cyanide compounds. In unconscious patients, after the institution of cardiopulmonary resuscitation (if indicated) and the administration of nitrite and thiosulfate, *all* contaminated clothing should be cut off the patient, and the victim should be *thoroughly* decontaminated with water.

The victim who suffers an acute dermal exposure to significant quantities of powdered or aqueous cyanide and remains alert should immediately undergo thorough water decontamination in a shower for several minutes and should immediately remove *all* clothing, including shoes and socks.

A person who only has inhaled HCN gas but has escaped to a safe environment without becoming seriously ill is not in danger of developing delayed onset of more serious symptoms (1).

BIOLOGIC MONITORING

Blood cyanide concentrations are generally used in the diagnosis of acute cyanide poisoning rather than in routine biologic monitoring. Urinary and plasma thiocyanate concentrations have been reported to be higher in workers exposed to cyanide than in control subjects. However, smoking and diet also influence thiocyanate concentrations in plasma and urine, making interpretation difficult (76). There are no studies clearly demonstrating that routine monitoring of blood cyanide levels, plama thiocyanate concentrations, or urinary thiocyanate excretions adds any information to that obtained from air cyanide concentrations and inspection of the worksite to ensure good housekeeping and work practices. In their recommended standard

for hydrogen cyanide and inorganic cyanide salts, NIOSH made no recommendations for biologic monitoring (4). The American Conference of Governmental Industrial Hygienists and the Occupational Safety and Health Administration (OSHA) also make no suggestions for biologic monitoring.

ENVIRONMENTAL MONITORING

Various manufacturers provide industry with real-time air cyanide monitors. Such monitors sound alarms when predetermined concentrations of cyanide in air are detected.

National Draeger provides Draeger Tubes that can be used for rapid, portable grab sampling. These tubes quantify air cyanide concentrations between 2 and 25 mg/m^3.

The recommended NIOSH method (112) for measurement of air cyanide concentrations involves drawing air through a cellulose-ester membrane filter and then through a bubbler containing 10 milliliters 0.1 N potassium hydroxide. Cyanide eluted from the filter with 0.1 N KOH and cyanide in the bubbler are quantified using an ion-specific electrode. This method does not distinguish between gaseous HCN and particulate cyanide salts.

EXPOSURE LIMITS

The American Conference of Governmental Industrial Hygienists (113) has set the TLV-TWA for sodium and potassium cyanide at 5 mg/m^3 (4.7 ppm) measured as cyanide. For HCN, the organization has set a ceiling limit of 10 ppm (11 mg/m^3 as HCN, or 10.6 mg/m^3 as CN).

OSHA has set a STEL (15-minute TWA) for HCN at 4.7 ppm (5 mg/m^3) measured as cyanide. The 8-hour TWA PEL for inorganic cyanide salts is 5 mg/m^3 (4.7 ppm).

NIOSH has recommended a 10-minute ceiling value for NaCN, KCN, Ca(CN)$_2$, and HCN of 5 mg/m^3 (4.7 ppm), measured as cyanide (4).

REFERENCES

1. Peden NR, Taha A, McSorley PD, et al. Industrial exposure to hydrogen cyanide: implications for treatment. Br Med J [Clin Res] 1986;293:538.

2. Gonzales ER. Cyanide evades some noses, overpowers others. JAMA 1982;248:2211.

3. Curry AS. Cyanide poisoning. Acta Pharmacol Toxicol 1963;20:291–294.

4. National Institute for Occupational Safety and Health. Criteria for a recommended standard . . . occupational exposure to hydrogen cyanide and cyanide salts. NTIS PB-266-230, NIOSH, U.S. Department of Health, Education, and Welfare, 1976.

5. Homan EF. Reactions, processes and materials with potential for cyanide exposure. In: Ballantyne B, Marrs TC, eds. Clinical and experimental toxicology of cyanides. Bristol: IOP Publishing, 1987:1–21.

6. Dugard PH. The absorption of cyanide through human skin in vitro from solutions of sodium cyanide and gaseous HCN. In: Ballantyne B, Marrs TC, eds. Clinical and experimental toxicology of cyanides. Bristol: IOP Publishing, 1987:127–137.

7. Muller-Hess B. [Intoxication caused by absorption of hydrocyanic acid through the skin] Muerch Med Wocheschr 1942;89:492.

8. Tovo S. [Poisoning due to KCN absorbed through skin.] Minerva Med 1955;75:158–161.

9. Thomas TA, Brooks JW. Accidental cyanide poisoning. Anaesthesia 1970;25:110–114.

10. Smith AR. Cyanide poisoning. NY Dept Labor Ind Bull 1932;11:169–170.

11. Young MA. Health hazards of electroplating. J Occup Med 1965;7:348–352.

12. Wright IH, Vesey CJ. Acute poisoning with gold cyanide. Anaesthesia 1986;41:936–939.

13. Stock PG, Monier-Williams GW. Preliminary report on the use of hydrogen cyanide for fumigation purposes. Reports on Public Health and Medical Subjects, no 19. London: Ministry of Health, 1923.

14. Cousineau A, Legg FG. Hydrocyanic acid gas and other toxic gases in commercial fumigation. Am J Public Health 1935;25:277–294.

15. Kleeman CR, Epstein FH, Rubini ME, et al. Initial distribution and fate of ferrocyanide in dogs. Am J Physiol 1955;182:548–552.

16. Gosselin RE, Smith RP, Hodge HC, eds. Clinical toxicology of commercial products. 5th ed. Baltimore: Williams & Wilkins, 1984:256.

17. McKelway JI. Three cases of poisoning by potassium cyanide. Am J Med Sci 1905;129:684–688.

18. Kreig A. Cyanide poisoning from metal cleaning solutions. Ann Emerg Med 1987;16:582–584.

19. Levine MS, Radford EP: Occupational exposures to cyanide in Baltimore fire fighters. J Occup Med 1978;20:53–56.

20. Jones J, McMullen J, Dougherty J. Toxic smoke inhalation: cyanide poisoning in fire victims. Am J Emerg Med 1987;5:318–321.

21. Wetherell HR. The occurrence of cyanide in the blood of fire victims. J Forensic Sci 1966;11:167–173.

22. Ballantyne B. Hydrogen cyanide as a product of combustion and a factor in morbidity and mortality from fires. In: Ballantyne B, Marrs T C, eds. Clinical and experimental toxicology of cyanides. Bristol: IOP Publishing, 1987:248–291.

23. Barcroft J. The toxicity of atmospheres containing hydrocyanic acid gas. J Hyg 1931;31:1–34.

24. Bonsall JL. Survival without sequelae following exposure to 500 mg/m³ of hydrogen cyanide. Hum Toxicol 1984;3:57–60.

25. Carmelo S. [New contributions to the study of subacute-chronic hydrocyanic acid intoxication in man.] Rass Med Ind 1955;24:254–271.

26. Drinker P. Hydrocyanic acid gas poisoning by absorption through the skin. J Ind Hyg 1932;14:1–2.

27. Walton DC, Witherspoon MG. Skin absorption of certain gases. J Pharmacol Exp Ther 1926;26:315–324.

28. Ballantyne B. Comparative acute toxicity of hydrogen cyanide and its salts. In: Lindstrom RE, ed. Proceedings of the fourth annual chemical defense bioscience review. Maryland: US Army Medical Research Institute of Chemical Defense, 1984.

29. Johnstone RT. Occupational medicine and industrial hygiene. St. Louis, CV Mosby, 1948:130–135.

30. Schulz V, Bonn R, Kindler J. Kinetics of elimination of thiocyanate in 7 healthy subjects and 8 subjects with renal failure. Klin Wochenschr 1979;57:243–247.

31. Sorbo B. Thiosulfate sulfurtransferase and mercaptopyruvate sulfurtransferase. In: Greenberg DM, ed. Metabolic pathways Vol VII. Metabolism of sulfur compounds. New York: Academic Press, 1975:433–456.

32. Westley J, Adler A, Westley L, et al. The sulfur transferases. Fundam Appl Toxicol 1983;3:377–382.

33. Ballantyne B. Toxicology of cyanides. In: Ballantyne B, Marrs TC, eds. Clinical and experimental toxicology of cyanides. Bristol: IOP Publishing, 1987:41–126.

34. Way JL, Sylvester D, Morgan RL, Isom GE, Burrows GE, Tamulinas CB, et al. Recent perspectives on the toxicodynamic basis of cyanide antagonism. Fundam Appl Toxicol 1984;4:S231–S239.

35. Vennesland B, Castric PA, Conn EE, et al. Cyanide metabolism. Fed Proc 1982;41:2639–2648.

36. Way JL. Cyanide intoxication and its mechanism of antagonism. Annu Rev Pharmacol 1984;24:451–481.

37. Piantadosi CA, Sylvia AL. Cerebral cytochrome a, a₃ inhibition by cyanide in bloodless rats. Toxicology 1984;33:67–79.

38. Vesey CJ, Wilson J. Red cell cyanide. J Pharm Pharmacol 1978;30:20–26.

39. McMillan DE, Svoboda AC. The role of erythrocytes in cyanide detoxification. J Pharmacol Exp Ther 1982;221:37–42.

40. Jouglard J, Nava G, Botta A, et al. A propos d'une intoxication aigue par le cyanure traitee par l'hydroxocobalamine. Marseille Med 1974;12:617–624.

41. Solomonson LP. Cyanide as a metabolic inhibitor. In: Vennesland B, Conn EE, Knowles CJ, et al. eds. Cyanide in biology. London: Academic Press, 1981:11–28.

42. Tursky T, Sajter V. The influence of potassium cyanide poisoning on the aminobutyric acid level in rat brain. J Neurochem 1962;9:519–523.

43. Krebs HG, Woods HG, Alberti KGMM. Hyperlactataemia and lactic acidosis. Essays Med Biochem 1975;1:81–103.

44. Mizock BA. Lactic acidosis. DM 1989;35:233–300.

45. Zilva JF. The origin of acidosis in hyperlactataemia. Ann Clin Biochem 1978;15:40–43.

46. Gevers W. Generation of protons by metabolic processes in heart cells. J Mol Cell Cardiol 1977;9:867–874.

47. Mizock BA. Controversies in lactic acidosis. JAMA 1987;258:497–501.

48. Johnston DG, Alberti KGMM. Acid-base balance in metabolic acidoses. Clin Endocrinol Metab 1983;12:267–285.

49. Ballantyne B. An experimental assessment of the diagnostic potential of histochemical and biochemical methods for cytochrome oxidase in acute cyanide poisoning. Cell Mol Biol 1977;22:109–123.

50. Wexler J, Whittenberger JL, Dumke PR. The effect of cyanide on the electrocardiogram of man. Am Heart J 1947;34:163–173.

51. DeBush RF, Seidl LG. Attempted suicide by cyanide. Calif Med 1969;110:394–396.

52. Graham DL, Laman D, Theodore J, et al. Acute cyanide poisoning complicated by lactic acidosis and pulmonary edema. Arch Intern Med 1977;137:1051–1055.

53. Brivet F, Delfraissy JF, Duche M, et al. Acute cyanide poisoning: recovery with non-specific supportive therapy. Intensive Care Med 1983;9:33–35.

54. Uitti RJ, Rajput AH, Ashenhurst EM, et al. Cyanide-induced parkinsonism: a clinicopathologic report. Neurology 1985;35:921–925.

55. Peters CG, Mundy JVB, Rayner PR. Acute cyanide poisoning. Anaesthesia 1982;37:582–586.

56. Flury F, Zernik F. HCN (hydrocyanic acid, prussic acid). In: Noxious gases—vapors, mist, smoke and dust particles. Berlin: Verlag von Jullius Springer, 1931:400–415.

57. McNamara BP. Estimates of the toxicity of hydrocyanide acid vapor in man. Edgewood Arsenal Technical Report EB-TR-76023, Department of the Army, August 1976.

58. Miller MH, Toops TC. Acute cyanide poisoning. Recovery with sodium thiosulfate therapy. J Indiana State Med Assoc 1951;44:1164.

59. Braddock WH, Tingle GR. So-called cyanide rash in gold mine mill workers. J Ind Hyg 1930;12:259–264.

60. Nolan JW. Potassium cyanide poisoning. JAMA 1908;50:365.

61. Wrangsjö K, Mårtensson A. Hydrazine contact dermatitis from gold plating. Contact Dermatitis 1986;15:244–245.

62. Mathias CGT. Contact dermatitis from cyanide plating solutions. Arch Dermatol 1982;118:420–422.

63. Elkins HB. The chemistry of industrial toxicology. 2nd ed. New York: John Wiley & Sons, 1959:94–95.

64. Barsky MH. Ulcerations of the nasal membranes and perforation of the septum in a copper plating factory—unusual and sudden incidence. NY State J Med 1937;37:1031–1034.

65. Cohen SR, Davis DM, Kramkowski RS. Clinical manifestations of chromic acid toxicity—nasal lesions in electroplate workers. Cutis 1974;13:558–568.

66. Blanc P, Hogan M, Mallin K, et al. Cyanide intoxication among silver-reclaiming workers. JAMA 1985;253:367–371.

67. Saia B, DeRosa E, Galzigna L. [Remarks on the chronic poisoning from cyanide.] Med Lav 1970;61:580–586.

68. Radojicic B. [Determining thiocyanate in urine of workers exposed to cyanides.] Arh Hig Rada Toksikol 1973;24:227–232.

69. Chandra H, Gupta BN, Bhargava SK. Chronic cyanide exposure—a biochemical and industrial hygiene study. J Anal Toxicol 1980;4:161–165.

70. Wollman SH. Nature of the inhibition by thiocyanate of the iodide concentrating mechanism of the thyroid gland. Am J Physiol 1956;186:453–459.

71. Wood JL. Biochemistry. In: Newman AA, ed. Chemistry and biochemistry of thiocyanic acid and its derivatives. New York: Academic Press, 1975:156–221.

72. Wuthrich F. [Chronic cyanide poisoning as industrial intoxicant.] Schweiz Med Wochenschr 1954 1954;84:105–107.

73. El Ghawabi SH, Gaafar MA, El-Saharti AA, et al. Chronic cyanide exposure: a clinical, radioisotope, and laboratory study. Br J Ind Med 1975;32:215–219.

74. Hartung R. Cyanides and nitriles. In: Clayton GD, Clayton FE, eds. Patty's industrial hygiene and toxicology. 3rd ed. Vol 2C. New York: John Wiley & Sons, 1982:4845–4900.

75. Howard JW, Hanzal RF. Chronic toxicity for rats of food treated with hydrogen cyanide. J Agric Food Chem 1955;3:325–329.

76. Maehly AC, Swensson A. Cyanide and thiocyanate levels in blood and urine of workers with low-grade exposure to cyanide. Int Arch Arbeitsmed 1970;27:195–209.

77. Monekosso GL, Wilson J. Plasma thiocyanate and vitamin B₁₂ in Nigerian patients with degenerative neurological disease. Lancet 1966;1:1062–1064.

78. Osuntokun BO, Wilson J, Langman MJS, et al. Report of a controlled

trial of hydroxocobalamin and riboflavin in the Nigerian ataxic neuropathy. J Neurol Neurosurg Psychiatry 1970;33:633–666.

79. Moore GRW, Traugott U, Scheinberg LC, et al. Tropical spastic paraparesis: a model of virus-induced, cytotoxic T-cell-mediated demyelination? Ann Neurol 1989;26:523–530.

80. Cruickshank JK, Rudge P, Dalgleish AG, et al. Tropical spastic paraparesis and human T cell lymphotropic virus type I in the United Kingdom. Brain 1989;112:1057–1090.

81. Doherty PA, Ferm V, Smith RP. Congenital malformations induced by infusions of sodium cyanide in the Golden hamster. Toxicol Appl Pharmacol 1982;64:456–464.

82. Ballantyne B. Artifacts in the definition of toxicity by cyanides and cyanogens. Fundam Appl Toxicol 1983;3:400–408.

83. Wilson J, Matthews DM. Metabolic inter-relationships between cyanide, thiocyanate and vitamin B_{12} in smokers and non-smokers. Clin Sci 1966;31:1–7.

84. Ballantyne B, Marrs TC. Post-mortem features and criteria for the diagnosis of acute lethal cyanide poisoning. In: Ballantyne B, Marrs TC, eds. Clinical and experimental toxicology of cyanides. Bristol: IOP Publishing, 1987:217–247.

85. Ballantyne B. In vitro production of cyanide in normal human blood and the influence of thiocyanate and storage temperature. Clin Toxicol 1977;11:173–193.

86. Symington IS, Anderson RA, Oliver JS, et al. Cyanide exposure in fires. Lancet 1978;8:91–92

87. Hall AH, Rumack B. Clinical toxicology of cyanide. Ann Emerg Med 1986;15:1067–1074.

88. Shragg TA, Albertson TE, Fisher CJ. Cyanide poisoning after bitter almond ingestion. West J Med 1982;136:65–69.

89. Johnson RP, Mellors JW. Arteriolarization of venous blood gases: a clue to the diagnosis of cyanide poisoning. J Emerg Med 1988;6:401–404.

90. Buchanan IS, Dhamee MS, Griffiths FED, et al. Abnormal fundal appearances in a case of poisoning by a cyanide capsule. Med Sci Law 1976;16:29–32.

91. Wesson DE, Foley R, Sabatini S, Wharton J, Kapusnik J, Kurtzman NA. Treatment of acute cyanide intoxication with hemodialysis. Am J Nephrol 1985;5:121–126.

92. Lasch EE, El Shawa R. Multiple cases of cyanide poisoning by apricot kernels in children from Gaza. Pediatrics 1981;68:5–7

93. Curry SC. Methemoglobinemia. Ann Emerg Med 1982;11:214–221

94. Chen KK, Rose CL. Nitrite and thiosulfate therapy in cyanide poisoning. JAMA 1952;149:113–119.

95. Kiese M, Weger N. Formation of ferrihaemoglobin with aminophenols in the human for the treatment of cyanide poisoning. Eur J Pharmacol 1969;7:97–105.

96. Vogel SN, Sultan TR, Ten Eyck RP. Cyanide poisoning. Clin Toxicol 1981;18:367–383.

97. Berlin CM. The treatment of cyanide poisoning in children. Pediatrics 1970;46:793–796.

98. Deleted in proof.

99. Moser P. Zur wirkung von nitrit auf rote blutzellen des menschen. Arch Exp Pathol Pharmakol 1950;210:60–70.

100. Hall AH, Doutre WH, Ludden T, Kulig KW, Rumack BH. Nitrite/thiosulfate treated acute cyanide poisoning: estimated kinetics after antidote. J Toxicol Clin Toxicol 1987;25:121–133.

101. Way JL, Leung P, Sylvester DM, Burrows G, Way JL, Tamulinas C. Methaemoglobin formation in the treatment of acute cyanide intoxication. In: Ballantyne B, Marrs TC, eds. Clinical and experimental toxicology of cyanides. Bristol: IOP Publishing, 1987:402–412.

102. Aw TC, Bishop CM. Letter. J Soc Occup Med 1981;31:173–175.

103. Friedberg KD, Shukla UR. The efficiency of aquocobalamine as an antidote in cyanide poisoning when given alone or combined with sodium thiosulfate. Arch Toxicol 1975;33:103–113.

104. Kruszyna R, Kruszyna H, Smith RP. Comparison of hydroxylamine, 4-dimethylaminophenol and nitrite protection against cyanide poisoning in mice. Arch Toxicol 1982;49:191–202.

105. Chen KK, Rose RL, Clowes GHA. Methylene blue (methylthionine chloride), nitrites and sodium thiosulphate against cyanide poisoning. Proc Soc Exp Biol Med 1933;31:250–251.

106. Weger NP. Treatment of cyanide poisoning with 4-dimethylaminophenol (DMAP)—experimental and clinical overview. Fundam Appl Toxicol 1983;3:387–396.

107. Dodds C, McKnight C. Cyanide toxicity after immersion and the hazards of dicobalt edetate. Br Med J [Clin Res] 1985;291:785–786.

108. Gurrows GE, Way JL. Antagonism of cyanide toxicity by phenoxybenzamine (abstract). Fed Proc 1975;36:534.

109. Way JL, Burrows GE. Cyanide intoxication: protection with chlorpromazine. Toxicol Appl Pharmacol 1976;36:1–5.

110. Way JL, End E, Sheehy MH, et al. Effect of oxygen on cyanide intoxication IV. Hyperbaric oxygen. Toxicol Appl Pharmacol 1972;22:415–421.

111. Callaghan JM, Halton DM. Solutions A and B: cyanide antidote or folklore myth? J Soc Occup Med 1988;38:65–68.

112. Eller PM, ed. NIOSH manual of analytical methods. NIOSH publication no. 84-100, NTIS PB85-179018. 3rd ed. Cincinnati, OH: NIOSH, 1984.

113. American Conference of Governmental Industrial Hygeinists. Documentation of the Threshold Limit Values and biological exposure indices, 5th Ed. Cincinnati, OH: ACGIH, 1986:153,314.

62

Hydrogen Sulfide

Jou-Fang Deng, M.D.

CHEMICAL AND PHYSICAL PROPERTIES

Hydrogen sulfide (H_2S; CAS registry number 7783-06-4) occurs in a variety of natural and industrial settings. It exists as a gas under normal conditions. However, it may be liquefied by reduced temperature or increased pressure. Synonyms for hydrogen sulfide include dihydrogen monosulfide, dihydrogen sulfide, hydrogen sulphide, hydrosulfuric acid, sewer gas, stink damp, sulfur hydride, and sulfuretted hydrogen (1).

Hydrogen sulfide is a colorless, irritant, and asphyxiant gas. It is generally stable when properly stored in cylinders at room temperature. However, in the air, it is flammable and explosive and may be ignited by static discharge. It does not polymerize. It may react with metals, oxidizing agents, and acids such as nitric acid, bromine pentafluoride, chlorine trifluoride, nitrogen triiodide, nitrogen trichloride, oxygen difluoride, and phenyldiazonium chloride. When heated to decomposition, it emits highly toxic sulfur oxide fumes. The general chemical and physical properties of hydrogen sulfide are listed in Table 63.1 (1–3).

SITES, INDUSTRIES, AND BUSINESSES ASSOCIATED WITH EXPOSURES

Hydrogen sulfide is one of the principal compounds involved in the natural cycle of sulfur in our environment. Natural sources constitute approximately 90% of the atmospheric burden of H_2S (4). It is found in the environment in volcanic gases, marshes, swamps, sulfur springs, and other geothermal sources, and as a product of bacterial action during the decay of plant and animal protein (2, 5, 6). Hydrogen sulfide generation can be expected whenever oxygen is depleted, and organic material containing sulfate is present (7). For example, in India and Sri Lanka, H_2S is produced as a byproduct in the process by which coconut fibers are separated from the husk. This procedure involves the decomposition of husks in shallow ponds, and H_2S is produced as a result of microbiologic decay. It occurs in most petroleum and natural gas deposits and also in many mines. As a result, it is a potential health hazard to workers involved in drilling, mining, smelting, or processing operations (2).

Hydrogen sulfide is used in the manufacturing of chemicals; in metallurgy; as an analytical reagent; as an agricultural disinfectant; as an intermediate for sulfuric acid, elemental sulfur, sodium sulfide, and other inorganic sulfides; as an additive in extreme pressure lubricants and cutting oils; and as an intermediate for organic sulfur compounds (1). Large quantities of H_2S are used in the production of heavy water, which is used as a moderator in some nuclear power reactors.

In other industries, hydrogen sulfide is produced as an undesirable byproduct. In manufacturing processes, it is formed whenever elemental sulfur or certain sulfur compounds are present with organic chemicals at high temperature (8). Examples include petroleum refineries, natural gas plants, petrochemical plants, coke oven plants, kraft paper mills, viscose rayon manufacture, sulfur production, iron smelters, food processing plants, and tanneries. In the tanning industry, H_2S is produced in the process by which hair or wool is removed from the hides.

In many instances, H_2S has been found together with other substances such as carbon disulfide, methane, sulfur dioxide; however, it could exist by itself. Generally, hydrogen sulfide is not found in high concentrations in the ambient air. Occasional catastrophic releases in processing and transport have exposed the general public to concentrations high enough to elicit toxic symptoms and death. Such accidents can be anticipated under the condition whenever sulfur containing chemicals react with acid (e.g., sodium sulfhydrate reacts with acid sewage) (9, 10).

The National Institute for Occupational Safety and Health (NIOSH) estimated in 1977 that approximately 125,000 employees in 73 industries were potentially exposed to hydrogen sulfide in the United States. The occupations of which employees may be exposed to H_2S are listed in Table 62.2 (2).

Since it is heavier than air, H_2S tends to accumulate in low-lying areas. This property is responsible for many of the poisonings occurring during oil drilling, manure sewage handling, and wastewater treatment processes. Most of the instances of H_2S poisonings are occupational. In the United States, H_2S is present in fatal concentrations in 4–14% of some natural gas at the wellhead; gas field leaks and resulting poisonings account for many of the fatalities related to H_2S exposures (2). In the high sulfur oil fields of Wyoming and western Texas, 26 persons died from exposure to H_2S between October 1, 1974, and April 28, 1976 (11). In addition to petroleum refining, other industries such as heavy water manufacturing, hide tanning, rubber vulcanizing, rayon manufacturing, pelt processing, manure refuse and sewage, fishing, hospital, and wastewater treatment have also reported H_2S poisonings (3). Acute H_2S poisoning is not solely an occupational hazard. Occasional community-wide accidents have also been reported. The most dramatic and

Table 62.1. Physical and Chemical Properties of Hydrogen Sulfide

Molecular formula	H_2S
Molecular weight	34.08
Boiling point	$-60.33°C$
Specific gravity, 0°C	1.54 g/l
Vapor pressure, 25°C	19.6 atm
Melting point	$-85.49°C$
Vapor density	1.19
Autoignition temperature	250°C
Explosive range in air	4.5–45.5%
Color	Colorless
Conversion factors	1 mg/m³ = 0.717 ppm
	1 ppm = 1.394 mg/m³

Adapted from references 1–3.

Table 62.2. Occupations with Potential Exposure to Hydrogen Sulfide

Animal fat and oil processors	Lead removers
Animal manure removers	Lithographers
Artificial-flavor makers	Lithopone makers
Asphalt storage workers	Livestock farmers
Barium carbonate makers	Metallurgists
Barium salt makers	Miners
Blast furnace workers	Natural gas production and
Brewery workers	processing workers
Bromide-brine workers	Painters using polysulfide
Cable splicers	caulking compounds
Caisson workers	Papermakers
Carbon disulfide makers	Petroleum production and
Cellophane makers	refinery workers
Chemical laboratory workers,	Phosphate purifiers
teachers, students	Photoengravers
Cistern cleaners	Pipeline maintenance workers
Citrus root fumigators	Pyrite burners
Coal gasification workers	Rayon makers
Coke oven workers	Refrigerant makers
Copper ore sulfidizers	Rubber and plastics processors
Depilatory makers	Septic tank cleaners
Dyemakers	Sewage treatment plant workers
Excavators	Sewer workers
Felt makers	Sheepdippers
Fermentation process workers	Silk makers
Fertilizer makers	Slaughterhouse workers
Fishing and fish processing	Smelting workers
workers	Soapmakers
Fur dressers	Sugar beet and cane processors
Geothermal power drilling and	Sulfur spa workers
production workers	Sulfur products processors
Gluemakers	Synthetic fiber makers
Gold ore workers	Tank gagers
Heavy metal precipitators	Tannery workers
Heavy water manufacturers	Textiles printers
Hydrochloric acid purifiers	Thiophene makers
Hydrogen sulfide production	Tunnel workers
and sales workers	Utility hole and trench workers
Landfill workers	Well diggers and cleaners
Lead ore sulfidizers	Wool pullers

Source: National Institute for Occupational Safety and Health, 1977.

serious event occurred in 1950 at Poza Rica, Mexico. The flare apparatus on a gas well malfunctioned and large quantities of H_2S were released into the atmosphere. Within 3 hours, 320 residents were hospitalized and 22 died (12).

CLINICAL TOXICOLOGY

Route of Exposure, Absorption, Metabolism, and Elimination

The kinetics of H_2S have been partially characterized in animal studies. In environmental and occupational exposures, the lung rather than the skin is the primary route of absorption (13, 14). The dermal absorption of H_2S is minimal (15, 16). Results from animal inhalation studies indicate that H_2S is distributed in the body to the brain, liver, kidneys, pancreas, and small intestine (17). With the body, H_2S is metabolized by oxidation, methylation, and reaction with metallo- or disulfide-containing proteins. Orally, intraperitoneally, and intravenously administered H_2S is primarily oxidized and directly excreted as either

Table 62.3. Physiologic Effects of Human Exposure to H_2S

Physiologic Effects	Concentration (ppm)
Odor intensity	
Threshold	0.02
Minimally perceptible	0.13
Faint but readily perceptible	0.77
Easily noticeable, moderate	4.6
Safe for 7-hour exposure	20
Strong, unpleasant but not	
intolerable	27
Eye and respiratory tract irritation is	
noticeable	50
Olfactory fatigue level	100
Olfactory nerve paralysis	150
Prolonged exposure may cause pulmonary	
edema	250
Dizziness, breathing ceases in few minutes	500
Unconscious quickly, death will result if not	
rescued promptly	700
Rapid collapse and respiratory paralysis	1000
Immenent death	5000

Adapted from CRC Crit Rev Toxicol 1984;13:25–97, with permission from CRC Press, Inc., Boca Raton, Florida.

free sulfate or conjugated sulfate in the urine (18). The importance of methylation in the detoxification processes of H_2S, however, is unknown (19). The reaction of H_2S with vital metalloenzymes such as cytochrome oxidase is the likely toxic mechanism of H_2S (7, 20). Reaction with nonessential proteins may also serve as a detoxification pathway (21, 22). Systemic poisoning occurs when the amount of H_2S absorbed exceeds that which can be detoxified and eliminated (14, 23). Because of its rapid oxidation in the blood, H_2S is not considered a cumulative poison (14, 24, 25). The fact that low concentrations of the gas, e.g., 20 ppm, can be tolerated for long periods without harm is also an indication that, at lower concentrations, potential cumulative action is unlikely (26).

There are no animal data available regarding the exhalation of H_2S after inhalation exposure. In animals, the excretion of H_2S by the lungs is minimal after parenteral administration of H_2S (26–28). However, because rescue personnel have developed H_2S poisoning shortly after starting mouth-to-mouth resuscitation on victims who had been poisoned, it is likely that significant H_2S is excreted from the lungs (9).

Acute Toxicity

PHYSIOLOGIC EFFECTS AND GENERAL TOXICOLOGY

Hydrogen sulfide is both an irritant and an asphyxiant gas. The physiologic and toxic effects associated with various concentrations of H_2S exposure are listed in Table 62.3, and can be summarized as follows:

Hydrogen sulfide is well-known by its characteristic odor of "rotten eggs." The perception threshold of this odor varies individually; however, 0.13 ppm has been generally accepted as the threshold. At concentration of 50 ppm, H_2S acts as an irritant on the mucous membranes of the eyes and the respiratory tract. Its irritant action on the eye produces keratoconjunctivitis, known as "gas eye." When inhaled, H_2S exerts an irritant action throughout the entire respiratory tract; the deeper structures suffer the greatest damage. The irritant action and odor of rotten eggs often provide the first warning of H_2S exposure. Unfortunately, above 150 ppm, the gas exerts a paralyzing effect on the olfactory apparatus. If an exposed person is not aware of this effect, it could jeopardize life. Prolonged exposure to moderate concentrations (250 ppm) may cause pulmonary edema. At concentrations over 500 ppm, drowsiness, dizziness, excitement, headache, unstable gait, and other systemic symptoms occur within a few minutes. Sudden loss of consciousness without premonition, anxiety, or sense of struggle are characteristic of acute exposure at concentrations above 700 ppm. At concentrations of 1000-2000 ppm, H_2S gas is rapidly absorbed through the lung into the blood. Initially hyperpnea occurs, followed by rapid collapse and respiratory inhibition. At higher concentrations, H_2S exerts an immediate paralyzing effect on the respiratory centers. When the concentration reaches 5000 ppm, imminent death almost always results. Generally speaking, imminent death due to asphyxia can happen at any time when the concentration reaches 1000 ppm or more, unless spontaneous respiration is reestablished or artificial respiration is promptly provided (3).

TARGET ORGAN TOXICITY

The main target organs or systems for H_2S include the olfactory apparatus, eyes, respiratory system, and nervous system. However, other organs such as the heart, digestive system, and endocrine system may also be affected (29–33). The organ-specific effects of H_2S exposure can be summarized as follows:

Effect on Olfactory Apparatus The typical "rotten eggs" odor of H_2S is detectable by olfaction at very low concentrations, between 0.02 and 0.13 ppm. However, the odor intensity may be perceived differently by different individuals when the ambient concentration is less than 30 ppm. Below this concentration, there is no known human health consequence related to the exposure. The characteristic odor of H_2S, as long as it is perceptible, provides a useful warning signal since the odor threshold is much lower than the toxic level. However, when the concentration reaches 100 ppm, olfactory fatigue occurs (2, 33, 34). Once the concentration reaches 150 ppm, H_2S exerts a paralyzing effect on the olfactory apparatus, and its natural signal of warning will be lost (24, 26, 32). These effects may occur gradually on exposure to small amounts of this gas or quite rapidly where lethal concentrations of the gas are present (35, 36). Therefore, odor of H_2S is an unreliable warning signal at elevated concentrations because of rapid paralysis of the olfactory apparatus (14, 23, 24).

Effect on Eyes The direct action of H_2S on mucous membranes is usually observed first by symptoms of eye irritation, resulting from local inflammation of the conjunctiva and cornea (3). Conjunctivitis or "gas eye" was first described by workers in the petroleum industry (3). Acute inflammation of conjunctiva accompanied by lacrimation and mucopurulent exudate is not uncommon. In severe cases, corneal erosion with blurred vision may also occur. Occasionally, corneal ulceration may occur, resulting in impaired vision (24). Since the cornea is affected together with the conjunctiva in many instances, keratoconjunctivitis rather than conjunctivitis more accurately describes the ophthalmologic effects of H_2S exposure (37–39). In general, irritation of the eyes occurs at a concentration of H_2S of 50 ppm; however, conjunctivitis or "sore eyes" have been observed upon exposures in the range of 5–100 ppm (40, 41).

Effect on Respiratory System At low concentrations, the irritant effects of H_2S are more prominent on the eyes and olfactory apparatus. However, prolonged exposure to concentrations as low as 50 ppm may cause inflammation and dryness of the respiratory tract (23, 24, 42). The irritant effect of H_2S extends rather uniformly throughout the entire respiratory tract, resulting in rhinitis, pharyngitis, laryngitis, bronchitis, and pneumonia (25). Cough, sore throat, hoarseness, runny nose, and chest tightness are the most common symptoms of exposure between 50 and 250 ppm. However, in acute massive exposure, symptoms of respiratory irritation may not appear, either because of the shortness of the exposure or because they are obscured by the more prominent, systemic effects. Apparently, irritating symptoms will vary with the duration and intensity of the exposures.

Pneumonia resulting from H_2S exposure is thought to partially result from impaired ciliary activity and alveolar macrophage dysfunction (43, 44). In an in vitro study, using sections of rabbit trachea exposed to H_2S in an environmentally controlled chamber, either 600 ppm for 5 minutes or 400 ppm for 10 minutes resulted in cessation of ciliary movement (43). In the rat, H_2S exposure to 45 ppm for 4 or 6 hours decreased the ability of the lungs to inactivate *Staphylococcus epidermidis* deposited by aerosol. The reduced *Staphylococcus* inactivation was considered to be due to an impaired alveolar macrophage function caused by the H_2S exposure (44). These findings may partially explain the mechanism of pneumonia occurring after H_2S poisoning. Since H_2S can penetrate the alveoli, pulmonary edema is not uncommon following prolonged exposure to H_2S in concentrations exceeding 250 ppm (23). In acute massive exposure, systemic poisoning by H_2S results in paralysis of the respiratory center of the brain. Upon acute exposures at concentrations above 1000 ppm, respiratory paralysis followed by imminent death may occur at any time (14, 23, 25). Autopsy findings from those individuals suffering an instantaneous death following H_2S exposure reveal no characteristic signs, indicating that asphyxia rather than a direct mucous membrane irritant effect predominates in an acute massive exposure of H_2S.

Effect on Nervous System The central nervous system effects of H_2S have been considered to be a result of enzyme poisoning at the cellular level. Following rapid absorption from the alveoli, H_2S is transported quickly to the brain. Central nervous system depression symptoms such as drowsiness, fatigue, and dizziness may occur with environmental exposure at 200 ppm. As the concentration reaches 500 ppm, headache, weakness of extremities, spasms, nausea, agitation, dizziness, and staggering may become more prominent. This may be followed by rapid loss of consciousness and respiratory paralysis as the concentration rises above 1000 ppm (24, 25). At higher concentrations of H_2S, rapid respiratory paralysis and death may occur at any moment without any warning symptoms. Delirium, coma, and convulsions along with other neurologic symptoms may also occur in certain conditions of acute exposures (9, 14, 24, 25, 31, 33, 45). Clinical observations show that many victims recover completely from an unresponsive status in the settings of acute massive H_2S poisoning. However, irreversible damage to the nervous system associated with prominent sequelae after H_2S poisoning is not uncommon (23, 24, 30, 31).

Effect on Other Organs or Systems Studies regarding the health effects of H_2S on the other organs or systems are limited. ECG tracings indicative of cardiac arrhythmia, myocardial ischemia, and myocardial infarction have been observed in cases of H$_2$S intoxication (10, 29, 30, 46, 47). Acute poisoning of rabbits with H$_2$S caused changes in ventricular repolarization, while subacute poisoning led to cardiac arrhythmia. A decrease in the reactivity of ATP phosphohydrolase and NADPH$_2$ oxidoreductase in myocardial cells was also noted, indicating a direct toxic effect of hydrogen sulfide on myocardial cells (48). These findings are predictable, since H$_2$S exerts its poisoning effects at the cellular level in a manner similar to cyanide. In H$_2$S poisoning, the gastrointestinal and endocrine systems may also be affected, producing symptoms of nausea, vomiting, diarrhea, abdominal cramps, gastric burning, and irregular menstruation (31–33, 49).

CLINICAL SYNDROME

The mechanism of H$_2$S poisoning is similar to that of other sulfides and cyanides. Similar to cyanide, H$_2$S is a potent inhibitor of cytochrome oxidase resulting in tissue hypoxia (50). In purified preparations of cytochrome oxidase, sulfide has proven more potent than cyanide (51).

Clinically, acute H$_2$S intoxication can be defined as the effects from a single exposure to massive concentrations of hydrogen sulfide that rapidly produce signs of unconsciousness and respiratory distress. Concentrations exceeding 700 ppm produce such acute effects. Subacute H$_2$S intoxication is the term applied to the effects of continuous exposure for up to several hours to concentrations ranging from 100–700 ppm. In this range of exposure, eye irritation is the most commonly observed effect. However, pulmonary edema may be a more important and potentially fatal complication of subacute H$_2$S intoxication (52). The following two cases illustrate typical presentations of acute massive and subacute intoxication by H$_2$S (52).

Case 1: Acute Massive Intoxication   "A 40-year-old healthy man collapsed immediately after having descended into a hot-spring reservoir for regular maintenance work to clean precipitant debris. The other four men who remained outside the manhole went down one by one to rescue him and also collapsed suddenly after smelling a strong odor of rotten eggs down at the bottom. . . . One died on the spot; the other four were resuscitated and sent to a hospital. They presented to the hospital emergency room with an odor of rotten eggs and were unconscious but agitated, vomiting, tachypneic, cyanotic, with clammy skin and gray-greenish sputum. During their hospitalization, aspiration pneumonia and keratoconjunctivitis were noted in three of them. They recovered completely without any significant sequelae" (52).

Case 2: Subacute Intoxication   "A 30-year-old man collapsed in a hot-spring reservoir after he and an 18-year-old man had been shovelling the precipitant debris at the bottom for 2 hours. . . . At emergency room, both presented with tachypnea. Diffuse rhonchi, rales, and wheezing were audible throughout their chests. Their chest films showed infiltrates characteristic of pulmonary edema, bilaterally. Both developed refractory respiratory failure and died within 12 hours after the exposure" (52).

The severity and variety of clinical manifestation and outcomes related to acute massive exposure of H$_2$S have been described extensively. The following acute clinical manifestations and outcomes are illustrated: (a) death due to acute respiratory arrest; (b) successful resuscitation from recurrent apnea and pulmonary edema; (c) initial unconsciousness followed by tachypnea and complete recovery; (d) recovery from simple pulmonary edema without systemic involvement; (e) unconsciousness followed by mild symptoms after recovery. One striking observation in the study was the predominance both in frequency and severity of the systemic neurologic manifestations over the local irritative effects. This finding is quite typical in the instances of acute massive H$_2$S intoxication (9). In 221 cases of exposure to H$_2$S associated with the oil, gas, and petrochemical industries in Canada, the overall mortality was 6%; three quarters of all victims experienced a period of unconsciousness, and 12% were comatose. A high proportion of patients had other neurologic signs and symptoms, including altered behavior patterns, confusion, vertigo, agitation, or somnolence. Respiratory tract effects were second in frequency only to neurologic manifestations. Forty percent of all patients required some form of respiratory assistance and 15% of all patients developed pulmonary edema. Less severely affected patients complained primarily of headache, sore eyes, or gastrointestinal upsets. Some clinical observations reported that victims of H$_2$S poisonings may survive with neurologic sequelae; however, Burnett et al. did not find any recognizable neurologic sequelae among survivors (31).

Chronic and Longterm Effects

The health effects of longterm exposures to low concentrations of H$_2$S are still uncertain. A preliminary study done in Rotorua, New Zealand—a major recreational center—showed that no chronic health impairment could be identified after longterm exposure to H$_2$S to 0.005–1.9 ppm (53). Other reports suggest that prolonged exposure to H$_2$S with concentrations below 50 ppm over long periods may produce a chronic form of poisoning (25, 54). Such a chronic intoxication is a subjective state, characterized by certain neurasthenic symptoms such as fatigue, headache, dizziness, and irritability (55). Some authors have suggested that chronic symptoms and signs actually reflect recurring acute or subacute toxic exposures (7).

CARCINOGENICITY, MUTAGENICITY, TERATOGENICITY, AND EFFECTS ON REPRODUCTION

There are no published reports of carcinogenesis, mutagenesis, or teratogenesis attributable to hydrogen sulfide exposure.

Management of Toxicity

TREATMENT

General Supportive Care   In acute H$_2$S intoxication, cessation of respiration is an immediate threat to life. Accordingly, the provision of artificially assisted respiration on an emergency basis is absolutely critical. Hence, moving the victim to fresh air and starting respiratory and cardiovascular support should be done immediately. Since many instances occurred in which the rescuers were overcome by H$_2$S, rescuers should wear a self-contained breathing apparatus. Mouth-to-mouth resuscitation is not recommended (9). After being moved away from the site, the victim needs to be monitored for respiratory distress and neurologic, ophthalmologic, and possible cardiovascular complications. If the victim is not breathing, cardiopulmonary resuscitation (CPR) should be started immediately. Since oxygen can enhance the metabolism of sulfide and may benefit the injured tissue, it should be supplied as quickly as possible.

Induction of Methemoglobinemia   Since the poisoning mechanism of H_2S is similar to that of cyanide, induction of methemoglobinemia by the nitrite antidote method, a common treatment for cyanide poisoning, has also been proposed in the treatment of H_2S poisoning (10, 56–58). In laboratory animals, the therapeutic induction of methemoglobinemia has been shown to have both protective and antidotal effects against sulfide as well as against cyanide (20). Clinically, several cases have been reported that were successfully treated by this method in conjunction with vigorous supportive care (10, 57, 58). Overall, however, the success rate of the nitrite antidote method for sulfide poisoning has not been as clearly established as for cyanide treatment, and the value of this method has been questioned (59). These authors feel that the methemoglobinemia protocol is too slow to detoxify the sulfides when compared with oxyhemoglobin. They suggest that breathing oxygen-enriched air is the only effective antidote.

To induce methemoglobinemia, the literature suggests beginning with a 3% sodium nitrite intravenous injection. However, if the sodium nitrite is not ready for injection, amyl nitrite by inhalation 15–30 seconds of every minute is recommended. Once 10 ml of 3% sodium nitrite is available, it can be injected intravenously over a 2–4 minute period for an adult. If signs and symptoms of systemic poisoning continue or recur, the nitrite injection should be repeated with half the dose. Cyanide antidote kits have been available in industrial and hospital settings for the purpose of methemoglobinemia induction. However, the thiosulfate solution contained in these kits has not been recommended in the treatment of H_2S poisoning.

Hyperbaric Oxygen Therapy   Recently, hyperbaric oxygen therapy has been proposed for severe H_2S poisoning (60, 61). Successful treatment by this regimen has been reported in two patients. The first patient was unconscious with pulmonary edema on presentation. After 300 milligrams sodium nitrite was injected, he could open and close his eyes on command but still showed decerebrate posturing of his right arm upon painful stimuli. He was extubated immediately after hyperbaric oxygen therapy (2.5 atmospheres absolute oxygen) for 90 minutes. Three hours after leaving the emergency room, he was eating a soft diet. He was discharged 48 hours later after another two sessions of hyperbaric oxygen therapy (60). The second patient was also unconscious on presentation. He received a total of 750 milligrams sodium nitrite by intravenous injection without clinical response. Hyperbaric oxygen therapy was started 10 hours after H_2S exposure. After the first hyperbaric oxygen therapy session, the patient was more alert and able to follow simple commands (61). It was proposed that hyperbaric oxygen therapy would increase oxyhemoglobin levels and tissue oxygen concentrations, thus allowing oxygen to better compete with sulfide for binding sites on the cytochrome oxidase system and also enhancing the catalytic oxidation of sulfide. Also, hyperbaric oxygen therapy could minimize the damage of injured tissue by optimum supportive care (61). Since hyperbaric oxygen therapy has been used only recently in the treatment of H_2S poisoning, more clinical evaluations are needed before drawing any conclusion. However, this method can be considered as an extension of the vigorous general supportive care that has been reemphasized by many investigators.

In 1985, 250 cases of exposure to H_2S in Alberta, Canada, were reviewed and compared with the study done in 1977 (62). It was found that (a) the fatality rate decreased from 6% to

Table 62.4.   Ambient Air Quality Standards for H_2S

State	Concentrations (ppm)	Averaging Time
California	0.03	1 hour
Connecticut	0.2	8 hours
Kentucky	0.01	1 hour
Massachusetts	0.014	24 hours
Montana	0.03	30 minutes
Nevada	0.24	8 hours
New York	0.10	1 hour
Pennsylvania	0.10	1 hour
Texas	0.08	30 minutes
Virginia	0.16	24 hours

Source: Environmental Protection Agency, 1986.

2.8%; (b) the unconsciousness rate at hospital arrival decreased from 13% to 2%; (c) the hospital admission rate fell from 51% to 22%; (d) and there was a relative decrease in the accident worker compensation claim rate (17.4%). These findings were consistent with an impact of increased awareness of the dangers of H_2S, improved first aid treatment at the site of exposure, and the vigorous supportive care in the clinic or hospital.

Although the Canadian study does not conclusively demonstrate the efficacy of vigorous general supportive care in the treatment of H_2S poisonings, its findings suggest that such an approach may be the most appropriate treatment.

DIAGNOSIS

The diagnostic criteria for environmental poisoning include: a history of exposure, an appropriate clinical syndrome, and the presence of the suspected chemical and/or its metabolites in body fluids. The diagnosis of H_2S poisoning relies primarily on the history of exposure, the presence of the smell of rotten eggs, and the fairly specific clinical syndrome. The presence of darkening of copper and silver coins in the pockets or of discolored jewelry provides supporting evidence of exposure to H_2S (2). The clinical picture of acute massive H_2S poisoning is usually very typical as the case above demonstrates. Since the plasma concentrations of sulfhemoglobin do not reflect the degree of H_2S exposure, their values in the clinical setting have never been confirmed. So far, there is no laboratory test considered valuable for diagnostic use in clinical practice. However, urinary thiosulfate and blood sulfide anion determination would be useful in a forensic setting (63).

EXPOSURE LIMITS, ENVIRONMENTAL AND BIOLOGIC MONITORING, AND MEDICAL SURVEILLANCE

Exposure Limits

No federal ambient air or emission standards for H_2S are presently in place in the United States. Several states, however, have standards, which are described in Table 62.4 (4).

The current Occupational Safety and Health Administration (OSHA) permissible exposure limit (PEL) for hydrogen sulfide is a ceiling concentration of 20 ppm for 15 minutes or a maximum allowable peak of 50 ppm for 10 minutes. NIOSH has recommended a reduced standard of 10 ppm ceiling for 10 minutes, and that work areas in which the concentration of hydrogen sulfide exceeds 50 ppm be evacuated. The American

Conference of Governmental Industrial Hygienists (ACGIH) recommends a Threshold Limit Value (TLV) of 10 ppm as a 8-hour time-weighted average (TWA) and a Short-Term Exposure Limit (STEL) of 15 ppm (1, 4).

Environmental Monitoring

Most H_2S poisonings have occurred in the places where it is commonly used or produced. Since these exposures are predictable and can be prevented, an environmental monitoring system may warn exposed workers of their overexposure and is valuable for prevention.

Hydrogen sulfide has lower and upper explosive limits of 4.3% and 45.5%, respectively, and an autoignition temperature of 260°C. Appropriate procedures and precautions must be taken to avoid the occurrence of fire and explosion. The storage and disposal of H_2S must comply with all local, state, and federal regulations. Efforts should be made to avoid or minimize the formation and/or accumulation of H_2S, for example, by the use of refrigeration on fishing boats, and maintenance of adequate air flow rates in sewers and storage areas.

Engineering controls should be used to keep airborne H_2S below concentrations at which it is hazardous to the health of workers. To confirm that H_2S concentrations are below the evacuation limit and to prevent worker exposure to H_2S at hazardous concentrations, a continuous real-time monitoring of workplace air will usually be required in addition to periodic personal breathing zone air sampling. For breathing zone air samples, NIOSH recommends that a midget impinger be used and that the methylene blue method be used for H_2S analysis (2). At the work site, a fixed hydrogen sulfide detector system must have a two-stage, spark-proof alarm with lower triggering level of 10 ppm to warn workers that H_2S is above the ceiling limit, and a higher triggering level of 50 ppm to signal workers to evacuate the area and to obtain respiratory protection for rescue or repair efforts or for carrying out contingency plans. Fixed H_2S monitors should also automatically trigger supplementary ventilation of the workplace. Portable H_2S monitors and/or detector tubes may also be supplementally used as needed. However, continuous monitoring can protect the workers only when it is combined with an alerting and alarm system, adequate ventilation, respiratory protection, and other appropriate measures. Respiratory protection (self-contained breathing apparatus) is needed when the engineering controls are in the process of being installed or when they fail and need to be supplemented. Such respirators may also be used for operations that require entry into tanks or closed vessels and in emergency situations. These respirators should be immediately accessible to employees in emergency situations. The workers must be advised of the hazards of exposure to H_2S and trained in the use of respiratory protective devices and in the administration of artificial respiration (2).

Biologic Monitoring

Biologic monitoring is not of value in preventing harmful effects of hydrogen sulfide exposure. Most of the effects that have been associated with hydrogen sulfide exposure are not cumulative but arise from sudden, comparatively brief exposures at high concentrations or from repeated exposures to individually bearable concentrations (2).

Medical Surveillance

NIOSH recommends that preplacement examinations be given to employees who are potentially exposed to H_2S (2). These examinations must specifically assess the worker's ability to use respiratory protection (64). These examinations should be made available at 3-year intervals to all workers exposed to H_2S at concentrations above the ceiling concentration limit. Individuals exposed to H_2S at concentrations above 50 ppm should be examined promptly by a physician (2).

REFERENCES

1. Environmental Protection Agency. Hydrogen sulfide. Chemical Profiles. Washington, DC: EPA. December 1985.
2. National Institute for Occupational Safety and Health. Criteria for a recommended standard...occupational exposure to hydrogen sulfide. DHEW Publication No. (NIOSH) 77–158, 1977. Washington, DC: U.S. Government Printing Office, 1977.
3. Beauchamp RO Jr, Bus JS, Popp JA, Boreiko CJ, Andjelkovich DA. A critical review of the literature on hydrogen sulfide toxicity. CRC Crit Rev Toxicol 1984;13:25–97.
4. Environmental Protection Agency. Health assessment document for hydrogen sulfide, review draft. PB 87-117420. Washington, DC: EPA, August 1986.
5. Cooper RC, Jenkins D, Young LY. Aquatic microbiology laboratory manual, TX: University of Texas, 1976.
6. Mercado SG. Geothermo-electric project of Cerro-Priete: contamination and basic protection. In: Proceedings of the second UN symposium on the development and use of geothermal resources. San Francisco: 1975:1386–1393.
7. National Research Council, USA Subcommittee on hydrogen sulfide. Hydrogen sulfide. Baltimore: University Park Press, 1979.
8. Macaluso P. Hydrogen Sulfide. In: Encyclopedia of chemical technology. 2nd ed. New York: John Wiley & Sons, 1969;19:375–389.
9. Kleinfeld M, Giel C, Rosso A. Acute hydrogen sulfide intoxication: an unusual source of exposure. Ind Med Surg 1964;33:656–660.
10. Peters JW. Hydrogen sulfide poisoning in a hospital setting. JAMA 1981;246:1588–1589.
11. Pettigrew GL. Preliminary report on hydrogen sulfide exposure in the oil and gas industry. Dallas: U.S. DHEW, Public Health Service, Dallas Regional Office, 1976.
12. McCabe LC, Clayton GD. Air pollution by hydrogen sulfide in Poza Rica, Mexico. An evaluation of the incident of Nov 24, 1950. Arch Ind Hyg Occup Med 1952;6:199–213.
13. Burgess WA. Potential exposures in industry: their recognition and control. In: Clayton GD, ed. Patty's industrial hygiene and toxicology. New York: John Wiley & Sons, 1978;1:1149–1222.
14. Yant WP. Hydrogen sulfide in industry: occurrence, effects and treatment. Am J Public Health 1930;20:598–608.
15. Laug EP, Draize JH. The percutaneous absorption of ammonium hydrogen sulfide and hydrogen sulfide. J Pharmacol Exp Ther 1942;76:179–188.
16. Walton DC, Witherspoon MG. Skin absorption of certain gases. J Pharmacol Exp Ther 1925;26:315–324.
17. Voigt GE, Muller P. The histochemical effect of hydrogen sulfide poisoning. Acta Histochem 1955;1:223–239.
18. Curtis CG, Bartholomew TC, Rose FA, Dodgson KS. Detoxication of sodium 35-S-sulfide in the rat. Biochem Pharmacol 1972;21:2313–2321.
19. Weisiger RA, Jakoby WB. S-Methylation: thiol S-methyltransferase. In: Jakoby WB, ed. Enzymatic basis of detoxification. New York: Academic Press, 1980;2:131.
20. Smith RP, Gosselin RE. Hydrogen sulfide poisoning. J Occup Med 1979;21:93–97.
21. Smith RP, Kruszyna R, Kruszyna H. Management of acute sulfide poisoning: effects of oxygen, thiosulfate, and nitrite. Arch Environ Health 1976;31:166–169.
22. Smith RP, Gosselin RE. The influence of methemoglobinemia on the lethality of some toxic anions. Toxicol Appl Pharmacol 1964;6:584–592.
23. Milby TH. Hydrogen sulfide intoxication: Review of the literature and report of unusual accident resulting in two cases of nonfatal poisoning. J Occup Med 1962;4:431–437.
24. Ahlborg G. Hydrogen sulfide poisoning in shale oil industry. Arch Ind Hyg Occu Med 1951;3:247–266.
25. Haggard HW. The toxicology of hydrogen sulfide. J Ind Hyg 1925;7:113–121.

26. Evans CL. The toxicity of hydrogen sulfide and other sulfides. J Exp Physiol 1967;52:231–248.

27. Gunina AI. Transformation of sulfur-35-labeled hydrogen sulfide introduced into blood. Dokl Akad Nauk SSSR 1957b;112:902–904.

28. Susman JL, Hornig JF, Thomas SC, Smith RP. Pulmonary excretion of hydrogen sulfide, methanethiol, dimethyl sulfide, and dimethyl disulfide in mice. Drug Chem Toxicol 1978;1:327–333.

29. Kaipainen WJ. Hydrogen sulfide intoxication: rapidly transient changes in the electrocardiogram suggestive of myocardial infarction. Ann Med Intern Fenn 1954;43:97–101.

30. Kemper FD. A near-fatal case of hydrogen sulfide poisoning. Can Med Assoc J 1966;94:1130–1131.

31. Burnett WW, King EG, Grace M, Hall WF. Hydrogen sulfide poisoning: review of five years' experience. Can Med Assoc J 1977;117:1277–1280.

32. Gafafer WM, ed. Occupational disease: a guide to their recognition. Publication no. 1097, Washington, DC: U.S. DHEW 1964:163.

33. Poda GA, Hydrogen sulfide can be handled safely. Arch Environ Health 1966;12:795–800.

34. Jones JP. Hazards of hydrogen sulfide gas (abstract). 23rd Annu Gas Meas Inst 1975;16.

35. Adelson L, Sunshine I. Fatal hydrogen sulfide intoxication. Arch Pathol 1966;81:375–380.

36. Johnstone RT, Saunders WB, eds. Occupational disease and industrial medicine. Philadelphia: WB Saunders, 1960.

37. Carson MB. Hydrogen sulfide exposure in the gas industry. Ind Med Surg 1963;32:63–64.

38. Nesswetha W. Eye damage through sulfur interactions. Arbeitsmed Sozialmed Arbeitshyg 1969;4:288–290.

39. Masure R. Keratoconjunctivitis of viscose rayon fibers: a clinical and experimental study. Rev Belge Pathol Med Exp 1950;20:297–341.

40. American Conference of Governmental Industrial Hygienists. Hydrogen sulfide. In: Documentation of the threshold limit values. 4th ed. Cincinnati, OH: ACGIH, 1980:225.

41. Elkins HB. Hydrogen sulfide. In: The chemistry of industrial toxicology. New York: John Wiley & Sons, 1950.

42. Mitchell CW, Yant WP. Correlation of the data obtained from refinery accidents with a laboratory study of H₂S and its treatment. U.S. Bureau of Mines Bull No. 231, 1925:59–79.

43. Cralley LV. The effect of irritant gases upon the rate of ciliary activity. J Ind Hyg Toxicol 1942;24:193–198.

44. Rogers RE, Ferin J. Effects of hydrogen sulfide on bacterial inactivation in the rat lung. Arch Environ Health 1981;36:261–264.

45. Henkin RI. Effects of vapor phase pollutants on nervous system and sensory function. In: Finkel AJ, Duel WC, eds. Clinical implications of air pollution research. Acton, MA: Publishing Sciences Group, 1976.

46. Ravizza AG, Carugo D, Cerchiari EL. The treatment of hydrogen sulfide intoxication: oxygen versus nitrites. Vet Hum Toxicol 1982;24:241–242.

47. Vathenen AS, Emberton P, Wales JM. Hydrogen sulfide poisoning in factory workers (letter). Lancet 1988;1:305.

48. Kosmider S, Rogala E, Pacholek A. Electrocardiographic and histochemical studies of the heart muscle in acute experimental hydrogen sulfide poisoning. Arch Immunol Ther Exp 1967;15:731–740.

49. Vasileva IA. Effect of small concentrations of carbon disulfide and hydrogen sulfide on the menstrual function of women and the estrual cycle of experimental animals. Gig Sanit 1973;7:24–27.

50. Albaum HG, Tepperman J, Bodonsky O. Spectrophotometric study of competition of methemoglobin and cytochrome oxidase for sulfide in vitro. J Biol Chem 1946;163:641–647.

51. Nicholls P. The effect of sulfide on cytochrome aa3, isosteric and allosteric shifts of the reduced A-peak. Biochim Biophys Acta 1975;396:24–35.

52. Deng JF, Chang SC. Hydrogen sulfide poisonings in hot-spring reservoir cleaning: two case reports. Am J Ind Med 1987;11:447–451.

53. Siegel SM, Penny P, Siegel BZ, Penny D. Atmospheric hydrogen sulfide levels at the Sulfur Bay Wildlife area, Lake Rotorua, New Zealand. Water Air Soil Pollut 1986;28:385–391.

54. Mitchell CW, Davenport SJ. Hydrogen sulfide literature. Public Health Rep 1924;39:1–13.

55. Illinois Institute for Environmental quality. Hydrogen sulfide health effects and recommended air quality standard. IIEQ Doc. no. 74–24, NTIS no. PB 233 843. Chicago: Environmental Resource Center, 1974.

56. Chen KK, Rose CL. Nitrite and thiosulfate therapy in cyanide poisoning. JAMA 1952;149:113–119.

57. Vannatta JB. Hydrogen sulfide poisoning: report of four cases and brief review of the literature. J Okla State Med Assoc 1982;75:29–32.

58. Stine RJ, Slosberg B, Beacham BE. Hydrogen sulfide intoxication: a case report and discussion of treatment. Ann Intern Med 1976;85:756–758.

59. Beck JF, Bradbury CM, Connors AJ, Donini JC. Nitrite as an antidote for acute hydrogen sulfide intoxication. Am Ind Hyg Assoc J 1981;42:805–809.

60. Whitcraft DD, Bailey TD, Hart GB. Hydrogen sulfide poisoning treated with hyperbaric oxygen. J Emerg Med 1985;3:23–25.

61. Smilkstein MJ, Bronstein AC, Pickett HM, Rumack BH. Hyperbaric oxygen therapy for severe hydrogen sulfide poisoning. J Emerg Med 1985;3:27–30.

62. Arnold IM, Dufresne RM, Alleyne BC, Stuart PJ. Health implication of occupational exposures to hydrogen sulfide. J Occup Med 1985;27:373–376.

63. Kangas J, Savolainen H. Urinary thiosulfate as an indicator of exposure to hydrogen sulfide vapor. Clin Chim Acta 1987;164:7–10.

64. National Institute for Occupational Safety and Health. Guide to industrial respiratory protection. DHHS Publication no. (NIOSH) 87–116, 1987. Washington, DC: U.S. Government Printing Office, 1987.

63

Benzene and Other Hemotoxins

Richard D. Irons, Ph.D.

INTRODUCTION

The cells of the blood fulfill a variety of critical functions for the individual including transport of oxygen, host resistance, and hemostasis. Toxic responses involving the blood often involve a reduction in the number of circulating cells, as a result of either direct destruction or decreased production and release. Among the most frequently encountered blood dyscrasias secondary to drug or chemical exposure are thrombocytopenias, which may result from direct destruction frequently as a result of drug-induced immune complex formation or decreased production resulting from bone marrow suppression. A characteristic of anemias or cytopenias associated with chemicals or drugs is that individual responses vary widely with respect to both the severity and the nature of abnormality encountered following toxic exposure. Most blood dyscrasias secondary to drug or chemical exposure are transient and are resolved upon withdrawal of the toxic stimulus. However, persistent and even fatal blood dyscrasias (e.g., cytopenias, myelodysplasias, and aplastic anemia) are not uncommon in cases of severe bone marrow depression and have a well-established tendency to progress to acute leukemia. When placed in historical perspective, a major criticism of the occupational regulatory process in recent years might be its singular preoccupation with the relationship between chemical exposure and cancer (e.g, leukemia) at the expense of more prevalent and equally morbid outcomes, such as aplastic anemia or myelodysplastic syndrome (MDS).

Hemopoiesis

Hemopoiesis is a process of cell amplification and differentiation in which a very small number of stem cells give rise to progressively more differentiated progenitor cells, which in turn give rise to mature blood cells. The earliest hemopoietic progenitor cell is the pluripotent stem cell (PSC), which can give rise to progenitor cells in all blood cell lineages but has very limited proliferative activity itself. After embryogenesis PSCs maintain exclusive responsibility for the production of blood cells throughout life. In the normal adult, hemotopoiesis occurs in the bone marrow and is largely restricted to scattered clusters of hemopoietic cells in the proximal epiphyses of the long bones, skull, vertebrae, pelvis, ribs, and sternum. Even under conditions of extreme hemopoietic stress, such as occurs following bone marrow transplantation, extramedullary hemopoiesis in spleen, liver, and lymph nodes occurs only rarely in humans. The hemopoietic precursor cells of the bone marrow and the mature cells of the blood exist in a dynamic equilibrium in which the senescence and destruction of mature blood cells are balanced by the production and release of new cells. In the average adult, destruction and replacement amount to between 200 and 400 billion cells per day. The rate of cell division in morphologically identifiable precursor cells in the

bone marrow approaches the maximum for mammalian cells. Therefore, significant and prolonged alterations in the production of blood cells must involve alterations in the differentiation of maturing precursors, the activation of an increased proportion of normally resting stem cell populations, or both.

EPIDEMIOLOGY

Leukemia

INCIDENCE AND PREVALENCE

In the United States there are approximately 24,000 new cases of leukemia a year, which represent about 3% of all malignancies. Acute myelogenous leukemia (AML) and its variants account for 46% of all leukemias; chronic myelogenous leukemia (CML), 14%; acute lymphatic leukemia (ALL), 11%; and chronic lymphatic leukemia (CLL), 29%. These numbers are generally comparable among Western countries. In adults AML constitutes almost 90% of all acute leukemias (1). All known etiologic agents together are responsible for a very small fraction of the overall incidence of leukemia, the vast majority of which arise de novo in the absence of any history of drug, radiation, or chemical exposure (2). Leukemia secondary to treatment of other malignant diseases, such as ovarian carcinoma, breast cancer, multiple myeloma, and chronic lymphocytic leukemia, is well-documented because of the ability to obtain detailed follow-up and accurate exposure histories in patients receiving previous radiation or alkylation therapy (3–8). Secondary AML is a well-established phenomenon and is by far the most predominant if not the only hemopoietic malignancy arising as a consequence of cancer treatment. Acute myelogenous leukemia has also been observed following immunosuppressive therapy for nonneoplastic disorders, although it should be noted that immunosuppressive therapy resulting in AML has frequently included multiple alkylating agents and/or radiation therapy (9). Isolated reports of other types of leukemia arising secondary to chemotherapy have appeared (10–12); however, in view of the very small numbers of cases and inconsistent pattern, it has been suggested that these represent coincidental occurrences (13). Chronic myelogenous leukemia has been observed following radiation and has been reported secondary to combined radiation-chemotherapeutic paradigms (14–16). However, it is noteworthy that, in over 1500 confirmed cases of leukemia secondary to radiation and/or chemotherapy reported in the world literature, CML has not been documented as occurring secondary to chemotherapy alone. In previous studies of Hodgkin's disease, treatment employing combined paradigms in which radiotherapy was followed by chemotherapy was particularly potent at inducing secondary AML, the cumulative risks of treatment approaching 10% (17–19). The frequency of occurrence of secondary AML varies depending on the treatment paradigms employed but generally ranges between 0.3% and 20% (13, 17–20).

PROBLEMS ENCOUNTERED IN THE STUDY OF LEUKEMIAS SECONDARY TO CHEMICAL EXPOSURE

Classification

There are a number of serious difficulties that frustrate attempts to study hemopoietic malignancies secondary to chemical exposure in addition to their relative scarcity. For years there has been growing recognition among hematologists and hematopathologists of the clinical and biologic importance of classifying hemopoietic and lymphoid neoplasms on the basis of individual cell types. At the same time there has remained a tendency on the part of epidemiologists to combine these relatively rare neoplasms into broad categories in order to have sufficient numbers to permit epidemiologic analysis. This tendency to combine or ''lump'' different nosologic categories together in order to derive sufficient analytical power can be misleading if the etiology and pathogenesis of the diseases are different. This problem is compounded by the major classification scheme of the International Classification of Diseases (ICD), which refers to only three major categories of lymphoid neoplasms (i.e., lymphosarcoma and reticulosarcoma, 200; Hodgkin's disease, 201; and lymphatic leukemia, 204). This scheme encourages the combination of acute and chronic myeloid leukemias (205) and frustrates efforts to use the morphologically based French-American-British Cooperative Group (FAB) classification of leukemias (21). Although the most recent edition (ICD-9) provides for increased subtyping, in part to accommodate more relevant nosology, the major classification scheme that forms the basis for most of the available epidemiologic literature remains biologically archaic.

Diagnosis

The advent of cell and molecular biology has led to increased classification and subtyping of hemopoietic and lymphoid neoplasms based on pheno- and genotypic analysis. In conducting retrospective studies, differences and ambiguities between the current and older literature will continue to serve as a source of frustration for several years to come. In the Western world, and for most of the developing world as well, variation in the diagnosis of AML does not represent a major source of confusion, differences in subtyping notwithstanding. However, as variations and improvements in diagnostic criteria have occurred, disparities with respect to disease classification have increased between the current and older literature and from one country or geographical region to another. CML, for example, is a malignant myeloproliferative disorder of the pluripotential stem cell that is characterized by the presence of the Philadelphia (Ph[1]) chromosome (22–24). The Ph[1] chromosome represents a shortened chromosome 22 (22q−) arising from a reciprocal translocation t(9;22)(q34;q11) and is present in over 95% of patients with CML. The molecular lesion is associated with the transposition of the *c-abl* gene from chromosome 9 to a specific segment of chromosome 22, known as the break cluster region (*bcr*) (25). Recent studies have indicated that even in the small number of patients with presumptive CML who are Ph[1]-negative, a significant number possess the *bcr-*

abl molecular rearrangements found in Ph[1]-positive CML (26–28). Because the morphologic and cytologic parameters of CML can be difficult or impossible to distinguish from myelodysplastic syndrome (MDS), cytogenetic analysis is important in the classification of patients with the disease. In one recent study of 25 cases originally classified as Ph[1]-negative CML, cytogenetic examination resulted in 24 being reclassified as MDS or other myeloproliferative disorders distinct from CML (29). Thus, comparisons of the incidence of CML and MDS between different populations and different studies is probably meaningless in the absence of detailed cytogenetic evaluation using banded chromosome analysis.

Study Design

Case reports are useful in drawing attention to a potential problem or suggesting a possible relationship between exposure and disease. A major strength of case reports is that the clinical diagnosis is usually well-documented. On the other hand, a major weakness is that a reliable exposure history is exceedingly difficult to obtain. As a result, details of exposure are usually circumstantial or anecdotal and not quantifiable. Rarely, *if ever*, is chemical exposure documented even remotely as well as the diagnosis (30). By definition, case histories or collections of case histories are cumulative, and the case selection process is not random. Therefore, it is impossible to assign with any certainty ''the denominator'' in comparing the incidence of an exposure-disease relationship relative to the general population. Case reporting is subjective and susceptible to such influences as the perception or suspicion of an association between a disease and exposure to a given agent and even the potential legal consequences of such an association (30). Such biases are not always subtle. There are instances where the authors have forthrightly admitted that the motivation for publishing a collection of case histories was to influence medicolegal proceedings (31), and there are ''collections'' of case histories with no more scientific justification than that they have been abstracted from court records (32).

Case reports, either isolated or collected, are important for suggesting a possible relationship between exposure and disease and for providing a rationale for the conduct of more rigorous and detailed studies. Yet despite their importance in this regard, they cannot be used to establish a causal relationship. Lack of accurate exposure data is often the factor limiting the value of quantitative epidemiologic studies. The virtual absence of reliable exposure data in case reports places even more severe restraints on their utility. Often the alleged exposure is isolated, transient, separated by months or years from the onset of the disease, or not characterized at all. Casual accounts of past chemical exposures are not an adequate substitute for personnel monitoring or industrial hygiene measurements.

Quantitative retrospective or prospective epidemiology studies have the advantage of being able to establish a causal association between a given exposure and disease. Nevertheless, individual epidemiology studies often lack sufficient sample size to be definitive on their own. If the incidence of the disease is rare in the study population, several independent studies may be necessary in order to establish a clear pattern between exposure to a specific agent and a particular disease. Under these conditions, meaningful comparisons between studies can often be obscured by inconsistency in the nosologic classifications used, differences in the assignment of subjects to exposure groups, or confounding exposures to different combinations of agents.

Although quantitative epidemiology studies can establish the relationship between occupational exposure and increased incidence of a disease, inability to reliably quantitate the exposure is often still a major weakness, especially in retrospective studies. Attempts to use job classification schemes as a surrogate for exposure often assume that risk is cumulative and that the product of duration and exposure concentration defines the risk of disease rather than specific exposure conditions, such as the regimen or frequency of exposure and dose-dependency. For some compounds, such as 2,4-dichlorophenoxyacetic acid (2,4-D) and benzene, there is evidence to suggest that cumulative assumptions may be inappropriate.

OCCUPATIONS, HEMOTOXICITY, AND LEUKEMIA

A number of chemicals have been evaluated for their potential to produce bone marrow toxicity or leukemia. However, associations between certain occupations and increased risk of leukemia or lymphoma have been observed for which the nature of the causative agent remains obscure. Increased incidence of leukemia in workers in the rubber and tire industry has consistently been reported in epidemiology studies (33, 34). In the absence of reliable exposure data, an assumed role for benzene served as a point of departure in a number of case reports and reviews, including one by this author (35). However, rubber and tire manufacture represents a complex setting in which simultaneous exposures to a variety of agents occur, and findings in subsequent studies have not proven to be consistent with the benzene hypothesis (36). Benzene exposure is associated with an increased risk of AML, whereas, in the rubber industry in particular, excesses are seen in lymphocytic as well as nonlymphocytic leukemias (37). Checkoway and coworkers evaluated the specific association of leukemia and solvent exposure in the rubber industry and found that risk of lymphocytic leukemia was stronger for other solvents (e.g., carbon tetrachloride and carbon disulfide) than for benzene (38). An increased incidence of leukemia, primarily AML, has been observed among welders (39–41), and an increased incidence of lymphatic/hemopoietic neoplasms has been reported among plumbers (42). Although metal fumes, solvents, and flux have been hypothesized to be involved, the causative agent(s) remain a mystery.

A particularly intriguing and potentially serious problem in occupational medicine relates to the effects of extended space flight on hematologic and immunologic function. A consistent observation on U.S. and Soviet space flights has been a postflight reduction in circulating red blood cell (RBC) mass and a decrease in cell-mediated immune function (43, 44). Crew members returning from Spacelab 1 experienced an average 13% decrease in RBC and nearly a 9% reduction in hemoglobin concentration. These changes were preceded by a precipitous depression in peripheral reticulocytes, which was less than half of normal by day 7 of the mission and reached a nadir of − 60.9% on landing day. This decrease in red cell mass, which is somewhat attenuated on longer missions, appears to involve both decreased erythrocyte lifespan and a suppression of erythropoiesis. Initial hypotheses to explain these effects included hyperoxia and a decrease in the production of erythropoietin by the kidney. Nevertheless, subsequent experiments have demonstrated that the clinical effects occur in the absence of elevated oxygen, and studies have failed to find a significant decrease in serum erythropoietin levels during space flight. Additional studies have provided evidence that hypogravity adversely influences lymphocyte function, including a decrease in cell density-dependent T lymphocyte response in vitro (45, 46). Lymphocyte activation requires cell-cell contact, lymphokine production and release, and receptor-lymphokine interactions that lead to cell proliferation. Regulation of hemopoietic precursor cells is known to involve similar interaction between growth factors and receptors present on growth factor-dependent cells. Therefore, hemopoietic cells as well are likely to be susceptible to a variety of influences in the space environment including: hypogravity, radiation, environmental contaminants, and microbial flora. However, the longterm biologic significance of these effects and the potential influence of the space flight environment on hemopoiesis and resistance to infectious disease remain unclear. Other occupations associated with potential exposure to hemotoxic chemicals will be discussed in the context of specific agents.

Cytopenias and Blood Dyscrasias

INCIDENCE AND PREVALENCE

In recent years a great deal of attention has been focused on leukemias secondary to chemical exposure. In contrast, relatively little concern has been paid to other blood dyscrasias arising under similar circumstances. This is a disturbing trend when one considers the relatively dismal prognosis of secondary aplastic anemia or MDS quite independent of the tendency of survivors to go on to develop acute leukemia. Until recently, reporting practices for hematologic dyscrasias have been much less uniform and reliable than for leukemias. If ascertaining the frequency of secondary leukemia is attended with serious difficulties, determining the incidence of other blood dyscrasias secondary to chemical exposure has been tantamount to impossible. Until very recently there have been no authoritative studies on the frequency of blood dyscrasias in the general population. However, Buffler and coworkers have recently completed a study of age-specific rates of MDS occurring in men over a 5-year period on the upper Texas Gulf Coast. Results of this study suggest that, while the age-adjusted rate of myelodysplasias is relatively low (i.e., 2–2.8/100,000), there are marked differences in the age-specific incidence, ranging from 0.061/100,000 for whites and Hispanics 20–29 years of age to 19.59/100,000 for the 70–79 age group (P. A. Buffler, personal communication).

Another source of confusion concerns variations in the nosologic criteria used to differentiate individual cytopenias, aplastic anemia, pancytopenia, hypoplastic anemia, aleukemic leukemia, MDS, and refractory anemia. For example, the incidence of MDS may be seriously underestimated by classifications employing the use of such terms as "Ph¹-negative" CML (29). In one ongoing follow-up study of approximately 2000 employees and retirees engaged in chemical manufacturing, the incidence of MDS cases appears to be about 36/100,000 (46a). Tentatively, these results suggest an elevation in the incidence of MDS in an occupational setting, if one employs age-specific incidence data obtained in the Buffler study as a denominator for comparison with the general population. Preliminary findings such as these illustrate the acute need for additional studies employing standardized nosology to determine if, indeed, there are occupationally related increases in MDS.

COMMON CHEMICALS AND TOXINS

Evidence for Hemotoxicity

On the basis of hard scientific evidence, benzene remains the only major industrial chemical for which a clear causal relationship with leukemia, specifically AML, has been established. Nevertheless, a number of agents have been reported to produce anemia, cytopenias, leukemia, or lymphoma for which the quality and quantity of supporting evidence varies widely. Among these are lead, arsenic, radium, ethylene oxide, pesticides (e.g., chlordane, heptachlor, and the phenoxy herbicides), ethylene glycol, trinitrotoluene (TNT), and 1,3-butadiene. For many of these chemicals the results of different studies are contradictory, and many suffer from weak methodology and inadequate statistical power. In this context, it appears that generalizations about the hemotoxicity of classes of compounds may be imprudent in the absence of more reliable information. An important consideration in study design is that the actual number of affected individuals is quite small. The gloomy predictions of current risk assessment notwithstanding, the actual demonstrated incidence of leukemia and blood dyscrasias does not represent a large proportion of the individuals exposed even in populations chronically exposed to a known human leukemogen, benzene. For virtually all other occupational or environmental agents, the incidence is much less.

LEAD

The changing patterns of lead (Pb) use in society have modulated the prevailing forms of Pb toxicity encountered in modern times. Lead poisoning was one of the most predominant hazards of past centuries; it has even been suggested to have contributed to the fall of the Roman Empire (47). Cases of moderate to severe Pb poisoning in which anemia is present have declined dramatically in recent years. However, chronic Pb poisoning as an occupational hazard is far from extinct. Painters exposed to Pb-contaminated dust pose a particular problem. The most significant effects of chronic Pb poisoning are those involving the central nervous system (CNS). For example, organic lead compounds, such as tetraethyl- and tetramethyllead, which have been widely employed as gasoline additives, are potent neurotoxins. Anemia, which can be clinically significant as well, is usually a late manifestation of chronic Pb intoxication and is moderate unless there is a severe hemolytic component. In both experimental and clinical experience, hematologic abnormalities associated with Pb toxicity are confined to the erythrocytes. Lead-induced anemia is brought about by two major mechanisms: interference with erythropoiesis by the inhibition of heme synthetase and δ-aminolevulinic acid (ALD) dehydrase, and direct binding of Pb to the erythrocyte membrane resulting in increased fragility. In many cases, the latter can be documented only with great difficulty. Pb is distinguished by its ability to produce selective suppression of erythropoiesis while generally sparing other cell lineages. In the bone marrow, there is a marked maturation arrest in erythropoiesis, accompanied by an increase in the number of erythroblasts. Polychromatophilic erythroblasts often exhibit basophilic stippling, which usually can be demonstrated in bone marrow cells even when not present in circulating erythrocytes. From a clinical point of view, it should be appreciated that basophilic stippling can be a prominent feature but is not as specific or sensitive for Pb poisoning as once thought, and, in fact, is uncommon in workers exposed to the current permissible exposure limit (PEL) (50 μg/m^3). The anemia associated with Pb poisoning can be moderately severe but is usually mild in industrial poisoning cases. Erythrocytes may be hypochromic but not hyperchromic, and there is usually a moderate reticulocytosis. A decrease in Fe utilization can usually be demonstrated. Elevations in bone marrow or erythrocyte porphyrin levels may occur early as a result of Pb toxicity to mitochondria, although their rise in urine usually is not an early indicator of Pb intoxication. Urinary ALD output is a useful diagnostic indicator in cases of suspected Pb poisoning, along with blood and urinary Pb measurements (48). The marginal evidence suggesting that Pb might be a human carcinogen has been the subject of debate (49–51). Surprisingly, there is no indication that exposure to Pb is associated with hemopoietic or lymphoid malignancies.

ARSENIC

Acute arsenic (As) poisoning is rarely occupational in origin and usually occurs via food or drink (52). Megaloblastic disturbances in hemopoiesis have been reported in acute arsenic poisoning, which may be accompanied by a marked reduction in leukocyte count (53). However, it would appear that hemopoietic toxicity is a relatively minor aspect of the multiple toxic effects of this metal. In cases of acute poisoning, elevations of As can be found in urine, which is the main route of excretion. It should be kept in mind that urinary excretion of As is rapid and the half-life of the metal in blood extremely short (~1–3 days). Arsenic determination in urine or blood can be a useful quantitative parameter when exposure is thought to have occurred. Urine concentrations correlate better with chronic exposure.

Increased mortality in workers occupationally exposed to arsenicals has been reported due to leukemia (unclassified) in one study (54) and to lymphoma and Hodgkin's disease—but *not* leukemia—in another (55). Taken together, these observations are by no means conclusive since the study results are inconsistent, the number of cases in each study is exceptionally small, and the likelihood of confounding exposures is great in both.

RADIUM

Occupational exposure to radium (Ra) no longer poses a significant health hazard, but Ra poisoning in the dial-painting industry during the first quarter of this century represents a classic but tragic episode in the history of occupational medicine. A landmark retrospective study of 634 women employed in this industry between 1915 and 1929 was reported by Polednak et al. (56). The affected population comprised virtually all women who were employed in the Ra dial industry prior to 1930. The major source of exposure was ingestion of Ra paint by workers who would lick the brushes used to paint luminous watch dials in order to maintain a fine point on the brush. Some inhalation of radon daughters and Ra dust is thought to have occurred as well. Depending on the age at first exposure, mortality ratios associated with "bone cancer" ranged between 81 and 250, reflecting the bone-seeking nature of ^{226}Ra. Excess deaths due to leukemia and "diseases of the blood and blood-forming organs" were also noted, with mortality ratios of 2.13 and 3.91 observed for each, respectively. Although the number of leukemias is small (i.e., 3), the pattern of ^{226}Ra deposition and the marked increase in bone-related cancers, together with reports of aplastic anemia, anemia, and leukopenia in earlier studies of Ra workers (50–53), suggest that a causal relationship may exist.

ETHYLENE OXIDE

Ethylene oxide is a direct acting epoxide and alkylating agent employed as an intermediate in chemical manufacture and used extensively as a gaseous sterilization agent. Exposures to ethylene oxide are most likely to occur in a hospital setting during the loading and unloading of sterilization chambers and the off-gassing of recently sterilized items. Ethylene oxide is clearly a biologically reactive agent, with chronic exposure associated with mutagenic and cytogenetic effects in humans and experimental animals (61). Even so, evidence in support of ethylene oxide as a human leukemogen must be viewed as extremely limited. In 1979 Hogstedt and coworkers reported two cases of leukemia and one lymphoma among a small group of Swedish workers exposed to ethylene oxide and potentially exposed to a variety of other agents as well (62, 63). Similarly, Theiss et al. reported a nonsignificant excess of deaths due to leukemia (i.e., 2 observed versus 1.1 expected) in potentially exposed workers (64). These results are contrasted by those of Morgan et al., who found no leukemia deaths among 767 worker with potential exposure to ethylene oxide (65). As noted by Austin and Sielkin, limitations inherent in all of these studies include inconsistent results, small cohort sizes, small numbers of observed and expected events, and inadequate quantitative exposure data (60).

GLYCOL ETHERS

The glycol ethers are a class of compounds that are used extensively in industry as solvents in the manufacture of varnishes, latex paints, dyes, inks, and antifreeze compounds. They are generally regarded as being of low toxicity. Previous case reports have suggested that glycol ethers may be hemotoxic to humans. In a cross-sectional survey of employees involved in glycol ether manufacture, no differences in hematologic parameters were observed between an exposed versus a control population (66). More recently, Welch and Cullen studied the effect of exposure to glycol ethers on shipyard painters (67). No significant differences in the means of hematologic variables were noted between exposed and nonexposed groups, and no correlation with cumulative exposure was established. However, a small proportion of the exposed group presented as anemic and granulocytopenic according to the criteria used in the study. In another study, motivated by the referral of a printer with aplastic anemia, Cullen et al. examined bone marrow injury in a small group of lithographers exposed to glycol ethers (68). Peripheral blood counts, including differential and platelet counts, were normal; yet bone marrow biopsies revealed various abnormalities including myeloid hypoplasia, stromal cell injury, and sideroblastosis in three of seven exposed workers. The lack of consistency between the results of these studies, together with the small number of exposed workers examined, provides an inadequate base upon which to draw any sweeping conclusions. While there is insufficient evidence to conclude that exposure to glycol ethers results in blood or bone marrow toxicity, common sense dictates that exposure of these agents should be minimized.

TRINITROTOLUENE (TNT)

Occupational exposure to TNT was historically associated with the munitions industry, and hemotoxicity resulting from wartime exposure to TNT has previously been reviewed by Scott et al. (69). The major route of exposure was via the skin and occurred during the hand loading of artillery shells. Although aplastic anemia has been reported as a consequence of TNT exposure, dermatitis, gastritis, toxic hepatitis, hemolytic anemia, and methemoglobinemia are all more common in cases of TNT poisoning.

AROMATIC SOLVENTS

An occasional misstatement in the secondary literature notwithstanding, benzene is the only primary aromatic solvent with hemotoxic properties. Neither the clinical nor the experimental literature will support an association between the alkylbenzenes, toluene, or xylenes and blood dyscrasias or leukemia. The explanation for such marked difference in the hemotoxicity of benzene and substituted benzenes is almost certainly related to major differences in the metabolism and bioactivation of these compounds. It is well established in experimental models that toluene, when present in relatively high concentrations, will actually protect against benzene-induced bone marrow toxicity by competing for primary metabolism.

1,3-BUTADIENE

1,3-Butadiene (BD) is a colorless gas used in the production of styrene-butadiene or polybutadiene rubber. Styrene-butadiene rubber was introduced as a substitute for natural rubber during World War II and has subsequently become a mainstay of the rubber industry. Early studies in experimental animals and in humans indicated very little acute or cumulative toxicity associated with exposure to BD. Subsequently, several epidemiology studies have studied the potential relationship between occupational exposure to BD and cancer; however, to date the results have proved to be illogical and contradictory. These studies show no consistent pattern with respect to either the duration of exposure or disease and in the aggregate fail to demonstrate an increase in hemopoietic neoplasms in butadiene-exposed workers. The first such study of synthetic rubber workers suggested that the incidence of leukemia was marginally increased in one of two plants, but only in workers with shortterm exposure, not longterm exposure (70). Another study of butadiene monomer workers revealed an increase in lymphosarcoma but *not* leukemia, again only in shortterm workers (71). Still, a third study found a deficit in lymphopoietic cancers compared with that expected in the total cohort and no increase in leukemia, but an increase in leukemia in a case-control study within the same cohort (71a; 71b; 72). At present, the contradiction between these two studies remains unexplained, although methodologic considerations are likely to play an important role. In the case-control study, the exposure status of cases was characterized as either ''never exposed'' or ''ever exposed'' to butadiene. Subsequent analysis has suggested that the statistical significance of the findings would disappear upon reassignment of exposure status for only one case (72a).

Studies of BD toxicity and carcinogenicity in experimental animals suggest that there are marked species differences in susceptibility to BD (73–76). Rats are relatively resistant to BD toxicity. The compound has proven to be carcinogenic in that species only at high exposure concentrations; there is no evidence of hemotoxicity in rats exposed to the chemical. On the other hand, subacute exposure to BD in mice results in a megaloblastic anemia, and chronic exposure results in an increased incidence of a variety of neoplasms, most spectacularly a 60% incidence of lymphatic leukemia. Additional studies reveal that BD exposure produces a marked increase in the replication of endogenous ecotropic retrovirus in the mouse and that the incidence of leukemia in different mouse strains may at least in part be influenced by their retroviral background. The relationship, if any, between these findings in experimental animals and potential health effects associated with BD exposure in humans are unknown at the present time.

CHLORDANE AND HEPTACHLOR

In recent years, the pesticide field has been plagued with an abundant but confusing literature that is confounded by exposure to multiple agents and replete with contradiction. Many of the apparent contradictions between studies may be explained by differences in the identification of chemicals involved, measures of exposure employed, and size of the cohorts examined.

Chlordane and heptachlor have received a great deal of attention because of their wide use as insecticides. Nevertheless, human studies are contradictory and fail to support a consistent association between these two agents and toxicity to the blood and bone marrow. The evidence suggesting that chlordane and heptachlor produce blood dyscrasias and leukemia is largely derived from a small number of case reports of aplastic and hypoplastic anemia for which the association of disease with exposure to these agents appears tenuous (57–60), together with a collection of cases assembled from the "nonscientific literature" (e.g., litigation records) (32, 77). These cases are taken from anecdotal sources (78). These are contrasted by quantitative epidemiology studies, both prospective and retrospective, as well as a case-control study of 60 cases of aplastic anemia (79), that have not found an increased incidence of leukemias or aplastic anemia in workers engaged in the production of application of these two chemicals (80–82). At the present time, it appears reasonable to conclude, both on the basis of the experimental and human literature, that an association between chlordane or heptachlor and hemotoxicity amounts to not much more than a hypothesis.

PHENOXY HERBICIDES

The chlorophenoxy herbicides are an important class of compounds, the principal examples of which are 2,4-dichlorophenoxyacetic acid (2,4-D), 2,4,5-trichlorophenoxyacetic acid (2,4,5-T) and 4-chloro-2-methylphenoxyacetic acid (MCPA). These compounds are among the most widely used herbicides in agriculture and first received wide notoriety in the 1960s as a result of the use of Agent Orange (a mixture of chlorophenoxy compounds) as a defoliant in the Vietnam War. An emotional controversy has surrounded the contamination of Agent Orange, as well as commercial preparations of some of these herbicides, with chlorinated dibenzodioxins, most significantly 2,3,7,8-tetrachlorodibenzo-p-dioxin (TCDD). A number of reviews have attempted to summarize the evidence concerning the potential leukemogenicity of the phenoxy herbicides. However, these have served only to highlight the difficulties in evaluating a group or class of compounds for which individual

representatives and/or their potential contaminants may have differing toxic profiles (83).

Following the first report by Hardell and Sandstrom in 1979, a number of case-control and retrospective cohort studies have attempted to examine the potential relationship between exposure to phenoxy herbicides and nonHodgkin's lymphoma (NHL) (84). The majority of studies have evaluated exposure to the phenoxyacetic acid herbicides as a group with largely inconsistent and contradictory results. Hardell et al. reported an increased risk of both Hodgkin's and nonHodgkin's lymphoma for the phenoxy herbicides, although no difference in risk was observed between those individuals exposed to products likely to contain TCDD as a contaminant and those not likely to contain TCDD (85). Woods et al. found a small increase in the risk of NHL among farmers but not in other occupations potentially exposed to 2,4-D (86). These studies were contrasted by the results of Pearce, who found no increase in NHL among New Zealand workers exposed to 2,4,5-T (87). A relatively large number of retrospective cohort studies of workers exposed to phenoxy herbicides have been reported over the last decade, which, when taken together, suggest no increase in NHL (83). However, two recent case-control studies of farmers in Kansas (88) and Nebraska (89) reveal a pattern that suggests that the use of 2,4-D in an agricultural setting increases the risk of NHL among persons frequently handling the chemical. These studies included histopathologic review of all cases. The Nebraska study further suggests that the risk of NHL increases with the degree of exposure to 2,4-D, as indicated by the application method and time spent in contaminated clothing, but not with the number of years of use. The small numbers of subjects in these studies is a limiting factor in evaluating the independent risks of 2,4-D, organophosphate insecticides, and fungicides, all of which are common use in the farming industry.

BENZENE

Sources and Production

Benzene (C_6H_6) is the simplest of the aromatic hydrocarbons and an important industrial compound, its production routinely ranking among the top 10 commodity chemicals. It is a clear, colorless, volatile liquid with a boiling point of 80.1°C and a vapor pressure of 100 mmHg. It is highly flammable and has a distinct aromatic odor. Benzene has limited solubility in water (1:1430 v/v) and is miscible with oils and alcohol. Benzene nomenclature can be a source of confusion. Benzol has been used as a synonym of benzene, especially in industrial settings. However, neither *benzene* nor *benzol* should be confused with *benzine*, which is found primarily in the European literature and refers to gasoline or petrol. Benzene was discovered by Faraday in 1825 and was first commercially produced from distillation of coal tar in 1849 (90). Since the 1940s, benzene has been reduced largely as a product of petroleum refining and is a major starting material in the production of styrene, cyclohexane, phenolics, and a variety of aromatic derivatives.

Sites, Industries, Businesses, and Behaviors Associated with Exposure to Benzene

OCCUPATIONAL EXPOSURE

Occupational exposure to benzene has been associated with its production and use as a synthetic intermediate and as a solvent.

In the past, workers in the painting, rotogravure, and certain rubber industries (e.g., Pliofilm) have represented a high risk group for exposure to benzene (91-93). Particularly high exposures have also been encountered as a consequence of the popular but short-lived use of benzene as solvent for adhesives used in the manufacture of shoes and leather goods (94, 95). Increasing recognition of the potential for bone marrow toxicity associated with benzene exposure has led to a sharp reduction in its use as a solvent and its replacement by far less toxic substitutes, such as toluene and xylenes that do not produce bone marrow toxicity.

Benzene is no longer available as a household solvent. Even so, it remains one of the most important commodity chemicals produced in the United States today. Potential sources of occupational exposure to benzene occur in the petroleum refinery, chemical and plastics industries, the transportation industry, gasoline stations, and, to a lesser extent, the iron, steel, pharmaceutical, and pesticide industries. In general, improvements in engineering and industrial hygiene practices over the last 40 years have led to a significant reduction in benzene exposure in the workplace. Nevertheless, work habits (i.e., precautions taken by individual workers) still influence the potential of occupational benzene exposure especially in situations involving the transfer of benzene and the repair and maintenance of chemical reactors, valves, fittings, and pipes.

ENVIRONMENTAL EXPOSURE

In addition to the potential for occupational exposure, benzene is ubiquitous in the environment. Benzene concentration in gasoline currently ranges from about 0.5–2%. It is a byproduct of combustion and is a constituent of fire smoke, automobile exhaust, and cigarette smoke. In addition, benzene has been reported to be a natural constituent of fruits, vegetables, meats, and dairy products with concentrations ranging from 2 μg/kg in canned beef to 2100 μg/kg for eggs (96). The importance assigned to environmental exposure to benzene today depends on the assumptions one makes with respect to the significance of cumulative low level exposure: If one assumes, as is the case with current regulatory risk assessments, that cumulative exposure to benzene dictates the risk of leukemia (i.e., that no exposure concentration is safe and that a simple product of concentration and exposure determines risk), then low level exposure from environmental sources represents a significant health hazard. If, on the other hand, one assumes that there is a threshold concentration below which benzene is not toxic, and that intermittent exposures to high concentrations present a much greater risk than low level exposure, then the overall health impact associated with environmental or "ambient" exposure is negligible.

BENZENE AND CIGARETTE SMOKING

Assumptions as to the significance of cumulative low level versus intermittent exposure are especially important in evaluating whether benzene in cigarette smoke constitutes a significant health hazard independent of its other myriad constituents (which include 1,3-butadiene and polyaromatic hydrocarbons, among countless other agents). According to EPA estimates, cigarette smoking represents the single most significant source of benzene exposure for about 50 million people in the United States, and on an integrated cumulative basis, this accounts for approximately half the total human exposure to benzene (98).

Cigarette smoke has been estimated to be 10,000 times more efficient as a source of benzene exposure than either auto exhaust or stationary source emissions, with the average smoker inhaling 10 times the average daily intake of the nonsmoker (97). The average urban inhabitant ingests daily an estimated 250 micrograms benzene in the diet and inhales 180 micrograms from the air. In contrast, the one-pack-a-day smoker inhales approximately 1800 μg/day in mainstream smoke (98). On the other hand, there is considerable evidence to suggest that there is a threshold concentration for benzene leukemogenesis. Accordingly, the absolute concentration of benzene in cigarette smoke probably presents a negligible risk compared with its other toxic constituents. A definitive end to the controversey will likely depend on mechanistic studies, since a resolution to this question is not likely to be forthcoming from the epidemiologic literature. The evidence for a small increase in leukemia incidence among smokers in some but not all studies is confounded by the presence of a veritable grab bag of toxic substances (99–104). While there is widespread concern over low level benzene exposure from such sources as petroleum refining and manufacturing, service stations, and from groundwater contamination, on a nationwide basis these appear to be relatively unimportant sources of *cumulative* benzene exposure for the general public and certainly are minimal compared with cigarette smoking (98).

Clinical Toxicity of Benzene

SIGNS, SYMPTOMS, AND SYNDROMES FROM TOXIC EXPOSURE

Benzene was introduced into commerce in the middle of the last century. Because of its superior solvent properties, it quickly gained popularity as a solvent for glues, inks, rubber, paints, and oils and as a starting material for the synthesis of pharmaceuticals and dyes. By the end of the 19th century, cases of occupational benzene poisoning were appearing with increasing frequency. These prompted a series of articles that dealt with the consequences of both acute and prolonged exposure to benzene at high concentrations (105–108). Acute effects were essentially limited to the CNS with prolonged exposure frequently associated with bone marrow depression, anemia, and pancytopenia.

Acute Toxicity

Acute toxicity associated with exposure to high concentrations of benzene involves the CNS and is manifested by excitement, convulsions, CNS depression, and death from cardiovascular collapse. In addition, petechial hemorrhaging has also been observed in some cases. Benzene exposure is rapidly fatal at concentrations approaching 20,000 ppm. Exposure to lower concentrations (3000–10,000 ppm) may be accompanied by euphoria, lightheadedness, headache, nausea, and unconsciousness, with individual responses varying dramatically. In general, acute symptoms are dependent on both the concentration and duration of exposure. Exposure to 7500 ppm for 30 minutes is life-threatening; 1500 ppm for 60 minutes produces significant symptoms; 50–150 ppm for 5 hours results in headache and weakness; whereas exposure to 25 ppm or less for 8 hours results in no demonstrable acute effect (109). If not initially fatal, recovery from acute exposure to benzene is usually complete. Recommended benzene exposure limits for military personnel in isolated emergency situations are 1000 ppm for 10 minutes, 500 ppm for 30 minutes, and 300 ppm for 60 minutes (110).

Chronic Toxicity

Toxicity arising from subacute or chronic exposure to benzene is almost exclusively limited to the hemopoietic and immune systems. The potential for benzene exposure to result in bone marrow toxicity was recognized as early as the beginning of the 20th century (106, 107). During the first quarter of this century, recognition of benzene as a bone marrow depressant actually led to its use as a chemotherapeutic agent for the treatment of CLL. Since that time, an impressive number of case reports have appeared linking chronic benzene exposure with bone marrow suppression. Clinical findings following chronic benzene exposure include: anemia, thrombocytopenia or lymphocytopenia, pancytopenia, and aplastic anemia, along with the signs and symptoms normally accompanying such disorders as weakness, petechiae, purpura, and increased frequency of infection. The most frequently reported finding is leukopenia with or without thrombocytopenia. In cases of chronic benzene poisoning, clinically significant decreases in circulating cells often occur in the presence of a hyperplastic bone marrow with maturation arrest in both erythroid and myeloid lineages (111, 112). Similarly, splenomegaly associated with myeloid metaplasia, which is usually inconsistent with a diagnosis of aplastic anemia, has been reported in a small number of cases of pancytopenia associated with benzene exposure (113). Greenberg, Goldwater, and colleagues conducted the first well-controlled, cross-sectional study of benzene toxicity in the printing industry and found that chronic exposure of rotogravure workers to high concentrations of benzene was associated with both a relative and absolute lymphocytopenia, which often preceded anemia or thrombocytopenia (92, 93). Granulopoiesis appears to be remarkably resistant to benzene toxicity, and granulocytopenia is only rarely encountered as an isolated finding in cases of chronic benzene exposure.

Reliable industrial hygiene data are lacking in much of the literature on benzene-induced hemotoxicity. There is no doubt that repeated exposure to high concentrations of benzene is hemotoxic, and symptomatology appears to be consistently associated with chronic exposures in excess of 100 ppm. However, determining with any precision the threshold for benzene hemotoxicity is problematic, since there is little reliable information associated with exposures to 50 ppm or less.

Benzene and Leukemia

HISTORY

Cases of leukemias attributed to benzene exposure have appeared in the literature since 1897 (114). However, compared with the spontaneous incidence of leukemias in the United States alone, the numbers appearing in early reports associated with benzene exposure were in and of themselves not impressive and represented a small proportion of blood dyscrasias secondary to benzene (69, 93, 112, 115, 116). Widespread acceptance of benzene as a potential leukemogen occurred as a result of two coinciding but independent events. General recognition that some bone marrow-suppressive agents could

produce leukemia occurred largely as a consequence of advances in cancer chemotherapy. Prior to the advent of intensive alkylation therapy for the treatment of Hodgkin's disease and other neoplasms during the 1960s, acute nonlymphocytic leukemia (ANLL) was not a natural complication of these diseases. However, by 1979 ANLL secondary to chemotherapy was well recognized along with the knowledge that exposure to bone marrow-suppressive agents could lead to the development of leukemia (117). Independently, a marked increase in the incidence of hemotoxicity among Turkish and Italian shoe and leather workers was observed as a consequence of the introduction of benzene-containing adhesives around 1960. Publication of a series of cases of AML in benzene-exposed workers in Turkey and Italy (94, 95) was instrumental in stimulating further quantitative epidemiology studies of the association between benzene exposure and AML. Since then, several epidemiology studies have evaluated the relationship between benzene exposure and leukemia. Although these studies are by no means consistent with respect to quality, cohort size, methodologies employed, or results, a pattern has emerged that supports a strong positive relationship between chronic benzene exposure and AML. Perhaps the most reliable quantitative evidence associating chronic benzene exposure with AML comes from a retrospective NIOSH study of rubber hydrochloride (Pliofilm) workers employed in two plants in Akron, Ohio, from 1940–1949 (91, 118, 119).

PATHOGENESIS AND DOSE RESPONSE

As previously discussed, regulatory controversy has centered on the nature and importance of the dose relationship between benzene exposure and the development of leukemia. Regulatory agency policy for cancer risk assessment assumes a cumulative relationship between exposure and risk, independent of the concentration to which an individual is exposed. Predicated on the assumption that carcinogenic processes differ from other toxic effects with respect to dose-dependency, the projected risk is determined by extrapolating the incidence observed at high exposure for some duration to that expected at some lower product of exposure and duration. The alternative view is that there is a threshold concentration for benzene exposure below which there is no significant bone marrow damage and consequently no increased risk of developing leukemia. There is a considerable body of clinical and experimental evidence to support the concept of a threshold for benzene leukemogenesis.

The results of the NIOSH benzene study form the basis for current risk assessments associated with benzene leukemogenesis. While it provides convincing evidence for a relationship between occupational benzene exposure and AML, the study suffers from a notable lack of accurate exposure data. The assumptions made by the authors of the NIOSH study, namely that the time-weighted exposures encountered from 1937–1975 were 50 ppm (120), have been repeatedly criticized for (a) underestimating the actual exposure history and (b) being inconsistent with available hematologic monitoring data on the study population. A review of U.S. Department of Labor records on health hazards in the rubber industry indicating the occurrence of fatal blood dyscrasias and CNS symptoms in this cohort, together with results of a longitudinal analysis of hematologic surveillance records from one of the original study sites, suggests that criticisms of the NIOSH benzene exposure estimates are well-founded (121–124).

Whether one can totally exclude the possibility of benzene-induced AML occurring in the absence of clinically demonstrated hemotoxicity is problematic, although it would certainly appear to be unlikely. As with all other secondary leukemias, the evidence linking benzene-associated AML with previous bone marrow damage is impressive. Numerous case reports have described the progression from pancytopenia, bone marrow depression or hyperplasia, and aplastic anemia to AML (112), and there do not appear to be any proven cases of benzene-induced leukemia in the absence of previous pancytopenia (125). In patients who have previously received chemo- or radiation therapy, abnormalities in hemopoietic stem cell regulation have been observed to persist years after peripheral blood parameters have begun to approach normal values (126). These findings suggest that peripheral blood parameters may not provide reliable evidence of bone marrow damage in all cases.

TYPES OF LEUKEMIA ASSOCIATED WITH BENZENE EXPOSURE

Questions as to which types of leukemia can occur as a result of benzene exposure have been heightened by a profusion of contradictions and inadequacies that are rife in the benzene epidemiology literature. Efforts to sort through the labyrinthine maze of case reports, case-control, and retrospective cohort studies are frustrated by marked discrepancies in study design, size, and reliability of exposure data. Significant confusion arises when attempting to superimpose a contemporary diagnostic framework on an older and unsystematic literature. Nevertheless, taken together, multiple studies have demonstrated a clear association between chronic benzene exposure and the development of AML (91, 95, 118, 127–129). Leukemias reported secondary to benzene exposure conform to define FAB subtypes of AML, including acute myeloblastic leukemia (M1, M2), monomyelocytic leukemia (M4), and erythroleukemia (M6); however, monoblastic leukemias (M5) are uncommon. The variant of AML most frequently reported as a consequence of chronic benzene toxicity is erythroleukemia (M6), which is frequently seen in patients secondary to chemotherapy as well. Because of its frequency in studies of benzene-exposed workers, the finding of erythroleukemia in a patient with a significant history of benzene exposure is probably diagnostic for benzene-induced leukemia. However, care must be taken to differentiate between compensatory erythroid hyperplasia accompanying another subtype and a true erythroleukemia.

A marked contrast exists between the strength of epidemiologic evidence linking chronic benzene exposure to AML and that suggesting an association with other leukemias. A small number of case reports and collected series have variously suggested a relationship between benzene and lymphoid leukemias, and even Hodgkin's disease (113). However, the number of cases reported is exceedingly small and the quantitative evidence linking ALL, CLL, or other lymphoid neoplasms to benzene exposure is even weaker than that reported secondary to chemotherapy. For example, the NIOSH study that establishes a positive association between benzene exposure and AML fails to demonstrate any relationship between benzene exposure and CML, CLL, or ALL (91). As previously discussed, an increased incidence of lymphoid neoplasms has been observed in the rubber and tire industry, although the pattern of disease observed does not correlate well with benzene ex-

posure (38). For CLL there is no known association with cytotoxic drugs, chemicals, or ionizing radiation. In the case of CML, there is in fact evidence to suggest that an association with benzene does not exist. The initial suggestion of a relationship between benzene and CML has come primarily from literature in which banded chromosome analysis was not employed as a diagnostic tool—principally older studies and case histories (116, 130, 131). The Yin China study represents the only quantitative epidemiology study indicating a significant increase in CML among workers exposed to benzene (129). Because of the predominant tendency of AMLs secondary to benzene to be preceded by MDS and other blood dyscrasias, the criteria for differential diagnosis of CML and MDS is specially critical. At present, extrapolation of the results of the Yin study with respect to leukemia subtypes is confounded by a lack of uniform diagnostic criteria, lack of cytogenetic analyses, and failure to use even the WHO disease classification system (132). In contrast, a relative decrease or absence of CML among leukemia cases associated with benzene exposure has been reported by Vigliani and coworkers (133, 134) and by Aksoy, who found a notable rarity of CML among benzene workers relative to unexposed populations (135). Even more impressive is the fact that, while CML is clearly a consequence of high level radiation, it has never been documented to occur secondary to chemical (i.e., chemotherapeutic) exposure alone. These findings are consistent with the observation that CML invariably arises in the PSC compartment, which is predominantly made up of cells at rest (23), whereas the target cell in AML appears most often to be a multilineage myeloid progenitor (23), which is a rapidly dividing cell and thus more susceptible to chemically induced damage.

Toxicology of Benzene

ABSORPTION, METABOLISM, AND DISTRIBUTION

By far the most significant route of occupational exposure to benzene is via inhalation. Although prolonged exposure or immersion of the skin in benzene or solutions containing a high concentration of benzene can result in a breakdown of the normal dermal barrier and significant absorption, intact skin does not normally constitute a major route of absorption for benzene vapor. Following inhalation, benzene is rapidly excreted unchanged via the lungs and as conjugated phenolic metabolites in the urine. Although the benzene molecule is geometrically simple, its metabolism is quite complex. It is now widely accepted that benzene metabolism is a requirement for bone marrow toxicity. Primary metabolism of benzene occurs predominantly in the liver via cytochrome P-450, the principal product being phenol. Phenol, in turn, undergoes further oxidation via cytochrome P-450 to produce the polyphenolic metabolites of benzene (principally hydroquinone), or alternatively, oxidation via peroxidases in extrahepatic tissues to form biphenols, hydroquinone, and its terminal oxidation product, p-benzoquinone (136, 137). Muconic acid has long been known to be a minor urinary metabolite of benzene, and its putative intermediate, trans, trans-muconaldehyde, has been shown to be hemotoxic and hypothesized to play a role in benzene toxicity (138, 139). However, for the present, the metabolic source of ring-opened products of benzene and their toxicologic significance remains unknown.

An important determinant in benzene bone marrow toxicity

appears to be the enzyme myeloperoxidase, which is a major constituent of bone marrow granulocytic cells (140) and catalyzes the oxidation of hydroquinone to 1,4-benzoquinone (139). Recent studies in experimental animals have demonstrated that benzene-induced myelotoxicity can be ameliorated by the simultaneous administration of indomethacin (141, 142). This suggests a role for prostaglandin synthetase (cyclooxygenase) in benzene-induced myelotoxicity. However, indomethacin also inhibits myeloperoxidase-mediated oxidation of hydroquinone (137), providing apt illustration that data obtained using "specific" inhibitors alone should be interpreted with caution.

MECHANISM OF ACTION

Bone Marrow Toxicity

Benzene appears to share characteristics in common with both cycle-specific and phase-specific agents. Cytotoxicity in bone marrow is cycle specific, dividing cells being targeted and arrested in G2 and mitosis (143). These findings are consistent with the remarkable sensitivity of the cytoskeleton (i.e., microtubules) to hydroquinone and p-benzoquinone, which interfere with GTP-dependent microtubule assembly by binding to sulfhydryl groups on the protein (144, 145). The effects of benzene metabolites are not entirely restricted to cells in G2 or M phases of the cell cycle, however. At nonlethal concentrations, the quinone metabolites of benzene can inhibit entry of cells into cycle in response to growth stimuli (146, 147).

Either as a result of the cycle-specific nature of benzene toxicity, its complex metabolism, or both, historically it has proven difficult to mimic benzene toxicity via administration of its individual metabolites to experimental animals. Certainly for many cycle- or phase-specific chemotherapeutic agents, the regimen of exposure is known to influence bone marrow toxicity. Shortterm repeated exposure to benzene results in a reduction in bone marrow cellularity that reaches a maximum between 3 and 10 days and is characterized by a loss of differentiating cells of intermediate maturity (143). An interesting aspect of the experimental toxicity of benzene and its quinone metabolites is the refractory nature of the bone marrow suppression observed in the face of continuing exposure. Treatment paradigms extending beyond 10–15 days are frequently accompanied by a gradual return to essentially normal bone marrow cellularity (148). Hydroquinone, for example, is a potent suppressor of bone marrow cell and lymphocyte growth in vitro (144, 146). Yet, it has proven exceedingly difficult to reproduce even transient benzene toxicity in vivo via the administration of hydroquinone, and even shortterm effects have required the use of massive doses of hydroquinone administered under nonphysiologic conditions (149). Although administration of phenol itself does not result in even transient bone marrow toxicity, the concomitant administration of hydroquinone and phenol (i.p.) has been demonstrated to result in significant bone marrow suppression and nondysjunctional events far and above that observed following administration of hydroquinone alone (137, 150). Consistent with the observed cycle-specific effects of benzene and its metabolites, interrupted exposure regimen (i.e., multiple exposure intervals interrupted by several days) are more effective in producing bone marrow suppression than repeated daily administration.

Leukemogenesis

How bone marrow toxicity relates to the development of secondary leukemogenesis in general is not yet understood, so consequently the mechanism by which benzene exposure leads to the development of AML is not known. It is has become increasingly obvious in recent years that cancer in general and leukemias in particular are clonal in origin and that the progression to clinical malignancy involves a complex sequence of multiple events that must occur in some order for the disease to manifest itself (151). The specific events required and their precise sequence are by no means known; however, a number of events have been variously hypothesized to play a role. These include: gene mutation resulting from point mutation or translocation; loss of a critical regulatory or suppressor gene that might occur as a result of deletion of part or all of a chromosome; activation of a proto-oncogene via mutation, translocation or deletion; or, perhaps, alterations in "gene dosage" as might occur in trisomy (152).

Two potential mechanisms of action most frequently invoked with respect to the possible role of benzene in the development of leukemia involve a potential mutation resulting from DNA adduct formation and, as an alternative, chromosomal deletion or aneuploidy arising as a consequence of a nondysjunctional event. Certainly, the chemistry of benzene and its known metabolites, as well as what is known about the cytogenetics of secondary leukemia, favor the latter hypothesis. In contrast to potent DNA-alkylating agents, benzene is not mutagenic, its metabolites are not mutagenic, and neither have they proven to be a teratogenic in multigeneration studies. Likewise, despite the great deal of effort that has been expended in the search for DNA adducts of benzene, the data implicating direct DNA alkylation as contributing significantly to its mechanism of action are not impressive. To date, results have largely been limited to deoxyguanosine adducts formed on incubation with benzene quinone metabolites, and their demonstration has only been accomplished in in vitro systems requiring artificial or nonphysiologic conditions, such as using purified, denatured, or mitochondrial DNA (153, 155). Although some reports have provided evidence suggestive of benzene DNA adduct formation in liver following injection of the compound in rats or rabbits, these have not been structurally characterized and benzene DNA adduct formation in bone marrow has not been reported (156–158). Results of at least one study suggest that DNA adducts derived from benzene metabolites are either not formed in vivo following benzene exposure or are formed at levels below detection (154).

On the other hand, the circumstantial evidence for a role for nondysjunctional events in benzene-leukemogenesis is substantial. Over 95% of cases examined of AML secondary to chemotherapy and/or irradiation examined demonstrate specific abnormalities in chromosomes with over 75% lacking part or all of chromosomes 5 and/or 7 (159). It is probably significant that several hemopoietic growth factors (e.g., IL-3, GM-CSF, and M-CSF) are localized to the long arm of chromosome 5 and are deleted in 5q− syndrome (160).

Available cytogenetic studies of benzene-related leukemias precede the advent of banded chromosome analysis; however, they also have reported the frequent incidence of aneuploidy and/or involvement of "C-type" chromosomes (i.e., chromosomes 5–7) (113). Benzene metabolites are well known sulfhydryl-alkylating reagents, effective at inhibiting spindle formation and arresting cells in G2/M (143–145).

Similarly, benzene metabolites give rise to chromosomal aberrations including aneuploidy and micronuclei representing predominantly whole chromosomes (161), and elevated frequencies of aneuploid cells have also been observed in peripheral blood cells of workers with occupational exposure to benzene (162—164).

Surveillance and Monitoring of Workers for Hematologic Disease

Opinions as to the adequacy of existing laboratory procedures for screening workers for evidence of hematologic disease differ and tend to reflect differences in training and perspective. Many hematologists feel that the routine complete blood count (CBC) provides an entirely adequate screening tool, especially since most patients with blood dyscrasias tend to present with overt clinical signs and symptoms. Alternatively, the occupational physician may find the value of the routine CBC as an early indicator of hemopoietic toxicity to be limited by the variability inherent in the general population as well as the number of situations in which CBC parameters may be altered (e.g., infection, drug use, menstruation). Oral contraceptives, alcohol, smoking habits, sex, race, and obesity are all known to influence WBC or RBC.

Because of the number of influences that have an impact on the kinetics of granulocyte release and margination of circulating granulocytes, the WBC in particular and the CBC in general have not proven to be a very sensible or reliable indicator of low level exposure to agents such as benzene or, for that matter, any form of early marrow damage (68, 121). A longitudinal study of workers employed in Pliofilm rubber production during World War II has demonstrated an impressive correlation between depressed WBC counts and estimated annual time-weighted average benzene exposures ranging from 60–137 ppm. However, the results suggest that routine hematologic surveillance is not useful for monitoring exposures below 50 ppm (121). As previously mentioned, essentially normal peripheral blood parameters may belie longterm underlying abnormalities in hemopoietic precursor cell regulation that are impossible to detect using routine laboratory methods (126).

Despite these limitations, the CBC remains the most accessible and widely used screening tool for evidence of hemotoxicity. For the monitoring of benzene workers, a number of alternative laboratory procedures have been variously recommended, although none have yet proven sensitive, specific, or useful enough for this purpose. For example, cytogenetic abnormalities are frequently observed in blood cells from patients exhibiting overt symptomatology of benzene hemotoxicity, yet they have not proven useful as a predictive tool and cannot be used to determine the likelihood of hematologic abnormalities in an asymptomatic individual (165). One sensitive but nonspecific parameter that is currently available with automated CBC instrumentation is the RDW, or coefficient of variation associated with the erythrocyte mean corpuscular volume (MCV). The size distribution of red cells, or Price Jones curve, is subject to any influence that can produce erythrocyte macrocytosis or microcytosis (e.g., reticulocytosis, folate deficiency, alcoholism, drug- or chemical-induced megaloblastic changes). Alterations in the coefficient of distribution will become evident before frank changes in the MCV are apparent. Determination of the underlying cause of this or any other change in peripheral blood parameters requires additional patient follow-up.

REFERENCES

1. Jandl JH. Blood. Boston: Little Brown, 1987:197–201.
2. Alderson M. The epidemiology of leukemia. Adv Cancer Res 1980;31: 1–76.
3. Karchmer RK, Amare M, Larsen WE, et al. Alkylating agents as leukemogens in multiple myeloma. Cancer 1974;33:1103–1107.
4. Canellos GP, Arseneau JC, DeVita VT, et al. Second malignancies complicating Hodgkin's disease in remission. Lancet 1975;1:947–949.
5. Catovsky D, Galton DA. Myelomonocytic leukemia supervening on chronic lymphocytic leukemia. Lancet 1971;1:478–479.
6. Pedersen-Bjergaard J, Nissen NI, Sorensen HM, et al. Acute nonlymphocytic leukemia in patients with ovarian carcinoma following long term treatment with Tresulfan (= dihydroxybusulfan). Cancer 1980;45:19–29.
7. Greene MH, Harris EL, Gershenson DM, et al. Melphalan may be a more potent leukemogen than cyclophosphamide. Ann Intern Med 1986;105:360–367.
8. Rosner F, Grunwald HW. Hodgkin's disease and acute leukemia. Am J Med 1975;58:339–353.
9. Grunwald HW, Rosner F. Acute leukemia and immunosuppressive drug use. Arch Intern Med 1979;139:461–466.
10. Falkson HC, Portugal MA, Falkson G. Leukaemia in Hodgkin's disease. S Afr Med J 1976;50:1429–1431.
11. Ali NO, Janes WO. Malignant myelosclerosis (acute myelofibrosis): report of two cases following cytotoxic chemotherapy. Cancer 1979;43:1211–1215.
12. Cuny G, Penin F, Guerci O, et al. Maladie de Hodgkin associee a une leucose aigue. Ann Med Nancy 1973;12:1103–1110.
13. Rosner F, Grunwald HW. Chemicals and leukemia. In: Henderson ES, Lister TA, eds. Leukemia. Philadelphia: WB Saunders, 1990:271–287.
14. Tucker MA, D'Angio GJ, Boice JD Jr, et al. Bone sarcomas linked to radiotherapy and chemotherapy in children. N Engl J Med 1987;317:588–593.
15. Tucker MA, Coleman CN, Cox RS, Varghese A, Rosenberg SA. Risk of second cancers after treatment for Hodgkin's disease. N Engl J Med 1988;31:76–81.
16. Mole RH. Ionizing radiations and human leukemia. In: Henderson ES, Lister TA, eds. Leukemia. Philadelphia: WB Saunders, 1990:253–269.
17. Coleman CN, Williams CJ, Flint A, Glatstein EJ, Rosenberg SA, Kaplan HS. Hematologic neoplasia in patients treated for Hodgkin's disease. N Engl J Med 1977;297:1249–1252.
18. Reimer RR, Hoover R, Fraumeni JF, Young RC. Acute leukemia after alkylating-agent therapy of ovarian cancer. N Engl J Med 1977;297:177–181.
19. Pedersen-Bjergaard J, Larsen SO. Incidence of acute non-lymphocytic leukemia, pre-leukemia, and acute myeloproliferative syndrome up to ten years after treatment of Hodgkin's disease. N Engl J Med 1982;307:965–971.
20. Bergsagel DE, Bailey AJ, Langley GR, MacDonald RN, White DF, Miller AB. The chemotherapy of plasma cell myeloma and the incidence of acute leukemia. N Engl J Med 1979;301:743–748.
21. World Health Organization. ICD-9, International Classification of Diseases for Oncology. 2nd ed. Geneva: NHO, 1990.
22. Nowell PC, Hungerford DA. A minute chromosome in human chronic granulocytic leukemia. Science 1960;132:1497.
23. Rowley JD. A new consistent chromosomal abnormality in chronic myelogenous leukemia identified by quinacrine fluorescence and Giemsa staining. Nature 1973;243:290–293.
24. Fialkow PJ, Denman AM, Jacobson RJ, and Lowenthal MN. Chronic myelocytic leukemia. J Clin Invest 1978;62:815–823.
25. Groffen J, Stephenson JR, Heisterkamp N, de Klein A, Bartram CR, Grosveld G. Philadelphia chromosomal breakpoints are clustered within a limited region, bcr, on chromosome 22. Cell 1984;36:93–99.
26. Kurzrock R, Blick MB, Talpaz M, et al. Rearrangement in the breakpoint cluster region and the clinical course in Philadelphia-negative chronic myelogenous leukemia. Ann Intern Med 1986;105:673–679.
27. Bartram CR, Kleihauer E, de Klein A, et al. C-abl and bcr are rearranged in a Ph[1]-negative CML patient. EMBO J 1985;4:683–686.
28. Kurzrock R, Gutterman JU, Talpaz M. The molecular genetics of Philadelphia chromosome-positive leukemias. N Engl J Med 1988;319:990–998.
29. Pugh WC, Pearson M, Vardiman JW, Rowley JD. Philadelphia chromosome-negative chronic myelogenous leukemia: a morphological reassessment. B J Hematol 1985;60:457–467.
30. Young NS. Drugs and chemicals as agents of bone marrow failure. In: Testa NG, Gale RP, eds. Hematopoiesis. New York: Marcel Dekker, 1988:131–157.
31. Girard R, Mallein, Fourel R, Tolot F. Lymphose et intoxication benzolique professionnelle chronique. Arch Mal Prof Med Trav Secur Soc 1966;27(10–11):781–786.
32. Epstein SS, Ozonoff D. Leukemias and blood dyscrasias following

exposure to chlordane and heptachlor. Teratog Carcinog Mutagen 1987;7:527–540.

33. Andjelkovic D, Taulbee J, Symons M. Mortality experience of a cohort of rubber workers, 1964–1973. J Occup Med 1976;18:387–394.

34. Delzell E, Monson RR. Mortality among rubber workers: V. Processing workers. J Occup Med 1982;24:539–545.

35. Irons RD. Benzene toxicology update. J Appl Toxicol 1982;2:57–58.

36. Monson RR, Fine LJ. Cancer mortality and morbidity among rubber workers. J Natl Cancer Inst 1978;61:1047–1053.

37. McMichael AJ, Spirtas R, Kupper LL, Gamble JF. Solvent exposure and leukemia among rubber workers: an epidemiologic study. J Occup Med 1975;17:234–239.

38. Checkoway H, Wilcosky T, Wolf P, Tyroler H. An evaluation of the associations of leukemia and rubber industry solvent exposures. Am J Ind Med 1984;5:239–249.

39. Silverstein M, Maizlish N, Park R, Mirer F. Mortality among workers exposed to coal tar pitch volatiles and welding emissions: an exercise in epidemiologic triage. Am J Public Health 1985;75:1283–1287.

40. Stern FB, Waxweiler RA, Beaumont JJ, et al. A case-control study of leukemia at a naval nuclear shipyard. Am J Epidemiol 1986;123:980–992.

41. Stern RM. Cancer incidence among welders: possible effects of exposure to extremely low frequency electromagnetic radiation (ELF) and to welding fumes. Environ Health Perspect 1987;76;221–229.

42. Kaminski R, Geissert K, Dacey E. Mortality analysis among plumbers and pipefitters. J Occup Med 1980;22:183–189.

43. Kimzey, S. The effects of extended spaceflight on hematologic and immunologic systems. J Am Med Woman's Assoc 1975;30:218–232.

44. Leach CS, Johnson PC. Influence of spaceflight on erythrokinetics in man. Science 1984;225:216–219.

45. Cogli A, Bechler B, Muller O, Hunzinger H. Effect of microgravity on lymphocyte activation. ESA SP-1091. European Space Agency. Feb 1988.

46. Steele KJ. Zero gravity and the immune system: a challenge to man's survival in space. Analog Science Fiction/Science Fact 1989;191:36–50.

46a. Coles S, Bennett J, Ross C. Medical surveillance for leukemia at a petrochemical manufacturing complex: four-year summary. J Occup Med 1991: in press.

47. Gilfillan SC. Lead poisoning and the fall of Rome. J Occup Med 1965;7:53–60.

48. Albahary C. Lead and hemapoiesis. Am J Med 1972;52:367–377.

49. Cooper WC, Gaffey WR. Mortality of lead workers. J Occup Med 1975;17:100–107.

50. Kang HK, Infante PF, Carra JS. Occupational lead exposure and cancer. Science 1980;207:935–936.

51. Cooper WC. Occupational lead exposure: what are the risks? Science 1980;208:129–131.

52. Landrigan PJ. Arsenic—state of the art. Am J Ind Med 1981;2:5–14.

53. Nordberg GF, Pershagen G, Lauwerys R. Inorganic arsenic—toxicological and environmental aspects. Odense, Denmark: Department of Community Health and Environmental Medicine, Odense University, 1979.

54. Axelson O, Dahlgren E, Jansson C-D, Rehnlund SO. Arsenic exposure and mortality: a case referent study from a Swedish copper smelter. Br J Ind Med 1978;35:8–15.

55. Ott MG, Holder BB, Gordon HL. Respiratory cancer and occupational exposure to arsenicals. Arch Environ Health 1974;29:250–255.

56. Polednak Ap, Stehney AF, Rowland RE. Mortality among women first employed before 1930 in the U.S. radium dial-painting industry. Am J Epidemiol 1978;107:179–195.

57. Martland HS, Conlon P, Knef JD. Some unrecognized dangers in the use and the handling of radioactive substances. JAMA 1925;85:1769–1776.

58. Martland HS. Microscopic changes of certain anemias due to radioactivity. Arch Pathol 1926;2:465–472.

59. Martland HS. Occupational poisoning in manufacture of luminous watch dials. JAMA 1929;92:466–473, 552–559.

60. Martland HS. The occurrence of malignancy in radioactive persons. Am J Cancer 1931;15:2435–2516.

61. Austin SG, Sielken RL. Issues in assessing the carcinogenic hazards of ethylene oxide. J Occup Med 1988;30:236–245.

62. Hogstedt LC, Malmquist N, Wadman B. Leukemia in workers exposed to ethylene oxide. JAMA 1979;241:1132–1133.

63. Hogstedt LC, Rohlen O, Berndtsson BS, Axelson O, Ehrenberg L. A cohort study of mortality and cancer incidence in ethylene oxide production workers. Br J Ind Med 1979;36:276–280.

64. Theis AM, Frentzel-Beyme R, Link R, et al. Mortality study on employees exposed to alkylene oxides (ethylene oxide/propylene oxide) and their derivatives. Proceedings of the Symposium on Prevention of Occupational Cancer 1981:Helsinki.

65. Morgan RW, Claxton KW, Divine BJ, et al. Mortality among ethylene oxide workers. J Occup Med 1981;23:767–770.

66. Cook RR, Bodner KM, Kolesar RC, et al. A cross-sectional study of ethylene glycol monomethyl ether process employees. Arch Environ Health 1982;37:346–351.

67. Welch LS, Cullen, MR. Effect of exposure to ethylene glycol ethers on shipyard painters: III. Hematologic effects. Am J Ind Med 1988;14:527–536.

68. Cullen MR, Rado T, Waldron JA, Sparer J, Welch LS. Bone marrow injury in lithographers exposed to glycol ethers and organic solvents used in multicolor offset and ultraviolet curing printing processes. Arch Environ Health 1983;38:347–354.

69. Scott JL, Cartwright GE, Wintrobe MM. Acquired aplastic anemia: an analysis of thirty-nine cases and review of the pertinent literature. Medicine 1959;38:119–172.

70. Meinhardt TJ, Young RJ, Hartle RW. Epidemiologic investigations of styrene-butadiene rubber production and reinforced plastics production. Scand J Work Environ Health 1978;4(suppl 2):240–246.

71. Divine BJ. An update on mortality among workers at a butadiene facility—preliminary results. Environ Health Perspect 1990; 86 (June):119–128.

71a. Matanoski GM, Schwartz L. Morality of workers in styrene-butadiene polymer production. J Occup Med 1987;29:675–680.

71b. Matanoski GM, Santos-Burga S, Zeger S, Schwartz L. Nested case-control study of lymphopoietic cancers in workers in the styrene-butadiene polymer manufacturing industry — revised final report. Baltimore: The Johns Hopkins University School of Hygiene and Public Health, 1989.

72. Matanoski GM. Environ Health Perspect 1990; 86 (June):107–117.

72a. Acquavella JF. The paradox of butadiene epidemiology. Exp Pathol 1989;37:114–118.

73. Irons RD, Stillman WS, Cloyd MW. Selective activation of endogenous ecotropic retrovirus in hematopoietic tissues of B6C3F1 mice during the preleukemic phase of 1,3-butadiene exposure. Virology 1987;161:457–462.

74. Irons RD, Smith CN, Stillman WS, Shah RS, Steinhagen WH, Leiderman LJ. Macrocytic-megaloblastic anemia in male NIH Swiss mice following repeated exposure to 1,3-butadiene. Toxicol Appl Pharmacol 1986;85:450–455.

75. Irons RD, Smith CN, Stillman WS, Shah RS, Steinhagen WH, Leiderman LJ. Macrocytic-megaloblastic anemia in male B6C3F1 mice following chronic exposure to 1,3-butadiene. Toxicol Appl Pharmacol 1986;83:95–100.

76. Irons RD, Cathro HP, Stillman WS, Steinhagen WH, Shah RS. Susceptibility to 1,3-butadiene-induced leukemogenesis correlates with endogenous ecotropic retroviral background in the mouse. Toxicol Appl Pharmacol 1989;101:170–176.

77. Infante PF, Epstein SS, Newton Jr WA. Blood dyscrasias and childhood tumors and exposure to chlordane and heptachlor. Scand J Work Environ Health 1978;4:137–50.

78. Furie B, Trubowitz S. Insecticides and blood dyscrasias: chlordane exposure and self-limited refractory megaloblastic anemia. JAMA 1976;235:1720–1722.

79. Wang HH, Grufferman S. Aplastic anemia and occupational pesticide exposure: a case-control study. J Med 1981;23:364–366.

80. Shindell S, Ulrich S. Mortality of workers employed in the manufacture of chlordane: an update. J Occup Med 1986;28:497–501.

81. Shindell S. Cancer mortality among workers exposed to chlordane. J Occup Med 1987;29:908–911.

82. MacMahon B, Monson RR, Wang HH, Zheng TZ. A second follow-up of mortality in a cohort of pesticide applicators. J Occup Med 1988;30:429–432.

83. Bond GG, Bodner KM, Cook RR. Phenoxy herbicides and cancer: insufficient epidemiologic evidence for a causal relationship. Fundam Appl Toxicol 1989;12:172–188.

84. Hardell L, Sandstrom A. A case control study: soft tissue sarcomas and exposure to phenoxyacetic acids or chlorophenols. Br J Cancer 1979;39:711–717.

85. Hardell L, Eriksson M, Lenner P, Lundgren E. Malignant lymphoma and exposure to chemicals, especially organic solvents, chlorophenols and phenoxy acids: a case-control study. Br J Cancer 1981;43:169–176.

86. Woods JS, Polissar L, Severson RK, Heuser LS, Kulander BG. Soft tissue sarcoma and non-Hodgkin's lymphoma in relation to phenoxyherbicide and chlorinated phenol exposure in Western Washington State. J Natl Cancer Inst 1987;78:899–910.

87. Pearce N. Phenoxy herbicides and non-Hodgkin's lymphoma in New Zealand: frequency and duration of herbicide use. Br J Ind Med 1989;46:143–144.

88. Hoar SK, Blair A, Holmes FF, Boysen CD, et al. Agricultural herbicide use and risk of lymphoma and soft-tissue sarcoma. JAMA 1986;256:1141–1147.

89. Zahm SH, Weisenburger DD, Babbitt PA, et al. A case-control study of non-Hodgkin's lymphoma and the herbicide 2,4-dichlorophenoxyacetic acid (2,4-D) in eastern Nebraska. Epidemiology, in press.

90. Purcell, WP. Benzene. In: Kirck RE, Othmer, DF eds. Encyclopedia of chemical technology. 3rd ed. Vol 3. New York: John Wiley & Sons, 1978:744–771.

91. Infante PF, Rinsky RA, Wagoner JK, Young RJ. Leukemia in benzene workers. Lancet 1977;2:76–78.

92. Greenburg L, Mayers MR, Goldwater L, Smith AR. Benzene poisoning in rotogravure printing. J Ind Hyg Toxicol 1939;21:395–420.

93. Goldwater LJ. Disturbances in the blood following exposure to benzol. J Lab Clin Med 1941;26:957–973.

94. Aksoy M, Erdem S, Dincol G. Leukemia in shoe-workers exposed chronically to benzene. Blood 1974;44:837–841.

95. Vigliani EC. Leukemia associated with benzene exposure. Ann NY Acad Sci 1976;271:142–151.

96. Gilbert D, Byrne M, Harris J, Steber W, Woodruff C. An exposure and risk assessment for benzene. Final draft Report 1982. Prepared by Arthur D. Little, Inc., for U.S. Environmental Protection Agency Office of Water and Waste Management, Washington, DC, EPA Contract No. 68-01-5949. Washington, DC: EPA, 1982.

97. Wallace LA. Major sources of benzene exposure. Environ Health Perspect 1989;82:165–169.

98. Wallace LA. The exposure of the general population to benzene. In: Benzene: occupational and environmental hazards. Scientific Update; Adv Modern Environ Toxicol 1989;16:113–130.

99. Austin H, Cole P. Cigarette smoking and leukemia. J Chronic Dis 1986;39:417–421.

100. Doll R, Peto R. Mortality in relation to smoking: 20 years' observations on male British doctors. Br Med J 1976;2:1525–1536.

101. Rogot E, Murray JL. Smoking and causes of death among U.S. veterans: 16 years of observation. Public Health Rep 1980;95:213–222.

102. Williams RR, Horm JW. Association of cancer sites with tobacco and alcohol consumption and socioeconomic status of patients: interview study from the Third National Cancer Survey. J Natl Cancer Inst 1977;58:525–547.

103. Kinlen LJ, Rogot E. Leukaemia and smoking habits among United States veterans. Br Med J 1988;297:657–659.

104. Wald N. Smoking and leukaemia. Br Med J 1988;297:638.

105. Lewin L. Die akute todlich Vergiftung durch Benzoldamaapf. Munch Med Wochenschr 1907;54:2377.

106. Santesson, CG. Uber chronische Vergiftung mit Steinkohlenteerbenzin; vier Todefalle. Arch Hyg Berl 1897;31:336–376.

107. Selling L. Preliminary report of some cases of purpura haemorrhagica due to benzol poisoning. Bull Johns Hopkins Hospital 1910;21:33–37.

108. Selling L. Benzol as a leucotoxin. Studies on the degeneration and regeneration of the blood and hematopoietic organs. Johns Hopkins Hospital Rep 1916;17:83–148.

109. Gerarde HW. Toxicology and biochemistry of aromatic hydrocarbons. Elsevier Monographs on Toxic Agents, Browning E, ed. Amsterdam: Elsevier, 1960:97–108.

110. Health effects of benzene: a review. Committee on Toxicology, Assembly of Life Sciences. National Research Council. National Academy of Sciences: Washington, DC, 1976.

111. Mallory TB, Gall EA, Brickley WJ. Chronic exposure to benzene (Benzol). III. The pathologic results. J Ind Hyg Toxicol 1939;21:355–377.

112. Hunter FT. Chronic exposure to benzene (Benzol). II. The clinical effects. J Ind Hyg Toxicol 1939;21:331–354.

113. Aksoy M. Benzene hematotoxicity. In: Aksoy M, Ed. Benzene carcinogenicity. Boca Raton, FL: CRC Press, 1988:59–151.

114. Le Noire, Claude. Sur un cas de purpura attribue a l'intoxication par le benzene. Bull Mem Soc Med Hop Paris 1897;14:1251–1260.

115. Hunter FT, Hanflig SS. Chronic benzol poisoning: a report of four cases. Boston Med Surg 1927;197:292–299.

116. Browning E. Toxicity and metabolism of industrial solvents. Amsterdam: Elsevier, 1965:3–50.

117. Casciato DA, Scott JL. Acute leukemia following prolonged cytoxic agent therapy. Medicine (Baltimore) 1979;58:32–47.

118. Rinsky RA, Young RJ, Smith AB. Leukemia in benzene workers. Am J Ind Med 1981;2:217–245.

119. Rinsky RA, Smith AB, Hornung R, et al. Benzene and leukemia. An epidemiologic risk assessment. N Engl J Med 1987;316:1044–1050.

120. White MC, Infante PF, Chu KC. A quantitative estimate of leukemia mortality associated with occupational exposure to benzene. Risk Anal 1982;2:195–204.

121. Kipen HM, Cody RP, Crump KS, Allen BC, Goldstein BD. Hema-

tological effects of benzene: a thirty-five year longitudinal study of rubber workers. Toxicol Ind Health 1988;4:411–430.

122. U.S. Dept. of Labor, Division of Labor Standards. Conference on health hazards in the rubber industry. Akron, Ohio, May 29, 1942.

123. Hornung RW, Ward E, Morris JA, Rinsky RA. Letter to the Editor. Toxicol Ind Health 1989;5:1153–1155.

124. Kipen HM, Cody RP, Goldstein BD. Use of longitudinal analysis of peripheral blood counts to validate historical reconstructions of benzene exposure. Environ Health Perspect 1989;82:199–206.

125. Goldstein BD. Hematoxicity in humans. J Toxicol Environ Health 1977;suppl 2:69–105.

126. Testa NG, Coutinho L, Chang J, Dexter TM. Use of long-term bone marrow cultures for autologous transplantation in acute myeloblastic leukemia. Proceedings of the 17th Annual Meeting of the International Society of Experimental Hematology, Houston, Texas, Aug 23, 1988, #250.

127. Vigliani EC, Saita G. Benzene and leukemia. N Engl J Med 1964;271:872–876.

128. Aksoy M, Dincol K, Erdem S, Dincol G. Acute leukemia due to chronic exposure to benzene. Am J Med 1972;52:160–166.

129. Yin S-N, Li G-L, Tain F-D, Fu Zl, Jin C, Chen YJ, et al. Leukaemia in benzene workers: a retrospective cohort study. Br J Ind Med 1987;44:124–128.

130. Tareef EM, Kontschalovskaya NM, Zorina LA. Benzene leukemias. Acta Unio Int Contra Cancrum 1963;19:751–755.

131. Goguel A, Cavigneaux A, Bernard J. Le leucemies benzeniques de la region Parisienne 1950 et 1065 (etudes de 50 observationes). Nouv Rev Fr Hematol 1967;7:465–480.

132. Wu W. Occupational cancer epidemiology in the People's Republic of China. J Occup Med 1988;30:968–974.

133. Vigliani EC, Forni A. Benzene and leukemia. Environ Res 1976;11:122–127.

134. Vigliani EC, Forni A. Chemical leukemogenesis in man. Ser Haematol 1974;7:211–223.

135. Aksoy M, Erdem S, Dincol G. Types of leukemia in chronic benzene poisoning. A study in thirty-four patients. Acta Haematol 1976;55:65–72.

136. Sawahata T, Neal RA. Horseradish peroxidase-mediated oxidation of phenol. Biochem Biophys Res Commun 1982;109:990–994.

137. Smith MT, Yager JW, Steinmetz KL, Eastmond DA. Peroxidase-dependent metabolism of benzene's phenolic metabolites and its potential role in benzene toxicity and carcinogenicity. Environ Health Perspect 1989;82:23–29.

138. Goldstein BD, Witz G, Javid J, Amoruso MA, Rossman T, Wolder B. Muconaldehyde, a potential toxic intermediate of benzene metabolism. Adv Exp Med Biol 1982;136A:331–339.

139. Witz G, Rao GS, Goldstein BD. Short-term toxicity of trans,trans-muconaldehyde. Toxicol Appl Pharmacol 1985;80:511–516.

140. Test ST, Weiss SJ. The generation and utilization of chlorinated oxidants by human neutrophils. Adv Free Rad Biol Med 1986;2:91–116.

141. Gaido KW, Wierda D. Suppression of bone marrow stromal cell function by benzene and hydroquinone is ameliorated by indomethacin. Toxicol Appl Pharmacol 1987;89:378–390.

142. Pirozzi SJ, Renz JR, Schlosser MJ, Kalf GF. Protection against benzene-induced myelo- and genotoxicity in mice by non-steroidal anti-inflammatory agents. Toxicologist 1988;8:281.

143. Irons RD, Heck Hd'A, Moore BJ, Muirhead K. Effects of short term benzene administration on bone marrow cell cycle kinetics in the rat. Toxicol Appl Pharmacol 1979;51:399–409.

144. Irons RD, Neptun DA, Pfeifer RW. Inhibition of lymphocyte transformation and microtubule assembly by quinone metabolites of benzene: evidence for a common mechanism. J Reticuloendothelial Soc 1981;30:359–372.

145. Irons RD, Pfeifer RW, Aune TM, Pierce CW. Soluble immune response suppressor inhibits microtubule function in vivo and microtubule assembly in vitro. J Immunol 1984;133:2032–2036.

146. Pfeifer RW, Irons RD. Inhibition of lectin stimulated agglutination and mitosis by hydroquinone: reactivity with intracellular sulfhydryl groups. Exp Mol Pathol 1981;35:189–198.

147. Wierda D, Irons RD. Hydroquinone and catechol reduce the frequency of progenitor B lymphocytes in mouse spleen and bone marrow. Immunopharmacology 1982;4:41–54.

148. Eastmond DA, Smith MT, Irons RD. An interaction of benzene metabolites reproduces the myelotoxicity observed with benzene exposure. Toxicol Appl Pharmacol 1987;91:85–95.

149. Wierda D, Irons RD, Greenlee WF. Immunotoxicity in C57BL/6 mice exposed to benzene and Aroclor 1254. Toxicol Appl Pharmacol 1981;60:410–417.

150. Barale R, Marrazzini A, Betti B, Vangelisti V, Loprieno N, Barrai I.

Genotoxicity of two metabolites of benzene: phenol and hydroquinone show strong synergistic effects in vivo. Muta Res 1990;244:15–20.

151. Nowell P. Molecular events in tumor development (editorial). N Engl J Med 1988;319:575.

152. Henderson ES. Etiology of leukemia: a persisting puzzle. In: Henderson ES, Lister TA, eds. Leukemia. Philadelphia: WB Saunders, 1990:205–206.

153. Rushmore T, Snyder R, Kalf G. Covalent binding of benzene and its metabolites to DNA in rabbit bone marrow mitochondria in vitro. Chem-Biol Interact 1984;49:133–154.

154. Reddy MV, Blackburn GR, Irwin SE, Kommineni C, Mackerer CR, Mehlmen MA. A method for the in vitro culture of rat Zymbal gland: use in mechanistic studies of benzene carcinogenesis in combination with $_{32}$P-postlabeling. Environ Health Perspect 1989;82:239–247.

155. Snyder R, Jowa L, Witz G, Kalf G, Rushmore T. Formation of reactive metabolites from benzene. Arch Toxicol 1987;60:61–64.

156. Lutz WK, Schlatter C. Mechanisms of the carcinogenic action of benzene: irreversible binding to rat liver DNA. Chem-Biol Interact 1977;18:241–245.

157. Arfellini G, Grill S, Colaci A, Mazzullo M, Prodi G. In vivo and in vitro binding of benzene to nucleic acids and proteins of various rat and mouse organs. Cancer Lett 1985;28:159–168.

158. Bauer H, Dimitriadis EA, Snyder R. An in vivo study of benzene metabolite DNA adduct formation in liver of male New Zealand rabbits. Arch Toxicol 1989;63:209–213.

159. Koeffler HP, Rowley JD. Therapy-related acute nonlymphocytic leukemia. In: Wiernik PH, Canellos GP, Kyle RA, Schiffer CA, eds. Neoplastic diseases of the blood. New York: Churchill Livingstone, 1985:357–381.

160. Le Beau MM, Enstein ND, O'Brien SJ. The interleukin 3 gene is located on human chromosome 5 and is deleted in myeloid leukemia with a deletion of 5q. Proc Natl Acad Sci USA 1987;84:5913–5917.

161. Yager JW, Eastmond DA, Robertson ML, Paradisin WM, Smith MT. Characterization of micronuclei induced in human lymphocytes by benzene metabolites. Cancer Res 1990;50:393–399.

162. Forni A, Cappellini A, Pacifico E, Vigliani EC. Chromosome changes and their evolution in subjects with past exposure to benzene. Arch Environ Health 1971;23:385–391.

163. Haberlandt VW, Mente B. Aberrationen der Chromosomenzahl und-struktur bei benzolexponierten Industriearbeitern. Zentralbl Arbeitsmed Arbeitsschutz 1971;21:338–341.

164. Ding X, Li Y, Ding Y, Yang H. Chromosome changes in patients with chronic benzene poisoning. Chin Med J (Engl) 1983;96:681–685.

165. Goldstein BD. Benzene toxicity. State Art Rev Occup Med 1988;3:541–554.

64

Halogenated Solvents

Donald G. Barceloux, M.D.

This review covers the health effects of the following halogenated solvents: 1,2-dichloroethane (ethylene dichloride), 1,2-dichloroethylene (acetylene dichloride), dichloromethane (methylene chloride), 1,2-dichloropropane (propylene dichloride), tetrabromoethane (acetylene tetrabromide), tetrachloroethane (acetyl tetrachloride), tetrachloroethylene (perchloroethylene), tetrachloromethane (carbon tetrachloride), 1,1,1-trichloroethane, trichloroethylene, trichloromethane (chloroform), and 1,1,2-trichloro-1,2,2-trifluoroethane (fluorocarbon 113).

Unfortunately, our knowledge of these chemicals and their health effects is not complete enough to delineate all the effects of exposure to these chemicals. Presently our knowledge is based on case reports of both single, acute, overdose, and chronic overexposure, epidemiology studies of workers, and animal experiments. The medicinal use of some of these solvents (e.g., trichloroethylene, tetrachloroethylene, tetrachloromethane, trichloromethane) provides limited data on the human effects of these chemicals. This collection of data must be interpreted both cautiously and critically in order to determine the health effects of these solvents. Case reports demonstrate only a temporal relation between exposure and health effects. This type of information depends heavily on the author's ability to exclude other causes of the illness.

Epidemiology studies attempt to associate a specific chemical with an illness. The validity of an epidemiologic study depends on the study design (type of study, adequate sample size, appropriate goals, and relevant individuals), assignment (response rate, dropout rate, selection bias), assessment (measures of outcome, information bias, confounding variables), interpretation (clinical importance, appropriate interpretation), and extrapolation (appropriate conclusion and range of data, direct applicability to new population). The lack of exposure data that provides actual concentrations and duration of exposure further limits epidemiologic studies. Even assuming that epidemiologic studies demonstrate a clear association between a chemical and the health effect, the determination of true causation depends on satisfying certain principles of causation. For example, early epidemiologic studies of malaria would have associated bodies of water with malaria; however, these studies would not necessarily differentiate between contaminated water, cultural practices (e.g., food sources, environmental factors), and mosquitoes.

Principles of causation include (a) consistency and volume of medical data, (b) biologic plausibility, (c) specificity of association, (d) temporal relationship, (e) strength of the association, and (f) dose-response relationship. Even though numerous, similar case reports make causation more tenable, only an epidemiologic study can confirm an association between a chemical and a health effect (1). Then, an analysis of these principals of causation is required to implicate the chemical as a cause of human illness. Unfortunately, none of these principles provides undisputable evidence for causation, and none is required for the determination of cause and effect (2).

Important questions in determining causation include: (a) Does the chemical produce a consistent pattern of dysfunction in humans? (b) Do animals develop similar dysfunction under comparable exposure conditions? (c) Are the animals' lesions reproducible, and do the pathologic changes satisfactorily account for the observed dysfunction? All of the desired data are never available and, therefore, the determination of causation depends on a careful analysis of existing medical data based on critiques of the validity of the human studies and the adequacy of animal data. The careful evaluation of the present accumulation of animal and human data on these halogenated solvents allows a determination of many, but not all, of the health effects of these chemicals.

INTRODUCTION

Medicinal History

Most of these halogenated solvents were discovered in the 1800s and were initially investigated as anesthetic agents. Flourens first used trichloromethane as an animal anesthetic in 1847, and later that year Simpson performed surgery on humans with trichloromethane anesthesia (3). Over the next 100 years trichloromethane was the anesthetic of choice until other drugs with less cardio- and hepatotoxicity replaced it after World War II. Halogenated solvents tested during the 1800s for use as an anesthetic and discarded included the following: 1,2-dichloroethane (excessive salivation, convulsive movements, postoperative blue-gray corneal opacities), tetrachloromethane (cardiac depression, prolonged recovery times), 1,1,1-trichloroethane (moderate hypotension, ventricular dysrhythmias during hypoxia and hypercarbia), dichloromethane (excessive clonic movements, lack of muscle relaxation), and 1,2-dichloroethylene (excessive flammability). Of these chemicals, only trichloromethane and tetrachloromethane were associated with the development of hepatorenal toxicity during use as an anesthetic.

Damage to the trigeminal nerve complicated the use of trichloroethylene as a narcotic in the early 1900s and led to the use of this agent for the treatment of tic douloureux. This treatment was suspended in the 1930s because of lack of efficacy, but cranial neuropathies appeared again following the use of trichloroethylene as an anesthetic in the 1940s. Otherwise, the incidence of adverse effects generally was low following the use of trichloroethylene as an anesthetic (4).

Hall introduced tetrachloromethane as an anthelmintic for the treatment of hookworm in 1921. For the next 10 years thousands of patients, particularly in the South Pacific, received small doses (3–10 milliliters in adults) of tetrachloromethane. Although this chemical was an effective agent, serious reactions occurred in a few patients, particularly alcoholics and poorly nourished children. These susceptible patients developed liver necrosis, renal damage, and gastrointestinal hemorrhage (5). Subsequently, tetrachloroethylene became a substitute for tetrachloromethane as a treatment for hookworm and pinworm. Over 50,000 cases of hookworm were treated with doses of tetrachloroethylene up to 8 milliliters (maximum average adult dose), with surprisingly few side effects other than giddiness and lightheadedness (6).

Tetrachloroethylene was not considered an adequate substitute for trichloromethane anesthesia because of its mucous membrane-irritating properties, poor volatility, and inadequate muscle relaxation (7). 1,1,2,2-Tetrachloroethane was not considered for medicinal use because the hepatotoxic properties of this compound were well-known in the United States by 1922. Willcox reported the development of a toxic hepatitis in airplane factory workers at the Hindon airplane factory in 1914 that was similar to the German experience where tetrachloroethane was a solvent for the cellulose acetate sprayed over the linen that covered the airplanes (8).

Chemistry

Table 64.1 lists the chemical data for each one of the halogenated solvents. Evaluation of the toxicity of each of these halogenated solvents should include an analysis of the toxicity of the respective isomers, which may differ substantially in their ability to cause human illness. The isomer 1,1-dichloroethane is approximately five times less toxic than 1,2-dichloroethane in subchronic animal studies (9) and is not commercially available in the United States.

Dichloroethylene exists in the following three forms: (a) 1,1-dichloroethylene, (b) cis-1,2-dichloroethylene, and (c) trans-1,2-dichloroethylene. Based on animal studies, 1,1-dichloroethylene possesses greater hepatotoxicity than the other chloroethylene compounds (10) and also produces a unique pattern of hepatocellular injury. The anesthetic action of the trans isomer appear twice as potent as the cis isomer of 1,2-dichloroethylene based on inhalation studies of rats (11).

The 1,1,2-isomer of trichloroethane produces more profound central nervous system depression than 1,1,1-trichloroethane, and the former probably is more hepatotoxic than 1,1,1-trichloroethane based on animal experiments that demonstrate a comparable degree of hepatotoxicity between 1,1,2-trichloroethane and tetrachloromethane (12).

Physicochemical Properties

Generally these chemicals are clear, colorless liquids that are nonflammable and possess characteristically sweet, chloroformlike odors and slight mucous membrane-irritating properties. They usually are highly volatile, slightly soluble in water, but highly miscible in most of the organic solvents. The exceptions to the poor flammability rule of these halogenated solvents are 1,2-dichloroethane, 1,2-dichloroethylene, and the thermal decomposition product of trichloroethylene, dichloroacetylene. Table 64.2 lists the odor properties of these chemicals. Generally, the odor warning properties of these chemicals are not sufficient to allow workers to detect levels above currently recommended workplace standards by olfactory means, but levels immediately dangerous to the health of workers usually can be detected by olfactory means.

Exposure

USES

All of these halogenated solvents have commercial applications in addition to those that result from their ability to dissolve

lipophilic material. Changes in the volume of the particular chemicals produced depend not only on their physicochemical properties but also on their recognized toxicity. Tetrachloroethylene replaced trichloroethylene as a dry cleaning and degreasing agent because of concern over hepatotoxicity and environmental contamination by the latter. Recently commercial production of 1,1,1-trichloroethane has increased substantially. This chemical is an excellent degreasing agent and probably produces less toxicity than other chlorinated hydrocarbons because of the minimal biotransformation of 1,1,1-trichloroethane in the human body. The United States Food and Drug Administration banned the use of trichloromethane as an active or inactive ingredient in human or drug products as of July 29, 1976. Similarly, domestic uses of tetrachloromethane were banned in the United States in 1970. Table 64.3 lists the commercial uses of these halogenated solvents.

IMPURITIES

Most technical and commercial grades of halogenated solvents contain impurities (e.g., other chlorinated hydrocarbons) and stabilizers (antioxidants and acid receptors). The concentration of these impurities rarely exceed 1–3% of the total liquid. Stabilizers present in 1,1,1-trichloroethane include nitromethane, butanols, 1,4-dioxane, butylene oxide, 1,3-dioxolane, and n-methylpyrrole. Stabilizers (amines, epoxides, esters) are added to tetrachloroethylene in order to prevent the formation of hydrochloric acid from moisture and light. Individual impurities rarely exceed 100 mg/kg of trichloroethylene, and total impurities usually do not exceed 1 g/kg trichloroethylene (13). Impurities include tetrachloromethane, trichloromethane, 1,2-dichloroethane, cis- and trans-1,2-dichloroethylene, pentachloroethane, 1,1,1,2-tetrachloroethane, 1,1,2,2-tetrachloroethane, 1,1,1-trichloroethane, 1,1,2-trichloroethane, 1,1-dichloroethylene, bromodichloroethylene, tetrachloroethylene, bromodichloromethane, and benzene.

REACTIONS

The formation of the toxic contaminant, dichloroacetylene, resulted from the use of trichloroethylene as an anesthetic agent in closed systems with alkali absorbers and as a cleaning solvent in submarines and space capsules. In the workplace, dichloroacetylene production resulted from the use of trichloroethylene on moist alkaline materials such as concrete (14). Significant decomposition of trichloroethylene into dichloroacetylene and phosgene occurs at temperatures above 60°C (15). In sunlight trichloromethane oxidizes to phosgene in strong oxidizing agents (e.g., chromic acid produced phosgene and chlorine gas from trichloromethane). Thermal decomposition of 1,1,1-trichloroethane occurs below 260°C, while large amounts of hydrogen chloride and trace amounts of phosgene form at temperatures above that level (16). Vapor formation and thermal oxidative degradation at high temperatures may produce phosgene, carbon monoxide, and hydrochloric acid from tetrachloroethylene. The addition of weak acids to tetrachloroethane produces trichloroethylene, whereas strong alkalis cause the formation of the flammable toxin, dichloroacetylene. Contact of dichloromethane with common metals at room temperatures usually produces no significant decomposition although prolonged heating with water at 180°F (79°C) causes the formation of methyl chloride, methanol, hydrochloric acid, formic acid, and some carbon monoxide. Thermal decomposition of products

Table 64.1. Chemical Data of Halogenated Solvents

Chemical Abstracts name	**1,2-Dichloroethane**
CAS registry number	107-06-2
NIOSH number	KI0525000
Structural formula	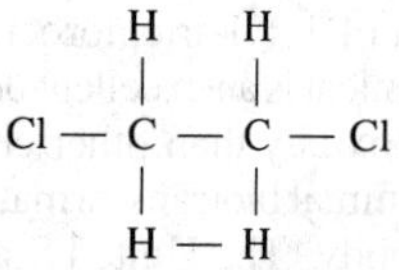

```
      H   H
      |   |
Cl — C — C — Cl
      |   |
      H — H
```

Synonyms	Alpha- or beta-dichloroethane, 1,2-bichloroethane, ethane dichloride, sym-dichloroethane dichloroethylene, ethylene chloride, ethylene dichloride, EDC, glycol dichloride
Trade names	Dutch liquid, Dutch oil, Freon 150, Brocide, ENT 1656, Borer-Sol, Destroxol, Gaze Olefiant, Dichlor-emulsion
Molecular formula	$C_2H_4Cl_2$
Molecular weight	98.9

Chemical Abstracts name	**1,2-Dichloroethene**
CAS registry number	540-59-0
NIOSH number	KV9360000
Structural formula	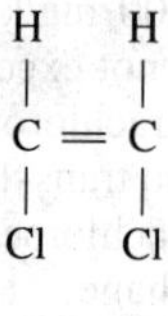

```
  H   H
  |   |
  C = C
  |   |
  Cl  Cl
```

Synonyms	1,2-Dichloroethylene, acetylene dichloride, sym-dichloroethylene, dichloro-1,2-ethylene (Fr), 1,2-dichloraethan (Ger), 1,2-DCE
Trade names	Dioform
Molecular formula	$C_2H_2Cl_2$
Molecular weight	96.95

Chemical Abstracts name	**Dichloromethane**
CAS registry number	75-09-2
NIOSH number	PA8050000
Structural formula	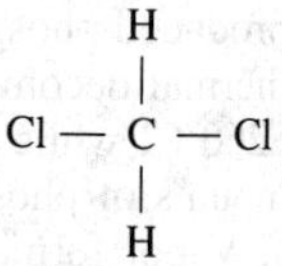

```
       H
       |
Cl — C — Cl
       |
       H
```

Synonyms	DCM, methane dichloride, methylene bichloride, methylene dichloride, methylene chloride
Trade names	Aerothene MM, Solmethine, Freon 30, Narkotil, Solaesthin
Molecular formula	CH_2Cl_2
Molecular weight	84.93

continues

Table 64.1. *Continued*

Chemical Abstracts name	**1,2-Dichloropropane**
CAS registry number	78-87-5
NIOSH number	TX9625000
Structural formula	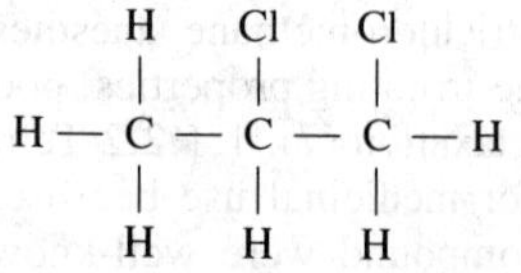

```
      H   Cl  Cl
      |   |   |
H — C — C — C — H
      |   |   |
      H   H   H
```

Synonyms	Alpha- or beta-dichloropropane, propylene chloride, propylene dichloride, 1,2-dichloropropane, bichlorure de propylene (Fr)
Trade names (pure compound)	ENT 15406, NCI-C55141
Trade names (insecticide formulations)	D-D (Shell Oil Company), Dorlone, Dowfume, Telone, Vidden D (Dow Chemical Company), Terr-o-cide (Great Lakes Chemical Corp.), Vorlex (Nor-Am Agricultural Products).
Molecular formula	$C_3H_6Cl_3$
Molecular weight	112.99

Chemical Abstracts name	**1,1,2,2-Tetrabromoethane**
CAS registry number	79-27-6
NIOSH number	KI8225000
Structural formula	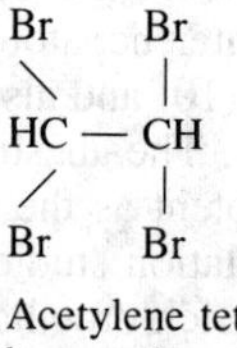

```
   Br     Br
    \      |
   HC — CH
    /      |
   Br     Br
```

Synonyms	Acetylene tetrabromide, sym-tetrabromoethane, 1,1,2,2-tetrabroomethaan (Dutch), 1,1,2,2-tetrabromoetano (Ital), 1,1,2,2-tetrabromaethan (Ger)
Trade names	Muthmann's liquid, AI3-08850
Molecular weight	345.7

Chemical Abstracts name	**1,1,2,2-Tetrachloroethane**
CAS registry number	79-34-5
NIOSH number	KI8575000
Structural formula	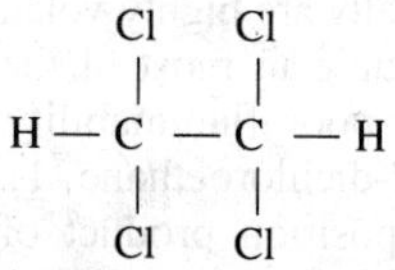

```
      Cl   Cl
      |    |
H — C — C — H
      |    |
      Cl   Cl
```

Synonyms	1,1,2,2-Tetrachloroethane, sym-tetrachloroethane, S-tetrachloroethane, acetylene tetrachloride, dichloro-2,2-dichloroethane, 1,1-dichloro-2,2-dichloroethane, 1,1,2,2-tetracloroetano (Ital), 1,1,2,2-tetrachloroethane (Fr), 1,1,2,2-tetrachloroaethan (Ger), 1,1,2,2-tetrachloorethaan (Dutch)
Molecular formula	$C_2H_2Cl_4$
Molecular weight	167.84

continues

Table 64.1. *Continued*

Chemical Abstracts name	**Tetrachloroethene**
CAS registry number	127-18-4
NIOSH number	KX3850000
Structural formula	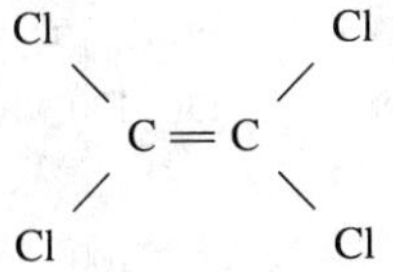

$$Cl \diagdown \qquad \diagup Cl$$
$$C = C$$
$$Cl \diagup \qquad \diagdown Cl$$

Synonyms	Carbon dichloride, ethylene tetrachloride, carbon bichloride, perchloroethylene, tetrachloroethane, 1,1,2,2-tetrachloroethylene, per, perc, perchlor
Molecular formula	C_2Cl_4
Molecular weight	165.8
Chemical Abstracts name	**Tetrachloromethane**
CAS registry number	56-23-5
NIOSH number	FG4900000
Structural formula	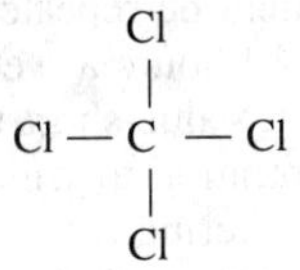

$$Cl$$
$$|$$
$$Cl - C - Cl$$
$$|$$
$$Cl$$

Synonyms	Carbona, tetrachlorocarbon, carbon chloride, carbon tet, methane tetrachloride, perchloromethane, tetrachlormethan (Ger), tetrachloure de carbone (Fr), tetrachlorometano (Ital)
Trade names	Freon 10, benzioform, univerm, tetrasol, fluikoids, fasciolin Halon 104, vermostricid
Molecular formula	CCl_4
Molecular weight	153.8
Chemical Abstracts name	**1,1,1-Trichloroethane**
CAS registry number	71-55-6
NIOSH number	KJ2975000
Structural formula	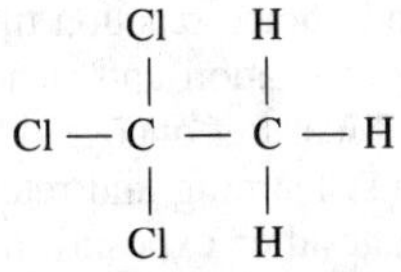

$$Cl \quad H$$
$$| \qquad |$$
$$Cl - C - C - H$$
$$| \qquad |$$
$$Cl \quad H$$

Synonyms	Alpha-trichloroethane, methyl chloroform, trielene, trichloroethane, methyl trichloromethane, 1,1,1-trichloroetano (Italian), 1,1,1-trichloraethan (German), 1,1,1-trichloorethaan (Dutch), aerothene TT, chloroethene, chlorothene NU, chlorothene VG alpha-T, TCEA, TCA, NCI-CA4626
Isomer	Ethane, 1,1,1-trichloro-1,1,2-trichloroethane, beta-trichloroethane, beta-T, NCI-C04579, vinyl trichloride)
Molecular formula	$C_2H_3Cl_3$
Molecular weight	133.41

continues

Table 64.1. *Continued*

Chemical Abstracts name	**Trichloromethane**
CAS registry number	67-66-3
NIOSH number	FS9100000
Structural formula	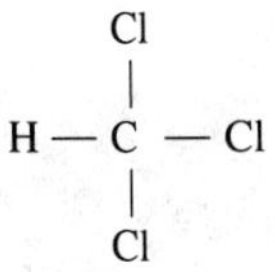

$$Cl$$
$$|$$
$$H - C - Cl$$
$$|$$
$$Cl$$

Synonyms	Chloroform, formyl trichloride methane trichloride, methenyl chloride, methenyl trichloride methyl trichloride, trichloroform, trichlorometano (Ital), chloroforme (Fr), chloroformio (Ital), trichloormethaan (Dutch)
Trade names	Freon 20, R20, R20 (refridgerant)
Molecular formula	$CH Cl_3$
Molecular weight	119.4
Chemical Abstracts name	**Trichloroethene**
CAS registry number	79-01-6
NIOSH number	KX450000
Structural formula	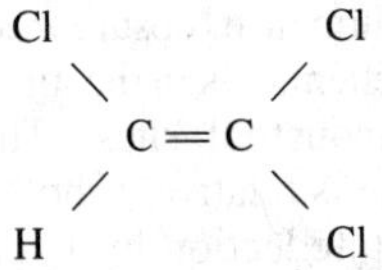

$$Cl \diagdown \qquad \diagup Cl$$
$$C = C$$
$$H \diagup \qquad \diagdown Cl$$

Synonyms	Acetylene trichloride, trichloroethylene, ethylene trichloride, ethenyl trichloride, TCE, Tri, 1,1,2-trichloroethylene, trichloroethylenum, trichloroethylen (German), trichloroethylene (French), trichloroetilene (Italian), trichlooretheen (Dutch)
Chemical formula	C_2HCl_3
Molecular weight	131.4
Chemical Abstracts name	**1,1,2-trichloro-1,2,2-trifluoroethane**
CAS registry number	76-13-1
NIOSH number	KJ4000000
Structural formula	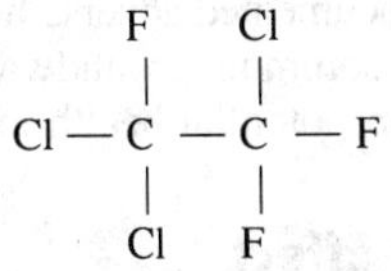

$$F \quad Cl$$
$$| \qquad |$$
$$Cl - C - C - F$$
$$| \qquad |$$
$$Cl \quad F$$

Synonyms	Trichlorotrifluoroethane, 1,1,2-trichloro-1,2,2-fluoroethane
Trade names	Freon 113, FC-113
Molecular formula	$C_2Cl_3F_3$
Molecular weight	187.37

Table 64.2.   Odor Properties

Solvent Chemical Name	Common Name	Levels (ppm) Threshold*	Levels (ppm) Obvious	Characteristics
1,2-Dichloroethane	Ethylene dichloride	6–110	180	Chloroform-like
1,2-Dichloroethylene	Acetylene dichloride	17		Acrid, ethereal
Dichloromethane	Methylene chloride	150–500	800	Pleasant, chloroform
1,2-Dichloropropane	Propylene dichloride	>0.25	130–190	Unpleasant, chloroform
Tetrabromoethane	Acetylene tetrabromide			Pungent, camphor
Tetrachloroethane	Acetylene tetrachloride	1.5		Pungent, chloroform
Tetrachloroethylene	Perchloroethylene	5–50	>100	Ethereal, chloroform
Tetrachloromethane	Carbon tetrachloride	100–200	250	Chloroform
1,1,1-Trichloroethane		16–400	800	Chloroform
Trichloroethylene	TCE	20–80	>100	Chloroform
Trichloromethane	Chloroform	50–200		Chloroform
1,1,2-Trichloro-1,2,2-trifluoroethane	FC-113	350–1000		Sweet

*Odor thresholds reported in the medical literature vary considerably based on the following variables: (1) chemical purity, (2) definition of odor response, (3) size and number of trials, (4) method of presentation of stimulus.

containing dichloromethane as a result of open flames include hydrogen chloride and, to a lesser extent, phosgene (17). 1,2-Dichloroethylene gradually decomposes under light, air, or moisture to form hydrochloric acid similar to 1,2-dichloroethane.

Environmental Fate

None of the halogenated solvents is a natural constituent of the environment. Human exposure occurs as a result of volatilization of these chemicals in the air or contamination of groundwater around industrial sites. The atmospheric lifetime of trichloroethylene is relatively short (approximately 10 days) as a result of photoreduction by hydroxy radicals (13), but the chemical decomposition of trichloroethylene in sealed water may be long (i.e., 25 years) based on in vitro studies. Consequently, the trichloroethylene released into the soil migrates readily to groundwater, where this chemical may remain for months to years. 1,1,2-Trichloro-1,2,2-trifluoroethane is very resistant to decomposition in the lower atmosphere (i.e., troposphere) and transport occurs slowly to the stratosphere, where the lifetime of this chemical ranges up to 100 years. With the exception of trichloroethane and tetrachloroethane, which possess atmospheric lifetimes of 5–10 years and over 2 years, respectively, the majority of these chemicals are photochemically degraded in the troposphere by hydroxy radicals before they can be transferred to the stratosphere. The contribution of trichloroethane, tetrachloroethane, and 1,1,2-trichloro-1,2,2-trifluoroethane to ozone depletion remains to be determined. Based on our present level of understanding, existing contamination of the environment by these halogenated solvents has not produced documented adverse health effects; however, these chemicals are common groundwater contaminants with unknown longterm potential health effects (see Chapter 27).

Acute Dose Effect

INHALATION

All of the halogenated solvents are central nervous system depressants that produce dose-related changes in mental function and consciousness depending on the individual chemical and the duration of exposure. Table 64.4 lists the environmental exposure levels considered safe by the Federal Occupational

Safety and Health Administration and the American Conference of Governmental and Industrial Hygienists. The Threshold Limit Value-time-weighted average (TLV-TWA) is the level at which an average worker may be repeatedly exposed day after day, 8 hours a day, and 40 hours a week, without adverse effect. The Threshold Limit Value-short term exposure limit (TLV-STEL) is the concentration to which workers can be exposed short term without suffering (a) sufficient narcosis to produce an increased incident of accidental injury or reduced work efficiency, (b) chronic or irreversible tissue damage, and (c) eye or upper respiratory tract irritation. The TLV-STEL is a supplemental acute exposure limit to the TLV-TWA, which primarily addresses chronic injury. The low TLV-TWA of 1,2-dichloroethane, tetrachloromethane, and trichloromethane result from their carcinogenic properties, whereas the low levels for tetrabromoethane and tetrachloroethane evolve from their potent hepatotoxicity. When the TLV-STEL is exceeded, neuropsychologic testing indicates that changes in psychomotor performance (i.e., manual dexterity) precedes decrements in cognitive performance (e.g., learning and memory). After an exposure to 300 and 500 ppm trichloroethylene lasting 3 hours, a reduction in manual dexterity appeared (18). After a 3-hour exposure to 800 ppm dichloromethane significant deficits in psychomotor tasks (e.g., simple and choice reaction times, reduced tapping speed, and impaired coordination and steadiness) developed in human volunteers (19). Measures of cognitive performance (reproduction of visual patterns, learning and retention of nonsense syllables) did not deteriorate after exposure for 2 hours to concentrations up to 1000 ppm dichloromethane (20). In general, mild exposures cause varying degrees of inebriation, headache, lightheadedness, weakness, irritability, and nausea, while exposure to higher levels produce slurred speech, incoordination, giddiness, confusion, lethargy, and ataxia, depending on the individual potency of the chemical and the duration of exposure. Levels of 10,000–25,000 ppm trichloroethane, trichloroethylene, trichloromethane, and dichloromethane produce coma in humans within a short period of time. Animal studies indicate that levels around 100,000–200,000 ppm 1,1,2-trichloro-1,2,2-trifluoroethane are required to produce coma and convulsions, but these concentrations are so high that asphyxia may contribute to central nervous system (CNS) changes (21).

DERMAL

Most of these chemicals do penetrate human skin but do so in insufficient quantities to substantially add to the body burden

Table 64.3. Commercial Uses of Halogenated Solvents

1,2-Dichloroethane	Vinyl chloride production**, chemical intermediate, lead scavenger, fumigant*, solvent*
1,2-Dichloroethylene	Low temperature extractant (caffeine, perfumes), solvent (fats, phenol, camphor, natural rubber, lacquer, thermoplastics)
Dichloromethane	Degreasing agent, paint/varnish remover, blowing agent for urethane foams; solvent extractant (drugs, coffee), fumigant (grain, fruits)
1,2-Dichloropropane	Soil fumigation (with dichloropropane), solvent, chemical intermediate (tetrachloroethylene, tetrachloromethane), lead scavenger, metal degreaser
Tetrabromoethane	Solvent, gauge fluid, flotation agent, catalyst, refractive liquid
Tetrachloroethane	Solvent, mothproofing textiles, paint/varnish/rust remover*, immersion liquid (crystallography)*, determination of theobromine in cacao*
Tetrachloroethylene	Grain fumigation, chemical intermediate (fluorocarbons), veterinary anthelmintic, heat exchange fluid
Tetrachloromethane	Chemical intermediate (Freon 11, Freon 12), fire extinguishing agent*, grain fumigant*, solvent*, metal degreaser*, flammability suppressant*, paint manufacturing*, gasoline additive*, semiconductor production*, refrigerant*
1,1,1-Trichloroethane	Cleaning solvent** (electrical machinery, plastics), textile spotting fluid, chemical intermediate, coolant, lubricant, inks, drain cleaners
Trichloroethylene	Vapor degreasing**, typewriter correction fluid, low temperature heat transfer fluid, fire retardant, chemical intermediate, polyvinyl chloride manufacturing, extractant, lacquer/adhesive
Tetrachloromethane	Chemical intermediate (Freon 22)**, cleansing agent*, insecticidal fumigant*, solvent*
1,1-2-Trichloro-1,2,2-trifluoroethane	Solvent (electrical, electronics)**, dry cleaning

*Minor use
**Major use

of the halogenated solvents. Exceptions to this generalization include tetrachloroethane and tetrachloromethane. The American Conference of Governmental and Industrial Hygienists adds a skin notation to these substances that refers to the potential contribution to the overall body burden from their percutaneous absorption.

ORAL

Data on the dose effect of ingestion of halogenated solvents are limited. Substantial variation may occur between individual subjects as a result of susceptibility (e.g., ethanol induced liver

disease, malnutrition). A 5½-year-old girl died from hepatorenal failure following the ingestion of 1 milliliter of tetrachloromethane (5), while a 29-year-old man survived a 100-milliliter ingestion of tetrachloromethane with supportive care and hemodialysis (22). Both 1,2-dichloroethane and 1,1,2,2-tetrachloroethane are highly toxic based on case reports. A fatal hepatorenal syndrome developed in a 14-year-old boy who ingested approximately 50 milliliters of dichloroethane (23). The ingestion of 28–57 milliliters of tetrachloroethane by a 20-year-old man resulted in coma, respiratory depression, and death occurring approximately 15 hours after ingestion (24). The estimated lethal oral dose in humans is approximately 3–5 milliliters (7 grams) of trichloroethylene per kilogram body weight, and a report in the Russian literature attributes a death to the ingestion of 50 milliliters of trichloroethylene (13). Based on case reports, ingestion of 0.5 milliliters of trichloroethylene per kilogram of body weight can produce significant CNS depression (25, 26). The ingestion of an estimated 8–10 ml of tetrachloroethylene in a 6-year-old, 22-kilogram boy induced coma requiring intubation for 5 days (27).

TOXICOKINETICS

Absorption

The pulmonary route is the main source of toxic exposures to the halogenated solvents. In general these chemicals are well-absorbed through both the lungs and gastrointestinal tract. The amount of absorption depends on the speed of transfer of the chemical through the pulmonary capillaries into the blood (i.e., blood/air partition coefficient) and the concentration of the chemical in the blood. This buildup depends primarily on the rate of metabolism because distribution of the solvents to lipid-rich tissue generally is slow. The greatest percentage of trichloroethylene is absorbed during the first few minutes although the absolute quantity absorbed increases with increasing ventilation. Rapid metabolism and a relatively high blood/air partition coefficient (approximately 15) explains the relatively complete absorption of trichloroethylene (28). Excellent absorption of tetrachloroethylene occurs across the capillary membranes of the pulmonary bed in part because of its extremely high blood/air partition coefficient (approximately 145). Peak blood levels are reached immediately after inhalation ceases (29). In human volunteers the lungs absorb approximately 25% of inhaled dose of trichloroethane at a level of 300 ppm trichloroethane for 6 hours (30). Following exposure to 100–200 ppm dichloromethane for 2–4 hours initial absorption of this solvent is rapid, but absorption reaches steady state conditions within 1–2 hours, probably because of the limited solubility of dichloromethane in the blood (31).

The low peak levels of fluorocarbons in the arteries compared with the total dose administered via inhalation suggests that absorption by the lungs is slow, as determined by animal studies (32). Case reports of human exposure and animal data suggest that oral absorption of trichloroethylene, trichloromethane, tetrachloroethylene, dichloromethane, dichloroethane, tetrachloroethane, and tetrabromoethane is rapid and substantial. In general, gastrointestinal absorption is less complete than pulmonary absorption. While 2–6 milliliters of tetrachloroethylene by mouth produces drowsiness, the inhalation of tetrachloroethylene vapors from approximately 5 milliliters produces anesthesia (7). The gastrointestinal absorption of trichloroethane and dichloroethylene appears less complete than other halo-

Table 64.4. Recommended Exposure Limits and Irritant Levels

	Federal OSHA			ACGIH		Eye/Upper Respiratory Tract Irritation
	TLV-TWA (ppm)	TLV-STEL (ppm)	Skin Designation	TLV-TWA	Skin Designation	
1,2-Dichloroethane	1*	2	–	10	–	NA
1,2-Dichloroethylene	200	–	–	200	–	NA
Dichloromethane	50	100	–	50	–	2300
1,2-Dichloropropane	75	110	–	75	–	NA
Tetrabromoethane	1**	none	–	–	–	1
Tetrachloroethane	1**	–	+	1	+	14–33
Tetrachloroethylene	25	–	–	50	–	100–600
Tetrachloromethane	2*	–	–	5	+	NA
Trichloroethane	350	450	–	350	–	1000
Trichloroethylene	50	200	–	50	–	400–1000
Trichloromethane	2*	–	–	10	–	4000
1,1,2-Trichloro-1,2,2-trifluoroethane	1000	1250	–	1000	–	NA

**Based on hepatorenal toxicity
*Based on carcinogenic properties
NA = not available; – = none; + = present.

genated solvents, and absorption of 1,1,2-trichloro-1,2,2-tri-fluoroethane is poor. The dermal absorption of most halogenated solvents is not sufficient to produce toxicity by itself, but the percutaneous absorption of tetrachloroethane and tetrachloromethane may contribute to the total body burden of these chemicals. Percutaneous absorption of dichloroethane (DCA) in guinea pigs produced a steadily increasing blood level of trichloroethylene that suggested the possibility of accumulating toxicity following cutaneous exposure to DCA (33).

Distribution

Once absorbed, halogenated solvents distribute rapidly to tissue based on their lipid content and individual tissue/blood partition coefficients. Generally the highest concentrations appear in the fat, brain, and blood. Peak blood levels occur soon after exposure ceases following inhalation, whereas peak levels following oral administration occur 1–2 hours after administration. Animal and human studies indicate that accumulation of these chemicals in fat generally is not substantial following chronic exposure unless concentrations are high. An exception is tetrachloroethylene, which does accumulate because of its markedly prolonged biologic half-life. Some of these halogenated solvents (e.g., trichloroethylene, trichloromethane, dichloroethane) do cross the placenta and may accumulate in the fetus.

Metabolism

The extent and type of metabolism varies substantially between the halogenated solvents. Substantial biotransformation of these chemicals occurs in the human body following exposure to dichloroethane, dichloropropane, tetrachloroethane, and trichloroethylene. This transformation generally occurs in the liver via the cytochrome P-450 oxidative pathway. Glutathione conjugation is an alternate common pathway. Animal studies indicate that the body extensively metabolizes dichloroethane depending on the amount administered. Although the exact intermediate has not been identified, recent evidence indicates that the episulfonium ion is the major toxic intermediary in vivo following biotransformation of this suspected carcinogen (34). The toxic intermediary of tetrachloroethane metabolism

has not been identified. Hydrolytic cleavage of the carbon chlorine bond via dichloroacetic acid to glyoxylic acid subsequently forms the end product, carbon dioxide. A minor pathway produces trichloroethylene and another one produces tetrachloroethylene. Figure 64.1 demonstrates the biotransformation of trichloroethylene. The cytochrome P-450 mixed function oxidase system converts trichloroethylene into an epoxide, which subsequently rearranges to trichloroacetylaldehyde and then chloral hydrate. Another pathway, which operates only at high doses, leads to the formation of dichloroacetyl chloride and dichloroacetic acid. Substantial species variation occurs in the ability to use these alternate pathways (35). Trichloroethane and tetrachloromethane undergo comparatively less transformation but produce toxic intermediates that probably produce hepatotoxicity by the formation of free radicals. The major metabolic pathway of dichloromethane involves formation of carbon monoxide by the hepatic microsomal cytochrome P-450 mixed function oxidase system (36). This reaction requires both molecular oxygen and reduced nicotinamide adenine dinucleotide phosphate (NADPH) to form formyl chloride, which then decomposes to carbon monoxide. Animal studies suggest that this pathway is easily saturable. The body metabolizes only small amounts of trichloromethane and tetrachloroethylene. The major metabolite of the former is trichloroethanol, while the major metabolites of the latter are trichloroacetic acid and oxalic acid. Trichloroethanol is a metabolic product of chloral hydrate and trichloroethylene as well as tetrachloroethylene and trichloroethane. Little if any metabolism of 1,1,2-trichloro-1,2,2-trifluoroethane occurs in the body.

Elimination

Pulmonary excretion and liver metabolism are the two major routes of elimination for halogenated solvents. Humans eliminate over 90% of an absorbed dose of trichloroethane unchanged through the lungs following an exposure to approximately 200 ppm trichloroethane (37). Similarly, rats excrete approximately 70–90% of an orally administered dose via the lungs within the first 72 hours as unchanged compound (29). The estimated elimination half-lives of unchanged trichloroethane and tetrachloroethylene are triexponential as a

Metabolism of Trichloroethylene

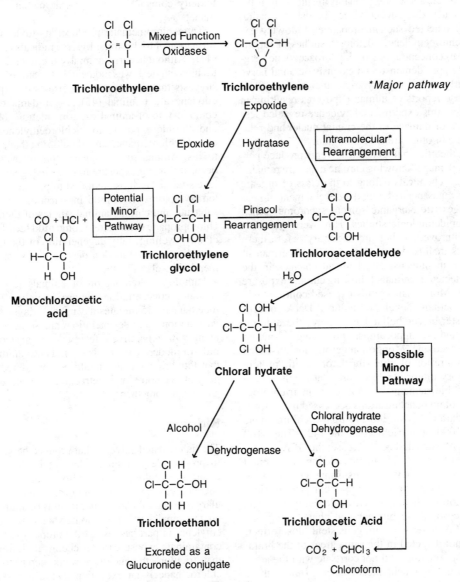

Figure 1.

result of excretion from the blood vessel-rich tissue, muscle tissue, and the fat compartment. Excretion from poorly perfused tissue (i.e., fat) averaged 53 hours for trichloroethane (30) and 55–65 hours for tetrachloroethylene (27). Following exposure to 200 ppm dichloromethane for 7.5 hours, human subjects eliminated approximately 30% of the absorbed dose of dichloromethane as carbon monoxide (38). The elimination of dichloromethane from the lungs is rapid, whereas the elimination of carbon monoxide from the air and carboxyhemoglobin from the blood is more gradual, probably because of the late release of dichloromethane from fat stores. At low doses the liver metabolizes approximately 70–90% of an absorbed dose of trichloroethylene, while the lungs excrete approximately 10–20% of the absorbed dose as unchanged trichloroethylene. Pulmonary excretion is less following the administration of an oral dose in animals. Following workplace exposures between 100 and 200 ppm trichloroethylene approximately 30–

50% of an absorbed dose appears in the urine as trichloroethanol and 10–30% as trichloroacetic acid (13).

PATHOPHYSIOLOGY

Central Nervous System

Central nervous system depression develops following exposure to high doses of all of the halogenated solvents, and most initial deaths result from respiratory depression and subsequent hypoxia. The exact mechanism of the central nervous system depression has not been delineated, but the most plausible explanation is a change in membrane fluidity that subsequently alters neural transmission. In general, pathologic examination of animals exposed to lethal concentrations of halogenated solvents do not demonstrate any significant histologic damage to the brain following acute overdose (39, 40). The cranial neuropathies that follow exposure to trichloroethylene as a degreasing agent or as an anesthetic probably resulted from the decomposition product, dichloroacetylene. To date no pathologic studies have detected such neuropathies following exposure to pure trichloroethylene. Histologic studies of rabbits and mice exposed to concentrations of dichloroacetylene ranging from 19 to 300 ppm demonstrated extensive cranial nerve damage, particularly in the sensory trigeminal nucleus (41). Compared with case reports of human exposures resulting in cranial neuropathies, this experimental evidence revealed less distinctive evidence of damage in the cranial nuclei and relatively more damage in other areas of the brain.

Whether any of the other halogenated solvents produce permanent neurologic damage following chronic exposure remains to be proven. These chemicals belong to the class of organic solvents that has been associated with the development of neurobehavioral changes (i.e., organic solvent syndrome) based on Scandinavian epidemiologic studies. However, better exposure data and improved studies are necessary before these chlorinated solvents are linked to the development of permanent neurologic changes in humans. Biochemical changes in the brain have been detected in animals following chronic exposure to trichloroethane. Mongolian gerbils exposed continuously to 70 ppm trichloroethane developed reduced DNA concentrations in the posterior cerebellar hemisphere, the anterior cerebellar vermis, and the hippocampus. Following a 3-month exposure to trichloroethane, Mongolian gerbils demonstrated an increased concentration of glial fibrillatory acetic protein (GFA) in the sensory motor cerebral cortex at levels of 210 and 1000 ppm trichloroethane but not 70 ppm trichloroethane. The S100 protein concentrations decreased in the frontal cerebral cortex after exposure to 210 ppm trichloroethane but not at 70 or 1000 ppm trichloroethane (42). The S100 protein is a marker of astroglial cell increase; the GFA protein is the main subunit of astroglial filaments and therefore found mainly in fibrillatory astrocytes. This same group found changes in the brains of Mongolian gerbils exposed to trichloroethylene, dichloromethane, and tetrachloroethylene. The clinical significance of these biochemical changes remains unclear because (a) there was no consistent dose-effect; (b) changes were not detected in the same areas of the brain; and (c) behavior abnormalities did not correlate with the areas of the brain demonstrating biochemical changes. Hence, these studies do not fulfill the principles of causation necessary to prove neurotoxicity. Further animal studies and epidemiologic data are necessary to delineate what permanent effects, if any, exposure to halogenated solvents at current workplace standards cause in the brain.

Liver

Tetrachloroethane, tetrachloromethane, and trichloromethane are classic hepatotoxins. Animal studies indicate that tetrachloroethane is relatively more toxic to the liver than either trichloromethane or tetrachloromethane (43). These hepatotoxins produce acute fatty infiltration, centrilobular necrosis, and cirrhosis in animals following chronic exposure. Those animal studies demonstrate substantial variability in both the binding and subsequent hepatotoxicity of trichloromethane depending on animal species, genetic strain, sex, and age, compared with the more consistent pattern of hepatotoxicity caused by tetrachloroethane and tetrachloromethane. This difference in animal toxicity correlates with the clinical experience in which tri-

chloromethane produced substantially fewer cases of hepatotoxicity compared with tetrachloroethane and tetrachloromethane.

Tetrachloromethane produces its toxicity as a result of the formation of trichloromethyl free radicals and lipid peroxidation (44). Although early animal experimentation suggested that trichloroethylene was moderately hepatotoxic, more recent work suggests that the hepatotoxic effects of exposure to trichloroethylene are minimal (45). Liver damage is an uncommon complication of animal experimentation following both acute and chronic exposure to trichloroethylene. Tetrachloroethylene, trichloroethane, and dichloromethane are weak hepatotoxins. Animal studies suggest that liver abnormalities would occur following exposure to these halogenated solvents only at levels far above those required to produce central nervous system symptoms (i.e., mild intoxication). Similarly, high dose subacute and chronic animal studies of dichloroethane and dichloropropane demonstrate some mild histologic changes (e.g., cloudy swelling, fatty degeneration of the liver) but no significant hepatic dysfunction despite doses far exceeding recommended levels (43, 46).

Pathologic examination of animals repeatedly exposed to saturated concentrations (approximately 50 ppm) of tetrabromoethane for 15 minutes/day up to 92 days revealed congestion, vacuolation, fatty degeneration, and some necrosis of the liver, along with reparative effects that suggested the possibility of mild to moderate cirrhosis (47). These animal studies indicate that tetrabromoethane should be considered in the same category of hepatotoxins as tetrachloroethane, tetrachloromethane, and trichloromethane.

Kidney

The halogenated solvents that produce hepatotoxicity also tend to produce less dramatic changes in the kidneys. The most common histologic abnormality following exposure to these chemicals is cloudy swelling of the tubular epithelium, particularly the convoluted tubule. Results of animal experimentation on the renal system are somewhat conflicting for trichloroethylene, in part because of the propensity for nephrotoxins to contaminate exposure to this chemical. Animal studies indicate that trichloroethylene is a weak nephrotoxin (48). 1,2-Dichloroethane is an exception to the general rule in that this chemical produces the most prominent histologic changes (slight degeneration to complete necrosis of the tubular epithelium, interstitial edema, and hemorrhage) in the kidney of rats following fatal exposures (49).

Cardiovascular System

The halogenated solvents are central nervous system depressants and are, therefore, capable of producing vasodilation and hypotension. Animal studies of trichloroethane indicate a two-phased depression of blood pressure following exposure to 8000–25,000 ppm trichloroethane. Initially there was a sharp decrease in both systolic and diastolic pressure, and a corresponding increase in myocardial contractility and cardiac output. A marked decrease in heart rate, myocardial contractility, and stroke volume characterize the terminal phase (50). Cardiac sensitization (multiple ventricular beats in excess of controls or ventricular fibrillation) developed in 3 of 18 dogs exposed to 5000 ppm trichloroethane following the intravenous injection of 8 milligrams of epinephrine per kilogram body weight, and in all dogs exposed to 10,000 ppm (51). Trichloroethylene and

1,1,2-trichloro-1,2,2-trifluoroethane, but not trichloromethane, demonstrate similar cardiac sensitization. The animal model of epinephrine-induced dysrhythmias has been used to explain sudden death in the workplace following exercise and exposure to halogenated solvents. However, this model does not duplicate sympathomimetic stimulation following stressful situations. In the latter situation the adrenal medula releases epinephrine and adrenergic transmitters (i.e., norepinephrine appears in the adrenergic terminals of the sympathetic nerves). Furthermore, the volume of sympathomimetic amines released following endogenous stimulation (e.g., approximately 0.004 mg/kg/minute in humans) and exogenous administration (e.g., 0.05 mg/kg/minute) is not equivalent (52). The development of ventricular dysrhythmias following halogenated solvent exposure are not well-documented in the workplace, but animal studies do suggest that dysrhythmias do occur following exposure to high doses (i.e., 5000 ppm) of these chemicals. The body does convert dichloromethane to carbon monoxide, and the resultant decrease in oxygen delivery may exacerbate preexisting cardiovascular disease (e.g., dysrhythmias, chest pain, myocardial ischemia) in workers. In animal studies high doses of dichloroethane or dichloropropane may produce adrenocortical hemorrhage (53) and, therefore, acute adrenal insufficiency may contribute to death in these animals.

Lungs

The halogenated solvents display varying degrees of upper respiratory tract irritation but seldom produce alveolar damage. Some animals (rabbits and rats) exposed to 1000 ppm dichloromethane for periods up to 6 months did develop gross pulmonary congestion, edema, and some focal necrosis of the lung (54). One study of rats gavaged with 0.25 milliliters of tetrachloromethane in mineral oil per kilogram body weight demonstrated intraalveolar fibrin, intramural clots, endothelial sluffing, and necrosis of granular pneumocyte in the exposed animals (55). These changes suggested a direct tetrachloromethane-induced toxicity to the authors, but their work has not been duplicated to exclude confounding factors such as mineral oil aspiration.

Eye

Generally these halogenated solvents produce mild chemical conjunctivitis in the eyes of animals given injections of these chemicals, depending on the concentration. Exposure to high concentrations of these chemicals in the air generally does not produce persistent changes. Blue-gray corneal opacities developed in dogs following the systemic, but not intraocular, administration of dichloroethane. No similar cases of corneal opacities have been reported in humans.

Post Mortem Findings

Postmortem examination of victims dying immediately of overexposure to halogenated solvents generally demonstrate only nonspecific findings. The most common finding on autopsy of victims dying of trichloroethane exposure is acute passive congestion of the viscera with petechial hemorrhages in the brain and lungs (56). Pathologic changes demonstrated on the autopsies of patients dying from hepatotoxicity after exposure to tetrachloromethane include fatty degeneration and centrilobular necrosis of the liver, degeneration of the proximal and

distal convoluted tubules and loops of Henle (i.e., acute tubular necrosis without involvement of the glomeruli), acute myocarditis, adrenal hemorrhage, gastrointestinal bleeding, pulmonary hemorrhage, and edema (57). Central nervous system changes usually reflect either underlying disease or the effects of hepatorenal failure (58). In contrast to animal studies, postmortem examination of suicidal poisonings from tetrachloroethane do not demonstrate significant hepatic or renal pathology. Generally death occurs approximately 10–20 hours after suicidal ingestion of a fatal amount of tetrachloroethane (24). Dissection and histologic examination of adrenals were not reported. These autopsy reports indicate that hepatorenal failure is not the etiology of death in acute tetrachloroethane-induced deaths, in contrast to those dying from chronic tetrachloroethane poisoning.

CLINICAL PRESENTATION

Acute Systemic Toxicity

All the halogenated solvents are classic CNS depressants that may produce some initial excitation followed by depression of the central nervous system. The type and onset of symptoms depends on the duration of exposure, concentration, previous exposure history, minute ventilation, and individual susceptibility. Following inhalation of high doses of these chemicals, the rapid onset of central nervous system depression may occur manifest by dizziness, ataxia, headache, fatigue, lethargy, nausea, and abdominal pain that progresses to stupor, apnea, coma, and death. Following exposure to high concentrations, symptoms may develop rapidly within minutes; and, similarly, following removal from exposure, recovery is rapid (i.e., 30 minutes unless hypoxic damage or trauma occurs). Exposure to tetrachloroethylene is an exception because of its prolonged elimination time. Neurologic signs and symptoms following ingestion of trichloroethylene or tetrachloroethylene may be delayed several hours and include mental confusion, disorientation, poor concentration, dysarthria, ataxia, incontinence, urinary retention, amnesia, dysphasia, and numbness. Prolonged coma may follow the ingestion of tetrachloroethylene (27), and delayed dysrhythmias (over 24 hours) may develop following the ingestion of large amounts of trichloroethylene in patients who display CNS depression (59). Dichloromethane possesses direct central nervous system effects independent of the production of carboxyhemoglobin. Furthermore, patients with cardiopulmonary disease may be particularly susceptible to the effects of dichloromethane-induced carboxyhemoglobinemia. A 66-year-old man developed an anterior myocardial infarction following a 3-hour exposure to a paint remover containing a concentration of 80% dichloromethane (60). Recovery is usually complete within 24 hours unless exposure produced secondary damage (i.e., myocardial ischemia, hypoxia), or the neurotoxin, dichloroacetylene, was present in the environment.

The hepatotoxic halogenated solvents (tetrachloroethane, tetrachloromethane, trichloromethane, tetrabromoethane, dichloroethane, dichloropropane) produce initial narcotic effects followed by the development of hepatorenal dysfunction. The exact presentation depends on the dose and individual susceptibility. Symptoms (vomiting, nausea, abdominal pain, edema, jaundice, fever, chills, diarrhea, anorexia, epistaxis, dyspnea) of the hepatorenal phase typically begin several days after exposure and progress depending on the severity of toxicity. Renal dysfunction typically occurs concurrently with hepatic damage, although rarely the severity of renal damage may exceed hepatic dysfunction. Surviving patients typically do not develop either hepatic or renal sequelae. The development of hepatic failure following exposure to other halogenated solvents is rare and poorly documented probably in part due to predisposing conditions that cause individual hypersensitivity. The ingestion of these chemicals, in particular, trichloroethylene, may produce substantial gastrointestinal irritation.

Pulmonary damage usually does not result from exposure to halogenated solvents unless known pulmonary irritants (e.g., phosgene, hydrogen chloride) contaminate the environment (61).

Central Nervous System

The lack of good exposure data and well-designed epidemiologic studies complicates the interpretation of the available data on the chronic neurologic sequelae of exposure to halogenated solvents. Although none of these pure chemicals is a recognized neurotoxin, early case reports and uncontrolled epidemiologic studies associated workplace exposure to trichloroethylene (62, 63), tetrachloroethylene (64, 65), and dichloromethane (66), with a high prevalence of nonspecific central nervous system symptoms (headache, irritability, emotionality, personality changes, fatigue, and anxiety). Furthermore, individual case reports associate the development of peripheral neuropathies with workplace exposure to trichloroethane (67), 1,1,2-trichloro-1,2,2-trifluoroethane (68), and trichloroethylene (69).

The present data on animal studies, case reports, and epidemiologic studies do not support a causal link between the development of chronic neurologic symptoms and exposure to halogenated solvents below established TLV concentrations. Determination of whether these neurologic complaints result from exposure to organic solvents (i.e., organic solvent encephalopathy) will depend on the results of work currently in progress on solving the problems with study design flaws and inadequate neuropsychiatric testing.

Gastrointestinal Tract

The replacement of hepatotoxic halogenated solvents with less toxic ones, along with improved industrial hygiene standards, led to a marked decrease in the number of reported cases of hepatotoxicity following exposure to the hepatotoxic halogenated solvents. Rare case reports have associated the development of hepatitis with exposure to trichloroethylene (70, 71), trichloroethylene and trichloroethane (72), and tetrachloroethylene (73). Liver biopsies typically demonstrate centrilobular necrosis in these cases, although fatty degeneration and necrosis of the midzonal areas also were present. Considering the large number of workers exposed to these halogenated solvents, the case reports of liver damage are exceedingly small. Occupational exposure to trichloroethylene also has been associated with the development of pneumatosis cystoides intestinalis (multiple gas-filled cysts within the intestinal wall) (74).

Skin

The halogenated solvents are defatting agents that may produce chronic irritation as a result of their defatting properties. They are not known to produce sensitization in the skin. A syndrome called degreaser's flush has been described and results from ethanol-induced vasodilation of superficial skin vessels. This skin response maximizes in approximately 30 minutes after exposure to trichloroethylene and resolves by approximately 60 minutes (75).

Reproductive Abnormalities

None of the halogenated solvents is a recognized teratogen but human data are inadequate to make final determinations. Evidence for teratogenesis independent of maternal toxicity following exposure to trichloromethane is limited in rats but absent in mice and rabbits (76). Although trichloroethylene crosses the placenta in animals, teratogenesis has not been demonstrated in either animals or humans to date. Similarly, trichloroethane passes the placental barrier and probably also distributes into the highly lipid breast milk, but exposure of rodents 7 hours daily on days 6 to 15 of gestation to 75 ppm trichloroethane produced no observable effects on implantation, litter size, fetal absorption, or incidence of skeletal or visceral malformations (77). This same study demonstrated no teratologic effects following exposure to 300 ppm tetrachloroethylene 7 hours daily during days 6 through 15 of gestation, but a significant increase in the incidence of resorptions among the fetal population appeared.

Carcinogenicity

The United States National Toxicology Program lists the following five halogenated solvents as suspected carcinogens: tetrachloromethane, 1,2-dichloroethane, dichloromethane, tetrachloroethylene, and trichloromethane. This category implies that these chemicals may be reasonably anticipated to be carcinogens based on (1) evidence of carcinogenicity from studies in humans that cannot exclude chance bias or confounding but appear credible; or (2) sufficient evidence of carcinogenicity from studies of animals which indicate an increased incidence of malignant tumors (a) in multiple species or strains, (b) in multiple experiments, or (c) to an unusual degree with regard to the incidence, site, or type of tumor.

Similarly, the International Agency for Research on Cancer lists these five chemicals in their Group B category—agents that are possibly carcinogenic in humans. This category applies to those chemicals for which there is limited evidence in humans and the absence of sufficient evidence in experimental animals, or there is sufficient evidence of carcinogenicity in experimental animals but inadequate evidence of carcinogenicity in humans.

The other agents are listed as chemicals not classifiable as to their carcinogenicity to humans. At the present time the rest of these halogenated solvents are not suspected carcinogens. Some controversy surrounds the classification of carcinogenicity to humans from exposure to trichloroethylene. A United States National Toxicology Program study using uncontaminated trichloroethylene at a dose of 1 gram of trichloroethylene per kilogram body weight demonstrated a significant increase in the incidence of hepatocellular carcinomas in B6C3F1 mice of both sexes (48). However, the failure to detect significant excesses of cancer in human epidemiologic studies may result from the fact that the metabolic pathways leading to the formation of proximate carcinogens are not activated at low doses where trichloroethylene follows first order kinetics (35).

LABORATORY

Biochemical Abnormalities

The most serious abnormalities of serum chemistry result from hepatorenal failure after exposure to the hepatotoxic halogenated solvents and include elevated serum hepatic aminotransferase, bilirubin, alkaline phosphatase, ammonia, creatinine, and lactate levels. A prolonged prothrombin time may lead to hemorrhage and a reduced hemoglobin level. Hypoglycemia may complicate liver failure. Maximum elevations of serum hepatic aminotransferase developed between 1 and 3 days after exposure in nonfatal cases and generally returned to normal within 2 weeks. Renal dysfunction is manifest by rising serum creatinine, and reduced urinary flow may accompany hepatic failure. The most sensitive indicator of hepatic dysfunction following exposure to trichloroethane is an elevation of the urinary bilinogen (78). Abnormalities may appear several days after exposure and remain a week after exposure.

Following large ingestions of trichloroethylene dysrhythmias may develop up to 24 hours after exposure. Premature ventricular contractions are the most common dysrhythmias; however, bradycardia, conduction disturbance, and serious ventricular dysrhythmias may occur during acute intoxication. Trichloroethylene and tetrachloromethane are radiopaque and appear on abdominal x-rays following ingestion (59, 79). Other blood abnormalities include hypercalcemia complicating the course of the ingestion of dichloroethane (23) and progressive monocytosis associated with chronic poisoning by tetrachloroethane (80).

Biochemical abnormalities following exposure to dichloromethane are unusual except those relating to the formation of carbon monoxide (i.e., carboxyhemoglobinemia, acidosis). Carboxyhemoglobin levels may not be a good indicator of toxicity, in part because the lungs excrete the carbon monoxide dissolved in venous plasma before it reaches the systemic (arterial) circulation (81). Furthermore, dichloromethane produces direct CNS depression independent of the carboxyhemoglobin level, and therefore CNS effects are not directly related to the carboxyhemoglobin level.

Analytical Methods

The method recommended for the determination of halogenated solvents in the occupational setting is the NIOSH activated charcoal method for collection and concentration, and subsequent solvent (carbon disulfide) extraction of the charcoal with gas chromatographic analysis of the extractant. Gas chromatography with electron capture has now largely replaced the Fujiwara colorimetry test for the determination of halogenated solvents in biologic samples. Either solvent extraction of samples or head space methods may be used. Use of the Fujiwara method may produce false positive results because of the presence of other halogens (chlorine, iodine, fluorine, and bromine). Photodetection with a halide meter possesses the same drawbacks. The biotransformation of trichloroethylene, tetrachloroethylene, and trichloroethane results in varying levels of trichloroacetic acid in the urine, and false positives may result if other chemicals, including chloral hydrate, are not excluded as potential sources of trichloroacetic acid.

Human Levels

Because of the ubiquitous presence of halogenated solvents in our environment, blood samples may contain detectable levels of these solvents without occupational exposure (82). Human data are too limited to establish definite dose-effect levels for these halogenated solvents. Some data are available from experimental human exposures to levels of halogenated solvents in the workplace. Additionally, some data from postmortem analysis of patients dying of suicidal and accidental overexposure to these chemicals are available (83, 84).

Health Surveillance

BIOLOGIC MONITORING

Table 64.4 lists the current workplace standards for environmental levels of the halogenated solvents. Workplace air monitoring evaluates the potential contaminants to which a worker is exposed but does not measure the actual dose received by the worker. The latter depends on work practices, protective equipment, and actual location in relation to the source of exposure. Biologic monitoring attempts to more accurately measure the dose the worker received although, because of individual variation, biologic monitoring should be applied to a group and not an individual. The American Conference of Governmental and Industrial Hygienists (ACGIH) developed biologic exposure limits as an aid to supplement environmental monitoring.

The concentration of tetrachloroethylene in exhaled air within the first hour represents recent exposure, while concentration the following morning and/or weekend more closely approximate the time-weighted average exposure (85). Following workplace exposure to tetrachloroethylene, the concentration of trichloroacetic acid rises in the blood for the first 24 hours and then declines with a half-life of approximately 80 hours (86). The ACGIH biologic exposure limit is 7 milligrams of trichloroacetic acid per liter of urine at the end of the work week.

The measurement of trichloroethane in exhaled air prior to the work shift (i.e., 16 hours after the cessation of exposure after at least 2 consecutive days) is the most specific biologic measure of trichloroethane exposure. The biologic exposure limit recommended by the ACGIH is 40 ppm trichloroethane; however, there is substantial individual variation. Measurement of urinary trichloroacetic acid is a less specific measure of trichloroethane dose in workers, but the urinary trichloroacetic acid is an accurate measure of the extent of trichloroethane exposure (87). The ACGIH recommended biologic exposure limit for trichloroethane in urine is 10 milligrams of trichloroacetic acid per liter voided at the end of the work week. This measurement is only a screening test and is not a specific measure of exposure because other chlorinated hydrocarbons produce trichloroacetic acid.

After exposure ceases, the end exhaled concentration of trichloroethylene also declines in a multiexponential fashion. Consequently, end exhaled air samples soon after exposure ceases indicate recent exposure while the level present in end exhaled air of trichloroethylene several hours after exposure ceases represents an average of the preceding several days. The ACGIH recommends an end exhaled air sample collected 16 hours after the last exposure to trichloroethylene of 0.4 ppm trichloroethylene or less. Trichloroethanol levels in exhaled air, blood, and urine are also indicators of the time-weighted average during the preceding several days because approximately 30–50% of an absorbed dose of trichloroethylene is biotransformed to trichloroethanol. The ACGIH recommends a concentration of 4 grams of free trichloroethanol per liter of blood collected at the end of the work week as a biologic limit of trichloroethylene exposure.

Blood carboxyhemoglobin levels probably should not exceed 5% in workers exposed to dichloromethane. This carboxyhemoglobin level approximates the concentration obtained following a workday exposure to 100 ppm dichloromethane in resting nonsmokers (88).

MEDICAL MONITORING

Preplacement physical examinations should focus on establishing a baseline for kidney and cardiac function as well as detecting preexisting conditions (arteriosclerotic heart disease, liver dysfunction, chronic skin conditions, alcoholism) that may predispose the worker to toxic effects of halogenated solvents. Periodic medical examinations should be designed to detect alterations in central nervous system function (e.g., impairment of perceptual speed, reaction time, and manual dexterity), hepatic dysfunction, gastrointestinal symptoms, and dermatitis. The extent of routine laboratory analyses (serum hepatic transaminases, urinalysis, serum creatinine) depends on the physician's judgment of the severity of exposure based on workplace practice, environmental monitoring, and biologic exposure limits.

TREATMENT
First Aid
DERMAL

Damage to the skin usually results either from prolonged skin contact or chronic defatting of the skin. Contaminated clothing should be removed and the affected area washed with soap and copious amounts of water.

EYE

Halogenated solvents are direct irritants to the epithelium of the eye, and installation of these compounds into the eye results in conjunctival erythema and damage to the corneal epithelium. Spontaneous recovery usually occurs. Corneal abrasions and some turbidity may result initially. Following direct installation of these chemicals into the eye, the eye should be irrigated thoroughly for at least 15 minutes and medical attention sought if erythema or irritation persists.

ORAL

Existing data are too limited on oral exposures to halogenated solvents to confidently predict the exact level at which decontamination measures should be instituted. Table 64.5 lists the recommended quantities of halogenated solvents at which syrup of ipecac is recommended. These guidelines apply only when the ingestion occurred less than several hours prior to initiation of treatment and the patient does not display a lack of gag reflex, coma, or convulsive activity. Following the administration of syrup of ipecac, the patient should be observed in the upright position to minimize the hazard of aspiration. To

Table 64.5.   Emesis Recommendations*

Solvent	Ingested Amount**
1,2-Dichloroethane	One swallow
1,2-Dichloroethylene	Large, intentional ingestion
Dichloromethane	Large, intentional ingestion
1,2-Dichloropropane	>One swallow
Tetrabromoethane	>Several swallows
Tetrachloroethane	One swallow
Tetrachloroethylene	Several swallows
Tetrachloromethane	One swallow
Trichloroethane	Large, intentional ingestions
Trichloroethylene	>One swallow
Trichloromethane	One swallow
1,1,2-Trichloro-1,2,2-trifluoroethane	Usually not necessary

*These recommendations are based on the limited data available and may change when better data become available. For contraindications, see text under First Aid.
**One swallow in a 2-year-old child and an adult is approximately 5 milliliter and 20 milliliter respectively. Large, intentional ingestions usually exceed 120–150 milliliter in adults. These levels are based on pure substances. For products containing more than one substance, the decision to induce emesis should be based on the most toxic substance present in the blend at a concentration exceeding 10–20%.

date, the indication of emesis following the ingestion of chlorinated hydrocarbons has not been associated with the development of aspiration pneumonitis. Dichloromethane is a mucous membrane irritant, and dilution with water or milk following ingestion should be initiated following the oral administration of small amounts of this chemical.

INHALATION

The immediate danger from large exposures to halogenated solvents is central nervous system and respiratory depression. The victim should be moved from the contaminated environment as soon as safely possible. The adequacy of respiration should be evaluated in the patient with altered mental status and oxygen and artificial ventilation begun as needed. For unconscious patients the pulse should be checked and cardiopulmonary resuscitation begun if the pulse is absent. Medical attention should be sought for any victim with alterations of mental status or respiratory difficulty.

Acute Management
STABILIZATION

The treatment of exposure to these chemicals is primarily supportive. Respiratory depression and dysrhythmias represent the greatest immediate danger to life following exposure. Initially the adequacy of oxygenation should be assessed and arterial blood gases drawn if indicated. Patients with altered mental status or those complaining of dyspnea should receive supplemental oxygen. Hypotension should initially be treated with volume expansion and then vasopressors as needed. Symptomatic patients should be monitored for the development of dysrhythmias. Although sympathomimetic drugs should be administered with caution, their use in the clinical setting should not be avoided if indicated. Sensitization of the myocardium occurs at levels above 5000 ppm in animal studies, and those levels are unlikely to occur in the clinical setting because of the rapid elimination of these solvents through the lungs. Lidocaine is the initial antiarrhythmic of choice with beta-blockers being a second line drug for ventricular ectopy. Hypertension usually responds to removal of the victim from exposure and initial volume repletion. Persistent hypertension necessitates a search for other causes (myocardial infarction, trauma, excessive volume depletion). Animal studies indicate that adrenal hemorrhage may occur following exposure to high concentrations of some halogenated solvents (i.e., dichloroethane, dichloropropane). Accordingly, acute adrenocortical insufficiency should be considered in any patient in whom hypotension or vascular collapse supervenes, or who does not respond to the usual supportive measures. The diagnosis of adrenal apoplexy should be confirmed by serum cortisol levels before treatment. Once a blood specimen has been collected, treatment should begin with intravenous hydrocortisone in a dose of 200–300 milligrams during the first 24 hours.

DECONTAMINATION

Table 64.5 lists the quantities of ingested solvents that require emesis. These levels are based on the best data available at the present time and may change as more data appear. Syrup of ipecac is the emetic of choice at a dose of 15 milliliters for 1- to 3-year-old children and 30 milliliters for patients over 10 years of age. The induction of emesis generally is not recommended beyond several hours because these compounds are rapidly absorbed. Contraindications to the use of syrup of ipecac include the presence of marked lethargy, loss of the gag reflex, coma, and convulsions. Lavage with saline is an alternative method of decontamination; however, the poor water solubility of these chemicals may limit the effectiveness of this method. No clinical studies are available to evaluate the efficacy of lavage. Activated charcoal probably does not absorb these chemicals and therefore is not indicated (89). There are no clinical studies to guide the clinical use of cathartics, and their use depends on clinical judgment in this setting.

ENHANCEMENT OF ELIMINATION

Because most of these chemicals are excreted through the lungs, good ventilation should be maintained. Hyperventilation (three times the normal minute volume) has been recommended for ingestions greater than 1.2 milliliters of tetrachloroethylene per kilogram body weight, or blood levels greater than 10 micrograms tetrachloroethylene per milliliter (27). In a 6-year-old boy this therapy reduced the rapid elimination half-life of tetrachloroethylene from 160 to 30 minutes but did not alter the slower terminal elimination half-life. Hemodialysis may be necessary for the development of renal failure; however, hemodialysis removes only small amounts of tetrachloromethane from the blood (90). To date, the elimination of other halogenated solvents by hemodialysis or hemoperfusion has not been studied. The high lipophilic characteristics of these solvents argue against the efficacy of hemodialysis.

Although the use of hyperbaric oxygen for 6 hours improved the survival of rats administered oral doses of tetrachloromethane (91) and a single case report noted a successful outcome following the use of hyperbaric oxygen (92), the use of hyperbaric oxygen in this setting remains experimental. A 32-year-old worker was found unconscious following exposure in a poorly ventilated area through a paint preparation containing approximately 25% dichloromethane (93). The initial carbox-

yhemoglobin level was 5.4% and rose to 13% despite 46 minutes of hyperbaric oxygen given 1 hour after admission. Although the authors felt that hyperbaric oxygen was beneficial, the clinical course did not correlate well with the carboxyhemoglobin level and probably resulted from the direct central nervous system effects of dichloromethane rather than the effects of carbon monoxide.

ANTIDOTES

A single case report documented the survival of a 61-year-old man following the ingestion of a lethal dose of 250 milliliters of tetrachloromethane after use of intravenous n-acetylcysteine (94). Theoretically this antidote repletes glutathione stores and prevents the formation of toxic intermediates; however, the clinical data at the present time are not adequate to support the use of n-acetylcysteine in this situation and, therefore, administration of n-acetylcysteine for tetrachloromethane overdose remains experimental. Although no antidotes have been studied for the treament of trichloromethane intoxication, the depletion of glutathione stores following overdose with this chemical suggests that n-acetylcysteine would be as effective as the administration of n-acetylcysteine following tetrachloromethane administration.

SUPPORTIVE CARE

Potential complications of exposure to halogenated solvents include cardiac dysrhythmias, aspiration pneumonia, chemical hepatitis (delayed), and hypoxic encephalopathy. Symptomatic patients should be monitored for the development of dysrhythmias, and patients who ingest large amounts of these compounds should be monitored for 24 hours to detect the delayed development of dysrhythmias. Patients exposed to high concentrations of these chemicals should receive a chest x-ray, arterial blood gas, electrocardiogram, and measurement of serum creatinine and hepatic transaminases. Profuse diarrhea may exacerbate electrolyte imbalance and predispose the patient to dysrhythmias. Consequently, generous intravenous fluid replacement should be given and serum electrolytes monitored at least daily. Patients exposed to large concentrations of the hepatotoxic halogenated solvents (dichloroethane, tetrabromoethane, tetrachloroethane, trichloromethane, tetrachloromethane) should be followed for at least 3 days to detect the development or progression of hepatorenal failure. Serial hematocrits and stool guaiac tests are necessary only for those patients who develop abnormalities in coagulation and therefore are predisposed to the development of gastrointestinal bleeding. Supportive care includes the treatment of renal failure with dialysis and hepatic failure with fresh frozen plasma, vitamin K, low protein diet, neomycin, lactulose, and careful fluid and electrolyte balance. These patients may benefit from total parenteral nutrition (22). Carboxyhemoglobin levels should be obtained from patients exposed to dichloromethane, but these levels do not necessarily accurately reflect the clinical status of the patient. The use of 100% oxygen or hyperbaric oxygen has not been well-studied following dichloromethane exposure but is a reasonable treatment method if the situation so dictates.

REFERENCES

1. Magos L. Thoughts on life with untested and adequately tested chemicals. Br J Ind Med 1988;45:721–726.

2. Hill AB. The environment and disease: association or causation? Proc R Soc Med 1965;58:295–300.

3. Gilman AG, Goodman LS, Rall TW, et al, eds. Goodman and Gilman's The pharmacological basis of therapeutics. 8th ed. New York: Macmillan, 1990:261.

4. Ostlere G. The role of trichloroethylene in general anesthesia. Br Med J 1948;1:195–196.

5. Lamson PD, Minot AS, Robbins BH. The prevention and treatment of carbon tetrachloride intoxication. JAMA 1921;90:345–349.

6. Lambert SM. Hookworm disease in the South Pacific, ten years of tetrachlorides. JAMA 1933;100:247–248.

7. Foot EB, Bishop K, Apgar V. Tetrachloroethylene as an anesthetic agent. Anaesthesiology 1943;4:283–292.

8. Willcox WH. An outbreak of toxic jaundice due to tetrachloroethane poisoning. A new type amongst aeroplane workers. Lancet 1915;1:544–547.

9. Hoffman HT, Birnstiel H, Jobst P. On the inhalation toxicity of 1,1- and 1,2-dichloroethane. Arch Toxicol 1971;27:248–265.

10. Reynolds ES, Moslen MT. Damage to hepatic cellular membranes by chlorinated olefins with emphasis on synergism and antagonism. Environ Health Perspect 1977;21:137–147.

11. Smyth HF. Hygienic standards for daily inhalation. The Donald E. Cummings Memorial lecture. Am Ind Hyg Q 1956;17:129–185.

12. Royal Society of Chemistry. Organo-chlorine solvents. Health risks to workers. Brussels Commission of the European Communities. Publication No. EUR 10531EN, 1986:131–146.

13. International Programme on Chemical Safety. Environmental health criteria 50 trichloroethylene. Geneva: World Health Organization, 1985.

14. Greim H, Wolff T, Hofler M, et al. Formation of dichloroacetylene from trichloroethylene in the presence of alkaline material. Possible cause of intoxication after abundant use of chloroethylene-containing solvents. Arch Toxicol 1984;56:74–77.

15. Firth JB, Stuckey RE. Decomposition of trilene in closed circuit anaesthesia. Lancet 1945;1:814–816.

16. Crummett WB, Stenger VA. Thermal stability of methyl chloroform and carbon tetrachloride. Ind Eng Chem Analyst (Edn) 1956;48:434.

17. National Institute for Occupational Safety and Health. Recommended standard for occupational exposure to methylene chloride. DHEW (NIOSH) Publication No. 76-138. Cincinnati, OH: Department of Health, Education and Welfare, 1976.

18. Stopps GJ, McLaughlin M. Psychophysiological testing of human subjects exposed to solvent vapors. Am Ind Hyg Assoc J 1967;28:43–50.

19. Winneke G. The neurotoxicity of dichloromethane. Neurobehav Toxicol Teratol 1981;3:391–395.

20. Gamberle F, Annwall G, Hultengren M. Exposure to methylene chloride II. Psychological functions. Scand J Work Environ Health 1975;1:95–103.

21. Hygenic Guide Series: 1,1,2-trichloro-1,2,2-trifluoroethane (trifluorotrichloroethane, fluorocarbon No. 113). Am Ind Hyg Assoc J 1968;29:521–525.

22. Fogel RD, Davidman M, Poleski MH, et al. Carbon tetrachloride poisoning treated with hemodialysis and total parenteral nutrition. Can Med Assoc J 1984;128:560–561.

23. Yodaiken RE, Babcock JR. 1,2-Dichloroethane poisoning. Arch Environ Health 1973;26:281–284.

24. Mant AK. Acute tetrachloroethane poisoning. A report on two fatal cases. Br Med J 1953;1:655–656.

25. Stephens JA. Poisoning by accidental drinking of trichloroethylene. Br Med J 1945;2:218–219.

26. Eichert H. Trichloroethylene intoxication. JAMA 1936;106:1952–1954.

27. Koppel C, Arendt U, Koeppe P. Acute tetrachloroethylene poisoning, blood elimination kinetics during hyperventilation therapy. Clin Toxicol 1985;23:103–115.

28. Monster AC. Differences in uptake, elimination and metabolism in exposure to trichloroethylene, 1,1,1-trichloroethane and tetrachloroethylene. Int Arch Occup Environ Health 1979;42:311–317.

29. Pegg DG, Zempel JA, Braun WH, et al. Distribution of tetrachloro(^{14}C)ethylene following oral and inhalation exposure in rats. Toxicol Appl Pharmacol 1979;51:465–474.

30. Nolan RJ, Freshour NL, Rick DL, et al. Kinetics and metabolism of inhaled methyl chloroform (1,1,1-trichloroethane) in male volunteers. Fundam Appl Toxicol 1984;4:654–662.

31. Divencenzo GD, Yanno FJ, Astill FJ. Human and canine exposures to methylene chloride vapor. Am Ind Hyg Assoc J 1972;33:125–135.

32. Shangel L, Koss R. Determination of fluorinated hydrocarbon propellants in blood of dogs after aerosol administration. J Pharm Sci 1972;61:1445–1449.

33. Jakobson I, Wahlberg JE, Holmberg B, et al. Uptake via the blood and elimination of 10 organic solvents following epicutaneous exposure of anesthetized guinea pigs. Toxicol Appl Pharmacol 1982;63:181–187.

34. International Programme on Chemical Safety. Environmental health criteria 62, 1,2-dichloroethane. Geneva: World Health Organization, 1987.

35. Kimbrough RD, Mitchell FL, Houk VN. Trichloroethylene: an update. J Toxicol Environ Health 1985;15:369–383.

36. Kubic VL, Anders MW. Metabolism of dihalomethanes to carbon monoxide III. Studies on the mechanism of reaction. Biochem Pharmacol 1978;27:2349–2355.

37. Humbert BE, Fernandez JG. Exposition au 1,1,1-trichlorethane; contribution à l'étude de l'absorption, de l'excrétion et du metabolisme sur des sujets humains. Arch Mal Prof 1977;38:415–425.

38. DiVincenzo GD, Kaplan CJ. Uptake, metabolism and elimination of methylene chloride vapor by humans. Toxicol Appl Pharmacol 1981;59:130–140.

39. Kranz JC Jr, Park CS, Ling JSL. Anesthesia LX. The anesthetic properties of 1,1,1-trichloroethane. Anaesthesia 1959;20:635–640.

40. Adams EM, Spencer HC, Rowe UK, et al. Vapor toxicity of trichloroethylene determined by experiments on laboratory animals. AMA Arch Ind Hyg Occup Med 1951;4:469–481.

41. Reichert D, Lieboldt G, Hanschlar G. Neurotoxic effects of dichloroacetylene. Arch Toxicol 1976;37:23–38.

42. Karkson JE, Rosengren LE, Kjellstrand P, et al. Effects of low dose inhalation of three chlorinated aliphatic organic solvents on deoxyribonucleic acid in gerbil brains. Scand J. Work Environ Health 1987;13:453–458.

43. Wright WH, Schaffer JM. Critical anthelmintic tests of chlorinated alkyl hydrocarbons and a correlation between the anthelmintic efficacy, chemical structure and physical properties. Am J Hyg 1932;16:325–428.

44. Kalf GF, Post GB, Synder R. Solvent toxicology. Recent advances in the toxicology of benzene, the glycol ethers, and carbon tetrachloride. Annu Rev Pharmacol Toxicol 1987;27:399–427.

45. Waters EM, Gerstner HB, Huff JE. Trichloroethylene 1. An overview. J Toxicol Environ Health 1977;2:671–707.

46. Heppel LA, Neal PA, Perrin TL, et al. The toxicity of 1,2-dichloroethane (ethylene dichloride): V. The effect of daily inhalations. J Ind Hyg Toxicol 1946;28:113–120.

47. Tray MG. Effect of exposure to the vapors of tetrabromoethane (acetylene tetrabromide). AMA Arch Ind Hyg Occup Med 1950;2:407–419.

48. United States National Toxicology Program. Technical report on the carcinogenesis studies of trichloroethylene (without epichlorhydrin) in F 344/n rats and BCF mice. NIH Publication No. 83-1979, NTP TR 243. Research Triangle Park, NC, 1983.

49. Spencer HC, Rowe VK, Adams EM, et al. Vapor toxicity of ethylene dichloride determined by experiments on laboratory animals. Arch Ind Hyg Occup Med 1951;4:482–493.

50. Herd PA, Lipsky M, Martin HF. Cardiovascular effects of 1,1,1-trichloroethane. Arch Environ Health 1974;28:227–233.

51. Reinhart CF, Mullins LS, Maxfield ME. Epinephrine-induced cardiac arrhythmia-potential of some common industrial solvents. J Occup Med 1973;15:953–955.

52. Back KC, Van Stee EW. Toxicology of halo alkane propellants and fire extinguishants. Annu Rev Pharmacol Toxicol 1977;17:83–95.

53. Heppel LA, Neal PA, Perrin TL, et al. The toxicity of 1,2-dichloroethane (ethylene) III. Its acute toxicology and the effect of protective agents. J Pharmacol Exp Ther 1945;84:53–63.

54. Heppel LA, Neal PA. Toxicology of dichloromethane (methylene chloride) III. Its effects on running activity in the male rat. J Ind Hyg Toxicol 1944;26:17–21.

55. Gould VE, Smuckler EA. Alveolar injury in acute carbon tetrachloride intoxication. Arch Intern Med 1971;128:109–117.

56. Hatfield TR, Mayleoski RT. A fatal methyl chloroform (trichloroethane) poisoning. Arch Environ Health 1970;20:279–281.

57. Moon HD. The pathology of fatal carbon tetrachloride poisoning with special reference to the histogenesis of the hepatic and renal lesions. Am J Pathol 1950;26:1041–1057.

58. Cohen MM. Central nervous system in carbon tetrachloride intoxication. Neurology 1957;7:238–244.

59. Thomas G, Baud FJ, Galliot M, et al. Clinical and kinetic study of 4 cases of acute trichloroethylene intoxication. Vet Hum Toxicol 1987;29(suppl 2) 97–99.

60. Stewart RD, Hake CL. Paint remover hazard. JAMA 1976;235:398–401.

61. English JM. A case of probable phosgene poisoning. Br Med J 1964;1:38.

62. Bardodej Z, Vyskocil J. The problem of trichloroethylene in occupational medicine. AMA Arch Ind Health 1956;13:581–592.

63. El Ghawabi SM, Mansoor MB, El Gamel AA, et al. Chronic trichloroethylene exposure. J Egypt Med Assoc 1973;56:715–724.

64. Coler HR, Rossmiller HR. Tetrachloroethylene exposure in a small industry. Arch Ind Hyg Occup Med 1953;8:227–233.

65. Gold J. Chronic perchloroethylene poisoning. Can Psychiatr Assoc J 1969;14:627–630.

66. Collier H. Methylene dichloride intoxication in industry. A report of two cases. Lancet 1936;1:594–595.

67. Liss GM. Peripheral neuropathy in two workers exposed to 1,1,1-trichloroethane. JAMA 1988;260:2217.

68. Raffi GB, Violante FS. Is freon 113 neurotoxic? A case report. Int Arch Occup Environ Health 1981;49:125–127.

69. Mitchell ABS, Parsons-Smith BG. Trichloroethylene neuropathy. Br Med J 1969;1:422–423.

70. Priest RJ, Horn RC. Trichloroethylene intoxication. A case of acute hepatic necrosis possibly due to this agent. Arch Environ Health 1965;11:361–365.

71. McCurrey RJ. Diverse manifestations of trichloroethylene. Br J Ind Med 1988;45:122–126.

72. Theile DL, Eigenbrodt EH, Ware AJ. Cirrhosis after repeated trichloroethylene and 1,1,1-trichloroethane exposure. Gastroenterology 1982;83:926–929.

73. Meckler LC, Phelps DK. Liver disease secondary to tetrachloroethylene exposure. A case report. JAMA 1966;197:144–145.

74. Sato A, Yamaguchi K, Nakajima T. A new health problem due to trichloroethylene: pneumatosis cystoides intestinalis. Environ Health 1987;42:144–147.

75. Stewart RD, Hake CL, Peterson JE. ''Degreaser's flush'' dermal response to trichloroethylene and ethanol. Arch Environ Health 1974;29:1–5.

76. Barlow SM, Sullivan FM. Reproductive hazards of industrial chemicals. London: Academic Press, 1982.

77. Schewtz TA, Leong BKJ, Gehring PJ. The effect of maternally inhaled trichloroethylene, perchloroethylene, methyl chloroform, and methylene chloride on embryonal and fetal development in mice and rats. Toxicol Appl Pharmacol 1975;32:84–96.

78. Stewart RD. Methyl chloroform intoxication. Diagnosis and treatment. JAMA 1971;215:1789–1792.

79. Bagnasco FM, Stringer B, Muslim AM. Carbon tetrachloride poisoning. NY State J Med 1978;78:646–647.

80. Minot GR, Smith LW. The blood in tetrachloroethane poisoning. Arch Intern Med 1921;28:687–702.

81. Langehennig PL, Seeler RA, Berman E. Paint removers and carboxyhemoglobin. N Engl J Med 1976;295:1137.

82. Hamijimiragha H, Ewers V, Jansen-Rosseck R, et al. Human exposure to volatile halogenated hydrocarbons from the general environment. Int Arch Occup Environ Health 1986;58:141–150.

83. Baselt RC. Disposition of toxic drugs and chemicals in man, 2nd ed. Davis, CA: Biomedical Publications, 1982.

84. Ellenhorn ME, Barceloux DG. Medical toxicology: diagnosis and treatment of human poisoning. New York: Elsevier, 1988.

85. Monster AC. Biological monitoring of chlorinated hydrocarbon solvents. J Occup Med 1986;28:583–588.

86. Monster AC, Boersma G, Steenweg H. Kinetics of tetrachloroethylene in volunteers; influence of workload and exposure concentration. Int Arch Occup Environ Health 1979;42:303–309.

87. Imbriani M, Ghittori S, Pezzagno G, et al. 1,1,1-Trichloroethane (methyl chloroform) in urine as biological index of exposure. Am J Ind Med 1988;13:211–222.

88. Astrand I, Ovrum P, Carlsson A. Exposure to methylene chloride. I. Its concentration in alveolar air and blood during rest and exercise and its metabolism. Scand J Work Environ Health 1975;1:78–94.

89. Laass W. Therapy of acute oral poisonings by organic solvents. Treatment by activated charcoal in combination with laxatives. Arch Toxicol 1980 (suppl 4) 406–409.

90. Nielson VK, Larsen J. Acute rneal failure due to carbon tetrachloride poisoning. Acta Med Scand 1965;178:363–374.

91. Burk RF, Reiter R, Lane JM. Hyperbaric oxygen protection against carbon tetrachloride hepatotoxicity in the rat. Association with altered metabolism. Gastroenterology 1986;90:812–818.

92. Truss CD, Killanberg PG. Treatment of carbon tetrachloride poisoning with hyperbaric oxygen. Gastroenterology 1982;82:767–769.

93. Rioux JP, Meyers RAM. Hyperbaric oxygen for methylene chloride poisoning: report on two cases. Ann Emerg Med 1989;18:691–695.

94. Mathieson PJ, Williams G, MacSweeney JE. Survival after massive ingestion of carbon tetrachloride treated by intravenous infusion of acetylcysteine. Hum Toxicol 1985;4:627–631.

65

Polychlorinated Biphenyls and Other Polyhalogenated Aromatic Hydrocarbons

Peter G. Shields, M.D.
John A. Whysner, M.D., Ph.D.
Kenneth H. Chase, M.D.

POLYCHLORINATED BIPHENYLS

Introduction

Polychlorinated biphenyls (PCBs) are a family of synthetic chlorinated organic compounds. In the United States, they were manufactured from 1929 to 1977 under the trade name Aroclor (1, 2). Manufacturers in other countries sold PCB mixtures under different trade names (Table 65.1). PCBs were widely used in the electrical utility industry as coolants for transformers and capacitors. They were also used as extenders in paints and pesticides, as lubricants in gas turbines, in hydraulic systems, textiles, sealants, carbonless copy paper, fluorescent light ballast, air conditioners, television sets, and other products (2). Ninety-five percent of capacitors were filled with PCBs, while the same was true for only 5% of transformers (2). PCBs were valued because of their fire resistance, chemical stability, and dielectric properties, allowing them to be used in areas where the risk of fire or explosion associated with other coolants was significantly greater.

Different Aroclor formulations vary by isomer composition and chlorine weight. Figure 65.1 shows the structure of a polychlorinated biphenyl compound with the numbering system for isomers. There are 209 theoretical isomers among 10 different congeners. Aroclors are classified by a 4-number system beginning with 12 and ending with the percentage, by weight, of chlorine; e.g., Aroclor 1260 is 60% chlorine by weight. The exception is Aroclor 1016, which was the most recently produced and which contained approximately 41% chlorine.

During the 1970s, concern regarding the continued unrestricted use of PCBs surfaced because of their persistence in the environment and toxicity in laboratory animals (3–5). Under the Toxic Substances Control Act, Congress banned further manufacture and limited the distribution of PCBs beyond 1979.

Absorption, Metabolism, and Excretion

A description of PCB pharmacokinetics in animals must take into consideration the complexity of various Aroclor compositions as well as genetically determined differences across species. PCBs can be absorbed through the skin, lungs, and gastrointestinal tract (6). They are transported by the blood stream to the liver and muscle, where they are redistributed to adipose tissue. An equilibrium is established whereby partitioning among tissues remains relatively constant for a given species.

PCBs are metabolized in the liver to form hydroxylated phenolic compounds, (presumably) via an arene oxide intermediate

(Fig. 65.2) (7, 8). They can be excreted as such or as methylsulfinyl metabolites via other metabolic pathways (9). Dechlorination also occurs. The rate of formation of metabolic products varies depending on the isomer (position and degree of chlorination) and animal species. Dogs and rodents metabolize PCBs relatively quickly compared with primates (8). Excretion is through biliary drainage to feces and urine. The half-life of PCBs in animals is shorter than in humans.

PCBs stimulate the activity of P-450 metabolic enzymes in animal liver, lung, and small intestine (10, 11). This enhances the metabolism of other chemicals. Steroid-like receptor bind-

Table 65.1. Commercial PCB Mixtures

Trade Name	Manufacturer	Country	Percent Chlorine by weight
Aroclor 1242	Monsanto Co.	U.S.A.	42
" " 1248	" "	" "	48
" " 1254	" "	" "	54
" " 1260	" "	" "	60
" " 1016	" "	" "	41
Clophen A30	Farbenfabricken Bayer	Germany	42
" " A50	" "	" "	54
" " A60	" "	" "	60
Kanechlor 300	Kanegatuchi Co.	Japan	42
" " 400	" "	" "	48
" " 500	" "	" "	53
" " 600	" "	" "	60
Pyralene 3010	Prodelec Co.	France	42
" " 1476	" "	" "	54
Apirolio	Caffarro Co.	Italy	42

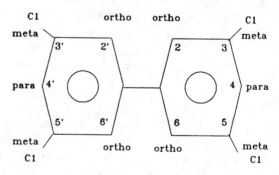

Figure 65.1. Structure of a PCB molecule. Chlorine substitution can occur at any numbered position. The structure shown is 3,5,3′5′-tetrachlorbiphenyl.

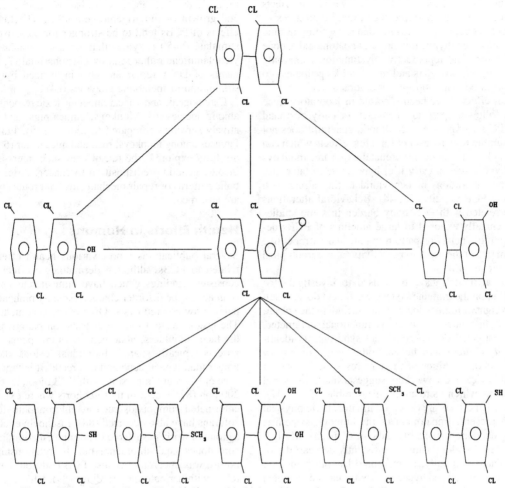

Figure 65.2. Metabolism of 2,4,2′,4′-tetrachlorbiphenyl has at least 7 metabolic excretion products.

ing proteins located in the cell cytoplasm moderate this effect (12–14). Different P-450 enzymes are induced depending upon the number and position of chlorine atoms within the PCB isomer, e.g., meta- and para- versus orthosubstitution. Metabolic stimulation varies widely across species (7, 9, 15, 16).

In humans, PCBs are also absorbed through the skin, lungs, and gastrointestinal tract (6). Dermal absorption is the major route in occupational groups (17), while ingestion is more important in environmental exposures (18–20). The latter occurs primarily through contaminated foods. PCBs have also been detected in placental cord blood (21) and breast milk (22–24).

Body burdens in humans depend on the route and length of exposure, place of residence, gender, age, and possibly extent of alcohol consumption (19, 25–29). Worldwide levels in various tissues have recently been summarized (30). The average PCB serum level for nonoccupationally exposed persons is approximately 7 ppb with a range of up to 30 ppb (27). In contrast, occupationally exposed persons can have PCB blood levels up to 3300 ppb (31). Adipose levels are generally less than 3 ppm, but levels up to 33 ppm have been reported (29, 31, 32). The National Human Adipose Tissue Survey found that levels above 3 ppm in the general population have been decreasing; however, the prevalence of any detectable level has been increasing (28). The partitioning coefficient between adi-

pose tissue and blood varies from 100–190:1 depending upon PCB body burdens (29, 32, 33, 34). Partitioning coefficients were also reported for brain:liver:fat of 1:3.5:81 in necropsy samples from Denmark (Kraul, 1976, cited in (6)).

Metabolism and excretion of PCBs in humans has not been adequately characterized (35). Human hepatic microsomes in vitro can metabolize 2,2′, 3,3′, 6,6′-hexachlorobiphenyl but not 2,2′, 4,4′, 5,5′-hexachlorobiphenyl (35). In a small group of occupationally exposed persons, the serum half-life was reported to be 6 to 7 months for Aroclor 1242 and 33 to 34 months for Aroclor 1260 (36). Children metabolize PCBs faster than their mothers as the half-life for the Japanese produced Kanechlor 500 (similar to Aroclor 1254) in blood was 2.8 years in children and 7.1 years in mothers (37). (Dilutional effects during growth might be responsible for this observation.) As in animals, metabolism of different isomers occurs at different rates. The mean half-life in blood for 2,4,5,3′,4′-pentachlorobiphenyl was 9.8 months, while the half-life for 2,3,4,3′,4′-pentachlorobiphenyl was 6.7 months (38).

Health Effects in Animals

PCBs produce relatively little acute toxicity. The dose required to produce death in 50% of treated animals ranges from 0.5 g/kg to 11.3 g/kg depending on the Aroclor and animal species (6).

Subacute and chronic exposures lead to a variety of effects in animals occurring as a syndrome. For example progressive weight loss, chloracne, alopecia, skin edema, swelling around the eyes, lymphoid and thymic involution, hepatomegaly, bone marrow depression, and reproductive dysfunction commonly occur together (6, 39, 40). Rats and mice, unlike primates, do not develop facial edema, alopecia, or chloracne.

Neurological effects have been reported in laboratory mice and monkeys following prenatal, neonatal, or early postnatal exposures to PCBs. Exposure in adulthood generally does not produce measurable toxicity except for a few effects which can be reversible (41, 42). Following prenatal exposure, monkeys can become hyperactive in early life, hypoactive in later life, and suffer other alterations of behavioral testing along with signs of clinical PCB toxicity (43, 44). Behavioral alterations have been correlated with PCB body burden in some studies (45). Mice prenatally exposed to large amounts of PCBs develop a "spinning" behavior pattern manifested as repetitive jerking movements of the head, hyperactivity, and stereotypical circular movements (46).

Several animal models have been used to investigate the effect of PCBs upon the immune system. Sufficient doses result in decreased weight of immunologic organs including the spleen, thymus, and lymph nodes. Numerous functional parameters have been investigated but no consistent syndrome is identifiable, and many studies contradict each other, e.g., some show enhancement and/or inhibition of immune responses. A recent study by Smialowicz and coworkers suggests that a threshold level exists below which there are no measurable effects (47). Furthermore, when effects are observed in vitro, toxic physical signs are also present. Impairment of the humoral system is manifested by decreased levels of antibodies, specifically IgA and IgM (48, 49). IgG levels are inconsistently decreased (50, 51). Cell-mediated immunity, as measured by mitogenic and vaccine responses or delayed hypersensitivity, can be inhibited (52–55) or enhanced (47). Mixed lymphocyte responses or cytotoxic lymphocyte responses are not affected at moderate doses (47). Finally, it has been reported that an increased incidence of infection may occur in some laboratory animals (54, 56, 57). Comparative studies of isomers suggest that those with substitution in the meta- or parapositions are more toxic (58, 59) and act through an aromatic hydrocarbon receptor (60).

The target organ for PCB tumorigenicity in animals is the liver. Three studies report that Aroclor 1260 or Clophen A60 induce hepatocellular carcinomas in laboratory mice and rats exposed to large doses over a lifetime (61–63). Aroclor 1254 and Kanechlor 500 at high doses also lead to a small incidence of hepatocellular carcinoma (64, 65). It should be noted that, in spite of the malignant morphologic appearance of the induced tumors, these lesions do not otherwise demonstrate malignant behavior. For example, animals with these tumors live longer than controls and metastases do not seem to occur (62, 63). Lesser chlorinated mixtures can also result in hepatomas, neoplastic nodules, and "preneoplastic" lesions (62, 63, 65–67). These latter lesions are reversible suggesting that they are not neoplastic (68).

Animal studies show that PCBs act as modifying agents following exposure to known carcinogens. They can act as tumor promoters or inhibitors (6, 7, 68–75). PCBs have been shown to promote hepatocellular tumors and preneoplastic lesions following ingestion of N-nitrosoamines (68, 70, 71, 76–78) and azo dyes (79). They also inhibit these same tumors if the animals are treated with PCBs prior to carcinogen exposure

(69, 72, 80, 81). PCBs can also inhibit the transplantability and growth of tumorigenic cells (82). The tumor-promoting effects of PCBs tend to be stronger for those isomers that can stimulate P-450 enzymes that are also stimulated by 3-methylcholanthrene rather than by phenobarbital (7, 83). Measurements of DNA repair are also influenced by the degree of stimulation of metabolic enzymes (84).

Carcinogenic and noncarcinogenic toxic responses vary widely among species (6). Monkeys, guinea pigs, and minks are relatively sensitive compared to rodents (85). Furthermore, differences among monkeys, rats, and mice occur (6, 86). Although not fully explored, the reasons for such interspecies variation include genetic predisposition to cancer, differences in metabolic patterns or repair mechanisms, and routes by which PCBs are absorbed.

Health Effects in Humans

Several publications report various health effects in humans related to PCBs, although dermatologic effects are the only consistent findings which have clinical relevance. Chloracne is an acne-type disorder characterized by pinhead to pea-sized, pale, straw-colored cysts. Often there is comedone formation. The lesions have a unique distribution pattern which includes the face, shoulders, abdomen, scrotum, penis, and ears. The nose is typically spared. Individual lesions also tend to last longer than typical acne and can recur. It is thought that chloracne only occurs in persons with PCB blood levels greater than 200 ppb (87) except in those cohorts where exposures to other chlorinated compounds such as chloronaphthylenes or dibenzofurans have also occurred (88). Fischbein et al. reported that a group of workers suffered hyperpigmentation, hyperkeratosis, comedones, and chloracne, but the relationship to PCB exposure was uncertain because PCB body burdens did not correlate with dermatologic findings (89). Chloracne has not been associated with environmental exposures (18, 90). PCBs can also cause transient dermatitis with contact.

Alterations in blood levels of liver-associated enzymes among groups of workers have been reported in several studies but not in parameters of liver function such as bilirubin, albumin, and prothrombin times (29, 31, 91, 92). It should be noted that, while differences were reported in the mean levels of serum alanine aminotransferase, aspartate aminotransferase, and gamma-glutamyl transpeptidase between exposed and unexposed workers, the group means and most individual levels were well within laboratory reference ranges (29, 31, 91, 92). The clinical significance of these findings also remains uncertain, as workers do not develop clinical manifestations of hepatitis or other liver disease. An Italian study of workers exposed to Pyralene, similar to Aroclor 1242, reported an unexpected incidence of hepatomegaly (93). This finding has not been reported by any other investigator. The ability to metabolize antipyrine was faster in five workers in one study (94) but normal in 47 workers in another (92).

Several studies correlate serum lipid levels with blood PCB levels. Chase et al. found a statistically significant age-adjusted positive correlation of plasma PCB levels with triglycerides but not cholesterol (29). Smith et al. investigated 228 workers and found a significant correlation with HDL cholesterol (31). Kreiss et al. (95) and Baker et al. (90) investigated groups of people who were environmentally exposed to both PCBs and DDT and reported correlation of serum PCB values with serum cholesterol and triglycerides. The cause and significance of these associations are unknown. While it has been postulated that PCBs cause abnormal lipid metabolism, more recent reports suggest that any correlation reflects PCB's affinity for serum lipids (34, 91, 92, 96, 97). Furthermore, cardiovascular disease, the major health effect that would be predicted from abnormal lipid levels, has not been shown to be increased in PCB-exposed cohorts (98–100).

Other PCB-related health effects have been suggested in the scientific literature. An association between PCB exposure and symptoms such as headache, fatigue, and nervousness has been reported in two studies that were not formally controlled (18, 101) and not corroborated in six others (29, 31, 32, 93, 102, 103). Neurologic findings were reported in one study (31) but not in others (29, 31, 104, 105). One study noted a positive association between serum PCB levels and blood pressure (106). However, this finding was not identified in 10 other studies (three specifically reported the results of blood pressure measurements, while numerous others report normal physical examinations) (29, 31, 32, 90, 93, 102–105, 107). Additionally, the original finding was later characterized by the same author as uncertain (27). Alterations in pulmonary function testing of workers exposed to PCBs have been reported in one study (108) but not duplicated in another that investigated the same group of workers (109), and they are not associated with symptoms or chest radiographic findings. Another study on a different group of workers also did not find pulmonary function abnormalities in relation to elevated PCB levels (92).

Reported reproductive effects in women occupationally or environmentally exposed to PCBs have included lower infant birth weight, smaller head circumference, shortened gestational age, and early impairment of psychomotor development (110–112). In all of these studies, however, the mean exposed and nonexposed differences between groups were quite small, and the authors concluded that the results were either not clinically important or the effects of PCBs would be minimal compared to other factors which affect growth. Clinical effects at 1 year of age were sought in children with environmental exposures, and no PCB-related effects could be identified (113). Maternal serum and cord blood PCB levels were not associated with premature rupture of fetal membranes (114).

In 1968 and again in 1978, persons in Japan and Taiwan, respectively, were exposed to large amounts of PCBs, polychlorinated dibenzofurans (PCDFs), quaterphenyls (PCQs), and terphenyls (PCTs) via accidental contamination of rice oil. These contamination cases are known as the Yusho and Yu Cheng episodes, respectively. In each case the oil was used for cooking and was consumed over several months. Various health effects were described including dermatological, neurologic, hepatic, and ocular manifestations (115–117). It has been determined that exposure to PCDFs and other compounds, rather than PCBs, were responsible for the toxic effects of the oil (118–122).

Epidemiologic studies have investigated causes of death in workers with longterm continuous exposure to *high* levels of PCB's (98–100). These reports fail to demonstrate consistently increased death rates either for all causes of death, cancer deaths, or any individual cause of death when compared to the expected number for the general population. One study reported an increased rate of hematologic neoplasms, but most of those individuals described had been exposed for a relatively short period of time prior to diagnosis, and no dose-response relationship could be identified (99). This finding was not duplicated in two other studies (98, 100). An increased rate of liver, biliary, and gallbladder cancer has also been reported (98), but

a dose-response relationship could not be identified, and other evidence suggests that these tumors should not be analyzed as a group.

Genotoxicity

The effects of PCBs at the genetic level have been widely investigated. The overwhelming evidence demonstrates that PCBs are not mutagenic (6, 7). DNA binding has been reported in crude studies, although a specific nucleotide adduct has not been identified (123, 124).

Regulatory Information

PCBs were banned for use in open systems in 1976 and in closed systems beyond 1979. Transformers which contain greater than 500 ppm are considered PCB transformers. Levels between 25 and 500 are considered "contaminated." Environmental and occupational exposures are regulated by several federal and state agencies. Exposure limit values are presented in Table 65.2.

POLYBROMINATED BIPHENYLS

Polybrominated biphenyls (PBBs) have been used primarily as flame retardants. Their structure is similar to PCBs (Fig. 65.1), but bromine, rather than chlorine, is substituted for hydrogen. With one exception, PBBs are not widespread environmental contaminants. This exception occurred in 1974 when PBBs (commercially produced as Firemaster) were accidentally mixed into livestock feed because of confusion with magnesium oxide (marketed as Nutrimaster) (3). Contamination was limited to persons living in Michigan. No human clinical illness has been causally linked to this PBB exposure (3). Although medical complaints and altered neurobehavioral studies were reported in presumably exposed Michigan residents versus Wisconsin controls, the symptoms and biologic studies were not correlated with body burdens (3, 125). Blood testing has similarly not revealed clinical abnormalities (3, 26). One occupational study reported chemical but not clinical evidence of hypothyroidism (126). Immune system parameters have been measured in Michigan residents and although several alterations have been reported in humoral and cell-mediated immunity, they were not correlated with PBB body burden (127). Other studies have assessed lymphocyte function in relationship to PBB levels and no correlations were found (128).

The effects of PBB exposure in laboratory animals are similar to the effects seen with PCBs (3). PBBs can cause hepatocellular carcinoma in rodents (129). It has also been reported that the major contaminant in the Firemaster mixture cited above is relatively nontoxic (130). PBBs, similar to PCBs, are tumor promoters (130). However, they have not been shown to be genotoxic.

CHLORINATED BENZENES

Chlorinated benzenes are a group of compounds that have been used as solvents, pesticides, herbicides, fungicides, and in a number of organic chemical syntheses. They are cyclic aromatic compounds with one to six substituted chlorine atoms. The structure appears in Figure 65.3. Exposure to these compounds occurs mainly in the occupational setting, but levels have been detected in a variety of environmental media in-

Table 65.2.   Regulatory Limit Values

Media	Agency	PCB	Limit	Comment	Reference
Food	Food and Drug Administration	Any Aroclor	0.2–3.0 ppm	Fish/shellfish	Federal Register (5/84)
			10 ppm	Packaging	EPA, 1987
Water	Environmental Protection Agency	Any Aroclor	0.5–.005 mcg/L		EPA, 1987
Air	National Institute of Occupational Safety and Health	Any Aroclor	1 mcg/m³	Occupational exposure	NIOSH Criteria Document 1977
	American Conference of Industrial Hygienists	Aroclor 1242	1 mg/m³	Skin; occupational exposure	ACGIH, 1990
		Aroclor 1254	0.5 mg/m³	Skin; occupational exposure	
	National Academy of Sciences	Any Aroclor	350 mcg/L	Suggested no adverse response level	NAS, 1977
	Occupational Safety and Health Administration	Aroclor 1242	1 mg/m³	Occupational exposure	Federal Register 29 CFR 1910.100
		Aroclor 1254	0.5 mg/m³	Occupational exposure	
Soil	Toxic Substances Control Act	Any Aroclor	50 ppm		
	Environmental Protection Agency	Any Aroclor	10–25 ppm		Federal Register (4/87)

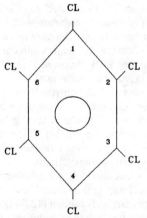

Figure 65.3.   Structure of Hexachlorbenzene.

cluding air, soil, food, and water. Higher degrees of chlorination result in lower water solubility, flammability, and volatility (131). Thus, the ability to become airborne or leach from soil is variable. Chlorinated benzenes are lipophilic so bio-accumulation in animal and human tissues occurs (although to a much lesser extent than other chlorinated aromatic hydrocarbons).

Limited information is available on the pharmacokinetics and toxicity of chlorinated benzenes in animals or humans. Animal studies indicate that, once absorbed into the body, P-450 metabolic enzymes in the liver convert the compounds into chlorinated phenols via an arene oxide intermediate (132, 133). The chlorophenols are excreted in the urine and feces as sulfur intermediates (134) or combine with cellular proteins after further detoxification (133, 135). Binding to cellular proteins allows for further metabolism and dechlorination (132, 135).

Human data for metabolism is essentially nonexistent. Chlorinated benzenes and metabolites have been detected in blood, adipose tissue, urine, and exhaled air of persons without known occupational exposures (28). The National Human Adipose Tissue Survey has reported detectable levels of chlorobenzene, 1,2-dichlorobenzene, and 1,4-dichlorobenzene in 96%, 63%, and 100%, respectively, of samples tested (136). For hexachlorobenzene, 100% of the samples had detectable levels with a median of 0.31 ppm in 1983 (28). Levels in humans have reportedly been decreasing over time. Retention time in humans has been predicted to be 15 years (137).

The major known health effect of chlorinated benzenes is the development of porphyria cutanea tarda (138). This was reported in the 1950s when persons in Turkey ingested grain contaminated with up to 0.2 g of hexachlorobenzene. Some of the ill health effects persisted up to 20 years. Occupational cohorts have not been reported to suffer porphyria cutanea tarda (131).

Isolated case reports and small studies exist for other health effects of chlorinated benzenes (131). A study on persons accidentally exposed to 1,2-dichlorobenzene used as a pesticide reported dizziness, headache, fatigue, nausea, and eye and mucous membrane irritation. The workers had a statistically significantly elevated number of clastogenic chromosomal alterations in peripheral leukocytes (8.9% vs 2% in controls) (139). Other studies have found clastogenic effects in persons exposed to 1,2,4,5-tetrachlorobenzene (140). Anecdotal cases exist linking chlorinated benzenes to aplastic anemia, chronic lymphocytic leukemia, acute myelogenous leukemia, hemolytic anemia, and methemoglobinemia (139).

An epidemiologic association between chlorinated benzenes and human cancer has not been established. Studies in animals noted an association of liver and kidney carcinoma as well as adrenal and parathyroid adenomas with hexachlorobenzene and dichlorobenzene but not with other chlorinated benzenes. Responses varied with species, with female rodents more susceptible. In vitro genotoxicity studies have been negative generally (141).

Acknowledgments

The authors would like to thank T. Michael McArdle and L. Ewick for their technical assistance.

REFERENCES

1. Lloyd JW, Moore RM, Woolf BS, Stein HP. Polychlorinated biphenyls. J Occup Med 1975;18:109.

2. Durfee RL. Production and usage of PCB's in the United States (Abstract). Proc Natl Conf PCB 1975;103–107.

3. Kimbrough RD. Human health effects of polychlorinated biphenyls (PCBs) and polybrominated biphenyls (PBBs). Annu Rev Pharmacol Toxicol 1987;27:87–111.

4. Kutz FW, Strassman SC. Residues of polychlorinated biphenyls in the general population of the United States meeting (Abstract). Proc Natl Conf PCB 1975.

5. Price HA, Welch RL. Occurrence of polychlorinated biphenyls in humans. Environ Health Perspect 1972;1:73–78.

6. ATSDR. Selected PCBs (Aroclor-1260, -1254, -1248, -1242, -1232, -1221, and -1016). Washington, DC: Agency for Toxic Substances and Disease Registry, U.S. Public Health Service, 1987:1.

7. Safe S. Polychlorinated biphenyls (PCBs): mutagenicity and carcinogenicity. Mutat Res 1989;220:31–47.

8. Sipes IG, Slocumb ML, Perry DF, Carter DE. 4,4′-Dichlorobiphenyl: distribution, metabolism, and excretion in the dog and monkey. Toxicol Appl Pharmacol 1980;55:554–563.

9. Sipes IG, Schnellmann RG. Biotransformation of PCBs: metabolic pathways and mechanisms. Environ Toxicol Ser 1987;1:97–109.

10. Taber PG, Chianale J, Florence R, Kim K, Wojcik E, Gumucio JJ. Expression of cytochrome P450b and P450e genes in small intestinal mucosa of rats following treatment with phenobarbital polyhalogenated biphenyls, and organochlorine pesticides. J Biol Chem 1988;263(19):9449–9455.

11. Ueng T, Alvares AP. Selective induction and inhibition of liver and lung cytochrome P-450-dependent monooxygenases by the PCBs mixture, Aroclor 1016. Toxicology 1985;35:83–94.

12. Lund J, Devereux T, Glaumann H, Gustafsson J. Cellular and subcellular localization of binding protein for polychlorinated biphenyls in rat lung. Drug Metab Dispos 1988;16:590–599.

13. McKinney JD, Chae K, McConnell EE, Birnbaum LS. Structure-induction versus structure-toxicity relationships for polychlorinated biphenyls and related aromatic hydrocarbons. Environ Health Perspect 1985;60:57–68.

14. Safe S, Bandiera S, Sawyer T, et al. PCBs: structure-function relationships and mechanism of action. Environ Health Perspect 1985;60:45–56.

15. Abdel-Hamid FM, Moore JA, Matthews HB. Comparative study of 3,4,3′,4′-tetrachlorobiphenyls in male and female rats, and female monkeys. J Toxicol Environ Health 1981;7:181–191.

16. McConnell EE. Comparative toxicity of PCBs and related compounds in various species of animals. Environ Health Perspect 1985;60:29–33.

17. Lees PSJ, Corn M, Breysse PN. Evidence for dermal absorption as the major route of body entry during exposure of transformer maintenance and repairmen to PCBs. Am Ind Hyg Assoc J 1987;48:257–264.

18. Humphrey HEB. Population studies of PCBs in Michigan residents. In: D'Itri FM, Kamrin MA eds. PCBs: human and environmental hazards. Lansing, MI: Ann Arbor Science, 1983:299–310.

19. Mussalo-Rauhamaa H, Raija Moilanen HP. Influence of diet and other factors on the levels of organochlorine compounds in human adipose tissue in Finland. J Toxicol Environ Health 1984;13:689–704.

20. Fiore BJ, Anderson HA, Hanrahan LP, Olson LJ, Sonzogni WC. Sport fish consumption and body burden levels of chlorinated hydrocarbons: a study of Wisconsin anglers. Arch Environ Health 1989;44(2):82–88.

21. Yakushiji T, Watanabe I, Kuwabara K, et al. Long-term studies of the excretion of polychlorinated biphenyls (PCBs) through the mother's milk of an occupationally exposed worker. Arch Environ Contam Toxicol 1978;7:493–504.

22. Frank R, Rasper J, Smout M, Braun H. Organochlorine residues in adipose tissue, blood and milk from Ontario residents, 1976–1985. Can J Pub Health 1988;79:150–158.

23. Yakushiji T, Watanabe I, Kuwabara K, Yoshida S, Koyama K, Kunita N. Levels of polychlorinated biphenyls (PCBs) and organochlorine pesticides

24. Mussalo-Rauhamaa H, Pyysalo H, Antervo K. Relation between the content of organochlorine compounds in Finnish human milk and characteristics of the mothers. J Toxicol Environ Health 1988;25:1–19.

25. Wolff MS, Fischbein A, Thornton J, Rice C. Lilis R, Selikoff IJ. Body burden of polychlorinated biphenyls among persons employed in capacitor manufacturing. Int Arch Occup Environ Health 1982;49:199–208.

26. Kreiss K, Roberts C. Serial PBB levels, PCB levels, and clinical chemistries in Michigan's PBB cohort. Arch Environ Health 1982;37:141–147.

27. Kreiss K. Studies on populations exposed to polychlorinated biphenyls. Environ Health Perspect 1985;60:193–199.

28. Mack GA, Mohadjer L. Baseline estimates and time trends for beta-benzene hexachloride, hexachlorobenzene, and polychlorinated biphenyls in human adipose tissue 1970–1983. Washington: United States Environmental Protection Agency, Office of Toxic Substances, Exposure Evaluation Division, 1985:i.

29. Chase KC, Wong O, Thomas D, Berney BW, Simon RK. Clinical and metabolic abnormalities associated with occupational exposure to polychlorinated biphenyls (PCBs). J Occup Med 1982;24(2):109–114.

30. Mes J. PCBs in human populations. In: Waid JS, ed. PCBs and the environment. Boca Raton, FL: CRC Press, 1987:39–61.

31. Smith AB, Schloemer J, Lowry LK, et al. Metabolic and health consequences of occupational exposure to polychlorinated biphenyls. Br J Ind Med 1982;39:361–369.

32. Emmett EA, Maroni M, Schmith JM, Levin BK, Jefferys J. Studies of transformer repair workers exposed to PCBs: I. study design, PCB concentrations, questionnaire, and clinical examination results. Am J Ind Med 1988;13:415–427.

33. Wolff MS, Thornton J, Fischbein A, Lilis R, Selikoff IJ. Disposition of polychlorinated biphenyl congeners in occupationally exposed persons. Toxicol Appl Pharmacol 1982;62:294–306.

34. Brown Jr JF, Lawton RW. Polychlorinated biphenyl (PCB) partitioning between adipose tissue and serum. Bull Environ Contam Toxicol 1984;33:277–280.

35. Schnellmann RG, Putnam CW, Sipes IG. Metabolism of 2,2′,3,3′,6,6′-hexachlorobiphenyl and 2,2′,4,4′,5,5′-hexachlorobiphenyl by human hepatic microsomes. Biochem Pharmacol 1983;32(21):3233–3239.

36. Steele G, Stehr-Green P, Welty E. Estimates of the biological half-life of polychlorinated biphenyls in human serum. N Engl J Med 1986;314:926–927.

37. Yakushiji T, Watanabe I, Kuwabara K, et al. Rate of decrease and half-life of polychlorinated biphenyls (PCBs) in the blood of mothers and their children occupationally exposed to PCBs. Arch Environ Contam Toxicol 1984;13:341–345.

38. Chen PH, Luo ML. Comparative rates of elimination of some individual polychlorinated biphenyls from the blood of PCB-poisoned patients in Taiwan. Food Chem Toxicol 1982;20:417–425.

39. Allen JR, Carstens LA, Barsotti DA. Residual effects of short-term, low-level exposure of nonhuman primates to polychlorinated biphenyls. Toxicol Appl Pharmacol 1974;30:440–451.

40. Allen JR, Abrahamson LJ, Norback DH. Biological effects of polychlorinated biphenyls and triphenyls on the subhuman primate. Environ Res 1973;6:344–354.

41. Seegal RF, Bush B, Brosch KO. Polychlorinated biphenyls induce regional changes in brain norepinephrine concentrations in adult rats. Neurotoxicology 1985;6(3):13–24.

42. Rosin DL, Martin BR. Neurochemical and behavioral effects of polychlorinated biphenyls in mice. Neurotoxicology 1981;2:749–764.

43. Bowman RE, Heironimus MP. Hypoactivity in adolescent monkeys perinatally exposed to PCBs and hyperactive as juveniles. Neurobehav Toxicol Teratol 1981;3:15–18.

44. Bowman RE, Heironimus MP, Barsotti DA. Locomotor hyperactivity in PCB-exposed rhesus monkeys. Neurotoxicology 1981;2:251–268.

45. Bowman RE, Heironimus MP, Allen JR. Correlation of PCB body burden with behavioral toxicology in monkeys. Pharmacol Biochem Behav 1978;9:49–56.

46. Tilson HA, Davis GJ, McLachlan JA, Lucier GW. The effects of polychlorinated biphenyls given prenatally on the neurobehavioral development of mice. Environ Res 1979;18:466–474.

47. Smialowicz RJ, Andrews JE, Riddle MM, Rogers RR, Luebke RW, Copeland CB. Evaluation of the immunotoxicity of low level PCB exposure in the rat. Toxicology 1989;56:197–211.

48. Loose LD, Pittman KA, Benitz K-F, Silkworth JB. Polychlorinated biphenyl and hexachlorobenzene induced humoral immunosuppression. J Reticuloendothel Soc 1977;22(3):253–271.

49. Bonnyns M, Bastomsky CH. Polychlorinated biphenyl-induced modi-

fication of lymphocyte response to plant mitogens in rats. Experientia 1976;32:522–523.

50. Hori S, Obana H, Kashimoto T, et al. Effect of polychlorinated biphenyls and polychlorinated quaterphenyls in cynomolgus monkey (Macaca fascicularis). Toxicology 1982;24:123–139.

51. Smith SH, Sanders VM, Barrett BA, Borzelleca JF, Munson AE. Immunotoxicological evaluation on mice exposed to polychlorinated biphenyls. Toxicol Appl Pharmacol 1978;45(1):330.

52. Vos JG, Driel-Grootenhuis LV. PCB-induced suppression of the humoral and cell-mediated immunity in guinea pigs. Sci Total Environ 1972;1:289–302.

53. Vos JG, Roij ThD. Immunosuppressive activity of a polychlorinated biphenyl preparation on the humoral immune response in guinea pigs. Toxicol Appl Pharmacol 1972;21:549–555.

54. Thomas PT, Hinsdill RD. Effect of polychlorinated biphenyls on the immune responses of rhesus monkeys and mice. Toxicol Appl Pharmacol 1978;44:41–51.

55. Thomas PT, Hinsdill RD. Perinatal PCB exposure and its effect on the immune system of young rabbits. Ann NY Acad Sci 1980;3:173–184.

56. Loose LD, Pittman KA, Benitz K-F, Mueller W. Impaired host resistance to endotoxin and malaria in polychlorinated biphenyl- and hexachlorobenzene-treated mice. Infect Immun 1978;20:30–35.

57. Imanishi J, Oku T, Oishi K, Kishida T, Nomura H, Mizutani T. Reduced resistance to experimental viral and bacterial infections of mice treated with polychlorinated biphenyl. Biken J 1984;27:195–198.

58. Silkworth JB, Grabstein EM. Polychlorinated biphenyl immunotoxicity: dependence on isomer planarity and the Ah gene complex. Toxicol Appl Pharmacol 1982;65:109–115.

59. Silkworth JB, Antrim L, Kaminsky LS. Correlations between polychlorinated biphenyl immunotoxicity, the aromatic hydrocarbon locus, and liver microsomal enzyme induction in C57BL/6 and DBA/2 mice. Toxicol Appl Pharmacol 1984;75:156–165.

60. Silkworth JB, Antrim L, Sack G. Ah receptor mediated suppression of the antibody response in mice is primarily dependent on the Ah phenotype of lymphoid tissue. Toxicol Appl Pharmacol 1986;86:380–390.

61. Kimbrough RD, Squire RA, Linder RE, Strandberg JD, Montali RJ, Burse VW. Induction of liver tumors in Sherman strain female rats by polychlorinated biphenyl Aroclor 1260. J Natl Cancer Inst 1975;55:1453–1459.

62. Norback DH, Weltman RH. Polychlorinated biphenyl induction of hepatocellular carcinoma in the Sprague-Dawley rat. Environ Health Perspect 1985;60:97–105.

63. Schaeffer E, Greim H, Goessner W. Pathology of chronic polychlorinated biphenyl (PCB) feeding in rats. Toxicol Appl. Pharmacol 1984;75:278–288.

64. Jones DCL. Bioassay of Aroclor 1254 for possible carcinogenicity. Washington, DC: National Institutes of Health, 1978:1.

65. Ito N, Nagasaki H, Makiura S, Arai M. Histopathological studies on liver tumorigenesis in rats treated with polychlorinated biphenyls. Gann 1974;65:545–549.

66. Kimbrough RD, Linder RE, Gaines TB. Morphological changes in livers of rats fed polychlorinated biphenyls. Arch Environ Health 1972;25:354–364.

67. Kimura NT, Baba T. Neoplastic changes in the rat liver induced by polychlorinated biphenyl. Gann 1973;64:105–108.

68. Oesterle D, Deml E. Promoting effect of polychlorinated biphenyls on development of enzyme-altered islands in livers of weaning and adult rats. J Cancer Res Clin Oncol 1983;105:141–147.

69. Makiura S, Aoe H, Sugihara S, Hirao K, Arai M, Ito N. Inhibitory effect of polychlorinated biphenyls on liver tumorigenesis in rats treated with 3′-methyl-4-dimethylaminoazobenzene, N-2-fluoroenylacetamide, and diethynitrosamine. J Natl Cancer Inst 1974;53:1233.

70. Nishizumi M. Effect of phenobarbital, dichlorodiphenyltrichloroethane, and polychlorinated biphenyls on diethylnitrosamine-induced hepatocarcinogenesis. Gann 1979;835–837.

71. Nishizumi M. Radioautographic evidence for absorption of polychlorinated biphenyls through the skin. Ind Health 1876;14:41–44.

72. Nishizumi M. Reduction of diethylnitrosamine-induced hepatoma in rats exposed to polychlorinated biphenyls through their dams. Gann 1980;71:910–912.

73. Deml E, Oesterle D, Wiebel FJ. Benzo[a]pyrene initiates enzyme-altered islands in the liver of adult rats following single pretreatment and promotion with polychlorinated biphenyls. Cancer Lett 1983;19:301–304.

74. Yoshimura H, Yoshihara S, Koga N, et al. Inductive effect on hepatic enzymes and toxicity of congeners of PCBs and PCDFs. Environ Health Perspect 1985;59:113–119.

75. Alvares AP, Kappas A. Heterogeneity of cytochrome P-450s induced by polychlorinated biphenyls. J Biol Chem 1977;252:6373–6378.

76. Preston BD, Van Miller JP, Moore RW, Allen JR. Promoting effects of polychlorinated biphenyls (Aroclor 1254) and polychlorinated dibenzofuran-free Aroclor 1254 on diethylnitrosamine-induced tumorigenesis in a rat. J Natl Cancer Inst 1981;66:509–515.

77. Pereira MA, Herren SL, Britt AL, Khoury MM. Promotion by polychlorinated biphenyls of enzyme altered foci rat liver. Cancer Lett 1982;15:185–190.

78. Oesterle D, Deml E. Dose-dependent promoting effect of polychlorinated biphenyls on enzyme-altered islands in livers of adult and weanling rats. Carcinogenesis 1984;5:351–355.

79. Kimura NT, Kanematsu T, Baba T. Polychlorinated biphenyls as a promotor in experimental hepatocarcinogenesis in rats. Z Krebsforsch 1976;87:257–266.

80. Hayes MA, Roberts E, Safe SH, Farber E, Cameron RG. Influences of different polychlorinated biphenyls on cytocidal, mitoinhibitory, and nodule-selecting activities of N-2-fluorenylacetamide in rat liver. J Natl Cancer Inst 1986;76:683–691.

81. Hori M, Fujita K, Yamashiro K, et al. Influences of polychlorinated biphenyls (PCB) and PCB-like chemicals on 20-methylcholanthrene-induced mouse skin carcinogenesis. Fukuoka Acta Med 1985;76:92–98.

82. Kerkvliet NI, Kimeldorf DJ. Antitumor activity of a polychlorinated biphenyl mixture, Aroclor 1254, in rats inoculated with Walker 256 carcinosarcoma cells. J Natl Cancer Inst 1977;59(3):951.

83. Buchmann A, Kunz W, Wolf CR, Oesch F, Robertson LW. Polychlorinated biphenyls, classified as either phenobarbital- or 3-methylcholanthrene type inducers of cytochrome P-450, are both hepatic tumor promoters in diethylnitrosamine-initiated rats. Cancer Lett 1986;32:243–253.

84. Kornbrust D, Dietz D. Aroclor 1254 pretreatment effects on DNA repair in rat hepatocytes elicited by in vivo or in vitro exposure of various chemicals. Environ Mutagen 1985; 1985;7:857–870.

85. Gillette DM, Corey RD, Helferich WG, et al. Comparative toxicology of tetrachlorobiphenyls in mink and rats. Fundam Appl Toxicol 1987;8:5–14.

86. Tryphonas L, Charbonneau S, Tryphonas H, et al. Comparative aspects of aroclor 1254 toxicity in adult cynomolgus and rhesus monkeys: a pilot study. Arch Environ Contam Toxicol 1986;15:159–169.

87. Ouw HE, Simpson GR, Siyali DS. Use and health effects of Aroclor 1242, a polychlorinated biphenyl, in an electrical industry. Arch Environ Health 1976;31:189–194.

88. Good CK. A cutaneous eruption in marine electricians due to certain chlorinated naphthalenes and diphenyls. Arch Dermatol Syphil 1943;48:251–257.

89. Fischbein A, Rizzo JN, Solomon SJ, Wolff MS. Oculodermatological findings in workers with occupational exposure to polychlorinated biphenyls (PCBs). Br J Ind Med 1985;42:126–130.

90. Baker EL, Landrigan PJ, Glueck CJ, et al. Metabolic consequences of exposure to polychlorinated biphenyls (PCB) in sewage sludge. Am J Epidemiol 1980;112:553–563.

91. Lawton RW, Ross MR, Feingold J, Brown Jr JF. Effects of PCB exposure on biochemical and hematological findings in capacitor workers. Environ Health Perspect 1985;60:165–184.

92. Emmett EA, Maroni M, Jefferys J, Schmith J, Levin BK, Alvares A. Studies of transformer repair workers exposed to PCBs: II. Results of clinical laboratory investigations. Am J Ind Med 1988;14:47–62.

93. Maroni M, Colombi A, Arbosti G, Cantoni S, Foa V. Occupational exposure to polychlorinated biphenyls in electrical workers. II. Health Effects. Br J Ind Med 1981;38:55–60.

94. Alvares AP, Fischbein A, Anderson KE, Kappas A. Alterations in drug metabolism in workers exposed to polychlorinated biphenyls. Clin Pharmacol Ther 1977;22(2):140–146.

95. Kreiss K, Zack MM, Kimbrough RD, Needham LL, Smrek AL, Jones BT. Cross-sectional study of a community with exceptional exposure to DDT. JAMA 1981;245:1926–1930.

96. Emmett EA. Polychlorinated biphenyl exposure and effects in transformer repair workers. Environ Health Perspect 1985;60:185–192.

97. Guo YL, Emmett EA, Pellizzari ED, Rohde CA. Influence of serum cholesterol and albumin on partitioning of PCB congeners between human serum and adipose tissue. Toxicol Appl Pharmacol 1987;87:48–56.

98. Brown DP. Mortality of workers exposed to polychlorinated biphenyls—an update. Arch Environ Health 1987;42:333–339.

99. Bertazzi PA, Riboldi L, Pesatori A, Radice L, Zocchetti C. Cancer mortality of capacitor manufacturing workers. Am J Ind Med 1987;11:165–176.

100. Gustavsson P, Hogstedt C, Rappe C. Short-term mortality and cancer incidence in capacitor manufacturing workers exposed to polychlorinated biphenyls (PCBs). Am J Ind Med 1986;10:341–344.

101. Fischbein A, Wolff MS, Lilis R, Thornton J, Selikoff IJ. Clinical

findings among PCB-exposed capacitor manufacturing workers. Ann NY Acad Sci 1979;320:703–715.

102. Takamatsu M, Oki M, Maeda K, Inoue Y, Hirayama H, Yoshizuka K. PCBs in blood of workers exposed to PCBs and their health status. Am J Ind Med 1984;5:59–68.

103. Stehr-Green PA, Welty E, Steele G, Steinberg K. Evaluation of potential health effects associated with serum polychlorinated biphenyl levels. Environ Health Perspect 1986;70:255–259.

104. Stehr-Green PA, Ross D, Liddle J. A pilot study of serum polychlorinated biphenyl levels in persons at high risk of exposure in residential and occupational environments. Arch Environ Health 1986;41:240–244.

105. Acquavella JF, Hanis NM, Nicolich MJ, Phillips SC. Assessment of clinical, metabolic, dietary, and occupational correlations with serum polychlorinated biphenyl levels among employees at an electrical capacitor manufacturing plant. J Occup Med 1986;28:1177–1180.

106. Kreiss K, Zack MM, Kimbrough RD, Needham LL, Smrek AL, Jones BT. Association of blood pressure and polychlorinated biphenyl levels. JAMA 1981;245:2505–2509.

107. Akagi K, Okumura M. Association of blood pressure and PCB level in Yusho patients. Environ Health Perspect 1985;59:37–39.

108. Warshaw R, Fischbein A, Thornton J, Miller A, Selikoff IJ. Decrease in vital capacity in PCB-exposed workers in a capacitor manufacturing facility. Ann NY Acad Sci 1979;320:277–283.

109. Lawton RW, Ross MR, Feingold J. Spirometric findings in capacitor workers occupationally exposed to polychlorinated biphenyls (PCBs). J Occup Med 1986;28:453–456.

110. Fein GG, Jacobson JL, Jacobson SW, Schwartz PM, Dowler JK. Prenatal exposure to polychlorinated biphenyls: effects on birth size and gestational age. J Pediatr 1984;105:315–320.

111. Gladen B, Rogan WJ, Hardy P, Thullen J, Tingelstad J, Tully M. Development after exposure to polychlorinated biphenyls and dichlorodiphenyl dichloroethene transplacentally and through human milk. J Pediatr 1988;113:991–995.

112. Taylor PR, Stelma JM, Lawrence CE. The relation of polychlorinated biphenyls to birth weight and gestational age in the offspring of occupationally exposed mothers. Am J Epidemiol 1989;129:395–406.

113. Rogan WJ, Gladen BC, McKinney JC, et al. Polychlorinated biphenyls (PCBs) and dichlorodiphenyl dichloroethene (DDE) in human milk: effects on growth, morbidity, and duration of lactation. Am J Public Health 1987;77:1294–1297.

114. Ron M, Cucos B, Rosenn B, Hochner-Celnikier D, Hadani-Ever P, Pines A. Maternal and fetal serum levels of organochlorine compounds in cases of premature rupture of membranes. Acta Obstet Gynecol Scand 1988;67:695–697.

115. Wong C, Chen C, Cheng P, Chen P. Mucocutaneous manifestations of polychlorinated biphenyls (PCB) poisoning: a study of 122 cases in Taiwan. Br J Dermatol 1982;107:317–323.

116. Lu Y, Wong P. Dermatological, medical, and laboratory findings of patients in Taiwan and their treatments. Am J Ind Med 1984;5:81–115.

117. Chia L, Chu F. Neurological studies on polychlorinated biphenyl (PCB)-poisoned patients. Am J Ind Med 1984;5:117–126.

118. Kunita N, Kashimoto T, Miyata H, Fukushima S, Hori S, Obana H. Causal agents of Yusho. Am J Ind Med 1984;5:45–58.

119. Kashimoto T, Miyata H, Kunita S, et al. Role of polychlorinated dibenzofuran in Yusho (PCB poisoning). Arch Environ Health 1981;36(6):321–326.

120. Masuda Y, Yoshimura H. Polychlorinated biphenyls and dibenzofurans in patients with Yusho and their toxicological significance: a review. Am J Ind Med 1984;5:31–44.

121. Nagayama J, Masuda Y, Kuratsune M. Determination of polychlori-

nated dibenzofurans in tissues of patients with 'Yusho.' Food Cosmet Toxicol 1977;15:195–198.

122. Kashimoto T, Miyata H, Kunita N. The presence of polychlorinated quaterphenyls in the tissues of Yusho victims. Food Cosmet Toxicol 1981;19:335–340.

123. Wong A, Basrur P, Safe S. The metabolically mediated DNA damage and subsequent DNA repair by 4-chlorobiphenyl in Chinese hamster ovary cells. Res Commun Chem Pathol Pharmacol 1979;24:543.

124. Morales NM, Matthews HB. In vivo binding of 2,3,6,2′,3′,6′-hexachlorobiphenyls and 2,4,5,2′,4′,5′-hexachlorobiphenyls to mouse liver macromolecules. Chem Biol Interact 1979;27:99–110.

125. Anderson HA, Lilis R, Selikoff IJ, Rosenman KD, Freedman S, Valciukas JA. Unanticipated prevalence of symptoms among dairy farmers in Michigan and Wisconsin. Environ Health Perspect 1978;23:217–226.

126. Bahn AK, Mills JL, Snyder PJ, et al. Hypothyroidism in workers exposed to polybrominated biphenyls. N Engl J Med 1980;302(1):31–33.

127. Bekesi JG, Roboz JP, Fischbein A, Mason P. Immunotoxicology: environmental contamination by polybrominated biphenyls and immune dysfunction among residents of the state of Michigan. Cancer Detect Prev Suppl 1987;1:29–37.

128. Silva J, Kauffman CA, Simon DG, et al. Lymphocyte function in human exposed to polybrominated biphenyls. J Reticuloendothel Soc 1979;26:341–347.

129. Kimbrough RD, Groce DF, Korver MP, Burse VW. Induction of liver tumors in femal sherman strain rats by polybrominated biphenyls. J Natl Cancer Inst 1981;66(3):535–540.

130. Sleight S. Effects of PCBs and related compounds on hepatocarcinogenesis in rats and mice. Environ Health Perspect 1985;60:35–39.

131. Environmental Protection Agency. Health assessment document for chlorinated benzenes—final report. Washington, DC: EPA Publication, 1985.

132. Stewart FP, Smith AG. Metabolism of the "mixed" cytochrome P-450 inducer hexachlorbenzene by rat liver microsomes. Biochem Pharmacol 1986;35:2163–2170.

133. Stewart FP, Smith AG. Metabolism and covalent binding of hexachlorobenzene by isolated male and female rat hepatocytes. Biochem Pharmacol 1987;36:2232–2234.

134. Tanaka A, Sato M, Tsuchiya T, Adachi T, Niimura T, Yamaha T. Excretion, distribution, and metabolism of 1,2,4-trichlorobenzene in rats. Arch Toxicol 1986;59:82–88.

135. Ommen BV, Adang AEP, Brader L, Posthumus MA, Muller F, Van Bladeren PJ. The microsomal metabolism of hexachlorobenzene. Biochem Pharmacol 1986;35:3233–3238.

136. Environmental Protection Agency. Broad scan analysis of FY82 -NHATS specimen vol II volatile organic compounds. In: EPA, ed. EPA-560/5-86-035-039. Washington, DC: EPA, 1986.

137. Burton MAS, Bennett BG. Exposure of man to environmental hexachlorobenzene (HCB)—an exposure commitment assessment. Sci Total Environ 1987;66:137–146.

138. Peters H, Cripps D, Gocmen A, Bryan G, Erturk E, Morris C. Turkish epidemic hexachlorobenzene porphyria. Ann NY Acad Sci 1986;514:183–190.

139. Zapata-Gayon C, Zapata-Gayon N, Gonzalez-Angulo A. Clastogenic chromosomal aberrations in 26 individuals accidently exposed to ortho dichlorobenzene vapors in the national medical center in Mexico City. Arch Environ Health 1982;37:231–235.

140. Kiraly J, Szentesi I, Ruzicska M, Czeize A. Chromosome studies in workers producing organophosphate insecticides. Arch Environ Contam Toxicol 1979;8:309–319.

141. Brusick DJ. Genotoxicity of hexachlorobenzene and other chlorinated benzenes (Abstract). Sci Pub 1985(77):393–397.

66

Polychlorodibenzodioxins and Polychlorodibenzofurans

John S. Andrews, Jr., M.D., M.P.H.

CHEMICAL AND PHYSICAL DESCRIPTION

Polychlorinated dibenzo-para-dioxins (dibenzo-p-dioxins or PCDDs) and polychlorinated dibenzofurans (PCDFs) each have a triple-ring structure as a nucleus. In PCDDs, two benzene rings are connected through a pair of oxygen atoms. In PCDFs, two benzene rings are connected through an oxygen atom and a carbon-to-carbon bond. A chlorine atom may be substituted for hydrogen on any carbon atom in the two benzene rings. Theoretically, 75 different PCDDs and 135 different PCDFs are possible. The general structures of these compounds and the numbering of their atoms are shown in Figure 66.1.

The chemical names of these compounds depend on the number and location of the chlorine atom substitutions for hydrogen atoms. The common name for the PCDDs is dioxins and the common name for PCDFs is furans, but from a toxicologic point of view there is a need to indicate the number and location of the chlorine atom substitutions because the toxicity in animals differs greatly from compound to compound. For example, the 2,3,7,8-tetrachlorodibenzo-p-dioxin (2,3,7,8-TCDD), which is the most toxic of the known congeners in animals, is an unusual molecule because it is symmetrical across both the horizontal and the vertical axes. It is a very stable, lipophilic compound that lacks reactive functional groups.

PCDDs and PCDFs may exist in relatively pure form, as contaminants of other products, and as contaminants adhering to particulates. None of these compounds is known to be made by living organisms. Because of the high lipid solubility of these compounds, they are easily incorporated into the lipid-containing tissues of fish, animals, and humans.

These compounds exist as solids at room temperature.

SITES AND MECHANISMS ASSOCIATED WITH EXPOSURE

Occurrence and Control in the Environment

These chemicals are not produced for commercial purposes, but chlorinated dibenzo-p-dioxins and chlorinated dibenzofur-ans occur as trace contaminants in several chemical processes, primarily during the synthesis of chlorinated phenols; for example, 2,3,7,8-TCDD is a byproduct in the synthesis of 2,4,5-trichlorophenol, an intermediate compound formed during the production of 2,4,5-trichlorophenoxyacetic acid and hexachlorophene. Trace levels of PCDDs and PCDFs are also formed during the bleaching of wood pulp to make white paper and white paper products, the incineration of chlorine-containing waste materials, and the combustion of leaded gasoline. PCDDs have also been found in cigarette smoke (1).

The Environmental Protection Agency (EPA) has listed dioxin-containing wastes as acute hazardous wastes, defined as "wastes that are so hazardous that they may, either through acute or chronic exposure, cause or significantly contribute to an increase in serious-irreversible or incapacitating-reversible illness regardless of how they are managed" (2, 3). Effective November 8, 1986, EPA has prohibited further land disposal of certain dioxin-containing hazardous wastes (3, 4).

Mechanisms and Processes Leading to Exposure

PCDDs and PCDFs have entered the environment by a variety of means, including the use of herbicides, bleaching, incineration, and combustion. Once there, they are remarkably stable, and many of these compounds, especially those that are substituted with chlorine at the 2,3,7,8 carbon positions, bioaccumulate in the human food chain. Sources of dioxin include food, milk (including human milk), air, the pesticide 2,4,5-trichlorophenoxyacetic acid, and dust that has been contaminated with PCDDs or PCDFs from waste disposal or incineration. PCDDs and PCDFs are not very water-soluble, but they tend to attach to particles. For these reasons, they are not often found in significant amounts in groundwater, surface water, or drinking water. However, due to the variety and ubiquitous sources of small amounts of PCDDs and PCDFs, these compounds can be found at parts per trillion levels in the lipid-

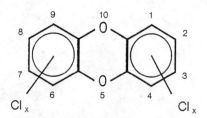

Polychlorinated Dibenzo-*p*-dioxins

Polychlorinated Dibenzofurans

Figure 66.1. General structures of polychlorinated dibenzo-p-dioxins (PCDDs) and polychlorinated dibenzofurans (PCDFs). The carbon atoms are numbered using standard nomenclature. Chlorine atoms (Cl$_x$) may be substituted for hydrogen atoms at any of the numbered carbon atoms.

containing tissues of humans, especially of persons living in industrialized countries (5–8).

CLINICAL TOXICOLOGY OF EXPOSURE

Route of Exposure (Ingestion, Inhalation, and Dermal Absorption)

Ingestion, inhalation, and dermal absorption are all thought to be routes of exposure to PCDDs and PCDFs. However, exposure for most individuals will be small, will come from a variety of sources, and will come through a variety of exposure routes. It is generally accepted that about 98% of human exposure comes from food (9). Exposure has also occurred from the use of hexachlorophene, from herbicide use, from exposure to PCDD- and PCDF-containing industrial wastes, and from industrial and transportation incidents. In occupational settings, exposure has occurred in chemical manufacturing processes and from handling the wastes from these processes.

Absorption

Data are incomplete on the absorption of PCDDs and PCDFs in humans from various routes of exposure. However, one animal study has shown that bioavailability is strongly influenced by the matrix in which the compound occurs (10). Although the absorption of 2,3,7,8-TCDD from the oily soil at Times Beach, Missouri, was shown to be greater than 50%, absorption from the nonoily New Jersey soil was less than 1% (11). Nonetheless, many risk assessments assume 100% absorption, which introduces a safety factor.

Metabolism

Little is known about the metabolism of these compounds in mammalian systems. The half-life of some of these compounds in humans can be measured not in hours, days, weeks, or months, but in years. Some animal studies of 2,3,7,8-TCDD have shown that a large proportion of the administered compound persists in an unmetabolized form in the liver, suggesting that toxicity is due to the compound itself and not a metabolite (12). Other metabolic studies in various species have shown that 2,3,7,8-TCDD gives rise to monohydroxy, dihydroxy, and monomethoxy metabolites. Administration of these metabolites from dogs to guinea pigs showed that the metabolites were at least 100 times less acutely toxic than 2,3,7,8-TCDD itself (13).

Elimination

Elimination of these compounds is generally assumed to occur slowly by loss of the lipid-containing materials to which the PCDDs and PCDFs are attached. The half-life of 2,3,7,8-TCDD in humans has been shown in two studies to be 7 years or more (14, 15); the primary route of elimination was the feces (15). McNulty et al. reported the half-life in the monkey to be 1 year (16). Rates of elimination of 2,3,7,8-TCDD in small animals following a single dose was found to range from 11 days (mouse) to 30 days (guinea pig) (17, 18).

SIGNS, SYMPTOMS, AND SYNDROMES OF TOXIC EXPOSURE

Acute Toxicity

The most toxic of these compounds that have been tested thus far in animals is 2,3,7,8-TCDD. Using 2,3,7,8-TCDD as a reference, the toxicity of the chlorinated dibenzo-p-dioxins and dibenzofurans decreases with both a decreasing and an increasing number of chlorine atoms. Compounds with chlorine substitutions at the 2,3,7,8 positions in each isomer group are the most toxic.

TARGET ORGAN TOXICITY

The most prominent acute manifestation of toxicity that has been shown in humans is chloracne, an acne-like condition that takes months or years to disappear (19–22). Clinically, this skin lesion is characterized by hyperplasia and hyperkeratosis of the interfollicular epidermis, hyperkeratosis of the sebaceous follicles, and squamous metaplasia of the sebaceous glands that form cysts and keratinaceous comedones in a typical distribution (23). Data are not yet available to determine the amount, route, or duration of exposure that is necessary to cause chloracne. Serum samples from exposed persons in Seveso, Italy, have shown that all children who had serum 2,3,7,8-TCDD levels greater than 11,000 parts per trillion (ppt) based on lipid content developed chloracne. A 16-year-old girl with serum levels of 800 ppt developed chloracne, whereas a 15-year-old boy with levels of 10,400 ppt did not. Chloracne was not seen in adults who had serum levels in the range of 1770–9140 ppt (24).

Other less consistently reported effects from dioxin exposure in humans include aesthenia, headaches, and pain in the extremities (22), peripheral neuropathy (25), ulcers (26), altered liver function (27), enzyme induction (28), altered lipid metabolism (29, 30), and abnormal urinary porphyrin patterns (31). Immune system dysfunction (32) and altered T-cell subsets (33, 34) have been reported by some investigators but have not been found by others (35, 36). Epidemiologic studies have shown an increase, associated with 2,3,7,8-TCDD exposure, in several liver enzymes, but these increases did not exceed what are considered normal values for these enzymes, and they disappeared over several years (37).

However, 2,3,7,8-TCDD has been shown to be extremely toxic in some animal species. For example, the range of oral LD_{50} in guinea pigs is 0.6–2.0 μg/kg (12), whereas in the hamster the LD_{50} is in the milligrams per kilogram range (3000 μg/kg). Other findings in animals include enzyme induction (38), altered liver function (39, 40), altered lipid metabolism (18, 41), porphyria (42, 43), and decreased thymus weight (44).

SYNDROMES

No syndromes associated with exposure to these polychlorinated compounds are known in humans. However, the most common finding after lethal exposure for animals is a loss of body weight and a "wasting away syndrome" (39). In Missouri, horses unintentionally exposed to 2,3,7,8-TCDD-contaminated waste oil exhibited a progressive deterioration in health including anorexia, listlessness, loss of body weight, dermatitis, emaciation, weakness, unsteady gait, and chronic cough (45). Similar findings were seen in dogs and cats (45).

Chronic and Longterm Effects

TARGET ORGAN EFFECTS

No specific chronic or longterm target organ effects are known in humans. In animals, 2,3,7,8-TCDD has been shown to be an inducer of microsomal enzymes and also to be immunotoxic (46). Doses as low as 0.25 μg/kg for 10 days in rats have been shown to be fetotoxic (47).

SYNDROMES

No syndromes from chronic exposure are known in humans.

TERATOGENESIS

The only teratogenic effect that has been suggested in humans is an increased prevalence of neural tube defects (48). However, 2,3,7,8-TCDD has been shown to be teratogenic in rats and mice (42, 49). In a study of birth defects carried out on 15,291 births in the Seveso, Italy, area from January 1, 1977, to December 31,1982 (50), 26 births were observed in the most highly contaminated area. None of the offspring showed any major structural defects, although two had mild defects (a female with a flat hemangioma 7 × 6 millimeters and a female with a small periurethral cyst). The data collected failed to demonstrate any increased risk of birth defects associated with 2,3,7,8-TCDD exposure, but the number of exposed pregnancies was small (2900 from exposed areas, of which only 461 were from the most highly contaminated areas). The results of a cytogenic study performed by Tenchini et al. on 25 induced abortions from women exposed to 2,3,7,8-TCDD showed no evidence of chromosomal aberrations (51).

CARCINOGENESIS

There is much debate about whether currently available data show that 2,3,7,8-TCDD is carcinogenic in humans. Two studies that are considered by some researchers to be important show a 5–7 times elevation in soft tissue sarcoma in persons with occupational exposure to phenoxy herbicides or chlorophenols (52, 53). These compounds were assumed to contain 2,3,7,8-TCDD. However, mortality studies of American Vietnam veterans who were exposed to 2,3,7,8-TCDD in Agent Orange have not shown any increase in carcinogenesis (54).

Although 2,3,7,8-TCDD has been shown to be carcinogenic in rats (0.1 μg/kg/day) and mice (0.5–2 μg/kg/week) (42, 55), these results do not resolve whether this compound acts as an initiator or a promoter. The majority of all carcinogenicity-type studies suggest that this compound is not genotoxic and that it is not likely, therefore, to be an initiator. However, no definite universal proof of this exists (56).

Management of Toxicity

CLINICAL EXAMINATION

Persons with recent exposure to PCDDs or PCDFs should have the chemicals removed from their skin as quickly as possible to prevent additional absorption of the compounds. Exposed persons should be asked for an exposure history, including onset of exposure, duration of exposure, and type of exposure.

Physical examinations, including a thorough examination of the skin, should be given. Routine blood and liver laboratory tests should be carried out. In most situations, however, evidence of exposure and disease relatable to the exposure will be lacking. Because chloracne is the only human effect documented thus far, no other specific abnormality can be considered pathognomonic for exposure.

TREATMENT

No specific treatments have been recommended for routine exposure.

LABORATORY DIAGNOSIS

No routine clinical test is available to measure PCDDs and PCDFs in sera or other human tissues.

SPECIAL DIAGNOSTIC TESTS

Serum levels of 2,3,7,8-TCDD and other PCDDs and PCDFs can be measured using gas chromatography/mass spectrometry (57, 58). Although in highly exposed persons 2,3,7,8-TCDD has been found in serum specimens as small as 1 milliliter, research laboratories usually need 250 milliliters of serum to give an accurate serum PCDD or PCDF level. These tests are currently expensive ($1000 or more) because much work must be done to rid specimens of interfering substances and considerable effort must be expended to ensure good quality control of the testing. The equipment necessary to test for these compounds in the parts per quadrillion range is also expensive, approaching $700,000.

BIOLOGIC MONITORING

There is no need to monitor persons for levels of PCDDs and PCDFs in their blood, serum, or adipose tissue unless they are thought to have been excessively exposed.

ENVIRONMENTAL MONITORING

Many laboratories can test soil, air, and water for PCDDs and PCDFs, but there is no evidence that routine environmental monitoring is indicated.

EXPOSURE LIMITS

No health advisories for levels of exposure to 2,3,7,8-TCDD are available. However, the EPA has said that a 10^{-4}–10^{-7} excess cancer risk exists (1 excess cancer case/10,000–10,000,000 persons) when 2.2×10^{-8}–2.2×10^{-11} mg/l of 2,3,7,8-TCDD is present in the water (59). The Food and Drug Administration (FDA) considers that no serious health concerns exist if levels in fish are below 25 ppt (3, 60). The National Institute for Occupational Safety and Health (NIOSH) considers 2,3,7,8-TCDD a potential occupational carcinogen that should be controlled to the fullest extent possible (3, 61). The EPA, the Centers for Disease Control (CDC), and the FDA have carried out risk assessments for 2,3,7,8-TCDD. The human intake values estimated by each agency as corresponding to an estimated cancer risk of 1×10^{-6} (1 excess cancer case/1,000,000 persons) are EPA, 6.4; CDC, 27.6, and FDA, 57.2

femtograms/kg/day (1,000,000,000,000,000 femtograms equals 1 gram) (3).

Toxic effects of PCDDs and PCDFs in humans are not so apparent. To detect any adverse effects, uniquely exposed populations have been examined. Several such incidents are described below.

Vietnam Veterans

During the period 1962–1970, the herbicide Agent Orange [a 1:1 mixture of 2,4-dichlorophenoxyacetic acid (2,4-D) and 2,4,5-trichlorophenoxyacetic acid (2,4,5-T) in diesel oil] was used as a defoliant in Vietnam. The herbicide was contaminated with from less than 1 to more than 20 ppm 2,3,7,8-TCDD (62). Many Vietnam veterans have expressed concern that their health may have been adversely affected by exposure to Agent Orange and its 2,3,7,8-TCDD contaminant. Several studies have been carried out. To date, these studies have not shown any specific pattern of disease that can be associated with 2,3,7,8-TCDD exposure. Analyses of serum samples from U.S. Army ground troops indicated that these troops were no more exposed to 2,3,7,8-TCDD in the Agent Orange than was a comparison group (62). However, preliminary results for U.S. Air Force members of Operation Ranch Hand indicate that some of them were unduly exposed (63). Results from studies of U.S. Air Force personnel who handled Agent Orange (Ranch Hand unit) have been reported (64, 65); follow-up studies are in progress. Analyses for 2,3,7,8-TCDD in serum samples from more than 900 of these personnel will be completed in 1990, at which time the relationship between findings of the physical examinations and Agent Orange exposure will be examined.

The states of Massachusetts (66) and New Jersey (67) are also conducting studies of Vietnam veterans. The Massachusetts study has reported results on 28 veterans and the New Jersey study, on 10 veterans. The results from both of these studies are similar to those found by the CDC and the U.S. Air Force (62, 63).

Occupational Exposure

PCDDs and PCDFs have been measured in persons with occupational exposure in several studies. In one study, 2,3,7,8-TCDD levels were measured in adipose tissue of exposed and unexposed persons in Missouri, some of whom had occupational exposure (8). In another study, levels of several PCDDs and PCDFs were measured in workers who had been exposed to 2,3,7,8-TCDD (68). NIOSH is carrying out an exposure and health effects study of 400 living workers who were employed at two plants in the United States that manufactured chemicals contaminated with 2,3,7,8-TCDD. An interim report on 143 of these workers and 54 control subjects has been presented (69). The laboratory measurements of PCDD and PCDF levels in all of the workers and control subjects for this study have been completed, and information on the correlation of the physical examination data and the measured PCDD and PCDF levels should be available in the near future.

Seveso, Italy

In July 1976, an explosion occurred at a factory in Meda, Italy, that produced 2,4,5-T, resulting in the contamination of parts of several nearby towns. Within 20 days of the explosion, Italian officials evacuated all families from the area immedi-

ately surrounding the explosion site and took measures to minimize exposure of nearby residents. Samples from a nearby resident who died from pancreatic adenocarcinoma unrelated to the explosion were found to contain, on a whole-weight basis, 6 ppt 2,3,7,8-TCDD in blood and 1840 ppt in adipose tissue (70). Recently, scientists at CDC tested 14 of the 30,000 serum samples that had been collected in 1976 from persons living in the nearby towns. Levels up to 27,800 ppt were measured on a lipid-adjusted basis (24). The potentially exposed populations and selected control subjects underwent physical examinations from 1976 to 1985. Although some liver function tests in some exposed groups showed slightly but significantly elevated activity, none of the groups had levels outside the normal range. Also, these differences disappeared over time (37). Thus, the only adverse, abnormal clinical finding has been chloracne (71). However, some adverse health effects, such as cancer, may have longer latency periods. Approximately 250 additional stored serum samples will be measured for 2,3,7,8-TCDD. These data will contribute to our knowledge of the half-life of 2,3,7,8-TCDD in men, women, and children; the extent of contamination surrounding the site; and the levels of 2,3,7,8-TCDD in persons who lived nearby.

ACKNOWLEDGMENTS

A special thanks to Dr. Charles Xintaras and Jeanne Bucsela who reviewed and edited drafts of this chapter. The preparation of this chapter was supported in part by funds from the Comprehensive Environmental Response, Compensation, and Liability Act (CERCLA) trust fund.

REFERENCES

1. Muto H, Takizawa Y. Dioxins in cigarette smoke. Arch Environ Health 1989;44:171–174.
2. Environmental Protection Agency. Hazardous waste management system: dioxin-containing wastes. Fed Reg 1985;50:1978-2006.
3. Agency for Toxic Substances and Disease Registry. Toxicological profile for 2,3,7,8-tetrachlorodibenzo-p-dioxin. Atlanta: Agency for Toxic Substances and Disease Registry, 1989.
4. Environmental Protection Agency. Hazardous waste management system: land disposal restrictions. Fed Reg 1986;51:40572–40677.
5. Schecter A, Ryan JJ, Gitlitz GL. Chlorinated dioxin and dibenzofuran levels in human adipose tissues from exposed and control populations. In: Rappe C, Choudhary G, Keith LH, eds. Chlorinated dioxins and dibenzofurans in perspective. Chelsea, MI: Lewis Publishers, 1986:51–65.
6. Ogaki J, Takayama K, Miyata H, Kashimoto T. Levels of PCDDs and PCDFs in human tissues and various foodstuffs in Japan. Chemosphere 1987;16:2047–2056.
7. Ryan JJ, Williams DT, Lau BP-Y, Sakuma T. Analysis of human fat tissue for 2,3,7,8-tetrachlorodibenzo-p-dioxin and chlorinated dibenzofuran residues. In: Keith LH, Choudhary G, Rappe C, eds. Chlorinated dioxins and dibenzofurans in the total environment II. Boston: Butterworth, 1984:205–214.
8. Andrews JS Jr, Garrett WA Jr, Patterson DG Jr, et al. 2,3,7,8-Tetrachlorodibenoz-p-dioxin levels in adipose tissues of persons with no known exposure and in exposed persons. Chemosphere 1989;18:499–506.
9. Beck H, Eckart K, Mathar W, Wittkowski R. PCDD and PCDF body burden from food intake in the Federal Republic of Germany. Chemosphere 1989;18:417–424.
10. Poiger H, Schlatter C. Influence of solvents and adsorbents on dermal and intestinal absorption of TCDD. Food Cosmet Toxicol 1980;18:477–481.
11. McConnell EE, Lucier GW, Rumbaugh RC, et al. Dioxin in soil: bioavailability after ingestion by rats and guinea pigs. Science 1984;223:1077–1079.
12. Esposito MP, Tiernan TO, Dryden FE. Dioxins. Washington, DC: Environmental Protection Agency, 1980; EPA publication no. EPA-600-2-80-197.
13. Poiger H, Weber H, Schlatter C. Special aspects of metabolism and kinetics of TCDD in dogs and rats. Assessment of toxicity of TCDD-metabolite(s) in guinea pigs. In: Hutzinger O, Frei RW, Merian E, Pocchiari F, eds. Chlorinated dioxins and related compounds. Impact on the environment. New York: Pergamon Press, 1982:317–325.

14. Pirkle JL, Wolfe WH, Patterson DG Jr, et al. Estimates of the half-life of 2,3,7,8-tetrachlorodibenzo-p-dioxin in Vietnam veterans of operation Ranch Hand. J Toxicol Environ Health 1989;27;165–71.

15. Poiger H, Schlatter C. Pharmocokinetics of 2,3,7,8-TCDD in man. Chemosphere 1986;15:1489–1494.

16. McNulty WP, Nielsen-Smith KA, Lay JO Jr, et al. Persistence of TCDD in monkey adipose tissue. Food Cosmet Toxicol 1982;20:985–986.

17. Gasiewicz TA, Olson JR, Geiger LE, Neal RA. Absorption, distribution and metabolism of 2,3,7,8-tetrachlorodibenzo-p-dioxin (TCDD) in experimental animals. In: Tucker RE, Young AL, Gray AP, eds. Human and environmental risks of chlorinated dioxins and related compounds. New York: Plenum Press, 1983:495–525.

18. Gasiewicz TA, Neal RA. 2,3,7,8-Tetrachlorodibenzo-p-dioxin tissue distribution, excretion, and effects on clinical parameters in guinea pigs. Toxicol Appl Pharmacol 1979;51:329–339.

19. Dunagin WG. Cutaneous signs of systemic toxicity due to dioxins and related chemicals. J Am Acad Dermatol 1984;10:688–700.

20. Crow KD. Chloracne and its potential clinical implications. Clin Exp Dermatol 1981;6:243–257.

21. Tindall JP. Chloracne and chloracnegens. J Am Acad Dermatol 1985;13:539–558.

22. Suskind RR. Chloracne and associated health problems in the manufacture of 2,4,5-T. In: Report to the Joint Conference of the National Institute of Environmental Health Sciences and International Agency for Research on Cancer. Lyon, France: World Health Organization, 1978.

23. Taylor JS. Environmental chloracne: update and overview. Ann NY Acad Sci 1979;320:295–307.

24. Centers for Disease Control. Preliminary report: 2,3,7,8-tetrachlorodibenzo-p-dioxin exposure to humans—Seveso, Italy. MMWR 1988;37:733–736.

25. Filippini G, Bordo B, Crenna P, Massetto N, Musicco M, Boeri R. Relationship between clinical and electrophysiological findings and indicators of heavy exposure to 2,3,7,8-tetrachlorodibenzo dioxin. Scand J Work Environ Health 1981;7:257–262.

26. Suskind RR, Hertzberg VS. Human health effects of 2,4,5-T and its toxic contaminants. JAMA 1984;251:2372–2380.

27. Poland AP, Smith D, Metter G, Possick P. A health survey of workers in a 2,4-D and 2,4,5-T plant with special attention to chloracne, porphyria cutanea tarda, and psychologic parameters. Arch Environ Health 1971;22:316–327.

28. Jaiswal AK, Nebert DW, Eisen HW. Comparison of aryl hydrocarbon hydroxylase and acetanilide 4-hydroxylase induction by polycyclic aromatic compounds in humans and mouse cell lines. Biochem Pharmacol 1985;34:2721–2731.

29. Oliver RM. Toxic effects of 2,3,7,8-tetrachlorodibenzo-1,4-dioxin in laboratory workers. Br J Ind Med 1975;32:49–53.

30. Axelson O. The health effects of phenoxy acid herbicides. In: Herrington JM, ed. Recent advances in occupational health. Edinburgh: Churchill Livingstone 1984:253–266.

31. Doss M, Sauer H, von Tieperman R, Colombi AM. Development of chronic hepatic porphyria (porphyria cutanea tarda) with inherited uroporphyrin decarboxylase deficiency under exposure to dioxin. Int J Biochem 1984:16:369–373.

32. Hoffman RE, Stehr-Green PA, Webb KB, et al. Health effects of long-term exposure to 2,3,7,8-tetrachlorodibenzo-p-dioxin. JAMA 1986;255:2031–2038.

33. Knutsen AP. Immunologic effects of TCDD exposure in humans. Bull Environ Contam Toxicol 1984;33:673–681.

34. Knutsen AP, Roodman ST, Evans RG, et al. Immune studies in dioxin-exposed Missouri residents: Quail Run. Bull Environ Contam Toxicol 1987;39:481–489.

35. Evans RG, Webb AP, Roodman ST, et al. A medical follow-up of the health effects of long-term exposure to 2,3,7,8-tetrachlorodibenzo-p-dioxin. Arch Environ Health 1988;43:273–278.

36. Webb KB, Evans RG, Knutsen AP, et al. Medical evaluation of subjects with known body levels of 2,3,7,8-tetrachlorodibenzo-p-dioxin. J Toxicol Environ Health 1989;28:183–93.

37. Mocarelli P, Marocchi A, Brambilla P, Gerthoux P, Young DS, Mantel N. Clinical laboratory manifestations of exposure to dioxin in children: a six-year study of the effects of an environmental disaster near Seveso, Italy. JAMA 1986;256:2687–95.

38. Poland A, Glover E. 2,3,7,8-Tetrachlorodibenzo-p-dioxin: a potent inducer of delta-aminolevulinic acid synthetase. Science 1973;179:476–477.

39. Courtney KD, Putnam JP, Andrews JE. Metabolic studies with TCDD (dioxin) treated rats. Arch Environ Contam Toxicol 1978;7:385–396.

40. Kociba R, Keyes DG, Beyer JE, Carreon RM, Gehring PJ. Long-term toxicologic studies of 2,3,7,8-tetrachlorodibenzo-p-dioxin (TCDD) in laboratory animals. Ann NY Acad Sci 1979;320:397–404.

41. Cunningham HM, Williams DT. Effect of tetrachlorodibenzo-p-dioxin on growth rate and the synthesis of lipids and proteins in rats. Bull Environ Contam Toxicol 1972;7:45-51.

42. Kociba RJ, Keyes DG, Beyer JE, et al. Results of a two-year chronic toxicity and oncogenicity study of 2,3,7,8-tetrachlorodibenzo-p-dioxin in rats. Toxicol Appl Pharmacol 1978;46:279–303.

43. Kociba RJ, Keeler PA, Park CN, Gehring PJ. 2,3,7,8-Tetrachlorodibenzo-p-dioxin (TCDD): results of a 13-week oral toxicity study in rats. Toxicol Appl Pharmacol 1976;35:553-574.

44. Vos JG, Moore JA. Suppression of cellular immunity in rats and mice by maternal treatment with 2,3,7,8-tetrachlorodibenzo-p-dioxin. Int Arch Allergy Appl Immunol 1974;47:777–794.

45. Case AA, Coffman JR. Waste oil: toxic for horses. Vet Clin North Am 1973;3:273–277.

46. Vos JG, Moore JA, Zinkl JG. Effect of 2,3,7,8-tetrachlorodibenzo-p-dioxin on the immune system of laboratory animals. Environ Health Perspect 1973;5:149–162.

47. Khera KS, Ruddick JA. Polychlorodibenzo-p-dioxins: Perinatal effects and the dominant lethal test in Wistar rats. Adv Chem Ser 1973;120:70–84.

48. Field B, Kerr C. Herbicide use and incidence of neural-tube defects. Lancet 1979;1:1341–1342.

49. Courtney KD, Moore JA. Teratology studies with 2,4,5-trichlorophenoxyacetic acid and 2,3,7,8-tetrachlorodibenzo-p-dioxin. Toxicol Appl Pharmacol 1971;20:396–403.

50. Mastroiacovo P, Spagnolo A, Marni E, Meazza L, Bertollini R, Segni G. Birth defects in the Seveso area after TCDD contamination. JAMA 1988;259:1668–1672.

51. Tenchini ML, Crimaudo C, Pacchetti G, Mottura A, Agosti S, De Carli L. A comparative cytogenetic study on cases of induced abortions in TCDD-exposed and nonexposed women. Environ Mutagen 1983;5:73–85.

52. Hardell L, Sandstrom A. Case-control study: soft tissue sarcomas and exposure to phenoxyacetic acids or chlorophenols. Br J Cancer 1979;39:711–717.

53. Ericksson M, Hardell L, Berg NO, Moller T, Axelson O. Soft-tissue sarcomas and exposure to chemical substances: a case-referent study. Br J Ind Med 1981;38:27–33.

54. Centers for Disease Control Vietnam Experience Study. Postservice mortality among Vietnam veterans. JAMA 1987;257:790–795.

55. National Toxicology Program (NTP). Carcinogenesis bioassay of 2,3,7,8-tetrachlorodibenzo-p-dioxin in Osborne-Mendel rats and B6C3F$_1$ mice (gavage study). Research Triangle Park, NC: National Toxicology Program, 1982; Technical Report Series no. 209 (NTP-80-31).

56. Shu HP, Paustenbach DJ, Murray FJ. A critical evaluation of the use of mutagenesis, carcinogenesis, and tumor promotion data in a cancer risk assessment of 2,3,7,8-tetrachlorodibenzo-p-dioxin. Regul Toxicol Pharmacol 1987;7:57–88.

57. Patterson DG Jr, Hampton L, Lapeza CR Jr, et al. High-resolution gas chromatographic/high-resolution mass spectrometric analysis of human serum on a whole-weight and lipid basis for 2,3,7,8-tetrachlorodibenzo-p-dioxin. Anal Chem 1987;59:2000–2005.

58. Nygren M, Hansson M, Sjostrom M, et al. Development and validation of a method for determination of PCDDs and PCDFs in human blood plasma. A multivariate comparison of blood and adipose tissue levels between Viet Nam veterans and matched controls. Chemosphere 1988;17:1663–1692.

59. Environmental Protection Agency. 2,3,7,8-Tetrachlorodibenzo-p-dioxins. Health advisory. Washington, DC: Office of Drinking Water, March 31, 1987.

60. Environmental Protection Agency. Health assessment document for polychlorinated dibenzo-p-dioxins. Washington, DC: Office of Health and Environmental Assessment, 1985; EPA report no. 600/8-84-014.

61. National Institute for Occupational Safety and Health. 2,3,7,8-Tetrachlorodibenzo-p-dioxin. Atlanta: U.S. Department of Health and Human Services, Public Health Service, Centers for Disease Control, National Institute for Occupational Safety and Health, 1984; Current intelligence bulletin 40.

62. Centers for Disease Control Veterans Health Studies Group. Serum 2,3,7,8-tetrachlorodibenzo-p-dioxin levels in US Army Vietnam-era veterans. JAMA 1988;260:1249–1254.

63. Centers for Disease Control. Serum 2,3,7,8-tetrachlorodibenzo-p-dioxin levels in Air Force health study participants—preliminary report. MMWR 1988;37:309–311.

64. Lathrop GD, Wolfe WH, Albanese RA, Moynahan PM. Air Force health study: An epidemiologic investigation of health effects in Air Force personnel following exposure to herbicides: Baseline morbidity study results. Brooks Air Force Base, TX: USAF School of Aerospace Medicine, 1984; National Technical Information Service no. AD-A-138-340.

65. Albanese RA. United States Air Force personnel and exposure to herbicide orange: interim report for period March 1984–February 1988. Brooks Air Force Base, TX: USAF School of Aerospace Medicine, 1988; USAFSAM-TR-88-3.

66. Schecter A, Constable J, Bangert JV. Isomer specific measurement of polychlorinated dibenzodioxin and dibenzofuran isomers in human blood from American Vietnam veterans two decades after exposure to Agent Orange. Chemosphere 1989;18:531–538.

67. Kahn PC, Gochfeld M, Nygren M, et al. Dioxins and dibenzofurans in blood and adipose tissue of agent orange-exposed Vietnam veterans and matched controls. JAMA 1988;259:1661–1667.

68. Patterson DG Jr, Fingerhut MA, Roberts DW, et al. Levels of polychlorinated dibenzo-p-dioxins and dibenzofurans in workers exposed to 2,3,7,8-tetrachlorodibenzo-p-dioxin. Am J Ind Med 1989;16:135–146.

69. Sweeney MH, Fingerhut MA, Patterson DG Jr, et al. Serum levels of 2,3,7,8-tetrachlorodibenzo-p-dioxin (2,3,7,8-TCDD) in New Jersey and Missouri chemical workers exposed to dioxin-contaminated processes: Interim report. Chemosphere 1990; in press.

70. Facchetti S, Fornari A, Montagna M. Distribution of 2,3,7,8-tetrachlorodibenzo-p-dioxin in the tissues of a person exposed to the toxic cloud at Seveso. Forensic Environ Appl 1981;1:1405–1414.

71. Caramaschi F, del Corno G, Favaretti C, Giambelluca SE, Montesarchio E, Fara GM. Chloracne following environmental contamination by TCDD in Seveso, Italy. Int J Epidemiol 1981;10:135–143.

67

Inorganic Acids and Bases

Christopher H. Linden, M.D.

SOURCES AND PRODUCTION

Definitions, Concepts, Common and Chemical Names

Acids and bases (or alkali) are classes of chemicals belonging to the more general category of substances known as corrosives or caustics. Inorganic (mineral) acids and inorganic bases, in contrast to their organic counterparts, do not contain carbon atoms. The term acid is derived from the Latin word for sour (acidis), which describes the taste of acidic compounds such as vinegar. Alkali is derived from the Arabic word for the ashes of a plant (al kali). A base was originally defined as a substance capable of reacting with an acid to form a neutral compound or salt.

The term corrosive originally referred to substances (primarily acids) which had the ability to attack (corrode) metals. It now denotes all compounds (acids, bases, and other classes of chemicals) which cause tissue injury as a result of nonspecific chemical reactions. Caustic, a term once used exclusively in reference to biologically toxic bases, is now considered synonymous with corrosive.

Knowledge of the chemistry of acids and bases is essential to understanding their toxicology. Only a brief review of relevant concepts is presented. The reader is referred to a basic chemistry text for further details.

The electrolytic dissociation theory, developed by Ostwald and Arrhenius in the 1880s, defines acids and bases as compounds that dissociate on solution in water to produce positively charged hydrogen ions (H^+ or protons) and negatively charged hydroxide ions (OH^-), respectively. A more comprehensive definition, proposed separately but almost simultaneous by both Bronsted and Lowry in 1923, defines an acid as a compound that has a tendency to donate (lose) a proton and a base as one that has a tendency to accept (gain) a proton.

Acids and bases can be classified as monobasic, dibasic, tribasic, etc., according to the number of dissociated H^+ or OH^- ions per molecule of the parent compound. A molar (M) solution contains one gram molecular weight of an acid or base per liter of water (or other solvent). Its normality (N), the number of gram equivalent weights of H^+ or OH^- in a liter, is 1 or more times the molarity depending on the basicity.

Acids and bases can also be classified according to their charge or lack of it. Molecular acids and bases are neutral (e.g., HCl, NaOH), cationic ones are positively charged (e.g., HSO_4^+), and anionic ones are negatively charged (e.g., HSO_4^-).

The acidity or alkalinity of a solution is commonly measured by one of two methods: determination of the pH or neutralization by titration. The pH, defined as the negative logarithm (base 10) of the H^+ ion concentration (pH = $-\log_{10} [H^+]$), can be calculated from the H^+ ion concentration (measured electrometrically by a hydrogen or glass electrode) or determined directly by an indicator dye which changes color at a known pH (e.g., litmus paper).

The pH of pure water is 7 at 25°C and defines a neutral pH. Solutions with a pH less than 7 are said to be acidic and those with a pH greater than 7 are considered basic. Solutions with extremes of pH (<2, >12) are said to be strongly acidic or strongly basic. Some common solutions and their pH values are shown in Table 67.1. It should be remembered that, because of the logarithmic transformation, solutions which differ by 1 pH unit have a 10-fold difference in H^+ ion concentration.

The second way to measure the acidity (or alkalinity) of an aqueous solution is to add incremental amounts of a known concentration (normality) of a strong acid or strong base (defined below) until a pH of 7 is reached. The number of equivalents of OH^- (or H^+) required for neutralization is called the titratable (or free) acidity or alkalinity. It represents the amount of acid or base (in charged or dissociated form) that is available for chemical reactions in a neutral solution.

Reactions between acids and bases can be expressed as equilibria with constants that define the position of the equilibrium. For the dissociation of an acid or base in water, the concentration of water is orders of magnitude higher than that of other reactants, and by convention, it is incorporated into the respective dissociation constants (K_a and K_b). In addition, since the extent of dissociation varies greatly between different acids and bases (K values range from less than 10^{-20} to more than 10^8), it is customary to express equilibrium constants in terms of their negative logarithm (base 10), the pK_a or pK_b. Loga-

Table 67.1. Approximate pH of Some Common Solutions

Solution	pH
Concentrated (37%) HCl	-1.1
1.0 M HCl	0
0.1 M HCl	1
0.01 M HCl	2
Gastric juice	1.2–3.0
Citrus juices	1.8–4
Carbonated beverages	2.5–3.5
Wines	2.8–3.8
Black coffee	5
Normal saline	5–5.5
Lactated Ringer's	6.5
Intracellular fluid	6.1–6.9
Distilled water	7.0
Blood	7.4
Interstitial fluid	7.4
Seawater	7.5
Tears	7.3–7.7
Bile	8
Limewater	10.5
Household ammonia	11.9
0.01 M NaOH	12
0.1 M NaOH	13
1 M NaOH	14
Saturated NaOH	15

rithmic transformation of equilibrium equations (i.e., the Henderson-Hasselbach equation) shows that the pK_a of an acid (or the pK_b of a base) is the pH (or pOH) at which equal concentrations of an acid (or base) and its conjugate or corresponding base (or acid) are present. The pK_a of a base is the pH at which equal concentrations of base and its conjugate acid are present, and it equals 14 minus the pK_b.

From a chemical perspective, strong acids and strong bases are those that are essentially completely dissociated in water. They have high dissociation constants (>1) and low (<0) or high (>14) pK_a values, respectively. Weak acids and conjugate acids of weak bases are incompletely dissociated in water, have intermediate dissociation constants, and have pK_a values between 0 and 14. Examples of each, in order of decreasing acid strength (increasing base strength) are shown in Table 67.2. Some common names for acids and bases are listed in Table 67.3.

Chemical Forms

Acids and bases exist as salts and anhydrides as well as in pure form. An acid or basic salt is a compound formed by replacing some, but not all, H^+ or OH^- ions of an acid or base by another ion or radical (e.g., $NaHSO_4$). An acid or basic anhydride is an oxide of a metalloid or a metal, respectively, which can combine with water to form an acid or base. In general, acid and basic salts and anhydrides have the same properties as the corresponding acid and base.

Chemical Reactions

Acids and bases, particularly the strong ones, are highly reactive compounds. With the exception of open reactions involving carbonic acid or bicarbonate, where the evolution of CO_2 gas results in cooling, reactions involving acids and bases generally produce heat. Neutralization reactions that involve strong acids and bases often produce large amounts of heat and can sometimes be violent. Similarly, the hydration of anhydrides tends to be highly exothermic (even explosive). The amount of heat generated when acids, bases, or their salts are added to water tends to be small but it can be great with the inverse (i.e., adding water to an acid or base), particularly when concentrated forms of strong acid or base are involved. When used as oxidizing or reducing agents, acids and bases may react violently with compounds or materials being treated. Acid reactions with metals may liberate hydrogen gas, potentially resulting in a fire or explosion. Hydrazine itself is highly flammable.

Chemical reactions involving acids are notorious for producing toxic gases. In addition, saturated or concentrated solutions of strong acids may release acid fumes, particularly when heated. Reactions involving aqueous solutions of the halogen acids may be accompanied by the evolution of a halogen gas (e.g., bromine, chlorine) as well as an acid gas. The actions of acids on sulfur-containing compounds (e.g., drain cleaning) may result in the liberation hydrogen sulfide and sulfur oxide gases. Reactions of acids with arsenic, phosphorous, and antimony compounds may liberate arsine (AsH_3), phosphine (PH_3), and stibine (SbH_3) gas, respectively. Mixing an acid with a cyanide salt can produce cyanide (HCN) gas. Combining bleach (sodium hypochlorite) with an acid may

Table 67.2 Inorganic Acids and Bases

Name	Chemical Formula	pK_a*
Strong acids (pK_a<0)		
Perchloric	$HClO_4$	
Permanganic	$HMnO_4$	
Bromic	$HBrO_3$	
Chloric	$HClO_3$	
Nitric	HNO_3	
Iodic	HIO_3	
Hydrobromic	HBr	
Hydrochloric	HCl	
Hydriodic	HI	
Sulfuric	H_2SO_4	
Pyrophosphoric	$H_4P_2O_7$	
Pyrosulfuric	$H_2S_2O_7$	
Chromic	CrO_3	
Weak acids		
Hypophosphoric	H_3PO_2	1.1
Periodic	HIO_4	1.6
Sulfurous	H_2SO_3	1.8
Sulfuric	HSO_4	1.9
Selenic	H_2SeO_4	1.9
Phosphoric	H_3PO_4	2.1
Arsenic	H_3AsO_4	2.3
Tellurous	H_2TeO_3	2.4
Selenious	H_2SeO_3	2.5
Phosphorous	H_3PO_3	2.7
Nitrous	HNO_2	3.3
Hydrofluoric	HF	3.4
Carbonic	H_2CO_3	6.5
Sulfurous	HSO_3	6.9
Hydrogen sulfide	H_2S	7.0
Hypochlorous	HClO	7.5
Telluric	$Te(OH)_6$	7.7
Ammonium ion	NH_4^+	9.2
Boric	H_3BO_3	9.2
Hydrocyanic	HCN	9.3
Silver ion	Ag^+	10.0
Hydrogen peroxide	H_2O_2	11.6
Water	H_2O	15.8
Weak bases		
Calcium carbonate	$CaCO_3$	5.7
Hydrazine	N_2H_4	8
Ammonia	NH_3	9.3
Ammonium hydroxide	NH_4OH	9.3
Magnesium hydroxide	$Mg(OH)_2$	10
Silver hydroxide	$Ag(OH)_2$	10
Arsenic trioxide	As_2O_3	10
Lead hydroxide	$Pb(OH)_2$	11
Zinc hydroxide	$Zn(OH)_2$	11
Calcium hydroxide	$Ca(OH)_2$	11.6
Barium hydroxide	$Ba(OH)_2$	11.7
Strong bases (pK_a >14)		
Cesium hydroxide	CsOH	
Lithium hydroxide	LiOH	
Potassium hydroxide	KOH	
Rubidium hydroxide	RbOH	
Sodium hydroxide	NaOH	
Calcium carbide	C_2Ca	
Calcium oxide	CaO	
Sodium carbonate	Na_2CO_3	
Potassium carbonate	K_2CO_3	
Sodium hypochlorite	NaClO	
Sodium hypophosphate	$Na_4P_2O_6$	
Sodium metasilicate	Na_2SiO_3	
Sodium silicate	$Na_2Si_3O_7$	
Trisodium phosphate	Na_3PO_4	

*Approximate values at 25°C. For bases, the pK_a is that of the conjugate acid and $pK_b = 14 - pK_a$.

Table 67.3. Common Names of Some Acids and Bases

Common Name	Chemical Name
Aquafortis	Nitric acid
Aqua regia (nitromuriatic acid)	Mixture of hydrochloric acid and nitric acid
Baking soda	Sodium bicarbonate
Bleach	Sodium hypochlorite
Caustic potash	Sodium hydroxide
Caustic soda	Potassium hydroxide
Chalk (Paris white)	Calcium carbonate
Lime	Calcium oxide
Limestone	Calcium carbonate
Lye	Sodium or potassium hydroxide
Muriatic acid	Hydrochloric acid
Oil of vitriol	Sulfuric acid
Slaked lime	Calcium hydroxide
Soda ash (washing soda)	Sodium carbonate
Soda lime	Mixture of sodium hydroxide and lime
Soluble glass (water glass)	Sodium silicate
Spirit of Hartshorn (ammonia water)	Ammonium hydroxide
Spirits of salts	Hydrochloric acid

produce chlorine gas (1, 2); combining it with ammonia may result in the evolution chloramine gases (NH_2Cl and $NHCL_2$) (3, 4).

Physical Forms

Most acids and bases are crystalline solids in pure form at room temperature. A few are gases (e.g., the halogen acids, hydrogen cyanide, hydrogen sulfide, and ammonia) or liquids (e.g., hydrazine). All exist as aqueous solutions. They can generally be stored in glass or plastic containers but not in metal or rubber ones. Acid and basic salts and anhydrides are primarily solids. Commercial products may contain combinations of acids or bases (or their derivatives) and other chemicals.

SITES, INDUSTRIES, AND BUSINESSES ASSOCIATED WITH EXPOSURE TO ACIDS AND BASES

Because of their chemical reactivity, the use of acids and bases is ubiquitous in industry, hobby pursuits, and in the home. Industrial activities involving potential exposure to acids and bases are listed in Table 67.4. Common household products containing these compounds are listed in Table 67.5.

There are over 80,000 exposures to acids and bases reported to poison centers in the United States each year (5). The actual number of exposures is probably several times greater. Industrial and avocational exposures are usually accidental and most commonly involve skin and eye contact followed by inhalational exposure. Ingestion may be accidental (e.g., environmental exploration by tasting in toddlers; misidentification of drinkable liquids by adults) or intentional (i.e., suicidal). Although once in vogue, the use of acid for murder (e.g., poisoned beverages) or malicious disfigurement (e.g., vitriol throwing) is now rare (6). Unfortunately, however, acids and bases have been used in recent incidents of product tampering (e.g., intentional adulteration of food and personal hygiene products).

Table 67.4. Industries, Occupations, and Processes Involving Potential Exposure to Acids and Bases

Acids
Acrylonitrile polymerization	Glue manufacturing
Astringent manufacturing	Jewelry manufacturing
Candle manufacturing	Mirror manufacturing
Chemical synthesis (Arsentates, chlorides, nitrates, phosphates)	Paper manufacturing
	Plumbing
Dental cement production and use	Nitroglycerin manufacturing
Disinfection/disinfectant manufacturing	Scale removal (boilers, gas and oil wells)
Electronics manufacturing	
Explosives manufacturing	Sugar refining
Felt hat production	Watch manufacturing
Fertilizer manufacturing	Woodworking
Glass making/working	

Bases
Baking powder manufacturing	Masonry
Case hardening	Optics manufacturing
Cement/mortar/plaster manufacturing	Printing
	Railroad shopwork
Compositors	Refrigeration
Degreasing	Soap manufacturing
Laundry working	

Both Acids and Bases
Aircraft manufacturing/ maintenance	Galvanizing
	Laboratory work
Automobile maintenance/ body work	Metal production/ working (cleaning, pickling, pitting, polishing, tempering)
Bleach manufacturing	
Bronzing	
Cellulose manufacturing	Mercerizing
Chemical manufacturing	Mordanting
Cloth preparation/ sizing	Oil drilling
	Ore drilling
Dye manufacturing	Painting
Electroplating	Petroleum refining
Enameling	Pharmacist
Engraving	Photograph developing
Etching	Rocket fuel production
Food presentation	Rubber manufacturing
Foundry work	Synthetic fiber manufacturing
Fur processing	
Furniture polishing	Tanning of leather
	Wiremaking

CLINICAL TOXICOLOGY OF EXPOSURE

Local Effects

Form the perspective of biologic toxicity, acids and bases are classified as primary irritants: they are capable of causing damage to all cells with which they come in contact. Because their ability to react with biologic tissue is high and nonselective, effects are generally limited to the sites of exposure: external or internal body surfaces such as the skin, eyes, and respiratory and gastrointestinal tracts. Pulmonary injury may result from the aspiration of ingested liquids as well as the inhalation of gases, dusts, and vapors. Surface injuries are often referred to as "chemical burns." Commercial products with corrosive activity may be classified and labeled according to their biologic potency or relative harmfulness (Table 67.6).

Pathologically, the gross appearance of tissue damaged by

Table 67.5. Some Household Products Containing Acids and Bases

Product	Active Ingredient
Batteries	
Automotive	Sulfuric acid
Alkaline	Hydroxides of alkali metals
Bleach	Chlorine/sodium hypochlorite
	Hydrogen peroxide
Cement	Calcium oxide
Clinitest® tablets	Sodium hydroxide
Denture cleaners	Hydrogen peroxide (generated from perborate and persulfate)
Dishwasher detergents	Sodium carbonates, phosphates and silicates
Drain cleaners	Sodium hydroxide
	Acids (nitric, sulfuric)
Dyes (hair)	Ammonia
Dyes/stains (wood, metal)	Acids (especially nitric)
Glass/metal cleaners	Acids (especially nitric)
	Ammonia
Mildew removers	Sodium hydroxide and hypochlorite
Oven cleaners	Sodium hydroxide
Paint removers	Sodium hydroxide
Roach insecticides	Boric acid
Rust removers	Acids, especially hydrofluoric
Toilet bowl cleaners	Ammonia
	Acids (hydrochloric, phosphoric, sodium bisulfate)
	Bases (sodium carbonate, silicates)

Table 67.6. Corrosive Classification of Commercial Products*

Class	Label/Signal Word	Definition
Weak irritant	"Caution"	Irritating to mucosa
Strong irritant	"Warning"	Irritating to mucosa and skin
Corrosive	"Danger"	May cause severe burns, permanent damage, or death—vapor harmful

*United States Consumer Safety and Protection Committee[7]

acids and bases is different. Acids typically produce coagulation necrosis with eschar formation, whereas bases cause liquefaction necrosis with tissue softening (8–19). With both acids and bases, epithelial sloughing with ulceration may ensue. In general, tissue injury begins within seconds of contact, progresses rapidly over the first few minutes, and continues slowly for a period of several hours to several days (20). Injured tissue first heals by way of granulation tissue formation (at several days to several weeks postexposure) and later by scar and stricture formation (beginning about 3 weeks postexposure).

Underlying biochemical reactions include protein precipitation (albuminate formation) in cases of acid injury and protein dissolution, lipid (membrane) emulsification, and fat saponification with injuries caused by bases. These reactions are accompanied by the production of heat and may result in concomitant thermal injury. The amount of thermal injury is usually small but tends to be greater with acids than with bases. Histologically, cell necrosis, microvascular thrombosis, and leukocyte and bacterial invasion is seen early in the course of injury by either agent. Later there is granulation tissue for-

mation followed by fibroblast proliferation, neovascularization, and connective tissue formation.

The extent of tissue destruction depends on the dose and formulation of acid or base involved as well as the duration of contact (8, 20). The greater the dose and the longer the exposure, the more severe the resultant injury. The dose is best expressed in terms of titratable acidity or alkalinity and depends on the identity of the acid or base as well as the concentration and volume of the solution. The identity of an acid or base determines its relative strength or potency. For a given molar concentration and volume, the greater the strength of an acid or base (i.e., the more extreme its pK_a), the greater its titratable acidity or alkalinity and the greater its biologic toxicity. And for a particular acid or base, as either the volume or the concentration (pH or pOH) increase, so does the titratable acidity or alkalinity and the biologic toxicity.

From a toxicologic perspective, acids and bases are considered strong (i.e., potent) if they have a pK_a of less than 2 or greater than 12 (Table 67.2) (16, 21). In practical terms, small volumes of solutions of strong acids and bases (even dilute ones), small volumes of solutions with extremes of pH (<2 or >12), large volumes of solutions of weak acids or bases, and large volumes of solutions of intermediate pH all have high titratable acidity or alkalinity and hence the potential for causing significant tissue damage. Household products containing ammonia, bleach, and hydrogen peroxide are generally less potent than their industrial counterparts, but they can sometimes cause severe injuries. Solid formulations tend to cause severe, localized injury, whereas liquid and gaseous agents tend to cause diffuse damage of variable severity.

Systemic Effects

As a rule, acids and bases are not absorbed into the systemic circulation, and their action is terminated by neutralization (reaction with tissue components) at the sites of exposure. Exceptions (i.e., absorbable agents) include the anions of some acids (e.g., arsenic and other heavy metals, cyanide, fluoride), ammonia, hydrazine, and perhaps large doses of ingested acids. The disposition and organ toxicity of specific acid anions are discussed in separate chapters. Systemic effects noted in patients with large ingestions of strong acids may be due to acid absorption and direct organ toxicity as well as to complications of local injury, such as hypoxia, shock, and intestinal ischemia or necrosis (22, 23). Although rare, systemic toxicity has also been reported following the ingestion of a base (24).

Ammonia may be absorbed from the lungs and the intestines (25–27). Blood ammonia levels may be transiently elevated following the inhalation or ingestion of large doses. They usually remain normal (<30 mg/dl), however, since absorbed ammonia is rapidly taken up by all metabolically active tissues (where it is used in amino acid transamination reactions), particularly the liver (where the excess is converted to urea). Small amounts of ammonia are excreted in expired air and urine, but hepatic metabolism is the primary route of elimination. Hyperammonemia asociated with liver failure and inborn errors of metabolism is primarily due to inability to metabolize ammonia which is normally produced in the gastrointestinal tract by way of bacterial action on nitrogenous wastes. The central nervous system is the principle target organ.

Hydrazine may be absorbed through the skin as well as through the respiratory and gatrointestinal tracts (28–32). It is widely distributed to tissues, but its metabolic fate is not clear. Target organs include the lungs, liver, kidneys, central nervous system (CNS), and possibly red blood cells, coagulation-fibrinolytic pathways and the immune system. Numerous enzymes, such as those involved in glucose, amino acid, ammonia, and lipid metabolism, are also affected. The antidotal activity of vitamin B_6 (pyridoxine) against CNS toxicity suggests that hydrazine inhibits enzymes requiring this agent as a cofactor [e.g., those involved in γ-aminobutyric acid (GABA) synthesis]. Hydrazine is eliminated from the blood with a half-life of about 2 hours. It is slowly excreted in the urine.

SIGNS, SYMPTOMS, AND SYNDROMES FROM TOXIC EXPOSURE

Acute Toxicity (Target Organ Toxicity)

The primary target organs for acids and bases are the eyes, the skin, and the respiratory and gastrointestinal tracts. Involvement of more than one target organ is not uncommon. Signs and symptoms depend on the site of exposure. Systemic toxicity may sometimes accompany surface injuries.

EYE EXPOSURE

Eye injury may result from contact with liquid, solid, mist, fume, or gaseous forms of an acid or base (33–37). Mild acid burns of the eye result in pain, photophobia, blepharospasm, tearing, and conjunctival injection. In moderate exposures, there may be local or diffuse clouding of the cornea and conjunctiva. Central corneal injuries (those along the visual axis) can result in decreased visual acuity. In severe cases, the entire thickness of the cornea as well as lens epithelium may be involved. Epithelial sloughing with corneal ulceration and perforation may occur. Uveitis, manifest by pain which is unrelieved with topical anesthetics and increases over time, decreased visual acuity, abnormal pupil size, shape, or reactivity, and a "cell and flare reaction" of the anterior chamber (leukocyte infiltration and smokey appearing aqueous humor), may develop several days after exposure.

Ophthalmic burns caused by bases tend to be more severe and progressive than those due to acids. The also have a greater tendency to result in late complications. Ammonium hydroxide is especially potent in its ability to penetrate corneal tissues. Mild alkali burns present as a chemical conjunctivitis similar to that described for acids. With moderate exposures, diffuse or localized vascular thrombosis and edema of the conjunctiva and sclera may give them a porcelain white appearance. Edema (clouding), softening (keratomalacia), sloughing, and ulceration of the cornea may be seen. Ulcerations may continue to progress for many days. As with acid injuries, those involving the central cornea or anterior chamber can result in decreased acuity of vision. In severe cases, corneal perforation, uveitis, increased intraocular pressure, and lens destruction may develop.

SKIN EXPOSURE

Corrosive burns of the skin may develop following exposure to solutions of acids or bases, liquid hydrazine, or high concentrations of acid or ammonia gas (25, 26, 30–32, 37–45). They may also occur when attempts are made to remove dry particulate matter from the skin by washing or flushing with water. Although the skin, because of its keratinization, is more resistant to corrosive injury than mucosal surfaces, all degrees of injury may be seen.

Mild to moderate (partial thickness) burns from both acids and bases generally resemble thermal burns and cause pain, tenderness, edema, and erythema. Blistering is uncommon, but sloughing may occur. Blanching may sometimes be noted with acid injuries.

Severe (full thickness) acid burns are characterized by a firmly adherent stiff or leathery eschar which is insensate. There may be an associated discoloration of the skin: typically white or gray with sulfuric acid, yellow-brown with nitric acid, and green with hydrochloric acid. Wounds may appear black if there is significant intradermal bleeding (due to red cell lysis and heme iron pigmentation). Spontaneous eschar separation usually occurs about 4 weeks after exposure. With severe alkali burns, the skin feels soapy and appears white to dark brown, and the eschar is initially pliant and soft. It may ulcerate or later become dry and friable.

Except for hydrofluoric acid, corrosive injury following skin exposure rarely penetrates beyond subcutaneous fat. Burns caused by anhydrous or liquid ammonia may be accompanied by frostbite (40). The use of hydrogen peroxide for wound irrigation has resulted in subcutaneous emphysema and systemic oxygen (gas bubble) embolism (46, 47).

INHALATIONAL EXPOSURE

Respiratory tract injury to the nose, mouth, pharynx, larynx, tracheobronchial tree, and pulmonary parenchyma may follow exposure to acid gases or fumes, ammonia gas, hydrazine fumes, and dusts of acids or bases (25, 26, 30–32, 39–41, 48–50, 57). Symptoms of mild injury include burning pain involving the nose, mouth, throat, and chest. In severe cases, dysphagia, hoarseness, coughing, dyspnea, weakness, dizziness, and syncope may be noted. Erythema and injection of mucosal surfaces may be seen in mild cases. Edema, stridor, and drooling indicate severe upper airway injury with potential or impending obstruction. A lateral soft tissue neck x-ray may reveal laryngeal or periglottic edema.

With mild inhalational exposures, lung sounds are usually normal. Wheezing, rales, rhonchi, and frothy or bloody sputum indicate moderate to severe pulmonary injury. Associated findings may include tachypnea, tachycardia, fever, hypoxia, and cyanosis. A chest x-ray may show diffuse or patchy infiltrates, atelectasis, or pulmonary edema with a normal size heart. Pneumomediastinum, pneumothorax, and pneumatoceles may also be seen. Pulmonary function testing may reveal evidence of small airway obstruction. Radioisotope (e.g., 133-xenon) lung ventilation scanning may show delayed washout of gas in areas of small airway destruction.

ASPIRATION

Aspiration may occur during the act of swallowing a liquid acid or base or upon the subsequent regurgitation or vomiting of ingested liquids (44, 56–73). The pulmonary pathology is similar to that seen after aspiration of gastric contents, but it is often more severe. All areas of the respiratory tract may be involved. Perhaps because bases generally have higher viscosity and lower volatility than acids, damage caused by their aspiration tends to be limited to the upper airway. Signs, symp-

Table 67.7. Endoscopic Grading of Esophageal and Gastric Injury

Grade	Depth	Appearance
I	Superficial	Mucosal hyperemia and edema
II	Transmucosal	Blistering, sloughing, or ulcerative lesions of mucosa with or without involvement of superficial muscle layers
III	Transmural	Ulcerative lesions extending into deep muscle layers, serosa, or beyond

toms, and ancillary test findings are the same as with inhalation exposure.

INGESTION

The ingestion of corrosives may cause injury to any area of the gastrointestinal (GI) tract from the mouth to the proximal small bowel (8–20, 56–114). One or more sites may be affected. Distal injuries may occur without coexistent oral lesions (89, 97, 105). Solids (tasted or ingested with a liquid) tend to stick to mucosal surfaces and cause severe injury to localized areas of the mouth, esophagus, and less often the stomach. Liquids generally cause more diffuse damage of variable severity.

Statistically, ingested bases tend to injure the esophagus more often and more severely than the stomach. With acids, the converse is true (9). There are so many exceptions, however, that these generalizations do not reliably predict toxicity in a particular individual. The limited amount of hydrochloric acid normally present in the stomach is insufficient to neutralize even small volumes of a strong or concentrated base. Conversely, the squamous epithelium of the esophagus, although slightly alkaline, offers little protection against the effects of strong or concentrated acid. And finally, although relatively resistant to injury, the acid-producing areas of the body of the stomach are not always spared from damage when strong or concentrated acids or bases are ingested.

Areas of the GI tract most prone to injury are those at (or immediately proximal to) points of anatomical narrowing: the cricopharyngeal, aortic/left mainstem bronchus (retrocardiac), and diaphragmatic/lower sphincter areas of the esophagus, and the antral/pyloric regions of the stomach.

Oropharyngeal burns cause pain, drooling, muffled or slurred speech, and dysphagia. Examination may reveal erythema, edema, ulcerations or white patches, particularly of the posterior mouth and pharynx. Symptoms of esophageal involvement may include chest pain, drooling, and dysphagia. Those of stomach and small bowel injury may include abdominal pain and tenderness (epigastric or generalized). Vomiting or regurgitation, sometimes with bloody emesis, may occur with either esophageal or gastric injuries.

The severity of esophageal and gastric burns is best assessed by endoscopy (Table 67.7). The extent (i.e., surface area) of injury may be small or large, patchy or diffuse, and may involve multiple anatomical sites. Accurate assessment of the depth of ulcerative lesions may be difficult because of adherent exudates. In addition, necrotic tissue may appear black (apparently due to iron pigmentation as a result of hemorrhage, erythrocyte hemolysis, and hemoglobin destruction).

Because of the greater risk of iatrogenic esophageal perforation associated with the use of a rigid endoscope, flexible fiberoptic endoscopy is the procedure of choice. In addition, the use of a flexible endoscope may obviate the need for general anesthesia. Finally, the admonition that the endoscope not be passed beyond the most proximal site of transmucosal (or deeper) esophageal injury because of the risk of causing a perforation originally arose in the era of rigid endoscopy and is no longer relevant. With carefully performed flexible endoscopy, the full extent of gastric and duodenal damage can often be safely assessed despite the presence of associated esophageal injuries.

Accurate assessment of the severity and extent of esophageal and gastric burns is important for prognostic purposes. Patients with superficial (Grade 1) burns are not at risk for stricture formation, whereas this complication has been noted in 40–100% of patients with transmural (Grade 3) lesions. Patients with transmucosal (Grade 2) burns may also develop strictures, but the risk appears to be low. Esophageal or gastric perforation occurs exclusively in patients with transmural burns (unless diagnostic or therapeutic interventions are causative or contributory).

The optimal timing of initial endoscopy is a matter of continued debate. If endoscopy is performed shortly after ingestion, the extent and severity of injuries may be underestimated. Conversely, if it is performed long after ingestion, the opportunity for maximal potential benefit of injury-specific therapy will be lost. The performance of endoscopy between 6 and 18 hours following ingestion is most often recommended and appears to be a reasonable compromise. In patients with severe symptoms, it is prudent to perform endotracheal intubation prior to endoscopy to avoid potential airway problems (e.g., aspiration). Repeat endoscopy may be useful in assessing the progression of injury and the effect of treatment.

Although contrast esophagography (cineofluoroscopy) may also identify esophageal injuries, it is less sensitive than endoscopy for accurate diagnostic assessment (95). Hence, it is used primarily as an adjunct to endoscopy. Serial radiographic studies are useful for following the course of injury and healing. Contrast esophagography and upper GI radiographs may also be used to confirm suspected perforation or stricture formation. Potential extravasation and lower tissue toxicity of water-soluble (ionic or nonionic) contrast agents make them preferable to barium for the evaluation of suspected perforations (despite their relative disadvantage in terms of x-ray clarity).

Findings on esophagography in patients with acute corrosive injury can be divided into those indicative of mucosal disruption and those indicative of a motility disorder (115, 116). Radiographic manifestations of mucosal injury include blurring or irregularities (e.g., scalloping or straightening) of esophagogastric margins due to superficial ulceration, sloughing, and pseudomembrane formation; linear or plaquelike retention of contrast due to deep ulceration; and extravasation of contrast in cases of perforation. Mucosal bullae may occasionally be visualized (117). Radiographic patterns indicating altered motility include atonic dilation, atonic rigidity with narrowing, and uncoordinated or otherwise abnormal peristaltic contractions. Only patients with the latter two patterns appear to be at risk for stricture formation.

The ingestion of large amounts of acid or base may result in shock with a rapid and thready pulse, hypotension, increased or decreased respirations, pallor, diaphoresis, and depressed sensorium. Shock may occur in the absence of gastrointestinal bleeding. Acute hemorrhage is, in fact, uncommon.

Esophageal and gastric perforation may result in mediastinitis or peritonitis. The former is suggested by fever, severe chest pain, respiratory distress, pleural rub, Hammond's crunch, and mediastinal widening with a pleural effusion (usually left-sided) on chest x-ray. Esophageal perforation may also result in pneumomediastinum or pneumothorax. Peritonitis is suggested by fever, abdominal tenderness, guarding, rebound, rigidity, and absent bowel sounds. Free air below the diaphragms on chest or abdominal x-ray may be noted in patients with stomach or bowel perforation. Gastrointestinal gangrene with intramural and intravascular gas (e.g., in portal veins and mesenteric arteries) has also been reported (118). Severe gastric and small bowel injuries often result in marked third-spacing of peritoneal fluid as manifest by abdominal distention and signs of hypovolemia. Rupture of the stomach (due to gastric distention caused by the evolution of carbon dioxide gas) may develop following the ingestion of sodium bicarbonate (119).

SYSTEMIC TOXICITY

Severe injuries caused by the ingestion of acids may be accompanied by metabolic acidosis, hemolysis, coagulopathy, hyponatremia, and renal toxicity (22, 92, 107). Metabolic acidosis may also occur in patients with severe GI damage caused by bases (24). Hyperphosphatemia and hypocalcemia have been reported following the ingestion of phosphoric acid (120). The systemic toxicity of acid anions (e.g., cyanide, heavy metals) is discussed in separate chapters. The intravenous injection of large amounts of bleach may cause acute hemolysis, hyperkalemia, hypoxia, and cardiopulmonary arrest (121, 122).

Coma, bradycardia, hypotension, pulmonary edema, acidosis, liver dysfunction and coagulopathy may be seen following the ingestion of large amounts of ammonia (27, 123). The serum ammonia, BUN, and amylase levels may be elevated. The inhalation of ammonia from ampules (smelling salts) initially causes decreased respirations, increased blood pressure, and sometimes bradycardia (124). Prolonged ammonia inhalation causes the blood pressure to decrease. Ammonia inhalation may also cause anaphylactoid reactions (125).

Hypotension, weakness, excited behavior, tremor, lethargy, ataxia, nystagmus, coma, fever, hyperglycemia, hypoglycemia, hepatitis (fatty degeneration), peripheral neuropathy, nephritis, and renal tubular necrosis may result from acute or chronic hydrazine exposure (28–32, 126–129). Seizures, hemolysis, and methemoglobinemia have been noted in animals but not in humans. The onset of systemic hydrazine toxicity may be delayed 14 hours or longer following skin exposure.

Chronic and Longterm Effects

TARGET ORGAN EFFECTS

Sequelae of severe acid burns of the eye include corneal vascularization, corneal scarring (cicatrix), and the formation of adhesions between the eyeball and eyelid (symblepharon) (34–36). Severe eye injury due to bases may result in vascularization, scarring, thickening (pannus), and persistent edema of the cornea, anterior chamber synechiae (adhesions between the iris and cornea or lens), cataracts, glaucoma, and symblepharon (33–36). Blindness may occur in both instances.

Full thickness skin burns may result in indolent ulcers and permanent scarring. They usually remain sterile until about 2–3 weeks after injury (44).

Severe inhalational injuries may cause persistent hoarseness, pulmonary fibrosis, bronchiectasis, and chronic obstructive airway disease (48, 50, 53).

Severe oral burns may result in chronic pain, ageusia or dysgeusia, and slurred speech. Severe gastrointestinal burns (i.e., those that are deep, circumferential, or extensive) may lead to esophageal strictures and pyloric stenosis. Esophageal strictures can be graded according to severity and extent (82).

Chronic skin exposure to low doses of corrosives, particularly bases, may result in a contact or eczematous dermatitis with erythema, drying, fissuring, and scaling. Electroplaters chronically exposed to acid fumes, particularly those of chromic acid, may develop ulcerations or perforations (''chrome holes'') of the nasal septum (130). Chromium compounds can also cause allergic or hypersensitivity dermatitis, asthma, and pneumonitis. Hydrazine as been reported to cause hypersensitivity dermatitis as well as a lupus erythematosus-like syndrome (30–32, 131).

TERATOGENESIS

There are no reported adverse effects of acids and bases on the human fetus. Hydrazine is mutagenic in a variety of in vitro test systems.

CARCINOGENESIS

Lung cancer has been associated with chronic exposure to chromium compounds (132). Epidermoid carcinoma of the nasal septum following direct contact with an ammonia-oil mixture has been reported (133). An increased incidence of pulmonary adenocarcinoma has been found in rodents, but not humans, exposed to hydrazine (134). Squamous cell carcinoma of the esophagus and stomach may occur 20–40 years after damage caused by ingested bases and acids, respectively (135–137).

Management of Toxicity

In order to prevent secondary casualties, corrosive or acid-resistant protective clothing (e.g., head gear, goggles, gloves, jumpsuits, boots) should be worn by rescuers of those involved in industrial accidents, particularly where explosion, fire, or significant chemical spills or leaks have occurred. Respiratory protection utilizing self-contained breathing apparatus may also be necessary. A positive pressure oxygen source (e.g., Scott Air Pack) is generally preferable to one utilizing a demand valve [e.g., minimum safety apparatus (MSA)]. Dilution or neutralization of spilled chemical material should never be performed without first investigating and excluding the possibility of precipitating a dangerous chemical reaction (e.g., explosion, toxic gas evolution).

CLINICAL EXAMINATION

Because the severity of injury caused by acids and bases relates directly to the duration of exposure, decontamination should initially take precedence over performing a detailed physical examination. Only resuscitative measures are of higher priority. Although most exposures result in immediate symptoms, a history of exposure is itself sufficient reason to initiate decontamination measures. Victims of industrial or transportational accidents should also be evaluated for injuries due to physical trauma.

Eye Exposure

The presence or absence of tearing and the appearance of the eyelids, their sulci, surrounding skin, conjunctivae, sclerae, corneas, and fundi should be noted. The location of any abnormalities should be clearly documented (i.e., by drawing a picture of the eye(s) or referring to the position on the corneal surface as if it were the face of a clock). Pupil size, shape, and reactivity, tear pH (e.g., via pHydrion paper testing of the lower conjunctival sulcus), and visual acuity should also be noted. Repeat examination of the eye surfaces under ultraviolet light following the instillation of fluorescein should be performed in all cases. Slit lamp examination of the anterior chamber should be performed in patients with corneal, pupillary, or visual abnormalities.

Skin Exposure

The location, size, color, texture, and sensibility of any visible burns or areas of discomfort should be noted. Assessment of patients with burns involving more than 10% of the body surface area should include complete vital signs, general physical examination, cardiac monitoring, and routine laboratory tests (e.g., blood count, coagulation profile, serum chemistries, urinalysis). The distal neurovascular status of extremities with circumferential or extensive burns should be documented.

Inhalation Exposure

Assessment of airway potency and respiratory function are of primary importance. Vital signs (especially the respiratory rate), skin color (e.g., the presence or absence of peripheral or generalized cyanosis), and ability to speak and swallow offered liquid as well as oral secretions should be noted. The physical examination should focus on the appearance of the oropharyngeal mucosa, the quality of the voice, and the presence of abnormal upper or lower airway and lung sounds. The oxygenation status should be assessed by oximetry or arterial blood gas analysis. The upper airway may be assessed by soft tissue neck radiographs in patients who do not require immediate intubation (see treatment section below). Patients with respiratory symptoms or abnormal breath sounds should have a chest x-ray and bedside pulmonary function testing (e.g., a peak flow by a Wright spirometer or an FEV_1 by a computerized spirometer). Patients with abnormal vital signs, chest pain, respiratory distress, or hypoxia should also be evaluated by a 12-lead ECG and routine laboratory studies.

Ingestion

Patients who have ingested acids or bases should be first assessed for the presence of concomitant respiratory tract injury as described under Inhalation Exposure. The location of any pain referable to the gastrointestinal tract, either spontaneous or associated with swallowing, should be noted. The appearance of oropharyngeal mucosa, the ability to swallow (both normal secretions and administered fluids), and a detailed abdominal exam should be documented. The patient should be checked specifically for neck or abdominal tenderness, bowel sounds, crepitus, and abdominal girth (distention). Patients with abnormal vital signs, inability to swallow, drooling, dysphagia, chest pain, respiratory symptoms, abdominal pain, or peritoneal signs should have cardiac monitoring, ECG, x-ray evaluation (e.g., neck, chest, abdomen), arterial blood gas analysis, routine laboratory studies (including coagulation studies, blood count, type and cross-match, routine chemistries, liver and renal function tests, and urinalysis), and endoscopy or radiographic contrast studies (see Acute Toxicity Section of this chapter).

Endoscopy should be used liberally. It is recommended in all patients with intentional ingestions of acids or bases which are chemically strong or have extremes of pH (i.e., less than 2 or greater than 12), and all patients with signs or symptoms of esophageal or gastrointestinal injury.

Systemic Toxicity

In addition to the focused examinations noted above, all patients, especially those with systemic complaints or exposures to corrosives that are known to cause systemic toxicity, should have a complete physical examination. Particular emphasis should be placed on the assessment of neurologic function and the exclusion of potential but possibly occult abnormalities by ancillary studies (e.g., ECG, laboratory testing, x-rays).

TREATMENT

Advanced life support measures should be instituted as necessary. As always, stabilization of the airway, breathing, and circulation are the highest priority. Decontamination is the next priority in management. Decontamination therapies are designed to limit local toxicity and are specific to the route of exposure. In some instances (e.g., exposure to hydrocyanic acid or acid anions containing heavy metals) the early institution of antidotal or enhanced elimination (i.e., chelation) therapy may also be necessary.

Eye Exposure

The involved eye(s) should immediately be irrigated with copious amounts of fluid (138). Patients at nonmedical facilities should be instructed to flush their eye(s) with tap water for 10–20 minutes. They should either pour water into the eye from a drinking glass or rinse the eye with slow running water from a faucet or shower head. If water is not available, milk or any clear, drinkable fluid may be used.

Patients who are at a medical facility should initially have their eye(s) irrigated with normal saline or lactated Ringer's solution (at least 2 liter per eye or for 20 minutes). Intravenous tubing with or without a scleral attachment is useful for this purpose. Intravenous tubing with or without a scleral irrigating solution should be allowed to flow by gravity. Since both normal saline and lactated Ringer's solutions are slightly acidic, they can themselves cause mild eye irritation. Lactated Ringer's solution tends to be better tolerated, perhaps because of its more physiologic pH (Table 66.1). Lactated Ringer's solution is also theoretically preferable to normal saline because it is buffered (i.e., resists changes in pH).

If possible, the tear pH should be determined prior to irrigation. Searching for pH paper should not, however, cause decontamination to be delayed. The instillation of a topical ophthalmic anesthetic such as proparacaine or tetracaine is often necessary, because patients are frequently unable to keep their eyes open to allow for successful irrigation unless anesthesia is provided. Any visible particulate material adherent to the surfaces of the eye should be manually removed (e.g., via cotton-tipped swab, eye spud, or forceps) prior to irrigation. After the initial irrigation, the tear pH should be checked or rechecked. If it falls outside the 5–8 pH range, continued irrigation is indicated.

Any patient with corneal, conjunctival, scleral, or lid lesions should be referred to an ophthalmologist for further evaluation and treatment. Specific treatment for corneal injuries may include the use of hydrophilic (gelatinous) contact lenses, eye patching, topical antibiotics, cycloplegics, mydriatics, drugs for the control of intraocular pressure, and topical or systemic therapy with agents which modulate collagen synthesis (e.g., ascorbic acid, citric acid, corticosteroids, calcium disodium EDTA, sodium EDTA, N-acetylcysteine, and D-penicillamine may be used for alkali injuries) (35, 36). Since many of these therapies are controversial or experimental, they should only be used by, or upon the direction of, an ophthalmologist.

Skin Exposure

Exposed skin should immediately be irrigated with saline, tap water, milk, or another clear drinkable liquid for a minimum of 10–20 minutes for acids and 30–60 minutes for bases. Any particulate material should be manually removed prior to wetting. Wound care (e.g., topical antibiotics, debridement, grafting) and intravenous fluid therapy is the same as that for thermal injuries.

Inhalation Exposure

Following removal of the victim from the source of exposure, cool, humidified, high-flow oxygen should be provided. The oxygen dosage can subsequently be adjusted according to the results of oximetry or arterial blood gas analysis. Patients with mild signs and symptoms can usually be treated with oxygen by face mask, whereas those with evidence of moderate to severe injury may require oxygen therapy by endotracheal tube (48, 50, 53). Patients with mild to moderate laryngeal edema may improve after the administration of racemic epinephrine (by aerosol inhalation). Indications for intubation include CNS depression (confusion or coma); respiratory distress with stridor, drooling, or cyanosis; hypoxia ($pO_2 < 60$) that is not rapidly correctable by oxygen [with or without continuous positive airway pressure (CPAP)]; and respiratory insufficiency ($pCO_2 > 50$). In patients with oropharyngeal or laryngeal edema, blind nasal intubation or the use of a fiberoptic laryngoscope may be successful when the glottis cannot be directly visualized. Cricothyroidotomy may be necessary if the trachea cannot otherwise be intubated. Positive end-expiratory pressure (PEEP) ventilation may be helpful in treating pulmonary edema, but diuretics should be avoided. Aggressive tracheal suctioning may also be necessary to remove secretions.

After patency of the upper airway and adequate oxygenation and ventilation are assured, pharmacologic therapy may be indicated. An early but brief course of systemic corticosteroids (e.g., 2 mg/kg/day of methylprednisolone i.v. in divided doses for 24–48 hours) may help reduce laryngeal edema. Patients with wheezing should be treated with standard asthma medications (e.g., beta-adrenergic agonists). Although steroids may be useful for refractory bronchospasm, they are not indicated solely for the treatment of pneumonitis or pulmonary edema.

Antibiotics should be used to treat documented pulmonary infection but not prophylactically. Pending the results of a gram stain and sputum culture, empiric therapy should include coverage for *Staphylococcus aureus* and Gram-negative organisms as well as oral flora. Cefazolin, cefoxitin, or cefuroxime are reasonable choices for the empiric treatment of patients with leukocytosis, fever, prurulent sputum, or infiltrates on chest x-ray.

Ingestion

Dilution of the ingested agent should be accomplished as soon as possible (13–19). Dilution is intended to decrease the concentration of acid or base and to minimize thermal injury. The administration of excessive amounts of fluid should be avoided because of the risk of inducing vomiting and reexposing the esophagus, whose wall is much thinner than that of the stomach, to gastric contents.

The awake, alert patient should immediately drink approximately 5 ml/kg of milk, tap water, or any clear, drinkable beverage (139, 140). For the dilution of bases, orange juice may be used, but lemon juice and vinegar should be avoided (141–142). Activated charcoal does not effectively adsorb acids or bases and will obscure endoscopic visualization and assessment of injury. Hence, unless an ingested agent is likely to cause systemic toxicity (e.g., hydrocyanic acid, hydrazine, acids or salts with heavy metal anions), charcoal administration is not recommended.

Orogastric nasogastric intubation for the purpose of gastric aspiration, lavage, or the administration of diluents to patients who cannot, or will not, drink them is controversial (13–19, 140). There is a theoretical risk of this procedure producing an iatrogenic esophageal or gastric perforation at the site of deep (transmural or transmucosal) lesions. The vast majority of iatrogenic perforations, however, occur during attempts at therapeutic dilation of stenoses. In over 4200 patients with corrosive ingestion (all the cases reported in the references cited in this chapter), only three perforations occurred sooner than 24 hours after ingestion. All of these were spontaneous, present at time of initial presentation, and none was due to the insertion of a gastric tube for decontamination. In addition, the author has noted extremes of gastric fluid pH as long as 12 hours after large ingestions (at the time of endoscopy). For these reasons, immediate gastric intubation followed by aspiration, dilution, and lavage is recommended for patients who have ingested more than one swallow of a strong acid or base in liquid form and present within 1 or 2 hours of ingestion. This approach has long been advocated for acid ingestions, but only recently for those involving bases (16, 140). Because solids may stick to mucosal surfaces and cause relatively greater local injury, the risk of perforation is theoretically higher. Hence, gastric intubation is not recommended for the decontamination of patients who have ingested solid acids or bases.

If gastric intubation is performed, a small-bore tube (e.g., 10 French in children and 18 French in adults) should be gently inserted in order to minimize mechanical trauma. One to two liters of milk or tap water are usually sufficient for gastric lavage. Because of the risk of water intoxication, normal saline is recommended for lavage in children under 2 years of age. The volume of lavage fluid aliquots should be kept small (about 5 ml/kg) in order to avoid regurgitation into the esophagus. Lavage should continue until the effluent has a pH of 5-7. Commercially available gastric tubes with a pH sensor (e.g.,

GrapHprobe) are ideal for this purpose. Alternatively, the pH of the lavage effluent can be determined by pH paper.

Following dilution and/or decontamination, management includes continued supportive care, symptomatic treatments, and measures intended to prevent complications (i.e., strictures and perforations). The efficacy of corticosteroids in preventing esophageal strictures remains controversial. Experimental studies suggest that steroids are effective in inhibiting collagen synthesis and preventing alkali-induced strictures if they are given prophylactically (143, 144). However, their efficacy when administered after the insult has not been clearly demonstrated. Only one controlled clinical trial has shown steroids to be beneficial (106), whereas two others have found them to be ineffective (68, 90). Strictures that develop in patients treated with steroids may be easier to subsequently dilate than those that develop in patients not treated with steroids (113). On the other hand, steroids may increase the incidence of perforation, infectious complications, and death (if antibiotics are not given concurrently), they may inhibit wound healing, and they may mask signs of mediastinitis and peritonitis (71, 113, 143). Hence, for optimal efficacy and minimal risk, steroids should be given as soon after ingestion as possible and they should not be used without concurrent antibiotic therapy or if there is a suspicion of esophageal or gastrointestinal perforation. The efficacy of steroids in preventing esophageal and gastric outlet strictures resulting from acid burns has not been studied.

Until further data become available, the following approach is suggested. Patients with suspected esophageal burns should be given an intravenous dose of a broad spectrum of antibiotic (e.g., ampicillin, cefazolin, or cefoxitin) as well as methylprednisolone (2 mg/kg) on presentation. These medications can be continued or discontinued depending on the degree and extent of esophageal injury noted on endoscopy and the preference of the specialist (e.g., gastroenterologist or general, pediatric, ear-nose-throat, or thoracic surgeon) who performs it. Even if a gastroenterologist does the endoscopy, surgical consultation is advisable. This will prevent delays in treatment should operative management become necessary.

Patients without visible injury on endoscopy, and those having only superficial (Grade 1) mucosal lesions or limited transmucosal (Grade 2) lesions are at negligible risk for perforation or stricture formation. Hence, antibiotics and steroids are not of potential benefit and should be discontinued. These patients can be discharged (with outpatient follow-up) or referred for psychiatric evaluation provided they are able to take oral fluids. Antacids, H2-blockers (e.g., ranitidine), analgesics, and sucrafate may be given for symptomatic relief.

Patients with extensive or circumferential transmucosal (Grade 2) lesions or shallow transmural (Grade 3) injury should be given nothing by mouth and provided with parenteral fluids or hyperalimentation until they are able to swallow their own secretions. Symptomatic therapy as mentioned above should be provided. Antibiotics should be continued for 3–5 days postingestion or until the patient is free of pain and able to swallow. Since these patients are at significant risk for stricture formation, corticosteroids may also be of benefit. Although the optimal dose is unknown, 2 mg/kg/day of intravenous methylprednisolone or oral prednisone, given in divided doses every 4–6 hours for 1 week and then tapered over the next 2 weeks, is often recommended.

Patients with deep or extensive transmural (Grade 3) lesions are at high risk for perforation as well as strictures and should not be given steroids. They should be given intravenous anti-biotics, analgesics, and H2-blockers such as cimetidine, but nothing by mouth. Patients with actual or suspected perforations and those with shock, acidosis, or peritoneal findings suggesting extensive tissue necrosis should be treated in a similar manner. They may also require operative management (i.e., drainage, debridement, diversion procedures, resection) and nutritional support via enteral (i.e., feeding jejunostomy) or parental hyperalimentation.

Other agents inhibit that collagen synthesis (e.g., β-aminopropionitrile, D-penicillamine, n-acetylcysteine) are effective in preventing strictures in experimental animals, but the clinical use of these agents has not yet been reported (145, 147). Similarly, mucosal protective agents such as sodium polyacrylate and sucrafate appear to limit tissue injury and prevent subsequent strictures in animal models, but their value in human poisoning remains unknown (147, 148).

Mechanical measures have also been used to prevent or treat strictures. Indwelling esophageal stents (Silastic tubes) may be placed at the time of endoscopy and left in place for about 2 weeks in an attempt to prevent stricture formation. Alternatively, nasogastric tubes or string may be placed in the esophagus to maintain a patent lumen and facilitate bouginage in the event that strictures subsequently develop (149, 151). The use of these procedures, however, may lead to reflux esophagitis and increase the risk of esophageal perforation, and their efficacy is controversial (12). Hence, their use cannot be routinely recommended.

Patients who go on to develop strictures can be treated by either bougienage or surgery (i.e., esophageal resection or replacement by colonic interposition). Dilation therapy should be delayed until at least 4 weeks after ingestion. If it is performed earlier, it is associated with a high incidence of iatrogenic perforations.

Systemic Toxicity

The treatment of systemic effects is primarily supportive: maintenance of physiologic, hematologic, and biochemical homeostasis by standard measures. In certain cases, agent-specific therapy may also be necessary. Treatments of cyanide, hydrogen sulfide, and heavy metal poisoning are discussed in other chapters.

The elimination of ammonia can be enhanced by hemodialysis, but this therapy is unlikely to be necessary in patients with normal liver and kidney function. Since hydrazine appears to cause a functional pyridoxine deficiency, patients with systemic hydrazine poisoning, particularly those with neurological dysfunction, should be given supplemental pyridoxine (vitamin B_6) (126, 127, 152). Although the optimal dose is unknown, 25 mg/kg i.v. is usually recommended. This dose can be repeated in several hours if there is an incomplete, transient, or no response.

LABORATORY DIAGNOSIS

When the history reveals the name of the offending agent, laboratory confirmation of its identity is not necessary for initial management. When the history fails to reveal the identity and symptoms suggest exposure to a corrosive, determining the pH of the agent involved may be helpful in identifying it as an acid or base. The diagnosis of systemic ammonia poisoning can be confirmed by measuring the serum ammonia level. Analytic methods for the identification and quantification of hy-

Table 67.8. Threshold Limit Values for Some Acids and Bases*

Substance	ACGIH TWAs		ACGIH STELs		NIOSH RELs		OSHA PELs	
	ppm	mg/m³	ppm	mg/m³	ppm	mg/m³	ppm	mg/m³
Ammonia	25	17	35	24	50	34.8 (C, 5 min)	50	35 (TWA, 8 hr)
Calcium carbonate	—	10	—	—	—	—	—	—
Calcium oxide	—	2	—	—	—	—	—	—
Chromic acid	—	—	—	—	—	0.025 (TWA, 10 hr)	—	0.1 (C, 0 min)
					—	0.05 (C, 5 min)		
Hydrazine	0.1	0.13	—	—	0.03	0.04 (C, 2 hr)	1	1.3 (TWA, 8 hr)
Hydrogen peroxide	1	1.4	—	—	—	—	—	—
Nitric acid	2	5.2	4	10	2	5 (TWA, 10 hr)	2	5 (TWA, 8 hr)
Potassium hydroxide	—	2(C)	—	—	—	—	—	—
Sodium bisulfite	—	5	—	—	—	—	—	—
Sodium hydroxide	—	2(C)	—	—	—	2 (C, 15 min)	—	2 (TWA, 8 hr)
Sulfuric acid	—	1	—	3	—	1 (TWA, 10 hr)	—	1 (TWA, 10 hr)

*Adapted from references 147 and 148.

ACGIH = American Conference of Governmental Industrial Hygienists; NIOSH = National Institute for Occupational Safety and Health; OSHA = Occupational Safety and Health Administration; TWA = time-weighted average; REL = recommended exposure limit; C = ceiling limit; STEL = short-term exposure limit; PEL = permissible exposure limit.

ACGIH TWAs are concentrations that produce no adverse effect on repeated exposure during an 8-hour workday and 40-hour workweek; STEL concentrations are the 15-minute TWAs that should not be exceeded; Cs denote the concentration that should not be exceeded at anytime. NIOSH and OSHA time limits for TWAs and Cs are noted in parentheses.

drazine are not routinely available. The utility of quantitative cyanide and heavy metal levels is discussed in other chapters.

Patients with intentional ingestions should generally have a toxicology screen (qualitative analysis of urine and serum) to rule out other exposures. Routine hematologic and biochemical laboratory studies should be performed on patients with moderate or severe skin, inhalation, or ingestion injuries and those with signs or symptoms of systemic poisoning.

Special diagnostic tests are not required. Biologic and environmental monitoring are not applicable to acids and bases.

EXPOSURE LIMITS

Workplace standards for atmospheric exposure limits are only defined for a small number of acids and bases (Table 67.8) (153, 154). Direct eye, skin, or gastrointestinal tract exposure to industrial or household products containing acids or bases (excluding small amounts present in foods, cosmetics, or toiletries) should be avoided completely.

REFERENCES

1. Gapany-Gapanavicius M, Yellin A, Almog S, Tirosh M. Pneumomediastinum: a complication of chlorine exposure from mixing household cleaning agents. JAMA 1982;248:349–350.
2. Reisz GR, Gammon RS. Toxic pneumonitis from mixing household cleaners. Chest 1986;89:49–52.
3. Pinkus JL. Monochloramine hazard from a mixture of household clean solutions. N Engl J Med 1965;272:1133.
4. Dooms-Goossens A, Gevers D, Mertens A, Vanderheyden D. Allergic contact urticaria due to chloramine. Contact Dermatitis 1983;9:319–320.
5. Litovitz TL, Schmitz BF, Holm KC. 1988 Annual Report of the American Association of Poison Control Centers National Data Collection System. Am J Emerg Med 1989;7:495–546.
6. Polson CJ, Green MA, Lee RM, eds. Clinical toxicology. 3rd ed. Philadelphia: JB Lippincott, 1984:243–259.
7. United States Consumer Protection Safety Committee. Report of the Toxicology Advisory Board. Washington, DC: TAB, USCPSC, 1982.
8. Dafoe CS, Ross CA. Acute corrosive oesophagitis. Thorax 1969;24:291–294.
9. Allen R, Thoshinsky M, Stallone R, Hunt TK. Corrosive injuries of the stomach. Arch Surg 1970;100:409–413.
10. Tewfik TL, Schloss MD. Ingestion of lye and other corrosive agents—a study of 86 infants and child cases. J Otolaryngol 1980;9:72–77.
11. Kirsh MM, Ritter F. Caustic ingestion and subsequent damage to oropharyngeal and digestive passages. Ann Thora Surg 1926;21:74–82.
12. Kirsh MM, Peterson A, Brown JW, Orringer MB, Ritter F, Sloan H. Treatment of caustic injuries of the esophagus: a ten year experience. Ann Surg 1978;188:675–678.
13. Bikhazi HB, Thompson ER, Shumrick DA. Caustic ingestion: current status. Arch Otolaryngol 1969;89:112–115.
14. Knopp R. Caustic ingestions. J Am Coll Emerg Phys 1979;329–336.
15. Tucker JA, Yarington CT. The treatment of caustic ingestion. Otolaryngol Clin North AM 1979;12:343–350.
16. Penner GE. Acid ingestion: toxicology and treatment. Ann Emerg Med 1980;9:374–379.
17. Friedman EM, Lovejoy FH. The emergency management of caustic ingestions. Emerg Med Clin North Am 1984;2:77–86.
18. Howel JM. Alkaline ingestions. Ann Emerg Med 1986;15:820–825.

19. Wason S. Coping swiftly and effectively with caustic ingestions. Emerg Med Rep 1989;10:25–32.

20. Leape LL, Ashcraft RW, Scarpelli DG, Holder DG. Hazard to health: liquid lye. N Engl J Med 1971;284,578–581.

21. Vancura EM, Clinton JE, Ruiz E, Krenzelok EP. Toxicity of alkaline solutions. Ann Emerg Med 1980;9:118–122.

22. Linden CH, Berner JM, Kulig K, Rumach BH. Acid ingestion: toxicity following systemic absorption (abstract). Vet Hum Toxicol 1983;25(suppl 1):66.

23. Grief F, Kaplan O. Acid ingestion: another cause of disseminated intravascular coagulopathy. Crit Care Med 1986;14:990–991.

24. Okonek S, Bierbach H, Atzpodien W. Unexpected metabolic acidosis in severe lye poisoning. Clin Toxicol 1981;18:225–230.

25. National Institute for Occupational Safety and Health (criteria document for a recommended standard): Occupational exposure to ammonia. DHEW 74-136. Washington DC: GPO, 1974:1–88.

26. International Programme on Chemical Safety: Ammonia. Environmental Health Criteria 54, Geneva: World Health Organization, 1986:1–210.

27. Linden CH, Rumack BH, Galle SJ. Systemic toxicity following household ammonia ingestion (abstract). Vet Hum Toxicol 1984;26(suppl 2):59.

28. Comstock CC, Lawson LH, Green EA, Oberst FW. Inhalation toxicity of hydrazine vapor. Arch Ind Hyg Occup Med 1954;10:476–490.

29. Clark DA, Bairrington JD, Bitter HL, et al. Pharmacology and toxicology of propellant hydrazines. Aeromedical review 11–68. Brooks Air Force Base, Texas: USAF School of Aerospace Medicine, Aerospace Medical Division, 1968:1–126.

30. National Institute for Occupational Safety and Health (Criteria document for a recommended standard). Occupational exposure to hydrazines. DHEW 78-172. Washington DC: GPO, 1978:1–269.

31. Reinhardt CF, Brittelli MR. Hetercyclic and miscellaneous nitrogen compounds. In Clayton GD, Clayton GD, eds, Patty's industrial hygiene and toxicology. New York: John Wiley & Sons, 1981:2791–2800.

32. International Programme on Chemical Safety. Hydrazine. Environmental Health Criteria 68. Geneva: World Health Organization, 1987:1–89.

33. Pfister KR, Koski J. Alkali burns of the eye: pathophysiology and treatment. South Med J 1982;75:417–422.

34. Tripathi RC, Tripathi BJ. The eye: chemical injuries, toxins, and poisons. In Riddell RH ed. Pathology of drug-induced and toxic diseases. New York: Churchill Livingston, 1982:432–456.

35. McCulley JP, Moore TE. Chemical injuries of the eye. In: Leibowitz HM, ed. Corneal disorders: clinical diagnosis and management. Philadelphia: WB Saunders, 1984:471–478.

36. Parrish CM, Chandler JW. Corneal trauma: chemical injuries. In: Kaufman HE, McDonald MB, Barron BA, Waltman SR, eds. The cornea. New York: Churchill Livingstone, 1988:608–644.

37. Vilogi J, Whitehead B, Marcus SM. Oven-cleaner pads: new risk for corrosive injury. Ann J Emerg Med 1985;3:412–414.

38. Girard LJ, Alford WE, Felman GL, Williams B. Severe alkali burn. Trans Am Acad Ophthalmol Otolaryngol 1970;74:788–803.

39. Helmers S, Top FH, Knapp LW. Ammonia injuries in agriculture. J Iowa Med Soc 1971;61:271–280.

40. Birken GA, Fabri PJ, Carey LC. Acute ammonia intoxication complicating multiple trauma. J Trauma 1981;21:820–822.

41. Arwood R, Hammond J, Ward GG. Ammonia inhalation. J Trauma 1985;25:444–447.

42. Early SH, Simpson RL. Caustic burns from contact with wet cement. JAMA 1985;254:528–529.

43. Skiendzielewski JJ. Cement burns. Ann Emerg Med 1980;9:316–318.

44. Sawhney CP, Kaushish R. Acid and alkali burns: considerations in management. Burns 1989;15:132–134.

45. Wang XW, Davies JWL, Sirvent RLZ, Robinson WA. Chronic acid burns and acute chronium poisonings. Burns 1985;11:181–184.

46. Bassan MM, Dudai M, Shalev O. Near-fatal systemic oxygen embolism due to wound irrigation with hydrogen peroxide. Postgrad Med J 1982;58:448–450.

47. Sleigh JW, Linter SPK. Hazards of hydrogen peroxide. Br Med J 1985;291:1706.

48. Close LG, Catlin FI, Cohn AM. Acute and chronic burns of the respiratory tract. Arch Otolaryngol 1980;106:151–158.

49. Walton M. Industrial ammonia gassing. Br J Ind Med 1973;30:78–86.

50. Montague TJ, Macneil AR. Mass ammonia inhalation. Chest 1980;77:496–498.

51. Flury KE, Dines DE, Rodarte JR, Rodgers R. Airway obstruction due to the inhalation of ammonia. Mayo Clin Proc 1983;58:389–393.

52. Sobonya R. Fatal anhydrous ammonia inhalation. Hum Pathol 1977;8:293–299.

53. O'Kane GJ. Inhalation of ammonia vapour: a report of the management of eight patients during the acute stages. Anaesthesia 1983;38:1208–1213.

54. Oberst FW, Comstock CC, Hackley EB. Inhalational toxicity of ninety percent hydrogen peroxide vapor-acute, subacute, and chronic exposures of laboratory animals. Arch Ind Hyg Occup Med 1954;10:319–327.

55. Kaelin RM, Kapaaci Y, Tschopp JM. Diffuse interstitial lung disease associated with hydrogen peroxide inhalation in a dairy worker. Am Rev Respir Dis 1988;137:1233–1235.

56. Moulin D, Bertrand JM, Buts JP, Nyakabasa M, Otte JB. Upper airway lesions in children after accidental ingestion of caustic substances. J Pediatr 1985;106:408–410.

57. Wason S, Gomolin I, Gross P, Mariam S, Lovejoy FH. Phosphorus tri-chloride toxicity: preliminary report. Am J Med 1984;77:1039–1042.

58. Giusti GV. Fatal poisoning with hydrogen proxide. Forensic Sci 1973;2:99–100.

59. Yarington CT. Ingestion of caustic: a pediatric problem. J Pediatr 1965;67:674–677.

60. Moore WR. Caustic ingestions: pathophysiology, diagnosis, and treatment. Clin Pediatr 1986;25:192–196.

61. Wasserman RL, Ginsburg CM. Caustic substance injuries. J Pediatr 1985;107:169–174.

62. Schild JA. Caustic ingestion in adult patients. Laryngoscope 1985;95:1199–1201.

63. Adam JS, Birck HG. Pediatric caustic ingestion. Ann Otol Rhinol Laryngol 1982;91:656–658.

64. Cardona JC, Daly JF. Management of corrosive esophagitis: analysis of treatment, methods, and results. NY State J Med 1964;64:2307–2313.

65. Feldman M, Iben AB, Hurley EJ. Corrosive injury to the oropharynx and esophagus: eighty-five consecutive cases. Calif Md 1973;118:6–9.

66. Borja AR, Ransdell HT, Thomas TV, Johnson W. Lye injuries of the esophagus: analysis of ninety cases of lye ingestion. J Thorac Cardiovasc Surg 1969;57:533–538.

67. Ferguson MK, Migliore M, Staszak VM, Little AG. Early evaluation and therapy of caustic esophageal injury. Am J Surg 1989;157:116–120.

68. Anderson KD, Rouse TM, Randolph JG. A controlled trial of corticosteroids in children with corrosive injury of the esophagus. N Engl J Med 1990;323:637–640.

69. Muhlendahl KEV, Oberdisse U, Krienke EG. Local injuries caused by accidental ingestion of corrosive substances by children. Arch Toxicol 1978;39:299–314.

70. Moazam F, Talbert JL, Miller D, Mollitt DL. Caustic ingestion and its sequelae in children. South Med J 1987;80:187–190.

71. Wason S. Coping swiftly and effectively with caustic ingestions. J Emerg Med 1985;2:175–182.

72. Oakes DD, Sherck JP, Mark JB. Lye ingestion clinical patterns and therapeutic implications. J Thorac Cardiovasc Surg 1982;83:194–204.

73. Middelkamp JN, Ferguson TB, Roper CL, Hoffman FD. The management and problems of caustic burns in children. J Thorac Cardiovasc Surg 1969;57:341–346.

74. Lopez GP, Dean BS, Krenzelok EP. Oral exposure to ammonia inhalants: a report of 8 cases (abstract). Vet Hum Toxicol 1988;30:350.

75. Ernest RW, Leventhal M, Luna R, Martinez H. Total esophagogastric replacement after ingestion of household ammonia. N Engl J Med 1963;268:815–818.

76. Norton RA. Esophageal and antral strictures due to ingestion of household ammonia: report of two cases. N Engl J Med 1960;262:10–12.

77. Chassin JL, Slattery LR. Jejunal stricture due to ingestion of ammonia. JAMA 1953;152:134–136.

78. Gonzalez LL, Zinninger MM, Altemeier WA. Cicatricial gastric stenosis caused by ingestion of corrosive substances. Ann Surg 1962;156:84–89.

79. Meyer CT, Brand M, DeLuca VA, Spiro HM. Hydrogen peroxide colitis: a report of three patients. J Clin Gastroenterol 1981;3:31–35.

80. Landau GD, Saunders WH. The effect of chlorine bleach on the esophagus. Arch Otolaryngol 1968;80:174–176.

81. French RJ, Tabb HG, Rutledge LJ. Esophageal stenosis produced by ingestion of bleach. South Med J 1970;63:1140–1144.

82. Pike DG, Peabody JW, Davis EW, Lyons WS. A re-evaluation of the dangers of Chlorox ingestion. J Pediatr 1963;63:303–305.

83. Yarington CT, Bales GA, Frazer JP. A study of the management of caustic esophageal trauma. Ann Otol Rhinol Laryngol 1964;73:1130–1135.

84. Okonek S, Reinecke HJ, Krienke EG, et al. Poisoning by hypochlorite-containing disinfectants: a retrospective analysis of 594 cases of poisoning (abstract). Dtsch Med Wochenschr 1984;109:1874–1877.

85. Fatti L, Marchand P, Crawshaw GR. The treatment of caustic strictures of the esophagus. Surg Gynecol Obstet 1956;102:195–206.

86. Davis LL, Raffensperger J, Novak GM. Necrosis of the stomach secondary to ingestion of corrosive agents: report of three cases requiring total gastrectomy. Chest 1972;62:48–51.

87. Adams JT, Skucas J. Corrosive jejunitis due to ingestion of nitric acid. Am J Surg 1980;139:282–285.

88. Abramson AL. Corrosive injury to the esophagus: result of ingesting

some denture cleanser tablets and powder. Arch Otolaryngol 1978;104:514–516.

89. Krenzelok EP, Clinton JE. Caustic esophageal and gastric erosion without evidence of oral burns following detergent ingestion. J Am Coll Emerg Phys 1979;8:5–7.

90. Cello JP, Fogel RP, Boland CR. Liquid caustic ingestion: spectrum of injury. Arch Intern Med 1980;140:501–504.

91. Subbarao KSVK, Kakar AK, Chandrasekhar V, Anathakrishnan N, Banerjee A. Cicatrical gastric stenosis caused by corrosive ingestion. Aust NZ J Surg 1988;58:143–146.

92. Soni N, O'Rourke I, Pearson I. Ingestion of hydrochloric acid. Med J Aust 1985;142:471–472.

93. Hawkins DB, Demeter MJ, Barnett TE. Caustic ingestion: controversies in management: a review of 214 cases. Laryngoscope 1980;90:98–109.

94. Stannard MW. Corrosive esophagitis in children: Assessment by esophagogram. Am J Dis Child 1978;132:596–599.

95. Mansson I. Diagnosis of acute corrosive lesions of the aesophagus. J Laryngol Otol 1978;92:499–504.

96. Cullen ML, Klein MD. Spontaneous resolution of acid gastric injury. J Pediatr Surg 1987;2:550–551.

97. Gaudreault P, Parent M, Mcguigan MA, Chicoine, Lovejoy FH. Predictability of esophageal injury from signs and symptoms: a study of caustic ingestion in 378 children. Pediatrics 1983;71:767–770.

98. Sugawa C, Mullins RJ, Lucas CE, Leibold WC. The value of early endoscopy following caustic ingestion. Surg Gynecol Obstet 1981;153:553–556.

99. Welsh JJ, Welsh LW. Endoscopic examination of corrosive injuries of the upper gastrointestinal tract. Laryngoscope 1978;88:1300–1309.

100. Postlethwait RW. Chemical burns of the esophagus. Surg Clin North Am 1983;63:915–924.

101. Buntain WL, Cain WC. Caustic injuries to the esophagus: a pediatric overview. South Med J 1981;74:590–593.

102. Steigmann F, Dolehide R. Corrosive gastritis. N Engl J Med 1956;245:981–986.

103. Symbas PN, Vlasis SE, Hatcher CR. Esophagitis secondary to ingestion of caustic material. Ann Thorac Surg 1983;36:73–77.

104. Aaron E, Taylor W, Mills LJ, Platt MR. Corrosive burns of the esophagus and stomach: a recommendation for an aggressive surgical approach. Ann Thorac Surg 1986;41:276–283.

105. Crain EF, Gershel JC, Mezey AP. Caustic ingestions: symptoms as predictors of esophageal injury. Am J Dis Child 1984;138:863–865.

106. Jordan FT. Diagnosis and treatment of acid gastric burns. New Phys 1976;25:70–74.

107. Warren JB, Griffin DJ, Olson RC. Urine sugar reagent tablet ingestion causing gastric and duodenal ulceration. Arch Intern Med 1984;144:161–162.

108. Fisher RA, Echhauser ML, Radivoyevitch M. Acid ingestion in an experimental model. Surg Gynecol Obstet 1985;161:91–99.

109. Webb WR, Koutras P, Ecker RR, Sugg WL. An evaluation of steroids and antibiotic in caustic burns of the esophagus. Ann Thorac Surg 1970;9:95–102.

110. Meredith JW, Kon ND, Thompson JN. Management of injuries from liquid lye ingestion. J Trauma 1988;28:1173–1180.

111. Cleveland WW, Chandler JR, Lawson RB. Treatment of caustic burns of the esophagus: early esophagoscopy and adrenocortical steroids. JAMA 1963;186:262–264.

112. Viscomi GJ, Beekhuis GJ, Whitten CF. An evaluation of early esophagoscopy and cortic osteroid therapy in the management of corrosive injury of the esophagus. J Pediatr 1961;59:356–360.

113. Haller JA, Andrews HG, White JJ, Tamer A, Cleveland WW. Pathophysiology and management of acute corrosive burns of the esophagus: results of treatment in 285 children. J Pediatr Surg 1971;6:578–581.

114. Klein J, Olson KRR, McKinney HE. Caustic injury from household ammonia. A J Emerg Med 1985;3:320.

115. Muhletaler CA, Gerlock AJ, de Soto L, Halter SA. Acid corrosive esophagitis: radiographic findings. Am J Radiol 1980;134:1137–1141.

116. Kuhn JR, Tunell WP. The role of initial cineesophagography in caustic esophageal injury. Am J Surg 983;146:804–806.

117. Levitt R, Stanley R, Wise L. Gastric bullae—an early roentgen finding in corrosive gastritis following alkali ingestion. Radiology 1975;115:597–598.

118. Fink DW, Boyden FM. Gas in the portal veins: a report of two cases due to ingestion of corrosive substances. Radiology 1966;87:741–743.

119. Mastrangelo MR, Moore EW. Spontaneous rupture of the stomach in a healthy adult man after sodium bicarbonate ingestion. Ann Intern Med 1984;101:650–651.

120. Caravati EM. Metabolic abnormalities associated with phosphoric acid ingestion. Ann Emerg Med 1987;16:904–906.

121. Froner GA, Rutherford GW, Rokeach M. Injection of sodium hypochlorite by intravenous drug users (letter). JAMA 1987;258:325.

122. Hoy RH. Accidental systemic exposure to sodium hypochlorite (chlorax) during hemodialysis. Am J Hosp Pharm 1981;38:1512–1514.

123. Schmidt FC, Vallencourt DC. Changes in the blood following exposure to gaseous ammonia. Science 1948;108:555–556.

124. Zitnik RS, Burchell HB, Shepherd JT. Hymodynamic effects of inhalation of ammonia in man. Am J Cardiol 1969;24:187–190.

125. Herrick RT, Herrick S. Allergic reaction to aromatic ammonia inhalant ampule. Am J Sports Med 1983;11:28.

126. Keirklin JK, Watson M, Bondoc CC, Burke JF. Treatment of hydrazine-induced coma with pyridoxine. N Engl J Med 1976;249:938–939.

127. Harati Y, Naikan E. Hydrazine toxicity, pyridoxine therapy, and peripheral neuropathy. Ann Intern Med 1986;104:727–729.

128. Sotaniemi E, Hirvonen J, Isomaki H, Takkunen J, Kaila J. Hydrazine toxicity in the human: report of a fatal case. Ann Clin Res 1971;3:30–33.

129. Reid FJ. Hydrazine poisoning. Br Med J 1965;2:1246.

130. Lindberg E, Hedensterna G. Chrome plating: symptoms, findings the upper airways, and effects on lung function. Arch Environ Health 38;367–374:1983.

131. Reidenberg MM, Durant PJ, Harris RA, DeBoccardo G, Lahita R, Steuzel KH. Lupus erythematosus-like disease due to hydrazine. Am J Med 1983;75:365–370.

132. Langard S, Vigander T. Occurrence of lung cancer in workers producing chromium pigments. Br J Ind Med 1983;40:71–74.

133. Shimkin MB, de Lorimier AA, Mitchell JR, Burroughs TP. Appearance of carcinoma following single exposure to a refrigeration ammonia-oil mixture. Arch Ind Hyg Occ Med 1954;9:186–193.

134. Wald N, Boreham J, Doll R. Bonsall J. Occupational exposure to hydrazine and subsequent risk of cancer. Br J Ind Med 1984;41:31–34.

135. O'Donnell CH, Abbott WE, Hirshfield JW. Surgical treatment of corrosive gastritis. Am J Surg 1949;78:251–255.

136. Appelqvist P, Salmo M. Lye corrosion carcinoma of the esophagus: a review of 63 cases. Cancer 45:2655–2658.

137. Parkinson AT, Haidak GL, McInerney RP. Verrucous squamous cell carcinoma of the esophagus following lye stricture. Chest 1970;57:489–492.

138. Rost KM, Jaeger RW, deCastro FJ. Eye contamination: a poison center protocol for management. Clin Toxicol 1979;14:295–300.

139. Rumack BH, Burrington JD. Caustic ingestions: a rational look at diluents. Clin Toxicol 1977;11:27–34.

140. Okada Y, Iway A, Kobayashi H. Gastric lavage solution for ingestion of corrosive agents. Jpn J Acute Med 1987;11:75–80.

141. Maull KI, Osmand AP, Maull CD. Liquid caustic ingestions: an in vitro study of the effects of buffer neutralization and dilution. Ann Emerg Med 1985;14:1160–1162.

142. Lacouture PG, Gaudreault P, Lovejoy FH. Clinitest table ingestion: an in vitro investigation concerned with initial emergency management. An Emerg Med 1986;15:143–146.

143. Haller JA, Bachman K. The comparative effect of current therapy on experimental caustic burns of the esophagus. Pediatrics 1964;34:236–245.

144. Knox WG, Scott JR, Zintel H, Guthrie R, McCabe RE. Bouginage and steroids used singly or in combination in experimental corrosive esophagitis. Ann Surg 1967;166:930–941.

145. Thompson JN. Corrosive esophageal injuries. II. An investigation of treatment methods and histochemical analysis of esophageal strictures in a new animal model. Laryngoscope 1987;97:1191–1202.

146. Lui A, Richardson M, Robertson WO. Effects of N-acetylcysteine on caustic burns (abstract). Vet Hum Toxicol 1985;28:316.

147. DiCostanzo J, Noirelerc M, Jouglard J, et al. New therapeutic approach to corrosive burns of the upper gastrointestinal tract. Gut 1980;21:370–375.

148. Ehrenpreis ED, Leiken JB, Ehrenpreis S, Goldstein JL. Use of sodium polyacrylate in rat gastrointestinal alkali burns. Vet Hum Toxicol 1988;30:135–138.

149. Mills LJ, Estrera AS, Platt MR. Avoidance of esophageal stricture following severe caustic burns by the use of an intraluminal stent. Ann Thorac Surg 1979;28:60–65.

150. Reyes HM, Lin CY, Schlunk FF, Replogle RL. Experimental treatment of corrosive esophageal burns. J Pediatr Surg 1974;9:317–327.

151. Wijburg FA, Heymans HS, Urbanns NA. Caustic esophageal lesions in childhood: prevention of stricture formation. J Pediatr Surg 1989;24:171–173.

152. Cornish HH. The role of vitamin B in the toxicity of hydrazine. Ann NY Acad Sci 1969;166:136–145.

153. American Conference of Governmental Industrial Hygienists: threshold limit values and biological exposure indices for 1990–1991. Cincinnati, OH: ACGIH, 1990.

154. Centers for Disease Control. MMWR 1986;35:1–33S.

68

Organic Acids and Bases

Hon-Wing Leung, Ph.D.
Dennis J. Paustenbach, Ph.D.

ORGANIC ACIDS

Organic acids constitute a very wide range of chemicals and have numerous industrial applications. Many are found naturally in the body and are biochemical intermediates in metabolic processes. The most common organic acids contain a dissociation hydrogen ion from a carboxyl (—COOH) functional group bound to an aliphatic (e.g., acetic acid), olefinic (e.g., acrylic acid), or aromatic hydrocarbon moiety (e.g., benzoic acid). Organic acids with the —COOH group are generally referred to as carboxylic acids. Longer chain aliphatic carboxylic acids are also known as fatty acids. Compounds containing a dissociable hydrogen ion from a hydroxyl group (—OH) may be classified as organic acid as well. However, their acid strength is generally much less than that of the carboxylic acid. Examples of organic acids containing the —OH group include the phenols (carbolic acid), glycols, naphthols, glycerols, and catechols (1).

Generally, chronic biologic effects are not a major concern with organic acids. Organic acids' primary adverse effects are irritation of the eyes, skin, and mucous membranes.

Industrial Uses

Carboxylic acids are usually prepared from oxidation of the corresponding aldehydes. For example, oxidation of acetaldehyde produces ethanoic acid. The higher carboxylic acids (fatty acids) are constituents of oil, fat, and waxes. Organic acids have a variety of industrial uses. They are employed in the production of fibers, resins, plastics, and dyestuffs. They are also important intermediates in the manufacture of pharmaceuticals, cosmetics, and food additives (2). Many of the carboxylic acids are generally recognized as safe (GRAS) and are used as food additives (3).

Routes of Exposure

The physical form of the organic acids may range from a liquid to a waxy solid. In general, the shorter chain organic acids are liquid at room temperature while the longer chain acids (greater than 10 carbons) tend to be solids. Table 68.1 shows the physicochemical properties of selected organic acids (4–7). Exposure through inhalation will be largely determined by the vapor pressure of the organic acids. Short chain organic acids such as formic, acetic, and propionic acid are more volatile, and as such they present a greater potential for inhalation exposure. Direct contact of organic acids with exposed body surfaces may produce primary irritation. The eyes, skin, and mucous membrane of the respiratory tract are particularly susceptible.

Predicting Irritation Potential

The ability of the organic acids to irritate tissue is a function both of molecular weight and of water solubility. As long as the compound is soluble in water, its potential to irritate increases with increasing molecular weight except for the first member of the aliphatic series, formic acid. As expected, at high molecular weights the acids are no longer water soluble and their irritation potential drops accordingly.

Organic acids that irritate the nose and mucous membranes can be expected to be skin irritants as well. The degree of irritation is predominantly governed by the strength of the acid, its water solubility, and its ability to penetrate the skin. The shorter chain organic acids are relatively strong acids and can produce corrosive effects (burns). Generally, substances with a pH below 2 are strong corrosives; however, pH alone is not the only determinant of severity. Important factors increasing the corrosive properties of an acid include concentration, molarity, and complexing affinity of the anion (8).

Metabolism

Aliphatic monocarboxylic acids are metabolized by beta-oxidation to acetate or butyrate, which are further metabolized to carbon dioxide and water via the citric acid cycle. In some cases, especially with medium chain carboxylic acids, metabolism may proceed by omega-oxidation, which produces dicarboxylic acid. Omega-oxidation does not normally occur with carboxylic acids with more than 12 carbons unless the capacity for beta-oxidation is saturated by a large dose or blocked because of substituents in the alpha or beta positions. Organic acids with alpha substituents are not readily metabolized and are eliminated in the urine after conjugation with glucuronide (9, 10).

Acute Toxicity

The acute oral toxicity of some common organic carboxylic acids (4, 11) are shown in Table 68.2. The most common toxic response resulting from acute exposure to organic acids is irritation. Irritation is a localized inflammatory reaction of the mucous membranes, epithelium, and other exposed areas of the body. It is characterized by the presence of erythema and edema. Exposure to some strong organic acids can produce a burning sensation to the eyes and respiratory tract. If the contact is with the skin, they can cause dermatitis. Severe dermal corrosion or ulceration with subsequent eschar formation may ensue in the case of prolonged exposure to some potent organic acids (12). The escharotic response is a result of the desiccating

775

Table 68.1. Physicochemical Properties of Organic Acids

Acid	CAS No.	Mol Wt	MP °C	BP °C	Solubility in Water	pKa1	pKa2	Vapor Pressure mm Hg	°C
(A) Saturated Acids									
Formic	64-18-6	46	8	100	Complete	3.75		35	20
Acetic*	64-19-7	60	17	118	Complete	4.76		11.4	20
Propionic*	79-09-4	74	−21	141	Complete	4.87		300	28
Butyric	107-92-6	88	−8	164	Complete	4.82		0.8	20
Isobutyric	79-31-2	88	−47	155	20%	4.86		1	15
Valeric	109-52-4	102	−34	186	3.3%	4.84		1	42
Isovaleric	503-74-2	102	−29	176	4.2%	4.78		1	34
Caproic	142-62-1	116	−5	205	1.1%	4.87		1	72
Isocaproic	646-07-1	116	−33	201	Slightly	4.84			
2-Methylvaleric	97-61-0	116		194	0.6%	4.78		0.02	20
2-Ethylbutyric	88-09-5	116	−31	194	Slightly	4.73		0.08	20
Heptanoic	111-14-8	130	−8	223	0.2%	4.88		1	78
Caprylic	124-07-2	144	18	240	Slightly	4.90		1	78
2-Ethylhexanoic	149-57-5	144		228	Slightly			0.03	20
Nonanoic	112-05-0	158	13	254	Insoluble			2	108
Capric	334-48-5	172	32	268	Insoluble			1	128
Undecylic	122-37-8	186	30	284	Insoluble			1	101
Lauric	143-07-7	200	44	225	Insoluble			1	121
Myristic	544-63-8	228	54	251	Insoluble			1	142
Palmitic	57-10-3	256	64	267	Insoluble			1	154
Stearic	57-11-4	284	69	291	0.03%			1	174
Oxalic	144-62-7	90	189	157	8.3%	1.46	4.40	0.54	105
Malonic	141-82-2	104	136		Very	2.80	5.85		
Succinic*	110-15-6	118	189	235	Slightly	4.17	5.64	0.03	47
Malic*	6915-15-7	134	131		Soluble	3.40	5.05		
Thiomalic	70-49-5	150	154		Soluble				
Tartaric*	87-69-4	150	171		Soluble	2.93	4.23		
Adipic*	124-04-9	146	153	338	Slightly	4.43	5.52	1	160
Citric*	77-92-9	192	153		Very	3.08	4.75		
Pimelic	111-16-0	160	106	272	Soluble	4.47	5.42		
Suberic	505-48-6	174	144	300	Slightly				
Propiolic	471-25-0	70	18	144	Complete	1.89		11	54
Acrylic	79-10-7	72	13	142	Complete	4.25		3	20
Crotonic	107-93-7	86	72	185	Very	4.69		0.2	20
Methacrylic	79-41-4	86	16	162	Slightly	4.66		0.7	20
Pentenoic	591-80-0	100	−23	188	Slightly	4.60		20	93
Hexenoic	1191-04-4	114	94			4.73		14	183
Sorbic*	110-44-1	112	134	228	Slightly	4.77			
Heptenoic	18999-28-5	129							
Undecylenic	112-38-9	184	24	275	Insoluble			10	160
Linolenic	1955-33-5	278	−11		Insoluble			0.05	125
Linoleic	2197-37-7	280	−5		Insoluble			16	229
Elaidic	112-79-8	282	45		Insoluble			100	288
Oleic	112-80-1	282	13		Insoluble			10	225
Ricinoleic	141-22-0	298	5		Insoluble			10	226
Arachidonic	506-32-1	304	−49		Insoluble				
Maleic	110-16-7	116	139		Very	1.83	6.09		
Fumaric	110-17-8	116	300		Slightly	3.03	4.44	1.7	165
Mesaconic	498-24-8	130	204		Slightly	3.09	4.75		
Citraconic	498-23-7	130	93		Very	2.29	6.15		
Itaconic	97-65-4	130	175		Slightly	3.85	5.45		
Aconitic	499-12-7	174	130	198	Slightly				

Data compiled and adapted from (4–7).
*Substances generally recognized as safe (GRAS) by the U.S. Food and Drug Administration (3).

action of the acid which causes a coagulation of the proteins in the superficial tissue. Unlike the liquefying necrosis of the strong bases, the coagulative necrosis of acid burns restricts the further penetration of the acids.

Death can occur from the inhalation exposure to organic acids, but this will only occur when escape is impossible, such as within confined spaces. Generally, the irritative effects of

organic acids provide sufficient warning properties to limit the exposure such that the only adverse effect elicited is temporary discomfort or annoyance. However, certain individuals may develop a tolerance for exposure to repeated high concentrations of organic acids. This phenomenon has been referred to in the medical literature as an adaptive response, desensitization, olfactory fatigue, as well as accommodation. Such unu-

Table 68.2. Median Lethal Oral Dose of Organic Acids in the Rat

Saturated Acids	mg/kg	Unsaturated Acids	mg/kg
Formic	1830	Propiolic	100–200
Acetic	3310–3530	Acrylic	340–3200
Propionic	2600–5760	Crotonic	400–1000
Butyric	2940–8790	Methacrylic	2260–9400
Isobutyric	280	Pentenoic	470
Valeric	1055–1844	Sorbic	3200–7360
Isovaleric	2000–<3200	Linolenic	>3200
Caproic	5970	Linoleic	>3200
Isocaproic	2050–<3200	Maleic	708
2-Methylvaleric	1600–3200	Fumaric	10700
2-Ethylbutyric	2033	Undecylenic	>2500
Heptanoic	7000		
Caprylic	1280–10080		
Ethylhexanoic	3000		
Capric	3320		
Lauric	12000		
Palmitic	>2000		
Stearic	>5000		
Oxalic	375–475		
Malonic	1310		
Propionic	2600–5760		
Succinic	2260		
Malic	>3200		
Thiomalic	800–1600		
Citric	11700		
Pimelic	7000		

Data compiled and adapted from Union Carbide Corporation unpublished data and (4, 11).

sual diseases as acid-etched teeth and perforated skin lesions are examples of this phenomenon (13). Although these diseases are only of historical interest in the United States, they may still exist in underdeveloped countries.

The irritation potency of organic acids is likely due to their acidity, i.e., their ability to produce or accept protons (hydrogen ions). The relative strength of an organic acid is measured by its respective equilibrium dissociation constant, K_a. Since K_a is usually a small number, it is more conveniently expressed as the negative decadic logarithm, denoted pK_a. For organic acids, the lower the pK_a, the stronger the acid, and vice versa. The presence of substituent groups on an organic acid may markedly affect its acidity. Electron-withdrawing substituents such as halogens (—FCl, —Br, —I) and nitro (—NO_2) group tend to disperse the negative charge and stabilize the anion, thus increasing acidity. In contrast, electron-releasing substituents such as alkyl and hydroxyl groups tend to intensify the negative charge, destabilize the anion, and thus decrease acidity (1). For this reason, chloroacetic acid and trichloroacetic acid are much stronger acids than acetic acid, while propionic and acetic acids are weaker acids than formic acid. A correlation between the strength of organic acids and their potential to cause irritation was recently established (14). A similar relationship of pK_a and acute skin irritation in humans for a homologous series of benzoic acid derivatives has also been reported (15).

Sensitization

Unsubstituted aliphatic acids do not sensitize humans, nor do they inhibit any enzyme systems as a primary toxic effect (16). Two examples of very active enzyme inhibitors are iodoacetic

and fluoroacetic acids. Iodoacetic acid has also been shown to be a sensitizer.

The first member of the aromatic homologues, benzoic acid, is a mild irritant and an occasional skin sensitizer. Since it is a solid at room temperature and has a low vapor pressure, it poses a lesser human health hazard compared to other more volatile chemical sensitizers.

Chronic Toxicity

With the exception of sensitization, organic acids rarely possess chronic toxic effects beyond those seen following acute exposure. None of these chemicals appears to have been positive in tests for mutagenicity or genotoxicity. This is not unexpected since the biologic activity of the organic acids is not usually due to systemic toxicity. In addition, their chemical structures are not ones that are likely to facilitate interaction with DNA or other macromolecules. For these reasons, these chemicals are not expected to have carcinogenic activity, and accordingly, have seldom been tested in chronic cancer bioassays.

METHANOIC ACID—1991 TLV: 5 PPM

Methanoic acid is commonly known as formic acid. It is also called formylic and hydrogen carboxylic acid. The major hazard of formic acid exposure is severe burns to the skin, eye, or mucosal surfaces. Lacrimation, increased nasal discharge, cough, throat discomfort, erythema, and blistering may occur depending on solution concentrations. Exposure to 0.3–42 ppm formic acid vapor for 1 hour was reported to be more irritating than the same concentration of formaldehyde (17). Formic acid was not teratogenic (4) or mutagenic (18). No histopathologic changes were noted in the skin of mice painted with 8% formic acid for 50 days (19). A worker accidentally splashed with formic acid developed severe dyspnea and dysphagia and died within 6 hours (20). Because formic acid can inhibit cellular respiration, workers with cardiovascular diseases are especially predisposed to the effects of formic acid (21).

ETHANOIC ACID—1991 TLV: 10 PPM

Ethanoic acid is commonly known as acetic acid. It is also called ethylic and methanecarboxylic acid. Rats given 390 mg/kg/day of acetic acid in the drinking water for 4 months were found to lose weight. No such effects were observed at a dose of 195 mg/kg/day (22). Gastric lesions were seen in rats fed 4.5 g/kg/day of acetic acid in the diet for 30 days. In a study of five workers exposed for 7–12 years to 80–200 ppm of acetic acid vapor, the principal findings were blackening and hyperkeratosis of the skin of the hands, conjunctivitis, bronchitis, pharyngitis, and erosion of the exposed teeth (23).

PROPANOIC ACID—1991 TLV: 10 PPM

Propanoic acid is commonly known as propionic acid. It is also called methylacetic and ethanecarboxylic acid. No remarkable changes were seen in rats fed 5% propionic acid for 110 days (24). A no observed effect level of 1 mg/kg/day was established in a study in rats fed propionic acid for 6 months (25). Propionic acid was not active in the in vitro mutagenicity assays (4).

BUTANOIC ACID—1991 TLV: NONE

Butanoic acid is commonly known as butyric acid. It is also called ethylacetic and 1-propanecarboxylic acid. Butyric acid is believed to be less irritating than propionic acid (26). No mortality was observed in rats exposed for 8 hours to air saturated with butyric acid vapor (27). No gastric lesions were found in rats fed 1–10% butyric acid for up to 500 days (24). Continuous inhalation of up to 200 mg/m^3 of butyric acid in rats for 7 months produced a slight reaction in the lung, but no other histologic changes were evident. The suggested maximum exposure concentration was 100 mg/m^3 (27).

PENTANOIC ACID—1991 TLV: NONE

Pentanoic acid is commonly known as valeric acid. It is also called propylacetic and 1-butanecarboxylic acid. No mortality occurred when rats were exposed for 8 hours to air saturated with valeric acid vapor (28). No significant changes were seen in rats with rabbits exposed to 200–300 mg/m^3 of valeric acid for 6 months (29). No remarkable change was observed in the glandular stomach of rats fed 5% valeric acid (24). Rats exposed continuously to valeric acid vapor for 97 days had no adverse changes. The recommended maximum permissible concentration was 6 mg/m^3 (30). The maximum allowable concentration (MAC) in the Soviet Union for valeric acid is 5 mg/m^3 (31).

HEXANOIC ACID—1991 TLV: NONE

Hexanoic acid is commonly known as caproic acid. It is also called n-hexoic and 2-butylacetic acid. Rats exposed to air saturated with caproic acid for 8 hours suffered no fatalities (32). No adverse changes were observed in rats fed 2–8% caproic acid in the diet for 3 weeks (33). The MAC in the Soviet Union for caproic acid is 5 mg/m^3 (31).

HEPTANOIC ACID—1991 TLV: NONE

Heptanoic acid is commonly known as heptylic acid. It is also called enanthic and 1-hexanecarboxylic acid. Mice receiving 125 mg/kg/day of heptylic acid by intraperitoneal injection died within 2–4 days after dosing (34).

OCTANOIC ACID—1991 TLV: NONE

Octanoic acid is commonly known as caprylic acid. It is also called n-octylic acid and 1-heptanecarboxylic acid. Caprylic acid is not mutagenic in the bacterial (*Salmonella typhimurium*) or the yeast (*Saccharomyces cerevisiae*) assays with or without metabolic activation (4). No reported exposure data are available.

NONANOIC ACID—1991 TLV: NONE

Nonanoic acid is commonly known as pelargonic acid. It is also called pelargic and 1-octanecarboxylic acid. Rats fed a diet of 4.17% pelargonic acid for 4 weeks had no discernible effects (35). A 12% solution of perlargonic acid in petrolatum produced no irritation or sensitization in humans (36).

DECANOIC ACID—1991 TLV: NONE

Decanoic acid is commonly known as capric acid. It is also called decylic and 1-nonanecarboxylic acid. No mortality was observed in rats exposed for 8 hours to saturated capric acid vapor (28). No gastric lesions were seen in rats fed 10% capric acid in the diet for 150 days (24). Capric acid (1% in petrolatum) did not produce irritation or sensitization when applied to human skin (37–38).

DODECANOIC ACID—1991 TLV: NONE

Dodecanoic acid is commonly known as lauric acid. It is also called duodecylic and 1-undecanecarboxylic acid. No adverse effects were seen in rats fed 10% lauric acid in the diet for 18 weeks (39). Rats fed a 10% lauric acid in the diet for 150 days developed no stomach lesions (24). Mice given subcutaneous injections of 1–5 mg of lauric acid three times per week for 24 months had no increased incidence of tumors (40).

TETRADECANOIC ACID—1991 TLV: NONE

The common name of tetradecanoic acid is myristic acid. It is also known as crodacid and 1-tridecanecarboxylic acid. Myristic acid was a moderate irritant when applied to human skin (41). Treatment of rats with 10% myristic acid in the diet for 33 days did not significantly alter body weight. However, there was evidence of increased erythrocyte fragility (42). Myristic acid was not carcinogenic (4).

HEXADECANOIC ACID—1991 TLV: NONE

The common name of hexadecanoic acid is palmitic acid. It is also known as cetylic and 1-pentadecane carboxylic acid. Rats fed 10% palmitic acid for 150 days developed no stomach lesions (24). Atherosclerotic lesions were noted in rats fed 6% palmitic acid for 16 weeks (43). No tumors were reported for mice treated with up to 5 mg of palmitic acid by subcutaneous injection three times per week (40).

OCTADECANOIC ACID—1991 TLV: NONE

Octadecanoic acid is commonly called stearic acid. It is also known as cetylacetic and 1-heptadecane carboxylic acid. Rats fed a diet containing 3000 ppm stearic acid had a somewhat erratic weight gain. There were, however, no pathologic lesions in all the organs examined (44). No sarcomas at the injection site were noted in mice given injections of 0.05 mg stearic acid once weekly for 6 months and observed for 21 months (45).

The toxicology of other aliphatic carboxylic acids are similar to those described for the saturated monocarboxylic acids. Generally, the health effects are characterized by low acute toxicity. The potential for irritation are much higher with the shorter chain members in the series, e.g., oxalic and malonic acids are relatively strong acids, whereas pimelic and sebacic acids are not irritants. The presence of a second carboxyl group in oxalic acid increases its acidity as compared with formic acid. The dicarboxylic acids are less extensively metabolized than the monocarboxylic acids. In fact, oxalic acid and malonic acid are excreted mainly unchanged. There have been reports that acrylic, crotonic, and methacrylic acids may have sensitization potential. There have been no reports suggesting any of the carboxylic acids are carcinogenic.

ORGANIC BASES

Chemical compounds classified as organic bases generally are amines. They contain one or more amino (—NH$_2$) functional groups which serve as proton acceptors, thus the basicity. They may be aliphatic amines (e.g., methylamine), aliphatic alcohol amines (e.g., ethanolamine), aromatic amines (e.g., aniline), or alicyclic amines (e.g., cyclohexylamine). The aliphatic amines can be further classified as primary, secondary, and tertiary amines depending on the number of alkyl side chains attached to the nitrogen of the amino moiety. Similar to the fatty acids, the longer chain aliphatic amines are called fatty amines. A variety of organic amines are naturally occurring. They are found in certain vegetables, fishes, cheeses, and bread (9–10).

Industrial Uses

Aliphatic and aromatic amines comprise a varied group of chemicals fundamental to industries producing explosives, pharmaceuticals, rubber chemicals, and dyes. They are also important intermediates in the synthesis of pesticides, plastics, and paints (2). The lower aliphatic amines are made by reacting ammonia with alcohols, aldehydes, or ketones. Alternatively, hydrogen cyanide is reacted with an alkene to yield an amide, which is then hydrolyzed to form the corresponding amine.

Routes of Exposure

The lower amines such as methylamine are gases or volatile liquids and are very soluble in water. They have a distinctive ammoniacal odor resembling that of decaying fish. The higher molecular weight amines are less volatile, odorless, and sparingly soluble in water. The physicochemical properties of selected organic amines (5–7, 46) are shown in Table 68.3.

Similar to the organic acids, the greatest potential for inhalation exposure to organic bases is with the shorter chain amines because of their greater volatility. Certain amines such as ethyleneamine have been shown to be respiratory sensitizers (47). Many of the amines can be absorbed through the skin and produce systemic effects. Aqueous solutions of organic amines are highly irritating, and prolonged contact can cause injury to the eyes, skin, and the respiratory tract. Ethyleneamine is also a skin sensitizer (48).

Metabolism

The amines are metabolized by the amine oxidases to ammonia and the corresponding aldehyde. The ammonia is converted to urea and excreted in the urine. The aldehyde is acted on by the enzyme aldehyde dehydrogenase to the respective carboxylic acid, which is further metabolized as discussed earlier in the chapter. The rate of deamination is faster with primary amines than secondary amines. The rate of oxidation appears to depend on the length of the alkyl chain, ranging from zero with the one-carbon methylamine to a maximum with hexylamine, and decreasing with further increase in chain length (9–10).

Toxicology

The acute oral toxicity of the organic amines ranges from slightly to moderately toxic (11, 46). The oral LD_{50} of selected amines in rats is shown in Table 68.4. Similar to the organic acids, the most significant acute effect of the organic amines is irritation. Exposure to concentrated vapor has produced severe inflammation of the respiratory tract and pulmonary edema in laboratory animals. Contact with the skin can cause burns re-

sulting in deep necrosis. Corneal damage resulting in blindness can occur to the eyes if the amines are allowed to remain in contact for prolonged period of time. The irritative effects of the amines are attributed to their alkalinity. Generally, the primary amines are more irritating than the secondary amines, which in turn are more irritating than the tertiary amines. The irritating potential tends to decrease as the alkyl chain length increases. The alkanolamines are less irritating than the corresponding alkylamines.

The alkylamines mimic the action of certain bioactive amines such as histamine and catecholamines, and may cause hemodynamic changes. The arylamines such as aniline produce methemoglobinemia (see Chapter 72). Secondary amines can react with nitrite to form nitrosamines which have been shown to be potent animal carcinogens. Certain polyamines especially ethylenediamine, diethylenetriamine, and triethylenetetramine are known to cause dermal and pulmonary allergic hypersensitization (47–49). Pathologic changes in the liver, kidneys, and heart have been observed in laboratory animals given high doses of the amines (50–51). However, in typical industrial exposures acute local effect of the amines, i.e., irritation, predominates.

ALKYLAMINES

The most important toxicities associated with the exposure to this class of organic bases are skin, eye, and respiratory tract irritation. Table 68.5 gives the current permissible exposure limits for these amines adopted by the United States Occupational Safety and Health Administration. As there is a paucity of longterm toxicity data on the alkylamines, the rationale of the exposure limits for these compounds is based largely on their irritative or other acute toxic effects in animals, and by analogy to one another.

ALICYCLIC AMINES

An important member of this class of amines is cyclohexylamine. Cyclohexylamine is known to have sympathomimetic effects mimicking that of the catecholamines (52). Humans acutely exposed to cyclohexylamine in industrial environment have reported symptoms of drowsiness, anxiety, and nausea (53). In a reproduction study mice fed a diet of 0.5% cyclohexylamine had growth retardation. The pregnancy rate, the number of live fetuses, and the fetal body weight were all reduced (54). In a multigeneration toxicity study, significant incidence of testicular atrophy and reduction of litter size were seen in rats given 150 mg/kg/day of cyclohexylamine (55). Cyclohexylamine has been widely tested for mutagenicity, teratogenicity, and carcinogenicity as it is a metabolite of the artificial sweetener sodium cyclamate. The data have been reviewed and no evidence of these effects has been demonstrated (56).

POLYAMINES

In addition to being an irritant, the polyamines typified by ethylenediamine (EDA), diethylenetriamine (DETA), and triethylenetetramine (TETA) have been reported to cause dermal and pulmonary sensitization. Most of the data on skin sensitization potential arose from the use of these compounds in topical pharmaceuticals, especially in Mycolog cream.

Table 68.3. Physicochemical Properties of Organic Bases

Name	CAS No.	Mol Wt	MP °C	BP °C	Solubility in water	VP mm Hg	°C	pKa1	pKa2
(A) Alkylamines									
Methylamine	74-89-5	31	−94	−6	Very	1500	25	10.7	
Dimethylamine	124-40-3	45	−93	7	Very	1500	10	10.7	
Trimethylamine	75-70-3	59	−117	3	Very	760	3	9.8	
Ethylamine	75-04-7	45	−81	16	Complete	400	3	10.7	
Diethylamine	119-89-7	73	−48	56	Complete	195	20	11.0	
Triethylamine	121-44-8	101	−115	89	Soluble	54	20	10.8	
Propylamine	107-10-8	59	−83	49	Soluble	400	31	10.6	
Di-n-propylamine	142-84-7	101	63	111	Soluble	30	25	11.0	
Isopropylamine	75-31-0	59	−101	34	Complete	460	20	10.6	
Diisopropylamine	108-18-9	101	−61	84	Slightly	70	20	11.0	
n-Butylamine	109-73-9	73	−50	77	Complete	72	20	10.7	
Di-n-butylamine	11-92-2	129	−60	160	Soluble	2	20	10.6	
Tri-n-butylamine	102-89-9	180	−70	214	Insoluble	20	100		
Isobutylamine	78-81-9	73	−85	68	Complete	100	19	10.8	
n-Amylamine	110-58-7	87	−55	104	Soluble				
Isoamylamine	107-85-7	87		95	Soluble				
n-Hexylamine	111-26-2	101	−19	133	1.2%	7	20	10.6	
n-Heptylamine	111-68-2	115	−18	157	Slightly				
2-Ethylhexylamine	104-75-6	130		142	0.25%				
Octadecylamine	124-30-1	270		232	Insoluble				
Allylamine	107-11-9	57		58	Complete			9.7	
Diallylamine	24-02-7	97	−88	111	8.6%			9.3	
Triallylamine	1102-75-9	137	−70	155	0.25%			8.3	
Cyclohexylamine	108-91-8	99		134	Soluble			10.7	
Dicyclohexylamine	101-83-7	181	20	254	Slightly				
N,N-Dimethylcyclohexylamine	98-94-2	127	−77	159	1.1%	3	25		
Ethylenediamine	107-15-3	60	9	116	Soluble	10	22	10.7	7.6
N,N-Diethylethylenediamine	100-36-7	116		145	Very	4	20	7.7	10.5
1,3-Propanediamine	109-76-2	74	−24	135	Soluble				
1,2-Propanediamine	78-90-0	74	−37	120	Complete	8	20	6.6	9.7
1,4-Butanediamine	110-60-1	88	27	158				9.2	10.8
1,3-Butanediamine	590-88-5	88		142					
1,5-Pentanediamine	462-94-2	102	9	178	Soluble				
1,6-Hexanediamine	124-09-4	116	41	204	Soluble			11.8	10.8
Diethylenetriamine	111-40-0	103	−3	207	Complete	0.2	20	4.4	9.2
Tetraethylene pentamine	112-57-2	189		340	Complete	<0.01	20	3.0	4.7

Name	CAS No.	Mol Wt	B.P. °C	Solubility in Water	pKa
(B) Alkanolamines					
Ethanolamine	141-43-5	61	170	Complete	9.5
Diethanolamine	111-42-2	105	268	96.4%	8.9
Triethanolamine	102-71-6	149	335	Complete	7.8
Propanolamine	156-87-6	75	187	Complete	
Isopropanolamine	78-96-6	75	160	Complete	
Triisopropanolamine	122-20-3	191	305	Very soluble	
Methylethanolamine	109-83-1	75	158	Complete	
Dimethylethanolamine	109-01-0	89	134	Complete	
Ethylethanolamine	110-73-6	89	169	Complete	
Diethylethanolamine	100-37-8	117	163	Complete	
Dibutylethanolamine	102-81-8	173	229	0.4%	
Methyldiethanolamine	105-59-9	119	247	Complete	
Ethyldiethanolamine	139-87-7	133	246	Complete	

Data compiled and adapted from (5–7, 46).

In a two-generation study of EDA, no reproductive toxicity was found in rats exposed to 0.5 g/kg/day (57). There was also no evidence of teratogenicity in rats fed up to 1 g/kg/day of EDA during organogenesis (58). EDA was not genotoxic in a variety of in vitro and in vivo mammalian test systems (59). A lifetime dermal bioassay established that EDA was not oncogenic (60).

The subchronic toxicity of DETA has been evaluated in a 90-day dietary study in the rats. Concentrations of 7,500 and 15,000 ppm DETA resulted in dose-related pathologic effects in the liver and kidney. A no observable effect level (NOEL) was 1,000 ppm (61). Both DETA and TETA have been tested for oncogenic potential in lifetime dermal painting studies in the mice and found to be not carcinogenic (62).

Table 68.4. Median Lethal Dose of Alkylamines and Alkanolamines in the Rat

Alkylamine	(g/kg)	Alkanolamine	(g/kg)
Methylamine	0.1–0.2	Ethanolamine	2.1
Dimethylamine	0.7	Diethanolamine	12.8
Ethylamine	0.4	Triethanolamine	8.0
Diethanolamine	0.54	Isopropanolamine	4.3
Triethanolamine	0.46	Triisopropanolamine	6.5
Propylamine	0.57	2-methylethanolamine	2.3
Dipropylamine	0.93	2-Dimethylethanolamine	2.3
Diisopropylamine	0.77	2-Ethylethanolamine	1.5
Butylamine	0.5	2-Diethyl	1.3
Dibutylamine	0.55	2-Dibutyl	1.1
Tributylamine	0.54	Propanolamine	2.8
Diisobutylamine	0.26	Ethylenediamine	1.5
Amylamine	0.47	1,3-Propanediamine	0.4
Dipentylamine	0.27	1,2-Propanediamine	2.2
2,2'-Diethyldihexylamine	1.64	1,3-Butanediamine	1.4
Allylamine	0.11	Diethylenetriamine	2.3
Diallylamine	0.58	Triethylenetetramine	4.3
Triallylamine	1.31		
2-Ethylbutylamine	0.39		
2-Ethylbutylamine	0.39		
Cyclohexylamine	0.71		
Dicyclohexylamine	0.37		

Data compiled and adapted from Union Carbide Corporation unpublished data and (11, 46).

Table 68.5. Permissible Exposure Limits for Alkylamines and Alkanolamines Adopted by the U.S. Occupational Safety and Health Administration

Amine	PEL (ppm)
Methylamine	10
Dimethylamine	10
Trimethylamine	10
Ethylamine	10
Diethylamine	10
Triethylamine	10
Isopropylamine	5
Diisopropylamine	5
Butylamine	5
Cyclohexylamine	10
Ethylenediamine	10
Diethylenetriamine	1
Ethanolamine	3
Diethanolamine	3

Source: OSHA. Air contaminant standards. Fed Reg 54 (Jan 19, 1989): 2232–2920.

ALKANOLAMINES

The most commonly used alkanolamines in industry are mono-ethanolamine (MEA), diethanolamine (DEA), and triethanolamine (TEA). The toxicologic properties of the alkanolamines generally resemble those of the corresponding alkylamines. The main biologic effects are local irritation of the skin, eye, and respiratory tract. The irritation potential decreases with increasing chain length. MEA is corrosive to the rabbit skin and eye, DEA causes minor irritation, and TEA is not irritating to the eye and skin (63–65).

Exposure of rats, guinea pigs, and dogs to 66–102 ppm of MEA for 24–30 days produced lung inflammation, liver, and kidney damage (66). Hepatotoxic effect was also reported in

a case of human poisoning to MEA (67). A recent report suggested that MEA given during period of organogenesis might produce embryopathic and teratogenic effects (68).

Studies conducted by the National Toxicology Program showed that rodents treated with DEA in drinking water and by dermal application for 90 days developed adverse effects in the liver, kidney, and heart (69–72). DEA appeared not to be mutagenic (73).

In a 90-day dermal study doses of TEA up to 2.3 g/kg/day produced only slight epidermal hyperplasia at the site of application but no other systemic effects (74). A recent dermal pharmacokinetic study suggested that the lack of systemic effects was not due to poor bioavailability following dermal administration of TEA (75). TEA was tested in a number of mutagenicity assays and found to be not genotoxic (76). A cancer bioassay in rats given drinking water containing up to 2% TEA for 2 years demonstrated that TEA was toxic to the kidneys but was not carcinogenic (77).

OCCUPATIONAL EXPOSURE LIMITS

Only a handful of the more than 100 organic acids and bases used in industry have occupational exposure limits (31). Although there is a great diversity among these groups of chemicals, the majority of them produce their adverse effects due to their acidity or alkalinity, i.e., the ability to produce or accept protons (hydrogen ions). Since the relative strength of an organic acid or base is measured by its respective equilibrium dissociation constant, K_a, this term should be useful in identifying acceptable levels of human exposure.

An approach for using the equilibrium dissociation constant to set preliminary occupational exposure limits was recently demonstrated (14). It was shown that the occupational exposure limits for organic acids and bases correlate well ($r \geq 0.80$) with the equilibrium dissociation constants (Figs. 68.1 and 68.2). This work is important and useful to clinicians since it showed that the higher the pK_a of an organic acid, the higher its exposure limit, i.e., less potential for irritation. Conversely, the higher the pK_a for an organic base, the lower the exposure limit, i.e., a greater tendency to be an irritant.

From this study (14), it was proposed that for organic acids and bases which have not yet had an occupational exposure limit (OEL) established, the following equation could be used to set a preliminary limit.

For organic acids: $\log \text{OEL } (\mu\text{mol/m}^3) = 0.43 \quad pK_a + 0.53$

For organic bases: $\text{OEL } (\mu\text{mol/m}^3) = -200 \, pK_a + 2453$

Table 68.6 shows the suggested occupational exposure limits calculated with these formulae for a variety of organic acids and bases.

The obvious shortcoming of this approach is that it does not take into account the direct biologic potency of the individual chemical. However, the advantages seem to clearly outweigh the potential disadvantages. For example, such an approach would reduce the number of laboratory animals that would be needed to screen chemicals. Second, such an objective and quantitative approach to setting OELs seems far more likely to yield an accurate result compared to more subjective approaches. Third, it offers an expedient way to set preliminary limits for the more than 90 organic acids and bases to which workers are occupationally exposed each day but for which there are no acceptable limits of exposure.

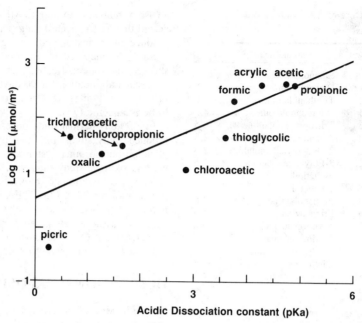

Figure 68.1. Correlation of occupational exposure limits with equilibrium dissociation constants of organic acids. The correlation coefficient, $r = 0.80$; $F_{1.8} = 7.5$; $0.01 < p < 0.05$. Reprinted with permission from: Leung, Hon-Wing, Paustenbach DS. Setting occupational exposure limits for irritant organic acids and bases. Appl Ind Hyg 1988;3(4):116–117.

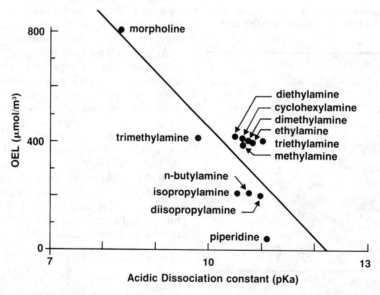

Figure 68.2. Correlation of occupational exposure limits with equilibrium dissociation constants of organic bases. The correlation coefficient, $r = -0.81$; $F_{1.10} = 21.17$; $p < 0.001$. Reprinted with permission from: Leung, Hon-Wing, Paustenbach DS. Setting occupational exposure limits for irritant organic acids and bases. Appl Ind Hyg 1988;3(4):116–117.

MANAGEMENT OF TOXICITY

The principal clinical manifestations of organic acid and base poisoning are irritation and corrosion. Exposure by ingestion causes severe burning pain to the mouth, pharynx, and stomach followed by vomiting and diarrhea which may be bloody. Asphyxia may occur from edema of the glottis. After initial recovery, onset of fever suggests mediastinitis or peritonitis from perforation of the stomach. Exposure by inhalation causes irritation of the respiratory tract which may be followed by pulmonary edema, tightness in the chest, dyspnea, and cyanosis.

Prolonged exposure may cause erosion of the teeth. Symptoms of skin contact are severe pain with dermal staining. The burn may penetrate the full thickness of the skin.

Exposure of the eyes can produce damage to the cornea, erythema, conjuctivitis, and iritis. The symptoms are tearing, pain, and photophobia (78). Generally, the damage to tissue by bases is more severe than by acids due to the solubilization of proteins, which allows deep penetration of the bases into tissues.

There are no specific antidotes for organic acid and base poisoning. Treatment involves the customary regimen of sta-

Table 68.6. Suggested Occupational Exposure Limits for Selected Major Organic Acids and Bases

Acid	mg/m^3	ppm	Base	mg/m^3	ppm
Acrylic	16	5	Allylamine	29	12
Butyric	35	10	Diallylamine	58	15
Caproic	49	10	Dibutylamine	43	8
Caprylic	62	10	Hexylamine	34	8
Crotonic	30	8.5	Isobutylamine	21	7
Heptanoic	55	10	Propylamine	20	8
Isobutyric	35	10	Triallylamine	109	20
Isocaproic	49	10			
Isovaleric	42	10			
Methacrylic	30	8.5			
Pentenoic	32	7.8			
Propiolic	1.5	0.5			
Valeric	42	10			

Exposure limits were calculated using the equations:

Acid: Log OEL (μmol/m^3) = 0.43 pKa + 0.53

Base: OEL (μmol/m^3) = −200 pKa + 2453

bilization, decontamination, and supportive care. Supportive care is necessary if airway complications arise. If the material is ingested, immediate dilution with milk or water within 30 minutes of exposure is indicated. However, neutralization with weak acids or bases should not be attempted since the exothermic reaction may aggravate the existing injury. Emesis is contraindicated because of reexposure of the esophagus. Activated charcoal is ineffective, since it does not absorb organic acids or bases. In the case of skin contact, remove all contaminated clothes and irrigate exposed skin copiously with water or normal saline. Exposed eyes should be irrigated with water for at least 30 minutes (2) (see Chapter 67).

REFERENCES

1. Neckers DC, Doyle MP. Organic chemistry. New York: John Wiley & Sons, 1977.
2. Gosselin RE, Smith RP, Hodge HC, Braddock JE. Clinical toxicology of commercial products. 5th ed. Baltimore: Williams & Wilkins, 1984.
3. Code of Federal Regulations. Vol 21, Part 582. Substances generally recognized as safe. Washington, DC: GPO.
4. Guest D, Katz GV, Astill BD. Aliphatic carboxylic acids. In: Clayton GD, Clayton FE, eds. Patty's industrial hygiene and toxicology. 3rd ed, Vol 2C. New York: John Wiley & Sons, 1982:4901–4987.
5. Weast TC, Astle MJ, Beyer WH, eds. CRC handbook of chemistry and physics. 70th ed. Boca Raton, FL: CRC Press, 1977.
6. Windholz M, Budavari S, Blumetti RF, Otterbein ES, eds. Merck Index. 10th ed. Rahway, NJ: Merck & Co, Ltd, 1983.
7. Dean JA, ed. Lange's handbook of chemistry. 13th ed. New York: McGraw-Hill, 1985.
8. Marzulli FN, Maibach HI. Dermatotoxicology. 3rd ed. New York: Hemisphere Publishing, 1989.
9. Lehninger A. Principles of biochemistry. New York: Worth Publishers, 1982.
10. Stryer L. Biochemistry. San Francisco: WH Freeman Publishing, 1981.
11. Registry of toxic effects of chemical substances. DHHS Publication no. 87-114. Washington, DC: National Institute of Occupational Safety and Health, 1987.
12. Adams RM. Occupational contact dermatitis. 2nd ed. Philadelphia: JB Lippincott Co, 1984.
13. Hunter D. The diseases of occupations. 6th ed. Boston: Little, Brown and Co, 1978.
14. Leung HW, Paustenbach, DJ. Setting occupational exposure limits for irritant organic acids and bases based on their equilibrium dissociation constants. Appl Ind Hyg 1988;4:115–118.
15. Berner B, Wilson DR, Guy RH, Mazzenga GC, Clarke FH, Maibach HI. The relationship of pKa and acute skin irritation in man. Pharm Res 1988;5:660–663.
16. Peterson JE. Industrial health. Englewood Cliffs, NJ: Prentice-Hall, 1977.
17. Amdur MO. Int J Air Pollut 1960;3:201–220.
18. Freese EB, Gerson J, Taber H, Rhaese J, Freese E. Inactivating DNA alterations induced by peroxides and peroxide-producing agents. Mutat Res 1967;4:517–531.
19. Frei JV, Stephens P. The correlation of promotion of tumour growth and of induction of hyperplasia in epidermal two-stage carcinogenesis. Br J Cancer 1968;22:83–92.
20. von Oettingen WF. The aliphatic acids and their esters—toxicity and potential dangers. AMA Arch Ind Health 1959;20:517–522.
21. Liesivuori J, Kettunen A. Farmer's exposure to formic acid vapor in silage making. Ann Occup Hyg 1983;27:327–329.
22. Sollman T. Studies of chronic intoxications on albino rats. III. Acetic and formic acids. J Pharmacol Exp Ther 1921;16:463–474.
23. Mori K. Production of gastric lesions in rats by acetic acid feeding. Gann 1952;43:433–466.
24. Mori K. Production of gastric lesions in the rat by the diet containing fatty acid. Jpn J Cancer Res 1953;44:421–427.
25. Shchepetova GA. Hygienic standards for propionic acid and sodium propionate in water bodies. Gig Sanit 1970;35:96–98.
26. Smyth HF, Carpenter CP, Weil CS. Range-finding toxicity data: list IV. Arch Ind Hyg Occup Med 1951;4:119–122.
27. Stasenkova KP, Kochetkova TA. Toxicologic characteristics of butyric acid. Toksikol Novykh Prom Khim Veshchestv 1962;4:19–28.
28. Smyth HF, Carpenter CP, Weil CS, Pozzani UC, Striegel JA. Range-finding toxicity data: list VI. Am Ind Hyg Assoc J 1962;23:95–107.
29. Egorov YL, Kasparov AA, Zakharov VM. Toxicology of synthetic fatty acids. Uchen Zap Mosk Nauchn-Issled Inst Gigieny 1961;9:40–46.
30. Dubrovskaya FI, Lukina IP. Effect of small concentrations of valeric acid vapors on experimental animals (white rats). Gig Salit 1966;31:7–10.
31. Cook WA. Occupational Exposure Limits—Worldwide. Akron, OH: American Industrial Hygiene Association, 1987.
32. Smyth HF, Carpenter CP, Weil CS, Pozzani UC. Range-finding toxicity data. Arch Ind Hyg Occup Med 1954;10:61–68.
33. Moody DE, Reddy JK. Hepatic peroxisome (microbody) proliferation in rats fed plasticizers and related compounds. Toxicol Appl Pharmacol 1978;45:497–504.
34. Fassett DW. Industrial Hygiene and Toxicology. 2nd ed. Vol II. Fassett DW, Irish DD, eds. New York: Wiley-Interscience, 1963.
35. Dryden LP, Hartman AM. Effect of vitamin B$_{12}$ on the metabolism in the rat of volatile fatty acids. J Nutr 1971;101:589–592.
36. Opdyke DLJ. Monographs of fragrance raw materials: pelargonic acid. Food Cosmet Toxicol 1978;16:839–841.
37. Opdyke DLJ. Monographs on fragrance raw materials: capric acid. Food Cosmet Toxicol 1979;17:735–742.
38. Stillman MA, Maibach HI, Shalita AR. Relative irritancy of free fatty acids of different chain length. Contact Derm 1975;1:65–69.
39. Fitzhugh OG, Schouboe PJ, Nelson AA. Oral toxicities of lauric acid and certain lauric acid derivatives. Toxicol Appl Pharmacol 1960;2:59–67.
40. Slern D, Wieder R, McDonough M, Meranze DR, Shimkin MB. Investigation of fatty acids and derivatives for carcinogenic activity. Cancer Res 1970;30:1037–1046.
41. Drill VA, Lazar P, eds. Cutaneous Toxicity. New York: Academic Press, 1977.
42. Elson CE, Voichick SJ. Dietary induced alterations in the fatty acids of rat bone marrow. Lipids 1970:698–701.
43. Relaud S. Thrombogenicity and atherogenicity of dietary fatty acids in rat. J Atheroscler Res 1968;8:625–636.
44. Deichmann WB, Radomski JL, MacDonald WE, Kascht RL, Erdmann RL. The chronic toxicity of octadecylamine. Arch Ind Health 1958;18:483–487.
45. Van Duuren BL, Katz C, Shimkin MB, Swern D, Weider R. Replication of low-level carcinogenic activity bioassays. Cancer Res 1972;32:880–881.
46. Beard RR, Noe JT. Aliphatic and alicyclic amines. In: Patty's industrial hygiene and toxicology. 3rd ed. Vol 2B. Clyston GD, Clayton FE, eds. New York: John Wiley & Sons, 1981.
47. Lam S, Chan-Yeung M. Ethylenediamine-induced asthma. Am Rev Respir Dis 1980;121:151–155.
48. Baer R, Ramsey DL, Biondi E. The most common contact allergens. Arch Dermatol 1973;108:74–78.
49. Echardt RE. Occupational and environmental health hazards in the plastics industry. Environ Health Perspect 1976;17:103–106.
50. Brieger H, Hodes WA. Toxic effects of exposure to vapors of aliphatic amines. AMA Arch Ind Hyg Occup Med 1951;3:287–291.
51. Pozzani UC, Carpenter CP. Response of rats to repeated inhalation of ethylenediamine vapors. Arch Ind Hyg Occup Med 1954;9:223–226.
52. Elchelbaum M, Hengstmann JH, Rost HD, Brecht T, Dengler HJ. Phar-

macokinetics, cardiovascular and metabolic actions of cyclohexylamine in man. Arch Toxicol 1974;31:243–263.

53. Watrous RM, Schulz HN. Cyclohexylamine, p-chloronitrobenzene, 2-aminopyridine: toxic effects in industrial use. Ind Med Surg 1950;19:317–320.

54. Kroes R, Peters PWJ, Berkvens JM, Verschuuren HG, De Vries T, Van Esch GJ. Long term toxicity and reproduction study (including a teratogenicity study) with cyclamate, saccharin and cyclohexylamine. Toxicology 1977;8:285–300.

55. Oser BL, Carson S, Cox GE, Vogin EE, Sternberg SS. Long term and multigeneration toxicity studies with cyclohexylamine hydrochloride. Toxicology 1976;6:47–65.

56. International Agency for Research on Cancer. Monographs on the evaluation of the carcinogenic risk of chemicals to man. Vol 22. Some non-nutritive sweetening agents. Lyons, France: IARC, 1980.

57. Yang RS, Garman RH, Weaver EV, Woodside MD. Two-generation reproduction study of ethylenediamine in Fischer 344 rats. Fundam Appl Toxicol 1984;4:539–546.

58. DePass LR, Yang RH, Woodside MD. Evaluation of the teratogenicity of ethylenediamine dihydrochloride in Fischer 344 rats by conventional and pair-feeding studies. Fundam Appl Toxicol 1987;9:687–697.

59. Slesinski RS, Guzzie PJ, Hengler WC, Watanbe PG, Woodside MD, Yang RSH. Assessment of genotoxic potential of ethylenediamine: in vitro and in vivo studies. Mutat Res 1983;124:299–314.

60. DePass LR, Fowler EH, Yang RSH. Dermal oncogenicity studies on ethylenediamine in male C3H mice. Fundam Appl Toxicol 1984;4:641–645.

61. Van Miller JP, Weaver EV, Negley JE, Gill MW. Ninety-day (subchronic) dietary toxicity study with the dihydrochloride salt of diethylenetriamine (DETA) in albino rat. Union Carbide Bushy Run Research Center Project Report 51-45. Export, PA: UCBRRC, 1988.

62. DePass LR, Fowler EH, Weil CS. Dermal oncogenicity studies on various ethyleneamines in male C3H mice. Fundam Appl Toxicol 1987;9:807–811.

63. Myers RC, Christopher SM. Monoethanolamine. Acute toxicity and primary irritancy studies. Union Carbide Bushy Run Research Center Project Report 51-86, Export, PA: UCBRRC, September 21, 1988.

64. Myers RC, Christopher SM. Diethanolamine. Acute toxicity and primary irritancy studies. Union Carbide Bushy Run Research Center Project Report 51-95, Export, PA: UCBRRC, September 21, 1988.

65. Myers RC, Christopher SM. Triethanolamine. Acute toxicity and primary irritancy studies. Union Carbide Bushy Run Research Center Project Report 51-94, Export, PA: UCBRRC, September 21, 1988.

66. Weeks MH, Downing TO, Musselman NP, Carson TR, Groff WA. The effects of continuous exposure of animals to ethanolamine vapors. Am Ind Hyg Assoc J 1960;21:374–381.

67. Jindrichova J, Urban R. Acute monoethanolamine poisoning. Pracov Lek 1971;9:314–317.

68. Mankes RF. Studies on the embryopathic effects of ethanolamine in Long Evans rats: preferential embryopathy in pups contiguous with male siblings in utero. Teratogenesis Carcinog Mutagen 1986;6:403–417.

69. Hejtmancik M, Persing R, Peters AC. The prechronic dermal study of diethanolamine in B6C3F1 mice. Final report to the National Toxicology Program. Columbus, OH: Battelle, July 1988.

70. Hejtmancik M, Ryan M, Peters AC. The prechronic dermal study of diethanolamine in Fischer 344 rats. Final report to the National Toxicology Program, Columbus, OH: Battelle, August 1988.

71. Hejtmancik M, Mezza L, Peters AC. The prechronic dosed water study of diethanolamine in Fischer 344 rats. Final report to the National Toxicology Program. Columbus, OH: Battelle, September 1988.

72. Hejtmancik M, Singer A, Peters AC. The prechronic dosed water study of diethanolamine in B6C3F1 mice. Final report to the National Toxicology Program. Columbus, OH: Battelle, October 1988.

73. Dean BJ, Brooks TM, Hodson-Walker G, Hutson DH. Genetic toxicology testing of 41 industrial chemicals. Mutat Res 1985;153:57–77.

74. DePass LR, Coleman JH. Ninety-day dermal toxicity study of triethanolamine in C3H/HeJ mice. Union Carbide Bushy Run Research Center Project Report 47-501, Export, PA: UCBRRC, June 8, 1984.

75. Waechter JM, Rick DL. The pharmacokinetics of triethanolamine in C3H/HeJ mice and Fischer 344 rats following dermal administration. Toxicologist 1989;9:84.

76. Inoue K, Sunakawa T, Okamoto K, Tanaka Y. Mutagenicity tests and in vitro transformation assays on triethanolamine. Mutat Res 1982;101:305–313.

77. Maekawa A, Onodera H, Tanigawa H, Furuta K, Kanno J, Matsuoka C, Ogiu T, Hayashi Y. Lack of carcinogenicity of triethanolamine in F344 rats. J Toxicol Environ Health 1986;19:345–357.

78. Ellenhorn MJ, Barceloux DG. Medical toxicology: diagnosis and treatment of human poisoning. New York: Elsevier, 1988.

79. OSHA. Air contaminats standards. Fed Reg 54 (Jan 19, 1989):2232–2920.

69

Hydrofluoric Acid

Edward P. Krenzelok, Pharm.D.

PROFILE OF HYDROFLUORIC ACID EXPOSURES

Hydrofluoric acid (HF) is a corrosive agent with unique chemical properties and has the potential to produce significant toxicity even following dermal exposure to seemingly small amounts and low concentrations. In contrast to most toxic exposures, nearly 90% of HF exposures result in the development of some toxic sequelae, and approximately 80% of patients require treatment in a health care facility (Table 69.1) (1–4). Although HF has a variety of industrial applications, exposures are not confined to the workplace, and over 60% of incidents occur in the home (5). Regardless of the location of the incident, most HF exposures occur from the failure to adhere to safety recommendations and to a lack of knowledge about the chemical itself.

SOURCES AND PRODUCTION

HF, known by a variety of synonyms (Table 69.2), is an inorganic acid produced when calcium-fluoride is reacted with sulfuric acid at high temperatures. Available as both a liquid and a gas, the liquid form is colorless and found in both the anhydrous and aqueous forms (Table 69.3). Anhydrous HF is highly reactive with water and boils at 19.4°C, whereas aqueous HF is not as reactive but will spontaneously fume at concentrations in excess of 48% (6). In all forms HF is 1000 times more undissociated than hydrochloric acid (7). The anhydrous and highly concentrated aqueous forms are considered to be strong acids, and the low concentration aqueous solutions are weak acids.

SITES, INDUSTRIES, AND BUSINESSES ASSOCIATED WITH EXPOSURES

Occupational Uses

HF was first used artistically to etch glass in 1670, and since then the use of HF has expanded to include a multitude of industrial applications (Table 69.4). The spectrum of industries using HF in industrial and commercial processes places a large number of workers at a substantial risk of being exposed to this highly toxic substance. HF exposure limits and workplace standards may be found in Table 69.5.

MECHANISMS, PROCESSES, REACTIONS LEADING TO EXPOSURE

HF is regarded as a hazardous chemical. However, the extensive toxicity profile, which is not universally appreciated, creates a high risk environment when HF is used in occupational applications. The failure to comprehend and recognize the basic physicochemical properties of HF, as well as human carelessness, are the primary epidemiologic factors which lead to exposures to HF.

Human Factors

Noncompliance with usage recommendations and precautionary information accounted for 62% of all HF exposures in one

Table 69.1. Composite National Hydrofluoric Acid Exposure Data 1985–88 (1–4)

All reported poisoning exposures	4.36 million
All reported hydrofluoric acid exposures	3,417 (0.08%)
Adults	87.4%
Accidental	98.8%
Treated in health care facility	78.6%
Outcome (severity)	
No effect	10.3%
Minor effect	57.8%
Moderate effect	29.6%
Major effect	2.2%
Fatalities	<0.1%

Table 69.2. Hydrofluoric Acid Synonyms

HF
Hydrogen fluoride solution
Hydrofluoric acid solution
Hydrofluoric acid
Aqueous hydrofluoric acid
Fluoric acid solution
CAS 7664-39-3
UN 1790
NIOSH/RTECS MW 7875000
STCC 4930022
Anhydrous hydrofluoric acid
HF
Anhydrous hydrogen fluoride
Anhydrous hydrofluoric acid
Hydrogen fluoride
CAS 7664-39-3
UN 1052
NIOSH/RTECS 7875000
STCC 4930024

Table 69.3. Liquid Forms and Common Concentrations of Hydrofluoric Acid

Form	Concentration
Anhydrous	100%
Aqueous	70%
Reagent grade	5–52%
Commercial products	0.5–70%
Household	8%

series (5). Workers commonly handle HF without taking safety precautions and wearing the appropriate safety equipment. This is best exemplified by the frequency of hand exposures, which occur when thin surgical-type latex gloves are used during HF application instead of heavier natural rubber, neoprene, nitrile, or PVC handwear, which are less likely to puncture and are more impervious to HF penetration. The failure to read and comply with product labels as well as the development of complacency which may occur during long temporal accident-free periods and the lack of continuing safety education by employers lead to HF exposure. Additional factors predisposing to exposures include inadequate ventilation at the site of use, placing HF solutions in improperly marked or unmarked containers, unauthorized use of industrial strength HF at home, and cottage industry applications such as ceramics where the craftsman may have little knowledge of HF's toxicity.

Physicochemical Factors

The majority of individuals who use HF are not chemists who are familiar with its chemical and toxic properties, but are

Table 69.4. Industrial Applications of Hydrofluoric Acid

Industry	Application
Aerosol	Propellants Solvents
Agriculture	Insecticide/fertilizer production
Aluminum industry	Manufacture of aluminum chloride Reduction of aluminum oxide
Atomic energy	Production of uranium tetrafluoride Purification of isotopes
Brewery	Control fermentation Cleaning
Ceramic	Etching and glazes
Foundries	Removal of sand/scale from castings
Glassware	Etching/frosting/polishing
Laundry/textile	Stain removal Trace metal removal
Leather	Tanning process
Masonry	Cleaning sandstone/marble/brick/etc.
Metal	Cleaning/polishing Stainless steel pickling Welding with fluoride-containing flux
Petrochemical	Production of high octane fuels
Pharmaceutical	Drug/dye production
Semiconductor industry	Wet etching of silicon wafers for microelectronic circuits and computer chips

Table 69.5. Hydrofluoric Acid Exposure Limits/Workplace Standards

Threshold limit value-ceiling (TLV-C)	3 ppm (2.5 mg/m^3)
Shortterm exposure limit (STEL)	3 ppm
Odor threshold	0.03 mg/m^3
Immediately dangerous to life and health value (IDLH)	20 ppm

workers who use it for a specific purpose. Their knowledge base regarding HF physicochemical properties is limited to a single application. Leakage may occur when HF is improperly stored in stoneware or steel containers, since HF dissolves silica found in stoneware and is corrosive to steel (8). Explosions may occur when HF is stored in improper containers, due to the accumulation of gaseous materials. Hydrogen gas evolves when HF is in contact with steel, and a gaseous form of silicon tetrafluoride may be produced when HF is stored in glass containers (8). Explosive potential can also be achieved when concentrated HF is admixed with alkali or aqueous substances.

Anhydrous HF must be stored under pressure or at low temperatures since it boils at 19.4°C and fumes at concentrations in excess of 48% (9, 10). Therefore, highly concentrated forms of HF easily produce vapors that can contaminate the workplace if the HF is not used under hoods or in appropriately ventilated areas. The ability to fume at moderate concentrations and relatively low temperatures creates ideal conditions after a spill for the development of extensive environmental hazards due to vapor cloud formation.

Industrial applications include the use of HF in concentrations from less than 1% to 100%. Although workers realize that concentrated HF is highly toxic, there is not equal appreciation of HF's ability to produce serious injury in concentrations of less than 10%. Therefore, when low concentrations are used, there is a tendency to not comply with safety precautions. The severity of injury from HF exposure is partially concentration-dependent, since concentrated HF generally produces more severe toxicity. However, it is essential that HF handlers understand the potential for toxicity at all concentrations and realize that there is no common percentage that can be relied on as safe!

CLINICAL TOXICOLOGY OF EXPOSURE

The severity of the toxic sequelae associated with HF exposures is dependent upon the extent, duration and route of exposure, concentrations of HF, temporal relationship of the exposure to decontamination and local and/or systemic treatment, and numerous other factors. Regardless of the influence of these factors, the clinical toxicology at the cellular level is the same.

Dermal Exposure

The majority of HF exposures are dermal, and over 70% of all HF exposures involve the hands and specifically the digits (5). HF is 1000 times less dissociated than hydrochloric acid. Being largely unionized, it is capable of penetrating the skin and proceeding through lipid barriers to deeper subcutaneous tissue, even bone. Concentrated HF has sufficient free hydrogen ions which produce immediate corrosive effects as well as penetrate to subcutaneous tissue (7, 11). Dilute solutions (<10–20%) rarely produce immediate external corrosive effects and manifest their toxicity in delayed fashion (up to 24 hours) after sufficient HF has penetrated to the subcutaneous tissue (7, 11). Once absorbed, HF distributes systematically, and fluoride ion dissociates from the hydrogen (12, 13). Free fluoride ion complexes with calcium and other cations such as magnesium, rendering them ineffective in their physiologic functions (14, 15, 16). Bone demineralization and necrosis occur, and as calcium becomes physiologically compromised potassium is released from nervous tissue, resulting in the development of severe pain (15, 17). Exposures to significant amounts of HF may produce hypocalcemia and effect cyclic adenosine monophosphate production sufficiently so as to produce arrhythmias and resultant hemodynamic compromise (17). These effects can occur from small surface area exposures to high HF concentrations or larger surface areas with low concentrations. It is all dependent on the total amount of HF absorbed. Therefore, dermal exposure can produce local effects as well as serious systemic toxicity, even fatalities.

Inhalation Exposure

The clinical toxicology of inhalation exposure parallels that of dermal exposures with two exceptions: the toxic effects have a rapid onset, and pulmonary compromise may develop. Inhalation exposures to HF are rare and are generally the result of an explosion or substantial spill. The likelihood of HF being an inhalation hazard (other than in an explosion) decreases in proportion to reductions in concentration below 50%, since the partial pressure decreases accordingly (8). HF is water soluble, and small amounts are effectively scrubbed out by the upper respiratory tract, thereby by preventing the extension of pathology beyond that region. These exposures are not likely to produce bronchospasm or pulmonary edema. However, since HF is so irritating, the inhalation of volatile fractions of concentrated HF can rapidly produce bronchospasm, chemical pneumonitis, and/or pulmonary edema, and can progress to death (8, 18, 19). Furthermore, systemic absorption of HF can produce complexation of calcium and magnesium and can result in cardiovascular compromise (17).

Ocular Exposures

Explosions and splash incidents commonly result in dermal as well as ocular exposures. The eye is exquisitely sensitive to acids, and HF has corrosive properties that are similar to other acids. Inorganic acids, with the exception of HF, rarely penetrate beyond the corneal stroma since they produce coagulation necrosis, which limits the extent of penetration in all but exposures to the most concentrated acids (20, 21). HF, being highly unionized, is able to penetrate ocular tissue, precipitate cations, and produce rapid opacification and severe damage to the anterior anatomy of the eye. Systemic toxicity is unlikely following exposure solely limited to the eye.

Ingestion

Occupational exposures to HF principally involve the dermal, ocular, and inhalational routes. Ingestions in this setting are rare, and the majority of reported cases are suicide attempts. The systemic clinical toxicology of ingested HF is the same as with the other routes of exposure. In addition to the established cellular toxicity, the corrosive nature of HF may produce superficial and/or transmural erosion of the oropharyngeal and gastric mucosa (14, 22). Aspiration may occur during the ingestion process and produce irritant effects in the pulmonary tree.

Toxicokinetics

ABSORPTION

As a highly unionized moiety, HF is able to penetrate through physiologic barriers and is systematically absorbed via any route of exposure. HF has a low pKa (3.8), which helps to maintain HF in the unionized state which further facilitates rapid gastric absorption (22, 23).

METABOLISM

After HF is absorbed via any route it eventually dissociates to free hydrogen and fluoride ions. Fluoride is not metabolized by any of the body's metabolic processes (23).

ELIMINATION

The elimination toxicokinetics of HF have not been established. Data on therapeutic doses of fluoride in healthy and osteoporotic patients indicate that approximately 50% of a daily dose of fluoride is eliminated via the urine, the feces account for 6–10%, and perspiration may account for the elimination of 13–23% of a daily dose (23). Renal compromise can occur within 30 minutes of exposure to highly concentrated HF, further reducing the elimination of HF (14, 18, 19). One patient with dermal exposure to anhydrous HF eliminated approximately 75% of the total renal excretion during the first 24 hours post exposure (24).

SIGNS, SYMPTOMS, AND SYNDROMES FROM TOXIC EXPOSURE

Acute Toxicity

A variety of factors influence the acute local and systemic toxicity of HF exposures. The most significant factor influencing acute systemic toxicity is the total amount of fluoride ion absorbed. In dermal exposures this is a function of the duration of the exposure, the total surface area affected, and the concentration of the HF. Fatalities have resulted following facial exposure (2.5% of the total body surface area) to anhydrous HF (25). Similarly, lower concentrations to larger surface areas or over prolonged periods may produce serious toxicity and even death (7, 26). The implementation of treatment may also influence patient outcome. Rapid decontamination of externally exposed patients may reduce the absorption of HF and reduce systemic and even local toxicity.

DERMAL TOXICITY

In 1943 the National Institutes of Health classified HF burns into three categories solely based on the concentration of HF (11). These guidelines do not take factors such as total affected surface area or the duration of the exposure into consideration. HF solutions not exceeding 20% may have a delay of up to 24 hours before producing erythema and pain. Burns from solutions with concentrations in the range of 20–50% are apparent within 1–8 hours after the exposure. Solutions of greater than 50% HF produce immediate pain and tissue destruction. Although these guidelines are old, there is general correlation between the concentration of HF and the onset of symtoms, especially with the highly concentrated solutions. However, symptoms from exposure to dilute solutions may occur more rapidly.

Exposures to dilute solutions which go untreated have the potential to produce serious tissue damage. Dilute solutions usually produce delayed severe pain with or without initial erythema. The pain may intensify and be characterized as a burning or throbbing sensation, and the affected area may suffer tissue destruction which may include the presence of whitish to black dessicated and hardened skin secondary to coagulation necrosis (7, 10, 15, 16). Single or coalescent bullae may develop, but this is the exception following the exposure to dilute solutions (7, 27). Concentrated solutions produce a more rapid onset of symptoms manifest by intense pain and rapid tissue destruction. Blister formation is common, and tissue destruction may result in the development of deep subcutaneous necrosis, destruction of fingernail beds, severe scar formation, and the necessity of amputation of an affected digit (7, 10, 15, 16). In significant hand exposures HF penetration may produce tendonitis and carpal tunnel syndrome. Serious systemic toxicity and death can result from dermal exposures.

INHALATION TOXICITY

HF is a respiratory irritant, and the inhalation of even low concentrations can produce minor irritation to the mucous membranes of the upper respiratory tract. The severity of irritation and the potential for severe toxic insults to the respiratory tract increases as the concentration of the inhaled HF increases. Concentrations in excess of 48% are known to fume, increasing the volatile fraction of HF which is capable of being inhaled. High concentrations may produce severe chemical pneumonitis, bronchospasm, bronchial swelling, which may obstruct the airway, hemorrhagic pneumonitis, and pulmonary edema (8, 16, 18, 19). Fatalities have been reported secondary to the inhalation of concentrated HF (18, 19). As with dermal exposures, HF inhalation may produce serious systemic toxicity.

OCULAR TOXICITY

Consistent with the dermal and inhalation routes of exposure, the severity of ocular toxicity is dependent on the concentration of HF and the length of the exposure. In rabbits mild conjunctival irritation occurs after exposure to 0.5% HF (20). Dilute solutions have produced delayed toxicity manifest as long as 4 days after the exposure and have the potential to produce severe ocular toxicity (21). Characteristically, ocular exposures to HF produce the immediate onset of severe pain, corneal erosion, and a conjunctival and corneal inflammatory response resulting in vascularization and scarring of the cornea (20, 21, 28, 29). The globe may perforate, and surrounding tissue including tear ducts and the eyelids may be adversely affected (29, 30). Systemic toxicity is an unlikely outcome.

INGESTION TOXICITY

HF has the potential to produce corrosive effects consistent with other acids. The corrosiveness increases as the concentration of the HF solution increases. Ingestion of HF produces pain and erosion of the mucous membrane of the mouth, esophagus, and stomach (31). The ingestion of a HF-containing rust remover available to consumers resulted in the development of spontaneous emesis, severe metabolic acidosis, hypotension, and death which occurred 90 minutes after the ingestion (22). The postmortem analysis revealed the presence of hemorrhagic pulmonary edema and diffuse hemorrhagic gastritis without the presence of ulceration. Systemic toxicity may occur in addition to the toxic local manifestations associated with HF ingestion.

SYSTEMIC TOXICITY

Only the ocular route has not been associated with the development of systemic toxicity from HF exposures. Electrolyte and acid-base abnormalities such as hypocalcemia, hypomagnesemia, hyponatremia, hyperkalemia, hyperphosphatemia, and metabolic acidosis may result from the absorption of HF (10, 14, 17, 22, 24, 25, 26, 31, 32, 33). The risk of developing hypocalcemia and the attendant electrolyte abnormalities is dependent on the degree of exposure to HF. The risk increases as the affected body surface area and HF concentration increase. The following conditions are thought to predispose the patient to the development of hypocalcemia: ≥1% surface area with ≥50% HF, >5% surface area with any concentration HF, and inhalation of ≥60% HF (33). The resultant effects of systemic fluorosis are cardiovascular insults such as hypotension, ventricular arrhythmias, and asystole (17, 23, 33). Renal toxicity has been reported (18, 19).

Chronic and Long-Term Effects

Chronic exposure to subacute amounts has a low index of toxicity (34, 35). Three men exposed on a daily basis to 80% HF to remove glass from the surface of platinum in a ventilated hood had increased urinary levels of fluoride but no evidence of systemic fluorosis (34). The repeated exposure and absorption of 10–80 mg of fluoride per day may produce systemic fluorosis initially manifest as increased bone density on radiographs due to fluoride deposition in bone, eventually leading to osteosclerosis due to the replacement of calcium by fluoride in the bone (23, 36). Ligaments and joints may calcify, restricting mobility and producing severe pain. This condition can be crippling. Other manifestations of chronic fluorosis include anorexia, nausea, vomiting, diarrhea or constipation, shortness of breath, stiffness and diffuse rheumatic pain, malaise, and headache (23, 36).

There is no evidence that HF is either teratogenic or carcinogenic.

MANAGEMENT OF TOXICITY

Paramount to the successful management of any HF exposure is cessation of the exposure by removing the patient from the toxic environment and decontamination. HF is rapidly absorbed, and any delay in decontaminating the patient will increase the severity of the exposure. Only in cases where life support is essential should decontamination be temporarily delayed.

Clinical Examination

Prior to the examination the treating physician and all assisting individuals should protect themselves from exposure to HF. Multiple layers of latex gloves, gowns, footwear covers, etc., should be used. All contaminated clothing should be placed in heavy plastic bags or containers and marked accordingly. Care should be taken to supervise these containers to prevent housekeeping personnel from being contaminated. Supportive care and decontamination should be instituted prior to performing the routine examination.

Affected areas should be examined for the presence of erythema, bullae, and burns. All contiguous anatomic regions should be examined, including skinfolds and areas covered by hair for evidence of toxicity. Dilute solutions may produce external evidence of toxicity in a delayed fashion. Therefore, the absence of burns does not rule out a toxic exposure unless the substance contained higher concentrations of HF. If sufficient time has passed, affected areas will be intensely painful, and palpation of those areas will not be necessary to elicit a response regarding the presence of pain. The affected area will generally be well demarcated, and that information should be descriptively and artistically documented.

Patients suffering from ocular exposures should have a slit lamp examination after their eyes have been thoroughly irrigated. An ophthalmologist should be consulted.

Patients with significant inhalation exposures will present with signs of respiratory compromise. The airway should be secured via endotracheal intubation if necessary. A thorough evaluation of respiratory function is essential. Pulmonary edema can be delayed, but it is unlikely to occur without the presence of severe upper respiratory tract irritation.

Ingestors of HF should have an extensive examination of the oropharyngeal cavity, and unless the solution is very dilute the patient's examination should include endoscopic evaluation of the esophagus and the stomach. These steps should be undertaken after sufficient dilution of the stomach contents with water or preferably milk. The rapid absorption of HF may produce early systemic toxicity, which may necessitate emergent life support and delay this examination.

Treatment

The focus of treatment is life support, decontamination, inactivation of the fluoride ion, and treatment of specific problems. As with all poisonings, if necessary, an airway must be secured, breathing supported, and the cardiovascular system maintained. Intravenous access should be established as soon as possible in patients with the potential to develop systemic toxicity. The patient should be thoroughly decontaminated. After successful completion of these initial steps, a regional poison information center should be consulted regarding the current therapy of HF exposures.

Dermal Exposures   All contaminated clothing must be removed, and the affected areas should be immediately and continuously irrigated with large volumes of lukewarm tap water for at least 15 minutes. After irrigation has been completed efforts should be made to prevent the absorption of any HF which remains on the skin. A variety of topical agents which allegedly complex with the fluoride ion have been used. They include the use of the cationic agent benzalkonium chloride, magnesium salts such as magnesium sulfate, and calcium gluconate. Benzalkonium chloride and magnesium salts have not been conclusively demonstrated to be more effective than thorough irrigation with water (28, 37). Some evidence exists to suggest that the liberal application of calcium gluconate gel to the affected area, immediately after irrigation is completed, may be efficacious (7, 16, 26). Topical therapies have limited usefulness, however, since they do not penetrate the skin and are unable to reverse the toxic subcutaneous effects of the fluoride ion. Dimethyl sulfoxide (DMSO) in combination with 10% calcium gluconate may be able to penetrate from the skin into the subcutaneous tissue (38). Patients presenting to emergency departments and suffering from the delayed onset of pain after the use of less concentrated solutions of HF may respond to the topical application of calcium gluconate gel. Patients who fail to respond as indicated by the relief or significant

reduction of pain within 45 minutes may need to be treated with parenteral administration of calcium gluconate.[7]

Two types of parenteral treatment exist—local infiltration therapy and intraarterial infusion. Local infiltration therapy is based on the principle of injecting small amounts of calcium gluconate into the affected subcutaneous tissue, usually a digit. The calcium allegedly precipitates the fluoride ion in the form of insoluble calcium fluoride. This inactivates the fluoride ion and stops both the tissue destruction and the associated pain. Calcium gluconate (10%) is injected into the subcutaneous tissue using a 25–30-gauge needle and not exceeding a total injected volume of 0.5 ml/cm^2 (7, 10, 16, 31). The procedure is painful and often difficult to perform in a patient who is already in a great deal of discomfort. The successful endpoint of treatment is the elimination of pain. To facilitate the injection process, local block anesthesia is often instituted. This is not recommended since it eliminates the resolution of pain as a goal of therapy. Subungual exposure is a common problem since 72% of all exposures involve the fingers (5). Infiltration therapy may not be effective, and nail removal may be necessary. However, patients who are exposed to less than 10% HF may not need nail removal (39). The pain may persist for several days, but there is evidence to suggest that there will not be any serious longterm sequelae. Properly performed, this procedure has gained widespread acceptance due to its success in resolving pain.

Improperly performed, local infiltration therapy has many attendant dangers. It is an extremely painful procedure which may result in patients refusing care and subsequently developing more toxicity. Care must be exercised to refrain from administering large amounts of calcium gluconate. Excessive administration may produce a compression syndrome which can result in vascular compromise, ultimately worsening the tissue destruction caused by the HF. Calcium chloride is very irritating to tissues and should never be used for local infiltration purposes (10).

Intraarterial calcium administration has been successful in the management of extremity exposures to HF (40, 41, 42). Compared with infiltration therapy it suffers from the disadvantages that it is not universally available, requires hospital admission, and is invasive. It requires that either calcium gluconate or calcium chloride be infused via the artery that provides the vascular supply to the affected area. After an arteriogram has confirmed which artery to use, the calcium salt is infused over a period of 4 hours using a parenteral infusion pump. A common treatment regimen recommends the administration of 10 ml of a 10% solution of either calcium gluconate or calcium chloride mixed in 50 ml of 5% dextrose solution (42). Pain generally resolves by the conclusion of the infusion. If the pain returns, the infusion should be repeated. If pain resolution does not occur, then another arteriogram should be performed to assess whether the cannulated artery is perfusing the affected tissue.

Ocular Exposures   Contact lenses should be removed if present. The affected eye(s) should be irrigated with large volumes of lukewarm tapwater or normal saline for a minimum of 15 minutes. A variety of antidotal irrigation solutions have been evaluated, and none has been found to be more efficacious than water or normal saline (20). Ointments and solutions containing benzalkonium chloride, calcium and magnesium salts have not been effective and have actually produced more severe ocular injury (20). Given the high affinity of calcium for fluoride, lactated Ringer's solution make have an application in ocular irrigation. Subconjunctival injection of calcium gluconate or calcium chloride has been both toxic and unsuccessful. Immediate aggressive irrigation (even exposures to dilute solutions of HF) is the most effective ocular treatment modality.

Inhalation Exposures Therapy should be directed at supportive care. Humidified oxygen should be administered. Since HF is a corrosive, primary consideration should be directed at maintaining an airway. Nebulized calcium gluconate has been suggested but there is no evidence that it is an effective therapy (16, 26).

Ingestion Exposures Immediate dilution with water or milk (may precipitate the fluoride) is essential. If the ingestion is within the previous 90 minutes and emesis has not occurred, gastric lavage with a small-bore nasogastric tube may be efficacious (31). This may prevent the absorption of inordinate amounts of HF and reduce systemic toxicity. Although lavage is generally not recommended when corrosives have been ingested, the nature of HF's systemic toxicity and its rapid absorption and often fatal outcome eliminate the contraindication of lavage. Syrup of ipecac-induced emesis is contraindicated, and there is no evidence to support the use of activated charcoal, which may actually obscure endoscopic evaluation of the patient.

Laboratory Diagnosis

Although fluoride levels may be obtained, the diagnosis of HF toxicity is largely historical and clinical since the dermal exposure syndrome is classical and in concert with a history of using HF. It is an easy diagnosis to make. Patients who are nonresponsive and have suffered dermal exposure to concentrated forms of HF may have obvious burns and the presence of hypocalcemia (reports of calcium levels as low as 2.2 mg/dl), hypomagnesemia, and hyperkalemia (25). Urine and blood fluoride levels are of little value in acute HF toxicity. They may identify individuals who have been chronically exposed with excessive fluoride exposure, subacute fluorosis, or overt fluorosis. Urinary fluoride monitoring should be intermittently conducted in individuals with chronic occupational exposure to HF.

REFERENCES

1. Litovitz T, Veltri JC. 1984 Annual Report of the American Association of Poison Control Centers National Data Collection System. Am J Emerg Med 1985;3:423–450.
2. Litovitz TL, Normann SA, Veltri JC. 1985 Annual Report of the American Association of Poison Control Centers National Data Collection System. Am J Emerg Med 1986;4:427–458.
3. Litovitz TL, Martin TG, Schmitz B. 1986 Annual Report of the American Association of Poison Control Centers National Data Collection System. Am J Emerg Med 1987;5:405–445.
4. Litovitz TL, Schmitz BF, Matyunas N, Martin TG. 1987 Annual Report of the American Association of Poison Control Centers National Data Collection System. Am J Emerg Med 1988;6:479–515.
5. El Saadi MS, Hall AH, Hall PK, Riggs BS, Augenstein WL, Rumack BH. Hydrofluoric acid dermal exposure. Vet Hum Toxicol 1989;31:243–247.
6. Mansdorf SZ. Anhydrous hydrofluoric acid. Am Ind Hyg Assoc J 1987;48:A452.
7. Edelman P. Hydrofluoric acid burns. State of the art reviews. Occup Med 1986;1:89–103.
8. Mayer L, Guelich J. Hydrogen fluoride (HF) inhalation and burns. Arch Environ Health 1963;7:445–447.
9. Shaw JB. Hydrofluoric acid. Dent Tech 1987;40:4–5.
10. Caravati EM. Acute hydrofluoric acid exposure. Am J Emerg Med 1988;6:143–150.
11. Division of Industrial Hygiene, National Institutes of Health. Hydrofluoric acid burns. Ind Med 1943;12:634.
12. Gutknecht J, Walter A. Hydrofluoric acid and nitric acid transport through lipid bilayer membranes. Biochim Biophys Acta 1981;644:153–156.
13. Craig RD. Hydrofluoric acid burns of the hands. Br J Plast Surg 1964;17:53–59.
14. Menchel SM, Dunn WA. Hydrofluoric acid poisoning. Am J Forensic Med Pathol 1984;5:245–248.
15. Anderson WJ, Anderson JF. Hydrofluoric acid burns of the hand: mechanism of injury and treatment. J Hand Surg 1988;13A:52–57.
16. MacKinnon MA. Hydrofluoric acid burns. Dermatol Clin 1988;6:67–74.
17. Mullett T, Zoeller T, Bingham H, Pepine CJ, Prida XE, Castenholz R, et al. Fatal hydrofluoric acid cutaneous exposure with refractory ventricular fibrillation. J Burn Care Rehabil 1987;8:216–219.
18. Braun J, Stob H, Zober A. Intoxication following the inhalation of hydrogen fluoride. Arch Toxicol 1984;56:50–54.
19. Watson AA, Oliver JS, Thorpe JW. Accidental death due to inhalation of hydrofluoric acid. Med Sci Law 1973;13:277–279.
20. McCulley JP, Whiting DW, Petitt MG, Lauber SE. Hydrofluoric acid burns of the eye. J Occup Med 1983;25:447–450.
21. Hatai JK, Weber JN, Doizaki K. Hydrofluoric acid burns of the eye: report of possible delayed toxicity. J Toxicol-Cut Ocular Toxicol 1986;5:179–184.
22. Manoguerra AS, Neuman TS. Fatal poisoning from acute hydrofluoric acid ingestion. Am J Emerg Med 1986;4:362–363.
23. Houts M, Baselt RC, Cravey RH. Fluoride. In: Courtroom toxicology. New York: Matthew Bender, 1985.
24. Burke WJ, Hoegg UR, Phillips RE. Systemic fluoride poisoning resulting from a fluoride skin burn. J Occup Med 1973;15:39–41.
25. Tepperman PB. Fatality due to acute systemic fluoride poisoning following a hydrofluoric acid skin burn. J Occup Med 1980;22:691–692.
26. Trevino MA, Herrmann GH, Sprout WL. Treatment of severe hydrofluoric acid exposures. J Occup Med 1983;25:861–863.
27. Shewmake SW, Anderson BG. Hydrofluoric acid burns: a report of a case and review of the literature. Arch Dermatol 1979;115:593–596.
28. Carney SA, Hall M, Lawrence JC, Ricketts CR. Rationale of the treatment of hydrofluoric acid burns. Br J Ind Med 1974;31:317–321.
29. Grant WM. Toxicology of the eye. 2nd ed. Springfield: Charles C Thomas, 1974:557–559.
30. Vaughan D, Asbury T. General ophthalmology. 11th ed. Los Altos: Lange, 1986:340.
31. Duffy JP. Hydrofluoric acid. In: Rumack BH, ed. Poisindex. Vol 60. Denver: Micromedex, 1989.
32. Mayer TG, Gross PL. Fatal systemic fluorosis due to hydrofluoric acid burns. Ann Emerg Med 1985;14:149–153.
33. Greco RJ, Hartford CE, Haith LR, Patton ML. Hydrofluoric acid-induced hypocalcemia. J Trauma 1988;28:1593–1596.
34. White DA. Hydrofluoric acid—a chronic poisoning effect. J Soc Occup Med 1980;30:12–14.
35. Brown MG. Fluoride exposure form hydrofluoric acid in a motor gasoline alkylation unit. Am Ind Hyg Assoc J 1985;46:662–669.
36. Waldbott GL. Toxicity from repeated low-grade exposure to hydrogen fluoride—case report. Clin Toxicol 1978;13:391–402.
37. Bracken WM, Cuppage F, McLaury RL, Kirwin C, Klaassen CD. Comparative effectiveness of topical treatments for hydrofluoric acid burns. J Occup Med 1985;27:733–739.
38. Zachary LS, Reus W, Gottlieb J, Heggers JP, Robson MC. Treatment of experimental hydrofluoric acid burns. J Burn Care Rehab 1986;7:35–39.
39. Roberts JR, Merigian KS. Acute hydrofluoric acid exposure (letter). Am J Emerg Med 1989;7:125–126.
40. Velvart J. Arterial perfusion for hydrofluoric acid burns. Hum Toxicol 1983;2:233–238.
41. Pegg SP, Siu S, Gillett G. Intra-arterial infusions in the treatment of hydrofluoric acid burns. Burns 1985;11:440–443.
42. Vance MV, Curry SC, Kunkel DB, Ryan PJ, Ruggeri SB. Digital hydrofluoric acid burns: treatment with intraarterial calcium infusion. Ann Emerg Med 1986;15:890–896.

70

Halogen Gases, Ammonia, and Phosgene

Ann Broderick, M.D.
David A. Schwartz, M.D., M.P.H.

Historically, we have understood the impact of the toxic inhalants through their use in war and accidental exposures. These events occur at unpredictable times, result in acute life-threatening symptomatology, and often involve large numbers of people. In World War I, phosgene was responsible for 80% of the fatalities from toxic inhalants (1). These wartime and accidental exposures have permitted the identification and evaluation of thousands of individuals exposed to toxic inhalants. Although the acute symptoms have been well described, the chronic sequelae of both single high dose and chronic low dose exposures have not been completely evaluated. These gases are predominantly used and found in highest concentration in the workplace. Exposures are, however, usually accidental and uncontrolled, resulting in potential risks to the surrounding community. This chapter will address the acute management of toxic inhalant exposure, specific chemical characteristics that predict the mechanism of injury, and chronic sequelae of acute and chronic exposure of ammonia, halogen gases, and phosgene.

The sources of these gases are largely industrial (Table 70.1). Over one-half million workers are exposed to these gases, with almost all of the workers having exposure to ammonia, largely because of the use of anhydrous ammonia as a source of nitrogen in fertilizer (2–4). Ammonia is also used in mining and in the manufacture of plastics, dyes, and explosives. Phosgene is generated by heating chlorinated hydrocarbons, which places firefighters, welders, and paint strippers at risk of exposure. It is also an intermediate in the production of isocyanates. Chlorine is used as a whitening agent in the paper and textile industries, as a disinfectant in sewage treatment, and in the production of organic chemicals for metal extraction; it is also a component of solvents, automotive fluids, and pharmaceuticals. Bromine and fluorine gases are widely used in the petrochemical industry. Bromine is commonly used as a fire retardant. In addition to exposures occurring in the workplace, the population at risk includes those living near industrial sites and transportation lines (railroads and highways).

CHEMICAL CHARACTERISTICS AND ACUTE MANAGEMENT

Ammonia

The chemical characteristics of each of these gases are helpful in understanding the mode of injury (Table 70.2). Ammonia is a highly water-soluble alkaline and colorless gas that has a pungent odor. It is transported as a liquid because 113 cubic feet of vapor can be condensed to one cubic foot of liquid. Most accidents occur in the transfer of connections from tank to equipment. Upon contact with the moist mucosal membranes such as the skin, eyes, and respiratory tract, ammonia reacts with water to form a strong alkali (ammonia hydroxide). This causes liquefaction of the surface and thereby exposes more tissue to the alkali. This process results in deep focal lesions or burns to the cornea, skin, and respiratory tract. If extensive, these lesions can cause edema and sloughing of the airway

Table 70.1. Sources of Occupational Exposure

Irritant Gas	Sources	No. of Persons with Occupational Exposure
Ammonia	Agriculture Mining Dyes Plastic/explosive manufacturing	500,000
Chlorine	Chemical industry Paper Textile Sewage treatment	15,000
Bromine	Petrochemical industry Fire retardant Sanitation Agricultural chemicals	20,000
Fluorine	Petrochemical industry Aluminum manufacturing Dye and ceramics Etching glass and enamel Flux for smelting Agriculture chemicals	20,000
Phosgene	Welding Paint stripping Fire fighting Pesticides Dyes Pharmaceuticals	10,000

Table 70.2. Chemical Characteristics and Standards

Irritant Gas	Water Solubility	Color	PEL* (ppm)	TLV**
Ammonia	High	None	50	25
Chlorine	Intermediate	Green-yellow	1.0	1.0
Bromine	High	Red-brown	1.0	0.1
Fluorine	Low	Yellow	0.1	1.0
Phosgene	Low	None	0.1	0.1

*Permissible exposure limits refer to the legal federal standards established by Occupational Safety and Health Administration (35).
**Threshold limit values refer to airborne concentrations of substances under which it is believed that all workers can be exposed all day without adverse effect. It is determined by the American Conference of Governmental Industrial Hygienists (36).

epithelia, which result in acute upper airway obstruction. Massive exposures can override the absorptive surface area of the upper respiratory tract and result in extensive injury to the lower airways and alveoli. Liquid ammonia ($-33°C$) can freeze the surface of the skin as well, causing thrombosis of surface vessels, ischemia, and necrosis.

A typical case history illustrates the time course and type of injury following a nonfatal acute ammonia exposure. A 61-year-old manager of an anhydrous ammonia company was accidentally sprayed in the face and chest with anhydrous ammonia when a valve malfunctioned. Immediate blepharospasm prevented him from moving away from the jet of ammonia. An employee led him to a water tank where he washed his face and chest for 15 minutes. He was taken to the local emergency room, arriving there 1 hour after the injury. Upon arrival he was aphonic and dyspneic with inspiratory stridor. He was coughing serosanguinous material. An emergency tracheostomy was performed. The chest radiograph was normal. He was treated with bronchodilators, steroids, and empiric antibiotics for treatment of second-degree burns over his thighs and chest. He recovered over a 15-day period with eventual removal of the tracheostomy. Serial chest radiographs were normal. His vision was unimpaired and he had no pulmonary complaints at the time of discharge.

The high solubility of ammonia in water makes it very important to flush the injured surfaces with water for 15–30 minutes. No ointments, including antibiotics to the eyes, should be used for at least 24 hours as they promote penetration of the ammonium hydroxide. If blepharospasm prevents access to the eye, 0.5% proparacaine optic solution should allow inspection and lavage (5). Inspection of the upper airway with either early intubation or tracheostomy is advocated in the presence of severe facial burns, because these lesions are invariably accompanied by extensive upper airway injury, including laryngeal sloughing, edema, and spasm. Laryngeal edema may occur in the absence of any visible lesion, and all patients with postexposure respiratory symptoms, increased alveolar-arterial difference, or hoarseness should be observed for at least 24 hours in the hospital. Bronchodilators, vigorous chest physiotherapy, and oxygen therapy can be used as necessary. Although the use of corticosteroids has not been tested in controlled, randomized trials, it has been used in the majority of the reported cases, presumably to reduce airway edema and bronchospasm (6–12). Treatment of burns will usually include fluids, antibiotics, and tetanus toxoid. An ophthalmologist should be involved in the management of the corneal injury.

Chlorine

Chlorine, a greenish-yellow gas, is less water soluble, and far less alkaline than ammonia. Chlorine injures cells by reacting with water and liberating hydrogen chloride and a free oxygen radical (13). Hydrogen chloride is highly soluble and causes irritation and inflammation of the eyes and upper respiratory tract. Hydrogen chloride alone cannot explain the extent of the airway injury seen in chlorine inhalation. Thus, oxygen radicals appear to be responsible for much of the epithelial cell injury to the lower respiratory tract. Although this gas was used in World War I, problems with uncontrollable drift and failure to vaporize at low ambient temperatures precluded its use as an effective poisonous gas. It was later replaced for this purpose by phosgene. Fortunately for those exposed, chlorine has a characteristic odor, is clearly visible, and is irritating to the

nasal mucosa. These features often limit the length of exposure. Like ammonia, chlorine is transported as a liquid under pressure with one liter of liquid chlorine producing 434 liters of chlorine at $25°C$. Clinically, acute exposure to chlorine may result in conjunctivitis, keratitis, blepharitis, and necrotizing tracheobronchitis. Pulmonary edema may develop within 6–24 hours of exposure.

The following case history will illustrate the clinical aspects of acute chlorine exposure in a nonfatal case. An 18-year-old woman presented to the emergency room with the acute onset of dyspnea while swimming. She recalled that a swimming pool employee added chlorine to the pool water while she was swimming laps. At one point, she turned her face for a breath and as she was inhaling deeply, she saw a green cloud hovering over the water. Within minutes, she became dyspneic, weak, and presyncopal. Her eyes were protected by goggles. She was transported to the emergency room where she complained of shortness of breath, chest tightness, and cough. Her respiratory rate was 28, otherwise, her physical exam was normal. Her arterial blood gas was remarkable for a mild respiratory alkalosis and a PaO_2 of 88 torr on 70% inspired oxygen. Figure 70.1 shows three chest radiograms: 1 month prior to exposure, on the day of exposure, and 1 month following exposure. Her chest radiograph on the day of exposure demonstrated new bilateral infiltrates primarily affecting the lower lobes that resolved within one month of exposure. She was treated with solumedrol and inhaled bronchodilators. She progressively improved and was discharged on steroids and inhaled beta agonists 4 days after the accident. Since discharge, she has had two exacerbations of her bronchospastic disease requiring corticosteroids. One and one-half years after the exposure, she has a normal chest radiogram, normal pulmonary function tests, and normal cardiopulmonary exercise test. However, she continues to have dyspnea on exertion that limits her exercise tolerance.

The management of acute chlorine exposure is largely supportive. Evaluation should include bedside examination of the oropharynx, a chest radiograph, and an arterial blood gas. Bronchodilator therapy may be most helpful directly after exposure. Some centers advocate the use of inhaled nebulized sodium bicarbonate to counteract the potential damage caused by HCl, however, no controlled trials have assessed the efficacy of this intervention. Admission to the hospital is warranted if any of the laboratory tests are abnormal or if respiratory symptoms do not abate 6 hours after exposure. Corticosteroids have not been tested in controlled studies. They are often used, however, in an effort to prevent the development of bronchiolitis obliterans. A single case report showed improved outcome in a patient who received steroids compared with her sister with identical exposure who had not received corticosteroids (14).

Bromine

Bromine is a dark red liquid that is widely distributed in the earth's crust and sea waters and is most easily recoverable from the hydrosphere. The largest use of bromine is as an additive to gasoline. It is also used as a fire retardant and as a disinfectant and is used in the manufacture of photographic film, paper, and dyes.

Bromine vapor is quite dangerous, and exposure to this agent has resulted in human fatalities. Brief exposure to bromine fumes can result in coughing, epistaxis, headache, gastrointestinal symptoms, and a diffuse dermatitis. Direct contact with the skin can result in the formation of vesicles and pustules

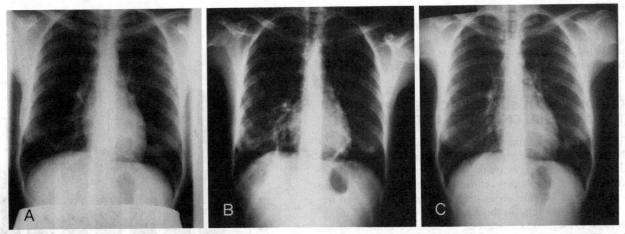

Figure 70.1.   Series of chest radiographs in a patient with acute chlorine exposure, 1 month prior to exposure (A), day of exposure (B), and 1 month after exposure (C). The chest radiograph on day of exposure shows bilateral alveolar infiltrates.

which may develop into deep, painful ulcers. Animal studies have shown that 3-hour exposures to bromine at 3 ppm can result in pulmonary edema and direct damage to the airway epithelia.

Fluorine

Fluorine is not found free in nature; however, many minerals contain small amounts of fluorine. Fluorspar, cryolite, and fluorapetite are the most common sources of fluorine. Fluorine is extremely reactive under pressure and is capable of causing burns to the skin. It is an irritating gas which can cause extensive upper and lower airway damage. Irritation of the eyes, nose, and throat occur at 5–10 ppm, and diffuse damage to the airways and parenchyma has been reported at 100 ppm. Brief exposures in human volunteers to 40 mg/m^3 were intolerable, and respiratory distress developed at 75 mg/m^3. Workers exposed to fluorine over a prolonged period of time were found to tolerate concentrations as high as 10 ppm for periods of 5–30 minutes without any acute effects (15). Exposure to fluorine gas is very unusual, and treatment should be directed at supportive measures only.

Phosgene

Phosgene (COCl) is a colorless, water-insoluble gas that has a sweet smell, much like freshly mown hay. Its water insolubility makes phosgene vapors only mildly irritating to the upper airway, eyes, and skin. Direct contact with liquid phosgene, however, can cause severe burns. Phosgene exerts its toxic effect through the evolution of HCl and CO_2 in the presence of water. The effect is delayed because the phosgene is slowly hydrolyzed to hydrochloric acid and carbon dioxide over 24 hours. Phosgene does not meet adequate water vapor for this reaction until it reaches the alveoli and terminal bronchioles. Yet, phosgene is considerably more toxic than equivalent concentrations of HCl, which usually damages the upper airway (16). It was proposed as early as 1920 in the studies that followed the World War I gassing that phosgene may actually diffuse into the tissues, react with water, and thereby exert the delayed tissue damage frequently seen with phosgene poisoning (16). The exposure to phosgene is frequently prolonged because the im-

mediate symptoms are mild and self-limited and the gas is not particularly offensive.

A classic case of a nonfatal phosgene poisoning occurred when methylene chloride containing paint removers was used in a poorly ventilated area. A 25-year-old woman refinished a desk in her basement with paint stripper containing methylene chloride. Shortly after starting her work, she had a slight burning sensation in her eyes and a dry cough. Two hours into the project, she felt a tightness in the chest and a dry, hacking cough. She walked up the stairs from the basement, felt dyspneic, and called to her husband who took her to the local emergency room. She was found to have an elevated temperature with a respiratory rate of 28. She had moist rales. Her arterial blood gas showed a mild respiratory alkalosis with moderate hypoxemia. Her chest radiograph showed diffuse pulmonary edema. She was started on oxygen therapy with symptomatic relief. She was managed with oxygen, bronchodilators, aminophylline, and corticosteroids. By the fifth hospital day, she was asymptomatic, with normal pulmonary function tests and normal chest radiographs (17).

Since there may be up to a 24-hour delay in the onset of symptoms, it is frequently difficult to clinically manage people with a suspected phosgene exposure. Diller (18) separates patients into three triage groups according to their initial symptoms: light exposure, serious exposure, and early pulmonary edema. The *light exposure* group can be identified as those who smelled phosgene but who had no initial symptoms. He recommends monitoring these patients for at least 8 hours, obtaining a chest radiogram 8 hours following exposure. Discharge would then be reasonable if the physical examination and chest radiogram were normal at that time. The *serious exposure* group is identified by the presence of initial ocular or pharyngeal irritation. These patients will probably require oxygen therapy. They should be monitored closely for the development of pulmonary edema. The *early pulmonary edema* group is identified by dyspnea upon presentation and needs to be transported emergently to an intensive care setting.

Although the initial management is complicated by a somewhat prolonged latency period, supportive measures, such as oxygen therapy, bronchodilators, and frequent suctioning, should be used as needed. Hypotension and pulmonary edema might be best managed with central venous monitoring. Steriods have been used empirically to reduce inflammation. Aminocaproic acid therapy has been advocated (18) because it has been shown to reduce pulmonary edema in rats with moderate phosgene poisoning (19, 20); however, there is no evidence that this is beneficial in humans and currently is not recommended as standard therapy.

CHRONIC SEQUELAE OF ACUTE EXPOSURE TO AMMONIA, CHLORINE, AND PHOSGENE

The data describing the chronic effects of acute exposure are largely from multiple case series. Since they all involve accidental exposures, there are no baseline values for pulmonary function, and few studies control for preexisting lung disease or smoking. All case series describe a tendency toward improvement over time in those who survive the initial insult. However, the longterm sequelae of exposure to these agents has not been thoroughly investigated. These agents appear to be capable of inducing bronchitis, chronic airflow obstruction, bronchiolitis obliterans, and peribronchial fibrosis. Since corticosteroids may play a role in preventing these chronic disorders, a therapeutic trial early following the exposure is indicated, especially among those with persistent airflow obstruction or restrictive lung function (21).

The chronic sequelae of inhalation injury have been best studied in cases of chlorine exposure. Jones et al., followed 113 people exposed to chlorine after a train derailment. Some were followed for 6 years. There were no significant declines in pulmonary function tests in 484 person-years of follow-up (22). Other studies have confirmed this return of pulmonary function (23–26). Schwartz et al. (27), however, recently observed a persistent loss in residual volume in 20 construction workers followed for an average of 8.5 years after an accidental exposure to chlorine in a pulp mill (Fig. 70.2). Following an initial elevation in the residual volume due to air trapping, there was a progressive loss of residual volume, with 67% of those tested 12 years after the exposure having abnormally low residual volumes (<80% predicted). The possible mechanism for the decrease in residual volume may be stiffening of the airways secondary to peribronchiolar fibrosis or mild interstitial fibrosis. A decline in residual volumes has also been observed by three other investigators (28–30). Although lung biopsies have not been performed in any of these case series, high resolution computed tomography of the chest was performed in a recent case of ammonia exposure. In this technique, the ultrastructure of the lung becomes more apparent because very thin (1 mm) sections are visualized. In a recent case of ammonia exposure, the high resolution scan clearly demonstrated peribronchial fibrosis in the distal airways (Fig. 70.3), indicating that the initial airway lesion probably resulted in a fixed fibrotic process primarily focused around the site of the initial injury.

No evidence is currently available to suggest that any of these agents or any other noxious gas has teratogenic or carcinogenic potential. However, given the anecdotal nature of these case reports and the relatively brief follow-up intervals, further data are needed to clarify these concerns.

CHRONIC SEQUELAE OF LONGTERM, LOW DOSE EXPOSURE

Few studies have investigated the relationship between specific measures of exposures and either symptoms or pulmonary func-

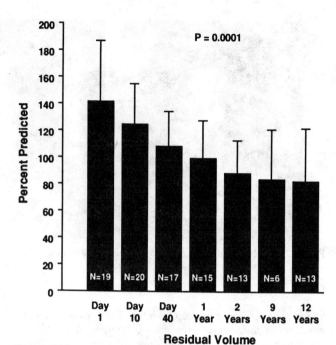

Figure 70.2. Progressive loss of residual volume seen in 20 construction workers during a 12-year period following accidental exposure to chlorine.

tion tests in workers exposed to irritant gases. Patil et al. evaluated the health of 382 diaphragm cell workers in 25 plants involved in the manufacture of chlorine (31). With few exceptions, the exposed workers had time-weighted averages less than the threshold limit value of 1 ppm. The workers were found to have normal pulmonary function tests. No dose-response was seen when workers were stratified according to amount of chlorine exposure. Ferris et al. conducted a prevalence study of chronic respiratory disease in a pulp mill with controls in a paper mill. No significant differences were found between the pulp and paper workers (32). Chester et al. also performed a prevalence study on 139 workers in a chlorine plant. No significant differences in pulmonary function were found between exposed and unexposed workers when stratified by smoking status (33). In their prevalence study of pulp mill workers, Enarson et al. (34) found that workers in the bleach and machine areas had no increase in respiratory symptoms or decline in pulmonary function when compared to workers with no exposure to chlorine. Similar studies have not been performed for either ammonia or phosgene gases.

Occupational hygiene for all three irritant gases might include tests for olfactory sense, use of impermeable gloves, eye protection, respirators if necessary, and availability of water where ammonia is used.

SUMMARY

Ammonia, chlorine, and phosgene gases represent significant hazards in the workplace and the surrounding communities. Of these exposures, ammonia is the most significant risk nationwide, particularly in farming areas. Successful treatment of ammonia injury depends on knowledge of its water solubility and the institution of immediate and copious washing of affected areas, with monitoring for laryngeal injury. Chlorine is

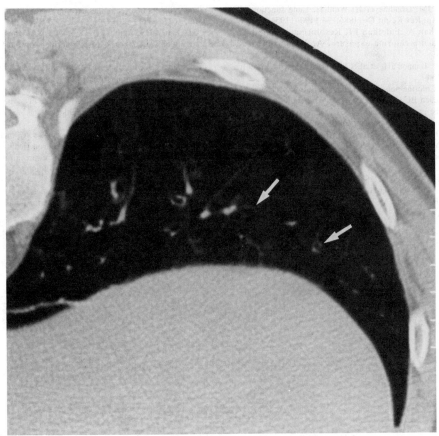

Figure 70.3.   A high resolution computed tomography of the chest demonstrates peribronchial fibrosis in the distal airways (arrow). This patient had been exposed to ammonia vapor in an industrial accident.

less instantaneous in its effect. There are no immediate control measures required in care of the acute exposure. Supportive care is the mainstay of therapy. The insidious nature of phosgene injury might lull an optimistic clinician into false hope. The clinically latent pulmonary edema may appear up to 24 hours after exposure. The exposed patient must be monitored for at least 8 hours. Understanding the mechanism of injury is critical toward appropriate treatment in all acute inhalational injuries.

REFERENCES

1. Fairhall LT. Industrial toxicology. 2nd ed. Baltimore: Williams & Wilkins, 1957:185–186.
2. National Institute of Occupational Safety and Health. Criteria for recommended standards: occupational exposure to ammonia. (NIOSH 74-136). Washington, DC: U.S. Department of Health, Education, and Welfare. Public Health Service. Centers for Disease Control. National Institute of Occupational Safety and Health, 1974.
3. National Institute of Occupational Safety and Health. Criteria for recommended standard: occupational exposure to chlorine. (NIOSH 76-170). Washington, DC: U.S. Department of Health, Education, and Welfare. Public Health Service. Centers for Disease Control. National Institute of Occupational Safety and Health, 1976.
4. National Institute of Occupational Safety and Health. Criteria for a recommended standard: occupational exposure to phosgene. (NIOSH 76-137). Washington, DC: U.S. Department of Health, Education, and Welfare. Public Health Service. Centers for Disease Control. National Institute of Occupational Safety and Health, 1976.
5. Helmers S, Top FH Sr, Knapp LW Jr. Ammonia injuries in agriculture. J Iowa Med Soc 1971;61:271–280.
6. Close LG, Catlin FI, Cohn AM. Acute and chronic effects of ammonia burns of the respiratory tract. Arch Otolaryngol 1980;106:151–158.
7. White ES. A case of near fatal ammonia gas poisoning. J Occup Med 1971;13:549–550.
8. Levy DM, Divertie MB, Litzow TJ, Henderson JW. Ammonia burns of the face and respiratory tract. JAMA 1964;190:95–98.
9. Taplin GV, Chopra S, Yanda R, Elam D. Radionuclidic lung-imaging procedures in the assessment of injury due to ammonia inhalation. Chest 1976;69:582–586.
10. Flury KE, Dines DE, Rodarte JR, Rodgers R. Airway obstruction due to inhalation of ammonia. Mayo Clin Proc 1983;58:389–393.
11. O'Kane GJ. Inhalation of ammonia vapor. Anesthesia 1983;38:1208–1213.
12. Conner EH, Dubois AB, Comroe JH. Acute chemical injury of the airway and lungs. Anesthesia 1962;23:538–547.
13. Adelson L, Kaufman J. Fatal chlorine poisoning: report of two cases with clinicopathologic correlation. Am J Clin Pathol 1971;56:430–442.
14. Chester EH, Kaimal PH, Payne CB Jr, Kohn PM. Pulmonary injury following exposure to chlorine gas. Chest 1977;72:247–250.
15. Hodge HC, Smith FA. Occupational fluoride exposure. J Occup Med 1977;19:12–39.
16. Winternitz MC. Collected studies on pathology of war gas poisoning. New Haven, CT: Yale University Press, 1920.
17. Gerritsen WB, Buschman CH. Phosgene poisoning caused by the use of chemical paint removers containing methylene chloride in ill-ventilated rooms heated by kerosene stoves. Br J Ind Med 1960;17:187–189.
18. Diller WF. Medical phosgene problems and their possible solution. J Occup Med 1978;20:189–193.
19. Boerner D, Ropertz S, Gruner G, Henschler D. Gerinnungsfoerdernde Stoffe zur behandlung toxischer Lungenoedems. Inaug Diss Wuerzburg, 1972.
20. Gruner G. Versuche zur Pharmakologie des toxischen lunge Lungenoedems. Inaug Diss Wuerzburg, 1972.
21. Schwartz DA. Acute inhalational injury. Occup Med 1987;2:297–318.

22. Jones RN, Hughes JM, Glindmeyer H, Weill H. Lung function after acute chlorine exposure. Am Rev Respir Dis 1986;134:1190–1195.

23. Hasan FM, Gehshan A, Fuleihan FJ. Resolution of pulmonary dysfunction following acute chlorine exposure. Arch Environ Health 1983;38:76–80.

24. Chasis H, Zapp JA, Bannon JH, et al. Chlorine accident in Brooklyn. Occup Med 1947;4:152–196.

25. Barret L, Faure J. Chlorine poisoning (letter). Lancet 1984;1:561–562.

26. Ploysongang Y, Beach BC, DiLisio. Pulmonary function changes after acute inhalation of chlorine gas. South Med J 1982;75:23–26.

27. Schwartz DA, Smith DD, Lakshminarayan S. Pulmonary sequelae associated with accidental inhalation of chlorine gas. Chest 1990. In press.

28. Charan NB, Lakshminarayan S, Myers GC, Smith DD. Effects of accidental chlorine inhalation on pulmonary function. West J Med 1985;143:333–336.

29. Kowitz TA, Reba RC, Parker RT, Spicer WS. Effects of chlorine gas upon respiratory function. Arch Environ Health 1967;14:545–558.

30. Weill H, George R, Schwarz M, Ziskind M. Late evaluation of pulmonary function after acute exposure to chlorine gas. Am Rev Resp Dis 1969;99:374–379.

31. Patil LRS, Smith RG, Worwald AJ, Mooney TF. The health of diaphragm cell workers exposed to chlorine. Am Ind Hyg Assoc J 1970;31:678–686.

32. Ferris BG Jr, Burgess WA, Worcester J. Prevalence of chronic disease in a pulp mill and a paper mill in the United States. Br J Ind Med 1967;24:26–37.

33. Chester EH, Gillespie DG, Krause FD. The prevalence of chronic obstructive pulmonary disease in chlorine gas workers. Am Rev Respir Dis 1969;99:365–373.

34. Enarson DA, Maclean L, Dybuncio A, et al. Respiratory health at a pulpmill in British Columbia. Arch Environ Health 1984;39:325–330.

35. Air contaminants-permissible exposure limits. Code of Federal Regulations. Title 29, Part 1910.1000. Washington, DC: Occupational Safety and Health Administration, 1989.

36. Threshold limit value and biological exposure indices for 1990–1991. Cincinnati: American Conference of Governmental Industrial Hygienists, 1991.

71

Sodium and Potassium

Edward P. Krenzelok, Pharm.D.

SOURCES AND PRODUCTION

Due to their highly reactive nature, neither sodium nor potassium is present in its elemental form in nature. Sodium is manufactured by the electrolysis of a molten mixture of the chloride salts of sodium and calcium (1). Whereas potassium production relies on the thermal reduction of potassium chloride with elemental sodium (1). In addition to the elemental forms, sodium is available as an amalgam with mercury. This form is said to be less reactive (2). Sodium and potassium are also produced as a combination alloy (NaK-78 (78% K)) containing both of the alkali metals (2, 3, 4). In their elemental forms they are relatively soft ductile metals with a bright silver appearance (1, 2). Specimens that appear to be a different color may be coated with highly reactive oxide compounds and should be properly disposed of or used only with extreme caution (5). Both sodium and potassium must be stored under airtight anhydrous conditions to prevent oxidation, which is a catalyst for reactivity. Sodium should be stored under oil and potassium under xylene (3, 4, 5). The synonyms for sodium and potassium are found in Table 71.1.

SITES, INDUSTRIES, AND BUSINESSES ASSOCIATED WITH EXPOSURES

Both of these elements have a multitude of occupational applications, and as salts they are ubiquitous in the food chain (Table 71.2). They are extremely important in a number of industrial processes. Combined with their highly reactive nature, the potential for human exposures and toxic sequelae is significant. Most occupational exposures occur when sodium and potassium are exposed to air and moisture through improper storage or while they are being used without taking the proper precautionary measures. The resultant reactions leading to these human exposures produce two toxic insults: thermal burns generated from an exothermic reaction and burns from caustic chemicals produced during the reaction (6).

Sodium

Sodium has an autoignition temperature of 115°C, which suggests that it will not ignite at room temperature (2). However, after the sodium is removed from its protective oil shroud, it is exposed to ambient air and moisture, which results in the oxidation of sodium and the external deposition of oxides and sodium hydroxide (2). These substances are hygroscopic, which results in the accumulation of more moisture and intensifies the production of oxides and hydrogen gas, which ultimately produces autoignition at room temperature. As the sodium bursts into flame it produces an intense yellow flame which is fueled by the continuous production of hydrogen during the combustion process (2, 5). Depending on the conditions, the ignition process may range from spontaneous combustion only resulting in flames to a violent explosive reaction.

A variety of occupational situations may produce hazardous conditions that terminate in a toxic exposure to sodium (5, 7). It should only be used in rooms that are warm and sufficiently dehumidified. Cold unheated rooms may contain significant ambient moisture. Sodium should be stored in rust-free metal or glass containers (7). If a glass container is used, it should be stored in an external metal container so that if the glass breaks, the spill is retained (7).

It is acceptable to cut sodium at room temperature under the

Table 71.1. Sodium and Potassium Synonyms

Sodium
  Elemental sodium
  Na
  Natrium
  Sodium
  Sodium, metal
  CAS 7440-23-5
  UN 1428
  NIOSH/RTECS VY 0686000
Potassium
  Elemental potassium
  K
  Potassium
  Potassium, metal
  CAS 7440-09-7
  UN 2257
  NIOSH/RTECS TS 6460000

Table 71.2. Industrial Applications of Sodium and Potassium

Industry	Application
Sodium	
Chemical	Detergent production
	Polymerization catalyst
	Chemical production
	Caustic soda
	Sodium peroxide
	Sodium cyanide
Electronics	Photoelectric cells
Metal	Titanium purification
	Hardened metallic alloys
Nuclear	Heat exchange medium with K in nuclear reactor
Petrochemical	Tetraethyl lead gasoline antiknock compounds
Potassium	
Chemical	Condensation, polymerization, and reduction catalyst
	Synthesis of organic chemicals
Nuclear	Heat exchange medium with Na in nuclear reactors
Solar	Heat transfer medium in solar collectors

following conditions. Both the sodium and the knife blade should be coated with mineral oil to prevent the formation of external oxidation products (7). The failure to follow these precautionary guidelines may lead to oxidation, resulting in autoignition of the sodium cake. Weighing sodium is another potentially hazardous situation. It can be removed from its protective oil environment for short periods of time to be weighed if the procedure is performed in a low humidity environment (7). It is best to weigh it in a beaker containing an inert hydrocarbon to prevent oxidation from occurring.

When minor spills occur it is commonplace to wipe them up with absorbent materials such as paper or cloth towels. This is extremely hazardous since the absorbent material absorbs the oil and exposes small sodium fragments to air, which may produce spontaneous combustion of the absorbent material.

Carelessness and lack of awareness about the reactive nature of sodium are responsible for the majority of toxic exposures. Exhaustive lists of other substances that react violently with sodium have been published (5, 8, 9).

Potassium

Potassium is the most reactive of the alkali metals and has the potential for autoignition at room temperature (2). As potassium becomes exposed to air and moisture, highly reactive superoxides are deposited on the potassium cake (2, 5, 9). Even minute amounts of superoxides can detonate the potassium, producing a violent and explosive reaction which results in the spattering of the potassium particles, affecting a large surface area and potentially several individuals. Potassium burns with a purple flame (2). The potassium and the superoxides react with a variety of organic and inorganic compounds (5, 8, 9).

Since potassium is even more reactive than sodium, greater care must be exercised during its use. It cannot be stored in aluminum containers because it reacts with aluminum to form potassium carbonate, which may corrode the container and lead to accidental exposures (5). Old potassium (identified by an external coating of yellow to orange potassium superoxide) should not be used for any application, since even normal contact may lead to autoignition (5). Reactions may occur when potassium is cut under other than ideal conditions. Many hydrocarbons such as kerosene react violently with potassium. It should only be cut utilizing forceps and anhydrous xylene (5).

Sodium and Potassium Fires

Alkali metal fires are extremely dangerous because of their explosive nature and the potential to inhale the corrosive metallic oxide byproducts of combustion. As with all fires they must be extinguished as expeditiously as possible. They are classified as Class D fires, which means that conventional extinguishers containing water, carbon dioxide, sodium bicarbonate, carbon tetrachloride, or soda acid must be avoided (2, 8). These agents would actually fuel the fire: halogenated hydrocarbons and carbon dioxide provide a source of combustible carbon. Sand should not be placed on potassium fires, because it produces a violent reaction (2). Class D fire extinguishers limited to those containing sodium carbonate (soda ash), sodium chloride, or graphite should be used (2, 6, 8, 9). Large amounts of sodium or potassium should not be stored in areas where sprinkler systems are installed, since water is detrimental in these fires.

CLINICAL TOXICOLOGY OF EXPOSURE

Burns are the primary sequelae associated with exposure to elemental sodium and potassium. The burns are a consequence of the reaction of sodium and potassium with the ambient environment or numerous chemicals. Most commonly the alkali react with moisture to produce a pronounced exothermic reaction and the evolution of either sodium or potassium hydroxide (6). The other feature to consider is the explosive nature of the reaction, which may cause the alkali to become imbedded in the skin or subcutaneous tissue (6).

Dermal exposure occurs when the alkali explodes. Heat will produce thermal burns; sodium or potassium hydroxide will produce liquefaction necrosis, and the imbedded particles will slowly be transformed to the corrosive hydroxide salt liberating heat and causing further thermal trauma in the process (6, 10). This cascade of events will continue until the source of sodium or potassium is exhausted or removed through surgical debridement.

Ocular exposures may also occur due to the spattering and explosive force associated with the reactions. The same exothermic and caustic processes can be expected to occur.

Toxic oxide, hydroxide, and carbonate salts are evolved during the combustion process (8, 11). As aerosolized particles of approximately one micron, they are respirable, can be deposited throughout the lower bronchial tree, and due to their irritant properties can produce pulmonary edema (11, 12).

MANAGEMENT OF TOXICITY

The basic management of all poisoning emergencies rests on the foundation of providing life support measures and decontamination of the patient. Normal external decontamination procedures for exposure to alkali include the removal of the contaminated clothing and thorough irrigation with copious amounts of water (10). Sodium and potassium exposures mandate the removal of any contaminated clothing, since the alkali impregnated in the clothing is no longer immersed in a protective hydrocarbon and is dangerously exposed to the air and water used for irrigation purposes. Water irrigation is absolutely contraindicated and **SHOULD NOT** be used to decontaminate the affected area since both sodium and potassium react violently with it.

Those caring for the victim with a dermal or ocular exposure to sodium or potassium must protect themselves from exposure. Protective eyewear, gowns, and dry surgical gloves must be worn. Care must be taken not to carelessly drop alkali fragments in the ambulance, the corridor leading to the emergency department, and the treatment suite. The alkali should only be handled with dry forceps and never touched even if gloves are being worn. All existing portions of the alkali must be placed into the appropriate medium to prevent additional reactions from occurring. Sodium debris can be placed in isopropyl alcohol containing no more than 2% water (9). Normal 70% isopropyl alcohol contains too much water and is not acceptable. Mineral oil is a suitable medium for sodium. Potassium specimens are extremely unstable and may even react in mineral oil. If available, pure tertbutyl alochol can be used to store potassium (5). Other alcohols such as ethanol and methanol, even in absolute forms, should not be used (5). "Dry" xylene is acceptable as a medium for potassium storage (5).

After removal of the patient's clothing the affected area should be covered with mineral or even cooking oil to prevent further exposure to air and moisture (6, 13). This may prevent oxidation and the exothermic reaction as well as the hydrolysis to the corrosive hydroxide. Even with the occlusive use of oil, water in the tissues may serve to catalyze the reaction of alkali fragments imbedded in the skin. Potassium reactivity may not be hindered even with the application of oil.

If the alkali metal is imbedded in the skin, the area must be surgically debrided, since the reactivity will not cease until the source is exhausted or removed (6). The removed fragments must be immediately placed into the nonreactive medium appropriate to that specific alkali metal to prevent further reactivity and subsequent harm to the patient and those providing patient care. Only after all evidence of the sodium or potassium are removed is it permissible to irrigate the area with water in a matter consistent with the treatment of alkali burns (6, 10).

The treatment of ocular burns should follow the same guidelines and precautions. The decontamination procedure should be performed as expeditiously as possible, since the eye is exquisitely sensitive to alkaline insults, and it is important to institute irrigation therapy as soon as the alkali debris is removed.

REFERENCES

1. Patty FA. Alkaline materials. In: Patty FA, ed. Industrial hygiene and toxicology. New York: John Wiley & Sons, 1963:859–869.
2. Meyer E. Chemistry of hazardous materials. Englewood Cliffs, NJ: Prentice-Hall, 1977:156–161.
3. Birch NJ, Karim AR. Potassium. In: Seiler HG, Sigel H, eds. Handbook on toxicity of inorganic compounds. New York: Marcel Dekker, 1988:543–547.
4. Birch NJ. Sodium. In: Seiler HG, Sigel H, eds. Handbook on toxicity of inorganic compounds. New York: Marcel Dekker, 1988:625–629.
5. Bretherick L. Handbook of reactive chemical hazards. 2nd ed. Worcester: Billing and Son, 1984:1024–1031, 1087–1095.
6. Clare RA, Krenzelok EP. Chemical burns secondary to elemental metal exposure: two case reports. Am J Emerg Med 1988;6:355–357.
7. Hawkes AS, Hill EF, Sittig M. Useful hints for sodium handling in the laboratory. J Chem Educ 1953;30:467–470.
8. Sax NI. Dangerous properties of industrial materials. 6th ed. New York: Van Nostrand Reinhold, 1984:2267–2268, 2406–2407.
9. The International Technical Information Institute. Toxic and hazardous industrial chemicals safety manual. Tokyo: The International Technical Information Institute, 1982:425–426, 465–466.
10. Temple AR. Corrosive-alkaline. In: Rumack BH, ed. Poisindex. Vol. 60. Denver: Micromedex, 1989.
11. Busch RH, McDonald KE, Briant JK, Morris JE, Graham TM. Pathologic effects in rodents exposed to sodium combustion products. Environ Res 1983;31:138–147.
12. Proctor NH. Setting health standards: toxicologic concepts. In: Proctor NH, Hughes JP, eds. Chemical hazards of the workplace. Philadelphia: JB Lippincott, 1978:3–9.
13. Stewart CE. Chemical skin burns. Am Fam Phys 1985;31:149–157.

72

Methemoglobin-Forming Chemicals

Donna L. Seger, M.D.

INTRODUCTION

In the differential diagnosis of the cyanotic patient, methemoglobinemia is occasionally encountered, rarely considered, and frequently misdiagnosed. Pathophysiologic concepts are the key to considering the diagnosis in the appropriate clinical setting.

Physiology and Pathophysiology

In the red blood cell (RBC), hemoglobin is continuously oxidized from the ferrous (Fe^{+2}) to the ferric (Fe^{+3}) state. Hemoglobin containing iron in the ferric state is termed methemoglobin. Normally, hemoglobin can transport oxygen only when iron is in the ferrous (Fe^{+2}) state. Oxyhemoglobin is the product of the reversible binding of oxygen to the ferrous iron of hemoglobin: $HgbFe^{+2}O_2 \leftrightarrow HbFe^{+3}O_2$. Oxyhemoglobin with iron in the ferric state differs from methemoglobin in that methemoglobin is formed from unoxygenated hemoglobin and cannot carry oxygen (1). Biochemical mechanisms exist within the RBC which continually convert methemoglobin to hemoglobin via reduction reactions. Physiologic concentrations of methemoglobin are less than 1% (2–5).

Tissue oxygenation occurs when an intact oxygen molecule is released from hemoglobin. Methemoglobin cannot transport oxygen nor carbon dioxide. Due to an electron shift prior to oxygen release, the deoxygenated hemoglobin molecule contains ferrous iron. Occasionally, an aberrant dissociation occurs in which oxygen takes an extra electron and forms a superoxide species (superoxo-ferriheme) (5). This superoxide species with iron in the Fe^{+3} state in a portion of the heme molecule induces conformational change in the oxyhemoglobin molecule which causes the ferrous ion in the hemoglobin tetramer to bind oxygen more tightly than normal. The tighter binding of oxygen decreases the amount of oxygen released at the tissue level. The methemoglobin concentration must be maintained at very low levels to ensure tissue oxygenation. High methemoglobin concentration decreases hemoglobin saturation and oxygen content of the blood. Arterial oxygen or carbon dioxide partial pressures (partial pressures are measurements of gas dissolved in solution) are not affected. Graphically, the oxyhemoglobin saturation curve is shifted to the left (2–5).

A steady state methemoglobin concentration of less than 1% is maintained by two physiologic mechanisms: (a) reduction of RBC oxidant compounds before they react with hemoglobin to form methemoglobin and (b) enzymatic reduction of methemoglobin to hemoglobin as soon as methemoglobin is formed. In these two systems the reducing agents (i.e., electron donors) are products of the anaerobic Embden Meyerhoff (EM) glycolytic pathway and the hexose monophosphate shunt (HMS). Energy is generated in the RBC by the EM and HMS as the RBC lacks the tricarboxylic acid cycle (TCA) and the cytochrome system (1, 4, 6).

Quantitatively, the most important RBC reductive system is the EM pathway, which accounts for 95% of the reducing activity in vivo (67% of the total reducing activity in vitro). Nicotine adenine dinucleotide (NADH) is the electron donor generated in the EM which reduces methemoglobin. NADH lacks full activity until 4 months of age (1, 6).

In the HMS, nicotine adenine dinucleotide phosphate (NADP) is enzymatically reduced by glucose-6-phosphate dehydrogenase (G-6-PD). NADPH (reduced NADP) reduces oxidized glutathione. In the presence of the enzyme glutathione peroxidase (GPX), reduced glutathione combines with oxidant compounds that convert hemoglobin to methemoglobin. NADPH also reduces methemoglobin to hemoglobin in the presence of both a cofactor and NADPH-methemoglobin reductase. NADP is regenerated in this process. Various other RBC substrates react differently with oxidants to reduce them and prevent them from oxidizing hemoglobin to methemoglobin. These reducing substrates and NADPH play a minor role in maintaining low levels of methemoglobin within the erythrocyte. However, a deficiency of reducing substrates may allow oxidants to cause a hemolytic anemia with Heinz body formation. Heinz bodies represent hemoglobin denaturation products. The mechanism by which oxidative agents cause hemoglobin denaturation and the relationship of denatured hemoglobin to methemoglobin is unclear (1, 3, 7).

An inherited defect of the HMS is G-6-PD deficiency. The deficiency of G-6-PD prevents the reduction of NADP to NADPH which normally provides reduced glutathione for combining with oxidants. The oxidants convert hemoglobin to methemoglobin and cause a hemolytic anemia with Heinz body formation (see Fig. 72.1). Clinical problems occur when the individual is subjected to an environmental stress such as an infection or is exposed to an oxidant drug or toxin. An acute hemolytic crisis may occur within hours of exposure to an oxidant. However, the reduction of oxidants plays little role in preventing methemoglobinemia in this situation (1, 3, 7).

Causes of Methemoglobinemia

Methemoglobinemia is a clinical syndrome in which greater than 1% of hemoglobin has been oxidized to the ferric form. It is either congenital or acquired. The majority of cases of methemoglobinemia are acquired and occur when drugs or toxins either oxidize hemoglobin directly in the circulation or facilitate hemoglobin oxidation. Congenital methemoglobinemia is caused by a congenital abnormal structure of the hemoglobin molecule (hemoglobin M disease) or congenital decreased activity of one of the reducing enzymes (8).

Congenital Methemoglobinemia

Hemoglobin M is an abnormal hemoglobin caused by substitution of amino acids on the alpha or beta chains of the hemoglobin molecule. In all the variants of this hemoglobinopathy, iron is maintained in the ferric form which causes methemo-

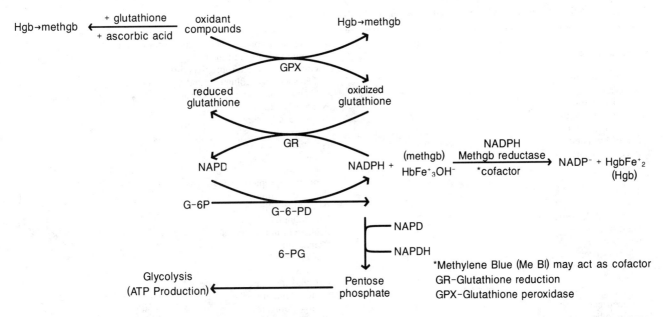

NADPH – 1. In HMS, reduces oxidized glutathione which subsequently combines with oxidant compounds in presence of GPX.
2. Reduces Methemoglobin (Methgb) to Hgb in presence of NADPH Methemoglobin reductase and cofactor

Figure 72.1. Role of NADPH in the hexose monophosphate shunt (HMS).

globinemia. Neither physiologic reducing mechanisms nor administered reducing agents (e.g., ascorbic acid, methylene blue) are able to reduce the methemoglobin. This condition is transmitted as a heterozygous autosomal dominant inheritance pattern. The homozygous mode of inheritance is incompatible with life, as all hemoglobin would be in the methemoglobin form. Patients with hemoglobin M are asymptomatic although they maintain methemoglobin levels of 25–30% and are clinically cyanotic (1, 3, 9).

Deficient enzyme activity is caused by deficient enzyme synthesis or production of a structurally abnormal enzyme. Congenital deficiency of the enzyme NADH methemoglobin reductase is the most common enzyme deficiency causing methemoglobinemia. Individuals with this enzyme deficiency have only the minor pathway of NADPH-methemoglobin reductase and nonenzymatic reducing agents to reduce methemoglobin to hemoglobin. This condition may be transmitted in either the homozygous or heterozygous inheritance pattern (1, 3, 4, 9).

Individuals with homozygous NADH reductase deficiency have methemoglobin levels of 10–50% and are therefore cyanotic. Although these individuals are usually asymptomatic, exertional dyspnea, easy fatigue, and headache may occur as methemoglobin levels approach 40%. (This is in contrast to patients with acquired methemoglobinemia who would be very symptomatic with similar levels.) Daily oral doses of methylene blue or ascorbic acid effectively maintain hemoglobin levels less than 10% (3).

Individuals with heterozygous NADH reductase enzyme deficiency maintain methemoglobin levels of 1–2% and are not cyanotic. Individuals with both heterozygous and homozygous NADH reductase deficiency are predisposed to acquired methemoglobinemia when exposed to oxidant substances (3).

Congenital deficiency of the enzyme NADPH reductase occurs infrequently. As this enzyme system is the minor methemoglobin reducing system, individuals with this condition do not suffer from methemoglobinemia. As stated previously,

individuals with G-6-PD deficiency have decreased levels of NADPH without the occurrence of methemoglobinemia (3, 9).

Acquired Methemoglobinemia

Acquired methemoglobinemia occurs when toxins oxidize hemoglobin at a rate that exceeds normal enzymatic capacity for hemoglobin reduction (6). Methemoglobin formation depends on the speed with which the substance is absorbed and enters the erythrocyte, the metabolites which may increase or decrease oxidizing potential, and the rate of excretion of the substance and its metabolites. The exact mechanism of acquired methemoglobinemia is poorly understood. Metabolites with free radical intermediates may be the methemoglobin-producing agents (1, 3, 10).

Etiologic Agents

A number of agents are known to cause methemoglobinemia (Table 72.1). A few of the more common methemoglobin-inducing agents will be discussed.

ANILINE

The chemicals that most frequently cause methemoglobinemia are nitrite and aniline derivatives. Although the mechanism of aniline-induced methemoglobinemia has not been elucidated, ingestion, inhalation, or dermal contact with aniline may rapidly cause severe methemoglobinemia. Aniline has also been reported to cause a Heinz body hemolytic anemia. This anemia may occur several days after aniline-precipitated methemoglobinemia is treated with methylene blue. Such patients should be monitored for delayed hemolysis (1, 11–13).

NITRITES

Nitrite is a common methemoglobin-forming agent, but the mechanism causing methemoglobin formation is unknown. The

Table 72.1. Agents Capable of Causing Methemoglobinemia (16, 20, 21)

Acetanilid	Well water contaminated with nitrites or nitrates
Acetophenetidin	Nitrate salts used in industry
Alloxans	Glyceryl trinitrate (nitroglycerin)
Alpha naphthylamine	Transdermal, sublingual, and oral nitrate/nitrite
Aminophenols	Contaminants from anaesthesia cannisters used with nitrous oxide
Ammonium nitrate	Nitrogen oxide
Aniline and derivatives	Nitrofurans
Chloromethylaniline	Nitroglycerin
Paradichlorlamine	Nitrophenol
Paranitroaniline	Ozone
Aniline dyes	Pamaquine
Anilinoethanol	Para-aminopropiophenone
Antipyrine	Para-bromoaniline
Arsine	Para-chloraniline
Benzene and derivatives	Para-toluidine
Dinitrobenzene	Pentaerythritol tetranitrate
Nitrobenzene	Phenacetin
Nitrosobenzene	Phenetidin
Benzocaine	Phenols
Chlorates	Phenylazopyridine
Chloranilines	Phenylenediamine
Chlorobenzene	Phenylhydrazine
Chloronitrobenzene	Phenylhydroxylamine
Cobalt preparations	Phenytoin (Dilantin)
Corning extract	Piperzaine
Crayons, wax (red or orange)	Plasmoquine
Dapsone	Prilocaine
Diaminodiphenylsulfone	Primaquine
Diesel fuel additives	Propitocaine
Dimethylamine	Pyridium
Dimethyl aniline	Pyrogallol
Dinitrophenol	Pyridine
Dinitrotoluene	Quinones
Hydrogen peroxide	Resorcinol
Hydroquinone	Shoe dye or polish
Hydroxylacetanilid	Sodium nitroprusside
Hydroxylamine	Spinach
Inks	Sulfonal
Kiszka	Sulfonamides
Lidocaine	Dapsone
Menthol	Prontosil
Meta-chloraniline	Sulfanilamide
Methylacetanilid	Sulfapyridine
Methylene blue	Sulfathiazole
Monochloroaniline	Sulfones
Naphthylamines	Tetranitromethane tetronal
Nitrites and nitrates	Tetralin
Amyl nitrite	Toluenediamine
Butyl/isobutyl nitrite	Toluidine
Sodium nitrite	Toluylhydroxylamine
Nitrite and nitrate preservatives in meat	Trichlorocarbanilide (TCC)
Vegetables (carrots and spinach) in infants	Trinitrotoluene
	Trional

nitrate ion is formed in soil, water, sewage, and the gastrointestinal tract. Organic nitrates may be reduced to inorganic nitrites by two mechanisms. In the liver, glutathione organic nitrate reductase catalyzes hydrolysis. In the bowel, intestinal microorganisms possess nitrate reductase systems, i.e., *Escherichia coli, Pseudomonas aeruginosa*, and *Acinetobacter*. The chief source of nitrate body burden is vegetables. Other sources include cured meats, fruits, juices, milk products, and bread (14–16).

Rural states continue to rely on well water high in nitrates.

High nitrate concentration often is due to poorly constructed wells, shallow wells which permit infiltration of surface water contaminated with nitrates from chemical fertilizer, or location of wells close to feed lots, barnyards, or septic tanks. Retrospective studies have determined that the maximal permissible nitrate level in drinking water is 45 ppm (NO_3) or 10 ppm (NO_3-N) (16).

Well water nitrates causing methemoglobinemia and infant cyanosis was first described by Comly in 1945. Infants are particularly susceptible to methemoglobin formation for a number of reasons. Infants have a decreased capacity to secrete gastric acid. The less acidic gastric pH is incapable of destroying bacteria that convert nontoxic nitrates to methemoglobin-producing nitrites. Infants also consume larger amounts of nitrate relative to total hemoglobin concentration. Additionally, NADH methemoglobin reductase activity levels remain low until 4 months of age. However, contrary to frequent reports, fetal hemoglobin has the same redox potential and rate of auto-oxidation as hemoglobin A and therefore does not contribute to methemoglobin susceptibility. Infants maintain a greater fluid intake per body weight and also per gram of hemoglobin, which increases the amount of ingested well water nitrates. Prior to feeding infants, water is frequently boiled, which concentrates nitrates (1, 3, 16–19).

NITROGLYCERIN

Nitroglycerin (NTG) has the potential to cause methemoglobinemia. Studies have shown that sublingual NTG in usual doses (4.8 milligrams over 25 minutes) (10) does not induce clinically significant methemoglobin levels (mean 0.55%). Similar results were found in patients admitted to coronary care units who were treated with isorbide dinitrate, NTG ointment, or a combination of the two. Although intravenous NTG administered in usual infusion ranges of 0.32–2.12 g/kg/min does not produce clinically significant methemoglobinemia, methemoglobinemia should be considered when intravenous NTG is administered in high doses for prolonged periods of time, or administered to patients with anemia, hepatic, or renal dysfunction (20–27).

Amyl nitrite, butyl nitrite, and other volatile nitrites are popular inhalants among certain populations. Users of these products claim they delay and prolong orgasm. Known as "rush," "poppers," and "snappers," these preparations can cause potentially fatal methemoglobinemia when inhaled or ingested. Inhalation of volatile nitrites can also cause massive hemolysis in the presence of an intrinsic RBC defect (i.e., G-6-PD deficiency) presumably due to nitrite ion-induced oxidative destruction of the RBC (20, 28–31).

DAPSONE

Dapsone (4, 4-diaminodiphenylsulfone) is a synthetic sulfone structurally similar to the sulfonamides. For years dapsone was used in the treatment of leprosy, and in dermatitis herpetiformis and malaria prophylaxis (combination drug Maolprim). Today, many dermatologists recommend dapsone for the treatment of pyoderma gangrenosum, pustular psoriasis, lichen planus, pemphigus, and subcorneal pustular dermatosis. Although dapsone may be poorly tolerated in patients with hypoxemia and anemia, it is currently being used in high doses in conjunction with sulfamethoxazole for treatment in *Pneumocystis carinii* pneumonia in patients with AIDS (32–34).

Toxicity of dapsone is due to the formation of a hydroxylated metabolite which is an oxidizing agent and thus capable of causing methemoglobinemia. Therapeutic-toxic dose ratio is low. Heinz body hemolytic anemia is present to a variable degree in most patients on greater than 200 mg/day. Elimination half-life is 10–50 hours, but after an overdose, half-life may be markedly prolonged. Prolonged methemoglobinemia following ingestion of dapsone may require repeated treatment with methylene blue. Continuous infusion of methylene blue

for 48 hours to treat the prolonged methemoglobinemia has been reported. Dapsone may also cause sulfhemoglobinemia and RBC hemolysis following an overdose. Hemolysis usually occurs 6–9 days after the afterdose. Fatalities have been reported, and most deaths occur 4–6 days after ingestion. Gastric emptying followed by repeated doses of activated charcoal may decrease the prolonged half-life that occurs following a toxic ingestion. Charcoal hemoperfusion, dialysis, and forced diuresis are not of proven benefit (32, 33, 35–37).

ANESTHETIC AGENTS

Lidocaine is not a direct oxidant, and the mechanism by which it produces methemoglobinemia is unknown. Therapeutic doses of intravenous lidocaine increase methemoglobin levels, but the level does not reach the toxic range. However, methemoglobinemia should be considered when lidocaine toxicity occurs (2).

Infant methemoglobinemia secondary to benzocaine administration has occurred following many routes of exposure. Use as a dermatologic ointment, anesthetic lubricant for rectal suppository, endotracheal tube, and esophageal stethoscope, topical teething preparation, and pharyngeal spray (Cetacaine) has been reported to cause methemoglobinemia in children. Methemoglobinemia has also been reported in adults following use of benzocaine as a pharyngeal topical anesthetic (38–42).

PHENAZOPYRIDINE

Pyridium, an azo dye, has been used as a genitourinary analgesic and antiseptic since the 1920s. Both methemoglobinemia and Heinz body hemolytic anemia have occurred in patients either on chronic pyridium or following acute toxic ingestions (7, 43).

Clinical Signs and Symptoms of Methemoglobinemia

Symptoms associated with methemoglobinemia are related to tissue hypoxia and are determined by the percentage of methemoglobin present in the RBC. The hallmark of methemoglobinemia is "chocolate brown cyanosis"—a bluish discoloration of the skin and mucous membrane—which is out of proportion to the severity and hypoxic symptoms. The lips and mucous membranes are more brown than blue as the skin becomes blue to purple with increasing serum levels of methemoglobin (4).

In assessing the cyanotic patient, the differentiation must be made between peripheral and central cyanosis. Peripheral cyanosis, a bluish discoloration observed in the nailbeds and the nose, is due to reduced perfusion in the extremities. Venous blood contains an excessive amount of reduced hemoglobin due to extensive oxygen extraction at the capillary level. As the blood is well-oxygenated, arterial blood is bright red. Central cyanosis, a bluish discoloration in the mucous membranes of the mouth, lips, and conjunctiva, is due to an excess amount of reduced hemoglobin in arterial blood. Arterial blood is not well-oxygenated and therefore is not bright red. Deoxyhemoglobin (5 g/dl), sulfhemoglobin (0.5 g/dl), or methemoglobin (1.5 g/dl) must be present to produce central cyanosis. Patients with methemoglobin levels less than 15% are usually asymptomatic. Major hypoxic symptoms occur with serum levels of

Table 72.2. Signs and Symptoms Associated with Methemoglobin Concentrations

Methemoglobin Concentration %	Signs and Symptoms
0–15	None
15–20	"Chocolate brown" blood; clinical cyanosis
20–45	Anxiety Exertional dyspnea Weakness Fatigue Dizziness Lethargy Headache Syncope Tachycardia
45–55	Decreased level of consciousness
55–70 (Inadequate tissue oxygenation)	Stupor Seizures Coma Bradycardia Cardiac arrhythmias
>70	Heart failure from hypoxia High incidence of mortality

55% or greater. Fortunately, methemoglobin levels seldom reach 70%, which is associated with a high mortality. Symptoms associated with specific serum levels are listed in Table 72.2 (43–46).

The most frequent cause of central cyanosis is cardiac or pulmonary disease. Therefore physical examination of the cyanotic patient must emphasize chest and cardiac exam. Diagnostic aids in the assessment of cardiac and pulmonary status are chest radiograph, electrocardiogram, and arterial blood gases. If these studies are normal, other causes of central cyanosis must be considered. Administration of 100% oxygen is indicated when cyanosis is present. Cyanosis unresponsive to the administration of 100% oxygen in a patient with normal or high arterial oxygen tension must make the clinician consider methemoglobin or sulfhemoglobinemia (43–46).

Sulfhemoglobinemia results from irreversible oxidation of hemoglobin by drugs or chemical agents. These agents form reversible methemoglobinemia in some instances and irreversible sulfhemoglobin in others. Sulfhemoglobin moves the oxyhemoglobin dissociation curve to the right, which increases oxygen delivery to the tissues. Profound cyanosis may be present, but dyspnea is minimal. Arterial blood has a lavender coloration. Sulfhemoglobinemia is not usually life-threatening. Sulfhemoglobinemia and methemoglobinemia tests reveal similar results. Spectrophotometry is necessary to differentiate the two conditions (1, 3, 8, 44).

LABORATORY TESTS

Bedside screening tests can rapidly confirm the diagnosis of methemoglobinemia. If greater than 15% methemoglobin is present in the serum, blood placed on filter paper will appear a classic chocolate brown color when compared with oxygen-

ated blood. A second screening test is to bubble oxygen through the patient's blood. Normal venous blood turns red when 100% oxygen is bubbled through it. Blood containing methemoglobin does not change color. A third screening test is to dilute venous blood with deionized water (1:100) and add a crystal of potassium cyanide (KCN). If methemoglobin is present, the blood will turn pink due to the formation of cyanomethemoglobin. Other indicators of methemoglobinemia include brown/black urine and/or the presence of protein and casts in the urine (1, 9, 35).

Arterial blood gas (ABG) analysis must be carefully interpreted. In most hospitals, ABG results are reported with a calculated oxygen saturation based on the measured partial pressure of oxygen (PaO_2). The PaO_2 (the amount of oxygen dissolved in the plasma) is unaffected by the presence of methemoglobin or other dysfunctional hemoglobins. Therefore oxygen saturation (SaO_2) will be falsely reported as normal even with very high levels of methemoglobin. Some oximeters measure fractional oxygen saturation, i.e., oxygen saturation is reported as a ratio of oxyhemoglobin to total hemoglobin (oxyhemoglobin, deoxyhemoglobin, methemoglobin, carboxyhemoglobin). When methemoglobin is present, the fractional oxygen saturation will be reported as appropriately low. Most oximeters, however, measure functional oxygen saturation, the ratio of oxyhemoglobin to the sum of oxyhemoglobin and deoxyhemoglobin. This measurement will report false normal oxygen saturation even with high levels of methemoglobin. Oxygen saturation reported on an ABG or by an oximeter that reports functional oxygen saturation are equally misleading (32).

Spectrophotometric methemoglobin analysis may not be readily available. Spectrophotometric analysis differentiates methemoglobinemia from sulfhemoglobinemia and reports methemoglobin concentration as a percentage of total hemoglobin. Falsely low levels may be reported if there is a delay between phlebotomy and laboratory analysis as the oxidation and reduction of methemoglobin continues at varying rates in vitro (16). Knowledge of total hemoglobin concentration is as important as knowing the percentage of hemoglobin in the methemoglobin form. Hypoxia will occur at lower methemoglobin levels in patients with anemia due to lower total oxygen carrying capacity (1, 3, 39).

TREATMENT

Treatment priorities for acquired methemoglobinemia include prevention of further absorption, enhancement of tissue oxygenation, administration of methylene blue in the symptomatic patient, and supportive care. Oxygen should be administered to all cyanotic patients. Dextrose (50%) and naloxone should be administered to any patient with a decreased level of consciousness. Gastric emptying should be considered and charcoal administered (20). If an industrial accident has occurred, clothes should be removed and the skin thoroughly washed (7, 10).

Treatment is indicated by the presence of hypoxia and systemic symptoms. Fluids and buffer administration will increase tissue perfusion and correct acidosis which is common in patients with significant hypoxia. Differentiation from other causes of cyanosis must be made. Even when blood is the classic chocolate brown in color and cyanosis is out of proportion to hypoxic symptoms, cardiopulmonary causes of cyanosis must be considered. Serum methemoglobin levels should be obtained. Hemoglobin electrophoresis and enzyme assays for G-

(From Hexose
Monophosphate Shunt)
NADPH + HbFe$^+_3$-OH   NADPH- MetHb reductase →   NADP$^-$
(5%-total reducing activity   *Cofactor   +HbFe$^+_2$
of RC)

(From Embden-Meyerhof
Pathway)
NADPH + HbFe$^+_3$-OH   NADPH- Met Hb reductase →   NADP$^+$+HbFe$^+_2$
(67%-total reducing activity
of RC)

*Methylene Blue (Me Bl) may act as cofactor

Figure 72.2. Enzyme systems for reduction of methemoglobin.

6-PD activity should be obtained to differentiate congenital from acquired methemoglobinemia (4).

The antidote for methemoglobin is methylene blue (tetramethylthionine chloride). Administration of methylene blue is indicated in symptomatic patients with methemoglobin levels greater than 30%. Treatment may be indicated in patients with levels less than 30% if they are anemic and symptomatic. As stated previously, normally 5% of methemoglobin is reduced by NADPH methemoglobin reductase. Methylene blue acts via cofactor substitution to transfer an electron from NADPH to form leukomethylene blue. Adequate NADPH must be present. Leukomethylene blue accelerates the reduction of ferric iron to ferrous iron in the hemoglobin molecule and reduces methemoglobin levels in 1–2 hours (Fig. 72.2). The oxidation reduction system between methylene blue and leukomethylene blue is reversible. When low levels of methylene blue are present, RBC reduction of methemoglobin occurs, but when high levels of methylene blue are present, the formation of methemoglobin is favored. If deficient G-6-PD is present, inadequate NADPH will prevent the reduction of methylene blue, and RBC hemolysis can occur. Consequently, NADPH methemoglobin reductase is ineffective. Methylene blue should be administered intravenously over a period of 5–10 minutes. The dose is 1–2 mg/kg (0.1–0.2 ml/kg) of a 1% solution in normal saline. It is not indicated in asymptomatic patients with methemoglobin levels less than 30%. Methemoglobinemia should resolve in these patients over the next 24–72 hours, provided absorption of the causative agent is not occurring. The patient may appear cyanotic even after symptoms disappear, as symptoms are usually not present when serum levels are less than 30% in nonanemic patients. Also, methylene blue is a dye which imparts a bluish coloration to the skin, so do not assume cyanosis is present based on skin discoloration after administration of methylene blue (1, 6, 18).

If symptoms of hypoxia have not disappeared at the end of 1 hour, administration of methylene blue should be repeated. However, before administering a second dose of methylene blue in an apparently refractory case, a second serum methemoglobin level should be obtained. Potential causes of continued hypoxia and lack of response to methylene blue include G-6-PD deficiency, NADPH-methemoglobin reductase deficiency and sulfhemoglobinemia. Recommendations for the total administered dose of methylene blue are inconsistent. Toxic dose reports range from 7–15 mg/kg. Toxicity occurs when methylene blue begins to act as an oxidant and methemoglobin levels are actually increased. Hemolysis with hyperbilirubi-

nemia, reticulocytosis, anemia, and rarely, hemolytic anemia with Heinz body formation may be a result. Repeated doses of methylene blue should not be withheld if they are necessary to clear the acquired methemoglobinemia. Continuous infusion of methylene blue has been reported to be beneficial in a patient with recurrent methemoglobinemia following a dapsone ingestion. Side effects of methylene blue administration include apprehension, dizziness, headache, mental confusion, nausea, vomiting, abdominal and precordial pain, tremors, and increased heart rate. Electrocardiographically, the T and R wave amplitude may decrease (1, 6, 7, 35).

Ascorbic acid reacts directly with oxidant compounds and reduces them within the RBC. It has no place in the treatment of acquired methemoglobinemia, as the rate at which it reduces methemoglobin is slower than the normal intrinsic mechanism. Ascorbic acid administration is indicated only when methemoglobinemia is caused by hereditary enzyme deficiency (1, 6, 7, 35, 39).

SUMMARY

Methemoglobinemia can be induced by a number of agents. Occasionally, this condition is congenital. As cyanosis due to methemoglobinemia does not respond to usual resuscitative measures, the diagnosis may be elusive. Rapid diagnosis and treatment with intravenous methylene blue may be lifesaving.

REFERENCES

1. Curry S. Methemoglobinemia. Ann Emerg Med 1982;11:214–221.
2. Weiss LD, Generalovich T, Heller M, et al. Methemoglobin levels following intravenous lidocaine administration. Ann Emerg Med 1987;16:323–325.
3. Hall AH, Kenneth W, Rumack BH. Drug-and chemical-induced methaemoglobinaemia. Toxicol Man Rev 1986;1:253–260.
4. Dolan MA, Luban NC. Methemoglobinemia in two children: disparate etiology and treatment. Pediatr Emerg Care 1987;3:171–175.
5. Mansouri A. Review: methemoglobinemia. Am J Med Sci 1985;5:22–209.
6. Goldfrank L, Price D, Kirstein R. Nitroglycerin (methemoglobinemia). In: Goldfrank L, Flominbaum N, Lewis N, Weisman R, Howland MA, eds. Goldfrank's toxicologic emergencies. New York: Appleton-Century-Crofts, 1990:391–396.
7. Green E, Zimmerman RC, Ghurabi WH. Phenazopyridine hydrochloride toxicity: a cause of drug-induced methemoglobinemia. J Am Coll Emerg Phys 1979;8:426–430.
8. Ludwig SC. Acute toxic methemoglobinemia following dental analgesia. Ann Emerg Med 1981;10:265–266.
9. Lukens J. The legacy of well-water methemoglobinemia. JAMA 1987;20:2793–2795.

10. Benjamin E, Iberti TJ. Methemoglobinemia and respiratory failure. Anesthesiology 1985;62:542–543.

11. Harvey JW, Keitt AS. Studies of the efficacy and potential hazards of methylene blue therapy in aniline-induced methaemoglobinaemia. Br J Haematol 1983;54:29–41.

12. Kearney TE, Manoguerra AS, Dunford JV. Chemically induced methemoglobinemia from aniline poisoning. West J Med 1984;140:282–286.

13. Harrison JH Jr, Jollow DJ. Contribution of aniline metabolites to aniline-induced methemoglobinemia. Mol Pharmacol 1987;32:423–431.

14. Murad F. Drugs used for the treatment of angina: organic nitrates, calcium-channel blockers, and β-adrenergic antagonists. In: Goodman, Gilman A, Rall T, Nies A, Taylor P. The pharmacological basis of therapeutics. 8th ed. New York: Pergamon Press, 1990:1764–1774.

15. Dixon DS, Reisch RF, Santinga PH. Fatal methemoglobinemia resulting from ingestion of isobutyl nitrite, a "room odorizer" widely used for recreational purposes. J Forensic Sci 1981;3:587–593.

16. Johnson CJ, Bonrud PA, Dosch TL, et al. Fatal outcome of methemoglobinemia in an infant. JAMA 1987;20:2796–2797.

17. Comly HH. Cyanosis in infants caused by nitrates in well water. JAMA 1987;20:2788–2792.

18. Fan AM, Wilhite CC, Book SA. Evaluation of the nitrate drinking water standard with reference to infant methemoglobinemia and potential reproductive toxicity. Regul Toxicol Pharmacol 1987;7:135–148.

19. May RB. An infant with sepsis and methemoglobinemia. J Emerg Med 1985;3:261–264.

20. Paris PM, Kaplan RM, Stewart RD, et al. Methemoglobin levels following sublingual nitroglycerin in human volunteers. Ann Emerg Med 1986;15:171–173.

21. Bojar RM, Rastegar H, Payne DD, et al. Methemoglobinemia from intravenous nitroglycerin: a word of caution. Ann Thorac Surg 1987;43:332–334.

22. Saxon SA, Silverman ME. Effects of continuous infusion of intravenous nitroglycerin on methemoglobin levels. Am J Cardiol 1985;56:461–464.

23. Marshall JB, Ecklund RE. Methemoglobinemia from overdose of nitroglycerin. JAMA 1980;4:330.

24. Robicsek F. Acute methemoglobinemia during cardiopulmonary bypass caused by intravenous nitroglycerin infusion. Brief Commun 1985;6:931–934.

25. Arsura E, Lichstein E, Guadagnino V, et al. Methemoglobin levels produced by organic nitrates in patients with coronary artery disease. J Clin Pharmacol 1984;24:160–164.

26. Zurick AM, Wagner RH, Starr NJ. Intravenous nitroglycerin, methemoglobinemia, and respiratory distress in a postoperative cardiac surgical patient. Anesthesiology 1984;61:464–466.

27. Kaplan KJ, Taber M, Teagarden JR, et al. Association of methemoglobinemia and intravenous nitroglycerin administration. Am J Cardiol 1985;55:181–183.

28. Toole JB, Robbins GB, Dixon DS. Ingestion of isobutyl nitrite, recreational chemical of abuse, causing fatal methemoglobinemia. J Forensic Sci 1987;6:1811–1812.

29. Laaban JP, Bodenan P, Rochemaure J. Amyl nitrite poppers and methemoglobinemia. Ann Intern Med 1985;5:804–805.

30. Bogart L, Bonsignore J, Carvalho A. Massive hemolysis following inhalation of volatile nitrites. Am J Hematol 1986;22:327–329.

31. Shesser R, Mitchell J, Edelstein S, et al. Methemoglobinemia from isobutyl nitrite preparations. Ann Emerg Med 1981;10:262–265.

32. Linakis JG, Shannon M, Woolf A, et al. Recurrent methemoglobinemia after acute dapsone intoxication in a child. J Emerg Med 1989;7:477–480.

33. Iserson KV. Methemoglobinemia from dapsone therapy for a suspected brown spider bite. J Emerg Med 1985;3:285–288.

34. Reiter WM, Cimoch PJ. Dapsone-induced methemoglobinemia in a patient with *P. carinii* pneumonia and aids. N Engl J Med 1987;27:1740–1741.

35. Berlin G, Brodin B, Hilden J. Acute dapsone intoication: a case treated with continuous infusion of methylene blue, forced diuresis and plasma exchange. Clin Toxicol 1985;22:537–548.

36. Dawson AH, Whyte IM. Management of dapsone poisoning complicated by methaemoglobinaemia. Med Toxicol 1989;5:387–392.

37. Endre ZH, Charlesworth JA, MacDonald GJ, et al. Successful treatment of acute dapsone intoxication using charcoal hemoperfusion. Aust NZ J Med 1983;13:509–512.

38. Kellett PB, Copeland CS. Methemoglobinemia associated with benzocaine-containing lubricant. Am Soc Anesthesiol 1983;59:463–464.

39. Gentile DA. Severe methemoglobinemia induced by a topical teething preparation. Pediatr Emerg Care 1987;3:176–178.

40. Seibert RW, Seibert JJ. Infantile methemoglobinemia induced by a topical anesthetic, Cetacaine. Laryngoscopy 1984;94:816–817.

41. Spielman FJ, Anderson JA, Terry WC. Benzocaine-induced methemoglobinemia during general anesthesia. J Oral Maxillofacial Surg 1984;42:740–743.

42. Buckley AB, Newman A. Methemoglobinemia occurring after the use of a 20% benzocaine topical anesthetic prior to gastroscopy. Gastrointest Endosc 1987;6:466–467.

43. Zimmerman RC, Green ED, Ghurabi WH. Methemoglobinemia from overdose of phenazopyridine hydrochloride. Ann Emerg Med 1980;9:147–149.

44. Mayo W, Leighton K, Robertson B. Intraoperative cyanosis: a case of dapsone-induced methaemoglobinaemia. Can J Anaesth 1987;34:79–82.

45. Jaffe ER. Methemoglobinemia in the differential diagnosis of cyanosis. Hosp Pract 1985;92–110.

46. Tada K, Tokaji A, Okaka Y, et al. A resuscitation puzzle: acute acquired methemoglobinemia. Crit Care Med 1987;6:614–615.

GASOLINE

"Gasoline" (mogas, motor spirit, petrol) is the generic name for the complex flammable mixture of paraffins, olefins, naphthenes, and aromatic hydrocarbons that serves as the principal fuel for the spark-activated internal combustion engine. Enormous quantities of gasoline are consumed annually, most of which is used to power the nearly half-billion motor vehicles driven in the world today (Table 73.1) (1–3). About one third of these are in the United States, where more than 1.25 trillion vehicle miles are traveled each year. In addition to motor vehicles, gasoline is the fuel for a host of other commercial, recreational, and household devices, including airplanes, motorbikes, snowmobiles, boats and personal watercraft, tractors, farm and garden equipment (mowers, cultivators, chain saws), and certain stationary engines (pumps and generators). Since gasoline, a commodity in commerce of immense economic consequence, is now virtually ubiquitous with humankind on the planet Earth, knowledge regarding its potential toxicity is essential for the disciplines of occupational, environmental, and emergency medicine.

CHEMICAL CHARACTERISTICS AND COMPOSITION

Gasoline is a complex mixture of hydrocarbons. The hydrocarbons are predominantly in the range C5-C10 (overall C4-C14), and include alkanes (paraffins), alkenes (olefins), naphthenes (cycloparaffins), and aromatics (4). The hydrocarbon classes found in gasoline are listed in Figure 73.1; the structural formula of a specific compound representative of each class is included. The wide ranges of hydrocarbon types normally present in the liquid phase of commercial gasoline are shown in Table 73.2, along with their approximate levels in the vapor phase. With respect to molecular composition, gasoline theoretically contains more than 1500 specific compounds (including isomers) (5). Analysis by gas chromatography and mass spectrometry generally results in the identification of 150–180 individual compounds (6,7). The most prominent compounds (2% by weight or greater) found in a typical U.S. commercial gasoline are shown in Table 73.3. From the toxicologic viewpoint, the low concentrations of benzene (1–2% in most U.S. gasolines, but somewhat higher, <4–5%, in certain reformulated and European gasolines) and n-hexane (<1–6%) are noteworthy (8,9). Only a few compounds (toluene, for example)

Table 73.1. Motor Gasoline Consumption

	Metric Tons (million)	Gallons (billion)
United States	305	115
Noncommunist world	633	235

approach or exceed 10% concentration; most of the 100+ specific chemicals occur at dilute levels of <1%.

While small quantities of Natural Gasoline (CAS number 8006-61-9) are sometimes separated during production of crude oil, commercial gasolines (no CAS number assigned) are manufactured in petroleum refineries by blending 4–8 component streams from processing units (Table 73.4) (4–6). Since gasoline is formulated to meet performance specifications (Table 73.5), its chemical composition and physical properties vary considerably, depending on the nature of the crude oil, refinery processing methods, and product qualities desired (10–12). A number of contaminants, including water, metals, particulate matter, and heterocyclics (nitrogen, sulfur, and oxygen compounds) are removed from the hydrocarbon streams to improve performance.

ADDITIVES

Gasoline also contains a number of additives; those commonly used and the purpose served are shown in Table 73.6 (6). Most additives are present in very dilute amounts (<5 pounds per 1000 barrels).

Lead alkyls (organolead compounds), which in the past were added to increase octane number and to suppress preignition, are currently limited to trace amounts in unleaded gasoline. Prior to 1985, gasoline contained tetraethyl/tetramethyllead at levels of 1.5–3.0 g/gallon (0.4–0.8 g/l). In 1985, the level was reduced to 0.5 (0.13 g/l), and in 1986, regulatory controls brought about a further reduction of 0.10 g/gallon (0.03 g/l). Today, unleaded gasoline contains 0.05 grams or less of lead per gallon (0.02 g/l).

Scavenging agents, ethylene dichloride (EDC) and ethylene dibromide (EDB), serve to prevent the accumulation of lead deposits in the engine. Former levels of EDC and EDB, which were 150–300 and 80–150 ppm, respectively, have been reduced, consequent to lower lead levels. Calculated airborne concentrations of lead and the scavengers EDC and EDB, based on the higher levels in use more than a decade ago, are shown in Table 73.2. Such levels no longer occur since organolead has been phased out.

Oxygenates may be added to gasoline as octane enhancers and antiknock agents. Such compounds as ethanol, methanol, tertiarybutyl alcohol, and methyl tertiarybutyl ether (MTBE) are now in use, particularly in reformulated gasolines. The amounts of oxygenates added are known to vary widely; MTBE at 10% concentration in liquid gasoline has been shown to result in a concentration of approximately 6% in the vapor phase.

In the processing of finished gasoline, organolead, EDB, EDC, MTBE, and other additives are blended in enclosed systems, so that worker exposures are unlikely to occur.

PHYSICAL PROPERTIES

Selected physical properties of motor gasoline are shown in Table 73.7 (10–12). The volatility of the hydrocarbon con-

Type	Name	Formula	Structure
Alkanes (Paraffins)	n-Octane	n-C_8H_{18}	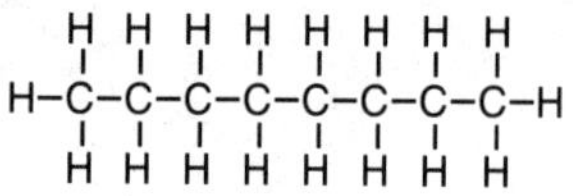
(Isoparaffins)	Iso-octane 2,2,4-Trimethylpentane	i-C_8H_{18}	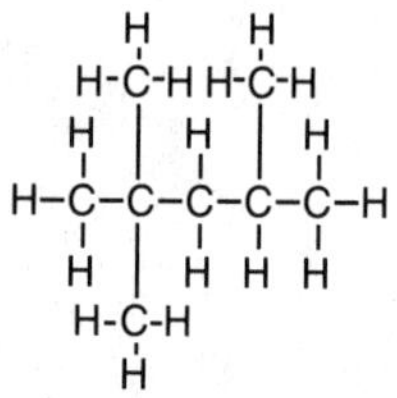
Alkenes (Olefins)	Hexene	C_6H_{12}	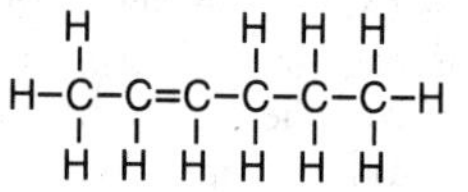
Naphthenes (Cycloparaffins)	Cyclohexane	C_6H_{12}	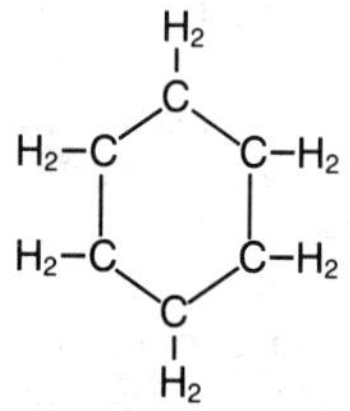
Aromatics	Toluene	C_7H_8	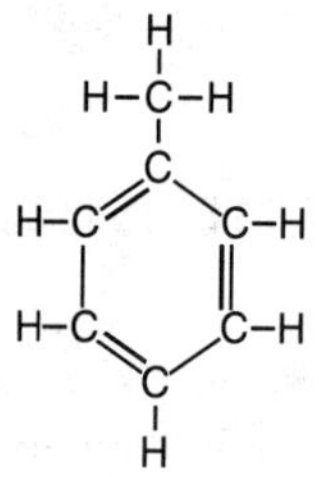

Figure 73.1.   Gasoline hydrocarbons: types and examples.

Table 73.2.   Composition of Gasoline [a]

	Liquid Phase (range)	Vapor Phase (approx. conc.)
Hydrocarbon class		
Alkanes/naphthenes	30–90%	90%
Aromatics	10–50%	2%
Alkenes	6–9%	9%
Additives		
1975 Organolead	±39/gallon	<0.004%[b]
Ethylene dichloride (EDC)	150–300 ppm	0.15 ppm
Ethylene dibromide (EDB)	80–150 ppm	0.08 ppm
1989 Organolead (EDC and EDB not used)	<0.05 g/gallon	0.004%[b]
Methyl tertiarybutyl ether	10%	6%

[a]By volume (except organolead).
[b]Undetectable

stituents is controlled by the nominal boiling point ranges. The octane number, which is adjusted in accordance with engine requirements and marketing strategies, is actually determined by a trial run of the gasoline sample in a specially constructed test engine. Approximate motor octane numbers are listed for typical regular and premium grade gasolines. The Reid vapor pressure is controlled to meet seasonal (temperature) and geographic (altitude) needs; the "high end" may be subject to regulatory limits [11 pounds per square inch (0.8 kg/cm^2) or less] to reduce vapor losses to the atmosphere.

With respect to solubility in water, the paraffinic hydrocarbons are highly insoluble, while certain aromatic compounds (benzene, for example) are somewhat soluble. Oxygenates (methyl tertiarybutyl ether, alcohols), present in certain blends, are miscible and will be extracted into a water column. Factors relevant to the explosion hazard of gasoline include: the ready volatility at ambient temperatures [1 gallon (3.7 liters) of liquid gasoline forms more than 20 cubic feet (0.56 cubic meters) of vapor at 15.5°C and 1 atmosphere], the explosive range of vapor (1–6 vol%), and the low flash point of the vapor. Other physical items listed in the table have the following exposure implications: liquid gasoline, being less dense than water, will float on an aquatic surface; gasoline vapor, with more than twice the density of air, will displace oxygen in a confined space; the low viscosity enhances evaporation by rapid spreading on (and running off) a surface. The odor threshold of gasoline is 0.06–0.08 ppm, with an odor recognition threshold of 0.15–0.2 ppm.

Table 73.3. Hydrocarbon Compounds Detected in U.S. Finished Gasoline at ≥2 wgt %

Chemical	Weight % Estimated Range	Weighted Average
Toluene	5–22	10
2-Methylpentane (+ isomers)	4–14	9
n-Butane	3–12	7
Iso-Pentane	5–10	7
n-Pentane	1–9	5
Xylene (3 isomers)	1–10	3
2,2,4-Trimethylpentane	<1–8	3
n-Hexane	<1–6	2
n-Heptane	<1–5	2
2,3,3-Trimethylpentane	<1–5	2
2,3,4-Trimethylpentane	<1–5	2
3-Methylpentane	<1–5	2
Benzene	<1–4	2
2,2,3-Trimethylpentane	<1–4	2
Methylcyclopentane	<1–3	2
2-Methyl-2-butene	<1–2	2

Table 73.4. Streams Used to Blend a Prototype Gasoline (API P5-6)

Stream	CAS Number	Volume %
Light catalytic cracked naphtha	64741-55-5	7.6
Heavy catalytic cracked naphtha	64741-55-4	44.5
Light catalytic reformed naphtha	64741-63-5	21.3
Light alkylate naphtha	64741-66-8	22.0

Table 73.5. Gasoline Performance Specifications

Compositional Feature	Function
Octane rating	Antiknock
Anti-icing	Minimize stalls of cold engine
Seasonal front-end volatility	Quick-starting
Full boiling range volatility	Warm-up acceleration
Back-end volatility	Complete combustion (limit engine deposits)
Oxidation stability	Storage life (minimize gum formation)

Table 73.6. Typical Additives Used in Motor Gasoline

Purpose	Agent
Antiknock	Tetraethyl-/tetramethyllead
Lead scavengers	Ethylene dichloride/dibromide
Detergents	Amines
Antirust agents	Sulfonates
Antioxidants	Aminophenols
Anti-icing	Alcohols, glycols
Upper cylinder lubricants	Light mineral oils
Oxygenates	Methyl tertiarybutyl ether (MTBE), Ethanol, methanol

GASOLINE VAPOR PHASE AND LIQUID PHASE

Important differences exist in the hydrocarbon composition of gasoline vapor as compared with liquid gasoline. The molecular

Table 73.7. Physical Properties of Commercial Motor Gasoline

Boiling point range	
U.S.	50–200°C
Europe	25–220°C
Aviation gasoline (Avgas)	25–170°C
Density	0.7–0.8 g/cm³
Kinematic viscosity (at 20°C)	1 centistokes
Reid vapor pressure	8-15 psi (0.4–0.9 atm)
Vapor density (air = 1)	2–5
Octane number regular grade	91–93
(ASTM) premium grade	96–99
Flash point	−46°C
Explosive/ignition range (vapor conc. in air)	1.3–6.0% by volume
Solubility in water	
Paraffinic hydrocarbons	Highly soluble
Aromatic hydrocarbons	Somewhat soluble
Oxygenates	Soluble

components of gasoline distribute into the volatile phase in relation to their individual boiling points and vapor pressures. During the process of evaporation from liquid to vapor phase, the low carbon-containing compounds (the "light" hydrocarbons with low boiling points, C3–C5) evaporate quickly to reach relatively high concentration in the vapor mixture, while the higher carbon compounds (with higher boiling points) evaporate slowly, resulting in low concentration levels. Overall, the vapor phase comprises principally alkanes and naphthenes (approximately 90% by volume), while the aromatics, which are potentially more toxic, are reduced to approximately 2% (Table 73.2, and Figs. 73.2 and 73.3) (13, 14). Following the addition of MTBE to gasoline, vapor phases will contain lower concentrations of MTBE.

Analysis of gasoline vapor during loading of tanker trucks at a U.S. bulk station revealed that C3–C5 compounds constituted more than 75% by volume of the total hydrocarbon vapor; similar studies at European work sites showed an average of 90% of C3–C5 compounds. These findings are particularly significant in evaluating the potentially toxic effects of gasoline vapor because of the low toxicity exhibited by the C3–C5 compounds. Benzene, a compound for which there is cause for concern, has levels in gasoline vapor that are usually less than 1 mg/m³ in U.S. samples and that may be somewhat higher in European samples (8, 9). Concentrations of organolead additives, along with the scavengers ethylene dichloride and ethylene dibromide, were too low to be detected in breathing zone air samples for tank truck loaders working with leaded gasoline (13). Analyses of other compounds with recognized toxic effects, n-hexane, toluene, and xylenes, revealed exposure levels well below their established exposure limits.

SITES, INDUSTRIES, AND BUSINESSES ASSOCIATED WITH EXPOSURE

While the operations of a modern petroleum refinery are highly complex, the processing methods involved in the manufacture of gasoline are well-characterized (4–6, 10, 11). Operational procedures are usually highly successful in maintaining refinery streams in a closed systems of pipes and vessels. Nevertheless, the refinery air contains low levels of hydrocarbon vapor, the result of fugitive emissions and multiple small releases, leaks, and spills. The same hydrocarbon compounds in gasoline are present in the refinery atmosphere, but their relative proportions

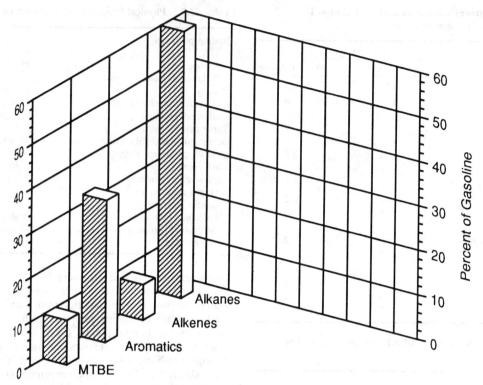

Figure 73.2.   Liquid phase of gasoline.

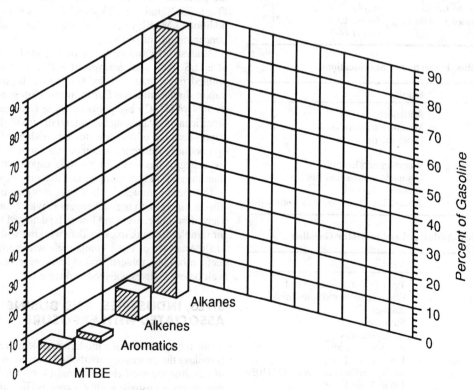

Figure 73.3.   Vapor phase of gasoline.

are different and variable to some degree throughout the refinery. Refinery workers are exposed to the mixture of hydrocarbons generally present in refinery air, and employee exposures to gasoline vapor potentially occur at any point downstream from the final blending site for the finished gasoline to the retail outlet (usually a gasoline pump in a service station).

There are approximately 300 petroleum refineries and 140,000 service stations and gasoline retail outlets in the United States

Table 73.8. Exposure to Airborne Gasoline Constituents in Selected US Operations and Occupations

Operation/Occupation	Total Mean Hydrocarbon Concentration 8-hr/TWA, mg/m³
Refinery workers	15
Driver/salesmen	39
Service station attendant	23
Marine loading	246
Loading of tanker trucks	
Top, no vapor recovery	46
Bottom, with vapor recovery	40
Gasoline truck drivers	46
Service station attendant	4

(15). Gasoline distribution systems utilize a wide variety of transport facilities and devices, including: pipelines, ocean-going tankers, barges, railway tank cars, tankerwagon trucks, drums, and canisters (including those carried by hand). Runion has identified the operating conditions during which access to hydrocarbon streams and vapors are prone to occur, with resultant employee exposures:

— operational start-ups, shutdowns, and mishaps
— turnarounds and other maintenance activities
— gauging, sampling, and analysis
— worker entry into tanks, vessels, and unit structures
— product, catalyst or process chemical transfer; loading and unloading
— waste treatment for handling activities (not closed processes) (16).

Extensive monitoring programs for workers potentially exposed to gasoline vapor have been reported (6, 14, 16–18). Exposures, expressed as total hydrocarbon for 8-hour time-weighted average (TWA) periods, are shown for selected petroleum worker assignments and worksites in Table 73.8. Overall, the highest exposures were measured during marine loading operations, intermediate levels were experienced by driver salespeople loading road tankers, while service station employees and refinery workers had low level exposures.

The application of industrial hygiene measures and engineering controls has resulted in significant reductions in worker exposures through the years. Incentives for even more use of controls include not only further reductions in worker exposures but also the prevention of vapor releases to the atmosphere (where certain hydrocarbon compounds contribute to the formation of photochemical smog) and provision of economic benefits by limiting product losses.

CLINICAL TOXICOLOGY OF EXPOSURE

Gasoline is the aggregate of myriad individual chemical substances, and consideration of its absorption, biotransformation, and excretion is exceedingly complicated. Consequently, observations pertinent to the clinical toxicology of gasoline focus on the whole gasoline, selected components (naphtha), or one or more specific compounds because of inherent toxicity (benzene) or as a "marker" (2,2,4-trimethylpentane) which serves as a surrogate for the whole complex mixture.

Routes of Exposure

Gasoline exposures occur by skin contact (with potential percutaneous absorption), ingestion (often associated with aspiration), and inhalation of the vapor (19). Of these various mechanisms, the inhalation route is by far the most important. Hydrocarbons in the C3–C10 range are transferred across the alveolar lining of the lungs quite readily, the mucosa of the gastrointestinal tract to a lesser degree, and the skin barrier least of all.

The disagreeable taste and odor generally serve to prevent the swallowing of gasoline or severely limit the quantity ingested. Unfortunately, the gagging and choking associated with the swallowing attempt often cause aspiration of the liquid gasoline into the respiratory tract, which is far more serious.

Exposure situations that result in skin contact with gasoline, usually from a spill or splash, invariably involve inhalation of vapor as well; the latter exposure is much more important with respect to systemic absorption. Experimental studies of the percutaneous absorption of benzene and isooctane demonstrate very limited transport across the skin (20, 21). Franz found absorption of benzene through the skin of palm and forearm of human volunteers following a brief (10–20 second) exposure to pure benzene to be 0.003 and 0.002 µl/cm², respectively. Topical application of isooctane in the monkey resulted in the absorption of 0.003 µl/cm²; similar application to human skin in vitro resulted in absorption of 0.006 µl/cm².

DISTRIBUTION, BIOTRANSFORMATION, AND EXCRETION

Because of high lipid solubility, hydrocarbons tend to accumulate in tissues in proportion to their fat content (principally brain, adrenal, bone marrow, and liver). Since hydrocarbons are relatively inert biochemically, most are excreted unchanged through the lungs; a small fraction may be excreted in urine, but this is restricted by the low solubility of the hydrocarbons in water. However, oxidative metabolism allows some aromatic hydrocarbons to be eliminated as water-soluble urinary biotransformation products conjugated with sulfuric acid, glycine, or glucuronic acid (22–24). (The oxidative pathway for n-hexane to a neurotoxic intermediate is well-documented; however, it deserves emphasis that this mechanism is unique and other hydrocarbons do not exhibit this form of neurotoxicity.

SIGNS, SYMPTOMS, AND SYNDROMES FROM TOXIC EXPOSURE

Knowledge of the toxicity of gasoline may be derived from the individual hydrocarbon compounds present in gasoline, from hydrocarbon mixtures that are components of gasoline (refinery streams, naphthas, solvents) or from the whole gasoline itself. While the importance of information derived from specific compounds and components is acknowledged, the following discussion relates to experimental studies and clinical observations on whole commercial gasoline and its vapor. Other fuels (liquefied natural gas and propane, alcohols, gasohols, and "reformulated" gasoline) whose end use is similar to that of gasoline are excluded from consideration. Except for the toxic effects resulting from organolead compounds following rather extraordinary exposure patterns to leaded gasoline, no distinctions of toxicologic significance are made regarding gasolines which differ with respect to additive packages, blends, grades, or commercial brands.

Experimental Studies in Animals

While toxicity studies in animals (rodents, for example) have limited applicability to humans, the usefulness of such studies in addressing clinical toxicity is widely recognized. Gasoline has been extensively investigated by standardized experimental procedures in laboratory animals. Key findings of the bioassay program conducted largely with technical and financial support of the American Petroleum Institute are summarized in Table 73.9 (25, 26).

Overall, a low order of toxicity for gasoline is demonstrated by various test procedures: the high oral dose (18 mg/kg) required to induce mortality (LD_{50}), absence of mortality on acute and subacute dermal exposures, minimal skin and eye irritation, absence of dermal sensitization, and the normal survival, clinical, and pathologic observations in subchronic and chronic inhalation studies. The slight increase in number of hepatocellular tumors in female mice in the chronic inhalation experiment is of questionable significance since this lesion is a rather common finding in bioassay studies with this species and sex. However, the induction of tubular nephropathy and renal cancers in male rats following chronic exposure to wholly vaporized gasoline by inhalation has been a subject of intense further investigation and warrants additional comment.

A metabolic pathway for hydrocarbons has been demonstrated which is unique for the male rat (27, 28). Branched chain alkanes (isoparaffins) with six or more carbon atoms are bound to a male rat-specific protein, alpha-2-microglobulin. The protein-hydrocarbon complex is deposited in cells in the proximal tubule of the kidney, leading to cellular degeneration and regeneration. The lesion is reversible, but if protracted as in the chronic inhalation exposure, continuing cell turnover ultimately results in nongenetic tumor promotion. This metabolic process is not operative in animals lacking the alpha-2-microglobulin (mice, dogs, guinea pigs, primates of either sex, and female rats). On this basis, the male rat model of renal carcinogenesis is deemed inappropriate for humans.

A large number of publications relating to experimental studies on hydrocarbons exist, and a critical review of findings reveals some disparities and even contradictions in results. Such discrepancies are not surprising in view of the variability of test substances (often ill-defined, sometimes inappropriate or nonrepresentative), test procedures and protocols, and levels of quality assurance used in conducting the research. Nevertheless, the bioassay studies provide an information base of considerable utility in evaluating the potential toxicity of gasoline in humans.

Clinical Observations

In 1941, Machle, in a review of gasoline intoxication, noted that, despite a paucity of reports, clinical cases of poisoning had occurred following the commercial use of petroleum distillates; he predicted that intoxications would become more frequent as a consequence of increasing opportunities for harmful exposure along with expanding distribution and use of gasoline (29). The following year, Professor Drinker of Harvard

Table 73.9. Bioassay Findings—Reference Gasoline

Test	Species	Results
Acute oral toxicity	Rat	LD_{50} = 18.85 ml/kg
Acute dermal toxicity	Rabbit	0% mortality at 5 ml/kg
Subchronic dermal toxicity	Rabbit	0% mortality at 8 ml/kg
Primary eye irritation	Rabbit	Nonirritating
Primary dermal irritation	Rabbit	Slightly irritating
Dermal sensitization	Guinea pig	Nonsensitizing
Mutagenesis assays		
Ames Salmonella	-----	Negative
In vitro lymphoma	Mouse	Negative
In vivo bone marrow cytogenetics	Rat	Negative
Reproductive assays		
(inhalation 400 and 1600 ppm)		
Dominant lethal teratogenesis	Mouse &	Negative
	Rat	Negative
Chronic dermal carcinogenicity	Mouse	No tumor induction
(50 μl twice/week/		No systemic effects
lifetime)		Mild skin irritation
Subchronic inhalation 0, 400, and	Rat	Survival, clinical, and pathology exams normal except:
1500 ppm, 6 hr/day, 5 days/week,	Monkey	tubular nephropathy in male rat
90 days		
Chronic inhalation 0, 67, 292, and	Rat &	Survival, clinical and pathology exams normal except:
2056 ppm 6 hr/day, 5 days/week,	Mouse	reduced wgt gain at highest dose
lifetime		nephropathic lesions and tumors, male rate
		increased number hepatic tumors, female mice
Immunoassays	Rat &	No treatment-related antigen and antibodies in sera, urine
30-day inhalation	Rabbit	
(1500 and 3000 ppm)		
Lung and kidney tissues from	Rat &	No antibasement membrane antibodies
chronic and subchronic inhalation	Monkey	
studies		

Table 73.10. Human Experience: Exposure to Gasoline Vapors

Concentration, ppm	Exposure Time	Effect
5,000–16,000	5 minutes	Lethal
10,000	4 minutes	Dizziness
10,000	10 minutes	Intoxication
3,000	15 minutes	Dizziness
1,000	1 hour	Dizziness, headache, nausea
1,000	30 minutes	Eye irritation only
500	1 hour	Eye irritation
160–270	8 hours	Eye irritation

School of Public Health, in evaluating the toxicity of gasoline vapor, described gasoline as a "very innocuous substance" (30). It is timely to update these pronouncements of nearly 50 years ago with a review of clinical experience with gasoline. In considering its harmful effects, it is important to distinguish the fires and explosion hazard and intoxications resulting from accidental spills and releases, inappropriate use, intentional misuse, and inhalation abuse from those occurring during manufacture, distribution, and intended use as a fuel for the internal combustion engine.

Acute Effects

FLAMMABILITY

The principal hazard of gasoline is clearly its flammability, unassociated with toxicity (11). Despite a formidable safety effort, flashes, fires, and explosions still occur. Whether due to an industrial accident in a refinery, the crash of a tanker truck on an expressway, the foolish misuse of gasoline as a firestarter for a barbecue, its criminal misuse in arson, the throwing of the infamous Molotov cocktail in a civil disturbance, or the blast of a flamethrower in war, a terrible toll in human suffering, scarring, disfigurement, disability, and death is taken in gasoline fires and explosions. Cole, Herndon, and colleagues have reported an "epidemic" of burns experienced by adolescents, many occurring in association with gasoline abuse ("sniffing") (31).

INHALATION: TOXICITY OF VAPOR

The inappropriate use of gasoline as a solvent for degreasing and cleaning purposes poses a frequent risk for shortterm vapor exposure. While the principal concerns for gasoline vapor relate to its irritant effects and its actions as a depressant for the central nervous system by way of its narcotizing (anesthetic) properties, the fact that high concentrations in a confined space may act as a simple asphyxiant by displacement of oxygen should not be overlooked.

The toxic effects of gasoline vapor are related to the inherent toxicity of the individual components, possible interactions (synergism, addition, or inhibition), their concentration in the vapor phase, and the duration of exposure. Human experience for exposures for various levels and periods are summarized in Table 73.10 (8, 29, 32). In general, exposures in the range 250–1000 ppm cause irritation to eyes, nose, and throat, as well as producing headache, dizziness, flushed face, dysphagia, slurred speech, nausea, anorexia, dullness, and mental confusion.

Exposure to 1000–5000 ppm for 15–60 minutes may cause central nervous system depression and feelings of anesthesia. More severe intoxication is associated with vomiting, miosis, delirium, cyanosis, coma, clonic convulsions, and respiratory depression. Inhalation exposure to greater than 5000 ppm may cause rapid loss of consciousness and death. Greater than 10,000 ppm may cause microhemorrhages and blood vessel damage in body organs.

Tetraethyllead absorption during exposure to leaded gasoline is not significant in acute exposures, and lead intoxication is not likely.

TOXICITY OF SCAVENGING AGENTS AND ADDITIVES

Ethylene dichloride (EDC)

Repeated exposures to EDC in an occupational environment have been associated with anorexia, nausea, vomiting, epigastric pain, irritation of mucous membranes, and liver and kidney dysfunction (33, 34). Hepatotoxicity can occur after inhalation exposure in humans. Marked fatty degeneration in monkeys was demonstrated at 400 ppm for 8–12 days. No effects in monkeys were demonstrated following exposure of 100 ppm up to 14 days. Guinea pigs exposed to 400 ppm for 14 days showed slight parenchymous degradation of the liver. Acute poisonings may occur with exposure concentrations of 75–125 ppm. Increases in hepatic enzymes have been observed in human exposure cases. Centrilobular hepatic necrosis has been observed in autopsy of one case of a 51-year-old man who died following an inhalation exposure in a confined space (34). This case was remarkable for the elevation of serum ammonia, serum transaminase (SGOT, SGPT), lactate dehydrogenase (LDH), and creatine kinase isoenzymes (MM-CPK). In addition, elevation of mitochondrial ornithine carbonyl transferase (OCT) and mitochondrial glutonic oxaloacetic transaminase was observed, which indicates that dichloroethane can cause mitochondrial damage.

Ethylene dibromide (EDB)

Exposures at concentrations of 10–40 ppm for 6 hours per day in rats and mice, 5 days per week for 105 days demonstrated increased tumors in the nasal cavity, respiratory tract, mammary glands, and spleen. There was also a decrease in fertility due to abnormal development of sperm (35).

Methyl tertiary butyl ether (MTBE)

MTBE has a fairly high water solubility and is one of the earliest ground contaminants after a spill. It has a boiling point of 131.4°F. MTBE has produced central nervous system depression, ataxia, and eye irritation in animal studies (36).

It deserves emphasis that the role of MTBE and other oxidants (methanol, ethanol) in reformulated gasoline continues to evolve, and the use of scavenging agents (EDC and EDB) has been discontinued due to the phase out of leaded gasoline in the United States (see section in this chapter on chemical characteristics and composition: additives).

FATALITIES FOLLOWING GASOLINE INHALATION

In data accumulated by the American Association of Poison Control Centers during 1989 (70 centers serving a population greater than 180 million with more than 1.5 million incidents resulting in 634 deaths), no deaths were attributed to gasoline; similarly, there were no gasoline fatalities recorded in 1988 (32, 37–39). The previous year (1987), two fatalities due to gasoline inhalation in teenage youths were reported; one was due to intentional abuse while the nature of the inhalation in the other was not identified (37–39).

The likely mechanism of sudden death is cardiac arrhythmia (ventricular fibrillation leading to asystole). Experimental studies suggest that myocardial irritability is induced as a direct toxic effect of volatile hydrocarbons, by release of catecholamines, and by interaction of the two processes. (Such fatal events have been noted more frequently as a consequence of ''sniffing'' solvents containing high concentrations of aromatic and halogenated hydrocarbons, rather than gasoline (40).

INHALATION ABUSE

Effects of extraordinary exposure levels and patterns experienced as a consequence of inhalation abuse warrant separate consideration. Inhalation abuse occurs commonly in teenagers and delinquent juveniles. While more than 50 publications relating to the subject have appeared during the last decade, no comprehensive investigation of the disorder has appeared, doubtless due to the elusive nature of the abusers. Exposure patterns in abuse cases vary widely; 4–6 inhalations of concentrated vapor (probably at levels of tens of thousands ppm) are reported to induce a ''high'' lasting a few to several hours; serious abusers may engage in the practice several times daily for protracted periods of time (41, 42).

NEUROTOXICITY IN ABUSERS

Sniffing and other forms of repeated overexposure can lead to central nervous system depression, hallucinations, encephalopathy, ataxia, Gilles de la Tourette disease, convulsions, retrobulbar neuritis, encephalitis, and conditions similar to multiple sclerosis. Neurologic manifestations reported in association with gasoline toxicity include vertigo, nystagmus, dementia, and peripheral neuropathy.

Well-documented cases of lead encephalopathy have been reported, the result of intense and persistent ''sniffing'' of leaded gasoline (43, 44). The clinical picture includes a variety of behavioral changes and central and peripheral neuropathies; abnormalities of neurologic evaluation and blood chemistries (parameters related to lead intoxication) are present. The syndrome is likely due to an admixture of severe and cumulative hydrocarbon and organic and inorganic lead toxicities and will predictably disappear when leaded gasoline is no longer available.

Both acute and chronic effects of gasoline toxicity in abusers are likely to be confounded by other factors leading to impaired health—malnutrition, chronic infection, emotional and psychiatric disorders, medical neglect, and stressful lifestyle. In view of the evidence indicating widespread practice of abuse, the apparent infrequency of occurrence of serious health effects suggests a remarkable tolerance for gasoline vapor on the part of the abusers.

INGESTION/ASPIRATION

The swallowing of gasoline occurs most frequently as an accident in children. Due to its unpalatability, adults rarely drink large amounts even in suicide attempts. Dysfunction of the swallowing reflex from vapor/liquid gasoline results in choking and gagging, so that aspiration is prone to occur. Hence, aspiration is properly considered an almost inevitable accompaniment of ingestion.

The most common cause of gasoline ingestion in adults is oral suction to initiate siphonage. A significant increase in such cases was reported during a period when gasoline was in short supply and during a severe blizzard (45, 46). (In the latter instance, the siphoned gasoline was needed for transfer to snowblowers and snowmobiles). In children, ingestion accidents occur as a result of improper storage of gasoline in beverage bottles (47).

Gasoline exhibits a low level of toxicity on the gastrointestinal tract. In contrast, entry of even a small amount (1 milliliter) into the respiratory tract causes severe pneumonitis; the low kinematic viscosity and surface tension facilitate spreading upon mucosal and alveolar surfaces which may be accentuated by gasping and coughing. The resulting chemical pneumonitis is severe and may be fatal, especially in infants and children.

Gasoline is relatively poorly absorbed from the intestinal tract; binding of hydrocarbons with food and intestinal contents and acceleration in transit time due to irritant effects may further reduce absorption. Machle noted the disparity in reports of a single oral dose fatal to humans (apparently about 7.5 g/kg), since deaths had been reported to occur from as little as 10 grams, but that recovery had followed ingestion of 250 grams (29). The disparity may have been due to the unrecognized presence and extent of aspiration pneumonitis.

A few cases of intravascular hemolysis have been reported as an uncommon systemic manifestation following ingestion of gasoline (48).

DERMAL EFFECTS

Ordinarily, skin contact with gasoline results from a splash or spill, which quickly spreads into a thin layer of liquid and promptly evaporates; this process produces no ill effects. In contrast, immersion incidents during which the skin is in prolonged contact with gasoline (an unconscious subject lying in a pool of liquid, for example) may result in a severe ''chemical burn.'' Such lesions involve partial or even full thickness of the skin, the effects being altogether similar to a thermal burn (49, 50). An occluded patch test with gasoline should never be carried out, since severe ulceration results from persistent skin contact with the liquid hydrocarbon under the patch.

Repeated skin contact with gasoline may cause a chronic dermatitis due to defatting of the skin. Such repeated contacts should not ordinarily occur, but are occasionally seen as a result of careless handling or inappropriate use of gasoline as a solvent (cleaning or degreasing agent). While skin sensitization to gasoline components is theoretically possible, contact dermatitis rarely occurs.

OCULAR EFFECTS

Exposure of the eyes to a splash of liquid gasoline or high vapor concentrations causes conjunctival irritation, but the effects are temporary.

Chronic and Long-Term Effects

The conventional view or assumption that longterm health effects due to gasoline were absent or negligible was based on many decades of experience, which included extensive health evaluation programs (including periodic examinations and surveillance of morbidity and mortality in petroleum workers) without evidence of occupationally related disease. However, it was recognized that conditions due to gasoline might exist but be obscured within the general ill health patterns afflicting populations at large. Such concerns focused particularly on the possibility of gasoline vapor exposures having a causal role in chronic renal disease and in cancer. The former issue has been addressed by health monitoring and the latter by epidemiologic studies in petroleum workers.

POSSIBLE RENAL EFFECTS

Gasoline vapor exposures in the occupational setting have been considered a possible cause of impaired renal function (51, 52). However, the studies linking renal disease (other than transitory urinary findings) to chronic gasoline vapor inhalation involve subjects with likely exposures to other known nephrotoxic agents (halogenated hydrocarbon solvents, metals, etc.). Such confounding is also noted in anecdotal reports attributing Goodpasture's syndrome to gasoline; an etiologic role for gasoline in Goodpasture's syndrome appears unlikely when serial cases are examined. Extensive periodic examination programs for gasoline workers have not disclosed evidence of impaired renal function, nor have uremia and end stage renal disease been reported as significant causes of death in the epidemiologic studies.

Following the report by MacFarland in 1984 on the induction of kidney tumors in male rats and increased liver tumors in female mice from wholly vaporized gasoline, concern was expressed that gasoline might be carcinogenic in humans (25). Further research indicates that the hyperplastic and neoplastic kidney lesions in male rats are due to accumulation of hyaline deposits in the proximal tubule of the kidney. This accumulation is secondary to alpha-2-microglobulin, a low molecular weight protein, which is synthesized in large amounts in the liver. This protein, which is unique to the male rat, binds to branched alkanes and is excreted by the glomerulus and reabsorbed, but the renal lysomal complex is unable to metabolize this compound and hyaline droplets accumulate (see section on experimental studies in animals).

Therefore, it is unlikely that this form of renal neoplasia is relevant in regard to human risk (26). The occurrence of liver tumors in the $B_6C_3F^1$ female mouse is also of questionable significance, as this mouse has a high frequency of spontaneous liver tumors.

EPIDEMIOLOGY STUDIES

More than 20 publications covering cohort mortality studies (including follow-up) in petroleum workers have appeared. Four articles have reviewed and evaluated these studies, the paper by Wong and Raabe presenting a metaanalysis of cancers by tumor site (53–56). Only one of the cohort studies focused on workers whose predominant exposure was gasoline (three distribution centers in the United Kingdom). The others involved general refinery workers, whose exposures were to volatile hydrocarbons present in the ambient air of refineries (which might serve as a surrogate for gasoline vapor). Since actual exposure levels were unknown, worker classification by job assignment provided a crude index of exposure.

In general, the findings in multiple epidemiologic investi-

gations demonstrated a "healthy worker effect" in refinery employees, with overall mortality rates considerably lower than comparison populations. Mortality from circulatory, respiratory, digestive, and genitourinary diseases were consistently lower among petroleum workers than in the general population.

While overall cancer death rates were low, some inconsistency is noted with respect to cancer incidence at certain specific sites; increased occurrence of tumors involving skin, brain, pancreas, prostate, kidney, and the hemopoietic system (leukemia) was reported in some, but not a majority of, cohorts. The International Agency for Research on Cancer, in assessing cancer occurrence in relation to gasoline exposure, concluded, "There is inadequate evidence for the carcinogenicity in humans of gasoline," and "Gasoline is possibly carcinogenic for humans" (6).

The general conclusions derived from clinical observations, health monitoring, and epidemiologic investigations are reassuring in that no definite evidence of occupationally related chronic health effects has been demonstrated in petroleum workers (and, by inference, in workers exposed to gasoline). The ultimate question of whether chronic low level exposure to gasoline vapor can cause disease (particularly cancer of specific sites) remains unresolved. Perhaps efforts to accumulate a sizable "downstream" gasoline worker population and more extensive case-control investigations will provide a more definitive answer.

MANAGEMENT OF GASOLINE INTOXICATION

Procedures selected for diagnostic examination and treatment depend on the nature of exposure and must be individualized for the particular case. Since no antidote or specific therapy exists for hydrocarbon intoxication, treatment is symptomatic and supportive. The following general measures warrant consideration and may be found useful as initial or early treatment in appropriate clinical situations:

Inhalation

Most patients overcome (anesthetized) by breathing high levels of gasoline vapor recover promptly upon removal from the contaminated site. Patients with more severe central nervous system depression may require resuscitation, oxygen, and breathing assistance. All patients should be observed for relapse and followed up for possible complications. In severe, chronic abuse cases with encephalopathy, the possibility of lead intoxication from inhaling leaded gasoline vapor must be considered since specific chelation therapy may be extremely important to expedite recovery.

Ingestion

Emesis should not be induced. Evacuation of stomach contents by gastric tube is not indicated because of the danger of aspiration unless the airway is protected by a cuffed endotracheal tube. If vomiting occurs, measures to minimize aspiration (Trendelenburg or left lateral decubitus position) should be used. The administration of activated charcoal slurry and a cathartic may be considered. Gasoline will also act as a cathartic. A chest x-ray and pulse oximetry can be useful in determining whether pulmonary aspiration has occurred. The chest x-ray may not show signs of infiltrates for several hours after aspiration. Aspiration pneumonitis is managed by standard accepted procedures and therapy.

Skin

Following contact with liquid gasoline (splash or spill), thorough cleansing with soap and water is all that is necessary. Chemical burns due to protracted immersion are treated as a thermal burn.

Eye

Irritation following exposure to liquid gasoline or its concentrated vapor is relieved by irrigation.

ENVIRONMENTAL MONITORING

In environmental monitoring for gasoline vapor exposure, sampling and analytical procedures are available to determine the concentration of total hydrocarbons and selected compounds collected at the sample site (57). Worksite or breathing zone air samples are drawn through a high volume collection tube where activated charcoal or polymer entraps the hydrocarbons present. The analytical procedure involves desorption followed by capillary gas chromatography with a flame ionization detector.

Exposure Limits

The adopted values established by the American Conference of Governmental Hygienists (ACGIH) are (58):

TWA 300 ppm (890 mg/m^3)
STEL 500 ppm (1480 mg/m^3).

Similar values have been established by the Occupational Safety and Health Administration (OSHA) (59):

TWA 300 ppm (900 mg/m^3)
STEL 500 ppm (1500 mg/m^3) (55).

BIOLOGIC MONITORING

The procedures used for environmental monitoring may be adapted for breath analysis. A qualitative pattern of hydrocarbon compounds can serve as a "fingerprint" for identification of gasoline exposure, and the quantitative determination of selected "marker" compounds can serve for derivation of an estimate of exposure severity. Similarly, the hydrocarbon content of blood and serum can be established, but with greater difficulty. These techniques have had rather extensive use in research, but their application to clinical and occupational settings has been limited.

PREVENTION OF HEALTH EFFECTS

During the normal course of manufacture, distribution, and use as a fuel, gasoline is largely contained within enclosed systems. While opportunities exist for release of liquid and vapor at a number of transfer points, exposures are controlled so that the likelihood of toxic reactions is negligible or nonexistent. Potentially hazardous exposures usually occur as a result of accidental spills and releases, improper containment, careless handling, inappropriate use, or intentional abuse. Obviously, education—perhaps assisted by additional regulation and enforcement—will have a major role in the further reduction of harmful exposures to gasoline.

REFERENCES

1. Statistical review of world energy. London: British Petroleum Company, 1988.

2. Basic petroleum data book. Petroleum industry statistics. Washington: American Petroleum Institute, Vol 9, 1989.

3. Petroleum supply monthly. Washington: Energy Information Administration Office of Oil and Gas. U.S. Department of Energy, February 1989.

4. Domask WG. Introduction to petroleum hydrocarbons. Chemistry and composition in relation to petroleum derived fuels and solvents. In: Mehlman MA, Hemstreet GP, Thrope JJ, Weaver NK, eds. Renal effects of hydrocarbon toxicology. Vol VII, Princeton, NJ: Princeton Scientific Publishers, 1984:1–27.

5. King RW. Petroleum: its composition, analysis and processing. In: Weaver NK, ed. State of the art reviews, occupational medicine in the petroleum industry. Philadelphia: Hanley & Belfus, 1988:409–431.

6. Gasoline. In: Occupational exposures in petroleum refining; crude oil and major petroleum fuels. IARC monographs on the evaluation of carcinogenic risks to humans. Lyon: International Agency for Research on Cancer, 1989:45:159–201.

7. Maynard JB, Sanders WN. Determination of the detailed hydrocarbon composition and potential atmospheric reactivity of full range motor gasolines. Air Pollut Control Assoc J 1969;19:505–527.

8. Runion HE. Benzene in gasoline. Am Ind Hyg Assoc J 1975;36:338–350.

9. CONCAWE. Developed by: Task Force on Exposure to Benzene. Exposure to atmospheric benzene vapor associated with motor gasoline. Report No. 2/81. Den Haag: The Oil Companies' International Study Group For Conservation of Clean Air and Water—Europe. 1981.

10. Bell HS. American petroleum refining. 3rd ed. New York: D. Van Nostrand Company, 1945.

11. Eckardt RE. Petroleum and petroleum products. In: Parmeggiani L, Tech. ed. Encyclopaedia of occupational health and safety. 3rd ed. Geneva: International Labour Office, 1983.

12. ASTM. Specifications for automotive gasoline. Annual book of ASTM standards. V. 05.01. (D439.) Philadelphia, PA: American Society for Testing and Materials, 1988.

13. McDermott JH, Killiany SE. Quest for a gasoline TLV. Am Ind Hyg Assoc J 1978;39:110–117.

14. CONCAWE. Developed by: Special Task Force CH (STF-14). A survey of exposure to gasoline vapor. Report No. 4/87. Den Haag: The Oil Companies' International Study Group for Conservation of Clean Air and Water—Europe. 1981.

15. Anderson RO. Fundamentals of the petroleum industry. Norman, OK: University of Oklahoma Press, 1984.

16. Runion HE. Occupational exposures to potentially hazardous agents in the petroleum industry. In: Weaver NK, ed. State of the art reviews, occupational medicine in the petroleum industry. Philadelphia: Hanley & Belfus, 1988:409–431.

17. Rappaport SM, Selvin S, Waters MA. Exposures to hydrocarbon components of gasoline in the petroleum industry. Appl Ind Hyg 1987;2:148–154.

18. Diakun R. Personal communication. Presentation to the U.S. Environmental Protection Agency, 1983.

19. Weaver NK. Gasoline toxicology—implications for human health. In: Maltcani C, Selikoff IJ, eds. Living in a chemical world. Occupational and Environmental Significance of Industrial Carcinogens. Vol 534. New York: The New York Academy of Sciences, 1988.

20. Blank IH, McAuliffe DJ. Penetration of benzene through human skin. J Invest Dermatol 1985;85:522–526.

21. Franz TJ. Absorption of petroleum products across the skin of monkey and man. API MBSD research publication 32-32749. Washington: American Petroleum Institute, 1984.

22. Gerarde HW, Gerarde DF. The ubiquitous hydrocarbons. Association of Food and Drug Officials of the U.S. 1961–1962;25–26:1–47.

23. Gerarde HW. Toxicology and biochemistry of aromatic hydrocarbons. Amsterdam: Elsevier (distributed by D. Van Nostrand, Princeton), 1960.

24. IPCS International Program on Chemical Safety. Environmental Health Criteria 20. Selected petroleum products. Geneva: World Health Organization, 1982.

25. MacFarland HN, Ulrich CE, Holdsworth CE, et al. A chronic inhalation study with unleaded gasoline vapor. J Am Coll Toxicol 1984;3:231–248.

26. Scala RA. Motor gasoline toxicity. Fundam Appl Toxicol 1988;10:553–562.

27. Short BG, Swenberg JA. Pathologic investigations of the mechanism of unleaded gasoline-induced renal tumors in rats. Research Triangle Park: Chemical Industry Institute of Toxicology. CIIT Activities, 1988;8:1–6.

28. Garg BD, Olson MJ, Li LC, Roy AK. Phagolysosomal alterations induced by unleaded gasoline in epithelial cells of the proximal convoluted tubules of male rats: effect of dose and treatment duration. J Toxicol Environ Health 1989;26:101–118.

29. Machle W. Gasoline intoxication. JAMA 1941;117:1965–1971.

30. Drinker P, Yaglow CP, Warren MF. The threshold toxicity of gasoline vapor. J Ind Hyg Toxicol 1943;25:225–232.

31. Cole M, Herndon DN, Desai MH, Abston S. Gasoline explosions, gasoline sniffing: an epidemic in young adolescents. J Burn Care Rehabil 1986;7:532–534.

32. Davis A, Schafer LJ, Bell ZG. The effects on human volunteers of exposure to air containing gasoline vapor. Arch Environ Health 1960;1:548–554.

33. USPHS. Toxicological profile for 1,2-dichloroethane. Agency for Toxic Substances and Disease Registry. U.S. Public Health Service, 1989.

34. Nouchi T, Miura H. Kanayama M, Mizuguchi O, Takano T. Fatal intoxication by 1,2-dichlorethane—a case report. Int Arch Occup Environ Health 1984;54:111–113.

35. Toxicology Update. Appl Toxicol 1989;9:203–210.

36. Page NP, Mehlman M. Health effects of gasoline refueling vapors and measured exposures at service stations. Toxicol Ind Health 1989;5;869–890.

37. Litovitz TL, Schultz BF, Holm KC. 1989 Annual Report of the American Association of Poison Control Centers National Data Collection System. J Emerg Med 1989;8:394–442.

38. Litovitz TL, Schultz BF, Holm KC. 1988 Annual Report of the American Association of Poison Control Centers National Data Collection System. J Emerg Med 1988;7:495–545.

39. Litovitz TL, Schultz BF, Holm KC. 1987 Annual Report of the American Association of Poison Control Centers National Data Collection System. J Emerg Med 1987;6:479–515.

40. Litovitz TL. Myocardial sensitization following inhalation abuse of hydrocarbons. In: Weaver NK, ed. State of the art reviews, occupational medicine in the petroleum industry. Philadelphia: Hanley & Belfus, 1988:567–568.

41. Watson JM. Solvent abuse by children and young adults: a review: Br J Addict, 1980;75:27–36.

42. Fortenberry JD. (Review). Gasoline sniffing. Am J Med 1985;79:740–744.

43. Edminster SC, Bayer MJ. Recreational gasoline sniffing: acute gasoline intoxication and latent organic lead poisoning. J Emerg Med 1985;3:365–370.

44. Coulehan JL, Hirsch W, Brillman J, et al. Gasoline sniffing and lead toxicity in Navajo adolescents. Pediatrics 1983;71:113–117.

45. Schwartz WK. (Letter) Gasoline ingestion. JAMA 1979;242:1968–1969.

46. Lacouture P, McGuigan M, Lovejoy FH. Gasoline ingestion after the great blizzard (Letter). N Engl J Med 1978;298:1037.

47. Banner W, Walson PD. Systemic toxicity following gasoline aspirations. Am J Emerg Med 1983;3:292–294.

48. Stockman JA. More on hydrocarbon-induced hemolysis (Letter). J Pediatr 1977;90:848.

49. Simpson LA, Cruse CW. Gasoline immersion injury. Plast Reconstr Surg 1981;67:54–57.

50. Hansbrough, JF, Zapata-Sirvent R, Dominic W, et al. Hydrocarbon contact injuries. J Trauma 1985;25:250–252.

51. Viau C, Bernard A, Lauwerys R, et al. A cross-sectional survey of kidney function in refinery employees. Am J Ind Med 1987;11:177–187.

52. Phillips SC, Petrone RL, Hemstreet GP. A review of the non-neoplastic kidney effects of hydrocarbon exposures in humans. In: Weaver NK, ed. State of the art reviews. Occupational medicine in the petroleum industry. Philadelphia: Hanley & Belfus, 1988:495–510.

53. Savitz DA, Moure R. Cancer risk among oil refinery workers: a review of epidemiologic studies. J Occup Med 1984;26:662–670.

54. Harrington JM. Health experience of workers in the petroleum manufacturing and distribution industry: a review of the literature. Am J Ind Med 1987;12:475–497.

55. Delzell E, Austin H, Cole P. Epidemiologic studies in the petroleum industry. In: Weaver HK, ed. State of the art reviews. Occupational medicine in the petroleum industry. Philadelphia: Hanley & Belfus, 1988:455–474.

56. Wong O, Raabe GK. Critical review of cancer epidemiology in petroleum industry employees with a quantitative meta-analysis by cancer site. Am J Ind Med 1989;15:283–310.

57. CONCAWE. Developed by: Analytical Working Group of the Special Task Force on Gasoline Vapor Exposure (H/STF-14). Method for monitoring exposure to gasoline vapor in air. Report No. 8/86. Den Haag: The Oil Companies' International Study Group for Conservation of Clean Air and Water—Europe. 1986.

58. American Conference of Governmental Industrial Hygienists. Threshold limit values and biological exposure indices for 1990–91. Cincinnati, OH: ACGIH, 1990:25.

59. Occupational Safety and Health Administration (OSHA). Air contaminants: final rule. Washington: Federal Register. Jan 15, 1989;54:2332–2983.

SOURCE/PRODUCTION/COMMON NAMES/ USES

Arsenic is mobilized from its natural sources by many activities. Most of these, such as ingestion of seafood or contaminated well water, opium inhalation, smelting of metals, and combustion of fossil fuels can result in chronic toxicity. Acute arsenic exposure can occur in cases of suicidal or homicidal ingestion, contamination of food and water supplies, or contamination of air. Large scale hazardous material incidents involving arsenic have not occurred in the United States. However, the potential for small or large scale exposures clearly exists, and the health effects could be severe as evidenced by the poisoning of 12,131 Japanese children who consumed arsenic-tainted dry milk. The incident caused 130 deaths (1).

The primary use of arsenic in the United States has been in insecticides, with the concentrated liquid forms having extreme potential toxicity to humans. The highest worker exposures in the insecticide industry have been reported to occur in the mixing, screening, drying, bagging, and drum-filling operations (2). Regulatory restrictions, especially for home products, have dramatically reduced this problem (3). Smelting of metals, especially copper, has produced high arsenic exposures (3, 4). Nearby populations have also been shown to have increased arsenic levels (5). Similarly, arsenic-containing products are used as herbicides, desiccants in the cotton industry, wood preservatives, and animal feed additives. Arsenic has also been utilized in chemical warfare agents (4). More recent industrial release of arsenic has occurred in the semiconductor industry (6). Arsenic is used as a dopant, speeding transmission in microcomputer chips used in communications equipment, scientific instruments, and the computer industry (7). It may be released from chips for hours after their manufacture (8). Gallium arsenide (GaAs) is a semiconductor that is replacing silicon in many applications. GaAs particulates are toxic in animal models, and arsine is used in GaAs production. The risks posed by this source are currently unknown. An extensive review of arsenic sources has been published (9).

Arsine (hydrogen arsenide, AsH_3) is a colorless, nonirritating, inflammable gas with slight garlic odor. Since it is present in many arsenic-containing ores, it may be generated in metal industries utilizing ores or if ores come in contact with acids (4). Arsine is also utilized in chip manufacture for the computer industry (7).

CHEMICAL/PHYSICAL FORMS

Arsenic has a molecular weight of 74.9 and is classified as a transition element or metalloid because it commonly complexes with metals but also reacts with carbon, hydrogen, and oxygen. Arsenic compounds are classified into three major groups: (a) inorganic arsenic compounds, (b) organic arsenic compounds, and (c) arsine gas. Arsenic compounds can also be classified by their valence state: trivalent (arsenic trioxide, so-

dium arsenite, and arsenic trichloride) or pentavalent (arsenic pentoxide, arsenic acid, and arsenate).

The most toxic form of arsenic is arsine gas (AsH_3). This is followed in generally decreasing order by inorganic trivalent arsenic compounds, organic trivalent compounds, inorganic pentavalent compounds, organic pentavalent compounds, and elemental arsenic (10). Trivalent arsenic (arsenite) is more toxic than pentavalent arsenic (arsenate). Both arsenite and arsenate forms are highly soluble in water. Most commercially available compounds containing arsenic are produced from arsenic trioxide (4). Organic arsenic-containing compounds include arsanilic acid, methylarsonic acid, dimethylarsinic acid (cacodylic acid), and arsenobetaine (3).

SITES, INDUSTRIES, AND BUSINESSES ASSOCIATED WITH EXPOSURES (see Table 74.1)

The microelectronics industry represents an increasing source of arsenic exposure. Both inorganic arsenic and arsine are used in the manufacture of computer chips used in communications equipment, scientific equipment, and computers. Several steps in manufacture could expose workers to arsenic, especially if equipment malfunctions occur. In such cases either air contamination or contamination of the person can occur. In addition, preliminary studies suggest that, in industrial gallium arsenide chip manufacture, air contamination by arsenic exceeds recommended limits and should be considered a source for arsenic toxicity (7).

The potential for hazardous material incidents exists in many of these industries. Accidents involving the source materials, i.e., arsine canisters or containers of arsenic oxide powders, may expose workers and the surrounding population. While mass exposures have not yet occurred, isolated deaths from industrial exposures have been reported (11).

CLINICAL TOXICOLOGY AND MANAGEMENT OF EXPOSURE

Routes of Absorption and Exposure

INHALATION

Airborne arsenic is usually in the As_2O_3 form (4). Documented biologic effects after respiratory exposure to arsenic concentrations previously thought to be benign raise serious questions about the safety of even minor inhalation exposure (3). Most arsenic is in particles that are deposited in the upper respiratory tract and cleared by mucociliary apparatus, thereby resulting in gastrointestinal absorption rather than pulmonary inhalation (3, 12). Further evaluation of this aspect of arsenic exposure is needed (3).

Inhalation of elemental arsenic, arsenic compounds, or arsine

Table 74.1. Sites, Industries, and Businesses Associated with Exposures

Business/Industry	Mechanism	Examples
Acute		
Pesticide spraying	Food and water contamination	Inorganic arsenicals
Microelectronic manufacture	Air contamination by gas or particulates	Arsine Arsenic oxides Gallium arsenide
Arsenical product production	Food and water contamination	Beer, soy water, milk
War gases	Air contamination	Lewisite, others
Chronic		
Microelectronic manufacture	Air contamination by gas or particulates	Arsine Arsenic oxides Gallium arsenide
Smelting of nonferrous ores	Air, water contamination	Gold, copper
Fossil fuel combustion	Air, water contamination	Coal, oil Shale
Phosphate detergents	Water, food contamination	Milk, others
Leaching of mine tailings and smelter	Water contamination	Residue piles
Copper leach liquors	Water contamination	Hazardous waste
Pesticide application	Air, water, food contamination	Agriculture
Arsenical manufacturing	Air, water contamination	Sheep dip factory Insecticides Herbicides Fungicides Algicides Wood Preservatives
Cotton harvesting	Air, water contamination	Cotton gin operation
Food additives		Poultry

can occur during several stages of semiconductor manufacture. Wafer manufacture requires handling of elemental arsenic. Arsenic oxides are produced during the heating process. Arsine gas is used as a dopant to introduce arsenic into the wafer. A worker can be exposed during accidents or by handling materials contaminated during the manufacturing process. High risk areas include ampule loading and breakout, ingot slicing and sandblasting, and epitaxial reactor loading and cleaning (7).

INGESTION

Over 90% of an ingested dose of inorganic trivalent or pentavalent arsenic is absorbed (4). Organic arsenic compounds in food and medication are also well absorbed (13, 14). Most reported cases of acute arsenic toxicity resulted from ingestion (3). In addition, particulate arsenic may be cleared by the pulmonary mucociliary apparatus, swallowed and become a source of gastrointestinal exposure.

SKIN ABSORPTION

Systemic absorption after dermal exposure has been reported and usually documented with elevated urinary arsenic levels (15). Little information is available concerning the chemical form, conditions for absorption, kinetics, or other information needed to evaluate the significance of skin absorption in specific populations (3).

Clinical Toxicology—Signs, Symptoms and Syndromes

ACUTE TOXICITY

Arsenic may injure multiple organs. Acute injury usually involves the blood, brain, heart, kidneys, and gastrointestinal tract. The bone marrow, skin, and peripheral nervous system may develop chronic toxicity after acute or chronic exposure. Thus, an acute ingestion may cause both acute and chronic syndromes.

Ingestion usually produces symptoms within 30 minutes, but onset may be delayed by ingestion with food. The clinical presentation generally reflects hypovolemia. Acute hypovolemia results from blood loss due to hemolysis and loss of intravascular volume due to increased vascular permeability. Systemic toxicity may include dehydration, intense thirst, vomiting, diarrhea, and electrolyte imbalance. Burning or dryness of mucous membranes may be noted. Gastrointestinal symptoms may include garlic or metallic taste, dysphagia, abdominal pain, vomiting, and diarrhea. Hematemesis, hematochezia, and melena may develop. The intestinal injury has been described as being caused by dilation of splanchnic vessels causing submucosal vesiculation. Rupture of vesicles may cause bleeding, rice water stools, and a protein-losing enteropathy. Besides ingestion and inhalation, arsenic compounds may be dermally absorbed (15).

Pulmonary symptoms of cough, dyspnea, and chest pain may develop, especially when exposure is by the pulmonary route (4). Acute respiratory failure may develop and require prolonged treatment. Pulmonary edema may occur, especially in cases of inhalation.

Altered neurologic status ranging from confusion to delirium, encephalopathy, seizures, and death may occur (16). The encephalopathy may become permanent. Chelation treatment has shown variable results on neurotoxicity (17). A delayed peripheral neuropathy may occur within a few weeks of exposure (18, 19, 20).

Few acute skin changes except flushing are found, although chronic skin changes from acute exposure may develop. Acute red blood cell hemolysis with accompanying hemoglobinuria and renal injury may occur (21). Hemolysis and hypovolemia may lead to acute renal failure (22).

A wide variety of hematologic defects have been described. Pancytopenia may develop after either acute or chronic poisoning (21, 23). Isolated defects such as leukopenia or anemia may also be seen. This may be normochromic, normocytic, or hypochromic, microcytic. Increased bone marrow vascularity, basophilic stippling, Rouleau formation, and thrombocytopenia have also been reported (21).

The ECG may show, in addition to tachycardia, QT interval prolongation, T-wave changes, ventricular fibrillation, or, rarely, atypical ventricular tachycardia (23, 24).

Arsine presents a much different clinical picture than that presented by the other arsenicals. It has a sudden onset of symptoms from 2–24 hours after exposure and includes nausea, abdominal colic, vomiting, dyspnea, followed by findings of

Table 74.2.   Manifestations of Acute Arsenic Poisoning

	Acute	Time of Onset
Systemic	Thirst	Minutes
	Hypovolemia-hypotension	Minutes to hours
Gastrointestinal	Garlic/metallic taste	Immediate
	Burning of mucosae	Immediate
	Nausea and vomiting	Minutes
	Diarrhea	Minutes to hours
	Abdominal pain	Minutes to hours
	Hemetemesis	Minutes to hours
	Hematochezia/melena	Hours
	Rice water stools	Hours
Hematologic	Red cell hemolysis	Minutes to hours
	Hematuria	Minutes to hours
	Isolated blood element decrease (i.e., lymphopenia)	Several weeks
	Pancytopenia	Several weeks
Pulmonary	Cough	Immediate
Primarily in inhalation exposures	Dyspnea	Minutes to hours
	Chest pain	Minutes to hours
	Pulmonary edema	Minutes to hours
Liver	Jaundice	Days
	Fatty degeneration	Days
	Central necrosis	Days
Kidneys	Proteinuria	Hours to days
	Hematuria	Hours to days
	Acute renal failure	Hours to days
Nervous system		
Central	Confusion/delirium	Hours
	Encephalopathy	Minutes to hours
	Seizures	Minutes to hours
Peripheral	Sensory and motor neuropathy	Several weeks

Table 74.3.   Manifestations of Chronic Arsenic Poisoning

	Effect
Systemic	Thirst
	Hypovolemia-hypotension
Skin/mucous membranes	Eczema
	Hyperkeratosis, palms and soles
	Warts
	Melanosis and/or vitiligo
	Mucous membrane irritation/ulceration
	Alopecia
	Squamous cell cancers
Gastrointestinal	Stomatitis
	Diarrhea
Hematological	Leukopenia
	Anemia
	Pancytopenia
	Acute myelogeneous leukemia
Kidneys	Acute renal failure
Nervous system	
Central	Confusion/delirium
	Encephalopathy
	Seizures
Peripheral	Sensory and motor neuropathy

acute intravascular hemolysis. These may include dark, bloody urine and jaundice. The triad of symptoms—abdominal pain, hematuria, and jaundice—are recognized as characteristic clinical features (26). Sudden death without development of the classic arsine gas syndrome may occur. Low level arsine exposure may also cause chronic arsenicalism (26). Table 74.2 lists the acute effects of arsenic exposure.

CHRONIC AND LONGTERM TOXICITY

The bone marrow, skin, and peripheral nervous system may become involved after acute or chronic exposure. Aplastic anemia has been documented. Acute myelogeneous leukemia has been reported after chronic exposure (23). Basal cell cancer and squamous cell cancer have been reported after prolonged exposure (27, 28). An excess of respiratory cancer in arsenic-exposed workers has been reported (29, 30), although recent additional monitoring of these patients no longer revealed a significant excess of lung cancer (31). The Occupational Safety and Health Administration (OSHA) has linked arsenic to cancer of skin, lungs, lymph glands, and bone marrow (32). It has also been associated with bladder, kidney, skin, prostate, lung, and liver cancer (33).

The skin is often involved in chronic exposure. Eczematoid lesions of variable severity may develop (4). Hyperkeratosis,

warts, and melanosis are common findings in chronically exposed patients (3, 4). Besides being a chemical irritant, arsenic may function as a contact allergen. Low, noncaustic skin exposures may result in vesiculation in sensitized people (3). Mucous membrane irritation and ulceration involving the face, cornea, nasal septum, and respiratory tract may also occur (34). The fingernails may become thin and brittle with transverse white striae called Mee's lines (35).

A sensorimotor peripheral neuropathy is common and begins 1–3 weeks after acute exposure (18, 20). Diffuse, symmetrical, painful neuritis begins in the peripheral extremities and progresses proximally over days to weeks (18, 20, 36). It also involves distinct muscle weakness and wasting and may be confused with Guillain-Barré syndrome (36). The patient may have diminished vibratory and position sense causing a gait disturbance. In the upper extremities the ulnar and median nerves are most commonly affected. In some cases, the neuropathy has persisted for years (4). In addition, prolonged central nervous system effects have been described. Cases of toxic encephalopathy associated with elevated arsenic levels slowly resolving over months to years have been described (17, 37).

Abnormal electrocardiograms and peripheral blood vessel damage have been reported in workers. Gangrene developed in some (38). Liver injury with elevation of transaminase enzymes has been noted in several reports (29, 39).

Elevated arsenic levels have been reported in the fetus born to a mother with acute ingestion of arsenic (40). Inorganic arsenic is teratogenic after administration of large doses in rodents. However, there is currently no evidence that toxic effects will be observed at permissible exposure limits (41).

Arsine causes chronic effects similar to the other arsenicals. Peripheral neuropathy has been reported, as have liver and renal injury (4). Table 74.3 lists the chronic effects of arsenic exposure.

TARGET ORGAN TOXICITY MEASUREMENTS

Bone marrow aspirate may show erythroid hyperplasia similar to pernicious anemia (42). Slowing of nerve conduction velocity and amplitude has been reported in exposed patients without evidence of slowed reflexes (19). Abnormal electromyograms have also been reported, although the clinical usefulness of this information has not been clarified (43). The rare, but well-documented arrhythmias suggest monitoring for cardiovascular arrhythmias during the entire course of acute toxicity.

Toxicology Management

CLINICAL MANAGEMENT

Ingestion As in all life-threatening emergencies, initial treatment should include maintenance of patent airway, adequate ventilation, and cardiovascular support. Aggressive monitoring of volume status should be performed in a critical care facility. Volume should be replaced as clinically indicated, first by isotonic crystalloid administration, then by specific blood products as indicated. Vasopressors are recommended for refractory hypotension; however, little evidence to support their use has been reported.

Arrhythmias should be treated according to standard guidelines. No data indicating specific antidotes to prevent arrhythmias have been reported.

Potential renal failure, in part due to hemoglobinuria, should be treated by appropriate volume repletion. Alkalinization of the urine is also recommended to prevent deposition of red cell breakdown products. Since arsenic and arsenic chelates are excreted in the urine, hemodialysis should be considered if oliguria or renal failure develop (44).

Chelation therapy is usually needed in symptomatic cases. Treatment should be initiated with British anti-Lewisite (BAL; dimercaprol) at 3–5 mg/kg/dose intramuscularly every 4–12 hours. As the patient improves this may be switched to penicillamine, 250 mg orally q.i.d. for 5 days. Generally, 24-hour urinary excretion of arsenic is followed before, during, and after chelation. Chelation may be restarted if urinary excretion of arsenic remains elevated or symptoms reappear. Dosages should be reduced in renal failure.

Reservations concerning BAL and penicillamine have recently been raised. In rabbits, treatment with BAL 1 hour after administration of arsenite was found to increase brain arsenic levels (45). Penicillamine's ability to effectively chelate arsenic has been described as ineffective or inferior to the water-soluble BAL analogs (46).

Newer dimercapto chelating drugs show great promise in effectively reducing the body burden of arsenic while avoiding the many side effects of BAL. Dimercaptosuccinic acid (DMSA) effectively treats experimental arsenic poisoning in animals and has been successfully utilized in humans (47, 48, 49). Accumulating clinical evidence suggests that it will be very useful in the treatment of acute arsenic poisoning. Accumulating evidence at the University of Arizona suggests that DMSA may also be useful in attenuating the effects of chronic exposure. Another dimercapto chelating agent, dimercaptopropanesulfonate (DMPS), has shown similar promise (50). Both have the advantages of being less toxic than BAL and of water solubility, making them effective after oral administration.

Prevention of Absorption In acute ingestions, emesis may remove unabsorbed compounds. Frequently, seriously exposed patients will have already vomited. After the stomach is emptied, activated charcoal (1 g/kg) and cathartic should be given to promote passage of gastrointestinal contents. A regional poison center should be consulted for details on these procedures.

Inhalation Acute toxicity by inhalation is unusual except in the case of arsine. Arsine inhalation is treated by removal from the source of exposure, making sure that rescue personnel are not exposed. Subsequent management is similar to other arsenic compounds, except that BAL chelation has not been shown to be helpful (4). In addition, standard management of intravascular hemolysis, such as alkalinization and maintenance of urine flow and transfusions, may be necessary.

The management of arsine exposures is directed at maintaining urine ouput and a satisfactory hematocrit. The use of exchange transfusion in severe cases of arsine exposure is the best therapy available (51). Hemodialysis until adequate renal function returns may also be needed (11).

LABORATORY DIAGNOSIS

Essentially all organ systems must be evaluated. Thus, laboratory tests should include complete blood count, liver and renal function tests, and blood and urine arsenic levels. An abdominal radiograph may show radiopaque contents after ingestion of arsenic.

SPECIAL TESTS

Monitoring of arsenic levels is complicated. Quantitative 24-hour collections are considered the most reliable. An unexposed individual should not excrete more than 100 μg/24 hours, even during chelation treatment. However, urinary concentrations may be transiently elevated after eating some seafoods (52).

Blood arsenic levels are highly variable. Blood arsenic will usually be elevated in acute exposure, but it is rapidly cleared. If there is a significant delay between ingestion and presentation, diagnosis based on blood arsenic levels may be erroneous. Blood levels are often normal in cases of chronic toxicity (4).

Determination of hair and nail arsenic levels has been attempted. Arsenic may begin to accumulate in these areas within hours of exposure (53). However, laboratories offering such tests to consumers have demonstrated inconsistent results (54). Utilizing pubic instead of scalp hair may be useful as this area is usually less exposed to environmental deposition of arsenic (16). Many authors discourage its use, but overall recommendations vary widely (4).

BASIC TREATMENT

Ingestion No specific treatment of ingestion has been suggested. Standard gastrointestinal decontamination procedures should be followed after acute ingestions of arsenic. Activated charcoal and cathartic may then be administered, but their efficacy is untested. Since arsenic is radiopaque, an abdominal radiograph may document ingestion of solid arsenic-containing compounds and allow assessment of efficacy of decontamination procedures.

Inhalation Supportive care of pulmonary injury is recommended. Some authors have recommended treatment with BAL for severe respiratory symptoms (4).

Dermal Exposure Clothing should be removed and the skin cleaned in all arsenic exposures. After decontamination of the skin, standard symptomatic skin care is used for dermatitis, ulcers, and other skin lesions (4).

BIOLOGIC MONITORING

Biologic monitoring offers the advantage of revealing an individual's exact exposure. However, the underlying concept is that the test performed accurately depicts the degree of toxicity the individual is experiencing. For some metals this correlation is good; in others it is poor. Blood arsenic levels have been shown to correlate poorly with arsenic exposure. However, urinary arsenic excretion correlates better with arsenic exposure. Correlation of urinary arsenic to airborne arsenic was demonstrated (55). Urinary arsenic excretion ranges from 0.01–1.0 mg/l. However, normal values in most laboratories range from 0.01–0.15 mg/l (56). This is affected by dietary intake of arsenic-rich foods. It can take 48 hours for urinary levels to return to normal after ingestion of arsenic-rich foods (56).

Instead of total arsenic determinations, which are highly influenced by recent arsenic ingestions such as seafood, levels of methylated derivatives of arsenic can be determined in the urine. Airborne inorganic arsenic is converted to methylated derivatives before urinary excretion (12). Monomethylarsonic acid (MMA) and dimethylarsinic acid (DMA) account for much of arsenic excretion (57). These levels are not influenced by the presence of organic arsenic from marine origin (7). Exposures below the NIOSH recommended level of 2 μg/m^3 will not increase urinary levels above background (7).

Analysis of hair or nail arsenic content exemplifies many of the problems involved in biologic monitoring of arsenic. Arsenic may accumulate during periods of exposure in these areas. Thus, it has been concluded that these are useful for monitoring arsenic toxicity. However, many pitfalls exemplify the problems involved in biologic monitoring of arsenic. First, it appears that arsenic prefers the sulfhydryl-rich environment of the hair and nails. Thus, accumulation may represent exposure, not toxicity. Second, environmental contamination of the exterior of these structures can lead to falsely high estimation of exposure. Third, the particular laboratory performing the analysis affects the reliability of results (58, 59). If specimens are properly collected and analyzed and the results appropriately interpreted, hair or nail arsenic levels may aid in the diagnosis of arsenic toxicity.

Arsenic levels are similar between men and women and among various hair colors. However, black women appear to have significantly increased arsenic content in the hair (59).

ENVIRONMENTAL MONITORING

Environmental monitoring of toxins is performed to identify workplace exposure without requiring direct sampling from the individual. Several concepts must be kept in mind when interpreting environmental monitoring. First, the results can only be as accurate as the sampling and analytical procedures used. Arsenic is often present in minute quantities that require processing and concentration procedures. Second, exposure and toxicity are not the same. An exposed individual may not develop toxicity, while another individual may develop toxicity to minimal exposures.

Choice of sample may be a major concern. Vegetation and other materials may have arsenic-containing dust on them. A decision must be made concerning inclusion or exclusion of the dust in the sample analyzed. Arsenic-containing solutions may have suspended material that may or may not need to be removed before analysis (3). Water, urine, and other aqueous samples should be analyzed within hours or frozen and stored.

Levels in natural waters decrease with time (60). Since trace concentrations are usually involved, preconcentration of the specimen may be necessary. Conversion of arsenic to arsine, coprecipitation with iron(III) hydroxide, distillation as arsenic(III) chloride, or extraction have been used (60). Oxidation to convert organic compounds to inorganic compounds may be necessary. In air samples arsenic is usually associated with small particulates. However, variable amounts of the arsenic in air samples may be volatile and not collected on sample air filters (60). In general, the analysis of arsenic in the environment should be carefully considered before sampling.

EXPOSURE LIMITS, TLV, PELS

Trivalent arsenic (arsinite) is much more toxic than pentavalent arsenic (arsenates). The pentavalent form may be converted to trivalent arsenic in vivo. Larger exposures of the pentavalent form are usually required to produce toxicity. The minimum lethal exposure reported has been 1 mg/kg of ingested arsenic in a child (61). Acute ingestion of 200 mg of arsenic trioxide may be fatal in an adult. The American Conference of Government and Industrial Hygienists (ACGIH) recommended TLV-TWA is 0.2 mg/m^3 with no STEL (62). OSHA PEL is 0.5 mg/m^3 (TWA) (63). The National Institute on Occupational Safety and Health recommended exposure standard is 0.002 mg/m^3 (64). For arsine gas the TLV-TWA is 0.05 ppm. Immediate death has occurred at 150 ppm (65).

SUMMARY

Always a serious threat to health, arsenic is becoming more threatening as its technologic applications increase. Experience in other countries shows that contamination of food and water can lead to severe, widespread consequences. As with many diseases, the diagnosis of arsenic toxicity often requires a suspicious mind on the part of the physician. This is particularly true of the neurologic manifestations which may only partially resolve with treatment. Once the diagnosis is made, effective therapy exists in the new dimercapto chelating agents.

REFERENCES

1. Yamashita N, Doi M, Nishio M. Recent observations of Kyoto children poisoned by arsenic tainted dry milk. Jpn J Hyg 1972;27:364.
2. Patty FA. Industrial hygiene and toxicology. 2nd ed. New York: John Wiley & Sons, 1962.
3. National Academy of Sciences. Medical and biologic effects of environmental pollutants, arsenic. Washington, DC: National Research Council, National Academy of Sciences, 1977.
4. Ishinishi N, Tsuchiya K, Vahter M, Fowler BA. Arsenic. In: Friberg L, Nordberg GF, Vouk V, eds. Handbook on the toxicology of metals. Amsterdam: Elsevier Science Publishers, 1986.
5. Baker EL Jr, Hayes CG, Landrigan PJ, Handke JL, Leger RT, Housworth WJ, Harrington JM. A nationwide survey of heavy metal absorption in children living near primary copper, lead, and zinc smelters. Am J Epidemiol 1977;106:261–273.
6. Webb DR, Sipes IG, Carter DE. In vitro solubility and in vivo toxicity of gallium arsenide. Toxicol Appl Pharmacol 1984;76:96–104.
7. Harrison RJ. Gallium arsenide. State of the art reviews. Occup Med 1986;1:49–58.
8. Ungers LJ, Jones JH, McIntyre AJ, McHenry CR. Release of arsenic from semiconductor wafers. Am Ind Hyg Assoc J 1985;46:416–420.
9. Buchanan WD. Toxicity of arsenic compounds. Amsterdam: Elsevier Publication Company, 1962.
10. Gorby MS. Arsenic poisoning. West J Med 1988;149:308–315.
11. Wald PH, Becker CE. Toxic gases used in the microelectronics industry. State of the art reviews. Occup Med 1986;1:105–117.

12. Smith TJ, Crecelius EA, Reading JC. Airborne arsenic exposure and excretion of methylated arsenic compounds. Environ Health Perspect 1977;19:89–93.

13. Crecelius EA. Changes in the chemical speciation of arsenic following ingestion by man. Environ Health Perspect 1977;19:147–150.

14. Bettley FR, O'Shea JA. The absorption of arsenic and its relation to carcinoma. Br J Dermatol 1975;92:563–568.

15. Garb LG, Hine CH. Arsenical neuropathy: residual effects following acute industrial exposure. J Occup Med 1977;19:567–568.

16. Jenkins RB. Inorganic arsenic and the nervous system. Brain 1966;89:479–498.

17. Fincher RME, Koerker RM. Long-term survival after acute arsenic encephalopathy. Am J Med 1987;82:549–552.

18. LeQuesne PM, McLeod JG. Peripheral neuropathy following a single exposure to arsenic. J Neurosci 1977;32:437–451.

19. Feldman RG, Niles CA, Kelly-Hayes M, Sax DS, Dison WJ, Thompson DJ, Landau E. Peripheral neuropathy in arsenic smelter workers. Neurology 1979;29:939–944.

20. Heyman A, Pfeiffer JB Jr, Willett RW, et al. Peripheral neuropathy caused by arsenical intoxication. A study of 41 cases with observations on the effects of BAL (2,3-dimercapto-propanol). N Engl J Med 1956;254:401–409.

21. Kyle RA, Pease GL. Hematologic aspects of arsenic intoxication. N Engl J Med 1965;273:18–23.

22. Gerhardt RE, Crecelius EA, Hudson JB. Moonshine-related arsenic poisoning. Arch Intern Med 1980;140:211–213.

23. Kjeldsberg CR, Ward HP. Leukemia in arsenic poisoning. Ann Intern Med 1972;77:935–937.

24. St. Petery J, Gross C, Victoria BE. Ventricular fibrillation caused by arsenic poisoning. Am J Dis Child 1970;120:367–371.

25. Peterson RG, Rumack BH. D-Penicillamine therapy of acute arsenic poisoning. J Pediatr 1977;91:661–666.

26. Fowler BA, Weissberg JB. Arsine poisoning. N Engl J Med 1974;291:1171–1174.

27. Jackson R, Grainge JW. Arsenic and cancer. Can Med Assoc J 1975;113:396–401.

28. Renwick JH, Harrington JM, Waldron HA, et al. Long-term effects of acute arsenical poisoning. J Soc Occup Med 1981;31:144–147.

29. Lee AM, Fraumeni JF. Arsenic and respiratory cancer in man: An occupational study. J Natl Cancer Inst 1969;42:1045–52.

30. Ott MG, Holder BB, Gordon HL. Respiratory cancer and occupational exposure to arsenicals. Arch Environ Health 1974;29:250–255.

31. Sobel W, Bond GG, Baldwin CL, Ducommun DJ. An update of respiratory cancer and occupational exposure to arsenicals. Am J Ind Med 1988;13:263–270.

32. Anonymous. Health hazards of inorganic arsenic. Washington, DC: OSHA, 1979.

33. Chen CL, Kuo TL, Wu MM. Arsenic and cancers. Lancet 1988;1:414–415.

34. Uhde GI. Arsenic eye burns. Am J Ophthalmol 1946;29:1090–1093.

35. Mees RA. The nails with arsenical polyneuritis. JAMA 1919;72:1337.

36. Donofrio PD, Wilbourn AJ, Albers JW, Rogers L, Salanga V, Greenberg HS. Acute arsenic intoxication presenting as Guillain-Barré-like syndrome. Muscle Nerve 1987;10:114–120.

37. Bolla-Wilson K, Bleecker ML. Neuropsychological impairment following inorganic arsenic exposure. J Occup Med 1987;29:500–503.

38. Tseng W-P. Effects and dose-response relationships of skin and blackfoot disease with arsenic. Environ Health Perspect 1977;19:109–119.

39. Axelson O, Dahlgren E, Jansson C-D, Rehnlund SO. Arsenic exposure and mortality: a case-referent study from a Swedish copper smelter. Br J Ind Med 1978;35:8–15.

40. Lugo G, Cassady G, Palmisano P. Acute maternal arsenic intoxication. Am J Dis Child 1969;117:328–330.

41. Council on Scientific Affairs. Effects of toxic chemicals on the reproductive system. JAMA 1985;253:3431–3437.

42. Selzer PM, Ancel MA. Chronic arsenic poisoning masquerading as pernicious anemia. West J Med 1983;139:219–220.

43. Hindmarsh JT, McLetchie OR, Heffernan LPM, Hayne OA, Ellenberger HA, McCurdy RF, Thiebaux HJ. Electromyographic abnormalities in chronic environmental arsenicalism. J Anal Toxicol 1977;1:270–276.

44. Vaziri ND, Upham T, Barton CH. Hemodialysis clearance of arsenic. Clin Toxicol 1980;17:451–456.

45. Hoover TD, Aposhian HV. BAL increases the arsenic-74 content of rabbit brain. Toxicol Appl Pharmacol 1983;70:160–162.

46. Kreppel H, Reichl FX, Forth W, Fichtl B. Lack of effectiveness of d-penicillamine in experimental arsenic poisoning. Vet Hum Toxicol 1989;31:1–5.

47. Aposhian HV, Carter DE, Hoover TD, Hsu C, Maiorino RM, Stone E. DMSA, DMPS and DMPA—as arsenic antidotes. Fundam Appl Toxicol 1984;4:858–870.

48. Graziano JH. Role of 2,3-dimercaptosuccinic acid in the treatment of heavy metal poisoning. Med Toxicol 1986;1:155–162.

49. Fournier L, Thomas G, Garnier R, Buisine A, Houze P, Pradier F, Dally S. 2,3-Dimercaptosuccinic acid treatment of heavy metal poisoning in humans. Med Toxicol 1988;3:499–504.

50. Hruby K, Donner A. 2,3-Dimercapto-1-propanesulphonate in heavy metal poisoning. Med Toxicol 1987;2:317–323.

51. Hesdorfer CS, Milne FJ, Terblanche J, Meyers AM. Arsine gas poisoning: the importance of exchange transfusion in severe cases. Br J Ind Med 1986;43:353–355.

52. Baselt RC. Disposition of toxic drugs and chemicals in man. CA, Davis: Biomed Publications, 1982:59–63.

53. Lander H, Hodge PR, Crisp CS. Arsenic in the hair and nails. J Forensic Med 1965;12:52–67.

54. Barrett S. Commercial hair analysis. Science or scam? JAMA 1985;254:1041–1045.

55. Nelson MK. Arsenic trioxide production. In: Carnow BW, ed. Health effects of occupational lead and arsenic exposure. Washington, DC: U.S. Government Printing Office, 1976.

56. Dickerson OB. Arsenic. In: Waldron HA, ed. Metals in the environment. New York: Academic Press, 1980.

57. Buchet JP, Lauwerys R, Roels H. Comparison of the urinary excretion of arsenic metabolites after a single oral dose of sodium arsenite, monomethylarsonate, or dimethylarsinate in man. Int Arch Occup Environ Health 1981;48:71–79.

58. Sky-Peck HH, Joseph BJ. The use and misuse of human hair in trace metal analysis. In: Brown SS, Savory J, eds. Chemical toxicology and clinical chemistry of metals. New York: Academic Press, 1983.

59. Savoie JY, Weber JP. Evaluating laboratory performance via an interlaboratory comparison program for toxic substances in blood and urine. In: Brown SS, Savory J, eds. Chemical toxicology and clinical chemistry of metals. New York: Academic Press, 1983.

60. Anonymous. Arsenic. Geneva: World Health Organization, 1981:27–30.

61. Woody NC, Kometani JT. BAL in the treatment of arsenic ingestion of children. Pediatrics 1948;1:372–378.

62. ACGIH. Threshold limit values and biological exposure indices for 1990–1991. Cincinnati, OH: American Conference on Government and Industrial Hygienists, 1990:25.

63. OSHA Occupational safety and health standards. Code of Federal Regulations. 1981;29 (Part 1910.1000):673–679.

64. NIOSH. Criteria for a recommended standard: occupational exposure to inorganic arsenic. Washington, DC: U.S. Dept of Health, Education, and Welfare, 1975.

65. Ellenhorn MJ, Barceloux DG. Medical toxicology. New York: Elsevier Science Publishing Company, 1988:1013.

Mercury

Douglas Campbell, M.D.
Melissa Gonzales, M.S.
John B. Sullivan, Jr., M.D.

INTRODUCTION

Mercury is a member of the class II family of metals along with zinc and cadmium. The chemical symbol, Hg, is derived from the Greek work hydrargyros, meaning ''water silver.'' This is perhaps its best description, as it is the only metal that is in the liquid state at room temperature. Mercury has an atomic weight of 200.6.

There are three basic forms of mercury: (a) elemental mercury, (b) inorganic, and (c) organic mercurial compounds. These three forms of mercury differ from each other in biologic and toxicologic activity. Elemental mercury (Hg) is also called quicksilver or hydrargyrum. Included in this category are any ionic compounds that can decompose into mercury vapor in the occupational setting. Inorganic mercury is found in either the mercurous form, Hg^{+1}, which is usually combined to form salts which dissociate slowly in water or body fluids to form Hg^{+2} and Hg^0 or the divalent mercuric form, Hg^{+2}. Organic mercury consists of two subcategories: long-chain alkyl and aryl mercurial compounds and short-chain alkyl compounds, which include methyl and ethyl mercury. The dialkyl derivatives of the short-chain group become toxic after the loss of one alkyl group. Table 75.1 lists the commonly found compounds in each of these three groupings.

SITES, INDUSTRIES, AND BUSINESSES ASSOCIATED WITH EXPOSURE

Approximately 70,000 workers are exposed to mercury yearly. The general population is exposed to mercury mainly via food such as fish (1). Release of mercury into the environment from human-related activities is estimated to be 2000–metric tons/year, mainly from mining and ore smelting (1).

Elemental mercury occurs as a part of the earth's natural geochemistry, comprising 0.5 μg/g of the earth's crust. Mercury is also released into the environment through mining and industrial discharge and the combustion of fossil fuels. In the atmosphere, mercury concentrations range from 3.9 ng/m³ over remote nonmineralized areas up to 50 ng/m³ over mineralized areas. Rocks and soils may contain 10–300 ng/g. Ocean water ranges from 3.0 ng/l in the open sea to 5–6 ng/l in coastal waters. The bulk of mercury in the oceans is apparently from natural sources such as volcanic eruptions and volatilization or solubilization of rocks, soils, and sediments (1).

Surface water contains less than 50.0 ng/l. Industrial and mining activities have increased the environmental flux of mercury from a concentration of 25,000 tons/year to 40,000 tons/year, with one third of this flux returning to land and two thirds to the oceans. Methylation of mercury by microorganisms such as *Methanobacterium* greatly increases the transport of mercury

in the environment, which also can eventually lead to the bioaccumulation of mercury in fish and thus eventually to humans.

World production of mercury is approximated 8000 tons/year. Two predominant extraction techniques are used in commercial production. Mercury can be extracted from cinnabar (mercury sulfide) by firing the ore in retorts with either lime or iron and collecting the liberated mercury vapor by condensation. In direct furnaces, sulfur dioxide formation releases mercury. Italy, Mexico, Spain, and the Soviet Union are the major producing countries. There are also ore deposits in Yugoslavia, Canada, Algeria, Japan, China, New Zealand, California, Oregon, Washington, and Nevada.

Mercury is predominantly used in the manufacture of electrical meters, industrial control instruments, and dry batteries, in the production of the chloralkali, in antimildew paints, as catalysts and fungicides, and, to a lesser degree, in pharma-

Table 75.1. Inorganic and Organic Mercurial Compounds and Their Uses

Inorganic	Ammoniated mercury ($HgNH_2Cl$)—antiseptic
	Mercuric acetate [$Hg(00C_2H_3)_2$]—catalyst in organic synthesis, pharmaceuticals
	Mercuric arsenate ($HgNH_3O_4$)—waterproof and antifouling paints
	Mercuric benzoate [$Hg(C_7H_5O_2)_2$]—antisyphilitic
	Mercuric bromide ($HgBr_2$)—medicinal use
	Mebromin (Mercurochrome—25% mercury + 20% bromine)—antiseptic cream mercurous chloride (calomel, mercury monochloride—Hg_2Cl_2)—a laxative
	Mercuric chloride (corrosive sublimate, mercury bichloride)—antiseptic solution
	Mercuric cyanate (fulminate of mercury, $Hg(CNO)_2$)—explosive
	Mercuric cyanide [$Hg(CN)_2$]—antiseptic, photography
	Mercuric oxide, red (red or yellow precipitate Hgo)—pigment, dry batteries
	Mercuric potassium cyanide silvering glass, in mirrors
	Mercuric sulfide—(cinnabar, red vermillion, Chinese red) used in tattoos, combined with cadmium sulfide
	Mercuric salicylate (salicylate mercury)—topical antiseptic
	Mercuric acetate [$Hg(OOC_2H_3)_2$]—
	Sublimate ($HgCl_2$)
Organic	Thimerosol (merthiolate—49% mercury)
	Alkyl mercury fungicides: dialkylmercury ethyl mercury (cresan, goanosan, lignasan)
	Phenyl mercury fungicides (Ph Hg +): phenylmercury (Gallotox, Merphenyl, Barbak, Corotrane)
	Alkoxyalkyl mercury fungicides: methoxyethylmercury (MetOEHg + Algalol, Aretan)
	Mercurial diuretics (Mersalyl, Chlormerodrin)

ceuticals and for general laboratory use. The largest number of exposed workers are in the health services, dental medicine, chemical products, electrial equipment manufacturing, chlor-alkali production, and mining (1).

Use in dental amalgams is declining, along with its usage as an explosive and as a slimicide in the paper and pulp industry. In the past, mercury was used in the felt hat industry and in fingerprinting. However, these uses are no longer practiced. Using mercury in the extraction of gold and silver has also become less common. The toxicity of organic mercury usually results from environmental contamination. Agricultural use as fungicides and seed dressings increases the potential for environmental contamination and for possible accidental ingestion. Organic mercurial compounds have also been used for medicinal purposes such as diuretics, external antiseptics, and laxatives. Table 75.2 lists some potential occupational exposures to the various forms of mercury.

REGULATORY AND ENVIRONMENTAL CONTROL

Mercury and mercury-containing compounds are on the list of toxic chemicals in Section 313 of the Emergency Planning and Community Right-to-Know Act of 1986. Table 75.3 summarizes the regulatory data with regard to all mercury compounds in the occupational and nonoccupational environment (2).

CLINICAL TOXICOLOGY

Mercury is a general protoplasmic poison. The general mode of toxicologic action involves the covalent binding of mercury to sulfhydryl groups, inactivating enzymes of cellular function and metabolism of carbohydrates at the pyruvic acid level (3). Binding also occurs to carboxyl, amide, amine, and phosphoryl groups. The high affinity of mercury for sulfhydryl groups as well as other biochemical moieties is the reason for its toxic manifestations and basic toxic mechanism.

Mercury toxicology is divided into elemental, inorganic, and organic poisoning. Elemental mercury is liquid at room temperature and readily vaporizes. In terms of inorganic mercury, the divalent mercuric salts are the most commonly encountered poison. The organic mercury compounds can be divided into those that are stable in living organisms and those that are broken down, such as phenyl mercury and methoxyalkyl mercury compounds (3).

Acute Elemental Mercury Toxicity

Due to a very low vapor pressure of 0.0012 mm Hg, elemental mercury is easily vaporized at room temperature, saturating the air at 13–18 mg/m^3 at 24°C (77°F). This physical property infers upon mercury an increased potential for inhalation intoxication that is not common to other metals. Mercury vapor is insoluble in water. Elemental mercury is readily oxidized in the presence of oxygen.

Exposure to elemental mercury predominantly occurs through inhalation of the vaporized metal. A small fraction of the inhaled dose is expired, but the majority of the mercury vapor quickly penetrates the alveolar membrane and is quickly absorbed into the circulation. The mercury is then oxidized to the divalent (Hg^{+2}) mercuric form after absorption into tissues and red blood cells. However, small amounts may persist in the elemental, more lipid soluble form for several minutes. During this time, the mercury quickly passes the blood-brain barrier, accumulating in the central nervous system (CNS), where it can injure sensory and motor neurons. Elemental mercury also accumulates in the kidney but rarely causes renal dysfunction. The mercuric ions do not significantly cross the blood-brain barrier, as they are not lipid soluble. Instead, the elemental form is oxidized in the CNS to the mercuric form,

Table 75.2.   Products and Industries with Potential Mercury Exposure

Elemental	Inorganic Mercurials	Organic Mercurials
Dental medicine	Disinfectants	Bactericides
Batteries	Paints and dyes	Embalming preparations
Barometers	Explosives	Paper manufacturing
Boiler makers	Fireworks manufacturing	Farmers
Calibration instruments	Fur processing	Laundry and diaper services
Caustic soda production	Ink manufacturing	External antiseptics
Carbon bush production	Chemical lab workers	Fungicides
Ceramics	Percussion caps and detonators	Insecticide manufacture
Chloralkali production	Spermicidal jellies	Seed handling
Ultrasonic amplifiers	Tannery workers	Wood preservatives
Direct current meters	Wood preservatives	Germicides
Infrared detectors	Tattooing materials	
Electrical apparatus	Taxidermists	
Electroplating	Vinyl chloride production	
Fingerprint detectors	Embalming preparations	
Silver and gold extraction	Mercury vapor lamps	
Jewelry	Antisyphilitic agents	
Fluorescent, neon, and mercury arc lamps	Thermoscopy	
Manometers	Silvering in mirrors	
Paints	Photography	
Paper pulp manufacturing	Perfumery and cosmetics	
Photography	Acetaldehyde production	
Pressure gauges		
Thermometers		
Semiconductor solar cells		

Table 75.3   Summary of Regulations Regarding Mercury and Mercury Compounds

Agency	Description	Value
	International	
WHO	Guideline for drinking water mercury (all forms)	0.001 mg/l
	Provisional tolerable weekly intake	0.3 mg total mercury (5 g/kg body weight), including a maximum of 0.2 mg methyl mercury, as mercury (3.3 g/kg body weight)
	National	
Regulations		
EPA	Listing mercury as a hazardous air pollutant	
	National Emission Standard for Mercury	
	Emissions from mercury ore processing facilities and mercury cell chloralkali plants	2300 g Hg maximum per 24-hour period
	Emissions from sludge, incineration plants, sludge drying plants, or a combination of these that process wastewater treatment plant sludges	3200 g Hg maximum per 24-hour period
OSHA	Permissible exposure limit (PEL)	
	Time-weighted average (TWA)	
	Organo mercury compounds	0.01 mg/m^3
	Mercury vapor	0.05 mg/m^3
	Ceiling limit	
	Mercury (aryl and inorganic)	0.01 mg/m^3
	Shortterm exposure limit Organo (alkyl mercury compounds)	0.03 mg/m^3
FD/	Permissible level in bottled water mercury	0.002 mg/l
EPA	Reportable quantity	
	Mercury	1 lb
	Mercury fulminate	10 lb
	Mercuric cyanide	1 lb
	Mercuric nitrate	10 lb
	Mercuric sulfate	10 lb
	Mercuric thiocyanate	10 lb
	Mercurous nitrate	10 lb
	Phenylmercuric acetate	100 lb
	Extremely hazardous substances	
	Threshold planning quantity (TPQ)	
	Mercuric chloride	500/10,000 lb
	Mercuric oxide	500/10,000 lb
	Ethylmercuric phosphate	10,000 lb
	Mercuric acetate	500/10,000 lb
	Methoxyethylmercuric acetate	500/10,000 lb
	Methylmercuric dicyanamide	500/10,000 lb
	Phenyl mercury acetate	500/10,000 lb
Guidelines		
NIOSH	Recommended Exposure Limit (REL) for occupational exposure to Mercury TWA	0.05 mg/m^3
	Immediately dangerous to life or health (IDLH) level	
	Mercury	28 mg/m^3
	Organo (alkyl) mercury compounds	10 mg/m^3
ACGIH	Threshold limit value (TLV)	
	TWA	
	Mercury as Hg (skin)	
	Alkyl compounds	0.01 mg/m^3
	All forms except alkyl vapor	0.05 mg/m^3
	Aryl and inorganic compounds	0.10 mg/m^3
	Shortterm exposure limit (STEL) mercury as Hg (skin)	
	Alkyl compounds	0.03 mg/m^3
EPA	Maximum contaminant level goal (MCLG) (proposed)	
	Mercury (inorganic)	0.002 mg/l
EPA	Ambient water quality criteria to protect human health:	144 ng/l
	Ingestion of water and aquatic organisms	146 ng/l
	Ingestion of aquatic organisms only	146 ng/l

continues

Table 75.3. *Continued*

Agency	Description	Value
EPA	Carcinogenic classification Oral reference dose (RfD)	Group D
	Mercury; inorganic only	3×10^{-4} mg/kg/day
	Mercury, alkyl and inorganic	3×10^{-4} mg/kg/day
	Methyl mercury	3×10^{-4} mg/kg/day
	Phenylmercuric acetate	8×10^{-5} mg/kg/day

State Regulations and Guidelines

Guidelines

Agency	Description	Value
State environmental agencies	Drinking water quality standards and guidelines for mercury for several states	
	Alabama	
	Alaska	0.0002 mg/l
	Arkansas	(for all listed states)
	California	
	Colorado	
	Connecticut	
	Delaware	
	Florida	
	Georgia	
	Idaho	
	Illinois	
	Iowa	
	Kansas	
	Kentucky	
	Maine	
	Maryland	
	Massachusetts	
	Minnesota	
	Mississippi	
	Missouri	
	Montana	
	Nebraska	
	Nevada	
	New Hampshire	
	New Mexico	
	New York	
	North Carolina	
	Oklahoma	
	Oregon	
	Pennsylvania	
	South Carolina	
	South Dakota	
	Tennessee	
	Texas	
	Virginia	
	Wisconsin	
State environmental agencies	Acceptable ambient air concentration standards and guidelines for mercury for several states	
	Connecticut	0.2 g/m^3 (8 hr avg)
	Kansas	0.024 g/m^3 (annual avg)
	Montana	0.08 g/m^3 (24 hr avg)
	Nevada	0.01 g/m^3 (annual avg)
	New York	1.19 g/m^3 (8 hr avg)
	North Carolina	0.167 g/m^3 (1 yr avg)
	Pennsylvania	3 g/m^3 (15 min avg)
	Virginia	(1 yr avg) 0.8 g/m^3 (24 hr avg)

Adapted with permission from: Toxicological profile for mercury, Agency for Toxic Substances and Disease Registry (ATSDR), U.S. Public Health Service and EPA, 1989.

which is primarily excreted in the urine and feces and to a lesser extent the salivary glands.

The lung is the primary target organ of elemental mercury vapor. Inhalation of high air concentrations can produce acute pneumonitis, erosive bronchitis, and bronchiolitis. Initial symptoms of acute mercury vapor inhalation include stomatitis, colitis, lethargy, confusion, fever and chills, shortness of breath, and a metallic taste in the mouth. The last four of these symptoms are characteristic of metal fume fever. Symptoms may resolve within 2–7 days or may progress into more serious pulmonary involvement. However, toxic pulmonary effects have resulted in the deaths of young children, most under 30 months of age, usually following an incident of mercury vaporization in the home. This difference in age-related outcome results from the direct effect of mercury vapor on the lung. Contact with the distal portion of the lung where absorption is almost complete can lead to exudative alveolar and interstitial edema. An obstruction from bronchial epithelium desquamation may develop and possibly result in severe ventilation/perfusion defects and hypoxemia. The obstruction is proportionately greater in infants than in older children and adults and results in alveolar dilation, interstitial emphysema, pneumatocele formation, pneumothorax, and mediastinal emphysema (4). In one case, a 22-year follow-up after aspiration of elemental mercury showed progressive fibrosis with pleural effusions, pulmonary granulomas, and bronchiectasis, probably resulting from the effects of local irritation. The fibrosis, however, may have minimized systemic absorption of sequestered mercury, since the patient showed no evidence of acute or chronic systemic toxic reaction (5).

In the elemental form, mercury is poorly absorbed from the gastrointestinal tract so that oral ingestion is seldom a clinically significant problem, unless massive doses are ingested (6). Ingestion is rarely an occupational hazard and is usually accidental or suicidal. Reports of ingestion of up to 204 grams of elemental mercury without systemic toxicity have been reported (6).

Mercury embolism in the lung is the greatest cause of fatality in suicide attempts from injection of metallic mercury. Renal damage is also possible with white blood cells appearing in the urine. This condition either can resolve itself spontaneously or may lead to renal failure. Other cases have survived injection without development of embolism or evidence of systematic poisoning (7, 8).

Chronic Elemental Mercury Exposure

The CNS is the primary target organ in chronic exposure to mercury vapor. Chronic exposure produces a classic triad of tremor, gingivitis, and erethism (insomnia, shyness, memory loss, emotional liability, nervousness, and anorexia). Depending on the dose absorbed, symptoms of mercurialism include vague feelings of weakness, fatigue, anorexia, weight loss, and gastrointestinal disturbances. The classic tremor associated with serious elemental mercury toxicity from high dose exposure appears as a fine tremor of the muscles that is interrupted by coarse shakes. Chronic low level exposure can also result in shortterm memory deficits, poor concentration, and decrements in performance of psychomotor skills. The regulatory limit for elemental mercury set by the Occupational Safety and Health Administration (OSHA) is 0.05 mg/m^3 for a time-weighted average (2).

Evidence of visual disturbances includes a brown light reflex

from the anterior capsule of the lens, opacities of the lens, and vascular changes at the corneoscleral junction (9). Peripheral neuropathy is common, but workers exposed to mercury vapor may also have subclinical reductions in sensory and peripheral nerve conduction (10). Parkinsonian states, dysarthria, and a syndrome resembling amyotrophic lateral sclerosis (ALS) have also been noted (9).

There is a correlation between mercury exposure and the urinary excretion of mercury. Occupational exposures of mercury that produce neurologic effects such as tremors are associated with urinary concentrations of mercury of 200 μg/l of urine (10). These symptoms are usually reversible following termination of exposure. Electromyography and nerve conduction studies may demonstrate impairment of peripheral nerves in workers chronically exposed to mercury vapor. Urine mercury concentrations greater than 200 μg/l have been associated with tremors and poor hand-eye coordination (11). Tremors have also been associated with a blood mercury concentration of 1–2 μg/dl (10).

A point of direct occupational exposure to mercury occurs in dental offices. The average dentist uses more than 1 kilogram of mercury each year in the preparation of amalgam fillings. CNS effects are prevalent in those dentists who frequently place amalgams. However, urine mercury levels were noticed to be only slightly elevated (11). Exposure to mercury vapor has been suggested as a factor leading to damage of the median nerve at the wrist. The potential for mercury exposure to the dental patient is evidenced by low levels of mercury release continuing for several years after the amalgam has been placed (12).

Mercury in the elemental form, once absorbed, also crosses the placenta and concentrates in the fetus. Once in the body, the elemental form is short-lived and is oxidized to the mercuric form. The elimination of mercury vapor is in the form of the mercuric ion.

Inorganic Mercury Toxicity

Ingestion, either accidental or intentional, is the primary route of toxicity for inorganic mercurial salts. Seven to fifteen percent of an oral dose is absorbed, while large amounts remain bound to the gastrointestinal mucosa. Insoluble compounds may be oxidized to more soluble compounds resulting in enhanced absorption. Very little traverses the blood-brain barrier. Alveolar and skin absorption represent additional routes of exposure. Once absorbed, inorganic mercury dissociates into mercuric ions, which accumulate in the kidney. The mercury ions are specifically concentrated in the terminal portion of the proximal renal tubule where they have a toxic effect on the cell membrane (13). Distribution throughout the rest of the body is uneven; there is some deposition in the liver and spleen with very low quantities in the brain. Inorganic mercury has a biological half-life of 40–60 days. Excretion is primarily in the feces and urine, with small amounts appearing in the saliva and sweat.

Two main problems arise from acute ingestion of inorganic mercury. The first is the local corrosive effects of the mercurial salts producing immediate necrotic damage on the mucosa of the mouth, throat, esophagus, and stomach (14). The patient may die within hours from shock and peripheral vascular collapse due to fluid and electrolyte losses (14). The second problem is the organ damage at the sites of excretion. The clinical manifestations of intoxication include gastroenteritis with abdominal pain due to precipitation of proteins by mercuric salts, nausea, vomiting, and hematochezia resulting in hypovolemia.

Renal excretion of mercuric ion initially results in a brief diuresis followed by acute tubular necrosis. Oliguria/anuria can develop within 24 hours in 50% of acute overdoses (14–17).

The full spectrum of inorganic mercury poisoning is seldom seen today, although any of its individual signs and symptoms can be encountered in occupationally exposed groups. The chronic effects of inorganic mercury exposure produce signs and symptoms similar to those seen with the chronic effects of elemental mercury. There is evidence of longterm behavioral impairment after low-level chronic exposure to inorganic mercury (18). Workers exposed to inorganic mercury have been shown to have subclinical psychomotor and neuromuscular changes which make it difficult to ascertain the full effects of chronic inorganic mercury intoxication (19, 20).

Mercury elimination from the body is mainly via urine and feces. Exposure to inorganic mercury can be determined by its measurement in blood or urine. Three different forms of mercury are described in the urine of exposed individuals: elemental mercury, mercury-cysteine complex, and a larger mercury complex (10).

Organic Mercury Toxicity

Although inorganic mercury toxicity has been known and described for centuries, organic mercury toxicity has only relatively recently been described. The first organic mercurials were used in chemical research. Diethyl mercury injections were used for the treatment of syphilis beginning in 1887, but soon abandoned because of severe CNS effects. Around 1913 organic mercury compounds were noted to induce a diuresis which led to the development of mercurial diuretics. These were used for more than 30 years before their replacement by less toxic drugs. Their antifungal and antibacterial properties prompted use as seed dressings and ointments. Misuse of treated seed has been the most common cause of poisoning from organic mercury.

Organic mercurials are used chiefly as preservatives and antiseptics. Methyl, ethyl, and phenyl compounds are used as seed dressings to inhibit fungal growth and delay germination. Examples include monomethyl mercury chloride (MMC), ethyl mercuric chloride, methyl mercuric iodide, and chloromethyl mercury. Mercurochrome, the first organic mercurial antiseptic, is still used routinely. Phenylmercuric acetate (PMA), phenylmercuric nitrate (PMN), phenylmercuric borate, thimerosol, and Mercurochrome are all mercurial antiseptics found predominantly in ophthalmic products like eye drops and contact lens solutions. They are also found in vaccines, immunoglobulins, nasal sprays, and lyophilized powders.

Mercury can form stable complexes with organic compounds to yield organic mercury. Additionally, microorganisms in soil and water can methylate inorganic mercury to form organic mercury. A nonenzymatic methylation of Hg(II) ions by methylcobalamine, a byproduct of bacterial synthesis, is the postulated mechanism.

Toxicologically, it is useful to classify organic compound into either short-chain alkyls (methyl and ethyl mercury), aryl (phenylmercuric acetate), or long-chain alkyls. In aryl compounds mercury is joined by a carbon link to an aromatic ring, such as benzene or toluene. The aryl- and long-chain mercury compounds behave like inorganic mercury toxicologically (10). Typical forms of organic mercury are:

methyl mercuric chloride: CH_3HgCl
ethyl mercury compounds: C_2H_5Hg

phenyl mercury acetate (PMA): $C_8H_8HgO_2$

Organic mercury exposure is primarily dietary. Ingestion of cereals treated with organic mercurial fungicides for planting and of fish from mercury-polluted streams and rivers are the sources. PMA is normally used in the powder form as a seed dressing and in paper manufacturing. Another seed dressing, methyl mercuric dicyanamide, is a liquid. Aerosolization can occur with either the dust or liquid forms.

Disinfectant makers, fungicide makers, seed handlers, farmers, lumberjacks, pharmaceutical industry workers, and wood preservers may be exposed to organic mercury compounds. In the paper industry organic compounds control slime. The largest number of cases of human poisoning from organic mercurials has resulted from ingestion of contaminated foods. Epidemics have occurred in Minamata Bay and Niigata, Japan, Iraq, Pakistan, Guatemala, Ghana, New Mexico, and the Soviet Union (21). Minamata Bay in 1956 and the Agano River, Niigata, Japan, in 1964 were polluted by the mercury effluent from factories using inorganic mercuric chloride catalysts in an acetaldehyde and vinyl chloride process. Inorganic mercury was methylated by the microflora of the bay and concentrated up the food chain. Methyl mercury was discovered in samples of the effluent, proving that the factory process itself methylated the inorganic mercury. Fish absorbed methyl mercury by eating contaminated food and directly through their gills. Fish have an excretion half-life of several hundred days, which allows the organic mercury to accumulate to concentrations a thousand times greater than surrounding water. This resulted in mercury levels as high as 50 ppm in fish and 85 ppm in shellfish. Affected individuals probably ingested up to 4 mg/day, which is 40 times the estimated safe daily intake, as fish was a dietary staple.

In northern Iraq in 1956 and central Iraq in 1960 people ate wheat grain treated with the fungicide, Granosan-M (7.7% ethyl mercury p-toluene sulfonanilide) intended for seed use (21). In Pakistan in 1961 and Guatemala between 1963 and 1965 people ate methyl mercury-treated seed (21). The largest epidemic occurred in Iraq in 1971–1972 from ingestion of homemade bread made from wheat seed treated with phenylmercuric acetate, methyl mercury dicyanamide, methyl mercury acetate, and ethyl mercury (21). This resulted in 6500 poisoning cases with 450 deaths. Three New Mexico children in 1969 developed organic mercury toxicity after consumption of meat from a hog feed seed grain treated with Panogen (cyanomethyl mercury guanidine).

Other sources of organic mercury compound exposure include food consumption and pharmaceutical product use. Consumption of game birds or their eggs from areas where methyl mercury fungicides are used can result in exposure. Vaginal contraceptive jellies and suppositories may contain PMA, PMN, or other organic mercurials which are easily absorbed. Thimerosal in ophthalmic products may cause blepharoconjunctivitis and punctate keratitis in contact lens users, but no systemic toxicity has been reported.

The short-chain alkyl mercury compounds are lipid soluble and volatile. Consequently, highly efficient absorption can occur through inhalation, ingestion, or dermal exposure. Furthermore, the most biologically significant short-chain alkyl, methyl mercury, crosses the placenta accumulating in the fetus and is excreted in toxic amounts in breast milk (22).

Latex paints may contain phenylmercuric acetate as a preservative. Beginning August 20, 1990, the Environmental Protection Agency announced no mercury-containing compounds could lawfully be added to interior latex paint. Paint produced before that time may still be sold, however.

Absorption and Distribution of Organic Mercury

Gastrointestinal (GI) absorption of organic mercurials is more complete than the inorganic compounds because of their increased lipid solubility. Over 90% of methyl mercury is absorbed from the GI tract compared with only 15% of inorganic mercury (11). Approximately 80% of inhaled short-chain mercury salt vapors are absorbed. Absorption of aerosols is dependent on particle size. Methyl mercury is distributed throughout the body because of its ability to cross all membranes easily. Blood levels equilibrate with tissue levels, making blood a good clinical indicator of exposure. About 90% of methyl mercury in whole blood is in the red blood cell, where it maintains a blood to plasma ratio of about 300:1. Although uniformly distributed, it concentrates in the liver, kidney, blood, brain, hair, and epidermis. Newly formed hair avidly incorporates methyl mercury in direct proportion to the blood concentration and, it is sometimes used as monitoring medium. The amount of methyl mercury in brain tissue, although less than in liver and kidney, is greater than in inorganic mercury poisoning. Tissue distribution of aryl and long-chain mercurials resembles methyl mercury initially. After 1 week, however, its tissue distribution is similar to inorganic mercurials (10).

Signs and symptoms of methyl mercury toxicity develop only after days to weeks of repeated exposure. Mercury has a strong affinity for the sulfhydryl groups of enzymes. Organic mercury covalently binds sulfur at very low concentrations to form mercaptides: RHg-SR′, where R is a protein. This results in inactivation of sulfhydryl enzymes, disrupting cellular metabolism. Cell membrane damage has also been noted in vitro and in vivo. Likewise, mercury can bind to primary and secondary amine, amide, carboxyl, and phosphoryl groups. Methyl mercury inhibits the sulfhydrylcontaining enzyme choline acetyltransferase which catalyzes the final step in acetylcholine's synthesis (10).

CNS EFFECTS

Target organ toxicity is confined almost exclusively to the central nervous system (10). This is attributed to methyl mercury's rapid access across the blood-brain barrier because of its lipid solubility. However, lipid-soluble complexes have not been detected. Probably, methyl mercury is secreted in bile conjugated to glutathion. It may then be transported across the blood-brain barrier as a complex with cysteine by a specific membrane carrier. This may be due to its resemblance to an endogenous substrate. The resultant neuronal damage is predominantly located within the cerebellar granular layer, the calcarine fissure of the occipital area, and the precentral gyrus.

DERMAL EFFECTS

Dermatitis consisting of erythroderma and pruritis initially of the hands, arms, and face followed by trunk and legs has been described in patients exposed to mercury during all three Iraqi epidemics. It was thought to occur from direct cutaneous contact. Blistering similar to second degree burns can occur from aryl mercury compounds. Cutaneous application of Mercuro-

chrome to burns has been associated with toxicity and death in children.

RENAL EFFECTS

Renal toxicity has not been observed in human methyl mercury poisoning. Interestingly, in the rat the predominant site of action of organic mercury compounds is the kidney with little CNS effect. Mercurial diuretics, methoxyethyl mercury, ethyl mercury, and phenyl mercury compounds have caused renal toxicity. Manifestations include nephrotic syndrome, albuminuria, and renal failure. An autoimmune response to a mercury-protein complex has been hypothesized.

RESPIRATORY EFFECTS

Organic mercurials are mucous membrane irritants. They may cause blistering of the oro- and nasopharynx. Significant absorption can occur via inhalation.

GASTROINTESTINAL EFFECTS

Ethyl mercury poisoning can produced nausea, vomiting, diarrhea, and abdominal cramps. Phenyl mercury may produce stomatitis and gum discoloration. Methyl mercury rarely produces GI effects.

HEMATOLOGIC EFFECTS

Mercurial diuretics have been associated with thrombocytopenia and agranulocytosis, while phenyl mercury has caused neutropenia.

Methyl Mercury

The Minamata Bay and Iraqi epidemics have better defined the clinical presentation of methyl mercury poisoning (10): (a) psychologic—difficult concentrating, short- and longterm memory loss, emotional volatility, depression, decreased intellectual abilities, and ultimately coma; (b) cerebellar—generalized ataxia with stumbling gait, dysdiadochokinesia, and uncoordination; (c) sensory numbness and stocking-glove paresthesias of distal extremities and mouth, deafness, tunnel vision, visual field constriction, scanning speech with slurring, dysphagia; (d) motor—spasticity, tremors of hands, face, or legs, and weakness proceeding to paralysis. The initial symptoms are fatigue and perioral/extremity paresthesias, followed by difficulty with hand movements. Sensation and visual disturbances occur next. Electrocardiographic abnormalities (S-T segment changes) were noted in about one third of cases from the last Iraqi poisoning. Important aspects of methyl mercury toxicity include its predisposition for the CNS, its insidious onset, and its poor prognosis for improvement.

Ethyl Mercury

Ingestion of ethyl mercury-treated seed resulted in the 1956 and 1960 Iraqi poisonings (21). Characterization of the clinical syndrome of the affected patients revealed distinct differences from methyl mercury toxicity. Involvement of the kidneys, GI tract, and skin were more representative of inorganic mercury toxicity. Patients suffered from polydipsia, polyuria, proteinuria, abdominal pain with nausea and vomiting, and pruritis, especially involving palms, soles, and genitals, often progressing to an exfoliative dermatitis. Although patients had slurred speech and ataxia, mentation was not affected. Deep musculoskeletal pains and frequent ECG changes (ST depression, T-wave inversion, prolonged Q-T and P-R intervals, and ectopy) were also reported.

Phenyl Mercury

This is an aryl mercury compound which is metabolized in vivo to inorganic mercury. It is much less toxic than methyl mercury because it is less volatile, crosses the placenta and blood-brain barrier more slowly, and is more rapidly excreted. Its toxicity resembles that of the inorganic mercurials.

Chronic and Longterm Effects of Organic Mercury

Signs and symptoms of both acute and chronic exposure are similar. The predominant symptoms are constriction of visual fields, sensory disturbances, muscular atrophy, and mental disturbances. Typically, symptoms worsen over 3–10 years, during which time cases may be misdiagnosed as other diseases. Since these cases were atypical of the Hunter-Russell syndrome, Harada named them chronic Minamata disease (23). Seven subtypes were described depending on the predominant symptoms. The delayed appearance of symptoms may be related to aging or the consumption of low levels of methyl mercury over a prolonged time.

Metabolism and Elimination of Organic Mercury Compounds

Organic mercury compounds can be subdivided into two classes based on mechanism of metabolism: short-chain alkyl mercury compounds, and aryl mercury and long-chain mercury compounds. Cleavage of the carbon-mercury bond occurs at differing rates after absorption. The aryl and long-chain mercury bonds are readily broken in vivo to yield inorganic mercury. Thus, aryl and long-chain mercury toxicity is similar to inorganic mercury. Short-chain mercurials have a strong, stable carbon-mercury bond which is cleaved slowly and the inorganic mercury does not play a role in the toxicity of alkyl mercury. All tissues biotransform organic mercury to an inorganic form except for muscle and blood. Inorganic mercury is oxidized to the divalent cation in the lungs, red blood cell, and liver. This in turn can be reduced to the elemental form to be exhaled as metallic mercury vapor.

The primary route of excretion of organic mercurials is fecal, with less than 10% appearing in the urine. Methyl mercury is secreted in the bile. A portion undergoes enterohepatic circulation while the remainder is converted to the inorganic form by intestinal flora. This internal recycling may account for the long biologic half-life of 70 days in human volunteers. This represents an excretion rate of 1%/day of the total body burden. Phenyl mercury is eliminated primarily fecally for the first few days, with some excretion of the parent compound in the urine. Later this shifts to predominantly urinary excretion of inorganic mercury. Organomercurials follow first order kinetics. There may be sex differences in elimination, with males being slower eliminators than females.

TERATOGENICITY

All forms of mercury cross the placenta into the fetal circulation. Elemental mercury passes more readily than inorganic mercury compounds, but organic alkyl mercury compounds pass with the greatest ease due to their relatively higher lipid solubility. Maternal exposure usually occurs from the consumption of foodstuffs treated with methyl mercury. However, inhalation and skin absorption are also possible routes of exposure to other forms of mercury. The fetotoxic effects of mercury were first noted when women who were undergoing treatment for syphilis with mercury were observed to frequently abort. Congenital damage has been reported in infants whose mothers were unaware of their exposure to methyl mercury during pregnancy because they suffered no ill effects. In contrast, some mothers have shown signs and symptoms of mercury intoxication while their infants did not, although abnormal neurologic signs in affected infants became more obvious with time.

The alkyl mercury concentrations in fetal red blood cells is 30% higher than in maternal red blood cells, and fetal tissue levels are twice the maternal tissue levels (10). Blood mercury levels of infants will be maintained by transmission of methyl mercury via maternal milk, which has 5% of the mercury concentration of maternal blood.

Methyl mercury is a teratogen in rats, mice, cats, hamsters, and humans. Organic mercury rapidly crosses the placental barrier, accumulating in the fetus (23). Twenty-five infants born during the Minamata epidemic had a cerebral palsy-like syndrome with severe mental retardation, cerebellar symptoms (ataxia, intention tremor, nystagmus, dysmetria), hypersalivation, hyperkinesia (chorea, athetasis), limb deformities, strabismus, and seizure disorders. Their mothers, although heavy fish eaters, had mild if any symptoms. Fetal hemoglobin, while increasing the fetus' susceptibility, may protect the mother by its stronger affinity for methyl mercury than the mother's hemoglobin. Moreover, congenital Minamata disease, as it is sometimes known, occurs at lower exposure levels of methyl mercury than those associated with adult toxicity. Autopsy data demonstrated cortical and cerebellar atrophy and hypoplasia, corpus callosum hypoplasia, and demyelination of the pyramidal tract (21, 23). This diffuse brain involvement differs from those changes seen in the adult. Microtubule-dependent neuronal migration and cell division may be inhibited. Methyl mercury appears to avidly bind the alpha- and beta-tubulin proteins, inhibiting the polymerization of microtubules. The observed arrest in late mitosis is consistent with microtubule inhibition. This inhibition is specific to small amounts of organic mercury (23).

MANAGEMENT OF MERCURY TOXICITY

Although occupational and exposure history is necessary, a complete physical examination including a thorough neurologic exam should also be performed. Patients should be evaluated for the presence of a tremor, pathologic reflexes, hyperreflexia, abnormal cerebellar function (especially ataxic gait, Rhomberg's sign, finger-to-nose), constriction of visual fields, nystagmus, dysarthric speech, short- and longterm memory, and impaired hearing. Nerve conduction studies as well as electromyography may reveal early neuropathy.

Hemoperfusion, hemodialysis, peritoneal dialysis, and forced diuresis do not remove significant amounts of either elemental, inorganic, or organic mercury. If renal failure develops, chelators can still be used.

Dimercaptopropanol (BAL, British anti-Lewisite), a parenterally administered dithiol, is traditionally used in severe elemental and inorganic mercury poisoning. It forms a complex (chelate) with the elemental mercury/inorganic mercury, which is renally eliminated. It is contraindicated in organic mercury poisoning because of experimental evidence in mice showing an increase in brain mercury levels. BAL is dosed in children and adults at 3–5 mg/kg im every 4 hours for the first 24 hours, then every 12 hours for the second 24 hours, then once a day for 3 days. A 2-day rest period followed by a treatment course of 5 days is repeated until 24-hour urinary excretion levels are less than 50 μg/l. The BAL-mercury chelate is dialyzable.

For less severe elemental and inorganic toxicity in adults, a 5-day course of d-penicillamine 250 mg orally every 6 hours (children use 100 mg/kg/day divided every 6 hours) has been traditionally used. N-Acetyl-D,L-penicillamine (NAP) has been used with mixed success in a small number of patients with acute and chronic inorganic and organic mercury toxicity. Unlike D-penicillamine, NAP has less effect on copper balance.

Newer water-soluble oral derivatives of BAL have been used to treat all forms of acute and chronic mercury toxicity. These include 2,3-dimercaptopropane-1-sulfonate (DMPS) and 2,3-dimercaptosuccinic acid (DMSA). In chronic methyl mercury animal studies, both drugs were more effective than BAL and NAP in increasing urinary excretion of mercury. DMSA (Chemet), a newly approved chelator for lead poisoning, has been successful in treating mercury poisoning. Animal and human studies support the increased efficacy, ease of administration, and lower side effect profile of DMSA and DMPS compared with BAL and penicillamine. DMSA is administered in doses of 10 mg/kg three times daily for 5 days, then twice daily for another 14 days. Monitoring of the clinical status and blood and urine mercury excretion is used to guide repeat dosing. Two weeks should be allowed between chelation therapies.

LABORATORY DIAGNOSIS

Laboratory evaluation of mercury poisoning should include a complete blood count, serum electrolytes, liver and renal function tests, and urinalysis. For acute oral ingestion of Hg salts, patients should be typed and crossed if hemorrhaging. A chest radiograph and electrocardiogram may be needed if a large exposure occurred from elemental mercury vapor. Urine and blood mercury levels are used to detect exposure. Attempts to correlate clinical symptoms and health effects with urine or blood levels show conflicting results. Some clinicians believe the best test for inorganic and elemental mercury is whole blood levels, while others use a 24-hour urinary mercury determination (10). Whole blood is the best medium for organic mercury, since it is concentrated in the red blood cells. Likewise, urine should provide a good measure of inorganic or elemental mercury since they tend to be renally excreted. Blood levels for mercury are normally less than 2 μg/dl and should not exceed 5 μg/dl. Paresthesias may develop above 20 μg/dl. Urinary mercury is normally less than 10 μg/l. A hazardous level for urine mercury in exposed workers is between 50–100 μg/l. For workers chronically exposed to mercury compounds, urinary excretion

over 50 μg/l is associated with an increased frequency of muscle tremors (10).

Special Diagnostic Tests

N-Acetyl glucosaminidase (NAG) and β-galactosidase are lysosomal enzymes in renal tubular cells which are being studied as sensitive indicators of renal dysfunction from inorganic mercury exposure. Urinary NAG levels correlated with the number of neuropsychologic symptoms among occupational workers exposed to inorganic mercury. Whether NAG is clinically useful as an indicator of kidney damage has not been determined.

Hair levels of mercury were used extensively in the investigation of the Minimata epidemic. Normally, hair mercury levels average 2–15 ppm, but those afflicted with the disease had levels between 100 and 700 ppm. Presently, due to concern about external contamination, hair analysis is not routinely used. Electromyography and nerve conduction velocities are useful in determining neurologic effects on peripheral nerves.

BIOLOGIC MONITORING

Occupational exposed individuals should undergo periodic physical examinations and 24-hour urinary mercury determinations every 6 months to a year. If air monitoring reveals mercury within the upper half of the TLV, employees should have a physical examination and a repeat urine mercury level. If the TLV is exceeded, the worker should have an immediate examination and urinary mercury determination. Hair analysis cannot be recommended at this time because of the concern with external contamination.

Blood level monitoring is the best measure of recent exposure to inorganic and elemental mercury. It is not a measure of the total body burden, however. Organic mercurials which are more lipid soluble than inorganic forms tend to concentrate in red blood cells. A plasma to RBC ratio of 1:1 is thought to be indicative of inorganic mercury; a plasma RBC ratio of 1:10 suggests organic mercury toxicity. Blood levels of less than 2 μg/dl may occur in occupationally exposed individuals (10). A history and physical examination help make a diagnosis of organic mercury intoxication. Symptoms may be seen with methyl mercury in the 3–5 μg/dl blood concentration range and with other mercurials at 20 μg/dl blood concentration.

Urine mercury concentrations may be significantly altered by disinfectants and other products. The upper limit of normal urinary excretion is 25 μg/l. Assessing the total body burden of mercury can be accomplished by a chelation challenge using d-penicillamine. A fourfold increase in a 24-hour mercury concentration over baseline indicates a significant body burden. There are abundant sulfhydryl groups in hair; thus mercury levels may be 250–300 times the RBC concentration.

ENVIRONMENTAL MONITORING

Prevention is the best management of toxicity in the occupational setting. Appropriate ventilation of work areas with dust, vapor, or aerosol exposure should prevent toxic accumulation. Personal and area air sampling of the environment should be routinely performed. Industrial hygiene surveys can be conducted to monitor levels of mercury. In enclosed areas and occupational settings, mercury vapor concentrations can be detected with electronic devices such as a mercury vapor analyzer. Ambient air concentrations can be detected at as low as 0.001 mg/m³. The National Institute for Occupational Safety and Health (NIOSH) recommends an air sampling method using a solid sorbent media, low flow rate, and flameless atomic absorption for detection of elemental mercury concentrations. The complete procedure for this analysis is outlined in Method 6000 of the *NIOSH Manual of Analaytic Methods*.

The mercury decontamination procedure for buildings includes removal of carpets, and several cleanings of floors, walls, and solid surfaces with a product containing a metallic mercury sulfide-converting powder, a chelating compound, and a dispersing agent. A polyurethane coating is then applied to all floor surfaces.

The recommended threshold limit value (TLV-TWA) for mercury vapor and for inorganic and nonalkyl organic mercurials is 0.05 mg Hg/m³ in the United States and the European Community. The ceiling value (TLV-C) for mercury vapor is 0.1 mg Hg/m³ in the United States and for methyl and ethyl mercury, the TLV-TWA is 0.01 mg Hg/m³. In the USSR, the TLV-C values are 0.01 mg/m³ for mercury vapor and 0.005 mg/m³ for alkyl mercury (2). It has been noted that an air concentration of mercury of 0.05 mg/m³ corresponds to a urinary concentration of approximately 50 µg/l and blood concentrations of around 30–35 µg/l (3).

The Environmental Protection Agency's suggested ambient air level for population exposure is <1 µg Hg/m³. Atmospheric discharges from industrial facilities are not to exceed 2.3 kg/day from chloralkali plants or smelters and 3.2 kg/day from sludge incineration and drying. Mercury discharge into waterways from chloralkali plants is regulated to the limit of 140 milligrams for every 1000 kilogram of product. The maximum allowable mercury concentration in fish is 1.0 mg/kg in the United States, Finland, and Sweden (2).

The maximum (ceiling limit) for methyl mercury which can not be exceeded at any time during the work period is 0.04 mg/m³. A separate area for eating and smoking should be provided. Respirators and protective clothing should be used during cleaning and maintenance operations and spills. Preemployment and periodic physical examinations should be conducted with emphasis on vision (especially visual fields), CNS, renal function, and skin.

The American Conference of Government Industrial Hygienists (ACGIH) makes yearly recommendations of airborne concentrations of substances to which workers can be repeatedly exposed day after day without adverse effects. These threshold limit values (TLV) can refer to a time-weighted average (TWA), a shortterm exposure limit (STEL), or a ceiling (C). The TLV-TWA is an average concentration for a normal 8-hour day and a 40-hour week which workers can be exposed to without adverse effect. The TWA-STEL is the maximum concentration that can occur during a 15-minute time period in an 8-hour day. This should occur no more than four times daily with an hour between exposures. A TWA-C is the maximum allowable airborne concentration at any time during the 8-hour work period which can not be exceeded. OSHA is entrusted with setting and enforcing workplace standards. OSHA receives guidance from NIOSH and ACGIH in formulating these levels. Permissible expo-

sure limits (PEL) are the legally mandatory guidelines established by OSHA. Usually, the TWA and PEL are the same. There may be differences, however, as TWA's are updated yearly, while PEL's are infrequently updated.

1991 Standards for Organic and Alkyl compounds are as follows:

NIOSH   0.01 mg/m³
ACGIH (TWA)   0.01 mg/m³
ACGIH (ceiling)   0.04 mg/m³
STEL   0.03 mg/m³
IDLH (immediately dangerous to life and health)   10 mg/m³.

1991 Standards for aryl and inorganic compounds are as follows:

ACGIH (10-hour TWA) 0.1 mg/m³.

REFERENCES

1. U.S.P.H.S. Potential for human exposure. Chapt 5 in: Toxicologic profile for mercury. Atlanta, GA: Agency for Toxic Substances and Disease Registry, U.S. Public Health Service, 1989:105.
2. U.S.P.H.S. Regulations and advsories. Chapt 7 in: Toxicologic profile for mercury. Atlanta, GA: Agency for Toxic Substances and Disease Registry, U.S. Public Health Service, 1989:123.
3. Berlin M. Mercury, Chapt 16 in: Friberg L, Nordberg G, Vouk V, eds. Handbook on the toxicology of metals, vol II. New York: Elsevier, 1986.
4. Jaffe KM, Shortleff DB, Robertson WO. Survival after acute mercury vapor poisoning: role of supportive care. Am J Dis Child 1983;137:749–751.
5. Dzau VJ, Szabos S, Chang YC. Aspiration of metallic mercury: a 22-year follow-up. JAMA 1977;238:1531–1532.
6. Wright N, Yoeman WB, Carter GE. Massive oral ingestion of elemental mercury without poisoning. Lancet 1980;1:206.
7. Hunter R, Rachman R. Soft tissue injection from a broken thermometer: a case report and review of the literature. Am J Clin Pathol 1974;61:296–300.
8. Bartolome C, Khan MA. Mercury embolization of the lung. N Engl J Med 1976;295:883–885.
9. Adams CR, Ziegler DK, Lin JT. Mercury intoxication simulating amyotrophic lateral sclerosis. JAMA 1983;250:642–643.
10. U.S.P.H.S. Health effects. Chapt 2 in: Toxicologic profile for mercury. Agency for Toxic Substances and Disease Registry, U.S. Public Health Service. Atlanta, GA: CDC, 1989:13–95.
11. Shapiro IM, et al. Neurophysiologic and neuropsychologic functions of mercury exposed dentists. Lancet May 22, 1982:1147–1150.
12. Wolf M, Osborne JW, Hanson AL. Mercury toxicity and dental amalgam. Neurotoxicology 1983;4:201–304.
13. Laundy T, et al. Deaths after peritoneal lavage with mercuric chloride solutions: case report and review of the literature. Br Med J 1984;289:96–98.
14. Winek CL, et al. Fatal mercuric chloride ingestion. Clin Toxicol 1981;18:261–266.
15. Leumann EP, Brandenberger H. Hemodialysis in patients with acute mercuric intoxication: concentrations of mercury in blood, dialysate, urine, vomitus and feces. Clin Toxicol 1977;11:301–308.
16. Tubbs R. Membranous glomerulonephritis associated with mercuric chloride solutions: case report and review of the literature. Br Med J 1982;77:409–413.
17. Datyner ME, Cox PA. Inorganic mercury poisoning. Anaesth Intensive Care 1981;6:266–269.
18. Williamson AM, et al. Occupational mercury exposure and its consequences for behavior. Int Arch Occup Environ Health 1982;50:273–286.
19. Miller JM, et al. Subclinical psychomotor and neuromuscular changes in workers exposed to inorganic mercury. Am Ind Hyg Assoc J 1975;(Oct):725–733.
20. Roseman KD, et al. Sensitive indicators of inorganic mercury toxicity. Arch Environ Health 1986;208–215.
21. Gerstner HB, Huff JE. Selected case histories and epidemology examples of human poisonings. Clin Toxicol 1977;131–150.
22. Amin-Zaki L, et al. Intrauterine methylmercury poisoning in Iraq. Pediatrics 1974;54:587–595.
23. Harda H. Congenital Minamata disease: intrauterine methlmercury poisoning. Teratology 1978;18:285–288.

CHEMICAL AND PHYSICAL PROPERTIES

Lead (atomic no. 82, atomic weight 207.21) is a gray, soft, heavy metal widely distributed in the earth's crust. It exists in nature as a mixture of three isotopes ^{206}Pb, ^{207}Pb, and ^{208}Pb. It forms compounds with a valence state of $+2$ and $+4$. Lead melts at a temperature of 327°C and boils at 1620°C. Because of its low melting point, it was one of the first metals smelted and used by ancient humans.

Lead is exploited commercially from a variety of ores, the most abundant of which is galena (PbS). When used as a metal, it is most commonly alloyed with tin, antimony, or arsenic. It forms a variety of inorganic compounds, many of which are brightly colored. Tetraethyllead and tetramethyllead are the only two organic compounds in common use (Table 76.1).

SITES, INDUSTRIES, AND BUSINESSES ASSOCIATED WITH EXPOSURE

World production of lead is approximately 9 million metric tons annually. In the United States, about 11 million metric tons of lead are consumed, about 5 million metric tons produced from mining and about 6 million metric tons recovered from scrap (principally from recycled batteries) (1). Sites, processes, and industries associated with lead exposures are presented in Table 76.2.

Lead is extracted from the ore first by a mechanical separation process involving flotation. The enriched ore is then smelted. After primary smelting, the lead bullion still contains significant amounts of other metals and undergoes a further step of refining.

Secondary lead smelters reclaim scrap lead. Storage batteries and lead-sheltered cable are the most commonly recycled products. Since the average lead storage battery has a useful life of only about 2 years, and 80% of the lead in batteries is recycled, this process of secondary smelting provides one third of the lead for new products each year. About half of all lead produced goes into lead storage batteries. Lead from the metal grids, and lead oxide (PbO) is used as a paste within the battery. Sheet lead is used to line chemical reaction vessels, for waterproofing and soundproofing, and for radiation shielding. Lead alloys are used as solders and to sheathe power and telephone cables from moisture.

Compounds of lead are used extensively for paints and coatings. The use of lead additives in residential pain was banned in the United States in 1977 because of the danger of childhood lead poisoning. Lead-containing pigments are still used for outdoor uses because of their bright colors and weather-resistant properties. "Red lead" (Pb_3O_4) is used extensively as a rust-proofer and primer for structural steel. Lead azide and lead stephenate are used in primers and explosives (2). Tetraethyllead and, to some extent, tetramethyllead are used as "anti-knock" additives to gasoline. Use has greatly declined in the United States, but leaded gasoline is still being used in other countries.

Dangerous exposures to lead occur when fumes or finely divided particles of lead are present in air or when contamination of food, drink, or hands leads to ingestion. This may occur at home, in the community, or at work.

Reduction in the use of leaded gasoline has reduced the largest source of general community exposure. Contamination of community and domestic water systems by the use of lead pipe or lead solder in pipe remains a problem in some areas. With the reduction of lead in air and the elimination of lead solder from food and beverage cans, food lead has greatly decreased during the 1980s in the United States. Contamination of household dust by indoor and outdoor use of lead-containing paint remains a major source of exposure for infants and toddlers (3).

The great diversity of lead-containing processes and products results in many ways workers can be exposed (Table 76.3). Regulation has reduced lead poisoning in major lead-using industries such as pigment manufacture and battery production but has had little impact in other areas such as demolition, scrap recovery, radiator repair, and home remodeling, which are characterized by smaller, unorganized workforces. Processes in which energy in the form of burning, blasting, grinding, or sanding is applied to lead-painted or -coated surfaces are the most common causes of uncontrolled exposures.

CLINICAL TOXICOLOGY

Absorption, Metabolism, and Excretion

As a fume or fine particulate, lead is readily absorbed through the lungs. It is relatively less well-absorbed from the gastrointestinal tract in adults (20–30%), but children absorb as much as 50% of dietary lead. Inorganic lead is not absorbed through intact skin, but organic lead compounds (tetraethyllead, tetramethyllead) can be. Absorption from the lungs is dependent on the size of the particulate. Particles in the 0.5–5.0-micron range are most likely to be deposited in the alveoli where they can be absorbed. Larger particles, which are entrapped in the larger airways, are likely to be swallowed and may lead to gastrointestinal absorption.

Absorption of ingested lead is influenced by its form, particle size, and iron and calcium absorption (4). After absorption into the bloodstream, almost all lead is carried bound to the red cell. Lead is distributed extensively throughout tissues, with highest concentrations in bone, teeth, liver, lung, kidney, brain, and spleen (2). With prolonged exposure over time, most absorbed lead ends up in bone. Lead appears to be substituted for calcium in the bone matrix and is not known to cause any deleterious effect on bone itself. Bone storage may act as a "sink," protecting other organs, but it is also a longterm storage depot which allows the chronic accumulation of lead in

Table 76.1. Lead Compounds

Lead Compound		Molecular Weight
Lead, metal	Pb	207.19
Lead acetate	Pb $(C_2H_3O_2)_2$	325.28
Lead arsenate	$Pb_3(AsO_4)_2$	899.4
Lead azide	$Pb(N_3)_2$	291.23
Lead carbonate (basic white lead)	$2PbCO_3Pb(OH)_2$	775.6
Lead chloride	$PbCl_2$	278.1
Lead chromate (chrome yellow)	$PbCrO_4$	323.18
Lead molybdate	$PbMoO_4$	367.13
Lead nitrate	$Pb(NO_3)_2$	331.2
Lead monoxide	PbO	223.19
Lead oxide (red)	Pb_3O_4	685.57
Lead sesquioxide	Pb_2O_3	462.38
Lead suboxide	Pb_2O	430.38
Lead peroxide	PbO_2	239.19
Lead oxychloride	$PbCl_2Pb(OH)_2^a$	519.29
Lead silicate	$PbSiO_3$	283.27
Lead sulfate	$PbSO_4PbO$	526.44
Lead sulfide	PbS	239.25
Lead stearate	$Pb(C_{18}H_{35}O_2)_2$	774.15
Tetraethyllead	$Pb(C_2H_5)_4$	323.44
Tetramethyllead	$Pb(CH_3)_4$	267.33

Table 76.2. Sites and Industries with Lead Exposure

Lead smelters
Battery manufacturing
Welding and cutting operations
Construction and demolition
Rubber industry
Plastics industry
Printing industry
Firing ranges
Radiator repair
Soldering of lead products
Production of gasoline additives
Zinc smelting
Solid waste combustion
Organic lead production
Copper smelting
Ore crushing and grinding
Frit manufacture
Paint and pigment manufacture

Table 76.3. Reported Cases of Adult Lead Poisoning by Industry
New York, New Jersey, California, Texas 1987

Industry (SIC code)	No. of Cases		No. of Cases With Blood Pb >70 μg/dl	
	No.	%	No.	%
Electric and electronic equipment (36)	462	35	15	21
Primary metal industries (33)	433	33	15	21
Chemical products (28)	87	7	0	0
Stone clay and glass (32)	83	6	2	2
Auto repairs (75)	47	4	4	5
Special trade contractors (17)	39	3	11	15
Heavy construction (16)	23	2	13	18
All others	153	10	11	18
Total	1327		71	

Data were available from only these four states which required reporting of elevated lead levels by laboratories in 1987.
Adapted from MMWR 1989;38:644.

μg/day by the kidney (6). With increasing body stores, this may rise considerably but is rarely more than 20 μg/day (7, 8). Excretion may be due both to glomerular filtration and in part to shedding of tubular epithelial cells where the lead tends to concentrate (9).

The extent of fecal excretion in humans is uncertain. Early lead balance studies by Kehoe (6) indicated that fecal lead nearly matched daily oral intake of lead. The extent to which this fecal lead content represents merely unabsorbed lead rather than excretion is not clear. In rats, bile has been shown to be a major route of excretion after intravenous administration of lead. The importance of this route in humans is unclear (10).

The kinetics of the uptake, distribution, and equilibration of lead in blood, bone, and soft tissue are complex (11). Models invoking three compartments, which correspond more or less anatomically to blood, soft tissue, and bone storage, are useful but not always satisfactory in predicting changes in tissue levels under all conditions. With initial exposure to a high dose, blood lead may rise and fall relatively quickly, but some of the decline in blood lead may be due to redistribution rather than excretion. Once a significant burden has been stored in bone, absorbed lead has a remarkably long half-life, as long as 10 years in some studies (12). In such a situation, blood lead (and presumably tissue levels as well) may remain elevated for decades after an exposure has ceased. While chelating agents increase urinary excretion, they may also alter the exchange between body compartments, for example across the blood-brain barrier (13). The clinical signs and symptoms of lead toxicity are summarized in Tables 76.4 and 76.5.

Acute Toxicity

Under conditions of extremely high respiratory exposure (for example, using oxyacetylene to cut lead-coated steel without respiratory protection) or with intravenous use of contaminated solutions (14), lead poisoning can manifest itself acutely. With large enough doses, an acute encephalopathy can develop, accompanied by renal failure and severe gastrointestinal symp-

the body and which can provide a source for remobilization of lead and continued toxicity after exposure has ceased.

Lead crosses the blood-brain barrier and concentrates in the gray matter of the brain. Lead also readily crosses the placenta. Because pregnancy is a period during which maternal calcium stores are mobilized, a significant amount of lead may be transferred to the developing fetus (5).

Lead is excreted by the adult at a rate of approximately 30

Table 76.4. General Signs and Symptoms of Lead Toxicity

Mild and moderate
Fatigue
Irritability
Lethargy
Paresthesias
Myalgias
Abdominal pain
Tremor
Headache
Vomiting
Weight loss
Constipation
Loss of libido

Severe
Motor neuropathy
Encephalopathy
Seizures
Coma
Severe abdominal cramping
Epiphyseal lead lines in children
Renal failure

Table 76.5. Symptoms of Lead Poisoning in Adults Spontaneous and Elicited Symptoms

Symptom	No. of Patients with This Complaint					
	Spontaneously Described		Elicited by Examiner		Total	
	No.	%	No.	%	No.	%
Headache	25	53	2	4	27	57
Irritability	15	32	13	28	28	60
Memory loss	4	9	14	29	18	60
Decreased memory span	2	4	9	19	11	23
Lassitude	22	47	2	4	24	51
Insomnia	8	17	5	11	13	28
Decreased libido	6	13	12	25	18	38
Anorexia	7	15	5	11	12	26
Nausea	8	17	3	6	11	23
Abdomen pain	9	19	3	7	12	26
Constipation	2	4	7	15	9	19
Arthralgias	14	30	8	17	22	47
Myalgias	10	21	4	9	14	30
Paresthesias	9	19	4	9	13	28
Motor weakness	5	11	2	4	7	15
Total patients					47	100

Symptoms from a series of 47 men presenting with elevated lead levels to the University of Maryland Occupational Health Project.

toms within a short time. In most cases, however, lead is absorbed more slowly over weeks to months, and the clinical course is subacute or chronic.

CHRONIC AND LONGTERM EFFECTS

Biochemical Basis of Toxicity

Absorbed lead is toxic to a variety of enzyme systems. Lead tends to have a particular affinity for sulfhydryl groups and may be particularly toxic to enzyme systems that are zinc-dependent. The heme synthesis pathway has had the most sys-

tematic study. Two enzymes are affected by lead: inhibition of δ-aminolevulinic acid dehydratase (ALA-D), a cytoplasmic enzyme, and ferrochelatase, a mitochondrial enzyme (15). Interference with ALA-D is dose-related and occurs at blood lead concentrations between 10 and 20 μg/dl. Interference with ALA-D is complete at blood lead concentrations of 70 and 90 μg/dl (15). Ferrochelatase catalyzes the transfer of iron from ferritin into protoporphyrin to form heme (15). Ferrochelatase inhibition by lead results in an increase in coproporphyrin excretion in urine and an increase in protoporphyrin in red blood cells (15). Erythrocyte protoporphyrin concentrations in adults will be elevated at blood lead concentrations of 25–30 μg/dl (15). Heme synthesis is essential not only to hemoglobin but to synthesis of cytochromes needed for all oxidative metabolism throughout the organism.

Lead has been shown to interfere with enzymes which are important in maintaining the integrity of membranes and to affect steroid metabolism (16). Concentrations of neurotransmitters have been shown to be affected in a number of studies (17). Vitamin D synthesis in renal tubular cells is affected by lead due to an interference with a heme-containing hydroxylase enzyme that converts 25-hydroxyvitamin D to 1,25-hydroxyvitamin D (18). The health effects of lead can range from subclinical to overt disease (Fig. 76.1, Tables 76.6 and 76.7).

Central Nervous System

Central nervous system (CNS) effects can develop after a brief intense exposure or more gradually with lower levels of exposure. Acute encephalopathy, characterized by diffuse pathologic changes and cerebral edema, is usually associated with high blood lead levels (over 150 μg/dl). A subacute or chronic encephalopathy affecting both cognitive function and mood is seen more commonly. Headaches and lassitude are common early symptoms of lead intoxication. Sleep disturbance, often with early morning awakening, irritability, and loss of libido are also frequently elicited by thorough history taking. Because of the nonspecific nature of these early CNS symptoms, patients frequently do not seek medical attention and when they do are often not correctly diagnosed. Cessation of exposure and chelation therapy often have a favorable effect on these symptoms, but in severe cases some level of symptoms may persist chronically.

CNS effects are not confined to those patients who become symptomatic. Studies of lead-exposed workers have shown abnormalities on psychometric testing, including cognitive difficulty and visuomotor problems (19–23). Baker and his colleagues (24, 25) demonstrated that workers exposed in a brass foundry whose blood lead levels were in the range of 40–60 μg/dl had impaired neurobehavioral function. The prevalence of abnormalities was correlated to an index of lead exposure integrated over time. When there was a striking reduction in lead exposure and blood lead levels in the workforce, there was a corresponding improvement in function among the exposed group but not the controls (24, 25). Mantere et al. (23) in Sweden showed that psychometric and nerve condition abnormalities developed in workers newly exposed to lead as blood lead levels rose above 30 μg/dl.

Very disturbing information about lead effects on CNS function in the young child has emerged from recent epidemiologic studies. Needleman and colleagues (26) evaluated a range of psychologic tests in a cohort of children from whom they excluded those with known lead poisoning. They collected de-

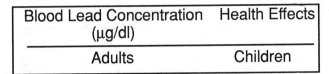

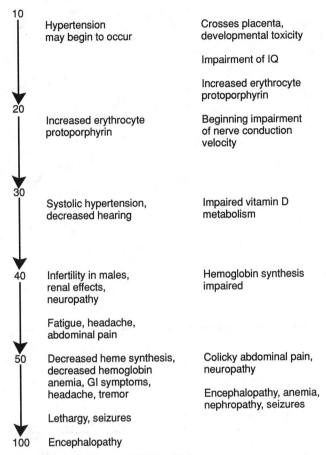

Figure 76.1.

ciduous teeth and analyzed their lead content, reasoning that this gave a fair estimate of cumulative lead exposure over the preschool years. Subsequent evaluation of the children's school performance, including assessment by teachers who were unaware of the children's lead status, was performed. Children with higher levels of lead absorption showed a marked deficit in school performance compared to children with lower levels of exposure (26). An 11-year follow-up study showed deficits in CNS functioning and a pattern of social failure that persisted into young adulthood in the children with higher lead exposures (27). More recently, the same group assessed the effect of in utero exposure to lead on cognitive development. Cord blood lead levels taken at birth were correlated with the results of developmental tests done at age 2 in 249 children. Blood lead levels had an inverse relationship with developmental scores, and this effect was seen at cord blood lead levels as low as the 10–20 µg/dl range (28). These studies have very disturbing implications, suggesting that lead absorption by children today not only may have irreversible effects on their development, but also may result in bone stores that will threaten the healthy growth of their children in turn.

Early after the introduction of tetraethyllead as a gasoline additive, numerous cases of severe encephalopathy developed among workers at tetraethyllead production facilities. The rapidity and severity of these intoxications were probably related both to dose absorbed, since organic lead can be readily absorbed through the skin, and can readily pass across the blood-brain barrier (29).

Peripheral Nerves

In the peripheral nervous system, lead causes a neuropathy which primarily affects the motor nerves and which appears to be principally axonal (17). Clinically, the neuropathy is more severe in the upper rather than lower extremity and may cause more severe effects on the dominant side. While the classic wrist drop of "painter's palsy" has become rare, subclinical neuropathy has been demonstrated in a number of populations of exposed workers, with effects beginning at levels of blood lead well within what had been regarded in the past as acceptable for industrial workers (23). Lead targets motor axons and produces axonal degeneration and segmental demyelination (15). Studies have demonstrated slowed conduction in small motor fibers of the ulnar nerve to be a sensitive marker of subclinical lead neurotoxicity (18, 30, 37). Decreases in ulnar nerve motor conduction velocity are seen at blood lead concentrations of 30–40 µg/dl. In addition to this form of polyneuropathy, lead absorption predisposes individuals to nerve entrapment, such as carpal tunnel and tarsal tunnel syndromes (22).

Hematologic

Anemia in lead poisoning results both from impairment of hemoglobin production previously discussed and from changes in red cell membranes. Hemoglobin levels may remain in a normal range despite moderately severe intoxication, since enzyme induction may compensate for the effects of lead. The effect of the intoxication may only become apparent when stress is placed on the erythrocyte, for example after blood donation (38). It is common to see a noticeable rise in hemoglobin concentration when lead intoxication resolves. With more severe intoxication, a normochromic, normocytic anemia develops, characterized by the presence of basophilic stippling of erythrocytes on smear. When anemia is severe, it is often because of the superimposition of a hemolytic process caused, presumably, by membrane changes (16).

Gastrointestinal

While gastrointestinal symptoms are quite prominent in the clinical presentation of lead toxicity, little is known about the mechanism by which pain and colic are produced. It is presumed to be related to effects on the autonomic ganglia of the gut. Transaminase elevations are occasionally reported in lead intoxication, but despite the relatively high concentration of lead in liver there seems to be little evidence of impaired function (16).

Renal

Lead exposure has for centuries been associated with the development of hypertension, renal failure, and gout (39). Studies of moonshine drinkers in Alabama have shown that gout, hypertension, and renal failure are a common outcome of lead

Table 76.6.   Summary of Lowest Observed Effect Levels for Key Lead-Induced Health Effects in Adults

Lowest Observed Effect Level (Blood Lead µg/dl)	Heme Synthesis and Hematologic Effects	Neurologic Effects	Renal Effects	Reproductive Effects	Cardiovascular Effects
100–120		Encephalopathic signs and symptoms			
80	Anemia	Encephalopathy symptoms	Chronic nephropathy		
60				Reproductive effects in females	
50	Reduced hemoglobin production	Overt subencephalopathic neurological symptoms			
40	Increased urinary ALA and elevated coproporphyrins	Peripheral nerve dysfunction (slowed nerve conduction)			
30				Altered testicular function	Elevated blood pressure (white men, aged 40–59)
25–30	Erythrocyte protoporphyrin (EP) elevation in males				
15–20	Erythrocyte protoporphyrin (EP) elevation in females				
<10	ALA-D inhibition				

Modified source: EPA 1986a.

Table 76.7.   Summary of Lowest Observed Effect Levels for Key Lead-Induced Health Effects in Children

Lowest Observed Effect Level (Blood Lead µg/dl)	Heme Synthesis and Hematologic Effects	Neurologic Effects	Renal Effects	Gastrointestinal Effects
80–100		Encephalopathic signs and symptoms	Chronic nephropathy (aminoaciduria, etc.)	Colic and other overt gastrointestinal symptoms
70	Anemia			
60		Peripheral neuropathies		
50				
40	Reduced hemoglobin synthesis	Peripheral nerve dysfunction (slowed NCVs)		
	Elevated coproporphyrin Increased urinary ALA	CNS cognitive effects		
30	Erythrocyte protoporphyrin elevation	Altered CNS electrophysiologic responses, effect on IQ	Vitamin D metabolism interference	
15	ALA-D inhibition	MDI deficits, reduced gestational age and birth weight (prenatal exposure)		
	Py-5-N[b] activity inhibition			
10				

[b]Py-5-N = pyrimidine-5′-nucleotidase.
Source: EPA 1986a (with updating).

intoxication by this route (40). Renal effects of lead have been extensively studied in humans and experimental animals. Lead accumulates in the proximal tubular cells, explaining the marked effect on urate excretion. In addition, Fanconi's syndrome (proteinuria, aminoaciduria, and phosphaturia) has been described. Inclusion bodies have been demonstrated in renal tubular cells on biopsy. These inclusions are thought by some to represent binding of lead by a renal binding protein which may mitigate the effects of lead on the cell's function (41). As toxicity progresses, a chronic interstitial nephritis may develop, in some cases progressing to end-stage renal failure.

Studies by Wedeen and his colleagues have shown increased body burdens of lead in a population of veterans with hypertension and renal failure. This has raised the possibility that some cases of unexplained renal failure may be caused by previously unrecognized lead poisoning. This finding was not duplicated in a study of members of a health maintenance organization in California (42, 43). Lead interferes with the renin-aldosterone system (16), and this may play a role in the development of hypertension that is seen as a sequela of lead poisoning.

Cardiovascular

Large scale mortality studies of individuals in the lead smelting and battery industries have strongly supported the link between lead and hypertension. In an American population, who worked between 1946 and 1970, most workers had mean blood levels in the range of 40–70 μg/dl. There was an increase in deaths from renal disease and from hypertensive cardiovascular disease (44). Mortality studies in the United Kingdom and Australia show a similar pattern (45, 46). Not all studies of occupational groups have shown an association between blood pressure and lead absorption (47). Little is known about the natural history of the development of hypertension in lead poisoning, its pathophysiology and relation to renal effects, and the effects of intervention.

Pulmonary

While a recent report has identified pneumoconiosis in lead miners, there are no reports of pulmonary dysfunction among other intoxicated populations, and the changes seen in miners may be due to silica in the ore (48).

Endocrine

Lead has been shown to cause decreased serum thyroxin levels, effects on adrenal hormones, and changes in vitamin D levels, but mechanisms and clinical significance have not been elucidated (16).

Reproductive Effects

FEMALE

Occupational exposure to lead, both maternal and paternal, has historically been associated with decreased fertility, spontaneous abortion, stillbirth, and increased infant mortality (49). There have been only a few modern epidemiologic studies of lead's effect on reproductive outcome in women. These studies suggest that the increase in spontaneous abortions seen among working populations may not be seen at the lower doses encountered in community exposure (50). Lead readily passes the placenta and accumulates in the fetus (5), and, as noted above, there is strong evidence that a mother's lead burden can cause serious effects on cognitive development of her child (28).

MALE

Effects on the males' reproductive system have been somewhat easier to study. Lancranjan et al. (51) showed that in battery plant workers there were decreased sperm counts and increased number of abnormal sperm. There was some evidence of an effect even among the plant's office workers who had blood leads that averaged 23 μg/dl. Workers also reported a marked increase in sexual dysfunction. A study among Italian battery workers showed similar findings and supported a direct toxic effect on spermatogenesis, rather than an effect mediated by endocrine changes (52).

MANAGEMENT OF TOXICITY IN CHILDREN

Awareness of the possibility of lead poisoning is critical to timely diagnosis. While children may be exposed in a variety of ways, most clinical intoxication is related to exposure to household dust containing high concentrations of lead from the use of lead paints. Children living in housing built before the Second World War are at greatest risk, although some interior use of lead paint continued until the last decade. While pica increases the risk, ordinary hand to mouth activity can provide enough lead intake to cause poisoning.

In children, lead poisoning manifests itself by irritability, apathy, anorexia, clumsiness, and loss of recently acquired behavioral skills. The child may complain of abdominal pain and constipation. The presence of vomiting, ataxia, and periods of lethargy and stupor herald the approach of frank encephalopathy. In severe cases, the patient may present with seizures and coma (53). The concomitant presence of anemia, particularly if basophilic stippling is present, may also be helpful in steering the physician to the correct diagnosis. On occasion, radiodense paint chips are seen in the gastrointestinal tract on x-ray, and there may be an epiphyseal "lead-line" on radiographs of long bones. Renal function should be assessed. Diagnosis is confirmed by measurement of blood lead and free erythrocyte protoporphyrin (FEP) or zinc protoporphyrin (ZPP). When some delay is involved in obtaining lab results, it may be necessary to begin therapy immediately on the presumptive diagnosis.

The management of pediatric lead poisoning has been described in detail by Chisolm (53, 54) and Piomelli et al. (55). With blood lead levels over 70 μg/dl or signs of encephalopathy, the child should be hospitalized and therapy begun with a combination of BAL (dimercaprol) (4–5 mg/kg i.m.) every 4 hours. Adequate urinary output should be established by hydration, and then calcium disodium ethylenediaminetetraacetic acid (CaNa$_2$-EDTA) 1500 mg/m^2/24 hours should be added to the treatment by continuous infusion in normal saline or dextrose and water. CaNa$_2$-EDTA may also be administered intramuscularly in divided doses every 4 hours. This combined therapy is continued for 5 days. Monitoring of liver and renal functions should be done during this combined therapy. A second course of therapy may be required if the blood lead concentration rebounds. This can best be assessed 2 days following combined therapy. At lower levels of blood lead, BAL can be omitted and CaNa$_2$-EDTA given at the lower dose of 1000 mg/m^2/day in divided doses intravenously or intramuscularly for 5 days. There may be a need for repeated courses of therapy, as lead levels often rebound when lead is mobilized from other compartments to replace the lead that has been chelated and removed. In up to 50% of patients treated BAL produces toxic or adverse side effects such as rash, fever, and hypertension. Children often experience febrile reactions to BAL. Other adverse effects include nausea, vomiting, and headache. Neither BAL nor CaNa$_2$-EDTA are ideal chelators. Two molecules of BAL bind one atom of metal. BAL is excreted mainly in the bile and can be administered if renal compromise is present. BAL penetrates the erythrocyte well.

D-Penicillamine is an oral chelator that effectively increases urinary lead excretion. It is administered in the form of either 125- or 250-mg dosage forms. The usual dose is 25–35 mg/kg/day in four divided doses. The typical adult dose is 250 mg four times a day by mouth for 10 days. Adverse effects of D-penicillamine include hypersensitivity reactions and renal toxicity. Blood dyscrasias such as leukopenia, thrombocytopenia, and eosinophilia have also occurred. Liver and renal functions should be monitored during therapy courses.

Asymptomatic children with elevated lead levels are often identified by investigation of siblings of a symptomatic child or during screening of high risk populations. It has been suggested that a CaNa$_2$-EDTA mobilization test showing a markedly elevated "chelatable" lead be used as a criterion for deciding on chelation therapy. Some concern has been raised about this approach because animal studies suggest CaNa$_2$-EDTA may facilitate redistribution of lead into the brain (13, 56). Indications for chelation therapy, especially for children, are under scrutiny at the present time, and they may change because of the concern about longterm consequences of lead body stores and with the development of better agents (57–60).

A newly approved oral chelating agent, dimercaptosuccinic acid (DMSA, Chemet, succimer) is now available in 100-milligram doses. DMSA has been approved as an orally effective chelating agent for lead poisoning in children for blood lead concentrations above 45 µg/dl. The recommended dose of DMSA for children is 10 mg/kg orally every 8 hours for 5 days (30 mg/kg/day). After 5 days, the dose is reduced to 10 mg/kg every 12 hours for the next 14 days. A course of treatment lasts 19 days. After this, a 2-week rest is recommended before resuming another course unless blood lead concentrations are remaining unacceptably high. DMSA will probably replace the other chelating agents as the drug of choice for treating lead poisoning.

DMSA is a water-soluble analog of dimercaprol (BAL) which has greater water solubility and limited lipid solubility and is effective orally. DMSA has been studied fairly extensively, both at the basic science and clinical levels, in China, the Soviet Union, and Japan. It was recently approved for use in lead poisoning in the United States. DMSA is well absorbed from the gastrointestinal tract and is orally administered as 100-milligram capsules.

In the United States, DMSA is primarily used for the treatment of lead poisoning, although much experience has been gained in its use in arsenic and mercury intoxication. DMSA is effective in mobilizing lead from soft tissue with large decrements in blood, brain, and kidney lead concentrations. Several studies on lead intoxication in humans have been performed showing the efficacy of DMSA for the treatment of lead intoxication. One study in children found that 1050 mg/m^2/day

Table 76.8.   Chelation of Lead in Adults and Children

Blood lead ≥100 µg/dl, severe symptoms and/or encephalopathy	*Dimercaprol (BAL) and CaNa$_2$ EDTA*—BAL 4–5 mg/kg i.m. every 4 hours or 300 mg/m^2 daily divided every 4 hours i.m. Plus CaNa$_2$-EDTA 1500 mg/m^2 daily administered every 4 hours i.v. or i.m. Both drugs are given for 5 days. If blood lead and clinical condition responds to therapy, then BAL may be eliminated in 2–3 days. The adult dose of CaNa$_2$-EDTA should not exceed 2000 mg/daily dose.
Blood lead <100 µg/dl mild to moderate symptoms, no encephalopathy	*DMSA (Chemet)*—Recommended for blood lead >45 µg/dl, in children 10 mg/kg orally t.i.d. (30 mg/kg/day) for 5 days, then same dose is administered b.i.d. for 14 days for a total course of 19 days. A repeat course is guided by blood lead levels and clinical response. A drug-free interval of 2 weeks should be allowed before repeating the course. *CaNa$_2$-EDTA*—1000 mg/m^2 daily in doses divided b.i.d. or t.i.d. by i.m. or i.v. route. Adult and pediatric doses are the same. A second course is based on blood lead response. A drug-free interval of 2–3 weeks should precede a repeat course.

Assure that there is no possible ongoing exposure before beginning chelation therapy!

of DMSA was significantly more effective than 1000 mg/m^2/day of intravenously administered CaNa$_2$-EDTA in reducing blood lead concentrations and restoring erythrocyte ALA-D activity (36).

DMSA has the advantage of being an oral agent which appears to be effective against several different heavy metals. Reports of toxicity have been rare and include an increase in urinary and concomitant decrease in plasma zinc concentrations, and a transient elevation in serum SGPT. The major adverse effect is gastrointestinal and includes nausea and vomiting. Rashes have been reported in 4% of patients (36). The strong sulfur odor of any of the thiol chelators makes the medication unpalatable to most patients. The course may be repeated if needed with an appropriate drug free interval of 2 weeks. Table 76.8 summarizes lead poisoning therapy.

Removal of the child from an environment where exposure may recur is critical. In some cases, this may necessitate prolonged hospitalization and the evaluation and removal of siblings to alternative living arrangements. In some cities, health authorities have developed "safe houses" where families can live until hazards are abated. Because removing lead-containing paint in a poorly controlled fashion can often leave the home more contaminated with lead dust than before, strict supervision of lead abatement is critical. Guidelines have been developed by the federal department of Housing and Urban Development (HUD) (61). Some local governments have developed regulations to guarantee that safe work practices are used, and that after removal of lead paint, living areas are carefully checked for residual dust (62). Even with appropriate management, the prognosis for complete recovery in severe cases is poor. Given the evidence of persisting neurologic problems in asymptomatic children with increased absorption (27), it is obvious that increased attention needs to be focused on prevention and early detection.

MANAGEMENT OF TOXICITY IN ADULTS

Recognition of lead poisoning in the adult depends on a high incidence of suspicion and careful history taking. The infrequency of diagnostic signs and the nonspecific nature of the symptoms frequently lead to misdiagnosis. Although lead poisoning usually has an insidious onset, symptoms may present suddenly and dramatically after a brief but intense exposure. Intense respiratory exposure can be produced by cutting or abrasive blasting of lead-coated steel or by use of powered sanding equipment on lead-painted surfaces. Severe acute disease has also been seen with ingestion of contaminated food (63) or other lead-containing products and is recently described from intravenous injection of contaminated methamphetamine (14). In this setting, patients may develop an acute encephalopathy which can mimic other neurologic or psychiatric illnesses. Acute colic may be mistaken for appendicitis or other intraabdominal catastrophe.

More commonly, symptoms develop insidiously over weeks to months as dose accumulates. The history may suggest any of a number of gastrointestinal, rheumatologic, or psychiatric illnesses. Diagnosis depends on careful history taking to reveal a possible source of exposure. In most cases, a worker in a primary lead-producing or -using industry will be aware of the exposure and may well be under medical surveillance. Workers in smaller industries and in construction where exposures are often uncontrolled are at great risk and may be totally unaware of their exposure. In this situation, the care with which the physician takes an occupational and environmental history is critical.

Processes that most commonly cause lead poisoning in adults are those involving disruption of painted or rustproofed surfaces. These can include burning or sanding of lead-containing paint, cutting or blasting structural steel, and welding or burning rustproofed steel. Secondary smelting, including the reclaiming of batteries and telephone cables, is frequently conducted by small businesses with little awareness of hazards to workers. Indoor firing ranges may have very high levels when ventilation is anything less than perfect. Hobbies, including stained glass work and ceramics, can also pose a risk. The use of lead-glazed pottery for food or beverages can also pose a threat that the patient may be unaware of.

Physical findings are usually of little help in diagnosis. Motor weakness may be detectable, and signs of peripheral nerve entrapment may be present. Gingival lead lines, which depend on the presence of some degree of pyorrhea to develop, are rarely seen. Routine lab work may reveal decreased hemoglobin and hematocrit, but severe anemia is not commonly seen. The classic sign of basophilic stippling is rarely seen. After the closure of the epiphyses, lead lines in bone no longer develop.

Environmental and Occupational Lead Exposure

Exposure of the general population to lead occurs from lead in air, water, food, and soil. Concentrations of lead in the air vary widely depending on the geographic location and the emission source (64). Air lead concentrations range from 0.000076 $\mu g/m^3$ in very remote areas to a high of greater than 10 $\mu g/m^3$ near direct emission sources such as a smelter (64). Urban

air sampling has revealed an average maximum concentration of 0.36 $\mu g/m^3$ from 147 sites in 1984 (64). With the introduction and use of non-lead-containing gasoline, the atmospheric content of lead has declined since 1983 (64). Unleaded gasoline contains 0.05 grams of lead per gallon compared with 0.1 grams in leaded gasoline.

Lead content of surface water in the United States varies between 5 and 30 $\mu g/l$ (64), with the higher concentrations in urban areas. Exposure of populations to lead in drinking water has been a concern. Sources of this lead are the use of lead solder in pipe joints, the use of lead pipes, or the effect of low pH water on the joints or pipe which subsequently leaches lead into the water (64). The Environmental Protection Agency (EPA) proposed to have a zero concentration of lead in drinking water. The EPA has proposed that the 50 $\mu g/l$ limit be lowered to 5 $\mu g/l$. It is estimated that 20% of the American population consume drinking water with lead concentrations exceeding 20 $\mu g/l$ (15). Lead occurs in foods such as dairy products, meat, fish, poultry, grains, and cereals (64). The baseline intake of lead on a daily basis by consuming food and water varies between 5 and 45 $\mu g/day$ for adults and 5–25 $\mu g/day$ for a 2-year-old child (64). The concentration of lead in soil results from both the natural occurrence of lead in crystal layers as well as human activities that produce lead. In urban areas, lead may be as high as 2000–10,000 $\mu g/g$ in soil near roads (64). Naturally occurring concentrations in soil range from less than 10 $\mu g/g$ to up to 30 $\mu g/g$ of lead (64). Near smelters, lead in soil may be as high as 60,000 $\mu g/g$ (64). Lead present in dust is a potential source of ingestion and inhalation. This is a particularly important source of lead for children, since children can consume 100 milligrams of dust per day (64).

Measurement of blood lead level and FEP or ZPP is the key to diagnosis. Because the test is technically difficult, use of a laboratory that routinely and regularly measures blood lead is important. Local health officials or the poison center may be of help in identifying the appropriate laboratory. OSHA maintains a list of laboratories certified to do measurements for medical surveillance.

Treatment of Lead Poisoning in Adults

The first step in treatment must be to identify the patient's exposure, to identify any other individuals (family members or coworkers) who may have also been exposed, and to intervene to stop the exposure. Involvement of local health officials may be essential to confirm the route of exposure and to identify and assess all those at risk. Lead excretion can be dramatically increased by the use of a number of chelating agents. $CaNa_2$-EDTA has been the mainstay of therapy in the past. Dimercaprol and penicillamine are also used in some situations; BAL as a supplement to $CaNa_2$-EDTA when lead levels are very high and pencillamine when an oral agent is necessary for longterm use. Both are limited by their side effects. In the presence of severe encephalopathy, or when blood lead levels exceed 100 $\mu g/dl$, treatment should begin with dimercaprol 4–5 mg/kg given intramuscularly every 4 hours, followed by $CaNa_2$-EDTA 2 g/day by continuous intravenous infusion for 5 days. Dimercaprol is thick and oily and must be administered by deep intramuscular injection. Up to 50% of patients will have some adverse reaction after receiving a dose of 4–5 mg/kg. Side effects include hypertension and tachycardia which is dose related. Rash is common along with nausea, vomiting, headache, and paresthesias. BAL is 50% excreted in bile and can be used if renal compromise is present.

CaNa$_2$-EDTA has low toxicity compared with BAL. Excretion is mainly urinary. Toxic effects of CaNa$_2$EDTA include renal tubular necrosis, which is reversible on discontinuation of therapy, rash, febrile reactions, fatigue, thirst, myalgia, chills, and rarely cardiac dysrhythmias. DMSA, an oral analog of dimercaprol, was approved by the Food and Drug Administration specifically for the use in children but is likely to play a major role in treating adults as well. DMSA has many advantages over other drugs.

Chelation therapy is indicated for the treatment of severe symptoms such as intractable headache, irritability, and other personality changes, myalgias or arthralgias, and abdominal colic. End organ damage, as evidenced by neuropathy or nephropathy, is also an indication for intervention. Even in the absence of symptoms, markedly elevated blood lead levels may be an indication for therapy. In some severe situations, it may be appropriate to institute therapy before test results return, as long as other treatable etiologies in the differential diagnosis have been considered.

At lower levels of blood lead, BAL is omitted and CaNa$_2$-EDTA or DMSA can be used alone. While DMSA is not yet approved for use in adults, it has proven to be an efficacious therapeutic agent in lead poisoning as well as in poisoning from arsenic and mercury. Approval for use can be obtained by request. While a variety of regimens are in use, it is unwise to exceed 2 grams of CaNa$_2$-EDTA daily in the adult. CaNa$_2$-EDTA should be given intravenously no more rapidly than 1 gram over an hour, and slower infusions are generally preferred to minimize the risk of hypercalcemia. Electrocardiographic monitoring is rarely indicated in the adult. Doses of CaNa$_2$-EDTA may need to be reduced in the presence of renal failure. While intramuscular injection of CaNa$_2$-EDTA is efficacious, it is exceedingly painful in adult doses. Oral CaNa$_2$-EDTA is not effective and may increase lead absorption.

Because repeated daily doses of CaNa$_2$-EDTA typically produce gradually decreasing amounts of urinary lead excretion, therapy is typically continued for 5 days and then interrupted to assess effect and watch for rebound. Blood levels should be assessed after each round of therapy and weekly thereafter to determine whether rebound is occurring and further therapy is warranted. Once a decision to undertake therapy has been made, it should be continued until symptoms have improved and lead levels remain at an acceptable level.

With a less acutely ill patient, a number of factors should be considered in deciding on the need for chelation. In cases with minimum symptoms no therapy other than cessation of exposure may be necessary. When the patient has persisting symptoms, history and laboratory values may provide information about prognosis. The magnitude of the blood lead level, which is sensitive to recent exposure, may be less useful than the FEP or ZPP, which sum up the effects of lead on the marrow over the preceding 2–3 months. Measurement of the "chelatable" lead burden by means of a test dose of EDTA can provide a better measure of lead body burden and may aid prognosis and influence decisions about treatment. Assessments of bone lead by x-ray fluorescence may eventually prove to have clinical utility in assessing body burden and in making therapeutic decisions (37). At any given blood lead level, the more slowly the dose has been accumulated and the greater the FEP or ZPP or chelatable lead, the longer the symptoms are likely to persist. Chelation therapy may shorten the symptomatic period in such

a situation, but repeated courses of treatment may be necessary. Because bone stores may be remobilized by therapy, blood lead levels often rebound after each course of treatment. As body burden is reduced, blood levels rebound more slowly, and to lower levels.

While chelation therapy has demonstrated its value in treating severe symptomatic intoxication, there are as yet no controlled studies of its effects on the outcome of other end organ effects. Controversy remains about its value in the setting of asymptomatic or mildly symptomatic intoxication. While removing lead as rapidly and as thoroughly as possible has theoretical attractiveness, it is possible that chelating agents may cause unintended harm by redistribution of lead into organs or organelles. Resolution of this issue may have to await controlled trials with the newer oral agents.

Chelation therapy should never be given prophylactically, nor be given to a patient in whom lead absorption may be continuing.

EXPOSURE LIMITS AND ENVIRONMENTAL MONITORING

Air

The EPA has established a national primary and secondary air quality standard of 1.5 μg/m^3 Pb as an arithmetic mean averaged over a calendar quarter (40CFR50.12).

Water

The Clean Water Act established a water quality criterion for lead at 50 micrograms Pb per liter for domestic water supply. The same limit is the National Primary Drinking Water Maximum Contaminant Level (MCL). The Safe Drinking Water Act requires suppliers of lead-contaminated water to notify customers of any lead content in their water and to describe the potential hazards of lead, what the water system is doing about it, and whether to seek alternative supply of water (52CFR41534). In most settings in the United States, the principal source of lead contamination of drinking water is not the source waters or the transmission system, but the use of lead-containing solder in domestic plumbing. Especially with acidic water, there can be substantial leaching as water sits in household pipes. Some states and municipalities have banned lead-containing solder for water supply pipes. The EPA has recommended that the 50-μg/l level be lowered to 5 μg/l.

Gasoline

The use of organic lead additives in gasoline has been nearly eliminated since the 1970s in the United States. Leaded gasoline is still permitted for farm equipment and some marine use. Since this was the single largest source of lead absorption to which the general population was exposed, the removal of lead from gasoline resulted in dramatic decreases in the average blood lead levels of the population.

Waste Disposal

Lead is treated as a hazardous waste under the Resource Conservation and Recovery Act (RCRA) (40CFR260).

Table 76.9.   Regulatory Limits for Lead Exposure

Agency	Sample or Medium	Concentration	Regulation
OSHA	Air	50 μg Pb/m³	Permissible exposure limit for an 8-hr workday
ACGIH	Air	150 μg Pb/m³	Time weighted average for 40-hr work week
EPA	Air	1.5 μg Pb/m³	3 month average
EPA	Water	50 μg Pb/l	Consideration being given to lowering this to 5 μg/l
OSHA	Blood	60 μg/dl	Removal from exposure
OSHA	Blood	40 μg/dl	Medical evaluation required
CDC (EPA)	Blood	10–15 μg/dl*	Level of concern in children

Adapted from ATSDR, U.S. Department of Health and Human Services, Public Health Service, 1990.
*Anticipated reduction for 1991.

Consumer Product Safety

Lead-containing paint and certain consumer products bearing lead-containing paint were banned by the United States Consumer Products Safety Commission. "Lead-containing" is defined by the presence of more than 0.06% Pb by weight of the paint or the dried surface (42CFR44199; 43CFR8515). Lead paint continues to be used in some exterior applications, and interior surfaces painted prior to 1975 should be suspect. Lead content can be checked from paint chips, from dust in window wells, or by the use of an x-ray fluorescence detector which can directly read from surfaces. Lead paint removal is regulated by HUD guidelines and by state and local regulations (61, 62).

OSHA REGULATIONS

The OSHA Lead Standard sets a Permissible Exposure Level for Pb of 50 μg/m³ air for an 8-hour time-weighted average (Table 76.9). An action level of 30 μg/m³ is also provided, above which an employer is obligated to provide training, protective clothing, washing facilities, and medical surveillance. The standard also requires the removal from exposure of workers whose lead levels are markedly elevated or who are felt by the physician to need such removal. Workers whose blood lead levels are ≥60 μg/dl must be immediately removed from the exposure. Workers whose blood lead levels exceed 40 μg/dl must have medical evaluations (64). Where it has been enforced, the lead standard has resulted in dramatic decreases in cases of intoxication and in average levels of blood lead among workers. The federal OSHA standard excluded agriculture and construction. Because some of the most severe cases of lead poisoning have occurred in industry, Maryland extended very similar regulations to construction, and other states may follow suit soon. Organic lead compounds were excluded from these regulations and are at present covered only by the older standard of 200 μg/m³ air.

OTHER PUBLIC HEALTH REGULATIONS

A number of states require the reporting of cases of lead poisoning in children or adults to health authorities. Encouraged by the National Institute of Occupational Safety and Health, a number of states are now requiring laboratories to report all elevated blood lead levels in order to begin a surveillance for excessive lead exposure and frank poisonings. Some local governments are continuing screening programs to detect elevated lead levels among children. Unfortunately, in most localities authorities take action to reduce the hazards of lead paint only after a poisoned child has been identified. This perpetuates a system that has traditionally relied on toddlers as biologic monitoring devices in order to avoid the costs of prospective inspections.

ACKNOWLEDGMENT

The author wishes to acknowledge the assistance and advice of Julian Chisolm, MD, Bruce Fowler, PhD, Ellen Silbergeld, PhD, and Liz Katz, BS, in the preparation of this chapter.

REFERENCES

1. Woodbury WD. Lead. In: Minerals yearbook 1987. Washington, DC: Bureau of Mines, United States Department of Commerce, 1987:541–567.
2. Stokinger HE. The metals. In: Clayton GD, Clayton FE, eds. Patty's industrial hygiene and toxicology. New York: Wiley Interscience, 1981:1687–1728.
3. Lead poisoning: strategies for prevention. Baltimore: Maryland Department of Health and Mental Hygiene, 1984.
4. Watson WS, Hume R, Moore MR. Oral absorption of lead and iron. Lancet 1989;(Aug. 2):236–237.
5. Barltrop D. Transfer of lead to the human foetus. In: Baltrop D, Burland WL, eds. Mineral metabolism in paediatrics. Philadelphia: FA Davis, 1968:135–150.
6. Kehoe RA. Toxicological appraisal of lead in relation to the tolerable concentration in the ambient air. J Air Pollut Cont Assoc 1969;19:690–700.
7. Forni A, Cambiaghi G, Secchi GC. Initial occupational exposure to lead. Arch Environ Health 1976;31:73–78.
8. Chisolm JJ, Barrett MB, Harrison HV. Indicators of internal dose of lead in relation to derangement in heme synthesis. Johns Hopkins Med J 1975;137:6–12.
9. Bennett WM. Lead nephropathy. Kidney Int 1985;28:212–220.
10. Arai F, Yamamura Y, Yamauchi H, Yoshida M. Biliary excretion of dimethyl lead after administration of tetraethyl lead in rabbits. Sangyo Igaku 1983;25:175–80.
11. Rabinowitz MB, Wetherill GW, Kopple JD. Kinetic analysis of lead metabolism in healthy humans. J Clin Invest 1976;58:260–270.
12. Christoffersson JO, Ahlgren L, Schute A, Skerfving S, Mattson S. Decrease of skeletal lead levels in man after end of occupational exposure. Arch Environ Health 1986;41:312–318.
13. Cory-Slechta DA, Weiss B, Cox C. Mobilization and redistribution of lead over the course of calcium disodium ethylene diamine tetraacetate chelation therapy. J Pharmacol Exp Ther 1987;243:804–813.
14. Chandler DB, Norton RL, Kauffman KW, et al. Lead poisoning associated with methamphetamine use, Oregon 1988. MMWR 1989;38:830–831.
15. Landigan P. Current issues in the epidemiology and toxicology of occupational exposure to lead. Environ Health Perspect 1990;89:61–66.
16. Cullen MR, Robins JM, Eskenazi B. Adult inorganic lead intoxication: presentation of 31 new cases and a review of recent advances in the literature. Medicine 1983;62:221–247.
17. Krigman MR, Bouldin TW, Mushak P. Lead. In: Spencer PS, Schaumberg HH, eds. Experimental and clinical neurotoxicology. Baltimore: Williams & Wilkins, 1980.
18. Goyer R. Lead toxicity: from overt to subclinical to subtle health effects. Health Perspect 1990;86:177–181.
19. Stollery BT, Banks HA, Broadbent DE, Lee WR. Cognitive function in lead workers. Br J Ind Med 1989;46:698–707.
20. Hogstedt C, Hane M, Agrell A, Bodin L. Neuropsychological test results and symptoms among workers with well defined long term exposure to lead. Br J Ind Med 1983;40:99–105.
21. Valciukas JA, Lilis R, Singer R, Fischbein A, Anderson HA, Glickman L. Lead exposure and behavioral changes: comparison of four occupational groups with different levels of lead absorption. Am J Ind Med 1980;1:421–426.
22. Bleecker ML, Agnew J, Keogh JP, Stetson DS. Neurobehavioral evaluation in workers following a brief exposure to lead. Adv Biosc 46:255–261.

23. Mantere P, Hanninen H, Hernberg S, Luukkonen R. A prospective follow-up study on psychological effects in workers exposed to low levels of lead. Scand J Work Environ Health 1984;10:43–50.

24. Baker EL, Feldman RG, White RA, et al. Occupational lead neurotoxicity: a behavioral and electro physiological evaluation. Br J Ind Med 1984;41:352–361.

25. Baker EL, Feldman RG, White RA, et al. Occupational lead in neurotoxicity: improvement in behavioral effects after reduction of exposure. Br J Ind Med 1985;42:507–516.

26. Needleman HL, Gunnoe C, Leviton A, et al. Deficits in psychological and classroom performance of children with elevated dentine lead levels. N Engl J Med 1979;300:689–695.

27. Needleman HL, Schell A, Bellinger D, Leviton A, Allred EN. The long term effects of exposure to low doses of lead in childhood. N Engl J Med 1990;322:83–88.

28. Bellinger D, Leviton A, Waternaux C, Needleman H, Rabinowitz M. Longitudinal analyses of prenatal and postnatal lead exposure and early cognitive development. N Engl J Med 1987;316:1037–1043.

29. Walsh TJ, Tilson HA. Neurobehavioral toxicology of the organoleads. Neurotoxicology 1984;5:67–86.

30. Seppalainen A, Hernsberg S, Kock B. Relationship between blood lead levels and nerve conduction velocities. Neurotoxicology 1979;1:313–332.

31. Seppalainen A, Hernsberg S. Subclinical lead neuropathy. Am J Ind Med 1989;1:413–420.

32. Seppalainen A, Hernsberg S, Vesanto R, Koch B. Early neurotoxic effects of lead exposure: a prospective study. Neurotoxicology 1983;4:181–192.

33. Goyer R. Transplacental transport of lead. Environ Health Perspect 1990;89:101–105.

34. Royce SE, Needleman HL. Case studies in environmental medicine: lead toxicity, San Rafael, CA. U.S. Department of Health and Human Studies, June 1990.

35. ATSDR. Toxicological profile for lead, Agency for Toxic Substances and Disease Registry. U.S. Public Health Service and EPA, by Oak Ridge National Laboratory DUE June 1990:7–44.

36. Graziano JH, Lolacono NJ, Meyer P. Dose-response study of oral 2,3-dimercaptosuccinic acid in children with elevated blood lead concentrations. J Pediatr 1992;113:751–757.

37. Wedeen RD. In vivo tibial XRF measurement of bone lead. Arch Environ Health 1990;45:69–71.

38. Grandjean P, Jensen BM, Sand SH, Jorgensen PJ, Antonsen S. Delayed blood regeneration in lead exposure: an effect on reverse capacity. Am J Public Health 1989;79:1385–1388.

39. Wedeen RP. Poison in the pot. Carbondale, IL: Southern Illinois University Press, 1984.

40. Morgan JM, Ball GV, Oh SJ, et al. Lead poisoning. South Med J 1972;65:278–288.

41. Goering PL, Fowler BA. Mechanisms of renal lead-binding protein protection against lead inhibition of delta-aminolevulinic acid dehydratase. J Pharmacol Exp Ther 1985;234:365–371.

42. Batumen V, Landy E, Maesaka JK, Wedeen RP. Contribution of lead to hypertension with renal impairment. N Engl J Med 1983;309:17–21.

43. Osterloth JD, Selby JV, Bernard BP, et al. Body burdens of lead in hypertensive nephropathy. Arch Environ Health 1989;44:304–310.

44. Cooper WC, Wong O, Kheifets L. Mortality among employees of lead battery plants and lead-producing plants, 1947–1980. Scand J Work Environ Health 1985;11:331–345.

45. Fanning D. A mortality study of lead workers, 1926–1985. Arch Environ Health 1988;43:247–251.

46. McMichael AJ, Johnson HM. Long term mortality profile of heavily exposed lead smelter workers. J Occup Med 1982;24:375–378.

47. Parkinson DK, Hodgson MJ, Bromet EJ, Dew MA, Connell MM. Occupational lead exposure and blood pressure. Br J Ind Med 1987;44:744–748.

48. Masjedi MR, Estineh N, Bahadori M, Alavi M, Sprince NL. Pulmonary complications in lead miners. Chest 1989;96:18–21.

49. Hamilton A, Hardy HL. Industrial toxicology. 2nd ed. New York: Harper, 1949:99–103.

50. Murphy MJ, Graziano JH, Popovac D, et al. Past pregnancy outcome among women living in the vicinity of a lead smelter in Kosovo, Yugoslavia. Am J Public Health 1990;80:33–35.

51. Lancranjan I, Popescu HI, Gavanescu O, Klepsch I, Serbanescu M. Reproductive ability of workmen occupationally exposed to lead. Arch Environ Health 1975;30:396–401.

52. Assennato G, Baser ME, Molinini R, et al. Sperm count suppression without endocrine dysfunction in lead exposed men. Arch Environ Health 1986;41:387–390.

53. Chisolm JJ. Treatment of lead poisoning. Mod Treatment 1971;8:593–612.

54. Chisolm JJ, Barltrop D. Recognition and management of children with increased lead absorption. Arch Dis Child 1979;54:249–262.

55. Piomelli S, Rosen JF, Chisolm JJ, Graef JW. Management of childhood lead poisoning. J Pediatr 1984;105:523–532.

56. Chisolm JJ. Mobilization of lead by calcium disodium edetate: a reappraisal. Am J Dis Child 1987;141:1256–1257.

57. Shannon MW, Graef JW, Lovejoy FH. Efficacy and toxicity of d-penicillamine in low level poisoning. J Pediatr 1988;112:799–804.

58. Shannon MW, Grace A, Graef JW. Use of penicillamine in children with small lead burdens (letter). N Engl J Med 1989;321:979–980.

59. Piomelli S. Use of penicillamine in children with small lead burdens (letter). N Engl J Med 1990;322:1887–1888.

60. Graziano JH. Use of penicillamine in children with small lead burdens (letter). N Engl J Med 1990;322:1888–1889.

61. U.S.H.U.D. Lead-based paint: interior guidelines for hazard identification and abatement. US Department of Housing and Urban Development. Fed Reg 1990;55:14556–14789 (April 18, 1990).

62. State of Maryland Department of the Environment Lead Abatement Regulations. COMAR 26.02.07.

63. Hershko C, Abrahamov A, Moreb J, et al. Lead poisoning in a West Bank Arab Village. Arch Intern Med 1984;144:1969–1973.

64. ATSDR. Toxicological profile for lead, prepared for Agency for Toxic Substances and Disease Registry U.S. Public Health Service, by Syracuse Research Corporation, June 1990.

77

Cadmium

Michael P. Waalkes, Ph.D.
Zakaria Z. Wahba, Ph.D.
Ricardo E. Rodriguez, Ph.D.

INTRODUCTION

Cadmium is a very toxic heavy metal; human exposure to cadmium has been and continues to be a major concern. A highly cumulative toxic agent, cadmium is estimated to have a biologic half-life in humans of approximately 20–30 years. Cadmium has been shown to have effects on a variety of tissues and biologic systems and has been associated with such diverse maladies as hypertension and carcinogenesis. Cadmium consumption increased markedly during the early 1900s and continues essentially unchanged at present. Very little cadmium is ever recycled. Thus the known and suspected effects of cadmium in humans as well as its continued industrial usage reinforce the view that cadmium poses a major threat to the human population and the environment (1–6).

PHYSICAL PROPERTIES, SOURCES, PRODUCTION AND USES

Physical Properties and Chemical Forms

Cadmium is a silvery, crystalline metal resembling zinc. It is only slightly tarnished by air or water. Metallic cadmium exists in a hexagonal close-packed arrangement (hcp) in which each atom has 12 nearest neighbors, six surrounding it in its own close-packed layer, three above and three below this layer. In this hcp structure each layer is a plane of symmetry, and the set of nearest neighbors of each atom has D_{3h} symmetry (7). Cadmium has oxidation states of 0, +1, and +2, with +2 the most common. Highly unstable but strongly reducing dimers of Cd^{+1} can be obtained by irradiation of aequous solutions.

The stereochemistry of cadmium is a direct result of the d shell configuration. There is no ligand field stabilization, since the outer d shell of cadmium is complete. Thus, the stereochemistry of cadmium compounds is determined solely by size, electrostatic forces, and covalent bonding forces. Cadmium has coordination numbers of 4 (tetrahedral), 5 (trigonal bipyramidal), and 6 (octahedral configuration). The coordination number of most cadmium-organo compounds is usually 2.

Cadmium is a member of Division A of Analytical Group II, which consists of the common metals whose ions form chlorides which are insoluble in dilute acid but whose sulfides are precipitated by hydrogen sulfide in 0.3 M hydrochloric acid. This property permits the separation and identification of cadmium from other heavy metals of Analytical Group II. Cadmium forms numerous divalent compounds including oxides, hydroxides, sulfides, selenides, tellurides, and halides. Complex anions can be formed with halides in aqueous solution. Complex cations with ammonia and amine ligands are well defined and are obtained as crystalline salts.

Natural Occurrence

Cadmium is found in the rare mineral elements greenockite (CdS), and otavite ($CdCO_4$). Both forms are found in zinc- and zinc-lead-rich ores. Other materials that contain cadmium are hawleyite (CdS), xanthrocroite ($CdS(H_2O)_x$), cadmoselite (CdSe), and monteporrite (CdO).

Production

Most of the cadmium produced comes from zinc smelters and from sludge obtained from electrolytic refining of zinc. Cadmium is recovered as a byproduct of refining. In 1973 world production of cadmium was 17 million kg, while U.S. production was 3.36 million kg (8).

There are several sources from which pure cadmium is produced including sintering of flue dusts and roasting of zinc ores, and as a byproduct of slag zinc. In the smelting of cadmium-containing zinc ores, the two metals are reduced together. Since cadmium is more volatile than zinc, the two compounds can be separated by fractional distillation. Cadmium is less active than zinc, and electrolytic separation can also be accomplished (9, 10).

Uses of Cadmium

A large part of the cadmium produced is used in electroplating metals such as iron and steel. Since cadmium is not easily corroded, it is an excellent protective agent against corrosion and much better than zinc. The most important application of cadmium electroplating is in the automotive and aircraft industries. Others include electronic parts, marine equipment, and industrial machinery (9).

A second large consumer of cadmium is the plastics industry. Cadmium salts of long-chain fatty acids admixed with barium salts serve as stabilizers for plastic. Substituted cadmium phosphonium chloride is utilized by the rubber industry as an additive.

The paint industry uses cadmium sulfide (CdS), cadmium selenide (CdSe), and cadmium oxide (CdO) in a mixture for use as pigments. Pure CdO is used in phosphors (6).

Cadmium is used to produce a number of alloys such as Woods metal (12.5% Cd) and Lipowitz alloy (10% Cd). Alloys containing a high proportion of cadmium in combination with nickel, silver, and/or copper are used for bearings where the high speeds and temperatures are excessive for tin or lead alloys. Other alloys varying in cadmium content from 10–95% are used for soldering aluminum. Low melting alloys are utilized in fire protection fusible links, fusible cores for foundry molds, bending pipes and thin sections, soldering, and sealing.

Cadmium is used as the negative electrode in long-lasting

cadmium-nickel batteries. These batteries are rechargeable and are very important in biomedical applications (9).

Cadmium is very important in the nuclear industry. Cadmium absorbs neutrons and is used in making neutron shields and rods that help control the chain reaction of nuclear reactors.

Production of Specific Cadmium Compounds and Industrial Uses

Cadmium acetate is produced by the reaction of cadmium nitrate with acetic anhydride. Its major uses include the production of iridescent effects on porcelains and pottery, as a reagent for the determination of sulfur, selenium and tellurium in cadmium electroplating, in dying and printing of textiles, and in purification of mercaptans from crude oils and gasolines.

Cadmium carbonate is produced by the reaction of cadmium hydroxide and carbon dioxide. Its uses include its application as a lawn and turf fungicide in the form of a wettable powder in combination with organic fungicides. Other uses include the preparation of high purity, specialized chemicals such as phosphors for use in monitors.

Cadmium chloride is produced by the reaction of cadmium metal, cadmium oxide or carbonate in hydrochloric acid. $CdCl_2$ is used in pesticides and nonpasture fungicides, as photographic material, as electronic coatings for vacuum tubes, and in manufacture of special mirrors and lubricants. $CdCl_2$ also has applications in dyeing, and calico printing of textiles.

Cadmium fluoroborate is produced by the reaction of aqueous fluoroboric acid and cadmium metal, carbonate, or oxide. Its primary use is in electroplating.

Cadmium fluoride is produced by the reaction of cadmium carbonate and hydrofluoric acid. It is used as an ingredient in glass and in nuclear reactor control rods.

Cadmium nitrate is produced by the reaction of cadmium oxide with nitric acid and used primarily in the manufacture of nickel-cadmium batteries and secondarily as turf fungicide.

Cadmium oxide is prepared by the distillation of cadmium metal from a graphite retort and subsequent reaction of vapor with air and is widely used in electroplating. Applications include the production of cadmium electrodes for alkaline batteries and the synthesis of other cadmium compounds.

Cadmium sulfate is produced by the reaction of cadmium metal, oxide, carbonate, with sulfide in sulfuric acid. The compound is used in the plastic (PVCs) manufacturing industry as a stabilizer because it enhances the stability of such products to heat and sunlight. $CdSO_4$ is also used in the production of pigments.

Cadmium sulfide is produced by the reaction of cadmium salts with hydrogen sulfide gas. It has several uses including as a pigment (yellow to deep maroon), as a heat stabilizer in plastics, as a colorizer of vulcanized rubber, and in epoxy resins. Cadmium sulfide is also used in printing inks for alkali resistance, in paints for resistance to hydrogen sulfide blacking, as a phosphor in cathode-ray tube screens, in phosphorescent tapes and markers, watch and instrument dials, and in x-ray fluorescent screens. Cadmium sulfide is also an active ingredient of certain shampoos designed for use in the treatment of seborrheic dermatitis of the scalp.

Table 77.1.   Businesses, Occupations, and Processes Associated with Cadmium Exposure

Primary production industries (cadmium smelting)
Lead and zinc smelting
Electroplating industry
Manufacture of cadmium-nickel batteries
Welding of cadmium-plated materials
Alloy production (copper-cadmium and silver-cadmium alloy manufacture)
Production of plastic stabilizers
Production of cadmium pigments
Jewelry manufacture
Electronic production industries

INDUSTRIES AND OCCUPATIONS ASSOCIATED WITH EXPOSURES

Businesses, Occupations, and Processes Associated with Cadmium Exposure

The major businesses associated with potential cadmium exposure are shown in Table 77.1. These include the primary production industries such as cadmium smelting (3). Lead and zinc smelting can also be a source of cadmium exposure. The electroplating industry is another primary source of exposure, as cadmium fumes can be generated during the electroplating process (3). The processing involved in manufacture of cadmium-nickel batteries can also lead to worker exposure due to formation of cadmium dusts (3). Cadmium fumes, generated by welding of cadmium-plated materials, are extremely dangerous and are the primary cause of acute fatal poisonings (3). In alloy production using cadmium, such as copper-cadmium and silver-cadmium alloy manufacture, significant exposures can occur (3). The production of plastic stabilizers and cadmium pigments also can lead to exposure (3). The production of jewelry using silver-based solder containing cadmium is another documented source of industrial exposure due to the generation of cadmium oxide fumes in the process (12). The use of cadmium in the rubber production may also lead to significant exposure.

Major anthropogenic environmental exposure sources include: the use of sewage sludge as fertilizer; manufacture and use of phosphate-based fertilizers; incineration of waste and wood; coal combustion; oil and gasoline combustion (2). Natural sources of environmental exposure include volcanogenic particles, wind-blown dust, and forest fires (2).

CLINICAL TOXICOLOGY OF CADMIUM EXPOSURE

Routes of Cadmium Exposure

Exposure to cadmium in human populations occurs both through the environment and in the work place. Though occupational exposure was in the past the most prominent form, significant exposure has occurred and continues to occur through the environment. Hence both types of exposure routes must be considered to be of relevance in clinical toxicology.

ENVIRONMENTAL CADMIUM EXPOSURE

Generally cadmium occurs naturally in the environment as sulfide deposits. Increased industrial use starting at the beginning of the present century gave rise to increases in production of cadmium from a few tons per year to nearly 18,000 tons in 1975 (2, 4). Cadmium is widely distributed and contamination of soil, water, and air has become increasingly widespread through mining, refining, and smelting operations. Other significant sources of environmental cadmium include the combustion of fossil fuels, municipal waste incineration, and agricultural practices including the use of phosphate fertilizers and sludge amendment for soils (2, 3). Use of cadmium in batteries, alloys, paints, and plastics also contributes to environmental levels and thus to human exposure (2, 3).

Oral exposure to cadmium is the major route in the nonindustrially exposed individual where food consumption constitutes the main environmental source of cadmium for the nonsmoking general population (2). The cadmium content of different foodstuffs ranges from 0.001 to 1.3 ppm and the average intake from food and water ranges from 10 to 30 μg daily (2). In highly polluted areas this level can rise to as high as 400 μg daily of cadmium intake (2, 4). Meat byproducts, especially liver and kidney, are high in cadmium. Shellfish and seafood can also be particularly high in cadmium in certain areas. Vegetable products generally contain greater levels of cadmium than meat-based foodstuffs (6). Exposure to cadmium by way of contaminated water that was used for irrigation of rice has been associated with Itai-Itai disease, a multisystem disorder with characteristic severe osteomalacia that occurred in Japan and affected primarily postmenopausal, multiparous women (2).

Inhalation of cadmium is another major source of cadmium intake for the general population. Average concentrations of cadmium in air are as follows: rural areas <1 to 6 ng/m^3, urban areas 5 to 50 ng/m^3, for industrial areas 20 to 700 ng/m^3 (4). Cadmium intake by inhalation in the general population averages 0.02 μg/day and can be as high as 2 μg/day in highly polluted areas. Thus, even with highly polluted atmospheric conditions, food is still the main cadmium source in the general population.

An additional source of respiratory cadmium intake is cigarette smoking, as the tobacco plant readily absorbs cadmium from polluted soils. It has been estimated that a one-pack-a-day smoker can potentially absorb 2 μg of cadmium daily in addition to other sources (4, 5). Thus cigarettes must be considered as an important additional source of human cadmium exposure.

OCCUPATIONAL CADMIUM EXPOSURE

Estimates indicate that approximately 1.5 million workers are potentially exposed to cadmium in the workplace in the United States. This includes primary cadmium industries, such as ore smelting, as well as secondary industries where exposure potential is less. Welding is a primary example of the latter.

The predominant route of exposure to cadmium in occupational settings is inhalation. Secondary oral exposure may occur under conditions of poor industrial hygiene, such as storage of food or eating in contaminated areas, but the exposure to cadmium from such sources is minor in comparison to inhalation. With the possible exception of organic compounds of cadmium used as stabilizers and catalysts in plastic production, dermal exposure under most conditions is probably not a significant factor, particularly where appropriate industrial hygiene is observed. Cigarette smoking must be considered a significant augmentation to industrial cadmium exposure. External con-

tamination of cigarettes with cadmium in the workplace can significantly increase worker exposure (4, 5).

Inhalation exposure can be to various chemical and physical forms of cadmium. Typically, exposure during ore smelting is to cadmium oxide fume, while exposure to mist and dusts of cadmium cyanate or cadmium chloride can occur during electroplating operations (4, 5).

Historically, air concentrations of cadmium in the workplace were very high, with values detected in the mg/m^3 range (4). Over the last several decades, with increased awareness of the toxic potential of cadmium and resultant improvements in industrial hygiene, these concentrations have dropped considerably and are typically below the federal occupational limit and even below the TLV. Despite this, however, cadmium intoxications resulting from inhalation under occupational conditions still occur (11, 12).

Absorption of Cadmium

Absorption of cadmium depends highly on the route of exposure and secondarily on the compound in question. Most salts of cadmium are absorbed poorly from the gastrointestinal tract. It is estimated that only about 5% of the cadmium that is ingested is absorbed, although various conditions, including dietary status and iron deficiency anemia, can elevate this proportion (2, 13). The absorption of cadmium from the gastrointestinal tract does not appear to be different in men or women (13). Cadmium has a relatively long transit time in the gastrointestinal tract, possibly due to uptake of cadmium by the mucosal cells (13).

Absorption from the respiratory system is, however, quite different. Whereas the gastrointestinal tract only absorbs approximately 5% of the cadmium presented to it, depending on the in vivo solubility of the inhaled compound, more than 90% of the cadmium deposited deep in the lung can be absorbed (4, 5). Thus the avid ability of the lung to absorb cadmium must be taken into consideration in assessing actual exposure levels. Furthermore cadmium absorbed from the pulmonary system will reach and can affect other distant organ systems. For instance, chronic nephrotoxicity is a well-documented result secondary to chronic inhalation of cadmium (2, 4).

Metabolism of Cadmium

Once absorbed, cadmium is bound to red blood cells and serum albumin. Serum cadmium is very rapidly taken up by soft tissues, primarily liver and kidney, and has a very high volume of distribution indicative of the rapid tissue concentration (1–3, 14). Typically over 50% of the body burden of cadmium will be found in the liver and kidney. The half-life of cadmium is thought to be very long, and accumulation occurs within these tissues (1). It is postulated that there is a critical concentration of cadmium within the kidney; once that is exceeded, cadmium-induced nephropathy will occur (1, 2). Human newborns have very low tissue levels of cadmium, and the placenta appears to be a somewhat effective barrier to cadmium, although the fetal exposure will occur with increasing maternal exposure (1, 15).

In the classical sense of the term, cadmium is not biotransformed. Furthermore cadmium, once absorbed, is only very slowly excreted. However, biological defense mechanisms to reduce the toxic potential of cadmium do exist. A key aspect of the metabolism of cadmium is the low-molecular weight, metal-binding protein metallothionein, which is synthesized in response to cadmium exposure (2). After synthesis, metallothionein will bind cadmium with a very high affinity and thus render it toxicologically inert (1, 2) when intracellular. Hence cadmium is detoxified by longterm storage rather than biotransformation or elimination. The liver and kidney are tissues with a high capacity for metallothionein synthesis (16), and soon after absorption most of the cadmium will be found predominantly in the liver and kidney (1, 2). Hence the metabolism of cadmium is intimately involved with metallothionein. Zinc treatment prior to normally toxic or lethal doses of cadmium in animals will prevent such effects (17, 18), due to its ability to induce metallothionein.

Indeed it appears that cadmium frequently will follow the biologic pathways of zinc metabolism, and to a lesser extent calcium. For instance, cadmium frequently will be taken up by cells through mechanisms normally devoted to zinc uptake (19–21). It is thought that on the molecular level many of the toxic effects of cadmium are due to its replacement of zinc in biologic systems. Zinc deficiency states modify cadmium distribution and potentially enhance cadmium toxicity (22).

Cadmium is stored in association with metallothionein for long periods. It is, however, felt that cadmium in association with metallothionein may be the actual toxic species to the kidneys. Cadmium-metallothionein is highly toxic to the kidney and will acutely induce a proximal tubular necrosis characteristic of longterm exposure to ionic forms of cadmium (23, 24). It appears that circulating cadmium-metallothionein is specifically taken up by the proximal tubule when it is degraded, and the cadmium is released in locally high concentrations. Rodents treated chronically with cadmium salts do not show nephropathy until after serum levels of cadmium-metallothionein are elevated (24). The source of cadmium-metallothionein is thought to be the liver, from which, with continued cadmium exposure, it is eventually lost. Monitoring serum cadmium-metallothionein may thus be a possible predictor of nephrotoxicity onset; however, this hypothesis has not been tested.

Cadmium Elimination

Once absorbed, cadmium is very poorly excreted. This observation is consistent with the very long biological half-life of cadmium, estimated at between 25 and 30 years in humans (2). Following absorption, the prominent route of cadmium elimination occurs via the urine; therefore, it is felt that urinary cadmium is a reflection of body burden (1, 2). After the onset of cadmium-induced nephropathy, there is a marked increase of urinary cadmium in the form of cadmium-metallothionein complex (2). Otherwise cadmium is eliminated unchanged.

Approximately 95% of ingested cadmium will be eliminated in the feces due to the poor level of cadmium absorption from the gastrointestinal tract. Thus fecal cadmium consists almost exclusively of unabsorbed cadmium. Although some cadmium that had been absorbed into the mucosa may be added to fecal cadmium through mucosal turnover, this would represent a very small portion of the total fecal content (13). In sufficient quantities oral cadmium is a very powerful emetic, and this too could be considered a form of elimination of unabsorbed cadmium.

SIGNS, SYMPTOMS, AND SYNDROMES FROM CADMIUM EXPOSURE

Acute Toxicity

ROUTES OF EXPOSURE AND TARGET ORGANS

Acute intoxication with cadmium can occur from either ingestion or inhalation. Such intoxication does, however, require relatively high concentrations. Acute cadmium exposure is typically most toxic to the tissue to which it is initially exposed, i.e., the lung (from inhalation) and gastrointestinal tract (from ingestion). Renal and hepatic involvement, however, can occur from either route of cadmium exposure.

ORAL EXPOSURE

Typical symptoms of oral intoxication with cadmium include nausea, vomiting, abdominal cramping and pain, diarrhea, increased salivation, tenesmus, and choking. Cadmium is also a very powerful emetic. Depending on the level of consumption, recovery from a single oral exposure can be rapid and apparently without longterm effects. This has been reported where intoxication occurred from consumption of contaminated drinks containing up to 16 mg of cadmium per liter (25). However, death has occurred with higher doses (25 mg of cadmium per kg body weight) (26). In addition to the above symptoms, hemorrhagic gastroenteritis, hepatic and renal (particularly cortical) necrosis, cardiomyopathy, and metabolic acidosis have been associated with high oral cadmium exposure (2, 26).

INHALATION EXPOSURE

Exposure to high levels of cadmium fumes by inhalation can also lead to intoxication (27–29). Signs and symptoms of acute cadmium poisoning following inhalation include (in order of frequency) nasopharyngeal irritation, chest pain, headache, dizziness, cough, dyspnea, vomiting, nausea, chills, weakness, and diarrhea (27). Sustained hyperpyrexia can occur in severe exposure cases and is typically associated with a poor prognosis (27). These symptoms are essentially those suggestive of metal fume fever. An antemortem diagnosis of cadmium intoxication rests on obtaining a knowledge of the conditions and agent (if possible) of exposure (28). An unpleasant metallic taste in the mouth, which is enhanced by cigarette smoking, occasionally occurs in exposed workers during or immediately following exposure (27). Cadmium fume pneumonitis is frequently accompanied by a pulmonary edema (occasionally hemorrhagic) of noncardiac origin (27). It is estimated that fully 20% of all cases of cadmium-induced chemical pneumonitis are fatal due to fulminant interstitial pulmonary edema (27, 28). Hepatic necrosis and bilateral renal cortical necrosis also occur in severe exposure cases (2, 29). Later pulmonary fibrosis can develop and result in a persistent restrictive ventilatory defect (27).

Chronic Toxicity of Cadmium

TARGET ORGANS AND SYSTEMS

The chronic toxic (noncarcinogenic) effects most clearly associated with cadmium exposure occur in the pulmonary system and in the kidney. Pulmonary system effects are exclusively associated with inhalation exposure, while renal effects appear after oral or inhalation exposures. Secondarily, chronic cadmium exposure has been associated with skeletal system toxicity, hypertension, and cardiovascular disease and carcinogenesis in the lung, prostate, kidney, and stomach, although these associations are less well established.

Pulmonary Effects   The chronic pulmonary effects of cadmium in humans typically are manifested as an obstructive lung disease (1, 2). A significant increase in deaths caused by respiratory disease in cadmium-exposed workers has been seen repeatedly in epidemiological studies (1, 2, 4, 5). The disease state results from a chronic bronchitis, progressive fibrosis of the lower airways, and alveolar damage resulting in emphysema (4). Pulmonary physiological assessment indicates a reduced vital capacity and an increased residual volume (4). Dyspnea is also a common complaint. The level of obstructive disease appears to be related to the duration and level of cadmium exposure (1, 2).

Less frequently, lung cancer has been associated with chronic cadmium inhalation, although not all epidemiologic studies have seen such an association (4, 5). Such studies are frequently complicated by such factors as concurrent exposure to metals other than cadmium and cigarette smoking. However, the recent production of malignant pulmonary tumors (adenocarcinomas) in rodents chronically exposed to cadmium via inhalation supports the available human data (5, 30).

Renal Effects   The chronic renal effects of cadmium are characterized by proximal tubular necrosis and dysfunction and can occur following chronic oral or inhalation exposure (1, 2). The manifestations of cadmium-induced nephropathy include low-molecular weight proteinuria, aminoaciduria, and glucosuria and are frequently accompanied by increased cadmium in the urine (1, 2). The lesions are most pronounced in the renal cortex. Cadmium complexed with metallothionein may be the exact etiologic agent (see section on metabolism above).

Nephropathy is thought to occur when the renal cortical cadmium concentration exceeds a "critical" level of 200 μg/g (2). The average level of cadmium in the renal cortex in nonoccupationally exposed individuals is approximately 15–30 μg at age 50; however, levels in nonpolluted areas of Japan range from 50–125 μg/g tissue (6). Cigarette smoking can double renal cortical cadmium concentration (6). Thus, even in the general population of nonoccupationally exposed individuals, a very small margin of safety exists for cadmium exposure and nephropathy.

The proteinuria induced by chronic cadmium exposure is characterized by low-molecular weight proteins that would normally be reabsorbed in the proximal tubular elements (1, 2). The most prominent protein found is β_2-microglobulin. Several other low-molecular weight proteins are present including retinol-binding protein and lysozyme (1, 2). Higher molecular weight proteins, such as albumin, indicative of glomerular effects in cadmium exposed workers are also occasionally present (31). The renal effects of cadmium are not exclusively seen in workers who have been exposed occupationally, and a low molecular weight proteinuria in the general population has been seen with environmental exposure to cadmium (32).

A single study has associated occupational cadmium exposure with renal cancer (23). This, however, has not been confirmed by other studies in human populations or in rodent

testing. Exposure to multiple agents of which cadmium was but one may have been an important factor in development of renal carcinogenesis (33).

Skeletal System   Cadmium intoxication can have dramatic effects on calcium homeostasis and metabolism and can increase calcium excretion. Osteomalacia and osteoporosis accompanied by bone pain are part of the syndrome, termed "Itai-Itai" (translated ouch-ouch) disease, that appears to have resulted from cadmium intoxication in a group of Japanese women in the 1940s (1, 2). The victims were typically postmenopausal and multiparous and presented with severe bone deformities and chronic nephropathy (1, 2). Beyond cadmium exposure, it is thought that nutritional deficiencies, particularly vitamin D deficiency, may also have contributed to this syndrome (1, 2).

Cardiovascular Disease   Hypertension following chronic cadmium exposure has been shown in rodent models (1, 2). The mechanism of this effect is unknown and could be linked to renal, cardiac, or direct vasoconstrictive effect of cadmium. In humans an increased rate of mortality from cerebrovascular disease has been detected in populations from cadmium polluted areas with cadmium-induced nephropathy (34).

Carcinogenesis and Teratogenesis   In several epidemiological studies cadmium exposure in the work place has been linked to carcinogenesis in various tissues including the lung, prostate, kidney, and stomach (4–6). One study has indicated an association between cadmium levels in the drinking water and prostatic cancer (35). Several epidemiologic studies are, however, negative in associating cadmium with human carcinogenesis (4–6). Evidence in animals indicates that cadmium can be a very potent carcinogen, and tumors of the lung (30), prostate, testes, and injection site (36, 37) are induced in rats and mice by cadmium injection.

Teratogenic effects of cadmium have not been observed in humans. Cadmium has been shown to be a potent teratogen in animal models. Its teratogenic effects mimic those produced by zinc deficiency.

Management of Toxicity

CLINICAL EXAMINATION

Signs and symptoms of cadmium intoxication depend on the route of exposure. Local irritation is one of the major signs of acute cadmium toxicity, whether it be irritation of the gastrointestinal tract following oral exposure or irritation of the respiratory system after inhalation.

Acute cadmium inhalation may cause irritation of the upper respiratory system, chest pains, nausea, and dizziness. In cases of excessive inhalation of cadmium fumes (usually cadmium oxide) and dusts, severe signs may develop such as loss of ventilatory capacity with a corresponding increase in residual lung volume, fatal pulmonary edema, or residual emphysema with peribronchial and perivascular fibrosis (38). Dyspnea is the most frequent complaint of patients with cadmium-induced lung disease.

In the case of acute intoxication after oral exposure, symptoms usually include some signs of irritation of the gastrointestinal tract, including nausea, vomiting, excessive salivation, diarrhea, and abdominal cramping. Death can result from hemorrhagic gastroenteritis (26). Acute high dose oral ingestion may also be accompanied by signs of liver and kidney damage, hypoproteinemia with hypoalbuminemia, and metabolic acidosis (26). Renal tubular dysfunction can occur following either chronic pulmonary or gastrointestinal exposure to the metal (1, 2). In fact renal dysfunction can occur long after withdrawal of cadmium exposure. A low molecular weight proteinuria indicative of proximal tubular damage is the hallmark of cadmium-induced renal dysfunction.

In advanced cases of cadmium intoxication secondary manifestations including severe osteoporosis and osteomalacia have occurred. This form of cadmium intoxication has been seen industrially after inhalation of cadmium and after longterm ingestion of contaminated food. Cadmium-induced bone diseases occur mainly at the later stages of cadmium poisoning. The patients are likely to have had kidney disease before the bone damage occurs. The diagnosis of osteoporosis and/or osteomalacia is based on blood analysis of calcium, phosphate, and alkaline phosphate and on x-ray of the skeleton, particularly the long bones, pelvis, and ribs (3). Severe bone pain is also common. Cadmium-induced bone loss is more frequently seen in postmenopausal women who have had multiple pregnancies.

TREATMENT

There are no clear data to support use of chelation therapy in humans as an effective means of therapeutic intervention in acute cadmium intoxication. However, it has been suggested that treatment with calcium disodium ethylenediaminetetraacetic acid ($CaNa_2EDTA$) may be effective when administered immediately after exposure to cadmium (39), as such treatment increases the urinary excretion of cadmium in rodents. The suggested dosage of $CaNa_2EDTA$ is 75 mg/kg/day in three to six divided doses for 5 days, and the total dose of $CaNa_2EDTA$ per 5-day course should not exceed 500 mg/kg (40). A second 5-day course may be given after at least 2 days without treatment following the first regimen (40). Standard precautions in the use of chelation therapy should be observed, and urinary cadmium content should be monitored.

In chronic exposure, the effectiveness of chelation therapy for cadmium poisonings is questionable. This is due to the long half-life of cadmium in humans (25–30 years) resulting from the ability of cadmium to induce and bind to metallothionein (41). It is thought that once metallothionein is synthesized in large amounts (24–48 hr after exposure), chelation will be ineffective. Experimental studies on animals have shown that the time period following cadmium exposure plays an important role in chelation therapy. As an alternative, to alleviate the problem of sites inaccessible to most chelators, a combination chelation therapy employing a water-soluble and lipid-soluble combination, namely 2,3-dimercaptopropanol (BAL) and diethylenetriamine pentaacetic acid (DTPA) (42), was used. In general, chelation therapy may be effective if the chelator is given very shortly after cadmium exposure, as there is a rapid decrease in the effectiveness of such therapy with increasing time following cadmium exposure. This is probably due to distribution of the metal to sites that are not reached by the chelators (43) as well as increased synthesis of the high affinity cadmium-binding protein metallothionein. Therefore, chelation therapy must take place as soon as possible after cadmium exposure.

In cases of Itai-Itai disease and some other cases of cadmium exposure, vitamin D was given to patients in large doses for long periods of time (months). This was primarily palliative therapy to alleviate some of the painful symptoms

due to bone loss (2, 44). An example of the dosage that was used is 100,000 IU of vitamin D_2 orally every day for 10 days (44). After discontinuation for 10 days, similar doses of vitamin D_2 were given again for 10 days. In addition, 300,000 IU of vitamin D_2 or vitamin D_3 were given eight times a year by intamuscular injection. Anabolic steroid was also given orally and intramuscularly. Total doses of vitamin D which were given for about 1 year were 14,000,000 IU of vitamin D_2, and 2,100,000 IU of vitamin D_3 parenterally (44). Treatment with large doses of vitamin D and anabolic steroids by oral and parenteral administration resulted in gradual clinical improvement. Thus, in cases of bone disease, treatment with calcium and vitamin D or its metabolite (Kalcitriol) can be helpful in restoration of bone function.

LABORATORY DIAGNOSIS

Among the critical target organs in cadmium exposure the most sensitive are the kidneys (45). Renal dysfunction is a common sign of cadmium toxicity due to accumulation of cadmium in the renal cortex (1–3). The concentration of cadmium in blood and urine may reflect the cadmium level in the whole body and predict the level of renal dysfunction. Renal function can be evaluated by determinating levels of urinary albumin, creatinine, β_2-microglobulin, and total protein.

The main biochemical finding in cadmium toxicity is proteinuria as a result of renal damage. It has been postulated that the proteinuria results from cadmium transport to proximal tubules by metallothionein (23, 24). The best indicator of cadmium-induced nephropathy appears to be β_2-microglobulin (1, 2). Recent attention has been given to studies of urinary levels of retinol-binding proteins as an indicator of cadmium exposure. The determination of retinol-binding proteins has certain advantages over that of β_2-microglobulin, as there is no interference from the pH of the urine (44).

In cases of Itai-Itai disease, radiographic examination of bone, particularly radius, ulna, femur, and humerus should be performed, especially if the patient suffers from generalized pain and deformities of the lower extremities (44).

SPECIAL DIAGNOSTIC TESTS

Specific diagnostic tests for detection of cadmium intoxication are essentially not available. Proteinuria and glycosuria appear to be the most common with renal disease due to industrial cadmium exposure. In addition, measurement of hypercalciuria, aminoaciduria, increased uric acid excretion with hypouricemia, and hypertension (1–3) have been used. Neutron capture γ-ray analysis using transportable measurement systems have been used to evaluate the amount of the metal that has been accumulated in liver and kidneys of workers employed in cadmium smelter plants (46, 47). However, this method is limited by its level of detection (48). It has been suggested that the critical level of cadmium in renal cortex may range from 215–390 μg/l (45, 48). Measurement of levels of metallothionein in urine has been recently proposed as a specific finding indicative of cadmium nephropathy and may prove of value in diagnosis of exposure to cadmium (49).

BIOLOGIC MONITORING

Monitoring of cadmium exposure in humans has generally involved the assessment of cadmium levels in the blood or urine.

It is thought that urinary cadmium does provide a good index of excessive cadmium exposure (1, 2). Blood concentrations of cadmium in nonexposed individuals are less than 10 μg/l. Cadmium in blood is more than 70% inside the red blood cell (49). In vivo neutron activation analysis has also been used to determine tissue burdens of cadmium, particularly in the liver and kidney, although this would not be sensitive enough to determine levels in the general population (1, 49). In the assessment of cadmium-induced nephropathy urinary levels of β_2-microglobulin are frequently used, although this is nonspecific and is rather a general indicator of renal dysfunction (49). Furthermore, urinary levels of β_2-microglobulin are only increased after the onset of renal pathology, and hence are not predictive. Blood cadmium concentrations in symptomatic workers with pulmonary and renal toxicity have varied between 18–73 μg/l (49). To accurately measure β_2-microglobulin, the urine pH must be greater than 5.5. β_2-Microglobulin degrades rapidly in acidic urine. Recently it has been proposed that urinary metallothionein levels should be monitored to assess cadmium exposure as these levels correlate with cadmium tissue levels (as determined by neutron activation) better than urinary levels of β_2-microglobulin (50). The predictive value of metallothionein determination is as yet unknown; however, it is a more specific test.

ENVIRONMENTAL MONITORING

Environmental surveying with stationary samplers have helped establish levels of various metals, including cadmium, in work place air and in ambient air (3). However, more accurate assessment of individual exposures is obtained by the use of personal samplers (3). Caution should be used with respect to personal sampler data with cadmium, because personal habits can lead to an inaccurate assessment of environmental exposure. Such habits included cigarette smoking which can result in oral contacts with contaminated hands and/or cigarettes and can cause substantially increased exposure in a manner that would not be detected by personal monitors (3).

EXPOSURE LIMITS

Most countries have not set legal limits for the maximum daily intake of cadmium from food consumption. The World Health Organization has recommended that total intake in foodstuffs be limited to 400 to 500 μg of cadmium per week (2). The United States has set the maximum concentration of cadmium in any foodstuff at 1 mg/kg and Japan uses the same concentration for rice (2).

Threshold limit values (TLVs) for cadmium in the United States are set at 50 μg/m³ (2). The World Health Organization has proposed a "health-based" permissible level of 10 μg/m³ (2).

REFERENCES

1. Goyer RA. Toxic effects of metals. In: Doull J, Klaassen CD, Amdur MO, eds. Casarett and Doull's toxicology: the basic science of poisons. New York: Macmillan, 1986:582–635.
2. Friberg L, Elinder C-G, Kjellstrom T, Nordberg GF, eds. Cadmium and health. Cleveland: CRC Press, 1986.
3. Friberg L, Nordberg GF, Vouk VB, eds. Handbook on the toxicology of metals. Amsterdam: Elsevier, 1986.
4. Waalkes MP, Oberdorster G. Cadmium Carcinogenesis. In: Foulkes EC, ed. Metal carcinogenesis. Boca Raton: CRC Press, 1990.
5. Oberdorster G. Airborne cadmium and carcinogenesis of the respiratory tract. Scand J Work Environ Health 1986;12:523–537.
6. IARC. IARC monographs on the evaluation of carcinogenic risk of chemicals to man; cadmium, nickel, some epoxides, miscellaneous industrial chemicals and general considerations on volatile anesthetics. Vol. 11. Lyon: IARC, 1976.
7. Cotton FA, Wilkinson G. Advanced inorganic chemistry: a comprehensive text. 4th edition. New York: Wiley, 1980.
8. Fairbridge RW, ed. The encyclopedia of geochemistry and environmental sciences. Vol. IV A. New York: Van Nostrand-Reinhold, 1974.
9. Nebergall WH, Schmidt FC, Holtzclaw HF Jr. College chemistry with analytical analysis. 5th ed. Lexington: Heath & Co, 1976.
10. IARC. IARC monographs on the evaluation of carcinogenic risk of chemicals to man; some inorganic and organometallic compounds. Vol. 2. Lyon: IARC, 1973.
11. Baker EL, Coleman C, Peterson WA, Landrigan PL, Holtz JL. Subacute cadmium intoxication in jewelry workers: an evaluation of diagnostic procedures. Arch Environ Health 1979;34:173–177.
12. Garry VF, Pohlman BL, Wick MR, Garvey JS, Zeisler R. Chronic cadmium intoxication: tissue response in an occupationally exposed patient. Am J Ind Med 1986;10:153–161.
13. Shaikh ZA, Smith JC. Metabolism of ingested cadmium in humans. In: Holmstedt B, Lauwerys R, Mecier M, Roberfroid M, eds. Mechanisms of toxicity and hazard evaluation. Amsterdam: Elsevier, 1980:569–574.
14. Klaassen CD. Pharmacokinetics in metal toxicity. Fundam Appl Toxicol 1981;1:353–357.
15. Kuhnert PM, Kuhnert BR, Bottoms SF, Erhard P. Cadmium levels in maternal blood, fetal cord blood, and placental tissues of pregnant women who smoke. Am J Obstet Gynecol 1982;142:1021–1025.
16. Waalkes MP, Klaassen CD. Concentration of metallothionein in major organs of rats after administration of various metals. Fundam Appl Toxicol 1985;5:473–477.
17. Gunn SA, Gould TC, Anderson WAD. Effect of zinc on cancerogenesis by cadmium. Proc Soc Exp Biol Med 1964;115:653–657.
18. Gunn SA, Gould TC, Anderson WAD. Specificity in protection against lethality and testicular toxicity from cadmium. Proc Soc Exp Biol Med 1968;128:591–595.
19. Waalkes MP, Poirier LA. Interactions of cadmium with interstitial tissue of the rat testes; uptake of cadmium by isolated interstitial cells. Biochem Pharmacol 1985;34:2513–2518.
20. Stacey NH, Klaassen CD. Cadmium uptake by isolated rat hepatocytes. Toxicol Appl Pharmacol 1980;55:448–455.
21. Failla ML, Cousins RJ, Mascenik MJ. Cadmium accumulation and metabolism by rat liver parenchymal cells in primary monolayer culture. Biochim Biophys Acta 1979;538:63–72.
22. Waalkes MP. Effects of dietary zinc deficiency on the accumulation of cadmium and metallothionein in selected tissues of the rat. J Toxicol Environ Health 1986;18:301–313.
23. Cherian MG, Goyer RA, Delaquerriere-Richardson L. Cadmium-metallothionein-induced nephropathy. Toxicol Appl Pharmacol 1976;38:399–404.
24. Dudley RE, Gammal LM, Klaassen CD. Cadmium-induced hepatic and renal injury in chronically exposed rats: likely role of hepatic cadmium-metallothionein in nephrotoxicity. Toxicol Appl Pharmacol 1985;77:414–426.
25. Nordberg GF. Cadmium metabolism and toxicity. Environ Physiol Biochem 1972;2:7–36.
26. Wiśniewska-Knypl JM, Jablońska J, Myślak Z. Binding of cadmium on metallothionein in man: an analysis of a fetal poisoning by cadmium iodide. Arch Toxicol 1971;28:46–55.
27. Dunphy B. Acute occupational cadmium poisoning: a critical review of the literature. J Occup Med 1967;9:22–26.
28. Barnhart S, Rosenstock L. Cadmium chemical pneumonitis. Chest 1984;86:789–791.
29. Patwardhan JR, Finckh ES. Fatal cadmium-fume pneumonitis. Med J Aust 1976;1:962–966.
30. Takenaka S, Oldiges H, Konig, Hochrainer D, Oberdorster G. Carcinogenicity of cadmium aerosols in Wistar rats. J Natl Cancer Inst 1983;70:367–373.
31. Bernard A, Roels H, Hubermont G, Buchet JP, Masson PL, Lauwerys RR. Int Arch Occup Environ Health 1976;38:19–30.
32. Shigamatsu I. Epidemiological studies on cadmium pollution in Japan. Proceedings of the First International Cadmium Conference. London: San Francisco Metal Bulletin, 1978.
33. Kolonel LN. Association of cadmium with renal cancer. Cancer 1976;37:1782–1787.
34. Nogawa K, Kobayashi, Honda R. A study of the relationship between cadmium concentrations in urine and renal effects of cadmium. Environ Health Perspect 1979;28:161–168.

35. Bako G, Smith ESO, Hanson J, Dewar R. The geographical distribution of high cadmium concentrations in the environment and prostate cancer in Alberta. Can J Public Health 1982;73:92–94.

36. Waalkes MP, Rehm S, Riggs CW, et al. Cadmium carcinogenesis in the male Wistar [Crl:(WI)BR] rats: dose-response analysis of tumor induction in the prostate and testes and at the injection site. Cancer Res 1988;48:4656–4663.

37. Waalkes MP, Rehm S, Riggs CW, et al. Cadmium carcinogenesis in the male Wistar [Crl:(WI)BR] rats: dose-response analysis of effects of zinc on tumor induction in the prostate and in the testes and at the injection site. Cancer Res 1989;49:4282–4288.

38. Zavon MR, Meadow CD. Vascular sequelae to cadmium fume exposure. Am Ind Hyg Assoc J 1970;31:180–182.

39. Cantilena LR, Klaassen CD. Decreased effectiveness of chelation therapy for Cd poisoning with time. Toxicol Appl Pharmacol 1982;63:173–180.

40. Klaassen CD. Heavy metals and heavy-metal antagonists. In: Gilman AG, Goodman LS, Rall TW, and Murad F, eds. Goodman and Gilman's the pharmacological basis of therapeutics. 7th ed. New York: Macmillan, 1986:1605–1627.

41. Vallee BL. Historical review and perspectives. In: Kagi JHR, Nordberg M, eds. Metallothionein. Experientia Suppl 1979;34:19–40.

42. Cherian MG, Rodgers K. Chelation of cadmium from metallothionein in vivo and its excretion in rats repeatedly injected with cadmium chloride. J Pharmacol Exp Ther 1982;222:699–704.

43. Waalkes MP, Watkins JB, Klaassen CD. Minimal role of metallothionein in decreased chelator efficacy for cadmium. Toxicol Appl Pharmacol 1983;68:392–398.

44. Nogawa K, Ishizaki A, Fukushima M. Studies on the women with acquired Fanconi syndrome observed in the Ichi River Basin polluted by cadmium. Environ Res 1975;10:280–307.

45. Roels H, Lauwerys R, Buchet JP, et al. In vivo measurement of liver and kidney cadmium in workers exposed to this metal: its significance with respect to cadmium in blood and urine. Environ Res 1981;26:217–240.

46. Al-Haddad IK, Chettle DR, Fletcher JG, Fremlin JH. A transportable system for measurement of kidney cadmium in vivo. Int J Appl Rad Isot 1981;32:109–112.

47. Thomas BJ, Harvey TC, Chettle DR, McLellan JS, Fremlin JH. A transportable system for the measurement of liver cadmium in vivo. Phys Med Biol 1979;24:432–437.

48. Roels H, Lauwerys R, Dardenne AN. The critical level of cadmium in human renal cortex: a reevaluation. Toxicol Lett 1983;15:357–360.

49. Carson B, Ellis H, McCann J. Toxicology and biological monitoring of metals in humans. Chelsea, MI: Lewis Publishers, 1987.

50. Tohyama C, Shaikh ZA, Nogawa K, Kobayashi E, Honda R. Elevated urinary excretion of metallothionein due to environmental cadmium exposure. Toxicology 1981;20:289–297.

78

Cobalt

Douglas M. Templeton, M.D.

PROPERTIES, SOURCES AND BIOLOGIC IMPORTANCE

Chemical Properties

Cobalt is a hard, bluish-white metal (atomic number 27, atomic weight 58.9332) of the first transition series. It has melting and boiling points of 1495°C and 2870°C, respectively, although some variation in the reported values results from the sluggish interconversion of two coexisting allotropes, designated α and β (1). Cobalt-59 is the single naturally occurring isotope; ^{60}Co is a γ-emitter of medical and technologic importance, having a half-life of 5.27 years. One of four ferromagnetic elements (the others being Fe, Ni, and Gd), Co has the highest Curie point (1131°C). Cobalt forms salts and compounds in oxidation states +2 and +3 (d^7 and d^6, respectively). In aqueous solution, reduction of $[Co(H_2O)_6]^{3+}$ to the cobaltous ion is favored by 1.84 V, although some ligands, notably NH_3, stabilize Co(III) in octahedral coordination.

Occurrence

Cobalt is the 30th most abundant element in the earth's crust, present on the average at 25 ppm (2). In nature, Co usually occurs with nickel (e.g., as the cobalt-nickel arsenide, smaltite) and often also with arsenic as $CoAs_2$, CoAsS (cobaltite), and $Co_3(AsO_4)_2 \cdot 8H_2O$ (erythrite). Most Co is recovered from deposits of copper, copper-nickel, or nickel ores. The copper/cobalt ore bodies of Zambia and Zaire are the major source of the world's Co, together accounting for more than one third of known Co resources. Zaire alone has about one half of the world's reserves which are presently extractable on an economic basis and supplies about half of the world's annual output (3). In these ores, Co occurs mainly as its sulfides and oxides. After roasting to water-soluble sulfate, it is leached and recovered by electrolysis. In the copper/nickel/iron sulfide deposits of the Soviet Union, Canada, and Australia, together accounting for about 20% of world production, Co frequently substitutes for Ni in numerous minerals.

The most important water-soluble salts are of the cobaltous ion, and include $CoCl_2 \cdot 6H_2O$, $Co(NO_3)_2 \cdot 6H_2O$, and $CoSO_4 \cdot 7H_2O$. The oxides and hydroxide [CoO, Co_2O_3, Co_3O_4, and $Co(OH)_2$], carbonate ($CoCO_3$), and sulfides (CoS, CoS_2, Co_2S_3, and Co_3S_7) are water-insoluble. A number of organic salts are also encountered in industry, including cobalt stearate, oleate, linoleate, resinate, and naphthenate. The Co carbonyls, used in preparation of high purity metal and as catalysts in olefin oxidations (4), are the most toxic forms of the element. The carbonyls $[Co(CO)_4]_2$ and $[Co(CO)_4]_3$ are low-melting solids, $Co(CO)_3NO$ is a liquid, and $HCo(CO)_4$ is a gas with high vapor pressure.

Biochemistry

Vitamin B_{12} (cyanocobalamin) is an organometallic tetrapyrrole having Co(III) coordinated by four nitrogen atoms of the corrin ring, by an intramolecular benzimidazole, and with an exchangeable CN in the final axial position. It is the only form of Co known to be biologically active in higher animals. It accounts for 10–20% of the element present in the body (5). In humans, vitamin B_{12} is required as a cofactor for the conversion of methylmalonic acid to succinic acid and in the synthesis of methionine. In the first reaction, deoxyadenosylcobalamin is the cofactor for methylmalonyl CoA mutase in the synthesis of succinyl CoA from methylmalonyl CoA. This reaction is important in the metabolism of fatty acids and aliphatic amino acids, and vitamin B_{12} deficiency leads to accumulation of abnormal lipids. In methionine synthesis, methylcobalamin is an intermediate in the methyl group transfer from N^5-methyltetrahydrofolate to homocysteine. Methionine-derived formate is necessary for purine metabolism and the production of folate, while S-adenosylmethionine plays a role in neuronal metabolism. These factors may account for the occurrence of megaloblastic anemia and neuropathy in vitamin B_{12} deficiency (6).

USES AND EXPOSURES

Uses

Approximately 80% of Co used worldwide is in metallic form, in one of several types of alloys, while the remainder is used as salts and compounds (4, 7). The special properties of the different classes of alloys suit them to specific end uses and in turn determine the major sources of industrial exposure. Since alloys are composite materials, exposures are seldom singular; multiple exposures to potentially toxic elements have somewhat hampered documentation of the effects of Co in the workplace.

In terms of absolute quantity, by far the most important use of Co is in production of the high temperature, so-called superalloys. These generally contain up to 60% Co, with 15–20% chromium (Cr), nickel (Ni), or tungsten (W). The stability of these alloys at high temperatures renders them invaluable in the fabrication of gas turbine engines and particularly in jet engines for aircraft, where higher operating temperatures enhance aircraft performance. Such alloys account for 35% of U.S. Co consumption, and the aircraft industry alone consumes 35% of end-use Co, amounting to 3.8 million pounds annually according to 1982 figures (3). The corrosion- and abrasion-resistant alloys, including stainless steels, Stellites (60% Co, 30% Cr, and lesser amounts of tungsten and carbon), and Tribaloy [50–60% Co, 30% molybdenum (Mo), with chromium (Cr) and silicon (Si)] are also important (8). These materials find general use in the manufacture of machine tools and construction equipment. Vitallium (65% Co, 30% Cr, and 5% Mo) is used for surgical and dental implants, due to its nonirritant nature and resistance to attack by biologic fluids (4).

Cobalt serves as the binder in cementing tungsten carbide and other metal carbides. The resulting wear-resistant "hard metal" accounts for about 10% of U.S. consumption. The nature of its fabrication process, as well as its end uses in mining equipment and industrial drilling and cutting tools, gives rise to an important constellation of signs and symptoms in exposed workers.

The ferromagnetic properties of Co are exploited in production of some of the best permanent magnets, for example the Alnico magnets, which combine Co with lesser amounts of aluminum (Al), Ni, and iron (Fe). Magnet steel is about 35% Co and may contain W and Cr. The soft magnets, such as Perminvar and Permendur, are also cobalt-based (8). These find a major use in the electronics industry, particularly in the manufacture of radio and television communications equipment (3).

Cobalt salts and compounds, generally supported on alumina, serve as important heterogeneous hydrogenation catalysts in a number of industrial processes. Organic complexes (linoleates, naphthenates, and resins) are used as drying agents in paints, varnishes, and inks and as bonding agents between rubber and metals or textiles, for example in tires. The color change from blue to pink upon hydration of many Co salts provides an indicator for use in desiccants. Addition of less than 2 ppm of cobalt oxide to glass masks the yellow tinge imparted by the presence of traces of iron oxides, while larger amounts produce a blue coloration in glass and ceramics (9). Additions of up to 0.5% provide the absorptive effect of welders' goggles. Mixtures of CoO with other oxides produce pigments ranging in color from blue, green, and violet to pink and brown, while $K_3Co(NO_2)_6$-based paints are yellow (8). Considering drying agents and pigments, the paint industries consume over two million pounds (about 20%) of Co annually in the United States. Cobalt sulfate is sometimes added to nickel plating baths to improve the surface characteristics of the deposit. The use of $CoSO_4$ or $CoCl_2$ as foam stabilizers in the brewing industry has been discontinued due to its toxicity (see below), and the use $CoCl_2$ in treating anemias has diminished. However, small amounts of $CoCl_2$ are added to livestock feeds, salt licks, and fertilizers in regions where the soil is deficient in Co. Vitamin B_{12} for medical purposes is extracted from animal livers or prepared microbiologically.

While the radiotoxicity of ^{60}Co is beyond the scope of this chapter, mention should be made of the important medical uses of the isotope as a source in the radiotherapy of cancer and for labeling vitamin B_{12} employed in the Schilling test. In addition, it is a source of γ-radiation for industrial sterilization.

Sources of Exposure

In terms of numbers of individuals exposed, greatest toxicologic importance can be attached to inhalation of Co fumes and cobalt-containing dusts and to skin sensitization from contact with cobalt-containing materials. Table 78.1 summarizes the potentially harmful exposures encountered in the major cobalt-related industries. Separation from ores and refining of Co, as well as secondary production (recycling) from discarded materials, presents a risk of inhalation of fumes. Milling of Co results in exposure to both dust and fumes from the electric furnace, and fumes from the molten Co prior to pelleting. Abrasion of polishing tools made of microdiamonds cemented in high purity (>99%) very fine Co has been associated with lung disease in exposed workers (10). These tools are used primarily in the diamond-finishing trade. Sites of production of compounds and salts and processing of CoO have also been investigated. In each of these industries, skin contact may contribute to or exacerbate sensitization in susceptible individuals.

The hard metal industry continues to be the subject of numerous studies on the occupational hazards of Co. Individuals involved in the grinding, presintering, and cutting phases of tungsten carbide production are exposed to cobalt-containing dusts, together with dusts of tungsten, titanium, and tantalum carbides, while the sintering and brazing processes produce fumes of high Co content (4). Final shaping and tool production result in further inhalational exposure to mixed dusts, while the abrasive nature of the dust appears to be a factor in sensitization from dermal exposure. In one recent study of the industry, exposed individuals included hard and soft grinders, shapers and machinists, and technical and clerical staff (11).

The potential for exposure in other end-use industries is highest in the paint, glass, ceramics, and rubber industries. When these environments are taken into account, more than one million workers in the United States are potentially exposed to Co in the workplace (7).

Toxicity from potential oral exposure in those handling cobalt-containing chemicals in a nonindustrial setting, for example, in artists using cobalt-based pigments or in those experiencing accidental exposure, has not to this author's knowledge been reported. Notorious incidences of ingestion of Co salts by heavy beer drinkers (12, 13) are not likely to be repeated, but serve as an important source of information on the toxic effects of oral Co salts in humans. The practice of therapeutic administration of $CoCl_2$ to patients with refractory anemia (14) seems largely to have been discontinued in the past decade. Appropriate administration of vitamin B_{12} carries no risk. Internal exposure to vitallium or stainless steel following surgical procedures has been associated with the development of skin sensitivity to Co, generally in combination with other metals (15).

TOXICOKINETICS

Uptake and Elimination

Questionable analyses of natural levels (see section on Biological Monitoring and Environmental Regulation) obscure the details of Co homeostasis. Individual daily intake probably varies widely, but is of the order of several hundred μg/day (4) or less (7), mostly from food. This includes both inorganic Co and vitamin B_{12}. Mean values of intake from balance studies reported by Schroeder et al. (16) are 300 μg/day from food and 6 μg/day from water, with outputs of 260, 40, and 6 μg/day in urine, feces, and sweat and hair, respectively. These widely quoted numbers should be scrutinized by current analytical methodologies, but may be of qualitative value. It is generally accepted that most of the daily intake is eliminated in the urine. Gastrointestinal absorption is dose dependent, but again the relationship is not clear. When ^{60}Co is given orally to humans as the chloride, absorption varies from 5% for 1 microgram of Co to 20% for 1.2 milligrams (17). However, Stokinger reports that oral doses of a few μg/kg are almost completely absorbed, the amount diminishing as dose increases (4). There is greater consensus regarding retention. Thirty percent of intravenous $^{60}CoCl_2$ was recovered in the first 24-hour urine collection following i.v. administration, with 9–16% retained for elimination with a half-life of at least 2 years (17). This slower phase of elimination is attributable to initial binding by plasma proteins. Similar whole body retention was observed following oral administration. In part, reported differences in absorption may be due to competition with other elements in

Table 78.1. Some Major Sources of Exposure to Cobalt and Its Compounds. The Widespread Use of Cobalt in Industrial Society Precludes an Exhaustive Listing (see References 4, 7, 20, and Specific Citations in This Chapter)

Activity	Cocontaining Compounds(s)	Significant Exposure
Occupation		
Metal production, refining	Co metal, fumes	Inhalation
	Carbonyls and hydrocarbonyl	
Chemical production	Co powder	Inhalation, dermal
	Soluble salts ($CoCl_2$, $CoSO_4$, ...)	
	Insoluble compounds (oxides, ...)	
Hard metal production	Co fumes, dusts	Inhalation,
	Cocontaining mixed dusts (e.g., tungsten carbide)	dermal, abrasion
Hard metal use (drilling, machining)	Mixed metal carbide dusts	Inhalation, dermal
Rubber industry (e.g., tire manufacture)	Organic Co salts	Dermal
Paint and varnish	Organic Co salts, soluble inorganic pigments	Dermal
Pottery	Co clay, soluble pigments	Dermal
Inks, offset printing	Organic Co salts	Dermal
Cement, construction	Soluble and insoluble compounds	Dermal
Diamond polishing	Co metal, powder	Inhalation, dermal
Dental technicians	Co alloys	Dermal
Nonoccupational		
Surgical implants	Co alloys	Internal
Dental prostheses	Co alloys	Oral, internal
Treatment of refractory anemia	$CoCl_2$	Oral
Metallic goods, jewelry, etc.	Co alloys	Dermal
Beer drinkers (formerly—see text)	Soluble Co salts	Oral

the gut. Iron and Co compete for absorption in perfused duodenum (18). Iron loading decreases Co uptake by isolated intestinal segments from the rat, while iron deficiency increases absorption (19). Evidence indicates that a pathway accounting for part of the total iron absorption is shared with Co, and perhaps several other trace elements (19). Diet also influences absorption. Cobalt binds to the sulfydryl groups of proteins and to amino acids, especially histidine. Protein-deficient diets may reduce binding in the gut and lead to greater absorption.

About 30% of inhaled inorganic Co is absorbed. Following occupational exposure, blood levels rise rapidly (20). Urinary excretion is again biphasic, with a rapid phase of about 2 days followed by a second phase of prolonged elimination (21). Significant exposures from air outside the workplace do not appear to have been documented; ecotoxicity is not a problem.

The recommended daily allowance of vitamin B_{12} is 3 micrograms, corresponding to 0.12 microgram of Co. The daily requirement is somewhat less, perhaps about 0.5 microgram of the vitamin (6). Typical daily intakes, mainly from red meat and dairy products are 5–45 micrograms (5, 20), and dietary deficiency is rare. Furthermore, the liver stores about 1 milligram of vitamin B_{12}, providing a reserve for several years. In healthy adults, about 70% of an oral dose of cobalamin is absorbed (20). This uptake requires the secretion of "intrinsic factor" (IF), a 50–60 kilodalton glycoprotein secreted by the gastric fundus. The absorption of the vitamin as its IF complex is mediated by specific receptors on the mucosal epithelium of the distal ileum. In the absence of IF, only about 2% of an oral dose of the vitamin is absorbed. Megaloblastic anemia resulting from vitamin B_{12} deficiency may be due to failure of the stomach to secrete IF (i.e. pernicious anemia), total gastrectomy, drug-related impairment of vitamin B_{12} absorption, or competition for the vitamin due to tapeworm infestation or bacterial overgrowth in the small intestine (22). The diagnosis of IF deficiency is made with the Schilling test. Labeled [^{60}Co]vitamin B_{12} is administered orally, while an excess of unlabeled material is given by intramuscular injection. The urinary excretion of ^{60}Co is then compared with and without oral co-administration of IF.

Distribution

The human body contains about 1 milligram of Co (5). Less than 0.2 milligram is stored in the form of vitamin B_{12}, mostly in liver (20). The remainder, in bones and soft tissues, is in inorganic form or bound to low molecular weight proteins. In plasma Co is mostly protein-bound to α_2-macroglobulin and albumin, the latter probably serving as the major transport form (5). Yamagata et al. (23) have reported a total body burden of 1.1 milligrams of the element, determined by neutron activation analysis. Of this, 14% is in bone, 43% in muscle, and the remainder in other soft tissues. After rats received ten daily subcutaneous injections of $CoCl_2$ (40 mg/kg), liver contained 11% of the administered dose, bone about 2.5%, and kidney, pancreas, spleen and blood together about 0.9% (14). Levels in body fluids are discussed below under Biologic Monitoring and Environmental Regulation.

Toxicity in Animals

ACUTE TOXICITY

Studies of the acute effects of administration to animals of metallic Co and its salts have been thoroughly summarized by Stokinger (4). The LD_{50} of metal powder administered i.v. or p.o. to small animals is about 100 mg/kg and 1.5 g/kg, respectively. In rodents, the value is 22–25 mg/kg for i.p. or intratracheal administration and has been reported as 112 mg/kg i.m. in the rat. For CoO, the LD_{50} is Co 1.7 g/kg in the rat, while following parenteral administration it is Co 135 mg/kg for rat and Co 800 mg/kg in the mouse. Other reported LD_{50}

values (with route of administration and species) are 5 g/kg (i.p., rat) for Co_2O_3, 1 g/m^2 (i.p., rat) for $CoCO_3$, Co 20 mg/kg (i.v., rat) and 165 mg/kg (percutaneous, guinea pig) for $CoCl_2$, 400 mg/kg (p.o., rabbit) for $Co(NO_3)_2$, and 54 mg/kg (i.p., mouse) for $CoSO_4$. Organic salts generally conform to these values. The LD_{50} of cobalt naphthenate is 3.9 g/kg (p.o.) in the rat, and of the lactate and albuminate Co approximately 10 mg/kg, parenterally, in rat and mouse.

Two patterns emerge: parenteral toxicity is greater than oral, and increased water solubility enhances toxicity. The former is explained by the fractional absorption of inorganic Co from the gastrointestinal tract, the latter by participation of cobaltous ion as the actively toxic species. In animal experiments, the LD_{50} of Co compounds is of the order of Co 10–20 mg/kg i.v., with oral toxicity about an order of magnitude lower (7). Oral toxicity in rats is decreased further when Co is administered with food, especially protein and the amino acid histidine (14).

Animals poisoned acutely with Co experience diarrhea and anorexia, and at higher doses albuminuria with anuria, vasodilation, hypotension, organ congestion, hemorrhages (especially in liver and the adrenals), hyperplastic marrow, alveolar thickening in lung, tubular degeneration in kidney, shrinkage of myocardial fibers, and pancreatic α-cell degeneration. The polycythemic dose of soluble Co salts in rats is about Co 40 mg/kg p.o. or 2.5 mg/kg parenterally. Intracheal administration of 150 mg of Co_3O_4 to guinea pigs showed no toxic effect, whereas a comparable dose of metallic Co resulted in pleural effusion, pneumonitis, and pericarditis.

Cobalt hydrocarbonyl and its decomposition products have a 30-minute LC_{50} for Co of about 165 mg/m^3 (24) and produce a chemical pneumonitis similar to that observed with $Ni(CO)_4$. Toxicity is less than with the nickel compound, however.

CHRONIC TOXICITY

Repetitive doses of Co metal or salts given to animals by various routes are often more toxic than a single dose, even when the latter is larger than the cumulative dose. This suggests cumulative toxicity. However, tolerance may also arise, the lethal dose increasing after multiple well-tolerated low level exposures. Effects of diet (greater toxicity results when Co is administered with milk) and counterion (greater tolerance is observed with Co citrate) must be considered. At 10 times the recommended human dose of $CoCl_2$, rats develop altered splenic architecture and hyperplastic bone marrow. Other toxic manifestations include thyroid hypofunction, degenerative changes in the myocardium, damage to pancreatic α-cells, hyperglycemia, abnormal liver function, renal tubular damage, deviations in lipid metabolism and hyperlipemia (elevations of triglycerides preceding those of cholesterol and free fatty acids), serum dysproteinemias, decreased platelet aggregation, and depressed heme synthesis (5, 20, 25).

Co inhalation by experimental animals for 3 years of 20 mg/m^3 as cobalt-containing mixed-metal carbide dust resulted in hyperplasia of the bronchial epithelium, focal pulmonary fibrosis, and granulomatous changes. Fumes of Co metal and oxides did not produce these changes after 2 years at Co levels of 1 mg/m^3. However, following 1 week of a sensitizing dose, miniswine showed decreased pulmonary compliance and increased collagen in alveolar septa after 3 months of daily exposure to 0.1 mg/m^3 of Co metal dust (26). This study was a factor in lowering of the Threshold Limit Values in several

countries. Chronic exposure to $HCo(CO)_4$ gives rise to biochemical and pathologic changes similar to those seen upon chronic inhalation of CoO.

MECHANISMS OF EXPERIMENTAL TOXICITY

Cobalt inhibits the decarboxylation of α-ketoacids by binding to dihydrolipoic acid, thus preventing conversion of pyruvate to acetyl CoA and blocking the tricarboxylic acid cycle (12, 14). The net result is a depression of oxidative phosphorylation. Inhibition of enzymes by binding of Co to sulfydryl groups may also contribute to disturbances in intermediary metabolism. These metabolic changes are probably responsible for the organ damage noted above. Lowering of the effective concentration of Ca ion in cytosol or mitochondria could lead to further electromechanical disturbances in the myocardium (12).

The effects of Co on lipid metabolism are complex and poorly understood. In addition to the involvement of vitamin B_{12} in relevant processes (see section on Biochemistry), inorganic Co decreases mitochondrial β-oxidation of long chain fatty acids (25) and inhibits lipoprotein lipase (14). The role of cobalt-induced pancreatic α-cell degranulation and glucagon release remains controversial (14).

The polycythemic effects of Co follow stimulation of erythropoietin release from kidney and give rise to an increased hematocrit and abnormal hemoglobin content in red cells (7). Erythropoietin release is apparently a result of depressed tissue respiration and renal hypoxia (14). Erythropoietin gene transcription begins in kidney nuclei 2–4 hr after subcutaneous injection of rats with 60 mg/kg $CoCl_2$ and parallels accumulation of the glycoprotein in plasma (27). Inhibition of δ-aminolevulinic acid synthetase by Co decreases hemes synthesis acutely (28), however, and lowers hepatic hemoproteins such as cytochrome P-450 (14). Interferences with platelet aggregation are probably mediated by fibrinogen outside the cell. Conformational changes in fibrinogen occur upon binding of Co (29). Abnormalities in plasma proteins include elevation of the α-globulin region, due in part to its constituents neuraminic acid (5) and α_1-antitrypsin (20).

Thyroid pathology occurs secondary to disturbances in iodine metabolism. Cobalt may decrease uptake of iodine by the thyroid (7) or may inhibit tyrosine iodinase (12), thereby reducing formation of thyroid hormone and causing excessive thyroid-stimulating hormone secretion.

Potential interactions with other trace elements are not well understood. The consequences of replacement of Zn by Co in some metalloproteins and of competition between Co and other essential elements for absorption in the gut are not known.

Toxicity in Humans

From the moderate toxicity demonstrated in acute animal experiments, it is to be expected that acute Co poisoning in humans seldom if ever occurs. Fatal intoxications have not been reported (7). In this section we will consider the toxic effects that have been observed in two human populations chronically exposed to Co salts, namely drinkers of cobalt-containing beer and those given $CoCl_2$ for therapeutic purposes. Both occurrences are of primarily historical interest and are described here for the light these inadvertent human "experiments" may shed on mechanisms of Co toxicity. Rare occurrences of human response to cobalt-containing implants are also described. To the medical practitioner and industrial hygienist, the importance of Co as a toxic agent is today confined almost exclusively to dermatitis and respiratory disease, which can occur following chronic inhalation and skin contact. More detailed description of these disorders is provided under Patterns and Management of Clinically Important Toxicity.

COBALT-BEER CARDIOMYOPATHY

In the 1960s, addition of Co salts to beer in concentrations of one or more ppm in Co was practiced in several local breweries in Canada, the United States, and Belgium (12, 13). The resulting Co ingestion of up to 10 mg/day by some heavy drinkers was associated with the development of an unusual cardiomyopathy. Elevated urinary Co excretion (up to 0.5 mg/day) was found in eight patients (30). Although blood levels were generally unavailable and the responsible beers were not analyzed (12), the absence of new cases after cessation of Co addition convincingly implicates the metal. Clinically, an abrupt onset of left-sided heart failure was followed by falling cardiac output, right-sided failure, cyanosis, hypotension, pericardial effusion, cardiomegaly, and cor pulmonale, with symptoms lasting from several days to more than 1 year. Electrocardiographic changes were present, with atrial flutter and fibrillation prominent. Myofiber hypertrophy or loss, accumulation of glycogen and connective tissue, and mitochondrial abnormalities were frequent findings on myocardial biopsy or autopsy. Mortality, 20–50% in the more seriously ill North American patients, was associated with cardiogenic shock and severe pyruvic and lactic acidoses, with arterial pH values as low as 6.9. Polycythemia was generally present. The severity of symptoms at an oral dose of less than 0.2 mg/kg/day may in part be due to altered nutritional status in the alcoholic and enhanced absorption of Co with a protein-deficient diet (12).

IATROGENIC Co TOXICITY

$CoCl_2$ Use for Refractory Anemia

Patients have been treated for refractory anemia with oral doses of Co of up to 37 mg/day as $CoCl_2$, for prolonged periods, with few adverse consequences. These amounts were sufficient to induce an erythropoietic response (14). Hypothyroidism and thyroid hyperplasia have been described in a pediatric population treated for sickle cell anemia with $CoCl_2$ (2.5 mg/kg/day) (31). Thyroid pathology was similarly noted in the cobalt-beer drinkers. Tolerance of these much higher doses of Co by many anemic patients, as compared with the alcoholics, may again relate to the poor nutritional status of the latter. The presence of ferrous sulfate in the pharmacologic preparation may also have competitively decreased the absorption of Co in the gut. However, the treatment is not without risk. Manifold et al. (32) describe a 17-year-old anephric girl with severe anemia persisting despite administration of iron and folate. She was given 25 milligrams $CoCl_2$ twice daily for 9 months, before dying in biventricular failure. At autopsy, gross cardiac enlargement was noted, with discrete patches of subepicardial necrosis, vacuolated fibers, and loss of striations. Neutron activation analysis found Co 8.9 µg/g dry weight in the myocardium, with a normal value said to be 0.2 µg/g.

Implantation of Cobalt-Containing Alloys

Tilsley and Rotstein (15) reported a case of painful exudative dermatitis over the site of implantation and a positive patch test for Co sensitivity in a patient who had 4 years earlier undergone tibial realignment with a vitallium plate. These authors describe two other cases of sensitivity after stainless steel implantation (one involving an exposed pacemaker lead) with patch tests positive for Co, Ni, and Cr. In addition to dermatologic manifestations, the sensitivity can produce bony necrosis and loosening of a prosthesis. Measurable release of Co from dental prostheses does not appear to increase significantly the daily oral intake of the element (33).

It has long been established that implantation of metallic Co into experimental animals can produce sarcomas at the site (34). In this regard Co differs little from a number of other metallic solids [e.g., Ni compounds (35)], and effects of local injury and irritation may be at least as important as biochemical interactions of slowly solubilized metal cations. At least 11 cases of local sarcomas occurring at the site of implantation of bone pins and plates have been reported in the human population (36). Here again interpretation is obscured by the multiplicity of exposure. Most implants would have contained nickel-cobalt-chromium alloys. Nickel (35, 37) and Cr(VI) (38) are well-established carcinogens and may account for these observations. However, participation of Co cannot be ruled out in view of its tumorigenic activity in experimental animals (34). No cancers at the sites of dental prostheses have been reported (39).

PATTERNS AND MANAGEMENT OF CLINICALLY IMPORTANT TOXICITY

Clinical Toxicity

RESPIRATORY DISEASE

Numerous studies have demonstrated an increased prevalence of respiratory pathology in hard metal workers. This may take the form of obstructive disease (occupational asthma or work-related wheezing) or interstitial lung disease (fibrosing alveolitis). In an American population of 290 tungsten carbide workers selected for long duration of exposure to high levels of cobalt-containing dust, obstructive disease was found in 5% of nonsmokers and interstitial infiltrates noted in 3.8% (40). A cross-sectional study of more than 1000 tungsten carbide workers at 22 sites identified work-related wheezing in 10.9% and a profusion of opacities on chest radiograms in 2.6% (11). Perhaps most significant, the relative odds of work-related wheeze was 2.1 when those with current workplace Co exposure exceeding 50 µg/m^3 were compared with those exposed to lower ambient concentrations, and the risk of profusion increased fivefold with average lifetime exposures above 100 µg/m^3. Exposure to Co alone is much more common than exposure to hard metal dust and gives rise to similar patterns of pathology (41). Diamond workers exposed to Co alone have developed a pattern of occupational asthma and fibrosing alveolitis termed "cobalt lung" (42, 43). These similarities have strengthened the argument for Co as the etiologic agent in hard metal dust.

The small percentage of exposed workers who develop interstitial lung disease and true occupational asthma has focused debate on the distinction between the sensitizing effects of Co and its direct cytotoxicity as causative. Compelling evidence for the importance of sensitization has recently appeared (44). Eight Japanese cases of confirmed occupational asthma related to hard metal dust were positive in inhalational provocation tests with nebulized aqueous $CoCl_2$. Specific IgE antibodies to a cobalt-human serum albumin complex were found in serum samples from four of these patients, but not in samples from 60 unexposed asthmatics or 25 nonasthmatic coworkers, and ^{57}Co was selectively bound by serum from seven (44).

Alternative nonimmune mechanisms may involve susceptibility of macrophages to activation by Co or reactivity of target cells to macrophage-derived mediators (10). Such processes probably underlie cobalt-induced interstitial lung disease. In this disorder, granulomatous change and lymphocytic infiltration, both characteristic of hypersensitivity pneumonitis, are seldom seen on biopsy (10), while the occurrence of unusual multinucleated giant cells is common (45). Clearly, the true mechanisms remain to be elucidated.

SKIN SENSITIVITY

Consistent with immunologic modes of action, allergic dermatitis has been reported in workers in numerous cobalt-related industries, including those in hard metal and Co alloy, paint, cement, and rubber industries (4, 46). An allergic dermatitis has been observed in Finnish potters handling Co clay (4). The dermatitis is of an erythematous maculopapular type (20) and is strongly associated with a history of eczema (47).

Management

Acute intoxication is rare and there has been little need for development of therapeutic modalities. Chelation with calcium-disodium EDTA has proven antidotal in experimental animals (4). Skin sensitivity with chronic exposure is treated as an allergic dermatitis and may occasionally require modification of work-related activities. When skin allergy is suspected, patch testing is performed with 1% of $CoCl_2$ in petrolatum. Testing for other sensitizing metals, such as nickel and chromate, should be included. When results are ambiguous, intradermal testing is helpful (48). When exposure to cobalt-containing dusts and fumes is frequent, annual medical evaluation, including a careful history of respiratory symptoms, chest x-ray, and lung function tests, is important for identifying the small population at risk for occupational asthma and interstitial lung disease. Blood samples should be drawn for erythrocyte count and hemoglobin content, plasma proteins, clotting times (evidence of decreased platelet aggregation), and serum lipids. Thyroid status should be carefully investigated by functional inquiry and physical examination. Any abnormalities require further evaluation by thyroid function tests, including ^{131}I concentrating capacity of the thyroid (5). Any evidence of systemic Co toxicity indicates careful monitoring of cardiac status on an ongoing basis. Prevention, with environmental monitoring and adherence to permissible exposures, is the most important aspect of management.

BIOLOGIC MONITORING AND ENVIRONMENTAL REGULATION

Reference Ranges and Monitoring

Reliable reference data for plasma Co concentration in healthy adults indicate a range of 0.1–0.2 ng/ml (49). This low level necessitates stringent control of contamination during sample collection, processing, and analysis. That values up to several orders of magnitude higher continue to be reported (50) indicates the difficulty of such control and the unreliability of many published data. Levels in erythrocytes are 1.5–2 times those in plasma (5). The scarcity of appropriate data limits the use of blood or serum levels for monitoring occupational exposure. Concentrations perhaps one order of magnitude higher in urine (5) render this fluid more amenable to analysis. Assessment of excretion is by no means routine, but urinary Co levels are the best and most accessible indicator of current exposure. In hard metal workers exposed to less than 100 $\mu g/m^3$, urinary Co was in the normal range at the beginning of the work week, and increased fourfold during the week (51). End-of-shift values on Monday correlated best with current exposure, those on Friday with past mean exposure. Levels of Co in blood and urine have been found to correlate with exposure and with each other, when hard metal workers were divided into 10 exposure groups and office workers were used as control subjects (52). Exposures varied from 28 ± 30 $\mu g/m^3$ for sintering workers to 367 ± 324 $\mu g/m^3$ for rubber press operators. Mean blood values taken during the shift were 18.7 ± 19.6 ng/ml for the rubber press operators, compared with 1.9 ± 1.1 ng/ml for the unexposed control subjects, while end-of-shift urine values for the two groups were 235 ± 182 and 2 ± 1 ng/ml, respectively. Based on such studies, monitoring of Co exposure by end-of-shift urine values can be recommended.

Analysis

The determination of Co in biologic and environmental matrices at the sub-ng/ml level is mainly by instrumental neutron activation analysis (INAA), electrothermal atomic absorption spectrometry (ETAAS), and voltammetry (7). A successful method for the determination of Co in plasma by inductively coupled plasma-mass spectrometry has recently been developed (Dr. Carlo Vandecasteele, personal communication). Other analytical techniques generally lack the required sensitivity or are subject to prohibitive interferences. INAA is generally the preferred method (53), the major drawbacks being the need for access to a nuclear reactor and the delay of about 1 month between irradiation and measurement. However, it is an excellent reference method for plasma (49) and has been used for Co analysis in a variety of body fluids, tissues, and foodstuffs. ETAAS offers detection limits of 0.004–1 ng/ml and the characteristic concentration is 0.03–1 ng/ml (53). Preconcentration is often employed; extraction has been achieved with methylisobutyl ketone, dithiocarbamates, nitroso- and pyridylazo-naphthols, tri-n-octylamine, and dithizone. Pyrolytically coated graphite tubes, high heating rates during atomization, and background correction are needed. Cobalt contamination from stainless steel blood collection and biopsy needles and from anticoagulant heparin solutions (53) is problematic. Deproteinization of serum and plasma samples can lead to underestimation of Co. Environmental monitoring of the workplace is usually achieved by deposition of dust on a filter, which is then ashed and analyzed by atomic absorption.

Exposure Limits

Threshold Limit Values (TLV) for metallic Co and Co dusts are 50 $\mu g/m^3$ in most countries. The U.S. value of 100 $\mu g/m^3$ is being revised downward to this standard. The corresponding values for Co carbonyls and hydrocarbonyl are 100 and 10 $\mu g/m^3$, respectively. It is important to note that numerous studies from Europe, Japan, and North America, in addition to those cited here, routinely document occupational exposures to Co exceeding 100 $\mu g/m^3$ for many workers. Standards for Co content of food and drinking water have not been established (7).

REFERENCES

1. Weast RC, ed. Handbook of chemistry and physics. 53rd ed. Cleveland: Chemical Rubber, 1972:B-11.

2. Klevay LM. Metals as nutritional factors. In: Brown SS, Kodama Y, eds. Toxicology of metals: clinical and experimental research. Chichester, UK: Ellis Horwood, 1987:5–18.

3. Blechman BM. National security and strategic minerals: an analysis of U.S. dependence on foreign sources of cobalt. Boulder, CO: Westview Press, 1985.

4. Stokinger H. Cobalt, Co. In: Clayton GD, Clayton FE, eds. Patty's industrial hygiene and toxicology, Vol 2a. 3rd ed. New York: John Wiley & Sons, 1981:1605–1619.

5. Tsalev DL, Zaprianov ZK. Atomic absorption spectrometry in occupational and environmental health practice, Vol I, analytical aspects and health significance. Boca Raton, FL: CRC Press, 1984:117–121.

6. Fairbanks VF, Klee GG. Biochemical aspects of hematology. In: Tietz NW, ed. Textbook of clinical chemistry. Philadelphia: WB Saunders, 1986:1495–1588.

7. Angerer J, Heinrich R. Cobalt. In: Seiler HG, Sigel H, eds. Handbook on toxicity of inorganic compounds. New York: Marcel Dekker, 1988:251–263.

8. Betteridge W. Cobalt and its alloys. Chichester, UK: Ellis Horwood, 1982.

9. Bamford CR. Colour generation and control in glass. Amsterdam: Elsevier, 1977.

10. Demedts M, Ceuppens JL. Respiratory disease from hard metal or cobalt exposure: solving the enigma. Chest 1989;95:2–3.

11. Sprince NL, Oliver LC, Eisen EA, Greene RE, Chamberlin RI. Cobalt exposure and lung disease in tungsten carbide production: A cross-sectional study of current workers. Am Rev Respir Dis 1988;138:1220–1226.

12. Alexander CS. Cobalt-beer cardiomyopathy: a clinical and pathologic study of twenty-eight cases. Am J Med 1972;53:395–417.

13. Morin Y, Daniel P. Quebec beer-drinkers' cardiomyopathy: etiological considerations. Can Med Assoc J 1967;97:926–928.

14. Taylor A, Marks V. Cobalt: a review. J Human Nutr 1978;32:165–177.

15. Tilsley DA, Rotstein H. Sensitivity caused by internal exposure to nickel, chrome and cobalt. Contact Dermatitis 1980;6:175–178.

16. Schroeder HA, Nason AP, Tipton IH. Essential trace metals in man: cobalt. J Chronic Dis 1967;20:869–890.

17. Smith T, Edmonds CJ, Barnaby CF. Absorption and retention of cobalt in man by whole-body counting. Health Physics 1972;22:359–367.

18. Thomson ABR, Valberg LS, Sinclair DG. Competitive nature of the intestinal transport mechanism for cobalt and iron in the rat. J Clin Invest 1971;50:2384–2394.

19. Barton JC, Conrad ME, Holland R. Iron, lead and cobalt absorption: Similarities and dissimilarities. Proc Soc Exp Biol Med 1981;166:64–69.

20. Elinder C-G, Friberg L. Cobalt. In: Friberg L, Nordberg GF, Vouk VB, eds. Handbook on the toxicology of metals, vol II. 2nd ed. Amsterdam: Elsevier, 1986:211–232.

21. Davison AG, Haslan PL, Corrin B, Coutts II, Dewar A, Riding WD, Studdy PR, Newman-Taylor AG. Interstitial lung disease and asthma in hard metal workers: bronchoalveolar lavage, ultrastructural, and analytical findings and results of broncheal provocation tests. Thorax 1983;38:119–128.

22. Wintrobe MM, Lee GR. Pernicious anemias and other megaloblastic anemias. In: Wintrobe MM, Thorn GW, Adams RD, Braunwald E, Isselbacher KJ, Petersdorf RG, eds. Harrison's principles of internal medicine. 7th ed. New York: McGraw-Hill, 1974:1585–1595.

23. Yamagata N, Murata S, Torii T. The cobalt content of the human body. J Radiat Res 1962;3:4–8.

24. Stokinger H. Metal carbonyls, $Me_x(CO)_y$. In: Clayton GD, Clayton FE, eds. Patty's industrial hygiene and toxicology, Vol 2a. 3rd ed. New York: John Wiley & Sons, 1981:1792–1807.

25. de Bruin A. Biochemical toxicology of environmental agents. Amsterdam: Elsevier North Holland, 1976.

26. Kerfoot EJ, Fredrick WG, Domeier E. Cobalt metal inhalation studies on miniature swine. Am Ind Hyg Assoc J 1975;36:17–25.

27. Schuster SJ, Badiavas EV, Costa-Giomi P, Weinmann R, Erslev AJ, Carao J. Stimulation of erythropoietin gene transcription during hypoxia and cobalt exposure. Blood 1989;73:13–16.

28. De Matteis F, Gibbs, AH. Inhibition of haem synthesis caused by cobalt in rat liver: evidence for two different sites of action. Biochem J 1977;162:213–216.

29. Smith AG, Smith AN. Effect of cobaltous chloride on aggregation of platelets from normal and afibrinogenemic human blood. Toxicol Lett 1984;23:349–352.

30. Sullivan JF, Egan JD, George RP. A distinctive myocardiopathy occurring in Omaha, Nebraska: clinical aspects. Ann NY Acad Sci 1969;156:526–543.

31. Gross RT, Kriss JP, Spalt TH. Haemopoietic and goitrogenic effects of $CoCl_2$ in patients with sickle cell anemia. Pediatrics 1955;15:284–290.

32. Manifold IH, Platts MM, Kennedy A. Cobalt cardiomyopathy in a patient on maintenance hemodialysis. Br Med J 1978;2:1609.

33. Stenberg T. Release of cobalt from cobalt chromium alloy constructions in the oral cavity of man. Scand J Dent Res 1982;90:472–479.

34. Heath JC. The production of malignant tumors by cobalt in the rat. Br J Cancer 1956;10:668–673.

35. Sunderman FW Jr. Recent research on nickel carcinogenesis. Environ Health Perspect 1981;40:131–141.

36. Waalkes MP, Rehm S, Kasprzak KS, Issaq HJ. Inflammatory, proliferative and neoplastic lesions at the site of metallic identification ear tags in Wistar [Crl:(WI)BR] rats. Cancer Res 1987;47:2445–2450.

37. Costa M, Heck JD. Perspectives on the mechanism of nickel carcinogenesis. Adv Inorg Biochem 1985;6:285–309.

38. Fan AM, Harding-Barlow I. Chromium. In: Fishbein L, Furst A, Mehlman MA, eds. Genotoxic and carcinogenic metals: environmental and occupational occurrence and exposure. Princeton, NJ: Princeton Scientific, 1987:87–125.

39. Lang BR, Morris HF, Razzoog ME, eds. International workshop: biocompatibility, toxicity and hypersensitivity to alloy systems used in dentistry. Ann Arbor: University of Michigan School of Dentistry, 1986.

40. Sprince NL, Chamberlin RI, Hales CA, Weber AL, Kazemi H. Respiratory disease in tungsten carbide production workers. Chest 1984;86:549–557.

41. National Institute of Occupational Safety and Health. Occupational hazard assessment: criteria for controlling exposure to cobalt. Cincinnati, OH: DHHS Publication 82-107, 1981:1–95.

42. Demedts M, Gheysens B, Nagels J, Verbeken E, Lauwerijns J, van den Eeckhout A, Lahaye D, Gyselen A. Cobalt lung in diamond polishers. Am Rev Respir Dis 1984;130:130–135.

43. Gheysens B, Auwerx J, van den Eeckhout A, Demedts M. Cobalt-induced asthma in diamond polishers. Chest 1985;88:740–744.

44. Shirakawa T, Kusaka Y, Fujimura N, Goto S, Kato M, Heki S, Morimoto K. Occupational asthma from cobalt sensitivity in workers exposed to hard metal dust. Chest 1989;95:29–37.

45. Anttila S, Sutinen S, Paananen M, Kreus K-E, Sivonen SJ, Grekula A, Alapieti T. Hard metal lung disease: a clinical, histological, ultrastructural and x-ray micro-analytical study. Eur J Respir Dis 1986;69:83–94.

46. Foussereau J, Cavelier C. Allergic contact dermatitis from cobalt in the rubber industry. Contact Dermatitis 1988;19:217–238.

47. Fischer T, Rystedt I. Cobalt allergy in hard metal workers. Contact Dermatitis 1983;9:115–121.

48. Möller H. Intradermal testing in doubtful cases of contact allergy to metals. Contact Dermatitis 1989;20:120–123.

49. Versieck J, Cornelis R. Trace elements in human plasma or serum. Boca Raton, FL: CRC Press, 1989;71–72.

50. Young, RS. Cobalt. In: Frieden E, ed. Biochemistry of the essential ultratrace elements. New York: Plenum Press, 1984:133–147.

51. Scansetti G, Lamon S, Talarico S, Botta GC, Spinelli P, Sulotto F, Fantoni F. Urinary cobalt as a measure of exposure in the hard metal industry. Int Arch Occup Environ Health 1985;57:19–26.

52. Ichikawa Y, Kusaka Y, Goto S. Biological monitoring of cobalt exposure, based on cobalt concentrations in blood and urine. Int Arch Occup Environ Health 1985;55:269–276.

53. Tsalev DL. Atomic absorption spectrometry in occupational and environmental health practice, Vol II, determination of individual elements. Boca Raton, FL: CRC Press, 1984:59–63.

79

Copper

Don Fisher, M.D., M.S.

SOURCES AND PRODUCTION

Chemical Forms

Copper (Cu) is a group IB metal which forms two series of compounds: copper(I) (cuprous) annd copper(II) (cupric) compounds. Metallic copper is quite resistant to corrosion and is not attacked by dry air, water, or nonoxidizing acid. Table 79.1 lists basic properties of copper. Copper(I) oxide (Cu_2O) occurs naturally as the reddish mineral cuprite. Copper(II) oxide is black and obtained by heating copper metal in air. In moist air copper becomes coated with green basic carbonate (1). Sulfide ores of copper, principally chalcopyrite ($CuFeS_2$) and chalcocite (Cu_2S), are the predominant forms mined and processed in the United States. The copper content of these ores is usually less than 1%. Table 79.2 lists the most common copper compounds, their common names, and predominant uses (1–4).

SITES, INDUSTRIES, AND BUSINESSES ASSOCIATED WITH EXPOSURES

Copper was the first metal used by man and appears to have been discovered on the island of Cyprus around 2500 B.C. (5). Copper salts have been used therapeutically for over 2000 years, and copper sulfate was a popular murder weapon and abortifacient in France in the mid 19th century (6). As of 1986, 1.26 million short tons were produced in the United States, primarily in Arizona, New Mexico, Missouri, and Montana. The United States produces 14% of world output, which exceeds 8.6 metric tons annually. Chile, Canada, and Peru are the principal producers (7). Mined ores of copper are concentrated by a flotation process and then refined. Smelting consists of applying sufficient heat (1100–1600°C) to concentrate the metal and fuse the remaining gangue (waste ore) into slag (8). Large quantities of copper are used in the manufacture of metallic items such as wire, rods, sheets, tubing, piping, roofing materials, cooking utensils, and coins. Numerous alloys of copper are used including bronze, brass, bell metal, gun metal, German silver, and beryllium-copper. Other alloys include aluminum, phosphor, manganese, and silicon bronzes. Compounds of copper are used as pigments, fungicides, insecticides, algicides, chemical reagents, pharmaceuticals, and intrauterine contraceptives and in electroplating. Table 79.3 is a list of occupations that encounter significant amounts of copper and copper compounds (9, 10).

Table 79.1. Properties of Copper

Atomic weight	63.5
Specific gravity	8.92
Melting point	1083° C
Boiling point	2567° C

CLINICAL TOXICOLOGY OF EXPOSURE

Routes of Exposure

Copper is an essential element in mammalian systems. Illness occurs when diet is deficient or intake is excessive. The principal route of exposure is through ingestion, but inhalation of copper dusts and fumes occurs in industrial settings. Toxicity has resulted from treatment of burns using topical copper compounds (11). Copper has been reported to be absorbed internally from prostheses, intrauterine devices, hemodialysis units using copper-containing equipment (11) and copper azide impregnation of the skin following an explosion (12).

Absorption

Adults ingest 1.2–5 mg/day, about half of which is absorbed (13). Following ingestion, maximum absorption of copper occurs in the duodenum. Absorption through the intestinal wall is facilitated by active transport, though the exact mechanism is unknown. Copper is initially bound in the serum to albumin, then later more firmly bound to ceruloplasmin, which binds over 95% of circulating copper. In acute poisoning, copper is also bound to metallothionein in the liver and kidney (14). Absorption is increased in copper deficiency and impaired in small bowel disease. Zinc and molybdenum inhibit the intestinal absorption of copper. Copper is distributed throughout the body but stored primarily in liver, muscle, and bone. Normal serum levels are around 1 μg/ml. Serum levels increase with age, but there are no increases in tissue stores (13).

Metabolism

Absorbed copper is initially bound to albumin and transported from the gastrointestinal tract to the liver. There it is transferred to ceruloplasmin, which is the primary transport vehicle for incorporating copper into the copper-dependent enzymes: tyrosinase, amine oxidases, and cytochrome oxidase. Copper is essential for hemoglobin formation and cross-linking collagen, elastin, and hair keratin (13, 15).

Elimination

The principal pathway for copper elimination is through the feces via excretion into the bile. Biliary copper is poorly absorbed. The plasma half-life for radiocopper (^{67}Cu) is 17–18 hours, whereas the half-life for whole-body ceruloplasmin-copper is 145 hours (15).

SIGNS, SYMPTOMS, AND SYNDROMES FROM TOXIC EXPOSURE

Acute Toxicity

Copper is an essential element, and, as with all essential elements, toxicity is uncommon. Acute copper toxicity is rare and

Table 79.2.   Common Copper Compounds and Uses

Compound (common names)	Uses
Cupric oxide (black copper oxide)	Catalyst, batteries, electrodes, desulfurizing oils, paints, insecticides, ceramic colorant, artificial gems, welding flux
Cuprous oxide (red copper oxide)	Fungicide, antifouling paint, photoelectric cells, catalyst, pigment for glass and glazes, in brazing paste
Cupric acetate, basic (verdigris)	In manufacture of pigments, fungicide, fabric dye, artificial flowers
Cupric acetoarsenate (Paris, French, emerald, Schweinfurt, parrot, or Vienna green)	Insecticide, marine pigment
Cupric arsenite (Swedish or Scheele's green)	Pigment, wood preservative, fungicide, insecticide, rodenticide
Cupric carbonate, basic (Bremen blue or green)	Seed treatment, fungicide, pyrotechnics, pigment, feed additive, in Burgundy mixture
Cupric chloride	Catalyst, mordant, petroleum desulfurizing and deodorizing agent, inks, electroplating, photography, pyrotechnics, pigments, wood preserving, disinfectant, feed additive
Cupric chromate (VI)	Fungicide, seed protectant, wood preserving, mordant, textile preservative
Cupric hydroxide (copper hydrate)	Manufacture of rayon, battery electrodes, other Cu salts; mordant, pigment, fungicide, insecticide, feed additive, catalyst, paper treatment
Cupric nitrate	Photocopying, colorant, mordant, finishing agent for copper, zinc, and aluminum metal, wood preservative, herbicide, fungicide, pyrotechnics; catalyst for solid rocket fuel and organic reactions
Cupric sulfate, pentahydride (bluestone, blue vitriol, Roman vitriol)	Fungicide, algicide, bactericide, herbicide, feed additive, in Bordeaux solution, mordant, dye preparation, tanning, wood preservative, electroplating, inks, pigments, photography, pyrotechnics
Cuprous cyanide	Electroplating, insecticide, fungicide, antifouling paints, polymerization catalyst
Cupric tungstate (VI) Cuprous selenide	Semiconductors

Table 79.3.   Partial List of Occupations with Exposure to Copper or Its Compounds

Asphalt makers
Battery makers
Copper smelting and smithing
Electroplating
Fungicide and insecticide workers
Gem colorers
Paint and pigment makers
Preservative manufacturers (wood, hides, rope)
Pyrotechnics workers
Rayon makers
Solderers
Textile finishers
Wallpaper manufacturers
Water treaters
Welders

usually not serious. Most reports of acute toxicity are from suicidal ingestion of copper sulfate. Fortunately, death is rare owing to copper sulfate's emetic properties. Mild forms of poisoning only produce nausea, vomiting, diarrhea, and malaise and have been described in patients poisoned by eating or drinking from copper-containing vessels (16, 17) or from a soft drink dispenser (18). Symptoms associated with severe poisoning usually follow the order of: metallic taste, nausea, vomiting (sometimes of blue-green vomitus), hematemesis, diarrhea, melena, hypotension, coma, oliguria, jaundice, and death (19–23).

Target Organ Toxicity

Skin   Contact dermatitis due to copper is rare (24). However, its occurrence can be substantiated by careful patch testing (25). Eczematous dermatitis (26) and urticaria (27) have been associated with use of copper intrauterine devices. Greenish discoloration of the hair has been seen in blond or lightly pigmented individuals exposed to copper dusts or copper-tainted water used for shampooing or swimming (6). Copper-8-quinolinolate and copper resinate (from rosin) are potential allergic sensitizers (24).

Eye   Impregnation of the eye with elemental copper or copper alloys is called chalosis. This is a brownish or greenish-brown discoloration of the cornea, lens, or iris which may occur following penetrating injuries with copper fragments. Copper sulfate, copper acetoarsenite, and verdigris (oxidized copper) cause irritation and inflammation but no permanent damage. Copper chloride and copper cyanide plating bath can cause severe reactions and permanent opacifications (28).

Respiratory   Chronic exposure to copper dusts and fumes in the industrial setting can lead to upper respiratory complaints and physical findings in workers. These include ulceration and perforation of the nasal septum and metal fume fever (10). No permanent lung changes have been reported from copper-related metal fume fever, and the illness does not return after cessation of exposure. Chronic exposure to sprayed copper sulfate solution (Bordeaux solution) has been reported to cause pulmonary interstitial disease and adenocarcinoma of the lung in vineyard sprayers—vineyard sprayer's lung (see the section below on syndromes for greater detail of metal fume fever and vineyard sprayer's lung).

Gastrointestinal   The predominant findings of acute copper sulfate poisoning are gastrointestinal. These include nausea, vomiting, diarrhea, hematemesis, melena, and jaundice. Patients who developed intense jaundice from centrolobular necrosis following massive acute copper sulfate poisoning had a more fulminant course than patients with milder jaundice from intravascular hemolysis (19). Workers who developed vineyard sprayer's lung also developed extensive liver pathology, including angiosarcoma. These pathologic findings are described in greater detail in the syndromes section.

Renal Renal abnormalities have been observed following copper sulfate ingestion. Hematuria, rising blood nitrogen (BUN), and oliguria were frequently observed in a large series of poisonings (19). A picture of acute tubular necrosis (ATN) was observed on urinalysis and renal biopsy. Intravascular hemolysis but not hypotension preceeded development of ATN. Oliguria occurred in all 14 patients with hematuria, and three died.

Neurologic Unlike insult found to the basal ganglia in Wilson's disease (see chronic and longterm effects section, below), there is no evidence of neurologic injury from acquired copper toxicity. Coma observed in acute copper sulfate poisoning probably results from uremia (10).

Hematologic Hemolytic anemia accompanies severe acute copper sulfate poisonings (19) and, additionally, follows burn treatment with copper sulfate and hemodialysis using copper-containing dialyzing equipment (29). Hemolytic anemia also occurs sporadically in Wilson's disease. The hemolysis is precipitous in these situations. Hemolysis alone probably leads to mild jaundice compared with those who develop centrolobular necrosis of the liver. A similar abrupt hemolytic crisis has also been seen in several animal species with acute and chronic copper poisoning (6).

Chronic and Longterm Effects

Acquired chronic copper toxicity, with the exception of vineyard sprayer's lung, has not been firmly established. Chronic disease from excessive copper storage is epitomized by Wilson's disease. It is an inherited, autosomal recessive error in copper metabolism. The disease is characterized by excess copper deposition in most organs, especially the liver, kidneys, brain, and eyes. Wilson's disease is also termed hepatolenticular degeneration, due to the prominent effects on the liver (cirrhosis) and eye (Kayser-Fleischer rings). Excellent therapeutic results are obtained following treatment with D-penicillamine to chelate excess copper (6). Indian childhood cirrhosis is a fatal disease of infants and children from the Vapi area of India. Excess dietary copper has been suggested as the cause (30–32). Further research is necessary to establish causation.

SYNDROMES

Metal Fume Fever Chronic recurrent inhalation of copper fumes and dust can lead to nasal septal perforation and a systemic illness, metal fume fever. This illness is characterized by nasal congestion, fever up to 39°C, chills, malaise, and shortness of breath. The symptoms generally develop after repeated exposure during the work week, tending to diminish toward the end of the week, only to return more prominently upon reexposure after the weekend. This phenomenon has led to the term "Monday morning fever" (2, 3). The illness is postulated to result from immune mechanisms (33), but there are no reports of chronic toxicity. All symptoms resolve following removal from exposure. A similar illness has been described in a patient undergoing hemodialysis. The symptoms resolved after a copper-containing part was removed from the dialysis unit (34).

Vineyard Sprayer's Lung This disease occurred when Bordeaux solution (1–2% solution of copper sulfate neutralized with lime) was chronically sprayed by Portuguese vineyard workers. These workers developed interstitial pulmonary disease, including histiocytic granulomas with associated nodular fibrohyaline scars containing abundant copper. The progression

toward pulmonary fibrosis was highly variable among individuals, and a high incidence of adenocarcinoma, particularly alveolar cell carcinoma, was observed. Extensive liver damage was also noted. Biopsies revealed fibrosis, micronodular cirrhosis, angiosarcoma, and portal hypertension (35, 36).

TERATOGENESIS

Copper ions cause irreversible immobilization of sperm in vitro, and intrauterine devices increase endometrial copper concentrations (37). High levels of copper given to mice during pregnancy caused increased fetal mortality and produced central nervous system malformations (38). No teratogenetic effects attributed to copper have been observed in humans.

CARCINOGENESIS

With the exception of adenocarcinoma of the lung and angiosarcoma of the liver seen in patients with vineyard sprayer's lung, there is no evidence of carcinogenesis from copper exposure (38). Excess lung cancer found in copper smelter workers has been shown to be caused by arsenic exposure (39).

Management of Toxicity

CLINICAL EXAMINATION

A careful history is essential in leading the practitioner to a suspicion of copper poisoning in acutely ill patients. The history should contain questions relevant to intentional poisoning with copper salts and to ingestion of food and drink, especially acidic beverages or alcohol prepared in copper-containing vessels. Persons acutely poisoned by copper (especially copper sulfate) should be evaluated initially for nausea, vomiting, and diarrhea. Blue-green vomitus is diagnostic. Investigation for abnormal liver and renal function as well as for hemolytic anemia should be conducted. Vital signs and urine output should be frequently monitored for hypotension and oliguria. The medical history is also the cornerstone of investigating dermatitis suspected to arise from copper. Inquiry as to exposure to copper salts at work, use of copper-containing jewelry, or use of a copper intrauterine device should be conducted. Patch testing may be necessary to confirm the diagnosis. A history of delayed onset of fever, chills, shortness of breath, and malaise following exposure to copper fumes should lead to the suspicion of metal fume fever. Fever, rigorous chills, diaphoresis, and wheezing may be noted on physical examination.

TREATMENT

Removal from exposure is generally sufficient to resolve most illnesses associated with copper toxicity. This is especially true for metal fume fever and dermatitis, though the latter may also require application of topical corticosteroid preparations (8).

In severe acute poisoning, induced emesis is rarely necessary, due to vomiting. Either intravenous calcium disodium EDTA or intramuscular dimercaprol should be given as soon as feasible. Exchange transfusions and corticosteroids have reportedly been useful (40, 41). Albumin-enriched peritoneal dialysis has been used together with exchange transfusions successfully in a 2-year-old boy (42). D-Penicillamine may be given after initial chelation treatment with dimercaprol (21).

Hemodialysis alone is not effective (38). Treatment of eye injuries includes vigorous irrigation with normal saline. Ophthalmologic referral is indicated for severe elemental copper, copper chloride, or copper cyanide plating bath injuries to the eye.

LABORATORY DIAGNOSIS

Laboratory findings in severe acute copper sulfate poisoning include: abnormal hepatocellular function, hyperbilirubinemia, (both direct and indirect), elevated BUN and creatinine, hematuria and cellular casts on urinalysis, anemia, positive stool guaiac, elevated serum copper, and ceruloplasmin.

Findings during episodes of metal fume fever include: leukocytosis, abnormal pulmonary function studies (small airways obstruction, reduced lung volumes and carbon dioxide diffusing capacity), peribronchiolar cuffing, and hazy infiltrates on chest x-ray, and elevated urine copper levels (43).

BIOLOGIC MONITORING: BLOOD, SERUM, AND URINE CONCENTRATIONS

Under conditions of extremely high copper dust levels (464 mg/m^3) urinary copper is elevated to approximately twice normal. However, at air concentrations near current exposure limits (1 mg/m^3) (44), biologic monitoring is not warranted (3).

Normal blood concentrations of copper are reported to be around 1 μg/ml (45). The mean value in women is slightly higher than in men. Copper concentration in serum or plasma varies with individuals, and diurnal variations can occur. One study reported plasma copper concentrations ranging from 0.89–0.37 μg/ml in healthy men and 0.87–1.53 μg/ml in healthy women (45). Ninety-five percent of the copper in plasma is in ceruloplasmin. The amount of copper bound to serum albumin ranges between 40 and 100 μg/l (45). Ceruloplasmin is one of the acute phase reactant proteins and increases in chronic inflammatory conditions (45). Estrogens and pregnancy also elevate ceruloplasmin. Erythrocytes also contain a significant portion of copper found in blood in the form of an enzyme superoxide dismutase (45).

Increased serum concentrations of copper are found in individuals with liver disease such as primary biliary cirrhosis and other cholestatic diseases (45). In tissues, the highest copper concentrations are found in the liver, brain, heart, and kidneys (45). The adult liver usually has 5–10 mg/kg of copper (45). Patients with Wilson's disease have increased liver concentrations of copper, reading 150–600 mg/kg of wet weight (45).

Copper excretion is mainly via the bile. Urinary excretion of copper is low in humans. Healthy adults have urinary concentrations less than 100 μg/24 hr (45). A daily intake of 2 mg of copper a day results in a urinary concentration between 11 and 48 μg/24 hr (45). Biliary excretion of copper is between 0.7–1.7 mg/day (45). Patients with Wilson's disease excrete copper at a much reduced rate even though they have elevated urinary copper concentrations (45) of around 90 μg/24-hr urine collection. Normal control subjects excrete about 20 μg/24-hr urine collection (45).

ENVIRONMENTAL MONITORING

Copper fume and dust levels should be measured to ensure compliance with Occupational Safety and Health Administration (OSHA) standards. Remonitoring should be performed for any changes in work practices or plant processes that could cause a rise in air concentrations.

EXPOSURE LIMITS

The OSHA Permissible Exposure Limit (PEL) and the American Congress of Government Industrial Hygienists (ACGIH) Threshold Limit Value (TLV) are 1 mg/m^3 for copper dusts and mists. The PEL and TLV for copper fume are 0.1 mg/m^3 and 0.2 mg/m^3, respectively.

REFERENCES

1. Winholz M, ed. The Merck index. 10th ed. Rahway, NJ: Merck and Co., 1983.
2. Stokinger HE. The metals. In: Patty FA, ed. Industrial hygiene and toxicology. 3rd ed. New York: Interscience Publishers, 1978.
3. Zenz CL. Occupational medicine, principles and practice. 2nd ed. New York: Elsevier, 1988.
4. Scheinberg HI. Copper, alloys and compounds. In: Encyclopedia of occupational health and safety. 2nd ed. Geneva: ILO Press, 1984.
5. Joralemon IB. Copper: the encompassing story of mankind's first metal. Berkeley, CA: Howell-North Books, 1973.
6. Owens CA. Copper deficiency and toxicity: acquired and inherited, in plants, animals, and man. Park Ridge, NJ: Noyse Publications, 1981.
7. Bureau of the Census. Statistical abstracts of the U.S., 1989. 109th ed. Washington, DC: U.S. Department of Commerce, 1989.
8. Wagner WL. Environmental conditions in U.S. copper smelters. Washington, DC: National Institute of Occupational Safety and Health, 1975.
9. National Institute of Occupational Safety and Health. Occupational diseases, a guide to their recognition. Washington, DC: U.S. Department of Health, Education, and Welfare, 1977.
10. Cohen SR. Environmental and occupational exposure to copper. In: Nriagu JO, ed. Copper in the environment. Part II: Health effects. New York: John Wiley and Sons, 1979.
11. Goyer RA. Toxic effects of metals. In: Klassen CD, Amdur MO, Doull J, eds. Toxicology: the basic science of poisons. 3rd ed. New York: Macmillan, 1986.
12. Bentur Y, Koren G, McGuigan M, Spielberg SP. An unusual skin exposure to copper; clinical and pharmacokinetic evaluation. Clin Toxicol 1988;26:371–380.
13. Owens, CA. Physiological aspects of copper: copper in organs and systems. Park Ridge, NJ: Noyse Publications, 1982.
14. Kurisaki E, Kuroda Y, Sato M. Copper-binding protein in acute copper poisoning. Forensic Sci Int 1988;38:3–11.
15. Marceau N. The use of radiocopper to trace copper metabolic transfer and utilization. In: Nriagu JO ed. Copper in the environment. Part II: Health effects. New York: John Wiley and Sons, 1979.
16. Ross AI. Vomiting and diarrhea due to copper in stewed apples. Lancet 1955;2:87–88.
17. Wyllie J. Copper poisoning at a cocktail party. Am J Public Health 1957;47:617.
18. Witherell LE, Watson WN, Giguere GC. Outbreak of acute copper poisoning due to soft drink dispenser. Am J Public Health 1980;70:1115.
19. Chuttani HK, Gupta PS, Gulati S, Gupta DN. Acute copper sulfate poisoning. Am J Med 1965;39:849–854.
20. Chugh KS, Sharma BK, Singhal PC, Das KC, Datta BN. Acute renal failure following copper sulphate intoxication. Postgrad Med J 1977;53:18–23.
21. Jantsch W, Kulig K, Rumack BH. Massive copper sulfate ingestion resulting in hepatotoxicity. Clin Toxicol 1984;22:585–588.
22. Akintonwa A, Mabadeje AFB, Odutola TA. Fatal poisonings by copper sulfate ingested from "spiritual water." Vet Hum Toxicol 1989;31:453–454.
23. Lamont DL, Duflou JAL. Copper sulfate: not a harmless chemical. Am J Forensic Med Pathol 1988;9:226–227.
24. Adams RM. Occupational skin disease. San Diego: Grune & Stratton, 1983.
25. Van Joost T, Habets JMW, Stolz E, Naafs B. The meaning of positive patch tests to copper sulfate in nickel allergy. Contact Derm 1988;18:101–102.
26. Barranco VP. Eczematius dermatitis caused by internal exposure to copper. Arch Dermatol 1972;106:386–387.
27. Barkoff JR. Urticaria secondary to a copper intrauterine device. Int J Dermatol 1976;15:594–595.
28. Grant WM. Toxicology of the eye. 3rd ed. Springfield, IL: Charles C Thomas, 1986.

29. Manzler AD, Schreiner AW. Copper-induced acute hemolytic anemia: a new complication of hemodialysis. Ann Intern Med 1970;73:409–412.

30. Adelson JQ. Indian childhood cirrhosis is a result of copper hepatotoxicity—in all likelihood. J Pediatr Gastrointerology Nutr 1987;6:491–492.

31. Abdulla M. Copper levels in Indian childhood cirrhosis. Lancet 1979;2:246.

32. Tanner MS, Bhaye SA, Kantarjian SH, et al. Early introduction of animal milk feeds as a possible cause of Indian childhood cirrhosis. Lancet 1983;2:992–995.

33. Andrews AC, Lyons TD. Binding of histamine and antihistamine to bovine serum albumin by mediation with Cu(II). Science 1957;126:561.

34. Lyle WH, Payton JC, Hui M. Hemodialysis and copper fever. Lancet 1973;1:1324–1325.

35. Pimentel JC, Marques F. "Vineyard sprayer's lung": a new occupational disease. Thorax 1969;24:678–688.

36. Pimental JC, Menezes AP. Liver granulomas containing copper in vineyard sprayer's lung: a new etiology of hepatic granulomatosis. Am Rev Respir Dis 1975;111:189–195.

37. Holland MK, White IG. Heavy metals and human spermatozoa III. The toxicity of copper ions for spermatozoa. Contraception 1988;38:685–695.

38. Agarqal K, Sharma A, Talukder G. Effects of copper on mammalian cell components. Chem Biol Interact 1989;69:1–16.

39. Lee AM, Fraumeni JF. Arsenic and respiratory cancer in man: an occupational study. J Natl Cancer Inst 1969;42:1045–1049.

40. Chowdbury AKR, Ghosh S, Pal D. Acute copper sulphate poisoning. J Indian Med Assoc 1961;36:330–336.

41. Gupta PS, Bhargava SP, Sharma ML. Acute copper sulphate poisoning with special reference to its management with corticosteroid therapy. J Assoc Phys India 1962;10:287–292.

42. Cole DEC, Lirenman DS. Role of albumin-enriched peritoneal dialysate in acute copper poisoning. J Pediatr 1978;92:955–957.

43. Armstrong C, Moore L, Hackler R, et al. An outbreak of metal fume fever, diagnostic use of urinary copper and zinc determinations. J Occup Med 1983;25:886–888.

44. American Congress of Government Industrial Hygienists. Threshold limit values and biological exposure indices for 1989–1990. Cincinnati, OH: ACGIH, 1989.

45. Aaseth J, Norseth T. Copper. Chapt 10, in: Friberg L, Nordberg G, Vouk V, eds. Handbook on the toxicology of metals. 2nd ed. New York: Elsevier Science Publishers, 1986:233–254.

SOURCES AND PRODUCTION

Chemical Forms

Zinc is a bluish-white soft metal placed in Group IIB of the periodic table. It is always divalent. Table 80.1 lists basic properties of zinc. In dry air it is highly resistant to attack except at temperatures above 225°C. In moist air, attach proceeds at room temperature. A light gray film of hydrated basic carbonate forms on the surface in the presence of CO_2 which protects the metal from further corrosion. When heated above 500°C, zinc volatilizes into small zinc oxide particles that rapidly flocculate as they cool, forming fumes. The principle mineral of zinc is sphalerite (ZnS). Zinc constitutes about 0.02% of the earth's crust and is widely distributed. It is a relatively poor conductor of electricity and heat (1–3).

SITES, INDUSTRIES, AND BUSINESSES ASSOCIATED WITH EXPOSURE

Zinc has been used as an alloy with copper and tin since ancient times but probably not recognized as a separate entity until the 15th century. Early Egyptian and other Mediterranian peoples may have used zinc as a topical ointment. Commercial production of zinc began in the 18th century (3). As of 1986, 224,000 short tons valued at $170 million were produced in the United States, chiefly in Tennessee, Missouri, New York, and Colorado. World production exceeded 6.8 million tons, of which the United States contributed 5%. Canada, Mexico, Honduras, and Peru are the principal producers. Zinc is considered a strategic metal, and 378,000 short tons are in inventory for national emergencies (4).

Zinc ore is processed by crushing and then concentrating to 50–60% metal by flotation. This concentrate is roasted to remove sulfur and then further processed by either smelting or electrolytic refining. Smeltered zinc contains impurities of other metals (lead, copper, and cadmium) and is suitable for galvanizing, spraying, annealing, and painting. Electrolytic refining produces high grade zinc (99.99 + %) suitable for alloys and diecasting (1–3, 5).

The principle use of metallic zinc is for galvanizing iron and steel to prevent corrosion and oxidation. Zinc metal is also diecast for automotive components, electrical equipment, tools, hardware, toys, and fancy goods. Alloys of zinc include combinations with lead, cadmium, iron, tin, copper, aluminum, magnesium, and titanium. Alloys generally inhance zinc's galvanizing and diecasting characteristics (1, 3). Table 80.2 lists important zinc compounds and their main uses. Of these compounds zinc oxide is the most widely used, primarily in the rubber industry, for compounding and vulcanizing, as a coolant, and as a sulfur scavenger. Zinc oxide is also used as a paint, a pigment, an ultraviolet light absorber, a mildew retardant, a fungicide, in the pharmaceutical industry for topical application, in cosmetics, in photocopying processes, and in ceramic glazes. Zinc chloride is important occupationally as a soldering flux, in wood preservation, in dry cell batteries, as a disinfectant, in oil refining, in dental cements, and in taxi-

Table 80.1. Properties of Zinc

Atomic weight	65.38
Specific gravity	7.14
Melting point	419.4°C
Boiling point	907°C

Table 80.2. Common Zinc Compounds and Uses

Compound (common names)	Uses
Zinc acetate	Wood preserving, mordant, glazes, reagent
Zinc carbonate	Pigment, feed additive, manufacture or porcelains, pottery, rubber
Zinc chloride	Deodorant, disinfectant, wood preservative, fireproofing, soldering flux, cement, mordant, petroleum refining, textile treatment, vulcanizing rubber, solvent for cellulose; manufacture of activated carbon, paper, glues, and dye
Zinc chromate (VI), hydroxide (zinc yellow, butter-cup yellow)	Pigment in paint, oil, varnish, linoleum, rubber.
Zinc cyanide	Electroplating, removing NH_3 from gas
Zinc fluoride	Fluoridination of organic compounds, glazes, enamels, wood preserving, electroplating; manufacture of phosphors for fluorescent lights
Zinc oxide (flower's of zinc, philosopher's wool, zinc white)	Pigments, cements, glass, tires, glue, matches, white ink, reagent, photocopy paper, flame retardant, semiconductor, fungicide, desulfurizing agent
Zinc phosphide	Rodenticide
Zinc silicate	Television screens, neon lights
Zinc stearate	Tablet and rubber manufacture; cosmetic and pharmaceutical powders; ointments, waterproofing, releasing agent in manufacture of plastics
Zinc sulfate (white vitriol, zinc vitriol)	Mordant, wood preserving, bleaching paper, reagent, manufacture of Zn salts
Zinc sulfide (zinc blende)	Pigment; manufacture of luminous dials, x-ray and television screens

Table 80.3. A Partial List of Occupations with Exposure to Zinc and its Compounds

Activated carbon makers
Alloy makers
Ceramic makers
Chemical synthesizers
Cosmetic makers
Dental cement makers
Deodorant makers
Disinfectant makers
Dry cell battery makers
Dye makers
Electronics workers
Electroplaters
Embalmers
Galvanizers
Laquer makers
Paper makers
Paint, pigment makers
Petroleum refinery workers
Pharmaceutical makers
Rubber workers
Taxidermists
Textile finishers
Welders, solderers
Wood preservers

dermy (1–3, 6). Table 80.3 lists some of the occupations with exposure to zinc and zinc compounds.

CLINICAL TOXICOLOGY OF EXPOSURE

Routes of Exposure

The most common route of exposure to zinc is through diet. Inhalation of zinc fume and dust occurs in some of the industrial settings mentioned above. Absorption occurs across broken epithelium when zinc oxide is applied to treat burns or wounds (3).

Absorption

Absorption of zinc occurs throughout the intestine but mainly in the second portion of the duodenum. The mechanism of passage through the gut mucosa is not completely understood but involves metallothionein binding or other zinc-protein complexes in lumenal cells. Absorption ranged from 25–90% following ^{65}Zn oral administration in humans and is influenced by dietary factors. Zinc absorption is decreased when consumed with some vegetable proteins, calcium, and phosphorus but increased when consumed with animal proteins (3).

Metabolism

Following oral administration of ^{65}Zn, measurable levels were found in the blood within 15–20 minutes, with peak levels in 2–4 hours. Plasma and serum levels were higher than whole blood. Zinc is stored primarily in skeletal muscle. Significant concentrations occur in the pancreas, prostate, liver, and retina (7).

Elimination

The biologic half-life exceeds 300 days. A total of 70–80% of ingested zinc is excreted in the feces. Urine and sweat excretion

together account for roughly 15%, but in hot climates 25% can be excreted by sweat alone. Breast milk also contains significant concentration of zinc (2, 3, 7).

SIGNS, SYMPTOMS, AND SYNDROMES FROM TOXIC EXPOSURE

Acute Toxicity

Acute symptoms of oral zinc poisoning are primarily gastrointestinal. Symptoms include nausea, vomiting, abdominal pain, diarrhea, and hematemesis. Fever is also reported. With supportive care zinc toxicity is usually self-limited, and resolution of symptoms occurs in a matter of hours or days.

TARGET ORGAN TOXICITY

Skin Due to its caustic action, zinc chloride can cause ulcerations and dermatitis of the exposed skin (8). Zinc pyrithione, a common constituent of shampoos, is also reported to cause dermatitis, confirmed by patch testing (9). Zinc oxide dust may give rise to papular, pustular eczema by blocking sebaceous glands (2).

Eye Both zinc chloride and zinc sulfate can cause significant eye injuries. Redness and persistent discomfort occur following exposure to concentrated solutions of either salt. Within 6 days a discrete stromal opacity of the cornea develops along with irregularity of the overlying epithelium. Lens opacities, iritis, and glaucoma may occur following splash of concentrated (50%) zinc chloride solution (10).

Respiratory Most zinc salts irritate mucous membranes of the upper respiratory tract after inhalation. Cough and dyspnea followed by the gradual onset of adult respiratory distress syndrome and death have been reported with inhalation of zinc chloride smoke from smoke bombs (11). Pulmonary toxicity is also seen in rats, mice, and guinea pigs exposed to varying levels of smoke from zinc oxide/hexachloroethane smoke bombs. A high incidence of adenocarcinoma of the lung was observed in the high dose group, but this was felt to be related to carbon tetrachloride generated by the smoke (12). Inhalation of zinc oxide dusts and fumes can produce metal fume fever; however, no changes in lung function occur between pre- and postshift values or between early and late work week values (13).

Gastrointestinal Gastrointestinal effects occur after ingestion of zinc chloride and zinc phosphide or from drinking acidic beverages from galvanized containers (2). These effects include abdominal pain, nausea, vomiting, diarrhea, and hematemesis. Zinc chloride has been found to cause esophagitis (14, 15) and mucosal burns of the stomach (16). The toxicity of zinc phosphide is probably due to release of phosphine, which occurs on contact with water and is accelerated by an acidic environment (17, 18). nausea, vomiting, and jaundice occur after intravenous zinc poisoning (19).

Renal Microhematuria has been reported following zinc chloride ingestion (14). Acute tubular necrosis, probably due to hypoxia, was found in soldiers following fatal adult respiratory distress syndrome caused by zinc chloride smoke inhalation (12). Oliguria and renal failure occurred following iatrogenic intravenous overadministration of zinc sulfate (19).

Neurologic Lethargy follows ingestion of zinc chloride (14–16, 20) and elemental zinc (20). Symptoms are reversible with treatment. Fatigue is associated with zinc metal fume fever (21).

Hematologic Chronic ingestion of high doses of supplemental zinc gives rise to anemia and leukopenia from induced copper deficiency. The anemia and leukopenia reversed with cessation of zinc supplements (22) and intravenous cupric chloride (23). Leukocytosis can occur in zinc metal fume fever (see below).

SYNDROMES

Metal Fume Fever Exposure to freshly generated zinc oxide fumes, usually from welding galvanized iron, commonly leads to metal fume fever. The syndrome consists of sweet metallic taste, dry cough, shortness of breath, fatigue, myalgias, fever, and chills beginning 4–12 hours after exposure. Other terms for the syndrome include: brass ague, brass chills, spelter shakes, zinc chills, and Monday morning fever. Fever may reach 40°C and is followed by profuse diaphoresis and rigorous shakes. The white cell count may reach 20,000 during the illness. Symptoms generally persist 1–3 hours, but even in severe cases total recovery occurs within 24–48 hours. No longterm sequelae are observed. Tolerance is gained rapidly after repeat exposures but also lost quickly such that a more pronounced manifestation of the illness occurs after short duration of nonexposure then reexposure, hence the term "Monday morning fever" (2, 5, 21).

Chronic and Long-Term Effects

Other than corneal and lens opacities after ocular zinc salt injury and anemia from zinc-induced copper deficiency, there are no known chronic effects of zinc toxicity.

TERATOGENICITY

Zinc toxicity appears not to be teratogenic, although zinc deficiency is (24).

CARCINOGENICITY

Testicular teratomas and seminomas as well as lung reticulosarcomas have occurred in birds and rodents when insoluble zinc salts in high concentrations are injected into these tissues. Zinc chromate is a suspect human carcinogen due to hexavalent chromium (25, 26). There is no evidence for zinc carcinogenicity in humans (24).

Management of Toxicity

CLINICAL EXAMINATION

Evaluating patients with acute onset of nausea, vomiting and abdominal pain following ingestion of solder flux, moss killer, or disinfectants should lead the clinician to suspect zinc chloride poisoning. Drinking acidic beverages from galvanized containers is a potential source of elemental zinc toxicity. Examination of the upper gastrointestinal tract should be conducted for mucosal burns and bleeding if hematemesis or guaiac-positive stools are encountered or if symptoms include abdominal or chest pain. Urine output must be monitored. When inhalation of zinc chloride or zinc phosphide is suspected, careful examination of the lungs and upper respiratory tract is warranted. Special consideration should be given to delayed onset pulmonary edema, which may not develop until several days after acute inhalation of zinc chloride smoke. In patients with microcytic-hemolytic anemia and normal iron stores, chronic abuse of zinc-containing multivitamins or zinc supplements should be considered.

TREATMENT

Treatment for acute zinc toxicity is supportive. Following oral ingestion of zinc or zinc salts, treatment should be directed toward control of nausea, vomiting, and diarrhea. Induced emesis and gastric lavage are usually unnecessary. In the case of zinc phosphide, water should not be given with ipecac or gastric lavage and activated charcoal should be mixed with sorbitol instead of water in order to minimize liberation of phosphine (17). Fluid and electrolyte imbalances must be corrected. Upper gastrointestinal mucosal burns should be treated with H_2 receptor antagonists, sucralfate, or antacids. Calcium disodium EDTA (13–15) and dimercaprol (19) have been successful in lowering serum zinc levels. N-acetylcysteine has been found superior to EDTA to lower elevated serum zinc levels in animals (27).

Experimental studies in animals have shown diethylenetriaminepentaacetic acid (DTPA) and cyclohexanediaminetetraacetic acid (CDTA) more effective in increasing urinary zinc excretion than Ca Na_2, EDTA or D-penicillamine (28).

Supportive care is also indicated for acute zinc chloride inhalation. This may require ventilatory support with positive end-expiratory pressure (PEEP), antibiotics, steroids, and maintenance of cardiac output. Inhalation of zinc oxide fumes and development of metal fume fever require nonspecific treatment other than removal from exposure, ensuring adequate engineering controls, or providing an appropriate personal protective device. Treatment of zinc-induced copper deficiency requires discontinuation of supplemental zinc and therapy with oral or intravenous copper.

LABORATORY DIAGNOSIS

Following acute zinc chloride ingestion, abnormal laboratory values have included elevations in serum zinc, glucose, amylase, lipase, and alkaline phosphatase. Serum zinc levels may be slightly elevated during bouts of metal fume fever (179 μg/dl, normal 55–150 μg/dl) (21). Metal fume fever also causes leukocytosis, up to 20,000, with left shift and may elevate LDH. Pulmonary function may be diminished and patchy infiltrates on x-ray may be seen during the episode. All findings return to normal during recovery (2, 5).

In zinc-induced copper deficiency anemia, serum copper, ceruloplasmin, hemoglobin, hematocrit, red cell indices, and reticulocyte count are depressed. Serum zinc may be normal or elevated. Serum iron and TIBC are normal. Ringed sideroblasts are seen on peripheral blood smears (22).

BIOLOGICAL MONITORING: BLOOD, PLASMA, URINE

For workers repeatedly exposed to zinc or zinc salts preplacement and periodic examinations should include a baseline history and physical examination, a complete blood count, liver and renal function tests, and spirometry.

Zinc concentrations in humans are highest in the prostate (100 mg/kg). High levels are also found in bone, kidney, mus-

Table 80.4. OSHA Permissible Exposure Limits for Zinc Compounds

Compound	TWA (mg/m³)	STEL (mg/m³)
Zinc chloride fume	1	2
Zinc chromate (as CrO₃)	0.01	-
Zinc oxide fume	5	10
Zinc oxide dust		
Total dust	10ᵃ	-
Respirable fraction	5	-
Zinc stearate		
Total dust	10ᵃ	-
Respirable fraction	5	-

ᵃTransitional value is 15 until 12/31/92.

cle, and pancreas (29). Concentrations of zinc in serum and plasma are around 1 μg/ml (100 μg/dl) (29). The zinc concentration in blood is fivefold higher than plasma, due to zinc concentration in erythrocytes (29).

Urinary excretion of zinc in humans not occupationally exposed is around 0.5 mg/24-hr urine collection (29). Occupational exposure to zinc can produce a plasma concentration of 1.4 μg/ml and urinary concentrations of 800 μg/g of creatinine (29).

ENVIRONMENTAL MONITORING

Workplace zinc fumes should be kept below 5 mg/m³ by engineering controls such as appropriate exhaust ventilation Use of personal protective devices (respirators) should be limited to short exposures that occur during unusual jobs (5). Monitoring should be done anytime there are changes in work process or procedure that may cause an increase in zinc fumes or dusts.

EXPOSURE LIMITS

Table 80.4 lists the Occupational Safety and Health Administration (OSHA) Permissible Exposure Limits (PEL), which include the 8-hour Time Weighted Average (TWA) and Short Term Exposure Limit (STEL), for zinc chloride, zinc chromate, zinc dust and fume, and zinc stearate dust and fume.

REFERENCES

1. Cumpston AG. Zinc, alloys and compounds. In: Encyclopedia of occupational safety and health. 2nd ed. Geneva: International Labour Office Press, 1984.
2. Stokinger HE. The metals. In: Patty FA, ed. Industrial hygiene and toxicology. 3rd ed. New York: Interscience Publishers, 1978.
3. National Research Council. Committee on medical and biologic effects of environmental pollutants. Zinc. Baltimore: University Park Press, 1979.
4. Bureau of the Census. Statistical Abstracts of the U.S., 1989. 109th ed. Washington DC: US Department of Commerce, 1989.
5. Zenz CL. Occupational medicine, principles and practice. 2nd ed. New York: Elsevier, 1988.
6. National Institute of Occupational Safety and Health. Occupational diseases, a guide to their recognition. Washington DC: US Department of Health, Education, and Welfare, 1977.
7. Prasad AS. Zinc metabolism. Springfield, IL: Charles C Thomas, 1966.
8. Adams RM. Occupational skin diseases. San Diego: Grune & Stratton, 1983.
9. Nigam PK, Tyagi S, Saxena AK, Misra, RS. Dermatitis from zinc pyrithione. Contact Derm 1988;19:219.
10. Grant WM. Toxicology of the eye. 3rd ed. Springfield, IL: Charles C Thomas, 1986.
11. Marrs TC, Colgrave HF, Edginton JAG, Brown RFR, Cross NL. The repeated dose toxicity of a zinc oxide/hexa-chloroethane smoke. Arch Toxicol 1988;62:123–132.
12. Hjortsø E, Qvist J, Thomsen JL, et al. ARDS after accidental inhalation of zinc chloride smoke. Intensive Care Med 1988;14:17–24.
13. Marquart H, Smid T, Heederik D, Visschers M. Lung function of welders of zinc-coated mild steel: cross-sectional analysis and changes over five consecutive work shifts. Am J Ind Med 1989;16:289–296.
14. Chobanian SJ. Accidental ingestion of liquid zinc chloride: local and systemic effects. Ann Emerg Med 1981;10:91–93.
15. Potter JL. Acute zinc chloride ingestion in a young child. Ann Emerg Med 1981;10:267–269.
16. Hedtke J, Daya MR, Nease G, Burton BT. Local and systemic toxicity following zinc chloride ingestion. (Abstract) American Academy of Clinical Toxicology annual meeting, Oct. 11–14, 1989. Atlanta.
17. Mack RB. A hard day's knight: zinc phosphide poisoning. NC Med J 1989;50:17–18.
18. Casteel SW, Bailey EM. A review of zinc phosphide poisoning. Vet Hum Toxicol 1986;28:151–154.
19. Brocks A, Reid H, Glazer G. Acute intravenous zinc poisoning. Br Med J 1977;1:1390–1391.
20. Murphy JV. Intoxication following ingestion of elemental zinc. JAMA 1970;212:2119–2120.
21. Noel NE, Ruthman JC. Elevated serum zinc levels in metal fume fever. Am J Emerg Med 1988;6:609–610.
22. Simon SR, Branda RF, Tindle BH, Burns SL. Copper deficiency and sideroblastic anemia associated with zinc ingestion. Am J Hematol 1988;28:181–183.
23. Hoffman HN, Phyliky RL, Fleming CR. Zinc-induced copper deficiency. Gastroenterology 1988;94:508–512.
24. Leonard A, Ferber GB, Leonard F. Mutagenicity, carcinogenicity and teratogenicity of zinc. Mutat Res 1986;168:343–353.
25. American Congress of Government Industrial Hygienists. Threshold limit values and biological exposure indices for 1989–1990. Cincinnati: ACGIH, 1989.
26. Dalager NA, Mason TJ, Fraumeni JF, Hoover R, Payne WW. Cancer mortality among workers exposed to zinc chromate paints. J Occup Med 1989;22:25–29.
27. Banner W, Koch M, Hopf S, Yates M, Goldstein J, Tong T. N-Acetylcystein in the chelation of zinc sulfate. (Abstract)
28. Domingo JL, Llobet JM, Paternain JL, Corbella J. Acute zinc intoxication: comparison of the antidotal efficacy of several chelating agents. Vet Hum Toxicol 1988;30:224–228.
29. Elinder C. Zinc, Chapter 28, in: Handbook on the toxicology of metals. 2nd ed. New York: Elsevier Science Publishers, 1986: 664–679.

81

Nickel

F. William Sunderman, Jr., M.D.

CHEMICAL AND PHYSICAL FORMS OF NICKEL

Common Names and Chemical Names

Nickel (Ni, atomic weight 58.71), the 24th element in order of natural abundance in the earth's crust, has no other common or chemical names.

Chemical Forms

Nickel exists in five major forms: (a) elemental Ni and its alloys, (b) inorganic, water-soluble Ni compounds, (c) inorganic, water-insoluble Ni compounds, (d) organic, water-insoluble Ni compounds, and (e) nickel carbonyl $Ni(CO)_4$. The oxidation states of Ni include $-1, 0, +1, +2, +3$, and $+4$. but the prevalent valences are 0 (e.g., in Ni metal, Ni alloys, and $Ni(CO)_4$ and $+2$ (e.g., in $NiCl_2$, $NiSO_4$, and NiO). Since Ni atoms contain unpaired electrons in two outer 3d orbitals, Ni can undergo redox reactions that involve transfers of one electron; as a consequence, Ni compounds participate in free-radical reactions that may contribute to Ni toxicity and carcinogenesis (1, 2).

Physical Forms

Nickel is a silver-white, lustrous, hard, malleable, ductile, ferromagnetic metal, resistant to corrosion in fresh- or seawater, as well as in many acids and alkalis. In crystalline compounds, Ni is usually found either in the α-form (with an hexagonal lattice) or in the β-form (with a cubic lattice). In aqueous solutions, Ni exists principally as the hexaquonickel ion, $Ni(H_2O)_6 2+$, which has an emerald green color. Nickel monoxide, NiO, occurs in two major forms with different properties: black NiO, which is chemically reactive and readily forms nickel salts on contact with mineral acids, and green NiO, which is relatively inert and refractory to solubilization in dilute acids. $Ni(CO)_4$ is a colorless liquid that boils at 43°C; the volatility and lipid solubility of $Ni(CO)_4$ are responsible for its extreme toxicity.

SITES AND INDUSTRIES ASSOCIATED WITH NICKEL EXPOSURES

Industries with Exposures to Nickel Compounds

The industries with particular exposures to Ni include (a) mining and refining of Ni ores and production of Ni alloys (e.g., stainless steel, Monel metal, nichrome); (b) electroplating; (c) welding; (d) fabrication of nickel-cadmium batteries; (e) production of glass bottles (owing to the common use of Ni molds); (f) making coins, jewelry, cutlery, and dental or medical implants; (g) chemical, pigment, and ceramic industries; (h) manufacture of magnetic tapes and computer components; (i)

production and use of Ni catalysts (e.g., Raney nickel) for hydrogenation of soaps, fats, and oils; (j) incineration of Ni-containing wastes; and (k) combustion of fossil fuels (3–6).

Mechanisms and Processes Leading to Nickel Exposures

In Ni refineries, atmospheric contamination by process dusts and aerosols (e.g., nickel subsulfide, αNi_3S_2; nickel hydroxide, $Ni(OH)_2$; nickel monoxide, NiO; nickel sulfate, $NiSO_4$ leads to inhalation exposures that can cause cancers of the respiratory tract. Accidental contamination of potable water or beverages with high concentrations of soluble Ni salts leads to oral exposures that may induce acute Ni toxicity. Use of jewelry, coins, and utensils that contain Ni alloys or have Ni-plated coatings leads to dermal contact that can induce hypersensitivity and dermatitis. Implantation of Ni-containing protheses or iatrogenic administration of Ni-contaminated medications (e.g., albumin, radiocontrast media, hemodialysis fluids) leads to parenteral exposures, causing acute toxicity, immunological disturbances, and possibly neoplasia. Industrial processes that involve nickel carbonyl (e.g., Mond reaction for nickel refining; Reppe reaction for synthesis of methacrylates, vapor-plating of electronics components) may lead to inhalation exposures to $Ni(CO)_4$ vapor, resulting in acute or chronic pulmonary injury.

CLINICAL TOXICOLOGY OF NICKEL EXPOSURE

Routes of Nickel Exposure

The *respiratory exposure route* is of paramount importance in nickel carcinogenesis. Epidemiologic studies have demonstrated increased incidence of cancers of the nasal cavities and lung in workers chronically exposed to inhalation of Ni refinery dusts (5). The *respiratory, oral,* and *parenteral exposure routes* are all important for acute nickel toxicity (e.g., inhalation of $Ni(CO)_4$; use of Ni-contaminated medications) (6-8). The *dermal exposure route* is primarily involved in nickel dermatitis, but evidence is growing that oral exposures to Ni can potentiate hand eczema in nickel-sensitive patients (9).

Absorption of Nickel

Inhaled nickel refinery dust is retained in the nasal sinuses and lungs for years after the cessation of exposure; some of the nickel is slowly absorbed, as evidenced by the sustained presence of hypernickelemia in retired refinery workers (10). Studies of acutely poisoned workers and animal experiments show that inhaled $Ni(CO)_4$ vapor is rapidly absorbed via the lung and enters erythrocytes, where the compound undergoes conversion to Ni^{2+} and carbon monoxide (11,12). Based on experiments in 10 human volunteers who received an oral dose of $NiSO_4$ (12–50 μg/kg body weight, added to drinking water or food), the alimentary absorption of Ni averaged 27% (SD ± 17) of the dose ingested in water after an overnight fast, compared with 0.7% (SD ± 0.4) of the same dose added to a standard American breakfast (i.e., a 40-fold difference) (13). During extracorporeal hemodialysis, traces of Ni^{2+} in hemodialysis fluid are absorbed into the plasma compartment, owing to the chelating action of plasma albumin (14).

Metabolism of Nickel

The metabolism and distribution of Ni^{2+} in humans has been fitted by a two-compartment toxicokinetic model (13). In human serum, Ni^{2+} is bound to albumin, nickeloplasmin (an $α_2$-macroglobulin), and ultrafiltrable constituents (e.g., histidine, glycine, aspartic acid) (15,16). Scanty data are available on the distribution of Ni in tissues of nonexposed persons. Based on analyses of autopsy tissues from 10 such subjects, mean Ni concentrations were ranked as follows: lung ⟩ thyroid ⟩ adrenal ⟩ kidney ⟩ heart ⟩ liver ⟩ brain ⟩ spleen ⟩ pancreas (17). Studies in rodents show that Ni^{2+} induces metallothionein synthesis in kidney and liver, but Ni^{2+} evidently does not bind to metallothioneins in these tissues (18).

Elimination of Nickel

Urine is the major route for elimination of absorbed Ni. In 50 healthy persons without occupational exposures, urine Ni excretion averaged 2.6 (SD ± 1.4) μg/day (19). In 10 volunteers who ingested $NiSO_4$, as described above, renal Ni elimination half-time averaged 28 (SD ± 9) hours; the renal clearance of Ni absorbed from drinking water averaged 8.3 (SD ± 2.0) ml/min/1.73 m^2 of body surface area (13). Approximately 99% of nickel in food remains unabsorbed in the alimentary tract and passes directly into the feces, averaging 208 (SD ± 146) μg/day (6, 13). Bile, sweat, saliva, gastric and intestinal secretions, hair, dermal detritus, milk, and menses are evidently minor routes for Ni elimination in humans (19).

SIGNS, SYMPTOMS, AND SYNDROMES FROM NICKEL EXPOSURES

Acute Nickel Toxicity

Two forms of acute Ni poisoning merit discussion: toxicity from inhalation of $Ni(CO)_4$ and toxicity from oral or parenteral exposures to Ni^{2+}.

Acute Nickel Carbonyl Poisoning Accidental inhalation of $Ni(CO)_4$ generally causes acute toxic effects in two stages, immediate and delayed. The immediate symptoms (e.g., headache, vertigo, nausea, vomiting, insomnia, irritability) usually last a few hours, followed by an asymptomatic interval of 12 hours to 5 days, before the onset of delayed pulmonary, cardiac, and neurological symptoms (e.g., tightness of the chest, non-productive cough, dyspnea, cyanosis, tachycardia, palpitations, sweating, visual disturbances, vertigo, weakness, and lassitude). The delayed symptoms can mimic viral pneumonia. In cases of severe $Ni(CO)_4$ poisoning, deaths have occurred 4–13 days postexposure. Autopsies have revealed pulmonary hemorrhage, protein-rich alveolar exudate, interstitial pneumonitis, damage to alveolar lining

cells, and denudation of bronchial epithelium. Pathological lesions (e.g., parenchymal degeneration, edema, punctate hemorrhages) have been noted in brain, liver, kidney, adrenals, and spleen. In survivors, the recovery period tends to be protracted, with lassitude and dyspnea persisting up to 6 months (20–23).

Acute Toxicity from Divalent Nickel Acute N^{2+} toxicity occurred when 32 electroplating workers accidently drank water contaminated with $NiSO_4$ and $NiCl_2$ (1.6 g Ni per liter) (24, 25). Twenty of the workers promptly developed symptoms (e.g., nausea, vomiting, abdominal discomfort, diarrhea, giddiness, lassitude, headache, cough, shortness of breath) that generally ceased within a few hours, but lasted 1–2 days in seven cases. In workers with symptoms, the Ni doses ranged from approximately 0.5–2.5 g. All of the subjects recovered rapidly, without evident sequelae and returned to work by the eighth day after exposure (25). Acute Ni^{2+} toxicity also occurred when 23 hemodialysis patients were accidently exposed to Ni-contaminated dialysis fluid, owing to leaching of a Ni-plated heating tank (26). Symptoms (e.g., nausea, vomiting, weakness, headache, palpitations) developed during and after the dialysis treatment and generally lasted a few hours, but persisted for 2 days in some subjects. No adverse sequelae were noted (26).

Chronic Nickel Toxicity

The chronic effects of exposures to Ni compounds primarily affect the immune system and the respiratory tract.

Immune system Hypersensitivity to Ni is a common cause of allergic contact dermatitis; positive dermal patch tests to Ni occur in 7–10% of women and 1–3% of men in the general population (9). Nickel dermatitis usually begins as a papulovesicular erythema of the hands, forearms, earlobes, or other areas of skin that contact Ni alloys and spreads secondarily to areas (usually symmetrical) that are distant from the contact sites. The erythematous lesions become eczematous and eventually undergo lichenification. Pompholyx (i.e., dyshidrotic eczema) is the predominant type of nickel-induced dermatitis, characteristically affecting the sides of the fingers, the palms, and sometimes the soles. Hypersensitivity to Ni can also cause pulmonary asthma, conjunctivitis, inflammatory reactions around Ni-containing dental implants or orthopedic prostheses, and anaphylactoid reactions after parenteral injection of Ni-contaminated medications (6, 19).

Respiratory Tract Chronic respiratory insufficiency may develop as a consequence of acute $Ni(CO)_4$ poisoning (23). In workers in Ni refineries, plating shops, and welding shops, chronic inhalation exposures to irritant Ni-containing dusts and aerosols may contribute to chronic respiratory diseases, including asthma, bronchitis, and pneumoconiosis (27). Ni-exposed workers can also develop hypertrophic rhinitis, sinusitis, nasal polyposis, and nasal septal perforations (27). The incidences of nonneoplastic respiratory diseases in Ni-exposed workers have not been thoroughly studied and the etiologic role of Ni may be debated, since affected workers are often exposed to sundry dusts and vapors, in addition to Ni compounds (6).

Nickel Carcinogenesis

Numerous studies have documented increased mortality rates from carcinomas of the lung and nasal cavities in nickel refinery workers, evidently as a result of chronic exposures to airborne Ni compounds (5, 7, 8, 27). Increased risks of other malignant tumors, including carcinomas of the larynx, kidney, prostate, and stomach, as well as soft tissue sarcomas, have occasionally been noted, but the statistical significance of these findings seems nil or dubious (28). Respiratory tract cancers in nickel refinery workers have been associated with inhalation exposures to Ni compounds with low aqueous solubility (e.g., αNi_3S_2, NiO), as well as soluble nickel compounds (e.g., $NiSO_4$).

Management of Nickel Toxicity

Diagnosis and Treatment of Acute Nickel Carbonyl Poisoning   After accidental exposure to $Ni(CO)_4$, the victim should be quickly transported to a hospital, following removal of any contaminated clothing, institution of life support measures, and administration of oxygen (12, 20, 21). The immediate therapy is similar to that for acute carbon monoxide poisoning. Hyperglycemia and glycosuria typically develop following exposure to $Ni(CO)_4$. An acute exposure to $Ni(CO)_4$ is classified as *mild* if the initial 8-hour urine collection has a Ni concentration <100 μg/liter; *moderate* if the Ni concentration in the initial 8-hour urine collection is >100 but <500 μg/liter and *severe* if the Ni concentration is >500 μg/liter. Patients in the *moderate* and *severe* categories of acute $Ni(CO)_4$ poisoning should be treated immediately with a chelating drug, sodium diethyldithiocarbamate (DDC) (20, 21). The beneficial effect of DDC in acute $Ni(CO)_4$ poisoning is attributed to marked diminution of the pulmonary Ni burden (29).

Diagnosis and Treatment of Divalent Nickel Toxicity   Presumptive diagnosis of acute Ni^{2+} poisoning derives from the clinical history and, if feasible, qualitative or quantitative analysis of Ni in the exposure medium (25). The immediate supportive treatment is to maintain body temperature, since Ni^{2+} impairs thermoregulation, and to administer i.v. fluids to induce diuresis, since Ni^{2+} is eliminated via the urine. Confirmation of the diagnosis rests upon quantitative determinations of Ni in body fluids, usually serum and urine.

In 19 electroplating workers who developed acute toxic symptoms after ingesting Ni^{2+-} contaminated water, serum Ni concentrations averaged 286 μg/liter (range 13–1340 μg/liter) and urine Ni concentrations averaged 5.8 mg/l (range 0.23–37 μg/liter) on the day after exposure (25). For comparison, the reference intervals for healthy, nonexposed persons are <0.05–1.1 μg Ni per liter of serum and 0.5–6.1 μg/liter in urine (19). The 10 most severely exposed workers were treated by i.v. infusion of isotonic sodium chloride solution at 150 ml/h for 3 days. The half-time for urinary elimination of Ni in these subjects averaged 27 hours (SD $\pm$ 7), which was significantly shorter than the mean half-time of 60 $\pm$ 11 hours in the subjects who did not receive i.v. fluid therapy. Transient hyperbilirubinemia, proteinuria, and reticulocytosis occurred in some patients, but all had rapid and uneventful recovery.

Hemodialysis would be the therapy of choice in acute Ni^{2+} poisoning, if renal function fails or cardiac or neurotoxicity becomes life-threatening. In contradistinction to acute $Ni(CO)_4$ poisoning, chelation treatment with diethyldithiocarbamate (DDC)

would be inadvisable in severe Ni^{2+} toxicity, since DDC enhances the cerebral uptake of Ni^{2+} (30, 31).

Biologic Monitoring of Exposures to Nickel   Urine and serum are the usual media for monitoring occupational, environmental, and iatrogenic exposures to Ni compounds. Urine specimens have the drawbacks of matrix variability and fluctuating specific gravity, but urine is generally preferable to serum, since collection of urine is noninvasive; collection of blood for Ni analysis, on the other hand, requires venipuncture with a plastic i.v. cannula (to avoid nickel contamination from steel needles), and Ni concentrations are approximately 8 times higher in urine that serum, enhancing the analytical accuracy and the sensitivity of monitoring (6, 19). Fecal analysis provides the most reliable index of oral exposures to Ni; expired breath may be useful for detection of $Ni(CO)_4$ after its inhalation. Analyses of Ni in other biological media, such as tissue samples obtained by biopsy or necropsy, and whole blood, saliva, sweat, milk, or hair are useful for investigative purposes (6, 19).

Readers are referred to reviews on Ni analysis for recommendations about specimen collection, transport, and storage, instrumental techniques, and quality assurance procedures (32-35). Electrothermal atomic absorption spectrophotometry (EAAS) and differential pulse absorption voltametry (DPAV) are the analytical approaches that have sufficient sensitivity to measure Ni concentrations in body fluids of nonexposed persons. The detection limits for Ni determinations by EAAS analysis with Zeeman background correction are approximately 0.5 μg/liter for urine, 0.1 μg/liter for whole blood, 0.05 μg/liter for serum, and 0.01 μg/g (dry weight) for tissues (6,34). Nickel analysis by DPAV with a dimethylglyoxime-sensitized mercury electrode provides detection limits as low as 1 ng/liter for Ni concentrations in whole blood, urine, saliva, and tissue homogenates (36). However, DPAV analyses are more cumbersome, difficult, and time-consuming than EAAS procedures. Nickel concentrations in body fluids and tissues from nonexposed persons are listed in Table 81.7 based on EAAS analyses in the author's laboratory (6, 13).

Studies in Ni refineries have demonstrated that biological monitoring programs can identify individual workers who fail to adhere to recommended work practices, as well as groups of workers with elevated Ni exposures (37, 38). Nickel concentrations in urine or serum specimens from workers with inhalation exposures to soluble Ni salts reflect the amount of Ni absorbed during the 1 or 2 preceding days. In contrast, in workers with inhalation exposures to Ni powders, alloys, and poorly soluble Ni compounds, Ni concentrations in urine and serum specimens reflect the combined influences of recent exposures and longterm accumulation, as well as the bioavailability of the Ni species (6, 19).

In persons exposed to soluble Ni compounds (e.g., $NiCl_2$, $NiSO_4$), Ni concentrations in body fluids are generally proportional to the exposure levels; absence of increased values usually indicates nonsignificant exposure and presence of increased values should be a signal to reduce the exposure. In persons exposed to poorly soluble Ni compounds (e.g., αNi_3S_2, NiO), increased concentrations of Ni in body fluids are generally indicative of significant Ni absorption and should be a signal to reduce the exposures to the lowest levels attainable by current technology; absence of increased values does not necessarily indicate freedom from the health risk (e.g., cancers of the nasal cavities and lungs) that have been associated with chronic exposures to such compounds (6, 19).

Table 81.1.   Nickel Concentrations in Body Fluids and Excreta of Healthy, Nonexposed Persons (6, 12).

Specimen	Subjects	Nickel Concentrations		Units
		mean ± SD	range	
Whole blood	30 (15m, 15f)	0.34 ± 0.28	<0.05–1.05	μg/liter
Serum	30 (15m, 15f)	0.28 ± 0.24	>0.05–1.08	μg/liter
Urine (random collection)	34 (18m, 16f)	2.0 ± 1.5	0.5–6.1	μg/liter
		2.0 ± 1.5	0.4–6.0	μg/g creatinine
Urine (24 hour collection)	50 (24m, 26f)	2.2 ± 1.2	0.7–5.2	μg/liter
		2.6 ± 1.4	0.5–6.4	μg/day
Feces (3 or 4 days)	20 (12m, 8f)	208 ± 146	69–540	μg/day

Special Diagnostic Tests   In addition to the analyses of Ni concentrations in biological samples discussed above, special diagnostic tests are employed to detect specific pathologic effects of Ni exposures (6, 9). These tests include (a) biopsy and cytological studies to detect respiratory tract dysplasia and neoplasia; (b) immunological tests for tumor antigens; (c) dermal patch test, lymphocyte transformation assay, and leukocyte procoagulant assay to detect Ni hypersensitivity; (d) β_2-microglobulin assay to detect nephrotoxicity; (e) pulmonary function tests; and (f) radiography of the chest and computerized axial tomography of the mediastinum and nasal cavities to detect chronic respiratory effects and tumors.

Environmental Exposures to Nickel   Nickel enters groundwater and surface water from dissolution of rocks and soils, from biologic cycles, from atmospheric fallout, and especially from industrial processes and waste disposal (1–5). Nickel leached from dump sites can contribute to nickel contamination of the aquifer, with potential ecotoxicity. Most inorganic Ni compounds are relatively soluble at pH values <6.5, whereas Ni exists predominantly as insoluble hydroxides at pH values >6.7. Therefore, acid rain has a pronounced tendency to mobilize Ni from soil and increase Ni concentrations in ground waters, leading eventually to increased uptake and potential toxicity for microorganisms, plants, and animals. Sea water contains 0.1–0.5 μg Ni per liter. Surface waters average 15–20 μg/liter and drinking water usually contains <20 μg Ni per liter. Drinking water samples occasionally contain much higher Ni concentrations, owing to pollution of the water supply or leaching from Ni-containing pipes or Ni-plated faucets. For example, Ni concentrations in municipal water samples collected at five locations in Sudbury, Ontario, Canada, averaged 109 μg/l (range 65–179 μg/L), attributable to the local deposits of Ni ore and pollution from Ni mines and smelters (39).

Nickel enters the atmosphere from natural sources (e.g., volcanic emissions and windblown dusts produced by weathering of rocks and soils), from combustion of fossil fuels, from the emissions of nickel mining and refining operations, from metal consumption in industrial processes, and from incineration of wastes. Atmospheric concentrations of Ni in urban areas are often related to the consumption of fossil fuels, since, for example, the Ni content of coal ranges from 4–24 mg/kg. Substantial atmospheric emissions of nickel are derived from fly-ash released from coal-fired power plants; nickel derived from petroleum is released into the environment in automotive exhaust fumes. In the USA, atmospheric Ni concentrations average 6 ng/m³ for nonurban areas, versus 17 ng/m³ (in summer) and 25 ng/m³ (in winter) for urban areas. In industrialized regions and large cities, atmospheric Ni concentrations as high as 170 ng/m³ have been recorded. Inhalation of Ni averages 0.2 μg/day (range 0.1–0.4 μg/day) for rural dwellers, com-

pared with 0.4 μg/day (range 0.2–1.0 μg/day) for urban dwellers (40). Cigarette smoking can increase inhaled Ni by as much as 4 μg/pack of cigarettes (41).

The average dietary intake of Ni by adult persons is approximately 165 μg/day, but may reach 900 μg/day in diets rich in oatmeal, cocoa, chocolate, nuts and soya products (1–5, 41).

Exposure Limits for Nickel   According to a recent tabulation of industrial regulations in 10 nations (42), the atmospheric limits for occupational exposures to nickel metal and sparingly soluble Ni compounds are as follows: 1 mg/m³—United Kingdom (UK), Japan, Netherlands, USA; 0.5 mg/m³—Denmark, Federal Republic of Germany (FRG), USSR, Sweden; 0.1 mg/m³—Norway; 0.01 mg/m³—Czechoslovakia. The corresponding atmospheric limits for occupational exposures to soluble Ni compounds are as follows: 1 mg/m³—Denmark, Japan, USA (OSHA); 0.1 mg/m³—Netherlands, Norway, Sweden, USA (ACGIH); 0.05 mg/m³—Czechoslovakia, FRG; 0.005 mg/m³—USSR. The limit value for Ni(CO)$_4$ for all countries except the FRG, where the limit is 0.07 mg/m³. In the FRG, Ni metal, nickel sulfides and sulfide ores, nickel oxides, and nickel carbonate, as they occur during production and use, are considered as carcinogens, so that no "MAK" limit has been established; only a technical guideline has been provided. The US Environmental Protection Agency is currently formulating regulations for Ni concentrations in drinking water; in the USSR, the maximum allowable concentrations for Ni are 200 μg/l in drinking water and 1 mg/l in wastewater directed to biologic treatment (43).

INFORMATION ON NICKEL TOXICOLOGY AND CARCINOGENESIS

For information on the toxicity and carcinogenicity of Ni compounds in experimental animals and the molecular mechanisms of Ni-induced genotoxicity, readers are referred to recent articles and reviews (44–52).

REFERENCES

1. Sunderman Jr, FW. Nickel. In: Seiler HG, Sigel H, eds. Handbook on toxicology of inorganic compounds. New York: Marcel Dekker, 1987.
2. Sunderman Jr, FW. Oskarsson A. Nickel. In: Merian E, ed. Metals and their compounds in the environment. Weinheim: VCH Verlag, 1990.
3. Sunderman Jr, FW. Sources of exposure and biological effects of nickel. In: O'Neill IK, Schuller P, Fishbein L, eds. Environmental carcinogens—selected methods of analysis. Lyon: International Agency for Research on Cancer, 1986;8:79–92.
4. Nriagu JO, ed. Nickel in the environment. New York: Wiley, 1980.
5. Sunderman Jr, FW, editor-in-chief. Nickel in the human environment. Lyon: International Agency for Research on Cancer, 1984.
6. Sunderman Jr, FW. Nickel. In: Clarkson TW, Friberg L, Nordberg GF,

Sager PR, eds. Biological monitoring of toxic metals. New York: Plenum Press, 1988.

7. Brown SS, Sunderman Jr, FW. Nickel toxicology. London: Academic Press, 1980.

8. Brown SS, Sunderman Jr, FW. eds. Progress in nickel toxicology. Oxford: Blackwells, 1985.

9. Maibach HI, Menné T, eds. Nickel and the skin: immunology and toxicology. Boca Raton, FL: CRC Press, 1989.

10. Torjussen W, Andersen I. Nickel concentrations in nasal mucosa, plasma, and urine in active and retired nickel workers. Ann Clin Lab Sci 1979;9:289–298.

11. Mikehyev MI. Distribution and excretion of nickel carbonyl. Gig Trud Prof Zab 1971;15:35–38.

12. Sunderman Jr, FW. A review of the metabolism and toxicology of nickel. Ann Clin Lab Sci 1977;7:377–398.

13. Sunderman Jr, FW, Hopfer SM, Sweeney KR, Marcus AH, Most BM, Creason J. Nickel absorption and kinetics in human volunteers. Proc Soc Exp Biol Med 1989;191:5–11.

14. Hopfer SM, Linden JV, Crisostomo MC, Catalanatto FA, Galen M, Sunderman Jr, FW. Hypernickelemia in hemodialysis patients. Trace Element Med 1985;2:68–72.

15. Sunderman Jr, FW. Kinetics and biotransformation of nickel and chromium. In: Stern RM, Berlin A, Fletcher Jr, AC, eds. Health hazards and biological effects of welding fumes and gases. Amsterdam: Excerpta Medica, 1986.

16. Nomoto S, Sunderman Jr, FW. Presence of nickel in alpha-2 macroglobulin isolated from human serum by high performance liquid chromatography. Ann Clin Lab Sci 1988;18:78–84.

17. Rezuke WN, Knight JA, Sunderman Jr, FW. Reference values for nickel concentrations in human tissues and bile. Am J Ind Med 1987;11:419–426.

18. Sunderman Jr, FW, Fraser CB. Effects of $NiCl_2$ and diethyldithiocarbamate on metallothionein in rat liver and kidney. Ann Clin Lab Sci 1983;13:489–495.

19. Sunderman Jr, FW, Aitio A, Morgan LG, Norseth T. Biological monitoring of nickel. Toxicol Ind Health 1986;2:17–78.

20. Sunderman FW, Sunderman Jr, FW. Nickel poisoning VIII. Dithiocarb: a new therapeutic agent for persons exposed to nickel carbonyl. Am J Med Sci 1958;236:26–31.

21. Sunderman FW. The treatment of acute nickel carbonyl poisoning by sodium diethyldithio-carbamate. Ann Clin Res 1971;3:182–185.

22. Vuopala U, Huhti E, Takkunen J, Huikko M. Nickel carbonyl poisoning. Report of 25 cases. Ann Clin Res 1970;2:214–222.

23. Shi Z. Acute nickel carbonyl poisoning: A report of 179 cases. Br J Ind Med 1986;43:422–424.

24. Daldrup T, Haarhoff K, Szathmary SC. Toedliche nickel-sulfate Intoxikation. Bericht Gerichtl Med 1983;41:141–144.

25. Sunderman Jr, FW, Dingle B, Hopfer SM, Swift T. Acute nickel toxicty in electroplating workers who accidently ingested a solution of nickel sulfate and nickel chloride. Am J Ind Med 1988;14:257–266.

26. Webster JD, Parker TF, Alfery AC, Smythe WR, Kubo H, Neal G, Hull AR. Acute nickel poisoning by dialysis. Ann Intern Med 1980;92:631–633.

27. Anon. Health Assessment Document for Nickel and Nickel Compounds. (Report #600/8-83/012FF) US Environmental Protection Agency. Washington, DC: EPA, 1986.

28. Doll R. Nickel exposure: a human health hazard. In: Sunderman Jr, FW, editor-in-chief. Nickel in the human environment. Lyon: International Agency for Research on Cancer, 1984:3–21.

29. Tjalve H, Jasim S, Oskarsson A. Nickel mobilization by sodium diethyldithiocarbamate in nickel-carbonyl-treated mice. Sunderman Jr, FW, editor-in-chief. Nickel in the human environment. Lyon: International Agency for Research on Cancer, 1984:311–320.

30. Oskarsson A, Tjalve H. Effects of diethyldithiocarbamate and penicillamine on the tissue distribution of ^{63}Ni in mice. Arch Toxicol 1980;45:45–52.

31. Belliveau JF, O'Leary GP, Cadwell L, Sunderman Jr, FW. Effect of diethyldithiocarbamate on nickel concentrations in tissues of $NiCl_2$-treated rats. Ann Clin Lab Sci 1985;15:349–350.

32. Stoeppler M. Analysis of nickel in biological materials and natural waters. In: Nriagu JO, ed. Nickel in the environment. New York: Wiley, 1980:661–882.

33. Sunderman Jr, FW. Determination of nickel in body fluids, tissues, excreta, and water. In O'Neill IK, Schuller P, Fishbein L, eds. Environmental carcinogens: selected methods of analysis. Lyon: International Agency for Research on Cancer, 1986;8:319–334.

34. Sunderman Jr, FW, Hopfer SM, Crisostomo MC. Nickel analysis by atomic absorption spectrometry. Methods Enzymol 1988;158:382–391.

35. Sunderman Jr, FW. Chemistry, analysis, and monitoring of nickel. In: Maibach HI, Menné T, eds. Nickel and the skin: immunology and toxicology. Boca Raton, FL: CRC Press, 1989:1–8.

36. Ostapczuk P, Valenta P, Stoeppler M, Nurnberg HW. Voltametric determination of nickel and cobalt in body fluids and other biological materials. In: Brown SS, Savory J, eds. Chemical toxicology and clinical chemistry of metals. London: Academic Press, 1983:61–64.

37. Hogetveit AC, Barton RT, Andersen I. Variations of nickel in plasma and urine during the work period. J Occup Med 1980;22:597–600.

38. Morgan LG, Rouge PJC. Biological monitoring in nickel refinery workers. In: Sunderman Jr, FW, editor-in-chief. Nickel in the human environment. Lyon: International Agency for Research on Cancer, 1984:507–520.

39. Hopfer SM, Fay WP, Sunderman Jr, FW. Serum nickel concentrations in hemodialysis patients with environmental exposure. Ann Clin Lab Sci 1989;19:161–167.

40. Bennett BG. Environmental nickel pathways to man. In: Sunderman Jr, FW, editor-in-chief, Nickel in the human environment. Lyon: International Agency for Research on Cancer, 1984.487–495.

41. Grandjean P. Human exposure to nickel. In: Sunderman Jr, FW, editor-in-chief, Nickel in the human environment. Lyon: International Agency for Research on Cancer, 1984:469–485.

42. Grandjean P. Health effects document on nickel. Toronto: Ontario Ministry of Labour, 1986.

43. Izmerov NF. Nickel and its compounds. Moscow: Center of International Projects, USSR State Committee of Science and Technology (GKNT), 1984.

44. Coogan TP, Latta DM, Snow ET, Costa M. Toxicity and carcinogenicity of nickel compounds. CRC Crit Rev Toxicol 1989;19:341–384.

45. Dostal LA, Hopfer SM, Lin SM, Sunderman Jr, FW. Effects of nickel chloride on lactating rats and their suckling pups, and the transfer of nickel through rat milk. Toxicol Appl Pharmacol 1989;101:220–231.

46. Fischer AB. The cellular toxicity of nickel. Life Sci Rep 1989;7:149–168.

47. Kasprzak KS. Nickel. In: Fishbein L, Furst A, eds. Genotoxic and carcinogenic metals: occupational occurrence and exposure. Princeton: Princeton Scientific Publications, 1987:145–183.

48. Kasprzak KS, Hernandez L. Enhancement of hydroxylation and deglycosylation of 2'-deoxyguanosine by carcinogenic nickel compounds. Cancer Res 1989;49:5964–5968.

49. Miura T, Patierno SR, Sakuramoto T, Landolph JR. Morphological and neoplastic transformation of C3H/10T½ Cl8 mouse embryo cells by insoluble carcinogenic nickel compounds. Environ Mol Mutagen 1989;14:65–78.

50. Sunderman Jr, FW. Lipid peroxidation as a mechanism of acute nickel toxicity. Toxicol Environ Chem 1987;15:59–69.

51. Sunderman Jr, FW. Mechanisms of nickel carcinogenesis. Scand J Work Environ Health 1989;15:1–12.

52. Sunderman Jr, FW. Toxicity to alveolar macrophages in rats following parenteral injection of nickel chloride. Toxicol Appl Pharmacol 1989;100:107–118.

82

Platinum and Related Metals: Palladium, Iridium, Osmium, Rhodium, and Ruthenium

Peter L. Goering, Ph.D.

INTRODUCTION*

Platinum (Pt) and the Pt metals, palladium (Pd), rhodium (Rh), ruthenium (Ru), iridium (Ir), and osmium (Os), are members of Group VIII of the Periodic Table of Elements. These elements, collectively referred to as the platinoids, are of high commercial value because of their great resistance to most corrosive agents. Alloys of platinum and the platinoids appear in chemical, petroleum, electrical, and automotive industries and in jewelry. Platinum salts are used as catalysts in automotive and chemical industries. The metals in this group are generally nontoxic in the metallic state, but the soluble halide salts, particularly of platinum, and osmium tetroxide (OsO_4) are highly reactive. Exposure to these elements results in hypersensitivity-allergy reactions in susceptible atopic individuals. Platinum is one of two heavy metals, along with gold, being used clinically: gold complexes for rheumatoid arthritis and platinum complexes for cancer chemotherapy. The platinum chemotherapeutic compounds, e.g., cisplatin, are used to treat testicular, ovarian, bladder, prostate, thyroid, head, and neck tumors that are unresponsive to standard chemotherapy. The use of these compounds is limited because renal, gastrointestinal, hematologic, and otologic toxicities may occur. The platinoids are not essential elements in mammals.

SOURCES AND PRODUCTION

Chemical Forms

Many complex salts of the platinum metals exist but the most common are: platinum chloride (platinum tetrachloride, platinic chloride, $PtCl_4$); platinum dichloride (platinous chloride, $PtCl_2$); platinum dioxide (platinic oxide, PtO_2); and platinum sulfate (platinic sulfate, $Pt(SO_4)_2$). Other salts, which are water soluble, include: ammonium and sodium chloroplatinates; sodium, potassium, and ammonium tetrachloroplatinates; and sodium, potassium, and ammonium hexachloroplatinates (1).

The platinoids form an important group of commercial metal alloys. Many of these alloys, such as Pt-Ir, are used for applications where high corrosion resistance is needed. Other alloys (uses in parentheses) include platinum black (catalyst), Pt-Co (permanent magnets), and Pt-Rh (catalyst) (2). In clinical medicine, the two most widely used chemotherapeutic platinum complexes are cis-diamminedichloroplatinum(II) (cisplatin, CDDP) and cis-diammine(1,1-cyclobutane dicarboxylato)platinum(II) (carboplatin, CBDCA).

The most biologically relevant oxidation states of platinum in chemical complexes are +2 (II) and +4 (IV). The coordination chemistry of Pt (II) complexes is square-planar, while that of Pt (IV) complexes is octahedral. These complexes are very stable, forming covalent attachments to various ligands which are relatively inert to ligand substitution (6). Others report that the square-planar, but not the octahedral, configuration is highly labile (7).

Other platinoids possess valence states ranging from +2 to +8. In biologic media, rhodium, ruthenium, and iridium, but not palladium and osmium, form stable compounds with a coordination number of 6 and an octahedral configuration. Simple salts such as chlorides, bromides, and sulfates and complex hexamine and tetramine salts of the platinoids are water soluble (7).

Ruthenium can exhibit valence states from +2 to +8, but +3 is the most common. $Ru(OH)_2$, $RuCL_4$, and RuO_2 are stable and water soluble, but generally the trivalent salts are not soluble. Rhodium forms salts with valence states +2, +3, and +4. Chloride, nitrate, sulfate salts, and the soluble hexachloro complexes are trivalent (7).

Palladium salts are water soluble and form di- and tetravalent salts. Palladium coordination complexes have not been demonstrated to be present in biologic systems. Iridium forms di-, tri-, and tetravalent compounds. Divalent halide and sulfate salts are water soluble, as are the anionic hexachloro- and hexaoxaloiridates (7).

Stable forms of osmium exhibit valences of +3, +4, and +8. The tri- and tetrahalides and tetroxides are water soluble, and OsO_4^{2-} is slightly soluble (7).

Physical Forms

Metallic platinum is available in several forms: powder (platinum black); single crystalline solids; wire (0.05–0.005 diameter); and other compositions used for electronics, metallizing, and decorating ceramics and metals (8). Powdered platinum black is finely divided metallic platinum and is flammable when exposed to air. Soluble salts exist and are the most toxic forms. The other platinoids exist as fumes and dusts in metallic form, and the soluble salts exist as crystalline solids (8).

SITES, INDUSTRIES, AND BUSINESSES ASSOCIATED WITH EXPOSURE

Sources and Uses

World production of new platinoid metals (not recycled) was reported in 1988 to be approximately 200 tons, of which greater than 90% was platinum and palladium (16). These elements are widely dispersed worldwide but the most economically significant deposits occur at parts per million levels in ores that contain significant deposits of copper and nickel. The main geographic sites for obtaining ore containing platinoid metals are in Sudbury, Ontario, Canada; the Bushveld Igneous Complex,

---

*The views stated in this chapter are not to be construed as official policy of the Food and Drug Administration.

Table 82.1.   Industries, Businesses, and Processes Associated with Platinoid Exposure

Primary production (mining and refining)
Recycling platinoid-containing products for extraction
Automotive
Electrical
Petroleum refining
Chemical
Ceramics, glass
Jewelry, arts
Dentistry
Pharmaceutical

South Africa; and near Norils'k, Siberia, Soviet Union, and in the Kola Peninsula, Soviet Union (6). The Soviet Union and South Africa produce 90% of all mined platinum. Other deposits are found in the Ural Mountains, in Colombia, and in some of the Western United States (9). Compound mineral species include sperrylite, $PtAs_2$; cooperite, PtS; and braggite, $(Pt, Pd, Ni)S$ (6, 9).

Table 82.1 lists the industries and businesses in which platinum and platinum metals are used with the percentage of total based on 1985 estimates (10): automotive (51%), electrical (13%), petroleum refining (10%), chemical (9%), ceramics and glass (3%), jewelry and arts (3%), dentistry (2%), and other (9%). The platinoids are of such value that end-products are recycled to extract these metals. Most of the commercial applications exploit the catalytic activities, nobility (resistance to oxidation), and strength (at high temperatures) of these elements. The chemical industry utilizes Pt-Rh catalysts for production of nitric acid and spinnerets for rayon, glass fiber, and Plexiglas manufacture. The pharmaceutical industry produces some drugs and vitamins with platinum catalysts, mostly in hydrogenation or dehydrogenation reactions. Platinum catalysts used in the automotive industry dominate use of this metal (approximately 50%) as a result of its being a component of catalytic converters for air pollution abatement (6, 8, 10).

Alloys of Pt-Ir are the most important commercial alloys because they are harder and more resistant to chemical attack than platinum alone. Such alloys are used for jewelry, electrical contacts, fuse wire, and hypodermic needles. Pt-Co alloys have been developed into powerful magnets and are used in hearing aids, self-winding watches, and dental alloys (11). Uses for other platinum alloys include dentistry, electroplating, and surgical wire (2). Palladium is also used in dental alloys (12, 13).

Research laboratories are the major consumers of osmium in the form of osmium tetroxide (OsO_4) which, when reduced, serves as a black tissue stain for electron microscopy. A potential new class of therapeutic agents, called osmarins, consist of osmium-carbohydrate polymers that are potent anti-inflammatory agents in experimental studies (14). Soluble salts of rhodium are used in electroplating and metallic Rh is used in the manufacture of high-reflectivity mirrors.

Mechanisms, Processes, Reactions Leading to Exposure

Most unintentional exposure to platinoid metals is due to poor industrial and occupational hygiene. Platinoid metals are mined, refined, and used as components in a number of commercial chemical processes; thus, workers can be exposed at any number of steps during production. In these production and man-

ufacturing steps, workers can be exposed through inhalation, dermal, and oral routes.

After mining, the ore is concentrated by crushing and flotation and then is smelted to produce a copper-nickel sulfide matte containing the platinoid metals. After further concentration processes, the metal-rich substance is refined in hydrochloric acid and chlorine. After distillation, platinum solutions are treated with ammonium chloride to precipitate ammonium hexachloroplatinate, which is redissolved and refined (15).

Industrial processing of platinoids may lead to inadvertent exposures. The petroleum industry uses platinum as a catalyst in a proprietary process known as "platforming," in which platinum catalyzes the isomerization of hydrocarbons in gasoline to increase its octane content. "Platfining" and "Platreating" are proprietary processes for the treatment of hydrocarbon mixtures to remove deleterious material such as sulfur and nitrogen to aid in the synthesis of hydrocarbons for petrochemical production (8).

Osmium poisoning occurs via inhalation of OsO_4, which readily vaporizes from aqueous solutions at room temperature. The alloy Os-Ir readily releases OsO_4 vapor at the high temperatures used for annealing processes (7).

Exposure to platinum complexes may occur in the clinical situation. Since its introduction into clinical practice in 1972, cisplatin administered alone or in combination with other chemotherapeutic agents has assumed a major role in the treatment of malignant testicular tumors (3, 4). Cisplatin has also exhibited major activity against ovarian cancer. Cisplatin may also be useful alone or in combination in the treatment of carcinomas of the bladder, lung, head and neck, endometrium, esophagus, and stomach. The compound has demonstrated some activity in the treatment of lymphomas and osteogenic sarcomas (3, 4). Recently the cisplatin analog, carboplatin, has been approved for use in the treatment of recurrent ovarian cancer (5). Carboplatin exhibits less toxic side effects than cisplatin but possesses comparable efficacy.

CLINICAL TOXICOLOGY OF EXPOSURE

Route of Exposure

There is a dearth of experimental reports available on the biochemistry and metabolism of the platinoids and their salts and even less literature dealing with clinical studies involving human exposures. The exceptions are the well-studied antitumor compounds cisplatin and carboplatin. Studies on the metabolism of platinoids are mostly of radioactive salts obtained from nuclear fission products. From the viewpoint of clinical toxicology, the most important routes of exposure for humans to the platinoids are inhalation and dermal, with oral exposure being much less significant. These exposures occur primarily in occupational settings. There is no evidence of human exposure to the platinoids as a result of environmental mobilization and excessive emissions due to mining and refining practices. The use of platinum and palladium as catalysts in automobile pollution abatement devices has not resulted in elevated concentrations of these elements near roads (16). When used in cancer chemotherapy, platinum compounds are administered intravenously.

Absorption

Oral absorption of the platinoids is very low. Generally, absorption of the platinoids via parenteral routes (s.c., i.m., i.p.)

other than i.v. is negligible, with significant retention of metal salts at the injection sites. Absorption of the platinoids from inhalation is much higher (7).

Metabolism

Following inhalation, a majority of the dose of platinoid metals and salts is retained in the lungs and respiratory tract. After i.v. injection, most platinoids distribute to soft tissues, mainly kidney, liver, muscle, and spleen (7). Very little evidence exists demonstrating longterm accumulation of the platinoids in these tissues, except for ruthenium, which is retained in bone.

Since cisplatin is not effective when administered orally, studies have been conducted using intravenous bolus injections. These studies have demonstrated that the drug has an initial plasma half-life of 25–50 min followed by a slower phase with a half-life of 58–73 hr. Approximately 90% of the Pt in blood is protein-bound 2–4 hr after administration (17). Concentrations of the non-protein-bound, or biologically active, form of cisplatin decline much more rapidly in plasma with the initial alpha phase half-life of 8–30 min and the slower phase from 40–48 min. By 4–5 hr, non-protein-bound drug accounts for less than 2–3% of total circulating platinum (18). Cisplatin distributes primarily to kidney, liver, intestines, and testes and a small percentage is capable of penetrating the central nervous system. Elevated levels of platinum persist in liver and kidney for 2–4 weeks (17, 18).

Cisplatin can react in a nonenzymatic manner with water in vivo to form monoaquo and diaquo species following dissociation of the chloride groups (3). These metabolites extensively bind to protein (>90%) and thus have minimal cytotoxicities but the non-protein-bound, ultrafilterable reactive species are cytotoxic.

The pharmacokinetic behavior of platinum administered as the cisplatin analog, carboplatin, is strikingly different compared with platinum administered as cisplatin. Carboplatin is well tolerated and does not induce nephrotoxicity. Thrombocytopenia is the major dose-limiting side effect. The pharmacokinetic differences between the two drugs are most likely related to the difference between the bidentate leaving group present in carboplatin as opposed to the two chlorine groups in cisplatin, the latter being more susceptible to hydrolysis (Fig. 82.1). In addition, carboplatin binds to plasma proteins much more slowly and less avidly than does cisplatin. Ultrafilterable (non-protein-bound) platinum in carboplatin has a much longer half-life (170 vs. 30 min) compared with cisplatin (19).

Excretion

Excretion of the platinoid salts after i.v. injection is mainly in urine. About 20–45% of the dose is excreted within 24 hours for platinum, rhodium, and ruthenium, and 80% of the dose is excreted in urine in 1 week. Orally administered platinoids are excreted primarily in feces (7).

Excretion of cisplatin is biphasic and occurs primarily via the urinary route. Approximately 20% of an intravenous bolus injection of cisplatin is excreted in urine during the initial 6 hours with 40–50% of the dose recovered in urine within 5 days. Elimination kinetics change when administered by infusion; the plasma half-life is reduced and more drug is excreted (17, 20). A higher percentage of a dose of carboplatin is ex-

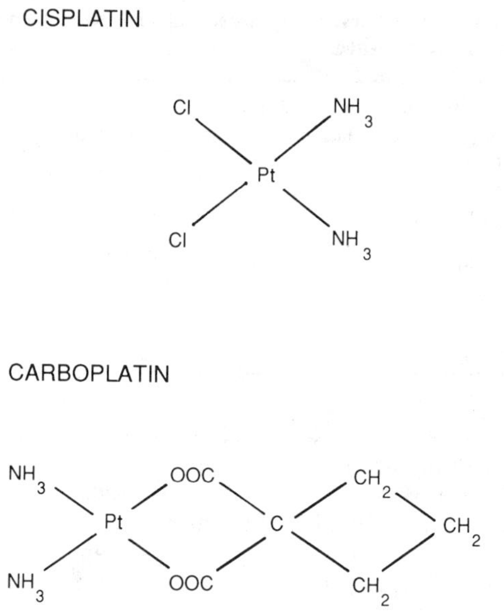

Figure 82.1. Basic structures of the chemotherapeutic platinum compounds, cisplatin and carboplatin.

creted in the urine than cisplatin (21) and most of the dose is excreted during the initial 24 hours after injection (22).

SIGNS, SYMPTOMS, AND SYNDROMES FROM TOXIC EXPOSURE

Acute Toxicity

After inhalation and dermal exposures, platinum oxides and soluble platinum salts can act as irritants or sensitizers (allergens). Ammonium tetrachloroplatinite(II) and ammonium hexachloroplatinate(IV) are the main occupational sensitizing agents. (Metallic elemental platinum seems to be inert, with an exception possibly being the very fine powdered form.) The latency period of sensitization may last for weeks or several months but could take years of working with Pt compounds prior to being sensitized (16).

Signs and symptoms of exposure by the inhalation and dermal routes after sensitization has occurred are conjunctivitis, urticaria, dermatitis, and eczema (see Table 82.2). A syndrome formerly termed "platinosis" can manifest the following symptomatology: lacrimation, sneezing, rhinorrhea, cough, dyspnea, bronchial asthma (from chloroplatinates), and cyanosis (23). The term platinosis is misleading in that it is suggestive of a pneumoconiosis and fibrosis, neither of which has been described as part of the platinum allergy syndrome. A more correct description for this syndrome is "allergy to platinum compounds containing reactive halogen ligands" (10, 15, 24). These symptoms described above may be mediated via an immediate (type I) hypersensitivity or a delayed (type IV, within 24 hours) hypersensitivity reaction. The common skin lesions are mainly between the fingers and in the antecubital fossae. The dermatitis reported in platinum refinery workers has been classified in the past as a type IV reaction (contact dermatitis); however, the dermatitis seen is of a primary irritant type, such as would follow exposure to strong acids and alkalis (24).

The allergic reaction described above is classified as a type I immediate hypersensitivity because it has been shown to be mediated by IgE, including release of histamine from mast cells. The platinum complexes are too small to be allergens

Table 82.2.   Clinical Signs and Symptoms of Platinum Allergy Following Inhalation, Dermal, and Ocular Exposure

Upper Respiratory	Lower Respiratory	Ocular
Rhinorrhea	Cough	Conjuctivitis
Sneezing	Dyspnea	Edema
Itching of nose, throat, palate	Asthmatic wheezing	Lacrimation
Nasal congestion	Cyanosis	Redness
		Itching
		Photophobia

Dermal	Systemic
Urticaria	Lymphocytosis
Angioedema	Eosinophilia
Eczema	
Contact dermatitis	
Pruritis	

Adapted from Boggs PB. Platinum allergy. Cutis 1985; 35:318–320.

and must combine with a large molecular weight carrier, such as human serum albumin, to form a hapten capable of eliciting specific antibodies. While IgE antibodies mediate the immediate reaction after reexposure, IgG antibodies are responsible for the delayed effects (16).

Cisplatin is a widely used antitumor agent of which the cytotoxic mechanism of action includes covalent binding to DNA and inhibition of DNA replication. Early clinical trials with cisplatin revealed that nephrotoxicity was the major dose-limiting effect, which occurred in about two thirds of patients. The incidence of this effect has been markedly reduced by the use of pretherapy hydration and diuretics and/or by altering the dosing regimen (51). In humans, acute tubular necrosis is evident in the third segment (pars recta) of the proximal tubule, the distal convoluted tubule, and the collecting duct. In animal and human studies, cisplatin nephrotoxicity is clinically manifested by elevations in blood urea nitrogen and serum creatinine; proteinuria; hyperuricemia; decreased creatinine clearance, glomerular filtration, and renal plasma flow; and increased urinary excretion of beta$_2$-microglobulin (3, 25).

The exact mechanism by which cisplatin-induced renal injury is produced is not clear. It is unclear what role the platinum atom itself plays in the nephrotoxic response. Administration of cisplatin and transplatin results in comparable renal concentrations of platinum; however, only the cis isomer is nephrotoxic (and has antitumor activity), indicating that the geometry of these complexes is important in the development of renal injury. Furthermore, the functional groups of the platinum complexes can significantly modify the nephrotoxic effect. These findings have supported the conclusion that cisplatin nephrotoxicity is related to the formation of an electrophilic metabolite such as an aquated and/or hydroxylated form of cisplatin (25). Evidence for several mechanisms exists including covalent binding of reactive metabolites to tissue macromolecules, such as proteins, lipids, or nucleic acids (25). Cisplatin has been shown to bind to sulfhydryl-containing cellular constituents, and toxicity may be related to decreases in cellular glutathione and/or formation of cytotoxic platinum-methionine complexes (26). Cisplatin toxicity may be related to production of free radicals, such as superoxide anion, and lipid peroxidation (27–29).

Other effects associated with shortterm cisplatin use are gas-

trointestinal disturbances, myelosuppression, allergic reactions, and electrolyte disturbances. Cisplatin will invariably induce gastrointestinal disturbances manifested as nausea and vomiting, but diarrhea is uncommon (51). Mild to moderate myelosuppression occurs in most patients with transient leukopenia and thrombocytopenia. Hypersensitivity reactions are rare but have been reported and range from skin rashes and facial edema to bronchoconstriction, tachycardia, and hypotension. The primary electrolyte alteration has been hypomagnesemia, which may be related to toxic action on kidney tubule ion transport processes (3, 17).

While possessing comparable antitumor efficacy, the recently approved cisplatin analog, carboplatin, has been shown to be less toxic except for myelosuppression (30, 31). Concomitant high-dose antiemetic treatment and extensive hydration are not necessary with carboplatin.

There has been a general paucity of reported cases of adverse human health effects associated with occupational or environmental exposure to ruthenium, rhodium, iridium, and palladium (16); however, ruthenium tetroxide fumes are highly injurious to both lungs and eyes. The compound can be classified as a respiratory irritant because nasal ulcerations and discoloration of respiratory mucous membranes can occur (7, 16). Industrial poisoning from rhodium is rare. It is generally accepted that exposure to rhodium compounds does not result in platinum-type allergic reactions (7, 16).

Metallic osmium is considered biologically inert; however, exposure to OsO_4 vapors in industrial and laboratory settings can result in extreme ocular and respiratory irritation and acute conjunctivitis. Other signs and symptoms include headache, bronchoconstriction, difficulty breathing, respiratory tract irritation, tracheal epithelium necrosis, bronchitis, and interstitial pneumonia (1, 4, 7, 16). Ocular irritation occurs at low vapor concentrations. Continuous or higher exposures may cause lacrimation and visual disturbances (appearance of rings around lights).

Chronic Toxicity

TARGET ORGAN EFFECTS

Chronic occupational exposure to platinum compounds may exacerbate platinum hypersensitivity reactions, especially in atopic individuals.

Reproductive toxicity is associated with longterm cisplatin use. Cisplatin used for chemotherapy alone and in combination with other chemotherapeutic agents has been shown to cause azoospermia in humans within 2 months after initiation of treatment (3). Recovery of sperm counts occurred in a majority of patients within 1.5–2 years after cessation of treatment.

Many heavy metals (lead, mercury, thallium, and gold) are known to be neurotoxic, and cisplatin is known to be toxic to the central and peripheral nervous systems (3, 17). Peripheral neuropathies (paresthesias) are the most common neurotoxicities and are reversible after discontinuation of treatment (3). Hematologic effects, which occur from 6–26 days after initiation of treatment, include hypomagnesemia, leukopenia, and thrombocytopenia (51). Ototoxicity caused by cisplatin is often irreversible and is manifested by tinnitus and hearing loss in the high-frequency (4000–8000 Hz) range (3, 17, 51). Longterm use of cisplatin may result in irreversible kidney damage.

While industrial palladium poisoning is considered rare, toxicity could occur by prolonged therapeutic use of palladium compounds (4, 7, 16). A colloidal form of palladium has been used in the clinical treatment of tuberculosis, gout, and obesity. Toxicity from these colloidal palladium compounds may be due to hemolysis (4, 7, 16). There have been some reports describing skin sensitization to palladium in the workplace, but it is generally held that these compounds do not pose a serious allergy problem similar to that associated with platinum salts (4, 7, 16). Recently, it has been shown that a palladium-protein conjugate does not have antigenic determinants similar to those of a platinum-protein conjugate (16). There are some reports of skin sensitization (a type IV hypersensitivity) to palladium due to exposure in a research laboratory and to dental alloys (13, 32).

OsO_4 has been used in Europe for 30–40 years for the treatment of rheumatoid arthritis, but its use is controversial. Chronic toxicity from osmium may occur after intraarticular injection, which results in osmium accumulation in liver, spleen, heart, and kidneys (14, 16).

TERATOGENESIS

The platinoids are not known to be teratogenic in humans or in experimental animal models. No information is readily available on whether experiments to test for this endpoint have been performed.

CARCINOGENESIS AND MUTAGENESIS

There are no reports of increased cancer risk from occupational exposure to platinum compounds. Although cisplatin is an effective chemotherapeutic agent in humans and experimental animals, it has been reported to increase the frequency of lung adenomas and induce skin papillomas and carcinomas in mice (4). In a lifetime exposure study, a minimally significant increase in malignant tumors primarily of the lymphoma-leukemia type were found in mice given access to 5 ppm rhodium and palladium (chloride salts) in drinking water (33).

Cisplatin is a strong mutagen in bacterial systems, including the salmonella typhimurium revertant tests (34). In in vitro studies, the compound induces chromosomal aberrations and increases in sister chromatid exchange (4). After hydrolysis of the cisplatin chloride groups to form activated species, the platinum complex can react with DNA, forming both intrastrand and interstrand cross-links. The N(7) group of guanine is highly reactive and the most readily demonstrated lesion resulting in cytotoxicity involves intrastrand cross-links between adjacent guanines (3, 17). Certain Pt(II), Pd(II), Rh(I), and Rh(III) complexes have been shown to be mutagenic in bacterial systems (35, 36).

Management of Toxicity

CLINICAL EXAMINATION

Clinical signs and symtoms (Table 82.2) of platinum exposure and toxicity via inhalation and dermal routes are those of classic allergic reactions and include irritation of the eyes and nose; cough, dyspnea, wheezing, and cyanosis; skin sensitization; and lymphocytosis (1, 10).

Careful clinical diagnosis is needed to differentiate an asthma-like attack due to platinum salts from other causes of asthma and from upper airway obstruction by tumor, laryngeal edema, endobronchial disease, acute left ventricular failure, and eosinophilic pneumonias. Sensitization dermatitis due to platinum salts must be differentiated from primary irritant dermatitis, nummular eczema, atopic dermatitis, pustular eruptions of the palms and soles, psoriasis, herpes simplex and zoster, drug eruptions, and erythema multiforme (1).

Signs and symtoms of OsO_4 exposure include: lacrimation, visual disturbances, conjunctivitis, headache, cough, dyspnea, and dermatitis. Diagnoses should be differentiated from other causes of conjuctivitis and mucous membrane irritation, such as viral infection of the upper respiratory tract and allergies. If involvement of the tracheobronchial tree is detected, the symptoms should be differentiated from cardiogenic pulmonary edema and viral or bacterial pneumonia (1).

TREATMENT

For treatment of excessive inhalation and dermal exposures to the platinoids, appropriate procedures should be initiated, such as removal from the source of exposure, irrigation of eyes, and washing of contaminated areas of skin with water. Treatments for contact dermatitis and bronchospasm may be initiated (1, 10, 24, 51).

Preventive measures which should be undertaken to limit inhalation and dermal exposures include adequate workplace ventilation; use of mechanical filter respirators, rubber gloves, and protective clothing; and better personal hygiene. Those individuals with allergies or sensitization should be removed from the source (23). Studies have demonstrated that, in general, atopic individuals, i.e., those sensitive to common environmental allergens, are sensitized to the platinoids more quickly than nonatopics (16). Workers in these facilities should be monitored on a regular basis through an industrial hygiene surveillance program. High standards of workplace isolation in platinum processing must be met so that no workers come into direct contact with a liquid, fume, dust, or solid containing platinum salts.

Use of antihistamines for platinum allergy is controversial but can provide temporary relief of some of the upper respiratory symptoms (10, 15). Bronchodilators can alleviate acute bronchospasm but are of no longterm benefit. In short, since platinum salt sensitivity is an allergy and symptoms develop only after exposure, the best treatment requires cessation of exposure (15).

To treat excessive exposure to OsO_4 vapors, the patient should be removed from exposure, eyes flushed with water, and skin washed thoroughly. For dermatitis, treatment modalities for contact dermatitis may be instituted. After severe exposure, hospitalization may be necessary for approximately 3–4 days to check for onset of delayed pulmonary edema. Treatment modalities for common respiratory irritants may be utilized (1).

During cisplatin therapy, all test values of renal and hematopoietic function, in addition to auditory acuity, should be monitored. Slow infusion of cisplatin can reduce toxicity while maintaining efficacy. When used alone, the usual intravenous dose is 100 mg/m^2 once every 4 weeks (17). The dosage must be reduced when given in combination with other chemotherapeutic agents. In order to prevent nephrotoxicity, hydration of the patient is recommended; infusion of 1–2 liters of fluid for 8–12 hours prior to treatment is appropriate. Hydration is continued to ensure that glomerular filtration and urinary output are adequate. Concurrent administration of a diuretic, such as furosemide or mannitol, has been advocated to maintain renal output (17).

Reduction of nephrotoxicity has been achieved via other intervention regimens. The coadministration of chloride salts to induce chloruresis may improve the therapeutic index of cisplatin via decreased renal activation of cisplatin chloride groups to cytotoxic hydroxyl and/or aquated species (37). Inducing chloruresis and maintaining hydration may allow for a doubling of the cisplatin dose, thus increasing antitumor efficacy and reducing dose-limiting nephrotoxicity; however, other systemic toxicities (myelosuppression, nausea, ototoxicity, and peripheral neuropathy) may still be present (38).

Other experimental renoprotective techniques utilize compounds with high affinities for heavy metals, such as the sulfhydryl-containing chelator, diethyldithiocarbamate (17). Dithiocarbamate analogs given prior to cisplatin can reduce the nephrotoxicity of cisplatin while not affecting antitumor efficacy, by a mechanism involving the shift of Pt excretion from the kidney to the biliary route (39). Sodium thiosulfate inhibits cisplatin nephrotoxicity when administered concomitantly to experimental animals (40) and may be effective clinically (41, 42).

LABORATORY DIAGNOSIS

In cases of asthma suspected to be induced by the platinoids, the following laboratory tests are recommended: electrocardiogram, sputum gram stain and culture, and differential white blood cell count (1). Lymphocytosis and eosinophilia have been reported (1, 10, 15). Arterial oxygen saturation (SaO_2) and arterial blood gases should be monitored. Lung function using spirometry should also be assessed (15, 24).

The major dose-limiting effect from use of cisplatin is nephrotoxicity; however, this can be controlled by varying dosing regimens and providing hydration (17). Kidney function tests will aid in the diagnosis of nephrotoxicity. The primary toxic effect associated with the newer cisplatin analog, carboplatin, is myelosuppression (30, 31). Thus, white blood cell counts should be monitored for potential toxicity related to cisplatin or carboplatin.

SPECIAL DIAGNOSTIC TESTS

In general, platinum allergy exists until proven otherwise when a worker exposed to platinum salts or chloroplatinic acid presents classic allergy symptoms (10). Several tests are available to confirm the diagnosis (10, 15, 24), including the skin prick test. Although no sensitization of workers due to repeated skin prick testing has been reported (15, 24) at the concentrations used (10^{-6}–10^{-3} g/ml) for the test, no study has been designed to confirm this claim. It cannot be overemphasized that occupational exposures should be controlled with proper clothing and ventilation so that routine invasive procedures are not necessary. The skin prick test uses three platinum salts: ammonium hexachloroplatinate [$(NH_4)_2PtCl_6$], sodium tetrachloroplatinate (Na_2PtCl_4), and sodium hexachloroplatinate (Na_2PtCl_6). A definite wheal and flare reaction is diagnostic. It is easily performed, rapid, and reproducible. A radioallergosorbent test (RAST) to identify serum IgE antibodies specific to platinum chloride complexes may be used (43). A bronchial challenge test is used occasionally.

BIOLOGICAL MONITORING

Determination of plasma concentrations of platinum may be useful for monitoring the therapeutic regimen and in preventing toxicity after cisplatin administration. The flameless graphite furnace atomic absorption spectro-photometric (GFAAS) methods are advantageous because of their high sensitivity, rapidity, and expediency (Table 82.3). A technique for platinum analysis using electrothermal atomic absorption spectrophotometry can be performed by injection of plasma samples (44, 45) directly into the graphite furnace. The sensitivity of the method is 0.07 μg/ml. Platinum is not detected in the plasma of normal subjects at the sensitivity level of this technique. Residue from the destruction of organic matter in the plasma may interfere with the analysis at lower platinum concentrations, but use of a deuterium background corrector reduces this effect. The matrix effect can be further reduced by dilution of plasma specimens with a detergent, such as 1% Triton X-100. This detergent reportedly aids in a more uniform drying of the sample while minimizing platinum loss during atomization. This technique was reported in an assay in which diluted plasma can be directly injected into the furnace with a total analysis time of less than 2 minutes. The assay is sensitive (0.05 μg/ml), precise (CV < 4.3%), and linear (r > 0.9922) in the ranges of 0.05–4 μg/ml for platinum in cisplatin (46).

A GFASS method (Table 82.3) is available for determining platinum in urine following dilution with dilute nitric acid (47). This same report describes the determination of platinum in urine by differential-pulse polarography (DPP) after dilution with boric acid-ethylene diamine buffer and adjustment to alkaline pH. The sensitivities of both methods are equal but the recoveries are low; 31 and 44% using DPP and GFASS, respectively. The low recovery is most likely due to the strong association of inorganic platinum with urinary constituents which are not broken down either through complexation (in DPP) or by acid digestion (in GFAAS).

In GFAAS, the proper conditions for drying, ashing, and atomization steps must be optimized. A gradual multistep drying program is necessary to ensure complete drying for reproducible absorbance. The ashing step must be carefully regulated so as to remove the effects of the matrix with minimal loss of platinum (46, 47).

In order to study the pharmacokinetics of ultrafilterable platinum (the cytotoxic and biologically active form) in plasma of patients receiving continuous infusion of cisplatin, an HPLC assay (Table 82.3) with high sensitivity (2.5 μg/ml) was developed using precolumn derivatization with diethyldithiocarbamate (48). The sample preparation requires minimal sample manipulation and a 20-fold increase in sensitivity over GFAAS methods can be achieved. A clinically useful high pressure liquid chromatography (HPLC) method has also been developed for measuring platinum as the parent drug or its metabolities in urine of patients administered platinum chemotherapeutic agents (49) which can circumvent many of the matrix interferences associated with other analytical techniques. The HPLC methods are advantageous because they are rapid, inexpensive, and require minimal sample preparation and are suited for analyzing large numbers of samples.

Determination of tissue platinum has been described (Table 82.3) using radiochemical neutron activation analysis (50). The method is an order of magnitude less sensitive than the GFAAS methods described above and is very time-consuming and tedious (sample preparation and irradiation can take up to 1 week). Although impractical for therapeutic monitoring, the

Table 82.3. Methods Used for Monitoring of Platinum in Biological Specimens

Technique	Matrix	Sensitivity (μg/ml or g*)	Precision (CV %)	Range of Linearity (μg/ml)	Recovery (%)	Reference
GFAAS	Plasma	0.07	8	0.2–2.0	NR	44
GFAAS	Plasma	0.05	2.8	0.05–4.0	81	46
GFAAS	Urine	0.4	NR	0.2–1.0	44	47
DPP	Urine	0.4	NR	0.2–1.0	31	47
HPLC	Plasma	0.0025	7.3	0.0025–1.0	100	48
HPLC	Urine	0.025	2.5	0.025–0.5	97	49
NAA	Tissue	0.3*	6	NR	NR	50

GFAAS, graphite furnace atomic absorption spectrophotometry; DPP, differential pulse polarography; HPLC, high performance liquid chromatography; NAA, neutron activation analysis; NR, not reported.

system allows for the determination of about 20 additional trace elements and thus the study of multielement interactions during platinum exposure is possible. Treatment with cisplatin has been shown to alter levels of some essential elements in plasma, e.g., magnesium is lowered (3, 17).

ENVIRONMENTAL MONITORING

To monitor the occupational environment for platinum, air is drawn through a 25-mm-diameter cellulose ester filter for approximately 2 hours. The filter is subsequently treated with hydrochloric acid to dissolve soluble platinum salts. The solution is analyzed for platinum by GFAAS or by inductively coupled plasma atomic emission spectroscopy (ICP-AES). Insoluble platinum salts and metal are then determined after dissolution in 50% aquaregia and evaporation to dryness several times with HCl followed by either analytical atomic method described above. The same procedure is followed for rhodium. Neutron activation analysis, IEC-AES, and GFAAS may be used to analyze the other platinoids (16).

EXPOSURE LIMITS

Current threshold limit values-time-weighted averages (TLV-TWA; 8 hr/day, 40 hr/week) for metallic platinum dusts and soluble platinum salts are 1.0 and 0.002 mg/m³, respectively (2, 52). The TLV for platinum salts was set at a level to prevent respiratory effects and is believed to provide protection against sensitization; however, it does not offer protection to a previously sensitized individual.

In 1984, the recommended TLV-TWA for rhodium metal and insoluble rhodium compounds (as rhodium) is 1.0 mg/m³ (52) and the TLV-TWA for soluble rhodium salts 0.01 mg/m³ (52). These TLVs were set at levels to prevent possible allergic effects; as of 1991, the TLVs have not changed.

Exposure to osmium tetroxide should not exceed 0.0016 mg/m³, as osmium (9, 52). This TLV-TWA was set at a level to prevent irritation of the eyes or respiratory tract. The threshold limit value-shortterm exposure limit (TLV-STEL) is 0.0048 mg/m³, as osmium (52).

No occupational exposure limits (TLVs) have been recommended for palladium, iridium, ruthenium, and their compounds.

REFERENCES

1. Proctor NH, Hughes JP, Fischman M. Chemical hazards of the workplace. Philadelphia: JB Lippincott Co., 1988:393–436.

2. Sax NI, Lewis RJ. Hawley's condensed chemical dictionary. 11th ed. New York: Van Nostrand Reinhold, 1987:926–928.

3. Loehrer PJ, Einhorn LH. Cisplatin. Ann Intern Med 1984;100:704–713.

4. Goyer RA. Toxic effects of metals. In: Klaassen CD, Amdur MO, Doull J, eds. Casarett and Doull's toxicology: the basic science of poisons. 3rd ed. New York: Macmillan, 1986:622–623.

5. Anonymous. Paraplatin approved for recurrent ovarian cancer. J Pharm Technol 1989;5:83.

6. McBryde WAE. Platinum and its compounds. In: Hampel CA, Hawley GG, eds. The encyclopedia of chemistry, 3rd ed. New York: Van Nostrand Reinhold, 1973:865–867.

7. Venugopal B, Luckey TD. Toxicity of group VIII metals. Chapt 8 in: Venugopal B, Luckey TD, eds. Metal toxicity in mammals—2. New York: Plenum Press, 1978:273–305.

8. Hawley GG. The condensed chemical dictionary. 9th ed. New York: Van Nostrand Reinhold, 1977:691–692.

9. Hammond CR. The elements. In: Weast RC, Astle MJ, Beyer WH, eds. CRC handbook of chemistry and physics. Boca Raton, FL: CRC Press, 1986–87:B5–B43.

10. Boggs PB. Platinum allergy. Cutis 1985;35:318–320.

11. Kawata Y, Shiota M, Tsutsui H, Yoshida Y, Sasaki H, Kinouchi Y. Cytotoxicity of Pd-Co dental casting ferromagnetic alloys. J Dent Res 1981;60:1403–1409.

12. Hermesch CB, Voss JE, Bales DJ, Mayhew RB. A clinical evaluation of a high-copper alloy containing palladium. J Indiana Dent Assoc 1982;61:13–15.

13. Van Ketel WG, Niebber C. Allergy to palladium in dental alloys. Contact Derm 1981;7:331–357.

14. Maugh TH. New ways to use metals for arthritis. Science 1981;212:430–431.

15. Jacobs L. Platinum salt sensitivity. Nurs RSA 1987;2:34–37.

16. Seiler HG, Sigel H. Handbook on toxicity of inorganic compounds. New York: Marcel Dekker, 1988:341–344, 501–574.

17. Calabresi P, Parks Jr, RE. Antiproliferative agents and drugs used for immunosuppression. In: Gilman AG, Goodman LS, Rall TW, Murad F, eds. Goodman and Gilman's the pharmacological basis of therapeutics. 7th ed. New York: Macmillan, 1985:1290–1291.

18. Balis FM, Holcenberg JS, Bleyer WA. Clinical pharmacokinetics of commonly used anticancer drugs. Clin Pharmacokinet 1983;8:202–232.

19. Curt GA, Grygiel JJ, Corden BJ, et al. A phase I and pharmacokinetic study of diamminecyclobutane-dicarboxylatoplatinum (NSC 241240). Cancer Res 1983;43:4470–4473.

20. Madias NE, Harrington JT, Platinum nephrotoxicity. Am J Med 1978;65:307–314.

21. Van Echo DA, Egorin MJ, Whitacre MY, Olman EA, Aisner J. Phase I clinical and pharmacologic trial of carboplatin daily for 5 days. Cancer Treat Rev 1984;68:1103–1114.

22. Egorin MJ, Van Echo DA, Tipping SJ, et al. Pharmacokinetics and dosage reduction of cis-diammine(1,1-cyclobutane dicarboxylate)platinum in patients with impaired renal function. Cancer Res 1984;44:5432–5438.

23. Plunkett ER. Handbook of industrial toxicology. New York: Chemical Publishing Co., 1976:341–342.

24. Hughes EG. Medical surveillance of platinum refinery workers. J Soc Occup Med 1980;30:27–30.

25. Goldstein RS, Mayor GH. Minireview—the nephrotoxicity of cisplatin. Life Sci 1983;32:685–690.

26. Tosetti F, Rocco M, Fulco RA, et al. Serial determination of platinum, protein content and free sulfhydryl levels in plasma of patients treated with cisplatin or carboplatin. Anticancer Res 1988;8:381–386.

27. Sodhi A, Gupta P. Increased release of hydrogen peroxide and superoxide anion by murine macrophages in vitro after cisplatin treatment. Int J Immunopharmacol 1986;8:709–714.

28. Sugihara K, Gemba M. Modification of cisplatin toxicity by antioxidants. Jpn J Pharmacol 1986;40:353–355.

29. Dobyan DC, Bull JM, Strebel FR, Sunderland BA, Bulger RE. Protective effects of O-(beta-hydroxyethyl)-rutoside on cisplatinum-induced acute renal failure in the rat. Lab Invest 1986;55:557–563.

30. Calvert AH, Harland SJ, Newell DR, et al. Early clinical studies with cis-diammine-1,1-cyclobutane dicarboxylate platinum(II). Cancer Chemother Pharmacol 1982;9:140–147.

31. Koeller JM, Trump DL, Tutsch KD, Earhart RH, Davis TE, Tormey DC. Phase I clinical trial and pharmacokinetics of carboplatin (NSC 241240) by single monthly 30-minute infusion. Cancer 1986;57:222–225.

32. Munro-Ashman D, Munro D, Hughes TH. Contact dermatitis from palladium. Trans St. John's Hosp Dermatol Soc 1969;55:196–197.

33. Schroeder HA, Mitchener M. Scandium, chromium(VI), gallium, yttrium, rhodium, palladium, indium in mice. Effects on growth and life span. J Nutr 1971;101:1431–1438.

34. Coluccia M, Correale M, Fanizzi FP, et al. Mutagenic activity of some platinum complexes: chemical properties and biological activity. In: Merian E, Frei RW, Hardi W, Schlatter C, eds. Carcinogenic and mutagenic metal compounds. New York: Gordon and Breach, 1985:467–474.

35. Warren G, Abbott E, Schultz P, Bennett K, Rogers S. Mutagenicity of a series of hexacoordinate rhodium(III) compounds. Mutat Res 1981;88:165–173.

36. Aresta M, Treglia S, Collucia M, Correale M, Giordano D, Moscelli S. Mutagenic activity of transition-metal complexes: Relation structure-mutagenic and antibacterial activity for some Pd(II), Pt(II) and Rh(I) complexes. In: Merian E, Frei RW, Hardi W, Schlatter C, eds. Carcinogenic and mutagenic metal compounds. New York: Gordon and Breach, 1985:453–466.

37. Earhart RH, Martin PA, Tutsch KD, Erturk E, Wheeler RH, Bull FE. Improvement in the therapeutic index of cisplatin (NSC 119875) by pharmacologically induced chloruresis in the rat. Canc Res 1983;43:1187–1194.

38. Corden BJ, Fine RL, Ozols RF, Collins JM. Clinical pharmacology of high-dose cisplatin. Cancer Chemother Pharmacol 1985;14:38–41.

39. Basinger MA, Jones MM, Gilbreath SG, Walker Jr, EM, Fody EP, Mayhue MA. Dithiocarbamate-induced biliary platinum excretion and the control of cis-platinum nephrotoxicity. Toxicol Appl Pharmacol 1989;97:279–288.

40. Uozumi J, Litterst CL. The effect of sodium thiosulfate on subcellular localization of platinum in rat kidney after treatment with cisplatin. Cancer Lett 1986;32:279–283.

41. Markman M, Cleary S, Howell S. Nephrotoxicity of high-dose intracavitary cisplatin with intravenous thiosulfate protection. Eur J Cancer Clin Oncol 1985;21:1015–1018.

42. DeBroe ME, Wedeen RP. Prevention of cisplatin nephrotoxicity. Eur J Cancer Clin Oncol 1986;22:1029–1031.

43. Murdoch RD, Pepys J, Hughes EG. IgE antibody responses to platinum group metals: a large scale refinery survey. Br J Ind Med 1986;43:37–43.

44. Baselt RC. Platinum. In: Baselt RC, ed. Analytical procedures for therapeutic drug monitoring and emergency toxicology. 2nd ed. Littleton, MA: PSG Publishing Co., 1987:238–239.

45. LeRoy AF, Wehling HL, Sponseller HL, et al. Analysis of platinum in biological materials by flameless atomic absorption spectrophotometry. Biochem Med 1977;18:184–191.

46. El-Yazigi A, Al-Saleh I. Rapid determination of platinum by flameless atomic absorption spectrophotometry following the administration of cisplatin to cancer patients. Ther Drug Monit 1986;8:318–320.

47. Shearan P, Smyth MR. Comparison of voltammetric and graphite furnace atomic absorption spectrometric methods for the direct determination of inorganic platinum in urine. Analyst 1988;113:609–612.

48. Reece PA. Sensitive high-performance liquid chromatographic assay for platinum in plasma ultrafiltrate. J Chromatogr 1984;306:417–423.

49. Bannister SJ, Sternson LA, Repta AJ. Urine analysis of platinum species derived from cis-dichlorodiammineplatinum(II) by high-performance liquid chromatography following derivatization with sodium diethyldithiocarbamate. J Chromatogr 1979;173:333–342.

50. Tjioe PS, Volkers KJ, Kroon JJ, DeGoeij JJM, The SK. Determination of gold and platinum traces in biological materials as a part of a multielement radiochemical activation analysis system. In: Merian E, Frei RW, Hardi W, Schlatter C, eds. Carcinogenic and mutagenic metal compounds. New York: Gordon and Breach, 1985:171–182.

51. Ellenhorn MJ, Barceloux DG. Medical toxicology—diagnosis and treatment of human poisoning. New York: Elsevier, 1988:1055–1056.

52. American Conference of Governmental Industrial Hygienists. Threshold limit values for chemical substances in the work environment. Cincinnati, OH: ACGIH, 1990–1991.

83

Beryllium

Lee S. Newman, M.D.

INTRODUCTION

Although discovered in the late 1700s, beryllium's value to industry and its pulmonary, dermatologic, and systemic toxicities have been recognized only in the past 60 years. As the fourth lightest element, with an atomic weight of 9.02, beryllium has low density, high melting point, high stiffness-to-weight ratio, and low coefficient of thermal expansion, making it especially attractive for high technology applications in aerospace, nuclear power, and electronics, not to mention dental prostheses and golf clubs.

While beryllium does occur naturally in soils and in coal, air concentrations are low even in major urban centers. Occupational exposures represent the major source of exposure that results in illness. Table 83.1 describes some of the major industries where beryllium exposure occurs. These industries include the extraction of beryllium from ore, production and use of beryllium alloys, beryllium ceramics manufacturing, electronics, nuclear reactors, atomic energy-related research, missile parts, tool and die manufacturing, dental laboratories, and nonferrous foundry operations including reclamation of precious metals. Historically beryllium was used in the fluorescent and neon lamp industries, although it was discontinued as the phosphor in the 1960s.

TOXICOLOGY

Deposition and Clearance of Beryllium

Beryllium causes injury to the lung, skin, and, to a lesser extent, other organs in at least two ways: through its effects on cellular immunity and by direct chemical toxic effects. Cutaneous inoculation with beryllium splinters can cause skin ulceration,

Table 83.1. Industries and Trades with Possible Beryllium Exposure

Aerospace
Automotive parts
Beryllium smelting/fabrication/extraction/metallizing
Ceramics
Computers
Dental technicians, supplies
Electronics
Foundries, nonferrous
Hazardous waste processing
Nuclear reactor manufacturing
Nuclear weapons production, development, and research
Plating
Refractories
Smelters, nonferrous
Telecommunications
Tool and die
Welding

granuloma formation, poor wound healing, and dermatitis, and has been seen with exposure to the metal salts and alloys. While skin contact can be a significant cause of morbidity, the principal source of toxicity comes through beryllium inhalation. Inhalational injury can be induced by exposure to either fume (beryllium oxides) or respirable dusts of beryllium salts, oxides, metal, or alloy.

Beryllium particles obey the basic principles of particle deposition in the lung, but it is apparent that the toxicity of beryllium is influenced also by the form in which it is inhaled. Critical properties include particle size, crystalline structure, and solubility, among other factors. The interaction of these factors with the respiratory and immune systems is poorly understood. Certain forms of beryllium are associated with greater risk of lung injury and have greater capability to induce a beryllium-specific immune response. For example, low temperature calcined beryllium oxide is more immunogenic than high calcined beryllium oxide. Fume exposure may be worse than dust; however, this remains conjecture. Most beryllium that is inhaled is cleared promptly by the phagocytic system in conjunction with the mucociliary escalator. Some of the beryllium inhaled is translocated from the airway to regional lymph nodes and interstitial space of the lung, where much of the immunologic response likely occurs. Beryllium is distributed principally to liver, bone, and kidney. Most excretion occurs in the urine. Species and individual differences also influence the rate of clearance and type of toxicity seen. As discussed below, susceptibility to the effects of beryllium can be both dose-dependent and dose-independent.

Exposure Limits and Monitoring

The history of the establishment of exposure limits for beryllium is intertwined with the history of beryllium's early employment in the development of nuclear weapons and nuclear power. Following World War II, the federal government, through the Atomic Energy Commission (AEC), was active in monitoring airborne beryllium and health hazards in factories of contractors. In 1949, the AEC established the air standards for beryllium that remain intact today. For occupational air exposures, a permissible level of 2.0 $\mu g/m^3$ was established based on an 8-hour time-weighted average. Peak level was set at 25 $\mu g/m^3$. The concentration of beryllium in air surrounding factories was not to exceed 0.01 $\mu g/m^3$. Studies of the epidemiology of beryllium disease have demonstrated that this standard, although arrived at somewhat arbitrarily, has been effective in eliminating most acute beryllium lung disease. However, the standard's impact on the incidence of chronic beryllium lung disease and cancer is less certain.

Industrial hygiene monitoring, while necessary and mandated under federal regulations, has been fraught with a number of limitations. First, it is often impossible to know until after the fact that major excursions in beryllium exposure have occurred. Second, there are technical limitations in the methods of air sampling and beryllium measurement employed. Area monitoring does not necessarily reflect the true inhalational exposure of an individual worker; however, this is still the most common type of monitoring performed. Accuracy and reproducibility of beryllium air-sampling measurements can vary greatly. Third, even with careful ventilatory controls and monitoring, the chronic form of beryllium lung disease continues to occur because it is due to a hypersensitivity to beryllium. Such hypersensitivity can develop in some individuals following even low level exposures that are well within the permissible exposure limits.

Animal Studies

Although humans were the first unwitting "animal models" of beryllium disease, toxic and immunologic effects of beryllium have been described in a wide number of species and cell types.

TOXICITY

When introduced intravenously, soluble beryllium salts form complexes with plasma proteins. Clearance of inhaled beryllium is discussed above. Beryllium is poorly absorbed through the gut, making the possibility of ingestion as a route of toxic exposure a less likely hazard. Beryllium induces changes in the structure and function of the liver, including interference with enzyme induction by the liver. Toxic effects on immune effector cells, including alveolar macrophages and lymphocytes, have also been demonstrated, as have alterations in fibroblast proliferation.

Neoplasms have been described in several animal models. This has included the production of osteosarcomas in rabbits and lung neoplasms in rats and monkeys. In this regard, it is noteworthy that beryllium has been shown to block the entry of cells into cell cycle, to produce alterations in the fidelity of DNA replication, and to alter hormone-regulated gene expression.

IMMUNOTOXICITY

Animal models have also been useful in demonstrating immunologic effects of beryllium as shown schematically in Fig. 83.1. The major conclusion of animal and human studies has been that beryllium induces a cellular immune response in which there is activation of berylium-specific T-lymphocytes. These T-cells accumulate and proliferate in the lung following inhalation exposure in beryllium-sensitized dogs and rats, among other species. The specificity of this response for beryllium has been confirmed by a demonstration of delayed-type hypersensitivity skin responses in animal models as well as by in vitro assays of cellular immune response including migration inhibition factor and lymphocyte transformation in response to beryllium salts. This latter test of T-lymphocyte response to beryllium has become a key tool in the diagnosis of human disease. Researchers have demonstrated that beryllium's ability to induce lung disease is influenced by genetic makeup. Guinea pig strains that vary only in their major histocompatibility complexes display different proclivity for beryllium lung disease. Our own work in murine models has focused on integrating the current understanding of chemical toxicologic effects of beryllium with the beryllium-specific immune response.

Population Studies

Acute and chronic beryllium disease occurred in epidemic form in the United States from 1945 to 1950 in beryllium extraction, alloy production, fluorescent lamp, and neon sign industries and in surrounding communities, until the identification of beryllium as an occupational and environmental hazard led to environmental control measures. The chronic disease was initially confused with sarcoidosis, a lung and multisystem disease of unknown etiology, from which it was clinically indistinguishable before the advent of current immunologic tests as discussed below. The United States Beryllium Case Registry was established in 1952 and includes over 600 cases of chronic beryllium disease. Sixty-five of these cases are attributed to ambient air pollution surrounding beryllium plants or to household dust brought home on work clothes. In the past decade, however, the Registry has laid dormant due to a lack of systematic reporting of cases, rather than due to any decline in chronic disease incidence. Although most clinicians are taught that beryllium disease is a "dinosaur," the chronic granulomatous form of disease is far from extinct. In fact, with increasing usage of beryllium in industry, the absolute number of cases can be expected to be increasing as well.

The epidemiology of chronic beryllium disease has been limited by misclassification of disease and of exposure status in the Registry. The Registry antedated the immunologic tests now available for beryllium disease, and therefore it is likely that some misclassification has occurred. Some cases of chronic beryllium disease may have been excluded from the Registry and some cases of sarcoidosis erroneously included. Therefore, limited conclusions can be drawn from the earlier studies published in the 1950s and 1960s with regard to beryllium disease prevalence. Prevalence estimates for chronic beryllium disease ranges from less than 1–5%. Although estimates of the number of workers in the United States with beryllium exposure range from 30,000–800,000, the size of the population at risk is unknown.

The epidemiology of acute beryllium disease suggests that, since the advent of improved environmental controls in industry, acute disease has been all but extinguished. But there still is potential for it to occur under upset conditions. Prevalence estimates in industry for acute beryllium disease range as high as 7% in the earlier literature.

The host factors that may influence an individual's susceptibility to the chronic lung disease, but not the acute pneumonitis, appear to be immunologic, although these are not well delineated at the present time. Cases of disease and sensitization to beryllium have been seen even with brief contact. The amount of exposure required to produce sensitization and disease in susceptible individuals is unknown, but may be independent of dose. Therefore, the surveillance net must be cast widely to avoid underdiagnosis. The population at risk of acute and chronic beryllium disease in the workplace probably should include all workers engaged in any job in which beryllium is used or produced. The possible exception may be the mining of beryl ore. No case has been described, although the mining industry has not been well studied.

Although cases of beryllium disease have occurred among residents living near beryllium refineries, none has been reported since the 1950s. While improved industrial hygiene standards for beryllium have prevented many cases of beryllium disease, research to date suggests that 1) enforcement of this peak standard is difficult, 2) disease is likely to occur even

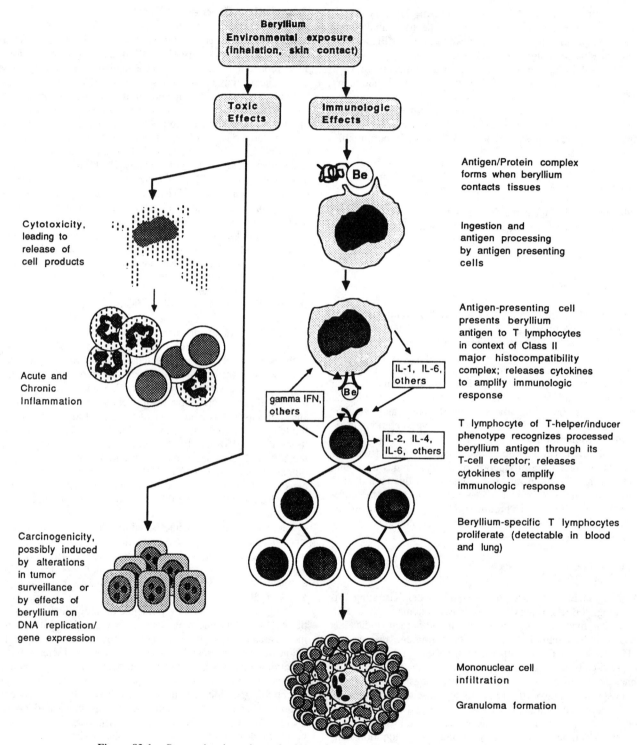

Figure 83.1. Proposed pathogenic mechanisms of acute and chronic disease. See text for details.

with maintenance of this standard, and 3) it is unknown whether a more stringent standard would prevent beryllium sensitization, chronic beryllium disease, or cancer.

BERYLLIUM DISEASE IN HUMANS

Beryllium's effect on humans can take several forms including skin disease, acute lung disease, chronic lung disease, and cancer. The major portion of this section will discuss chronic beryllium disease, as this continues to be the most common health effect of beryllium exposure.

Skin Disease

Skin contact with beryllium salts can cause dermatitis and sensitization to subsequent beryllium exposure. The dermatitis usually resolves with cessation of exposure. The acute dermatologic findings can be associated with conjunctivitis and upper respiratory tract involvement as discussed below.

Inoculation with beryllium either by metal splinter or by imbedding of particles in the skin through wound contamination can produce chronic ulceration of the skin. Biopsies of such lesions generally demonstrate the presence of noncaseating granulomas. Resolution is achieved only by aggressive, recurrent debridement or by excision of the lesion. Without treatment, poor wound healing is the rule, although the degree of active inflammation can wax and wane.

Pulmonary Disease

The inhalational effects of beryllium in humans exist on a continuum from an acute chemical pneumonitis to a chronic granulomatous process of insidious onset. It is noteworthy that there have been many cases of acute disease which have progressed into the chronic form of disease.

ACUTE PULMONARY EFFECTS

Acute inhalational exposure, generally to high levels of beryllium, has been associated with acute nasopharyngitis, tracheobronchitis, and chemical pneumonitis. Upper respiratory symptoms include epistaxis, sensation of facial fullness, and pain. The nasopharyngeal region is found to be edematous and hyperemic with punctate areas of bleeding on examination. With persistence of exposure or in the absence of treatment, ulceration and fissures can form, in some cases resulting in nasal perforation. With removal from exposure, improvement in the nasopharyngeal symptoms and signs occur in most cases over a span of 4–6 weeks.

TRACHEOBRONCHITIS

Acute tracheobronchitis frequently accompanies the chemical pneumonitis. The onset of the tracheobronchitis can be abrupt or gradual, most likely related to the dose of exposure, solubility and other properties of the beryllium compound. Symptoms include chest pain, dry nonproductive cough, and shortness of breath. Objective findings include rhonchi on pulmonary auscultation along with hyperemia of the upper respiratory tract. Chest radiograph may show an increase in peribronchial markings. With removal from exposure, recovery generally occurs within the span of 1 month, although it may also evolve into a chronic bronchitis as seen with the chronic form of beryllium lung disease.

ACUTE BERYLLIUM PNEUMONITIS

Exposure to concentrations of beryllium in the range of 100 μg/m^3 even of short duration can result in the onset of acute chemical pneumonitis. The symptoms, physical findings, lung function abnormalities, and radiographic changes resemble those seen in other forms of acute chemical pneumonitis. Most common symptoms include dyspnea, cough with sputum production, hemoptysis, substernal chest pain, fever, fatigue, and weight loss. Physical findings include rales, cyanosis, tachypnea, and tachycardia. The radiographic findings in acute beryllium pneumonitis range from near normal chest radiographs to diffuse bilateral infiltrates resembling viral pneumonitis to bilateral pulmonary edema involving all lung fields.

Pulmonary function tests are notable for low lung volumes. Arterial blood gases reveal room air hypoxemia.

Pathologic changes found on autopsy in patients with acute beryllium pneumonitis include severe bronchitis and alveolitis with intraalveolar inflammation and edema, as well as inflammatory infiltrates throughout the lung parenchyma that are nongranulomatous in appearance. None of the clinical, physiologic, or roentgenographic findings are pathognomonic of acute beryllium pneumonitis. The diagnosis relies on the establishment of beryllium exposure with a compatible clinical picture. Demonstration of beryllium in urine as a marker of exposure in such cases is of limited value because of the relatively slow excretion of beryllium and the many technical problems with the assay.

Cases often are complicated by the presence of severe pulmonary edema and can result in sustained morbidity and significant mortality. Most patients who survive the acute pneumonitis will have symptoms of several months duration. Bronchiectasis can be a longterm sequela. According to data from the United States Beryllium Case Registry, approximately 17% of patients with acute disease subsequently develop chronic beryllium lung disease.

Depending on the severity of the case, treatment involves removal from exposure, bed rest, and corticosteroid therapy and may in some cases require oxygen supplementation and even endotracheal intubation for respiratory failure. Fortunately, acute beryllium pneumonitis has become rare since the improvement of ventilatory controls in industry. Cases of acute beryllium pneumonitis can still occur during upset conditions.

Some individuals develop a less severe, subacute form of the chemical pneumonitis due to beryllium exposure but may be misdiagnosed as having viral or other pulmonary infection. The identification of such subacute cases of beryllium disease is obviously problematic unless the clinician is aware of the patient's history of current or recent beryllium exposure.

CHRONIC BERYLLIUM DISEASE

Clinical Symptoms Chronic beryllium disease, also known as chronic berylliosis, is a granulomatous disease which manifests itself principally in the lung, although systemic involvement can occur. Unlike the acute pneumonitis, magnitude of exposure does not appear to be an important factor in the development of chronic beryllium disease because it is a hypersensitivity reaction to beryllium, which acts as an antigen or hapten. Recent studies suggest that the chronic disease occurs even at low levels of exposure and even with short duration of exposure. Estimates of chronic disease prevalence range from 1–5% in most series. There is usually a latency period of several months to 30 years from the time of first beryllium exposure to the development of clinical illness. The average latency is 6–10 years, although this may change as medical surveillance improves.

Dyspnea on exertion is the most common initial symptom. It is frequently accompanied by chest pain and cough and in more severe cases by arthralgias, fatigue, and weight loss. Findings on physical examination may include bibasilar dry rales on ausculation, cyanosis, digital clubbing, lymphadenopathy, and skin lesions. Signs of right heart failure and cor pulmonale may be detected in advanced cases.

Although granulomatous involvement of the lung is the typical finding in chronic beryllium disease, noncaseating granulomas can also be found in other organs including the liver, spleen, regional lymph nodes, myocardium, skeletal muscle, kidney, salivary glands, bone, and skin with attendant symptoms referable to the organs of involvement. Skin involvement which is not the result of direct skin inoculation with beryllium can occur in association with chronic beryllium disease. These are nodular skin lesions that show noncaseating granulomas on biopsy. Hepatomegaly has been observed in approximately 10% of patients. Rare reports of splenomegaly, central nervous system involvement, and cardiomyopathy have also been described. Renal calculi, hypercalcemia, and hypercalciuria are all associated with beryllium disease, although the mechanism for nephrolithiasis and altered calcium metabolism is as yet poorly understood.

Biochemical abnormalities in the blood include nonspecific elevations of serum immunoglobulins, elevations of uric acid, and liver enzyme abnormalities if hepatic involvement has occurred. While there is disagreement in the literature as to the value of serum angiotensin-converting enzyme (ACE) levels in this disease process, it has been our experience that ACE levels are frequently not elevated in cases of chronic beryllium disease.

Pulmonary Physiology Pulmonary function abnormalities in chronic beryllium disease take several forms including 1) a predominantly obstructive pattern found in approximately one third of patients; 2) a restrictive defect seen in one quarter of the patients; and 3) reduced diffusing capacity for carbon monoxide (DLCO) with normal lung volumes and normal air flow in one third of cases. Overlap of obstructive plus restrictive physiology also occurs. Some individuals may have normal lung volumes, normal air flow, normal DLCO, and normal resting arterial blood gases, but on exercise physiology testing will demonstrate marked widening of the alveolar-arterial oxygen gradient (A - a)DO$_2$, marked oxygen desaturation, and a ventilatory limitation. This gas exchange abnormality may be the earliest detectable physiologic change. Another subset of patients are normal on every measure of pulmonary physiology, but have granulomas in the lung and demonstrate beryllium-specific immunologic responses by lung lavage lymphocytes. It is not yet known what the clinical outcome will be for these patients with subclinical involvement.

Radiographic and Imaging Abnormalities Chest radiographs in chronic beryllium disease range from completely normal to showing diffuse bilateral infiltrates with hilar adenopathy. Although classically described as having mid and upper lung field predominance of small irregular opacities, parenchymal involvement can be seen in any or all lung fields on chest radiograph (Fig. 83.2). Pleural involvement has also been described in approximately 10% of cases. Our preliminary research suggests that high resolution CT scans may have improved resolution over conventional chest radiographs. Gallium scans are probably of limited value, usually adding little to either the diagnosis or clinical assessment of disease activity beyond the information gained with other tests.

Pathology Pathologic alterations seen at autopsy or via open lung biopsy or transbronchial lung biopsy include noncaseating granulomas, diffuse mononuclear cell infiltration of the interstitium of the lung, with varying degrees of pulmonary fibrosis (Fig. 83.3). Some individuals have a predominantly granulomatous pattern, while others have a more mononuclear infiltrative pattern with fewer or no granulomas on biopsy. Lung biopsy cultures and special stains for acid-fast bacilli and fungi are negative. Findings on bronchoalveolar lavage include high white cell counts, increased lymphocyte percentage, and

elevated ratio of T-helper lymphocytes (CD4 +) to T-suppressor lymphocytes (CD8 +).

Diagnostic Evaluation Figure 83.4 illustrates our current recommendation for the evaluation and diagnosis of beryllium disease. It hinges on the highly specific and sensitive beryllium lymphocyte transformation test (LTT) and on access to lung biopsy specimens through bronchoscopy. With fiberoptic bronchoscopy, transbronchial lung biopsy, and bronchoalveolar lavage it is now possible for clinicians to make a specific, accurate diagnosis of chronic beryllium disease. Transbronchial biopsies confirm the presence of noncaseating granulomas and/or mononuclear cell infiltrates with a yield of greater than 90%. The bronchoalveolar lavage cells are used 1) to identify the presence of lymphocytic alveolitis (which correlates with the pathologic changes on biopsy) and 2) to test for lymphocyte responses to beryllium salts—the LTT, which is discussed below.

The diagnostic criteria in Figure 83.5 represent the first significant departure from the first criteria which were proposed in the 1950s. The criteria employed by the Case Registry required at least four of the following six features and inclusion of at least one of the first two: 1) epidemiologic evidence of significant beryllium exposure; 2) presence of beryllium in lung tissue, lymph nodes, or urine; 3) evidence of lower respiratory tract disease and consistent clinical course; 4) radiographic evidence of interstitial disease; 5) evidence of restrictive and/or obstructive ventilatory abnormality or decreased carbon monoxide diffusing capacity; 6) pathologic alterations consistent with beryllium disease on examination of lung tissue and/or lymph nodes.

Under the old criteria, sarcoidosis was difficult to distinguish from chronic beryllium disease because the pathologic, clinical, radiographic, and physiologic features of the two diseases are virtually identical. The only differentiating factor under the old diagnostic schema was the history of beryllium exposure or the demonstration of beryllium in biologic specimens as a marker of exposure.

With the development of specific and sensitive immunologic tests for beryllium disease, the problem of differentiating these two diseases has receded. Recent studies have validated the LTT which, when taken in conjunction with transbronchial biopsy, allows excellent discrimination of chronic beryllium disease from the wastebasket term "sarcoidosis."

Immunologic Markers of Disease The beryllium lymphocyte transformation test (Fig. 83.6) is an in vitro test of beryllium-specific cell-mediated immunity. It was first developed in the early 1970s, but its value as a diagnostic tool became realized in the 1980s when it was first applied to lung lymphocytes obtained by bronchoalveolar lavage. It had long been known that beryllium hypersensitivity occurs in patients with the disease. In the 1950s, a beryllium patch test was developed, proving that delayed-type hypersensitivity was common in patients with chronic beryllium disease. However, the patch test itself was plagued by false negatives, false positives, induction of beryllium sensitivity in previously unexposed individuals, and exacerbation of symptoms in patients with previous exposure or disease. For these reasons, the patch test is no longer used.

The lymphocyte transformation test is a safe alternative method of detecting the beryllium-specific, cell-mediated immune response. It is performed on blood or lavage cells exposed to beryllium salts in culture. If T-lymphocytes are present which possess "memory" for beryllium as an antigen, then those cells will start to proliferate in vitro. Alternatively, if the pa-

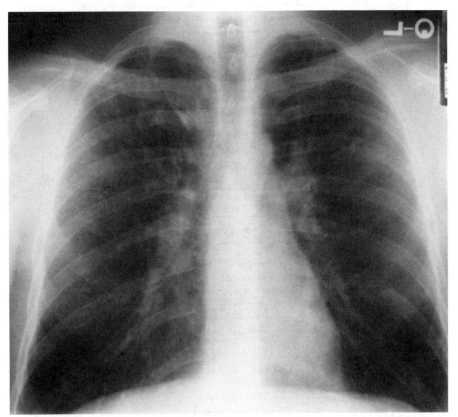

Figure 83.2. Chest radiograph from a 44-year-old white male ceramics engineer with a history of exposure to beryllium oxide dust and fumes 10 years previously. Radiograph shows bilateral interstitial infiltrates, somewhat worse in the upper lung zones, and hilar adenopathy consistent with chronic beryllium disease.

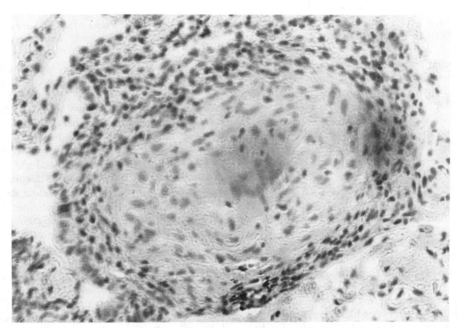

Figure 83.3. High power photomicrograph from transbronchial lung biopsy of a 35-year-old white male machinist with chronic beryllium disease shows noncaseating granulomas and mononuclear cell interstitial infiltration.

tient's cells have never "seen" beryllium as an antigen before, they will ignore it and not proliferate. Proliferation is assessed by adding a radiolabeled DNA precursor such as tritiated thymidine to the cell culture. The more radioactivity that is detected in the cells, the more proliferation that has occurred in response to beryllium. Patients with sarcoidosis and other gran-

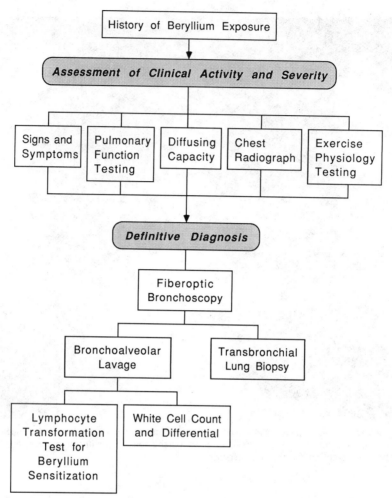

Figure 83.4. The goals of the evaluation in suspected cases of beryllium disease are twofold: 1) to evaluate the level of impairment (usually due to lung involvement) and 2) to make a definitive diagnosis (with the aid of the beryllium LTT and transbronchial lung biopsies).

ulomatous diseases who have never been exposed to beryllium have uniformly negative lymphocyte responses to beryllium.

The use of lavage lymphocytes, rather than blood lymphocytes, for the beryllium LTT has been advocated by some researchers because 1) some individuals have a negative blood LTT response but a positive lung LTT response; 2) the magnitude of the lung lymphocyte response is generally greater than the blood response; 3) bronchoscopy will generally be performed anyway in order to obtain biopsies for histologic confirmation, so the lavage usually will not require a separate procedure. However, recent research has shown that the less invasive blood version of the test is nearly as sensitive as the lavage LTT.

In cases in which granulomatous lung disease has already been demonstrated and the clinician is wondering in retrospect whether the patient has beryllium disease, the blood LTT can clinch the diagnosis. A negative blood LTT result should not be used alone to exclude the diagnosis of beryllium disease, until the technical differences between blood and lavage LTT results are resolved, but positive blood LTT results correlate well with positive lavage LTT results. Although the beryllium LTT is not widely available, both blood and lavage can be shipped by overnight courier to a laboratory which routinely performs this assay.

The blood LTT can be useful in screening beryllium-exposed worker populations. In our experience this test is more sensitive than the routine screening tools of chest radiograph, clinical exam, and pulmonary function testing. It identifies 1) individuals who are sensitized to beryllium but who do not have disease, 2) individuals with subclinical pulmonary granulomatous involvement, and 3) patients with clinical illness.

This lymphocyte response in blood and lavage is of interest not only as a diagnostic tool and screening test, but also for the information which it provides about the immunologic underpinnings of chronic beryllium disease. A proposed mechanism of chronic beryllium disease pathogenesis is shown in Figure 83.1. Following inhalation of beryllium, the lung becomes the battleground for a chronic inflammatory response. Macrophages ingest the beryllium particles and "present" them to lung lymphocytes. A marked increase in the number of lung lymphocytes occurs as those cells recognize the foreign invader. The proliferating lymphocytes are mainly T-helper cells (CD4 + phenotype). This explains why bronchoalveolar lavage in beryllium disease yields large numbers of inflammatory cells, which are mainly lymphocytes of T-helper phenotype. The cells from this lymphocytic "alveolitis" proliferate when they "see" beryllium in the LTT, confirming that they are on this pulmonary battlefield with the mission of specifically containing

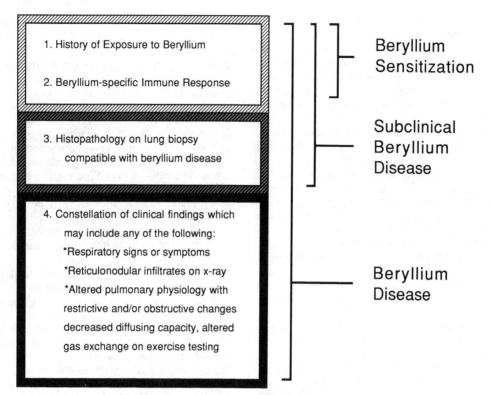

Figure 83.5. Current diagnostic criteria for chronic beryllium disease take into account the role of the immune system in pathogenesis. Some individuals are sensitized to beryllium but have no signs of disease. Others are sensitized, have biopsy-proven granulomas in the lung, but are asymptomatic and unimpaired. A third category has what is classically referred to as "chronic beryllium disease" with the attendant signs, symptoms, and radiographic/physiologic changes.

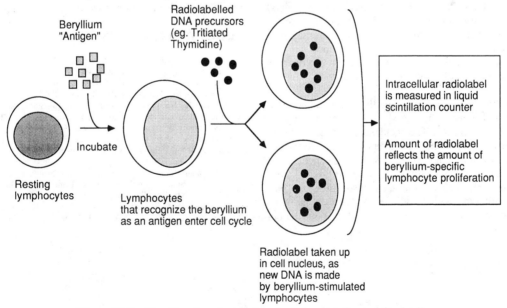

Figure 83.6. Beryllium lymphocytic transformation test. See text for details.

the beryllium onslaught. The outcome is a pulmonary parenchyma scarred by granulomas and strewn with infiltrates of macrophages and lymphocytes.

Prognosis and Treatment The clinical course of chronic beryllium disease is extremely variable. Some patients remain stable for many years, only later in life developing significant clinical deterioration. Others advance more precipitously, with respiratory embarrassment occurring in their 20s and 30s. In several reports, patients have improved without treatment, although this is more the exception than the rule. There still is little hope for cure or remission. Clinical progression is usually very gradual. The majority of patients experience a slow, inexorable decline in lung function, with respiratory failure and right heart failure occurring in approximately 35% of affected individuals if left untreated. Based on a case series from the first decades of recognized chronic beryllium disease, the mortality associated with chronic beryllium disease was estimated at approximately 30%. That figure may improve now that earlier diagnosis and earlier intervention is possible using the LTT and bronchoscopy.

Although there have been no controlled trials, corticosteroids are considered the treatment of choice for chronic beryllium disease. Generally, low dose cortiocosteroid therapy is sufficient (5–20 mg prednisone daily or alternate day dosing). This is associated with improvement in the signs, symptoms, radiographic abnormalities, and gas exchange and pulmonary function test abnormalities. Treatment is usually lifelong, because patients frequently will develop clinical exacerbation with withdrawal of cortiosteroids. Our clinical impression is that corticosteroid therapy favorably alters the course of this disease by reducing chronic inflammation. However, steroid treatment is not associated with longterm cure. Other immunomodulatory agents have not been investigated in treatment of chronic beryllium disease.

As in other pulmonary diseases, supplemental oxygen therapy can usually improve hypoxemia. Treatment of right heart failure and pulmonary hypertension may require the addition of diuretics. Antibiotic treatment of secondary bacterial tracheobronchitis and pneumonia may be required. Patients should be immunized to prevent influenzal and pneumococcal infections.

CARCINOGENESIS

Beryllium has been shown to cause malignancies in several species, by several routes of administration. These include development of lung cancer in monkeys and rats and osteosarcoma in rabbits. There may to be some species differences, in that other researchers have shown that guinea pigs do not develop malignancy following either injection or inhalation of beryllium.

Although it has been controversial, there is evidence that beryllium-exposed workers have a slight but significantly increased risk of lung cancer. The incidence of lung cancer in beryllium-exposed workers may be inversely related to the duration of their exposure. The excess risk of lung cancer is not explained by smoking habits and is not synergistic with smoking-related cancer risk. There is no clear association of a particular tumor cell type with beryllium exposure in humans. Clearly a great deal more information is needed about the be-

ryllium carcinogenesis issue. However, based on existing data, it should be considered a probable human carcinogen.

MEDICAL SURVEILLANCE AND PREVENTION

While the occurrence of acute beryllium disease has been reduced greatly by the improvements in industrial control over beryllium air concentrations, cases of chronic beryllium disease continue to be identified in many industries. No clear dose-response relationship has ever been found for chronic beryllium disease. As discussed, most evidence suggests that this is an immunologically mediated process in which exposure to even low levels of beryllium are sufficient to induce sensitization and disease. At this time, there is no way of prescreening individuals in order to determine susceptibility. However, there are ways of screening exposed workers for subclinical disease so that earlier medical interventions can be made if clinical decline begins to occur.

The traditional medical surveillance standard in the industry has included annual physical examination, chest radiograph, spirometry, and, in some cases, diffusing capacity. These tools are relatively insensitive and nonspecific. Recent work has shown that the addition of the blood LTT to the screening armamentarium enhances the ability of clinicians to identify individuals who are sensitized to beryllium, as well as individuals who already have granulomas in their lungs at subclinical and early clinical stages. Although we do not know at this time whether early diagnosis and removal from ongoing exposure will lead to a better clinical outcome, medical prudence dictates that such individuals be removed from exposure. In light of the role of beryllium as a probable carcinogen, efforts should still be made in industry to bring exposure levels even lower than those recommended by the current standard.

SUGGESTED READINGS

1. Cullen MR, Cherniack MG, Kominsky JR. Chronic beryllium disease in the United States. Semin Respir Med 1986;7:203–209.

2. Kreibel D, Brain JD, Sprince NL, Kazemi H. The pulmonary toxicity of beryllium. Am Rev Respir Dis 1988;137:464–473.

3. Kreiss K, Newman LS, Mroz M, Campbell PA. Screening blood test identifies subclinical beryllium disease. J Occup Med 1989;31:603–608.

4. Newman LS, Kreiss K, King Jr, TE, Seay S, Campbell PA. Pathologic and immunologic alterations in early stages of beryllium disease: reexamination of disease definition in natural history. Am Rev Respir Dis 1989;139:1479–1486.

5. Rossman MD, Kern JA, Elias JA, et al. Proliferative response of bronchoalveolar lymphocytes to beryllium. Ann Intern Med 1988; 108:687–93.

6. Sprince NL. Beryllium disease. In: Merchant JA, ed. Occupational respiratory disease. U.S. Department of Health and Human Services (NIOSH) Publication No. 86-102. Washington, DC: DHHS, 1986;385–99.

84

Chromium

Robert J. Geller, M.D.

SOURCE/ PRODUCTION/ COMMON NAMES/ USES

As mined, chromium occurs as chromium oxide complexed with iron in the form FeO $= CR_2O_3$. Chromite ore typically also contains aluminum and magnesium oxides and may in addition have titanium and/or vanadium oxides in varying quantities (1). Chromium is present in its trivalent state in chromite ore.

Chromium compounds are widely used in industry, with the majority used in pigments (33% of chromium use), metal surface plating (25%), leather tanning (25%), and textile production (10%). Photographic processes and catalyst production also are prominent uses.

CHEMICAL/PHYSICAL FORMS

Chromium has a molecular weight of 52. It is generally present as a solid, one notable exception being chromyl chloride, a hexavalent chromium compound which is a fuming liquid.

The chemical and toxicologic properties of chromium differ markedly depending on the valence state of the metal. Chromium occurs in its metallic state (valence 0) and in valence states $+2$ through $+6$, but only the trivalent ($+3$) and hexavalent ($+6$) states are commonly found forms. Chromium in its $+2$ state frequently oxidizes rapidly to the $+3$ form, and the $+4$ and $+5$ states are found only as intermediates in the conversion between the $+3$ and $+6$ states.

Some of the chromium compounds of industrial significance are included in Table 84.1.

SITES, INDUSTRIES ASSOCIATED WITH EXPOSURE

A compilation of data provided by the National Institute for Occupational Safety and Health (2) and the articles cited in

Table 84.1. Some Common Chromium Compounds

Divalent (Cr^{+2})	
Chromous chloride	$CrCl_2$
Chromous sulfate	$CrSO_4$
Trivalent (Cr^{+3})	
Chromic oxide	Cr_2O_3
Chromic sulfate	$Cr_2[SO_4]_3$
Chromite ore	$FeO \cdot Cr_2O_3$
Hexavalent (Cr^{+6})	
Chromium trioxide	CrO_3
Chromic acid	H_2CrO_4
Chromic acid anhydrides:	
Sodium chromate	Na_2CrO_4
Potassium chromate	K_2CrO_4
Dichromates:	
Sodium dichromate	$Na_2Cr_2O_7$
Potassium dichromate	$K_2Cr_2O_7$
Ammonium dichromate	$(NH_4)_2Cr_2O_7$

this discussion include the industries in Table 84.2 as a partial list of those involved in chromium use.

Chromium toxicity has been studied frequently in the chrome-plating and chromium chemical manufacture industries. These studies, because of their cohort design, inherently involve occupational settings which most likely had higher exposure levels than are presently allowable. Also, the studies did not always distinguish between similar though not identical jobs. Hard chrome plating (intended for protection of the surface) involves the application of a more dense chrome finish than bright chrome plating (intended for application of a bright decorative surface), yet the two were not always studied separately.

CLINICAL TOXICOLOGY

Routes of Absorption and Exposure

INHALATION

Metallic chromium, chromous or chromic salts (valences 0, $+2$, $+3$) are minimally absorbed following inhalation. Local pulmonary deposition of these salts has been reported following exposure, but without evidence of adverse systemic effects (2, 3).

Inhalation of highly water-soluble hexavalent chromium salts, such as chromic acid, sodium dichromate, and potassium dichromate, may result in systemic absorption. Less water-soluble salts are unlikely to produce systemic effects but may produce pulmonary effects (1).

INGESTION

Trivalent chromium salts are absorbed following ingestion, but only 1–25% of the dose ingested is absorbed (4). The extent of absorption varies with the particular salt ingested and the circumstances of ingestion.

Hexavalent salts are converted by gastric juices to the trivalent form prior to absorption (5).

DERMAL ABSORPTION

Trivalent salts are generally poorly absorbed through intact skin (1). Once the dermal barrier is broken, however, absorption may occur.

Hexavalent salts are generally topically well absorbed, even through intact skin.

Clinical Toxicology—Signs/Symptoms

ACUTE

Hexavalent Chromium Compounds

Following oral or dermal exposure, hexavalent chromium compounds, including chromic acid, the chromates, and dichro-

Table 84.2. Industries Likely to Use Chromium Compounds

Anodizing
Color TV picture tube manufacture
Copper etching
Glass working
Lithography
Metal plating
Metal working
Oil purification
Photoengraving
Photography
Portland cement use
Stainless steel grinding
Textile production
Welding

mates, are potentially the most toxic of the chromium compounds commonly encountered. Ingestion of dichromates has proven fatal in six of 13 cases collected in one review (6); the oral lethal dose is estimated to be 0.5–5 g (7).

Dermal Hexavalent chromium compounds may be absorbed percutaneously, even through intact skin. On contact with skin, hexavalent chromium compounds act as both irritants and sensitizers. Following local exposure to either airborne particles or contact with contaminated surfaces, chromate dust or chromic acid mist has caused nasal lesions which progress in some cases to frank ulceration (''chrome ulcers'') and even perforation of the nasal septum (8,9). These initial lesions have been described as ''discrete areas of nasal irritation which burned intensely when the affected nostril was manually collapsed'' (8). More severe lesions present an erythematous weeping and crusted appearance. In one study of chromic acid workers, the incidence and severity of nasal injury was related both to length of exposure and to the laxity of industrial hygiene practiced by the individual worker (8).

Following cutaneous exposure to chromic acid, burns or erosions of the skin may occur. These ''chrome holes'' initially appear as papular lesions, either singly or grouped, with central ulceration. With progression, adjacent soft tissues become eroded as well (8).

Allergic contact dermatitis to chromates has been widely observed. Following exposure of sensitive individuals to even low levels of chromates, dermatitis may develop (10). Furthermore, chromate sensitivity has proven quite persistent once developed (11,12). In one study, 92% of the study patients with dichromate sensitivity induced by exposure to Portland cement continued to display contact dermatitis 10 years following the initial development of symptoms (11).

Chromate sensitivity, once induced, may produce difficulty in multiple settings. Contact with textiles colored with chromate-based pigments can be sufficient to exacerbate the dermatitis. The wearing of leather shoes tanned with chromates can produce dermatitis of the feet if the feet are allowed to remain sweaty. ''Housewives' eczema'' may be largely a chromate sensitivity phenomenon, as detergents and bleaches in some areas contain more than trace amounts of chromate salts (10).

Gastrointestinal Following ingestion, gastric secretions convert hexavalent chromium to trivalent chromium, which is more readily absorbed from the gastrointestinal tract (5). In this process, however, the gastric and intestinal mucosa are in grave danger of severe erosive injury. Even small ingestions

of dichromates have resulted in hemorrhagic gastroenteritis and death (13, 14).

Renal Acute renal failure is common following large oral ingestions of hexavalent chromium compounds as well as following dermal exposures (15). Acute renal failure can occur following a dermal burn of 10% body surface area or less. A 28-year-old white man, while at work, suffered a burn to the left calf with a concentrated chromic acid solution. The area was immediately irrigated with water; however, full thickness burns covering 1% of body surface area developed over the next few days. He developed nausea and vomiting within 1 hour of exposure and complete anuria within 24 hours. Laboratory evaluation 4 days post-exposure were remarkable for a blood urea nitrogen of 82 mg/dl and serum creatinine of 14.7 mg/dl. The sodium was 132 mEq/l, potassium 4.9 mEq/l, calcium 9.1 mg/dl, phosphorus 5.0 mg/dl, and uric acid 7.6 mg/dl. The white blood count was $12.4/mm^3$, platelets 240,000, hemoglobin 15.5 g/dL, hematocrit 46%, and lactate dehydrogenase 1274 Units/l. A renal ultrasound showed no evidence of obstruction. A diagnosis of acute tubular necrosis secondary to acute chromium intoxication was made. Two weeks after exposure, the patient required hemodialysis three times a week.

This case illustrates the potential for serious chromium intoxication and acute renal failure following chromic acid burns. The smallest burn previously reported in the literature to result in acute renal failure covered 10% of the body surface area. This patient's burn covered only 1% of the body surface area, 10 times smaller than that previously reported to result in acute chromium intoxication (16).

Pulmonary Inhalation of hexavalent chromium salts may result in pulmonary sensitization (2). Inhaled concentrated chromic acid mist has been reported to result in pulmonary edema, which may be delayed up to 72 hours following exposure. Chronic inhalation of hexavalent chromium presents an increased risk of lung cancers, which will be further discussed under the heading of chronic exposure.

Adult respiratory distress syndrome (ARDS) has been reported following substantial ingestion (14).

Hepatic Hepatic dysfunction has uncommonly been observed following exposure to chromic acid (2).

Trivalent Chromium

Trivalent chromium is poorly absorbed by inhalation and through intact skin, resulting in a low order of systemic toxicity. However, should trivalent chromium gain access to the systemic circulation, toxic effects may develop. For example, a 70% total body thermal burn from hot chromic sulfate mixed with sulfuric acid produced chromium poisoning with acute renal failure (17).

Pulmonary Inhalation of trivalent chromium salts can cause occupational asthma. In one case, IgE antibodies to chromic sulfate was demonstrated (18). Pneumoconiosis has also been observed following exposure to chromite ore dust (4, 19).

CHRONIC/LONGTERM TOXICITY

Chronic inhalation of hexavalent chromium presents an increased risk of lung cancers, with the degree of risk varying depending on the particular salt(s) and their solubility under

Table 84.3. Ascorbic Acid Dosage for Therapy of Hexavalent Chromium Ingestion

Salt	Dose of Ascorbic Acid per Gram of Chromium Salt Ingested
Chromic acid, chromic trioxide	3.85g ascorbic acid/g
Sodium dichromate	2.9g ascorbic acid/g
Potassium dichromate	2.62g ascorbic acid/g
Ammonium dichromate	3g ascorbic acid/g

biologic conditions, the circumstances of exposure, and concomitant risk factors such as cigarette smoking. Calcium, lead, and zinc chromates are generally accepted as pulmonary carcinogens (1, 20).

Much discussion of the carcinogenic potential of other chromium compounds has occurred in the recent literature, with little consensus. Many authors maintain that the other hexavalent salts, trivalent salts, and metallic chromium are not potential carcinogens, and the reader is referred to several excellent reviews for further details of this debate (20–27).

Toxicology Management

CLINICAL MANAGEMENT

No matter what the route(s) of exposure, the initial approach to the patient must of course include assessment of the patient's clinical status, followed by support of basic cardiopulmonary functions. Once the airway has been stabilized, and cardiopulmonary support instituted as indicated, further measures can be considered.

Ingestion

Decontamination *Emesis* should generally *not* be induced, due to the potential corrosive effects of the chromium compound and the potential for rapid deterioration of the patient.

Ascorbic acid should generally be administered orally or nasogastrically, if the patient is seen while the chromium compound is still in the stomach. Ascorbic acid has been shown to ameliorate the effects of topical human exposure to chromates (28), and to reduce toxicity following ingestion in rats if given within 2 hours of exposure (28). Ascorbic acid functions to chemically reduce Cr^{+6} to Cr^{+3}, the form less toxic to the gastric and intestinal mucosa. The dosage of ascorbic acid recommended for several hexavalent salts is shown in Table 84.3 (15).

Dilution of the ingested agent is appropriate, particularly if its pH is quite low (e.g., chromic acid) or quite high (eg., ammonium dichromate). Dilution may be accomplished with water or with fluids which also serve as demulcents, such as milk. The use of demulcent compounds (such as antacids, corn starch, or milk) in addition to those used for dilution has been recommended (15) and seems reasonable but has not been formally studied.

Gastric lavage to reduce the dose ingested should be utilized if chromium is still present in the stomach. A soft tube is preferable due to the possibility of injury to gastric mucosa already having occurred. Lavage using antacids such as magnesium hydroxide has been suggested, but no studies have been carried out to demonstrate its relative efficacy to the use of water.

Activated charcoal has not been experimentally studied in the treatment of chromate poisoning but would not be anticipated to be of benefit because charcoal does not bind other metals well.

Elimination enhancement *Exchange transfusion* was effective in reducing blood chromium levels 67% in one case, using 10.9 liters of blood (17). Existing evidence does not allow the conclusion that exchange transfusion should generally be employed, however.

Hemodialysis and *charcoal hemoperfusion* do not substantially enhance chromium removal from the body if renal function remains normal (14, 29). However, if renal failure ensues, hemodialysis may be necessary for management of the renal failure itself.

Treatment *Fluid balance* must be maintained carefully. The patient should be monitored carefully for evidence of gastrointestinal bleeding, methemoglobinemia, hemolysis, coagulopathy, seizures, or pulmonary dysfunction, and appropriate supportive measures should be employed as indicated. If hemolysis develops, gentle *alkaline diuresis* may be indicated to reduce the possibility of further renal injury. If methemoglobinemia exceeding 30% is observed, treatment with methylene blue should be employed.

Chelation with calcium disodium EDTA and BAL does not seem to confer clinical benefit (13,30). *N-Acetylcysteine* (NAC) increased chromium clearance and reversed oliguria in rats poisoned with potassium dichromate, but there is no human published experience using NAC (30).

Inhalation

Following inhalation of hexavalent or trivalent chromium compounds, patients should be removed from further exposure and carefully assessed. If respiratory distress or cyanosis is noted, oxygen should be administered. Bronchospasm should be treated with bronchodilators; selective beta-2 agonists such as albuterol or terbutaline may be the agents of initial choice.

If the inhaled agent was concentrated chromic acid, continued observation and assessment for the delayed development of pulmonary edema should be considered. Similar precautions following the inhalation of other concentrated hexavalent, highly soluble chromium compounds are prudent.

Dermal

The skin should be copiously irrigated with water. The affected area should be evaluated for the presence of chemical or thermal burns, and treatment should be provided as indicated.

The topical application of a freshly made 10% ascorbic acid solution (28, 31), or of a barrier cream containing 2% glycine and 1% tartaric acid (32) has proven beneficial in some industrial settings in reducing the consequences of topical exposure to hexavalent chromium compounds.

LABORATORY STUDIES

Specific measurement of chromium or chromate levels following exposure has not been shown to have prognostic or therapeutic value. However, they may serve to further document exposure and assess the efficacy of measures used to enhance elimination (1).

BIOLOGIC MONITORING

Routine biologic monitoring of employees in chromium industries has not been shown to be of benefit. In selected cases, where biologic monitoring of individual employees is desired, comparing chromium levels in urine samples before and after exposure has been suggested (1). Confounding factors must be addressed prior to institution of any biologic monitoring. These factors include the difficulty of accurate and precise laboratory measurement and the possibility of sample contamination during collection and storage.

EXPOSURE LIMITS/TLVS/PELS

The U. S. Occupational Safety and Health Administration, as its final rule permissible exposure limits, on a time-weighted average basis (PEL-TWA) (33), and the American Council of Government and Industrial Hygienists (ACGIH), as its threshold limit values (TLV) (34) on a time-weighted average basis, recommend the following limits:

Chromium Compound	OSHA PEL	ACGIH TLV
Metallic chromium	1 mg Cr/m^3	0.5 mg Cr/m^3
Divalent chromium compounds	0.5 mg Cr/m^3	0.5 mg Cr/m^3
Trivalent chromium compounds	0.5 mg Cr/m^3	0.5 mg Cr/m^3
Hexavalent chromic compounds, and chromic acid	0.1 mg CrO$_3$/m^3	0.05 mg CrO$_3$/m^3
Chromite ore	—	0.05 mg Cr/m^3

The National Institute of Occupational Safety and Health states the following air concentrations are Immediately Dangerous to Life and Health (IDLH limits) (35):

Metallic chromium	500 mg Cr/m^3
Insoluble chromium salts	500 mg Cr/m^3
Soluble divalent salts	250 mg Cr/m^3
Soluble trivalent salts	250 mg Cr/m^3
Hexavalent chromium compounds, and chromic acid	30 mg CrO$_3$/m^3

SUMMARY

Chromium toxicity varies with the particular chromium compound. Metallic chromium, divalent, and trivalent chromium is relatively harmless. Hexavalent chromium compounds are dangerous following acute large exposures and may also be hazardous following chronic exposure to lower concentrations.

The optimal treatment for chromium toxicity lies in its prevention, with the use of good industrial hygiene practices and utilization of proper workplace industrial controls. Once toxicity develops, however, the ideal therapy has not yet been found.

ACKNOWLEDGMENT

The author wishes to recognize the special contribution of Antonio Muniz in the review and retrieval of the published literature pertaining to chromium toxicity.

REFERENCES

1. Sawyer HJ. Chromium and its compounds. In: Zenz C, ed. Occupational medicine: principles and practical applications. 2nd ed. Chicago: Year Book Medical Publishers, 1988:531–539.

2. Tabershaw IR, Utidjian HMD, Kawahara BL. Chromium and its Compounds. In: Kay MM, et al. eds. Occupational diseases: a guide to their recognition. Rev. ed. Washington, DC: National Institute of Occupational Safety and Health, 1977:352–354.

3. Proctor NH, Hughes JP, Fischman ML et al. Chromium. In: Proctor NH, Hughes JP, Fischman ML et al. Chemical hazards of the workplace. 2nd ed. Philadelphia: Lippincott, 1988:155–158.

4. Baselt RC, Cravey RH. Disposition of toxic drugs and chemicals in man. 3rd ed. Chicago: Year Book Medical Publishers, 1989:190–192.

5. DeFlora S, Badolati GS, Serra D et al. Circadian reduction of chromium in the gastric environment. Mutat Res 1987;192:169–174.

6. Bader TF. Acute renal failure after chromic acid injection. West J Med 1986;144:608–609.

7. Kaufman DB, DiNicola W, McIntosh R. Acute potassium dichromate poisoning. Am J Dis Child 1970;119:374–376.

8. Cohen SR, Davis DM, Kramkowski RS. Clinical manifestations of chromic acid toxicity. Cutis 1974;13:558–568.

9. Lee HS, Goh CL. Occupational dermatosis among chrome platers. Contact Derm 1988;18:89–93.

10. Fisher AA. Blackjack disease and other chromate puzzles. Cutis 1976;18:21–22, 35.

11. Burrows D. Prognosis in industrial dermatitis. Br J Dermatol 1972;87:145–148.

12. Breit R, Turk RBM. The medical and social fate of the dichromate allergic patient. Br J Dermatol 1976;94:349–351.

13. Ellis EN, Brouhard BH, Lynch RE et al. Effects of hemodialysis and dimercaprol in acute dichromate poisoning. J Toxicol Clin Toxicol 1982;19:249–258.

14. Iserson KV, Banner W, Froede RC et al. Failure of dialysis therapy in potassium dichromate poisoning. J Emerg Med 1983;1:143–149.

15. Sharma BK, Singhal PC, Chugh KS. Intravascular hemolysis and acute renal failure following potassium dichromate poisoning. Postgrad Med J 1978;54:414–415.

16. Stoner RS, Tong TG, Dart RC, Sullivan JB. Acute chromium intoxication with renal failure after 1% body surface area burns from chromic acid [Abstract]. Presented at the AAPCC/AACT/ABMT/CAPCC Annual Scientific Meeting, Baltimore, Maryland, October 1–4, 1988.

17. Kelly WF, Ackrill R, Day JP et al. Cutaneous absorption of trivalent chromium: Tissue levels and treatment by exchange transfusion. Br J Ind Med 1982;39:397–400.

18. Novey HS, Habib M, Wells ID. Asthma and IgE antibodies induced by chromium and nickel salts. J Allergy Clin Immunol 1983;72:407–412.

19. Mancuso TF, Hueper WC. Occupational cancer and other health hazards in a chromate plant. Ind Med Surg 1951;20:358–363.

20. DeFlora S, Bagnasco M, Serra D et al. Genotoxicity of chromium compounds: a review. Mutat Res 1990;238:99–172.

21. Abe S, Ohsaki Y, Kimura K et al. Chromate lung cancer with special reference to its cell type and relation to the manufacturing process. Cancer 1982;49:783–787.

22. Braver ER, Infante P, Chu K. An analysis of lung cancer risk from exposure to hexavalent chromium. Teratogen Carcinog Mutagen 1985;5:365–378.

23. Farkas I. WHO—coordinated international study on the health effects of occupational exposure of welders to chromium and nickel. Nutr Revs 1985;suppl 1:683–689.

24. Hayes RB, Sheffet A, Spirtas R. Cancer mortality among a cohort of chromium pigment workers. Am J Ind Med 1989;16:127–133.

25. Langard S. One hundred years of chromium and cancer: a review of epidemiological evidence and selected case reports. Am J Ind Med 1990;17:189–215.

26. Norseth T. The carcinogenicity of chromium and its salts. Editorial. Br J Ind Med 1986;43:649–651.

27. Svensson BG, Englander V, Akesson B et al. Deaths and tumors among workers grinding stainless steel. Am J Ind Med 1989;15:51–59.

28. Samitz MH. Prevention of occupational skin diseases from exposure to chromic acid and chromates: Use of ascorbic acid. Cutis 1974;13:569–574.

29. Behari JR, Tandon SK. Chelation in metal intoxication. VIII. Clin Toxicol 1980;16:33–40.

30. Banner W, Koch M, Capin DM et al. Experimental chelation therapy in chromium, lead, and boron intoxication with N-acetylcysteine and other compounds. Toxicol Appl Pharmacol 1986;83:142–147.

31. Milner JE. Ascorbic acid in the prevention of chromium dermatitis. J Occup Med 1980;22:51–52.

32. Romaguera C, Grimalt F, Vilaplana J et al. Formulation of a barrier cream against chromate. Contact Derm 1985;13:49–52.

33. Occupational Safety and Health Administration, Department of Labor. Air contaminants, final rule; 29 CFR Part 1910. Fed Reg 1989;54(12):2332–2983.

34. American Conference of Government and Industrial Hygienists. Threshold limit values and biological exposure indices for 1990–1991. Cincinnati: ACGIH, 1990.

35. National Institute for Occupational Safety and Health, Department of Health and Human Services. Pocket guide to chemical hazards. Fifth Printing. Washington, DC: DHHS, 1985.

85

Manganese and Magnesium

David A. Gilmore, Jr., M.D.
Alvin C. Bronstein, M.D.

MANGANESE SOURCES AND PRODUCTION

Manganese (Mn—molecular weight 54.9) is a reddish-gray or silvery, soft metal, member of group VII of the periodic table. Manganese is the 10th most abundant metal in the earth's crust at an average concentration of 1000 ppm. It is the 19th most abundant seawater metal at 1 ppb (1). Various ores contain manganese: pyrolusite, braunite, manganite, hausmannite, and psilomelane, oxides; hauserite, a sulfide; manganesespat, a carbonate; and tephroite, a silicate (1). The most commercially important of these is pyrolusite, which is made up primarily of manganese dioxide (2).

The average adult contains about 12 milligrams of manganese. The skeletal system contains about 43%, with the rest in soft tissues including liver, pancreas, kidneys, brain, and central nervous system (1). The mean whole blood adult manganese concentration, with most bound in the erythrocyte porphyrin complex, is 9 μg/l (range 3.9–15.0). Mean serum manganese concentration is 1.8 μg/l (range 0.9–2.9) (3).

Manganese is predominantly used in the production of steel alloys such as ferromanganese, silcomanganese, manganin, and spielgeleisen. Ferromanganese (approximately 80% manganese) and spielgeleisen (15–30% manganese) are examples of manganese iron alloys. Silcomanganese (between 65–68% manganese) alloys silicon and manganese (4). Because manganese is moderately reactive and brittle it is found in Heusler alloys (18–25% manganese) with copper and aluminum or zinc. Many iron and steel manufacturing processes require the addition of manganese to molten iron to reduce the iron oxide content by the formation of manganese oxide. Manganese oxide dissolves readily in molten slag and is easily separated from the iron. Manganese is also used to reduce the oxygen and sulfur content of molten steel to increase ductility. Fourteen kg of manganese is required for each ton of steel produced (5).

Iron and steel alloys made with manganese demonstrate increased durability and corrosion resistance. Steel manganese alloys are more malleable when forged than others. Manganese may be produced from ferrous scrap used in the production of electric and open-hearth steel (4).

Manganese and manganese compounds are used in the manufacture of dry cell batteries as a depolarizer, and also in paints and varnishes, inks, dyes, matches and fireworks, bleaching agents, laboratory reagents, motor oils, fertilizers, disinfectants, welding rods, and in the synthesis of hydroquinone, the green-colored potassium manganate and the purple-hued potassium permanganate. Manganous acetate is used in dyeing, leather tanning, and fertilizers and as a drier for linseed oil (1). It also used as a decolorizer and coloring agent in the manufacture of glass and ceramics. Manganese carbonate is found in the pigment manganese white. Manganese sulfate is a red pottery glaze and fertilizer for vines and tobacco. Manganese ethylene-bis-dithiocarbamate (Maneb), which has been shown

to cause thyroid hyperplasia and fetal abnormalities in rats, is a commercial fungicide. Manganese is soluble in water and dilute acid. Manganese easily dissolves in groundwater. Concentrations greater than 1320 g/l have been observed in drinking water (6). Manganese can be found as manganous and manganic salts, manganese sulfate, and oxides of manganese.

Manganese is mostly found in Australia, Brazil, Canada, Chile, China, Cuba, India, Gabon, Ghana, Morocco, South Africa, and Russia. Low grade deposits are found in the United States. Solid ore, powder, dust, or fumes are found as sulfides and oxides.

An essential trace element, manganese, is necessary for the functioning of many enzyme systems: pyruvate carboxylase—a metalloenzyme, arginase, phosphatase, and lipid and mucopolysaccharide synthetases (1). It is found in nuts, grain, meats, poultry, infant formulas, and parenteral nutrition preparations. The average adult ingests between 4 and 10 mg/day (2,8). The National Research Council (7) has set maximum daily requirements for dietary manganese (Table 85.1).

SITES, INDUSTRIES, AND BUSINESSES ASSOCIATED WITH EXPOSURES

The most common sources of manganese exposure are dust from steel manufacturing, welding (9), mining, and ore extracting facilities. Toxic exposures have been reported from ingestion of contaminated drinking water by mining operations and the improper discarding of lead-acid batteries. Manganese is transferred across the placenta (8) and can be transferred in breast milk (10). The mean concentration in breast milk is 7–120 μg/l (10). It is a trace nutrient added to all prepared infant formulas.

Methylcyclopentadienyl manganese tricarbonyl (MMT) has been tried as a replacement additive in unleaded fuels for the antiknock ingredient tetraethyl lead. MMT is one of several organomanganese compounds which have been proposed for this use (1, 11). MMT is used as an additive in machine, diesel, and fuel oils (12).

Table 85.1. The National Research Council Has Set The Following Maximum Daily Requirements for Dietary Manganese:

Age	Years	MDR
Adults		2.0–5.0 mg/day
Adolescents	11.0+	2.0–5.0
Children	7.0–10.0	2.0–3.0
Children	4.0–6.0	1.5–2.0
	1.0–3.0	1.0–1.5
Infants	0.5–1.0	0.6–0.7
	0.0–0.5	0.3–0.6

CLINICAL TOXICOLOGY OF EXPOSURE

Since manganese and its compounds are found readily as dusts, fumes, and solutes in ground water, the primary routes of manganese exposure are inhalation and oral ingestion. There does not seem to be significant dermal absorption, although contact dermatitis has been reported. The mechanism of absorption of manganese from the gastrointestinal tract has not been clearly elucidated, although there exists a specific beta-1 globulin protein used for serum transport—transmanganin (1, 12, 13). Only the Mn^{+3} cationic form of manganese seems to be well absorbed. Ingested Mn^{+2} is oxidized to Mn^{+3} in the alkaline medium of the duodenum (13). Some absorbed Mn^{+3} is conjugated with bile in the liver and excreted in the intestine with reuptake in the enterohepatic circulation (8). After intestinal uptake, manganese complexes with the beta-1 globulin, transmanganin (13). No definitive studies have been performed to demonstrate active or passive transport systems in the gastrointestinal tract (13).

Iron deficiency states and low protein dietary states have been associated with increased absorption of oral manganese (8, 14–16). Increased dietary calcium or phosphorus decreases manganese absorption (8). Alveolar absorption is possible by passive diffusion into the capillary vascular system. However, it has been shown that inhalation of radiolabeled manganese is transferred to the gut and absorbed there, demonstrating significant gastrointestinal absorption even with inhalation exposures (17).

Manganese does not appear to pass through the cytochrome P-450 or glucuronidation pathways and elimination does not require active metabolism. In general, the higher the oxidation state of manganese, the more toxic the compound. The exception is Mn^{+2}, which is 2.5–3 times more toxic than Mn^{+3}. The anion in a manganese salt also acts as a predictor of toxicity, with manganese citrate being more toxic than (in descending order) manganese chloride, sulfate, or acetate (1). Manganese is also found in hair, which serves as a minor excretory pathway (18). Assays of hair manganese concentration do not correlate with exposure or poisoning symptoms (19).

Absorbed manganese (Mn^{+3}) rapidly appears in bile fluid and undergoes enterohepatic circulation followed by excretion. Small amounts of manganese can be found in pancreatic fluid with only extremely small amounts detectable in urine (approximately 6% of absorbed dose). The major route of manganese excretion is via the feces (13, 17).

SIGNS, SYNDROMES, AND SYMPTOMS FROM TOXIC EXPOSURE

Acute Toxicity

Acute exposure to manganese may produce a collection of flu-like symptoms, termed metal fume fever or manganese pneumonitis (20). Metal fume fever is caused by the inhalation of the finely divided powder of manganese oxides (20). Manganese pneumonitis has been described in workers exposed to manganese ore, dry cell battery, and potassium permanganate manufacturing processes (19, 21). The pneumonitis appears to be due to direct damage to respiratory epithelium as well as an immunodepressant action (21). Manganese dioxide has been shown to depress humoral immunity, alveolar macrophage function, and phagocytic activity (22, 23).

Metal fume fever is usually self-limiting and appears to be more of an immune system reaction rather than due to cellular damage or bacterial process. The syndrome is characterized by fever, chills, nausea, coughing, and congestion. It usually manifests itself after the worker has gone home and at the beginning of the work week with symptoms remitting by the weekend. Episodes are usually self-limiting and require supportive treatment. Many industrial processes such as welding or metal cutting can produce manganese oxides (20).

Manganese pneumonitis may be relatively more severe and require antibiotic and bronchodilator therapy (21). Episodes of manganese pneumonitis put workers at risk for developing hyperreactive airways disease with longterm sequelae and chronic pulmonary disease (24).

Due to poor solubility characteristics, the occurrence of acute central nervous system toxicity has not been reported. Manganese appears to be the least acutely CNS toxic of the metals requiring longterm, continuing exposure for CNS toxicity (3).

Chronic Toxicity

Reports in the literature date back as far as Dr. John Couper's description of 1837 (25), and exposures ranging from 6 months to 24 years have been documented (26, 27). The most comprehensive review of manganese poisoning has been by Mena et al. (17, 27, 28), including a review of clinical presentations, pathophysiology, and possible treatment modalities among exposed children miners.

Manganese concentrates in mitochondrial-rich tissues, and the highest concentrations are found in (in descending order) brain, kidney, pancreas, and liver (8). Isolated reports of liver dysfunction have been reported, but there is no confirmatory evidence for chronic liver toxicity. Elevated liver enzymes with eosinophilia have been reported in past literature but these were due to coexistent parasitic infection. There have been no documented cases of nephrotoxicity associated with manganese toxicity (8, 19).

Increased exposure to manganese can lead to significant calcium loss stool via result and in lowered serum calcium levels. Metabolic activation of chondroitin sulfate synthetase, polysaccharide polymerase, and galactotransferase has been described in manganese excess (29).

Interference with hematopoiesis has been reported but not confirmed from large group studies. Decreases in spermatogenesis and sperm motility with decreases in succinic dehydrogenase in cat seminiferous tubules resulting in reduction of glucose-6-phosphate dehydrogenase activity producing decreased cellular metabolism have been demonstrated (30, 31).

The central nervous system effects of manganese have been the ones most closely studied. The major effects, well reported in the literature, are associated with both psychiatric and neurologic dysfunction. Tissue burden and serum concentrations of manganese do not correlate with symptomatology. Mena and colleagues found higher tissue burdens in unaffected versus affected Chilean miners in a large group study (17, 27, 28). This raises the question of a possible genetic and/or metabolic defect in the handling of manganese, which remains to be elucidated. This is in contrast to Wilson's disease or lead encephalopathy, where serum levels do serve as markers for the degree of illness or as confirmatory evidence for diagnosis. It is theoretically possible for continued exposure to produce incremental damage to the CNS without obvious elevations in serum manganese concentration (18,19). This is most likely because the miners with chronic manganese central nervous system poisoning had left the workplace by the time blood manganese concentrations were obtained. Manganese had cleared the blood, and the body burden was located in tissue deposits (18, 19).

Rat studies indicate a slow accumulation of manganese in brain tissue. The accumulation seems to cause a deterioration in the globus pallidus and corpus striatum of the basal ganglia, unlike Parkinson's disease where the lesion is in the substantia nigra. Decreased levels of catecholamines and serotonin in the corpus striatum and depletion of dopamine by manganese-mediated oxidation catalysis of dopamine seem to be the basic pathophysiologic defect (30, 31).

Chronic manganese poisoning may be divided into three phases: prodromal, intermediate, and established (19). The psychologic and neuromotor manifestations, known as "locura manganica" or manganese madness described in the literature, display a wide degree of variability in both intensity and duration (27). Most often the evidence of cognitive dysfunction and emotional disturbance begins to occur prior to severe motor and neurologic dysfunction—prodromal phase. These symptoms include asthenia, anorexia, nonspecific muscular pain, nervousness, irritability, uncontrolled violent outbursts, insomnia, decreased libido, impotence, and labile affect (19). The intermediate phase is marked by the beginning of compulsive inappropriate laughter or crying, clumsiness of movement, exaggeration of reflexes in lower limbs, speech disorders, masque manganese, visual hallucinations, sialorrhea, and confusion. Reports of visions, chasing cars, and unexplained physical violence are common. In all cases the patients understood they were behaving irrationally, but were unable to correct their own dysfunctional states (8, 17, 19, 25, 26, 29).

During the established phase, subjective and objective symptoms intensify. One of the most common physical complaints is a generalized muscular weakness followed by difficulty in walking, stiffness, and impaired speech (up to and including muteness). The difficulty in walking includes impairment of propulsion and retropulsion, often noted when the patient is walking downhill. The patient may characteristically continue to accelerate and can only stop himself/herself by striking an obstacle. Malingering may be ruled out by the striking degree of retropulsion such that, if the patient is pushed from the front, he/she will completely collapse without attempting to protect himself/herself from a backward fall (18, 19). The most common neurologic signs are a "masklike" expressionless face, decreased postural reflexes, increased muscle tone, and a slow and shuffling forward gait without associated arm movement, accompanied by an anteriorly flexed trunk. Samples of handwriting demonstrate marked micrographia. Tremors may be noted, which are often fine, small amplitude resting tremors usually seen with hyperextension of the arms and hands, which become exaggerated on movement (17, 19).

Manganese interferes with reproductive function by inhibiting energy synthesis in the seminiferous tubules of the testis (32). There does not seem to be any effect on steroidogenesis (32, 33, 34). Extensive studies in the Australian literature of the Gryoote islanders of New South Wales chronically exposed to high levels of environmental manganese have described malformations and motor disorders in that population, including stillbirth, talipes equinovarus, cleft lip, imperforate anus, cardiac defects, pulmonary defects, syndactyly, and deafness (14, 35).

There has been one reported case of carcinogenesis with carcinoma of the lung following manganese exposure, but there does not seem to be evidence for widespread induction of carcinogenesis among large group populations (36).

Management of Toxicity

CLINICAL EXAMINATION

Acutely exposed patients should be removed from the source of the exposure and decontaminated as the exposure and condition warrants (37). Rescue personnel should wear appropriate gloves, boots, and goggles. Special attention should be directed to the respiratory system with monitoring of airway, breathing, and circulatory status. Supplemental oxygen and intravenous fluids should be administered as necessary.

Chronically exposed patients require a complete toxicologic history and physical examination with special attention to the neurologic system. A comprehensive occupational history should be obtained. Acute treatment for metal fume fever and pneumonitis is based on the clinical status of the patient. Metal fume fever patients usually require only removal from the exposure and supportive treatment. Manganese pneumonitis may necessitate antibiotic therapy with bronchodilator treatment as needed. The patients' chest x-ray and pulmonary functions should be followed. Patients require monitoring for the development of reactive airways disease.

There is no effective treatment for chronic central nervous system manganese poisoning. Various therapeutic agents have been suggested. Levodopa (L-dopa), a dopamine precursor, and 5-OH-tryptophan, a serotonin precursor, have been proposed (38, 39). Promising therapeutic benefits have been shown with varying L-dopa regimens up to a maximal dose of 8 g/day in six divided doses with the range being 4.8–8 g/day (38). One patient developed increased hypotonia, weakness, and tremor with a 3-gram L-dopa dose. Symptoms improved markedly with the institution of a 3-gram dose of 5-OH-tryptophan. This was felt to be due to an imbalance in the dopamine and serotonin receptors triggered by L-dopa (38). Low protein diets have also been suggested to improve symptoms of chronic manganese poisoning (40).

LABORATORY DIAGNOSIS

Patients acutely exposed to manganese should have a full biochemical serum magnesium and calcium analysis including liver profile, blood urea nitrogen (BUN), creatinine, complete blood count, and urinalysis. Chronically exposed patients also require a thyroid profile, vitamin B_{12} and folate determination to assist in the differential of other neurologic diseases. A computerized axial tomographic (CAT) or magnetic resonance imaging (MRI) scan of the brain and EEG may be necessary to rule out other possible central nervous system disease states which could mimic chronic manganese poisoning symptom complexes.

SPECIAL DIAGNOSTIC TESTS

Serum manganese concentration should be obtained, although toxicity does not seem to correlate with serum concentration. Workers suspected of experiencing high risk manganese exposure require yearly medical monitoring, since blood or tissue monitoring has no prognostic value.

Most patients suspected of chronic manganese poisoning should have a complete neuropsychological evaluation. The testing battery is usually constructed from existing neuropsychological tests, the diagnostic utility and validity of which have been proven (41). A modified Halstead-Reitan test battery is frequently used. This examination should be conducted by a neuropsychologist with experience in toxicologic syndromes.

ENVIRONMENTAL MONITORING

Air samples for manganese air concentration determinations should be analyzed by the inductively coupled plasma (ICP) method as described in the *NIOSH Manual of Analytical Methods, Vol III* (NIOSH 77-157-C)(42).

MANGANESE EXPOSURE LIMITS

The OSHA established permissible exposure limit (PEL) for inhalation exposure to manganese compounds measured as manganese is 5 mg/m^3 (42). This is a ceiling air concentration limit. This means that this ceiling air concentration should never be exceeded during any part of the work day. If instantaneous air monitoring is not available, then the ceiling value must be assessed as a 15-minute time-weighted average (TWA).

The NIOSH recommended exposure limit (REL) for manganese compounds measured as manganese is 1 mg/m^3 (42). The NIOSH shortterm exposure limit (STEL) is 3 mg/m^3 (42). An immediately dangerous to life or health (IDLH) concentration has not been established for manganese (42).

The American Association of Governmental and Industrial Hygienists (ACGIH) Threshold Limit Value-time-weighted average (TLV-TWA) for manganese dust is 5 mg/m^3 (43). There is no ACGIH STEL value. The ACGIH TLV-TWA for manganese fume is 1 mg/m^3 with a STEL level of 3 mg/m^3 (43). The ACGIH TLV-TWA for MMT as manganese skin exposure is 0.1 mg/m^3 (43). No ACGIH STEL for MMT currently exists. Neither OSHA nor NIOSH have specific values established for MMT.

High levels of manganese salts in water impart a bitter taste and give the water a brackish look (6). The public drinking water standard for manganese is 0.5 mg/l (6). This is based on aesthetic changes in water purity and not according to established levels of toxicity (6). There is no clearly defined level of toxic exposure in drinking water determined in the literature at this time.

MAGNESIUM SOURCES AND PRODUCTION

Magnesium (Mg—molecular weight 24.3) is a bright silvery colored metal that lies in group IIA of the periodic table. Magnesium is the eighth most abundant element, making up about 2.5% of the earth's crust. Magnesium is obtained from a variety of ores such as brucite, dolomite, carnallite, kieserite, magnesite, olivine, and periclase (44). The most important of these commercially is dolomite. Seawater contains about 0.13% magnesium. Magnesium is produced either by thermal reduction extraction from roasted dolomite or from seawater using an electrolytic process. Approximately 80% of magnesium is produced from seawater extraction. Magnesium is a component found in the various amphibole and serpentine hydrated silicates that collectively are known as asbestos. The serpentine fiber, chrysotile asbestos [$Mg_6Si_4O_{10}(OH)_8$], is the most common form of asbestos.

Magnesium, which is one-third lighter than aluminum, is used in a variety of manufacturing areas for its light weight and strength. Magnesium metal may be produced in chip, powder, pellet, turnings, or ribbon form (44). In finely divided forms it is easily ignited and burns with an intense white flame producing a dense white smoke (45). Finely divided metal (less than 3 millimeters) reacts easily with water to liberate hydrogen, a flammable gas. This reaction is not as vigorous as that produced by sodium or lithium with water; nevertheless firefighters should not use water to extinguish a magnesium fire. Dry concrete, sand, graphite, soda ash, powdered sodium chloride, or suitable powder should be used (46). Magnesium is insoluble in water and ordinary solvents (44). Carbon tetrachloride, carbon dioxide, or foam fire extinguisher should not be used due to reactions (45).

Magnesium is the second most plentiful intracellular fluid divalent cation in both plants (chlorophyll) and animals involved in a number of enzymatic reactions that entail protein synthesis and carbohydrate metabolism (47). Magnesium is an essential cofactor for neuromuscular transmission (48).

Industrial uses include aircraft fuselages, ship building, engine components, hand tools, batteries, sporting goods, luggage, ladders, and furniture. It is also used as a reducing agent in the manufacture of metallic beryllium, titanium, uranium, and zirconium and the manufacture of fireworks and flares.

Magnesium compounds include magnesium carbonate, magnesium chloride, magnesium oxide (MgO) fume (magnesia fume), and magnesium sulfate. Magnesium oxide fume is a finely divided particulate dispersed in air. Magnesium oxide fume is found in mineral dusts and as a byproduct of welding and smelting. It may be produced when magnesium metal is burned, thermally cut, or welded (45). Inhalation of magnesium oxide may cause "metal fume fever" (49–51).

Magnesium has a variety of medical uses. The most common preparations are for use as oral cathartics and antacids; magnesium sulfate (Epsom salts), magnesium hydroxide (milk of magnesia), and magnesium citrate. These agents are classified as osmotic laxatives. Magnesium may also stimulate duodenal secretion of cholecystokinin, which may stimulate fluid secretion and gastrointestinal motility (52). Although magnesium is poorly absorbed, individuals with impaired renal function may develop toxic serum concentrations and frank magnesium toxicity (53–56). Even in patients with normal renal function, hypotension and hypoventilation has been reported (57).

Magnesium sulfate is also administered as an intravenous preparation for the prevention of seizures associated with eclampsia of pregnancy. Magnesium is added to parenteral hyperalimentation solutions as an essential nutrient necessary for phosphorylation reactions.

SITES, INDUSTRIES, AND BUSINESSES ASSOCIATED WITH EXPOSURE

Magnesium may be found in multiple compounds: magnesium aluminum phosphide, magnesium arsenate, magnesium carbonate, magnesium chloride, magnesium nitrate, magnesium oxide, magnesium perchlorate, magnesium peroxide, and magnesium sulfate. Industrial processes that liberate magnesium oxide fumes may produce inhalation exposures resulting in acute symptoms. Magnesium oxide is found in cement, insulation, rubber, fertilizers, rayon processing, and paper manufacturing processes. Severe skin burns can result from skin exposure to the metal.

Magnesium aluminum phosphide is a crystalline gray flammable solid. It reacts with water to form magnesium and aluminum hydroxide and phosphine (PH_3), a flammable poisonous gas that will ignite spontaneously in air. Magnesium carbonate is used in the production of ceramics, glass, inks, fertilizers, insulation, and certain chemical compounds and rubber. Magnesium chloride is used as a flocculating agent, in fire resistance treatments, and as a drying preventative in ceramics and paper, and in the production of metallic magnesium. Magnesium hydroxide is used in medicines, sugar refining, uranium processing, and pulp manufacture. Magnesium oxide is used in the making of cement, insulation, rubber, fertilizers, and paper, and in rayon processing. Magnesium sulfate (Epsom salts) is used in the manufacture of cement, ceramics, explosives, matches, and pharmaceuticals, as well as in leather tanning and textile dyeing.

Health care facilities are common settings for hypermagnesemia from administration of magnesium sulfate or magnesium oxide to patients with renal or intestinal disease (58, 59).

CLINICAL TOXICOLOGY OF EXPOSURE

The major source of occupational exposures is via inhalation of magnesium oxide dusts. There is minimal absorption from topical dust exposure (44). Contact dermatitis may result from high concentration secondary to fume or dust exposure.

Overexposure in health care facilities results from the oral, parenteral, urinary tract, or rectal administration in medicinal preparations (58–64).

Approximately 15–30% of an oral dose is absorbed in the small intestine with a very small amount exchanged across the mucosal surface of the colon (65). The average adult has a dietary ingestion of 10–20 mmol/day. Approximately 1800 mg of magnesium ion is filtered by the glomerulus daily (48). Magnesium is not metabolized after absorption. It is filtered at the glomerulus with up to 95% being resorbed at the proximal tubule (66). Renal tubular reabsorption seems to be by an active transport mechanism. This process obeys zero order kinetics and therefore, when the T_{max} is exceeded, excess magnesium is excreted (66). The renal elimination rate can exceed the maximal rate of gastrointestinal absorption. Therefore hypermagnesemia in patients with normal renal function is rare. Hypomagnesemia is common in patients with glomerular filtration rates below 30 ml/min. Renal excretion of magnesium is increased in hypercalcemic and hypernatremic states (48). Calcium appears to antagonize magnesium ion absorption in the small intestine. Normal plasma magnesium concentrations range from 0.75–1.1 mM (1.5–2.2 mEq/l) (48). Approximately one third is bound to plasma proteins with the rest free. There is 1000 mM (2000 mEq) in the average 70-kilogram person with 50% distributed in bone, 45% intracellular, and 5% extracellular. Intracellular concentrations range from 2.5–15 mM (5–30 mEq/l) (47). There is rapid range absorption from inhalation across the alveolar capillary membrane resulting in systemic absorption and local tissue injury. Intracellular concentrations range from 2.5–15 mM (5–30 mEq/l) (47). There is rapid absorption from inhalation across the alveolar capillary membrane resulting in systemic absorption and local tissue injury.

SIGNS, SYMPTOMS, AND SYNDROMES FROM TOXIC EXPOSURES
Acute Toxicity

Acute central nervous system (CNS) toxicity is manifested as depression progressing to lethargy and coma (64, 66). Neu-

romuscular paralysis, hypotonicity, and hyporeflexia are seen. Cardiac conduction abnormalities include prolongation of PR, QRS, and QT intervals. Interventricular conduction delays, atrioventricular block, and asystole are found as symptoms progress.

Inhalation may produce local pulmonary irritation resulting in pulmonary edema and respirator paralysis due to primary muscle paralysis (49).

Gastrointestinal effects include hypomotility and possibly fluid sequestration. Effects on the endocrine system have been observed in neonates. Decreased parathyroid hormone activity and end organ response have been found in neonates (67).

Magnesium oxide produces a metal fume fever respiratory syndrome similar to that produced by zinc oxide. Typically seen in workers in smelting or welding operations, metal fume fever usually is seen on a Monday morning with symptoms subsiding throughout the rest of the work week (68). Symptoms usually manifest at air concentrations of magnesium oxide greater than 10 mg/m^3. The symptoms of metal fume fever usually begin after the worker goes home and include chills, sometimes preceded by a metallic taste in the mouth, dry throat, cough, dyspnea, general malaise, muscular ache, fever, nausea, and sometimes emesis. Fever of 38–39°C has been reported. Symptoms usually resolve within 12–24 hours. Symptoms are associated with a leukocytosis. Chest x-ray may show increased bronchovascular markings or be normal. The symptom complex is thought to be immunologic although the exact mechanisms have not been determined.

Chronic Effects of Magnesium Poisoning

The abnormalities associated with systemic hypermagnesemia have not been documented to persist after the hypermagnesemic state has been corrected. Chronic pulmonary dysfunction associated with pulmonary edema and exposure to fumes and dusts have not been documented with longterm controlled follow-up. Chronic use of magnesium antacid has caused renal failure from precipitating of magnesium phosphate in the kidney. Neonates born to mothers treated with intravenous magnesium sulfate have shown decreased end organ response to parathyroid hormone (67). There are no other documented cases of teratogenic effects. There is no evidence that hypermagnesemic stats or exposure to dust and fumes results in an increase in carcinogenesis.

Management of Toxicity

A patient exposed to magnesium should be removed from the hazardous material scene and decontaminated. Any magnesium should be gently brushed off first before any water is used to decontaminate the patient. Physical examination should be especially directed to the CNS, cardiac and respiratory systems. Sudden respiratory arrest may occur; therefore, airway control is paramount. An intravenous line should be started and the patient placed on a cardiac monitor (69). Initial treatment is therefore supportive.

Laboratory testing should include complete blood count, serum electrolytes, blood glucose, blood urea nitrogen, creatinine, calcium, and magnesium levels. Twenty-four hour urine collection for magnesium yields a more accurate clinical correlation than serum concentration. The serum magnesium concentration does not always correspond with clinical effect as it does not correlate with intracellular levels (48). In acute situations rapid serum monitoring is therefore preferable although it may not give a complete picture of total body burden.

In general, symptoms of toxicity increase with increasing serum concentrations:

3–9 mEq/l: cutaneous vasodilation producing erythema, nausea, vomiting, bradycardia, hypotension, hyporeflexia, sedation, lethargy

10 mEq/l: muscle paralysis, hypoventilation, stupor, cardiac conduction abnormalities, ventricular arrhythmias

14–15 mEq/l: cardiac arrest (asystole)—corresponds to approximately 30-mg/kg oral dose (70, 71).

Plasma magnesium at which complete heart block occurs may be variable.

Treatment

Gastric decontamination with syrup of ipecac or gastric lavage may be of benefit if performed within 4 hours of ingestion. Sodium cathartics should not be used. Activated charcoal has not been shown to be effective in reducing magnesium levels or as a magnesium binder (70).

Patients may develop acute respiratory arrest at relatively minimal toxic serum concentrations. Therefore, careful monitoring is important. Pulmonary edema may be treated by supportive care and positive end-expiratory pressure (PEEP) as indicated. Fever and myalgia associated with metal fume fever are usually treated with salicylates or other non steroidal antiinflammatory medication.

Cardiac conduction abnormalities and acute hypotension may be treated with intravenous calcium as a magnesium antagonist. Hypotension should initially be treated with normal saline and pressor agents if necessary. Refractory hypotension will often respond to calcium gluconate given as 10 millimeters of a 10% solution slow i.v. push over 3–5 minutes (70). This dose may be repeated depending on clinical status. If more than one dose of calcium gluconate is given, the calcium and magnesium serum levels should be rechecked. Serum calcium levels should be monitored as the hypermagnesemic state may be associated with either hypo- or hypercalcemia. Symptomatic patients with serum magnesium levels greater than 5 mEq/l should be treated.

Hemodialysis is an effective mode for removing magnesium. Magnesium is a small positively charged atom that freely passes across the dialysis membrane. Symptomatic patients with magnesium levels greater than 8 mEq/l are recommended for hemodialysis (48, 59).

Reports of up to 200-gram ingestion in a hypothermic patient did not result in significant cardiovascular effect despite a serum level of 19 mEq/l (63). Respiratory depression has been reported in patients with renal impairment after receiving Hemiacidrin (urinary irrigation solution) and magnesium citrate.

Magnesium fires are explosive and extremely dangerous as they produce a billowing noxious cloud of magnesium oxide and hydrogen. Full respiratory protective equipment (self-contained breathing apparatus) (72) along with protective clothing and goggles must be used because of the potential for airway irritation and pulmonary edema. Eye and skin damage can result from flying, burning magnesium particles. Powder forms of magnesium may form an explosive mixture with air and be ignited by a spark. Magnesium may react with water, acids, bromine, chlorine, iodine, or oxidizing agents (46).

Air samples for magnesium air concentration determinations should be analyzed by the inductively coupled plasma (ICP) method as described in the *NIOSH Manual of Analytical Methods, Vol. III*, (NIOSH 77-157-C) (72). The OSHA established permissible exposure limit (PEL) for magnesium oxide is 10 mg/m³ (72). The ACGIH Threshold Limit Value-Time Weighted Average (TLV-TWA) is also 10 mg/m³ (73). No Short Term Exposure Limit (STEL) currently exists. NIOSH has not set a Recommended Exposure Limit (REL) because it concluded that available literature was inadequate to support the 10-mg/m³ (72) PEL. More study is clearly needed on workplace magnesium limits.

REFERENCES

1. Venugopal B, Luckey TD. Toxicity of group VII metals. Metal toxicity in mammals. Vol 2. Chemical toxicity of metals and metalloids. New York: Plenum Press, 1978:261–271.

2. Sittig M. Handbook of toxic and hazardous chemicals and carcinogens. 2nd ed. Park Ridge, NJ: Noyes Publications, 1985:559–560.

3. Baselt RC, Cravey RH. Disposition of toxic drugs and chemicals in man. 3rd ed. Chicago: Year Book Medical Publishers, 1989:392.

4. Saric M, Markicevic A, Hrustic O. Occupational exposure to manganese. Br J Ind Med 1977;34:114–118.

5. Penalver R. Manganese poisoning. Ind Med Surg 1955;24:1–7.

6. Kondakis XG, Makris N, Leotsinidis M, Prinou M, Papapetropoulos T. Possible health effects of high manganese concentration in drinking water. Arch Environ Health 1989;44:175–178.

7. Food and Nutrition Board. National Research Council. Recommended dietary allowances. 10th ed. Washington, DC: National Academy of Sciences, 1989.

8. Cotzias GC. Manganese in health and disease. Physiol Rev 1958;38:503–532.

9. Clausen J, Rastogi SC. Heavy metal pollution among autoworkers. II. Cadmium, chromium, copper, manganese and nickel. Br J Ind Med 1977;34:216–220.

10. Vuori E. A longitudinal study of manganese in human milk. Acta Paediatr Scand 1979;68:571–573.

11. Lynam, DR. Environmental assessment of MMT fuel additives. Sci Total Environ 1990;40:49–50.

12. Sandstead HH. Some trace elements which are essential for human nutrition: zinc, copper, manganese and chromium. Prog Food Nutr Sci 1975;1:371–391.

13. Cotzias GC. Manganese versus magnesium: why are they so similar in vitro and so different in vivo? Fed Proc 1961;20:98–103.

14. Kilburn CJ. Manganese malformations and motor disorders: findings in a manganese exposed population. Neurotoxicology 1987;8:421–430.

15. Pollack S, George JN, Reba RC, Kauman RM, Crosby WH. The absorption of nonferrous metals in iron deficiency. J Clin Invest 1965;44:1470–1473.

16. Gruden N. Iron-59 and manganese-54 retention in weanling rats fed iron fortified milk. Nutr Rep Int 1982;25:849–858.

17. Mena I, Horiuchi K, Barke K, Cotzias GC. Chronic manganese poisoning. Individual susceptibility and absorption of iron. Neurology 1969;19:1000–1006.

18. Cotsias GC, Horiuchi K, Fuenzalida S, Mena I. Chronic manganese poisoning: clearance of tissue manganese concentrations with persistence of the neurological picture. Neurology 18:376–382.

19. Rodier J. Manganese poisoning in Moroccan mines. Br J Ind Med 1955;12:21–35.

20. Piscator M. Health hazards from inhalation of metal fumes. Environ Res 1976;11:268–270.

21. Davis TAL. Manganese pneumonitis. Br J Ind Med 1946;3:111–135.

22. Bergstrom R. Acute pulmonary toxicity of manganese dioxide. Scand J Work Environ Health 1977;3(suppl 1): 1–41.

23. Adkins BN, Luginbuhl GH, Miller FJ, Gardner DE. Increased pulmonary susceptibility to streptococcal infection following inhalation of manganese oxide. Environ Res 1980;23:110–120.

24. Brooks SM, Weiss MA, Bernstein IL. Reactive airways dysfunction syndrome (RADS). Persistent asthma syndrome after high level irritant exposures. Chest 1985;88:376–384.

25. Couper, J. On the effects of black oxide of manganese when inhaled into the lungs. Br Ann Med Pharmacol 1837;1:41–42.

26. Casamajor L. An unusual form of mineral poisoning affecting the nervous system: manganese? JAMA 1913;60:646–49.

27. Mena I, Marin O, Fuenzolida S, Cotzias GC. Chronic manganese poisoning: clinical picture and manganese turnover. Neurology 1967;17:128–136.

28. Mena I. The role of manganese in human disease. Ann Clin Lab Sci 1974;4:487–491.

29. Burch RE, Hahn HKJ, Sullivan JF, Aspects of the roles of zinc, manganese, copper in human nutrition. Clin Chem 1975;21:501–520.

30. Florence TM, Stauber JL. Neurotoxicology of manganese. Lancet 1988;1:363.

31. Parenti M, Rusconi L, Cappabianca V, Parati EA, Groppetti A. Role of dopamine in manganese neurotoxicity. Brain Res 1988;473:236–240.

32. Laskey JW, Rehnberg GL, Hein JF, Carter SD. Effects of chronic manganese (Mn$_3$O$_4$) exposure on selected reproductive parameters in rats. J Toxicol Environ Health 1982;9:677–687.

33. Iman Z, Chandra SV. Histochemical alterations in rabbit testis produced by manganese chloride. Toxicol Appl Pharmacol 1975;32:534–544.

34. Magnus O, Brekke I, Abyholm T, Purvis K. Effects of manganese and other divalent cations on progressive motility of human sperm. Arch Androl 1990;24:159–66.

35. Cawte J. Emic accounts of a mystery illness: the Groote Eylandt syndrome. Aust N Z J Psychiatry 1984;18:179–187.

36. Rab S. Squamous cell lung cancer in dry battery worker. J PMA 1990;40:49–50.

37. Bronstein AC, Currance PL. Emergency care for hazardous material exposures. St. Louis: CV Mosby, 1988:191–192.

38. Mena I, Court J, Fuenzalida S, Papavasiliou PS, Cotzias GC. Modification of chronic manganese poisoning: treatment with L-dopa or 5-OH tryptophane. N Engl J Med 1970;282:5–10.

39. Cotzias GC, Papavasiliou S, Ginos J, Steck A, Duby S. Metabolic modification of Parkinson's disease and of chronic manganese poisoning. Annu Rev Med 1971;22:305–326.

40. Mena I, Cotzias GC. Protein intake and treatment of Parkinson's disease with levodopa. N Engl J Med 1975;292:181–184.

41. Hartman DE. Neuropsychological toxicology. New York: Pergamon Press, 1988:37.

42. NIOSH. NIOSH Pocket Guide to Chemical Hazards. Cincinnati, OH: National Institute for Occupational Safety and Health, 1990. DHHS publication (PHS) 90-117:138–139.

43. American Conference of Governmental and Industrial Hygienists. 1990–1991 Threshold Limit Values for chemical substances and physical agents and biological exposure indices. Cincinnati, OH: ACGIH, 1990:25.

44. Sittig M. Handbook of toxic and hazardous chemicals and carcinogens. 2nd ed. Park Ridge, NJ: Noyes Publications, 1985:551.

45. Association of American Railroads. Emergency handling of hazardous materials in surface transportation. Washington, DC: AAR, 1987:425.

46. National Fire Protection Association. Fire protection guide on hazardous materials, NFPA Standard 480: magnesium. Quincy, MA: NFPA, 1987.

47. Mudge GH, Weiner IM. Water, salts, ions: agents affecting volume and composition of body fluids. In Gilman AG, Rall TW, Nies AS, Taylor P, eds. The pharmacological basis of therapeutics, 8th ed. New York: Pergamon Press, 1990:704.

48. Mordes JP, Wacker WEC. Excess magnesium. Pharmacol Rev 1978; 29:273–300.

49. Finkel AJ, Hamilton A, Hardy HL. Hamilton and Hardy's industrial toxicology. 4th ed. Littleton, MA: Year Book Medical Publishers, 1983:146–148.

50. Piscator M. Health hazards from the inhalation of metal fumes. Environ Res 1976;11:268–270.

51. Mueller EJ, Seger DC. Metal fume fever. A review. J Emerg Med 1985;2:271–275.

52. Harvey RF, Read AE. Mode of action of the saline purgatives. Am Heart J 1975;89:810–812.

53. Wecker WEC, Parsi AF. Magnesium metabolism. N Engl J Med 1968;278:658–663, 712–717, 772–776.

54. Cato AR, Tulloch AGS. Hypermagnesemia in a uremic patient during renal pelvis irrigation with Renacidin. J Urol 1974;111:313–314.

55. Jenny DB, Goris GB, Urwiller RD. Hypermagnesemia following irrigation of renal pelvis. Cause of respiratory depression. JAMA 1978;240:1378–1379.

56. Mordes JP. Extreme hypermagnesemia as a cause of refractory hypotension. Ann Intern Med 1975;83:657–658.

57. Fassler CA, Rodriguez RM, Badesch WJ, et al. Magnesium toxicity as a cause of hypotension and hypoventilation. Occurrence in patients with normal renal function. Arch Intern Med 1985;145:1604–1606.

58. Smilkstein MJ, Steedle D, Kulig KK, Marx JA, Rumack BH. Magnesium levels after magnesium-containing cathartics. Clin Toxicol 1988;26:51–56.

59. Bronstein AC, Worley S, Rumack BH. Life threatening hypermagnesemia successfully treated with hemodialysis. Abstract B-2, AAPCC/AACT/ABMT/CAPCC Annual Scientific Meeting, October 7–12, 1984, San Diego, California.

60. Morton AR. Severe hypermagnesemia after magnesium sulfate enemas. Br Med J 1985;291:516.

61. Collinson PO. Severe hypermagnesemia due to magnesium sulfate enemas in patients with hepatic coma. Br Med J 1986;293:1013–1014.

62. Aucamp AK, Van Auchtenbergh SM, Theron E: Potential hazards of magnesium sulfate administration. Lancet 1981;2:1057.

63. Garcia-Webb P, Bhagat C, Oh T, et al. Hypermagnesemia and hypophosphatemia after ingestion of magnesium sulphate. Br Med J 1984;288:759.

64. Gerard SK, Hernandez C, Khayam-Bashi H. Extreme hypermagnesemia caused by an overdose of magnesium-containing cathartics. Ann Emerg Med 1988;17:728–731.

65. Shils ME. Magnesium in health and disease. Annu Rev Nutr 1988;8:429–460.

66. Massry SG. Pharmacology of magnesium. Annu Rev Pharmacol Toxicol 1977;17:67–82.

67. Donovan FF. Neonatal hypermagnesemia; effect on parathyroid hormone and calcium homeostasis. J Pediatr 1980;96:305–310.

68. Armstrong CW. An outbreak of metal fume fever. J Occup Med 1983;23:886.

69. Bronstein AC, Currance PL. Emergency care for hazardous material exposures. St. Louis: CV Mosby, 1988:95–96.

70. Graber TW, Yee AS, Baker FJ. Magnesium: physiology, clinical disorders and therapy. Ann Emerg Med 1981;10:49–57.

71. Randall RE, Cohen D, Spray CC, Rossmeisl EC. Hypermagnesemia in renal failure. Ann Intern Med 1964;61:73–88.

72. NIOSH pocket guide to chemical hazards (DHHS publication (PHS) 90-117:138–139). Cincinnati, OH: National Institute for Occupational Safety and Health, 1990.

73. American Conference of Governmental and Industrial Hygienists. 1990–1991 Threshold Limit Values for chemical substances and physical agents and biological exposure indices. Cincinnati, OH: ACGIH, 1990:25.

86

Vanadium, Titanium, and Molybdenum

John G. Benitez, M.D.

INTRODUCTION

This chapter will describe the sources, methods of exposure, and clinical toxicology of three unrelated metals: vanadium, titanium, and molybdenum. Although frequently used together in the steel and alloy industries, they are unrelated, and frequently used in different chemical compounds for different industries, and will therefore be described separately.

VANADIUM TOXICITY

Sources and Production

Vanadium is one of the most common trace elements in nature, found as relatively insoluble salts usually in the trivalent state (7). It is extracted from the following mineral deposits: carnotite, phosphate rock, titaniferous magnetite, and vanadiferous clays. It exists in fossil fuels in variable small amounts (1, 8). Vanadium is an essential trace element for normal human growth and nutrition. Vanadium deficiency results in increased hematocrits, increased blood and bone marrow iron, and decreased blood lipid levels (2, 6).

In order to produce vanadium, it must first be extracted from the ores, slags, and boiler residues which contain vanadium in a low state of oxidation. Conversion to water-soluble vanadate ($NaVO_3$) requires that the ores, slags, and residues be roasted with salt, soda ash, or sodium sulfate. The resultant product is then leached with water or soda ash solution, and sometimes followed by a further leaching with dilute acid. Ores which exist with oxidized vanadium, such as carnotite, may be leached with acid directly without roasting. The resulting precipitate is sodium polyvanadate and can be treated by solvent extraction or ion exchange to separate any impurities present. With titaniferous magnetite the roasting and leaching process may be used, but a common procedure used in the Soviet Union and South Africa is to smelt the magnetite and produce a pig iron containing vanadium. After the pig iron is blown with oxygen, the vanadium is recovered in the slag as vanadium pentoxide. The slag can then be roasted and leached as previously described or used directly to produce ferrovanadium. Purification of vanadium is achieved by various other procedures in which vanadium pentoxide, vanadium trichloride, or vanadium trioxide are reduced with other elements such as calcium, magnesium, sodium, carbon, or aluminum, To produce pure metal (99.95%), impure grades of vanadium are refined by an electrolytic process (1).

Vanadium forms compounds in either a bi-, tri-, tetra-, or pentavalent states. Its chemistry is similar to phosphorus (2). Pentavalent vanadium is commonly seen as the oxide V_2O_5, and it reacts with halides to form pentavalent halides such as, $VOCl_3$, VOF_3, and $VOBr_3$. Reaction of the metal with fluorine yields the trivalent halide VF_3. Reduction of vanadium pentoxide with ammonia forms the tetravalent oxide, VO_2. Dissolution of VO_2 in acids makes salts such as $VOSO_4$ and $VOCl_2$. Vanadium tetrachloride, VCl_4, is made by chlorination of vanadium at 300°C. When vanadium pentoxide is reduced with ammonia or hydrogen at 650° C, the trivalent oxide, V_2O_3, is formed. The chloride is made by reduction of VCl_4. Bivalent vanadium oxide is prepared by the reduction of vanadium pentoxide with hydrogen at 1700° C (1).

Sites, Industries, and Businesses Associated with Exposures

Vanadium is found in several industries. Common ones include the mining and production of vanadium, steel and steel-alloy making, and in the chemical industries. See Table 86.1 for further details.

Exposure to vanadium pentoxide is the most common form of vanadium exposure studied. Other exposures happen much less frequently, and as a result data are limited on other chemical forms of vanadium. The usual route of entry is by inhalation of dusts, although dust entry through the gastrointestinal tract can also occur. Direct ingestion or parenteral exposure is uncommon but has occurred in experimental situations. Workers who use vanadium pentoxide are at risk when inhaling fine dusts as fine particulate matter may penetrate deeper into the tracheobronchial tree (1, 5). Exposures in industries occur with liberation of dusts during the mining and processing of ores, the cleaning and maintenance of furnaces and boilers, the use in the chemical industries, and the use during the manufacture of steels and alloys (12).

Clinical Toxicology of Exposure

Foods, both plant and animal sources, incorporate variable amounts of vanadium. Seafoods tend to incorporate vanadium to a greater extent. Foods contain vanadium in the range of a few parts per billion and probably play no part in acute toxicity (1). Industrial

Table 86.1. Industries Using Vanadium

Industry	Compound Used
Steel and alloy making	Ferrovanadium; aluminum/vanadium alloy
Iron/steel industries	Vanadium carbides
Flame cutting/brazing/welding	Steel/titanium/vanadium alloys
Chemical production (catalyst)	Vanadium pentoxide
Dye manufacture	Vanadium salts; ammonium metavanadate
Polymers/synthetic rubbers/ceramics/electronics	Vanadium oxychloride, tetrachloride, triacetylacetonate
Boiler repair/cleaning	Vanadium pentoxide
Pacemaker batteries	Vanadium pentoxide

Source: References 1, 9.

exposure to vanadium is through the respiratory system (8, 9). Some vanadium is ingested orally through the trapping of dusts in the oro- and nasopharynx.

Salts are poorly absorbed in the intestine; only about 1% is absorbed (1). Of the vanadium that is absorbed, only a small amount enters bone and is mobilized slower than in other tissues. Vanadium is detected in several tissues: liver, lung, kidney, bone, spleen, thyroid, brain, fat, hair, bile, blood, urine, lower small and large intestines, and omentum (1, 2). No vanadium has been detected in the human aorta, brain, muscle, ovary, or testis (1). The normal human serum concentration is 0.67 ng/ml (range 0.26–1.3). Vanadium is rapidly excreted through the urine (91%), with 60% of an absorbed amount excreted within 24 hours. The remainder is excreted in the feces (9%) (1, 2).

Signs, Symptoms, and Syndromes from Toxic Exposure

ACUTE TOXICITY

Acute exposure to vanadium oxide dusts is associated with acute upper and lower airway irritation (11). Conjunctivitis, rhinitis, and pharingitis commonly occur within 0.5 hour of exposure and up to 12 hours after the exposure. Cough, wheezing, dyspnea, and substernal soreness occur with more severe exposures (2, 5, 8, 9). A green-black discoloration of the tongue occurs with some exposures. The discoloration occurs from simple exposure of the tongue mucosa to vanadium powder (9).

Reversible airway disease occurs with exposure to vanadium dust. Airway narrowing with decreases in the forced vital capacity (FVC) and the forced expiratory volume (FEV_1) can be detected within 24 hours of exposure. Complete reversal of these pulmonary function tests occurs in 8 to 10 days and no long term changes in pulmonary function tests have been observed (8–10).

Although vanadium interferes with the Na-K pump, causing renal dysfunction in animals, no studies or case reports support this effect in humans (7).

CHRONIC TOXICITY

No chronic pulmonary effects have been demonstrated to date (1). Vanadium is both mutagenic and clastogenic in animal studies, although no human effect has been shown (4, 8).

MANAGEMENT OF TOXICITY

Vanadium pulmonary toxicity is difficult to differentiate from infection of allergy of the respiratory tract in that presenting signs and symptons are similar. Specific vanadium exposure history must be elicited. Examination may reveal a patient with clear watery discharge from the eyes and nose. Mucosal surfaces may be erythematous. Auscultation of lung fields will reveal ronchi or wheezing.

Treatment is supportive and patient counseling may be necessary to assure that no permanent damage will develop (1). Experimental animal data show that some chelators may help remove the body burden of vanadium, although dialysis has not been clinically necessary after vanadium exposure (3).

The laboratory is not helpful in determining or verifying exposure. Complete blood cell counts and chest x-rays are

Table 86.2. Permissible Exposure Limits (PEL) for Vanadium

Agency	Limits
ACGIH TLV	0.05 mg/m³ respirable dusts or fumes
OSHA TWA	0.5 mg/m³ dust ceiling
	0.1 mg/m³ fumes
NIOSH	0.05 mg/m³ 15-minute ceiling

usually normal (11). Measuring urine vanadium concentration may be helpful, especially if the exposure was recent (less than 2 weeks). Monitoring of these levels over 5 to 7 days should be sufficient to notice a decrease if the patient was removed from the source or the source controlled (8, 9, 12, 13).

Monitoring of particle size and concentration should be undertaken to monitor the working environment. Personal monitor sampling should also be performed when possible (1).

Protection of the environment should include measures to decrease dust formation, minimizing skin and eye contact, and preventing dust accumulation. Warning labels on all containers used for vanadium products should include warnings indicating skin, eye, and respiratory irritation hazards. Ventilation protection should be required (11–13).

Permissible Exposure Limits are listed in Table 86.2.

TITANIUM

Sources and Production

Titanium is one of the most common components of the earth's crust, being ninth in abundance. Titanium occurs naturally as ilmenite (iron titanate) and rutile (titanium dioxide) (14, 15).

Titanium forms four distinct oxides: titanium monoxide (TiO), dititanium trioxide (Ti_2O_3), titanium dioxide (TiO_2), and titanium trioxide (TiO_3). In construction, titanium alloys are used with aluminum, iron, manganese, chromium, molybdenum, or vanadium (14).

Titanium slag is produced by smelting ilmenite (iron titanate) in an electric furnace. Titanium dioxide content is typically 70–85%. Titanium dioxide is made by chlorinating ore at temperatures of 850°–1000°C. Impurities are removed chemically and through fractional distillation. The resulting titanium tetrachloride is converted to titanium dioxide by burning titanium tetrachloride in air or oxygen at temperatures of 1200°–1370°C. Aluminum chloride is added to assure near-total conversion to rutile titanium dioxide (15).

Sites, Industries and Businesses Associated with Exposures

Titanium is commonly used in titanium alloys for military and commercial airplane parts. In addition, titanium frequently is used as a white pigment for a wide range of paints, paper, inks, plastics, etc. (Table 86.3).

Exposure occurs by breathing titanium dioxide dusts. Because of lack of human data with other forms of titanium, the discussion will be limited to titanium dioxide. Exposure may occur at any stage: in the mining of ores, in the preparation of titanium oxide, and in any of the industries listed where the powder is stored and used.

Clinical Toxicology of Exposure

Titanium dioxide inhalation is the most common route of exposure. Ingestion is certainly possible when some dust accu-

Table 86.3.   Industries Using Titanium

Industry	Compound Used
Military hardware (planes/missiles)	Titanium alloy
Commercial airplane parts	Titanium alloy
White pigment for paints/papers/inks/plastics/ceramics/cosmetics	Titanium dioxide
Organic chemicals production (catalyst)	Titanium tetrachloride (anhydrous)
Flame retardant for wood	Titanium dioxide

Source: References 14, 15, 20.

mulates on mucosal surfaces of the oro- and nasopharynx. Pulmonary retention of titanium dioxide particles is well documented in several studies (15). No data are available on the amount of titanium that may be absorbed orally. However, titanium dioxide is found in the lymphatics and regional nodes that drain the lungs, indicating a slow removal by this process (15). Titanium and other metals dissolve into surrounding tissues from metal alloy implants. No clinical significance has been demonstrated (19).

Signs, Symptoms, and Syndromes from Toxic Exposure

ACUTE TOXICITY

Titanium dioxide is an irritant to the upper airway, like other nuisance dusts (20). There is no evidence that it induces an acute inflammatory reaction at exposure concentrations commonly seen (16). Inhalation of titanium tetrachloride may lead to inhalation injury resulting in a chemical pneumonitis and airway irritation. However, this injury most likely results from the halide ion (5). In workers with preexisting chronic obstructive airway disease, titanium dioxide inhalation may exacerbate their symptoms (20).

CHRONIC TOXICITY

Titanium dioxide dust is retained in the lungs. Titanium dioxide dust particles are also found in the regional nodes draining the lungs, suggesting that these particles are slowly cleared by the lymphatics (15). There is little evidence that titanium dioxide promotes a chronic inflammatory reaction in the lungs (16). However, in a case report, hypersensitivity to titanium was demonstrated. This patient had granulomatous disease of the lungs, and particulate matter was found consisting of aluminum, titanium, zinc, nickel, and silicates. Causal relation between the titanium and the granulomatous disease was not proven (17). There is inconclusive evidence demonstrating an increased incidence of chronic bronchitis and loss of ventilatory function (5, 15). Titanium dioxide dust inhalation is currently considered to be a nuisance dust that only results in upper airway irritation (16).

No data are available on human genetic effects, and very limited epidemiological data on carcinogenicity are available. Inconclusive results on carcinogenicity most likely result because workers are exposed to other chemicals (asbestos, silica) either prior to or during their current job. Pulmonary fibrosis seen in some of these workers may be due to the presence of

Table 86.4.   Permissible Exposure Limits (PEL) for Titanium

Agency	Limits
OSHA TWA	15 mg/m^3 total dust
ACGIH TLV	10 mg/m^3

silicon compounds (15). Recent animal data support the conclusion that titanium dioxide is a nuisance dust and does not produce any increased incidence of cancer rates (18).

MANAGEMENT OF TOXICITY

The patient may complain of irritated eyes and pharynx, and examination of the patient will reveal inflamed mucosal surfaces. Coughing is a frequent finding, although ronchi and rales are usually absent unless there is underlying pulmonary or cardiac disease. Because titanium dioxide is an irritant dust, management of exposure is supportive. The worker should be removed from the environment and supportive pulmonary care should be provided. Most laboratory tests are not helpful, with the exception that serum and urinary titanium levels help identify recent exposure (20).

Good industrial hygiene and monitoring of the environment should limit dust exposure to employees. If the employee must work in an environment high in titanium dioxide dust and poor ventilation, respirators should be used (20).

Permissible Exposure Limits are listed in Table 86.4.

MOLYBDENUM

Sources and Production

Molybdenum is obtained from ores such as molybdenite (MoS_2), wulfenite ($PbMoO_4$), and powellite [$Ca(MoW)O_4$]. Molybdenite is the most common and is obtained directly by mining and also as a byproduct in some copper mining operations. Molybdenite is roasted to molybdic oxide (MoO_3). Molybdic oxide is then converted to ammonium molybdate ([NH_2]Mo_2O_7). Several molybdenum products can be produced since molybdenum forms compounds with various valence states: 0, +2, +3, +4, +5, and +6. Examples of these products are: molybdenum dioxide and trioxide; molybdenum pentachloride ($MoCl_5$); and nitrogen, sulfur, and oxygen chelates (14).

Differences in toxicity occur if compounds are more soluble than others. Insoluble molybdenum compounds include metallic molybdenum, molybdenum disulfide (MoS_2), and lead molybdate ($PbMoO_4$). Soluble compounds include molybdenum trioxide (MoO_3), ammonium molybdate, ammonium paramolybdate [$(NH_4)_6Mo_7O_{24}\cdot4H_2O$], calcium molybdate ($CaMoO_4$), and sodium molybdate, dihydrate ($Na_2MoO_4\cdot2H_2O$) (21, 22).

Sites, Industries, and Businesses Associated with Exposures

Common uses of molybdenum include metallurgy, including the use in alloys, and as catalysts for the chemical industry. Exposure commonly occurs in the mining and processing of ores. See Table 86.5 for further details.

Molybdenum and its compounds may be inhaled by breathing dust and may also be absorbed by skin contact. The more soluble the compound, the more toxic its manifestations are.

Table 86.5. Industries Using Molybdenum

Industry	Compounds Used
Powder metallurgy or vacuum-arc-cast metal	Molybdic oxide or ammonium molybdate
Catalysts and their manufacture	Molybdenum powder or molybdenum acetylacetonate
Feedstock	Molybdenum powder
Dry lubricant	Molybdenum sulfide
Molybdenum coatings	Molybdenum pentachloride
Alloy manufacture	Molybdenum
Pigment manufacture	Zinc molybdate

Source: References 14, 21, 24.

Exposure may occur during the liberation of dusts from mining and the processing of ore, the grinding of metals or alloys, in oxyacetylene cutting, and from dusts of its various compounds (14, 21, 22).

Clinical Toxicology of Exposure

Exposure to molybdenum and related compounds usually occurs by the inhalation of dusts. If these compounds are water-soluble, absorption is increased and toxicity may be greater than non-water-soluble compounds. Because of this property, skin absorption may occur (14). Gastrointestinal absorption is about 50% of an ingested amount and depends on the water solubility of the compound involved (14).

Molybdenum is contained principally in liver, kidney, fat, and blood. The major portion contained in the liver is contained in a nonprotein cofactor bound to the mitochondrial membrane. It may be moved to an apoenzyme, transforming it into an active enzyme (26). Molybdenum is primarily excreted (greater than 50%) renally. It may also be excreted through the bile when excess molybdenum is present (14, 26).

Signs, Symptoms, and Syndromes from Toxic Exposure

ACUTE TOXICITY

Molybdenum products may cause acute toxicity in humans, but adequate studies are lacking. Workers involved in producing molybdenum oxide had a higher rate of headaches, backaches, aching joints, and nonspecific skin and hair changes. Increases in serum uric acid and ceruloplasmin are also noted (14, 24). Fumes from arcing molybdenum metal causes respiratory irritation in animals. Molybdenum trioxide may cause irritation to mucous membranes (eyes, nose, throat). It has also caused weight loss and digestive disturbances in animals, but human data are minimal (21, 22).

CHRONIC TOXICITY

Data are extremely limited on chronic toxicity from molybdenum and its compounds. Some workers had x-ray changes suggesting pneumoconiosis, but no longterm effects have been found that can be attributed directly to molybdenum (14, 21). Vitallium, an alloy of chromium, cobalt, and molybdenum, is implicated in producing pneumoconiosis in dental technicians. They are exposed by working with this alloy in the molding, cutting, and polishing of prosthetic parts. However it is difficult

Table 86.6. Permissible Exposure Limits (PEL) for Molybdenum

Agency	Limits
OSHA TWA	5 mg/m^3 soluble compounds 15 mg/m^3 insoluble compounds
ACGIH TLV	5 mg/m^3 soluble compounds 10 mg/m^3 insoluble compounds

to attribute pulmonary fibrotic changes to a specific metal or combination of metals in these cases (25). Kidney disease and liver dysfunction are reported in animals but not in humans (21, 22). No changes in tissue growth rates are noted with alloys containing molybdenum (23). In summary, molybdenum may cause a pneumoconiosis in susceptible individuals, but definitive data are lacking.

MANAGEMENT OF TOXICITY

Persons exposed to hazardous concentrations of molybdenum should be removed from further exposure. Treatment is symptomatic and there is no specific therapy for removal of molybdenum from tissues. Treatment of joint complaints is supportive. Laboratory measurement of serum and urine molybdenum levels may be performed, but levels do not correlate with signs or symptoms. Serum uric acid and ceruloplasmin levels may be elevated (24).

Prevention of exposure is the mainstay in preventing toxicity. For soluble or insoluble compounds, good process enclosures with general dilution ventilation and with local exhaust ventilation is adequate. Workers exposed to insoluble molybdenum compounds should wear personal protective equipment designed to limit dust, mist, or fume inhalation. Workers exposed to soluble compounds need impervious clothing, gloves, face shields, and other appropriate clothing as necessary to prevent skin contact (21, 22).

Permissible Exposure Limits are listed in Table 86.6.

REFERENCES

1. Zenz C. Vanadium and its compounds. In: Zenz C, ed. Occupational medicine, principles and practical applications. 2nd ed. Chicago: Year Book Medical Publishers, 1988:630–638.
2. Hosokawa S, Yoshida O. Vanadium in chronic hemodialysis patients. Int J Artif Organs 1990;13:197–199.
3. Domingo JL, Gomez M, Llobet JM, Corbella J. Chelating agents in the treatment of acute vanadyl sulphate intoxication in mice. Toxicology 1990;62:203–211.
4. Owusu-Yaw J, Cohen MD, Fernando SY, Wei CI. An assessment of the genotoxicity of vanadium. Toxicol Lett 1990;50:327–336.
5. Nemery B. Metal toxicity and the respiratory tract. Eur Respir J 1990;3:202–219.
6. Hopkins LL, Mohr HE. Vanadium as an essential nutrient. Fed Proc 1974;33:1773–1775.
7. Phillips TD, Nechay BR, Heidelbaugh ND. Vanadium: chemistry and the kidney. Fed Proc 1983;42:2969–2973.
8. Kiviluoto M. Observations on the lungs of vanadium workers. Br J Ind Med 1980;37:363–366.
9. Lees REM. Changes in lung function after exposure to vanadium compounds in fuel oil ash. Br J Ind Med 1980;37:253–256.
10. Musk AW, Tees JG. Asthma caused by occupational exposure to vanadium compounds. Med J Aust 1982;1:183–184.

11. Levy BS, Hoffman L, Gottsegen S. Boilermakers' bronchitis. Respiratory tract irritation associated with vanadium pentoxide exposure during oil-to-coal conversion of a power plant. J Occup Med 1984;26:567–570.

12. NIOSH and OSHA. Occupational health guideline for vanadium pentoxide dust. In: Occupational health guidelines for chemical hazards. Cincinnati, OH: National Institute for Occupational Safety and Health and Occupational Safety and Health Administration, 1978.

13. NIOSH and OSHA. Occupational health guideline for vanadium pentoxide fume. In: Occupational health guidelines for chemical hazards. Cincinnati, OH: National Institute for Occupational Safety and Health and Occupational Safety and Health Administration, 1978.

14. Rowe DM, Solomayer JA, Zenz C. Other metals. Chapt 45 in: Zenz, C, ed. Occupational medicine, principles and practical application. 2nd ed. Chicago: Year Book Medical Publishers, 1988.

15. Titanium dioxide. IARC Monogr Eval Carcinog Risks Hum 1989;47:307–326.

16. Driscoll KE, Lindenschmidt RC, Maurer JK, et al. Pulmonary response to silica or titanium dioxide: inflammatory cells, alveolar macrophage-derived cytokines, and histopathology. Am J Respir Cell Mol Biol 1990;2:381–390.

17. Redline S, Barna BP, Tomashefski JF, Abraham JL. Granulomatous disease associated with pulmonary deposition of titanium. Br J Ind Med 1986;43:652–656.

18. Bernard BK, Osheroff MR, Hofmann A, Mennear JH. Toxicology and carcinogenesis studies of dietary titanium dioxide-coated mica in male and female Fischer 344 rats. J Toxicol Environ Health 1990;29:417–429.

19. Sunderman FW. Carcinogenicity of metal alloys in orthopedic prostheses: clinical and experimental studies. Fundam Appl Toxicol 1989;13:205–216.

20. NIOSH and OSHA. Occupational health guideline for titanium dioxide. In: Occupational health guidelines for chemical hazards. Cincinnati, OH: National Institute for Occupational Safety and Health and Occupational Safety and Health Administration, 1978.

21. NIOSH and OSHA. Occupational health guideline for molybdenum and insoluble molybdenum. In: Occupational health guidelines for chemical hazards. Cincinnati, OH: National Institute for Occupational Safety and Health and Occupational Safety and Health Administration, 1978.

22. NIOSH and OSHA. Occupational health guideline for soluble molybdenum compounds (as molybdenum). In: Occupational health guidelines for chemical hazards. Cincinnati, OH: National Institute for Occupational Safety and Health and Occupational Safety and Health Administration, 1978.

23. Goldring SR, Flannery MS, Petrison KK, et al. Evaluation of connective tissue cell responses to orthopedic implant materials. Connect Tissue Res 1990;29:77–81.

24. Walravens PA, Moure-Eraso R, Solomons CC, et al. Biochemical abnormalities in workers exposed to molybdenum dust. Arch Environ Health 1979;34:302–308.

25. De Vuyst P, Vande Weyer R, De Coster A, et al. Dental technician's pneumoconiosis, a report of two cases. Am Rev Respir Dis 1986;133:316–320.

26. Goyer RA. Toxic effects of chemicals. In Klassen CD, Amdur MO, Doull J, eds. Casarett and Doull's toxicology. 3rd ed. New York: Macmillan Publishing Co, 1986:582–635.

John B. Sullivan, Jr., M.D.

SOURCES AND PRODUCTION

Thallium (Tl), which belongs to the aluminum family of metals, was first discovered in 1861 by William Crookes. Thallium toxicity was recognized in 1863 (1) and is toxicologically related to divalent lead (1). Thallium is found in the United States and Brazil in the form of minerals of lorandite and crookesite. Thallium is a byproduct of cadmium production and is recovered from lead and zinc flue dust smelting (2). Thallium is found in nature as the sulfate salt form and is found also in potash, lead and zinc ores, and fossil fuels.

CHEMICAL AND PHYSICAL FORMS

Thallium, atomic number 81, has an atomic weight of 204.4 and is a crystalline, blue-white metal (2). It has oxidation states of 1+ and 3+ and is generally used as the salt form. Following exposure to air, the elemental metal forms a brownish-black oxide (2). Thallium is a highly reactive metal and is soluble in acids. Thallium forms monovalent and trivalent salts. Thallium is present in the earth's crust, and there are at least 18 thallium compounds known, among which are elemental thallium, thallium oxide, thallium acetate, thallium carbonate, thallium chloride, thallium selenide, thallium selenite, thallium nitrate, and thallium sulfate. Thallium salts are colorless, odorless, and tasteless when dissolved in water (3). It is mainly found in the sulfate salt form (Tl_2SO_4).

SITES AND INDUSTRIES ASSOCIATED WITH EXPOSURES

The main sites for thallium environmental contamination are cement factories, coal-burning power plants, and smelters. The public is exposed to thallium via coal-burning power plant emissions, copper, zinc, cadmium, and lead smelters. Drinking water contamination with thallium may occur in the area of smelting operations (2). Atmospheric thallium is present as the elemental form, oxide, or sulfate. Thallium is commonly used in semiconductors and electrical switching devices.

Thallium salts were first introduced as pesticides in Germany in 1920 (1). These initial compounds contained about 2% thallium sulfate (4). The persistence of thallium in the environment along with its cumulative effect as a poison made it an ideal rodenticide. Human and animal poisonings with thallium have been reported since the use of thallium in pesticides and rodenticides. In the late 19th century, thallium was widely used as a therapeutic agent for syphilis, tuberculosis, and dysentery, and as a depilatory agent (1, 3, 4).

Thallium salts have been used mainly as rodenticides and pesticides, although their use was restricted in 1965 in the United States, developing countries continue to make thallium-containing pesticides available for use. Thallium is also used in the manufacturing of optical lenses, fireworks, dyes, and

pigments. The use of thallium has become an important metal in the superconductor industry (5).

Compounds containing 3.5–5% thallium sulfate were available in the 1950s in the southeastern United States for control of ants and roaches. In 1965 household use of thallium preparations were banned by the U.S. Department of Agriculture. Thallium-containing rodenticides in the United States typically contained between 1 and 3% thallium sulfate in the 1960s.

Thallium sulfate was widely used as a rodenticide in the 1920s. The United States banned its use in 1965. However, many other countries continue using thallium as a rodenticide. The majority of thallium used in the United States is employed in the electronics industry for photo-electric cells, lamps, scintillation counters, and semiconductor manufacturing (2). Thallium is also used as a catalyst in organic chemical processes. It is used in optical lenses and infrared spectrometers and for coloring glass (2). Thallium is used as a myocardial imaging agent in medicine. Recently, thallium has found great utility and promise in the superconductor industry (5). Thallium as the cation in a tetragonal crystalline form and as thallium oxide has found use in the superconductor materials (5). Thallium's main use is in the production of optical lenses and imitation jewelry.

The resurgence of thallium in the United States and other countries as a metal catalyst in organic synthesis and as a metal used in the superconductor industry reinforces the need to understand its clinical toxicology. Also important is the need to know how to manage poisonings from thallium due to both accidental and intentional ingestions where it continues to be used as a rodenticide (such as Mexico and Turkey).

Inhalation of contaminated air or ingestion of contaminated fruit are the main sources of low level human exposure. Because thallium is a cumulative poison and can be absorbed through the skin as well as the gastrointestinal tract, knowledge of environmental exposure is necessary.

Thallium exposures can occur from accidental and suicidal ingestions of the salt forms. Exposure also occurs from inhalation in a work area or ingestion of contaminated foods. Exposure to flue dusts from pyrite roasting, lead, copper, zinc, and cadmium smelting (2) can result in dermal contamination as well as inhalation of dusts containing thallium. Absorption of thallium occurs through inhalation, ingestion, and dermal contact.

CLINICAL TOXICOLOGY OF EXPOSURE

Absorption, Metabolism, Distribution, and Elimination

Thallium is absorbed by the intact skin, by inhalation, and by the gastrointestinal route. Absorption in animal models has been demonstrated to be very rapid following dermal, oral, or inhalation routes of exposure, and almost 100% bioavailability

Table 87.1. Thallium Toxicity

Acute toxicity
  Coma
  Ataxia
  Tremor
  Muscular atrophy
  Paralysis
  Cranial nerve neuropathy
    Ptosis, ophthalmoplegia, retrobulbar neuritis, facial neuritis
  Psychosis
  Seizures
  ECG changes
  Nausea
  Vomiting
  Abdominal pain
  GI bleeding

Subacute toxicity
  Distal neuropathy
  Distal paresthesias
  Distal motor weakness
  Ascending neuropathy
  Polyneuritis
  Ataxia
  Fatigue
  Psychosis
  Emotional changes
  Dermatitis
    Erythema, nail changes, scaly skin, Mee's lines
  Elevated liver enzymes
  Constipation

occurs within 1 hour following. Concentrated thallium is clearly dangerous when handled by inexperienced people.

Absorption via the gastrointestinal tract is almost 100%. Following absorption, thallium is widely distributed intracellularly, with the kidneys having the highest concentrations, mainly in the renal medulla (2). Concentrations are also found in cardiac tissue and liver. Thallium also concentrates in hair. The concentration of thallium in adipose tissue and brain tissue is low or none (6). Thallium enters the cell and concentrates intracellularly (6). Thallium distributes equally between red blood cells and plasma (6). Thallium also crosses the placenta into the fetus but in much smaller amounts than present in the maternal tissues.

Thallium elimination is mainly via the gastrointestinal tract and kidneys. Thallium is slowly eliminated by first order kinetics by these routes. The excretion of thallium in urine is associated with the urinary excretion of potassium (6). Potassium and thallium are known to replace each other in the NaK-ATPase pump; thus thallium accumulates intracellularly. The elimination of thallium in urine is low, lasting weeks, despite the concentration of thallium in the kidneys (6).

Biologic half-times for thallium in humans have been estimated to be 30 days (2). Thallium plasma concentrations generally remain low despite high urine and fecal content. In human cases of poisoning the excretion of thallium occurs very slowly over several weeks to months.

Acute Toxicity

Thallium is a potent neurotoxin (Table 87.1). Following acute exposure, usually by the oral route, the initial manifestations are nausea and vomiting (7). These gastrointestinal symptoms

may subside and be followed in about 7–14 days by further gastrointestinal disturbances such as pain, constipation, bloating sensation, and bleeding. Coma, delirium, hallucinations, gastrointestinal bleeding, and seizures may occur early if the exposure is severe.

The clinical manifestations of thallium poisoning appear gradually over the course of a few weeks. Neurologic symptoms occur after the first week and consist of paresthesias and neuritis, particularly in the lower extremities. After the second week, polyneuritis is usually evident (7). Alopecia may occur by 1–3 weeks after the exposure (8). Ataxia, tremors, and painful neuritis of the lower extremities may be severe. The neuropathy shows multiple sites of nerve involvement on electrophysiology studies. Muscle stretch reflexes are usually present until late in the clinical course. Cranial nerves may be involved, and the patient may manifest ptosis, facial paralysis, retrobulbar neuritis, and disconjugate gaze (8). Psychologic and emotional changes can occur with intense depression and psychosis. Recovery is slow and requires months.

Vagal nerve damage may result in tachycardia, paralytic ileus, and slight hypertension (7). Electrocardiographic changes are similar to those seen in hypokalemia (7). Constipation is commonly seen in thallium poisoning. Death may occur due to cardiac dysrhythmias, shock, coma, and renal failure.

Dermal changes include erythema, anhidrosis, and injury to sebaceous glands (7, 8). Diaphoresis may occur late in the course. A scaliness of the skin is also common in thallotoxicosis. Nail growth is interfered with for several weeks, and Mee's lines (white stripes across the nails) may be seen (7).

Elevation of liver enzymes is commonly seen in thallotoxicosis (7). In addition, renal function can be impaired, and proteinuria may be noted.

Chronic and Longterm Effects

Recovery from thallotoxicosis can require many months. Residual neuropathy can occur. Chronic exposure to thallium is rare, and cases reported usually involved weakness in the legs, hair loss, painful legs, and psychologic disturbances. Alopecia may not occur for months following occupational exposure to thallium (7).

DIAGNOSIS AND BIOLOGIC MONITORING

Diagnosis can be difficult without appropriate history. Certain signs and symptoms are characteristic of thallium poisoning, such as alopecia and polyneuritis. Concentrations of thallium can be confirmed in blood and urine. Urine thallium concentrations are higher than blood concentrations. Since renal excretion is one of the main elimination routes for thallium, a 24-hour urine sample quantitating thallium is the most helpful in ascertaining exposure. The urine concentration of thallium poisoning will be greater than 300 μg/l (2). Levels of thallium in the urine of workers has ranged from 50–100 μg/l (2).

The administration of 40 milliequivalents of potassium chloride orally to a patient prior to a 24-hour urine collection will increase the urinary excretion of thallium and help confirm the diagnosis (8).

MANAGEMENT OF TOXICITY

Treatment of thallium intoxication is surrounded by some controversy; however, there are clear guidelines that can be applied to achieve success in therapy. First, there is no effective chelating agent for thallium. None of the traditional chelating agents—dimercaprol (BAL), calcium disodium EDTA, D-penicillamine, nor dimercaptosuccinic acid (DMSA)—has shown any efficacy in thallotoxicosis or increasing the elimination of thallium in poisoning cases. Diethyldithiocarbamate (dithiocarb) and diphenylthiocarbazone (dithizone) have been studied as potential thallium-chelating agents in animals (9–11). Following these animal studies and in some cases, human trials, these chelators were discarded as nonefficacious. In fact, some patients demonstrated clinical deterioration with increasing coma and electroencephalographic changes following dithiocarb administration in thallotoxicosis (11, 12). Dithiocarb apparently formed a lipophilic complex with the thallium ion, which allowed for increased central nervous system concentration of thallium.

Due to the fact that animal and human studies have shown that administration of potassium resulted in an increase in urinary excretion of thallium as well as increases in plasma thallium concentrations, current therapy for thallotoxicosis involves a combination of the oral administration of potassium chloride plus activated charcoal (9). Potassium and thallium are interchangeable metals across the cell membrane. Thallium can replace potassium in the NaK-ATPase pump. Thus administration of potassium will help push thallium from its intracellular site into the extracellular area and plasma, making urinary and fecal excretion possible (7, 9). Potassium alone may result in a worsening of clinical symptoms despite a decrease in thallium half-life due to redistribution of thallium from plasma (7).

Potassium ferric-cyanoferrate II (Prussian blue) has also been found to be efficacious in thallotoxicosis (13–15). Prussian blue, an inorganic pigment, has been orally administered in doses of 250 mg/kg daily dose dissolved in 50 milliliters of 15% mannitol divided twice a day (10 grams twice daily has been administered for cases of thallium poisoning) (2, 13, 14). Prussian blue is not absorbed by the gastrointestinal tract. The potassium in Prussian blue substitutes for thallium, and the thallium is then adsorbed by the remaining Prussian blue lattice in the gut which is fecally excreted. Prussian blue thus acts as an ion exchange medium for thallium.

Due to the fact that the administration of potassium and activated charcoal has been successful in increasing the total body elimination of thallium, and since Prussian blue may not be easily obtained, the administration of a combination of oral potassium chloride and activated charcoal is recommended. This therapy has proven to be successful in two severe thallium cases managed by the author. The dose of potassium chloride is 20 milliequivalents four times per day with activated charcoal 20–30 grams four times per day. A cathartic is usually also required due to the constipating effect of thallium. This therapy may proceed for several weeks to several months while monitoring clinical improvement and decreasing urinary thallium concentrations.

TERATOGENICITY AND CARCINOGENICITY

Thallium crosses the placenta and distributes to the fetus, but in small amounts compared with maternal concentrations. The teratogenic effect of thallium compounds has been demonstrated in animals. Achondroplastic malformations in chickens, reduced fetal body weight, hydronephrosis, and vertebral body absence in rats have been noted. Thallium has not been classified as a carcinogen in animals or humans.

EXPOSURE LIMITS

The American Conference of Governmental Industrial Hygienists as well as the Occupational Safety and Health Administration have adopted a threshold limit value of 0.1 mg/m^3 for thallium. The acceptable daily intake of thallium is calculated to be 15.4 mg/day according to the Environmental Protection Agency.

REFERENCES

1. Bendl BJ. Thallium poisoning: report of a case successfully treated with dithizone. Arch Dermatol 1969;100:443–445.
2. Kazantzis G. Thallium. In: Handbook on the toxicology of metals. 2nd ed. Friberg L, Nordberg GF, Vouk V, eds. Amsterdam: Elsevier Science Publishers, 1986:549–567.
3. Papp JP, Gay PC, Dodson VN, Pollard MH. Potassium chloride treatment in thallotoxicosis. Ann Intern Med 1969;71:119–123.
4. Chamberlain PH, Stavinoha WB, Davis H, Kniker WT, Panos TC. Thallium poisoning. Pediatrics 1958;22:1170–1182.
5. Sleight AW. Chemistry of high-temperature super-conductors. Science 1988;242:1519–1527.
6. Lund A. Distribution of thallium in the organism and its elimination. Acta Pharmacol Toxicol 1956;12:251–259.
7. Saddique A, Peterson CD. Thallium poisoning: a review. Vet Hum Toxicol 1983;25:16–22.
8. Smith DH, Doherty RA. Thallotoxicosis: report of three cases in Massachusetts. Pediatrics 1964;34:480–480.
9. Lund A. The effect of various substances on the excretion and the toxicity of thallium in the rat. Acta Pharmacol Toxicol 1956;12:260–268.
10. Boak RL, Schmidtke RP, Wallach JD, Davis LE, Niemeyer KH. Thallium intoxication: a specific antidote, supportive therapy and clinical evaluation. Vet Med 1965;Dec:1227–1231.
11. Kamerbeek HH, Rauws AG, ten Ham M, van Heijst ANP. Dangerous redistribution of thallium by treatment with sodium diethyldithiocarbamate. Acta Med Scand 1979;189:149–154.
12. Special communication: thallium poisoning. Clin Toxicol 1972;5:89–93.
13. Van Der Merwe CF. The treatment of thallium poisoning: a report of 2 cases. S Afr Med J 1972;2:960–961.
14. Kamerbeek HH, Rauws AG, ten Ham M, van Heijst ANP. Prussian blue in therapy of thallotoxicosis. Acta Med Scand 1971;189:321–324.
15. Heydlauf Horst. Ferric-cyanoferrate (II): an effective antidote in thallium poisoning. Eur J Pharmacol 1969;6:340–344.

88

Selenium

David J. Thomas, Ph.D.

SOURCES AND PRODUCTS

Overview—Aspects of Selenium Biochemistry

The diverse biological effects of selenium (Se) contributes to continuing interest in this element (1), and three aspects of its biochemistry warrant special attention. First, Se is an essential element for mammals (2), being present in selenocysteine at the active site of glutathione peroxidase (3) (EC 1.11.1.9). Se deficiency in humans has occurred endemically in some areas of China (4; Keshan disease and Kaschin-Beck disease) and occasionally during courses of total parenteral nutrition and in low birthweight infants (5–8). Second, Se is a modifier of the response to a number of toxins. Se treatment can reduce metal toxicity (9–11), and Se nutriture can potentiate or attenuate the toxicity of organic agents (12). Some of these effects may be due to influence of Se status on glutathione metabolism (13) or on activities of xenobiotic metabolizing enzymes (14). In addition, Se nutriture affects the development and progression of many types of cancer. Third, Se is acutely and chronically toxic.

Sources and Distribution of Se in the Biosphere

Selenium (atomic number 34) is a metalloid of atomic mass 78.96 that exists in at least four oxidation states in nature. Selenate ($+6$), selenite ($+4$), elemental selenium (0), and selenide (-2) are all found in soils and vary in availability for translocation and incorporation into plants. Commercially, Se is extracted from copper refinery slimes (15).

Concentrations of Se in soils varies from 0.03 ppm to more than 30 ppm in regions with seleniferous soils (15, 16). Regions with seleniferous soils include the upper Great Plains (northeastern Nebraska and southeastern South Dakota in the United States and Enshi County, Hubei province in the People's Republic of China. Plants of genera *Astragalus*, *Haplopappus*, *Machaeranthera*, and *Stanleya* are primary Se bioaccumulators, and their presence may identify regions of increased soil Se concentrations (15). Concentrations of Se in groundwater are usually quite low; however, regions with seleniferous soils often have elevated Se levels in water. Irrigation drainage water can contain extremely high concentrations of Se (17). Air concentrations of Se are generally quite low and derive at least in part from burning of Se-containing fossil fuels (16). In general, the contribution of respired Se to the body burden of Se is small. However, inhalation of gaseous Se or Se-laden aerosols can produce acute or chronic toxicity.

OCCUPATIONAL AND ENVIRONMENTAL EXPOSURE TO SE

Table 88.1 (18–21) lists occupational uses and environmental conditions in which excessive Se exposure might occur. Al-

though Se exposure is usually well controlled in industrial settings, the potential for Se intoxication exists. Exposure to excessive amounts of Se by ingestion of Se-contaminated food or by inhalation of Se-containing aerosol can also occur. Excessive exposure to Se by ingestion of Se supplements (21, 22) or by use of a Se-containing shampoo (19) are unusual but documented events.

Chronic Se poisoning has been described in North American and Chinese populations. During the 1930s, the health status of individuals residing in regions of Nebraska, South Dakota, and Wyoming with seleniferous soils was examined (23). Common signs and symptoms found in individuals with the highest levels of Se in urine (>200 μg per liter) were icteroid discoloration of skin, changes in fingernails, gastrointestinal disorders, and discoloration and decay of teeth. Notably, "alkali disease," chronic Se intoxication of horses, pigs, and cows, also occurred in this area.

Chronic Se intoxication has also occurred in Enshi County, Hubei Province, in the People's Republic of China and was most severe in the early 1960s (4, 24). In this region, the Se-rich stony coal used for heating and cooking was the major source of Se exposure. Release of Se by coal burning increased respiratory exposure to Se and resulted in widespread Se intoxication. Hair loss, sloughing of nails, reddish skin lesions, and increased dental caries were the most common signs of intoxication. More severe signs of intoxication (peripheral anesthesia, acroparesthesia, and hemiplegia) also occurred. Reduced use of Se-containing coal, improved ventilation and an

Table 88.1. Possible Occupational and Environmental Sources of Se Exposure[a]

Occupational	
Glass manufacturing	Se used as decolorizer and pigment
Pigment and glaze production	Se used as colorant in dyes and glazes
Printing and etching processes	Se-containing inks used
Plastic production	Se used as colorant
Steel production and machinery	Se used in alloying of steel and in copper-based alloys
Electrical devices and insulation	Se used in photoelectric cells and rectifiers and as a gaseous electrical insulator (SeF_6)
Rubber production	Se used as antioxidant and accelerator
Inhalation of hydrogen selenide	Potential exposure to gas during transfer and use
Copper refining	H_2Se production in refining of copper

Environmental
Ingestion of Se-containing plant and animal material
Inhalation of Se-containing gases or aerosol

Iatrogenic
Self medication with Se-containing supplements
Use of Se-containing antidandruff shampoo

[a]Data (4, 15, 18–21)

overall improvement in diet have resulted in reduction of chronic Se poisoning in China (25).

CLINICAL TOXICOLOGY OF EXPOSURE

Exposure and Absorption

Organic Se compounds (e.g., selenomethionine) are the most bioavailable in humans; selenite and selenate are less well absorbed. It appears that large differences in dietary Se intake have little effect on the extent of gastrointestinal absorption of this element. Up to about 80% of dietary Se is absorbed under conditions of either low or high Se levels in diet. At extremes, daily intake of Se in diet ranges from 10 to 20 μg/day in areas where Se deficiency has been recognized up to about 5000 μg/day in seleniferous regions. A "safe and adequate" dietary intake of Se probably ranges from about 50 to 200 μg/day (26), and this intake is probably achieved by most individuals in the United States. Absorption of Se from the respiratory tract has been examined. For a Se aerosol with a 0.5 μm median mass aerodynamic diameter, the rate of clearance is 0.48 m^3 of air per hr (27). The solubility of respired Se-compounds apparently affects the rate of lung absorption. Longterm occupational exposure to elemental Se dust can lead to very high concentrations of Se in the lung (28). Selenide is a reactive species and can form hydrogen selenide (H$_2$Se), a toxic gas. Because H$_2$Se decomposes rapidly in air to produce elemental Se and water, the risk of exposure to this gas is minimal (29). Chronic Se poisoning has occurred after prolonged inhalation of Se released by coal burning (25).

Skin absorption of Se has not been extensively studied. In rats, a skin absorption rate for a sodium selenite solution of 10% per hr has been reported (30). Some Se compounds (e.g., Se oxychloride) are potent vesicants, producing severe burns at the site of application (31), and dermal application of Se oxychloride can be lethal in the dog (32). A case report of signs and symptoms consistent with Se poisoning in a woman using a Se sulfide-containing shampoo suggests that dermal absorption occurred (19). Eye irritation can occur with chronic exposure to H$_2$Se (20).

Metabolism and Elimination

In addition to similarities between the metabolism of Se and sulfur (33), the most striking aspects of Se metabolism are the reduction of selenate (+6) and selenite (+4) to selenide (−2) and the subsequent clearance of selenide-containing compounds. In a glutathione-dependent process, a series of Se-containing glutathione analogs are formed with the resulting production of Se (−2). At least two reactions in this reductive pathway are catalyzed by glutathione reductase (EC 1.6.4.2) and require NADPH. Selenide is a reactive species that forms stable complexes with metals. Selenide can be metabolized to dimethylselenide, a volatile compound which is lost in expired air. Dimethylselenide has a distinctive garlic-like odor, and exhalation of this agent accounts for the garlicky breath characteristic of Se intoxication. Selenide is also metabolized to trimethylselenonium ion, which is a major form of Se excreted in urine (34).

The systemic kinetics of Se in humans have been described (35–38). Urinary loss is the major route for excretion of selenium. A depletion-repletion study in young men showed that

a dietary intake of about 70 μg of Se is required to maintain body Se stores (39).

SIGNS, SYMPTOMS, AND SYNDROMES FROM TOXIC EXPOSURE

Teratogenicity, Mutagenicity, and Carcinogenicity of Se

There are few data on the teratogenicity of Se in mammals. In mallards high dietary concentrations of selenite (10 ppm) or of selenomethionine (25 ppm) reduced egg yield and inhibited embryonic growth. Selenomethionine was relatively more teratogenic and more readily tranferred from hen to egg than was selenite (40). In aquatic birds exposed to high enviornmental Se levels at Kesterson Reservoir in northern California, similar patterns of congenital malformations have been noted (41). Selenite is mutagenic in bacteria (42) and genotoxic in yeast (43).

Se has been characterized as a carcinogen or a tumor promoter and as an anticarcinogen (44). A number of animal studies demonstrate that various Se compounds are carcinogens (45). The potential of Se as a tumor promoter is demonstrated by the interaction of dietary Se level with dietary fat intake in development of pancreatic cancer in mice (46). Se also inhibits development of chemically and virally induced tumors (47, 48). In human populations, the relation between Se intake and cancer risk remains unclear. Ecologic studies of Se contents of foodstuffs and prevalence of certain tumors suggested an inverse relation between these variables (49). Prospective studies of cancer risk and Se status have yielded inconsistent results (50–54). Given current interest in the reduction of cancer risk by dietary modification, further studies of the relation between Se status and cancer incidence can be expected.

Toxic Effects and Management of Toxicity

Table 88.2 (55–60) summarizes the course, treatment, and outcome of cases of acute or chronic Se intoxication. Although most signs and symptoms are nonspecific, the presence of a garlicky odor of the breath may be an important clue of excessive Se exposure, particularly in cases of chronic Se intoxication (61). However, other possible causes of the garlic odor which must be considered of differential diagnosis are excessive exposure to phosphorous, tellurium, arsenic, lewisite, pyridine, dimethyl sulfoxide, or garlic (55). Treatment of Se intoxication is largely symptomatic. Sources of exposure must be identified and steps taken to control exposure. Although dimercaptopropanol (BAL) has been used to treat acute selenate poisoning (60), use of chelating agents is not generally supported. BAL treatment may increase the toxicity of Se (57). Use of glutathione to detoxify Se may have some therapeutic value, but futher studies are needed.

Laboratory diagnosis of Se intoxication involves determination of the concentration of Se in blood or urine. A variety of studies have examined the relation among Se intake, the concentration of Se in blood, and the excretion of Se in urine (62). An early study in selenium refinery workers led to the recommendation of 100 μg of Se per liter as a maximum allowable concentration in urine (63). However, based on more recent results obtained in seleniferous areas of China and the U.S., urinary output of Se in the range of 600–1000 μg/day

Table 88.2. Examples of Selenium Intoxication in Humans

Exposure	Signs and Symptoms	Treatment and Clincial Course	Reference
Hydrogen selenide inhalation (generation of hydrogen selenide in metal etching and printing operation; exposure for about 1 month)	Nausea and vomiting, metallic taste in mouth, dizziness, fatigue, garlic odor on breath	Se-containing ink replaced in printing operation; signs and symptoms resolved	18
Hydrogen selenide inhalation (chronic and intermittent for 1 year)	Chronic diarrhea with lower quadrant abdominal pain; bitter metallic taste and garlic odor on breath, granular conjunctivitis, and dental caries	Exposure ended; signs and symptoms resolved	55
Hydrogen selenide inhalation (acute)	Severe dyspnea with pneumomediastinum; restrictive and obstructive airway disease with impaired function at 3 yrs after exposure	Symptomatic treatment only with oxygen theophylline and hydrocortisone	56
Selenium metal fume and dust inhalation (50-year employment in Se refinery)	Reddish orange hair and reddish fingernails; high Se concentrations in lungs, hair, and nails at autopsy		28
Selenious acid ingestion (Ingestion of gun-blueing solution by 3-year-old boy)	Coma, hypotension, excessive salivation; strong garlic odor on breath	Gastric intubation and aspiration and mechanical ventilation; death about 2 hours after ingestion of gun blueing	57
Selenious acid ingestion (ingestion of gun blueing solution by 2-year-old girl)	Vomiting, diarrhea, muscle spasm/restlessness, excessive salivation, hypertension, tachycardia	Parenteral fluids; complete recovery	58
Selenious acid ingestion (ingestion of gun blueing solution by 2-year-old boy)	Second-degree burn of esophagus and stomach, comatose, metabolic acidosis, hemoconcentration, hyperglycemia, leukocytosis, cardiomyopathy, intestinal distension	Vomiting induced and mechanically ventilated; condition much improved at 4 days after ingestion, then developed acute respiratory distress; lung function deteriorated with *Legionella dumofii* infection which was not responsive to treatment; patient died at 17 days after ingestion	59
Sodium selenate ingestion (ingestion of sheep drench by 15-year-old girl)	Strong garlic odor on breath, diffuse T-wave ECG flattening; increased SGOT and serum alkaline phosphatase activities	Vomiting induced with gastric lavage and forced diuresis; vitamin C, BAL and diazepam given; complete recovery; discharged on 17th hospital day	60
Dietary selenium supplement ingestion (self-medication with an over-the-counter preparation—13 cases occurred in U.S.)	Nausea, abdominal pain, diarrhea, hair and nail changes; peripheral neuropathy, fatigue/irritability	Se-containing preparation improperly compounded and contained 182 times as much Se as labeled	21
Endemic selenium intoxication (ingestion of plant food grown on seleniferous soils in Enshi county, Hubei province, People's Republic of China)	Sloughing of nails, hair loss, skin lesions with increased reddish pigmentation, increased dental caries, peripheral anesthesia, acroparesthesia, hemiplegia	Change in food supply to reduce Se consumption	24

may indicate overexposure (62). Urinary output of Se increases with increasing daily intake of Se, suggesting that monitoring of urinary Se concentration would provide data on exposure (64, 65). It has been suggested that a blood Se concentration greater than 0.6 μg/ml is evidence of increased exposure. In a case of fatal acute selenious acid poisoning in a 2-year-old boy (59), a plasma Se concentration of 2.85 μg/ml was detected. Hence, a reliable report of high plasma or blood Se concentration should trigger immediate concern and intervention. Hair is a biologic medium which might be of use in monitoring Se exposure. A high correlation between blood and hair Se concentrations has been reported (24), but the correlation between hair Se concentration and tissue concentrations of Se is less well understood (66). "Normal" Se concentration

in serum is lower in young children than in adults, and it reaches adult levels at about 10 years of age (67, 68). This observation may be of importance in assessing the significance of a particular blood or serum Se concentration in a child.

Measurement of erythrocyte or plasma glutathione peroxidase activity is probably not useful as an indicator of excessive Se exposure. The activity of this enzyme is near maximal at normal levels of Se intake (69). Reduced whole blood glutathione peroxidase activity has been associated with high dietary intake of Se (64), and in acute selenious acid poisoning only a small increase in plasma glutathione peroxidase activity accompanied a very high plasma Se concentration (58).

Based on presently available data, the TLV-TWA for Se and its compounds is 0.2 mg/m³ and 0.05 ppm for Se hexafluoride and hydrogen selenide (70). Primary emphasis in setting these TLVs is to prevent irritation of eyes and mucous membranes.

REFERENCES

1. Oldfield JE. The two faces of selenium. J Nutr 1987;117:2002–2008.
2. Schwarz K, Foltz CM. Selenium as an integral part of factor 3 against dietary necrotic liver degeneration. J Am Chem Soc 1957;79:3292–3293.
3. Rotruck JT, Pope AL, Ganther HE, et al. Selenium: biochemical role as a component of glutathione peroxidase. Science 1973;179:585–590.
4. Guang-Qi Y. Research on selenium-related problems in human health in China. In: Combs GF, Levander OA, Spallholz JE, Oldfield JE, eds. Selenium in biology and medicine, Part A. New York: Van Nostrand Reinhold, 1987:9–32.
5. Johnson RA, Baker SS, Fallon JT, et al. An occidental case of cardiomyopathy and selenium deficiency. N Engl J Med 1981;304:1210–1212.
6. Kien CL, Ganther HE. Manifestations of chronic selenium deficiency in a child receiving total parenteral nutrition. Am J Clin Nutr 1983;37:319–328.
7. Vinton NE, Dahlstrom KA, Strobel Ct, Arment ME. Macrocytosis and pseudoalbinism: manifestations of selenium deficiency. J Pediatr 1987;111:711–717.
8. Lockitch G, Jacobson B, Quigley G, Dison P, Pendray M. Selenium deficiency in low birth weight neonates: an unrecognized problem. J Pediatr 1989;114:865–870.
9. Stillings BR, Lagally H, Bauersfeld D, Soaves J. Effect of cysteine, selenium and fish protein on the toxicity and metabolism of methyl mercury in rats. Toxicol Appl Pharmacol 1974;30:243–254.
10. Flora SJS, Behari JR, Ashquin M, Tandon SK. Time-dependent protective effect of selenium against cadmium-induced nephrotoxicity and hepatotoxicity. Chem-Biol Interact 1982;42:345–351.
11. Magos L, Clarkson TW, Sparrow S, Hudson AR. Comparison of the protection given by selenite, selenomethionine and biological selenium against the renotoxicity of mercury. Arch Toxicol 1987;60:422–426.
12. Combs GF, Combs SB. Selenium effects on drug and foreign compound toxicity. Pharmacol Ther 1987;33:303–315.
13. Hill KE, Burk RF, Lane JM. Effect of selenium depletion and repletion on plasma glutathione and glutathione-dependent enzymes in the rat. J Nutr 1987;117:99–104.
14. Wendel A, Reiter R. Modulation of xenobiotic metabolism in mouse liver by dietary seleniun. In: Combs GF, Spallholz JE, Levander OA, Oldfield JE, eds. Selenium in biology and medicine, Part A. New York: Van Nostrand Reinhold, 1987:283–290.
15. Committee on Medical and Biologic Effects of Environmental Pollutants. Division of Medical Sciences Assembly of Life Sciences National Research Council. Selenium. Washington, DC: National Academy of Sciences 1976:1–40.
16. Bennett BG, Peterson PJ. Assessment of human exposure to environmental selenium. In: Combs GF, Levander OA, Spallholz JE, Oldfield JE, eds. Selenium in biology and medicine, Part B. New York: Van Nostrand Reinhold, 1987:608–618.
17. Fan AM, Book SA, Neutra RR, Epstein DM. Selenium and human health implications in California's San Joaquin Valley. J Toxicol Environ Health 1988;23:539–559.
18. Buchan RF. Industrial selenosis. Occup Med 1947;3:439–456.
19. Ransome JW, Scott NM, Knoblock EC. Selenium sulfide intoxication. N Engl J Med 1961;264:384–385.
20. Robin JP. Safety and health aspects of selenium and tellurium in a copper refinery. In: Proc Int Symp Ind Uses Selenium Tellurium, 3rd ed. Darien, Connecticut. Selenium-Tellurium Development Association, 1984:28–56.
21. Helzlsouer K, Jacobs R, Morris S. Acute selenium intoxication in the United States. Fed Proc 1985;44:1670.
22. Jensen R, Closson W, Rothenberg R. Selenium intoxication—New York. MMWR 1984;33:157–158.
23. Smith MI, Franke KW, Westfall BB. The selenium problem in relation to public health. Public Health Rep 1936;51:1496–1505.
24. Yang G, Wang S, Zhou R, Sun S. Endemic selenium intoxication of humans in China. Am J Clin Nutr 1983;37:872–881.
25. Whanger PD. China, a country with both selenium deficiency and toxicity: some thoughts and impressions. J Nutr 1989;119:1236–1239.
26. Levander OA. The global selenium agenda. In: Hurley LS, Keen CL, Lonnerdal B, Rucker RB, eds. Trace elements in man and animals. Vol 6. New York: Plenum 1988:1–6.
27. Medinsky MA, Cuddihy RG, Griffith WC, Weissman SH, McClellan RO. Projected uptake and toxicity of selenium compounds from the environment. Environ Res 1985;365:181–192.
28. Diskin CJ, Alper JC, Fliegel SE. Long-term selenium exposure. Arch Intern Med 1979;139:824–826.

29. Glover JR. Selenium and its industrial toxicology. Ind Med Surg 1970;39:50–54.
30. Dutkiewicz T, Dutkiewicz B, Balcerska I. Dynamics of organ and tissue distribution of selenium after intragastric and dermal administration of sodium selenite. Bromatol Chem Toksykol 1972;4:475–481.
31. Cerwenka EA, Cooper C. Toxicology of selenium and tellurium and their compounds. Arch Environ Health 1961;3:161–200.
32. Moxon AL. Selenium poisoning. Physiol Rev 1943;23:305–337.
33. Levander OA. Selected aspects of the comparative metabolism and biochemistry of selenium and sulfur. In: Prasad AS, Oberleas D, eds. Trace elements in human health and disease. Vol II. New York: Academic Press, 1976:135–163.
34. Ganther HE. Metabolism of hydrogen selenide and methylated selenides. In: Draper HH, ed. Advances in nutritional research. New York: Plenum Press, 1979:107–129.
35. Thomson CD, Stewart RDH. The metabolism of (^{75}Se) selenite in young women. Br J Nutr 1974;32:47–57.
36. Griffiths NM, Stewart RDH, Robinson MF. The metabolism of (^{75}Se) selenomethionine in four women. Br J Nutr 1976;35:372–382.
37. Stewart RDH, Griffiths NM, Thomson CD, Robinson MF. Quantitative selenium metabolism in normal New Zealand women. Br J Nutr 1978;40:45–54.
38. Janghorbani M, Christensen MJ, Nahapetian A, Young VR. Selenium metabolism in healthy adults: quantitative aspects using the stable isotope $^{74}SeO_3{}^{2-}$ Am J Clin Nutr 1982;35:647–654.
39. Levander OA, Sutherland B, Morris VC, King JC. Selenium balance in young men during selenium depletion and repletion. Am J Clin Nutr 1981;34:2662–2669.
40. Hoffman DJ, Heinz GH. Embryotoxic and teratogenic effects of selenium in the diet of mallards. J Toxicol Environ Health 1988;24:477–490.
41. Ohlendorf HM, Kilness AW, Simmons JL, et al. Selenium toxicosis in wild aquatic birds. J Toxicol Environ Health 1988;24:67–92.
42. Kramer GF, Ames BN. Mechanisms of mutagenicity and toxicity of sodium selenite (Na_2SeO_3) in Salmonella typhimurium. Mutat Res 1988;201:169–180.
43. Anjaria KB, Madhvanath U. Genotoxicity of selenite in diploid yeast. Mutat Res 1988;204:605–614.
44. Birt DF. Update of the effects of vitamins A, C, and E and selenium on carcinogenesis. Proc Soc Exp Biol Med 1986;183:311–320.
45. Woo Y-T, Lai DY, Arcos JC, Argus MF, eds. Chemical induction of cancer: structural bases and biological mechanisms. In: Natural, metal, fiber and macromolecular carcinogens. Vol IIIC. New York: Academic Press, 1988:439–502.
46. Birt DF, Julius AD, Runice CE, et al. Enhancement of BOP-induced pancreatic carcinogenesis in selenium-fed Syrian golden hamsters under specific dietary conditions. Nutr Cancer 1988;11:21–33.
47. Milner JA. Effect of selenium on virally induced and transplantable tumor models. Fed Proc 1985;44:2568–2572.
48. Birt DF, Lawson TA, Julius AD, Runice CE, Salmasi S. Inhibition by dietary selenium of colon cancer induced in the rat by bis(2-oxypropyl)nitrosamine. Cancer Res 1988;42:4455–4459.
49. Schrauzer GN, White DA, Schneider CJ. Cancer mortality correlation studies: III. Statistical associations with dietary selenium intakes. Bioinorg Chem 1977;7:23–34.
50. Willett WC, Polk BF, Morris JS, et al. Prediagnostic serum selenium and risk of cancer. Lancet 1983;2:130–134.
51. Salonen JT, Alfthan G, Huttunen JK, Puska P. Association between serum selenium and the risk of cancer. Am J Epidemiol 1984;120:342–349.
52. Salonen JT, Salonen R, Lappeteläinen R, et al. Risk of cancer in relation to serum concentrations of selenium and vitamins A and E: matched case-control analysis of prospective data. Br Med J 1985;290:417–420.
53. Burney PG, Comstock GW, Morris JS. Serologic precursors of cancer: serum micronutrients and the subsequent risk of pancreatic cancer. Am J Clin Nutr 1989;49:895–900.
54. Virtamo J, Valkeila E, Alfthan G, et al. Serum selenium and risk of cancer. A prospective follow-up of nine years. Cancer 1987;60:145–148.
55. Adlerman LC, Bergin JJ. Hydrogen selenide poisoning: an illustrative case with review of the literature. Arch Environ Health 1986;41:354–358.
56. Schecter A, Shanske W, Stenzler A, Quintilian H, Steinberg H. Acute hydrogen selenide inhalation. Chest 1980;77:554–555.
57. Carter RF. Acute selenium poisoning. Med J Aust 1966;1:525–528.
58. Lombeck I, Menzel H, Frosch D. Acute selenium poisoning of a 2-year-old child. Eur J Pediatr 1987;146:308–312.
59. Nantel AJ, Brown M, Dery P, Lefebvre M. Acute poisoning by selenious acid. Vet Hum Toxicol 1985;27:531–533.
60. Civil IDS, McDonald MJA. Acute selenium poisoning: Case report. NZ Med J 1978;87:354–356.

61. Hogberg J, Alexander J. Selenium. In: Friberg L, Nordberg GF, Vouk VB, eds. Handbook on the toxicology of metals. 2nd ed. Amsterdam: Elsevier 1986:482–520.

62. Magos L, Berg GG. Selenium. In: Clarkson TW, Friberg L, Nordberg GF, Sager PR, eds. Biological monitoring of toxic metals. New York: Plenum 1988:383–405.

63. Glover JR. Selenium in human urine: a tentative maximum allowable concentration for industrial and rural populations. Ann Occup Hyg 1967;10:3–14.

64. Valentine JL, Faraji B, Kang HK. Human glutathione peroxidase activity in cases of high selenium exposures. Environ Res 1988;45:16–27.

65. Elinder CG, Gerhardsson L, Oberdoerster G. Biological monitoring of toxic metals—overview. In: Clarkson TW, Friberg L, Nordberg GF, Sager PR, eds. Biological monitoring of toxic metals. New York: Plenum 1988:63–65.

66. Cheng YD, Zhuang GS, Tan MG, et al. Preliminary study of correlation of Se content in human hair and tissues. J Trace Element Exp Med 1988;1:19–21.

67. Lockitch G, Halstead AC, Wadsworth L, et al. Age and sex-specific pediatric reference intervals and correlations for zinc, copper, selenium, iron, vitamins A and E, and related proteins. Clin Chem 1988;34:1625–1628.

68. Lloyd B, Robson E, Smith I, Clayton BE. Blood selenium concentrations and glutathione peroxidase activity. Arch Dis Child 1989;64:352–356.

69. Rea HM, Thomson CD, Campbell DR, Robinson MR. Relation between erythrocyte selenium concentrations and glutathione peroxidase (EC 1.11.1.9) activities of New Zealand residents and visitors to New Zealand. Br J Nutr 1979;42:201–208.

70. American Conference of Governmental Industrial Hygienists, Inc. Hydrogen selenide. In: Documentation of the threshold limit values and biological exposure indices. 5th ed. Cincinnati, OH: ACGIH, 1986:517—518.

89

Intermetallic Semiconductors and Inorganic Hydrides

Dean E. Carter, Ph.D.
John B. Sullivan, Jr., M.D.

SOURCES AND PRODUCTION

In the microelectronics industry, the substrate predominantly used for semiconductor devices is silicon. However, other semiconductor materials have been introduced into the market which have an increasing number of applications. These materials include the III–V intermetallic semiconductor substrates.

The intermetallic semiconductors described here are composed of equimolar ratios of group III and group V elements. The most commonly used intermetallic semiconductor is gallium arsenide (GaAs), followed by gallium phosphide (GaP) and indium phosphide (InP). However, any combination of the group III elements aluminum (Al), gallium (Ga), and indium (In) with the group V elements phosphorus (P), arsenic (As), and antimony (Sb) should be semiconductors as long as they are in a 1:1 molar ratio of group III: group V (e.g., AlGaAs) and research in this area may yield a variety of semiconductors with special applications.

The III–V intermetallic semiconductors are all crystalline solids of high density. They can be prepared by condensing vapors of the elemental forms of the metalloids, and, thus, gallium arsenide can be characterized as Ga(0)As(0). The chemical form of the intermetallic does not appear to be as important for toxicology as the chemical forms of its dissolution products.

The inorganic hydrides also include some of the group III and group V elements because these elements are used as dopants for silicon based semiconductors. The materials to be described include: arsine (AsH_3), phosphine (PH_3), stibine (SbH_3), diborane (B_2H_6), and silane (SiH_4).

In addition to their common names, they also can be described as the hydride of the element (e.g., antimony hydride). These materials are all gases at room temperature. Phosphine, diborane, and silane can autoignite in air at elevated temperatures, and they may represent a hazard from explosion or combustion. All of these compounds may react rapidly with oxidants, and the possibility of explosive reactions after accidental release must be considered. The hydrides of phosphorus, arsenic, and presumably antimony can be formed from nascent hydrogen and the metallic phosphide, arsenide, and stilbide, respectively. It is also generally thought that arsine can be formed when arsenides like gallium arsenide react with acids, but recent work from our laboratories (Carter) has shown that arsine is only formed when gallium arsenide reacts with concentrated hydrochloric acid (1). Other common acids such as sulfuric, nitric, or perchloric acids did not form arsine.

Phosphine can be formed during the machining (e.g., cutting, grinding, and polishing) of phosphides like GaP and InP when water-cooled processes are used (2). It can also be produced when GaP and InP are annealed in hydrogen atmospheres and alkaline media. Stibine gas may be formed during annealing of InSb type semiconductors in a hydrogen atmosphere and during processing of InSb with nonoxidizing acids. Although all the conditions which might form toxic hydrides like phosphine, arsine, and stibine have not been completely investigated, their formation should always be considered when etching processes are involved

SITES, INDUSTRIES, AND BUSINESSES ASSOCIATED WITH EXPOSURES

These materials are used primarily in the microelectronics industry. GaAs has been most often used for optoelectronic devices over the past two decades. GaAs devices include: light-emitting diodes (LEDs), optical communications transmitters, and solid-state semiconductor lasers. GaAs may find use as a photovoltaic solar cell material. Several favorable properties as compared with silicon-based devices suggest that GaAs may find applications in military, space, telecommunications, and supercomputing systems. Potential applications include high frequency microwave and millimeter wave telecommunications, satellite communications, ground- and space-based radar, electronic warfare, and intelligent weapons. Other applications could include cellular telephones, high definition television, and automobile and aircraft instrument displays and controls (3).

The manufacture of GaAs components has four major steps: ingot growth, wafer processing, epitaxial growth, and device fabrication. In one process, GaAs is formed by heating stoichiometric quantities of elemental gallium and arsenic in a sealed quartz ampule. Crystal growth is achieved in a reactor by one of several techniques. Exposure to GaAs can occur during ampule breakout when the quartz tube is broken and particles released, during cleaning and maintenance operations for quartz glassware, and during cleaning of the reactors. The large crystal (called an ingot) has its ends cropped, the ingot is lathed, and then it is mounted onto a holder for wafer slicing. Once sliced, the wafers are lapped to a desirable thickness, chemically cleaned, and polished. Exposure to GaAs particles may be expected during these cropping, slicing, lapping, polishing, backlapping, and wafer-saving steps.

Epitaxial growth processes form thin layers of GaAs during the manufacture of the device. These processes involve the chemical reaction of gallium and arsenic species to form GaAs on the surface of the wafer. For example, vapor phase epitaxy utilizes the reaction at high temperature between gallium halides and arsine (or arsenic halides). Exposure to particles can occur during epitaxial reactor cleaning and maintenance. GaAs device fabrication includes nitride and silox deposition, photolithography, plasma and/or wet etching, diffusion, metallization, backlapping, and final test (3). Some of these processes may generate solutions containing soluble gallium and arsenic products. Contact with these would result in exposure to gallium and arsenic salts.

The inorganic hydride gases may be used in a large number of the manufacturing processes for electronic devices. It should be recognized that these gases are commonly found in microelectronic manufacturing facilities, and they are usually presented in substantial quantities. In addition, there are cases in which arsine has been liberated when nascent hydrogen was formed in materials containing arsenic (4). Many metal ores contain arsenic as an impurity, and, thus, arsine may be generated in metal industries, in nonferrous metal refineries and in the manufacture of silicon steel when the ores come into contact with acid.

TOXICOLOGY OF EXPOSURE

The toxic effects from the intermetallic semiconductors appear to occur primarily after inhalation exposure, although oral exposure to high doses may also result in some toxicity. Only GaAs has been studied in any detail, and those studies are in experimental animals. A dose of 30 mg/kg of GaAs introduced into the lung by intratracheal administration produced enzymatic changes in the body characteristic of soluble arsenic compounds; equivalent changes were observed only when 1000 mg/kg GaAs was given by oral administration (5). The cumulative absorption of GaAs from the lung as measured by the amount of arsenic found in blood and urine was approximately 10–20% of the administered dose, and this appeared over a period of several days (6). This absorption was fairly constant over the dose range of 10–100 mg/kg (5). After oral administration, the amount absorbed appeared to depend on dose in the range 10–1000 mg/kg; at 1000 mg/kg, less than 1% was absorbed, but the percentage of the dose absorbed rose to almost 10% at the 10-mg/kg dose. These results are all based on arsenic data because no gallium was detected in either blood or urine. Lung and fecal analyses found more gallium than arsenic, suggesting that gallium was more poorly absorbed from the lung than was arsenic and greater amounts of gallium were cleared from the lung by mucociliary mechanisms and subsequently swallowed. Dermal absorption of GaAs does not appear to be a problem, but GaAs exposure to the conjunctival sac of the eye caused a reaction in the mucous membranes (7).

The absorption of GaAs appeared to be accompanied by the formation of arsenic oxide. The urinary metabolites of GaAs in the hamster were the same as those found after inorganic arsenic exposure (arsenite, arsenate, monomethylarsonic acid, and dimethylarsinic acid), and the quantities found were intermediate to those found after arsenite and arsenate administration (6).

Excretion of arsenic absorbed from GaAs is probably as rapid as that found after inorganic arsenic administration; about 35% of the soluble sodium arsenite was excreted within 48 hours in humans (4). GaAs is absorbed slowly from the lung, so arsenic excretion is expected to continue for several weeks after GaAs exposure. GaAs remaining in the lung is eliminated slowly; a single intratracheal dose of 100 mg/kg was excreted in about 3 months and had a half-life in the range of 2 weeks.

Little is known about the bioavailability, metabolism, or excretion of the other III–V intermetallic compounds. Their bioavailability should be dependent on their dissolution rates in water as well as chemical properties which would govern their oxidation rates. Experiments with GaAs showed the presence of oxides of arsenic on the surface of the GaAs crystal after exposure to aqueous solutions, suggesting that oxidation may be necessary for the dissolution of these compounds (8).

Exposure to the hydride gases (phosphine, arsine, stibine, silane, and diborane) is mainly via the inhalational route. Absorption of arsine should be quite efficient due to its substantial solubility in water (1, 8). Arsine is apparently absorbed unchanged after inhalation since it has unique effects on the red blood cell, but it eventually breaks down to release inorganic arsenic in the body (9). Little appears to be known about the bioavailability, metabolism, or excretion of these compounds. Controlled studies on these compounds have been complicated by their toxic nature.

The III–V intermetallic compounds have a low order of acute lethality after oral or intratracheal administration in animals. The oral LD_{50} of GaAs in mice and rats was reported to be greater than 15 g/kg (10). The threshold for acute effects after intragastric administration was reported as 7.0 g/kg (7). A threshold for acute effects of inhalation of GaAs aerosol for 4 hours was 152.5 mg/m^3 using a variety of toxic indicators (7). A dose of 200 mg/kg GaAs has been given to rats by intratracheal instillation without having lethal effects (11). Roschina (1966) reported an LD_{50} of 3.7 g/kg for indium antimonide powder when given to white mice by intraperitoneal administration in peach oil (12). The oral LD_{50} for indium arsenide was stated to be greater than 15 g/kg and the threshold for acute effects after a single 4-hour inhalation exposure was 139 mg/m^3 (10, 13). Tarasenko and Fadeev reported an oral LD_{50} of 8 g/kg for gallium phosphide in mice (7, 14).

Lung changes appear within a week after a single exposure to GaAs. A dose of 100 mg/kg GaAs given by intratracheal instillation to rats resulted in type II pneumocyte hyperplasia, alveolar proteinosis, and interstitial pneumonia as determined from histopathologic examination (15). An inflammatory response was also indicated by enzyme activity changes in bronchopulmonary lavage studies. Significant increases were found in total lung weight and lung lipid, protein, and DNA content. Similar, but less severe, effects were seen at 30 mg/kg, and at 2.5 mg/kg the biochemical effects were essentially absent. Indium antimonide has been reported to cause desquamative and interstitial pneumonia in the lungs after 25 mg were administered by intratracheal instillation to unspecified animals and for an unspecified duration (12).

CLINICAL TOXICOLOGY

Gallium Arsenide and Arsine

Arsine gas (AsH_3) is very toxic and can be generated from gallium arsenide by the action of hydrogen on arsenic such as would occur with acidic solutions. It is a colorless, nonirritating gas with a garlic odor. The fatality rate from arsine gas exposure is reported to be as high as 25% (16). Signs and symptoms of arsine poisoning include headache, nausea, abdominal pain, dyspnea, and hemolysis from 2–24 hours after inhalational exposure (17). Severe toxicity is manifest by red blood cell hemolysis and secondary multiple organ effects such as acute renal failure and pulmonary edema. A triad of hemolysis, abdominal pain, and hematuria is classic for arsine poisoning (16). Arsine is soluble in blood and plasma and complexes with red blood cells. A massive release of arsine into a work environment can potentially produce numerous casualties.

Clinically, the signs and symptoms of acute poisoning are those consistent with acute and massive hemolysis. Initially, there is painless hemoglobinuria, dizziness, weakness, nausea, vomiting, abdominal cramping, and tenderness. After a latent period, usually 2–24 hours, jaundice accompanied by anuria or oliguria may occur. Evidence of bone marrow depression has also been reported. Individuals with preexisting renal or cardiac disease, or hypersensitivity to hemolytic agents resulting from a congenital deficiency of reduced erythrocyte glutathione (GSH), are potentially more sensitive to the effects of arsine.

Acute high dose exposure to arsine is associated with rapid hemolysis of red blood cells and subsequent renal failure. Experimental evidence indicates that the hemolytic activity of arsine is due to its ability to effectively reduce erythrocyte glutathione (GSH) concentrations. The hemolysis associated with acute arsine exposure is characterized by a latent period the length of which is inversely proportional to the extent of exposure. Inhalation of 250 ppm of arsine is quickly lethal, inhalation of up to 50 ppm for 30 minutes may produce death, and 10 ppm can be lethal after a longer exposure period.

These data are consistent with a mechanism of toxicity involving oxidant injury and depletion of erythrocyte GSH, which is critical for the maintenance of the structural integrity of the erythrocyte membrane. If erythrocyte GSH synthesis is equal to the exposure, then significant acute hemolysis is not observed. However, if arsine doses exceed GSH resynthesis, then acute fulminant hemolysis can be produced. If significant but nondepleting exposure occurs, biochemical evidence of low to moderate hemolysis is produced. These observations confirm a strong inverse correlation between the GSH erythrocyte concentration and the extent of hemolysis in arsine-exposed erythrocytes.

Treatment of arsine toxicity consists of immediate removal of the individual from the exposure. Clinical evaluation for hemolysis by examination of plasma for elevation of free hemoglobin, hematuria, and fragmentation of erythrocytes should be done. Alkalinization of the urine may help prevent acute renal failure in the event of hemolysis. Exchange transfusion may also be helpful should hemolysis occur. The use of heavy metal chelators is not of value. The arsine-hemoglobin complex is not dialyzable, and thus exchange transfusion represents the only real definitive therapy (16). Exchange transfusion is recommended if hemolysis is occurring and there is an elevated free plasma hemoglobin above 1.5 mg/dl (16). Recovery is dependent on the supportive care rendered, extent of exposure, and secondary pathology due to the hemolysis.

A Threshold Limit Value-time-weighted average (TLV-TWA) for workplace exposure to arsine is 0.05 ppm. This is the concentration to which nearly all workers can be repeatedly exposed to, on an 8 hour time-weighted average (TWA) basis, during a working lifetime without adverse effect. This TLV was adopted by the American Conference of Governmental Industrial Hygienists (ACGIH) in 1977. The Federal Occupational Safety and Health Administration (OSHA) also uses 0.05 ppm as the permissible exposure level (PEL). Notably, the documentation for this value provides little human exposure-response information. There are multiple reasons for this lack of documentation: (a) arsine is colorless, nonirritating and odorless below 1–2 ppm; (b) at intermediate doses, there is a significant latency period between exposure and hemolytic response. Thus, exposure may be undetected, and airborne concentrations remain undetermined.

Chronic, low level exposure to arsine may result in higher than usual excretion of urinary arsenic in workers of greater than 50 µg/l of urine (16), even when dietary intake is considered. A correlation has been found between urinary arsenic excretion and chronic exposure to arsine gas well below accepted regulatory standards. Further investigation is required regarding the longterm health hazards of chronic, low level arsine gas exposure.

The animal database associated with the TLV provides little quantitative dose-response information on the hemolytic effects of arsine exposure. Lethality in mice exposed to arsine concentrations ranging from 8–800 ppm has been evaluated. Hematologic responses were evaluated in mice exposed to 5–26 ppm arsine for 1 hour. The results range from a no-effect level of 5 ppm to a lethal concentration of 26 ppm. This concentration range is extremely narrow and represents less than a tenfold difference for the 1-hour exposure studied. Systemic effects from the arsenic formation absorbed from the lung into the general circulation should be expected. Gallium arsenide administered to the lung caused some changes indicating toxicity to the liver and kidney; blood aminolevulinic acid dehydratase (ALAD) was decreased within 3 days of administration, liver and kidney ALAD was inhibited, and urinary aminolevulinic acid was increased 3–6 days after exposure (11). Effects in kidneys, liver, and spleen were also noted after indium antimonide administration, but no details were described (12).

Phosphine

Phosphine is produced by the reaction of hydrogen with metallic phosphides, such as aluminum phosphide, zinc phosphide, or gallium phosphide. Aluminum and zinc phosphides are fumigants. Phosphine is a colorless gas with a fish-like odor at air concentrations greater than 2 ppm (16). Phosphine is acutely toxic and is difficult to detect in dangerous amounts even though its odor threshold is 0.03 ppm (18). The TLV recommended by OSHA is 0.3 ppm, with a shortterm exposure limit of 1 ppm (16).

Symptoms of phosphine exposure to average concentrations less than 10 ppm include diarrhea, nausea and vomiting, tightness of the chest and cough, dyspnea, paresthesias, tremor, ataxia, headache, and dizziness. More severe poisoning results in pulmonary edema, cardiovascular collapse, jaundice with elevated liver enzymes, myocardial injury with elevated MB-creatine phosphokinase fraction of cardiac enzymes, and cardiac dysrhythmias. Mortality from severe poisoning is high.

A death was reported from exposure to concentrations of 8 ppm phosphine for 1–2 hr/day (19). Death attributed to phosphine poisoning occur after ingestion of aluminum phosphide for suicide attempts. Doses equivalent to 2 or more grams of phosphine gas taken orally has caused deaths. Clinical signs consisted of gastritis, altered sensorium and vascular failure, and cardiac arrhythmia in some cases (20). Postmortem examination showed pulmonary edema, gastrointestinal mucosal congestion, and petechial hemorrhages on the surface of liver and brain. Histopathologic changes included desquamation of the epithelium of the bronchioles, vacuolar degeneration of hepatocytes, dilation and engorgement of hepatic central veins, and sinusoids and areas showing nuclear fragmentation.

The mechanism of phosphine toxicity is not understood. There are local irritating and systemic effects of the toxin. Treatment is supportive and there is no definitive therapeutic intervention.

Stibine

Stibine gas (SbH_3) antimony hydride, is produced by the action of hydrogen on metallic antimony. It is a colorless gas with an OSHA TLV of 0.1 ppm. Stibine exposure by inhalation produces red blood cell hemolysis. It is also a lung irritant and causes subsequent injury to the kidney and liver. Signs and symptoms of poisoning include hemolysis, hemoglobinuria, hematuria, nausea, vomiting, jaundice, shock, and renal failure. Treatment is supportive. The use of exchange transfusion would be recommended along the same guidelines as with arsine toxicity if hemolysis is occurring.

Diborane and Higher Boron Hydrides

Boron hydrides have been used as high energy sources and are very reactive compounds. Decaborane, $B_{10}H_{14}$, has been used as a rocket propellant, and its toxicity is mainly central nervous system with excitation and depression (21). The boron hydrides are in general very reactive, strong reducing agents and readily react with organic amines, alcohols, ketones, halogenated hydrocarbons, and unsaturated hydrocarbons (22). Diborane is the only boron hydride that is a gas at normal pressures and temperature (22). Boranes are soluble in hydrocarbons and slightly soluble in water. Diborane hydrolyzes rapidly in water to hydrogen and boric acid. Amine boranes are very stable. Pentaborane and decaborane hydrolyze very slowly (22). Boranes are fuels sources, fuel additives, initiators of rubber vulcanization, fungicides and bactericides, and initiators of ethylene, styrene, vinyl, and acrylic polymerization (22).

Diborane (B_2H_6) is a gas under normal temperature and pressure. It is produced by reacting lithium aluminum hydride with boron fluoride. Diborane is a colorless gas with a nauseating odor detectable at 2–4 ppm (16). Diborane is a fire and explosive hazard and may autoignite in air above temperatures of 104–120°F (40–45°C) (16).

Inhalational exposure to diborane results in hydrolysis to boric acid and hydrogen. The upper airway would be expected to be a main target of diborane. However, systemic toxicity, with pulmonary edema, also can occur. In addition, when diborane contacts air, higher hydrides are formed which will have toxicity different from boric acid.

Acute toxicity of diborane produces respiratory irritation, pneumonitis, and, if exposure is severe, pulmonary edema. Human health effects from subacute exposure to diborane have been reported in occupational settings and have included chest tightness, cough, headache, nausea, chills, dizziness, extreme fatigue, and obtundation after a relatively small exposure to the gas (22). These symptoms may occur soon after exposure or be delayed for up to 24 hours. Exposure may also result in fever, tremors, and muscle fasciculations. Animals exposed to toxic concentrations die a respiratory death (22). Hypotension, bradycardia and cardiac dysrhythmias were noted in animal studies. On autopsy, the lungs of the animals showed pulmonary edema and hemorrhage (22). Diborane has a distinctive rotten egg type odor that alerts workers to the exposure. The odor threshold is reported to be around 3 ppm. The TLV for diborane is 0.1 ppm. Therefore, if the odor is detected, the TLV could be violated. Massive inhalational exposure of diborane can be expected to produce pulmonary damage, pneumonitis, pulmonary edema, and maybe other systemic organ effects on the heart, liver, and kidneys. Treatment is mainly supportive care.

The other boranes, pentaborane (B_5H_9) and decaborane ($B_{10}H_{14}$), have toxicity which is different than diborane. Decaborane is a white solid, and pentaborane is a liquid. Pentaborane has a detectable odor of garlic-like at 0.8 ppm. Decaborane has an odor threshold which is described as "chocolate-like

and unpleasant" at 0.7 ppm (22). Both pentaborane and decaborane can produce toxicity via inhalation, ingestion, or dermal exposure. Both are soluble in hydrocarbons, but not water. Decaborane does not hydrolyze readily to boric acid. A direct negative inotropic cardiac effect has been demonstrated in animals secondary to decaborane (22). Other animal studies have demonstrated hypotension following decaborane exposure. Apparently, the reducing power of the borane hydrides parallels their toxicity. Pentaborane produces acute animal toxicity consisting of tremors, convulsions, ataxia, corneal opacities, coma, and death (22). Decaborane also produces seizures in animal models.

Clinical human cases of higher borane hydride toxicity have involved stupor, seizures, dizziness, disorientation, hyperexcitability, leucocytosis, hyperglycemia, elevated blood urea nitrogen, and liver damage (22). Dizziness, headache, fatigue, muscle spasm, and drowsiness appear to be common symptoms appearing early in humans following exposure to these compounds. It is of interest to note that symptoms may occur early or be delayed for as long as 24 hours (22). Symptoms may last 1–3 days. Muscle spasm may be prominent and involve large muscle groups. Renal and liver toxicity has been mild in the reported cases (22).

Changes in neurotransmitter concentrations with inhibition of norepinephrine, dopamine, and serotonin metabolism have been attributed to decaborane and pentaborane (23). Neurologic and neuropsychologic symptoms occurring following pentaborane exposure include confusion, impaired concentration, and recent memory deficits and may persist for days after exposure (23). Mild cognitive defects on neuropsychometric examinations have been reported following pentaborane exposure (23).

Silane

Silane (SiH_4) is a carrier gas used in the microelectronics industry. The main hazards of silane gas are asphyxiant conditions in confined spaces, fire, and explosions.

CHRONIC AND LONGTERM HEALTH EFFECTS

Not much is known about the longterm effects of exposure to III–V intermetallic compounds. Inhalation of GaAs aerosol by rats and guinea pigs at 12 mg/m³ for 4 months showed some fibrosis, epithelial degeneration in the kidney and convoluted tubules, and fatty degeneration of the liver (7, 10). Based on results from single dose studies, these changes are reasonable. Other longterm effects which might be expected would be those resulting from the dissociation of the intermetallic into its corresponding oxides. Thus, repeated exposure to gallium arsenide would be expected to show longterm effects associated with low doses of gallium oxide and arsenic oxide. Gallium oxide does not appear to show systemic toxicity after repeated inhalation or oral exposure, but the longterm effects of arsenic oxides are well known and described elsewhere in this volume.

The longterm effects of the hydrides have not been well-studied either. Phosphine does not appear to have cumulative effects, but there are no well-controlled repeated dose studies which have examined longterm effects. Chronic arsine exposure results in a progressive decline in the red blood cell number and in the hemoglobin. Mice and rats exposed to concentrations as low as 0.5 ppm for 90 days (6 hr/day, 5 days/week) produced a regenerative anemia secondary to the hemolysis. Increased concentrations of methemoglobin were found in mice exposed to 2.5 ppm arsine for 90 days (24). Mice exposed to levels as low as 0.5 ppm for 14 days showed that arsine inhalation had marked effects on the murine immune system, and these effects implicated the T-cell as a sensitive target (25). The results of these animal studies must be considered when the effects of human exposure are evaluated.

BIOLOGIC MONITORING

There are no well-characterized biologic monitors which are specific for any of these compounds. Those containing antimony (e.g., indium antimonide, stibine) should be able to use the biologic monitors for absorbed antimony; however, the absorbed antimony may not be able to be accurately related to the lung burden of intermetallic compounds. Blood and urine analyses are used as biologic monitors for antimony. Values for normal subjects have been reported for blood (3 μg/l), serum (0.3 μg/l), and 24-hr urinary excretion (0.5–2.6 μg/l). Levels above these may indicate exposure to antimony, although quantitative data relating exposure to urinary levels are incomplete (26).

Urinary arsenic levels are generally used as a biologic monitor for arsenic exposure if care is taken to eliminate the exposure to "seafood" forms of arsenic. Large quantities of arsenic in the form of arsenobetaine may be ingested with seafood, and, although arsenobetaine contributes to the total arsenic levels, it has a low toxicity and does not originate from the exposure to inorganic arsenic. Workers are usually asked to refrain from eating seafood 3–4 days before being tested for arsenic and the levels determined reflect workplace exposure to inorganic arsenic compounds. Inorganic forms of arsenic and their metabolites can be analyzed separately, but these analyses are difficult and are still being reduced to routine practice. Urinary levels from normal inorganic arsenic exposure should be less than 50 μg/l (26).

No definitive data exist with regard to the biologic monitoring of gallium or indium (27).

EXPOSURE LIMITS

No specific exposure limits have been formulated for any of the III–V intermetallic compounds. The National Institute of Occupational Safety and Health (NIOSH) issued an alert and recommended the exposure to gallium arsenide be controlled by observing the NIOSH Recommended Exposure Limit (REL) for inorganic arsenic (2 μg/m³ of air as a 15-minute ceiling) (27). NIOSH also recommended that the concentration of gallium arsenide in air be estimated by determination of arsenic. For antimony and compounds a TLV of 0.5 milligrams of antimony per cubic meter was recommended by ACGIH in 1980 (19).

For phosphine a TLV of 0.3 ppm (approximately 0.4 mg/m³) and a STEL of 1 ppm (approximately 1 mg/m³) were recommended (ACGIH, 1980). A TLV of 0.05 ppm (0.2 mg/m³) as arsenic is recommended by ACGIH for arsine (19). NIOSH has recommended the arsenic standard described above, and the OSHA standard for exposure to arsine is 0.05 ppm (0.2 mg/m³ of air) as a TWA in any 8-hour work shift of a 40-hour week. A TLV of 0.1 ppm (approximately 0.5 mg/m³) and a STEL of 0.3 ppm (approximately 15 mg/m³) were recommended by ACGIH for stibine (19).

REFERENCES

1. Scott N, Carter DE, Fernando Q. Reaction of gallium arsenide with concentrated acids: formation of arsine. Am Ind Hyg Assoc J 1989;50:379–381.

2. Knizek M. Toxicology risks during manufacture and processing of AIII-BV type semiconductors. Electrotchnike Cas 1978;29:152–157.

3. McIntyr AJ, Sherin BJ. Gallium arsenide processing and hazard control. Solid State Technol 1989;(July):101–104.

4. Ishinishe N, Tsuchiya K, Vahter M, Fowler BA. Arsenic. In: Friberg L, Nordberg GF, Vouk VB, eds. Handbook on the toxicology of metals. Vol II. Amsterdam: Elsevier Publishers, 43–83.

5. Webb DR, Sipes IG, Carter DE. In vitro solubility and in vivo toxicity and gallium arsenide. Toxicol Appl Pharmacol 1984;76:96–104.

6. Rosner MH, Carter DE. Metabolism and excretion of gallium arsenide and arsenic oxides by hamsters following intratracheal instillation. Fundam Appl Toxicol 1987;9:730–737.

7. Fadeev AI. Materials on substantiation of the MAC for gallium arsenide in the air of workplaces. Gig Tr Prof Zabol 1980;3:45–47.

8. Pierson B, Van Wagenen S, Nebesny K, Fernando Q, Scott N, Carter DE. Dissolution of crystalline gallium arsenide in aqueous solutions containing complexing agents. Am Ind Hyg Assoc J 1989;50:455–459.

9. NIOSH Arsine (Arsenic Hydride) poisoning in the workplace. Current Intelligence Bulletin 32. U.S. Department of Health, Education and Welfare, National Institute for Occupational Safety and Health, DHEW (NIOSH) Publication No. 79–142, 1979.

10. Fadeev AI. Toxicity of some compounds of arsenic with rare metals. Aktual Probl Gig Tr 1978;32–35.

11. Goering PL, Maronpot RR, Fowler BA. Effect of intratracheal gallium arsenide on delta-aminolevulinic acid dehydratase in rats: relationship to urinary excretion of aminolevulinic acid. Toxicol App Pharmacol 1988;92:179–193.

12. Roschina TA. Toxicological characteristics of indium antimonide and gallium arsenide: new semiconducting materials. Gig Tr Prof Zabol 1966;10(5):30–33.

13. Fadeev Ai, Borobeva RS, Akinfieva TA. Toxicity of intermetallic compounds. Met Gigien Aspekty Otseni i Ozdorovleniya Okruzh Sredy M 1983;246–251.

14. Tarasenko NY, Fadeev AI. Occupational health problems related to the industrial use of gallium and indium compounds. Gig Sanit 1980;45(10):13–16.

15. Webb DR, Wilson SE, Carter DE. Comparative pulmonary toxicity of gallium arsenide, gallium (III), oxide and arsenic (III) oxide intratracheally instilled into rats. Toxicol Appl Pharmacol 1986;82:405–416.

16. Wald P, Becker C. Toxic gases used in the microelectronics industry. State of the art reviews: Occupational Medicine 1986;1(1):105–117.

17. Landrigan P, Costello R, Stringer W. Occupational exposure to arsine. Scand J Work Environ Health 1982;8:169–177.

18. Fluck E. The odor threshold of phosphine. J Air Pollut Contr Assoc 1976;26:795.

19. ACGIH. Documentation of the threshold limit values. 4th ed. Cincinnati, OH: American Conference of Governmental Industrial Hygienists, 1980.

20. Misra UK, Tripathi AK, Pandey R, Bhargwa B. Acute phosphine poisoning following ingestion of aluminum phosphides. Hum Toxicol 1988;7:343–345.

21. Naeger L, Leibman K. Mechanisms of decaborane toxicity. Toxicol Appl Pharmacol 1972;22:517–527.

22. Rousch G. The toxicology of the boranes, J Occup Med 1959;1:46–52.

23. Hart R, Silverman J, Garretson L, Schulz C, Hamer R. Neuropsychological function following mild exposure to pentaborane. Am In Med 1984;6:37–44.

24. Blair PC, Bechtold M, Thompson MB, Moorman CR, Moorman MP, Fowler BA. Evidence for oxidative damage to erythrocytes in rats and mice induced by arsine gas. Toxicologist 1988;8:19.

25. Rosenthal GJ, Fort MM, Germolec DR, Ackermann MF, Blair P, Lamm KR, Luster MI. Effects of subchronic exposure to arsine on immune functions and host resistance. Toxicologist 1988;8:19.

26. Elinder CG. Gerhardsson L, Oberdoerster G. Biological monitoring of toxic metals—overview. In: Clarkson TW, Friberg L, Nordberg GF, Sager, PR, eds. Biological monitoring of toxic metals. New York: Plenum Press, 1–71.

27. NIOSH 1988: Reducing the potential risk of developing cancer from exposure to gallium arsenide in the microelectronics industry. DHHS Publication No. 88–100. Publications Dissemination, DSDTT, Cincinnati, OH: NIOSH, 1987.

28. Elinder CG, Friberg L. Antimony. Friberg L, Nordberg GF, Vouk VB, eds. Handbook on the toxicology of metals. Vol II. Amsterdam: Elsevier Publishers, 1986:26–42.

90

Metal Oxides

Francis J. Farrell, M.D.

Metal oxides produce four types of lung disease: metal fume fever, chemical pneumonitis, hypersensitivity pneumonitis, and occupational asthma (1). This chapter will concentrate primarily on metal fume fever produced by metal oxides.

Metal fume fever, a common acute industrial disease, is caused by the inhalation of oxides of metals, especially zinc. The first description was published by Potissier in 1822 (2). It was first described in England in 1831 by Thackrah among brass founders (3). Gardner in 1848 gave the first report in the United States (4). It is also known as brazier's disease, spelter shakes, brass chills, zinc chills, welder's ague, copper fever, Monday fever, foundry fever, ''the smothers'', and ''galvo'' (5–12) (see Table 90.1). Various metal oxides can cause this syndrome, but the most common ones are those of zinc, aluminum, selenium, antimony, cadmium, iron, copper, magnesium, nickel, silver, and tin (13–21) (see Table 90.2). Of welders aged 20–59 years, 31% have had metal fume fever (18). Zinc oxide is extremely volatile at relatively low temperatures, and therefore a large amount of zinc oxide fume (powder) is produced during welding on galvanized metal and in the smelting process. The zinc oxide particles formed range in size from 0.2–1 μm, and these are inhaled. The small particle size allows the zinc oxide to pass into the smaller bronchoalveolus. Typically, the syndrome begins 4–12 hours after sufficient exposure to freshly formed fumes of zinc oxide (22). It is manifested initially by a metallic taste in the mouth, dryness, and throat irritation.

The attacks have been described as resembling a flu-like illness or acute malaria (23). Subsequently, shaking chills, weakness, muscle and joint aches, sweating, and high fever occur (24). Coughing, weakness, fatigue, and shortness of breath may also be present. The episode runs its course in 24–48 hours. Leukocytosis may occur during the acute period. Physical examination may reveal rales and wheezing (5, 25). There is a temporary period of tolerance for a day or two afterward, hence the name Monday fever. There are usually no longterm complications, and many authors think that it can recur frequently without major physiologic damage; however, this is somewhat controversial (26, 27). Arterial blood gas analyses frequently show hypoxemia, depending on the severity of exposure. The chest radiograph usually is normal but, in severe exposure, may show pneumonitis or pulmonary edema. Pulmonary function studies frequently show a decrease in forced vital capacity (FVC) but rarely obstruction (28). Occasionally, the diffusing capacity of carbon monoxide is decreased (29).

INDUSTRIAL EXPOSURES

Metal fume fever occurs most commonly among welders. However, it also may occur among zinc smelters, brass solderers, brass foundry workers, chrome electroplaters, chrome welders (from hexavalent chromic oxide fumes), iron galvanizers, molten metal fabricators, metal grinders, manufacturers of steel alloys, and those who work near electric furnaces which are used to melt metals (see Table 90.3).

Welding

Welding is a process for joining metals in which adherence is produced by heating the metals to the appropriate temperature. Brazing is also a form of welding. There are a number of other similar techniques such as oxygen cutting and arc-gouging. The latter is used for removing metal. There are several types of welding (see Table 90.4).

ARC WELDING—MMA (MANUAL METAL ARC)

''Arc welding occurs when the arc electrode is brought in contact with the work piece. A high temperature arc is thus initiated between them. The heat generated by the arc is controlled by current and the length of the arc. When these two are correct, the tip of the electrode and the base metal beneath it are melted. As the electrode tip melts, globules are pinched off, passing through the arc to be deposited in the molten puddle of the base metal. At the same time, the (flux) coating also melts to stabilize the arc and provide a gaseous shield against atmospheric contamination caused by oxygen and nitrogen. The cooling liquefied flux also provides a shield against contamination of the weld bead'' (30).

MMA is a form of electric arc welding which uses a flux-coated consumable stick electrode. This is also called ''stick welding.'' The part to be welded and the consumable wire electrode represent two electrodes that are attached to an AC or DC power supply. When the electrodes are near one another, the electric arc is established. The metal bead is deposited, and joining occurs. Vaporization of the electrode constituents produces a complex particulate fume by condensation. Also, the electrode itself and the flux both produce fume. Fumes are solid particles generated by condensation from the gaseous state, generally after volatization from molten metals and often accompanied by a chemical reaction such as oxidation. Fumes flocculate and sometimes coalesce (31).

The flux-coated electrode has an antioxide effect, which

Table 90.1. Synonyms for Metal Fume Fever

''The Smothers''
''Galvo''
Welders ague
Foundry fever
Brass chills
Monday fever
Brazier's disease
Spelter shakes
Copper fever
Zinc shakes
Zinc chills

allows the welds to have physical properties equal to or exceeding those of the parent metal (30). The flux or coating materials on the electrode provide an automatic cleansing and deoxidizing action on the molten weld. As the coating burns in the arc it releases a gaseous inert atmosphere that protects the molten end of the electrode as well as the molten weld pool (30).

MMA fume consists of chains and clusters of submicron particles and glassy coated spheres up to 10 microns in diameter (32). Approximately 20% of MMA fume is deposited initially in the lungs of laboratory animals, and the balance is exhaled, depending on particle size (32).

ARC WELDING—MIG (METAL INERT GAS)

The next kind of electric arc welding uses a gas-shielded consumable wire electrode, and is called metal inert gas welding (MIG). The welding torch has a center of consumable wire. Next to this electrode on the torch is a flow of inert gas such as helium, argon, carbon dioxide, or a blend of these gases (33). This results in high metal fume concentrations. The gas is used to prevent the formation of oxides and nitrides with the weld metal, which weakens the weld ductility and tensile strength.

In MIG fume, there is no flux, and hence the fume is less complex. Chains are formed by condensation, which are submicron in diameter and may be as long as 100 μm (32). These chains are made up of oxide encapsulated metals.

Table 90.2. Metals That Cause Metal Fume Fever

Most common	Zinc, copper, brass (copper and zinc alloy), magnesium
Less common	Manganese, antimony, silver, tin, selenium, aluminum, nickel, vanadium, chromium, stainless steel, cadmium, lead, iron, cobalt, mercury, arsenic

Table 90.3. Industrial Exposures

Welders
Zinc smelters
Brass solderers
Brass foundry workers
Chrome electroplaters
Chrome welders
Galvanizers of iron
Fabricators of molten metals
Metal grinders
Electric furnace workers who melt metals
Steel alloy manufacturers

Table 90.4. Types of Welding

Arc welding
MMA (manual metal arc) or "Stick Welding;" A consumable wire electrode, flux-coated, is used
MIG (metal inert gas)
Consumable electrode with *no* flux and inert gas
Gas welding
Oxygen-fuel system generates a torch flame; flux on rod

GAS WELDING

In gas welding, the torch flame is generated by oxygen-gas as a fuel. Filler rods with flux on them release metal fumes. Electrodes may be made of stainless steel, copper, brass, bronze, aluminum, or lead. Bronze is an alloy of copper and tin to which other metallic substances, especially zinc, are sometimes added. It is hard, sonorous, and sometimes brittle. It is used for statues, bells, and cannons, the proportions of the respective ingredients being varied to meet the particular requirements. Brass, on the other hand, is a yellowish metal that is essentially an alloy of copper and zinc. The type of electrode depends upon the type of metal being welded.

ABSORPTION, METABOLISM, AND ELIMINATION

When zinc or its alloys are heated above 930°F particles of zinc up to one micron in diameter are formed (34). Trace particles less than one micron in diameter when inhaled cause the acute febrile illness known as metal fume fever. It is common in welders who work on various types of nonferrous metals or ferrous metals alloyed with or coated with other metals. Zinc fume from galvanized coatings is the commonest cause. However, aluminum, antimony, nickel, selenium, silver, and tin metal fumes are produced in all high temperature industrial operations such as welding. The submicron particles are deposited in different parts of the respiratory tract, but up to 50% of the inhaled particles are deposited in the lower regions (35). Individual variations occur depending on the breathing rate and tidal volume and whether inhalation is by nose or mouth. Metals are either stored in the lung, cleared, go to the gastrointestinal tract, or pass through the pulmonary tissues via the blood or lymph, and thus systemic absorption occurs (35). Zinc is used to retard corrosion and impart a desirable surface texture. The zinc coating (galvanizing) is applied either by dipping the metal piece in a bath of molten zinc or by electroplating (30). Because the zinc oxide is highly volatile at relatively low temperatures, operations involving molten metals and galvanized metal can produce large amounts of zinc oxide fume, which is a dense white smoke.

Exposure to *cadmium* should always be considered in the differential diagnosis of metal fume fever, because of its potential seriousness. Cadmium is a lustrous white metal and has broad industrial uses ranging from electroplating to solder used in welding and brazing (36). It is a ubiquitous trace element nonessential for human nutrition which is present in the environment, especially in sea water, drinking water, meat, certain grains, and many dairy products (37). Over 10 million pounds of cadmium are used industrially in the United States each year. The metal is used in the manufacture of electrical conductors, bearings, ceramics, pigments, vapor lamps, dental prosthetics, storage batteries, and rustproofing of tools and other steel articles, and as a component in various alloys. The photographic plating, rubber, motor, aircraft, and battery industries all use cadmium, and it is a byproduct in zinc smelting (38). It is highly resistant to corrosion. Oxyacetylene burning and welding or soldering of cadmium-containing metal is especially hazardous where ventilation is not adequate. This has become a common health hazard. For example, coppersmiths and plumbers soldering copper tubing may be heavily exposed to cadmium. Serious problems may occur without recognition, because most workers are not aware of the potential toxicity of cadmium and take no precaution (37). In addition to this, the initial symptoms are usually not severe enough to cause them to seek medical attention. The acute inhalation of cadmium fumes can cause both metal fume fever and chemical pneumonitis. Patterson described three stages of lung damage in rats after inhalation of cadmium oxide: 1) acute pulmonary edema within 24 hours and lasting 3 days, 2) proliferative interstitial pneumonitis 3–10 days after exposure with epithelial and fibroblastic proliferation in lung parenchyma, and 3) permanent lung damage consisting of perivascular and peribronchial fibrosis (39). Initially, acute exposure symptoms resemble metal fume fever, but after 24 hours, instead of improving, pulmonary edema and chemical pneumonitis occur. It may resolve over 7 days, but in 20% of the cases the dyspnea is progressive and may be accompanied by wheezing or hemoptysis; in these cases death occurs 5–7 days after exposure (35, 36, 38). After inhalation of cadmium oxide, it may take months for pulmonary function studies to return to normal. Chronic poisoning may also produce disease, including emphysema (38). The vapor pressure at its melting point (320°C) is very significant, and hence a concentration of 50,000 times the safe limit can be easily produced when cadmium is melted. The current Occupational Safety and Health Administration (OSHA) standard for cadmium dust is 200 $\mu g/m^3$ as an 8-hour TWA and 600 $\mu g/m^3$ as a maximum ceiling. The American Conference of Governmental Industrial Hygienists (ACGIH) recommended a ceiling limit for cadmium oxide fumes of 50 $\mu g/m^3$ in an 8-hour TWA standard for cadmium dust and salts (as cadmium) of 50 $\mu g/m^3$ (25). The OSHA and LTV limits for 1980 for zinc oxide and zinc chloride are 5 and 1 mg/m^3, respectively (25).

SIGNS, SYMPTOMS, AND SYNDROMES FROM TOXIC EXPOSURE

The onset of metal fume fever occurs 4–6 hours after the exposure and usually lasts less than 48 hours. The initial presenting symptoms are a metallic or sweet taste in the mouth, frequently accompanied by dryness and thirst. There is throat irritation, dyspnea with occasional coughing, and wheezing (40). On occasion, there are pleuritic chest pains and rarely paresthesias (6). A macular rash has been reported (5). Rales may be present (40).

There is occasional hoarseness, vomiting, headache, shaking chills, fever, myalgia, weakness, lethargy, sweating, and joint pain (Table 90.5). The episode runs its course in 24–48 hours, and there may be a temporary period of tolerance for a day or two afterward, hence the name Monday fever. No longterm complications are usually present, and many authors think that it can recur frequently without major physiologic damage. *Physical findings* usually reveal a low grade fever, and, while the chest may be clear, there also may be rales or wheezing present. There is usually coughing, some sweating, and rarely bradycardia or tachycardia. A macular rash rarely is present.

Laboratory: Leukocytosis usually occurs with an increase in band cells. Arterial blood gases may show hypoxemia. The chest radiograph is usually normal but may show pneumonitis or pulmonary edema after severe exposure. Pulmonary function studies may be normal or show a decrease in forced vital capacity, but rarely show an obstructive pattern. Diffusion capacity of carbon monoxide (DLCO) may be decreased. In some cases, LDH has been elevated (40). Serum zinc may be increased, and determination of urinary zinc levels is usually not

helpful. Urinary copper may be increased if copper exposure is the cause. In general, serum or urinary metal determinations are of little help in the diagnosis. There may be evidence of pulmonary shunting (5) (Table 90.6).

Since there are no specific laboratory or physical findings to establish a diagnosis, a careful history must be relied upon. The symptoms may resemble a flu-like illness, malaria, or septicemia (Table 90.7). Hence, the diagnosis may escape early detection. Frequently, because of the incubation time, symptoms occur *after work* and no medical attention is sought. The best clues to early diagnosis are a history of exposure, a metallic taste, and nasal irritation (40).

TREATMENT

The treatment of metal fume fever is supportive. Intravenous steroids may be given in severe cases, as well as intravenous theophylline and inhaled bronchodilators for wheezing. Oxygen is helpful, but antibiotics have proven to be of little value. Observation is generally recommended for a 24-hour period (Table 90.8). The pulmonary function usually reverts to normal, but on occasion may remain abnormal for long periods of time (6). There is one case report of a "disabling pneumopathy" occurring after recurrent metal fume fever (41). My-

Table 90.5. Symptoms of Metal Fume Fever

Onset—4–6 hours after exposure
Duration—less than 48 hours
Metallic or sweet taste in mouth
Nasal irritation
Mouth dryness and thirst
Throat irritation
Coughing, wheezing, chest tightness
Hemoptysis and pleuritic chest pains (rare)
Paresthesias (rare)
Joint pain
Hoarseness
Nausea and vomiting
Headache
Shaking chills
Sweating
Fever
Myalgia
Weakness
Lethargy

Table 90.6. Lab Findings

Leukocytosis
Hypoxemia on arterial blood gases
Chest radiograph—usually normal, but may show pneumonitis or pulmonary edema after severe exposure.
Spirometry—lowered FVC (restrictive); rarely obstructive
DL_{CO}—decreased
Increased LDH level
Urinary or serum metals—usually not helpful but may be elevated
Pulmonary shunting

Table 90.7. Differential Diagnosis

"Flu"
Malaria
Septicemia

ocardial and skeletal muscle injury has been reported in one case (42).

PATHOPHYSIOLOGY

The exact cause of metal fume fever is unknown. However, there have been some interesting immunologic associations, although it is generally thought that this syndrome does not have an immunologic basis because prior exposure is not required (2) (Table 90.9). One theory states that the presence of finely divided and dispersed metallic oxide in the lung destroys the microorganisms of the lower respiratory passages, thereby liberating endotoxins into the alveolar capillaries and causing an acute febrile response. Once this "sterilization" has occurred, it renders the lower respiratory tract "immune" to further fume exposure until sufficient time has elapsed for the reaccumulation of organisms (21). It has also been demonstrated in rats that the zinc particles accumulate in the alveoli and resident macrophages to result in metal fume fever and eventually pulmonary fibrosis (45).

It is well known that the macrophage produces interleukin-1 (IL-1) in a response to a variety of nonspecific stimuli including immune complexes, lipopolysaccharides, leukotrienes, and interleukin-2 (IL-2) (48). Synonyms for interleukin-1 (IL-1) include: endogenous pyrogen, hemopoietin-1, and catabolin. IL-1 is an inflammatory cytokine produced primarily by macrophages. Interleukin-1-alpha is membrane bound and Interleukin-1-beta is secreted. Therefore, IL-1 secretion's net effect is to contain invaders. It represents a primitive protective system, but too much secretion can result in disease. For example, massive infection can cause shaking chills and fever, that resemble septicemia or metal fume fever. Hence, metal fume fever may be due to the nonspecific protective action of stimulated macrophages producing IL-1. Although no one knows exactly how long it takes for the macrophage to recover after discharge, it is tempting to speculate that this time period would represent the refractory interval seen in metal fume fever.

Table 90.8. Treatment Guidelines for Exposure to Metal Fumes

Terminate exposure
Administer oxygen by mask
Supportive pulmonary care
Inhalation therapy with bronchodilators if indicated for bronchospasm
Theophylline loading and maintenance may be necessary for adjunct management of bronchospasm
Observation for 24 hours in symptomatic individuals
Corticosteroids may be helpful in severe cases
Antibiotics are of no value except in secondary infection
Check CPK and cardiac enzymes as indicated

Table 90.9. Pathophysiology

Theories

Modification of lung proteins with absorption, foreign protein reaction, endotoxins, a nonspecific response to IL-1 (19, 20, 21, 43)
Immune complex disease (29, 44)
Metal particles accumulate in alveolar macrophages and interfere with phagocytosis (45)
Hypersensitivity pneumonitis (1, 46)
Delayed IgE reaction (47)

Amdur suggested that metal fume fever was caused by a modification of lung protein due to the zinc fumes, which was then absorbed, and produced a foreign protein reaction (20, 43, 45).

Mueller suggested the possibility that immune complexes were formed resulting in the symptoms (29).

Migally demonstrated that zinc particles accumulate in the alveoli and resident macrophages and suggested that this results in metal fume fever and eventually pulmonary fibrosis (45).

Other authors have speculated that metal fume fever is possibly a form of hypersensitivity pneumonitis (1, 46). While hypersensitivity pneumonitis is a flu-like illness occurring 6–8 hours after exposure, usually to organic dust, it has been reported after exposure to cobalt and beryllium (49) (Table 90.10). It has also been reported after exposure to zinc (1, 46). The symptoms are very similar.

Hypersensitivity pneumonitis (extrinsic allergic alveolitis) represents a group of lung diseases affecting the small airways, the alveoli, and interstitium. They are caused by a variety of inhaled organic dusts, but also other causes (Table 90.10). Sensitization to the particular antigen, which may be animal or plant proteins, microorganisms, fungi, organic dust, and occasionally low molecular weight chemicals as well as metals, occurs. There are several forms: acute, subacute, and chronic. It is usually associated in the acute stage with precipitating antibodies to the particular antigen. The classic acute features begin with fever, myalgia, and lethargy 4–8 hours after exposure to the antigen. This is usually accompanied by chest tightness or wheezing, a dry cough, and dyspnea. Usually the symptoms improve within 24 hours in the absence of additional exposure. The physical exam reveals fever, tachycardia, and dyspnea. Occasionally, there are rales or wheezes, but usually auscultation of the chest is clear. Leukocytosis may occur. Pulmonary function studies reveal a restrictive defect. On repeated exposure, chronic interstitial lung disease may develop.

The chest x-ray is variable but may show a pattern that resembles pulmonary edema. There is an increase in activated T-cells in the bronchial-alveolar lavage fluid. Pathologically, there may be numerous noncaseating sarcoid-like granulomata usually associated with giant cells (2). There may be infiltration with monocytes such as lymphocytes, plasma cells, and histiocytes. Aveolar macrophages are increased. Some patients may have hypersensitivity pneumonitis and have no precipitins, and some patients have precipitins but no disease. The exact immune mechanism is unknown, although complement activation is thought to play a part, and in some cases it may be due to immune complex formation. The alternate complement pathway may be activated. However, the complete pathogenesis is not entirely understood. Hence, one can readily see the common features between hypersensitivity pneumonitis and metal fume fever.

Farrell reported a case of angioedema and urticaria as acute and late-phase reaction to zinc fume exposure (47). The patient also had associated metal fume fever-like symptoms. Hives and angioedema developed immediately and in a delayed fashion in a 34-year-old man after he had welded zinc at his job and resulted in an associated metal fume fever-like reaction, 6–8 hours later. The author found it conceivable that a delayed type IgE mechanism was involved. Mast cell degranulation in human skin causes both immediate and late-phase allergic reactions (50–52). The mediators released cause an influx of neutrophils and eosinophils at the site, which in turn initiates a more chronic inflammatory reaction of mononuclear cells

Table 90.10.   Types of Hypersensitivity Pneumonitis

Antigen	Antigen Source	Name of Disorder
Thermophilic actinomycetes		
Micropolyspora faeni	Moldy hay	Farmer's lung
	Mushroom compost	Mushroom worker's lung
Thermoactinomyces vulgaria	Moldy sugarcane	Bagassosis
	Moldy hay	Farmer's lung
	Mushroom compost	Mushroom worker's lung
Thermoactinomyces sacchari	Moldy compost	Mushroom worker's disease
	Bagasse	Bagassosis
Thermoactinomyces candidus	Contaminated home humidifier and air conditioning ducts	Humidifier lung
Thermoactinomyces viridis	Cattle	Fog fever
	Moldy cork	Suberosis
	Vineyards	Vineyard sprayer's lung
	Ventilation system	
True fungi		
Aspergillus clavatus	Moldy malt	Malt worker's lung
	Moldy barley	Farmer's lung
Aspergillus fumigatus	Moldy cheese	Cheese washer's lung
	Moldy hay	Farmer's lung
Cryptostroma corticale	Moldy maple logs	Maple bark disease
	Maple bark	Maple bark stripper's lung
Graphium sp.	Moldy wood dust (especially redwood)	Sequoiosis
Pullularia sp.	Moldy wood dust	Sequoiosis
	Water and steam	Sauna taker's lung
Alternaria sp.	Moldy wood pulp	Wood pulp worker's disease
Mucor stolonifer	Moldy paprika pods	Paprika slicer's lung
Penicillium caseii	Cheese mold	Cheese worker's lung
	Humidifier water	Humidifier lung
Cephalosporium sp.	Humidifier water	Humidifier lung
Penicillium frequentans	Moldy cork dust	Suberosis
Aspergillus versicolor		Dog house disease
Lycoperdon		Lycoperdonosis
Animal causes		
Furrier's lung		
Pigeon serum proteins	Pigeon droppings	Pigeon breeder's disease
Duck proteins	Feathers	Duck fever
Turkey proteins	Turkey products	Turkey handler's disease
Parrot serum proteins	Parrot droppings	Budgerigar fancier's disease
Chicken proteins	Chicken products	Feather plucker's disease
Bovine and porcine proteins	Pituitary snuff	Pituitary snuff taker's lung
Rat serum protein	Rat urine	
Bat serum protein	Bat droppings	Bat lung
Insect products		
Ascaris siro (mite)	Dust	
Sitophilus granarius (wheat weevil)	Contaminated grain	Miller's lung
Amoebae		
Naegleria gruberi	Contaminated water	
Acanthamoeba polyphaga	Humidifier water	Humidifier lung
Acanthamoeba castellani		
Vegetable products		
Unknown	Sawdust (redwood, maple, red cedar)	Sequoiosis
	Cereal grain	Grain measurer's lung
	Dried grass and leaves	Thatched roof disease
	Tobacco plants	Tobacco grower's disease
	Tea plants	Tea grower's disease
	Cloth wrappings of mummies	Coptic disease
Chemicals, drugs, metals		
Toluene diisocyanate	Urethane foam	
Nitrofurantoin	Iatrogenic	
Sodium cromolyn lung	Iatrogenic	
Hydrochlorothiazide	Iatrogenic	
Hard metal disease		
Zinc		
Beryllium		
Pauli's reagent lung		
Thermotolerant bacteria		
Bacillus subtilis enzymes	Detergent	Detergent worker's lung
Bacillus cereus	Humidifier water	Humidifier lung

(53). It has been postulated that basophils attracted to the site during the immediate allergic reaction rather than mast cells, are stimulated to degranulate during the late-phase reaction (54). Also, mast cells might be restimulated to release additional mediators during the late-phase reaction. Human neutrophil-derived histamine releasing activity (HRA-N) as described by White and Callender (1985) is released spontaneously by neutrophils and is capable of doing this (55). Only certain IgE molecules interact with HRA-N to produce the late-phase reaction, and this heterogeneity explains why some patients have a late-phase reaction and others do not (55, 56). Kaplan and Zelichman reported a case of a welder who developed dyspnea and hives within 15 minutes after acetylene welding with a rod containing iron, carbon, manganese, phosphorus, sulfur, silicon, chromium, and vanadium. This was proven by challenge testing. An interesting aspect of the case was that the patient had a history of metal fume fever previously, but did not develop metal fume fever symptoms after the challenge. This was also suggestive of an immunologic reaction (17).

Animal studies in metal fume fever revealed that guinea pigs exposed to the current TLV of zinc at 5 mg/m³ for 3 hours on 6 consecutive days had lung and pulmonary function changes 72 hours after exposure, but there were no similar findings after a single exposure to 8 mg/m³. Functional, morphologic, and biochemical changes indicative of an inflammatory reaction involving mainly the peripheral airways were noted (57). Infiltration of the proximal portion of the alveolar ducts in the adjacent alveoli was noted, characterized by interstitial thickening, increased pulmonary macrophages, and neutrophils. There was a mixed cellular infiltrate of macrophages, lymphocytes, and neutrophils. Pulmonary flow resistance increased and remained increased for 24 hours. Compliance decreased below the control for 48 hours, and the resistance increased. The latter was felt to be due to abnormalities in the small airways. Edema and premature closing of the small airways was thought to contribute to the decreased compliance. Lung volumes were decreased following exposure, probably due to edema and cellular infiltration. This also was felt to explain the decrease in DLCO and the resultant hypoxemia. Exposure to zinc fumes is not felt to be teratogenic or carcinogenic.

In conclusion, biologic monitoring should be undertaken as well as strict adherence to the PELs and TLVs, and adequate ventilation should be ensured to prevent metal fume fever. Cadmium chemical pneumonitis should always be considered because of its potential seriousness.

ACKNOWLEDGMENT

I thank Lark Grove for her secretarial help and typing skill in the preparation of this manuscript.

REFERENCES

1. Malo JL, Cartier JA. Occupational asthma due to fumes of galvanized metal. Chest 1987;92:375–377.
2. Morgan WKC, Seaton A. Occupational lung disease. 2nd ed. Philadelphia: W.B. Saunders Co, 1984:575.
3. McMillan G. Metal fume fever. Occup Health 1986;May:148–149.
4. Zenz C. Other metals. In: Zenc C, Occupational medicine. 2nd ed. Chicago: Year Book Medical Publishers, 1988:645–646.
5. Dula D. Metal fume fever. J Am Coll Emerg Phys 1978;7:448.
6. Anseline P. Zinc fume fever. Med J Aust 1972;2:316–318.
7. Asher F. Hamilton & Hardy's industrial toxicology. 4th ed. Littleton, Co: PSG Publishers, 1983:146–148.
8. Papp J. Metal fume fever. Postgrad Med 1968;43:160–163.
9. Stake J. Metal fume fever in ferro-chrome workers. Cent Afr J Med 1977;23:25–28.
10. Smith C. Metal fume fever—a case review. Occup Health Nurs J 1980;28:23–25.
11. Fishburn CW, Zenz C. Metal fume fever—a report of a case. J Occup Med 1969;11:142–144.
12. Hopper W. Case report—metal fume fever. Postgrad Med 1978;5:123–124.
13. Drinker P. Certain aspects of the problem of zinc toxicity. J Ind Hyg 1922;8:177–197.
14. Hammond JW. Metal fume fever in the crushed stone industry. J Ind Hyg Toxicol 1944;24:117–119.
15. Glass WI. Mercury metal fume fever. NZ Med J 1970;71:297–298.
16. Drinker K, Drinker P. Metal fume fever V—results of the inhalation by animals of zinc and magnesium oxide fumes. J Ind Hyg Toxicol 1928;10:56.
17. Kaplan I, Zelichman I. Urticaria and asthma from acetylene welding. Arch Dermatol 1963;88:188–194.
18. Ross R. Welders metal fume. J Soc Occup Med 1974;24:125–129.
19. Sayers RR. Metal fume fever and its prevention. Public Health Rep 1938;24:1080–1086.
20. Koelsch F. Metal fume fever. J Ind Hyg 1923;8:87–97.
21. Kuh J, Collen M, Kuh C. Metal fume fever. Permanente Found Med Bull 1946;4:145–151.
22. Key MM, Henschel AF, Butler J, Ligo RN, Tabershaw IR. Occupational diseases: a guide to their recognition. United States Dept. of Health, Education, and Welfare. Washington, DC: Government Printing Office 1977:408–410.
23. Doig AT, Challen PJR. Respiratory hazards in welding. Ann Occup Hyg 1964;7:223–231.
24. Sturgis CC, Drinker P, Thomson RM. Metal fume fever. Vol I. Clinical observations on the effect of the experimental inhalation of zinc oxide by two apparently normal persons. J Ind Hyg 1927;9:88–97.
25. Rom W. Environmental and occupational medicine. Boston: Little Brown and Co, 1983:503.
26. Drinker P, Thomson RM, Finn JL. Metal fume fever. Vol IV. Threshold doses of zinc oxide, preventive measures, and the chronic effects of repeated exposures. J Ind Hyg 1927;9:331–345.
27. Roto P. Asthma, symptoms of chronic bronchitis and ventilatory capacity among cobalt and zinc production workers. Scand J Work Environ Health 1980;6 (suppl 1):1–49.
28. Anthony JS, Zamel N, Aberman A. Abnormalities in pulmonary function after brief exposure to toxic metal fumes. Can Med Assoc J 1978;119:586–588.
29. Mueller EJ, Seger DL. Metal fume fever—a review. J Emerg Med 1985;2:271–274.
30. Arc electrode manual. 4th ed. Lake Zurich: Jefferson Publications:13.
31. Levy BS, Wegman DH. Occupational health. Boston: Little Brown and Co, 1983:471.
32. Hewitt PJ, Gray CN. Some difficulties in the assessment of electric arc welding fume. Am Ind Hyg Assoc J 1983;44:727–732.
33. Burgess WA. Potential exposures in industry—their recognition and control. In: Clayton G, Clayton F, eds. Patty's industrial hygiene and toxicology. New York: John Wiley & Sons, 1978:1172–1178.
34. Stokinger HE. Industrial hygiene and toxicology. 2nd ed. New York, NY: John Wiley & Sons, 1967:1183, 1186, 1187.
35. Piscator M. Health hazards from inhalation of metal fumes. Environ Res 1976;11:268–270.
36. Barnart S, Rosenstock L. Cadmium chemical pneumonitis. Chest 1984;86:789–791.
37. Johnson J, Kilburn K. Cadmium-induced metal fume fever—results of inhalation challenges. Am J Ind Med 1983;4:533–540.
38. Louria D, Joselow MM, Browder AA. The human toxicity of certain trace metals. Ann Intern Med 1972;76:307–319.
39. Patterson JC. Studies on toxicity of cadmium: pathology of cadmium poisoning in man and experimental animals. J Ind Hyg Toxicol 1947;29:294–301.
40. Armstrong CW, Moore LW, Hackler RL, Miller Jr. GB, Strouble RB. An outbreak of metal fume fever—the diagnostic use of urinary copper and zinc determinations. J Occup Med 1983;12:886–888.
41. Hartman AL, Hartman W, Buhlmann AA. Magnesium oxide as a cause of metal fume fever. Schueizerische Med Worhensch 1983;113:776–770.
42. Shusterman D, Neal E. Skeletal muscle and myocardial injury associated with metal fume fever. J Fam Pract 1986;23:159–160.
43. Amdur MO, McCarthy JF, Gill MW. Respiratory response of guinea pigs to zinc oxide fume. Am Ind Hyg J 1982;43:887–889.
44. McCord C. Metal fume fever—an immunologic disease. Ind Med Surg 1960;29:101–107.
45. Migally N, Murphy RC, Doye A, Zambernad J. Changes in pulmonary

alveolar macrophages in rats exposed to oxide of zinc and nickel. J Submicrosc Cytol 1982;14:621–626.

46. Trudeau C, Malo JL, Cartier A (Montreal, Canada). Hypersensitivity pneumonitis after exposure to zinc (Abstract #6). American Academy of Allergy and Immunology Annual Meeting 1989:173.

47. Farrell FJ. Angioedema and urticaria as acute and late-phase reaction to zinc fume exposure, with associated metal fume fever-like symptoms. Am J Ind Med 1987;12:331–337.

48. Strober W, James S. The interleukins. Pediatr Res 1988;24:111–119.

49. Mandel J, Baker B. Recognizing occupational lung disease. Hosp Pract 1989:21–30.

50. Lemanske RF, Jr., Kaliner M. Mast cell-dependent late phase reactions. Clin Immunol Rev 1981–82;1:547–548.

51. Lemanske RF, Jr, Kalinger MA. Late phase allergic reactions. Int J Dermatol 1983;22:401–409.

52. Lemanske RF, Jr, Guthman DA, Oertel H, Barr L, Kaliner M. The biologic activity of mast cell granules. Vol VI. The effect of vinblastine-induced neutropenia on rat cutaneous late phase reactions. J Immunol 1983;130:2837–2842.

53. Kaliner MA. Late phase reactions. N Engl Regional Allergy Proc 1986;7:236–240.

54. Naclerio RM, Proud D, Togias AG, et al. Inflammatory mediators in late antigen-induced rhinitis. N Engl J Med 1985;313:65–70.

55. Warner JA, Pienkowski MM, Plaut M, Norman PS, Lichtenstein LM. Identification of histamine releasing factor(s) in the late phase of cutaneous IgE-mediated reactions. J Immunol 1986;136:2583–2587.

56. Orchard MA, Kagey-Sobotka A, Proud D, Lichtenstein LM. Basophil histamine release induced by a substance from stimulated human platelets. J Immunol 1986;136:2240–2244.

57. Lam HF, Conner MW, Rogers AE, Fitzgerald S, Amdur MO. Functional and morphologic changes in the lungs of guinea pigs exposed to freshly generated ultrafine zinc oxide. Toxicol Appl Pharmacol 1978;78:29–38.

91

Organometals and Reactive Metals

Claus-Peter Siegers, M.D.
John B. Sullivan, Jr., M.D.

WATER REACTIVE AND PYROPHORIC METALS

Metals and compounds of metals that react violently with water, ignite spontaneously in air, or that are flammable, present clear health hazards. Materials that spontaneously combust on exposure to air are termed pyrophoric. Highly reactive metallic compounds include organometals and a variety of elemental metals represented by the alkali metals (lithium, potassium, sodium), metals of groups IIb of the Periodic Table (cadmium, zinc, mercury), IIIa (aluminum), IVa (lead and tin), group Va (arsenic), group IIa (magnesium), and cesium, rubidium, thorium, titanium, uranium, plutonium, and zirconium (1).

Metals that are combustion hazards in a solid state are cesium, rubidium, sodium, lithium, and potassium. Metals that are explosive and combustible when mixed with air as a dust include: aluminum, beryllium, titanium, magnesium, and cadmium (2). Hazards related to organometallic compounds and reactive metals are derived from their inherent toxicity, high degree of explosivity, and flammability when exposed to water or air and toxic byproducts of their reactions.

ORGANOMETALS

Organometals are volatile, flammable liquids with unique toxicity and high chemical reactivity. Organometals are compounds that contain a metal bound to the carbon of an organic group in the form of (1): (a) metals covalently bound to the carbon atom of an alkyl organic group, (b) alkyl or aryl metallic compounds of electropositive metals forming an ionic compound, (c) compounds containing metals that are bound to aromatic rings, alkenes, or alkynes. The organic group attached to a metal atom depends on the valence state of the metal. Carbonyl compounds contain the carbonyl group, $C = O$, which imparts increased acidity and also provides a site for nucleophilic addition (3). The activity of a carbonyl group toward nucleophils is due to the presence of the oxygen in the carbonyl group which imparts a tendency for a negative charge (3).

Organometals are hazardous materials due to their toxicity and highly reactive, combustible properties. Those compounds that are relevant as environmental and occupational human health risks are listed in Table 91.1. As a group, organometallic toxicity is due to interaction with sulfhydryl (SH) groups. Also, most of these compounds are highly reactive with water in addition to being pyrophoric.

The clinical toxicity of organometals differs markedly from their inorganic counterparts. Due to the organic nature of these compounds they can penetrate the central nervous system. The shorter chain alkyl organometallic compounds appear to be more toxic than the longer chain compounds. Also, the body may metabolize these substances differently, attempting to cleave the metal-carbon bond. An example of this is given by the alkylmercury compound in which methylmercury is much more

stable than ethylmercury. The conversion of methylmercury to the inorganic mercury does not appear to be a mechanism of toxicity of this compound. The aryl and alkoxyalkylmercury compounds are less toxic than the alkyl compound due to their conversion to inorganic mercury.

The toxicity of the metal in question can be altered by the ligand formation. As the organometal is absorbed systematically, it must dissociate into the free cation or exist in its complexed form.

Organometals are used in a variety of chemical reactions in synthetic procedures as well as in polymerization reactions. There are approximately 50 organometallic compounds commercially used. The Department of Transportation lists organometals as hazardous materials for transportation under the classification of pyrophoric liquids or solids (2). Most organometals are shipped as regulated hazardous materials. As an example, organoaluminum compounds all react violently with water. Tetraethyllead (C_2H_5) is a flammable liquid but does not react with water. Due to the fact that most organometallic compounds are pyrophoric liquids, they are shipped as solutions in organic solvents.

Diethyl zinc and ethyl sodium react with water to produce ethane, a very flammable gas. Water reactive organometallic compounds such as ethyl sodium and the organoaluminum compounds increase a fire's intensity when water is applied (2). Carbon dioxide is usually employed to extinguish fires involving organometallic compounds. Also, sand or graphite can be used to help extinguish organometallic fires (2).

ORGANOLEAD COMPOUNDS

Sources, Production, and Exposure

Tetraethyllead, also known as tetraethylplumbane or lead tetraethyl, has a formula of $C_8H_{20}Pb$ and a molecular weight of 323.45. Tetraethyllead does not occur naturally. It is prepared by the reaction of $PbCl_2$, with ethyl zinc or Grignard reagent, by heating C_2H_5Cl and sodium-lead alloy in an autoclave (4–7). Tetraethyllead can also be produced from ethylene and hydrogen using triethylaluminum. Alternate syntheses use nonhalide compounds.

Tetraethyllead is a colorless, flammable liquid which burns with an orange-colored flame with a green margin. It is insoluble in water and soluble in benzene, ether, and gasoline, and slightly soluble in alcohol. It does not react with water. The tetraalkyllead compounds tetraethyllead and tetramethyllead are used as a gasoline additive to prevent "knocking" in motors.

Exposure to tetraethyllead is greatest for workers in refineries and gas stations and for mechanics and other members of the automobile industry. Ubiquitous exposure results from gasoline exhaust.

Table 91.1. Organometals

Organometal	Physiochemical Properties and Reactivity
Nickel carbonyl (C_4NiO_4)	Colorless, volatile liquid; oxidizes in air and is explosive
Tetraethyllead (C_8H_20Pb)	Flammable colorless liquid, not pyrophoric, does not react with water
Methyl mercury (C_2H_6Hg)	Colorless, volatile, flammable liquid; insoluble in water
Iron pentacarbonyl (C_5FeO_5)	Colorless to yellow, oily liquid; pyrophoric in air; insoluble in water
Trimethylaluminum $Al(CH_3)_3$	Liquid which undergoes spontaneous combustion in air, explosive, decomposes violently in water
Tri(isobutyl)aluminum $Al(C_4H_9)_3$	Colorless liquid; unstable above 165°F; pyrophoric, violently reacts with water
Triethylaluminum $AL(C_2H_5)_3$	Colorless liquid; ignites when exposed to air; reacts violently with water; used as incendiary munition
Chlorodiethylaluminum $(C_2H_5)_2AlCl$	Colorless to light volatile liquid; ignites when exposed to air; reacts violently with water to form HCl gas and aluminum oxide
Ethyldichloroaluminum $AL(C_2H_5)_2 Cl_2$	Colorless volatile liquid; ignites when exposed to air; reacts violently with water to form HCl gas, aluminum oxide
Dimethylcadmium $(CH_3)_2 Cd$	Colorless liquid; explosive and decomposes above 212°F; pyrophoric and decomposes in water
Tetramethyltin $Sn(CH_3)_4$	Colorless liquid, highly volatile, insoluble in water; thermally stable up to 750°F
Diethylzinc $(C_2H_5)_2Zn$	Highly flammable in air; extremely disagreeable odor; highly reactive with water
Ethylsodium (C_2H_5Na)	Highly reactive with water and forms flammable ethane
Dimethylarsine Chloride $(CH_3)_2 ASCl$	Highly flammable, colorless liquid; produces highly toxic vapor on exposure to air; offensive odor
Tributyltin $SN (C_4H_9)_3H$	Highly irritating to skin, eyes, and mucous membranes; can produce chemical burns on prolonged contact
Dibutyltin $SN (C_4H_9)_2H_2$	Thymic atrophy in animal studies; immunotoxin; reactive with water and can produce chemical burns
Trimethyltin $Sn (CH_3)_3H$	Reactive with water; colorless liquid; may produce chemical burns on contact
Triphenyltin $SN (C_6H_5)_3$	Colorless liquid; reactive with water
Tetraphenyltin $SN (C_6H_5)_4$	Colorless liquid; minimal fire hazard
Diethyltin $SN (C_2H_5)_2H_2$	Colorless liquid; reactive with water; thymic atrophy in animal studies; immunotoxin
Ethyl lithium C_2H_5Li	Colorless liquid; violently reacts with water to generate heat and LiOH; spontaneously flammable in air
Phenyl lithium C_6H_5Li	Colorless liquid; reacts violently with water to form LiOH and heat; spontaneously flammable in air
Methyllithium CH_3Li	Colorless liquid; spontaneously flammable in air; reacts violently with water to form heat plus LiOH
Trimethylphosphine $(CH_3)_3P$	Spontaneously flammable in air

Clinical Toxicology

The toxic effects and organ distribution of alkyllead compounds are different from those of inorganic lead. Tetraethyllead and tetramethyllead are rapidly dealkylated by the liver to the tri- alkyl metabolites which are responsible for clinical toxicity. The trialkyl intermediates are only slowly biodegraded to inorganic lead (8–11).

In contrast to inorganic lead, the alkyl compounds are rapidly absorbed by inhalation or by the intact skin and distributed to the central nervous system. Inhalational abuse of leaded fuel is a cause of alkyllead-induced encephalopathy (8–11).

Symptoms of Toxic Exposure

The toxic effects of alkyllead in the form of trimethyl or triethyl compounds present as neuropsychiatric or neurobehavioral manifestations as compared with inorganic lead. Acute intoxication is characterized by symptoms of hallucinations, delusions, excitement, or insomnia, which may progress to convulsions and delirium in fatal cases (8–11). Alopecia may also occur in some cases. Toxic effects of chronic exposure to alkyllead are similar to those of inorganic lead compounds (8–11).

Management of Toxicity

Treatment of organolead intoxication includes the administration of metal chelating agents which increase urinary lead excretion. However, chelation therapy may not influence central nervous system symptoms.

Oral ingestion of fuel containing tetraethylead must be treated as an ingestion of organic solvents. Pulmonary aspiration may occur secondary to ingestion. Gastric lavage should only be attempted if the airway can be adequately protected with a cuffed endotracheal tube. Cathartics may aid in gastrointestinal elimination acutely.

Biologic monitoring of environmental or occupational exposure to alkyllead compounds is the same as for inorganic lead.

ORGANOMERCURY COMPOUNDS

Sources, Production, and Exposure

Methylmercury (dimethylmercury) has a chemical formula of C_2H_6Hg and a molecular weight of 230.66.

Dimethylmercury is an environmental contaminant found together with monomethyl mercury compounds in fish and birds (12, 13). Dimethylmercury is a colorless, volatile, flammable liquid. It is soluble in ether and alcohol and insoluble in water. Methylmercury is the most toxicologically important organomercury compound. Other members of these compounds include ethylmercury, phenylmercury, and the alkoxyalkylmercury compounds.

Exposure to organic mercury results from handling alkylmercury-containing fungicides in the agricultural industry, medical use of alkylmercury-containing ointments or diuretics which are obsolete, or from food, mainly fish contaminated with organomercurial fungicides as a result of enrichment in the food chain (12–14).

Clinical Toxicology

Inhalation of alkylmercury vapor is the main cause of acute intoxication. Chronic exposure results from ingestion of alkylmercury-contaminated food.

In contrast to elemental mercury, organic mercury compounds are rapidly and completely absorbed by the lungs, gastrointestinal tract, and the skin because of their high lipid solubility. The absorption of methylmercury, even mixed with food, is about 95% in adults.

A major difference among the organomercurials is that the

stability of the carbon-mercury bond in vivo varies considerably. Thus, the alkylmercury compounds are much more resistant to biodegradation than either phenylmercury or alkoxyalkylmercuric compounds.

The biodistribution of organic mercury compounds, in particular short-chain alkylmercuries, is unlike that of inorganic mercury. Although both forms of mercury distribute preferentially to the kidney, the concentration in brain and blood is substantially higher for methylmercury. As a consequence, toxic manifestations of inorganic mercury are renal, whereas those for methylmercury are referable to the central nervous system.

Methylmercury is eliminated mainly in the feces as a result of biliary excretion and exfoliation of intestinal epithelial cells. Intestinal reabsorption occurs due to hepatobiliary recirculation. The enterohepatic recirculation of methylmercury can be interrupted by the oral application of a polythiol resin, which increases fecal excretion.

Symptoms of Toxic Exposure

The highest concentration of mercury occurs in the kidney, regardless of the chemical form of exposure. However, the kidney is the primary target organ for toxicity only in the case of inorganic mercury. The toxic effects of exposure to short-chain alkylmercury compounds is on the central nervous system. Central nervous system toxicity includes tremors, confusion, hallucinations, and delusional activity (15–18).

Tremor is also seen in inorganic mercury toxicity. Neuropsychiatric symptoms occur in methylmercury intoxication as well as in toxicity from inorganic mercury. Symptoms also include paresthesias and visual field constriction. At higher exposure levels, other sensory defects occur, such as loss of hearing and vestibular function and defects in smell and taste. Other neurologic effects of toxic exposure to methylmercury are incoordination, paralysis, and abnormal reflexes (15–18). Moreoever, behavioral abnormalities, including spontaneous fits of laughter and crying as well as intellectual deterioration, are specific for methylmercury poisoning (15–18).

Mercury readily crosses the placenta into the fetal tissue regardless of the chemical form of exposure. Fetal intoxication by way of the mother has been documented in cases of methylmercury poisoning (19).

Management of Toxicity

Metal chelating agents can be used to aid in elimination of mercury. Dimercaprol (BAL) is contraindicated in organic mercury intoxication, because it favors the uptake of mercury into the brain. D-Penicillamine, or better, its N-acetyl derivative, has been recommended as more effective and less toxic in the treatment of methylmercury poisoning. The more water-soluble and less toxic derivative of dimercaprol, 2,3-dimercapto-1-propanesulfonate (DMPS), has been shown to be more effective in methylmercury poisoning than several other chelators currently used. 2,3-Dimercaptosuccinic acid (DMSA) is also efficacious as a chelator in treating toxicity from mercury. DMPS was used to treat the 1971 victims of methylmercury poisoning in Iraq (20). The half-life of methylmercury was 10 days during DMPS therapy, as opposed to 26 days for those receiving D-penicillamine and 17 days for those receiving N-acetyl-DL-penicillamine (20).

In measurements of the half-life of methylmercury in blood, the fastest elimination rate was achieved by DMPS. Despite being effective in removing mercury from the blood, the clinical efficacy of chelators in the treatment of methylmercury poisoning that results in a neuropsychiatric syndrome is not very impressive. However, therapy is recommended.

ORGANOALUMINUM COMPOUNDS

Sources, Production, and Exposure

Organoaluminum compounds include trimethylaluminum, triethylaluminum, triisobutylaluminum, chlorodiethylaluminum, and dichloroethylaluminum. Trialkylaluminum compounds are colorless liquids at room temperature, sensitive to oxidation and hydrolysis in air, are very reactive when exposed to water, and are used as incendiary agents for military purposes.

Alkylaluminum halides of industrial importance are chlorodiethylaluminum and dichloroethylaluminum. The halides are colorless, volatile liquids or low-melting solids; they are less sensitive to oxidation upon exposure to air. The halogen aluminum bonds are cleaved by water and alcohol. Alkylaluminum compounds are used as catalysts in polymerization processes and occur as intermediates in organic syntheses. Exposure to alkyl aluminum may occur in workers by inhalation or dermal contact. The trialkylaluminum compounds are pulmonary irritants following inhalation and are corrosive to the skin and mucosal membranes.

Symptoms of Toxic Exposure

Dermal or mucosal contact with trialkylaluminum can cause severe corrosive injury. Following inhalation of vapor, irritation of the bronchoalveolar mucosa occurs. In severe cases pulmonary edema may develop, often after a delay of several days.

After eye contact, immediate rinsing with clear water is necessary to prevent ocular injury. Pulmonary toxicity is managed symptomatically.

ORGANOARSENIC COMPOUNDS

Sources, Production, and Exposure

These include dimethylarsine (also known as cacodyl, from the Greek word "caco" meaning bad or ill), cacodylic acid, arsenic trimethyl, aryl and alkylarsenic halides, and arsenphenolamine. Dimethylarsine is a highly flammable, colorless liquid that produces a highly toxic vapor with an offensive odor on exposure to air.

Arsenphenolamine (arsaminol, arsphenamine, Salversan) was historically used as an antisyphilitic drug and is no longer a therapy. It is a light yellow, hygroscopic powder. It oxidizes on exposure to air, becoming darker and more toxic.

Diphenylchloroarsine (Clark I), diphenylcyanarsine (Clark II), methyldichloroarsine, ethyldichloroarsine, bis(2-chlorovinyl)chloroarsine (Lewisite), and bis(2-chloroethyl)sulfide (Lost) were used in World War I as poison gases. Among the cacodyls, hydroxydimethylarsine oxide has been used as an herbicide.

Arsenical poison gases for military use are condemned by most nations of the world; nevertheless, exposure might be possible during the production of such gases, in handling, or in decontamination of hazardous worksites. Cacodylic acid and its salts used as herbicides may give rise to intoxications following inhalation or dermal contact.

Clinical Toxicology

Acute intoxication is a result of inhalation of arsenic-containing poison gases. Chronic exposure to alkylarsenic compounds can result from ingestion of food contaminated with herbicides. Inhalation of arsenical gases produces immediate irritation of the bronchoalveolar mucosa and, in severe cases, the development of acute pulmonary edema. Dermal and ocular injury also occur with blistering of the skin. Arsenical gases have a garlic-like odor and are less toxic than the arsenic halides. Chronic exposure to arsenical gases in herbicide-contaminated food intake may give rise to symptoms of chronic arsenic intoxication: gastrointestinal disorders, paresthesias, rashes, hyperpigmentation, peripheral neuropathy, and blood dyscrasias.

Management of Toxicity

Acute intoxication with arsenical gases or cacodyls are managed similarly to other pulmonary irritants. Drug therapy of acute or chronic poisoning with organic arsenicals is the same as with inorganic arsenic compounds. Dimercaprol (BAL), 2,3-dimercaptosuccinic acid (DMSA), and 2,3-dimercaptopropane-1-sulfonate (DMPS) are effective in therapeutic chelators.

NICKEL CARBONYL

Sources, Production, and Exposure

Nickel tetracarbonyl has a molecular weight of 170.73 and a chemical formula of $Ni(CO)_4$. It is a colorless, yellow to clear volatile liquid which oxidizes in the air and can ignite. It is soluble in alcohol, benzene, chloroform, acetone, and carbon tetrachloride. Nickel carbonyl is highly flammable and volatilizes at room temperature (21). Nickel carbonyl is formed by nickel or its compounds in the presence of carbon monoxide; it is an intermediate in nickel refining. It is shipped in compressed gas cylinders. It reacts with oxidizers, chlorine, nitric acid, oxygen, butane, and explosively with liquid bromine. Its vapor is heavier than air and can travel along floors to ignition sources (vapor density = 5.9) (21).

Occupational exposure to nickel carbonyl may occur during the process of refining nickel. The routes of exposure are mainly inhalation and absorption of the liquid following dermal contact. Nickel carbonyl and its vapor is decomposed by heat to carbon monoxide and nickel. Nickel carbonyl is highly explosive, and vapors in air can explode at 20°C (21). Vapors can explode in a closed space, and containers can explode if heated (21). Nickel carbonyl reacts slowly with air to produce nickel oxide.

Clinical Toxicology

Following inhalation, nickel carbonyl is rapidly absorbed by the lung and binds to erythrocytes and plasma albumin. It is distributed to various tissues, including muscle, fat, bones, connective tissue, intestine, liver, brain, and blood (21, 22). After dietary exposure, excretion of nickel is mainly in the feces. Inhalation of nickel carbonyl results in the appearance of high amounts of urinary nickel; only minor amounts appear in the stools. Biodegradation of nickel carbonyl to nickel and carbon monoxide is important with respect to symptoms of toxicity after exposure. Nickel carbonyl has a musty odor with an odor threshold of 1 ppm. The OSHA permissible exposure limit (PEL) is 0.001 ppm. This is also the concentration that is immediately dangerous to life and health (IDLH) (21).

Nickel carbonyl is the most toxic of the nickel compounds. An atmospheric exposure of 30 ppm for 30 minutes has been estimated to be lethal in humans (21–23). Initial symptoms of toxicity are giddiness, headache, vomiting, and shortness of breath. Delayed symptoms occurring in 12–24 hours are dyspnea, cyanosis, leukocytosis, hyperthermia, and acute chemical pneumonitis (21–23). Delirium and other central nervous symptoms may also appear. Death from a toxic exposure may occur between 2 and 13 days (21–23). Pathotoxicologic alterations found in the lungs include interstitial edema, fibroblast immigration, and capillary injury. Hepatic injury can also occur (21–23). Vapors are irritating to the eyes and mucous membranes. Dermal contact with the liquid can produce dermatitis and burns resulting in absorption of the compound and systemic toxicity (21–23).

Chronic exposure to nickel carbonyl has been implicated in cancer of the lungs and nose. These epidemiologic findings have been confirmed by inhalation exposure in experimental animals. Tobacco smoke may also contain significant amounts of nickel carbonyl.

An increased incidence of carcinomas of the lungs in nickel carbonyl-exposed workers has been detected only in England and was not confirmed by epidemiological data from other countries (Germany, United States, Canada, France, Finland, Soviet Union). This has been explained by a coexposure of workers in England to arsenic-containing sulfuric acid. However, based on the experimental data, nickel carbonyl must be classified as carcinogenic for humans. It is likely that nickel itself is carcinogenic and not just in its carbonyl state.

The increase of nickel in the urine has been used clinically to confirm an exposure (24). Urinary concentrations above 0.5 mg/l are considered to be serious. Monitoring of carboxyhemoglobin in blood may also be relevant to explain signs of toxicity, since nickel carbonyl is metabolized to carbon monoxide (24).

Management of Toxicity

Acute intoxication with nickel carbonyl can be managed by metal complexing agents like dimercaprol or, better, diethyldithiocarbamate trihydrate (dithiocarb) (25, 26). Daily oral doses of 25–50 mg/kg dithiocarb or 3 mg/kg dimercaprol every 4 hours are recommended in cases of severe intoxication (25, 26). Otherwise, management is symptomatic.

Nickel carbonyl exposure can be monitored by measuring urinary levels of nickel (>0.5 mg/l); environmental exposure is monitored by gas detector tubes.

IRON PENTACARBONYL

Sources, Production, and Exposure

Iron carbonyl (pentacarbonyliron), C_5FeO_5, has a molecular weight of 195.90 and is a colorless yellow oily liquid. It is pyrophoric in air and burns to F_2O_3 and decomposes by light to $Fe_2(CO)_9$ and CO. It is practically insoluble in water, readily soluble in most organic solvents (ether, acetone, ethyl acetate), and slightly soluble in alcohol.

Iron carbonyl is prepared from iron, iron compounds, and CO. Iron carbonyl is used in the manufacture of powdered iron cores for high frequency coils used in the radio and television industry. It is also used as an antiknock agent in motor fuels and as a catalyst in organic reactions.

The risk of exposure to iron pentacarbonyl is mainly for workers in the chemical industry. Routes of exposure are by inhalation or dermal contact. As a lipid-soluble compound it is rapidly absorbed and may decompose to iron and carbon monoxide.

Clinical Toxicology

Acute toxicity of iron pentacarbonyl is similar to that of nickel carbonyl. Chronic exposure may result in iron overload with the consequence of secondary hemochromatosis. Iron pentacarbonyl as a lipophilic compound is rapidly absorbed after dermal contact.

Iron pentacarbonyl is a pulmonary irritant and can produce pulmonary edema on inhalation. It also affects the central nervous system and may cause liver and kidney damage.

Management of Toxicity

In acute intoxication, the treatment of pulmonary edema and shock is of primary importance. Iron overload may be reduced by treatment with desferoxamine, an iron-chelating agent. The intravenous dose should not exceed 15 mg/kg/hour. Environmental or occupational exposure to iron pentacarbonyl is monitored by gas detector tubes. The exposure TLV is 0.1 ppm with a short term exposure limit (STEL) of 0.2 ppm.

ORGANOTIN COMPOUNDS

Organotin toxicity ranges from the very toxic trialkyltins to the lesser toxic dialkyl and monoalkyltin compounds. Tributyltin is a fungicide used in exterior paint (27). Tributyltin oxide is both a solid and a liquid, and human exposures can occur from inhalation as well as skin absorption. The organotin compounds produce irritation of the eyes, mucous membranes, throat, and skin (28).

Exposure to tributyltin can produce irritation of the eyes, throat, conjunctivitis, and mucous membrane. Dermal contact of a solution or a solid can produce chemical burns and necrosis (27, 28).

Tributyltin has been shown to cause immunosuppression, anemia, and weight loss in animals. Due to the toxic effects of tributyltin, it is used as a biocide in exterior paints only, not in interior paints (27, 29).

The organotin compounds are biocides in many products and processes that require preservation such as wood, leather, paper, paint, and textiles (27). Tributyltin, triphenyltin, and tetraorganotin are incompatible with strong oxidizers. All organotin compounds, especially tributyl and dibutyltins, produce severe dermal injury and burns. Intense itching, inflammation, and erythema can occur upon exposure. The lesions that develop are generally diffuse, erythematous, and heal quickly after exposure is terminated. Exposure to the eyes can produce lacrimation, conjunctivitis, and conjunctival edema (28, 30, 31).

Trialkyl and tetra alkyltin compounds are neurotoxic and can cause headache, dizziness, photophobia, vomiting, muscle weakness, and flaccid paralysis (30, 31). Triphenyltin is a hepatotoxin (31). The typical organotins are triethyltin, dibutyltin, tributyltin, and triphenyltin. These compounds are in the form of triethyltin iodide, dibutyltin chloride, tributyltin chloride, triphenyltin acetate, and bistributyltin oxide. Trimethyltin and triethyltin are the most toxic of alkyltin compounds and produce specific neurotoxicity (28, 30, 31). Animals receiving injections of trialkyltin compounds develop aggressive behavior within 48 hours of dosing (31). Lesions are found in the hippocampus, pyriform cortex, amygdaloid nucleus, and cortex (31). In addition to aggressive behavior, animals developed irritability and tremor (31). Cerebral edema occurs in some animals following dosing with triethyltin (31).

Triethyltin can produce neurological symptoms of severe headache, vertigo, photophobia, visual disturbances, abdominal pain and vomiting, urinary retention, paralysis, and psychic disturbances upon ingestion (28, 30, 31). Persistent neurological sequelae include diminished visual acuity, focal anesthesia, flaccid paralysis, incontinence, and cerebral edema.

Triphenyltin is a hepatotoxin and in some occupational exposures has produced hepatic damage with hepatomegaly and elevated liver enzymes (31). Triphenyltin is also a dermal irritant and can produce other effects such as headache, nausea, vomiting, and blurred vision on toxic exposure (28).

Trimethyltin has produced hyperexcitability, and neurologic and behavioral changes in animals, as well as seizures in some animal studies. In humans, triemthyltin toxicity has been manifested with memory loss, anorexia, confusion, decreased vigilance, disorientation, and seizures (28, 30, 31).

The organotin compounds are known to have immunotoxic properties in animals (29). Dialkyltin compounds produce decreased thymus weight and decrease in thymocytes in animals administered the compound. Trimethyltin dichloride has shown histopathologic changes in the organ weight of the thymus and spleen of 50–60% (29). Also, in animal studies, there was a decrease in T-cell dependent antibody response and B-cell lymphocyte proliferation of 60–80% (29). In addition, trimethyltin affected cellular immunity and was shown to have an 80% decrease in T-lymphocyte proliferation from mitogen stimulation (29). Tributyltin has immunotoxic effects in animal species. Rats fed tributyltin oxide orally showed decreases in the lymphoid organ weight such as the thymus (thymic atrophy) and spleen as well as decrease in white blood cell count and decreased lymphocyte counts. Animals fed triphenyltin also show immunotoxic effects such as decreases in the weight of thymus, spleen, and lymph nodes as well as a decrease in B-cell lymphocyte proliferation, delayed hypersensitivity reactions, and decrease in T-cell lymphocyte proliferation response to mitogen, as well as a decreased host resistance (27, 29).

REACTIVE METALS

Many elemental metals are highly reactive with air or water and explode, combust, or release hazardous byproducts of their reaction. In addition to their intrinsic toxicity, health hazards from these compounds occur due to their reactivity (2). Table 91.2 summarizes hazard properties of these metals.

Alkali Metals

The alkali metals of sodium, potassium, and lithium are highly reactive. These three metals are used extensively in industry and have multiple commercial applications. The general chemical reactivity characteristics of the alkali metals are:

—They react violently with water and generate hydrogen gas which may combust or explode, thus intensifying a fire.

—They may spontaneously combust on contact with air.

—They react with halogenated hydrocarbons to further combustion.

—They react with carbon dioxide.

—Their byproducts of combustion are highly toxic and extremely caustic.

Sodium and potassium are much more reactive compared to lithium. When lithium burns, it does so with an intense white flame and generates lithium oxide. If water is applied to burning lithium, an explosive reaction occurs due to generation of highly flammable hydrogen gas. Lithium also reacts with nitrogen gas (2).

Sodium, used in numerous synthetic processes, can spontaneously ignite in air at room temperature. Exposed to air, sodium becomes gray-white in color due to the deposition of a coating of sodium hydroxide and sodium oxide. Sodium hydroxide absorbes moisture from the air which can lead to combustion of the metal (2). On contact with water, sodium violently decomposes and rapidly generates explosive hydrogen gas and sodium hydroxide. Sodium burns with a yellow flame in air to form sodium oxide and burns in pure oxygen to form sodium peroxide (2). Sodium oxides are strong irritants to eyes, mucous membranes, and respiratory tract.

Potassium is a silvery-white metal that is more reactive than sodium (2). Potassium will spontaneously ignite in room air at room temperatures. It burns with a violet flame. This combustion releases toxic potassium oxide (K_2O) and potassium peroxide (K_2O_2) (2). Potassium explodes on contact with liquid bromine. Potassium violently reacts with water in an explosive manner to form potassium hydroxide (KOH) and hydrogen gas. Potassium forms superoxide on contact with pure oxygen (KO_2) which hydrolyzes to oxygen and hydrogen peroxide as well as KOH. The superoxide of potassium will react explosively with organic solvents and other organic matter (2).

Cesium and Cerium

Cesium is one of the most reactive of all metals and will combust on contact with air. Cesium reacts explosively with cold water, generating combustible hydrogen gas. Cesium is a highly caustic metal and will cause necrosis of all tissues on contact. It burns without a visible flame (2, 32). Cerium will ignite if scratched and can rapidly decompose in hot water.

Sodium-Potassium Alloy

A metal alloy of sodium-potassium (NAK) forms a very unstable compound and has been used as an effective heat exchange medium in nuclear reactors (2). This alloy reacts violently with air, water, halogenated hydrocarbons, and carbon dioxide. NAK alloy in contact with organic matter creates an explosive combination.

Rubidium and Plutonium

Other pyrophoric metals igniting spontaneously in air are rubidium and plutonium (2, 32). Rubidium reacts violently with water, forming caustic byproducts that can cause tissue necrosis on contact. Rubidium can be liquid at room temperature and is a soft, silver-white metal. Rubidium forms four oxides: Rb_2O, Rb_2O_2, RB_2O_3, Rb_2O_4 (32). Rubidium is easily ionized, and both cesium and rubidium are considered for use in "ion-engines" for space travel (32). Naturally occurring rubidium contains Rb^{87}, a β particle emitter with a half-life of 5×10^{11} years.

Table 91.2.   Reactive Metals

Metal	Physiochemical Properties and Reactivity
Aluminum (Al)	Atomic weight 26.98, atomic number 13, M.P. 660.37°C. Pure aluminum is a silvery-white metal with high thermal conductivity and corrosion resistance. It is flammable in dust state, powder, or flakes. Dust suspended in air can explode. Aluminum dust in contact with carbon tetrachloride can explode. When mixed with water, burning aluminum generates explosive hydrogen gas.
Antimony (Sb)	Atomic weight 121.75, atomic number 51, M.P. 630.74°C. The explosive form of Sb contains small amounts of halogens. It is a poor thermal conductor. It is a blue-silvery, brittle, white metal and burns with a blue flame. In a molten condition, antimony will react with water and release hydrogen which then reacts with the antimony to form toxic stibine vapors (SbH_3). When heated, it releases toxic stibine fumes and stibine oxide (Sb_2O_3).
Beryllium (Be)	Atomic weight 9.012, atomic number 4, M.P. 1278°C. Very light metal. Metal powder can be explosive in air. Dust can produce acute and chronic pulmonary injury.
Boron (B)	Atomic weight 10.81, atomic number 5, M.P. 2079.9°C. Sublimes at 2550°C. Amorphous boron is used in pyrotechnic flares and burns with a green flame. Used as an ignition source in rockets.
Cadmium (Cd)	Atomic weight 112.41, atomic number 48, M.P. 320.9°C. Soft, bluish-white metal, easily cut. Metal dusts of cadmium mixed with air can be explosive. Cadmium dust inhalation can cause acute and chronic pulmonary disease.
Cerium (Ce)	Atomic weight 140.12, atomic number 58, M.P. 799°C. A very abundant rare earth metal. It is an iron-gray metal. Decomposes rapidly in hot water and slowly in cold water. Pure cerium can ignite if scratched. Cerium is used in "self-cleaning" ovens, glass manufacturing, glass polishing, carbon-arc lighting, and in nuclear industry.
Cesium (Cs)	Atomic weight 132.90, atomic number 55, M.P. 28.4°C. Silvery, soft metal. Very alkaline element. It has a high affinity for O_2. Cesium hydroxide is the strongest base known. Used in atomic clocks and rocket propulsion. Highly reactive metal with air (pyrophoric) or water. Reacts explosively with cold water and generates hydrogen and burns without a flame. Very caustic to tissue and will produce rapid tissue necrosis on contact.
Lithium (Li)	Atomic weight 6.941, atomic number 3, M.P. 180.54°C. Soft silvery metal. Very light in weight and floats in hydrocarbon solvents. Reacts with water to evolve hydrogen. Requires an ignition source due to absorption of heat and hydrolysis by lithium metal. The pure metal does not react spontaneously in air. Lithium reacts with oxygen in air at 400°F (200°C) to form lithium oxide (Li_2O). Lithium combines directly with nitrogen to form lithium nitride (Li_3N). At its melting point, lithium ignites and burns with a very intense white flame. Burning lithium will react violently and explosively with water to form lithium hydroxide. Lithium burns in air, nitrogen, carbon dioxide.
Magnesium (Mg)	Atomic weight 24.305, atomic number 12, M.P. 648.8°C. Light, silvery-white metal. In the dust form, it can explode on contact with ignition source. Magnesium chips and ribbons ignite easily. Water applied to burning magnesium will cause an explosive reaction due to the release of hydrogen gas.
Potassium (K)	Atomic weight 39.09, Atomic number 19, M.P. 63.25°C. Silvery-white metal. More reactive than sodium. Reacts explosively on contact with water and generates hydrogen and KOH. To prevent reaction in air, potassium is stored in a hydrocarbon such as kerosene. Burns in air at room temperature with purple flame producing K_2O and K_2O_2. Forms superoxide on contact with pure oxygen (KO2). The potassium superoxide can detonate on contact with organic solvents and organic matter.
Plutonium (Pu)	Atomic weight 244, atomic number 94, M.P. 641°C. Isotope Pu^{239} has a half-life of 24,900 years. Plutonium is a product of nuclear reactions involving uranium. Plutonium is extremely hazardous due to its emission of alpha particles. Plutonium is absorbed by bone marrow. Plutonium is warm to the touch due to its intense alpha decay. The metal releases enough heat to boil water. It can cause tissue necrosis on contact.
Rubidium (Rb)	Atomic weight 85.46, atomic number 37, M.P. 38.89°C. Soft, silvery-white metal with high degree of electropositivity. It is the second most alkaline element. Ignites spontaneously in air. It reacts violently with water and liberates hydrogen which combusts. Rubidium reaction with water forms caustic hydroxides that can cause tissue necrosis on contact.
Ruthenium (Ru)	Atomic weight 101.07, atomic number 44, M.P. 2310°C. Hard, white metal. Does not react with cold or hot acids. However, will explode when mixed with potassium chlorates. Used as a metal hardener.
Sodium (Na)	Atomic weight 22.98, atomic number 11, M.P. 97.81°C. Waxy appearing silver metal. Exposed to air, sodium becomes coated with a gray layer of sodium hydroxide and sodium oxide which can absorb moisture, thus causing combustion. Sodium can spontaneously ignite in room air and at room temperature. Exposure to water produces an explosive combustion releasing hydrogen gas.
Strontium (Sr)	Atomic weight 87.62, atomic number 38, M.P. 769°C. Strontium is stored in kerosene to prevent oxidation. It is a silvery metal that turns yellow in air forming an oxide. Metal dust in air spontaneously ignites. Strontium salts are used in pyrotechnics to produce a crimson color. Strontium[90] is a product of nuclear fallout with a half-life of 28 years and is a radiological health hazard.
Sulfur (S)	Atomic weight 37.06, atomic number 16, M.P. 112.8°C. Light yellow, brittle solid. Sulfur can be in a crystalline form or amphorous form. A component of black gunpowder. Sulfur dust in air can ignite and explode.
Tellurium (Te)	Atomic weight 127.60, atomic number 52, M.P. 449.5°C. Tellurium is used as an ingredient of blasting caps. Burns with blue-green flame forming dioxides. Toxicity manifested by peripheral neuropathy, seizures, tremor, coma, liver damage, kidney damage. Gases produce pulmonary irritation. Exposed individuals can develop garlic odor to breath, sweat, and urine.

continues

Table 91.2. *Continued*

Metal	Physiochemical Properties and Reactivity
Thorium (Th)	Atomic weight 232.04, atomic number 90, N.P. 1750°C. Thorium is a source of nuclear fuel. Silver-white, soft metal in a pure state. Pyrophoric in a dust state. Commonly used in mantles, in portable gas lighters and burns with a bright, white light.
Titanium (Ti)	Atomic weight 47.88, atomic number 22, M.P. 1660°C. When pure, it is a lustrous white metal. Titanium burns in both air and nitrogen. It resists corrosive effects of acids. Titanium is stronger and lighter than steel. Titanium tetra-chloride ($TiCl_4$) is used in incendiary munitions and produces thick smoke when exposed to moisture in air.
Uranium (U)	Atomic weight 238, atomic number 92, M.P. 1132°C. Uranium is a heavy, silver-white metal. It is pyrophoric in a dust state in air. Uranium is dissolved by acid but not by alkalis.
Yttrium (Y)	Atomic weight 88.9, atomic number 39 M.P. 1522°C. Silvery metal which ignites in air in dust state. Yttrium oxide, the most common form of the metal, is used in color television tubes to impart the red color.
Zinc (An)	Atomic weight 65.38, atomic number 30, M.P. 419.58°C. Zinc dust can ignite in air and produce white fumes of zinc oxide.
Zirconium (Zr)	Atomic weight 91.22, atomic number 40, M.P. 1852°C. Zirconium is a gray-white lustrous metal. In a dust state it can spontaneously ignite in air. Zirconium is used in nuclear reactors, explosive primers, flash bulbs, lamp filaments, and as an alloy with steel in surgical instruments.

Plutonium is a byproduct of uranium use in nuclear reactors with the most important isotope being Pu^{239} with a half-life of 24,900 years (32). Plutonium is specifically absorbed by bone marrow and produces radiologic toxicity by intense α particle emissions (32). As a metal, it can produce enough heat to boil water. Plutonium is highly dangerous radiologic hazard. Plutonium is highly chemically reactive and can cause necrotic damage to tissues and dermal burns (32).

Metal Dusts

The powdered or dust forms of pure thorium, sulfur, aluminum, strontium, magnesium, titanium, uranium, yttrium, zinc, and zirconium can ignite and explode spontaneously in air (2, 32). The combustion hazard of these dusts is diminished greatly if the metals are not in a pure state. Once the metal oxide forms as an outside coating around the metal, the hazard is reduced. Combustion also depends on metallic particle size and the dispersion of these in air (2).

Magnesium

Magnesium dust is explosive when mixed with air. Solid magnesium can also burn with an intense white flame. Water directly applied to flaming magnesium will produce an explosive reaction. Burning magnesium produces very irritating magnesium oxide fumes (MgO) which can seriously injure the lungs (2).

Aluminum

Aluminum dust is explosive when mixed with air and upon contact with an ignition source (2, 32). Burning aluminum will react with water, forming aluminum oxide (Al_2O_3) and explosive hydrogen gas (2). Zinc dust also is an explosive hazard when mixed with air and reacts slowly with water to generate hydrogen gas (2, 32).

Titanium

Titanium, in a pure state, will ignite in air as a dust. It will also burn in nitrogen. It is very resistant to the corrosive effects of acids and alkalis (32).

Titanium tetrachloride ($TiCl_4$) reacts with water or with moisture in air to form an irritating, corrosive, thick smoke. Its hydrolysis products include hydrochloric acid, titanium hydroxide, $Ti(OH)_4$, and $TiOCL_2$. All of these are irritants of the respiratory tract and skin.

Tellurium

Tellurium is an ingredient of blasting caps. It is a silvery-white brittle metal. Tellurium is a unidirectional semiconductor metal whose conductivity increases on exposure to light (32). Tellurium burns with a green-blue flame, forming dioxides. Tellurium is toxic to humans and animals and produces central nervous symptoms of tremors and convulsions (33). Tellurium exists in a powdered form and crystalline form. Amorphous tellurium is a black powder, whereas the crystalline form is silver-white. Toxicity can be produced by elemental tellurium, as well as the gases hydrogen telluride, tellurium hexafluoride, tellurium dioxide, and acid forms (32, 33). Tellurium vapors are respiratory irritants. Clinical toxicity is manifested by peripheral and central neurotoxicity and liver and kidney damage (33).

Peripheral neuropathy, seizures, and tremor can occur following absorption (33). Exposed individuals also have a garlic-odor breath, sweat, and urine (37). Acute exposure to toxic gases produces weakness, cough, stupor, coma, and garlic odor to breath and urine (33). Tellurium has a TLV of 0.1 mg/m^3.

REFERENCES

1. Vouk V. General chemistry of metals, Chap 2 in: Handbook of the toxicology of metals, Vol I. Friberg L, Nordberg G, Vouk V. New York, NY: Elsevier, 1986:14–35.
2. Meyer E. Chemistry of hazardous materials, Englewood Cliffs, NJ: Prentice-Hall, 1977.
3. Morrison R, Boyd R. Organic chemistry. 2nd ed. Boston, MA: Allyn and Bacon, 1966.
4. Beattie AD, Moore MR, Goldberg A. Tetraethyl-lead poisoning. Lancet 1972;2:12–15
5. Gething J. Tetramethyl lead absorption: a report of human exposure to high level of tetramethyl lead. Br J Ind Med 1975;32:329–333.
6. Lehnert G, Mastall H, Szadkowski D, Schaller KH. Berufliche Bleibelastung durch Autoabgase in Großstadtstraßen. Dtsch Med Wochenschr 1970;95:1097–1099.

7. Maruna RFL, Maruna H. Die Bleibelastung von Taxilenkern durch den Nachweis der Delta-Aminolävulinsäure im Harn. Wien Med Wochenschr 1975;125:615–620.

8. Millar JA, Thompson GG, Goldberg A, Barry PS, Lowe EH. δ-Aminolevulinic acid dehydrase activity in the blood of man worling with lead alkyls. Br J Ind Med 1972;29:317–320.

9. Seshia SS, Rajani KR, Boeckx RL, Chow PN. The neurological manifestations of chronic inhalation of leaded gasoline. Dev Med Child Neurol 1978;20:323–334.

10. Schmidt D, Sansoni B, Kracke W, Dietl F, Bauchinger M, Stich W. Die Bleibelastung der Münchner Verkehrspolizei. Münch Med Wochenschr 1972;114:1761–1763.

11. Stevens CP, Feldhake CJ, Kehoe RA. Isolation of triethyllead-ion from liver after inhalation of tetraethyllead. J Pharmacol Exp Ther 1960;128:90–94.

12. Eyl ThB. Methyl mercury poisoning in fish and human beings. Clin Toxicol 1971;14:291–296.

13. Rivers JB, Pearson JE, Schultz CD, Total and organic mercury in main fish. Bull Environ Contam Toxicol 1972;8:257–267.

14. Swensson A, Ulfarsson V. Toxicology of organic mercury compounds used as fungicides. Occup Health Rev 1963;15:5–11.

15. Pierce PE, Thompson JF, Likosky WH, Nickey LN, Barthel WF, Hinman AR. Alkyl mercury poisoning in humans. J Am Med Assoc 1972;220:1439–1442.

16. Somjien GG, Herman SP, Klein R, Brubaker PE, Briner WH, Goodrich JK, Krigman MR, Haseman JK. The uptake of methyl mercury (^{203}Hg) in different tissues relates to its neurotoxic effects. J Pharmacol Exp Ther 1973;187:602–611.

17. Kershaw TG, Dhahir PH, Clarkson TW. The relationship between blood levels and dose of methylmercury in man. Arch Environ Health 1980;35:28–36.

18. Kojima K, Fujita M. Summary of recent studies in Japan on methylmercury poisoning. Toxicology 1973;1:43–62.

19. Amin-Zaki L, Elhassani S, Majeed MA, Clarkson TW, Doherty RA, Greenwood MR. Studies of infants postnatally exposed to methylmercury. J Pediatr 1974;85:81–84.

20. Clarkson T, Magos L, Cox C, et al. Tests of efficacy of antidotes for removal of methylmercury in human poisoning during the Iraq outbreak. Pharmacol 1981;218:74–83.

21. Dangerous properties of industrial materials report Nov/Dec 8(6):8–16, 1988.

22. Jones CC. Nickel carbonyl poisoning. Arch Environ Health 1973;26:245–248.

23. Sundermann FW, Kincaid JF. Nickel poisoning. Studies on patients suffering from acute exposure of vapors of nickel compounds. J Am Med Assoc 1954;1565:889–894.

24. Ludewigs JH, Thiess AM. Arbeitsmedizinische Erkenntnisse bei der Nickelcarbonylvergiftung. Zbl Arbeitsmed Arbeitsschutz 1970;20:329–339.

25. Kasprzak KS, Sunderman Jr FW. Metabolism of nickel-carbonyl-^{14}C. Toxicol Appl Pharmacol 1969;15:295–303.

26. Sundermann Jr FW. The treatment of acute nickel carbonyl poisoning with sodium diethyldithiocarbamate. Ann Clin Res 1971;3:182–185.

27. Sundermann FW, Sundermann Jr FW. Nickel poisoning VIII. Dithiocarb: a new therapeutic agent for persons exposed to nickel carbonyl. Am J Med Sci 1958;236:26–31.

28. Morbidity and Mortality Weekly Report, 1991;40:280–281.

29. Proctor N, Hughes J, Fischman N. Chemical hazards of the workplace. 2nd ed. Philadelphia, PA: J.B. Lippincott, 1988.

30. Descotes J. Immunotoxicology of drugs and chemicals. New York, NY: Elsevier, 1986.

31. Sittig M. Handbook of toxic and hazardous chemicals. Park Ridge, NJ: Noyes Publications, 1981.

32. Magos L. Tin. Chap 23 in: Friberg L, Nordberg G, Vouk V, eds. Handbook on the toxicology of metals. Vol II. New York, NY: Elsevier, 1986.

33. Weast R, Astle M, Beyer W, eds. CRC handbook of chemistry and physics. Boca Raton, FL: CRC Press Inc., 1986.

34. Gerhardsson L, Glover J, Nordberg G, Vouk V. Tellurium, Chap 21 in: Friberg L, Nordberg G, Vouk V, eds. Handbook on the toxicology of metals. New York, NY: Elsevier, 1986.

92

Phosphorus and Phosphorus Compounds

Heeten Desai, M.D.

SOURCES AND PRODUCTION

Phosphorus is a compound whose toxicity is manifested by elemental and various inorganic forms, including white or yellow elemental phosphorus; phosphoric acid; chloro and sulfide compounds of phosphorus; phosphine and metal sulfides. The free element does not occur in nature; however, its significant use in industry and potential sources of exposure necessitates an understanding of its toxicology and effects on human health. Although inorganic compounds cause human toxicity, phosphates and phosphoric acid are used more extensively in industry (Table 92.1).

Historically, phosphorus (white) was used in the production of matches. Its use was eventually abolished in 1906 after a causal relationship between the occupational disease "phossy jaw," a necrosis of the bone, and phosphorus was determined.

Table 92.1. Uses of Phosphorus and Phosphorus Compounds

Substance	Uses
Phosphorus	Rat poisons, smoke screens, fireworks, gas analysis, explosives, raw material for industrial production of PCl_3
Phosphoric acid	Manufacture of phosphates (salts, detergents), acid catalyst, rustproofing of metals, fertilizers, soft drinks, water treatment, pickling
Phosphorus trichloride	Chlorinating agent, manufacture of other phosphorus chloride compounds, ingredient of textile finishing agents
Phosphorus pentachloride	Chlorinating and dehydrating agent, catalyst in manufacture of acetylcellulose, dyes
Phosphorus pentasulfide	Safety matches, ignition compounds, introducing sulfur into organic compounds, insecticides, flotation agents
Metal phosphides (zinc, aluminum, calcium)	Rodenticides, insecticides, grain fumigation
Phosphine	Acetylene gas (welding), ferrosilicon, from contact of water with metal sulfides, doping agent for electronic components
Phosphorus oxychloride	Plasticizers, hydraulic fluids, gasoline additives, fire-retarding agents, chlorinating agent, catalyst

The compound phosphorus sesquisulfide was later used in the production of matches, since it was a non-toxic substitute (1).

CHEMICAL AND PHYSICAL FORMS OF PHOSPHORUS

Phosphorus (P_4) exists in two forms: red phosphorus, which is insoluble, nonabsorbable, and nonvolatile; and white or yellow phosphorus, which is typically pale yellow, or colorless crystals which darken on light exposure (2,3).

Phosphoric acid (H_3PO_4, orthophosphoric acid) can exist as crystal or clear liquid. Phosphorus oxychloric acid can exist as crystal or clear liquid. Phosphorus oxychloride ($POCl_3$) is a colorless liquid with a pungent smell. It is degraded by water vapor in air, creating fumes, while hydrochloric and phosphoric acids are formed.

Phosphorus trichloride (PCl_3, phosphorus chloride) is a colorless clear fuming liquid, which is a product of the incomplete chlorination of phosphorus. The vapor can hydrolyze in humid air, resulting in explosive mixtures. Decompostion by water produces phosphoric and hydrochloric acid.

Phosphorus pentachloride (PCl_5, phosphoric chloride, phosphorus perchloride) exists in crystalline form with a pale yellow or green color and has an acrid odor.

CLINICAL TOXICOLOGY OF EXPOSURE

Due to the variety of compounds and forms in which phosphorus exists, that is, solid, liquid, and gas phases, exposure can occur via several routes. Phosphorus can cause burns to skin and mucous membranes. Inhalation can occur from fumes released by contact of phosphorus with air (spontaneous combustion) or from fumes released in the workplace from phosphorus-containing compounds. Ocular, oral, and parenteral exposure remain as other mechanisms of contact with phosphorus compounds.

Absorption, Metabolism, and Elimination

The elemental form of phosphorus is insoluble in water but is soluble in fat and bile and is therefore absorbed from the intestine. Toxic quanitities can be inhaled from vapors as well as absorbed from the skin. The exact metabolic fate of phosphorus is not clear. However, it appears that it is metabolized to hypophosphoric acid via oxidation. Excretion of these metabolic products occurs via the kidney, as harmless acids and via the lungs as unchanged phosphorus in the expired air.

Occupational and Environmental Exposure

Table 92.2 is a list of the various types of occupations in which exposure to phosphorus and phosphorus compounds may occur. This encompasses a wide variety of tasks and functions per-

Table 92.2. Occupations in Which Exposure to Phosphorus and Phosphorus Compounds May Occur (11)

Occupation	Exposure Limits (ACGIH)
Military personnel, munition and firework makers	TLV 0.1 mg/m³ STEL 0.3 mg/m³
Various production workers	TLV 1 mg/m³ STEL 3 mg/m³
Production workers	TLV 0.5 ppm (3 mg/m³)
Production workers	TLV 0.1 ppm (1 mg/m³)
Production workers	TLV 1 mg/m³ STEL 3 mg/m³
Manufacturers of pesticides, fumigators	
Workers involved with the production of acetylene,	TLV 0.3 ppm (0.4 mg/m³) STEL 1 ppm (1 mg/m³)
Production workers	TLV 0.1 ppm (0.6 mg/m³) STEL 0.5 ppm (3.0 mg/m³)

formed by many people, and exposure can occur at any stage of the process. Included are threshold limit values for the different compounds. Chloro compounds of phosphorus present a pollution hazard when present in water, but little information is available regarding magnitude as well as correlation of toxicity with levels.

Signs, Symptoms, and Syndromes from Toxic Exposure

Acute Toxicity

Phosphorus (white/yellow) is regarded as a general protoplasmic poison. Oral exposure is most often from rat poisons either intentional or accidental (children) and not from occupational exposure (4). Poisoning has been divided into three stages of toxicity. The first stage is characterized by gastrointestinal symptoms consisting of abdominal pain, nausea, vomiting, and diarrhea, which can lead to significant volume depletion and shock. Cutaneous burns may also be present. The poisoned individual has often been characterized as having a garlic-like odor with phosphorescent vomitus and feces, although the absence of these features does not exclude phosporus poisoning (5,6). In McCarron et al.'s review, only a small percentage actually had the characteristic odor and phosphorescence of vomitus and stool (6). Presentation of these symptoms occurred any time from several minutes up to 24 hours after exposure. If the patient survives, the second stage is characterized by a quiescent period lasting on the average from 1–3 days. Stage 3 is characterized by multisystem involvement. Gastrointestinal symptoms include abdominal pain and vomiting (often blood streaked) with liver involvement. Pathologically the liver shows extensive fatty degeneration, and shortly thereafter liver failure may ensue with all its associated problems. Fatty degeneration also occurs in the heart, kidneys, and voluntary muscle. Renal failure, arrhythmias, seizures, coma, and cardiovascular collapse can all occur, eventually leading to death (5). Fumes of yellow phosphorus are an irritant to the respiratory tract and eyes, causing lacrimation, blepharospasm, and photophobia.

Solid phosphorus contamination of the eye can produce severe injury.

Phosphorus burns present a special problem since the burns can be deep and, painful with vesiculation and necrosis. As phosphorus contacts the skin, the burn will progress until all the phosphorus is consumed and its progression is halted by the deprivation of oxygen, such as immersion in water. Healing is often poor and slow. Liver and kidney failure may ensue from absorption from the burn site (7).

Phosphoric acid exposure occurs via inhalation. The mist is an irritant of the respiratory tract, eyes, and skin, causing cough, tearing, and blepharospasm. The higher the concentration of acid, the greater the symptoms. The risk of pulmonary edema is very small (8). There is no evidence that phosphorus poisoning occurs from phosphoric acid exposure (8). Phosphorus pentasulfide is an irritant to the eyes, skin, and respiratory tract. Interestingly, hydrogen sulfide gas and phosphoric acid are the result of hydrolysis of this compound in the presence of moisture. Theoretically these products could cause significant toxicity, although it apears that hydrogen sulfide poisoning has not been reported from this mechanism (3).

The chloro compounds of phosphorus, including phosphorus trichloride and phosphorus pentachloride, produce fumes and vapors, which cause toxicity from inhalational exposure. Phosphorus trichloride is produced by the treatment of molten phosphorus with chlorine gas. Similarly, phosphorus pentachloride is produced by treating the trichloride compound with chlorine in excess. The primary toxic effects of these compounds are on the skin, mucous membranes, and respiratory tract. Characteristic findings upon exposure include conjunctival irritation with photophobia and lacrimation. Pain in the throat, rhinitis, cough, and dyspnea may be followed by respiratory symptoms ranging from mild bronchial spasm to severe respiratory distress and pulmonary edema (9, 10). These symptoms may be delayed, although in significant exposures symptoms usually appear quite promptly. Bronchitis and bronchopneumonia can occur following irritation of the upper airway. In a report by Wason et al., exposure due to a phosphorus trichloride spill was described. Although 450 patients were evaluated in local hospitals, 17 patients returned for assessment. The most frequent symptoms reported were eye irritation, nausea, vomiting, subjective wheezing, lacrimation, and dyspnea (in decreasing order). Pulmonary function tests showed changes in large and small airway resistance correlating with distance from the spill, as well as duration of exposure (10).

Phosphine poisoning is another important source of phosphorus toxicity, albeit rare. The sources of this exposure stem from the action of water on calcium phosphide, which liberates phosphine, acetylene gas welding, and ferrosilicon as well as rodenticides and grain fumigants. Effects include severe gastrointestinal symptoms of nausea, vomiting, and pain, diarrhea, central nervous system depression, headache, ataxia, convulsions, and coma. A delayed pulmonary edema may also occur (1).

CHRONIC AND LONGTERM EFFECTS

Chronic exposure to phosphorus may result in a condition termed "phossy jaw," although this is probably more of historical significance. Recognition of this condition and its association with phosphoris as well as stricter controls on exposure have virtually eliminated the incidence of this occupational disease. Chronic inhalation of phosphorus as well as chloro compounds of phosphorus causes damage to bony tissue. These compounds can penetrate through enamel and act on the periosteum, causing thickening. Bacteria can then invade the bone, causing a periostatis with eventual necrosis of the bone. This condition causes painful swelling of the mandible. The time course of this disease can be over a prolonged period (1).

Exposure to fumes of phosphorus trichloride and pentachloride may result in a chemical bronchitis with a chronic cough and/or wheezing. In an animal study of chronic exposure to the oxychloride, trichloride, and pentachloride of phosphorus, morphologic changes were demonstrated in the liver, bone, kidneys and lungs. Pathology in the respiratory passages consisted of desquamative rhinitis, tracheitis and bronchitis. After cessation of exposure for a number of months most changes reverted except those of the respiratory tract (9). Human effects have been less well-documented.

Skin contact may lead to a dermatitis. Teratogenic or carcinogenic effects from exposure to phosphorus-containing compounds have not been documented in humans, although, in the same above-mentioned study by Roschin et al., mutagenic effects were demonstrated in rats from exposure to the oxychloride of phosphorus (9).

MANAGEMENT OF TOXICITY

Appropriate management and treatment of exposure involves a knowledge of the toxic effects of the chemicals to which the worker is exposed. Prevention and safety measures are of paramount importance. All workers who will come in contact with phosphorus and its compounds should have a comprehensive preplacement examination including a careful examination of the oral cavity. Preexisting conditions, particularly of respiratory and gastrointestinal tract (liver), should be noted.

Treatment of acute phosphorus exposure should consist of initial stabilization with attention to airway/respiratory distress and shock, if present. Personnel involved in treatment of poisoned victims must adhere to adequate precautions to protect themselves as well. Protective respiratory gear should be worn in circumstances where continued exposure to gas, vapors, or fumes may occur. Gown and gloves need to be worn, as rescuers or health personnel may come in contact with particles causing burns and toxicity. Treatment of burns involves application of a 2–3% solution of copper sulfate, which will cause formation of an insoluble salt, thereby preventing further absorption and damage. This treatment, however, has been questioned by some authors, due to potential toxicity with copper. Alternatively, a 2–3% silver nitrate solution has been used on the theory that silver granules precipitating on the skin will prevent absorption of the phosphorus compound (10).

Oral exposure should be treated with gastric decontamination. Use of oils will promote absorption of phosphorus from the gastrointestinal tract and should be avoided. Hypovolemia secondary to nausea, vomiting, and diarrhea should be aggressively treated with crystalloid until normovolemia is restored. Close attention should be paid to hepatic and renal function. Adequate urine output should be maintained, and sequelae of liver failure such as coagulopathies and nutritional deficiency should be treated as the need arises with the appropriate measures.

Treatment for exposure to the chloro compounds consists of removal from the source, removal of any clothing contaminated with the compounds, and observation and treatment of any respiratory complication such as bronchospasm and pulmonary edema that may arise. Ocular splash or injury requires copious irrigation and examination with slit lamp to assess degree of injury, and ophthalmologic consultation if indicated.

Laboratory investigation for determination of phosphorus toxicity is not particularly useful. Serum levels of phosphorus can be measured but may be either increased, decreased, or normal. Parameters such as hemoglobin, blood electrolytes, renal and liver function, and coagulation profile are necessary to follow the course of illness and guide treatment.

In summary, diagnosis and treatment is facilitated by a thorough knowledge of the effects of phosphorus and phosphorus-containing compounds and the circumstances under which work-related exposure can occur. Prevention of this exposure, adequate safety measures, and education complete the necessary requirements for a safe work environment.

REFERENCES

1. Finkel AJ, ed. Hamilton and Hardy's industrial toxicology. 4th ed. John Wright, PSG, 1983:116–118.
2. NIOSH. NIOSH/OSHA: Pocket guide to chemical hazards. Washington, DC: National Institute of Occupational Safety and Health (NIOSH 78–210), 1985.
3. Proctor NH, Hughes JP, Fischman M. Chemical hazards of the workplace. JB Lippincott, 1988:417–418.
4. Gosselin RE, Smith RP, Hodge HC, eds. Clinical toxicology of commercial products. 5th ed. Baltimore: Williams & Wilkins, 1984:348–352.
5. Chretin TE. Acute phosphorus poisoning. N Engl J Med 1945;232:247–249.
6. McCarron MM, Gaddis GP. Acute yellow phosphorus poisoning from pesticide pastes. Clin Toxicol 1981;18:693–711.
7. Ben-Hur N. Phosphorus burns. Prog Surg 1978;16:180–181.
8. Lewis RJ Sr, Sweet DV, eds. Registry of toxic effects of chemical substances (RTECS). DHHS (NIOSH) pub no 84-101–106, 1984.
9. Roshchin AV, Molodkina NN. J Hyg Epidemiol Microbiol Immunol 1977;4:387–394.
10. Wason S, et al. Phosphorus trichloride toxicity: preliminary report. Am J Med 1984;77:1039–1042.
11. American Conference of Governmental Industrial Hygienists. Threshold limit values and biological exposure indices 1990–1991. Cincinnati, OH: ACGIH, 1990.

93

Acrylamide

Marianne Cloeren, M.D., M.P.H.

CHEMICAL AND PHYSICAL PROPERTIES

Acrylamide (CH₂CHCONH₂, CAS registry number 79-06-1) is an odorless white crystalline solid at room temperature. Synonyms are propenamide, acrylic amide, and akrylamid. Acrylamide is an vinyl monomer produced from the hydration of acrylonitrile and sulfuric acid (84.5%), followed by neutralization. It is stable in solution, and is soluble in polar solvents such as water, ethanol, and acetone. Table 93.1 lists the general chemical and physical properties of acrylamide (1–3).

Acrylamide polymer has a wide range of applications; the major use of acrylamide monomer, a skin irritant and neurotoxin, is in the production of polymer, which is believed to be nontoxic (4, 5). Acrylamide has two major functional groups, an amide group conjugated with a vinyl group; it undergoes reactions at both of these groups:

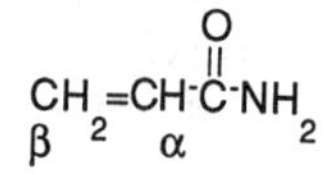

$$CH_2=CH\text{-}\overset{\overset{\textstyle O}{\|}}{C}\text{-}NH_2$$
$$\beta \qquad \alpha$$

It reacts easily at the beta position with hydroxy, amino, and thiol groups, but its most important reaction from an industrial standpoint is vinyl-type polymerization:

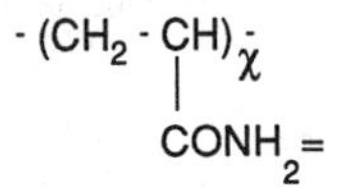

$$\text{-}(CH_2\text{-}CH)_{\overset{}{x}}$$
$$|$$
$$CONH_2$$

In the industrial polymerization of acrylamide, solutions of 8–30% acrylamide monomer are placed in a reactor vessel with one component of a redox system (e.g., sodium bromate/sodium sulfite) while the other component is gradually added. Metal ions are sometimes used as cocatalysts (4). The gelatinous solid polyacrylamide, which is impermeable to water, is then poured out, washed and dried, cut up, ground, and sold as the granulated solid polymer (6).

SITES, INDUSTRIES, AND BUSINESSES ASSOCIATED WITH EXPOSURES

Monomeric acrylamide was first made in Germany in 1893, patented in the United States in 1935 by Rohm and Haas Company, and first produced commercially in the 1950s by American Cyanamid Company (7).

There are three major U.S. manufacturers of acrylamide with a total production capacity as of January 1984 of 215 million pounds per year (8). Acrylamide monomer production has been estimated at 15–20 million pounds in 1966, 40 million in 1973, and 86 million in 1983 (7, 8), and industry projections for 1991 put U.S. production at 95–100 million pounds.

Acrylamide polymers were first used as flocculators (used to separate solids from aqueous solution) in sewage and wastewater treatment and in some mining operations. This is still their major use, but there are many other applications of acrylamide, with the list growing rapidly. Polyacrylamide has long been used in the paper and pulp industry to strengthen paper and board. It is used in the treatment of drinking water and in the oil industry to help bring oil to the surface of a well. Acrylamide polymers will break oil-in-water emulsions, dissipate fog, and stabilize soil. A major use of acrylamide is as a grouting agent; the liquid monomer, together with a catalyst and a cross-linking agent, is pumped into soil, clay, or stone walls of excavations, where it polymerizes to produce a watertight seal. It is used in this way in the construction of dams, foundations, tunnels, roadways, and sewer systems. In biomedical research, polyacrylamide gels are used for chromatography and electrophoresis. Other applications are in photography, metal coatings, ceramics, plastics, paints, adhesives, and binders and in the textile industry (dyes, sizing, and permanent press fabrics) (1, 4, 9). The National Institute for Occupational Safety and Health (NIOSH) estimated in 1976 that 20,000 U.S. workers were potentially exposed to acrylamide (7). Table 93.2 lists industries with exposure to acrylamide.

There have been about 50 cases of human acrylamide intoxication reported in the literature, all occupationally related except one Japanese family of five poisoned by contaminated well water (7, 10). Although acrylamide polymer is widely used, the polymer is nontoxic and poses a health risk only from the small amount of monomer allowed to contaminate it (up to 2% in some applications) (4, 5). All cases of occupational intoxication reported thus far occurred in workers involved in

Table 93.1. Physical and Chemical Properties of Acrylamide[a]

Appearance	White crystalline solid
Odor	None
Molecular formula	CH₂=CHCONH₂
Molecular weight	71.08
Melting point	84.5°C
Boiling point	125°C at 25 mmHg
Density	1.222 g/ml at 30°C
Heat of polymerization	19.8 kcal/mol

[a]Adapted from *The Condensed Chemical Dictionary* (1) and *NIOSH* (7).

Table 93.2. Industries with Potential Exposure to Acrylamide

Acrylamide manufacture
Adhesive tape manufacture
Ceramics plants
Construction (waterproofing of dams, sewers, roads, tunnels)
Flocculator production
Metal coating operations
Mining
Oil wells
Paint factories
Papermaking
Synthetic fiber manufacture
Textile mills, in sizing, dyes, and permanent press fabrics

the polymerization of monomeric acrylamide (7), either in factories where polymers were produced (6, 11) or during grouting operations (12, 13).

CLINICAL TOXICOLOGY

Routes of Exposure, Absorption, Metabolism, and Elimination

Acrylamide is very soluble in water and easily absorbed following all routes of administration, except inhalation, which has not been closely examined. It has similar neurotoxicity whether administered orally, intravenously, intraperitoneally, subcutaneously, intramuscularly, or dermally in aqueous solution (14, 15). Dermal contact and ingestion have been the major routes of exposure in humans, but there are no data on the possible contribution of inhalation of airborne acrylamide. Garland and Patterson (6) suggested that inhalation is an unimportant route of acrylamide exposure, since the monomer is heavy and forms no dust; they noted that there were no cases of acrylamide poisoning at the factories they visited where skin protection was rigidly enforced.

Studies on radionuclide-labeled acrylamide administered intravenously to rats show that it is distributed within a few minutes throughout the total body water. Its serum concentration then decreased exponentially with a half-life of less than 2 hours. Though freely distributed, the majority is bound to tissues and circulating proteins, especially hemoglobin. At one day after injection, the highest levels of free and protein-bound label were found in whole blood, with decreasing levels found in kidney, liver, brain, spinal cord, and sciatic nerve. By 14 days after injection, the free label had disappeared, but the protein-bound label remained at 25% of its day 1 level, except in whole blood, where it remained at 100% of its day 1 level (16, 17). This persistence of tissue-associated radiolabel may represent either protein binding or incorporation of *metabolic* fragments of acrylamide into proteins (18).

The major route of biotransformation of acrylamide is conjugation with glutathione, a reaction which appears to be detoxifying. After enzymatic and nonenzymatic reaction with glutathione, acrylamide is eventually excreted in the urine as N-acetyl-S-(3-amino-3-oxypropyl)cysteine. Acrylamide inhibits the enzyme activity of glutathione-S-transferase in vitro and in vivo; thus it may inhibit its own detoxification via this route (16, 18).

Acrylamide also undergoes biotransformation via the microsomal cytochrome P-450 system, as evidenced by increased clearing of acrylamide in homogenates from animals whose cytochrome P-450 levels have been elevated by pretreatment with phenobarbital (19); however, delay of acrylamide-induced neuropathy by pretreatment with phenobarbital shown in one study (19) has not been reproduced (16, 20), and in another study the opposite effect was shown (21).

SIGN, SYMPTOMS, AND SYNDROMES FROM TOXIC EXPOSURE

General Toxicology

Acrylamide monomer has been recognized as a potent neurotoxin since the 1950s, when it was first produced commercially.

After several poorly documented cases of neurotoxicity in workers handling acrylamide, numerous animal studies have confirmed its neurotoxicity. Although its neurologic effects predominate, weight loss is a consistent finding in animal studies and is not due to reduced food intake, since acrylamide-intoxicated animals gained less weight than control rats fed to match the intake of the study of rats (22). Weight loss has also been described in human cases (6, 11). In addition, acrylamide causes a contact dermatitis, which may be the only sign of acrylamide exposure but often precedes development of neurologic symptoms (6, 11–13, 23, 24).

Neurotoxicity of Acrylamide

Acrylamide is best known for its peripheral (motor and sensory) polyneuropathy; however, it also affects the central and autonomic nervous systems. Acrylamide neuropathy falls into the category of "dying-back polyneuropathies," characterized by degeneration of axons proceeding distally to proximally and affecting fibers in both the peripheral and central nervous systems.

Acute Toxicity

Human Cases   There has only been one reported episode of acute acrylamide poisoning in humans, which probably occurred over several days of exposure. Igisu and colleagues (10) describe a family in Japan poisoned by acrylamide after it leached into their well water from nearby sewer grouting work. The family used the well water for bathing, cooking, and drinking. Acrylamide was subsequently measured at 400 ppm in the well water (a level which, when fed to rats daily, caused paralysis in 24 days (14)). Symptoms appeared about 3.5 weeks after the sewer work occurred. The symptoms in three adults, who were more severely affected than the two children, were gait disturbance, delirium, and hallucinations (visual only in two; visual, auditory, and tactile in one). All three had slurred speech, and two had horizontal nystagmus. One had urinary retention. On initial exam there was no sensory deficit, weakness, or decreased deep tendon reflexes; however, these findings developed in all three patients 2–4 weeks later, after mental status had returned to normal. Electroencephalogram on initial presentation showed only excessive sleepiness. Blood hematology and chemistry tests were normal. At the time that sensory deficits appeared, motor nerve conduction tests were normal, but sural sensory nerve conduction tests showed decreased velocity in all three patients. The three adults had recovered within 4 months.

Of the two children, the 13-year-old was more affected than the 10-year-old, with drowsiness and truncal ataxia, but no other findings on exam. He had recovered within 2 weeks. The 10-year-old had only peculiar behavior, which lasted only 3 days. The difference in effect in the children may be related to lower cumulative dose (they were at school during the day) or may be due to the relative protection of youth shown in some animal studies (25, 26).

Table 93.3 lists the signs and symptoms of acute acrylamide poisoning. An interesting point about this family is that none of the patients demonstrated signs of dermatitis (seen consistently in occupational cases), despite some probable contribution of dermal exposure through bath water. It is likely that ingestion of acrylamide played a greater role in these cases than in the occupational cases.

Animal Experiments   Acute toxicity of acrylamide was

studied in cats in 1958 by Kuperman (15), who found that the development of neurotoxicity was independent of the route of administration and that the effects were cumulative if given in divided doses; therefore, the same total dose was required to produce a given effect. The effects in cats were primarily ataxia and tremor, which were reversible when acrylamide was discontinued. Kuperman also found that very high doses caused convulsions and death.

McCollister (14) in 1964 studied the toxicity of acrylamide in various animals. He found the LD_{50} for a single oral dose to be 150–180 mg/kg in rats, guinea pigs, and rabbits, and 100–200 mg/kg in cats and monkeys. In one monkey given a total of 200 mg/kg in two divided doses, the monkey was unable to stand on day 3 but had some strength and was able to crawl. It died the same day, and pathology showed congestion of lungs and kidneys and focal necrosis in the liver. Histologic examination of the liver showed congestion of the sinusoids with fatty degeneration and necrosis. Kidneys showed degeneration of the convoluted tubules and glomeruli. Peripheral nerves were not examined but no central nervous system pathology was seen. Sign of toxicity in rats, cats, and monkeys were, progressively, stiffness and/or weakness of the hindquarters, loss of ability to control the hindquarters, urinary retention, ataxia of the forelimbs, and inability to stand. McCollister verified Kuperman's finding that the effects depended on the cumulative dose and were independent of route of administration.

Chronic Toxicity

Human Cases There have been about 50 cases of acrylamide poisoning in humans reported in the literature (7). All of these cases, with the exception of the previously discussed Japanese family, occurred over weeks to months in an occupation requiring handling of the monomer in the course of polymerization. Typically, a dermatitis occurs first and may be the only symptom. Patients describe peeling skin and red or blue discoloration of the skin where contact with acrylamide occurred (usually hands and arms). They describe excessive sweating, especially of the palms and soles. Following or concomitant with the skin changes is usually gait disturbance, then paresthesiae, numbness, and weakness in the distal extremities. Sometimes there is slurred speech and overflow incontinence due to neurogenic bladder. There may be weight loss. Physical examination is notable for truncal ataxia, variable sensory deficits, distal weakness, absent deep tendon reflexes, and some-

times distal small muscle wasting. On cessation of exposure, all patients improved, but most required several months to return to baseline, and some had not fully recovered after 1 year (7, 13). Table 93.4 lists the signs and symptoms of chronic acrylamide intoxication in the six patients described by Garland and Patterson (6), which are typical cases; these six patients worked at three different factories where flocculators were produced.

Fullerton (27) looked at the nerves of patients 1, 4, and 5 of Garland and Patterson (6) during recovery from acrylamide intoxication and found disproportionate slowing of conduction distally in muscle fibers and decreased sensory action potentials. Histologic examination of the sural nerve of the patient most recently exposed to acrylamide (2.5 months) showed some axonal degeneration, decreased density of large fibers, and evidence of nerve regeneration.

Animal Experiments Numerous studies have looked at chronic acrylamide toxicity in animals. Chronic acrylamide intoxication in animals produces predominantly a peripheral neuropathy. Signs appear distally initially and slowly progress proximally, as is typical of the dying-back polyneuropathies. Animals develop hindlimb unsteadiness with loss of upper and lower deep tendon reflexes (28); this progresses to gross ataxia, then paralysis and finally complete paralysis; bladder distention is also common (29). Hindlimb signs appear before forelimb signs. Reaction to painful stimuli is preserved even when the animals are paralyzed (28, 30). Cessation of exposure is always followed by improvement and usually complete recovery, although this may take months. An anamnestic response has been noted; animals become more vulnerable to later repeat doses than they originally were (29, 31). Kaplan and Murphy suggest that this response may be due to reinjury of nerves which have only partially regenerated (31).

Electrophysiologic studies on acrylamide-intoxicated animals show no abnormalities until symptoms are present, and then show a small reduction in nerve conduction velocity (30). In severely intoxicated animals, nerve conduction velocity is reduced 20–50% in distal regions (26, 30, 32). Hindlimbs are more affected than forelimbs (30) and both velocity and amplitude reduction are more marked in sensory conduction than in motor (32). The reduction in maximal nerve conduction velocity is thought to be secondary to degeneration of the largest diameter, fastest conducting nerve fibers (9). The early demise of large long axons has been confirmed by quantitative histologic studies (26, 28, 33).

Table 93.3. Signs and Symptoms of Acute Acrylamide Poisoning in a Japanese Family[a]

Patient	Mother	Father	Grandmother	Son	Daughter
Age	40	42	65	13	10
Initial presentation					
Ataxia	+	+	+	+	—
Hallucinations	+	+	+	—	—
Disorientation	+	+	+	—	—
Slurred speech	+	+	+	—	—
Nystagmus	—	+	+	—	—
Drowsiness	—	—	+	+	—
Later findings					
Decreased sensation	+	+	+	—	—
Paresthesiae	+	+	—	—	—
Absent DTRs	+	—	—	—	—

[a]Table adapted from the text of the original article by Igisu H, Goto I, Kawamura Y, Kato M, Izumi K, Kuroiwa Y. Acrylamide encephaloneuropathy due to well water pollution. J Neurol Neurosurg Psychiatry 1975;38:581–584.

Table 93.4. Signs and Symptoms of Chronic Acrylamide Poisoning in Six Factory Workers

	1	2	3	4	5	6
Age	19	23	30	56	59	57
Exposure (weeks)	6	12	12	8	60	4
Excessive sweating	+	+		+	+	
Peeling skin	+	+		+		
Difficulty walking	+					
Paresthesiae		+		+	+	+
Weight loss	+					
Lethargy/fatigue	+		+	+	+	+
Slurred speech	+			+		
Decreased sensation	+	+	+	+	+	+
Temperature		+		+		
Vibration	+		+			+
Pin prick		+				
Light touch		+				
Position			+			
+Romberg's sign	+	+	+		+	+
Absent DTRs	+	+	+	+	+	+
Muscle weakness	+	+	+	+	+	+
Muscle wasting	+					+
Other	a			b		
Time to recovery (months)	>6	8	? ("quick")	>6	?	>4

*a*Tremors
*b*Urinary incontinence
Adapted from Garland TO, Patterson MWH. Six cases of acrylamide poisoning. Br Med J 1967;4:134–138.

Histopathologic studies in animals were at first unrewarding. The early light microscopic studies did not look at peripheral nerves, and found no central nervous system abnormalities (14, 15). In 1966, Fullerton and Barnes established acrylamide toxicity as a dying-back neuropathy by showing degeneration of distal axon of long peripheral nerves (26).

Studies on baboons confirmed distal axonal degeneration in large diameter nerves, and also showed some paranodal changes thought to be due to Schwann cell response to degeneration axons (28).

Electron microscopy allowed more detailed examination of affected nerves. Prineas (34) discovered that an increase in distal axonal neurofilaments preceded degeneration, and that small axons in the spinal gray matter and axons in the gracile nucleus were affected along with large peripheral nerves. The earliest detectable morphologic changes in cats intoxicated with acrylamide were found by Schaumburg and colleagues (35) to occur in the Pacinian corpuscles in the toe pads. First filopod axon processes were lost, axolemmas disappeared, and axoplasm was phagocytosed by inner core cells. These change were found before any clinical signs of toxicity. The next changes were degeneration of adjacent primary annulospiral endings of muscle spindles in hind foot muscles, then degeneration of secondary muscle spindle endings of the motor nerve terminals supplying nearby extrafusal muscle fibers. Accumulation of neurofilaments occurred in these sensory and motor terminals as early degeneration began. Degeneration proceeded proximally and was accompanied by adaxonal Schwann cell ingrowths and swollen paranodal regions. Unmyelinated fibers were found to be relatively resistant; however, Post and McLeod (33, 36) found involvement of unmyelinated nerves, with larger diameter fibers degenerating more than smaller ones. They also showed that the sympathetic and parasympathetic nervous systems are damaged by acrylamide in the same way as the peripheral nervous system.

Similar, though less marked, changes have been found in the central nervous system, in the gracile nucleus and fasciculus gracilis (34), in the cerebellar vermis (37), and in the pineal gland (38), as well as in the distal ends of spinal cord fibers (34).

Following chronic intoxication of rats with acrylamide, there is evidence of regeneration of nerve fibers, even in animals still receiving acrylamide in their diet (26). Regenerating nerve fibers were also seen in a sural nerve taken from a patient with acrylamide poisoning with evidence of regeneration at the time of exposure (27). Although regeneration occurs in the presence of acrylamide, it is impaired (39, 40). This impaired regeneration was studied by Griffin and coworkers (40), who found that [^{3}H]leucine was incorporated normally into sensory ganglia during regeneration, but that the radioactivity was carried less rapidly beyond the crush than in controls. They noted that the label accumulated in abnormal growth sprouts, and felt that the cause of delayed transport was this trapping of protein, not a primary defect in fast axonal transport.

The biochemical event (or events) responsible for the distal retrograde degeneration seen in acrylamide poisoning has not been determined, but recent studies have investigated the possibility that degeneration is caused by a perturbation in energy metabolism in the axon (41–46). Other studies have looked at axonal transport, especially alterations in retrograde axonal transport, which could conceivably disrupt biofeedback to the perikaryon regarding metabolic needs at the distal end (18, 47). Other hypotheses argue for primary axon damage by local toxic action (35) or for metabolic damage to the perikaryon, making it unable to meet the metabolic demands of the distal axon (18, 34, 35). Elucidation of the biochemical mechanisms of acrylamide neurotoxicity may lead to treatment of similar distal retrograde neuropathies seen in some natural diseases, such as amyotrophic lateral sclerosis, Werdnig-Hoffmann's disease and Friedrich's ataxia.

Acrylamide Analogues

Some attention has been paid to analogues of acrylamide, in the hope that studying them will shed light on the biochemical mechanisms of neurotoxicity. Several analogues were found to be neurotoxic, but none more so than acrylamide. Reduction of the double bond or deletion of the nitrogen atom were found to eliminate neurotoxicity. The acrylyl moiety (CH_2CHCO-) was found to be essential for neurotoxicity, and there was no relation between reactivity with sulfhydryl groups and neurotoxicity 918). N-Hydroxymethylacrylamide, N,N-diethylacrylamide, N-methylacrylamide, and N-isopropylacrylamide all caused some neurotoxicity at higher doses than were required for acrylamide (16, 20, 48–50). These and several nonneurotoxic analogues were all metabolized by glutathione and by microsomal enzymes (51). The neurotoxic analogues had negligible breakdown to acrylamide; thus their neurotoxicity is not secondary to acrylamide itself (16). One analogue, methylene-bis-acrylamide, was not neurotoxic but caused weight loss (20). There have been, as yet, no published data on human poisonings with analogues of acrylamide.

Teratogenicity and Reproductive Effects

In rodent studies, acrylamide crosses the placenta to reach significant concentrations in the fetus, causing neurotoxic effects (tibial and optic nerve degeneration) in the neonates at levels that were nontoxic to the mother. The lowest observed effect level for developmental toxicity in mice was 20 mg/kg/day.

Acrylamide affects reproductive ability by causing decreased copulatory performance in male rats, decreased fertility in male mice, and degeneration of testicular epithelial tissue in mice. The lowest observed effect level and no observed effect level for reproductive effects in mice were 2 and 0.5 mg/kg/day, respectively. Acrylamide also causes dominant lethal effects by loss of total embryos implanted per litter and by increased resorption of embryos (8).

Carcinogenicity

Acrylamide studies in rats and mice have shown increased incidence of benign and malignant tumors, qualifying acrylamide as an animal carcinogen. Although the very limited epidemiologic data (52, 57) do not show any increased mortality from cancer in humans exposed to acrylamide, the American Conference of Governmental Industrial Hygienists has assigned acrylamide an A2 rating (suspected human carcinogen) and the Occupational Safety and Health Administration (OSHA) is now implementing stricter standards on workplace exposure to reduce the risk of cancer (53).

Management of Toxicity

Diagnosis Clinical examination should focus on the skin and neurologic system. No laboratory evaluation of blood or urine has proved useful in diagnosing or monitoring acrylamide intoxication. Suspicion of acrylamide poisoning, if occupational, warrants removal of the patient from the job and investigation of worksite conditions. Abnormal sensory and motor nerve conduction tests may be helpful in documenting deficits and monitoring recovery; however, it should

be kept in mind that, in acute or subacute intoxication, these tests may not become abnormal until many days after the initial presentation.

Although there are no routine laboratory tests helpful in diagnosing acrylamide intoxication, some experimental methods have been suggested. Poole and coworkers (54) detected acrylamide in nerve tissue homogenates from intoxicated animals using eletron-capture gas chromatography. Bailey and associates (55) suggested monitoring exposure to acrylamide by determination of S-(2-carboxyethyl)cysteine in hydrolyzed hemoglobin; acrylamide exposure causes formation of covalently bound reaction product with cysteine residues in hemoglobin, with a dose-response relationship between acrylamide dose and production of hemoglobin adduct.

Treatment There is no treatment for acrylamide intoxication. Most patients gradually recover following cessation of exposure. Patients may be more susceptible to repeat injury from acrylamide if they return to an exposed situation before complete recovery. There are no good data on when (or whether) patients should return to an exposed job.

Exposure Limits and Environmental Monitoring As of March 1, 1989, a new permissible exposure limit (PEL) for acrylamide was set by OSHA. The previous PEL was 0.3 mg/m^3 as a time-weighted average (TWA) concentration for up to a 10-hour work day, 40-hour work week. The new PEL, effected to reduce risk of cancer, is an 8-hour TWA PEL of 0.03 mg/m^3 with "skin" notation. A study by the EPA showed that most worker exposures were already less than this PEL (53).

Skin protection is mandatory for all acrylamide workers, including (as needed) gloves, aprons, long-sleeved overalls, footwear, and safety goggles and/or face shields. The Edmond Snorkel vinyl-coated glove has been reported to have low permeability to acrylamide, whereas some polyvinyl chloride-coated gloves are more permeable. Protective clothing and gloves should be tested prior to use for permeability to acrylamide; both gloves and clothing should be cotton lined for comfort. Respiratory protection is only recommended in nonroutine or emergency situations that may result in exposure concentrations higher than the PEL, and then should consist of air-supplied respirators, the use of which workers should be instructed in during training. In case of eye contact, eyes should be flushed for at least 15 minutes with low-pressure flowing water. Skin contact should be treated with immediate and copious washing with soap and water. In case of ingestion, vomiting should be induced if the worker is conscious, and a physician should be contacted. All employees should have basic instruction on the hazards of acrylamide and prevention of exposure. NIOSH also recommends regular physical examinations of acrylamide workers with attention to skin and neurologic function, as well as weekly examinations by trained personnel of fingertips and other potentially exposed skin for evidence of peeling.

For worksite monitoring, NIOSH recommends that a midget impinger be used to sample the breathing zone of all locations and operations in which there is exposure to acrylamide. Gas chromatography is used to analyze the sample. Differential pulse polarography has also been used to analyze acrylamide concentrations (7, 56).

Ideally, engineering advances will allow totally enclosed systems; then workers will no longer need to handle the toxic monomer, except as needed for maintenance and repair of enclosed systems (and then with protective clothing and respirators) (7).

REFERENCES

1. Hawley GG, ed. The condensed chemical dictionary. 10th ed. New York: Van Nostrand Reinhold, 1981:16.

2. MacWilliams DC. In: The Kirk-Othmer concise encyclopedia of chemical technology. New York: John Wiley & Sons, Inc., 1985:22–23.

3. Rom WN, ed. Environmental and occupational medicine. Boston: Little, Brown & Co., 1983:603.

4. Spencer PS, Schaumburg HH. A review of acrylamide neurotoxicity. Part I: properties, uses and human exposures. Can J Neurol Sci 1974;1:143–150.

5. McCollister DD, Oyen F, Rowe VK. Toxicologic investigations of polyacrylamides. Toxicol Appl Pharmacol 1965;7:639.

6. Garland TO, Patterson MWH. Six cases of acrylamide poisoning. Br Med J 1967;4:134–138.

7. National Institute for Occupational Safety and Health. Criteria for a recommended standard . . . occupational exposure to acrylamide. Oct 1976. DHEW (NIOSH) Publications No. 77–112.

8. Dearfield KL, Abernathy CO, Ottley MS, Brantner JH, Hayes PF. Acrylamide: its metabolism, developmental and reproductive effects, genotoxicity, and carcinogenicity. Mutat Res 1988;195:45–77.

9. LeQuesne PM. Acrylamide. In: Spencer PS, Schaumburg HH, eds. Experimental and clinical neurotoxicology. Baltimore: Williams & Wilkins, 1980:309–325.

10. Igisu H, Goto I, Kawamura Y, Kato M, Izumi K, Kuroiwa Y. Acrylamide encephaloneuropathy due to well water pollution. J Neurol Neurosurg Psychiatry 1975;38:581–584.

11. Davenport JG, Farrell DF, Sumi SM. ''Giant axonal neuropathy'' caused by industrial chemicals: neurofilamentous axonal masses in man. Neurology 1976;26:919–923.

12. Auld RB, Bedwell SF. Peripheral neuropathy with sympathetic overactivity from industrial contact with acrylamide. Can Med Assoc J 1967;96:652–654.

13. Kesson CM, Baird AW, Lawson DH. Acrylamide poisoning. Postgrad Med J 1977;53:16–17.

14. McCollister DD, Oyen F, Rowe VK. Toxicology of acrylamide. Toxicol Appl Pharmacol 1964;6:172.

15. Kuperman AS. Effects of acrylamide on the central nervous system of the cat. J Pharmacol Exp Ther 1958;123:180–192.

16. Edwards PM. Distribution and metabolism of acrylamide and its neurotoxic analogues in rats. Biochem Pharmacol 1975;24:1277–1282.

17. Hashimoto K, Aldridge WN. Biochemical studies on acrylamide, a neurotoxic agent. Biocem Pharmacol 1970;19:2591–2604.

18. Miller MS, Spencer PS. The mechanisms of acrylamide axonopathy. Annu Rev Pharmacol Toxicol 1985;25:643–666.

19. Kaplan ML, Murphy SD, Gilles FH. Modification of acrylamide neuropathy in rats by selected factors. Toxicol Appl Pharmacol 1973;24:564–579.

20. Edwards PM. Neurotoxicity of acrylamide and its analogues, and effects of these analogues and other agents on acrylamide neuropathy. Br J Ind Med 1975;32:31–38.

21. Srivastava SP, Seth PK, Das M, Mukhtar H. Effects of mixed-function oxidase modifiers on neurotoxicity of acrylamide in rats. Biochem Pharmacol 1985;34:1099–1102.

22. Gipon L, Schotman P, Jennekens FGI, Gispen WH. Polyneuropathies and CNS protein metabolism. I. Description of acrylamide syndrome in rats. Neuropathol Appl Neurobiol 1977;3:115.

23. Pegum JS, Medhurst FA. Contact dermatitis from penetration of rubber gloves by acrylamide monomer. Br Med J 1971;2:141–143.

24. Lambert J, Matthieu L, Dockx P. Contact dermatitis from acrylamide. Contact Derm 1988;19:65.

25. Suzuki K, Pfaff LD. Acrylamide neuropathy in rats. Acta Neuropathol 1973;24:197–213.

26. Fullerton PM, Barnes JM. Peripheral neuropathy in rats produced by acrylamide. Br J Ind Med 1966;23:210–221.

27. Fullerton PM. Electrophysiologic and histologic observations on peripheral nerves in acrylamide poisoning in man. J Neurol Neurosurg Psychiatry 1969;32:186.

28. Hopkins A. Effect of acrylamide on the peripheral nervous system of the baboon. J Neurol Neurosurg Psychiatry 1970;33:805–816.

29. Spencer PS, Schaumburg HH. Review of acrylamide neurotoxicity. II: Experimental animal neurotoxicity and pathologic mechanisms. Can J Neurol Sci 1974;1:152–169.

30. Leswing RJ, Ribelin WE. Physiologic and pathologic changes in acrylamide neuropathy. Arch Environ Health 1969;18:23.

31. Kaplan ML, Murphy SD. Effect of acrylamide on rotarod performance and sciatic nerve beta-glucuronidase activity of rats. Toxicol Appl Pharmacol 1972;22:259.

32. Hopkins AP, Gilliatt RW. Motor and sensory conduction velocity in the baboon; normal values and changes during acrylamide neuropathy. J Neurol Neurosurg Psychiatry 1971;34:415–426.

33. Post EJ, McLeod JG. Acrylamide autonomic neuropathy in the cat: 1. Neurophysiological and histological studies. J Neurol Sci 1977;33:353.

34. Prineas J. The pathogenesis of dying-back neuropathies II. An ultrastructural study of experimental acrylamide intoxication in the cat. J Neuropathol Exp Neurol 1969;28:598–621.

35. Schaumburg HH, Wisniewski HM, Spencer PS. Ultrastructural studies of the dying-back process. 1: Peripheral nerve terminal and axon degeneration in systemic acrylamide intoxication. J Neuropathol Exp Neurol 1974;33:260–284.

36. Post EJ, McLeod JG. Acrylamide autonomic neuropathy in the cat: 2. Effects on mesenteric vascular control. J Neurol Sci 1977;33:375.

37. Ghetti B, Wisniewski HM, Cook RD, Schaumburg HH. Changes in the CNS after acute and chronic acrylamide intoxication [abstract]. Am J Pathol 1973;70:78A.

38. Schmidt RE, Plurad SB, Clark HB. Acrylamide induced sympathetic autonomic neuropathy causing pineal degeneration. Lab Invest 1987;56:505–517.

39. Morgan-Hughes JA, Sinclair S, Durston JHJ. The pattern of peripheral nerve regeneration induced by crush in rats with severe acrylamide neuropathy. Brain 1974;97:235.

40. Griffin JW, Price DL, Drachman DB. Impaired axonal regeneration in acrylamide intoxication. J Neurobiol 1977;8:355.

41. Schotman P, Gipon L, Jennekens FGI, Gispen WH. Polyneuropathies and CNS protein metabolism. II: Changes in the incorporation rate of leucine during acrylamide intoxication. Neuropathol Appl Neurobiol 1977;3:125.

42. Schotman P, Gipon L, Jennekens FGI, Gispen WH. Polyneuropathies and CNS protein metabolism. III: Changes in protein synthesis rate induced by acrylamide intoxication. J Neuropathol Exp Neurol 1978;37:820.

43. Brimijoin WS, Hammond PJ. Acrylamide neuropathy in the rat: effects on energy metabolism in the sciatic nerve. Mayo Clin Proc 1985;60:3–8.

44. Howland RD. Biochemical studies of acrylamide neuropathy. Neurotoxicology 1985;6(4):7–16.

45. Sharma RP, Obersteiner EJ. Acrylamide cytotoxicity in chick ganglia cultures. Toxicol Appl Pharmacol 1977;42:149.

46. Johnson EC, Murphy SD. Effect of acrylamide intoxication on pyridine nucleotide concentration and functions in rat cerebral cortex. Biochem Pharmacol 1977;26:2151.

47. Miller MS, Miller MJ, Burks TF, Sipes IG. Altered retrograde axonal transport of nerve growth factor after single and repeated doses of acrylamide in the rat. Toxicol Appl Pharmacol 1983;69:96–101.

48. Tanii H, Hashimoto K. Neurotoxicity of acrylamide and related compounds in rats: effects on rotarod performance, morphology of nerves and neurotubulin. Arch Toxicol 1983;54:203–213.

49. Barnes JM. Observations on the effects on rats of compounds related to acrylamide. Br J Ind Med 1970;27:147–149.

50. Hashimoto K, Sakamoto J, Tanii H. Neurotoxicity of acrylamide and related compounds, and their effects on male gonads in mice. Arch Toxicol 1981;47:179–189.

51. Tanii H, Hashimoto K. Studies on in vitro metabolism of acrylamide and related compounds. Arch Toxicol 1981;48:157–166.

52. Sobel W, Bond GG, Parsons TW, Brenner FE. Acrylamide cohort mortality study. Br J Ind Med 1986;43:785–788.

53. Federal Register. Jan 19, 1989. Vol 54, no. 12, 2674.

54. Poole CF, Sye WF, Zlatkis A, Spencer PS. Determination of acrylamide in nerve tissue homogenates by electron—capture gas chromatography. J Chromatogr 1981;217:239–245.

55. Bailey E, Farmer PB, Bird I, Lamb JH, Peal JA. Monitoring exposure to acrylamide by the determination of S-(2-carboxyethyl)cysteine in hydrolyzed hemoglobin by gas chromatography-mass spectrometry. Anal Biochem 1986;157:241–248.

56. McLean JD, Mann JR, Jacoby SA. A monitoring method for determining acrylamide in an industrial environment. Am Ind Hyg Assoc J 1978;39:247.

57. Collins JJ, Swaen SMH, Marsh GM, Utidjian HMD, Caporossi JC, Lucas LJ. Mortality patterns among workers exposed to acrylamide. J Occup Med 1989;31:614–617.

94

Isocyanates

Karen K. Phillips, M.D., M.P.H.
John M. Peters, M.D., Sc.D.

INTRODUCTION

Since the early 1950s, United States manufacturers have used isocyanates primarily as starting materials for a variety of plastic products including rigid and flexible polyurethane foams, urethane-based coatings such as paints and electrical wire insulation, and elastomers and spandex fibers. The main health effects of isocyanates involve the lung, but other organ systems may be affected. Most reported toxic effects have been due to toluene diisocyanate (TDI) because of its widespread use. Although slightly different in their properties, other isocyanates cause similar problems under appropriate conditions.

USES OF ISOCYANATES

Toluene diisocyanate (TDI; CAS no. 26471-62-5) is a combination of 2,4-toluene diisocyanate (CAS no. 584-84-9) and 2,6-toluene diisocyanate (CAS no. 91-08-7), usually found in an 80:20 mixture of the isomers. TDI is required for the manufacture of flexible foam used in a variety of products including mattresses, upholstery cushions, automobile seats, and packaging materials. Methylene diphenyl diisocyanate (MDI) has replaced TDI in the production of rigid foams because it is less hazardous owing to its lower volatility. Rigid foam is used as insulation in home refrigerators and ovens, while spray-in foam is used for railroad cars, truck trailers, and boats. As protective coatings, polyurethanes are applied to electrical wiring where their insulating properties are of value. They are used as two-part paints and floor, concrete, and wood finishes where their hardness and durability are advantageous. Aircraft, truck, and other coatings are often composed of diisocyanate prepolymer systems. Isocyanates are also used as adhesives and as elastomers in automobile bumpers, printing rolls, liners for mine and grain elevator chutes, shoe soles, coated fabrics, and spandex fibers. MDI is used as part of a no-bake binder system for casting molds in foundries. Other diisocyanates such as hexamethylene diisocyanate (HDI) (a common component of paints), naphthalene diisocyanate (NDI), isophorone diisocyanate (IPDI), polymethylene polyphenyl isocyanate (PAPI), and dicyclohexyl methane diisocyanate (hydrogenated MDI or HMDI) also have commercial uses. Representative trade names for isocyanate products can be found in Table 94.1. Methylisocyanate (MIC) is used in the manufacture of carbamate pesticides. The 1984 Bhopal, India, tragedy where more than 2000 people died and 100,000 were affected was due to the release of methylisocyanate into the surrounding community.

SYNTHESIS OF ISOCYANATES AND POLYURETHANE

Isocyanates are readily reactive compounds because of their chemical configurations. They contain $-N=C=O$ groups, which react with active hydrogens in compounds such as water, acids, and alcohols but can also react with themselves to form dimers or other polymers. Uncontrollable polymerization and heat formation occur when mixed with bases, such as caustic soda and tertiary amines (1).

Isocyanates are manufactured from the reaction of primary aliphatic or aromatic amines such as 2,4- and 2,6-toluenediamine (TDA) and phosgene in a solvent such as mono-or dichlorobenzene or xylene. This reaction occurs rapidly to form hydrogen chloride and an intermediate which is converted to TDI upon heating. TDI is a colorless to pale yellow liquid with a sharp, pungent odor.

In the manufacture of polyurethane foams, isocyanate (part A) is typically added to polyether or polyester polyols along with combustion-retarding agents, catalysts, and blowing agents (part B or resin) to form polyurethane. The addition of water causes the generation of CO_2 gas with subsequent foam formation. Without the addition of water, the polyurethane mixture can be used as a coating material. Commercially, polyurethane adhesives and coatings may be available as two-component systems that react together and must be mixed just prior to use or as one-component systems that require reaction with oxygen or moisture after application for curing.

CLINICAL TOXICOLOGY OF EXPOSURE

A National Institute of Occupational Safety and Health (NIOSH) survey in 1974 estimated that between 50,000 and 100,000 workers in the United States are regularly exposed to diisocyanates at any one time (2). Exposure to isocyanates can occur anywhere from the initial manufacture of the isocyanates to their final use in the production of foams and other polyurethane products. Exposure can also occur from the application of polyurethane paints and coatings, from the handling and machining of foams, and from combustion of these materials (3). (Table 94.2)

Inhalation of isocyanates as vapors or aerosols is the main risk to the health of the worker. Dermal contact may also expose the worker to the effects of isocyanates. TDI and HDI, the more volatile isocyanates, cause problems at room temperature

Table 94.1. Representative Trade Names of Isocyanates

Centari
Desmodur
Hylene
Imron
Isonate
Mondur
Nacconate
Niax
Rubinate

Table 94.2. Occupations Associated with Isocyanate Exposure

Adhesive workers
Aircraft builders
Appliance makers
Boat makers
Cushion makers
Foam blowers
Insulation workers
Isocyanate workers
Lacquer workers
Life preserver makers
Mine tunnel coaters
Painters
Plastic foam makers
Plastic molders
Polyurethane foam makers
Rubber workers
Shipbuilders
Ship welders
Textile processors
Upholstery workers
Varnishers
Wire-coating workers

while the less volatile isocyanates, MDI and NDI, are less likely to cause respiratory problems except when heated or inhaled as an aerosol. HMDI rarely causes respiratory sensitization even when heated but seems to elicit more dermal reactions. Of considerably less importance than isocyanates in causing health effects are the additives or solvents used in the production of polyurethane. Catalysts such as metal salts (e.g., organotin compounds) or tertiary amines may be used. Combustion-retarding agents and blowing agents may also be added to the preparation and are usually organic phosphates or phosphonates and may contain chlorine or bromine. Methylene chloride or chlorofluorocarbons have been used as blowing agents in the manufacture of polyurethane foams (4).

Exposure to isocyanates is likely to be higher in the initial steps of polyurethane and other isocyanate-using productions than at the end. TDI exposures in the flexible polyurethane foam industry are higher on foam lines, in the maintenance department, and in research and development where exposure to raw TDI is more likely compared to the finishing areas (5).

Although most exposure occurs during the manufacture and use of isocyanates, finished products may contain some residual amounts of unreacted monomers, which may be released in small amounts (1). The application of polyurethane coatings, such as paints and varnishes, can cause exposure to diisocyanates. Single-component coatings exist in a prepolymerized form and so are less likely to be inhaled than two-component products which contain unreacted isocyanates. Exposure has also been demonstrated from handling and machining polyurethane foam. Although reversal of dimerization can occur at high temperatures, thermal decomposition products of polyurethanes consist mainly of carbon monoxide, benzene, toluene, nitrogen oxides, hydrogen cyanide, acetaldehyde, acetone, propene, carbon dioxide, alkenes, and water vapor (4).

MECHANISM OF ACTION CAUSING TOXICITY

A variety of mechanisms have been proposed to explain the toxicity of isocyanates. Immunologically, both humoral (IgE-mediated) and cellular mechanisms have been evaluated. Iso-

cyanates are highly reactive with amino groups and can readily haptenize with plasma proteins producing neoantigens. IgE-mediated hypersensitivity mechanisms appear possible in the etiology of isocyanate-induced asthma, especially when symptoms occur immediately after exposure. Investigators have demonstrated isocyanate-specific IgE antibodies in the sera of exposed workers. The prevalence, however, of these antibodies approximates 20% in some studies, suggesting that this may not be the major mechanism of isocyanate asthma. Furthermore, specific IgE antibodies have been detected in the sera of exposed, asymptomatic individuals (6). Epidemiologic studies have also failed to show a correlation between isocyanate asthma and atopy, further indicating that the disease is probably not entirely IgE-mediated. A possible role of cellular mechanisms has been shown through the production of a leukocyte inhibitory factor by lymphocytes from sensitized individuals (3).

TDI has also been found to suppress the increase of intracellular cyclic adenosine monophosphate (cAMP) by the beta-agonist isoproterenol in peripheral blood lymphocytes indicative of a pharmacologic mechanism of action (7). Research data suggest that isocyanates may cause nonspecific inhibition of a variety of membrane receptors and enzyme systems. Both immunologic and nonimmunologic mechanisms appear to be involved (8). Although much research has been directed toward the mechanism of isocyanate-induced disease, the complete pathophysiology remains unknown.

SIGNS, SYMPTOMS, AND SYNDROMES FROM TOXIC EXPOSURE

Isocyanates cause varied effects due to exposure. TDI can act as a direct irritant to mucous membranes, skin, and the respiratory system. It can also act as a sensitizer capable of causing such adverse effects as TDI-induced asthma and bronchial hyperreactivity to nonspecific agents and can cause lung function decline in individuals not sensitive to the specific isocyanate.

Respiratory Effects

The principal patterns of respiratory response to TDI are: (a) chemical bronchitis (following high doses); (b) isocyanate asthma and nonspecific bronchial hyperreactivity (symptomatic variable airflow obstruction in sensitized subjects); (c) acute nonspecific airway disease (acute asymptomatic deterioration in lung function during a workshift); (d) chronic nonspecific airway disease (chronic deterioration in lung function with prolonged low levels of exposure); and (e) hypersensitivity pneumonitis (3).

CHEMICAL BRONCHITIS

Acute exposure to isocyanates can cause respiratory and mucous membrane irritation. Symptoms such as eye, nose, and throat burning or irritation with rhinitis, laryngitis, or bronchitis may occur upon inhalation. Cough with chest pain or tightness may also occur, frequently at night. Transitory changes in lung function may develop. High exposures may result in chemical pneumonitis and pulmonary edema. Changes in lung function seem to improve within 1–2 years in most cases, although they may persist. Chronic bronchitis has also been reported to be more frequent in workers exposed to high concentrations or repeatedly to low concentrations of TDI (9).

ISOCYANATE ASTHMA

Asthma occurring from exposure to isocyanates in a polyurethane manufacturing plant was first recorded in 1951 by Fuchs and Valade (10). Isocyanate asthma presents clinically with symptoms of wheezing, cough, and shortness of breath, often at night; these symptoms improve on weekends and vacations. Possible predisposing factors for isocyanate asthma include exposure to large or multiple isocyanate spills and upper respiratory tract infections, although usually there is no explanation (11). It is estimated that 5% of exposed workers develop clinically apparent asthma due to isocyanate sensitization, although values of up to 30% have been reported depending on exposure levels and criteria used to define sensitivity (3).

Although varying periods of isocyanate exposure (one day to years) may exist before the development of asthma, isocyanate asthma more often develops within the first few months of exposure. The duration and concentration of isocyanate exposure triggering sensitivity are unknown. Exposure to even low levels of isocyanates can cause asthma. Once sensitized, exposure to even smaller amounts can produce asthmatic episodes. Sudden death has occurred in sensitized subjects inadvertently exposed to relatively low concentrations of TDI (3). Workers who are found to be sensitized to isocyanates must be removed to jobs where no further isocyanate exposure will occur. Many patients with occupational asthma due to TDI continue to have persistent asthma months or years after removal from exposure (12). In some subjects, the asthma may progress even if they are no longer exposed.

Workers who develop isocyanate asthma may also have hypersensitivity to other environmental allergens. This nonspecific bronchial hyperreactivity does not always accompany specific sensitivity to isocyanates. Nonspecific hyperreactivity cannot be predicted from the presence of atopy or from the initial degree of airflow obstruction (13). Like isocyanate asthma, nonspecific hyperreactivity can be lost over time. It may persist, however, for prolonged periods following cessation of exposure to isocyanates. Decreases in isocyanate sensitivity and nonspecific hyperreactivity have occurred after removal from exposure but appeared again upon reexposure.

Asthma due to isocyanate sensitization can be of immediate, late, or dual onset. Smooth muscle contraction is thought to be the mechanism for immediate asthmatic responses induced by isocyanates, since they quickly reverse after bronchodilators or spontaneously (14). By contrast, bronchodilators do not prevent late asthmatic responses induced by isocyanates. Asthmatics without a history of exposure to isocyanates, even those with methacholine sensitivity, do not respond to TDI inhalation challenge, indicating an isocyanate-specific response. Prednisone has been shown to prevent both late asthmatic reactions and the associated increase in airway responsiveness. Prednisone has also been found to have no effect on the early component in those with dual responses. Elevated levels of inflammatory cells are found in TDI-sensitive individuals experiencing late or dual asthmatic episodes but not in those experiencing only immediate reactions. Late asthmatic reactions to TDI and the associated increase in airway responsiveness may be linked to an acute inflammatory process in the airways of sensitized subjects.

Paggiaro and coworkers studied 114 subjects with asthma induced by TDI (15). Bronchial provocation with TDI elicited immediate responses in 24 subjects, late responses in 50, and dual responses in 40 subjects. Those with dual responses had a longer duration of symptoms and a greater prevalence of airway obstruction with a lower mean FEV_1. A methacholine challenge was performed on 27 subjects; those with dual responses showed greater nonspecific bronchial hyperresponsiveness than those with only late or early responses. Mapp and associates found bronchial hyperreactivity diagnosed by positive methacholine inhalation challenge to occur in TDI asthmatics with dual or late but not immediate responses (16). In addition, six workers with a clinical history suggestive of TDI sensitivity had initial methacholine challenges which were negative but 8 hours after a TDI inhalation challenge developed positive methacholine responses (17). Cross-reactivity to other diisocyanates by challenge testing has been seen in some people with TDI asthma who have no history of previous exposure to diisocyanates other than TDI.

In one study only one fourth of the subjects with isocyanate asthma recovered completely within 10 months after exposure ended (12). In those that recovered, methacholine responsiveness returned to normal, indicating that airway hyperresponsiveness is not a predisposing factor for the occurrence of isocyanate-induced asthma. Some subjects with early or dual responses totally recovered, while some with dual responses lost only their immediate reactions becoming late responders. None with only late responses recovered.

It is possible to produce "allergic skin sensitization" of guinea pigs and mice with solutions of TDI. Dermal contact with TDI may result in respiratory tract hypersensitivity, as has been shown in guinea pigs (3).

MDI has also been reported to cause asthma and hypersensitivity pneumonitis (18, 19). Only a small proportion of patients demonstrate IgE antibodies to MDI-protein conjugates. It is likely that most isocyanates react similarly and will eventually be shown to cause respiratory problems much like TDI.

ACUTE NONSPECIFIC AIRWAY DISEASE

Several studies have shown that workers exposed to TDI experience asymptomatic airflow obstruction during the course of a workshift (3). The degree of this acute change is correlated with longterm changes in pulmonary function and severity of exposure. Exposure to low levels of TDI has been shown to cause a dose-related acute loss of pulmonary function. At the same dose, chronic deterioration in FEV_1 has been seen. Therefore, it has been proposed that excessive longterm changes in lung function may be predicted in individuals from the daily change, which may provide a means of identifying susceptible subjects.

CHRONIC NONSPECIFIC AIRWAY DISEASE

A dose-response relationship between prolonged low levels of exposure to isocyanates and chronic deterioration in lung function has been demonstrated. Wegman and coworkers found that exposure to low levels of isocyanates in a polyurethane manufacturing plant produced a dose-response decrease in FEV_1 when exposed for more than 2 years to ≥ 0.002 ppm of TDI (20). Groups of workers exposed to higher concentrations had larger average annual decrements in FEV_1 than those exposed to lower concentrations. Subjects showing the largest acute responses are likely to show the greatest chronic changes. These effects were seen in subjects exposed to levels of TDI below the existing permissible exposure limit (PEL).

Diem and associates prospectively studied a plant manufacturing TDI to evaluate the respiratory function of its workers (21). Personal air samples showed frequent excursions of TDI above 0.020 ppm. After 2 years there was no exposure-related decline in pulmonary function. Over 5½ years, those who spent ≥15% of their time working in an environment with ≥0.005 ppm TDI showed a greater decline in FEV_1 than other subjects. Nonsmokers had an annual excess loss of 38 ml of FEV_1 equal to a total loss of 1.5 liters over a 40-year working lifetime. Smoking and TDI effects on lung function were found not to be additive. There was no effect in current or previous smokers. The potential exists for longterm declines in pulmonary function in workers exposed to low levels of isocyanates.

HYPERSENSITIVITY PNEUMONITIS

Hypersensitivity pneumonitis or extrinsic allergic alveolitis has been linked to isocyanate exposure. Generally, symptoms of hypersensitivity pneumonitis include fever, chills, malaise, dyspnea, and a nonproductive cough. Chest radiographs may show diffuse patchy infiltrates or discrete nodules or may be normal even in symptomatic subjects. Pulmonary function testing may show a restrictive pattern and impaired diffusion capacity. Steriods have been shown to be effective in treating the illness, but further exposure must be avoided to prevent recurrence.

Pulmonary opacities resulting from exposure to diisocyanates have also been reported accompanied by airflow obstruction (3). In one case, acute asthma followed hypersensitivity pneumonitis in a worker challenged with MDI in the laboratory.

Exposure to toluene diisocyanate has also been reported to cause chronic restrictive pulmonary disease (1).

Other Effects

Direct exposure to solutions of isocyanates is irritating to the skin and mucous membranes and may cause contact dermatitis. Erythema, edema, and blistering are possible. Exposure to aerosols may cause ocular irritation, rhinitis, and sore throat.

Neurological symptoms including a feeling of drunkenness, numbness, and loss of balance have been described as occurring immediately after a single severe exposure to TDI by firemen in a burning polyurethane foam factory, with some symptoms persisting up to 4 years (2). They also reported nausea, vomiting, and abdominal pain, which were transitory. Whether these complications resulted from the neurotoxic effects of isocyanates, hypoxia from respiratory reactions, or other simultaneous chemical exposure is not known.

CARCINOGENESIS

In animal studies, commercial grade TDI given by gavage has produced tumors in rats and mice in a dose-response relationship. After contact with water, TDI is converted to toluene diamine, which is carcinogenic to both mice and rats (3). This may explain the carcinogenicity by gavage. 2,4-Diaminotoluene, the hydrolysis product of 2,4-TDI, caused similar tumors when tested in rats and mice (1).

The International Agency for Research on Cancer (IARC) determines there is sufficient evidence for the carcinogenicity of toluene diisocyanate to experimental animals but inadequate evidence to determine its carcinogenicity to humans (1). However, in the absence of adequate data in humans, it is reasonable to regard chemicals for which there is sufficient evidence of carcinogenicity in animals as if they represented a carcinogenic risk to humans. NIOSH recently released information classifying TDI and TDA as potential occupational carcinogens (22). Teratogenesis and reproductive effects have not been studied in animals or human populations.

MANAGEMENT OF TOXICITY

Clinical Examination

Medical history may reveal symptoms of cough, shortness of breath, nocturnal wheezing, and chest pain in workers with respiratory symptoms due to isocyanates. Symptoms may worsen with continued TDI exposure. Depending on the type of respiratory response elicited, physical examination may reveal pulmonary wheezes, coarse rales, or a normal lung exam. Irritation of mucous membranes may be present, including redness and swelling. Dermal reactions consisting of mild irritation to erythematous blisters may be seen.

Treatment

Immediate treatment of direct contact with eyes or mucous membranes should include irrigation with saline or water. Skin should be washed with soap and water and then with alcohol. Inhalation requires immediate removal to fresh air. Ingestion of TDI requires the giving of large quantities of water and inducing vomiting, unless the person is unconscious.

Bronchodilators are useful in ameliorating immediate asthmatic episodes. Theophylline partially inhibits both the immediate and late reactions of asthma induced by TDI, but does not affect the increase in airway responsiveness, apparently affecting a bronchoconstrictor component of the late asthmatic reaction rather than the inflammatory component (23). Prednisone or high dose inhaled beclamethasone are useful in preventing both late asthmatic episodes and the increase in nonspecific bronchial hyperreactivity induced by TDI.

Laboratory Diagnosis

Specific IgE antibodies to monofunctonal isocyanates have been reported in sensitized workers but specific IgE to diisocyanate conjugates have not been identified (3). In one study, p-tolyl monoisocyanate (TMI) conjugated to human serum albumin was used to identify specific IgE antibodies in three of four subjects sensitized to TDI but was not found in exposed but nonsensitized subjects (7). There appeared to be a dose-response relationship between exposure concentration and number with a positive titer. Others have found only 0–16% of sensitized subjects with specific IgE antibodies to TMI. Specific IgE has also been shown to occur in exposed workers without asthma (6).

Special Diagnostic Tests

Spirometry testing may reveal normal pulmonary function or airway obstruction in subjects with isocyanate asthma. Upon inhalation challenge, immediate, late, or dual asthmatic reactions may develop, defined as a 20% decrease in FEV_1. Challenge testing may be indicated in carefully selected cases although the risk of this is apparent. A diagnosis of isocyanate asthma can usually be made without the need to do an inhalation challenge. Isocyanate asthma may be diagnosed if the worker has reversible airflow obstruction associated with exposure to low levels of isocyanates. The doses of TDI used for inhalation challenges do not cause immediate or late bronchoconstriction in normal subjects or in asthmatic subjects not sensitized to TDI, even if they have hyperresponsive airways (24).

Biologic Monitoring

Medical surveillance should be provided to all workers exposed to diisocyanates in the workplace. Preplacement examinations including a comprehensive medical and work history, with special emphasis on preexisting respiratory conditions and smoking history should be performed (2). A physical exam with emphasis on the respiratory system, chest x-ray, and baseline spirometry should be included. The worker must also be judged fit to use a respirator. Annual periodic exams consisting of interim medical and work histories, a physical exam, and pre- and postshift or workweek spirometry should be performed. If medical conditions are found that could be directly or indirectly aggravated by exposure to diisocyanates, for example, respiratory allergy, chronic upper or lower respiratory irritation, or chronic obstructive pulmonary disease, the worker should be counseled on the increased risk from working with these substances. If evidence of sensitization is found, provisions must be made to remove the worker from further exposure.

It has not been shown that preplacement assessment is useful in the prediction of employees who will develop TDI-induced lung disease. Atopy and asthma unrelated to isocyanates do not predispose to isocyanate asthma. Not all subjects who have specific sensitivity to TDI have increased nonspecific bronchial hyperreactivity. Isocyanates in low concentrations have no effect on hyperreactive airways. Therefore, methacholine testing is not likely to identify those who will develop TDI asthma (25). Baseline methacholine testing is similar in subjects who develop immediate, dual, or late responses.

The available evidence indicates that serial measurement of the FEV_1 is a useful means of identifying acute and longterm effects of isocyanates in a workforce. Peters and Wegman demonstrated a correlation between acute and chronic effects of TDI, which may provide a way of identifying subjects who are at risk of developing longterm declines in FEV_1 (3). An annual decrement in FEV_1 of 0.020 liters in an adult nonsmoker would be anticipated from aging alone. It has been suggested that all subjects should have preemployment measurements and subsequent measurements at least annually or more often if symptoms arise. Workshift decrements of 0.3 liters or greater and annual decrements of 5% or 0.2 liters should be cause for evaluation and more frequent testing since these decrements may be associated with eventual chronic airflow obstruction or representative of asthma, which may become intractable.

Environmental Monitoring

The NIOSH criteria document defines occupational exposure to diisocyanates as exposure to airborne levels above one-half the recommended time-weighted average (TWA) occupational exposure limit or above the recommended ceiling limit (2). Adherence to all provisions of the standard is required at this level including periodic medical exams, respiratory protection, and personal monitoring.

Environmental monitoring of the workplace where diisocyanates are present should be conducted annually or after any process changes to determine whether there is exposure. If exposure is found to be present, personal monitoring is to be used in calculating the exposure of each employee occupationally exposed to diisocyanates. Area and source monitoring may be utilized to supplement personal monitoring. Samples from each operation in each work area and each shift should be taken at least once every 6 months. Records of environmental exposures applicable to an employee must be included in the employee's medical record.

Air levels of TDI can be measured by a variety of methods (3). The Marcali method and its derivatives, also called wet colorimetric methods, are the oldest and have been the reference for newer methods. They involve collecting air samples in a midget impinger by bubbling workplace air through an acid absorption medium. The intensity of the colored derivative is measured spectrophotometrically.

Tape methods, or dry colorimetric methods, for measuring isocyanates were initially developed by Reilly. Dry colorimetic methods are based on color-forming reactions that occur when chemically impregnated paper tape is exposed to air containing isocyanates. After monitoring, the tape is passed through a reflectance meter for quantification.

Chromatographic methods [gas chromatography, thin layer chromatography, and high performance liquid chromatography (HPLC)] are the most sensitive for measuring and distinguishing between isocyanates but are technically difficult and expensive. The current NIOSH-approved analytical method forms urea derivatives that can be measured quantitatively by HPLC with ultraviolet spectrometric detection (1).

Exposure Limits

The current Occupational Safety and Health (OSHA) PEL for TDI is 0.005 ppm (0.04 mg/m^3) as an 8-hour TWA with a shortterm exposure limit (STEL) of 0.02 ppm (0.15 mg/m^3) for any 15-minute period (26). The American Conference of Governmental Industrial Hygienists (ACGIH) threshold limit value (TLV) for TDI is 0.005 ppm (0.036 mg/m^3) as an 8-hour TWA and STEL Value at 0.02 ppm (0.14 mg/m^3) (27). Engineering controls should be the first approach for protecting workers. However, in special cases where this is not practical, personal protective equipment must be used to prevent skin and eye contact. Rubber, polyvinyl chloride, or other materials resistent to penetration by diisocyanates should be used. Workers should wear face shields with goggles, gloves, aprons, suits, boots and suitable respiratory equipment. Type C supplied-air respirators with full facepieces should be used above the recommended limit while engineering controls are being installed. Safety showers and eyewash stations should be readily available at operations involving TDI and TDA.

REFERENCES

1. International Agency for Research on Cancer. IARC monographs on the evaluation of the carcinogenic risk of chemicals to humans: some chemicals used in plastics and elastomers, 1986;39:287–323.
2. U.S. Dept. of Health, Education and Welfare/National Institute for Occupational Safety and Health. Criteria for a recommended standard: occupational exposure to diisocyanates (DHEW/NIOSH Pub. no. 78–215). Washington, DC: U.S. Government Printing Office, 1978.
3. Musk AW, Peters JM, Wegman DH. Isocyanates and respiratory disease: current status. Am J Ind Med 1988;13:331–349.
4. Woolrich PF. Polyurethanes and polyisocyanurates. In: Cralley LV, Cralley LJ, eds. Industrial hygiene aspects of plant operations. New York: Macmillan, 1982;1:423–439.

5. Rando RJ, Abdel-Kader H, Hughes J, Hammad YY. Toluene diisocyanate exposures in the flexible polyurethane foam industry. Am Ind Hyg Assoc J 1987;48:580–585.

6. Butcher BT, O'Neil CE, Reed MA, Salvaggio JE. Radioallergosorbent testing with *p*-tolyl monoisocyanate in toluene diisocyanate workers. Clin Allergy 1983;13:31–34.

7. Chan-Yeung M, Lam S. Occupation alasthma. Am Rev Respir Dis 1986;133:686–703.

8. Bernstein, IL. Isocyanate-induced pulmonary diseases: a current perspective. J Allergy Clin Immunol 1982;70:24–31.

9. McKerrow CB, Davies HJ, Jones AP. Symptoms and lung function following acute and chronic exposure to tolylene diisocyanate. Proc R Soc Med 1970;63:376–378.

10. Fuchs S, Valade P. Etude clinique et experimentale sur quelques cas d'intoxication par le desmodur T (diisocyanate de tolylene 1-2-4 et 1-2-6). Arch Mal Prof 1951;12:191–196.

11. Banks DE, Butcher BT, Salvaggio JE. Isocyanate-induced respiratory disease. Ann Allergy 1986;57:389–396.

12. Mapp CE, Corona PC, Fabbri L. Persistent asthma due to isocyanates. Am Rev Respir Dis 1988;137:1326–1329.

13. Lam S, Wong R, Yeung M. Nonspecific bronchial reactivity in occupational asthma. J Allergy Clin Immunol 1979;63:28–34.

14. Fabbri LM, Boschetto P, Zocca E, et al. Bronchoalveolar neutrophilia during late asthmatic reactions induced by toluene diisocyanate. Am Rev Respir Dis 1987;136:36–42.

15. Paggiaro PL, Innocenti A, Bacci E, Rossi O, Talini D. Specific bronchial reactivity to toluene diisocyanate: relationship with baseline clinical findings. Thorax 1986;41:279–282.

16. Mapp CE, Di Giacomo GR, Omini C, Broseghini C, Fabbri LM. Late, but not early, asthmatic reactions induced by toluene-diisocyanate are associated with increased airway responsiveness to methacholine. Eur J Respir Dis 1986;69:276–284.

17. Mapp CE, Dal Vecchio L, Boschetto P, De Marzo N, Fabbri LM. Toluene diisocyanate-induced asthma without airway hyperresponsiveness. Eur J Respir Dis 1986;68:89–95.

18. Zammit-Tabona M, Sherkin M, Kijek K, Chan H, Chan-Yeung M. Asthma caused by diphenylmethane diisocyanate in foundry workers. Am Rev Respir Dis 1983;128:226–230.

19. Malo JL and Zeiss CR. Occupational hypersensitivity pneumonitis after exposure to diphenylmethane diisocyanate. Am Rev Respir Dis 1982;125:113–116.

20. Wegman DH, Peters JM, Pagnotto L, Fine LJ. Chronic pulmonary function loss from exposure to toluene diisocyanate. Br J Ind Med 1977;34:196–200.

21. Diem JE, Hones RN, Hendrick DJ, et al. Five-year longitudinal study of workers employed in a new toluene diisocyanate manufacturing plant. Am Rev Respir Dis 1982;126:420–428.

22. NIOSH. Toluene diisocyanate (TDI) and toluenediamine (TDA); evidence of carcinogenicity. Cincinnati, OH: US Department of Health and Human Services, Public Health Service, CDC, 1990: Current intelligence bulletin #53. DHHS Publication no. (NIOSH) 90–101.

23. Mapp C, Boschetto P, Dal Vecchio L, et al. Protective effects of anti-asthma drugs on late asthmatic reactions and increased airway responsiveness induced by toluene diisocyanate in sensitized subjects. Am Rev Respir Dis 1987;136:1403–1407.

24. Paggiaro P, Bacci E, Talini D, et al. Atropine does not inhibit late asthmatic responses induced by toluene-diisocyanate in sensitized subjects. Am Rev Respir Dis 1987;136:1237–1241.

25. Mapp CE, Boschetto P, Dal Vecchio L, Fabbri LM. Occupational asthma due to isocyanates. Eur Respir J 1988;3:273–279.

26. 29 CFR 1910.1000, Table 2-1-A. Washington, DC: GPO.

27. ACGIH. 1990–1991. Threshold limit values for chemical substances and physical agents and biological exposure indices. Cincinnati, OH: American Conference of Governmental Industrial Hygienists, 1991:35.

95

Acrylates and Methacrylates

Barbara Scolnick, M.D.

Exposure to acrylate and methacrylate monomers and polymers occurs in plastic manufacturing, printing, dentistry, surgery, and, when considering implants, even patients' bodies. Because of their use in medicine, these materials have been subject to a great deal of study for pharmacologic, toxicologic, and biocompatibility considerations. From the experience of the last 50 years, it is clear these are extremely useful chemicals. However, with regard to occupational health, some areas of real concern have emerged, and many areas of theoretical risk have also become apparent.

SOURCES AND PRODUCTION

The term acrylates includes the derivatives of acrylic acid and methacrylic acid. Acrylic acid, also known as propionic acid has the chemical formula $C_3O_2H_4$, $CH_2{=}CH{-}COOH$. Methacrylic acid differs by having a methyl group rather than the alpha hydrogen: $C_4O_2H_6$: $CH_2{=}C(CH_3){-}COOH$. These acids are of commercial interest because some derivatives, especially their esters, easily combine with each other to form polymers. By beginning with various monomers, polymers of great variability can result from tough plastics to clear rubbers and have found extensive use in our modern world.

Commercially the most important monomer of both series is methyl methacrylate:

$C_5O_2H_8$: $CH_2{=}C(CH_3){-}\overset{\displaystyle O}{\overset{\|}{C}}{-}O{-}CH_3$. The polymethyl methacrylate polymer has some unique characteristics. It transmits light well at wavelengths of 360–1000 nanometers (wavelengths of visible light are 400–700). It is a tough, hard plastic that is weather and moisture resistant. It is thermoplastic, i.e., when heated above its Tg (glass transition temperature), it is easily bent or molded into complex shapes. It is often recognized by its brand names, Plexiglas or Lucite.

The commercial history of these monomers dates from the 1930s. Although Redtenbacker had described the production of acrylic acid by oxidizing acrolein in 1843, it was Otto Rohm's doctoral thesis in 1901 that described the tough, clear plastic prepared from polymers of ethyl methacrylate (1). In 1909, he and Otto Haas began a company to manufacture "organic glass," finding its first use in creating safety glass. Rohm & Haas Germany and Rohm & Haas USA remain major producers.

The monomers are derived from basic petrochemicals. Since 1970, a propylene oxidation process involving the oxidation of propylene to acrolein and subsequent oxidation of acrolein to acrylic acid is used (2).

The monomers of commercial interest are all liquids with a pungent odor, and all have a tendency for "spontaneous" polymerization and must be handled with care. They are usually stabilized with minimal amounts of inhibitors. The inhibitors most frequently used are hydroquinone or monomethylether of hydroquinone (MEHQ). For most applications, inhibitors do not have to be removed. If necessary, they can be removed with ion exchange resins. Washed uninhibited monomers are not stable and should be used promptly. In any case, monomers should always be used within 1 year.

The chemical formulas, synonyms, and Chemical Abstract Service (CAS) code numbers of some of the commercially important monomers of the acrylic acid series are summarized in Table 95.1.

The liquid monomers are polymerized in one of several processes: bulk, solution, emulsion, or suspension. The ensuing polymer is either sheet plastic, liquid, or powder. The lower molecular weight esters are soluble in aromatic hydrocarbons; those of higher molecular weight are soluble in aliphatic hydrocarbons. Polymerization can be initiated either in a heat curing process, requiring addition of heat, a UV process, requiring the addition of a chemical that absorbs UV light into the system, or a "cold curing" process requiring a chemical accelerator to start the polymerization (3).

SITES, INDUSTRIES, AND BUSINESSES

The major uses of the acrylates and methacrylates are in the following industries:

Paints

Acrylic esters undergo polymerization with water to form emulsion polymers. When the emulsion such as paint or adhesive is applied to a surface, the water evaporates, leaving a tough film. The acrylate polymers form a coating that is resistant to water, sunlight, and weather. They are known as latex paints.

Paper

Emulsions of acrylic polymers are coated onto paper to make it more water resistant and receptive to ink. They also can be added to paper pulp to make the paper resistant to grease and oil.

Table 95.1. Names and Formula of Common Acrylates

Compound	Synonyms	Formula	CAS #
Acrylic acid	Propene acid Acroleic acid	C3H4O2	79-10-7
Ethyl acrylate	Acrylic acid ethyl ester	C5H8O2	140-88-5
Methyl acrylate	Acrylic acid methyl ester	C4H6O2	96-33-3
Methacrylic acid		C4H6O2	79-41-4
Methyl methacrylate	Methacrylic acid methyl ester	C5H8O2	80-62-6

Adhesives

Acrylic emulsions are used as resin adhesives on envelopes, labels, and decals. Sealants are also used for bathtub caulk, baseboard seams, and glazing.

Textiles

Methylacrylate is used primarily as a comonomer with acrylonitrile in the preparation of acrylic fibers. They generally contain 85% acrylonitrile.

Building Materials

Polymethyl methacrylate sheets are used in building panels, bathroom fixtures, and plumbing. As a glazing, it is used for bank teller windows, police cars, enclosures for swimming pools, domes for tennis courts, skylights, and telephone booths.

Automotive

Polymethyl methacrylate is used for dials, instrument panels, medallions, taillights, and backup lights.

Toy Industry

High performance colorful methacrylates are used extensively in the toy industry.

Oil Additives

Long chain polymethacrylates are used as additives to increase the viscosity of automobile oils.

Leather

Emulsion acrylate polymers bind to leather to improve appearance, prevent cracking, and add scuff resistance.

Cosmetics

Ethylacrylate has been used as a fragrance additive in some soaps and creams at levels of 0.001–0.01%. It smells somewhat like pineapple. There are reports of it being identified in the volate component of fresh pineapple. This is the only natural source of any acrylate (4).

Printing

"Solventless technology" in printing involves a system of synthetic resins, acrylate monomers, and UV light. When UV light is shown on the system, the monomers almost instantly bind and cross-link the polymers causing "curing." These monomers are more complex than the low molecular weight "traditional" acrylates and are known as multifunctional acrylic monomers (MFA). The most common are pentaerythrinitrol triacylate (PETA), trimethylpropane triacylate (TMPTA), and hexanedioldiacrylate (HDODA) (Figure 95.1).

Dentistry

Polymethyl methacrylate began to be used in denture bases in 1946. This is the portion of the denture that rests in the mouth

Figure 95.1.   Structure of multifunctional acrylic monomers (MFA).

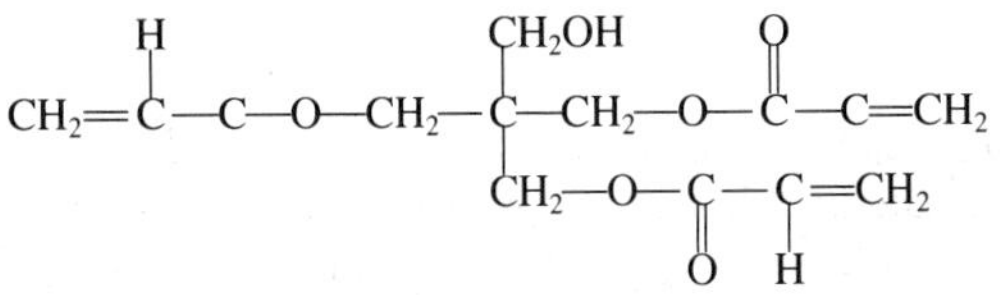

Pentaerythritol triacrylate (PETA)

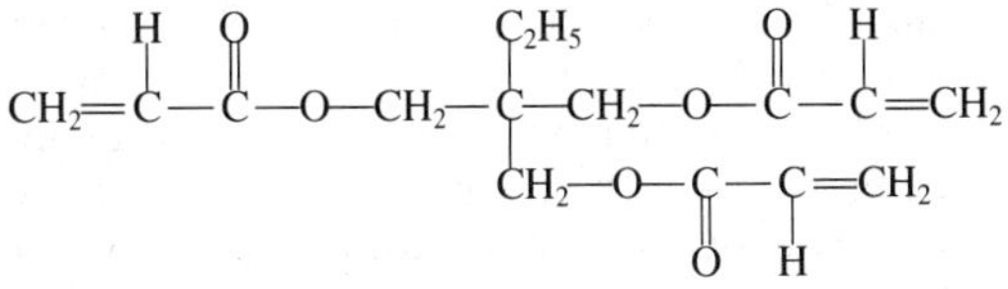

Trimethylolpropane triacrylate (TMPTA)

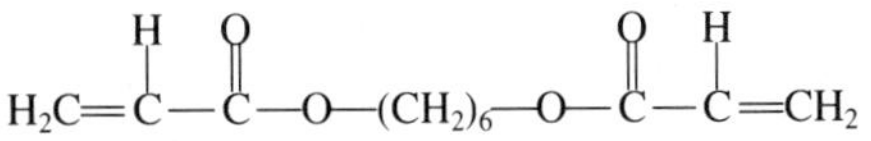

1,6-Hexanediol diacrylate (HDODA)

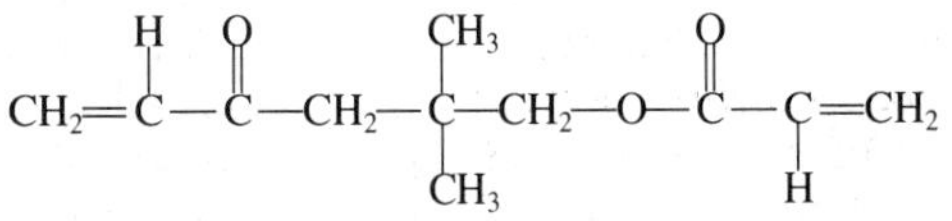

Neopentylglycol diacrylate (NPGDA)

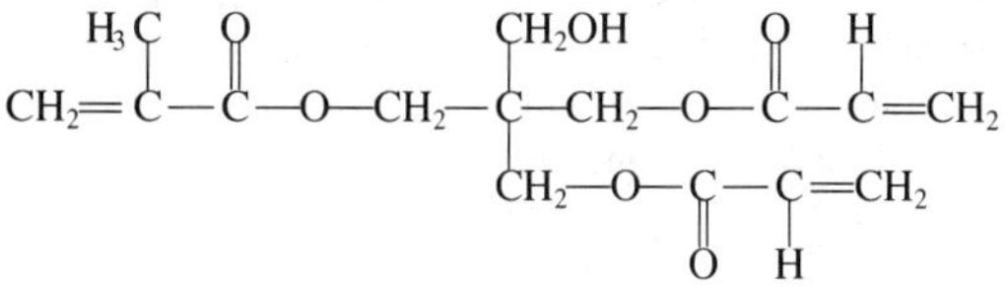

Trimethylolpropane trimethylacrylate (TMPTMA)

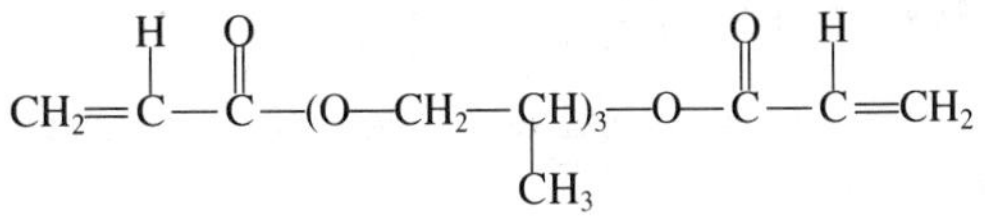

Tripropyleneglycol diacrylate (TRPGDA)

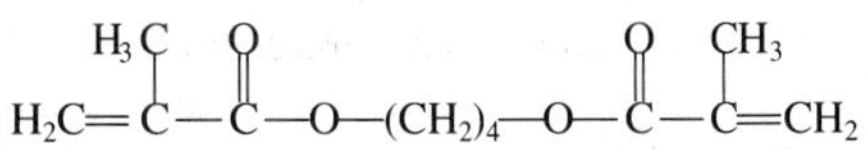

Tetraethyleneglycol dimethacrylate (TTEGDMA)

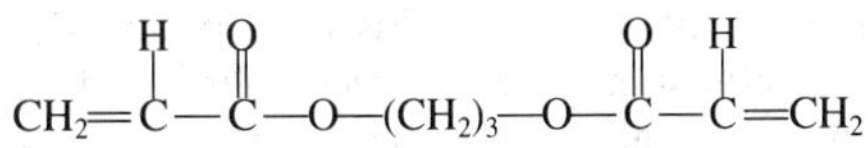

Triethyleneglycol diacrylate (TREGDA)

and retains the artificial teeth. The most common resin is a liquid/powder type, wherein the liquid monomer is combined with the powder polymer into a doughlike consistency, packed into a mold which conforms to the patient's mouth, and cured by heat curing, UV light, or cold curing. Another use in dentistry is as filling material when combined with inorganic materials to form composite resins (5).

Medicine

Methyl methacrylate resins are used to repair cranial defects and in plastic surgery. The major use of methyl methacrylate, however, is in orthopedics. In 1959 Sir John Charnley revolutionized hip replacement surgery by using cold curing polymethyl methacrylate as a bony cement to anchor metallic hip prosthesis (6). Although refinements have been made over the ensuing 31 years, the basic system of cold curing the methyl methacrylate monomer liquid and a polymer powder remains the same. In the operating room the orthopedist kneads the mixture into the proper rubbery consistency and injects it into the joint. After extensive use in the United Kingdom in the 1960s bony cement was approved in the United States in 1969. Currently 140,000 total joint replacements are performed annually (7).

Optics

The concept of replacing eyeglasses with lenses in direct contact with the cornea was conceived in the 1800s but delayed because glass was obviously not suitable. After World War II, Ridley, an ophthalmologist, noted that fragments of airfighter canopies constructed of polymethylmethacrylate (PMMA) were tolerated well in the eyes of injured pilots (8). This led to its use in contact lenses. "Hard contact lenses" are still made of polymethacrylate. The hydrophobic nature of PMMA causes problems with comfort. A newer acrylic polymer is based on the monomer 2-hydroxyethyl methacrylate (HEMA). By replacing the methyl group with a hydroxyethyl (C—C—OH) group, the monomer becomes hydrophilic and can absorb a great deal of water, although it does not dissolve in water. This is the monomer used for "soft" contact lenses.

CLINICAL TOXICOLOGY

Route of Exposure

Exposure to acrylate and methacrylate monomers occurs through skin absorption and inhalation.

Metabolism

In humans undergoing total hip replacement surgery both methyl methacrylate (MMA) and methacrylic acid were found in the circulation (9). Methacrylic acid as the coenzyme A ester is a normal intermediate in the catabolism of valine. In rats, over 80% of an administered dose of carbon-14-labeled MMA is respired as CO_2 within 5–6 hours (10). This supports the idea that MMA is metabolized via intermediate metabolism and the citric acid cycle. Thus it is unlikely the metabolites would be reactive dangerous particles.

The acrylates behave differently. Studies in rats have found that methyl acrylate and ethyl acrylate are enzymatically hydrolyzed by plasma and homogenates of rat liver, lung, and kidney (11). However, the acrylates ester also reacted with glutathione in vitro and decreased tissue nonprotein sulfhydryl groups in vivo. The carboxylase inhibitor triorthotolyl phosphate (TOTP) potentiated the toxicities of the acrylates. This implies that carboxyesterases are important in the detoxification of acrylates. There must exist competition between the glutathione conjugation system and carboxylesterases. The conjugation system could potentially result in dangerous alkylating agents (12).

SIGNS, SYMPTOMS, AND SYNDROMES OF TOXIC EXPOSURES

Acute Toxicity

The liquid monomers all have a pungent corrosive odor and are irritating to the mucous membranes in high concentration. Most of the monomers are severe eye irritants when instilled into rabbit eyes. Methacrylates tend to be less irritating than acrylates. If a liquid monomer from either series is inadvertently splashed in the eye, the eye must be irrigated with copious amounts of water.

The acrylates and methacrylates affect the skin in two ways. They cause a contact irritant dermatitis and an allergic dermatitis.

In 1954, Fisher reported on allergic eczematous dermatitis affecting the hands of dentists who worked with the liquid methacrylate (13). Patch tests were positive, and the condition cleared when the monomer was avoided.

In the late 1960s there were outbreaks of dermatitis associated with artificial acrylic nails. Some of these cases were extreme, with onycholysis, nail dystrophy, and eczema around the nail bed. The Food and Drug Administration received sufficient complaints from consumers that, after litigation on July 3, 1974, the District Court in Chicago issued an injunction prohibiting the further manufacture of a product called "Long Nails," which contained a MMA monomer (14).

In 1971 Pegum and Medhurst reported the case of an orthopedic surgeon who developed an allergic contact dermatitis from bony cement (15). This was the first time it was noted that the monomer readily passes through rubber gloves.

In the 1970s, as polyfunctional acrylic monomers began to find extensive use in ultraviolet polymerizing systems, reports of contact dermatitis have come from the printing trade (16–18). The most widely used multifunctional acrylic momomers, pentaerythritol (PETA), trimethylol propane triacrylate (TMPTA), and hexanediol diacrylate (HDODA), have been shown to be irritants as well as allergens. From these reports, it is evident that an individual can have a negative patch test to MMA, the most frequently tested, yet be allergic to other acrylates.

Any estimate of the incidence of skin reactions is difficult. Spiechowicz reports that 10% of dental technicians after 2–14 years exposure develop MMA sensitization (19).

All acrylates should be handled with minimal skin contact. If an already sensitized individual must continue to be exposed, heavy-gauge rubber or polyvinyl chloride gloves should be used.

Possible Cardiopulmonary Toxicity

Early toxicological studies of acrylates were performed by Deichman in 1941, Spealman in 1945, and Treon in 1949 (20–22). These established the oral LD_{50} and inhalation LC_{50} in the guinea pig, rabbit, and rat. The results are summarized in Table 95.2. When toxic quantities of acrylates were absorbed, the

Table 95.2. LD$_{50}$ and LC$_{50}$ for Common Acrylates

Route	Species	Compound	Dose (LD$_{50}$ or LC$_{50}$)
Oral	Rabbit	Methyl acrylate	7 ml/kg
Oral	Rabbit	Ethyl acrylate	4–6 ml/kg
Oral	Rabbit	Butyl acrylate	7–10 ml/kg
Oral	Rats	Methyl acrylate	8 ml/kg
Oral	Rats	Ethyl acrylate	14.8 ml/kg
Inhalation	Rats	Methyl acrylate	1000 ppm
Inhalation	Rats	Methyl methacrylate	4000 ppm

animals developed accelerated respiration, followed by motor weakness, decreased respiration, and finally coma.

Early reports appeared in the literature of severe hypotension occurring in patients undergoing total hip replacement (THR) surgery (23–26). Occasionally there was cardiac arrest and patient death (27, 28). This phenomena has been extensively studied, but the culprit remains unknown. Some investigators have implicated fat and bone marrow emboli caused by reaming the femoral cavity. Others have questioned the heat effect from the exothermic polymerization, and many think the residual monomer is toxic (29, 30).

Mir, Lawrence, and Autian studied the effects on blood pressure, heart rate, ECG, and respiration in anesthetized dogs following intravenous administration of methacrylic acid and 12 of its esters (31). They found they all decreased heart rate, increased respiratory rate, produced ECG changes, and affected blood pressure by causing hypotension, hypertension, or a biphasic response. The same investigators perfused isolated rabbit heart with solutions containing methacrylate esters at concentrations of 1:1,000, 1:10,000, and 1:100,000, and found significant reduction in cardiac rate and force of contraction (32).

The question for patients is whether free MMA in the circulation ever reaches concentrations that are toxic. In THR, where exposure is greatest, venous blood can reveal MMA levels of 1 mg/100 ml (33). Clinically, MMA is being used extensively, and for the time being the profession is cautiously approving it.

No case reports have implicated any acrylate as a cardiovascular toxin in any occupationally exposed population. There have only been a few epidemiology studies of occupational exposure to methacrylates. In 1976, National Institute on Occupational Safety and Health (NIOSH) studied 91 workers in five plants manufacturing polymethyl methacrylate sheets, where the average 8-hour time weighted average was 4–49 ppm (34). These individuals were compared with 43 nonexposed workers at the same plants. The authors found no effect over the work shift in blood pressure, pulse, or symptoms. A few unexpected differences were found that may be statistical "red herrings" or may be significant. The high exposure group had different mean values for glucose, cholesterol, albumin, bilirubin, and more frequent complaints referable to the nervous system than the control group.

Possible Neurotoxin

Several reports in the Russian literature suggest that MMA causes vague central nervous system symptoms such as fatigue, headache, and loss of appetite (34, 35). All these studies suffer from lack of a control group. The NIOSH 1976 study found that complaints of dizziness, shakiness, and drowsiness were more common in the exposed (46%) than control (23%) groups. Innes and Tansy studied the effect of MMA vapors on the EEG and neuronal discharge rates of rat brains (36). At a concentration of 400 ppm, four times the threshold limit value, MMA monomer vapor produced a rapid, reversible reduction in neuronal discharge rates in the lateral hypothalamus and ventral hippocampus of rats as compared to control animals.

MMA has been implicated as a neurotoxin on peripheral nerves. Many of the reports of allergic dermatitis comment on the finger and palmar paresthesias that accompany the skin breakdown (37). The paresthesias often take 2–3 months to heal after the skin has recovered. Seppalainen and Rajaniemi studied nerve conduction velocities on 20 dental hygienists and 18 control subjects (38). Dental technicians had significantly slower distal sensory conduction velocities from the digits I, II, and III on the right hand, and also from the radial aspects of the digits II and III on the left hand, than did the controls. Findings are considered to represent mild axonal degeneration in the area with closest and most frequent contact with MMA.

Chronic Effects on Metabolism

Borzelleca and associates administered ethyl acrylate and MMA to rats at doses 6–2000 ppm for 2 years (39). At the highest level (2000 ppm) of ethyl acrylate, there was a definite decrease in weight in the females over the course of the study.

Tansey found that rats receiving daily 8-hour exposures to 116 ppm MMA vapor for 3 months had lower body weight than controls. They also found that individual oxygen consumption measurements made for exposed rats were 45% increased over controls (40). At necropsy there was no gross or microscopic pathology to the heart, GI tract, or liver.

Lawrence and Autian demonstrated that animals exposed to MMA and ethylmethacrylate increased their sleeping time (41). It is unclear whether this is an effect on enzymes or the central nervous system.

Tansay and others have found that MMA vapors produce transient slowing of the small bowel in rats and dogs (42). In vitro studies of isolated guinea pig ileum demonstrated prompt inhibition of contraction when the intestine was bathed in a solution containing methacrylate esters (43).

The significance of these studies on occupationally exposed humans is unclear. Anecdotally, many dental students when working with MMA complain of nausea and anorexia (44). An operating room nurse who developed a generalized hypersensitivity to bony cement complained of anorexia that lasted several hours after each THR case (45). McLaughlin reported that during three THR the concentration of the monomer vapor in the operating room never rose above 280 ppm. This concentration was measured within 15 seconds after mixing the cement. It quickly dropped to 50 ppm in 2 minutes and to about 2 ppm within 6 minutes, where it remained constant for 11 minutes (46).

Acrylates as Possible Teratogens

There are no case reports or epidemiology studies on humans which address the issues of acrylates as teratogens.

There are several different animal studies, and results have been both positive and negative. Singh et al., treated pregnant rats with i.p. injections of monomers of five methacrylate esters on days 5, 10, and 15 of gestation (47). On the 20th day of gestation these rats as well as a control group which had received cottonseed oil, water, or saline as i.p. injection were killed. At one or more of the doses used, each compound produced some or all of the following effects: resorption, gross skeletal malformations, fetal death, and decreased fetal size. This study has been criticized for using i.p. exposure. Murray et al. exposed Sprague-Dawley pregnant rats to inhaled ethyl acrylate for 6 hr/day on day 6–15 of gestation at doses 0, 50, and 150 ppm (48). They found no effect at 50 ppm, but at 150 ppm maternal toxicity marked by decreased body weight and decreased food consumption was noted. McLaughlin et al. exposed pregnant mice to MMA vapor at concentration 1330 ppm on days 5–15 for 2 hr/day and found no evidence of fetal toxicity (46). Merkle and Klimish exposed pregnant Sprague-Dawley rats by inhalation to n-butyl acrylate a 0, 25, 135, or 250 ppm for 6 hr/day on gestation day 7–16 (49). At 135 and 250 ppm postimplant, deaths were increased, but no teratogenic response was found.

Acrylates as Possible Carcinogens

Polymerized acrylates and methacrylates are presumed to be innocuous materials except for any residual monomer. The one exception is the possible oncogenic role of PMMA when used in implants. Oppenheimer et al. placed subcutaneous implants in Wistar rats (50). Eleven of the 25 rats developed sarcomas. Similar results have been found by other investigators, and the term ''solid state'' oncogenesis for the induction of tumors by solid materials in experimental animals at the implantation site has been defined. It seems that the physical properties of the foreign body are more important than the chemical nature. The literature on solid state carcinogenesis is reviewed by Williams (51). PMMA appears to be safe in humans. Assuming 25 years for induction of cancers in humans, we would be seeing the rising tide of malignancies from the early total hip replacement surgeries. There are no reports of malignant degeneration around the implant site.

The liquid monomers, both older monofunctional and newer multifunctional acrylates, have been subject to much study in animal experiments.

DePass et al. studied the dermal oncogenic potential of acrylic acid, ethyl acrylate, and butyl acrylate by painting them on the dorsal skin of mice three times weekly for their entire lifetimes (52). They used a negative control of acetone and a positive control of 3-methylcholanthracene. They found no carcinogenic activity of any of these acrylates.

The same investigators studied dermal oncogenic potential of some newer acrylates used in photocurable coatings with the same experimental system. The NPGDA and EA (see Fig. 95.1) -treated mice showed the development of tumors. There were eight and six, respectively, as compared with 34 in the positive anthracene control group and zero in the acetone group (53).

Celanese Corporation studied eight multifunctional acrylates (MFAs) in dermal tests on C3H/Hej mice (54). Fifty animals were treated twice weekly for 80 weeks with a concentration determined to be only minimally irritating. Five of theses MFAs showed no increase in tumors. These were: TMPTA, TMPTMA, HDODA, TRPGDA, and TTEGDMA. Three MFAs, PETA, TREGDA, and TTEGDA, showed an increased number of tumors. TTEGDA caused severe skin damage and skin tumors. PETA and TREGDA showed increased numbers of skin cancers and disturbingly induced an increased incidence of lymphomas in treated animals.

Table 95.3. Exposure Limits for Common Acrylates

Compound	ACGIH TLV	OSHA PEL
Acrylic acid	10 ppm	none
Ethyl acrylate	5 ppm	25 ppm
Methyl acrylate	10 ppm	10 ppm
Methacrylic acid	20 ppm	none
Methyl methacrylate	100 ppm	100 ppm

The National Toxicology Program has studied methyl methacrylate exposure by oral route in F344/N rats and B6C3F1 mice and found no induction of tumors (55).

The National Toxicology Program studied ethyl acrylate by oral administration to mice and rats (56). Fifty male and female mice were fed ethyl acrylate in doses 100 mg/kg bodyweight (bw) and 200 mg/kg bw by five times weekly for 103 weeks. Significant increases of squamous cell papillomas and carcinomas of the stomach were noted in both species.

Miller studied ethyl acrylate by inhalation in mice and rats (57). Groups of 105 female and male mice (B6C3F1) and rats (Fischer 344) were exposed to ethyl acrylate at concentrations of 25, 75, 225 ppm for 6 hr/day, 5 days/week for 27 months. There was no increased incidence of tumors in the exposed groups. In the highest exposed groups, the mean body weight was lower, and nonneoplastic lesions of the olfactory mucosa were noted in both species.

Summarizing the data, the International Agency for Research on Cancer has concluded there is sufficient evidence for the carcinogenicity of ethyl acrylate in experimental animals. With respect to methyl acrylate and n-butyl acrylate, there is inadequate evidence. They did not evaluate the data for the multifunctional acrylates (4).

Recently a study of workers at a Rohm & Haas plant exposed to both ethyl acrylate and MMA reported a significant excess of colorectal cancers (Standardized Mortality Ratio 1.67 52 obs/31.2 exp) (58). A standardized mortality ratio study of 2671 men exposed to MMA at two American Cyanamid plants followed 1951–1981 found no excess incidence of cancer (59).

Exposure Limits

Table 95.3 summarizes the limits recommended by the American College of Industrial Hygienists in terms of threshold limit values (TLV) based on an 8-hour day, 40-day work week, and mandated by the Occupational Safety and Health Administration in terms of permissible exposure limits (PEL) (60).

The acrylates and methacrylates are exceedingly useful chemicals. They are strong skin sensitizers and irritants. They are also irritating to the eye, and their pungent odor irritates the nasal passages (61). The chronic toxicity is not fully evaluated. The newer multifunctional acrylates and ethyl acrylate have been implicated as causing cancer in some rodent tests.

ACKNOWLEDGMENT

I wish to thank Dr. Robert Pressberg for his help in preparing this chapter.

REFERENCES

1. Glavis FS, Woodman JF. Rohm & Haas Co. Methacrylate compounds. In: Stnader A, ex. ed. Kirk-Othmer encyclopedia of chemical technology. 2nd ed. Vol 13. New York: John Wiley & Sons, 1967:331–363.

2. Kine BB, Novak RW. Rohm & Haas Co. Methacrylic polymers. In: Grayson M, ex. ed. Kirk-Othmer encyclopedia of chemical technology. 3rd ed. Vol 15. New York: John Wiley & Sons, 1981:377–398.

3. Kine BB, Novak RW. Rohm & Haas Co. Acrylic polymers. In Grayson M, ed. Kirk-Othmer encyclopedia of chemical technology. 3rd ed. Vol 1. New York: Wiley & Sons, 1978:386–408.

4. World Health Organization. International Agency for Research on Cancer. IARC Monographs on the Evaluation of the Carcinogenic Risk of Chemicals to Humans. Some chemicals used in plastics and elastomers. Vol 39. This publication represents the views and expert opinions of an IARC Working Group on the Evaluation of the Carcinogenic Risk of Chemicals to Humans which met in Lyon, 11–18 June, 1985. Distributed for IARC by the Secretariat of the WHO. Printed in Switzerland:81–98.

5. Bever MB. Encyclopedia of material science and engineering. Massachusetts Institute of Technology. Oxford: Pergamon Press, Ltd, 1986. Combe EC. Acrylic dental polymers: formulation and synthesis. Cambridge, MA: MIT Press, 1986;1:51–56.

6. Charnley J. Anchorage of the femoral head prosthesis to the shaft of the femur. J Bone Joint Surg Br 42;1960:28.

7. Wijn JR, van Mullen PJ. Biocompatibility of acrylic implants. In: Williams D, ed. Biocompatibility of clinical implant materials. Vol II. Boca Raton, FL: CRC Press, 1981:99–126.

8. Ridley, H. Intraocular lenses; recent development in surgery of cataract. Br J Ophthalmol 1952;36:113.

9. Crout HG, Corkill JA, James ML, Ling RSM. Methylmethacrylate metabolism in man. Clin Orthop Rel Res 1979;141:90–95.

10. Bratt H, Hathaway HDE. Fate of methyl methacrylate in rats. Br J Cancer 1977;36:114–119.

11. Silver EH, Murphy SD. Potentiation of acrylate ester toxicity by prior treatment with the carboxylesterase inhibitor triorthotolyl phosphate (TOTP). Toxicol Appl Pharmacol 1981;57:208–219.

12. Delbressine LPC, Seutter-Berlage F, Seulter E. Identification of urinary mercapturic acids formed from acrylate methacrylate and crotonate in the rat. Xenobiotica 1981;11:241–247.

13. Fisher AA. Allergic sensitization of the skin and oral mucosa to acrylic denture materials. JAMA 1954;156:238.

14. Fisher AA, Franks A, Glick H. Allergic sensitization of the skin and nails to acrylic plastic nails. J Allergy 1957;28:84.

15. Pegum JS, Medhurst FA. Contact dermatitis from penetration of rubber gloves by acrylic monomer. Br Med J 1971;ii:141.

16. Nethercott JR. Skin problems associated with multifunctional acrylic monomers in ultraviolet curing inks. Br J Dermatol 1978;98:541–552.

17. Emmett EA. Contact dermatitis from polyfunctional acrylic monomers. Contact Derm 1977;3:245–248.

18. Nethercott JR, Jakubovic HR, Pilger G, Smith JW. Allergic contact dermatitis due to urethane acrylate in ultraviolet cured inks. Br J Ind Med 1983;40:241–250.

19. Spiechowicz E. Experimental studies on the effect of acrylic resin on rabbit skin. Berufsdeamatosen; 1971;19:132–144.

20. Deichmann W. Toxicity of methyl, ethyl and n-butyl methacrylate. J Ind Hyg Toxicol 1941;23:343.

21. Spealman CR, Main RJ, Haag HB, Larson PS. Monomeric methyl methacrylate. Ind Med 1945;14:292–298.

22. Treon JR, Sigman H, Wright H, Kitzmiller KV. The toxicity of methyl and ethyl acrylate. J Ind Hyg Toxicol 1949;31:317–326.

23. Phillips H, Cole PV, Lettin AW. Cardiovascular effects of implanted acrylic bone cement. Br Med J 1971;3:460.

24. Cohen CA, Smith TC. The intraoperative hazard of acrylic bone cement; a report of a case. Anesthesiology 1971;35:547.

25. Gresham GA, Kuczmski A. Cardiac arrest and bone cement. Br Med J 1970;3:465.

26. Hyland J, Robbins RHC. Cardiac arrest and bone cement. Br Med J 1970;4:176.

27. Kepes ER, Underwood PS, Becsey L. Intraoperative death associated with acrylic bone cement. JAMA 1972;222:576.

28. Herndon JH, Bechtol CO, Crikenberger DP. Fat embolism during total hip replacement: a prospective study. J Bone Joint Surg Am 1974;56:1350.

29. Feith R. Side effects of acrylic cement implanted into bone. Acta Orthop Scand Suppl 1975:161.

30. Mir GN, Lawrence WH, Autian J. Toxicological and pharmacological actions of methylacrylate monomers. III. Respiratory and cardiovascular functions of anesthetized dogs. J Pharm Sci 1974;63:376.

31. Mir GN, Lawrence WH, Autian J. Toxicological and pharmacological actions of methacrylate monomers. I. Effects on the isolated perfused rabbit heart. J Pharm Sci 1973, 62:778.

32. Homsy CA, Tullos HS, Anderson MS, Differante NM, King JR. Some physiological aspects of prosthesis stabilization with acrylic cement. Clin Orthop. 1972;83:317.

33. Cromer J, Kronoveter K. A study of methyl methacrylate exposures and employee health. Publication No. DHEW (NIOSH) 77-119. US Department of Health, Education, and Welfare, National Institute for Occupational Safety and Health, Washington DC: GPO, 1976:1–43.

34. Blagodatin VM, Golova IA, Blagodatkina NK, et al. Issues of industrial hygiene and occupational pathology in the manufacture of organic glass (Russ). Gig Tr Prof Zabol (Russ) 1976;14:11–14.

35. Karpov BD. The effect of small concentrations of methyl methacrylate vapors on the inhibition and stimulation process of the cortex of the brain. Trad Lenigr Sanit Gig Med Inst (Russ) 1953;14:43–8.

36. Innes DL, Tansy MF. Central nervous system effects of methyl methacrylate vapor. Neurotoxicity 1981;2:515–522.

37. Blair FI, Fisher AA, Salvati EA. Contact dermatitis in surgeons from methylmethacrylate bone cement. J Bone Joint Surg Am 2 1975;57:547.

38. Seppalainen AM, Rajaniemi R. Local neurotoxicity of methylmethacrylate among dental technicians. Am J Ind Med 1984;5:471–477.

39. Borzelleca JF, Larson PS, Hennigar GR, Huf EG, Crawford EM, Smith RB. Studies of chronic oral toxicity of monomeric ethyl acrylate and methyl methacrylate. Toxicol Appl Pharmacol 1964;6:29–36.

40. Tansy MF, Kendall FM. Update on the toxicity of inhaled methylmethacrylate vapor. Drug Chem Toxicol 1979;2:315–330.

41. Autian J. Structure toxicity relationships of acrylic monomers. Environ Health Perspect 1975;ii:141–152.

42. Tansy MF, Martin JS, Benhagen S, Sandin WE, Kendall FM. GI motor inhibition associated with acute exposure to methylmethacrylate vapor. J Pharm Sci 1977;66:613–618.

43. Mir GN, Lawrence WH, Autian J. Toxicological and pharmacological actions of methacrylate monomers. Vol II. Effects on isolated guinea pig ileum. J Pharm Sci 1973;62:1258–1261.

44. Tansy MF, Benhagem S, Probst S, et al. The effects of methylmethacrylate vapor on gastric motor function. J Am Dent Assoc 1974;89:372–6.

45. Scolnick B, Collins J. Systemic reaction to methylmethacrylate in an operating room nurse. J Occup Med 1985;28:196–198.

46. McLaughlin RE, Reger SI, Barkalow BS, Allen MS, Di Fazio CA. Methylmethacrylate: a study of teratogenicity and fetal toxicity of the vapor in the mouse. J Bone Joint Surg Am 1978;60(30):355–358.

47. Singh AR, Lawrence WH, Autian J. Embryonic fetal toxicity and teratogenic effects of a group of methacrylate esters in rats. J Penet Res 1972;51:1632–1638.

48. Murray JS, Mille RR, Deacon TR, et al. Teratological evaluation of inhaled ethyl acrylate in rats. Toxicol Appl Pharmacol 1981;60:106–111.

49. Merkle J, Klimisch HR. n-Butyl acrylate: prenatal inhalation toxicity in the rat. Fund Appl Toxicol 1983;3:443–447.

50. Oppenheimer BS, Oppenheimer ET, Stout AP, Danishefsky I. Malignant tumors resulting from embedding plastics in rodents. Science 1953;118:305.

51. Williams DF, Roaf S, eds. Implants in surgery. London: WB Saunders, 1973:274.

52. DePass LR, Fowler EH, Meckley DR, Weill CS. Dermal oncogenicity bioassays of acrylic acid, ethylacrylate, and butyl acrylate. J Toxicol Environ Health 1984;14:115–120.

53. DePass LR, Maronpot RR, Weil CS. Dermal oncogenicity bioassays of monofunctional and multifunctional acrylates and acrylate based oligomers. J Toxicol Environ Health; 1958;16:55–60.

54. Andrews LS, Clary JJ. Review of the toxicity of multifunctional acrylates. J Toxicol Environ Health 1986;19:149–164.

55. Chan PC. National toxicology program technical report on the toxicology and carcinogenesis studies of methylmethacrylate in F344/N rats and B6C3F1 mice. NIH publication No. 86-2570 NTP TR 314. US Department of Health and Human Services. Washington, DC: GPO, 1985.

56. NTP Technical Report on the carcinogenesis studies of ethylacrylate (CAS no. 140-88-5) in F344/N rats and B6C3F mice (gavage studies). Bethesda, MD: U.S. Dept. of Health and Human Services, Public Health Service, National Institutes of Health; (Springfield, VA: National Technical Information Service, distributor), 1983. National Toxicology Program technical report series no. 259 NIH publication no., 83-2515. Ethyl Acrylate. National Toxicology Program. August 1983. NTP-82-077. US Public Health Service. National Toxicology Program.

57. Miller RR, Young RJ, Kociba DG. Chronic toxicity and oncogenicity bioassay of inhaled ethylacrylate in Fischer 344 rats and B6C3F1 mice. Drug Chem Toxicol 1985;8:1–42.

58. Maher K, De Fonso L. Unpublished data, 1984.

59. Collins JJ, Page LC, Caporossi JC, Utidijian HM, Saipher JN. Mortality patterns among men exposed to methyl methacrylate. J Occup Med 1989;31:41–6.

60. US Occupational Safety and Health Administration (1976) Occupational safety and health standards, subpart Z—toxic and hazardous substances. 29 USC 17 C1910.1000; 31:8303.

61. Cooke FW (Clemson University, Clemson South Carolina, USA) Acrylics as biomedical materials 1:59–65. In: Bever MB, Ed-in-Chief. Massachusetts Institute of Technology. Oxford: Pergamon Press Ltd. Distributed by the MIT Press, Cambridge, MA, 1986.

INTRODUCTION

Ozone (O_3) is a naturally occurring colorless or light blue gas with a pungent ''electrical'' odor (1, 2). As a reactive oxidizing agent that is slightly soluble in water, ozone is a potent respiratory tract irritant. Since ozone is the principal oxidant found in photochemical smog, exposure occurs most commonly by breathing air in urban and suburban environments. Currently over half of the U.S. population lives in areas that have not met the federal ambient air quality standard for ozone (3). The continued failure to attain this clean air objective means that millions of people are intermittently exposed to ozone concentrations that would violate the occupational standard if such exposures were to occur in the workplace (See Table 96.1). Although ozone exposure may occur in a wide variety of occupational settings, published reports of accidental industrial intoxication are uncommon.

SITES, INDUSTRIES, AND BUSINESSES ASSOCIATED WITH EXPOSURE

Ozone occurs in the environmental and occupational settings listed in Table 96.2.

Mechanisms of Formation and Related Industrial Processes

Ozone in ambient air is formed by the action of ultraviolet solar radiation on nitrogen oxides and reactive hydrocarbons, both of which are emitted by motor vehicles and many industrial sources. Although the overall chemistry is complex, the basic reaction sequence involves the photodissociation of nitrogen dioxide (NO_2) into nitric oxide (NO) molecules and oxygen atoms. The latter react with oxygen (O_2) to form ozone. Because the reactions are driven by UV radiation, ozone formation tends to be greatest on warm, sunny days. The daily pattern of ambient ozone formation in heavily populated areas is typically characterized by a broad peak lasting from the late morning until the late afternoon or early evening (3). Ozone is also formed by the effect of lightning on oxygen in the atmosphere and at high altitudes by the action of ultraviolet light on oxygen.

Indoor ozone tends to reflect outdoor concentrations, but at substantially lower levels, owing to its ready destruction on indoor surfaces (7). The most common nonindustrial indoor sources are photocopying machines and electrostatic air cleaners (3). Electronic irradiation of air is used to manufacture ozone used commercially. Because of the high cost of shipping ozone, it is usually manufactured on-site (1). The most common occupational exposures to ozone have been reported to occur in electric arc welding, in industries using ozone as an oxidizing agent, and in aircraft cabins (8–10). However, during the 1980s

Table 96.1. Exposure Limits and Guidelines

Environmental

National Ambient Air Quality Standard	0.12 ppm (1-hr avg)
Recommended Episode Criteria (Smog Alert Levels)	
Stage 1 (Alert)	0.20 ppm (1-hr avg)
Stage 2 (Warning)	0.40 ppm
Stage 3 (Emergency)	0.50 ppm
Emergency Exposure Limit (NAS)	1 ppm (1-hr avg)

Occupational

Threshold Limit Value (ACGIH)	0.10 ppm (8-hr TWA)
Permissible exposure limit (OSHA)	0.10 ppm (8-hr TWA)
Short-term exposure limit (OSHA)	0.30 ppm (15-min avg)
Immediately dangerous to life and health (NIOSH)	10 ppm (30-min avg)

Sources: 40 Code of Federal Regulations 50 (1989); 29 Code of Federal Regulations 1910.1000 (1989); American Conference of Governmental Industrial Hygienists. Documentation of threshold limit values and biological exposure indices. 5th ed. Cincinnati, OH: 1986:453; National Research Council, Committee on Toxicology. Emergency and continuous exposure limits for selected airborne contaminants. Vol 1. Department of Health and Human Services, Public Health Service. NIOSH pocket guide to chemical hazards. Washington, DC: US Government Printing Office, 1990:172.

Table 96.2. List of Sites, Uses, and Occurrence of Ozone

Environmental

Stratosphere (up to 10 ppm from UV effect on oxygen)
Troposphere (photochemical smog, electrical storms)

Occupational

Oxidizing agent in chemical manufacturing
Peroxide manufacturing
Disinfectant (drinking water, food in cold storage rooms, sewage treatment)
Deodorizing agent (air, sewer gas, feathers)
Industrial waste treatment
Bleaching agent (paper pulp, oils, textiles, waxes, flour, starch, sugar)
Aging of liquor and wood
Contamination of high altitude aircraft cabins
Mercury vapor lamps
Photocopy machines
Electric arc welding
High voltage electrical equipment
Linear accelerators
X-ray generators
Indoor ultraviolet sources
Electrostatic air cleaners

Sources: Sax NI, Lewis RJ. Hawley's condensed chemical dictionary. 11th ed. New York: Van Nostrand Reinhold Company, 1987; National Research Council, Committee on Indoor Pollutants. Indoor pollutants. Washington, DC: National Academy Press, 1981; Key MM, Henschel AF, Butler J, Ligo RN, Tabershaw IR. Occupational diseases. A guide to their recognition. Washington, DC: U.S. Department of Health, Education, and Welfare, National Institute for Occupational Safety and Health, 1977:428–430.

aircraft ozone exposures were drastically reduced as airlines installed ozone converters in ventilation systems and began listing tropopause heights in flight plans (to alert pilots to modify flight paths, if necessary, to avoid cabin ozone contamination; personal communication, Dr. William Wells, United Air Lines). Given the magnitude of the ozone air pollution problem, persons in outdoor occupations, particularly those requiring physical exertion (see ''Absorption,'' below), may also receive overtly toxic exposures.

CLINICAL TOXICOLOGY

Route of Exposure

Due to its high chemical reactivity, the half-life of ozone gas in liquid or solid media is negligible (11). Thus, ozone uptake is generally limited to anatomical sites of air-liquid interface (e.g., the mucous membranes of the respiratory tract and eye).

Absorption

Ozone is a strong irritant, and its relatively low solubility facilitates delivery to the lower respiratory tract, the principal target site. Still, ozone is absorbed throughout the respiratory tract. Although systemic absorption is limited by ozone's reactivity, a small fraction of inhaled ozone is absorbed into the blood, resulting in increased red blood cell fragility and alterations in blood chemistry (12).

Approximately 40–50% of inspired ozone is taken up in the nasopharynx, while about 90% of the ozone reaching the lower respiratory tract is removed (13, 14). Oral or oronasal (contrasted with exclusively nasal) breathing and a lower ventilation rate result in small, but statistically significant, increases in extrathoracic uptake of ozone in tidal-breathing human subjects. Similar modest increases in intrathoracic removal efficiency are associated directly with concentration and inversely with breathing rate (14). One model of ozone dosimetry predicts tissue penetration throughout the lung, with the greatest tissue dose occurring at the junction of conducting airways and gas exchange parenchyma, and a minute fraction absorbed into the blood (15, 16). These predictions are consistent with the distribution of lesions observed in several animal species. Recent work involving real-time measurements in the posterior pharynx of ozone-exposed volunteers suggests that reduction of tidal volume, a common functional response to ozone exposure, results in a significant decline in lower respiratory tract uptake of ozone, which is in reasonable quantitative agreement with the prediction of the above-noted model (17).

The magnitudes of symptomatic and functional responses to acute ozone exposure are roughly proportional to the effective dose delivered to the lung (i.e., concentration × duration of exposure × minute ventilation) (18, 19). There has been extensive documentation of enhanced responses to ozone associated with increasing concentration and ventilation (20). Only recently, however, has the importance of duration of exposure been quantified. Chamber studies involving exposures up to 6.6 hours in length with moderate exercise (ozone concentrations were ≤0.12 ppm) demonstrate a progressive increase in respiratory symptoms and a concomitant decline in pulmonary function indices (21, 22).

Metabolism

A potent oxidant, ozone is capable of reacting with many types of biological molecules and tissues, making it difficult to identify a characteristic critical biochemical effect. However, ozone's toxicity has been attributed primarily to oxidation of: (a) amino acids and sulfhydryl groups in enzymes and other proteins; and (b) polyunsaturated fatty acids to fatty acid peroxides, resulting in free radical formation (20). Cellular membranes contain both protein and lipid, and are thought to be the major site of action of ozone toxicity (23). Free radicals react with molecular oxygen to form organic peroxy free radicals, which in turn react with phospholipids in the cellular plasma membrane, resulting in denaturation of unsaturated fatty acid side chains and the creation of additional organic free radicals. Peroxidation of membrane structural lipids results in predictable toxic effects: increased permeability across the membrane, leakage of essential electrolytes and enzymes, inhibition of intracellular metabolic chains, and swelling and disintegration of mitochodria, lysozomes, and other organelles (24). Consistent with these observations, increased airway epithelial permeability due to ozone exposure has been reported in experimental animals and in human volunteers (25, 26). Severe damage results in cell lysis and necrosis, which has been observed in ozone-exposed experimental animals.

SIGNS, SYMPTOMS, AND SYNDROMES OF TOXIC EXPOSURE

Acute Toxicity

SYMPTOMS AND SIGNS OF ACUTE OZONE EXPOSURE

The most common respiratory symptoms caused by exposure to ambient levels of ozone are cough, substernal pain or soreness on deep inspiration, shortness of breath, chest tightness, dry throat, wheeze, and dyspnea (3). Nonrespiratory symptoms reported in controlled exposures of volunteers also include headache, nausea, and malaise. These effects are unlikely to occur in individuals at rest when ambient ozone concentrations are less than 0.30 ppm. However, as noted above, increasing the ventilation rate or duration of exposure can provoke symptoms at ozone concentrations as low as or even lower than the current federal ambient air quality standard (0.12 ppm, averaged over 1 hour) (21, 27). Earlier occupational case reports and a controlled study representative of occupational but not ambient exposures suggest a more severe spectrum of pulmonary and extrapulmonary effects, including (in addition to the above-noted symptoms) somnolence and extreme fatigue, dizziness, insomnia, decreased ability to concentrate, cyanosis, pulmonary edema, acrid taste and smell, and eye irritation (see below) (2, 28–31). Animals exposed to higher concentrations of ozone (3.2–12 ppm) for 4 hours die from pulmonary edema and hemorrhage (28, 32). In view of the dearth of published reports of severe respiratory outcomes in humans, however, exposures sufficient to induce them must be quite rare.

Substantial interindividual variability in sensitivity to ozone is common, but preexisting respiratory disease per se does not necessarily entail heightened toxic responses. For instance, in an investigation involving controlled 2-hour exposures to ozone and to filtered air, subjects with a history of allergic rhinitis did not differ from normal subjects in ozone-related symptoms or pulmonary function changes, with the exception of a slightly greater increase in specific airway resistance (33). In contrast, several epidemiologic studies suggest that ozone concentrations found in urban air can provoke asthmatic episodes (34–36). Interestingly controlled exposure studies suggest that mild asthmatics do not appear to be markedly more sensitive to the effects of ozone than healthy individuals (37, 38, 38a). Nor does chronic obstructive pulmonary disease appear to enhance respiratory sensitivity to ozone (39, 40).

Ozone has also been well documented to significantly impair the ability to perform sustained exercise (41–43). Inspiratory discomfort is thought to be the principal reason for the diminution of exercise performance (44, 45).

Acute exposure to ozone also produces marked effects on pulmonary mechanics and bronchial reactivity. Established consequences of ozone exposure in chamber studies include decreases in inspiratory capacity, FVC, FEV_1, peak flow, and tidal volume, and increased specific airway resistance and frequency of respiration (20, 21, 32, 46, 46a). Some, but not all, of these responses can be blocked by pretreatment with atropine, and thus are thought to be mediated by the parasympathetic nervous systems possibly through reflex inhibition of inspiratory muscle contraction (46, 46a, 47). Increased airway reactivity after ozone exposure is associated with significant increases of arachidonic acid metabolites and neutrophils in the airways, indicating the potential importance of inflammation as both a consequence and a mediator of ozone toxicity in humans and experimental animals (48–50). There is considerable interindividual variability in functional responsiveness to ozone, with 5–25% of study populations demonstrating markedly greater effects than other subjects (20). That the functional changes are highly reproducible over periods from 3 weeks to 14 months suggests the existence of an intrinsic responsiveness to ozone (51, 52).

Several field studies of children suggest that exposure to ozone concentrations at or below the federal ambient air quality standard is associated with transient decrements in lung function (53, 54). In one study of an air pollution episode lasting several days, during which maximum daily ozone concentrations ranged between 0.12 and 0.185 ppm, peak flow decrements in some children lasted up to a week after termination of the episode (55). In a few controlled exposure studies, children appear to experience declines in pulmonary function comparable in magnitude to those observed in adults, but they do not report symptoms to the same extent (56–58). Although this apparent difference in symptom reporting between children and adults may represent real differences in somatic perception, it may also be the result of the relatively low mean ozone concentrations to which the children were exposed.

In some individuals, acute symptomatic and functional responses to ozone become attenuated with repeated daily exposures. In controlled chamber studies, maximum responses are observed on the second day of exposure, but on subsequent days there may be little or no ozone-related effect (59). In a laboratory setting, "adaptation" to ozone toxicity typically persists for up to 1 week following cessation of exposure but may last up to about 3 weeks (60–62). Repeated real-world exposures appear to induce longer periods of attenuated responses (62a).

Eye irritation that occurs during smog episodes is due mainly to other photochemical oxidants, such as peroxyacetylnitrate, not to ozone (20, 63–64). However, in industrial settings, eye and nasal irritation may occur (65). Concentrations greater than 2 ppm have been reported to be irritating to normal human eyes within minutes (66).

Numerous studies of mice exposed even briefly (2–3 hours) to ozone concentrations at or below the current federal ambient air quality standard (0.12 ppm) have shown significantly decreased resistance to bacterial but not viral respiratory infections (67–72). A limited number of epidemiologic and clinical studies have, in general, failed to detect an effect of ozone or oxidant air pollution on respiratory infections in humans, although this issue has not been adequately investigated (73–76).

PATHOLOGY

Ozone may damage tissues throughout the respiratory tract, depending on the pattern of breathing and the exposure concentration and duration. At high concentrations, ozone may cause desquamation of the airways and pulmonary edema (77). At sublethal concentrations (up to 1.0 ppm), airway epithelial cells are also damaged, but the principal site of injury is the central portion of the pulmonary acinus. Type I alveolar and ciliated bronchiolar cells appear to be particularly susceptible to ozone toxicity, with damage evident as early as four hours of exposure (78). Inflammatory responses at the junction of the conducting airways and the gas exchange zone have been reported consistently in studies of rodents, dogs, and nonhuman primates (20). Continued exposure over several days results in replacement of type I by type II cells as well as hypertrophy and hyperplasia of nonciliated cuboidal cells in the bronchiolar epithelium (79, 80). When animals are allowed to recover in clean air from acute and subacute exposures, these lesions all appear to be reversible (79, 80).

Although microscopic examination of airway damage from acute ozone exposure has not been performed in humans, several investigators have measured markers of inflammation in ozone-exposed volunteers. Bronchoalveolar lavage fluid from these subjects showed large increases in polymorphonuclear cells (up to 8.2-fold over control levels), other inflammatory mediators, and protein concentrations consistent with a transudation of serum (48, 81). The latter finding suggests increased pulmonary vascular permeability, one of the hallmarks of inflammation, and tends to corroborate earlier work demonstrating increased permeability of the respiratory epithelium, as measured by ^{99}Tc-labeled DTPA clearance (25). Although these data are somewhat limited, they indicate that the inflammatory effects of ozone repeatedly demonstrated in animals also occur in the human lung.

Chronic Toxicity

One of the principal uncertainties about ozone toxicity is the relationship between repeated exposures and chronic respiratory disease. Exposure of guinea pigs and rats to a relatively high ozone concentration (approximately 1.0 ppm) for 268 days caused a chronic bronchiolitis, with bronchiolar fibrosis, pneumonitis, "mild to moderate" emphysema, and occasional epithelial lesions in the trachea and major bronchi (82). Exposure of rats to substantially lower concentrations (between 0.12 and 0.25 ppm) resulted in less severe but still significant changes in the terminal bronchioles and alveolar septa, as well as a distribution of inflammation similar to that observed in acute exposures (83, 84). Chronic exposures of monkeys showed changes in nasal epithelial secretory product, respiratory bronchiolitis (with inflammatory thickening of the bronchiolar wall and hypertrophy and hyperplasia of nonciliated cuboidal cells in the bronchiolar epithelium), and other changes, including the development of hyperplastic nodules that persisted after the cessation of exposure (85–87). It is noteworthy that in a 3-month study of nonhuman primates, the degree of inflammation after 90 days was less than that observed after 7 (85). This may be a consequence of the greater resistance of the altered epithelial cell population to environmental insults.

These animal experiments demonstrate that chronic exposure to ozone concentrations found in typical urban air results in centriacinar inflammation and small airway structural changes. Other lines of evidence support the notion that repeated ozone exposure may result in chronic lung disease, including the observations that ozone inactivates human alpha-1 antiproteinase inhibitor and appears to cause the synthesis and deposition of abnormal collagen in rat lung (88, 89). Recent epidemiologic studies suggest the existence of significant associations of photochemical oxidant exposure with an accelerated decline in lung function and with symptoms of chronic respiratory disease in nonsmokers (90, 91). Problems in longterm measurement of ozone or oxidant exposure and the high covariation between ozone and particulate air pollution, however, limit the interpretation of these investigations.

Genetic Toxicity and Carcinogenicity

Ozone is genotoxic in a variety of assay systems, but results of different experiments are inconsistent (20). Effects reported include bacterial mutations, plasmid DNA strand breakage, sister chromatid exchange, and chromatid and chromosome breaks in lymphocytes (92). For example, a threefold increase in chromatid-type aberrations persisted for up to 6 weeks in subjects exposed to 0.5 ppm ozone for 6–10 hours (93). In contrast, no significant changes in chromosome or chromatid breaks were observed in lymphocytes of subjects exposed to 0.4 ppm ozone for 4 hours (94). More recently, cultured human epidermal cells exposed to 5 ppm ozone for 10 minutes showed no indication of any DNA strand breakage (95). Although ozone's ability to cause free radical formation gives grounds for suspicion that it may be genotoxic in humans, this issue has not been extensively explored (95a).

Short (5-minute) exposure to 5 ppm ozone induces neoplastic transformation in hamster embryo cells and mouse fibroblasts (96). Although some studies suggest that chronic ozone exposure may cause the development of murine pulmonary adenomas and other hyperplastic nodules in the lungs of nonhuman primates, this compound has not been adequately tested for carcinogenicity (86, 97). However, because exposure to ozone is so common and because there is some experimental documentation of oncogenicity, the U.S. National Toxicology Program has selected ozone to be tested in a 2-year carcinogenesis bioassay, which is ongoing at the time of this writing.

Management of Toxicity

Avoidance of exposure is obviously the best management strategy. In the occupational setting this means providing adequate engineering controls (e.g., entirely enclosed processes or local exhaust ventilation), thorough worker education about appropriate work practices (use of personal protective equipment, such as an ozone-decomposing respirator, when adequate ventilation is impractical) and recognition of ozone-related symptoms, and strict adherence to health and safety rules. In the context of environmental exposures, individuals should be advised to avoid doing aerobic exercise during peak ozone hours (typically late morning until early evening in many urban areas) and to pay attention to the health advisories accompanying the declaration of a smog alert. However, it should be borne in mind that signs and symptoms of ozone toxicity have been repeatedly demonstrated to occur in exercising adults at ozone concentrations lower than the current recommended stage 1 smog alert level (0.20 ppm) (21, 22, 32).

Diagnosis of ozone-related toxicity is based on a history of exposure and recognition of symptoms compatible with exposure. Because ozone symptomatology may mimic several cardiorespiratory illnesses, the differential diagnosis includes influenza, the common cold, sinusitis, asthma, bronchopneumonia, pulmonary embolism, and myocardial infarction (30). Asthmatic episodes triggered by ozone should be treated according to standard protocols. Although ozone is theoretically capable of causing pulmonary edema in humans, the scarcity of published reports indicates that it is historically rare. Severe industrial overexposure should be managed like other acute inhalational injury, with supportive treatment. Except in these unusual instances, ozone-related symptoms are self-limited after termination of exposure, with recovery in milder cases generally occurring within hours. Symptomatic treatment would include analgesics for headache and chest pain and cough suppressants if indicated. Some reports of industrial ozone toxicity indicate a more prolonged convalescence, with resolution of symptoms occurring over 1–2 weeks (30).

REFERENCES

1. Sax NI, Lewis RJ. Hawley's condensed chemical dictionary. 11th ed. New York: Van Nostrand Reinhold Company, 1987.

2. Jaffe LS. The biological effects of ozone on man and animals. Am Ind Hyg Assoc J 1967;28:267–277.

3. Lippmann M. Health effects of ozone: a critical review. J Air Pollut Control Assoc 1989;39:672–695.

4. National Research Council, Committee on Indoor Pollutants. Indoor pollutants. Washington, DC: National Academy Press, 1981.

5. Perkins PJ, Holdeman JD, Nastrom GD. Simultaneous cabin and ambient ozone measurements on two Boeing 747 airplanes, vol. I. Washington DC: U.S. Department of Transportation, Federal Aviation Administration, Report No. FAA-EE-79-05, 1979.

6. Key MM, Henschel AF, Butler J, Ligo RN, Tabershaw IR. Occupational diseases. A guide to their recognition. Washington, DC: U.S. Department of Health, Education, and Welfare, National Institute for Occupational Safety and Health, 1977:428–430.

7. Graedel TE. Ambient levels of anthropogenic emissions and their atmospheric transformation products. In: Air pollution, the automobile and public health. Health Effects Institute, Washington, DC: National Academy Press, 1988:133–160.

8. Morgan WKC, Seaton A. Occupational lung diseases. 2d ed. Philadelphia: W.B. Saunders Co., 1984:625–626.

9. Schwartz DA. Acute inhalational injury. In: Rosenstock L, ed. State of the art reviews: occupational pulmonary disease. Philadelphia: Hanley & Belfus, 1987:305.

10. Reed D, Glasser S, Kaldor J. Ozone toxicity symptoms among flight attendants. Am J Ind Med 1980;1:43–54.

11. World Health Organization. Ozone and other photochemical oxidants. In: Air quality guidelines for Europe. Copenhagen, Denmark: World Health Organization Regional Office for Europe, 1987:315–326.

12. Buckley RD, Hackney JD, Clark K, et al. Ozone and human blood. Arch Environ Health 1975;30:40–43.

13. Miller FJ, et al. Nasopharyngeal removal of ozone in rabbits and guinea pigs. Toxicology 1979;14:273–281.

14. Gerrity TR, Weaver RA, Berntsen J, House DE, O'Neil JJ. Extrathoracic and intrathoracic removal of ozone in tidal breathing humans. J Appl Physiol 1988;65:393–400.

15. Miller FJ, Overton Jr JH, Jaskot RH, Menzel DB, et al. A model of the regional uptake of gaseous pollutants in the lung. 1. The sensitivity of the uptake of ozone in the human lung to lower respiratory tract secretions and exercise. Toxicol Appl Pharmacol 1985;79:11–27.

16. Overton JH, Graham RC, Miller FJ. A model of the regional uptake of gaseous pollutants in the lung. II. The sensitivity of ozone uptake in laboratory animal lungs to anatomical and ventilatory parameters. Toxicol Appl Pharmacol 1987;88:418–432.

17. Gerrity TR, McDonnell WF. Do functional changes in humans correlate with the airway removal efficiency of ozone? In: Schneider T, Lee SD, Wolters GJR, Grand LD, eds. Atmospheric ozone research and its policy implications. Proceedings of the 3rd US-Dutch International Symposium, Nijmegen, the Netherlands, May 9–13, 1988. Amsterdam: Elsevier, 1989:293–300.

18. Silverman F, Folinsbee LJ, Barnard J, Shephard RJ. Pulmonary function changes in ozone—interaction of concentration and ventilation. J Appl Physiol 1976;41:859–864.

19. Adams WC, Savin WM, Christo AE. Detection of ozone toxicity during continuous exercise via the effective dose concept. J Appl Physiol 1981;51:415–422.

20. U.S. Environmental Protection Agency. Air quality criteria for ozone and other photochemical oxidants (5 vols). Research Triangle Park, NC: EPA Rept. No. 600/8-84/020 a-eF, 1986.

21. Folinsbee LJ, McDonnell WF, Horstman DH. Pulmonary function and symptom responses after 6.6 hour exposure to 0.12 ppm ozone with moderate exercise. J Air Pollut Control Assoc 1988;38:28–35.

22. Horstman DH, Folinsbee LJ, Ives PJ, Abdul-Salaam S, McDonnell WF. Ozone concentration and pulmonary response relationships for 6.6-hour exposures with five hours of moderate exercise to 0.08, 0.10 and 0.12 ppm. Am Rev Respir Dis 1990;142:1158–1163.

23. Menzel DB. Ozone: an overview of its toxicity in man and animals. J Toxicol Environ Health 1984;13:183–204.

24. Man SFP, Hulbert WC. Airway repair and adaptation to inhalation injury. In: Loke J, ed. Pathophysiology and treatment of inhalation injuries. New York: Marcel Dekker, 1988:1–47.

25. Kehrl HR, Vincent LM, Kowalsky RJ, et al. Ozone exposure increases respiratory epithelial permeability in humans. Am Rev Respir Dis 1987;135:1124–1128.

26. Miller PD, Gordon T, Warnick M, Amdur MO. Effect of ozone and histamine on airway permeability to horseradish peroxidase in guinea pigs. J Toxicol Environ Health 1986;18:121–132.

27. McDonnell WF, Horstman DH, Hazucha MJ, et al. Pulmonary effects of ozone exposure during exercise: dose-response characteristics. J Appl Physiol 1983;54:1345–1352.

28. Stokinger HE. Ozone toxicology: a review of research and industrial experience: 1954–1964. Arch Environ Health 1965;10:719–731.

29. Griswold SS, Chambers LA, Motley HL. Report of a case of exposure to high ozone concentrations for two hours. Arch Ind Health 1957;15:108–110.

30. Nasr AN. Ozone poisoning in man: clinical manifestations and differential diagnosis. A review. Clin Toxicol 1971;4:461–466.

31. Kleinfeld M, Giel CP. Clinical manifestations of ozone poisoning: report of a new source of exposure. Am J Med Sci 1956;231:638–643.

32. Stokinger HE. Evaluation of the hazards of ozone and oxides of nitrogen. Arch Ind Health 1957;15:181–197.

33. McDonnell WF, Horstman DH, Abdul-Salaam S, Raggio LJ, Green JA. The respiratory responses of subjects with allergic rhinitis to ozone exposure and their relationship to nonspecific airway reactivity. Toxicol Ind Health 1987;3:507–517.

34. Whittemore AW, Korn EL. Asthma and air pollution in the Los Angeles area. Am J Public Health 1980;70:687–696.

35. Holguin AH, Buffler PA, Contant Jr CF, et al. The effects of ozone on asthmatics in the Houston area. In: Lee SD, ed. Evaluation of the scientific basis for ozone/oxidants standards. (APCA International Specialty Conference Transactions: TR–4). Pittsburgh, PA: Air Pollution Control Association, 1985:262–280.

36. Schoettlin CE, Landau E. Air pollution and asthmatic attacks in the Los Angeles area. Public Health Rep 1961;76:545–548.

37. Koenig JG, Covert DS, Morgan MS, et al. Acute effects of 0.12 ppm ozone or 0.12 ppm nitrogen dioxide on pulmonary function in healthy and asthmatic adolescents. Am Rev Respir Dis 1985;132:648–651.

38. Linn WS, Buckley RD, Spier CE, et al. Health effects of ozone exposure in asthmatics. Am Rev Respir Dis 1978;117:835–843.

38a. Kreit JW, Gross KB, Moore TB, Lorenzen TJ, D'Arcy J, Eschenbacher WL. Ozone-induced changes in pulmonary function and bronchial responsiveness in asthmatics. J Appl Physiol 1989;66:217–222.

39. Kehrle HR, Hazucha MJ, Solic JJ, Bromberg PA. Responses of subjects with chronic obstructive pulmonary disease after exposures to 0.3 ppm ozone. Am Rev Respir Dis 1985;131:719–724.

40. Solic JJ, Hazucha MJ, Bromberg PA. The acute effects of 0.2 ppm ozone in patients with chronic obstructive pulmonary disease. Am Rev Respir Dis 1982;125:664–669.

41. Schelegle ES, Adams WC. Reduced exercise time in competitive simulations consequent to low level ozone exposure. Med Sci Sports Exerc 1986;18:408–414.

42. Wayne WS, Wehrle PF, Carroll RE. Oxidant air pollution and athletic performance. JAMA 1967;199:151–154.

43. Gong Jr. H, Bradley PW, Simmons MS, Tashkin DP. Impaired exercise performance and pulmonary function in elite cyclists during low-level ozone exposure in a hot environment. Am Rev Respir Dis 1986;134:726–733.

44. Adams WC. Effects of ozone exposure at ambient air pollution episode levels on exercise performance. Sports Med 1987;4:395–424.

45. Folinsbee LJ, Silverman F, Shephard RJ. Decrease of maximum work performance following ozone exposure. J Appl Physiol 1977;42:531–536.

46. Golden JA, Nadel JA, Boushey HA. Bronchial hyperirritability in healthy subjects after exposure to ozone. Am Rev Respir Dis 1978;118:287–294.

46a. Hazucha MJ, Bates DV, Bromberg PA. Mechanism of action of ozone on the human lung. J Appl Physiol 1989;67:1535–1541.

47. Beckett WS, McDonnell WF, Horstman DH, House DE. Role of the parasympathetic nervous system in acute lung response to ozone. J Appl Physiol 1985;59:1879–1885.

48. Seltzer J, Bigby BG, Stulbarg M, et al. O₃-induced change in bronchial reactivity to methacholine and airway inflammation in humans. J Appl Physiol 1986;60:1321–1326.

49. Hulbert WM, McLean T, Hogg JC. The effect of acute airway inflammation on bronchial reactivity in guinea pigs. Am Rev Respir Dis 1985;132:7–11.

50. Holtzman MJ, Fabbri LM, O'Byrne PM, et al. Importance of airway inflammation for hyperresponsiveness induced by ozone. Am Rev Respir Dis 1983;127:686–690.

51. McDonnell WF, Horstman DH, Salaam SA, House DE. Reproducibility of individual responses to ozone exposure. Am Rev Respir Dis 1985;131:36–40.

52. Gliner JA, Horvath SM, Folinsbee LJ. Pre-exposure to low ozone concentrations does not diminish the pulmonary function response on exposure to higher ozone concentrations. Am Rev Respir Dis 1983;127:51–55.

53. Kinney PL, Ware JH, Spengler JD, Dockery DW, Speizer FE, Ferris BG. Short-term pulmonary function change in association with ozone levels. Am Rev Respir Dis 1989;139:56–61.

54. Spektor DM, Lippmann M, Lioy PJ, et al. Effects of ambient ozone on respiratory function in active normal children. Am Rev Respir Dis 1988; 137:313–320.

55. Lioy PJ, Vollmuth TA, Lippmann M. Persistence of peak flow decrement in children following ozone exposures exceeding the national ambient air quality standard. J Air Pollut Control Assoc 1985;35:1068–1071.

56. Avol EL, Linn WS, Shamoo DA, et al. Respiratory effects of photochemical oxidant air pollution in exercising adolescents. Am Rev Respir Dis 1985;132:619–622.

57. Avol EL, Linn WS, Shamoo DA, et al. Short-term respiratory effects of photochemical oxidant exposure in exercising children. JAMA 1987;37:158–162.

58. McDonnell WF, Chapman RS, Leigh MW, Strope GL. Respiratory responses of vigorously exercising children to 0.12 ppm ozone exposure. Am Rev Respir Dis 1985;132:875-879.

59. Farrell BP, Kerr HD, Kulle TJ, Sauder LS, Young JL. Adaptation in human subjects to the effects of inhaled ozone after repeated exposure. Am Rev Respir Dis; 1979:725–730.

60. Linn WS, Medway DA, Anzar UT, et al. Persistence of adaptation to ozone in volunteers exposed repeatedly for six weeks. Am Rev Respir Dis 1982;125:491–495.

61. Horvath SM, Gliner JA, Folinsbee LJ. Adaptation to ozone: duration of effect. Am Rev Respir Dis 1981;123:496–499.

62. Kulle TJ, Sauder LS, Kerr HD, Farrell BP, Bermal MS, Smith DM. Duration of pulmonary function adaptation to ozone in humans. Am Ind Hyg Assoc J 1982;43:832–837.

62a. Linn WS, Avol EL, Shamoo DA, et al. Repeated laboratory ozone exposures of volunteer Los Angeles residents: an apparent seasonal variation in response. Toxicol Ind Health 1988;4:505–520.

63. Wilson KW. Survey of eye irritation and lachrymation in relation to air pollution. La Jolla, CA: Copley International Corporation. (Prepared for the Coordinating Research Council, Inc., New York) 1974.

64. Hammer DL, Hasselblad V, Portnoy B, Wherle PF. Los Angeles student nurse study: daily symptom reporting and photochemical oxidants. Arch Environ Health 1974;28:255–260.

65. Challen PJR, Hickish DE, Bedford J. An investigation of some health hazards in an inert-gas tungsten-arc welding shop. Br J Ind Med 1957;15:276–282.

66. Grant WM. Toxicology of the eye. 3rd ed. Springfield, Il: Charles C Thomas Publisher, 1986:693–694.

67. Selgrade MJK, Illing JW, Starnes DM, Stead AG, Menache MG, Stevens MA. Evaluation of effects of ozone exposure on influenza infection in mice using several indicators of susceptibility. Fundam Appl Toxicol 1988;11:169–180.

68. Wolcott JA, Zee YC, Osebold JW. Exposure to ozone reduces influenza disease severity and alters distribution of influenza viral antigens in murine lungs. Appl Environ Microbiol 1982;44:723-731.

69. Coffin DL, Blommer EJ. Alteration of the pathogenic role of streptococci group C in mice conferred by previous exposure to ozone. In: Silver IH, ed., Aerobiology. Proceedings of the Third International Symposium held at the University of Sussex, England. London: Academic Press, 1970:54–61.

70. Ehrlich R, Findlay JC, Gardner DE. Effects of repeated exposures to peak concentrations of nitrogen dioxide and ozone on resistance to streptococcal pneumonia. J Toxicol Environ Health 1979;5:631–642.

71. Gardner DE. Oxidant-induced enhanced sensitivity to infection in animal models and their extrapolations to man. J Toxicol Environ Health 1984;13:423–439.

72. Miller FJ, Illing JW, Gardner DE. Effect of urban ozone levels on laboratory-induced respiratory infections. Toxicol Lett 1978;2:163–169.

73. Pearlman ME, Finklea JF, Shy CM, Van Bruggen J, Newill VA. Chronic oxidant exposure and epidemic influenza. Environ Res 1971;4:129–140.

74. Wayne WS, Wehrle PF. Oxidant air pollution and school absenteeism. Arch Environ Health 1969;19:315–322.

75. Durham WH. Air pollution and student health. Arch Environ Health 1974;28:241–254.

76. Henderson FW, Elliott DM, Orlando GS. The immune response to rhinovirus infection in human volunteers exposed to ozone. In: Lee SD, Mustafa MG, Mehlman MA, eds. International symposium on the biomedical effects of ozone and related photochemical oxidants. Princeton, NJ: Princeton Scientific Publishers, 1983:253–254.

77. Coffin DL, Stokinger HE. Biological effects of air pollutants. In: Stern AC, ed. Air pollution. 3rd ed. Vol II. London: Academic Press, 1977:231–360.

78. Evans JM, Oxidant gases. Environ Health Perspect 1984;55:85–95.

79. Plopper CG, Chow CK, Dungworth DL, Brummer M, Nemeth TJ. Effects of low levels of ozone on rat lungs. II Morphological responses during recovery and reexposure. Exp Mol Pathol 1978;29:400–411.

80. Chow CK, Hussain MZ, Cross CE, Dungworth DL, Mustafa MG. Effect of low levels of ozone on rat lungs. I. Biochemical responses during recovery and reexposure. Exp Mol Pathol 1976;25:182–188.

81. Koren HS, Devlin RB, Graham DE, et al. Ozone-induced inflammation in the lower airways of human subjects. Am Rev Respir Dis 1989;139:407–415.

82. Stokinger HE, Wagner WD, Dobrogorski OJ. Ozone toxicity studies. III. Chronic injury to lungs of animals following exposure at a low level. Arch Ind Health 1957;16:514–522.

83. Barry BE, Miller FJ, Crapo JD. Effects of inhalation of 0.12 and 0.25 parts per million ozone on the proximal alveolar region of juvenile and adult rats. Lab Invest 1985;53:692–704.

84. Crapo JD, Barry BE, Chang LY, Mercer RR. Alterations in lung structure caused by inhalation of oxidants. J Toxicol Environ Health 1984;13:301–321.

85. Eustis SL, Schwartz LW, Kosch PC, Dungworth DL. Chronic bronchiolitis in nonhuman primates after prolonged ozone exposure. Am J Pathol 1981;105:121–137.

86. Fujinaka LE, Hyde DM, Plopper CG, Tyler WS, Dungworth DL, Lollini LO. Respiratory bronchiolitis following long-term ozone exposure in bonnet monkeys: a morphometric study. Exp Lung Res 1985;8:167–190.

87. Harkema JR, Plopper CG, Hyde DM, St. George JA, Dungworth DL. Effects of an ambient level of ozone on primate nasal epithelial mucosubstances. Am J Pathol 1987;127:90–96.

88. Johnson DA. Ozone inactivation of human alpha$_1$-antiproteinase inhibitor. Am Rev Respir Dis 1980;121:1031–1038.

89. Rieser KM, Tyler WS, Hennessy SM, Dominiguez JJ, Last JA. Long-term consequences of exposure to ozone. II. Structural alterations in lung collagen of monkeys. Toxicol Appl Pharmacol 1987;89:314–322.

90. Detels R, Tashkin DP, Sayre JW, et al. The UCLA population studies of chronic obstructive lung disease. 9. Lung function changes associated with chronic exposure to photochemical oxidants; a cohort study among never-smokers. Chest 1987;92:594–603.

91. Euler GL, Abbey DE, Hodgkin JE, et al. Chronic obstructive pulmonary disease symptom effects of long-term cumulative exposure to ambient levels of total oxidants and nitrogen dioxide in California Seventh-Day Adventist residents. Arch Environ Health 1988;43:279–285.

92. Recommendation for an ambient air quality standard for ozone. Berkeley, CA: California Department of Health Services, 1987.

93. Merz T, Bender MA, Kerr HD, Kulle TJ. Observations of aberrations in chromosomes of lymphocytes from human subjects exposed to ozone at a concentration of 0.5 ppm for 6 and 10 hours. Mutat Res 1975;31:299–302.

94. McKenzie WH, Knelson JH, Rummo NJ, House DE. Cytogenetic effects of inhaled ozone in man. Mutat Res 1977;48:95–102.

95. Borek C, Ong A, Cleaver JE. DNA damage from ozone and radiation in human epithelial cells. Toxicol Ind Health 1988;4:547–553.

95a. Steinberg JJ, Gleeson JL, Gil D. The pathobiology of ozone-induced damage. Arch Environ Health 1990;45:80–87.

96. Borek C, Zaider M, Ong A, Mason H, Witz G. Ozone acts alone and synergistically with ionizing radiation to induce in vitro neoplastic transformation. Carcinogenesis 1986;7:1611–1613.

97. Hassett C, Mustafa MG, Coulson WF, Elashoff RM. Murine lung carcinogenesis following exposure to ambient ozone concentrations. J Natl Cancer Inst 1985;75:771-777.

Oxides of Nitrogen and Sulfur

Michael Lipsett, M.D.

INTRODUCTION

Exposures to oxides of nitrogen and sulfur commonly occur in industry and, at lower concentrations, in the general environment. Both classes of compounds are toxic by inhalation. The principal sites of toxicity and mechanisms of action are different for nitrogen oxides and sulfur oxides. Most of the following discussion will focus on the dioxides (NO_2 and SO_2, respectively), which are the most harmful to humans and have been extensively characterized toxicologically.

NITROGEN OXIDES: CLASS MEMBERS AND PROPERTIES

Nitrogen oxides are reactive substances commonly understood to encompass nitric oxide (NO), nitrogen dioxide (NO_2), and nitrogen tetroxide (N_2O_4), referred to together under the general label "NO_x" (in air pollution literature) or "nitrous fume" (in the older occupational literature). This chapter follows the conventional categorization, and therefore other compounds that are members of the larger family of nitrogen oxides, such as the anesthetic nitrous oxide (N_2O), peroxyacetyl nitrates, nitrites, nitroso compounds, and nitrogen-containing acids, are not discussed, nor are the unstable compounds nitrogen peroxide (N_2O_2) and dinitrotrioxide (N_2O_3).

Nitrogen tetroxide is the dimer of nitrogen dioxide, and increasing temperature favors formation of the latter at equilibrium. At ambient temperatures and concentrations, small quantities of NO_2 are likely to be present as N_2O_4 (1). Nitric oxide is oxidized in ambient air to form nitrogen dioxide, which is therefore always present when nitric oxide is detected. Numerous chemical reactions can interconvert the nitrogen oxides. Some relevant physical characteristics of these compounds are presented in Table 97.1.

Although NO_2 is a liquid below 21° C, inhalation of the gas is the most common route of toxic exposure and is the only one considered in this chapter.

SOURCES OF EXPOSURE TO NITROGEN OXIDES

Occupational settings commonly associated with exposures to nitrogen oxides involve production, transportation, and use of nitric acid (Table 97.2) (2). Contact of this acid with organic material or certain metals (e.g., in acid dipping) produces nitrogen dioxide. Combustion of nitrogen-containing materials in enclosed spaces, such as diesel or other fossil fuels (or less commonly dynamite in underground mines) can also result in the accumulation of toxic quantities of NO_2. Gas or electric arc welding causes the formation of nitrogen oxides through the oxidation of atmospheric nitrogen. It is common to burn propane or kerosene to add heat and carbon dioxide to the air in greenhouses: NO_x concentrations can reach 3.5 ppm in this environment (3). "Silo-filler's disease" is caused by nitrogen dioxide formed when crops (such as corn or alfalfa) to be used as feed for livestock are stored in a silo or pit. Within a few hours of filling the silo, carbohydrates in the crop begin to ferment, resulting in (among other things) oxidation of nitrates to NO_2, which can attain lethal levels (4).

Nitrogen oxides are also important pollutants of indoor and outdoor air, but generally at lower levels than can be detected in occupational contexts. High temperature combustion of fossil fuels in motor vehicles and industry (particularly in the generation of electricity) is the main source of nitrogen oxide pollution in ambient air. Nitrogen in these fuels reacts with atmospheric oxygen and, at high combustion temperatures, nitrogen and oxygen in the air combine to form nitric oxide, which is then further oxidized to nitrogen dioxide (5). These oxides of nitrogen participate in the photochemical generation of ozone and other oxidants. Maximal outdoor half-hour and 24-hour averages of NO_2 have been reported to be 0.45 and 0.21 ppm, respectively, while annual urban averages are typically much lower (0.01–0.05 ppm) (3). Motor vehicle emissions near busy streets and intersections and roads can result in high local NO_x concentrations. The typical diurnal NO_x pattern consists of a low background concentration

Table 97.1. Names and Properties of Nitrogen Oxides

Compound	Formula	Color	Odor	B.P. (°C)	Solubility (g/100 g H_2O)
Nitric oxide Nitrogen monoxide Mononitrogen monoxide	NO	None	None	−151.7	0.006
Nitrogen dioxide	NO_2	Reddish-brown to yellow	Acrid, irritating	Liquid is mainly N_2O_4	Reacts with water to form HONO and HNO_3
Nitrogen tetroxide Dinitrogen tetroxide	N_2O_4	None as gas, yellowish-brown as liquid	Same as NO_2	21.1	Same as NO_2

Source: National Research Council. Nitrogen Oxides. Washington, DC: National Academy of Sciences, 1977:4–19.
[a]Under conditions involving exposure to gas, equilibrium favors formation of NO_2.

Table 97.2. Exposures and Sites of Occurrence of Nitrogen Oxides

Occupational
  Combustion of fossil fuels (e.g., automobile garages, ice resurfacing machines in skating rinks, other internal combustion engines, boilers)
  Electric arc fixation of nitrogen
  Decomposition of aqueous nitrous acid
  High temperature oxidation of ammonia
  Nitric acid production and transportation
  Manufacture of lacquers and dyes
  Other chemical manufacturing uses (nitrating agent, oxidizing agent, catalyst, inhibitor of acrylate polymerization)
  Manufacture or use of explosives
  Missile fuel oxidizer
  Agriculture (silo filling)
  Mining (diesel exhaust; shot-firing at coal seams)
  Arc welding
  Firefighting (involving exposure to smoke from plastics, shoe polish, nitrocellulose film or fossil fuels)

Nonoccupational
  Gas- and oil-fired household appliances
  Kerosene heaters
  Motor vehicle exhaust
  Cigarette smoke
  Ice skating rinks
  Industrial boilers

Sources: Sax NI, Lewis RJ. Hawley's Condensed Chemical Dictionary. 11th ed. New York, NY: Van Nostrand Reinhold Company, 1987; Yockey CC, Eden BM, Byrd RB. The McConnell missile accident:clinical spectrum of nitrogen dioxide exposure. JAMA 1980;244:1221–1223; Leaderer BP. Air pollutant emissions from kerosene space heaters. Science 1982;218:1113–1115; Schwartz DA. Acute inhalational injury. In: Rosenstock L, ed. Occupational pulmonary disease. Philadelphia, PA: Hanley & Belfus, Inc., 1987:297–318; Tse RL, Bockman AA. Nitrogen dioxide toxicity. Report of four cases in firemen. JAMA 1970;212:1341–1344.

with morning and late afternoon spikes resulting from rush-hour traffic (3).

Although regulatory attention has focused on outdoor concentrations of NO_x, greater human exposure occurs indoors (6, 7). Gas burning appliances, such as unvented furnaces, stoves, and water heaters, are the chief sources of nitrogen oxides indoors, although tobacco smoke and kerosene space heaters can also be contributing factors, as can penetration of outdoor NO_2 from motor vehicle exhaust (8–10). When a gas stove is used for cooking, peak 1-hour NO_2 kitchen concentrations can approach or even exceed 1 ppm (3).

Nitric oxide is also synthesized endogenously from L-arginine by macrophages and neutrophils, as well as endothelial, neural, and other cell types. Nitric oxide appears to have multiple physiologic roles, including vasorelaxation, inhibition of platelet adhesion and aggregation, and modulation of neurotransmission (11, 12).

CLINICAL TOXICOLOGY OF EXPOSURE

As noted above, inhalation represents the only important route of exposure to nitrogen oxides, although occasionally missile fuel accidents may result in dermal and mucous membrane contact with liquid nitrogen tetroxide (13).

Absorption

Brief exposures of healthy volunteers to 0.55–13.5 mg/m³ (0.29–7.2 ppm) NO_2 resulted in absorption of between 81% and 90%,

when NO_2 was measured in inhaled and exhaled air (14). More recently, Bauer et al. reported 72% absorption of inhaled NO_2 (0.30 ppm) in asthmatic volunteers exposed at rest via a mouthpiece, increasing to 87% with exercise (15). Although nitric oxide is poorly soluble in water, it is efficiently (>80%) absorbed via inhalation and recently it has been proposed as a test gas for alveolar-capillary diffusion (16, 17).

Metabolism

The metabolic transformations and tissue reactions of NO_x have not been extensively characterized, but it is likely that inhaled NO_2 reacts with intrapulmonary water to form nitric (HNO_3) and nitrous (HNO_2) acids (18). In an experiment involving short (7–9 minutes) exposures of rhesus monkeys to radiolabeled NO_2, pulmonary ^{13}N radioactivity remained virtually unchanged during the immediate postexposure period (21 minutes), while during the same interval ^{125}Xe activity declined nearly to baseline levels, indicating binding of NO_2 or its derivatives to respiratory tissues (18). NO_2 causes radical formation, resulting in auto-oxidation of unsaturated fatty acids (19). In an in vitro experiment with perfused rat lung, most absorbed NO_2 was converted to nitrite ion (NO_2^-), presumably via formation and subsequent dissociation of HNO_2 (20).

NO has an affinity for hemoglobin that is several thousand times higher than that of carbon monoxide (17). On absorption into the blood it rapidly forms nitrosylhemoglobin, which is then converted into methemoglobin, nitrite (NO_2^-) and nitrate (NO_3^-) (16, 17). Most inhaled NO is excreted as nitrate in the urine (16).

SIGNS, SYMPTOMS, AND SYNDROMES FROM NITROGEN OXIDE EXPOSURE

Acute Toxicity

The relatively low solubility of the nitrogen oxides results in minimal mucous membrane or upper respiratory irritation, with the principal site of toxicity being the lower respiratory tract. The odor of NO_2 is detectable at 1–3 ppm, while mucous membrane irritation does not generally occur at concentrations less than 13 ppm (21). Individuals unfamiliar with the visual or olfactory characteristics of nitrogen dioxide or in whom olfactory fatigue develops may unwittingly inhale large volumes of this gas, putting them at risk for delayed-onset lower respiratory toxicity (22). The severity of the clinical effects depends primarily on the concentration of nitrogen oxides inhaled and less on the duration of exposure. Mild intoxication may induce transient nonspecific symptoms, including dyspnea, cough, headache, fatigue, nausea, vertigo, and somnolence, which dissipate over the following hours to days, but may persist up to 2 weeks without clinically detectable pulmonary findings. Exposure to massive concentrations of nitrogen oxides may cause sudden death from laryngospasm, bronchospasm or asphyxiation (23).

Between these extremes of exposure is a multiphasic course of disease that can be fatal if untreated. An individual may experience a variety of acute symptoms, including dyspnea, cough, wheeze, chest pain, palpitations, weakness, diaphoresis, nausea, vomiting, headache, and eye irritation during or shortly after exposure. Exposed individuals have described a "choking" or "smothering" sensation (24). Removal to fresh air often brings symptom alleviation or even disappearance, which may induce the individual not to seek medical care. After an interval of a few hours (usually 4–12), the exposed individual may present with chemical pneumonitis or frank pulmonary edema, with dyspnea, tachypnea, cyanosis, cough, hemoptysis, substernal pain, and tachycardia (21, 22, 25–30). Bilateral rales, rhonchi, and wheezes can be heard at this stage (26, 29, 30). A chest radiograph taken soon after nitrogen oxide exposure may be normal and does not rule out the subsequent development of pulmonary edema.

The arterial hypoxemia observed at this stage is due not only to an impaired diffusion capacity secondary to alveolar edema, but also to ventilation-perfusion defects and, in some cases, to methemoglobinemia resulting from the reaction of nitrite ions with hemoglobin (23). Whereas the normal limit for methemoglobinemia is less than 1%, concentrations of 2–3% have been reported among arc welders and up to 44% among silo fillers (31). Metabolic acidosis may be present, the result of lactic acid formation in response to hypoxemia and of the entry into the circulation of nitric and nitrous acids created by the reaction of NO_2 with water. Although systemic hypotension can be caused by the vasodilatory effects of nitrates and nitrites, this finding is not commonly reported. The early appearance of findings characteristic of pulmonary edema is indicative of severe exposure and a worse prognosis. Although most individuals receiving appropriate, timely therapy survive NO_2-induced pulmonary edema, the case fatality rate has historically been reported to be substantial (29%) (23).

After apparent recovery from the acute illness, some patients may subsequently develop bronchiolitis obliterans approximately 10–30 days after the exposure. This delayed manifestation of severe respiratory symptoms may also occur in the absence of a prior episode pulmonary edema (25, 30, 32). Often this symptomatic relapse is heralded by fever and chills with rapid deterioration of the patient's condition. Other presenting symptoms may include fatigue, progressive shortness of breath and dyspnea, tachypnea, cough, hemoptysis, chest tightness, and cyanosis (21, 23, 27, 30). Auscultation reveals bilateral inspiratory rales and expiratory wheezes, although occasionally there may be minimal or no unusual findings (21, 32). Laboratory findings include a neutrophilic leukocytosis and an elevated sedimentation rate (32). Chest x-rays may show a patchy distribution of pneumonitis or, more commonly, diffuse, nodular infiltrates similar to those seen in miliary tuberculosis, with confluence of nodules in severe cases (2, 22, 32). Pathologic examination of open lung biopsy as well as autopsy specimens demonstrates an inflammatory exudate with fibrinous organization, which may eventually occlude the lumen of small bronchi and bronchioles (30, 32, 33).

Exposure to NO_2 in nonoccupational settings carries less dramatic (but still potentially serious) consequences than those described above. Some epidemiologic studies suggest that use of gas stoves may be associated with an increased incidence of respiratory illnesses in preschool children, decrements in lung function in school-aged children, and exacerbation of respiratory symptoms in asthmatic adults (34, 35). Controlled studies of mild asthmatics indicate that exposure to as low as 0.20–0.30 ppm NO_2 transiently enhances exercise-induced bronchoconstriction and causes subsequent bronchial hyperreactivity, as measured by challenge with methacholine or cold air (15, 36, 37). However, NO_2-induced changes in pulmonary function and reactivity in other asthmatic study populations have not been consistent findings (38, 39).

Acute and subacute exposures to NO_2 (at concentrations usually in excess of 5 ppm) increase susceptibility to infection in experimental animals after challenge with respiratory pathogens, including bacteria, viruses, and mycoplasma (40–42). In immunotoxicologic investigations involving animal models and, more recently, analyses of bronchoalveolar lavage fluid of human volunteers, NO_2 has been reported to affect a variety of host defenses against infection. Anatomic and physiologic effects include stunted cilia in fewer numbers, decreased ciliary beat frequency and motility, changes in macrophage function and morphology, depressed intrapulmonary killing of microorganisms, and changes in serum immunoglobulin responses to specific antigens (40–48). Several epidemiologic studies and one recent clinical investigation suggest that NO_2 may also increase the susceptibility of children and adults to respiratory illnesses, whereas others have not found such an effect (34, 49–52).

Chronic Toxicity

Severe, symptomatic NO_2 intoxication after acute exposure has on occasion been linked with persistent respiratory impairment, with symptoms of chronic bronchitis, and with spirometric evidence of an obstructive or restrictive defect (13, 23, 24, 53, 54). Lingering nonrespiratory symptoms from acute overexposure to NO_x are infrequent; however, several survivors of a massive rocket fuel spill reported headache and other subjective neuropsychiatric complaints for up to 1 year after the accident (13). As noted below, prolonged exposure to concentrations of nitrogen dioxide well in excess of current exposure limits results in focal emphysema in experimental animals: the evidence regarding whether such an effect may also occur in humans exposed occupationally is meager and mixed (55, 56). In this connection it is interesting to note that acute exposure of healthy nonsmokers to 3 or 4 ppm NO_2 for several hours resulted in a 45% reduction of alpha-1-protease inhibitor activity in bronchoalveolar lavage fluid, though this finding could not be replicated at lower concentrations (1.5 ppm continuously for 3 hours or 0.05 ppm with three 2 ppm spikes) (57, 58).

Epidemiologic studies of the respiratory effects of repeated indoor exposure of the general population to NO_2 suggest an association with intercurrent respiratory illness and pulmonary function deficits. However, inconsistent results among different study populations indicate that any such association is likely to be of small magnitude (34, 50, 52, 59). Outdoor exposures (which occur at substantially lower levels than indoors) are even less likely to demonstrate an effect of chronic exposure (60).

Repeated exposures to NO_2 may carry systemic consequences. Nitrogen dioxide has been demonstrated to cause a variety of effects on the immune system (61, 62). In an interesting series of reports, low level exposure to NO_2 was shown to facilitate the development of melanoma metastases in the lungs of mice, probably through capillary endothelial cell injury, formation of microthrombi, and effects on the immune response (63–65). Furthermore, nitrogen dioxide generates free radical reactions and is genotoxic in vitro, and may therefore be potentially carcinogenic or cocarcinogenic, although direct evidence to support this proposition is lacking (66–68).

MECHANISM OF RESPIRATORY TOXICITY AND PATHOLOGY

The toxicity of NO_2 is thought to be due to initiation of lipid peroxidation and to oxidation of cellular proteins and reducing substances (69). NO_2 can oxidize a variety of biologic molecules, generating free radicals that can undermine the structural and functional integrity of cell membranes, enzymes and other proteins (particularly those containing thiol groups), nucleic acids, and other biomolecules. Vitamin E, a membrane-associated free radical scavenger, can diminish NO_2-induced lipid peroxidation (70). As is also seen in ozone toxicity, peroxidation of the cell membrane causes effects that have been well characterized: increased membrane permeability, leakage of essential electrolytes and enzymes, inhibition of cellular metabolism, and swelling and disintegration of intracellular organelles including mitochondria, lysozomes, and endoplasmic reticulum (71). Consistent with the notion that the cell membrane is the principal site of NO_2 toxicity is the observation of increased paracellular permeability, which may be due in part to this substance's effect on intracellular tight junctions. Increased paracellular permeability has several pathologic consequences, including easier access to irritant nerve endings (possibly altering bronchial reactivity), and facilitation of the passage of toxic particles to the mucosa or submucosa (71).

The histopathologic events involving acute lung injury by NO_2 have been summarized by Evans (72). Cells sustaining the greatest damage from sublethal (2–17 ppm) concentrations of NO_2 are type I alveolar and ciliated cells in the bronchiolar epithelium, principally at the junction of the terminal airways and the gas exchange tissue. In the continued presence of NO_2, repair processes result in hyperplasia of cuboidal epithelial cells derived from type II cells, clearance of cellular and amorphous debris, interstitial thickening, and an inflammatory response. The new cells have a substantially lower surface-to-volume ratio and are more resistant to the effects of NO_2. These histologic changes are all reversible if animals are allowed to recover in clean air (72).

Animal experiments involving low level (2 ppm or less) exposures for durations of weeks to several years demonstrate a constellation of findings that are relatively consistent among several species, representing various degrees of tissue damage and repair. As is true of acute sublethal lung injury, the site of greatest injury is the junction of the airways and the alveoli. Typical changes include evidence of lipid peroxidation, type I cell damage with type II cell proliferation, increased alveolar permeability, and increased production of antioxidant enzymes (73, 74). Continuous exposure for several weeks to higher concentrations (30 ppm) produces a transient acute bronchiolitis and alveolitis, which subsequently evolve into a patchy centriacinar emphysema, with remodeling of alveoli and small airways and mild interstitial fibrosis (75, 76). The development of focal emphysema may be attributable to the accumulation of a significant elastase burden in the lung secondary to neutrophil recruitment and degranulation (75).

Management of Toxicity

PREVENTION

Given the potential severity of overexposure to nitrogen oxides, the best management strategy is prevention, principally through engineering controls and work practices, but also through worker education. In particular, workers should learn to seek medical attention even if the exposure did not seem excessive, because (as noted above), delayed onset of severe lower respiratory injury may occur in the absence of symptoms concurrent with

or shortly after exposure. Other preventive measures will depend on the context. For example, welders should be provided adequate ventilation or protective respiratory equipment. Entry into a silo within 1–2 weeks after filling should be avoided or, if this is not possible, the silo should be vented prior to entry. Farm workers should be educated about the hazards of entering a recently filled silo, including not only appropriate safety practices, but also visual and olfactory cues to the recognition of NO_2, as well as symptoms due to exposure to silo gas. Warning notices should be prominently posted, and children should never be permitted to play near a silo (4).

TREATMENT

Management of NO_2 inhalation is complicated by the occurrence of similar symptoms of respiratory distress (dyspnea, tachypnea, cough, and hypoxemia) that represent three stages of disease due to three separate pathophysiologic phenomena (acute bronchospasm, pulmonary edema, and bronchiolitis obliterans), which may be observed in sequence or alone (28). In the initial acute phase, the diagnosis may not be obvious, and will depend on eliciting a history suggestive of nitrogen oxide exposure. Carbon monoxide toxicity may complicate the management if the individual was exposed in a setting involving combustion. In an agricultural context, "acute farmer's lung" (which is due to hypersensitivity to thermophilic actinomycetes and often presents as an influenza-like illness) can usually be distinguished from NO_2 intoxication by a history indicating that the silo air was dusty and that the crop had not been recently ensiled (4). Other elements of the differential diagnosis would include asthma, pulmonary emboli, myocardial infarction, and respiratory infection. Once an appropriate diagnosis has been made, the management of the acute phase consists mainly of supportive care as for any toxic inhalation: oxygen, bronchodilators, and ventilatory support, as needed, and close observation to detect any deterioration in the patient's respiratory status. If methemoglobinemia is present, it may exacerbate hypoxemia and should be treated with methylene blue (2 mg/kg) (31).

The mainstays of therapy of the phases of pulmonary edema and a later relapse (bronchiolitis obliterans) involve treatment with oxygen (as dictated by the patient's blood gas profile) and corticosteroids. The pulmonary edema is of the increased permeability type, and should generally be treated as other acute lung injury (77). Although there have been no controlled clinical trials testing the efficacy of steroid administration, numerous case reports indicate that such treatment results in dramatic improvement, whereas death from progressive respiratory failure may otherwise occur (2, 25, 30, 32, 53, 78). Some authors recommend continuation of oral steroids for 6–8 weeks after a severe initial episode to retard or abort the proliferative cellular phase of bronchiolitis (21, 23).

EXPOSURE LIMITS

Various occupational and environmental limits are presented in Table 97.3.

SULFUR OXIDES: CLASS MEMBERS AND PROPERTIES

The remainder of this chapter will focus primarily on the toxicity of sulfur dioxide (SO_2), which is also referred to as sulfurous

Table 97.3. Nitrogen Oxides Exposure Limits

Nitric oxide	
Threshold Limit Value (ACGIH 8-hr TWA)	25 ppm
Permissible exposure limit (OSHA 8-hr TWA)	25 ppm
Immediately dangerous to life and health	
(NIOSH 30-min avg)	100 ppm
Nitrogen dioxide	
Threshold Limit Value (ACGIH 8-hr TWA)	3 ppm
Permissible exposure limit (OSHA ceiling 15-min)	1 ppm
Immediately dangerous to life and health	
(NIOSH 30 min)	50 ppm
National Ambient Air Quality Standard	
(EPA annual average)	.053 ppm

Sources: 40 Code of Federal Regulations 50 (1989); 29 Code of Federal Regulations 1910.1000 (1989); American Conference of Governmental Industrial Hygienists. Documentation of Threshold Limit Values and Biological Exposure Indices. 5th ed. Cincinnati, OH:1986; National Research Council, Committee on Toxicology. Emergency and Continuous Exposure Limits for Selected Airborne Contaminants. Vol 1. Washington, DC: National Academy Press, 1984; U.S. Department of Health and Human Services, Public Health Service. NIOSH Pocket Guide to Chemical Hazards. Washington, DC: US Government Printing Office, 1990:162, 164.

Table 97.4. Uses and Sites of Occurrence of Sulfur Oxides

Sulfur dioxide	
Chemical manufacturing (sulfuric acid, sulfites, thiosulfates, hydrosulfites, sulfonation of oils and other uses)	
Recovery of volatile materials	
Reducing agent and anti-oxidant	
Paper manufacturing	
Metal and ore refining	
Portland cement manufacture	
Disinfectant and fumigant	
Food preservative (to inhibit bacterial growth, browning, and enzyme-catalyzed reactions)	
Soybean protein	
Solvent extraction of lubricating oils	
Derived from:	
Combustion of sulfur-containing fuels (particularly in power plants and oil refineries)	
Purification (and compression) of SO_2 gas from smelting	
Roasting pyrites	

Sources: Sax NI, Lewis RJ. Hawley's Condensed Chemical Dictionary. 11th ed. New York, NY: Van Nostrand Reinhold Company, 1987; Anonymous. Sulfur dioxide exposure in Portland cement plants. MMWR 1984;33:195–196.

anhydride or sulfurous oxide. Sulfur trioxide (SO_3, also known as sulfuric anhydride) forms sulfuric acid when in the presence of water, and its toxicity is therefore identical to that produced by exposure to the latter (see Chapter 67). SO_2 is a highly irritating, colorless, soluble gas with a pungent odor and taste. In contact with water it forms sulfurous acid, which accounts for its significant irritancy to eyes, mucous membranes, and skin.

SOURCES OF SULFUR OXIDE EXPOSURE

In 1974, the National Institute for Occupational Safety and Health (NIOSH) estimated that approximately 500,000 workers were potentially exposed to sulfur dioxide (79). Sources of exposure to SO_2 are listed in Table 97.4, and various exposure limits are presented in Table 97.5.

As an outdoor air pollutant, the principal source of SO_2 is the combustion of sulfur-containing fuels, particularly in power

plants. In ambient air, sulfur dioxide can be oxidized at a rate of 0.5–10.0%/hr to sulfur trioxide, which can be hydrated to form sulfuric acid (3). Although SO_2 has been suspected as a major cause of illness and death in several air pollution catastrophes in this century, much of the toxicity may have been due to the particles with which it was associated. Concern about SO_2 as an air pollutant has focused recently on its capacity to induce bronchoconstriction in asthmatics and other sensitive individuals and on its role as a precursor in the formation of acid aerosols (80). In nonoccupational settings, SO_2 is generally found at substantially lower concentrations indoors than outside; however, the use of kerosene space heaters can generate significant indoor concentrations (9, 81).

CLINICAL TOXICOLOGY OF EXPOSURE

Absorption

Sulfur dioxide is soluble in water and thus tends to be efficiently absorbed in the upper respiratory tract. Two factors affecting the efficiency of absorption are the mode of breathing (oral versus oronasal) and ventilation rate. The nose filters out most inhaled SO_2, preventing its passage to sensitive irritant receptors at and below the larynx (82, 83). At rest, most people (about 85%) breathe through the nose, providing protection against SO_2 toxicity (84). Mouth breathing, particularly at higher airflow rates, substantially increases the fraction of SO_2 reaching the lung (82). Thus, voluntary hyperventilation or exercise at a level of exertion requiring oronasal breathing lowers the threshold for SO_2-induced respiratory symptoms and bronchomotor responsiveness (84–86). Deep lung penetration and toxicity are enhanced by oxidation and adsorption to submicron acidic particles (87).

Distribution and Metabolism

Water rapidly dissolves SO_2 to form ions of hydrogen (H^+), bisulfite (HSO_3^-) and sulfite ($SO_3^=$) which exist in equilibrium as follows:

$$SO_2 + H_2O \leftrightarrow HSO_3^- + H^+ \qquad pK_a = 1.86$$
$$HSO_3^- \leftrightarrow SO_3^= + H^+ \qquad pK_a = 7.2 \qquad (88)$$

Table 97.5. Sulfur Dioxide Exposure Limits

Threshold limit value (ACGIH) (8-hr TWA)	2 ppm
(15-min ceiling)	5 ppm
Permissible exposure limit (OSHA 8-hr TWA)	2 ppm
NIOSH recommendation	0.5 ppm
Immediately dangerous to life or health	
(NIOSH 30-min avg)	100 ppm
National Ambient Air Quality Standard (EPA)	
(24-hr average)	0.14 ppm
(annual average)	0.03 ppm

Sources: 40 Code of Federal Regulations 50 (1989); 29 Code of Federal Regulations 1910.1000 (1989); American Conference of Governmental Industrial Hygienists. Documentation of Threshold Limit Values and Biological Exposure Indices. 5th ed. Cincinnati, OH: 1986; National Research Council, Committee on Toxicology. Emergency and Continuous Exposure Limits for Selected Airborne Contaminants. Vol 1. Washington, DC: National Academy Press, 1984; U.S. Department of Health and Human Services, Public Health Service. NIOSH Pocket Guide to Chemical Hazards. Washington, DC: US Government Printing Office, 1990:200.

Direct effects of SO_2 on the respiratory tract cannot be easily studied in the absence of water; although hydrolysis occurs rapidly, the toxicity of SO_2 may be due to the gas itself, bisulfite, sulfite, and hydrogen ions (89). At the airway surface the ratio of bisulfite to sulfite ions is likely to be about 5:1, and recent work suggests that bisulfite is a more potent bronchoconstrictor (in asthmatics) than sulfite ion (89, 90). Bisulfite ion reacts with many biological molecules via nucleophilic substitution, and sulfur-containing free radicals may also produce cellular damage (88). The quantities of hydrogen ion produced during inhalation of SO_2 are less than the acid concentrations required to produce bronchoconstriction in asthmatics (90). At higher concentrations that would be more characteristic of occupational than environmental exposures, however, hydrogen ion may play a more prominent role in causing toxicity.

Radiolabeled sulfur dioxide is absorbed from the respiratory tract of experimental animals in the blood and is distributed throughout the body, concentrating in the liver, spleen, esophagus, and kidneys (91, 92). It is metabolized to a variety of sulfur-containing compounds and is excreted principally via the urine as sulfate (91). Significant quantities of SO_2 may be retained for a week or more in the lungs and trachea of experimental animals (92).

SIGNS, SYMPTOMS, AND SYNDROMES OF EXPOSURE

Acute Toxicity

Because of the high solubility of SO_2, it is extremely irritating to the eyes and upper respiratory tract, warning the exposed individual to escape before serious damage occurs. The odor is detectable at 0.5 ppm, while concentrations above 6 ppm produce instantaneous mucous membrane irritation (93). Symptoms include ocular irritation and lacrimation, rhinorrhea, cough, shortness of breath, chest tightness or discomfort, and a choking sensation. The lower respiratory symptoms are often associated with SO_2-induced bronchoconstriction.

Numerous controlled exposure investigations have demonstrated that SO_2 increases specific airway resistance. There is a wide variability in responsiveness to this substance: some asthmatics and atopics appear to be much more susceptible than other populations tested (94–96). Studies in animals and nonasthmatic humans indicate that SO_2 induces vagal reflex bronchoconstriction; however, in asthmatics and others who are sensitive to the effects of SO_2, additional mechanisms appear to operate (89, 94, 95, 97, 98). Exercise (or voluntary oral hyperventilation) and low humidity augment the responses observed in asthmatics (86, 99–102). With moderate exercise or hyperventilation, lower respiratory symptoms and/or bronchomotor effects have been consistently observed in asthmatics after short (several minutes) exposures to SO_2 concentrations of 0.5 ppm and above, and in some cases in the range of 0.2–0.3 ppm, all of which are substantially below the current TLV (96, 101, 103, 104). Recently it has been reported that preexposure to a low concentration of ozone (0.12 ppm) for 45 minutes potentiates the bronchoconstrictive effect of an otherwise subthreshold dose of SO_2 in adolescent asthmatics, suggesting the potential for interaction with other pollutants commonly found in urban environments (105).

There are occasional reports of industrial accidents in which severe pulmonary injury occurred from relatively brief exposure to high concentrations of SO_2. Charan et al. (106) reported that an accident in a paper mill resulted in death within minutes for two workers, whose lungs were found to have extensive sloughing of bronchial and bronchiolar mucosa, as well as hemorrhagic alveolar edema. Galea (107) reported a case of a pulp and paper mill employee who died 17 days after 15–20-minute exposure to sulfur dioxide fumes. Initially this worker's symptoms consisted of ocular irritation and pain on inspiration, which both subsided within a few days. However, 1.5 weeks later, he presented with a productive cough, dyspnea, wheeze, and bilateral rales, which progressed despite aggressive therapy. Autopsy findings included extensive tracheobronchitis, mucus hypersecretion, bronchiolitis obliterans, and diffuse alveolar damage.

Woodford et al. (108) described a clinical course reminiscent of severe intoxication by nitrogen dioxide in an individual exposed to SO_2 in an enclosed space for about 15–20 minutes. Within 2 days this individual developed pulmonary edema, which improved with treatment. Two weeks after the accident, he experienced respiratory symptoms consistent with bronchiolitis obliterans (no confirmatory biopsy was obtained).

Chronic Toxicity

Prolonged exposure of dogs to high concentrations of SO_2 (200 ppm) causes a syndrome similar to human chronic bronchitis, involving chronic airway obstruction, airway inflammation, and symptoms of cough and mucus hypersecretion. However, unlike human disease, in this animal model there is decreased airway responsiveness to inhaled bronchoconstrictor agents, which appears to be associated with chronic airway inflammation (109, 110). When exposed to 15 ppm using the same experimental protocol, none of these effects is evident (110). With few exceptions, chronic exposure of animals to SO_2 does not produce observable adverse effects at concentrations lower than 20 ppm (79, 89).

In humans, survivors of massive sulfur dioxide exposure have shown a chronic, obstructive defect in serial pulmonary function studies, along with bronchial hyperreactivity (106, 108, 111, 112). The extent to which recurrent occupational or environmental exposures to SO_2 produce adverse effects in humans is not clear, however, in part because in both contexts there are usually confounding exposures to particulates or other irritants. Although some investigations suggest that occupational SO_2 exposure (even at levels below the current TLV) is associated with increased upper and lower respiratory symptoms and decrements in various spirometric indices, others have not (79, 113–115).

Somewhat more puzzling are the results of some community studies, which indicate that SO_2 is associated not only with increased respiratory symptoms and with decrements in pulmonary function, but also with increased daily mortality (116–120). Such effects appear even at 24-hour SO_2 averages less than 0.10 ppm. In these situations, SO_2 is likely to be an indicator for a complex mixture of pollutants, including perhaps acid sulfates and other particles; however, a few studies suggest effects related to SO_2 but not particulates (117, 119).

Management of Toxicity

Fortunately, severe injury by SO_2 is rare, owing perhaps to its strong intrinsic warning properties. Treatment is symptomatic: topical administration of sodium bicarbonate solution aerosol may alleviate eye or respiratory mucous membrane irritation

(2). Respiratory support may be indicated in cases where the exposed individual was trapped or was otherwise unable to escape the exposure. Systemic corticosteroids can be beneficial in acute SO_2-induced lung injury, although there is less published evidence to support their use than in the case of NO_2 (J. Balmes, personal communication: 112). In experimental settings, SO_2-induced bronchospasm in asthmatics often appears to be reversible within a half-hour even without treatment, but may require bronchodilator administration.

REFERENCES

1. National Research Council. Nitrogen oxides. Washington, DC: National Academy Press, 1977:4–19.

2. Seaton A, Morgan WKC. Toxic gases and fumes. In: Morgan WKC, Seaton A, eds. Occupational lung diseases. 2nd ed. Philadelphia, PA: W. B. Saunders Co., 1984:609–642.

3. World Health Organization. Air quality guidelines for Europe. Copenhagen: WHO Regional Publications, European Series No. 23, 1987.

4. Douglas WW, Hepper NGG, Colby TV. Silo-filler's disease. Mayo Clin Proc 1989;64:291–304.

5. Seinfeld JH. Atmospheric chemistry and physics of air pollution. New York, NY: John Wiley & Sons, 1986:79–86.

6. Spengler JD, Duffy CP, Letz R, Tibbetts TW, Ferris BG. Nitrogen dioxide inside and outside 137 homes and implications for ambient air quality standards and health effects research. Environ Sci Tech 1983;17:164–168.

7. Marbury MC, Harlos DP, Samet JM, Spengler JD. Indoor residential NO_2 concentrations in Albuquerque, New Mexico. J Air Pollut Control Assoc 1988;38:392–398.

8. Lindvall T. Health effects of nitrogen dioxide and oxidants. Scand J Work Environ Health 1985;11 (suppl 3):10–28.

9. Leaderer BP. Air pollutant emissions from kerosene space heaters. Science 1982;218:1113–1115.

10. Borland C, Higenbottam T. Nitric oxide yields of contemporary UK, US and French cigarettes. Int J Epidemiol 1987;16:31–34.

11. Nathan CF, Stuehr DJ. Does endothelium-derived nitric oxide have a role in cytokine-induced hypotension? J Natl Cancer Inst 1990;82:726–728.

12. Griffith T, Randall M. Nitric oxide comes of age. Lancet 1989;2:875–876.

13. Yockey CC, Eden BM, Byrd RB. The McConnell missile accident: clinical spectrum of nitrogen dioxide exposure. JAMA 1980;244:1221–1223.

14. von Nieding G, Wagner M, Krekeler H, Smidt U, Muysers K. Absorption of NO_2 in low concentrations in the respiratory tract and its acute effects on lung function and circulation. In: Second International Clean Air Congress at the Union of Air Pollution Prevention Association, Washington, DC, December 6–12, 1970.

15. Bauer MA, Utell MJ, Morrow PE, Speers DM, Gibb FR. Inhalation of 0.30 ppm nitrogen dioxide potentiates exercise-induced bronchospasm in asthmatics. Am Rev Respir Dis 1986;134:1203–1208.

16. Yoshida K, Kasama K. Biotransformation of nitric oxide. Environ Health Perspect 1987;73:201–206.

17. Meyer M, Piiper J. Nitric oxide (NO), a new test gas for study of alveolar-capillary diffusion. Eur Respir J 1989;2:494–496.

18. Goldstein E, Goldstein F, Peek NF, Parks NJ. Absorption and transport of nitrogen oxides. In: Lee SD, ed. Nitrogen oxides and their effects on health. Ann Arbor, MI: Ann Arbor Science Publishers, 1983:143–160.

19. Pryor WA. Mechanism and detection of pathology caused by free radicals. Tobacco smoke, nitrogen dioxide, and ozone. In: McKinney JD, ed. Environmental health chemistry. The chemistry of environmental agents as potential human hazards. Ann Arbor, MI: Ann Arbor Science Publishers, Inc., 1981:445–466.

20. Postlethwaite EM, Bidani A. Pulmonary disposition of inhaled NO_2-nitrogen isolated rat lungs. Toxicol Appl Pharmacol 1989;98:303–312.

21. Tse RL, Bockman AA. Nitrogen dioxide toxicity. Report of four cases in firemen. JAMA 1970;212:1341–1344.

22. Lindquist T. Nitrous gas poisoning among welders using acetylene flame. Acta Med Scand 1944;119:210–243.

23. Horvath EP, doPico GA, Barbee RA. Dickie HA. Nitrogen dioxide-induced pulmonary disease. Five new cases and a review of the literature. J Occup Med 1978;20:103–110.

24. Leib GMP, Davis WN, Brown T, McQuiggan M. Chronic pulmonary insufficiency secondary to silo-filler's disease. Am J Med 1958;24:471–474.

25. Jones GR, Proudfoot AT, Hall JI. Pulmonary effects of acute exposure to nitrous fumes. Thorax 1973;28:61–65.

26. Hirotani T, Maenaka Y, Yamamoto S, Kobayashi K. Adult respiratory distress syndrome caused by inhalation of oxides of nitrogen. Keio J Med 1987;36:315–320.

27. Milne JEH. Nitrogen dioxide inhalation and bronchiolitis obliterans. J Occup Med 1969;538–547.

28. Guidotti TL. The higher oxides of nitrogen: inhalation toxicology. Environ Res 1987;15:443–472.

29. Fleming GM, Chester EH, Montenegro HD. Dysfunction of small airways following pulmonary injury due to nitrogen dioxide. Chest 1979;75:720–721.

30. Moskowitz RL, Lyons HA, Cottle HR. Silo filler's disease. Am J Med 1964;36:457–462.

31. Rom WN, Barkman H. Respiratory irritants. In Rom WN, ed. Environmental and occupational medicine. Boston: Little, Brown, 1983:273–283.

32. Lowry T, Schuman LM. ''Silo-filler's disease''—a syndrome caused by nitrogen dioxide. JAMA 1956;162:153–160.

33. McAdams AJ. Bronchiolitis obliterans. Am J Med 1955;19:314–322.

34. Speizer FE, Ferris B, Bishop YM, Spengler JD. Respiratory disease rates and pulmonary function in children associated with NO_2 exposure. Am Rev Respir Dis 1980;121:3–10.

35. Ostro BD, Lipsett MJ, Wiener M, Selner JS. Asthmatic responses to acid aerosols. Am J Public Health (in press).

36. Koenig JQ, Covert DS, Smith MS, Van Belle G, Pierson WE. The pulmonary effects of ozone and nitrogen dioxide alone and combined in healthy and asthmatic adolescent subjects. Toxicol Ind Health 1988;4:521–532.

37. Roger LJ, Horstman DH, McDonnell W, et al. Pulmonary function, airway responsiveness and respiratory symptoms in asthmatics following exercise in NO_2. Toxicol Ind Health 1990;6:155–171.

38. Mohsenin V. Airway responses to nitrogen dioxide in asthmatic subjects. J Toxicol Environ Health 1987;22:371–380.

39. Avol EL, Linn WS, Peng RC, Valencia G, Little D, Hackney JD. Laboratory study of asthmatic volunteers exposed to nitrogen dioxide and to ambient air pollution. Am Ind Hyg Assoc J 1988;49:143–149.

40. Rose RM, Fuglestad JM, Skornik WA, et al. The pathophysiology of enhanced susceptibility to murine cytomegalovirus respiratory infection during short-term exposure to 5 ppm nitrogen dioxide. Am Rev Respir Dis 1988;137:912–917.

41. Parker RF, Davis JK, Cassell GH, et al. Short-term exposure to nitrogen dioxide enhances susceptibility to murine respiratory mycoplasmosis and decreases intrapulmonary killing of Mycoplasma pulmonis. Am Rev Respir Dis 1989;140:502–512.

42. Pennington JE. Effects of automotive emissions on susceptibility to respiratory infections. In: Watson SY, Bates RR, Kennedy D, eds. Air pollution, the automobile, and public health. Washington, DC: National Academy Press, 1988:499–518.

43. Schlesinger RB. Comparative toxicity of ambient air pollutants: some aspects related to lung defense. Environ Health Perspect 1989;81:123–128.

44. Suzuki T, Ikeda S, Kanoh T, Mizoguchi I. Decreased phagocytosis and superoxide anion production in alveolar macrophages of rats exposed to nitrogen dioxide. Arch Environ Contam Toxicol 1986;15:733–739.

45. Frampton MW, Smeglin AM, Roberts NJ, Finkelstein JN, Morrow PE, Utell MJ. Nitrogen dioxide exposure in vivo and human alveolar macrophage inactivation of influenza virus in vitro. Environ Res 1989;48:179–192.

46. Jakab GJ. Modulation of pulmonary defense mechanisms by acute exposures to nitrogen dioxide. Environ Res 1987;42:215–228.

47. Dawson SV, Schenker MB. Health effects of inhalation of ambient concentrations of nitrogen dioxide. Am Rev Respir Dis 1979;120:281–292.

48. Heller RF, Gordon RE. Chronic effects of nitrogen dioxide on cilia in hamster bronchioles. Exp Lung Res 1986;10:137–152.

49. Goings SAJ, Kulle TJ, Bascom R, et al. Effect of nitrogen dioxide on susceptibility to influenza A virus infection in healthy adults. Am Rev Respir Dis 1989;139:1075–1081.

50. Koo LC, Ho JHC, Ho CY, et al. Personal exposure to nitrogen dioxide and its association with respiratory illness in Hong Kong. Am Rev Respir Dis 1990;141:1119–1126.

51. Jacobsen M, Smith TA, Hurley JF, Robertson A, Roscrow R. Respiratory infections in coal miners exposed to nitrogen oxides. Health Effects Institute Research Report Number 18; 1988; 64 pp.

52. Samet JM, Marbury MC, Spengler JD. Health effects and sources of indoor air pollution. Part I. Am Rev Respir Dis 1987;136:1486–1508.

53. Becklake MR, Goldman HI, Bosman AR, Freed CC. The long-term effects of exposure to nitrous fumes. Am Rev Tuberc 1957;76:398–409.

54. Muller B. Nitrogen dioxide intoxication after a mining accident. Respiration 1969;26:249–261.

55. Kennedy MCS. Nitrous fumes and coal-miners with emphysema. Ann Occup Hyg 1972;15:285–300.

56. Robertson A, Dodgson J, Collings P, Seaton A. Exposure to oxides of

nitrogen: respiratory symptoms and lung function in British coalminers. Br J Ind Med 1984;41:214–219.

57. Mohsenin V, Gee JBL. Acute effect of nitrogen dioxide exposure on the functional activity of alpha-1-proteinase inhibitor in bronchoalveolar lavage fluid of normal subjects. Am Rev Respir Dis 1987;136:646–650.

58. Johnson DA, Frampton MW, Winters RS, Morrow PE, Utell MJ. Inhalation of nitrogen dioxide fails to reduce the activity of human lung alpha-1-proteinase inhibitor. Am Rev Respir Dis 1990;142:758–762.

59. Fischer P, Remijn B, Brunekreef B, van der Lende R, Schouten J, Quanjer P. Indoor air pollution and its effect on pulmonary function of adult non-smoking women: II. Associations between nitrogen dioxide and pulmonary function. Int J Epidemiol 1985;14:221–226.

60. Euler GL, Abbey DE, Hodgkin JE, Magie AR. Chronic obstructive pulmonary disease symptom effects of long-term cumulative exposure to ambient levels of total oxidants and nitrogen dioxide in California Seventh-Day Adventist residents. Arch Environ Health 1988;43:279–285.

61. Azoulay-Dupuis E, Bouley G, Moreau J, Muffat-Joly M, Pocidalo J. Evidence for humoral immunodepression in NO_2-exposed mice: influence of food restriction and stress. Environ Res 1987;42:446–454.

62. Kuraitis KV, Richters A. Spleen cellularity shifts from the inhalation of 0.25–0.35 ppm nitrogen dioxide. J Environ Pathol Toxicol Oncol 1989;9:1–11.

63. Richters A. Effects of nitrogen dioxide and ozone on blood-borne cancer cell colonization of the lungs. J Toxicol Environ Health 1988;25:383–390.

64. Richters A, Richters V. Nitrogen dioxide (NO_2) inhalation, formation of microthrombi in lungs and cancer metastasis. J Environ Pathol Toxicol Oncol 1989;9:45–51.

65. Richters A, Richters V, Alley WP. The mortality rate from lung metastases in animals inhaling nitrogen dioxide (NO_2). J Surg Oncol 1985;28:63–66.

66. Gorsdorf S, Appel KE, Engeholm C, Obe G. Nitrogen dioxide induces DNA single-strand breaks in cultured Chinese hamster cells. Carcinogenesis 1990;11:37–41.

67. Victorin K, Busk L, Cederberg H, Magnusson J. Genotoxic activity of 1,3-butadiene and nitrogen dioxide and their photochemical reaction products in Drosophila and in the mouse bone marrow micronucleus assay. Mutat Res 1990;228:203–209.

68. Witschi HP. Ozone, nitrogen dioxide and lung cancer: a review of some recent issues and problems. Toxicology 1988;48:1–20.

69. Sagai M, Ichinose T. Lipid peroxidation and antioxidative protection mechanism in rat lungs upon acute and chronic exposure to nitrogen dioxide. Environ Health Perspect 1987;73:179–189.

70. Calabrese EJ, Horton HM. The effects of vitamin E on ozone and nitrogen dioxide toxicity. World Rev Nutr Diet 1985;46:124–147.

71. Man SFP, Hulbert WC. Airway repair and adaptation to injury. In: Loke J., ed. Pathophysiology and treatment of inhalation injuries. New York: Marcel Dekker, 1988:1–47.

72. Evans MJ. Oxidant gases. Environ Health Perspect 1984;55:85–95.

73. Crapo JD, Barry BE, Chang LY, Mercer RR. Alterations in lung structure caused by inhalation of oxidants. In: Miller FJ, Menzel DB, eds. Fundamentals of extrapolation modeling of inhaled toxicants: ozone and nitrogen dioxide. Washington, DC: Hemisphere Publishing Corporation, 1984:301–321.

74. Morrow PE. Toxicological data on NO_x: an overview. In: Miller FJ, Menzel DB, eds. Fundamentals of extrapolation modeling of inhaled toxicants: ozone and nitrogen dioxide. Washington, DC: Hemisphere Publishing Corporation, 1984:205–227.

75. Glasgow JE, Pietra GG, Abrams WR, Blank J, Oppenheim DM, Weinbaum G. Neutrophil recruitment and degranulation during induction of emphysema in the rat by nitrogen dioxide. Am Rev Respir Dis 1987;135:1129–1136.

76. Freeman G, Crane SC, Stephens RJ, Furiosi NJ. Pathogenesis of the nitrogen dioxide-induced lesion in the rat lung: a review and presentation of new observations. Am Rev Respir Dis 1968;98:429–443.

77. Flick MR. Pulmonary edema and acute lung injury. In: Murray JF, Nadel JA, eds. Textbook of respiratory medicine. Philadelphia, PA: W.B. Saunders Company, 1988:1359–1409.

78. Gailitis J, Burns LE, Nally JB. Silo-fillers disease. Report of a case. N Engl J Med 1958;258:543–544.

79. National Institute for Occupational Safety and Health. Criteria for a recommended standard . . . occupational exposure to sulfur dioxide. 1974:16, 20–26.

80. U.S. Environmental Protection Agency. Review of the national ambient air quality standards for sulfur oxides; updated assessment of scientific and technical information. Addendum to the 1982 OAQPS staff paper. Research Triangle Park, NC: EPA 450/05 86-013, 1986:9–21.

81. Godish T. Air quality. Chelsea, MI: Lewis Publishers, Inc., 1985:294.

82. Frank NR, Yoder RE, Brain JD, Yokoyama E. SO_2 absorption by the mouth and nose under conditions of varying concentration and flow. Arch Environ Health 1969;18:315–322.

83. Speizer FE, Frank NR. The uptake and release of SO_2 by the human nose. Arch Environ Health 1966;12:725–728.

84. Kleinman MT. Sulfur dioxide and exercise: relationships between response and absorption in upper airways. J Air Pollut Control Assoc 1984;34:32–37.

85. Bethel RA, Erle DJ, Epstein J, Sheppard D, Nadel JA, Boushey HA. Effect of exercise rate and route of inhalation on sulfur-dioxide-induced bronchoconstriction in asthmatic subjects. Am Rev Respir Dis 1983;128:592–596.

86. Sheppard D, Saisho A, Nadel JA, Boushey HA. Exercise increases sulfur dioxide-induced bronchoconstriction in asthmatic subjects. Am Rev Respir Dis 1981;123:486–491.

87. Amdur MO. Aerosols formed by oxidation of sulfur dioxide. Review of their toxicology. Arch Environ Health 1971;23:459–468.

88. Neta P, Huie RE. Free-radical chemistry of sulfite. Environ Health Perspect 1985;64:209–217.

89. Sheppard D. Mechanisms of airway responses to inhaled sulfur dioxide. In Loke J, ed. Pathophysiology and treatment of inhalation injuries. New York, NY: Marcel Dekker, 1988:49–66.

90. Fine JM, Gordon T, Sheppard D. The roles of pH and ionic species in sulfur dioxide- and sulfite-induced bronchoconstriction. Am Rev Respir Dis 1987;136:1122–1126.

91. Yokoyama E, Yoder RE, Frank NR. Distribution of ^{35}S in the blood and its excretion in urine of dogs exposed to $^{35}SO_2$. Arch Environ Health 1971;22:389–395.

92. Balchum OJ, Dybicki J, Meneely GR. The dynamics of sulfur dioxide inhalation, absorption, distribution, and retention. Arch Ind Health 1960;21:564–569.

93. Schwartz DA. Acute inhalational injury. In Rosenstock L, ed. Occupational pulmonary disease. Philadelphia, PA: Hanley & Belfus, 1987:297–318.

94. Sheppard D, Wong WS, Uehara CF, Nadel JA, Boushey HA. Lower threshold and greater bronchomotor responsiveness of asthmatic subjects to sulfur dioxide. Am Rev Respir Dis 1980;122:873–878.

95. Snashall PD, Baldwin C. Mechanisms of sulphur dioxide induced bronchoconstriction in normal and asthmatic man. Thorax 1982;37:118–123.

96. Linn WS, Avol EL, Peng RC, Shamoo DA, Hackney JD. Replicated dose-response study of sulfur dioxide effects in normal, atopic, and asthmatic volunteers. Am Rev Respir Dis 1987;136:1127–1134.

97. Nadel JA, Salem H, Tamplin B, Tokiwa Y. Mechanism of bronchoconstriction during inhalation of sulfur dioxide. J Appl Physiol 1965a;20:164–167.

98. Nadel JA, Salem H, Tamplin B, Tokiwa Y. Mechanism of bronchoconstriction during inhalation of sulfur dioxide: reflex involving vagus nerves. Arch Environ Health 1965;10:175–178.

99. Sheppard D, Eschenbacher WL, Boushey HA, Bethel RA. Magnitude of the interaction between the bronchomotor effects of sulfur dioxide and those of dry (cold) air. Am Rev Respir Dis 1984;130:52–55.

100. Linn WS, Shamoo DA, Anderson KR, Whynot JD, Avol EL, Hackney JD. Effects of heat and humidity on the responses of exercising asthmatics to sulfur dioxide exposure. Am Rev Respir Dis 1985;131:221–225.

101. Linn WS, Venet TG, Shamoo DA, et al. Respiratory effects of sulfur dioxide in heavily exercising asthmatics. Am Rev Respir Dis 1983;127:278–283.

102. Bethel RA, Sheppard D, Epstein J, Tam E, Nadel JA, Boushey HA. Interaction of sulfur dioxide and cold dry air in causing bronchoconstriction in asthmatic subjects. J Appl Physiol 1984;57:419–423.

103. Horstman D, Roger LJ, Kehrl H, Hazucha M. Airway sensitivity of asthmatics to sulfur dioxide. Toxicol Ind Health 1986;2:289–298.

104. Balmes JR, Fine JM, Sheppard D. Symptomatic bronchoconstriction after short-term inhalation of sulfur dioxide. Am Rev Respir Dis 1987;136:1117–1121.

105. Koenig JQ, Covert DS, Hanley QS, Van Belle G, Pierson WE. Prior exposure to ozone potentiates subsequent response to sulfur dioxide in adolescent asthmatic subjects. Am Rev Respir Dis 1990;141:377–380.

106. Charan NB, Myers CG, Lakshminarayan S, Spencer TM. Pulmonary injuries associated with acute sulfur dioxide inhalation. Am Rev Respir Dis 1979;119:555–560.

107. Galea M. Fatal sulfur dioxide inhalation. Can Med Assoc J 1964;91:345–347.

108. Woodford DM, Coutu RE, Gaensler EA. Obstructive lung disease from acute sulfur dioxide exposure. Respiration 1979;38:238–245.

109. Shore SA, Kariya ST, Anderson K, et al. Sulfur-dioxide-induced bronchitis in dogs. Effects on airway responsiveness to inhaled and intravenously administered methacholine. Am Rev Respir Dis 1987;135:840–847.

110. Scanlon PD, Seltzer J, Ingram RH, Reid L, Drazen JM. Chronic ex-

posure to sulfur dioxide. Physiologic and histologic evaluation of dogs exposed to 50 or 15 ppm. Am Rev Respir Dis 1987;135:831–839.

111. Harkonen H, Nordnam H, Korhonen O, Winblad I. Long-term effects of exposure to sulfur dioxide. Am Rev Respir Dis 1983;128:890–893.

112. Rabinovitch S, Greyson ND, Weiser W, Hoffstein V. Clinical and laboratory features of acute sulfur dioxide inhalation poisoning: two-year follow-up. Am Rev Respir Dis 1989;139:556–558.

113. Archer VE, Gillam JD. Chronic sulfur dioxide exposure in a smelter. II. Indices of chest disease. J Occup Med 1978;20:88–95.

114. Osterman JW, Greaves IA, Smith TJ, Hammond SK, Robins JM, Theriault G. Respiratory symptoms associated with low level sulphur dioxide exposure in silicon carbide production workers. Br J Ind Med 1989;46:629–635.

115. Rom WN, Wood SD, White GL, Bang KM, Reading JC. Longitudinal evaluation of pulmonary function in copper smelter workers exposed to sulfur dioxide. Am Rev Respir Dis 1986;133:830–833.

116. Dockery DW, Ware JH, Ferris BG, Speizer FE, Cook NR, Herman SM. Change in pulmonary function in children associated with air pollution episodes. J Air Pollut Contr Assoc 1982;32:937–942.

117. Charpin D, Kleisbauer JP, Fondarai J, Graland B, Viala A, Gouezo F. Respiratory symptoms and air pollution changes in children: the Gardanne coal-basin study. Arch Environ Health 1988;43:22–27.

118. Derrienic F, Richardson S, Mollie A, Lalloch J. Short-term effects of sulphur dioxide pollution on mortality in two French cities. Int J Epidemiol 1989;18:186–197.

119. Hatzakis A, Katsouyanni K, Kalandidi A, Day N, Trichopoulos D. Short-term effects of air pollution on mortality in Athens. Int J Epidemiol 1986;15:73–81.

120. Groupe Cooperatif PAARC. Pollution atmospherique et affections respiratoires chroniques ou a repetition. II. Resultats et discussion. Bull Eur Physiopathol Respir 1982;18:101–116.

John J. Clary, Ph.D.
John B. Sullivan, Jr., M.D.

SOURCES AND PRODUCTION

Common Names and Chemical Names

Formaldehyde has been manufactured commercially for nearly 100 years and is presently produced worldwide. Common names for formaldehyde include BFV, Fannoform, Formalith, Formol, Fyde, Ivalon, Lysoform, Morbicid, and Superlysoform. Chemical names include formaldehyde, formaldehyde gas, formaldehyde solution, formalin, formalin 40, formalin 100%, formic aldehyde, methaldehyde, methanal, methyl aldehyde, methylene glycol, and methylene oxide.

Chemical Forms

Formaldehyde (HCHO) production is reported in terms of formalin, which is a 37% aqueous solution and the most common chemical form of formaldehyde. Formalin contains methanol at a concentration of 0.5–15% to prevent polymerization of formaldehyde to cyclic trimers or to paraformaldehyde. Formalin is a slightly acidic, clear solution with a strong pungent odor. Formaldehyde is also available as its linear low molecular weight homopolymer, paraformaldehyde, or as a cyclic trimer, trioxane (1).

Physical Forms

Pure formaldehyde is a colorless gas which condenses to form a liquid at high vapor pressure. Formaldehyde also exists in the powdered and liquid state, which is usually in the form of an aqueous solution. Liquid formaldehyde, which has a boiling point of $-19°C$ and a melting point of $-118°C$, is miscible with water, acetone, benzene, diethyl ether, chloroform, and ethanol (1). Trioxane, the cyclic trimer of formaldehyde, is a solid which is used as a fuel source since it burns easily.

SITES, INDUSTRIES, AND BUSINESSES ASSOCIATED WITH EXPOSURE

Table 98.1 lists occupations associated with formaldehyde exposure, and Table 98.2 gives airborne formaldehyde concentrations monitored in Finland (2, 3).

Mechanisms, Processes, and Reactions Leading to Exposure

Formaldehyde is produced by the oxidation of methanol with air in the presence of a silver or an iron oxide-molybdenum oxide catalyst. The majority of formaldehyde in the United States is used for plastics and resin manufacture. Formaldehyde is also used for the production of intermediates. Urea-formaldehyde resins, which are used primarily as adhesives in the manufacture of particle board, medium density fiberboard, and hardwood plywood, consume more formaldehyde than any other resins. Phenolic resins and polyacetal resins also use formaldehyde. Phenolic resins are used principally as adhesives in water-resistant plywood and as binders in fiberglass insulation. Polyacetal resins, produced from formaldehyde or its trimer, tiroxane, are used as unreinforced thermoplastic resins in a variety of applications where they can replace metals in mechanical working parts (e.g., automobiles, trucks, consumer articles, plumbing, industrial machinery, and appliances (4, 5).

Formaldehyde is used for the production of chemical intermediates. An example of this is in the manufacture of acetylenic chemicals. This synthesis involves the reaction of two molecules of formaldehyde with acetylene to produce 2-butyne-1,4-diol, which is then hydrogenated to 1,4-butanediol (5).

ROUTE OF EXPOSURE

Dermal

The use of formalin solutions in hospitals, pathology laboratories, and funeral homes to fix or preserve tissues can lead to both dermal and inhalation exposure. Low levels of dermal exposure are also possible in the general population from the use of cosmetics and personal health care products containing formaldehyde as a preservative (6). Dermal exposure in the workplace can occur if an individual handles solid paraformaldehyde or liquid formaldehyde products or materials that generate formaldehyde such as trioxane. Permanent press clothing is treated with formaldehyde resin systems, and there have been reports of dermal exposure to formaldehyde from these garments. However, the residual formaldehyde levels in clothing have been reduced significantly over the last few years (7).

Inhalation

Formaldehyde is a gas at room temperature, and exposure by inhalation can occur. Low concentrations of airborne formaldehyde are always found in the ambient air, primarily as a result of burning organic fuels such as wood, coal, gas, oil, gasoline, or diesel (6). In 1978, formaldehyde generated from automobile exhaust in the United States was estimated to be 660,000,000 pounds per year. Concentrations found in the air under certain conditions can be relatively high (up to several hundred ppb) in areas such as unvented parking garages or tunnels with slowly moving traffic (1).

Inhalation exposure to formaldehyde can be found in the workplace wherever formaldehyde or formaldehyde resin systems are used. Polyacetal resins (plastic made from formaldehyde) can release formaldehyde vapors during the heating phase of the molding process. The use of formaldehyde generators such as hexamethylenetetramine and tirioxane can also

Table 98.1. Potential Occupational Exposures to Formaldehyde*

Anatomists
Agricultural workers
Bakers
Biologists
Bookbinders
Botanists
Crease-resistant textile finishers
Deodorant makers
Disinfectant makers
Disinfectors
Dress-goods shop personnel
Dressmakers
Drug makers
Dye makers
Electrical insulation makers
Embalmers
Embalming-fluid makers
Ethylene glycol makers
Fertilizer makers
Fireproofers
Formaldehyde resin makers
Formaldehyde employees
Foundry employees
Fumigators
Fungicide workers
Fur processors
Glass etchers
Glue and adhesive makers
Hexamethylenetetramine workers
Hide preservers
Histology technicians (assumed to include necropsy and autopsy
   technicians)
Ink makers
Lacquerers and lacquer makers
Medical personnel (assumed to include pathologists)
Mirror workers
Oil well workers
Paper makers
Particle board workers
Pentaerythritol makers
Photographic film makers
Plastic workers
Resin makers
Rubber makers
Soil sterilizers and greenhouse workers
Surgeons
Tannery workers
Taxidermists
Textile mordanters and printers
Textile waterproofers
Varnish workers
Wood preservatives

*From National Institute for Occupational Safety and Health (1976)

produce formaldehyde vapors. Resin systems are used as glues in the manufacturing of wood products such as furniture and paneling and could also release measurable formaldehyde vapors. Formaldehyde resin systems are also used in several textile applications such as the manufacture of carpets and permanent press clothing (7).

Urea formaldehyde foam was injected into walls of homes in the past to reduce air leakage and reduce the heating cost. Under certain conditions where installation was faulty, this led to an excess release of formaldehyde vapors into the homes.

Due to the controversy surrounding this application, this material is not used in the United States for retrofitting housing at the present time.

Cigarette smoking is also a source of airborne formaldehyde. The smoking of a cigarette will produce up to 50 micrograms of formaldehyde. The side stream of tobacco smoke is reported to contain up to 40 ppm of formaldehyde (1).

Oral Route

There is also potential exposure by the oral route. Many foods have measurable levels of formaldehyde. Smoked foods and food prepared on a grill can have as high as 1000 ppm formaldehyde. Formaldehyde is also very common in foods such as fruits (apples, tomatoes, etc.). It is also found in dairy products, vegetables, and baked goods (Table 98.3). Agents which release formaldehyde, such as hexamethylenetetramine, are sometimes used as a food preservative as well as a drug. The most common drug use of hexamethylenetetramine is for urinary tract infections. Normal use of this drug can release up to 4000 milligrams of formaldehyde into the body. Oral exposure is also possible from the use of certain personal care products (mouthwashes, toothpaste, etc.) where formaldehyde is used as a preservative (6). Formaldehyde exposure in drinking water is thought to be extremely low, although there have been claims that plastic fittings used in plumbing may release some formaldehyde into the water (1).

ABSORPTION, METABOLISM, AND DISTRIBUTION

Formaldehyde is readily absorbed from the respiratory and oral tract, and to a much lesser degree from the skin (1). Formaldehyde is the simplest aldehyde and reacts readily with macromolecules such as proteins and nucleic acids. Inhalation exposure has been reported to result in almost complete absorption. Dermal absorption due to contact with formaldehyde-containing materials such as textiles, perma-press clothing, cosmetics, or other materials is of low order of magnitude.

Formaldehyde is a normal metabolite of the body involved in methylation reactions through the tetrafolate mechanism; normal blood levels of formaldehyde in humans and animals are approximately 2.5 ppm (2.5 mg/l). Formaldehyde is rapidly metabolized with a half-life in the blood of approximately 1.5 minutes (8). This half-life is based primarily on primate data although available human data are consistent with this observation of a very short half-life. Data from other species suggest that the half-life of formaldehyde is fairly similar in many species. Formaldehyde's normal blood levels and short half-life, as well as the assumption that the levels of water soluble formaldehyde in the blood are in equilibrium with the body fluids pool, lead to a calculation that an adult human body normally produces and metabolizes (detoxify or utilizes) over 50,000 milligrams of endogenous formaldehyde per day. Formaldehyde is either converted to carbon dioxide by the formate pathway and then exhaled or incorporated into the one carbon pool. Radioactivity following exposure to ^{14}C-formaldehyde is found throughout the body and supports the concept of rapid incorporation and metabolism. (Fig. 98.1) shows an overview of the general metabolic production and fate of formaldehyde in the body.) The high endogenous production and use by the body of formaldehyde is of importance in understanding the potential action of formaldehyde in the body and is consistent

Table 98.2. Airborne Formaldehyde Concentrations in Occupational and Nonoccupational Environments*

Environment	Number (years of measurements)	Formaldehyde Concentration (mg/m^3)		Number of Measurements	Source
		Arithmetic Mean	Range		
Textile plants	2 (1977–1979)	0.2	0.1–0.5	16	Finishing and dyeing substances
Shoe factories	1 (1977)	1.9	0.9–2.7	4	Formalin spraying
Particle board plants	3 (1977–1979)	1.15	0.1–4.9	220	Urea and melamine resins
Wooden furniture manufacturing plants	19 (1977–1979)	1.35	0.1–5.4	134	Adhesives, lacquers, paints
Plywood plants	6 (1977–1979)	0.35	0.1–1.2	91	Phenolic and urea resins
Adhesive plants	1 (1977)	1.75	0.8–3.5	17	Urea-formaldehyde resins
Foundries	10 (1972–1975)	2.7		43	Furan resin
	3 (1977–1979)	0.6	0.05–2.0	8	
Welding and machine shops	3 (1977–1980)	0.5	0.05–1.2	9	Plastic tape, paints, corrosion prevention
Construction sites	7 (1974–1975)	2.8	0.5–7.0	10	Lacquer
Hospital clinics	7 (1977–1979)	0.7	0.05–3.5	25	Formaldehyde disinfectant
Office, schools	4 (1977–1980)	0.24	0.05–0.77	12	Insulation foam, adhesive, lacquer
Workshops manufacturing electrical machinery: soldering, lacquering, treatment of plastic	10 (1977–1979)	<0.1 / 0.35	0.2–0.5	47 / 8	Solder, lacquer, melamine formaldehyde plastic

*From Niemela R, Vainio H. Formaldehyde exposure in work and the general environment. Occurrence and possibilities for prevention. Scand J Work Environ Health 1981;7:95–100.

Table 98.3. Level of Formaldehyde in Foods

Food Source	mg/kg	Food Source	mg/kg	Food Source	mg/kg
Dairy		Vegetable		Smoked foods	
Milk	0.3–3.3	Carrots	0.3–10.0	Wurst	1.26
Yogurt	0.3–3.3	Cucumber	2.3	Herring	0.65
Butter	0.1	Cauliflower	6.6	Kerring filets	1.09
Cheese	0.3–1.2	Cabbage	4.7–5.3	Meats[a]	Trace
Eggs	0.2–1.2	Radish	3.7–4.4	Vacuum-packed meats	0.7–2.8
Yolks	5.5	Spinach	3.3–25.0	Smoked bacon	
Provolone cheese	3.14–56.84	Onions	13.3–26.3	Inner layer	0.8–11.5
Fruit		Meat/fish		Outer layer	3.5–52.0
Apples	1.7–22.3	Raw sausage		Smoked ham	
Pears	6.0–38.7	Filling	2.0–30.6	Outer layer	224–267
Grapes	2.9–3.3	Skin	34.0–214	Boiled smoked sausage	0.7–32.2
Tomatoes	5.7–16.7	Raw marine fish	6.5–13.6	Smoked marine fish	3.5–20.0
Breads and cereals		Raw freshwater fish	0.7–0.8	Smoked freshwater fish	1.5–8.8
Crust/crumb		Fresh haddock	20		
Method of baking		Kipper	50,–1,000	Other	
Straight	2.0–9.9	Raw meat			
Sponge	2.0–9.8	Beef	0.7–3.4	Maple syrup	up to 2
No time	1.7–8.6	Veal	0.7–3.4	Beer	0.009
Preferment	1.4–10.2	Pork	0.7–3.4	Soy bean	tr–0.1
		Mutton	0.7–3.4		
		Chicken	2.3–5.7		

[a]Calabrian sausage, smoked pork fat, speck, lard, Hungarian salami, puriser.

with the idea that formaldehyde is not a systemic toxicant. Exogenous exposure is so low when compared with the endogenous production that measured formaldehyde levels in the blood and tissues do not change following either inhalation exposure (15 ppm) or ingestion of foods containing high levels of formaldehyde (9). Conversion of formate to carbon dioxide is a rate limiting step in the direct breakdown of formaldehyde in primates, including humans. The rodent, on the other hand, is much more efficient in the conversion of formate to carbon dioxide and as a result it is very difficult to demonstrate formate buildup in a rodent. Formate accumulation can be observed in humans or primates under certain conditions (i.e., oral ingestion of high levels of methanol which is metabolized to formaldehyde).

Formaldehyde is normally converted and excreted as carbon dioxide in the air, as formic acid in the urine, or as one of many breakdown products from one carbon pool metabolism. Because of rapid absorption by both the oral and inhalation route and the rapid metabolism, little or no formaldehyde is excreted unmetabolized. Rats exposed to ^{14}C-formaldehyde by inhalation had 40% of the radiolabel excreted in the air and 20% in the urine and feces; 40% remained in the carcass.

CLINICAL TOXICOLOGY—ACUTE EXPOSURE

Formaldehyde solutions (greater than 2%) are dermal irritants (10). Concentrated formaldehyde solutions can be corrosive to

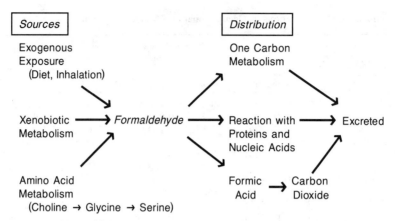

Figure 98.1. Sources and fate of formaldehyde in the body.

Table 98.4.   LD50 Values for Formaldehyde in Various Species

Species	Route	LD_{50}	Reference
Rat	Oral	800	Smyth et al. (1941)
	s.c.	420	Skog (1950)
	i.v.	87	Langecker (1954)
Mouse	s.c.	300	Skog (1950)
Rabbit	Dermal	270	Lewis and Tatkin (1980)
Guinea pig	Oral	260	Smyth et al. (1948)

the eye and cause chemical burns to the skin in animals as well as in humans. The dermal sensitization potential to formaldehyde has been estimated to be as high as 5% in the general population (10). Dermal sensitization in animals has also been adequately demonstrated. Formaldehyde gas causes mucous membrane and ocular irritation as well as upper respiratory tract irritation at concentrations above 1 ppm in the general population (11). This sensory irritation becomes unacceptable at high concentrations, and therefore tends to serve as a warning of excessive exposure. Normal body defense mechanisms, such as tearing of the eyes and mucociliary action in the nasal cavity, are actually part of the body's protective mechanism and serve to prevent tissue exposure at levels below 1 ppm. Some individuals appear to be hypersensitive to airborne formaldehyde and react to vapor exposures much less than 1 ppm. Bronchial spasms and asthmatic-like reactions have been reported in certain individuals exposed to airborne formaldehyde, although asthmatics do not appear to be any more sensitive than the normal population to formaldehyde vapors. A very few isolated cases of respiratory sensitization in humans have been reported, although no respiratory sensitization has been demonstrated in any animal species. Many other responses such as headaches and nausea have been reported in humans and related to formaldehyde vapor exposures. However, in many cases, these complaints cannot be directly related to formaldehyde but to indoor air pollution in general. The acute lethal dose by various routes in animals is presented in Table 98.4.

Inhalation exposure to high concentrations are reported to produce tissue damage in the nasal cavity of various experimental species (12).

CHRONIC AND LONGTERM EXPOSURE STUDIES

Because of the high metabolic production rates and rapid breakdown in the body of endogenous formaldehyde, it is expected that no systemic effects would be observed following formaldehyde exposure either in the workplace or from foods. This expectation in humans is borne out by experimental animal data. No responses have been seen in animal experiments at sites distant from the site of contact. Formaldehyde at high concentrations only causes local tissue effects such as the squamous metaplasia and hyperplasia found in the nasal cavity in rodents and nonhuman primates exposed by inhalation. Tissue damage to the nasal cavity of rodents exposed to high airborne levels of formaldehyde has not been demonstrated in humans. This is not unexpected because the levels necessary to produce damage in rodents are high and very unpleasant and irritating to humans. Humans would tend to remove themselves from these types of environments. Formaldehyde action appears to be more concentration than total dose dependent (concentration × time) (11). Anatomical differences between rodents and humans in the structure of the nasal cavity and the fact that humans tend to breath through their mouths when exposed to irritating material (a rodent is an obligatory nose breather) help explain the difference in the response between species. The response in humans to repeated exposure, particularly by inhalation, has been sensory irritation (discomfort); no tissue damage has been demonstrated histologically. It is thought under repeated exposure that humans can adapt to some degree to formaldehyde's sensory irritating properties and develop a tolerance.

Chronic oral exposure to high levels of formaldehyde (2000 ppm) also resulted in squamous metaplasia and hyperplasia in the forestomach of rodents. This is the primary site of contact, but no cancer occurred. The forestomach is not an organ found in humans. The significance of the forestomach response from the oral exposure is of questionable relevance to humans (13).

CANCER

High levels of inhalation (15 ppm) exposure have resulted in the production of squamous cell carcinomas in the nasal cavity (site of tissue damage) in rats and mice but not the hamster exposed up to 10 ppm (14). No treatment-related tumors have been seen in rodents chronically exposed to formaldehyde orally or dermally. It is postulated that the squamous cell carcinomas in the rat are related to tissue damage caused by high levels of airborne formaldehyde. The mechanism of cancer production in the rat nasal cavity is thought to be related to overcoming normal defense mechanisms (mucociliary protection) and producing local tissue damage (15). This results in

Table 98.5. Incidence of Squamous Cell Carcinomas in Fischer 344 Rats and B6C3F1 Mice Exposed to Formaldehyde Vapor*

| | Dose (ppm) | | | | | | |
| | 0 | | 2.0 | | 5.6 | | 14.3 |
	M	F	M	F	M	F	M	F
Rat	0	0	0	0	1	1	51**	52**
Mouse	0	0	0	0	0	0	2+	0

*Number of tumor-bearing animals; number of nasal cavities examined was between 115 and 120 for males and females of each species.
**Statistically significant in life-table test for positive trend with dose (p<0.0167) and life table comparison of control group versus 14.3 ppm.
+Not statistically significant by life-table analysis nor by the Fisher exact test. From Kerns WD, Donofrio DJ, Pavkov, KL. The chronic effects of formaldehyde in rats and mice: a preliminary report. Chapter 11 in Gibson JE. ed. Formaldehyde Toxicity. New York, NY: Hemisphere Publishing, 1983.

increased cell turnover, more single-stranded DNA (formaldehyde will only react with single-stranded DNA), and less time for the normal DNA repair mechanisms to operate. The repeated tissue damage then serves as a promoting event, which could lead to carcinoma in the nasal cavity of rats. Formaldehyde is weakly genotoxic in vitro, but in vivo tests fail to demonstrate activity. This in vivo response is not unexpected considering the high body burden and turnover of endogenous formaldehyde.

Table 98.5 shows the number of squamous cell carcinomas in rats and mice seen in a 2-year study (approximate lifetime of rats). A pronounced species difference is noted in the study as well as a very steep dose-response curve with a 50-fold increase in tumor response seen with a 2.5-fold increase in dose in rats. No treatment-related tumors were seen at 2 ppm in the rats or 2 and 6 ppm in the mice.

TERATOGENESIS

Potential teratogenicity has been studied in rodents following exposure to formaldehyde. In a study where pregnant mice received formaldehyde by gavage at several doses (the highest dose resulting in death to several of the pregnant mice), no evidence of any treatment-related malformation was observed (16). Another study exposing rats to 10 ppm formaldehyde, 6 hr/day during the organogenesis period (6–15 days) showed no evidence of treatment-related malformations (17). The results are consistent with the lack of systemic toxicity suggested by the high normal production and metabolism of formaldehyde in the body.

There are no reports of teratogenic effects in humans following formaldehyde exposure. In a study of nurses exposed to formaldehyde and ethylene oxide, an increase in spontaneous abortions was observed that was shown to be related to exposure to ethylene oxide but not to formaldehyde.

HUMAN CANCER

There have been over 30 epidemiologic studies done to address the potential carcinogenicity in humans. The largest studies, which covered large industrial cohorts, were conducted by the National Cancer Institute in the United States (18), and by the MRC in the United Kingdom (19). These studies concluded that there is no evidence that formaldehyde caused cancer in humans. Many of the other studies were more limited. Some

suggest that formaldehyde may cause cancer in humans even though concomitant exposure to wood dust is mentioned. Wood dust is a known producer of nasal cancer in humans. Excess brain tumors in another study were later related to diagnostic and social economical factors. A panel of expert epidemiologists was established and chaired by Dr. John Higginson, former head of the International Agency for the Research on Cancer. This panel evaluated all of the studies and reached the following conclusion: a) "There is no convincing evidence of a relationship with formaldehyde exposure for any malignancy in man." b) "If a relationship does exist, the excess risk in absolute terms must be small." These conclusions are further supported by the lack of any consistent pattern of response in the studies which they evaluated (20).

Tumors other than at the site of contact are unlikely when one considers the normal metabolism of formaldehyde in the body. The irritant properties of formaldehyde provide warning of excessive exposure, and this could also play a role in the response seen in humans. Normal defense mechanisms such as mouth breathing and mucociliary clearance and the lack tissue damage and cell proliferation at levels of exposure up to 3 ppm of formaldehyde suggest that formaldehyde is not a carcinogenic hazard.

TOXICOLOGY MANAGEMENT

Clinical Examination

Skin—Formaldehyde will penetrate the skin and produce allergic dermatitis. Formaldehyde at 1–3 ppm or greater induces clinical irritation. There are no indications that formaldehyde causes photoirritation. Contact urticaria has been reported in several cases.

Oral—Ingestion of formaldehyde can cause sloughing of the gastric epithelium with gastric bleeding. Metabolic acidosis from formation of formic and lactic acid can occur.

Inhalation—Sensory irritation (eye, nose, and throat) is seen following inhalation exposure at a level of 1 ppm and higher (11). Higher levels produce severe upper respiratory tract irritation and cough.

Eye—Formaldehyde splashed into the eye can cause burning and corneal injury.

Laboratory Diagnosis

Skin Reaction—A positive patch test indicates an allergic hypersensitivity type IV skin reaction (21). An open skin test using less than 1–2% formalin will demonstrate immunologic contact urticaria by showing a wheal and flare response. Intradermal tests of formaldehyde for type I allergies are useless in humans. If radioimmunoassay for formaldehyde were developed, it would be useful to demonstrate if asthma or respiratory complaints are due to formaldehyde allergy. There is no evidence of a type IV reaction involved in respiratory allergies to formaldehyde. Pulmonary function test may be useful, although only small transient effects have been noted following high levels of exposure to formaldehyde or mixed exposures. Hyperactive airway syndrome has been demonstrated in standard tests using methacholine and histamine challenge; these tests have limited value in evaluating formaldehyde exposure as do bronchial provocation tests (21).

Blood levels of formaldehyde and urinary formic acid have been suggested as tests to biologically measure exposure. Because of the high natural body production of formaldehyde, neither of these indicators is of any value in assessing formaldehyde exposure. They would be useful if very high oral ingestion had taken place.

Basic Treatment

Skin—Treated as any burn to prevent allergic contact dermatitis, exposure to formaldehyde or formaldehyde-containing products should be minimized.

Inhalation—Patients should be removed from exposure. If symptoms persist, hospitalization may be required. Very high levels (100 ppm) may be lethal. Pulmonary damage may occur.

Oral—High concentrations of formaldehyde may be irritating to the gastrointestinal tract. Ingestion can result in metabolic responses similar to methanol poisoning. Hemodialysis is efficacious just as in methanol poisoning and should be considered if metabolic acidosis occurs.

Biologic Monitoring

No useful biologic monitoring has been developed. Blood formaldehyde levels and urinary formate have been suggested as biologic indicators of exposure, but the high normal body burden of formaldehyde (blood 2.5 ppm) and complete, rapid metabolism make these tests useless as a biologic monitor.

Environmental Monitoring

There are several methods for collecting and measuring airborne formaldehyde. Sampling is done with a bubbler, inpringer, solid sorbent, or passive dosimeter. Concentrations are determined by colorimetric, polarographic, high performance liquid chromatographic, gas chromatographic, or direct instruments (electrochemical, colorimetric, infrared, or photionization). Most passive technique is based on an impinger with 1% sodium bisulfite that uses chromotropic acid to develop color. The reported limit of detection of this method is 0.02 ppm, but the technique is sensitive to 0.01 ppm. The American Industrial Hygienists Association Occupational Exposure and Work Practice Guidelines for Formaldehyde published in 1989 detail analytical methods including limitations (22).

Exposure Limits—See Table 98.6.

LOW LEVEL OCCUPATIONAL AND ENVIRONMENTAL EXPOSURES

Health effects from formaldehyde exposure have been a controversial area for years (23). Acute local effects secondary to exposure such as mucous membrane irritation, ocular irritation, and dermatitis are well known. Controversial health effects revolve around systemic reactions such as immunologic alterations, cancer, and sensitization (23, 24). Health effects secondary to chronic exposure to low concentrations of formaldehyde vapors have been associated with multiple medical complaints (25–27). Much debate has centered around low level exposure to formaldehyde in the home and occupational environment and subsequent health complaints.

Current Occupational Safety and Health Administration standards set a time-weighted average (TWA) of 1 ppm. However, people have reported symptoms of eye irritation, throat irri-

tation, fatigue, headache, and nausea at environmental air concentrations between 0.1 and 1 ppm (24–27). Formaldehyde vapors between 0.8 and 1.0 ppm have also been associated with respiratory symptoms and ocular irritation (24–27). Other studies have reported increased frequency of mucous membrane irritation among individuals occupationally exposed to air concentrations ranging around 1 ppm (24).

Actual changes in respiratory functions following chronic low level exposure has been difficult to document. Despite an increased frequency in mucous membrane irritation symptoms among workers exposed to 1–3 ppm formaldehyde, there was no decrease in $FEV_{1.0}\%$ or FVC % (24). Other investigations have confirmed the lack of pulmonary impairment in home or work environments at low level concentrations up to 3 ppm where individuals experienced nonspecific symptoms (25). Formaldehyde vapor concentrations in mobile homes and other home environments may have concentrations typically ranging from 0.1–0.5 ppm.

Studies of control exposure to formaldehyde have shown a variety of subjective responses to low air concentrations. However, it is important to realize that rarely is formaldehyde the sole irritant in an environment. Numerous other chemicals can be present at low concentrations which can add to the irritant effect experienced by individuals.

The association of asthma and formaldehyde has been investigated (28–30). Formaldehyde is very water soluble and is mainly absorbed in the upper airway and thus usually does not reach the lower bronchial or alveolar areas in the lungs. Investigations involving individuals with asthma or symptoms of wheezing thought to be exacerbated by formaldehyde have demonstrated that vapor concentrations up to 3 ppm did not cause bronchospasm (28–30).

Formaldehyde Controlled Chamber Studies

Human sensory response to formaldehyde is seen under many different conditions. These conditions can be divided into three general types: controlled chamber studies, workplace studies, and environmental complaint-type studies. All have advantages as well as disadvantages. The controlled chamber studies where exposure levels are carefully controlled are the best to establish dose response correlation with sensory irritation. No confounding factors such as other chemicals or dust being present or changes in exposure levels during the observation period are found in controlled studies. In most controlled studies unacclimatized individuals are used. This may be a drawback, but these subjects are usually more sensitive than acclimatized individuals. Some individuals can develop a tolerance to the sensory irritation potential of formaldehyde.

Controlled studies of formaldehyde in test subjects' responses to formaldehyde levels ranging up to 4.0 ppm for periods up to 37 minutes have been conducted. Blink rate was found to increase statistically above 1.7 ppm, and the average irritation threshold was between 1 and 2 ppm. The response was greater if the exposure was intermittent rather than continuous demonstrating some tolerance (31).

In another controlled study, a small decrease in mucous flow rate was reported by some subjects exposed at 0.25, 0.42, or 1.6 ppm, but not at 0.83 ppm. The lack of dose response makes this observation of questionable significance. Fifteen of 16 subjects reported slight discomfort in the form of eye irritation at 0.83 ppm formaldehyde. A few individuals reported eye discomfort at lower levels (32).

Table 98.6. Occupational Exposure Limits*
It is to be noted that all of these OELs are subject to revision.

OEL/C	0.3 ppm	Denmark
OEL/ST	0.5 mg/m³	German Democratic Republic
OEL/TWA	0.5 mg/m³	Union of Soviet Socialist Republics
	1 mg/m³	Hungary, Yugoslavia
OEL/C	1 ppm	Finland, Norway, Sweden
OEL/TWA	1 ppm	American Conference of Governmental Industrial Hygienists (ACGIH TLV), Australia, Austria, Federal Republic of Germany, Italy, The Netherlands, Switzerland
OEL/TWA	1 ppm	Occupational Safety and Health Administration (OSHA)
	1.6 ppm	Brazil, Chile
OEL/ST	1 mg/m³	Bulgaria
OEL/C	2 ppm	Australia, Belgium, India, Japan, Venezuela
OEL/ST	2 ppm	ACHIH (TLV), Argentina, France, The Netherlands, United Kingdom
OEL/ST	2 ppm	OSHA
	2 mg/m³	Hungary
OEL/TWA	2 mg/m³	Czechoslovakia, Poland
OEL/TWA	2 ppm	Argentina, Mexico, United Kingdom
OEL/TWA	3 mg/m³	People's Republic of China
OEL/C	4 mg/m³	Rumania
OEL/C	5 mg/m³	Czechoslovakia
OEL/C	5 ppm	Indonesia
OEL/TWA	5 ppm	Egypt, Republic of China

*OEL, occupational exposure limit; C, ceiling; ST, Shortterm exposure limit; TWA, time-weighted average.

Bender (1983) selected a population that was sensitive to formaldehyde eye irritation. About half of his volunteers were rejected because either they reported eye irritation from clean air (air movement) or were unresponsive in the test system. Volunteers were exposed to controlled formaldehyde levels ranging from 0.35–1.0 ppm for 6-minute periods. At formaldehyde levels below 1.0 ppm the reported eye irritation was not significantly different from clean air. At 1.0 ppm 20 of 27 reported slight to moderate eye irritation (33).

Nineteen nonsmoking subjects were exposed to 0.5, 1.0, 2.0, or 3.0 ppm formaldehyde for 3-hour periods (34). Nasal flow resistance was observed at 3.0 ppm, but not lower. At 0.5 ppm none of the subjects reported eye irritation, while four of 19 reported eye irritation at 1.0 ppm. Odor was detected by four of nine at 0.5 ppm. Odor was correlated with eye irritation response at higher doses. No significant decrement in pulmonary function or increase in bronchial reactivity to methacholine was noted at any test dose. The average subjective response to irritation at 1.0 and 2.0 ppm was described as ''mild, present but not annoying.'' At 3.0 ppm eye irritation was classified as moderate (annoying) (34).

These control chamber studies demonstrate that eye irritation is the first sign of sensory irritation seen in unacclimatized subjects as the formaldehyde concentration is increased. The threshold for slight eye irritation is around 1.0 ppm. This eye response serves as a warning of exposure and helps prevent the upper respiratory tract irritation that is seen at higher concentration. No effect on pulmonary function was seen in any of these studies where exposure was just to formaldehyde (up to 3.0 ppm) and not to other confounding factors such as dust.

In summary, environmental exposure to low concentrations of formaldehyde has been associated with health complaints. Objective decrements in pulmonary function do not appear to occur with exposures less than 1 ppm. Bronchospasm and urticaria can occur following exposure but are uncommon events.

REFERENCES

1. NCR (National Research Council). Formaldehyde and other aldehydes. Washington, DC: National Academy Press, 1981.
2. NIOSH (National Institute for Occupational Safety and Health). Criteria for a recommended standard . . . occupational exposure to formaldehyde (DHEW NIOSH Publ. No. 77-126). Washington, DC, GPO, 1976.
3. Niemela R, Vainio H. Formaldehyde exposure in work and the general environment. Occurrence and possibilities for prevention. Scand J Work Environ Health 1981;7:95–100.
4. Gerberich HR, et al. Formaldehyde. In: Kirk RE, Othmer DF eds. Encyclopedia of chemical technology. 3rd ed. New York, NY: John Wiley & Sons, 1985;11:231–250.
5. IARC (International Agency for Research on Cancer), 29:345–389. 1982 Monographs on the evaluation of the carcinogenic risk of chemicals to humans.
6. Hart RW, Terturro A, Neimeth L. Consensus workshop in formaldehyde. Environ Health Perspect, 1984;58:323–381.
7. Code of Federal Regulations 29, Part 1910–1926. Washington DC: GPO, 1987.
8. Celanese Corporation. Pharmacokinetics and metabolism of formaldehyde, 1987.
9. Heck H, Casanova-Schmitz M, Dodd PB, et al. Formaldehyde concentrations in the blood of humans and Fischer-344 rats exposed to formaldehyde under controlled conditions. Am Ind Hyg Assoc J 1985;46:1–3.
10. Maibach H. Formaldehyde: effects on animal and human skin. In: Gibson JE, ed. Formaldehyde toxicology. New York: Hemisphere Publishing Co., 1983:166–174.
11. Clary JJ. Risk assessment for exposure to formaldehyde. In: Gibson JE, ed. Formaldehyde toxicity. New York, NY: Hemisphere Publishing Co., 1983.
12. Rusch GM, Clary JJ, Rhinehart WE, Bolte HF. A 26-week inhalation toxicity study with formaldehyde in the monkey, rat, and hamster. Toxicol Appl Pharmacol 1983;68:329–343.
13. Til HP, Woutersen RA, Feron VJ, Hollanders VHM, Falke HE. Two-year drinking water study of formaldehyde in rats. Food Chem Toxicol 1989;27:77–87.
14. Starr T, et al. Estimating human cancer risk from formaldehyde: critical issues. In: Formaldehyde: analytical chemistry and toxicology. Washington, DC: American Chemical Society, 1983;210:299–334.
15. Feron VJ, Woutersen RA. Role of tissue damage in nasal carcinogenesis. In: Feron VJ, Basland MC, eds. Nasal carcinogenesis in rodents: relevance to human health risk. Proceedings of the TNO-CIVO/NYU Symposium, Veldhoven, Netherlands, October 24–28, 1988. 1989, 76.
16. Marks TA, Worthy WC, Staples RE, et al. Influence of formaldehyde and sonacide (potentiated acid glutaraldehyde) on embryo and fetal development in mice. Teratology 1980;22:51–58.

17. Robinson, et al. A teratological study of inhaled formaldehyde in the rat. Bio-Research Laboratories Ltd., Project No. 81581. (Sponsored by the Formaldehyde Council of Canada), 1985.

18. Blair A, Stewart P, O'Berg M, et al. Mortality among industrial workers exposed to formaldehyde. J Natl Cancer Inst 1986;76:1071–1084.

19. Acheson ED, Gardner MJ, Pannett B, et al. Formaldehyde in the British chemical industry—an occupational cohort study. Lancet 1984;1:611–616.

20. Universities Associated for Research & Education in Pathology. Epidemiology of chronic occupational exposure to formaldehyde: report of the ad hoc panel on health aspects of formaldehyde. Toxicol Ind Health 1988;4:77–90.

21. Imbus HR. Clinical evaluation of patients with complaints related to formaldehyde exposure. J Allergy Clin Immunol 1985;76:831–840.

22. AIHA (American Industrial Hygienists Association). Occupational exposure and work practice guidelines for formaldehyde, 1989.

23. Bardana EJ, Montanaro A. The formaldehyde fiasco: a review of the scientific data. Immunol Allergy Prac 1987;9:11–24.

24. Main DM, Hogan TJ. Health effects of low-level exposure to formaldehyde. J Occup Med 1983;25:896–900.

25. Bracken MJ, Leasa DJ, Morgan WKC. Exposure to formaldehyde: relationship to respiratory symptoms and function. Can J Public Health 1985;76:312–316.

26. Kilburn KH, Warshaw R, Boylen CT, et al. Pulmonary and neurobehavioral effects of formaldehyde exposure. Arch Environ Health 1985;40:254–260.

27. Imbus HR. Clinical evaluation of patients with complaints related to formaldehyde exposure. J Allergy Clin Immunol 1985;76:831–840.

28. Alexanderson R, Kolmodin-Hedman B, Hedenstierna G. Exposure to formaldehyde: effects on pulmonary function. Arch Environ Health 1982;37:279–284.

29. Frigas E, Filley WV, Reed CE. Bronchial challenge with formaldehyde gas: lack of bronchoconstriction in 13 patients suspected of having formaldehyde-induced asthma. Mayo Clin Proc 1984;59:295–299.

30. Hendrick DJ, Rando RJ, Lane DJ, Morril MJ. Formaldehyde asthma: challenge exposure levels and fate after five years. J Occup Med 1982;24:893–897.

31. Weber-Tschopp A, Fischer T, Grand JE. Reizuirkungen des formaldehyde (HCHO) auf den Menschen. Arch Occup Environ Health 1977;39:207–218.

32. Anderson I. Formaldehyde in the indoor environment—health implications of setting standards. In: Fanger PO, Valbjorn O, eds. Proc First International Indoor Climate, 1979:66–87.

33. Bender JR, Mullin LS, Graepel GJ, Wilson WE. Eye irritation response of humans to formaldehyde. Am Ind Hyg Assoc J 1983;44:463–465.

34. Kulle TJ, Sauder LR, Hebel JR, Green DJ, Chatham MD. Formaldehyde dose-responses in healthy nonsmokers. J Air Pollut Contr Assoc 1987;39:919–924.

Jacob L. Pinnas, M.D.
Geraldine C. Meinke, Ph.D.

THE ALDEHYDES

Concern about the health hazards due to exposure to potentially carcinogenic or immunotoxic substances in the environment has increased significantly in recent years. Indeed, one of the most controversial issues in medicine today is the problem of chemical sensitivities (1–5). The number of people at risk of exposure to irritating and sensitizing chemicals appears to be growing, and no geographic area is unaffected.

Aldehydes are highly reactive chemical compounds which are not only synthesized for industrial use but also occur naturally within our bodies and within our environment (6, 7). Aldehydes are recognized irritants, particularly the low molecular weight and halogen-substituted aldehydes. Inhaling aldehyde vapors can lead to chemical bronchitis, pneumonitis, and pulmonary edema. In general, the toxicity of aldehydes decreases with increasing molecular weight, while the presence of a double bond in aliphatic aldehydes considerably enhances their toxicity. Higher molecular weight, complex aldehydes are used in fragrances and may occasionally sensitize. Dialdehydes are uncommon in industry, but one might expect them to be more reactive based upon their chemistry. Aromatic or substituted aromatic groups which replace hydrogen on the aliphatic chain of aldehydes usually do not add to their toxicity (8, 9).

Aldehydes are characterized by the presence of the formyl (CHO) functional group. They are considered to be one of the major classes of industrial chemicals. While the construction industry is the principal consumer, aldehydes are also important to agriculture, garment, pharmaceutical, and rubber industries. Higher molecular weight aldehydes are used as flavors and fragrances in essential oils and perfumes (8).

Aldehydes which have been shown to present problems to humans because of their irritating, toxic, or immunologic effects include acetaldehyde, acrolein, cinnamaldehyde, formaldehyde, and glutaraldehyde. Other aldehydes that may pose some minor problems include: butyraldehyde, chloracetaldehyde, crotonaldehyde, and furfural. Acrolein, crotonaldehyde, and formaldehyde appear to be more toxic than acetaldehyde (8–10).

ACETALDEHYDE

Synonyms: Acetic Aldehyde, Ethanal, Ethyl Aldehyde

Acetaldehyde (CH_3CHO) is widely distributed in the human environment. It is classified as a mild eye and mucous membrane irritant and at high concentrations causes narcosis in animals (8, 9, 11). It occurs in the atmosphere partly as the consequence of wood combustion and incomplete combustion cof fuels and is a major component in the gas phase of tobacco smoke (12–16). It is used to manufacture acetic acid and many other chemicals (17) as well as in the manufacture of products such as plastics, synthetic phenolic and urea resins, disinfectants, drugs, dyes, explosives, flavorings, perfumes, photographic chemicals, rubber accelerators, antioxidants, varnishes, vinegar, and yeast (18). It is an important compound in the agricultural and food industry. Acetaldehyde is a product of most hydrocarbon oxidations; it is a normal intermediate product in the respiration of higher plants; it occurs in traces in all ripe fruits and may form in wine and other alcoholic beverages after exposure to air (6).

Besides industrial and agricultural uses, acetaldehyde is also formed in the body during the metabolism of many endogenous and foreign compounds. Acetaldehyde is formed within the body during normal metabolism and, to a large extent, as an oxidative metabolite of ethanol by the enzyme alcohol dehydrogenase (19). It is a highly reactive, freely diffusible molecule which can be found in the peripheral blood of patients abusing alcohol (20, 21) in much higher concentrations than control populations. Low to moderate air concentrations of acetaldehyde (50–200 ppm) cause eye irritation and upper respiratory discomfort. High blood concentrations of the chemical can cause dyspnea and central nervous system depression. Acetaldehyde is toxic to the cilia of the respiratory epithelium and may represent a major cause of damage by cigarette smoke. Its irritant potential in the workplace is usually not a great problem since it is only about one-tenth as strong of an irritant as formaldehyde (8, 9, 22–24). Exposure to large amounts, however, may affect the eyes, liver, skin, and lung (21). If liquid acetaldehyde contacts skin for a prolonged period, it results in erythema and may cause burns; repeated contact may result in dermatitis due to either primary irritation or sensitization.

New employees who may be exposed to acetaldehyde should be examined prior to and periodically after beginning work with careful attention to the eyes, skin, and respiratory system. Protective garments should be worn to prevent skin and eye contact. For accidental exposures, eye wash and shower equipment should be provided in work areas. Chest radiographs and screening pulmonary function studies can provide useful baseline information. In transporting or storing acetaldehyde, precautions must be taken to prevent leaks and to ensure safe conditions, because this aldehyde boils at room temperature. When mixed with air, it is highly flammable and reacts to form acetic acid, highly explosive peroxides, and other products. The occupational exposure limits for acetaldehyde in different countries vary between 25 and 200 ppm, which is roughly equivalent to concentrations of 40–400 µg/l of air. Acetaldehyde content of cigarette smoke from a single cigarette is up to 1 milligram, of which 20 µg/minute has been estimated to reach the blood circulation within the lung (25). Contribution to daily acetaldehyde production and release into the environment occurs from automobile emissions, which can exceed 100 milligrams of acetaldehyde per mile (26).

In vitro cellular studies demonstrated that acetaldehyde produces cross-linking of DNA, induction of sister chromatid exchanges especially late in the G1 phase of the cell cycle following repeated or continuous exposure (27–32). While acetaldehyde has been shown to be toxic to cilia and chromosomes in plant and lower animal systems, mutagenicity and carcinogenicity testing in higher animals has been negative to date. In addition to the capacity of acetaldehyde to cross-link DNA by chemically reacting with nucleic acid bases, it may cross-link proteins by reacting primarily with lysine groups to form Schiff bases. Recent evidence suggests that the combination of acetaldehyde with albumin is an example of hapten-carrier complex which can serve as an antigen inducing antibodies to the hapten even when a nonimmunogenic self-protein such as rabbit serum albumin is used when immunizing rabbits (33). The titer and incidence of these antibodies appear to be increased in chronic alcoholics (34–36). Whether environmental or industrial exposure to acetaldehyde can similarly induce antibodies against acetaldehyde has not yet been studied.

ACROLEIN

Synonyms: Acrylaldehyde, Propenal, Allyl Aldehyde, Ethylene Aldehyde, Aqualin

Acrolein (CH_2=CHCHO) is a three-carbon, unsaturated, highly reactive, highly volatile aldehyde that is a major component of wood, cotton, polyethylene, and cigarette smoke (37–41) as well as diesel fuel exhausts and photochemical smog (42–44). It occurs as a metabolite of glycerol, alkyl formate, and alkyl alcohol (45), and it is used in the manufacture of pharmaceuticals, perfumes, food supplements, and resins. It is also used as a biocide and fungicide. This unsaturated aldehyde is a severe pulmonary irritant and lacrimating agent with a piercing, disagreeable, acrid odor. It is ciliastatic and capable of causing direct tissue damage similar to that reported for formaldehyde (47–49). Due to its high aqueous solubility and high chemical bioreactivity, acrolein has a relatively short half-life and exerts its greatest effects on the upper and lower respiratory tract (50, 51). It is felt by some to be a significant contributor to smoke-induced inhalation, injury, and death.

The toxic effects of acrolein exposure include sensory irritation, enzymatic inhibition, elevated liver alkaline phosphatase, protein synthesis inhibition, weight loss, and death (52). Acrolein is a suspected carcinogen because of its 2,3-epoxy metabolite and its weak mutagenic activity in the Salmonella screen (47, 53). Acrolein is also a weak sensitizer and may elicit asthmatic-type reactions. There are some indications that acrolein may possess immunotoxic potential. At air concentrations of 20 ppm, acrolein can rapidly induce pulmonary edema. Exposure to 150 ppm for 10 minutes can be lethal in humans (54, 55). In other organ systems, acrolein is believed to cause tissue damage by the mechanism of release of toxic O_2 radicals via activation of arachidonic acid cascade, by binding to sulfhydryl groups, and by protein damage (57–59). Acrolein induces lacrimation (60). Lacrimators in general are known to be powerful skin irritants and acrolein exposure causes painful dermatitis and chemical burn injury on longer exposure (61).

CINNAMIC ALDEHYDE

Cinnamaldehyde, Cinnamal, β-phenylacrolein, 3-Phenylpropenal, and V-phenylacrolein

Cinnamic aldehyde (C_6H_5CH=CHCHO), a constituent of cinnamon, is an aromatic aldehyde with a burning taste responsible for the typical odor and flavor of the spice. It is a skin irritant and has been reported to be a strong skin irritant and sensitizer and a urticariogenic agent in most atopic and nonatopic individuals. Delayed contact dermatitis caused by this substance has been described by many investigators (62–67).

Cinnamaldehyde is a common ingredient in household products such as deodorizers, detergents, soaps, and cosmetics. It is frequently used as a flavoring agent in mouthwashes, dentifrices, cough mixtures, throat lozenges, candy, soft drinks, chewing gum, ice cream, baked goods, condiments, and meats. Cinnamaldehyde and related chemicals present in cinnamon are also used extensively in perfumes, hair tonics, and lotions (67).

As a perfume ingredient, cinnamaldehyde is considered a frequent allergen (68–73). This aromatic aldehyde has been implicated in occupational dermatitis in bakers, confectioners, and chemists (74). Cinnamaldehyde in dentifrices may produce irritant, stinging sensations and allergic cheilitis and stomatitis (75–80). Cinnamic alcohol and aldehyde in perfume facial tissue and sanitary napkins can produce allergic dermatitis. Because of its presence in such an extensive number of products it is one of the more common causes of contact urticaria both nonimmunologic and immunologic and may even produce a delayed systemic, eczematous contact dermatitis (84, 85). Once sensitization to cinnamon occurs, cross-reactions may occur with balsam of Peru, balsam of Tolu, cassia oil, and patchouli oil, benzoin (86, 87). The cinnamon oil used commercially is usually obtained from *C. cassia*. As much as 68% of the oil consists of cinnamic aldehyde. Powdered cinnamon contains only about 1% of the aldehyde and is not an irritant under ordinary circumstances.

Cinnamaldehyde has been shown to possess antifungal activity (88–90). Cinnamaldehyde, benzaldehyde, and various aliphatic aldehydes all inhibit protein synthesis in a variety of *in vitro* systems (91–96).

GLUTARALDEHYDE

Synonyms: Glutaric Dialdehyde, 1,5-Pentanedial

Glutaraldehyde [HCO$(CH2)_3$CHO] is an aliphatic dialdehyde with a molecular weight three times that of formaldehyde. It is a moderately irritating dialdehyde which readily polymerizes and is available most frequently as a 50% aqueous solution. In the United States, glutaraldehyde is the second most commonly used aldehyde next to formaldehyde, and it has been estimated that approximately 35,000 employees are occupationally exposed (97). In a buffered alkaline solution (pH 7.5–8.5) it is a highly effective microbiocidal agent (98–106) (sporicidal, bactericidal, viricidal, fungicidal). Alkaline glutaraldehyde is widely used in cold sterilization of medical, surgical, and dental equipment and instruments and for home sterilization of artificial kidney machines (103, 104, 107–109). Alkaline glutaraldehyde is also used a biocide in contaminated water, cooling towers, and air conditioners (110). Besides its use as a biocide, glutaraldehyde is also used as a therapeutic agent for warts (111, 112), bullous disease (113, 114), and hyperhidrosis (115–120), onychomycosis (121–122), as a tanning agent for leather (123, 124), as a fixative in histochemistry and electron microscopy (125), as a cross-linking agent in the preparation of microcapsules (126) and implantable collagen, and in preparation of some antigens as reagents (127, 128). Glutaraldehyde increases the water resistance of wallpaper and hardens photographic gelatin (129); it is used as an intermediate in the manufacture of resins and dyes and as a preservative in cosmetics and household cleaning products (130, 131).

Although glutaraldehyde is a weak allergen, the vapors from glutaraldehyde may act as an irritant to bronchial and laryngeal mucous membranes, and prolonged exposure could produce localized edema and other symptoms suggestive of an allergic response. Occupational exposure to health care workers is common. Recent reports have implicated glutaraldehyde exposure as a cause of occupational asthma (132), and recently it has been reported to cause asthma in endoscopy personnel exposed to glutaraldehyde cleaning solutions (133–135).

Glutaraldehyde is a known sensitizer (136), and case reports of occupational contact dermatitis from glutaraldehyde have been described (115, 137–140). Sensitization has occurred mainly through its use as a cold sterilizing solution in hospitals and dental clinics where medical and allied professionals including x-ray film handlers may be exposed to activated glutaraldehyde in concentrations of 0.13–2%.

Activated glutardehyde buffered to a pH of 7.5–8.5 is reported to be a stronger irritant than inactivated glutaraldehyde solutions which have weak acidity (141, 142). The National Institute of Occupational Safety and Health (NIOSH) recommended a ceiling limit for glutaraldehyde of 0.2 ppm, and OSHA has recently adopted this as a permissible exposure level (143). Studies in hospital environments with cold sterilization using glutaraldehyde solutions by NIOSH demonstrated airborne concentrations of glutaraldehyde of 0.4 ppm. A 2% glutaraldehyde sterilizing solution can produce airborne concentrations that exceed the newly set OSHA limit of 0.2 ppm if proper hood ventilation is not provided when the solution is left uncovered. Containment of vapors and prevention of skin contact are important industrial hygiene principles to help avoid sensitization of the skin and respiratory irritation and/or asthma. Proper skin protection must be provided as well as ventilation controls. Neoprene or butyl rubber gloves are protective. Latex rubber gloves are not as protective. Concomitant sensitization to other occupational contactants, such as rubber components and formaldehyde, appears to be common, and there appears to be a tendency for hand eczema associated with glutaraldehyde to persist even when known sources of exposure to glutaraldehyde are avoided (138–140).

OTHER ALDEHYDES

Chloroacetaldehyde (C_2H_3ClO) is a liquid with an irritating odor used as a fungicide and a tree bark remover. It is an irritant of the eyes, mucous membranes, and respiratory tract (144). It has a ceiling TLV of 1 ppm (3 mg/m^3). Due to its strong irritancy properties, the liquid can cause eye and skin burns following splash exposure. Exposure to the vapors can produce irritation of eyes, skin, and airway. High concentrations of the vapor can cause pulmonary edema (144). It has an immediately dangerous to life and health (IDLH) level of 250 ppm (144).

Crotonaldehyde ($CH_3CH{=}CHCHO$) is a liquid with a strong, irritating odor and is also very flammable (144). It has a TLV of 2 ppm (6 mg/m^3). Due to the potent irritant properties of crotonaldehyde, eye and skin contact with the liquid can result in severe burns. Its vapors are highly irritating to the eyes, mucous membranes, and respiratory system. Clinical cases of sensitization have occurred (11). Crotonaldehyde vapors may produce pulmonary edema at high concentrations. Vapors can

also cause lacrimation, skin irritation, and respiratory irritation (11).

Furfural ($C_5H_4O_2$) is a colorless, oily liquid used in refining of lubricating oils, gas oils, diesel fuels, vegetable oils, resins, and other organic materials (11, 145). It is an aromatic heterocyclic aldehyde used in the production of insecticides, fungicides, and germicides (145), and as a reagent in analytic chemistry. It is produced from a variety of agricultural byproducts, including corncobs, oat hulls, rice hulls, bagasse, cottonseed hulls, and papermill waste. It is a skin, eye, and mucous membrane irritant. Although the vapor is a potent irritant, the liquid has a relatively low volatility so that inhalation by workers of significant quantities is unlikely. Exposure of workers to air concentrations of from 2–14 ppm caused complaints of eye and throat irritation and headache (144). The liquid is irritating to the skin and contact can cause dermatitis. The TLV is 2 ppm (8 mg/m^3) and the IDLH level is 250 ppm.

Benzaldehyde (C_6H_5CHO) is the simplest aromatic aldehyde. It is a colorless or yellowish liquid found in oil of bitter almond, preservatives, and biologics and has been reported to cause contact urticaria. Benzaldehyde is found in dyes, pharmaceuticals, perfumes, and flavoring agents.

Among the higher aliphatic aldehydes, propionaldehyde is used primarily as a chemical intermediate in the production of 1-propanal, propionic acid, and trimethylolethane. Butyraldehydes are used a chemical intermediates in the production of 1-butanol, 2-butanol, 2-ethyl-1-hexanol, and a wide variety of specialty chemicals.

In summary, aldehydes are potentially irritating toxic reactive compounds which under certain circumstances can sensitize animals and humans. Although formaldehyde has been most studied, other aldehydes, particularly the dialdehyde, glutaraldehyde, are emerging as problems, especially in factory and health care workers.

REFERENCES

1. Bardana Jr EJ, Montanaro A. Chemically sensitive patients: avoiding the pitfalls. J Respir Dis 1989;10:32–45.
2. Lewtas J. Toxicology of complex mixtures of indoor air pollutants. Annu Rev Pharmacol Toxicol 1989;29:415–439.
3. National Research Council. Complex mixtures. Washington, DC: National Academy Press.
4. Selner JC. Workup of the chemically sensitive patient. Masters in Allergy 1989;1:8–16.
5. Cullen MR, ed. Workers with multiple chemical sensitivities. Occupational medicine: state of art reviews 2, 1987.
6. Schauenstein E, Esterbauer E, Zollner H. Aldehydes in biological systems. Their natural occurrence and biological activities. London: Pion Ltd., 1977:205.
7. S.R.I. International. Class study report. Aldehydes. Menlo Park, CA: SRI International, for National Cancer Institute, Chemical Selection Working Group, 1978.
8. Steinhagen WH, Barrow CS. Sensory-irritation structure—activity study of inhaled aldehydes in B6C3F1 and Swiss-Webster mice. Toxicol Appl Pharmacol 1984;72:495–503.
9. Raffle PAB, Lee WR, McCallum RJ, Murray R. Hunter's diseases of occupations. Aromatic and aliphatic compounds: aldehydes, ketones, ethers, acetals. Boston: Little Brown, 1987:321–326.
10. Brabec MJ. Aldehydes and acetals. In: Clayton GD, Clayton FE, eds. Patty's industrial hygiene and toxicology. Vol. 2A. Toxicology. New York: Wiley, 1981:2621–2669.
11. Proctor NH, Hughes J, Fischman M. Chemical hazards of the workplace. Philadelphia: J.B. Lippincott, 1988.
12. Salem H, Cullumbine H. Inhalation toxicities of some aldehydes. Toxicol Appl Pharmacol 1960;2:183–187.
13. Stedman RL. The chemical composition of tobacco and tobacco smoke. Chem Rev 1968;68:153–207.
14. Harke H-P, Boors A, Frahm B, Peters H, Schultz C. The problem of

passive smoking. Concentration of smoke constituents in the air of large and small rooms as a function of number of cigarettes smoked and time. Int Arch Arbeitsmed 1972;29:323–339.

15. Jermini C, Weber A, Grandjean E. Quantitative determination of various gas-phase components of the side-stream smoke of cigarettes in the room air as a contribution to the problem of passive smoking. Int Arch Occup Environ Health 1976;36:169–181.

16. Groedel TE. Chemical compounds in the atmosphere. New York: Academic Press, 1979:440.

17. Hester AS, Hemmler K. Chemicals from acetaldehyde. Ind Engl Chem 1959;51:1424–1430, 1T11.

18. Sitting M. Handbook of toxic and hazardous chemicals and carcinogens. 2nd ed. Park Ridge, NJ: Noyes Publications, 1981:21.

19. Lindrios KO. Acetaldehyde—its metabolism and role in the actions of alcohol. In: Israel Y, Glaser FB, Kalart H, Popram RE, Schmidt W, Smart RG, eds. Research advances in alcohol and drug problems, 1978:1111–1176.

20. Lynch C, Lim CK, Thomas M, Peters TJ. Assay of blood and tissue aldehydes by HPLC analysis of their 2,4-dinitrophenyl-hydiazine adducts. Clin Chim Acta 1983;130:117–122.

21. Kozsten MA, Matsuzaki S, Feinman L, Leiber CS. High blood acetaldehyde levels after ethanol administration. N Engl J Med 1975;292:386–389.

22. Auerback C, Moutschen-Dahmen M, Moutschen J. Genetic and cytogenetical effects of formaldehyde and related compounds. Mutat Res 1977;39:317–362.

23. Fishbein L, Flamm WG, Falk HL. Chemical mutagenes. New York: Academic Press, 1970:211–212.

24. International Agency for Research on Cancer. IARC Monographs on the evaluation of the carcinogenic risk of chemicals to humans: allyl compounds, aldehydes, epoxides & peroxides. 36:101–132, Lyon: International Agency for Research on Cancer, 1985.

25. Guerin MR. Chemical composition of cigarette smoke. In: Gori GB, Bock FG, eds. A safe cigarette? Banbury Reports. Vol 3. Coldspring Harbor, NY: Coldspring Harbor Laboratory, 1980.

26. Lipari F, Swarin SJ. Determination of formaldehyde and other aldehydes in automobile exhaust with an improved 2,4-dinitrophenylhydrazine method. J Chromatogr 1982;247:297–306.

27. Lambert B, He SM. DNA and chromosome damage induced by acetaldehyde in vitro. Ann NY Acad Sci 534: Living in a chemical world. New York, NY: New York Academy of Sciences, 1988.

28. He SM, Lambert B. Induction and persistence of SCE-inducing damage in human lymphocytes exposed to vinyl acetate and acetaldehyde in vitro. Mutat Res 1985;158:201–208.

29. Hemminki K, Suni R. Sites of reaction of glutaraldehyde and acetaldehyde with nucleosides. Arch Toxicol 1984;35:186–190.

30. Norppa H, Tursi F, Pfäffli P, Mäki-Paakanen J, Järventaus H. Chromosome damage induced by vinyl acetate through in vitro formation of acetaldehyde in human lymphocytes and Chinese hamster ovary cells. Cancer Res 1985;45:4816–4821.

31. Obe G, Ristow H. Mutagenic cancerogenic and teratogenic effects of alcohol. Mutat Res 1979;65:229–259.

32. Obe G, Natarajan AT, Meyers M, Den Hertog A. Induction of chromosomal aberrations in peripheral lymphocytes of human blood in vitro and of SCEs in bone-marrow cells of mice in vitro by ethanol and its metabolite acetaldehyde. Mutat Res 1979;68:291–294.

33. Fleisher JH, Lung CC, Meinke GC, Pinnas JL. Acetaldehyde-albumin adduct formation: possible relevance to an immunologic mechanism in alcoholism. Alcohol Alcohol 1988;23:133–141.

34. Lin RC, Lumeng L, Shshidi S, Kelly T, Proud D. Protein-acetaldehyde adducts in serum of alcoholic patients. Alcoholism: Clin Exp Res 1990;14:438–443.

35. Niemela O, Klajner F, Orrego H, Vidins E, Blendis L, Israel Y. Antibodies against acetaldehyde modified protein epitopes in human alcoholics. Hepatology 1987;7:1210–1214.

36. Hoerner M, Behrens UJ, Warner T, Lieber CS. Humoral immune response to acetaldehyde adducts in alcoholic patients. Res Commun Chem Pathol Pharmacol 1986;54:3–12.

37. Hales CA, Barkin PW, Jung W, Trautman E, Lamborghini D, Herrig N, Burke J. Synthetic smoke with acrolein but not HCl produces pulmonary edema. J Appl Physiol 1988;64:1121–1133.

38. Morikawa T. Acrolein. Formaldehyde and volatile fatty acids from smoldering combustion. J Combust Toxicol 1976;3:135–151.

39. USDHEW. Smoking & health. Report of the Advisory Committee to the Surgeon General of the Public Health Service. (USPHS Publication 1103). Washington, DC: U.S. Dept. of Health, Education & Welfare, 1964.

40. Ayer HE, Yeager DW. Irritants in cigarette smoke plumes. Am J Public Health 1982;72:1283–1285.

41. Newsome JR, Norman V, Keith CH. Vapor phase analysis of tobacco smoke. Tobacco Sci 1965;9:102–110.

42. Pattle RE, Burgess F, Sinclair K, Edington JAG. The toxicity of fumes from a diesel engine under four different running conditions. Br J Ind Med 1957;14:47–52.

43. Altshuler AP, McPherson SP. Spectrophotomeric analysis of aldehydes in the Los Angeles atmosphere. J Air Pollut Control Assoc 1963;13:109–111.

44. Kane LE, Alorie Y. Sensory irritation to formaldehyde and acrolein during single and repeated exposures in mice. Am Ind Hyg Assoc J 1977;38:509–522.

45. Izard C, Liberman C. Acrolein. Mutat Res 1978;47:115–138.

46. Dahlgren SE, Dalen H, Dalhamn T. Ultrastructural observations on chemically induced inflammation in the guinea pig trachea. Virchows Arch Abt B Zellpathol 1972;11:211.

47. Denine EP, Robbins SL, Kensler CJ. The effects of aerolein inhalation on the tracheal mucosa of the chicken. Toxicol Appl Pharmacol 1971;19:416.

48. Kensler CJ, Battista SP. Components of cigarette smoke with ciliary-depressant activity. Their selective removal by filters containing activated charcoal granules. N Engl J Med 1963;269:1161.

49. Beauchamp Jr RO, Morgan KT, Kilgerman AD, Andelkobich DA, Heck HA. A critical review of the literature on acrolein toxicity. CRC Crit Rev Toxicol 1985;14:309–380.

50. Egle Jr, JL. Retention of inhaled formaldehyde, propionaldehyde and acrolein in the dog. Arch Environ Health 1972;25:119–124.

51. Leikauf GD, Leming LM, O'Donnell JR, Doupnik GA. Bronchial responsiveness and inflammation in guinea pigs exposed to acrolein. J Appl Physiol 1989;66:171–178.

52. Astray AL, Jakab GL. The effects of acrolein exposure on pulmonary antibacterial defenses. Toxicol Appl Pharmacol 1983;67:49–54.

53. National Toxicology Program, Fiscal Year 1982. Review of current research related to toxicology, NTP-82-040. Washington, DC: NTP, 1982.

54. Leach CL, Hatorum NS, Ratajczah HV, Gerbart JM. The pathologic and immunologic effects of inhaled acrolein in rats. Toxicol Lett 1987;39:189–198.

55. National Research Council. Vapor-phase organic pollutants, volatile hydrocarbons & oxidation products. Washington, DC: National Academy of Sciences, 1976:191–192.

56. American Conference of Governmental Industrial Hygienists. Acrolein documentation of TLVs for substances in workroom air. 3rd ed. Cincinnati, OH: ACGIH, 1976.

57. Dawson JR, Norbeck K, Anundi I, Maldeus P. The effectiveness of N-acetylcysteine in isolated hepatocytes against the toxicity of pacetamol, acrolein and paraquat. Arch Toxicol 1984;55:11–15.

58. Grundfest CC, Chang J, Newcombe D. Acrolein: a potent modulator of lung macrophage arachidonic acid metabolism. Biochim Biophys Acta 1982;713:149–159.

59. Zitting A, Heinomen T. Decrease of reduced glutathione in isolated rat hepatocytes caused by acrolein, acrylonitrate and the thermal degradation products of styrene copolymers. Toxicology 1980;17:333–341.

60. Grant WM. Toxicology of the eye. 2nd ed. Springfield, IL: Charles C Thomas, 1974:91–92.

61. Hazardous chemicals data book 1986. 2nd ed. Park Ridge, NJ: G. Weiss Noyes Data Corporation, 1986:52.

62. Calnan CD. Cinnamon dermatitis from ointment. Contact Derm 1976;2:167.

63. Aretander, S. Perfume & flavor chemicals (aroma chemicals). Vols I & II. Montclair, NJ: S. Aretander, 1969.

64. Bonnevie P. Some experiences of wartime industrial dermatoses. Acta Derm Venereol 1948;28:231–237.

65. Fisher AA. Contact dermatitis. 2nd ed. Philadelphia: Lea & Febiger, 1973.

66. Fisher AA. Dermatitis due to cinnamon and cinnamic aldehyde. Cutis 1975;16:383.

67. Collins TW, Mitchell JC. Aroma chemicals. Reference sources for perfume and flavor ingredients with special reference to cinnamic aldehyde. Contact Derm 1975;1:43.

68. Rudzki E, Grzywa Z. Two types of contact urticaria and immediate reactions to patch-test allergens. Dermatologica 1978;157:110.

69. Schorr WF. Cinnamic aldehyde allergy. Contact Dermatitis 1975;1:108.

70. Ogier M, Duverneuil G. Dermites allergiques a l'aldéhyde cinnamique. Arch Mal Prof Med Trav Secur Soc 1977;38:835.

71. Hjorth N. Eczematous allergy to balsams, allied perfumes and flavoring agents. Acta Derm Venereol 1961;41;46:1–216.

72. Mathias CGT, Chappler RR, Maicbach HI. Contact urticaria from cinnamic aldehyde. Arch Dermatol 1980;116:74.

73. Calnan CD. Cinnamon dermatitis from an ointment. Contact Dermatitis 1976;2:167.

74. Malten KE. Four bakers showing positive patch tests to a number of fragrance materials which can be used in flavors. Acta Dermatol Vernereol (Stock) 1979;59:117.

75. Magnusson B, Wilkinson DS. Cinnamic aldehyde in toothpastes, 1. Clinical aspects and patch tests. Contact Dermatitis 1975;1:70.

76. Kirton V, Wilkinson DS. Sensitivity to cinnamic aldehyde in a toothpaste, 2. Further studies. Contact Dermatitis 1975;1:77.

77. Drake TE, Maibach HI. Allergic contact dermatitis & stomatitis caused by cinnamic aldehyde flavored toothpaste. Arch Dermatol 1976;112:202.

78. Anderson KE. Contact allergy to toothpaste flavors. Contact Dermatitis 1978;4:195.

79. Miller J. Cheilitis from sensitivity to oil of cinnamon present in bubble gum. JAMA 141;116:131–132.

80. Laubach JL, Malkinson FD, Ringiose, EJ. Cheilitis caused by cinnamon (cassia) oil in toothpaste. JAMA 1953;152:404–405.

81. Guin JD. Contact dermatitis to perfume in paper products. J Am Acad Dermatol 1981;4:733.

82. Keith I, Erich W, Bush IM. Toilet paper dermatitis [Letters to the Editor]. JAMA 1969;209:269.

83. Larsen WG. Sanitary napkin dermatitis due to perfume. Arch Dermatol 1989;115:363.

84. Fisher AA. Systemic eczematous ''contact-type'' dermatitis medicamentosa. Ann Allergy 1966;24:415.

85. Kern AB. Contact dermatitis from cinnamon. Arch Dermatol 1960;81:599.

86. Leifer W. Contact dermatitis due to cinnamon recurrence of dermatitis following oral administration of cinnamon oil. Arch Dermatol 1951;64:53.

87. Nearing H, van Ketel WG. Allergy from spices used in Indonesian cooking. International Symposium on Contact Dermatitis, Gentofte, Denmark: 1974.

88. Bullerman LW, Liew FY, Seier SA. Inhibition of growth and aflatoxin production by cinnamon and clove oils. Cinnamic aldehyde and eugenol. J Food Sci 1977;42:1107-1109.

89. Kurita N, Miyaji M, Kurane R, Takahara Y, Ichimura K. Antifungal activity and molecular orbital energies of aldehyde compounds from oils of higher plants. Agric Biol Chem 1981;45:945-952.

90. Kurita N, Miyaji M, Kurane R, Takahara Y. Antifungal activity of components of essential oils. Agric Biol Chem 1981;45:945-952.

91. Moon KH, Pack MY. Cytotoxicity of cinnamic aldehyde on leukemia L1210 cells. Drug Chem Toxicol 1983;6:521-535.

92. Petterson EO, Ronning W, Nome O, Oftebro R. Effects of benzaldehyde on protein metabolism of human cells cultivated in vitro. Eur J Cancer Clin Oncol 1983;19:935-940.

93. Guidotti GG, Loreti L, Ciaranfi E. Studies on the antitumor activity of aliphatic aldehydes-I. The mechanism of inhibition of amino acid incorporation into protein of Yoshida ascites hepatoma cells. Eur J Cancer Clin Oncol 1965;1:23-32.

94. Sessa A, Scalabrino G, Arnaboldi A, Perin A. Effects of aliphatic aldehyde metabolism on protein and thiol compounds in rat liver and hepatoma induced by 4-dimethyl-aminoazobenzene. Cancer Res 1977;37:2170-217.

95. Ciaranfi E, Loreti L, Borghetti A, Guidotte GG. Studies on the antitumor activity of aliphatic aldehydes-II. Effects on survival of Yoshida ascites hepatoma-bearing rats. Eur J Cancer Clin Oncol 1965;1:147-151.

96. Dornish JM, Patterson EO, Oftebro R. Synergistic cell inactivation of human NHIK 3025 cells by cinnamaldehyde in combination with cis-diamminedichloroplatinum(II). Cancer Res 1988;48:938-942.

97. National Research Council Committee on Aldehydes. Formaldehyde and other aldehydes. Washington, DC: National Academy of Sciences Press, 1981.

98. Gorman SP, Scott EM, Russell AD. A review: antimicrobial activity, uses and mechanism of action of glutaraldehyde. J Appl Bacteriol 1980;48:161-190.

99. Snyder RW, Cheatle EL. Alkaline glutaraldehyde an effective disinfectant. Am J Hosp Pharm 1965;22:321-327.

100. Stonehill AA, Knop S, Borick PM. Buffered glutaraldehyde: a new chemical of sterilizing solution. Am J Hosp Pharm 1963;20:458-465.

101. Borick PM, Donershine FH, Chandler VL. Alkylized glutaraldehyde: a new antimicrobial agent. J Pharmacol Sci 1984;57:1273.

102. Pepper RE, Chandler VL. Sporocidal activity of alkaline alcoholic saturated dialdehyde solutions. Appl Microbiol 1963;11:384.

103. Blough HA, Selective inactivation of biological activity of myxoviruses by glutaraldehyde. J Bacteriol 1966;92:226.

104. O'Brien HA, Mitchell JD, Haberman S, Rowan DF, Winford TE, Pellet J. The use of activated glutaraldehyde as a cold sterilizing agent for urological instruments. J Urol 1966;95:429.

105. Sabel FL, Hellman A, McDade MJ. Glutaraldehyde inactivation of virus in tissue. Appl Microbiol 1969;17:645.

106. Dabrowa N, Landau JW, Newcomer VD. Antifungal activity in vitro. Arch Dermatol 1972;105:555.

107. Boucher RMG. Potentiated acid 1,5-pentanedial—a new chemical sterilizing and disinfecting agent. Am J Hosp Pharm 1974;31:546.

108. Snyder RW, Cheatle EL. Alkaline glutaraldehyde: an effective disinfectant. Am J Hosp Pharm 1965;22:321.

109. Meeks CH, Pembleton WE, Hench ME. Sterilization of anesthesia apparatus. JAMA 1967;199:276.

110. Clark EG. Risk of isothiazolinones. J Soc Occup Med 1987;37:30-31.

111. London ID. Buffered glutaraldehyde solution for warts. Arch Dermatol 1971;104:440.

112. London ID. Twenty-five percent Glutaraldehyde solution for warts. Arch Dermatol 1971;104:440.

113. DesGroseillers JP, Brisson P. Localized epidermolysis bullosa. Report of two cases and evaluation of therapy with glutaraldehyde. Arch Dermatol 1974;109:70.

114. Gordon HH. Glutaraldehyde therapy for epidermolysis bullosa. Arch Dermatol 1974;110:297.

115. Goncalo S, Brandao M, Pecequeiro M, Morena A, Sousa I. Occupational contact dermatitis to glutaraldehyde. Contact Dermatitis 1984;10:183-184.

116. Juhlin L, Hansson H. Topical glutaraldehyde for plantar hyperhidrosis. Arch Dermatol 1968;97:327-330.

117. Gordon HH. Hyperhidrosis: treatment with glutaraldehyde. Cutis 1972;9:372.

118. March R, Quermonne MA. Inhibition of palmar skin conductance in mice by antiperspirants. J Soc Cosmet Chem 1976;27:333.

119. Naginton J, Rook A, Highet A. Virus and related infection. Chapt 20 in Rook A, Wilkinson D, Ebling F, et al., eds. Textbook of dermatology, Vol 1. Boston: Blackwell Scientific, 1986.

120. Gordon BI, Mailbach HI. Eccrine anhydrosis due to glutaraldehyde, formaldehyde and ionotophoresis. J Invest Dermatol 1969;53:436.

121. Grand LV. A further look at the treatment of onychomycosis with topical glutaraldehyde. J Am Podiatry Assoc 1974;64:158-160.

122. Suringa DWR. Treatment of superficial onychomycosis with topically applied glutaraldehyde a preliminary study. Arch Dermatol 1970;102:163.

123. Filachione EM, Korn AH, Ard JS. The ultra-violet absorption of protein bound glutaraldehyde. J Am Leather Chem Assoc 1967;62:480.

124. Fisher A. Contact dermatitis. 3rd ed. Philadelphia: Lea & Febiger, 1986:157.

125. Russel AD, Hopwood D. The biological uses and importance of glutaraldehyde. In: Ellis GP, West GB, eds. Progress in medicinal chemistry. Vol 13. Amsterdam: North-Holland Publishing Co, 1976:271.

126. Wade MJ, Friedman L, Ross VC. Biochemical and toxicological aspects of glutaraldehyde. FDA BY-Lines no.1. Washington, DC: Food and Drug Administration, 1982.

127. Doina O, Lenkie R, Ghetic V. Immunogenicity of glutaraldehyde-treated homologous albumin in rabbits. Immuno Chem 15;687-693:1978.

128. Payne JW. Polymerization of proteins with glutaraldehyde soluble molecular-weight markers. Biochem J 1973;135:867-873.

129. Cronin E. Contact dermatitis. NY: Churchill Livingstone, 1980:796.

130. Meltzer N, Henkin H. Glutaraldehyde—a preservative for cosmetics. Cosmet Toiletr 1977;92-95.

131. Weaver JE, Mailbach HI. Dose response relationships in allergic contact dermatitis: glutaraldehyde-containing liquid fabric softener. Contact Dermatitis 1977;3:65.

132. Nicewicz JT, Murphy DMF, Welsh JP, Sualli H. Occupational asthma caused by glutaraldehyde exposure. Immunol Allergy Prac 1986;8:272.

133. Benson WG. Exposure to glutaraldehyde. J Soc Occup Med 1984;34:63-64.

134. Corrado OJ, Osman J, Davies, RJ. Asthma and rhinitis after exposure to glutaraldehyde in endoscopy units. Hum Toxicol 1986;5:325-328.

135. Norback D. Skin and respiratory symptoms from exposure to alkaline glutaraldehyde in medical services. Scand J Work Environ Health 1988;14:366-371.

136. Ballantyne B, Berman B. Dermal sensitizing potential of glutaraldehyde: a review of recent observations. J Toxicol Cut Ocula Toxicol 1984;3:251-262.

137. Nethercott JR, Holness DL, Page E. Occupational contact dermatitis due to glutaraldehyde in health care workers. Contact Dermatitis 1988;193-196.

138. Nethercott JR, Gallant C. Disability due to occupational skin disease. Occupational Medicine: State of the Art Reviews 1986;1:199-203.

139. Nethercott JR, Holness DL. Contact dermatitis in funeral service workers. Contact Dermatitis 1988;18:263-267.

140. Berdazzi F, Melino M, Alagna G, Geronesi S. Glutaraldehyde dermatitis in nurses. Contact Dermatitis 1986;14:319-320.

141. American Conference of Government Industrial Hygienists. Threshold limit values and biological exposure indices, 1990–1991. Cincinnati, OH: ACGIH, 1990.

142. National Research Council Committee on Aldehydes. Formaldehyde and other Aldehydes. Washington, DC: National Academy of Science Press, 1981.

143. Documentation of the threshold limit values. 4th ed. Department of Health and Human Services National Institute for Occupational Safety and Health. Cincinnati, OH: American Conference of Governmental Industrial Hygienists, 1985.

144. Sittig M. In: Handbook of toxic and hazardous chemicals. Park Ridge, NJ: Noyes Publications, 1981.

145. Dunlop AP. Furfural and other furan compounds. In: Standen A, Kirk-Othmer encyclopedia of chemical technology. 2nd ed. Vol 10. New York, NY: Wiley-Interscience, 1966:237-251.

100

Military Munitions and Antipersonnel Agents

Charles E. Stewart, M.D.
John B. Sullivan, Jr., M.D.

CHEMICAL MUNITIONS

Poison gases have been used as early as 428 BC, when burning wax, pitch, and sulfur were used in wars between the Athenians and Spartans (1). Chemical warfare was used extensively in World War I with devastating effects against unprepared and unprotected troops. Mustard gas, for example, produced five times as many casualties as either high explosives or shrapnel (2). These agents were more incapacitating than lethal, with death from chemical weapons found in only 7% of casualties. This is about 4 times lower than the death to casualty ratio seen with conventional munitions.

Since some potential military adversaries maintain large stocks of these agents and train under realistic conditions with these agents, it is likely that they could be used in future conflicts. Indeed, there is evidence that mustard gas was used in the 1980–88 Iran-Iraq war and a strong possibility that a new agent (yellow rain) was used in the Afghanistan conflict with the USSR.

More important to the civilian physician and the poison control center is the possibility that these agents might be employed by a terrorist group. Chemical warfare agents are easily synthesized from readily available chemicals and could be employed by or on behalf of a country intent on terrorist operations. Modern pesticide producing plants can manufacture nerve agents, while ethylene and sulfurated petrochemicals may be combined in the Levinstein process to produce sulfur mustard gas (3).

Lethal Agents

These include cyanide, vesicants, nerve agents, and choking agents. The organophosphate anticholinesterase compounds are widely used in agriculture. A less common use of these agents is as lethal agents in war. This lethal use may be to destroy and demoralize the enemy or may be to deny an area of operations to the enemy (Table 100.1).

CYANIDE

Cyanide-containing compounds have been stocked by some nations for use as a chemical warfare agent. Cyanide was used in World War I, but did not prove to be as successful as chlorine, because of high volatility. Potassium cyanide poisoning of food and water supplies is an ancient terrorist tactic.

The military designators for the cyanide compounds used in warfare are:

AC (hydrogen cyanide HCN)
CK (cyanogen chloride CNCL)

These agents may be delivered by munitions from artillery, mortars, bombs, or simply released from cannisters. Like all of the chemical warfare agents, area of action is weather- and wind-dependent.

Cyanogen chloride has a similar action to that of hydrogen cyanide. It is not lethal at lower concentrations, but it also possesses potent pulmonary irritant and lacrimator effects.

The military incorrectly refers to these agents as "blood agents." The correct site of action is at the tissue level, and the blood is unaffected.

The cyanide compounds are among the most rapidly acting of war gases. They act by binding the iron component (ferric) of the cytochrome "c" oxidase system, since the cytochrome system is necessary for cellular respiration and transport of oxygen.

Inhalation of cyanide agents may cause:

1. Dryness and burning of the throat
2. Air hunger
3. Hyperpnea
4. Apnea
5. Seizures and coma
6. Cardiovascular collapse

The diagnosis of hydrogen cyanide poisoning is difficult without a history of exposure. Particularly in the field, without laboratory support, these agents are difficult to identify. The odor of bitter almonds is perceptible by only 50% of the population. Symptoms as noted above are quite nonspecific. Arterial blood gases may show a metabolic acidosis, normal PaO_2 and O_2 saturation. Oxygen cannot be used at the tissue level, so venous blood is often bright red in appearance.

Table 100.1. Chemical Warfare Agents

Category	U.S. Code	Common Name
Lethal agents		
Nerve agents	GA	Tabun
	GB	Sarin
	GD	Soman
	VX	
Vesicant agents	HD	Mustard
	L	Lewisite
	CX	Phosgene oxime
	T	Bis-2-chloroethylsulfide
Blood agents	AC	Hydrogen cyanide
	CK	Cyanogen chloride
Choking agents	CG	Phosgene
	CL	Chlorine
Generally nonlethal agents		
Vomit agents	DM	
	DA	
Tear gas	CR	
	CS	
	CN	
	CA	

The success of therapy of acute cyanide intoxication depends primarily on the speed with which the cellular oxygen utilization is restored. The patient should be immediately removed from the contaminated atmosphere.

The definitive treatment of cyanide intoxication differs in various countries, but only one method is approved for use in the United States.

The United States military currently advocates the use of nitrites and thiosulfate for treatment of cyanide intoxication. Sodium nitrite (10 milliliters of 3% solution) is used intravenously followed by sodium thiosulfate (50 milliliters of 25% solution). The sodium nitrite forms methemoglobin. Cyanide binds preferentially to the methemoglobin to form cyanmethemoglobin and is then converted by the thiosulfate to the much less toxic thiocyanate ion and excreted.

During this therapy, the patient's respiration and oxygenation should be adequately supported. Blood agents are summarized in Table 100.2.

NERVE AGENTS

Nerve gases in current use, storage, or production include tabun (GA), sarin (GB), soman (GD) [''G'' for German—found in German military stores after World War II], and VX (Fig. 100.1). The first three agents, the so-called ''G'' agents, are highly toxic organophosphate compounds that were developed between World War I and World War II. The vapor pressures of the ''G'' agents make them significant inhalation hazards in any warm climate or with droplet aerosols. VX is an oily liquid that persists on scene for weeks or longer. It is considered a ''persistant nerve agent.'' All four of the agents may be well-absorbed through the skin. Nerve gases irreversibly inhibit acetylcholinesterase.

Nerve agents kill by a sequence of effects. These agents combine with acetylcholine to prevent the synaptic transmitter functions of acetylcholine at the neuromuscular junction (5). Acetylcholine will accumulate at neuromuscular junctions and cause a loss of function at those junctions. This explains the peripheral and central effects of these agents, but no direct evidence exists unequivocally relating the nerve agent toxicity solely to acetylcholinesterase inhibition (6).

The importance of nerve agent's peripheral effects is paramount. These include the simulation of the endings of the parasympathetic nerves at the smooth muscle of the iris, the ciliary body, the bronchial tree, gastrointestinal tract, bladder, and blood vessels (7). This also includes the activation of secretory glands of the respiratory tract and stimulation of the cardiac muscle. Sympathetic stimulation includes nerves to the sweat glands. These are the characteristic muscarine-like signs and symptoms associated with cholinergic excess (muscarinic effects).

Salivation, lacrimation, and defecation result from these effects of the nerve agent on muscarinic end organs. Bronchoconstriction, laryngospasm, and airway obstruction may likewise contribute to the lethality of the agents from the muscarinic effects.

The accumulation of acetylcholine at the endings of the motor nerves to voluntary muscles and the autonomic ganglia results in nicotinic-like signs and symptoms. For muscle, this would mean the following sequence of events would occur:

1. Spontaneous activation of myofibrils (fasciculations) as acetylcholine accumulates and paralyzes random neuromuscular junctions

2. Tremors and twitching as entire muscle groups are lost
3. Flaccid paralysis as the entire muscle group loses the effective function of the neuromuscular junction

Finally, the accumulation of excessive acetylcholine in the brain and spinal cord is thought to result in central nervous system symptoms of twitching, jerking, staggering gait, convulsions, and coma. Objective changes in the electroencephalogram may be demonstrated (8).

Individuals poisoned by a nerve agent display similar symptoms regardless of exposure route. The intensity and sequence of the symptoms is, however, influenced by the route of absorption:

Rhinorrhea
Bronchial secretions
Tightness of the chest
Bronchospasm
Dimness of vision
Miosis
Dyspnea
Drooling and excessive sweating
Nausea
Vomiting, cramps, and involuntary defecation and urination
Twitching, jerking, and staggering gait
Headache, confusion, coma, and convulsions
Respiratory depression and respiratory arrest

Skin exposure may produce localized sweating and fasciculations as the first effect. Eye exposure may produce miosis and dimness of vision as first effects.

Other effects and complications include hypoxia, ischemia, acidosis, hyperthermia, hypothermia, peripheral neuropathy, and cerebral edema. These have been seen in patients who have received convulsive doses of nerve agents (9). It is obvious that many of the longer term effects are directly related to the problems of providing adequate ventilation to the contaminated, seizing patient who has copious airway secretions.

A summary of organophosphate-induced muscarinic and nicotinic symptoms are shown in Table 100.3.

Nerve agents may be delivered in either vapor, droplet, or both forms. Any artillery or mortar capable of delivering a chemical munition is suitable. M55 rockets and M23 land mines are two such munitions. Low flying missiles or aircraft that deliver a droplet spray are ideal. The Soviets have adapted SCUD missiles to ''splatter'' these agents with a small explosive charge. Finally, release of the vapor or droplets from pressurized containers in aerosol forms can be accomplished. Delivery patterns will be dependent on the munition, capacity of the chemical container and weather patterns.

Symptoms appear much more slowly from absorption through the skin than from respiratory exposure. Although skin absorption of a lethal dose may occur within 1–2 minutes, it may take up to 1–2 hours for death to occur. If inhaled or absorbed through eye or mucous membranes, the agents kill in 1–10 minutes. If food or water contaminated with nerve agents is ingested, the victim may experience symptoms in about 0.5 hour.

When systemic symptoms are produced, no matter by what route of exposure, the red blood cell and/or plasma cholinesterase activity will be depressed, usually to below 30% of baseline levels. As a guide, in the absence of other causes, a cholinesterase activity of less than 50% of baseline would in-

Table 100.2. Blood Agents

Hydrogen cyanide
Chemical name—Hydrogen cyanide or hydrocyanic acid
Formula—HCN
Molecular weight—27.02
Vapor density (compared with air)—0.93
Liquid density—0.687
Boiling point—25.7°C

Decomposition temperature—Above 65.5°C (Forms explosive polymer on standing. Stabilized material can be stored up to 65°C.)

Rate of hydrolysis—Low under field conditions.

Stability in storage—Unstable except when very pure. May form explosive polymer on long standing. Can be stabilized by addition of small amounts of phosphoric acid or sulfur dioxide.

Action on metals or other materials—Little or none.

Odor—Similar to bitter almonds.

Clinical effects—Binds to cytochrome oxidase enzyme system and interferes with cellular respiration. Produces seizures, metabolic acidosis, hypotension, cardiovascular collapse, respiratory failure.

Median lethal dosage (MLD_{50})—Median lethal dosage varies widely with concentration because of the rather high rate at which AC is detoxified by the body. For example, at 200 mg/m^3 concentration, the lethal dosage is approximately 2000 mg/min/m^3, whereas at 150 mg/m^3 the lethal dosage is approximately 4500 mg-min/m^3.

Median incapacitating dosage (ICt_{50})—Varies with the concentration.

Dermal effects—Dermatitis.

Rate of action—Very rapid. Death occurs within 15 minutes after a lethal dosage has been received.

Protection required—Protective mask and protective clothing.

Persistency—Short; the agent is highly volatile, and in the gaseous state it dissipates quickly in the air.

Cyanogen chloride (CK)
Chemical name—Cyanogen chloride
Formula—CNCl
Molecular weight—61.48
Vapor density (compared with air)—2.1
Liquid density—1.18 at 20°C
Boiling point—12.8°C
Decomposition temperature—Above 100°C

Rate of hydrolysis—Very low

Hydrolysis products—HCl and CNOH

Stability in storage—Stable at 65°C for 30 days.
Tends to undergo condensation or polymerization in storage to form the solid compound 2,4,6-trichloro-s-triazine, $C_3N_3Cl_3$ (cyclic). Impurities promote polymerization which may occur with explosive violence.

Action on metals or other materials—None if CK is dry.

Odor—Its irritating and lacrimatory properties are so great that the odor can go unnoticed.

Median concentration detectable (by lacrimatory effect)—12 mg/m^3

Median lethal dosage (MLD_{50})—11,000 mg-min/m^3

Median incapacitating dosage (ICt_{50})—7000 mg-min/m^3

Rate of detoxification—0.02–0.1 mg/kg/min

Clinical effects—It is assumed that the effect of CK arises from its conversion to cyanide in the body. In general, CK may be considered a rapid-acting chemical agent with clinical toxic effects like cyanide.

Protection required—Protective mask. CK will break or penetrate a protective mask canister or filter element more readily than most other agents. A very high concentration may overpower the filter; high dosages will break down its protective ability.

Persistency—Short. Vapor may persist in jungle and forest for some time under suitable weather conditions.

Arsine (SA)
Chemical name—Arsenic trihydride, arsine
Formula—AsH$_3$
Molecular weight—77.93
Vapor density (compared with air)—2.69
Liquid density—1.34 at 20°C
Boiling point—−62.5°C
Decomposition temperature—280°C
Rate of hydrolysis—Rapid, but an equilibrium condition is reached quickly. (Under certain conditions, SA forms a solid product with water which decomposes at 30°C)

Hydrolysis products—Arsenic acids and hydride

Stability in storage—Not stable in uncoated metal containers. Metals catalyze decomposition of arsine.

Action on metals and other materials—Reacts slowly with copper, brass, and nickel. May also be decomposed by contact with other metals.

Odor—Mild garlic-like odor

Median lethal dosage (MLD_{50})—5000 mg-min/m^3. It is estimated that 2 milligrams of SA per kilogram of body weight would be lethal to a human.

Median incapacitating dosage (ICt_{50})—2500 mg-min/m^3

Rate of detoxification—Not rapid enough to be of importance

Toxic effects—Rapid red blood cell hemolysis with potential subsequent renal failure and other target organ failure.

Rate of action—Effects are delayed from 2 hours to as much as 11 days.

Reprinted with permission: U.S. Army FM3-9, U.S. Air Force 355-7.

dicate exposure to an anticholinesterase agent. This measurement is not readily available in the field.

The most common cause of death after acute exposure to nerve agents is respiratory arrest, originally thought to be due to the flaccid paralysis of the respiratory muscles. Respiratory arrest will often occur prior to neuromuscular blockade and is not always due to muscle paralysis. Multiple animal studies have shown that the respiratory depression occurs before the neuromuscular blockade and the bronchoconstriction have

reached significant proportions (10). These studies support the contention that a major contribution to respiratory failure is central nervous system rather than peripheral toxicity.

Nerve gases also result in a number of delayed toxicities. The inhibition of cholinesterase enzymes is irreversible, so effects are prolonged. Until the tissue cholinesterase enzymes are restored to normal levels, there is a period of increased susceptibility to another exposure of any nerve agent. This regeneration of enzyme levels may take as long as 2–3 months.

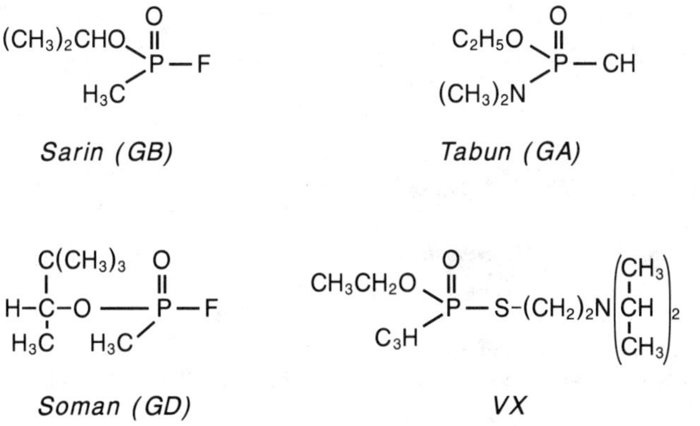

Figure 100.1. Nerve agents commonly stored or produced. Reprinted with permission from Rickett D, Glenn J, Houston W. Medical defense against nerve agents, a new direction. Milit Med 1987;152:35–41.

During this period of regeneration of enzyme, the effects of repeated exposures are cumulative.

Among these delayed effects are sudden cardiac failure in patients who have apparently recovered from the effects of organophosphate exposure (11).

Organophosphate exposure can produce both central and peripheral nervous system signs and symptoms if the patient survives the respiratory failure and other immediately lethal events. The symptoms may include impaired memory, hallucinations, fatigue, confusion, concentration deficits, and fatigue (12, 13). Signs may include both central and peripheral neuropathies and late seizures.

There is animal evidence that prolonged nerve agents-induced toxic convulsions produce irreversible brain damage. Benzodiazepine anticonvulsants appear to reduce the morbidity associated with these convulsions.

Table 100.3.   Acute Physiologic Effects of Nerve Agents

Site of Action	Signs and Symptoms
Nicotinic effects	
Striated muscle	Fatigue, weakness, twitching, fasciculations, muscle cramps, and paralysis
Sympathetic ganglia	Pallor and occasional hypertension
CNS	Tension, anxiety, restlessness, difficulty concentrating, confusion, slurred speech, ataxia, weakness, coma, absence of reflexes, Cheyne-Stokes respirations, convulsions, depression of circulatory and respiratory centers, death
Muscarinic effects	
Pupils	Miosis, usually pinpoint, occasionally unequal
Ciliary body	Headache, difficulty focusing, dimness of vision
Mucous membranes	Hyperemia, rhinorrhea, conjunctivitis, increased salivation and lacrimation
Bronchial tree	Tightness in chest, wheezing, bronchoconstriction, increased secretions, pain in chest, dyspnea, cough, pulmonary edema
Gastrointestinal	Nausea, vomiting, abdominal cramps, diarrhea, tenesmus
Sweat glands	Increased sweating

Recent work has proposed that the sole toxic effect of the nerve agents is not just the inactivation of acetylcholinesterase. Albuquerque and associates have described agonistic effects at the nicotinic cholinesterase receptor sites from tabun, sarin, and soman (14). These agents are capable of activation of the ionic channel in a manner similar to acetycholine. He also noted that VX prevents ionic conductance through the channel, even if acetylcholine binds to the nicotinic receptor site. This means that there is no single site of treatment for an antidote.

Therapy

For over 40 years, the standard therapy for emergency treatment of anticholinesterase agents has been atropine sulfate. This treatment was proposed within weeks after the capture of German stocks of nerve agents in World War II. Atropine will reverse the muscarinic effects of nerve agent poisoning such as bronchospasm, excessive respiratory secretions, and intestinal hypermotility. Atropine provides no protection for the effects of the organophosphates on the nicotinic receptors such as neuromuscular junctions.

Large doses of atropine may be required for reversal of the muscarinic effects of nerve agents. Although the military issues 1-milligram autoinjectors, this is an inadequate dose for field treatment. Well-documented exposures requiring 20–40 milligrams of atropine are not unusual with exposure to these agents. Doses of more than 2000 mg/day have been required in organophosphate poisoning (15). It would be likely that these doses would not be unusual in the treatment of exposure to the more powerful military agents.

In 1951, the oximes (pralidoxime) were first proposed as a treatment of poisoning by the nerve agents. These drugs were used to reactivate acetylcholinesterase bound by the nerve agent. However, there is no oxime available that is effective in reactivation of acetylcholinesterase that has been bound to all four of the nerve agents. Secondly, after a variable period (called the aging period), reactivation is very difficult (16). For commercial organophosphates, aging occurs after 24–48 hours. For GD, this aging period is about 2 minutes. Even self-administered oxime, given at the first symptoms of GD exposure, would not be completely effective. Other oximes have been studied for efficacy in treating organophosphate toxicity: Obidoxime and asoxime (17). Asoxime shows promise in reversing toxic effects of soman (17). Also asoxime has fewer adverse side effects compared with other oximes.

Currently the United States Army uses pralidoxime chloride (2-PAM) to reactive cholinesterase (Fig. 100.2). It is not completely effective and is least effective against GD. VX, on the other hand, has an aging period of several *hours* and use of 2-PAM is helpful in the treatment of this agent. United States soldiers carry three pralidoxime chloride autoinjectors, each containing 600 milligrams of the oxime, and three atropine autoinjectors, each with 2 milligrams of atropine. They are trained to administer 1 injector of each agent through protective clothing and undergarments if any symptoms of exposure occur.

Animal data suggest that a serum pralidoxime level of about 4 μg/ml may be the minimal level to offer protection against the toxic effects of organophosphates (18, 19). Current therapeutic guidelines suggest administration 1 gram of pralidoxime chloride every 4–6 hours—which may be inadequate for treatment of these warfare agents. Infusions (0.5 g/hr) provide serum levels of about 15 μg/ml in a steady-state simulation in adults and may provide better therapy (20). The addition of diazepam

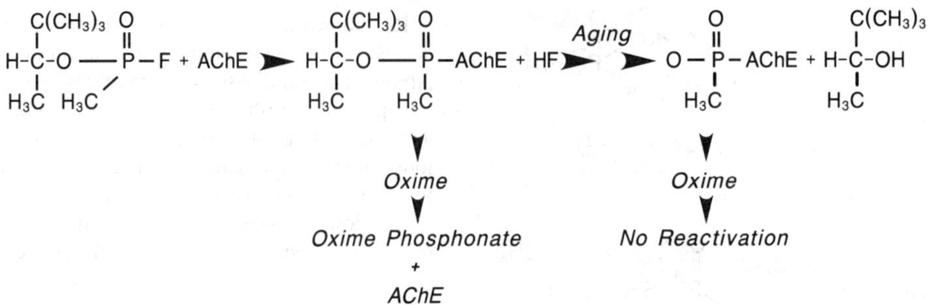

$$
\begin{array}{c}
\underset{\substack{|\\H_3C\quad H_3C}}{\overset{\substack{C(CH_3)_3\quad O\\|\qquad\quad||}}{H\text{-}C\text{-}O\text{---}P\text{-}F}} + AChE
\quad\blacktriangleright\quad
\underset{\substack{|\qquad\quad|\\H_3C\qquad H_3C}}{\overset{\substack{C(CH_3)_3\quad O\\|\qquad\quad||}}{H\text{-}C\text{-}O\text{---}P\text{-}AChE}} + HF
\quad\overset{Aging}{\blacktriangleright\blacktriangleright}\quad
\underset{\substack{|\\H_3C}}{\overset{\substack{O\\||}}{O\text{-}P\text{-}AChE}} +
\underset{\substack{|\\H_3C}}{\overset{\substack{C(CH_3)_3\\|}}{H\text{-}C\text{-}OH}}
\end{array}
$$

$$
\begin{array}{ccc}
& \blacktriangledown & \qquad\qquad \blacktriangledown \\
& Oxime & \qquad\qquad Oxime \\
& \blacktriangledown & \qquad\qquad \blacktriangledown \\
& Oxime\ Phosphonate & \qquad No\ Reactivation \\
& + & \\
& AChE &
\end{array}
$$

Figure 100.2.   The binding of an organophosphate to acetyl cholinesterase enzyme and reversal of process by oxime therapy. Reprinted with permission from Rickett D, Glen J, Houston W. Medical defense against nerve agents, a new direction. Milit Med 1987;152:35–41.

to the treatment protocol is recommended because diazepam helps protect against seizures. In addition, diazepam has improved morbidity and mortality of soman poisoning independent of anticonvulsant effects (17).

Since atropine/oxime antidote therapy has limitations, another approach is to competitively inhibit the nerve agent with a "pretreatment" drug. This drug must be relatively nontoxic and easily tolerated and must compete with nerve agents for acetylcholinesterase. The most effective current therapeutic agents are the carbamates, which reversibly bind to acetylcholinesterase. After the nerve agent has bound to some of the remaining acetylcholinesterase, the carbamate-bound enzyme can reactivate spontaneously and continue the essential neurotransmission.

Humans can tolerate carbamylation of 20–30% of their acetylcholinesterase. A high dose of nerve agent may permanently inactivate all remaining acetylcholinesterase and cause death. A lower, but otherwise lethal, dose may be protected by the reversible carbamylated acetylcholinesterase. The current carbamylate of choice is pyridostigmine (a relative of physostigmine). It has a wide therapeutic margin of safety and appears to have no longterm toxicity to humans. Pyridostigmine has been used in the United States for years as a therapy for myasthenia gravis and is readily available in 30 milligram tablets. The usual "pretreatment" dose is 30 milligrams orally every 8 hours, starting 6–8 hours prior to exposure (21).

Data show that the use of atropine and 2-PAM (pralidoximine) will protect an animal for about 1.6 times the median lethal dose. With the addition of pretreatment, the protective ratio was increased to well over 20 times the median lethal dose. A human who survives a multiple exposure with the use of this combination therapy may require weeks to recover full function.

The major problem with pretreatment is that it does not protect the individual against nerve agent-induced convulsions. Again, one expects multiple casualties from the combinations of convulsions, copious secretions, and decreased respiratory effort. Benzodiazepine will help protect against these convulsions but cannot be effectively administered as a "pretreatment."

Human monoclonal antibodies to the various nerve agents have been proposed as passive protection prior to nerve agent exposure. These antibodies are promising but require more research before field use (22).

The cardinal principles of therapy for nerve agent intoxication are:

1. Protect self—Not only should the medical provider be wearing full protective gear, but he/she should be pretreated with pyridostigmine bromide.
2. Terminate exposure by removing the individual from the area.
3. Assist ventilation (**NOT** mouth to mouth).
4. Administer atropine—The dose depends on the symptoms. Initial therapy of mild to moderate symptoms will require at least 2 milligrams i.m. or i.v. and may well require up to several milligrams over a period of time.
5. Decontaminate the patient.
6. Reactivate enzymes with an oxime—2-PAM, 500–1000 milligrams i.v. as an initial dose. This is repeated every 4–6 hours as needed.
7. Confirm the diagnosis by assaying red blood cell acetylcholinesterase and/or plasma acetylcholinesterase.

Local decontamination of these agents may be accomplished with soap and water. Most of these agents will decompose with time; therefore area decontamination may neither be feasible nor safe. Since these are lethal agents, ANY decontamination should be accomplished in complete protective gear with self-contained breathing apparatus if available. Charcoal inserts for protective masks have only limited life span and should be carefully checked and replaced promptly. The military has several detection devices for these agents. All health care providers must be in full protective gear at all times during care for the patient until an environmental health specialist who is trained to detect these agents can "clear" the patient. Severely intoxicated patients may remain unconscious for hours or days. Characteristics of nerve gas agents are summarized in Table 100.4.

Tabun

Tabun or GA is ethyl N,N-dimethylphosphoroamidocyanidate. It has a faintly fruity order and is an anticholinesterase agent. The median lethal dose is about 200 mg/min/m^3 via inhalation and about 20–40,000 mg/min/m^3 via percutaneous absorption. GA has a half-life in the environment of about 1 to ½ days. It is effectively detoxified on humans by bleach or soapy water. Equipment may be effectively detoxified with a dilute alkali solution, steam and ammonia, or bleach solution.

Sarin

Sarin or GB is isopropyl methylphosphonofluoridate. It has no odor when pure. It is an anticholinesterase. The medial lethal dose is between 70 and 100 mg/min/m^3 for inhalation and about

Table 100.4. Nerve Gas Agents

Tabun (GA)—A colorless to brownish liquid giving a colorless vapor

Chemical name—Ethyl N,N-dimethyl-phosphoroamidocyanidate.

Formula—$C_2H_5OP(O)(CN)N(CH_3)_2$

Molecular weight—162.3
Vapor density (compared with air)—5.63
Liquid density—1.073 at 25°C
Vapor pressure—0.070 mm Hg at 25°C
Decomposition temperature—Complete decomposition in 3¼ hours at 150°C

Rate of hydrolysis—Reacts slowly with water but rapidly with strong acids or alkalies; self-buffering at pH 4–5. Autocatalytic below pH 4, due to presence of HCN. Half-life, 7 hours at pH 4–5. Hydrolysis catalyzed by phosphate.

Hydrolysis products—HCN
Stability in storage—Stable in steel containers at ordinary temperatures. No activity on metals or other materials.

Odor—Faintly fruity; none when pure.

Median concentration detectable (by eye effects)—3.2 mg/m³

Median lethal dosage (MLD_{50}) (respiratory).
Approximately 200–400 mg/min/m³ for resting individuals

Median incapacitating dosage (ICt_{50}) (respiratory)
Approximately 300 mg/min/m³ for resting individuals

Approximately 300 mg/min/m³ for resting individuals.

Clinical effects—very high toxicity; rapid acting, much greater toxic effects through eye than through skin. Vapor causes miosis resulting in decreased vision. Irreversibly inhibits acetylcholinesterase enzyme.

Dermal effect—LD_{50} (liquid), 1–1.5 g/person. Liquid decontamination of smallest drop is essential. Vapor penetrates skin readily. Skin LCt_{50} of vapor is not known—probably between 20,000 and 40,000 mg/min/m³.

Protection required—Protective mask and protective clothing. Ordinary clothing may degas vapors for about 30 minutes after contact with vapor. Immediately remove all liquid from clothing.

Decontaminants—Soap and water wash.

Persistency—Depends upon munitions used and the weather. Heavily splashed liquid persists 1–2 days under average weather conditions.

Sarin (GB)—A colorless liquid; vapor is colorless.
Chemical name—Isopropyl methyl phosphonofluoridate

Formula—Molecular—$CH_3P(O)(F)OCH(CH_3)_2$

Molecular weight—140.10

Vapor density (compared with air)—4.86

Liquid density—1.0887 at 25°C

Boiling point—158°C

Decomposition temperature—Complete decomposition after 2.5 hours at 150°C

Rate of hydrolysis—Variable with pH. Half-life 7.5 hours at pH 1.8; 30 hours in unbuffered solution. Rapidly hydrolyzed in alkaline solutions.

Hydrolysis products—Hydrofluoric acid under acid conditions; isopropyl alcohol and polymers under alkaline conditions.

Stability in storage—Fairly stable in steel containers at 65°C. Stability improves with increasing purity.

Action on metals or other materials—Slightly corrosive on steel.

Odor—Almost none in pure state.

Median lethal dosage (LCt_{50}) (respiratory). 70–100 mg/min/m³ for resting men; 35 mg/min/m³ for men engaged in mild activity.

Median incapacitating dosage (ICt_{50}) (respiratory). 75 mg/min/m³ for resting men; 35 mg/min/m³ for men engaged in mild activity.

Rate of detoxification—Low detoxification rate; cumulative.

Clinical effects—Very high toxicity and rapidly acting toxin; much greater through eye than through skin. Vapor causes miosis and decreased vision. Irreversible inhibition of acetylcholinesterase.

Dermal effect—LD_{50} is 1.7 g/person. Liquid does not injure skin but penetrates it rapidly. Immediate decontamination of the smallest drop is essential. Vapor penetrates skin also. Skin MLD_{50} of vapor is approximately 12,000 mg/min/m³ for naked man, and 15,000 mg/min/m³ for man in ordinary combat clothing. Median incapacitating dosage from vapor skin in approximately 8000 mg/min/m³ with ordinary clothing.

Persistency—Evaporates at approximately the same rate as water. Depends upon munitions used and the weather.

Soman (GD)—GD is a colorless liquid which gives off a colorless vapor.
Chemical name—Pinacolyl methyl phosphonofluoridate

Formula—$CH_3P(O)(F)OCH(CH_3)$

Molecular weight—182.178

Vapor density (compared with air)—6.33

Liquid density—1.0222 at 25°C

Boiling point—198°C

Decomposition temperature—Unstabilized—decomposes in 4 hours at 130°C. Stabilized—decomposes in 200 hours at 130°C.

Rate of hydrolysis—Varies with pH; complete in 5 minutes in 5 percent NaOH solutions. Half-life at pH 6.65 and 25°C is 45 hours.

Hydrolysis products—Hydrofluoric acid

Stability in storage—Less stable than GA or GB

Odor—Fruity; with impurities, odor of camphor

Median lethal dosage (MLD_{50}) (respiratory)—70–100 mg/min/m³

Median incapacitating dosage—(ICt_{50}) GB, GA range

Rate of detoxification—Low detoxification rate; essentially cumulative

Clinical effects—Very high toxicity and rapidly acting toxin; vapor causes miosis with decreased vision. Toxicity much greater through eye than through skin. Irreversibly binds to acetylcholinesterase.

Dermal effect—Extremely toxic by skin absorption. Liquid does not injure skin, but penetrates it rapidly. Immediate decontamination of the smallest drop is essential. Skin LCt_{50} of vapor is not known.

Rate of action—Very rapid. Death usually occurs within 15 minutes after fatal dosage is absorbed.

Protection required—Protective mask and protective clothing. Ordinary clothing degasses vapor for about 30 minutes after contact with vapor. This should be considered before unmasking. Immediately remove all liquid from clothing.

continues

Table 100.4. *Continued*

Persistency—Depends upon munitions used and the weather. Heavily splashed liquid persists 1–2 days under average weather conditions.

V-Agents—The standard V-agent is VX. VX is an odorless amber colored liquid similar in appearance to motor oil.
Formula—$C_{11}H_{26}NO_2PS$
Molecular weight—267.38
Vapor density (compared with air)—9.2
Liquid density—1.0083 g/cc at 25°C
Freezing point—Below −51°C; −39°C calculated
Boiling point—298°C (calculated) decomposes
Vapor pressure—0.0007 mm Hg at 25°C
Decomposition temperature—Half-life: 36 hours at 150°C, 1.6 hours at 200°C; 4 minutes at 250°C; 36 seconds at 295°C

Rate of hydrolysis—Half-life at 25°C. pH 2–3 100 days; pH 13 16 minutes; pH 14 1.3 minutes.

Hydrolysis products—Diethyl methylphosphonate, 2-diisopropyl-aminoethyl mercaptan, ethyl hydrogen methyl-phosphonate, bis(ethylmethylphosphonic)anhydride, bis *S*-(2-diisopropyl-aminoethyl)methylphosphonodithioate. (Toxic hydrolysis products form at pH 7–10.)

Stability in storage—Relatively stable at room temperature. Unstabilized VX of 95 percent purity decomposed at a rate of 5% a month at 71°C.

Action on metal or other material—Negligible on brass, steel, and aluminum.

Median lethal dosage (MLD_{50})—30 mg/min/m³.

Median incapacitating dosage (ICt_{50})—50 mg/min/m³.

Rate of detoxification—Low; essentially cumulative.

Dermal and ocular toxicity—Extremely toxic by skin and eye absorption. Liquid does not injure the skin or eye, but penetrates rapidly. Immediate decontamination of the smallest drop is essential.

Rate of action—Very rapid. Death usually occurs within 15 minutes after fatal dosage is absorbed.

Protection required—Protective masks and protective clothing.

Persistency—depends upon munitions used and the weather. Heavily splashed liquid persists for long periods of time under average weather conditions.

Reprinted with permissions: U.S. Army FM3-9, U.S. Air Force 355-7.

12,000–15,000 mg/min/m³ for percutaneous absorption. Sarin may persist for as long as 5 days. It is effectively detoxified on humans by bleach or soapy water. Equipment may be effectively detoxified with a dilute alkali solution, steam and ammonia, or bleach solution.

Soman

Soman, GD, or pinacolyl methylphosphonofluoridate is a colorless liquid which has a fruity or camphor odor. Its mechanism of action is similar to GB. By inhalation, the median lethal dose is 70 mg/min/m³, while absorption of only 0.35 grams is the median lethal percutaneous dose for 70-kilogram man. This is essentially the same median lethal dose as GB. The onset time of symptoms is about the same as GB. It is considered a relatively persistent agent, midway between GB and GA.

VX

The most toxic of the nerve agents is VX or O-ethyl S-(2-diisopropylaminoethyl) methylphosphonothiolate. It is more stable, less volatile, and more efficient at penetration of intact skin. It is thought to be 100 times as toxic as GB for humans by the percutaneous route. By inhalation, VX is about twice as toxic as GB. The median lethal dose by inhalation is about 30 mg/min/m³, while the percutaneous absorption makes the median lethal dose by that route as low as 6 mg/min/m³. The physiologic effects and onset times of symptoms are similar to GB.

Most importantly to medical providers, VX is more difficult to decontaminate than the G agents. Since VX has a low volatility, the straw or clear liquid drops on the skin do not evaporate and will be absorbed more readily. It is a relatively persistent agent and lasts between 2 and 6 days in soil. Decontamination of humans may be done with hot soapy water, while equipment may be decontaminated with 5–10% solutions of Na_2CO_3 or bleach.

Binary Agents

In 1980, the United States proposed production of a "new" variant of nerve agent—the binary munition. In this, the concept is to fill munitions with one of two agents, transport them to the battlefield, and load a second compartment in the projectile prior to use. When the projectile or bomb is fired or exploded, the two compartments rupture and the two agents combine. The product of the resulting reaction is a nerve gas such as sarin of VX. The munition is delivered in the usual fashion from mortar, plane, or artillery piece. The advantage is safety in transport and storage. There is no advantage in dissemination or decontamination. Many of these nerve agents are stored at sites around the United States (Fig. 100.3).

CHOKING AGENTS

The choking agent group is characterized by pronounced irritation of the upper and lower respiratory tract. These agents are treacherous because they have a latent period following exposure. A victim with dyspnea and mild chest discomfort may progress in severity over a few hours after exposure.

Chlorine

Chlorine is a slightly water-soluble, yellowish gas that is about 2.5 times heavier than air. The use of 498 tons of chlorine released from 20,730 cylinders on April 22, 1915, was the cause of more than 7000 casualties at Ypres, Belgium. This agent has fallen into military disfavor because it is quite easy to detect and protect against. Millions of tons of chlorine are used for bleaching, water purification, chemical processes, and swimming pools. It is probably the cause of more cases of accidental industrial toxic exposure than any other single agent.

Adding chlorine bleach to an acidic cleaning agent will produce free chlorine gas. The extent of the resulting injury depends on the concentration and duration of the exposure. Symptoms begin in moments, and no delayed symptoms are noted. Clinical effects are noted in Table 100.5.

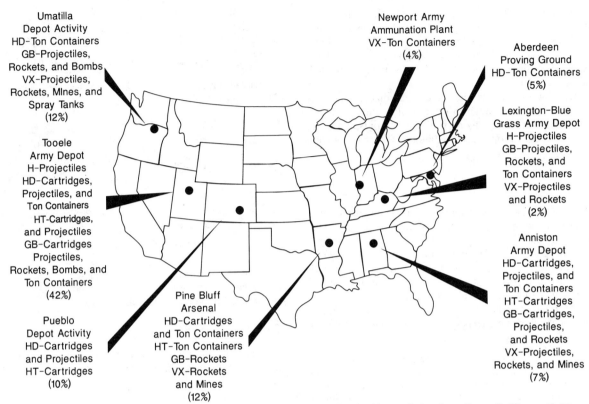

Figure 100.3. Storage sites of chemical munitions in the United States. Reprinted with permission from Carnes S, Watson P. Disposing of the U.S. chemical weapons stockpile. JAMA 1989; 262:653–659.

Table 100.5. Clinical Effects of Various Concentrations of Chlorine Gas

Concentrations	Effects
0.002 ppm	Odor detection threshold
1 ppm	US TLV—TWA limit
1–3 ppm	Mild mucous membrane irritation. US short term exposure is limited to 3 ppm
5–15 ppm	Moderate mucous membrane and upper respiratory tract irritation. Lacrimation, conjunctival, irritation, and rhinorrhea
30 ppm	Chest pain, dyspnea, cough, severe upper respiratory tract irritation, headache, and vomiting. Laryngeal edema may produce hoarseness.
40–60 ppm	Pulmonary damage—ulcerative tracheobronchitis, laryngeal edema, pneumonitis, and pulmonary edema. Corneal abrasions and burns. Cutaneous burns may be present in moist areas.
430 ppm	Potentially lethal for exposure of about 30 minutes
1000 ppm	Fatal within minutes

Chlorine gas is heavier than air and may be delivered by bomb, artillery, or mortar round, or simply released from a cannister. It will follow the curves of the hills and will flow into caves, trenches, and hollows. During World War I, in Ypres, Belgium, the German military released the agent from pressurized canisters.

Chlorine forms both hydrochloric (HCL) and hypochlorus acid on contact with water. Hypochlorus acid will sponta-neously decompose to hypochloric acid and free oxygen radicals. Free chlorine and all of the combination products of chlorine and water will disrupt cellular proteins. Molecular chlorine is about 10–30 times more toxic than the combination products (23).

Chronic effects are usually related to the extent of pulmonary damage. The typical pulmonary pattern of those exposed to a moderate concentration of chlorine gas is an increased airway resistance with normal diffusion capacity. Pulmonary function tests will return to normal in most patients within months (24). As might be expected, patients with worse subjective complaints tended to have a slower resolution than those with simpler complaints such as cough (25).

Decontamination of the victim should begin with copious irrigation of irritated areas. Following irrigation of the patient and removal of the patient's clothing, the medical provider needs no special contamination protection for pure chlorine exposure.

The victim of chlorine inhalation should be treated as if the patient has suffered a severe smoke inhalation. High flow humidified oxygen should be immediately instituted. The patient should be carefully evaluated for potential airway obstruction.

Treatment is symptomatic for limited exposures. Eyes should be copiously irrigated and checked for corneal burns. Humidification of the air or oxygen will help the cough and sore throat. Cutaneous burns should be treated as all caustic acid injuries, with copious irrigation with high flow low pressure tap water. Symptomatic treatment can include nebulized inhalation of a mixture of 2 ml 8.4% $NaHCO_3$ with 2 ml of normal saline.

Patients who are symptomatic longer than 4 hours after exposure should be monitored in the hospital. Humidified oxygen should be continued until symptoms abate. Those with respiratory distress or stridor should be intubated. Arterial blood gases, chest x-ray, and pulmonary function tests should be obtained in all of these patients. Bronchospasm may be treated with bronchodilators.

Treatment of the chlorine-induced noncardiac pulmonary edema is also supportive. Intubation and positive end expiratory pressure may reduce the pulmonary edema. Steroids appear to offer no advantage. Prophylactic antibiotics are of no proven value.

Phosgene

Phosgene ($COCl_2$ or carbonylchloride) is a chemical intermediate in production of plastics, dyestuffs, and insecticides. The military designator for this agent is CG, and the similar and related diphosgene is DP. Organochlorine compounds may decompose to phosgene when heated. This includes polyvinyl chloride plastics, Teflon, and carbon tetrachloride. It is one of the most deadly of the chemical war munitions.

Erich Maria Remarque in *All Quiet on the Western Front* eloquently described the effects of phosgene gas during World War I:

We found one dugout full of them, with blue heads and black lips. Some of them in a shell hole took off their masks too soon; they did not know that the gas lies longest in the hollows; when they saw others on the top without masks, they pulled off theirs too and swallowed enough to scorch their lungs. Their condition is hopeless, they choke to death with hemorrhages and suffocation.

Phosgene is a colorless, heavier than air, chemical agent designed to cause pulmonary damage and asphyxia. It has a characteristic odor of new-mown hay, but this is not a sufficient warning to prevent toxicity. It does not cause immediate damage and thus often has a lengthy and deep exposure. During World War I, it was responsible for over 60–80% of the "gas" deaths.

The average lethal dose is 500–800 ppm/min. This means that a 10-minute exposure to only 50–80 ppm would likely be lethal. Mild symptoms occur at 3–5 ppm.

Initial exposure to low concentration can cause pharyngitis, cough, chest tightness, and dyspnea. Nausea, headache, and lacrimation may also be present. These symptoms clear within a short time. Severe mucous membrane irritation associated with phosgene occurs from a high level exposure and produces serious toxicity. After a latent period of about 2–24 hours, pulmonary edema develops, with production of large amounts of frothy sputum (26).

This pulmonary edema is a direct toxic effect on the alveoli and does not respond to furosemide, intravenous nitrates, or morphine. The exact site of action has not yet been determined (27). Extensive fluid loss into the lungs may cause hypovolemic shock. Phosgene may also cause vasoconstriction within the lung.

Phosgene decomposes to carbon monoxide and hydrochloric acid in the presence of moisture. Decontamination with copious amounts of water will sufficiently decompose this agent. Medical providers in decontamination stations should be protected with charcoal filter respirators. Decontamination stations should be well-ventilated, and much of decontamination is accomplished by simple aeration.

The basic approach to the pulmonary damage caused by

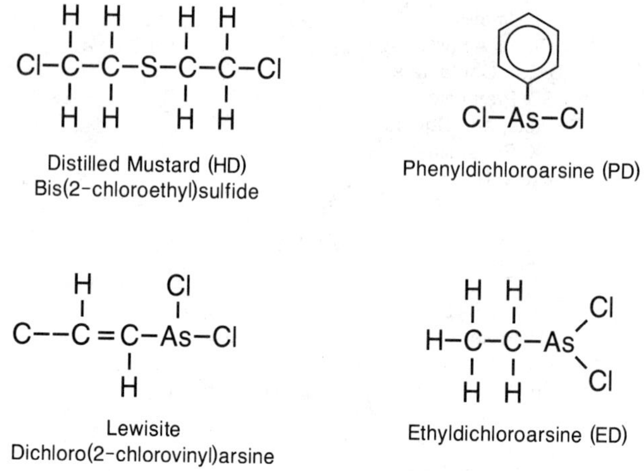

Figure 100.4. Blister agents.

phosgene is supportive. There is no antidote. The use of steroids is suggested by many authorities, but is controversial and not substantiated by good clinical data.

VESICANT GASES

These are blistering agents that are toxic to lungs, eyes, and mucous membranes. In some cases their effects may be delayed.

Mustard

Mustard gas [bis-(2-chloroethyl)sulfide] was used for the first time in Ypres, Belgium, in 1915 during World War I. It was most recently employed during the Iran-Iraqi conflict (28). It is representative of the vesicant or "blister" agents (Fig. 100.4). Other similar agents include sulfur mustard (HD), nitrogen mustard (HN), agent T, and phosgene oxime (CX).

These agents may be delivered by bomb, by artillery or mortar round, or by release from cannisters. Missiles are readily adapted to deliver this agent in large quantities.

Very little information is available on the longterm toxicity of agent T which has a much lower volatility than mustard. Agent T may be mixed with mustard for increased inhalation injury (this may be referred to as agent HT). For practical purposes, agents T and HT will be considered as close variants of mustard.

Mustard-Lewisite mix (HL) is a combination of both mustard and Lewisite with the rapid effects of the Lewisite and the delayed effects of the mustard. Decontamination and detection are similar to HD (mustard). Medical providers require protective mask and clothing for casualty management.

Nitrogen mustard [methylbis(β-chloroethyl)amine] is an oily, pale yellow to colorless liquid that is freely soluble in organic solvents but insoluble in water. Mustard is easily vaporized by heat and quickly spreads by wind, where it smells like garlic. Mustard is a primary tissue irritant and has no significant allergic component to the injury. Mustard vapor injury is markedly enhanced by high humidity in a hot environment. Topical nitrogen mustard has been used in therapy in the treatment of mycosis fungoides (29). Mustard gases will go through ordinary clothing without burning it and attacks only living tissue; the reaction is manifested only after several hours have passed (30). Between 80 and 90% of the mustard penetrates the skin and enters the circulation.

Early recognition of vesicant agent exposure is difficult because the initial effects may be only irritation of mucous membranes, similar to that found with either the choking agents or the tear gases. The dermal damage is complete in moments, but the manifestations of injury may take a latent period of 1–12 hours to appear.

In most patients, lesions are primarily cutaneous, but respiratory, ocular, and gastrointestinal manifestations may occur. In Requena and associates' (31) study of eight unprotected Iranian mustard victims, all had conjunctivitis, and two had serious corneal injuries. Three had respiratory distress.

Inhalation of mustard vapor produces a serious upper respiratory tract irritation. Cough, bloody sputum, and dyspnea are all likely. If the patient has a protective mask, only cutaneous manifestations are likely. Pulmonary edema is much less common with mustard gas than with the choking agents. Bronchopneumonia is a common complication in inhalation injuries due to mustard and Lewisite.

The area of exposure becomes erythematous and progresses into widespread bullae, similar to those of toxic epidermal necrolysis (31). The affected areas may turn black.

There is no antidote for this agent. Treatment is supportive. Protection of the staff and decontamination of the patient are the first priorities. (In Heully and Gruninger's description of a mustard shell explosion, 11 victims were from family and medical staff who attended the three patients.) Droplets of the oily agent should be removed by blotting and then cleansing with soap and water. Scrubbing and hot water should be avoided, as both activities enhance the absorption of the agent.

Steroids have been used, without confirmation of efficacy. Prophylactic antibiotic therapy is not recommended.

Topical measures have included cleansing with povidone-iodine solution and application of silver sulfadiazine cream.

The blister and vesicant war agents are summarized in Table 100.6.

Arsenic (Lewisite)

Lewisite is dichloro(2-chlorovinyl)arsine. Like mustard, arsenical vesicants are designed to be irritating. If ocular exposure occurs, they cause immediate pain, blepharospasm, and rapid formation of eyelid edema.

Lewisite is differentiated from the mustards by immediate pain upon skin contact. A skin contact of only 5 minutes will cause a chemical burn that results in a deep ulceration. Lewisite may also cause somewhat more nasal irritation than mustard gases.

British anti-Lewisite (BAL) was developed as an antidote to Lewisite and as an ointment was applied to the skin with some success. Exposed skin may be decontaminated by flushing with cool water. Neither scrubbing nor hot water is appropriate because they will enhance the absorption and toxicity. Blisters should be opened and drained of fluid. Further treatment should be similar to that of thermal burns with replacement of fluid losses and relief of pain.

The intramuscular administration of dimercaprol (BAL) has provided some relief. Since the agent continues to burn until removed or detoxified, the first dose should be given as soon as possible. The dose of dimercaprol is 4 mg/kg i.m. every 4 hours for 3–4 days.

Intravascular hemolysis and subsequent hemolytic anemia may complicate the clinical picture. In extreme cases, these hemolytic manifestations may cause renal failure.

Arsenicals increase capillary permeability and cause extensive interstitial fluid losses (''third-space'' shifts). If the patient is hypotensive, hypovolemia should be presumed and corrected before the use of sympathomimetics.

Infrequently Used Blister Agents

Phenyldichloroarsine (PD) is a variant of Lewisite, is very irritating to eyes and mucous membranes, and causes rapid blister formation on exposed skin (0.5–1 hour). Exposure to this agent can cause nausea and vomiting.

Casualty management requires protective mask with charcoal inserts and protective clothing. Decontamination of closed areas may be accomplished with bleach or bicarbonate solutions. No decontamination of open areas is needed.

Ethyldichloroarsine (ED) produces a vapor harmful only on long exposure. The liquid form causes blisters with exposures of less than 1 minute. Immediate irritation occurs with delayed formation of bullae. If liquid droplets are inhaled, pulmonary edema and respiratory damage may occur. Eye injury occurs on exposure.

Medical providers should be provided with both protective masks and overgarments. Decontamination in closed spaces may be accomplished with bleach. No decontamination is needed in open areas as the substance decomposes rapidly.

Methyldichloroarsine (MD) is another rapidly acting blister agent with effects, decontamination, and detection similar to ED.

Nonlethal Agents

Perhaps the most information available to the public exists about the nonlethal agents. This is simply because they are in current use by many law enforcement agencies in the United States and other countries. Some of these agents may be encountered by an emergency physician. Most of these agents are entirely unclassified, and access to data about them is easily obtained.

LACRIMATOR AGENTS

Lacrimator agents (''tear gas'') have been extensively used by law enforcement agents, and the military. They have gained widespread acceptance as a means of nonlethal control of crowds, riots, and for subduing barricaded criminals (Fig. 100.5). They are also sold as hand-held self-defense weapons (chemical Mace and cogeners) in some states.

Proponents of the use of lacrimator agents feel that, if used correctly, the noxious exposure is transient and of no significant longterm consequence. This view is certainly not universally held (32). The very nature of a crowd means that the exposure to the weapon will be difficult to control and the effects will be indiscriminate.

With the ubiquitous use of these agents by police and law enforcement departments, it is quite likely that these agents will be treated in a civilian emergency department. Widespread area use may cause many casualties and disrupt the function of several emergency departments. Medical personnel can be exposed to residual agent on the victim's skin or clothes.

The munitions themselves are not innocuous. Projectiles may cause lethal injury from kinetic or explosive effects if either the projectile or fragments strike the victim. This is not only true in tear gas projectiles but in munitions designed for military

Table 100.6. Blister Agents

Blister agents primarily affect eyes, lungs, and skin.
Effects may be immediate or delayed depending on the agent.

Distilled mustard (HD)
  HD is H more purified and has less odor and a slightly greater blistering power than the more impure mustard chemical. It is also more stable in storage.

  Chemical name—Bis(2-chloroethyl) sulfide
  Formula—$(ClCH_2CH_2)_2S$

  Molecular weight—159.08
  Vapor density (compared to air)—5.4
  Liquid density—1.2685 at 25°C
  Boiling point—217°C calculated; decomposition temperature—149° to 177°C

  Rate of hydrolysis—Half-life is 8.5 minutes in distilled water at 25°C and 60 minutes in salt water at 25°C

  Hydrolysis products—Hydrogen chloride and thiodiglycol

  Stability in storage in steel or aluminum containers

  Very little action on metals or other materials when pure

  Garlic odor

  Median lethal dosage (MLD_{50}):
    Inhalation—1500 mg/min/m^3
    Skin absorption (masked personnel)—10,000 mg/min/m^3

  Ocular injury—200 mg/min/m^3

  Dermal absorption—(masked personnel)—2000 mg/min/m^3. Wet skin absorbs more mustard than dry skin. For this reason HD exerts a casualty effect at lower concentrations in hot humid weather, since the body is moist with perspiration. The dosage given above for skin absorption applies to temperatures of approximately 21°–27°C, as the body would not be perspiring excessively at these temperatures. Above 27°C, perspiration causes increased skin absorption. The incapacitating dosage drops rapidly as perspiration increases; at 32°C, 1000 mg/min/m^3 could be incapacitating.

  Rate of detoxification—Very low. Even very small, repeated exposures are cumulative in their effects or more than cumulative due to sensitization. This has been shown in the post-war case histories of workers in mustard-filling plants. Exposure to vapors from spilled HD causes minor irritative symptoms. Repeated severe exposure to such vapors can produce pulmonary damage.

  Clinical effects—Eyes are very susceptible to low concentrations; higher concentrations are required to produce incapacitating effects on skin.

  Rate of action—Delayed—usually 4–6 hours until first symptoms appear. (Latent periods have been observed, however, up to 24 hours and, in rare cases, up to 12 days.)

  Protection required—Protective mask and permeable protective clothing for vapor and small droplets; impermeable clothing for protection against large droplets, splashes, and smears.

  Persistency—Depends upon munition used and the weather. Heavily splashed liquid persists 1–2 days in concentrations that can cause casualties under average weather conditions, and a week to months under very cold conditions.

Nitrogen mustard (HN-1)
  Chemical name—2,2-Dichlorotriethylamine
  Formula—$(ClCH_2CH_2)_2NC_2H_5$
  Molecular weight—170.08

  Vapor density—(compared to air)—5.9
  Liquid density—1.09 at 25°C

Decomposition temperature—Decomposes before boiling point is reached.

Rate of hydrolysis—Slow due to low solubility in water

Hydrolysis products—Hydroxyl derivatives and condensation products. (Intermediate products, all of which are toxic, are produced during hydrolysis.)

Stability in storage—Polymerizes slowly and stable enough for munition use.

Action on metals or other materials—Slight corrosion of steel at 65°C.

Odor—Faint fishy or musty odor.

Median lethal dosage (MLD_{50})—
  Inhalation—1500 mg/min/m^3
  Skin absorption (masked personnel)—20,000 mg/min/m^3

Median incapacitating dosage (ICt_{50})—
  Ocular injury—200 mg/min/m^3

Dermal absorption (masked personnel)—9000 mg/min/m^3

Rate of detoxification—Not detoxified; cumulative

Clinical effects—Eyes are susceptible to low concentration; higher concentrations are required to produce incapacitating effects by skin absorption. Toxicity may be delayed 12 hours or longer.

Protection required—Protective mask and permeable protective clothing for vapor and small droplets; impermeable clothing for protection against large droplets, splashes, and smears.

Persistency—Depends on munitions used and the weather. Somewhat shorter than duration of effectivness for HD, whose heavily splashed liquid persists 1–2 days under average weather conditions, and a week or more under very cold conditions.

Nitrogen mustard (NH-2)
  Highly unstable and is no longer seriously considered for use as a military chemical agent. It is more toxic than NH-1.

  Chemical name—2,2'-Dichloro-N-methyldiethylamine
  Formula—$(ClCH_2CH_2)_2NCH_3$
  Molecular weight—156.07
  Vapor density (compared with air)—5.4
  Liquid density—1.15 to 20°C
  Boiling point—75°C at 15 mm Hg. At atmospheric pressure, HN-2 decomposes below boiling point

  Decomposition temperature—Decomposes before boiling point is reached. Instability of HN-2 is associated with its tendency to polymerize or condense; the reactions involved could generate enough heat to cause an explosion.

  Rate of hydrolysis—Hydrolysis is slow except where alkali is present. Dimerizes rapidly in water

  Hydrolysis products—Complex condensates or polymers

  Stability in storage—Not stable

  Action on metals or other materials—None

  Odor—In dilute form like soft soap. In high concentrations fruity.

  Median lethal dosage (MLD_{50}) (by inhalation)—3000 mg/min/m^3

  Median incapacitating dosage (ICt_{50})—
    Ocular injury—100 mg/min/m^3
    Dermal absorption (masked personnel)—Somewhere between the values given for HN-1 and HN-3.

  Rate of detoxification—Not detoxified

continues

Table 100.6. *Continued*

Clinical effects—Dermal and ocular toxicity mainly. HN-2 has the greatest blistering power of the nitrogen mustards in vapor form, but is intermediate as a liquid blistering agent. Toxic eye effects are produced more rapidly than HD. Skin effects may be delayed 12 hours or longer.

Protection required—Protective mask and permeable protective clothing for vapor and small droplets; impermeable clothing for protection against large droplets, splashes, and smears.

Persistency—Depends on munitions used and the weather. Somewhat shorter than duration of effectiveness for HD, whose heavily splashed liquid persists 1–2 days under average weather conditions, and a week or more under very cold conditions.

Nitrogen mustard (HN-3)
The most stable in storage of the three nitrogen mustards.

Chemical name—2,2'2''-trichlorotriethylamine
Formula—$N(CH_2CH_2Cl)_3$
Molecular weight—204.54
Vapor density (compared with air)—7.1
Liquid density—1.24 at 25°C
Boiling point—256°C calculated, decomposes. At atmospheric pressure, HN-3 decomposes below boiling point.

Decomposition temperature—Decomposes before boiling point is reached; relatively high.

Rate of hydrolysis—Very slow due to low solubility in water.

Hydrolysis products—$N(CH_2CH_2OH)_3$ and hydrogen chloride in dilute solutions. Dimer formation in higher concentrations.

Stability in storage—Stable enough for use as a munition even under tropical conditions. However, the agent darkens and deposits a crystalline solid in storage.

Action on metals or other materials—None if HN-3 is dry.

Odor—None when pure

Median lethal dosage (MLD_{50}):
Inhalation—1500 mg/min/m³
Dermal absorption (masked personnel)—10,000 mg/min/m³

Median incapacitating dosage (ICt_{50})
Ocular injury—200 mg/min/m³
Dermal absorption (masked personnel)—2,500 mg/min/m³. This information is based on estimates and indicates that HN-3 closely approaches HD in vapor toxicity and that it is the most toxic of the nitrogen mustards.
Rate of detoxification—Not detoxified; cumulative.

Rate of action—Most symptoms are delayed 4–6 hours (as after exposure to HD) but, in some cases, lacrimation, eye irritation, and photophobia develop immediately.

Protection required—Protective mask and permeable protective clothing for vapor and small droplets; impermeable clothing for protection against large droplets, splashes, and smears.

Persistency—Considerably longer than for HD (See HD).

Mustard-T mixture (HT)
A mixture of 60% HD and 40% T, sulfur and chlorine compound similar in structure to HD. It is a clear yellowish liquid with an odor similar to that of HD. HT has a strong blistering effect, has a longer duration of effectiveness, is more stable, and has a lower freezing point than HD. Its low volatility makes effective vapor concentrations in the field difficult to obtain. Properties are essentially the same as those of HD.

Clinical effects—Causes blisters, irritates the eyes, and is toxic when inhaled
Protection required—Protective mask and permeable protective clothing for vapor and small droplets; impermeable protective clothing for protection against large droplets, splashes, and smears.

Decontaminants—bleach

Persistency—Depends on munitions used and the weather. Somewhat longer than duration of effectiveness of HD, whose heavily splashed liquid persists 1–2 days under average weather conditions, and a week or more under very cold conditions.

Phosgene oxime (CX)
Dichloroformoxime-CCL_2NOH

CX may appear as a colorless, low-melting point (crystalline) solid or as a liquid. It has a high vapor pressure, slowly decomposes at normal temperatures (depending on temperature and humidity), boils at 53° to 54°C at 28 mm Hg, melts at 39° to 40°C, and is readily soluble in water. It has a disagreeable odor.

Clinical effects—CX is a powerful irritant which produces immediate pain varying from a mild irritancy sensation to severe local pain. Severe irritation of the mucous membranes. When CX comes in contact with the skin, the area becomes blanched in 30 seconds and is surrounded by erythema. A wheal forms in about 30 minutes and the blanched area turns brown in about 24 hours, scab formation in a week. The scab generally falls off in about 3 weeks. Itching may be present throughout healing which, in some cases, may be delayed beyond 2 months.

Protection required—A proper fitting protective mask protects the respiratory system; the remainder of the body can be protected by a complete set of protective clothing.

Decontaminants—Because of the rapid reaction of CX with the skin, decontamination will not be entirely effective after pain occurs. Nevertheless, decontamination should be accomplished as rapidly as possible by flushing the area with large amounts of water to remove any agent that has not reacted with the skin.

Lewisite (L)
Chemical name—Dichloro(2-chlorovinyl)arsine
Formula—$ClCH:CHAsCL_2$
Molecular weight—207.35
Vapor density (compared with air)—7.1
Liquid density—1.89 at 20°C
Boiling point—190°C
Decomposition temperature—Above 100°C

Rate of hydrolysis—Rapid for vapor and dissolved Lewisite. Low solubility in water limits hydrolysis.

Hydrolysis products—Hydrogen chloride and chlorovinyl-arsenious oxide. The latter is a nonvolatile blister-forming solid not readily washed away by water. Alkaline hydrolysis destroys these blister-forming properties.

Stability in storage—Stable in steel or glass container

Action on metals or other materials—None if L is dry

Odor—very little when pure

Median lethal dosage (MLD_{50})—Inhalation—1200–1500 mg/min/m³

Dermal absorption (masked personnel)—100,000 mg/min/m³. When the humidity is high, it hydrolyzes rapidly and it is difficult to maintain a concentration sufficient to blister bare skin. This difficulty is still further increased by the high vapor pressure and short duration of effectiveness of Lewisite.
Median incapacitating dosage (ICt_{50})—
Ocular injury (from vapor)—Below 300 mg/min/m³
Dermal absorption (masked personnel)—Over 1500 mg/min/m³. Lewisite irritates the eyes and skin and gives warning of its presence.

Clinical effects—Mainly dermal and ocular toxicity. An exposure of 1500 mg/min/m³ produces severe corneal damage to the eyes. It has the same blistering action on the skin as HD, even though the lethal dosage for lewisite is much higher.

Rate of action—Rapid

continues

Table 100.6. *Continued*

Protection required—Protective mask and permeable protective clothing for vapor and small droplets; impermeable protective clothing for protection against large droplets, splashes and smears.

Persistency—Somewhat shorter than for HD. Very short duration under humid conditions.

Mustard-Lewisite mixture (HL)

Mustard-lewisite mixture is a variable of HD and lewisite which provides a low-freezing mixture for use in cold weather operations or as high-altitude spray. Properties are listed for the eutectic mixture (the mixture having the lowest possible freezing point), which is 63% Lewisite and 37% HD by weight. Other mixtures, such as 50-50, may be prepared to meet predetermined weather conditions and have advantages over the eutectic mixture because of the increased HD content.

Molecular weight—186.4 (calculated on basis of eutectic mixture 63% L and 37% HD)

Vapor density (compared with air)—6.5

Liquid density—Between the densities of the components; approximately 1.66 at 20°C.

Boiling point—Indefinite, but below 190°C

Decomposition temperature—Above 100°C

Rate of hydrolysis—Lewisite is rapidly hydrolyzed in the liquid or vapor state; HD hydrolyzes slowly at ordinary temperatures.

Hydrolysis products—Hydrogen chloride, thiodiglycol, and chlorovinylarsenious oxide. Alkaline hydrolysis destroys the blistering properties.

Stability in storage—Stable in lacquered steel containers.

Action on metals and other materials—Little or none if dry.

Median lethal dosage (MLD$_{50}$)—
Ocular injury—About 200 mg/min/m^3
Dermal absorption—1500–2000 mg/min/m^3

Odor—garlic

Clinical effects—Dermal and ocular toxicity are very high. Produces immediate burning and irritation of skin and erythema within 30 minutes; blistering delayed about 13 hours.

Protection required—Protective mask and permeable protective clothing for vapor and small droplets; impermeable protective clothing for protection against large droplets, splashes, and smears.

Persistency—Depends on munitions used and the weather. Somewhat shorter than that of HD, whose heavily splashed liquid persists 1–2 days under average weather conditions and a week or more under very cold conditions.

Phenyldichloroarsine (PD)

Although phenyldichloroarsine is classed as a blister agent, it also acts as a vomiting compound.

Chemical name—Phenyldichloroarsine
Formula—$C_6H_5AsCl_2$
Molecular weight—222.91
Vapor density (compared with air)—7.7
Liquid density—1.65 at 20°C
Boiling point—252–255°C

Decomposition temperature—Stable to boiling point

Rate of hydrolysis—Rapid

Hydrolysis products—Hydrogen chloride and phenylarsenious oxide

Stability in storage—Very stable

Action on metals or other materials—None

Odor—None

Median concentration detectable (by nasal and throat irritation)—0.9 mg/m^3

Median lethal dosage (MLD$_{50}$) (by inhalation)—2,600 mg/min/m^3

Median incapacitating dosage (ICt$_{50}$)—16 mg/min/m^3 as a vomiting agent; 1800 mg/min/m^3 as a blistering agent.

Rate of detoxification—No specific information, but like related arsenicals, PD is probably rapidly detoxified in sublethal dosages.

Clinical effects—Dermal and ocular toxicity—About 30 percent as toxic to the eyes as HD; that is 633 mg/min/m^3 would produce casualties by eye injury. On bare skin PD is about 90 percent as blistering as HD, but is decomposed immediately by wet clothing. Immediate effect on eyes; effects on skin delayed 30 minutes to 1 hour

Protection required—Protective mask and permeable protective clothing for vapor and small droplets; impermeable protective clothing for protection against large droplets, splashes, and smears.

Persistency—Depends on munitions used and the weather. Somewhat shorter than that of HD under dry conditions; Short duration when wet. (Heavily splashed liquid HD persists 1–2 days under average weather conditions, and a week or more under very cold conditions.)

Ethyldichloroarsine (ED)

Ethyldichloroarsine was introduced by the Germans in March 1918 in an effort to produce a volatile agent with a short duration of effectiveness that would be quicker acting than DP or HD and that would be more lasting in its effects than PD

Chemical name—Ethyldichloroarsine
Formula—$C_2H_5AsCl_2$
Molecular weight—174.88
Vapor density (compared with air)—6.0
Liquid density—1.66 at 20°C
Boiling point—156°C
Decomposition temperature—Stable to boiling point

Rate of hydrolysis—Rapid

Hydrolysis products—Hydrogen chloride and ethylarsenious oxide

Stability in storage—Stable in steel

Action on metals or other materials—None on steel; attacks brass at 50°C; destructive to rubber and plastics

Odor—Fruity, but biting and irritating

Medial lethal dosage (MLD$_{50}$)—
Inhalation—3000–5000 mg/min/m^3, depending on the period of exposure. Since ED is detoxified by the body at an appreciable rate, the product of concentration and time is not a constant. As "time" increases, "concentration" does not decrease proportionately. For example, exposure to 40 mg/m^3 for 75 minutes might have an effect similar to that produced by exposure to 30 mg/m^3 for 166 minutes.

Skin absorption—100,000 mg/min/m^3
Median temporarily incapacitating dosage (ICt$_{50}$) by inhalation—5 to 10 mg/min/m^3

Clinical effects—Dermal and ocular eye toxicity. Vapor is irritating but not harmful to eyes and skin except on prolonged exposure. Liquid ED has approximately one-twentieth the blistering action of liquid lewisite. Irritating effect on nose and throat, is intolerable after 1 minute at moderate concentrations; blistering effect is less delayed than with HD, whose skin effects may be delayed 12 hours or longer.

Protection required—Protective mask and permeable protective clothing for vapor and small droplets impermeable protective clothing for protection against large droplets, splashes, and smears.

Persistency—Short

Reprinted with permission: U.S. Army FM3-9, U.S. Air Force 355-7.

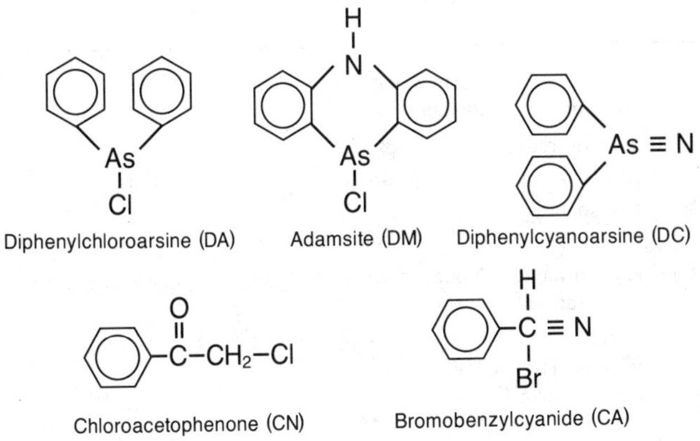

Diphenylchloroarsine (DA)　　Adamsite (DM)　　Diphenylcyanoarsine (DC)

Chloroacetophenone (CN)　　Bromobenzylcyanide (CA)

Figure 100.5. Riot control agents.

and civilian grenade launchers. Smaller devices are frequently aimed at the face, and both ocular and facial trauma may result.

Hand-held "gas grenades" are usually pyrolytic smoke generators, and not bursting devices. As such, burn victims may result from either direct contact with the grenade or secondary fires. Once aerosolized in this manner, prevailing atmospheric conditions determine the path of the agent. This dependence on air flow may lead to substantial toxicity in enclosed areas. Common lacrimator agents are listed in Table 100.7:

Lacrimator Agents

CA—Bromobenzylcyanide
CS—Ortho-chlorobenzylidenemalononitrile
CR—Dibenoxazepine
CN—2 Chloroacetophenone
CNC—Chloroacetophenone in chloroform
CNS—Chloroacetophenone and chloropicrin in chloroform
　　Bromacetone
　　Benzyl bromide
　　Ethyl bromoacetate

General Principles of Therapy

Patients with respiratory distress should receive oxygen, and the airway evaluated for edema. An intravenous line and cardiac monitoring are appropriate, but may not be possible when faced with mass exposure to these agents. Most of these patients will recover without sequelae with only decontamination as therapy. In these situations, medical care should be reserved for those who are in objective distress. All patients with exposure to a lacrimator agent will be in subjective distress.

In severely symptomatic patients, arterial blood gases and chest x-rays should be obtained. Bronchospasm may be treated with usual bronchodilator therapy.

The second priority is decontamination and removal from exposure. Significant decontamination may be achieved by simply undressing and showering the patient even if the agents are not completely water-soluble. Contaminated skin should be cleansed with soap and water. Showers may sweep hair contaminants onto eyes and skin and transiently reactivate symptoms.

The eyes should be examined and treated with topical antibiotics and mydriatics as needed. Topical antibiotics may be helpful while irrigating the eye, but need not be dispensed with the patient. Eyes should not be patched in a chemical injury. Vesiculations and bullae should be treated as a second-degree

chemical injury and skin should be copiously irrigated with saline. Patients with respiratory distress after exposure is terminated should be observed for the development of bronchospasm. Pneumonia and pulmonary edema are late complications. Prophylactic antibiotics and steroids are controversial and probably not efficacious.

CS

CS (o-chlorobenzylidene malonitrile) is the standard riot control agent used by the United States armed forces. It is available in a variety of munitions designed for both small and large area dispersion. CS is insoluble in water, and soluble in alcohol, ether, and carbon disulfide. It is effective as aerosolized particles generated by pyrolytic generators. An aerosolized spray may also be generated by Freon or similar propellants (Paralyzer).

The "effective" concentration of CS is about 5 mg/m^3. The estimated lethal dose is about 6000 mg min/m^3, but this is based on animal studies. Ocular symptoms may be found with concentrations as low as 4 μg/m^3.

Symptoms of exposure to CS include profuse nasal and ocular discharge, photophobia, a burning sensation of all exposed mucous membranes, and conjunctival irritation. A longer exposure may produce tightness in the chest, shortness of breath, malaise, and a feeling of suffocation. A headache is not uncommon after even relatively brief exposure, and both malaise and headache may persist for several hours. Panic reactions are quite commonly provoked by an intense desire to escape from the agent.

When applied directly to the skin, it produces extreme irritation and erythema. Moistened skin will have a burning sensation and bullae may be produced with high concentrations and longer duration of exposure. When humidity is higher, the skin lesions produced are more severe, but this is most likely related to opening of sweat ducts in the increased humidity. In addition to the direct irritant effects, an allergic eczema reaction may also be produced. Gross contamination of eyes with concentrated material may lead to structural damage.

Exposure to CS spray is usually harmless, but skin manifestations such as ulcerations, facial edema, and allergic dermatitis have been reported (33). Characteristically, the areas of greatest exposure will develop redness and burning on the first day. On the following day edema may occur with diffuse facial swelling.

CN

CN (2-chloroacetophenone) is the standard tear gas used by local law enforcement agencies and is the active ingredient in many hand-held tear gas projectors. It is considered by most authorities to be similar in effects to CS, but somewhat milder. The median incapacitating dose is slightly higher than for CS, and the clinical effects are less pronounced.

CN is toxic at 35–40 mg/m^3 (34). The maximum safe dosage for shortterm inhalation is 500 mg/m^3. At least five deaths have resulted from exposure to higher concentrations, primarily in enclosed areas (35, 36). The lethal dose has been calculated at about 1000 mg/m^3 from animal studies.

Allergic contact dermatitis requiring treatment with steroids has been noted after multiple exposures (37). Rarely, blistering and symptoms similar to those seen with CS are noted.

CN is a relatively volatile agent and produces a blue-white

Table 100.7. Lacrimators

These agents cause increased lacrimation and irritation of the skin. Since tear compounds produce only transient casualties, they are widely used for riot control, and for situations where longterm incapacitation is unacceptable. When released indoors, they can cause serious illness or death.

Chloroacetophenone (CN)
  Chemical name—Chloroacetophenone
  Formula—$C_6H_5COCH_2Cl$
  Molecular weight—154.59
  Vapor density (compared with air)—5.3
  Liquid density—1.187 at 58°C
  Boiling point—248°C

Decomposition temperature—Stable to boiling point

Rate of hydrolysis—Not readily hydrolyzed

Hydrolysis products—Hydrogen chloride and a hydroxyacetophenone

Stability in storage—Stable

Action on metals or other materials—Tarnishes steel slightly

Odor—Fragrant; similar to that of apple blossoms

Median lethal dosage (MLD50)—7000 mg/min/m³, dispersed from solvent; 14,000 mg/min/m³ dispersed from thermal grenade.

Median incapacitating dosage (ICt50)—80 mg/min/m³

Rate of detoxification–Rapid; effects disappear in minutes. High concentrations may cause skin irritation which usually disappears within a few hours.

Clinical effects—Dermal and ocular toxicity. Irritating; not toxic in concentrations likely to be encountered in the field. Rapidly acting.

Protection required—Protective mask

Persistency—Short, because the compounds are disseminated as an aerosol.

CNC
  Chemical name—None; solution of chloroacetophenone in chloroform
  Formula—Chloroform–CHCl₃ (70 parts by weight)
  CN—$C_6H_5COCH_2Cl$ (30 parts by weight)
  Molecular weight—128.17 (on basis of components)
  Vapor density (compared with air)—4.4
  Liquid density—1.40 at 20°C

Boiling point—Variable. Increases as chloroform boils off and approaches the boiling point of pure CN (60 to 247°C).

Volatility—This is an indeterminant value under field conditions because the vapor pressure of chloroform is high and the vapor pressure of CN is low. Therefore, there is no true volatility as in the case of a pure compound.

Decomposition temperature—Stable to the boiling point.

Rate of hydrolysis—Not readily hydrolyzed.

Hydrolysis products—Hydrogen chloride and a hydroxyacetophenone.

Stability in storage—Adequate

Action on metals or other materials—Slight

Odor—Similar to that of chloroform

Median lethal dosage (MLD50)—The active ingredient is CN; therefore, with allowance for the diluting action of the chloroform vapor, the median lethal dosage would be similar to that of CN, about 11,000 mg/min/m³.

Median incapacitating dosage (ICt50)—About 80 mg/min/m³

Rate of detoxification—Rapid for sublethal exposure

Clinical effects—Dermal and ocular toxicity. Irritating; Instantaneous acting.

Protection required—Protective mask

Persistency—Short, because the compound is disseminated as an aerosol.

CNS
  Chemical name—None; mixture of chloroacetophenone, chloropicrin, and chloroform.
  Formula—
    CN—$C_6H_5COCH_2Cl$ (23%)
    Chloropicrin (PS)—$C(NO_2)Cl_3$ (38.4%)
    Chloroform—CHCL₃ (38.4%)
  Molecular weight—141.78 (on basis of components)
  Vapor density (compared with air)—About 5.0
  Liquid density—1.47 at 20°C

Boiling point—No fixed temperature; varies from 60° to 247°C

Decomposition temperature—Stable to boiling point

Rate of hydrolysis—Not readily hydrolyzed

Hydrolysis products—Hydrogen chloride and a hydroxyacetophenone

Stability in storage—Stable

Action on metals or other materials—Very little

Odor—Like flypaper

Median lethal dosage (MLD50)—11,400 mg/min/m³

Median incapacitating dosage (ICt50)—60 mg/min/m³

Dermal and ocular toxicity—Irritating; not toxic

Rate of action—Instantaneous

Clinical effects—In addition to having effects described under CN, CNS also has the effects of chloropicrin (PS), which acts as a vomiting compound, a choking agent, and a tear compound. CNS may cause lung effects similar to those of CG and also may cause nausea, vomiting, colic, and diarrhea which may persist for weeks. The lacrimatory effects of PS are much less marked than those of CN and are relatively unimportant for CNS, as shown by the fact that these effects are no greater than with CNC, which contains no PS. Effects of CNS may be prolonged for weeks.

Protection required—Protective mask

Persistency—Short

CNB
  CNB was adopted in 1920 and remained in use until it was replaced by CNS. The advantage claimed for CNB was that its lower chloroacetophenone content made it more satisfactory than CNS for training purposes. Actually, the same result can be obtained with CNC merely by using a lower concentration.

Chemical name—None; solution of chloroacetophenone in benzene and carbon tetrachloride

Formula—
  CN—$C_6H_5COCH_2Cl$ (10 parts by weight)
  Carbon tetrachloride—CCl₄ (45 parts by weight)
  Benzene—C_6H_6 (45 parts by weight)
Molecular weight—119.7 (on basis of components)
Vapor density (compared with air)—Approximately 4
Liquid density—1.14 at 20°C

Boiling point—Varies from 75° to 247°C as the two solvents are vaporized

Decomposition temperature—Above 247°C

Rate of hydrolysis—None

continues

Table 100.7. *Continued*

Hydrolysis products—None

Stability in storage—Adequate

Action on metals or other materials—Very slight

Odor—like benzene

Median lethal dosage (MLD$_{50}$)—No specific data, but about the same as for CN (11,000 mg/min/m^3)

Median incapacitating dosage (ICt$_{50}$)—80 mg/min/m^3

Rate of detoxification—Rapid, if poisonous amounts of solvents have been inhaled

Clinical effects—Dermal and ocular toxicity. Not toxic. Instantaneous acting.

Protection required—Protective mask

Persistency—Short

Bromobenzylcyanide (CA)
   Chemical name—Bromobenzylcyanide
   Formula—C$_6$H$_5$Ch(Br)CN
   Molecular weight—196.0
   Vapor density (compared with air)—6.7
   Liquid density—1.47 at 20°C
   Boiling point—242°C, but with decomposition

Decomposition temperature—Decomposes slowly at 60°C; more rapidly as the temperature increases. Decomposes completely at 242°C. Hydrobromic acid and dicyanostilbene are formed.

Rate of hydrolysis—Very slow

Hydrolysis products—Complex condensation products

Stability in storage—Fairly stable in glass, leadlined, or enamel-lined containers

Action on metals or other materials—Vigorous corrosive action on all common metals except lead. Reaction with iron may be explosive

Odor—Like soured fruit, but not unpleasant

Median lethal dosage (MLD$_{50}$)—Estimated 8000–11,000 mg/min/m^3. Volatility is too low to permit attaining a lethal dosage in the field. Lethal dosage may be obtained in enclosed places.

Median incapacitating dosage (ICt$_{50}$)—About 30 mg/min/m^3

Rate of detoxification—Rapidly detoxified at the low concentrations ordinarily encountered

Clinical effects—Dermal and ocular irritation.

Rate of action—Instantaneous

Protection required—Protective mask

Persistency—Depends on munitions used and the weather. Heavily splashed liquid persists 1–2 days under average weather conditions.

O-chlorobenzylidene malononitrile (CS)
   For riot control CS exists as a family of three forms: CS, CS1, and CS2. CS identifies the white crystalline form. It has a minimum purity of 96 percent; it is insoluble in water and ethanol, but is soluble in methylene chloride. CS is thermally dispersed as a solid aerosol. CS1 is a mixture consisting of 95% crystalline CS blended with 5 percent silica aerogel to reduce agglomeration, and micropulverized to 3- to 10-micron size to achieve the desired respiratory effects when dispersed as a solid aerosol. CS2 is CS containing a hydrophoric compound, Cab-O-sil, which improve the physical characteristics of CS by reducing agglomeration and hydrolysis.

Chemical name—O-chlorobenzylidene malononitrile

Formula—ClC$_6$H$_4$CHC(CN)$_2$
Molecular weight—188.5
Density—1.04 g/ml crystalline density; 0.24–0.26 g/ml bulk density

Boiling point—310–315°C (with decomposition)

Decomposition temperature—Unknown

Rate of hydrolysis—Rapid for dissolved CS. CS is only slightly soluble in water (about 0.008 weight percent at 25°C); thus solid CS in water is hydrolyzed relatively slowly.

Hydrolysis products—O-chlorobenzaldehyde and malononitrile

Stability in storage—Stable

Action on metals—Very slight action on steel

Odor—Pepper-like

Median lethal dosage (MLD$_{50}$)—61,000 mg/min/m^3 (M7A3 grenade)

Median incapacitating dosage (ICt$_{50}$)—10–20 mg/min/m^3

Rate of detoxification—Quite rapid. Incapacitating dosages lose their effects in 5–10 minutes.

Clinical effects—Highly irritating

Rate of action—Very rapid

Protection required—Protection is provided by the protective mask and ordinary field clothing secured at the neck, wrist, and ankles. Personnel handling CS should wear rubber gloves for additional protection.

Persistency—Varies, depending upon amount of contamination

Reprinted with permission: U.S. Army FM3-9, U.S. Air Force 355-7.

powder on release. Since the agent is volatile, aeration and vacuuming are usually sufficient for decontamination. If this is not sufficient, CN can be decomposed with a 5% bicarbonate solution.

Chloroacetophenone can be dissolved in chloroform for use as a spray (CNC). It is the same as CN in all aspects. CNC is the active ingredient in chemical mace and similar sprays. A similar compound, chloroacetophenone and chloropicrin in chloroform (CNS), is also suitable for use as a spray but longer lasting due to the chloropicrin additive. Chloroacetophenone in benzene and carbon tetrachloride (CNB) is another agent that is similar in effects to CN, but is more potent.

These agents should be decontaminated and treated as if they were CN or CS. Protection from them is the same as for CN.

Detection of the agents is the same as CN, since a major portion of active agent is CN.

CR

CR, or dibenoxazephine, is a potent lacrimator agent developed in Great Britain in 1962 as an alternative to CS and CN (38). Despite greater potency (10 times that of CS), toxic effects are less common with this agent. CR is a crystalline powder that is the parent compound to the antipsychotic drug loxapine. It is capable of being deployed as either an aerosol or as a liquid. The estimated "effective" concentration of CR is about 1 mg/m^3. There have been no known lethalities, but the estimated lethal dose is greater than 100,000 mg min/m^3. Eye irritation in volunteers occurs at a concentration of 2 μg/m³. Exposure to even weak concentrations of CR produces an intense lacrimator reaction with bleopharospasm. Contact with skin may produce the customary irritation, pain, and erythyma, but skin sensitization is unusual. Areas exposed to CR may become painful during showers (or other water contact) 24–48 hours after exposure (39). General decontamination principles with water shower and soap should be used for skin decontamination. Conjunctival irritation may require topical anesthesia and copious irrigation with saline solution.

CA

Bromobenzylcyanide (CA) is a highly irritating agent similar to CN. It has been used as a riot control and "tear gas" agent. Protective mask and garments are similar to CN. Decontamination in open and closed spaces is also similar to that used for CN. CA may be detected by the military M-nitrobenzene detector kit.

VOMIT AGENTS

This is a class of riot control chemicals summarized in Table 100.8. These agents are normally solids which vaporize on heating and then condense to form aerosols.

DM

DM, also known as "nausea gas" or Adamsite, is not commonly used in the United States. It produces both the respiratory and skin irritant effects of the lacrimating agents and profound nausea. It is substantially more toxic than the other lacrimator agents and is not used by civilian law enforcement agents. Exposure to this agent is unlikely to be found in a civilian emergency department.

The standard charcoal insert protective mask will work well for inhalation protection. The skin irritation is relatively minor, and ordinary clothing will adequately protect against this agent.

No decontamination is needed in the field. Bleach solution is appropriate for decontamination.

DC

Diphenylcyanoarsinine (DC) is an irritating agent with rapid onset of rhinorrhea and lacrimation symptoms associated with headache, nausea, and severe vomiting.

The standard charcoal insert protective mask will work well for inhalation protection. The skin irritation is relatively minor and ordinary clothing will adequately protect against this agent.

No decontamination is needed in the field. Alkali solution or DS2 will suffice for decontamination in confined areas.

DA

Diphenylchloroarsinine (DA) $(C_6H_5)_2AsCl$ is an agent with a very rapid onset of both respiratory and skin irritation effects combined with a severely nauseating effect. This agent has been used in riot control and training but is not thought to be produced or currently stocked.

The standard charcoal insert protective mask will protect against inhalation. Skin irritation is minor, and ordinary cloth-

ing will usually protect against this. Dilute bleach solution is adequate for field decontamination.

INCAPACITATING AGENTS

Plans for incapacitating of troops without harming them have fascinated military commanders for ages. In the early 1960s the addition of lysergic acid diethylamide (LSD) to water supplies of troops was suggested. Scientists have experimented to accomplish the same purpose with other agents including LSD, mescaline, psilocybin, psilicine (40). Only one chemical agent has had documented production and use. Undoubtedly, other classified agents exist and have probably been produced in restricted amounts.

BZ

BZ (benzilate) is a delayed onset (1–4 hours after exposure) incapacitation agent. It caused fast heartbeat, dizziness, vomiting, dry mouth, blurred vision, stupor, confusion, and random activity. A shrub within the vicinity may appear as an immense danger and a threat. The affected soldier may react as if drunk, may just sit quietly, or may become belligerent to those about him. As such, it is ideal to incapacitate troops without wounding or killing them. Of course, if the exposed person is attempting to drive a tank or an aircraft the effects of such an agent could produce accidents and injury.

Protective mask with charcoal absorptive filters is adequate to protect medical providers. The compound is not absorbed through the skin.

Decontamination may be accomplished with water and soap wash or with dilute bleach.

Any poison would be used for incapacitation or sabotage. Poisons which have delayed effects (latency) that are stable in both humid and hot environments and that have no specific syndrome are not easily diagnosed. If the poison is highly toxic, so that only a small amount leads to disease or death, it may be added to a water supply or food source. One such poison proposed for military use is fluoroacetic acid, which will inhibit the tricarboxylic acid cycle. Symptoms of poisoning may include muscle twitching, visual disturbance, motor restlessness, seizures, fecal and urinary incontinence, coma, cardiac dysrhythmias, cardiogenic shock, and finally death through respiratory or cardiac depression. The latency period is 30 minutes to 6 hours after ingestion (41).

EXPLOSIVE DEVICES

An explosive is a "stable" material that will rapidly change from solid (or liquid) to an expanding gas, upon detonation or combustion. The rapid increase in pressure by the expanding gas causes an explosion. Although many substances can be exploded in one form or another, only those substances that are intended to produce an explosion are categorized as such.

Explosives are generally selected for their use on the basis of velocity of detonation. For example, an explosive having a rapid detonating velocity is generally used for cutting and breaching, while that of a lower velocity will be used for cratering and quarrying.

Explosives produce voluminous quantities of products of combustion that may be dangerous. It is difficult to calculate the relative danger of these combustion products in open air,

Table 100.8. Vomiting Agents

Vomiting compounds cause great discomfort to victims; when released indoors, they can cause serious illness or death.

Diphenylchloroarsine (DA)
  Chemical name—Diphenylchloroarsine
  Formula—$(C_6H_5)_2AsCl$
  Molecular weight—264.5
  Vapor density (compared with air)—Forms no appreciable vapor
  Liquid density—1.387 at 50°C
  Boiling point—333°C with decomposition

Decomposition temperature—300°C

Rate of hydrolysis—Slow in mass but rapid when finely divided

Hydrolysis products—Diphenylarsenious oxide and hydrogen chloride. The oxide is very poisonous if taken internally.

Stability in storage—Stable when pure

Action on metals or other materials—None when dry

Odor—None

Median lethal dosage (MLD_{50})—15,000 mg/min/m^3 (estimated)

Median incapacitating dosage (ICt_{50})—12 mg/min/m^3 if received over 10 minute periods; probably higher for shorter time.

Clinical effects—Dermal and ocular toxicity, vomiting. Very rapid acting, within 2 or 3 minutes after 1 minute exposure.

Protection required—Protective mask

Persistency—Short, because compound is disseminated as an aerosol.

Adamsite (DM)
  Chemical name—Diphenylaminochloroarsine (also phenarsazine chloride)
  Formula—$C_6H_4(AsCl)(NH)C_6H_4$
  Molecular weight—277.57
  Vapor density (compared with air)—Forms no appreciable vapor
  Solid density—1.65 at 20°C
  Boiling point—410°C calculated
  Vapor pressure—Negligible

Decomposition temperature—Above melting point

Rate of hydrolysis—Quite rapid when in aerosol form. When solid DM is covered with water, a protective oxide coating is formed hindering further hydrolysis.

Hydrolysis products—Diphenylarsenious oxide and hydrogen chloride. The oxide is very poisonous if taken internally.

Stability in storage—Stable when pure

Action on metals or other materials—Slight when dry

Odor—No pronounced odor

Median lethal dosage (MLD_{50})—15,000 mg/min/m^3

Median incapacitating dosage (ICt_{50})—22 mg/min/m^3 for one 2 minute exposure, 8 mg/min/m^3 for 60 minute exposure

Rate of detoxification. Quite rapid in small amounts. Incapacitating amounts lose their effects after about 30 minutes.

Clinical effects—Dermal and ocular toxicity. Irritating; relatively nontoxic. Rapidly acting in about 1 minute is required for temporary incapacitation at a concentration of 22 mg/min/m^3.

Protection required—Protective mask

Persistency—Short, because compounds are disseminated as an aerosol.

Diphenylcyanoarsine (DC)
  Chemical name—Diphenylcyanoarsine
  Formula—$(C_6H_5)_2AsCN$
  Molecular weight—255.0
  Vapor density (compared with air)—Does not form appreciable vapor
  Liquid density—1.3338 at 35°C
  Boiling point—350°C with decomposition

Decomposition temperature—about 25% decomposed at 300°C. Largely decomposed as a result of dispersing blast.

Rate of hydrolysis—Very slow

Hydrolysis products—Hydrogen cyanide and diphenylarsenious oxide

Stability in storage—Stable at all ordinary temperatures

Action on metals or other materials—None

Odor—Similar to a mixture of garlic and bitter almonds

Median lethal dosage (MLD_{50})—10,000 mg/min/m^3. It would be nearly impossible to build up a vapor concentration of DC which would be lethal within a practicable time.

Median incapacitating dosage (ICt_{50})—30 mg/min/m^3 for 30-second exposure; 20 mg/min/m^3 for 5 minute exposure.

Rate of detoxification—Rapid. Incapacitating amounts lose their effect after about 1 hour

Clinical effects—Dermal and ocular toxicity. Irritating; Very rapid acting. Higher concentrations are intolerable in about 30 seconds

Protection required—Protective mask

Persistency—Short, because the compound is disseminated as an aerosol

Reprinted with permission: U.S. Army FM3-9, U.S. Air Force 355-7.

but in closed spaces, the products may be very toxic. Gases from the explosion can include carbon monoxide, hydrogen sulfide, and oxides of nitrogen.

Explosives can be divided into two general categories:

Low Explosives or Propellant Explosives

Low grade explosives are ignited and then burn quite rapidly. Black power, developed by the Chinese in the 10th century, is the prototype of these explosive agents. A major effect of the "low" explosive agents is the force produced by rapidly expanding gases. Nitrocellulose and smokeless gunpowder are common propellant explosives. Many other specialized propellant explosives have been developed as rocket propellants.

High Explosives or "Detonating" Explosives

Detonating or "secondary" explosives detonate. The detonation occurs as the parent compound undergoes a rapid change into several gaseous byproducts. Detonating explosives are somewhat more stable than low grade explosives, and the explosive process can be initiated only by trauma or shock. The archetype high explosive is nitroglycerine, discovered by the Italian, Ascanio Soberro. Alfred Nobel made it much safer to use in the formulation of dynamite (a combination of nitroglycerine, ammonium nitrate, and fuller's earth or wood pulp). Some modern detonating explosives are listed in Table 100.9.

Initiating or "primary" explosives are a separate class of very sensitive high explosives that require a mild shock to detonate. Fulminate of mercury, lead styphnate, and lead azide are examples of initiating explosives that have been used as primer material in shells or blasting caps to initiate another explosive. Detonators are considered to be such a small portion of the explosion that no specific effects are attributable solely to the detonator.

Fuel-air explosives are designed to have a rapid propagation of combustion in a gaseous mix. These munitions either vaporize a liquid or release a gas into the air. Alternatively both a fuel and an oxidizer may be simultaneously released. The

Table 100.9   Common Explosives

Aluminum containing polymeric propellant
Aluminum ophorite
Amatex
Amatol
Ammonal
Ammonium nitrate explosive mixtures
Aromatic nitro-compound explosive mixtures
Ammonium perchlorate
Ammonium picrate
ANFO (ammonium nitrate-fuel oil mixture)
Baratol
Baronol
BEAF [1,2-bis(2,2-difluoro-2-nitroacetoxyethane)]
Black powder
Blasting powder
Blasting gelatin
BTNEC [bis(trinitroethyl)carbonate]
BTNEN [bis(trinitroethyl)nitramine]
BTTN (1,2,4-butanetriol trinitrate)
Butyl tetryl
Calcium nitrate
Cellulose hexanitrate
Chlorate explosive mixtures
Composition A and variations
Composition B and variations
Composition C and variations
Copper acetylide
Cyanuric triazide
Cyclotrimethylenetrinitramine (RDS, Cyclonite, hexogen)
Cyclotetramethylentetranitramine (HMX, Octogen)
Cyclotol
DATB (diaminotrinitrobenzene)
DDNP (diethyleneglycol dinitrate)
Dimethylol dimethyl methane dinitrate
Dinitroethyleneurea
Dinitroglycerine
Dinitrophenol
Dinitrophenolates
Dinitrophenyl hydrazine
Dinitroresorcinol
Dinitrotoluene-sodium nitrate
DIPAM
Dipicryl sulfone
Dipicylamine
DNDP (dinitropentano nitrile)
DNPA (2,3-dinitropropyl acrylate)
Dynamite
EDDN (ethylene diamine dinitrate)
EDNA
Ednatol
EDNP (ethyl 4,4-dinitropentanoate)
Erythritol tetranitrate
EGDN (ethylene glycol dinitrate)
Ethyl tetryl
Fulminate of mercury
Fulminate of silver
Fulminate of gold
Guanyl nitrosamino guanyl tetrazene
Guanyl nitrosamino guanylidene hydrazine
Guncotton
Heavy metal azides
Hexanite
Hexanitrodiphenylamine
Hexanitrostilbene
Hexolites
Hydrazoic acid

KDNBF [potassium dinitrobenzo-furoxane]
Lead azide
Lead mannite
Lead mononitroresorcinate
Lead picrate
Lead stypinate
Magnesium ophorite
Mannitol hexanitrate
MDNP (methyl 4,4-dinitropentanoate)
MEAN (monoethanolamine nitrate)
Mercury fulminate
Mercury oxalate
Mercury tartrate
Metriol trinitrate
Minol-2 (40% TNT, 40% ammonium nitrate, 20% aluminum)
MMAN (Monoethylamine nitrate)
Mononitrotoluene-nitroglycerin mixture
NIBTN (nitroisobutametriol trinitrate)
   (virtually any nitrated organic mixture)
Nitric acid and carboxylic fuels
Nitrocellulose
Nitrogelatin
Nitrogen trichloride
Nitrogen tri-iodide
Nitroglycerin (NG, RNG, Nitro, glyceryl trinitrate, trinitroglycerin)
Nitroglycide
Nitroglycol (EGDN)
Nitroguanidine
Nitroparaffins
Nitronium perchlorate
Nitrostarch
Nitrourea
Octol (75% HMX, 25% TNT)
Organic aminine nitrates
Organic nitramines
PEX (RDX and plasticizer)
Penthrinite
Pentolite
PYX [2,6-bis(picrylamino)-3,5-dinitropyridine)]
PETN [Nitropentaerythrite, pentaerythrite tetranitrate, pentaerythritol tetranitrate]
Picramic acid and its salts
Picramide
Picrate of potassium
Picratol
Picric acid
Picryl chloride
Picryl fluoride
PLX (95% nitromethane, 5% ethylenediamine)
Polynitro aliphatic compounds
Polyolpolynitrate-nitrocellulose gels
Potassium chlorate and lead sulfocyanate
Potassium nitrate
Potassium nitroaminotetrazole
Silver acetylide
Silver azide
Silver oxalate
Silver syphanate
Silver tartarate
Silver tetrazene
Sodatol
Smokeless powder
Sodium azide
Sodium dinitro-ortho-cresolate
Sodium picramate
Tacot (tetranitro-2,3,5,6-dibenzo-1,3a,4,6a-tetrazapentalene)

continues

Table 100.9. *Continued*

TATB (triaminotrinitrobenzene)	Trimethylolethane trinitrate-nitrocellulose
TEGDN (triethylene glycol dinitrate)	Trimonate
Tetrazene	Trinitroanisole
Tetranitrocarbazole	Trinitrobenzene
Tetryl (2,4,6-tetranitro-N-methylaniline)	Trinitrobenzoic acid
Tetrytol	Trinitrocresol
TMETN (trimethylolethane trinitrate)	Trinitro-meta-cresol
TNEF (trinitroethyl formal)	Trinitronaphthalene
TNEOC (trinitroethyl orthoformate)	Trinitrophenol
TNEOF (trinitroethyl orthoformate)	Trinitrofluoroglucinol
TNT (trinitrotoluene, trotyl, tilite, triton)	Trinitroresorcinol
Torpex	Trinitrol
Tridite	Urea nitrate
Trimethylol ethyl methane trinitrate composition	

(Per Firearms and Explosives Operations Branch, Bureau of Alcohol, Tobacco, and Firearms)

This is a list of many of the explosives used in industry. As mentioned previously, many other mixtures and compounds may be explosively detonated but are not normally used or classified as explosives. This list does not include all explosive mixtures; and blasting caps, ignitors, and caps are not included.

Higgins SE. Commerce in explosives; list of explosive materials. Fed Reg 1990;55(9):1306–1307.

idea is to approximate the ideal fuel-vapor/oxidizer mixture so that combustion is propagated as an explosive wave. The toxic effects would be limited to the primary fuel and oxidizer prior to an explosion and the products of combustion of the fuel and oxidizer after an explosion. Liquified petroleum gas, hydrogen, and vaporized petroleum products have all been proposed for these munitions.

Current United States Military and Civilian Explosives

HIGH EXPLOSIVES

The following are common high explosives:

Ammonium nitrate Most widely used raw material in commercial explosives and may be present in up to 96% concentration.

Amatol 80/20 (mixture of ammonium nitrate and TNT)—it is a widely available commercial explosive.

RDX (cyclotrimethylenetrinitramine)

TNT (trinitrotoluene)

Nitroglycerine Very sensitive to both stock and vibration.

PETN—pentaerythritetetranitrate (used in detonating cord and blasting caps)

Composition B (TNT and RDX mixture)

Composition C-3 (obsolete)

Composition C-4 (RDX plus plasticizer)

Tetrytol

Tetryl

Picric acid

Dynamite (multiple compositions)*

Gelatin dynamite (multiple compositions)*

Ammonia dynamite (multiple compositions)*

Commercial dynamites are classified according to the percentage of nitroglycerine (by weight) they contain; for example, 50% straight dynamite contains 50% nitroglycerine. Ammonia and gelatine dynamite are named for the equivalency to straight dynamite; 40% ammonia dynamite is as strong as 40% straight dynamite (It doesn't necessarily contain 40% nitroglycerine). Ammonia dynamite contains both ammonium nitrate and nitroglycerine in different compositions.

LOW EXPLOSIVES

The following is a listing of low explosive compounds:

Nitrostarch

Nitrocellulose

"Smokeless" gunpowder These may contain either nitrocellulose or nitroglycerin or both. In addition, some contain nitroguanidine.

Black powder

Most solid rocket fuels Compositions of specific rocket fuels are generally proprietary or classified and are available on a "need to know" basis.

Fireworks Compositions of fireworks are generally proprietary information and not available. Strontium, barium, cobalt, and copper salts are commonly found agents which add color to a blast.

Nitroglycerine

Nitroglycerine solution is readily absorbed through the skin and by inhalation. Toxic effects include headache, dizziness, syncope, and hypotension (42).

The exposure limit for nitroglycerine is 0.5 ppm. There is no documented record of any toxic effect other than headache at these present-day industrial exposure levels to nitroglycerine and dynamite. Chronic exposure to TNT and dinitrobenzene from production of munitions has been associated with both toxic hepatitis and aplastic anemia (43, 44, 45). Munitions workers have also been noted to have an excess number of ischemic heart disease deaths (46). There is additional evidence that these agents should be considered as possible carcinogens (47). Monitoring of blood pressure is important.

The vasodilator effect of nitroglycerine is due to smooth muscle relaxation. Intracranial and meningeal vessel vasodilation causes a headache. Nitroglycerine does not induce methemoglobinemia.

Other Explosive Agents

Pentaerythritetetranitrate (PETN) may cause skin rashes and gastrointestinal distress. RDX (cyclonite, hexogen, or cyclotrimethylenetrinitramine) is toxic to the nervous system, liver, and kidneys. Acute exposure can cause nausea, vomiting, convulsions, and coma. Chronic toxicity can cause liver and kidney damage. Tetrazene, an initiating explosive used in percussion caps, may lead to asthma or dermatitis in workers who are exposed (48).

INCENDIARY DEVICES

Incendiaries can produce injury or death by thermal radiation and by direct contact burns. Incendiary agents cause combustion of flammable materials and thermal damage or degradation of nonflammable materials. Both flame and incendiary agents are employed against personnel and material targets. Incendiary agents usually contain additives and metals to increase their generated temperatures. Depletion of oxygen and cargon monoxide production are additional causes of incapacitation or lethality to personnel (49).

Flame Agents

Flame agents are based primarily on hydrocarbon fuels and may be either gasoline or blends of gasoline with fuel oil of any type. All hydrocarbons including fuel and diesel oils, jet fuel, kerosene, and automotive and aviation gasoline can be modified with thickeners and gellants for use as flame agents. Recent advances have placed primary emphasis on thickened metal alkyls in encapsulated form with the favored flame agent being thickened triethylaluminum (TEA). For field use, almost any grade of hydrocarbon, usually gasoline, can be used in the preparation of flame agents (49).

UNTHICKENED FUEL

Because oil burns much more slowly than gasoline, oil-gasoline mixtures are used in flame throwers. Increase in proportion of oil increases the range and reduces the amount of fuel burned in flights to the target. However, portable flame throwers are being phased out with the acquisition of encapsulated flame system using TEA as its agent. These encapsulated agent flame systems are effective at significantly longer ranges and are also more accurate (49).

MIXTURES

Mixtures of fuel oils and gasoline may be used. Mixtures are purely a matter of choice, and ingredient proportions need not be exact. Regardless of the proportions of oil and gasoline used, such mixtures are still referred to as unthickened fuels (49).

Unthickened fuel is used only in portable flame throwers and may be used when thickened fuel is not available.

THICKENED FUEL

Thickened fule increases the range of flame throwers, imparts slower burning properties, gives clinging qualities, and causes flames to rebound off walls or other surfaces and to go around corners. It is used in fire bombs, flame throwers, and flame field expedients. The target on which the fuel is employed and the means of dispersion used must be known for determination of the optimum mixture. More thickener is used in thickened fuel for fire bombs and mechanical flame throwers than for portable flame throwers (49).

NAPALM

Napalm is a prime incendiary munition. Napalm is specifically defined as the aluminum salt or soap of a mixture of naphthenic and aliphatic carboxylic acids that is used to thicken gasoline (49). The napalm formula is about 50% mixed acids derived from coconut oil, 25% oleic acid (carbolic acids), and mixed naphthenic acids from petroleum to form the remainder. The gelling agent is usually aluminum hydroxide. Commonly, the name is used to refer to the product of thickened gasoline used as an incendiary (49).

Napalm is designed to burn vigorously and to "stick" to burning objects. It is used against both objects and personnel. Thickened gasoline has a combustion temperature of 675°C.

A similar product is a combination of petroleum fuel plus rubber polystyrene as a gel. These formulas may also contain powdered magnesium and sodium nitrate as gelling agents. Typical combustion temperatures are about 1000°C (49).

THICKENERS

M1 thickener (Napalm)—M1 thickener, known as Napalm, is mixed aluminum soap in which approximately 50% of the organic acids are derived from coconut oil and 25% from oleic acid. It is issued as small granular particles, variable in color from light tan to brown (49). The thickening qualities also vary. An undesirable feature of M1 thickener is that it absorbs moisture rapidly from the air; the moisture degrades the gelling properties so that the thickener may become unusable. When M1 thickener is stirred into gasoline at temperatures ranging from 16–29°C, it swells until the entire volume of gasoline becomes a more or less homogeneous gel. The gel may vary in consistency from a fluid to a rubbery material, depending on the amount of thickener added. If allowed to set undisturbed: this compound becomes a semirigid jelly-like form. If the gel is shaken violently, stirred vigorously, or forced through a small opening under pressure, it becomes almost liquid again, but resumes a jelly-like form upon standing. The percentage of M1 thickener used in thickening fuels ranges from 4% for portable flame thrower fuels to 12% for the highest consistency likely to be required (49).

M2 THICKENER (NAPALM)

M2 incendiary oil thickener is a mixture of 95% M1 thickener and 5% devolatilized silica aerogel or other approved antiagglomerant. Moisture content may vary between 0.4–1.0%. M2 thickener is an improvement over M1 thickener for use in fire bombs because its free flowing and faster setting characteristics allow its use in continuous mechanical mixers. M2 is less suitable than M1 for use in flame thrower fuels because it results in decreased firing range. M2 thickener is not suitable for gelling jet fuels (49).

M4 THICKENER (IS0)

M4 incendiary oil thickener is a di-acid aluminum soap of isooctanoic acids derived from isooctyl alcohol or isooctyl aldehyde obtained from the oxidation of petroelum. M4 thickener is a very fine white granular material. Moisture content is no more than 1.2% with chlorides not exceeding 0.3% and sulfate not exceeding 1.5%. It contains 2% Santocel C or Attasorb clay which serves as an antiagglomerant. M4 thickener is much less susceptible to moisture in the air and has a higher density than the other thickeners. For thickened fuels of comparable consistency, about one-half as much M4 thickener as M1 thickener is required, and the mixing time for M4 thickener is about one-half to one-tenth of that for M1 thickener. Peptizers are needed with M4 thickener at about 0°F. Compared with fuels prepared with other available thickeners, fuels prepared with M4 thickener are superior in flame thrower firing performance with respect to range, burning, and target effects. M4 thickener is preferred over other thickeners (49).

OTHER THICKENERS

Natural rubber and isobutyl methacrylate (polymer AE) are effective thickeners but are much more difficult to use than M1, M2, and M4 thickener. IM incendiary oil, type I, is an example of the use of isobutyl methacrylate, polymer AE. The type mixture has the following composition (49):

Ingredient	Percent
Stearic acid	3.0
Isobutyl methacrylate, polymer AE	5.0
Calcium	2.0
Gasoline	88.75
Water	1.25

Three additional IM incendiary oil mixtures are obtained by varying the above ingredients (49).

PEPTIZERS

A peptizer is any substance that hastens or facilitates the dispersal of a colloidal material in a dispersion medium. In addition, the peptizer lowers the final viscosity of the thickened fuel and facilitates the formation of a gel at lower temperatures than would otherwise be possible. At temperatures below 60°F, M1 and M2 thickeners fail to disperse in gasoline or blended fuel, and either the fuel must be warmed or a peptizer must be employed. Usually it is much easier and safer to use a peptizer than to warm the fuel. Cresylic acid and octoic acid (2-ethylhexoic acid) are the most common peptizers, cresylic acid (mixtures of xylenols and cresols) is preferred for use with M1 and M2 thickeners, and 2-ethylhexoic acid is preferred for use with M4 thickener. There are wide variations in the properties and behavior of the several ingredients of thickened fuel (49).

In most cases, munitions containing thickened hydrocarbon fuels are equipped with white phosphorus igniters to insure ignition because the bursting charge may or may not cause ignition. Since ignition of white phosphorus is prevented by water, a sodium igniter is used in a thickened fuel munition to be dropped over water. Both thickened fuels in the portable flame thrower are ignited by a red phosphorus-tipped metal match which scratches an igniting mixture (49).

NAPALM B

Napalm B is a special fire bomb fuel formulation developed by the Air Force. It was originally composed of a solution containing 50% polystyrene, 25% benzene, and 25% gasoline by weight (49). This composition was later revised to 46% polystyrene, 21% benzene, and 33% gasoline by weight. Napalm B withstands high velocity impact dissemination more effectively than M2-thickened gasoline gels, resulting in less burned en route, and more fuel delivered on target. Because the original composition did not burn efficiently at moderately low temperatures, the formula was revised to improve the combustion characteristics at such temperatures (49).

METAL INCENDIARIES

Metal incendiaries include those consisting of magnesium in various forms and powdered or granular aluminum mixed with powdered iron oxide. Magnesium is a soft metal which, when raised to its ignition temperature, burns vigorously in air. In either solid or powdered form it is used as an incendiary filling; in alloyed form it is used as the casing for small incendiary bombs such as the M126 which has a casing of the following composition: 4.45% aluminum, 1.25% zinc, and 94.31% magnesium. This alloy has an ignition temperature of between 548–598°C (49).

Magnesium Incendiaries

Chemical symbol—Mg
Atomic weight—24.32
Melting point—651°C
Boiling point—1,110°C
Ignition temperature—623°C
Burning temperature—1982°C—Burning temperature is variable, as it depends upon rate of heat dissipation, rate of burning, and other factors
Density—1.74 at 5°C
Combustion product—magnesium oxide (MgO)

BURNING CHARACTERISTICS

Magnesium burns with a blinding white flame. It melts as it burns; and the liquid metal, burning as it flows, drops to lower levels, igniting all combustible materials in its path. Burning stops if oxygen is prevented from reaching the metal or is cooled below its ignition temperature. Magnesium does not have the highest heat of combustion of the metals, but none of the other metals has been successfully used singly as an air-combustible incendiary. Certain other metals may be alloyed with magnesium without affecting its ignitability. The alloyed metal has strength to withstand distortion, whereas pure magnesium does not. In massive form, magnesium is difficult to ignite. This problem is overcome by packing a hollow core in the bomb with thermite, an easily ignited mixture which supplies its own oxygen and burns at a very high temperature (49).

Thermite and Thermate Incendiaries

Thermite is essentially a mixture of powdered iron oxide (Fe_2O_3) and powdered or granular aluminum. The aluminum has a higher affinity for oxygen than iron has and, if a mixture of iron oxide and aluminum powder is raised to the combusion temperature of aluminum, an intense reaction occurs (49):

$$Fe_2O_3 + 2Al \rightarrow Al_2O_3 + 2Fe + heat$$

Under favorable conditions, the thermite reaction produces temperatures of about 2200°C (3992°F). This is high enough to turn the newly formed metallic iron into a white hot liquid which acts as a heat reservoir to prolong and to spread the heat or igniting action (49).

Thermite is composed of approximately 73% ferric oxide

and 27% fine granular aluminum. The thermate mixture composed of thermite with various additives is used as a component in igniter compositions for magnesium bombs. A number of such compositions were developed before World War II. Three of these were Therm-8, Thermate-Th2 (formerly Therm-8-2), and Thermate-TH3 (formerly Therm-64-C) (49). Therm-8 was the precursor of later and improved igniting formulations. TH2 differed from Therm-8 in that it contained no sulfur and slightly less thermite. TH3 was found to be superior in either Therm-8 or TH2 and was adopted for use in the incendiary magnesium bombs. The composition by weight of TH3 is as follows (49):

INGREDIENT	Percent
Thermite	68.7
Barium nitrate	29.9
Sulfur	2.0
Oil (binder)	0.3

The TH3 core is ignited by the primer; this burning core then melts and ignites the magnesium alloy body. The incendiary action is localized since there is little scattering action (49).

TH4

Another thermate (TH4) filling has been developed to replace the original thermite (TH1) used since 1943 (49). The action of TH4 is essentially the same as that of TH1. The principal differences are in the percentages of the basic ingredients, the addition of an oxidizer (barium nitrate), and the substitution of polyester resin for sodium silicate as a binder. The composition of TH4 is (49):

Ingredient	Percent
Iron oxide, magnetic	51
Barium nitrate	22
Aluminum, granular	19
Aluminum, grained	3
Polyester grained (Laminac 4116)	5

OIL AND METAL INCENDIARY MIXTURES

PT1 is a complex thick mixture of magnesium dust, magnesium oxide, and carbon with a sufficient amount of petroleum distillate and asphalt to form the paste (49).

PTV is an improved oil and metal incendiary mixture with the following compositions (49):

INGREDIENTS	Percent
Polybutadiene	5.0 ± 0.1
Gasoline	60.0 ± 1.0
Magnesium	28.0 ± 1.0
Sodium nitrate	6.0 ± 0.1
P-aminophenol	0.1

Incendiary bombs containing PT1 or PTV mixture are easily ignited since they contain many combustible ingredients. These formulations contain both metal and an oxidizer (49).

WHITE PHOSPHORUS MUNITIONS AND PYROPHORIC FUELS

White phosphorus is a waxy translucent substance that ignites spontaneously on contact with air. It is usually preserved under water and becomes a liquid at 44°C. White phosphorus is used extensively in the construction of military weapons and fireworks and is a component of insecticides and rodenticides.

Following an explosion of a white phosphorus munition, flaming droplets of white phosphorus are flung widely about and dense clouds of white smoke with a typical "garlic-like" smell are produced. The flaming pieces of phosphorus cause thermal tissue damage but may also cause high-speed projectile injuries (50). The smoke is produced by the oxidation of phosphorus to acid, which can damage lungs and skin. Some "tracer" bullets have white phosphorus as a major component. This may lead to absorption of retained phosphorus fragments after either an explosion of a phosphorus-based shell or after a bullet wound with a tracer bullet (51).

Flaming white phosphorus should be extinguished by immersing the pieces in water. Surface particles and particles embedded in clothing should be promptly removed. During transport, the medical providers should cover the burned areas with moistened cloths to prevent further burning.

The military recommends washing these wounds with a 1% copper sulfate solution which combines with the phosphorus to form copper phosphate, which can be readily identified as black particles (52). These black pieces can be easily be debrided. If the particles are not debrided, they will be absorbed, and systemic effects may occur.

Once debridement is completed, then no further copper sulfate solution is needed. The copper sulfate solution should not be used for a prolonged period because of the risk of systemic copper poisoning manifested by vomiting, diarrhea, oliguria, intravascular hemolysis, hematuria, hepatic necrosis, and cardiovascular collapse. The hemolysis is thought to be due to copper's inhibition of the erythrocyte hexose monophosphate shunt.

To minimize copper absorption, the wound may be irrigated with a solution of 5% sodium bicarbonate and 3% copper sulfate suspended in 1% hydroxyethyl cellulose (53). Wet dressings of copper sulfate in any form should never be applied to the wound (54). Following debridement, the wound should be irrigated with copious amounts of water to remove the copper salts.

Phosphorus is highly fat-soluble and is easily absorbed from particles in the subcutaneous tissues or from the gastrointestinal tract if ingested. The two most common systemic effects are hepatotoxicity and renal damage, but changes in blood phosphorus and calcium levels may also be noted. ECG changes with prolongation of the QT interval, ST segment depression, T-wave changes, and bradycardia can also be noted (55). Sudden death has been reported in patients with reversed calcium-phosphorus ratios (56). Monitoring for electrocardiographic abnormalities and changes in serum calcium and phosphorus is appropriate for patients with significant wounds. In cases where systemic absorption is suspected, blood urea nitrogen, creatinine, serum phosphorus, and liver enzymes should be assessed frequently.

Phosphorus pentoxide, the white smoke associated with white phosphorus munitions, presents the same clinical picture as phosgene exposure. A patient can progress to pulmonary edema following the inhalation of phosphorus pentoxide smoke. This is managed symptomatically as phosgene toxicity.

Pyrophoric Fuels

Pyrophoric fuels are spontaneously flammable and combustible in air.

WHITE PHOSPHORUS (WP) AND EUTECTIC WHITE PHOSPHORUS (EWP)

White phosphorus, which is used primarily as a smoke agent, can also function as an antipersonnel flame compound capable of causing serious burns. Eutectic white phosphorus is a solution of 45% P_2S_5 in white phosphorus and is liquid at temperatures as low as $-40°F$. The dissemination efficiency of either form as flame is very low, as both are unthickened.

TRIETHYLALUMINUM (TEA)

Triethylaluminum thickened with polyisobutylene is a thickened pyrophoric agent. TEA reacts when it is disseminated in the atmosphere by spontaneously combusting.

White Phosphorus (WP)

During World War II, white phosphorus was used as a screening smoke and an incendiary. In attacks on fortified positions, the M15 WP hand grenade forced enemy abandonment after other methods had failed.

Chemical name—White or yellow phosphorus
Formula—P_4
Molecular weight 124.11
Density of solid—1.83 at 20°C
Boiling point—290°C
Vapor pressure and volatility—Not applicable
Decomposition temperature—None

Stability in storage—Stable if kept in an oxygen-free environment

Action on metals—None

Odor—like matches

Physiologic action—Burning solid or liquid WP burns the flesh; such burns heal very slowly. Vapors of WP are poisonous, producing bone decay. (No vapors are found in smoke.)

Protection required—None against smoke; flameproof clothing against burning particles

Plasticized White Phosphorus (PWP)

PWP is prepared by a series of steps. First, WP is melted and stirred into cold water; granules about 0.5 millimeter in diameter are produced. Then, the slurry of granules and water is mixed with a very viscous solution of synthetic rubber (40% GRS rubber in an organic solvent.) All of the granules become coated with a film of rubber and are thereby separated from each other. The mass is then folded, stretched, and refolded until the composition is homogeneous. This rubbery mass is dispersed by an exploding munition but does not break up to such an extent as WP; therefore, pillaring with PWP is much less marked than with WP.

Magnesium Munitions

Magnesium munitions are exclusively employed as flares. Burning magnesium metal produces magnesium oxide and heat. These munitions can also be used as incendiary devices.

Injuries that result from these munitions may combine the effects of both a caustic injury from the magnesium oxide and a thermal injury. The injury should be copiously irrigated to ensure that there is no caustic material remaining in the wound.

SMOKE GENERATING AGENTS

Methods of smoke generation, developed just prior to World War II, made it feasible to use screening smokes extensively in both offensive and defensive operations in World War II. Screening smokes were used to conceal movements and installations. The obscuring action of screening smokes is largely due to reflection and refraction of light rays by the individual suspended solid or liquid particles of which the smoke is composed (49). This obscuring action occurs to the greatest extent in the absence of light-absorbing particles such as carbon; white smokes, therefore, have the greatest screening action. Actually, white smokes are composed largely of colorless particles, and the white appearance is due to reflection and refraction of all the visible light rays. The fewer undeviated light rays which pass through the smoke particles, the more effective the smoke screen becomes. Smoke particles exhibit irregular individual motions which cause the smoke to diffuse and spread; larger particles settle out. The life persistency of a smoke cloud is determined chiefly by wind and convection currents in the air. Ambient temperature also plays a part in the disappearance of fog oils smoke.

A fume is a suspension of microscopic oxidized metallic particles 0.02–0.25 microns in diameter. This size of metal particle is ideal to penetrate into the lung with inhalation of the smoke (49). Metal fume fever can occur in those exposed for significant times to fumes from incendiary smoke munitions (49).

Tracheobronchitis and a mild pneumonitis are the most common manifestations of this illness. The patient may complain of fever, headache, cough, and chest discomfort. These symptoms generally resolve without residual effects.

Airway and parenchymal lung injury and pulmonary edema are less common, but may occur after exposure to smoke agents. Acute renal cortical necrosis may follow inhalation of some of the metals.

Treatment for this syndrome is the same as for metal fume fever. Since most cases resolve spontaneously without further therapy, only those with significant symptoms should be hospitalized. No special decontamination is necessary.

Water vapor in the air plays an important role in the formation of most smokes; for this reason, high relative humidity improves the effectiveness of most smokes. The water vapor exerts its effects not only through hydrolysis, but also by assisting the growth to effective size of hygroscopic smoke particles by hydration. If these particles are too small, they do not effectively scatter light rays and thus do not assist the screening action. Optimum size of smoke particles is 10^{-4} centimeters (1 micron) (49).

Smoke may be generated by mechanical or thermal means or by a combination. Screening smokes composed of solids are usually disseminated by a thermal method. This method can also be used for liquids. Subsequent cooling condenses the vapor of the solid or liquid into minute particles, which form the smoke. A chemical reaction may accompany the thermal process; for example, hexachloroethane (HC) is disseminated by the thermal process but smoke is not formed until certain chemical reactions take place.

Smoke may be injurious if very heavy concentrations are

inhaled for even a short time. (This is particularly true of HC smoke.) (49)

Titanium Tetrachloride (FM)

Traces of moisture cause FM to solidify; making it difficult to handle in spraying apparatus. Also the acidity of the smoke causes health effects (49).

Chemical Name—Titanium tetrachloride
Formula—$TiCl_4$
Molecular weight—189.73
Vapor density—Not applicable
Liquid density—1.7 at 20°C
Boiling point—135°C

Decomposition temperature—Above the boiling point

Rate of hydrolysis—Reacts immediately with water or water vapor.

Hydrolysis products—Solid $TiOCl_2$ and HCl, chiefly, but also $Ti(OH)_4$ if sufficient water is present.

Stability in storage—Stable in steel containers if FM is dry

Action on metals or other materials—None on steel if FM is dry; vigorous action if FM is moist. FM smoke is definitely corrosive.

Odor—Acrid

Protection required—None for ordinary smoke clouds; protective mask for heavy concentrations

Sulfur Trioxide-Chlorosulfonic Acid Solution (FS)

FS was developed during 1929 and 1930 to replace the more expensive and less effective FM. FS was used in the final phase of the Luzon Campaign (World War II), when smoke screens without fire hazard were desired (49).

Chemical name—None: solution of sulfur trioxide (SO_3) dissolved in chlorosulfonic acid ($ClSO_3H$)

Formula—55 parts by weight of SO_3 and 45 parts by weight of $ClSO_3H$

Molecular weight—96.47 (based on components)

Vapor density—Not applicable since FS does not exert its effect in vapor form

Liquid density—1.9 at 20°C
Boiling point—About 80°C (Decomposes)
Rate of hydrolysis—Instantaneous

Hydrolysis products—Sulfuric acid is produced by hydration rather than by hydrolysis of sulfur trioxide. Chlorosulfonic acid is hydrolyzed to form hydrogen chloride and sulfuric acid.

Stability in storage—Adequate if dry

Action on metals or other materials—None on metals if FS is dry; however, it is corrosive in the presence of moisture. Since FS smoke is made up of acid components, it will destroy any material that is decomposed by acids. An example of such a material is nylon. Drops of FS of sufficient size will decompose the nylon plastic and weaken or sever the fibers at the points of contact. FS is also highly injurious to many types of paint. Therefore, FS should not be used where possible damage to nylon or vehicle finishes may occur.

Odor—Acrid

Physiologic action—Liquid FS is highly irritating to the skin. The smoke causes a prickling sensation on the skin because of the minute acid particles of which it is composed. Splashes of liquid FS in the eye produce extremely painful acid burns. Exposure to heavy concentrations or prolonged exposure to ordinary concentrations may cause severe irritation of eyes, skin, and respiratory tract.

Protection required—None for ordinary smokes; protective mask for high smoke concentration. Heavy rubber gloves should be worn for handling the liquid.

HC Mixture (HC)

During World War I, the greatest single advance in smoke was probably made by Captain Berger of the French Army when he developed a pyrotechnic mixture in which carbon tetrachloride (CCl_4) and a metal (Zn) reacted to produce a volatile hygroscopic chloride as a dense smoke (49). While neither the United States nor Great Britain used the Berger mixture during World War I, American scientists later improved it by adding an oxidizer for the carbon so that it would not darken the smoke.

At the beginning of World War II, a mixture of another composition was prepared and was designated HC smoke mixture. In this mixture, CCl_4 was replaced by solid hexachloroethane. Ammonium chloride as a reducing agent and a perchlorate as an oxidizing agent were added. In 1940 after the fall of France, perchlorates were not available and chlorates were tested. Chlorates proved to be hazardous, however, because they often caused formation of free chloric acid which ignited the smoke mixture spontaneously. Further experimentation led to the development of the present HC smoke mixture (type C) which consists of zinc oxide, aluminum, and hexachloroethane (49).

As the HC mixture burns, intense heat and smoke are produced. By far the greater proportion of the smoke is zinc chloride, which rapidly absorbs moisture from the air to form particles of effective size. Most of the aluminum remains behind as solid aluminum oxide. During the process of smoke formation, small amounts of volatile aluminum, chloride and hexachloroethane are lost as vapor (49).

Stability—HC smoke mixture (type C) having a total moisture content of 0.6% is reasonably stable.

Physiologic action—As normally encountered, HC smoke has no physiologic action. It has a slightly acrid odor. In high concentrations such as might be encountered very near an operating munition, in an enclosed space, during exposure to dense HC screens, and during prolonged exposure to ordinary field concentrations, a sufficient concentration of zinc chloride may be encountered to produce toxic effects and the protective mask should be worn (49).

Oil Smoke

During World War II, a method of smoke generation was developed, based on production of minute oil particles by use of purely physical means (49). The most desirable drop size of these particles range from 0.5 to 1.0 micron (1 micron = 0.001 millimeter; 1 inch = 25.4 millimeters). The small drops of oil scatter light rays and produce a smoke which appears to be white. Actually, an individual drop would be transparent under magnification. These drops are produced as soon as the vaporized oil passes through the nozzle of a generator and is cooled by surrounding air. The air cools the oil vapor so quickly that only very small drops are able to form. The average size of the final drops is controlled by the concentration of the condensing vapor and the rate of cooling. If the oil vapor emerges from the nozzle at high velocity, large volumes of air are sucked into the vapor stream by the rushing vapor. The resulting dilution and cooling produces an enormous number of condensation nuclei. Unless the cooling effect is rapid, the larger drops tend to pick up the vapor lost by the small drops which vaporize more quickly than the larger drops. This tendency disappears as soon as the drops are cooled because fog oil has negligible vapor pressure at ordinary temperatures. Thus, the whole process depends upon a high temperature followed by quick cooling. The final oil smoke cloud is stable, and the life of the cloud is determined almost solely by meteorological conditions (49).

Physiologic action of oil smoke—Average field concentrations of oil smoke are harmless to personnel regardless of length of exposure. Breathing a high concentration of oil smoke for even extended periods produces no immediately apparent symptoms, but chest pains may develop later on. Oil in the lungs may be a causative factor in development of pneumonia and possibly other diseases. Operating personnel exposed to prolonged high concentrations of oil smoke should wear protective masks as much of the time as possible (49).

SIGNALING SMOKES

Smoke signals were utilized in ancient times in circumstances when hand and flag signals were not visible and where sound of voice or horn was not audible. However, during the black gunpowder era when battlefields were always enveloped in a thick haze, smoke could not be used for signaling. With the advent of smokeless powder, smoke signals again became feasible and are now an important means of communication. By prearrangement, colored smoke can be used to identify friendly units; to control the laying and lifting of artillery, mortar, and small arms fire; to identify targets; and to coordinate fire and maneuver of combat arms engaged in local assault operations. Colored smoke is nontoxic in ordinary field concentrations (49).

Means of Producing Signaling Smokes

Of four possible methods for producing signaling smokes, only one has been found feasible—that of volatilizing and condensing a mixture containing an organic dye. Of the dyes tested, the most satisfactory ones are the general types of azo, antraquinone, azine, or diphenylmethane dyes (49). The filling for a colored smoke munition is essentially a pyrotechnic mixture of fuel and a dye, with a cooling agent sometimes added to prevent excessive decomposition of the dye. The heat produced by the fuel volatilizes the dye, which then condenses outside the munition to form the colored smoke. The fuel is made up of a mixture of an oxidizing agent, such as potassium chlorate ($KClO_3$) and a combustible material such as sulfur or sugar. The burning time can be regulated by adjusting the proportions of oxidant and combustible material, and by use of coolants such as baking soda. Pyrotechnic mixes of colored smoke are

filled in cartridges, hand grenades, and canisters for use with projectiles such as the 105 millimeters (49).

BIOLOGIC WEAPONS

Biologic agents of war can be divided into two categories—live agents and biotoxins. Live biologic agents can be subdivided into four different categories:

DEBILITATION AGENTS

These diseases would cause a transient disease that temporarily incapacitates the military or selected portions of the civilian population. Delivery systems would be designed to affect the target populations such as military, air traffic controllers, or policemen, and other spread would be incidental.

A short-term disease that rapidly conferred immunity would be superb for this role. Diseases such as influenza, encephalitis, psittacosis, or salmonella, or staphyloccocal food poisoning are models for these agents. These diseases would be expected to cause relatively few fatalities.

INTERMEDIATE DISEASES

Diseases such as brucellosis, psittacosis, or tularemia may be employed with the intention of simply incapacitating the enemy for long periods of time. Part of the incapacitation would be the overloading of the medical system to deny its use for more conventional casualties. Terror and panic would obviously aid the effects of these agents. There would be substantial overlap between the first two categories in agents used in this role.

FATAL DISEASES

These diseases are designed to demoralize the population and kill. Diseases such as anthrax and plague are representative of these diseases. A major factor in the use of this type of weapon would be to panic both the military and the civilian population. A rapidly spreading disease with a highly visible component and abundant symptoms would enhance the terror of the biologic weapon to the civilian population.

DENIAL AGENTS

If the aggressor wished to deny all use of area such as airfields, oil wells, or other fixed emplacements, a very long-acting agent with a spore formation would be appropriate. In this regard, anthrax already had been both contemplated and tested for use in World War II by the British.

Biologic Weaponry Use

In 1972, over 50 nations, including the United States and the USSR signed the Biological Weapons Convention (57) that condemn the use or even development of biologic warfare agents. However, research in the area of biologic agents continues.

Current biotechnology may allow the development of organisms resistant to all known drugs or vaccines. Tailored bacteria or viruses would be unlike any current agents. Antibiotics and immunization may be completely useless against these agents. Tailoring could include a limited life span or a further genetic alteration after a given number of replications.

There is a practical reason that biologic agents are not used in warfare. Biologic agents rely on dispersal systems that are too random to use in a tactical environment. These infecting agents can spread unexpectedly.

Once released, the biologic agent is not easily controllable. Spread of the agent by wind and water can occur. A single person can carry the agent outside the target area and infect other areas of populations.

Possible Biologic Agents

These diseases have been proposed as possible biologic agents. Almost any disease that has or can be imagined could be used as a biologic agent.

POSSIBLE DISEASE AGENTS

These biologic agents have all been proposed or have been actively used in the past as war agents in one respect or another:

Anthrax
Brucella (brucellosis)
Encephalitis (various types) viruses
Clostridium perfringens
Influenza virus
Yersinia pestis (plague)
Chlamydia psittaci (Psittacosis)
Coxiella burnetti (Q fever)
Rift Valley fever virus
Smallpox virus
Trypanosoma parasites
Francisella tularensis (tularemia)
Yellow fever virus

DELIVERY SYSTEMS

Biologic agents can be delivered in multiple ways. Often advocated is an aerosolized spray. This can be done from a hand-held pressurized tank, low-flying aircraft, cruise missile, or even a spray bottle. The agents may also be dispersed in liquid form in many types of shells or missiles.

ANTHRAX

Anthrax is a disease produced by the *Bacillus anthracis* bacteria. Anthrax spores can be used as a biologic warfare agent and are easily disseminated by projectile. Anthrax can produce dermal lesions through cutaneous innoculation via skin breaks. Dermal pustules appear in 12–24 hours following the innoculation. The pustules develop into larger, erythematous based lesions with a central necrotic area. Systemic infection can follow as well as widening areas of necrosis. Death may occur in 5–6 days if untreated. Bacilli can be found in the exudate of lesions. Inhalation of anthrax spores can produce the pulmonary form of the disease which is a severe pneumonia. The organism is sensitive to penicillin.

BOTULINUM TOXIN

This is the clostridium botulinum exotoxin formed by the botulinum bacillus. Through repeated purification procedures, it has been obtained in a crystalline form and is one of the most lethal toxins known. There are at least six distinct types: A, B, C, D, E, and F. Types A, B, E, and F are known to be toxic to man; types C and D are toxic to animals but very rarely to humans.

Botulism is an acute, often fatal disease. It is characterized by vomiting, constipation, thirst, general weakness, headache, fever, dizziness, double vision, and dilation of the pupils. Paralysis is the usual cause of death. Muscular weakness and disturbance of vision are early symptoms. There is loss of accommodation, dimness of vision and double vision, accompanied frequently by roving of the eyes, and dizziness as a result of paralysis of the eye muscles. Difficulty in talking and swallowing and lack of coordination are striking features and in severe cases there is respiratory paralysis which is the immediate cause of death. There are no sensory changes. Gastrointestinal symptoms are variable and minor and consist of early nausea and vomiting, sometimes with diarrhea. Later there is persistent constipation. The fatality rate depends on the amount of the toxin ingested and other factors. Recovery is very slow; disturbances of vision and weakness may last for months.

Sources of the toxin are the bacteria *Clostridium botulinum* and *Cl. parabotulinum*, which are rodshaped, slightly motile, sporulating, gram-positive, anaerobic bacilli. The principal reservoir of these bacteria is soil. The bacteria grow and form their toxin under anaerobic conditions, usually in improperly preserved canned foods such as meats, seafoods, corn, string beans, spinach, and olives. Growth requires a neutral to moderately alkaline medium. Its resistance to sterilization by heat is reduced at low pH, which helps explain why preserved acid fruits are never implicated in outbreaks.

Transmission is through eating uncooked or improperly cooked food contaminated with botulinum toxin. Fresh, well-cooked foods are not involved, as heat destroys the toxin. The bacteria do not grow or reproduce in the human body; poisoning is due entirely to the toxin already formed in the ingested material. The toxin could possibly be introduced through breaks in the skin or by inhalation, as in the case of laboratory accidents.

Symptoms of poisoning usually do not appear until 12–72 hours after food containing the preformed toxin has been consumed; the length of time depends on the amount of toxin contained in the food consumed.

All persons are susceptible to the poisoning. The few who recover have an active immunity of uncertain duration and degree.

The disease has worldwide distribution; it may occur wherever improperly canned food products are consumed. Most cases of botulinum are caused by food that has received some preliminary treatment, such as canning, smoking, or pickling. Home-processed foods are usually responsible because the temperature of canning is not sufficient to kill the spores, and the foods are sometimes too old when canned. Foods packed in tin cans and contaminated with *C. botulinum* may produce gas, giving the appearance of "swells" (bulging of the can), but this is not always the case.

The mortality rate is approximately 65% in the United States, where the disease is usually produced as a result of eating contaminated canned foods. In Europe, the disease is usually produced as a result of eating contaminated smoked, salted, or spiced meats; and the mortality rate is about 25%.

The disease is not common enough to justify widespread immunization; however, active immunization with botulinum toxoid is of proven protective value for high risk groups such as laboratory technicians.

Treatment is mainly supportive. Antitoxin therapy is of

doubtful value, particularly where large doses of the toxin have been consumed. When a case of botulism is recognized, immediate search should be made for all other persons who may have eaten the suspected food; they should receive a prophylactic dose of polyvalent botulism antitoxin. Treatment after symptoms have appeared is of little avail. The gastrointestinal tract should be emptied to get rid of unabsorbed toxin; polyvalent antitoxin should be administered; and, if respiratory paralysis occurs, the use of a respirator may be helpful.

The toxin is stable for a week in nonmoving water. It persists for a long time in food when not exposed to air. The toxin is destroyed by boiling for 15 minutes or, when in food, by cooking for 30 minutes at 80°C (176°F). Botulinum spores resist boiling at atmospheric pressure for 6 hours; however, pressure cooking will destroy the spores. Botulinum toxin differs from other bacterial toxins in that it is not destroyed by gastrointestinal secretions.

STAPHYLOCOCCUS TOXIN (STAPHYLOCOCCUS FOOD POISONING)

This toxin is produced in food by certain strains of staphylococci. Since this toxin has a specific action on the cells of the intestinal mucosa, it is called an enterotoxin.

Staphylococcus food poisoning is produced following the ingestion of food in which various strains of staphylococci are growing. It is usually characterized by sudden, sometimes violent, onset of severe nausea; vomiting; stomach cramps; severe diarrhea; and prostration. Patients usually feel normal 24 hours after the attack begins.

Modes of transmission include consumption of contaminated custard-filled pastries, processed meats (particularly ham), and contaminated pasteurized milk from cows with infected udders. Improper food handling is responsible for many outbreaks.

Onset of symptoms may be up to 4 hours; however, usually 2–4 hours elapse between consumption of contaminated food and the appearance of symptoms.

The microorganisms that produce this toxin are distributed worldwide and are probably the principal cause of acute food poisoning. Fatalities are extremely rare. No immunization is available. Treatment is supportive.

Food poisoning is not contagious. Most outbreaks are small and confined to persons who have eaten from the same contaminated food supply.

The toxin is resistant to freezing, to boiling for 30 minutes, and to potable quantities of chlorine. The organisms that develop the toxin remain viable after 67 days of refrigeration.

REFERENCES

1. Hu H, Fine J, Epstein P, Kelsey K, et al. Tear gas—harassing agent or toxic chemical weapon? JAMA 1989;262:660–664.
2. Clarke R. The silent weapons. New York: David McKay, 1968.
3. Murphy S. Chemical warfare: the present position. Med War 1985;1:31–39.
4. Recommendations for protecting human health against potential adverse effects of long term exposure to low doses of chemical warfare agents. MMWR 1988;37:72–74.
5. Harris LW, Heyl WC, Stitcher DL, et al. Effects of 1,1'-oxydimethylene bis-(4-tertbutylpyridinium chloride) (SAD-128) and decamethonium on reactivation of soman and sarin-inhibited cholinesterase by oximes. Biochem Pharmacol 1978;27:757–761.
6. Rickett DJ, Glenn JF, Houston WE. Medical defense against nerve agents: new directions. Milit Med 1987;152:35–41.
7. Rengstorff RH. Accidental exposure to sarin: vision effects. Arch Toxicol 1985;56:201–203.
8. Duffy FH, Burchfiel JL, Bartels PH, et al. Long term effects of an organophosphate upon the human electroencephalogram. Toxicol Appl Pharmacol 1979;47:161–176.
9. McLeod CG. Pathology of nerve agents: perspective on medical management. Fund Appl Toxicol 1985;5:S10–S16.
10. DeCandole CA, Douglas WW, Lovatt-Evans C, et al. The failure of respiration in death by anticholinesterase poisoning. Br J Pharmacol Chemother 1953;8:466–475.
11. Ludomirsky A, Hlein HO, Sarelli P, et al. Q-T prolongation and polymorphous ("Torsade de Pointes") ventricular arrhythmias associated with organophosphorus insecticide poisoning. Am J Cardiol 1982;49:1654–1658.
12. Abou-Donia M. Organophosphorus ester-induced delayed neurotoxicity. Annu Rev Pharmacol Toxicol 1981;21:511–548.
13. Laskowski MB, Olson WH, Dettbarn WD. Ultrastructural changes at the motor end-plate produced by an irreversible cholinesterase inhibitor. Exp Neurol 1976;47:290–306.
14. Albuquerque EX, Akaike A, Shaw K-P, et al. The interaction of anticholinesterase agents with the acetylcholine receptor-ionic channel complex. Fundam Appl Toxicol 1981;1:183–192.
15. Du Toit P, Muller F, Van Tonder W, et al. Experience with the intensive care management of organophosphate insecticide poisoning. S Afr Med J 1981;60:227–229.
16. Dunn MA. Pretreatment for nerve agents. Unpublished US Army Information Paper, 1987;AFZC-DMD.
17. Kusic R, Jovanovic D, Randjelovic D, et al: HI-6 in man: Efficacy of the oxime in poisoning by organophosphorus insecticides. Hum Exp Toxicol 1991;10:113–118.
18. Sundwall A. Minimum concentrations of N-methylpyridinium-2-aldoxime methane sulfonate (P2S) which reverse neuromuscular block. Biochem Pharmacol 1961;8:413–417.
19. Crook JW, Goodman AL, Colburn JL, et al. Adjunctive value of oral prophylaxis with the oximes 2-PAM lactate and 2-PAM methanesolfonate to therapeutic administration of atropine in dogs poisoned by inhaled sarin vapor. J Pharmacol Ex Ther 1962;136:397–399.
20. Hoidal CR, Hall Kulig KW, et al. Pralidoxime chloride continuous infusions [letter]. Ann Emerg Med 1987;16:831.
21. Pyridostigimine pretreatment for nerve agents. U.S. Army Academy of Health Sciences Field Circular 8-48, March 26, 1987.
22. Dunn MA, Sidell FR. Progress in medical defense against nerve agents. JAMA 1989;262:649–651.
23. Barrow CS, Alarie Y, Warrick JC, et al. Comparison of the sensory irritation response in mice to chlorine and hydrogen chloride. Arch Environ Health 1977;32:68–76.
24. Kaufman J, Burleons D. Clinical roentgenologic and physiologic effects of acute chlorine exposure. Arch Environ Health 1971;23:39–34.
25. Hasan FM, Gehshan A, Fuleihan FJD. Resolution of pulmonary dysfunction following acute chlorine exposure. Arch Environ Health 1983;38:76–80.
26. Diller WF. Medical phosgene problems and their possible solutions. J Occup Med 1975;32:271–277.
27. Frosolono MF, Pawlowski R. Effects of phosgene on rat lungs after single high level exposure. II. Ultrastructure changes. Arch Environ Health 1977;32:278–283.
28. Report of the specialists appointed by the Secretary General to investigate allegations by the Islamic Republic of Iran concerning the use of chemical weapons. New York: Security Council of the United Nations, 1986; Document S/16433.
29. Van Scott EJ, Kalmanson JD. Complete remission of mycosis fungoides lymphoma induced by topical nitrogen mustard (NH2). Cancer 1973;32:18–30.
30. Heully F, Gruninger M, et al. Collective intoxication caused by the explosion of a mustard gas shell. (Trans US Army) Annales d Medicine Legale 1956;36:195–204.
31. Requena L, Requena C, Sanches M, et al. Chemical warfare: cutaneous lesions from mustard gas. J Am Acad Dermatol 1988;19:529–536.
32. Hu H, Fine J, Epstein P, et al. Tear gas—harassing agent or toxic chemical weapon? JAMA 1989;262:660–663.
33. Petersen KK, Schroeder HM, Eiskjaer SP. CS taregasspray som skadevoldende middel. Kliniske aspecter. Ugeskr Laeger 1989;151:1388–1389.
34. Beswick FW. Chemical agents used in riot control and warfare. Hum Toxicol 1983;2:247–256.
35. Stein AA, Kirwan WE. Chloroacetophenone (tear gas) poisoning: A clinico-pathologic report. J Forensic Sci 1964;9:374–382.
36. Chapman AG, White C. Death resulting from lacrimatory agents. J Forensic Sci 1978;23:527–530.
37. Fuchs T, Ippen H. Kontaktallergie auf CN und CS-Tranengas Derm Beruf Umwelt 1986;34:12–14.

38. Fine KC Bassin RH, Stewart MM. Emergency care for tear gas victims. J Am Coll Emerg Phys 1977;6:144–146.

39. Holland P. The cutaneous reactions produced by dibenzoxazepine (CR). Br J Dermatol 1974;90:657–659.

40. Weger NP. Therapy of chemical warfare agent poisoning. Med Bull US Army, Europe. 1981;38(7/8):30–32.

41. Weger NP. Therapy of chemical warfare agent poisoning 1981;38 (7/8):30–32. Med Bull US Army, Europe. 1981;38(7/8):30–32.

42. Twibell JD, Home JM, Smalldon DW, Higgs DG. Transfer of nitroglycerine to hands during contact with commercial explosives. J Forensic Sci 1982;27:783–791.

43. Hathaway JA. Trinitrotoluene: a review of the reported dose-related effects providing documentation for a workplace standard. J Occup Med 1977;19:341–345.

44. McConnell WJ, Flinn RH. Summary of 22 trinitrotoluene fatalities in World War II. J Ind Hyg Toxicol 1946;28:76–86.

45. Crawford MA. Aplastic anemia due to trinitrotoluene intoxication. Br J Med 1954;2:430–437.

46. Levine RJ, Andjelkovich DA, Kersteter SL, et al. Heart disease in workers exposed to dinitrotoluene. J Occup Med 1986;28:811–816.

47. National Institute for Occupational Safety and Health. Current Intelligence Bulletin 44. Washington, DC: U.S. Government Printing Office, 1985. Publication 85–109.

48. Burge PS, Hendy M, Hodgson ES. Occupational asthma, rhinitis, and dermatitis due to tetrazene in a detonator manufacturer. Thorax 1984;39:170–471.

49. U.S. Army FM3-9, U.S. Air Force 355-7.

50. Konjoyan TR. White phosphorus burns: case report and literature review. Milit Med 1983;148:881–884.

51. Stewart C. Environmental emergencies. Baltimore: Williams & Wilkins, 1989.

52. Dempsy WS. Combat injuries of the lower extremities. Clin Plast Surg 1975;2:585–614.

53. Ben-Hur N, Appelbaum J. Biochemistry, histopathology and treatment of phosphorus burns. Isr J Med Sci 1973;9:40–48.

54. Stewart CE. Chemical skin burns. Am Fam Physician 1985;31:151–157.

55. Bowen TE, Whelen TJ Jr, Nelson TG. Sudden death after phosphorus burns: experimental observations of hypocalcemia, hyperphosphatemia and electrocardiographic abnormalities following production of a standard white phosphorus burn. Ann Surg 1971;174:779–784.

56. Bowen TE, Whelen TH, Nilson TG Sudden deaths after phosphorus burns: experimental observations of hypocalcemia, hyperphosphatemia,, and electrocardiographic abnormalities following induction of a standardized white phosphorus burn. Ann Surg 1970;174:779–784.

57. Lambert RW, Mayer JE: International Negotiations on the Biological Weapons and Toxin Convention. Washington, DC: US Arms Control and Disarmament Agency, 1975.

101

Organophosphate and Carbamate Insecticides

John B. Sullivan, Jr., M.D.
Jamie Blose, Pharm.D.

SOURCES AND PRODUCTION

Organophosphate and carbamate pesticides are widely used for the control of insects. Exposures occur in agricultural industries, among pesticide applicators, in manufacturing of pesticides, and in home use. Pesticide use to control insects had improved agricultural output. Included among the compounds grouped as pesticides are herbicides, rodenticides, food preservatives, and plant growth regulators. Insecticides can be categorized into four different groups: (a) synthetic organic insecticides: chlorobenzene derivatives (dichlorodiphenyltrichloroethane, DDT), cyclodienes (chlordane, aldrin, dieldrin), benzenehexachlorides (lindane), carbamates, and organophosphates; (b) inorganic chemical-type insecticides, such as arsenic, thallium, and cyanide compounds; (c) biologic insecticides, such as pheromones, insect-specific bacteria and viruses; and (d) insecticides from botanical sources, such as nicotine and pyrethrin (1). Organophosphorous compounds have been in existence since 1854 but weren't recognized as having toxic potential until the 1930s (1). The first organophosphate insecticide discovered was tetraethyl-pyrophosphate (TEPP) and was developed in Germany as a substitute for the botanical insecticide nicotine which was in short supply before and during the second World War. It was at this time that the chemical warfare nerve agents tabun and sarin were developed. Although TEPP is an effective insecticide, its highly toxic profile and the fact that it can be rapidly inactivated by hydrolysis in the presence of moisture, left researchers looking for more stable compounds (1). In 1944, parathion and its oxygen analogue, paraoxon, were developed. Parathion has been recognized as one of the most successfully used compounds. It has a wide range of insecticidal activity and a good physiochemical profile including low volatility and stability in water and mild alkalinity. Despite parathion's popularity, its potential for toxicity has led to the development and use of less hazardous compounds.

Chemical Forms

Organophosphate insecticides are normally esters, amides, or thiol derivatives of phosphoric, phosphonic, phosphorothioic or phosphonothioic acids (Fig. 101.1) (1). Both organophosphates and carbamates inhibit acetylcholinesterase enzymes in tissues, blood, and plasma. The basic chemical structure of carbamates is shown in Fig. 101.2. A general listing of common organophosphates and carbamates is given in Tables 101.1 and 101.2. At least 100 compounds have now been reviewed by the World Health Organization (WHO) for consideration as agents for the control of disease vectors (1).

Sites and Situations Associated with Exposures

Organophosphates and carbamates have many uses including controlling insects on food and crops as well as infestations on man or animals and buildings. Soman, sarin, and tabun are very toxic cholinesterase inhibitors and are used as chemical warfare agents. Most exposures to organophosphates and carbamates occur as a result of agricultural use, pesticide application in homes and businesses, and by accidental or intentional ingestion or exposure.

Organophosphates and carbamates are available as emulsified concentrates or wettable powder formulations for reconstitution as liquid sprays, but also as granules for soil application (1). A limited number are also available as fogging formulations, smokes, impregnated resin strips for use indoors, or animal or human pharmaceutical preparations (1). There are two main methods of delivering large volumes of pesticides in the agricultural world. These include land-based delivery and aerial spraying. In land-based delivery, generally, the pesticide concentrates are mixed and loaded into tractor-powered or knapsack sprayers. For tractor spraying, the concentrated pesticide is diluted after loading, but for knapsack sprayers it is loaded from large drums as a premixed, diluted solution, thereby reducing the need to handle the concentrate (2).

Newer methods of application include ultralow volume-controlled droplet applicators which produce small drops from a spinning disc. The object is to use less pesticide and to target it more accurately, but the active chemical is much more concentrated than in conventional spraying and, in practice, has a greater potential for human toxicity (3). A more effective means

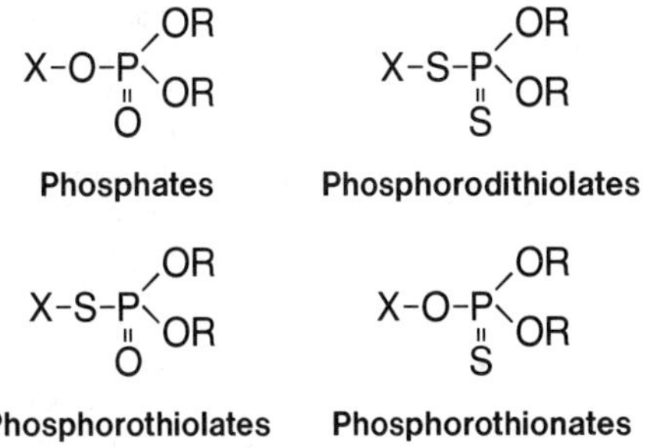

Phosphates   **Phosphorodithiolates**

Phosphorothiolates   **Phosphorothionates**

Figure 101.1. Basic structures of organophosphates. X = Miscellaneous structure of the organophosphate; R = Alkyl structure. Adapted from Minton N, Murray V. A review of organophosphate poisoning. Med Toxicol 1988;3:350–375.

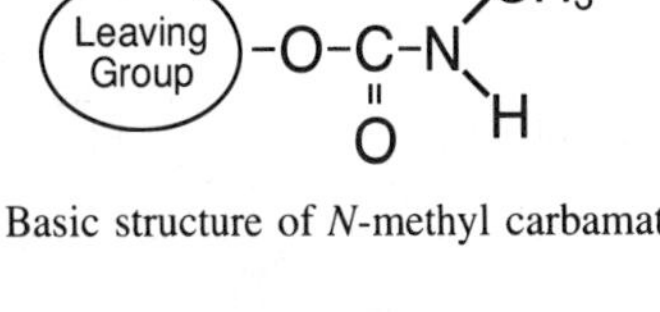

Figure 101.2. Basic structure of *N*-methyl carbamate insecticides.

Table 101.1.   Cross Reference for Some of the Cholinesterase-Inhibiting Organophosphate Pesticide Trade Names

Trade Name	Chemical Name	Trade Name	Chemical Name
Aflix	formothion	Dimecron	phosphamidon
Afos	mecarbam	Dimethogen	dimethoate
Agrisil	trichloronate	Dipterex	trichlorfon
Agritox	trichloronate	Di-Syston	disulfoton
Agrothion	fenitrothion	Disyston S	oxydisulfoton
Alkron	parathion	Dithione	sulfotepp
Alleron	parathion	Dylox	trichlorfon
Amiphos	DAEP	E-605	parathion
Anthio	formothion	Easy Off-D	folex
Anthon	trichlorfon	Ectoral	ronnel
Appex	Gardona+	Ekatin	thiometon
Asuntol	coumaphos	Ekatin M	morphothion
Azodrin	monocrotophos	Ektafos	dicrotophos
Basudin	diazinon	Elsan	phenthoate
Baymix	coumaphos	Emmatos	malathion
Bayrusil	diethquinalphione	Entex	fenthion
Baytex	fenthion	Equinno-Aid	trichlorfon
Baythion	phoxim	Ethyl Parathion	parathion
Betasan	bensulide	Etilon	parathion
Bidrin	dicrotophos	Etrolene	ronnel
Bilobran	monocrotophos	Exothion	endothion
Birlane	chlorfenvinphos	Filariol	bromophos ethyl
Bladafume	sulfotepp	Folidol E-605	parathion
Bladen	parathion	Folidol M	methyl parathion
Borinox	trichlorfon	Folithion	fenitrothion
Bromex	naled	Fostion MM	dimethoate
Carbicron	dicrotophos	Frumin Al	disulfoton
Carfene	azinphos-methyl	Fujithion	DMCP
Cidial	phenthoate	Fyfanon	malathion
Citram	amiton	Gardentox	diazinon
Co-Ral	coumaphos	Garrathion	carbophenothion
Corothion	parathion	Gusathion M	azinphos-methyl
Cvgon	dimethoate	Guthion	azinphos-methyl
Cythion	malathion	Hercules AC527	dioxathion
Dagadip	carbophenothion	Karbofos	malathion
Dalf	methyl parathion	Klimite 40	TEPP
Dasanit	fensulfothion	Korlan	ronnel
Daphene	dimethoate	Lebaycide	fenthion
Dazzel	diazinon	Malamar	malathion
Dedevap	dichlorvos	Malaspray	malathion
De-Fend	dimethoate	Maretin	naphthalaphos
De-Green	DEF	Meldane	coumaphos
Delnav	dioxathion	Menite	mevinphos
Diazajet	diazinon	Metasystox	demeton methyl
Diazide	diazinon	Metasystox-R	oxydemeton-methyl
Diazol	diazinon	Metron	methyl parathion
Dibrom	naled	Mintacol	paraoxon
Di-Captan	dicapthon	MLT	malathion
Mocap	prophos	Tamaron	monitor
Morphotox	morphothion	Tanone	phenthoate
Murfotox	mecarbam	Tartan	cyanthoate
Muscatox	coumaphos	Task	dichlorvos
N-2790	dyfonate	Tekwaisa	methyl parathion
Nankor	ronnel	Terracur P	fensulfothion
Neragan	bromphos ethyl	Tetrachlorvinphos	gardona
Neguvon	trichlorfon	Tetraethyl Pyrophosphate	TEPP
Nialate	ethion	Tetram	amiton
Niram	parathion	Tetron	TEPP
Nitrox	methyl parathion	Thimet	phorate
No Pest	dichlorvos	Thiocron	amidthion
Novathion	fenitrothion	Thiodemeton	disulfoton
Nuvacron	monocrotophos	Thiophos	parathion
Nuvanol	fenitrothion	Thiotepp	sulfotepp
Orthophos	parathion	Tiguvon	fenthion
Ortho Phosphate Defoliant	DEF	Timet	phorate

continues

Table 101.1. *Continued*

Trade Name	Chemical Name	Trade Name	Chemical Name
Panthion	parathion	Trichlorophon	trichlorfon
Parathene	parathion	Trimetion	dimethoate
Parawet	parathion	Trinox	trichlorfon
Patron M	methyl parathion	Trithion	carbophenothion
Perfekthion	dimethoate	Trolene	ronnel
Pestan	mecarbam	Tugon	trichlorfon
Pestox III	schradan	Valexon	phoxim
Phosdrin	mevinphos	Vapona	dichlorvos
Phosfene	mevinphos	Vaponite	dichlorvos
Phoskit	parathion	Vapotone	TEPP
Phosphopyran	endothion	Viozene	ronnel
Phosvit	dichlorvos	Volaton	phoxim
Phytosol	trichloronate	Zithiol	malathion
rolate	imidan	Zolone	phosalone
Rabon	Gardona⁺		
Rampart	phorate		
Rawetin	naphthalaphos		
Resistox	coumaphose		
Rhodiatox	parathion		
Rogor	dimethoate		
Roxion	dimethoate		
Ruelene	crufomate		
Ruphos	dioxathion		
Sapecron	chlorfenvinphos		
Solverex	disulfoton		
Soprathion	parathion		
Spectracide	diazinon		
Stathion	parathion		
Sumithion	fenitrothion		
Supona	chlorfenvinphos		
Systox	demeton		
Sytam	schradan		

of application is the aerial spraying method using either helicopters or fixed-wing aircraft. The chemicals used are in a higher concentration, and therefore particular attention should be given to the possibility of an accidental human or environmental exposure. Some specific factors to keep in mind when using this method include (1–4): (a) winds which disperse organophosphates in open areas; (b) temperature variations in hot climates; volatility may increase leading to high vapor concentrations; (c) rain which could increase the spread or area covered by the chemicals; and (d) fluvial and tidal flow which will affect water-borne spread and contamination; and (e) residues remaining on crops and in soil.

Most statistics of pesticide poisoning are based on the World Health Organization's estimates: in 1972, there were approximately 500,000 cases noted annually from statistics gathered in 19 countries with a mortality estimate of 5,000; in 1977, 20,640 deaths were reported annually from nine different countries; in 1981, approximately 750,000 cases were reported annually; and in 1983, a maximum of 2,000,000 cases were reported annually of which approximately 40,000 could be fatalities (1). The incidence of exposure also seems to be increasing (1).

MECHANISM OF TOXIC ACTION

Both organophosphates and carbamates inhibit acetylcholinesterase. The pharmacologic effects of acetylcholinesterase inhibition are due to stimulation of muscarinic receptors, nicotonic receptors, and central nervous system receptors by acetylcholine which accumulates (5).

Normally, acetylcholine, the chemical neurotransmitter at autonomic and neuromuscular synaptic junctions, is hydrolyzed into acetic acid and choline by the enzyme acetylcholinesterase (Fig. 101.3). Acetylation of the enzyme occurs at the esteratic site; an electrostatic linkage between the choline portion of acetylcholine and the anionic site serves to "anchor" the neurotransmitter so that hydrolysis can occur. Acetylcholine hydrolysis prevents synaptic buildup of the neurotransmitter thus maintaining normal synaptic function. When an organophosphate reacts at the esteratic site of acetylcholinesterase, it forms an extremely stable phosphorous-enzyme bond. The phosphorylation process leads to inactivation of the enzymes, producing depressed activity of cholinesterase in neuronal and nonneuronal tissues, red blood cells, and serum.

Carbamates react in a similar fashion, although the binding that occurs is spontaneously reversible. Due to this reversibility, toxicity and treatment vary from organophosphates to some degree.

CHOLINESTERASE ENZYMES

Two major forms of cholinesterase exist in invertebrates which hydrolyze acetylcholine: acetylcholinesterase ("true cholinesterase"), found primarily in nervous tissue and erythrocytes

Table 101.2. Cross Reference for Some of the Cholinesterase-Inhibiting Carbamate Pesticide Trade Names

Trade Name	Chemical Name	Trade Name	Chemical Name
A363	Matacil	Methiocarb	Mesurol
Ambush	Aldicarb	Metmercaptron	Mesurol
Aminocarb	Matacil	Minacide	Promecarb
Aphox	Pirimicarb	Mos 78	Mobam
Arprocarb	Baygon	MXMC	Mesurol
Bay 9010	Baygon	NC 6897	Ficam
B-37344	Mesurol	NIA 10242	Carbofuran
Bay 39007	Baygon	Nudrin	Methomyl
Bay 44646	Matacil	OMS 716	Promecarb
Bay 70142	Carbofuran	Ortho 5353	Bufencarb
Bendiocarb	Ficam	PHC	Baygon
Blattenex	Baygon	Pirimor	Pirimicarb
Bux	Bufencarb	PP 062	Pirimicarb
Carbamult	Promecarb	Propoxur	Baygon
Carbanolate	Banol	Ravyon	Carbaryl
Carpolin	Carbaryl	Romate	Dichlormate
Carzol	Formetanate (Hydrochloride)	Rowmate	Dichlormate
		Schering 34615	Promecarb
CIBA 8353	Dioxacarbe	Schering 36056	Formetanate (Hydrochloride)
Curaterr	Carbofuran		
D-1221	Formetanate (Hydrochloride)	Sendran	Baygon
		Septene	Carbaryl
D-1410	Oxamyl	Sevin	Carbaryl
Dicarol	Formetanate (Hydrochloride)	Sirmate	Dichlormate
		Snip	Dimetilan
Dowco 139	Mexacarbate	Sok	Banol
Draza	Mesurol	Suncide	Baygon
Elocron	Dioxacarb	Temik	Aldicarb
ENT 27164	Carbofuran	Tendex	Baygon
ENT 27300	Promecarb	Tricarnam	Carbaryl
EP 316	Promecarb	UC 9880	Promecarb
EP 332	Formetanate (Hydrochloride)	UC 21149	Aldicarb
		UC 22463	Dichlormate
Famid	Dioxacarb	UC 7744	Carbaryl
FMC 10242	Carbofuran	Unden	Baygon
Furadan	Carbofuran	Vydate	Oxamyl
G-22870	Dimetilan	Yaltox	Carbofuran
G-13332	Dimetilan	Zectron	Mexacarbate
Hexavin	Carbaryl		
IPMC	Baygon		
Karbaspray	Carbaryl		
Lannate	Methomyl		
Maz	Mexacarbate		
MCA-600	Mobam		
Mercaptodmethur	Mesurol		
Metalkamate	Bufeneath		

and butyrylcholinesterase (''pseudocholinesterase''), present in plasma and nonneuronal tissues (6). The pathotoxicological effects of organophosphate and carbamate toxicity result from inhibition of neuronal (true) acetylcholinesterase. Butyryl-cholinesterase also hydrolyzes succinylcholine (6).

The sites and types of synapses affected by organophosphates lead to specific pathophysiologic effects in poisoned patients. Different receptors for acetylcholine exist on the postganglionic neurons within the autonomic ganglia and at the postjunctional autonomic effector sites. Receptors within the autonomic ganglia and adrenal medulla are stimulated by nictone (''nicotinic receptors'') and those on autonomic effector cells by the alkaloid muscarine (''muscarinic receptors''). Excessive amounts of acetylcholine initially excite and then ''paralyze'' normal function of these synapses, producing characteristic muscarinic, nicotinic, and central nervous system effects (Table 101.3).

CLINICAL TOXICOLOGY

Acute Toxicity

The rapidity and sequence of muscarinic effects due to organophosphate and carbamate poisoning depend on the route of exposure, the toxicity of the compound, and prior status of acetylcholinesterase activity (4). Organophosphates are readily absorbed through the skin and through contaminated clothes. In patients accidentally exposed to vapors of insecticides, the first effects are usually ocular and respiratory. These include miosis, ocular pain, congestion of the conjunctivae, spasm of the ciliary muscle, dimness of vision, and rhinorrhea. Respiratory symptoms occur in the form of dyspnea and chest tightness. These initial signs and symptoms may be followed by bronchoconstriction and excessive amounts of tracheobronchial

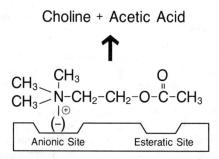

Figure 101.3. Acetylcholinesterase. Hydrolysis of acetylcholine by acetylcholinesterase. Anionic portion of molecule is attacted to anionic binding site, positioning organophosphate for hydrolysis at enzyme active site.

Table 101.3. Clinical Effects of Acetylcholinesterase Inhibitors (Acetylcholine Excess)

Site of Action	Physiologic Effects
Muscarinic Effects	
Sweat glands	Sweating
Pupils	Constricted pupils
Lacrimal glands	Lacrimation
Salivary glands	Excessive salivation
Bronchial tree	Bronchospasms
Gastrointestinal	Pulmonary edema
	Cramps, vomiting, diarrhea
Cardiovascular	Bradycardia
Ciliary body	Blurred vision
Bladder	Urinary incontinence
Nicotinic Effects	
Striated muscle	Fasciculations, cramps, weakness, twitching, paralysis, respiratory depression and respiratory distress, respiratory arrest, cyanosis
Sympathetic ganglia	Tachycardia, elevated blood pressure
Central nervous system effects	Anxiety, restlessness, ataxia, convulsions, insomnia, coma, absent reflexes, Cheyne-Stokes respirations, respiratory and circulation depression

secretions. Victims who ingest organophosphate compounds usually present with complaints related to the gastrointestinal tract, such as anorexia, nausea, vomiting, abdominal cramps, and diarrhea. In patients with percutaneous local exposure to liquid organophosphate compounds or gases, localized excessive sweating and muscular fasciculations may be the earliest manifestations.

Nicotinic effects of organophosphate and carbamate poisons are more likely to prove immediately life-threatening because of the respiratory depressant effects (5). Initial manifestations of anticholinesterase blockade at myoneural junctions of skeletal muscle usually include muscle fatigue and generalized muscular weakness. Patients may develop muscle fasciculations or muscle twitchings. Subsequently, muscle weakness and paralysis occur followed by apnea due to paralysis of respiratory muscles. In untreated patients, these nicotinic effects, together with bronchoconstriction and excessive tracheobronchial secretions, can produce a rapidly fatal clinical course.

Central nervous system manifestations due to organophosphate compound poisoning encompass a wide clinical spectrum. In carbamate poisonings, the central nervous system signs are not as prominent as those produced by organophosphates. In the less severe forms of poisoning, confusion, ataxia, slurred speech, and loss of tendon reflexes occurs. With more severe involvement, patients develop Cheynes-Stokes respirations, generalized convulsions, coma, and central respiratory paralysis. Medullary vasomotor and other cardiovascular centers may also be affected, causing potentially lethal disruption of cardiorespiratory function (5).

The classic presentation of organophosphate and carbamate poisoning relates to the excessive stimulation of muscarinic and nicotinic receptor sites by excess acetylcholine with subsequent receptor exhaustion. However, the clinical syndrome can have different manifestations, depending on the age of the patient, dose, and nature of the pesticide. A number of unrelated conditions may also mimic clinical features of organophosphate poisoning such as gastroenteritis, Guillain-Barre syndrome, and pontine infarction (5–9). A careful history and physical examination serves not only to pinpoint the etiology but also the severity of poisoning.

Important data to obtain include the specific organophosphate, route of exposure, amount, concentrations, and the time elapsed since exposure.

A classification of organophosphate compounds based upon their degree of toxicity to humans and their distribution in various commercial products is in Table 101.4. The most toxic organophosphate compounds are agricultural insecticides such as parathion and disyston. Malathion and diazinon are organophosphates frequently utilized in household insecticide sprays and have much lower toxicity.

Physical examination of patients with suspected organophosphate poisoning should focus on identifying severity of toxicity for purposes of therapy. The organophosphate-containing diluent of many pesticides possesses a typical kerosene-like odor. Patients who have consumed such compounds frequently demonstrate this odor. Contamination of the skin and clothes with organophosphate containing liquid also gives rise to the typical hydrocarbon odor and systemic toxicity via dermal absorption.

Mild organophosphate poisoning may present a syndrome of headache, nausea, vomiting, abdominal cramps, and diarrhea. In patients with moderate organophosphate poisoning, generalized muscle weakness, skeletal muscle fasciculations, dysarthria, miosis, excessive secretions, shortness of breath, chest tightness, and dyspnea may found. Severely poisoned patients may present with seizures, coma, miotic pupils, fasciculations, skeletal muscle paralysis, pulmonary edema, and respiratory failure.

Certain features of organophosphate poisoning may also occur in other disease states. In some patients, for instance, symptoms arising from oral ingestion may be mistaken for an episode of gastroenteritis. Patients with muscle weakness may simulate Guillain-Barre syndrome, especially in patients with diazinon and chlorpyrifos poisoning, who may present with a predominance of nicotinic manifestations. The small-sized pupils may erroneously suggest opiate poisoning, or even pontine infarction. Excessive tracheobronchial secretions and bronchospasm may mimic an attack of acute bronchial asthma.

Other unusual features of organophosphate poisoning can occur from selective inhibition of either red blood cell cholinesterase or plasma cholinesterase. Certain organophosphates may selectively inhibit plasma cholinesterase or RBC cholinesterase following an acute exposure. Mevinphos has been known

Table 101.4.   Samples of Organophosphate Insecticides

Common Name	Chemical Name
High Toxicity	
TEPP	Tetraethylpyrophosphate
parathion	O,O-diethyl O-*p*-nitrophenyl phosphorothioate
phosdrin	dimethyl-O-(1-methyl-2-carbomethoxyvinyl phosphate)
disyston	dimethyl S-(4-oxo-1,2,3,-benzotriazinyl-3-methyl phosphorodithioate)
Intermediate Toxicity	
ronnel	O,O-dimethyl O-(2,4,5-trichlorophenyl) phosphorothioate
coumaphos	diethyl-O-(3-chloro-4-methyl-7-coumarinyl) phosphorothioate
chlorpyrifos (dursban)	O,O-diethyl-O-(3,5,6-trichloro-2-pyridyl) phosphorothioate
trichlorfon	dimethyl trichlorohydroxy-ethyl phosphonate
Low Toxicity	
malathion	dimethyl-S-(1,2-bis-carbo-ethyl phosphorodithioate
diazinon	diethyl-O-(2-isopropyl-6-methyl-4-pyrimidyl) phosphorothioate
dichlorvos, DDVP	O,O-dimethyl-O-2,2-dichlorovinyl phosphate

to selectively depress plasma cholinesterase over RBC cholinesterase following an acute exposure (9). Phosmet,*N*-(mercaptomethyl) phthalamide *S*-(O,O-dimethyl-phosphoro-dithiolate), has been known to selectively depress RBC cholinesterase over plasma cholinesterase in the case of a poisoned child (10). Chlorpyrifos exposure in children has also depressed plasma cholinesterase selectively (10). Dimethoate, a phosphorotrithioate, selectively depressed RBC cholinesterase in a clinical case (10). Also, some organophosphates that require metabolism to a toxic intermediate such as parathion, malathion, and dimethoate may present with delayed symptoms.

Pediatric patients and some adult patients may present with a predominance of nicotinic effects manifesting mainly neuromuscular weakness. This neuromuscular weakness can be overlooked in a small child who may appear very quiet and still. In children, normal or abnormal muscle tone should be confirmed. Of note should be the fact that tachycardia and generalized tonic-clonic seizures are frequently seen in the pediatric pesticide exposures and are rarely reported in adult poisoning unless a massive exposure has occurred (11).

Occupational and Chronic Exposure

Occupational exposure to organophosphate and carbamates occur mainly in agricultural workers who mix pesticides, apply pesticides, or who work with crops containing pesticide residues. Illness can occur from any of these exposures and may be insidious, making the diagnosis difficult. Exposure in occupational settings is primarily inhalational or dermal. Cali-

fornia is the only state that requires medical surveillance of those who handle or apply organophosphates (9).

Cholinesterase values can be used to monitor exposed workers; however, the range of normal plasma and RBC cholinesterase values varies greatly. Occupational exposure to organophosphates can result in a decline in cholinesterase values that might be 50% lower than the upper limits, but yet is still within normal limits. This decline can be accompanied by mild to moderate symptoms of toxicity which include nausea, headache, dizziness, blurred vision, abdominal pain, vomiting, chest tightness, and shortness of breath. Symptoms may be present for several months before the syndrome is identified. Studies of field workers exposed to pesticides have shown that a 30% decrease in RBC cholinesterase can be associated with symptoms of moderate organophosphate toxicity (12). This same study indicated that a rise in plasma cholinesterase of 15–20% occurred following discontinuation of a significant exposure. This rise in plasma cholinesterase is consistent with the rapid rate of recovery of the enzyme in plasma (12).

A continued increase in plasma cholinesterase after discontinuation of exposure helps to further confirm the toxicity. RBC cholinesterase values should be monitored until they stabilize before sending someone back to work. RBC cholinesterase normally varies 10% (12). An increase in RBC cholinesterase of less than 10% over a previous value is not indicative of poisoning (12), whereas an increase of RBC cholinesterase of greater than 10% suggests regeneration of enzyme and a toxic effect.

Workers who have a longterm exposure to organophosphates may have chronically depressed cholinesterase values yielding a falsely low baseline on medical surveillance (13).

Dimethoate, an agricultural pesticide, is an indirect-acting anticholinesterase. It is converted in the liver to active metabolites (14). Phosphorothioates, like dimethoate, require metabolic oxidation of the phosphorous-sulfur (P=S) bond before producing toxicity. Due to this oxidation step, these substances can exhibit a slower onset of symptoms as compared to compounds possessing a direct-acting P=O bond (14). Dimethoxon, an active metabolite of dimethoate, is thought to be 75–100 times more potent than dimethoate for the inhibition of rat brain cholinesterase (14). Phosphorothioates are generally lipophilic and therefore concentrate in the body fat and are released over a relatively long period of time. This phenomena can be responsible for reappearance of acute clinical effects observed in an acute exposure following therapy.

Dimethoate is poorly absorbed through the skin but rapidly absorbed by the oral route (15). Because of its low vapor pressure, the vapor hazard of dimethoate is minimal, although there may be considerable hazard from dust or mist produced during various application methods. Erythrocyte acetylcholinesterase is more sensitive to inhibition by dimethoate than plasma pseudocholinesterase (15).

LABORATORY DIAGNOSIS OF TOXICITY

The laboratory diagnosis of organophosphate poisoning is based on depression of plasma and red blood cell cholinesterase activity. Routine laboratory tests are usually unremarkable with a few notable exceptions. Hyperglycemia and glucosuria have occasionally been observed (8). The increase in serum glucose is believed to be secondary to the release of catecholamines from the adrenal medulla, which is activated by hyperactivity of the sympathetic ganglia (8). Hypokalemia has also been noted occasionally and is speculated to be secondary to an alteration of the distribution of potassium between intracellular and extracellular membranes, which in turn is used to augment circulating catecholamines (16, 17). Leukocytosis, both with and without a left shift, was a common finding in a number of studies (8). Elevated serum amylase secondary to pancreatic injury because of parasympathetic overstimulation and hypersecretion has been observed (18). Proteinuria has also been noted (19).

As essential prerequisites to accurate diagnosis, clinicians should know the potential limitations of these laboratory aids, chiefly of cholinesterase estimation, as well as the utility of a "therapeutic test" in equivocal cases of organophosphate poisoning.

Although not routinely available in most clinical laboratories, red blood cell cholinesterase activity estimation is the most specific diagnostic test for organophosphate poisoning. There are four laboratory techniques most commonly used for quantitative determinations of both plasma and RBC acetylcholinesterase activities. These are the electrometric (Michel), the titrimetric (pH stat), the colorimetric (Ellman) and gas chromatographic (Cranmer) methods (Table 101.5).

Most of the organophosphates and carbamates inhibit both plasma and red blood cell cholinesterase. Although, as previously noted, there are a few exceptions that are known (Table 101.6). Ideally, clinicians should estimate "true" cholinesterase, which indicates the extent of inhibition of synaptic cholinesterase which is best reflected in red cell cholinesterase activity levels. However, plasma cholinesterase is an easier test to obtain and is more available. More importantly, clinicians must draw the required blood sample before administration of the antidote pralidoxime.

In most cases, the depressed cholinesterase activity levels correspond to the severity of poisoning. Thus, symptomatic patients frequently have more than 50% depression of serum cholinesterase (8). Twenty to fifty percent of normal cholinesterase activity often signifies mild poisoning, while 10–20% of normal values usually indicate moderately severe poisoning, and less than 10% cholinesterase activity points to severe poisoning (Table 101.7) (9). This correlation proves valid only in the initial stage of acute poisoning, however. A greater degree

of inhibition occurs in patients with repeated exposures, in whom depressed values may persist even after symptomatic recovery. In severe poisoning, serum cholinesterase may not normalize for about 4 weeks after the exposure. Red cell cholinesterase activity may take 90–120 days to return to normal.

Although a normal erythrocyte cholinesterase activity effectively rules out organophosphate poisoning in most cases, evaluation of lowered values can often prove problematic (12). Moderately severe symptoms may occur, for instance, even in patients whose erythrocyte cholinesterase activity is only 33% inhibited (12). Another limitation stems from reliance on a laboratory "normal range" of cholinesterase activity to evaluate a given patient's status. Since the normal range is wide, patients with baseline "high" normal values may have less than 50% of cholinesterase activity, a value within the normal range (12), and be symptomatic.

Clinicians should also remember that depression of serum cholinesterase activity is not unique to organophosphate poisoning. Low activity levels may also occur in a number of other states, especially in parenchymal liver disease, such as viral hepatitis, cirrhosis, congestion due to cardiac failure, and metastatic carcinoma. Low values may also occur in patients with malnutrition, acute infections, anemia, myocardial infarction, and dermatomyositis (Table 101.8). In a small fraction of patients, about 3% of the general population, low cholinesterase levels occur due to a genetic variant. Also, plasma cholinesterase with a normal RBC cholinesterase can be found in patients who are pregnant or who are taking birth control pills (20–21). In pregnancy, the plasma cholinesterase values have been known to fall well below the lower normal values (20).

PHARMACOTHERAPY AND MANAGEMENT

In patients who do not exhibit clear-cut features of organophosphate poisoning, clinicians may find the effect of atropine and/or pralidoxime useful for confirming the diagnosis (5). Since patients with organophosphate poisoning are usually resistant to atropine, a small dose of 0.5–1 mg of atropine given parenterally does not result in characteristic anticholinergic effects such as tachycardia or mydriasis. However, if such signs develop soon after administering a small dose of atropine, pa-

Table 101.5. Laboratory Techniques for Plasma and RBC Acetylcholinesterase Activity

Laboratory Method	Procedure	Normal Values
Electrometric method (Michel method)	Plasma and red cells are incubated with acetylcholine for 1 hour. The drop of the pH is due to the formation of acetic acid and is directly proportional to the cholinesterase activity.	Plasma 0.53–1.24 pH units Red Blood Cells 0.57–0.98 pH units
Titrimetric method (pH stat method)	Plasma and red cells are incubated with acetylcholine for 3 minutes, and the acid formed is titrated with a base. The amount of base used is directly proportional to the cholinesterase activity.	Plasma 3.6–6.8 μM/ml/min Red Blood Cells 11.1–16.0 μM/ml/min
Colorimetric method (Ellman method)	Plasma and red cells are incubated for 10 minutes with acetylthiocholine, and the resultant thiocholine produces a yellow color in the presence of 5:5-dithiobid-(2-nitrobenzoic acid). The concentration of the yellow complex is directly proportional to the amount of cholinesterase present.	Plasma 5.8–16.6 M-SH/ml/3min
Gas chromatographic method (Cramer method)	Plasma and red cells are reacted for 30 minutes with a compound that is similar to acetylcholine. The product formed, dimethyl butanol, is quantitated using a gas chromatograph.	Plasma 2.1–4.6 μM/ml/min Red Blood Cells 8.1–11.8 μM/ml/min

Table 101.6. Organophosphates and Selective Inhibition of Acetylcholinesterase

Organophosphate	Selective Cholinesterase Inhibition
Phosdrin	Plasma cholinesterase
Phosmet	RBC cholinesterase
Chlorpyrifos	Plasma cholinesterase
Dimethoate	RBC cholinesterase

These organophosphates may selectively depress the activity of either RBC or plasma cholinesterase in clinical situations.

Table 101.7. Summary of Specific Antidote Treatment for Acute Organophosphate Poisoning

Level of Poisoning	Clinical Features	Red Cell Cholinesterase (% normal)
Subclinical	No symptoms or signs	>50%
Mild	Tiredness, dizziness, headache, nausea, vomiting, diarrhea, abdominal pain, salivation, wheezing.	20–50%
Moderate	Symptoms of mild poisoning plus weakness, inability to walk, muscle fasciculations, dysarthria, miosis.	10–20%
Severe	Symptoms of moderate poisoning plus coma, flaccid paralysis, cyanosis, pulmonary edema, and respiratory distress. Marked miosis with loss of pupil reflexes.	<10%

Used with permission from: Minton W, Murray V. A review of organophosphate poisoning. Med Toxicol 1988;3:365.

Table 101.8. States Affecting Cholinesterase Activity

Cholinesterase	State
Plasma	
Low	Parenchymal liver disease, hepatic metastases
	Malnutrition (protein or thiamine)
	Chronic debilitating conditions
	Acute infections
	Some anemias
	Myocardial infarction
	Pregnancy
	Birth control pills
Normal	Uncomplicated obstructive jaundice
	Myasthenia gravis
	Hyperthyroidism
	Asthma
	Hypertension
	Epilepsy
	Diabetes mellitus
Raised	Nephrotic syndrome
Red Cell	
Raised	Reticulocytosis due to anemias, hemorrhage, and treatment of metabloblastic/pernicious anemias

A plasma cholinesterase may be reduced in debilitated patients with these conditions.
Adapted with permission from: Minton W, Murray V. A review of organophosphate poisoning. Med Toxicol 1988;3:363.

tients either have not been exposed to organophosphates, have a very mild form of poisoning, or may have a predominance of the nicotinic effect which can be seen with certain organophosphates in both adults and children. Intravenous injection of 1 g of pralidoxime also produces symptomatic amelioration, chiefly in the form of improved muscle strength.

Optimum management of organophosphate poisoning demands more than the administration of specific antidotes. To ensure a favorable outcome, clinicians must also pay attention to decontamination measures, provide adequate cardiorespiratory support, treat convulsions, and prevent specific complications. Finally, clinicians should formulate a rational approach to monitor patients who are occupationally exposed on a chronic basis.

Decontamination measures attempt to reduce or eliminate further exposure via dermal, ocular, and gastrointestinal routes in affected patients. Begin by removing all exposed clothing, and thoroughly cleanse the patient with large amounts of water and soap. Avoid causing further damage to the skin which may lead to increased absorption of the poison. Contaminated or potentially contaminated clothing must be placed in plastic bags. Emergency care personnel should wear disposable gloves during the decontamination procedures and immediately bag or destroy patients' clothing. Other frequently overlooked contaminated sites such as the hair and nails must also be decontaminated.

Ocular exposure may not only cause severe discomfort to the patient, but also create confusion during the course of treatment. When organophosphate-containing aerosols or vapors directly affect the eyes, patients develop a severe degree of miosis that may last hours or days despite systemic therapy (9). Use large amounts of sterile saline—up to 1 liter per eye—for 10–15 minutes to flush out the incriminated chemical from the eyes. If saline is not available, clean tap water may be utilized.

In patients who have ingested organophosphate compounds either accidentally or with suicidal intent, carefully assess the state of consciousness prior to gastric evacuation. Since many of these pesticides have a solvent diluent, pulmonary aspiration with subsequent pneumonitis can occur. To eliminate unabsorbed poison, administer activated charcoal, beginning with 30 g in adults. In patients who are unconscious, insert a nasogastric or orogastric tube and perform gastric lavage with appropriate precautions to protect the airway, such as placing the patient in the lateral decubitus position or perform intubation.

Patients with organophosphate toxicity are susceptible to cardiac asystole due to sinus arrest or ventricular fibrillation. Hypoxia and a direct toxic effect often results in a hyper-irritable myocardium (5, 9).

Appropriate respiratory support not only proves immediately life-saving, but also critically influences the outcome of organophosphate poisoning. Atropine may also lead to ventricular fibrillation in hypoxic, acidotic patients. Adequate control of the airway with proper ventilation to correct acidosis and restore tissue oxygenation as soon as possible, is important to reduce ventricular ectopy hazard. Depending on the degree of respiratory distress, patients may require a combination of atropine, airway suctioning with or without tracheal intubation, positive airway pressure and mechanical ventilations. After restoring adequate respiratory function, cardiovascular support frequently necessitates expansion of blood volume prior to utilization of inotropic agents such as dopamine.

Convulsions may arise as an effect of the poisoning, cerebral hypoxia, or the presence of another poison. In patients whose convulsions stem from cerebral hypoxia, improved cardiopulmonary function subsequent to controlling the acute episode with anticonvulsants is essential. In addition to optimum cerebral perfusion, seizures can be controlled with intravenous diazepam, up to 20 mg in adults, administered slowly until seizures stop. For children under 12 years of age, use 0.1–0.2 mg/kg of the drug. Lorazepam may be used in children at the dose of 0.03–0.05 mg/kg up to a maximum of 4 mg every 6 hours. In all cases, watch carefully for hypotension and respiratory depression, both of which are especially likely to occur in such patients. The use of diazepam in organophosphate poisoning has been shown to improve mortality and morbidity in animal studies independent of its anticonvulsant effects (5).

Pharmacologic treatment of organophosphate poisoning relies on concurrent or sequential administration of the anticholinergic agent atropine and the cholinesterase "activator" pralidoxime. While atropine counters the muscarinic and central nervous system manifestations of organophosphate compound poisoning, pralidoxime reverses both the muscarinic effects, and unlike atropine, the nicotinic adverse effects of the poison as well.

Atropine

Atropine blocks muscarinic receptors and reverses muscarinic receptor stimulation, thus reversing many symptoms of poisoning. Atropine does not, however, block nicotinic receptors and because of this, a poisoned patient may have respiratory depression even if fully atropinized. Due to the fact that atropine is a tertiary amine, it crosses the blood-brain barrier and lowers the level of cerebral acetycholine.

The concept of proper dosing of atropine (atropinization) is vital. The endpoint of atropine therapy is to reverse and dry all secretions. For adults, most authorities recommend a dose of 1–2 mg of the drug every 10–15 minutes intravenously until full atropinization occurs (5). Clinicians can gauge this effect primarily by drying of secretions, in addition to other signs such as tachycardia, dry mouth, and mydriasis. For children under 12 years of age, give 0.05–0.10 mg/kg of atropine in a similar regimen. Only a few such doses may be required in less severely affected patients, while continuous intravenous infusion of atropine sulfate, 0.4 mg/ml at 0.01–0.03 mg/kg/min—or even more may be required in patients who have been severely poisoned.

Atropine is also quite effective by the intramuscular route, although its anticholinergic effects ensure more promptly following intravenous administration.

Pulse rate and pupillary size may not prove absolutely reliable as monitoring indices during anticholinergic therapy. Tachycardia per se is a nonspecific sign, and dilated or even unequal pupils have occurred, though rarely, in organophosphate poisoning. Cholinesterase inhibition may cause either bradycardia or tachycardia, depending upon factors such as resting vagal tone, and also whether organophosphate toxicity produces predominantly muscarinic effects (bradycardia) or nicotinic effects (tachycardia) via cardiac sympathetic ganglia. A normal or slow pulse rate to begin with, increasing after introduction of atropine usually indicates anticholinergic effect, however, especially at rates above 120–140 per minute. Similarly, baseline normal or small-sized pupils which subse-

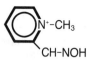

Figure 101.4. Pralidoxime. Cholinesterase reactivating oxime used in the treatment of organophosphate poisoning.

quently dilate on anticholinergic administration indicate atropinization.

Atropine administration should not be suddenly terminated if a patient is being treated for days. Instead, allow for progressively increasing intervals of time between successive doses, keeping a close watch on patients for return of cholinergic features, such as miosis, excessive lacrimation or salivation, or depressed respiration. In many patients, such signs may prove quite subtle and include recurrence of small airway obstruction (wheezing) and rales. Such patients may, in fact, require further anticholinergic drug administration.

The decision to stop administration of atropine must remain individualized in patients. In general, however, experts advise that occupational exposure with dermal contact and/or inhalation usually need full atropinization for at least 12–24 hours, after ensuring thorough dermal decontamination. In patients who have ingested the poison, intensive atropinization for several days is essential, with total administration of many grams of atropine. Also, patients exposed to toxic doses of fat-soluble organophosphates such as fenthion should be atropinized for 3–4 days to prevent recurrence of symptoms. Two laboratory estimations, if available, may help in reducing atropine dosage—rising levels of blood cholinesterase activity and elimination of organophosphate metabolites from patients' urine. Clinically, pupillary size, heart and pulse rate are also useful monitoring indices.

Patients with significant exposure to organophosphate compounds usually demonstrate a large degree of tolerance to atropine. Hence, despite frequent administration of very large doses, atropine toxicity rarely occurs in such patients. Occasionally, however, in mildly poisoned patients given excessively large doses of atropine, symptoms and signs such as delirium, hyperpyrexia, and muscle fasciculations may occur. Mild degrees of atropinization merely prove discomforting to patients and do not require specific treatment.

Oximes

Severe degrees of organophosphate poisoning, especially in patients demonstrating muscle fasciculations and neuromuscular weakness, mandate use of Pralidoxime chloride (PAM) (Fig. 101.4). Pralidoxime chloride proves efficacious in such patients through a combination of three major biochemical effects. Of these, the most important is cleavage of the phosphate bond from cholinesterase, which reactivates the cholinesterase enzyme. In addition, pralidoxime may also directly react with and detoxify the organophosphate molecule, and also possesses an anticholinergic "atropine-like" effect. Unlike atropine, however, pralidoxime administration reactivates cholinesterase enzyme at neuromuscular junctions and postganglionic autonomic neurons. Thus, pralidoxime helps counter muscular weakness in sites such as thoracic muscles, alleviating respiratory dysfunction. Although pralidoxime is a quarternary ammonium compound and presumably does not cross into the central nervous system, it may mediate a beneficial effect at this level and should, therefore, be tried (5).

Pralidoxime should be administered regardless of the type of organophosphate involved. The effectiveness of pralidoxime depends on the length of the postexposure period and the specific organophosphate compound involved. For optimum effects, pralidoxime should be administered immediately after poisoning. Inhibited acetylcholinesterase becomes difficult to reactivate with time, due to a process known as "aging" (also termed the Straver reaction). The organophosphorous moiety on the inhibited enzyme becomes dealkylated, which prevents reaction with the oxime. The rate of aging varies greatly among the different organophosphorous compounds. In patients administered the drug more than 36 hours after exposure, significant reactivation of cholinesterase may not occur. However, administration of pralidoxime should occur in these late cases in hopes of obtaining some effect. In some cases, pralidoxime has successfullly reversed toxicity of diazinon and chlorpyrifos days after exposure (personal data). Treatment also proves effective in poisoning due to other cholinesterase inhibitors such as TEPP and mevinphos.

In patients with normal renal function, pralidoxime can be administered in the dose of 1 g intravenously every 4–6 hours for adults, and 25–50 mg/kg of body weight per dose in children. The drug should be given over 20 minutes in an intravenous infusion, with each dose in 100–200 ml 5% glucose in dextrose and water. In very severe poisoning, the dose can be doubled. Recovery of consciousness and amelioration of muscle weakness and fasciculations usually occur within 10–40 minutes of administration. Continuous infusion is preferable to repeated injections. In severely poisoned patients, an initial combination of atropine and pralidoxime may prove more effective. Serial determination of plasma or RBC cholinesterase may also help judge the efficacy of pralidoxime administration.

In most patients, few side effects occur with therapeutic doses of pralidoxime. Adverse effects include excitement, mania, confusion, tachycardia, dizziness, headache, blurred vision, impaired accommodation, diplopia, muscle weakness, and rigidity. Excessively rapid administration of pralidoxime may also cause temporary worsening of cholinergic manifestations, an effect possibly related to the moderate anticholinesterase activity of oximes. Rarely, acute hypersensitivity reactions may occur following pralidoxime therapy.

Although pralidoxime is currently the most commonly used oxime for use in humans, other oximes such as obidoxime, trimedoxime, and asoxime have also been shown to have potent enzyme reactivating properties (22, 23). Unlike pralidoxime, obidoxime is able to cross the blood-brain barrier and reactivate brain cholinesterases; however, this may not confer additional benefits over peripheral cholinesterase reactivators. Work with asoxime suggested that it has less side effects than prolidoxime (23). Asoxime, also termed HI-6, has demonstrated efficacy against soman, a military nerve agent (23). Asoxime has also been shown to be effective in treating commercial insecticide poisonings with less side effects in humans (23). Also, asoxime produced clinical improvement before RBC-cholinesterase values rose thus indicating a direct pharmacologic effect (23).

CARBAMATES AND PRALIDOXIME USE

Organophosphates and carbamates have similar modes of action as well as similar toxic effects. Despite these similarities, pralidoxime does not have the popularity in treating carbamate poisonings as it does in organophosphate poisonings. Reasons for this include the fact that carbamates are generally shorter

acting and 2-PAM is thought to have a potential additive inhibitory effect on cholinesterase in carbamate poisoning.

There is no reported evidence in humans that pralidoxime is unsafe as adjunctive therapy with atropine in a critically ill, carbamate-poisoned patient. Unfortunately, there are no published cases of dual therapy, probably because a serious life-threatening carbamate intoxication is likely to have had several treatments administered simultaneously, making it difficult to determine if the pralidoxime made the patient better or worse.

Complications and Longterm Sequelae of Exposure

The most frequent complications of organophosphate poisoning are aspiration pneumonia, chemical pneumonitis due to aspiration, complications of multiple seizures, and target organ effects of hypoxemia. Vigorous respiratory management is therefore crucial in all patients with organophosphate poisoning.

Delayed neurological complications are rare and result from inhibition of an esterase termed neurotoxic esterase (24–27). This delayed sensorimotor neuropathy commences peripherally and proceeds proximally. Symptoms include lower extremity parasthesias which may progress to weakness and ataxia, with occasional progression of symptoms to the arms (24–27). In the classical presentation, these ataxic symptoms usually occur 6–21 days after an acute nonlethal exposure (24–27). The early administration of pralidoxime and atropine does not seem to prevent this complication. In general, longterm recovery has been slow with symptoms persisting for months to years.

Prognosis

Untreated patients usually die within 24 hours after complications occur. The more severely poisoned victims may succumb to complications after a period of a few days. In all other cases, provided cerebral hypoxia has been successfully prevented or treated, clinicians can expect total symptomatic recovery within 7–10 days.

Biological Monitoring

In view of their potentially serious toxicity, strict adherence to certain precautions is necessary for those exposed to organophosphate compounds at the workplace, especially for agricultural workers. Mandatory measures include strict personal hygiene, thorough cleansing of contaminated clothes, wearing of protective gloves and clothing at all times, and limiting dermal contact (28, 29).

In persons likely to be continually or frequently exposed to organophosphates, such as farm workers, a baseline red blood cell cholinesterase estimate may prove helpful. Intermittent estimation may also be useful, since cholinesterase inhibition often occurs before symptomatic poisoning. Workers with significant reductions in cholinesterase values should avoid further exposure and await normalization of cholinesterase enzyme activity.

Patients without prior cholinesterase estimates may present with a history of exposure, cholinesterase features, and "low normal" cholinesterase levels. Such patients should return to work only after repeat cholinesterase estimates 3–5 days later. If significant exposure has occurred, repeat estimates will reveal increases of 15–20% in cholinesterase activity (12, 13).

REGULATION OF PESTICIDES

The Federal Insecticide, Fungicide, and Rodenticide Act (FIFRA), enacted in 1947, remains the primary statute regulating pesticide manufacturing, use, and distribution. FIFRA has been amended in 1972, 1975, and in 1978. The Environmental Protection Agency has been responsible for regulation of pesticide use since 1970 (30).

Pesticide regulation first occurred under the Insecticide Act of 1910. This early act was a consumer protection measure against mislabeling and distribution of ineffective pesticides (30). FIFRA eventually replaced this act. Pesticides are also regulated by the Environmental Protection Agency under the following:

1. Federal Environmental Pesticide Control Act
2. Resource Conservation Recovery Act of 1972 (RCRA)
3. Comprehensive Environmental Response, Compensation, and Liability Act (Superfund)
4. Toxic Substances Control Act (TSCA)
5. Clean Water Act
6. Safe Drinking Water Act

A pesticide is defined under FIFRA as ''any substance or mixture or substances intended for preventing, destroying, repelling, or mitigating any pest, and . . . any substance or mixture of substances intended for use as a plant regulator, defoliant, or dessicant (30).'' Pesticides include insecticides, fungicides, herbicides, rodenticides, dessicants, disinfectants, defoliants, and nematocides (30). FIFRA requires all pesticides sold or distributed to be registered with the EPA. Once registered, FIFRA classifies the use of a pesticide as general or resticted. The application and use of pesticides is tightly controlled by the EPA under FIFRA.

FIFRA prohibits the sale of unregistered pesticides, the production of pesticides by unregistered manufacturers, the use of adulterated pesticides, and the use of a pesticide in a manner inconsistent with its labeling. The EPA has the authority to enforce FIFRA by legal sanctions including civil penalties, criminal fines, injunctions, product seizure, termination of product sales, or recalls (30). When evidence indicates that a particular pesticide may be a significant health hazard, the appropriate regulatory agency or agencies can take any of the following actions (31):

1. Issue permissible exposure limits for the workplace,
2. Cancel registration and order withdrawal of the product from the market,
3. Place restrictions on use or application of the compound,
4. Set tolerance limits for pesticide residues on foodstuffs,
5. Cancel registration,
6. Establish maximum permissible contamination levels for the pesticides in drinking water.

In addition to the regulation of pesticide use and application, FIFRA requires the pesticide manufacturer to be registered with the EPA. The EPA, under agreement with the Food and Drug Administration, establishes pesticide tolerances for raw foods and produce (30). Pesticides that might be considered food additives are controlled by the EPA under the Food, Drug, and Cosmetic Act (30). It is of interest that once a pesticide is discarded, it becomes a hazardous waste and is then under regulation by RCRA and not FIFRA.

The 1978 amendment to FIFRA allows manufacturers of pesticides to have a waiver on submission of data demonstrating efficacy of their product, except where the product has a direct relation to or effect on public health. In addition, the 1978 amendment allows for public disclosure of the safety and health data regarding pesticide regulation (30). The 1978 amendment also transfers to states the responsibility to enforce pesticide use regulations if they can demonstrate that they possess the means to do so. The EPA reserves the right to revoke any state's responsibility for pesticide regulation if that state is unable or unwilling to enforce the regulations (30).

Regulation of a pesticide suspected to be a carcinogen is not uniformly applied by all federal agencies (31). However, these agencies have been consistent in regulating a substance when it is expected to cause an increase of more than four cases of cancer per 1000 persons (31). If the expected increase in cancer is less than one in a million, then regulation is unlikely (31). Cost-effectiveness of regulation is also considered. If the cost of regulation is anticipated to be less than $2 million per life saved, then it is called for (31).

REFERENCES

1. Minton N, Murray V. A review of organophosphate poisoning. Med Toxicol 1988;3:350–375.
2. Smith DM. Modern farming. In: Harrington JM, ed. Recent advances in occupational health. Leith Walk, Edinburgh: Churchill Livingstone, 1987:55–73.
3. Wolfe HR, et al. Exposure of workers to pesticides. Arch Environ Health 1967;14:622–633.
4. Kahn E. Pesticide related illness in California farm workers. J Occup Med 1976;18(10):693–696.
5. McDonough J, Jaax N, Crowley R et al. Atropine and/or diazepam therapy protects against soman-induced neural and cardiac pathology. Fundam Appl Toxicol 1989;13:256–276.
6. Chatonnet A, Lockridge O. Comparison of butylcholinesterase and acetylcholinesterase. Biochem J 1989;260;625–634.
7. Fisher J. Guillain Barre syndrome following organophosphate poisoning. JAMA 1977;238:1950.
8. Mellar D, Fraser I, Kruger M. Hyperglycemia in anticholinesterase poisoning. Can Med Assoc J 1981;124:745–747.
9. Coye M, Barnett P, Midtling J, Velasco A, et al. Clinical confirmation of organophosphate poisoning of agricultural workers. Am J Ind Med 1986;10:399–409.
10. Personal data of Dr. John B. Sullivan, University of Arizona, Health Sciences Center, Tucson, Arizona.
11. Zwiener RJ, Ginsburg CM. Organophosphate and carbamate poisoning in infants and children. Pediatrics 1988;81:121–126.
12. Midtling JE, Barnett PG, Coye MJ, et al. Clinical management of field worker organophosphate poisoning. West J Med 1985;142:514.
13. Ames RG, Brown SK, Mengle DC, Kahn E, Stratton JW, Jackson RJ. Cholinesterase activity depression among California agricultural pesticide applicators. Am J Ind Med 1989;15:143–150.
14. Sanderson D, Edson E. Toxicological properties of the organophosphate insecticide dimethoate. Br J Ind Med 1964;21:52–64.
15. Hayes W. Pesticides studied in man. Baltimore, MD: Williams & Wilkins, 1982:2884–435.
16. Mackey C. Anticholinesterase insecticide poisoning. Heart Lung 1982;11:479–484.
17. Hui K. Metabolic disturbances in organophosphate insecticide poisoning (letter). Arch Pathol Lab Med 1983;104:154.
18. Haubenstock A. More on the triad of pancreatitis, hyperamylasemia, and hyperglycemia. JAMA 1983;249:1563.
19. Hayes M, VanDer Westhuizen N, Gelfand M. Organophosphate poisoning in Rhodesia. S Afr Med J 1978;53:230–234.
20. Robson N, Robertson I, Whittaker M. Plasma cholinesterase changes during the puerperium. Anesthesia 1986;41:243–249.
21. Whittaker M, Charlier AR, Ramaswamy S. Changes in plasma cholinesterase isoenzymes due to oral contraceptives. J Reprod Fertil 1971;26:373–375.
22. Das Gupta S, Ghosh AK, Moorthy MV, et al. Comparative studies of pralidoxime, trimedoxime, obidoxime and diethyxime in acute fluostigmine poisoning in rats. Pharmazie 1982;37:605.
23. Kusic R, Jovanovic D, Randjelovic S, et al. HI-6 in man: Efficacy of

the oxime in poisoning by organophosphorus insecticides. Hum Exp Toxicol 1991;10:113–118.

24. Lotti M, Becker CE, Aminoff MJ. Organophosphate polyneuropathy: pathogenesis and prevention. Neurology 1984;34:658–662.

25. Gordon JJ, Inns RH, Johnson MK, Leadbeater L, Maidment MP, Upshall DG, Cooper GH, Rickard RL. The delayed neuropathic effects of nerve agents and some other organophosphorus compounds. Arch Toxicol 1983;52:71–82.

26. Senanayake N, Johnson MK. Acute polyneuropathy after poisoning by a new organophosphate insecticide. Med Intell 1982;306:155–159.

27. Cherniack M. Organophosphorous esters and polyneuropathy. Ann Int Med 1986;104:264–266.

28. Hayes AL, Wise RA, Weir FW. Assessment of occupational exposure to organophosphates in pest control operators. Am Ind Hyg Assoc J 1980;41(Aug):568–575.

29. US Department of Health, Education, and Welfare (NIOSH). Criteria for a recommended standard occupational exposure during the manufacture and formulation of pesticides. DHEW (NIOSH) Pub. No. 78. Cincinnati, OH: NIOSH, 1977.

30. Casto KM. Environmental health law. Chapt 8 in: Blumenthol DS, ed. Introduction to environmental health. New York, NY: Springer Publishing, 1985:215–247.

31. Council of Scientific Affairs. Cancer risks of pesticides in agricultural workers. JAMA 1988;260(7);959–966.

102

Organochlorine Pesticides

Mark Van Ert, Ph.D., C.I.H.
John B. Sullivan, Jr., M.D.

INTRODUCTION

Chlorinated hydrocarbon pesticides encompass a wide range of chemical compounds as represented by the following general categories (Table 102.1):

1. DDT, DDE, and DDD
2. Hexachlorocyclohexane (HCH) and isomers, including lindane (gamma-HCH)
3. Cyclodiene compounds: chlordane, heptachlor, aldrin, dieldrin, endrin, endosulfan, isobenzan
4. Chlordecone, kelevan, and mirex
5. Toxaphene
6. Dicofol and methoxychlor

The general toxicity of chlorinated hydrocarbon insecticides is central nervous system stimulation and/or central nervous system depression, depending on the compound and dose. Cyclodienes, hexachlorocyclohexanes, and toxaphene pesticides inhibit gamma aminobutyric acid (GABA)-induced chloride influx in the CNS and thus interfere with GABA receptor function (1, 2). This mechanism of inhibition is consistent with the clinical symptoms of CNS excitation and seizures seen in acute toxicity from organochlorine pesticides. In general, aldrin, dieldrin, lindane, toxaphene, endrin, and chlordane can cause seizures, muscle tremors, confusion, agitation, and coma as common manifestations which can occur via oral, dermal, and inhalational exposure routes.

DDT, DDE, and DDD

DDT (dichlorodiphenyl trichloroethane or 1,1,1-trichloro-2,2-bis(p-chlorophenyl) ethane) was one of the most popular chem-

Table 102.1. Organochlorine Pesticides

DDT
DDE
DDD (Rothane)
Aldrin
Dieldrin
Endrin
Endosulfan
Isobenzan (telodrin)
Chlordane
Heptachlor
Hexachlorocyclohexane (technical grade)
Lindane (gamma-hexachlorocyclohexane)
Chlordecone (Kepone)
Kelevan
Mirex (Dechlorane)
Dicofol (Kelthane)
Methoxychlor (Marlate)
Toxaphene

icals used for controlling insects in agricultural areas and also in the control of typhus- and malaria-carrying insects. Technical DDT is a mixture of three forms: p,p'-DDT, o,p'-DDT, and o,o'-DDT. These analogs of DDT are odorless, white crystalline solids. DDE (dichlorodiphenyl-dichloroethylene, 1,1-dichloro-2,3-bis (p-chlorophenyl) ethylene) and DDD (1,1-dichloro-2,2-bis (p-chlorophenyl) ethane) are minor contaminants found in technical DDT (3). DDT is no longer used as a pesticide in the United States. However, it is still widely applied in several areas of the world for the control of insects and insect disease vectors.

Chemical and Physical Properties

The chemical structures and technical names of these compounds are shown in Figures 102.1–3. Technical DDT is formed by condensing chloral hydrate with chlorobenzene in the pres-

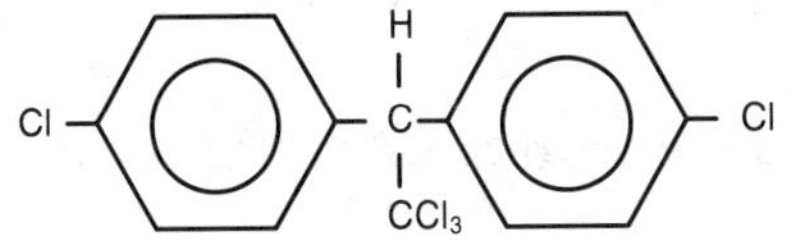

Chemical formula	$C_{14}H_9Cl_5$
Chemical name	p,p'-DDT
Synonyms	1,1,1-trichloro-2,2-bis(p-chlorphenyl) ethane; Dichlorodiphenyl trichloroethane
Trade name	Genitox, Anofex, Detoxen, Pentachlorin, Dicophane, Chlorophenothane

Figure 102.1. DDT. Reprinted with permission from USPHS. Toxicological profile for p,p'-DDT, p,p'-DDE, p,p'-DDD Agency for Toxic Substances and Disease Registry, U.S. Public Health Service, Government Printing Office, December 1989:1.

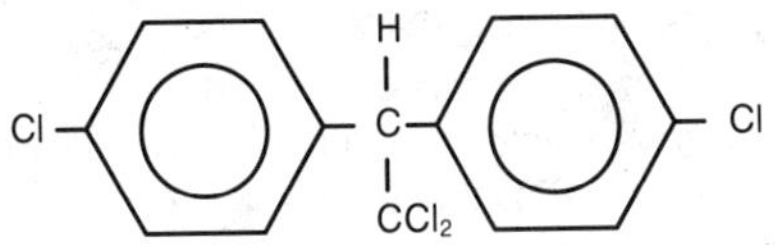

Chemical formula	$C_{14}H_8Cl_4$
Chemical name	p,p'-DDE
Synonyms	DDT dihydrochloride; Dichlorodiphenyldichloroethylene; 1,1-Dichloro-2,2-bis(p-chlorophenyl) ethylene

Figure 102.2. DDE. Reprinted with permission from USPHS. Toxicological profile for p,p'-DDT, p,p'-DDE, p,p'-DDD Agency for Toxic Substances and Disease Registry, U.S. Public Health Service, Government Printing Office, December 1989:1.

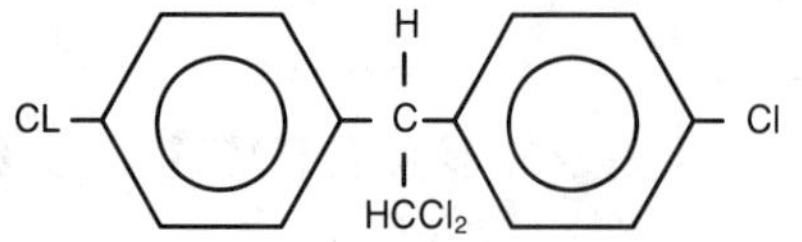

Chemical formula	$C_{14}H_{10}Cl_4$
Chemical name	p,p'-DDD
Synonyms	1,1-bis(4-chlorophenyl)-2,2-dichloroethane; 1,1-dichloro-2,2-bis(p-chlorophenyl) ethane
Trade name	DDD; Rothane; Dilene

Figure 102.3. DDD. Reprinted with permission from USPHS. Toxicological profile for p,p'-DDT, p,p'-DDE, p,p'-DDD Agency for Toxic Substances and Disease Registry, U.S. Public Health Service, Government Printing Office, December 1989:1.

ence of sulfuric acid (4). DDT was first synthesized in 1874, and its insecticide properties were discovered in 1939 (4). In 1972, the EPA banned the use of DDT within the United States except in cases of public health emergencies. However, exportation of DDT continued from the United States, and in 1985 producers exported over 300,000 kilograms of DDT (4). In 1972 between 4–7 million kilograms of DDT were utilized in the agricultural areas of the United States (4). Most of this DDT used in 1972 was on cotton crops. Peak usage of DDT occurred in 1963 when 80 million kilograms of DDT were applied to agricultural areas within the United States (4).

Human Exposure to DDT, DDE, and DDD

Despite being banned in the United States in 1972, DDT is still used heavily in other areas of the world for control of disease-transmitting insects. Concerns regarding DDT use include: (*a*) Does DDT or its metabolites cause human cancer? (*b*) Does the bioaccumulation of DDT, DDE, and DDD pose some unknown health effect to future generations? (*c*) Does the persistency of DDT and its metabolites in the environment pose environmental health risks to animals and humans? DDT persists for long periods of time following its application to soil and is converted to DDE, which persists even longer. DDT, DDE, and DDD may leach into water supplies from soil and crops. DDT and DDE bioaccumulate, and concentrations tend to increase as the food chain advances from plants to animals. Human exposure results primarily from ingestion of meat, fish, poultry, and vegetables (5, 6).

DDT and its primary metabolites, DDE and DDD, have been found at hazardous waste sites on the National Priorities List in the United States. DDT and its metabolites are ubiquitous in the environment and are constantly being transformed and redistributed. Volatilization of DDT and DDE account for losses from soil and water (5, 6). DDD is less volatile than either DDT or DDE. DDT, DDE, and DDD are highly lipid soluble and thus concentrate in human and animal adipose tissue. The long environmental half-life of these compounds coupled with their lipophilic properties results in bioaccumulation.

Photo-oxidation and biodegradation of DDT can occur in air, soil, and water. DDT and DDE are slowly degraded to CO_2 and hydrochloric acid by solar radiation (5, 6). Environmental concentrations of DDT, DDE, and DDD worldwide have tended to remain relatively constant despite widespread continued ap-

plication due to their continuous bio-oxidation by ultraviolet light (6).

The loss of DDT from soils is primarily through volatilization, water runoff, and chemical transformation. Some biodegradation occurs by aerobic and anaerobic microorganisms. Aerobic metabolism results in a conversion of DDT to DDE. Anaerobic conditions result in conversion of DDT to DDD. DDT conversion to DDE is slower than its conversion to DDD. The DDE and DDD metabolites of DDT are resistant to further transformation, and the half-life estimates for biodegradation of DDT in soil range from 2–15 years (5, 6). Human exposures occur mainly through diet via bioaccumulation up the food chain and from breast feeding.

Low levels of DDT and its metabolites will be present in the environment for decades, given the fact that other countries are still applying the chemical. Due to the partitioning of DDT and DDE into human breast milk, breast fed infants will receive DDT and DDE from the mother. Exposure to DDT and its metabolites by inhalation is negligible.

Due to the ban on use of DDT in this country, only those involved in its manufacture have the potential for exposure to high concentrations.

Distribution of DDT in the Environment

DDT and its analogs can easily be detected and identified by gas chromotography/mass spectrometry in both environmental samples and human tissues. DDE, the primary metabolite of DDT, is commonly found in samples of human adipose tissue.

Regulations relating to DDT and its analogs are presented in Table 102.2. DDT, DDE, and DDD are also listed in the Toxic Chemicals Section 313 of the Emergency Planning and Community Right to Know Act of 1986 Superfund Amendment Reauthorization Act (SARA Title III).

Airborne concentrations of DDT have been found to range from 1.4–1560 ng/m^3 and DDE from 1.9–131 ng/m^3 (5). Since the ban on DDT use, air concentrations have been declining. Over the period 1974–1975, the arithmetic mean DDT air concentration decreased from 11.9 ng/m^3–7.5 ng/m^3 (5). Air samples collected in the Gulf of Mexico in 1977 showed a DDT range of 0.010–0.078 ng/m^3 (5).

The United States National Soils Monitoring Program has followed the soil pattern concentration of DDT since its ban. DDT and DDE residues in soils have been steadily declining since the 1972 ban. In 1970, soil DDT concentrations averaged 0.18 ppm, decreasing to 0.02 ppm by 1972 (5).

The concentrations of DDT and DDE also declined in foods between 1965–1975. This overall and continuing decline in DDT and DDE levels in foods is attributable to the ban on DDT use (5).

Monitoring of DDT and its residues in water has been extensive. The median concentration of DDT and DDE in ambient water samples in the United States is approximately 1 part per trillion (ppt) (5). Industrial effluents have shown concentrations of 10 ppt of DDT, DDE, and DDD. Overall, the concentrations of DDT and its residues appear to be decreasing in the environment since its ban in 1972.

Absorption, Metabolism, and Excretion of DDT and Its Metabolites

DDT and its metabolites, DDE and DDD, are found in samples of human blood, adipose tissue, human breast milk, umbilical

Table 102.2. Regulations Applicable to DDT, DDE, or DDD

Agency	Description	Value
WHO	Conditional acceptable daily intake in food	0.005 mg/kg
WHO	Evidence of human carcinogenicity	no data
OSHA	TWA	1 mg/m^3
EPA	Maximum contaminant level in drinking water	
EPA	Reportable quantity	1 lb (proposed)
EPA	Listing as a hazardous waste substance	no data
EPA	Listing as toxic pollutant	no data
	Listed in RCRA Appendix IX for groundwater monitoring	no data
EPA	TSCA chemical substance inventory	no data
EPA	Recommended action levels for sum of residues	
	Range	0.05 (grapes, tomatoes)—3.0 (carrots) ppm
	Most fruits & vegetables	0.1 ppm—0.5 ppm
	Eggs	0.5 ppm
	Grains	0.5 ppm
	Milk	0.05 ppm
	Meat	5 ppm
EPA	Reference dose (oral)	5.0×10^{-4} mg/kg/day
	Potency factor (oral, inhalation)	3.4×10^{-1} mg/kg/day (DDT, DDE)
		2.4×10^{-1} mg/kg/day (DDD)
FIFRA	Most uses cancelled in 1972	
Guidelines		
NIOSH	IDLH	no data
	TWA (air and skin)	1 mg/m^3
ACGIH	TWA	1 mg/m^3
NAS	Suggested no-adverse-response-level (SNARL)	no data
	7-day	no data
	24-hour	no data
EPA	Ambient water quality criteria to protect human health	2.85 µg/L (DDT)
		(DDD) no data
		(DDE) no data
EPA	Carcinogenic classification	B2
	Water and fish and shellfish ingestion	0.0024 ng/L (DDT) (risk level corresponding to 10^{-7})
		2.6×10^{-6} µg/L for concentrations $\langle\, 1 \times 10^3$ µg/L (DDD)
	Fish and shellfish consumption only	0.0024 ng/L (DDT) (risk level corresponding to 10^{-7})

State Regulations and Guidelines

State Environmental Agencies	Drinking water quality standards and guidelines for DDT and several states	
	Alabama	No special or state rule
	Alaska	No special or state rule
	Arizona	No special or state rule
	California	No special or state rule
	Colorado	No special or state rule
	Connecticut	No special or state rule
	Delaware	No special or state rule
	Florida	No special or state rule
	Georgia	No special or state rule
	Hawaii	No special or state rule
	Idaho	No special or state rule
	Illinois	50 µg/L
	Indiana	No special or state rule
	Iowa	No special or state rule
	Kansas	0.42 µg/L (DDT)
		2.4×10^{-5} µg/L (DDE)
		2.4×10^{-5} µg/L (DDD)
	Kentucky	No special or state rule
	Maine	0.83 µg/L
	Maryland	No special or state rule
	Massachusetts	No special or state rule
	Minnesota	1.0 µg/L
	Mississippi	No special or state rule

continues

1030 Part 5, Specific Toxins

Table 102.2. *Continued*

Agency	Description	Value
	Missouri	No special or state rule
	Montana	No special or state rule
	Nebraska	No special or state rule
	Nevada	No special or state rule
	New Hampshire	No special or state rule
	New Mexico	No special or state rule
	New York	No special or state rule
	North Carolina	No special or state rule
	Ohio	No special or state rule
	Oklahoma	No special or state rule
	Oregon	No special or state rule
	Rhode Island	No special or state rule
	South Carolina	No special or state rule
	South Dakota	No special or state rule
	Tennessee	No special or state rule
	Texas	No special or state rule
	Utah	No special or state rule
	Vermont	No special or state rule
	Virginia	No special or state rule
	West Virginia	No special or state rule
	Wisconsin	No special or state rule
State Environmental Agencies	Acceptable ambient air concentrations standards and guidelines for DDT for several states	
	Connecticut	$5~\mu g/m^3$ (8 hr)
	Kansas	$2.381~\mu g/m^3$ (DDT) (annual)
		$2.4 \times 10^{-5}~\mu g/kg$ (DDE) (guideline)
		$2.4 \times 10^{-5}~\mu g/L$ (DDD) (guideline)
	Nevada	$0.04~\mu g/m^3$ (8 hr)
	Philadelphia, Pennsylvania	$1.8~\mu g/m^3$ (DDT) (1 yr)
		$1.8~\mu g/m^3$ (DDE)
	Virginia	$16~\mu g/m^3$ (24 hr)

EPA weight of evidence classification scheme for carcinogens: A—Human Carcinogen, sufficient evidence from human epidemiologic studies; B1—Probable Human Carcinogen, limited evidence from epidemiological studies and adequate evidence from animal studies; B2—Probable Human Carcinogen, inadequate evidence from epidemiologic studies and adequate evidence from animal studies; C—Possible Human Carcinogen, limited evidence in animals in the absence of human data; D—Not Classified as to human carcinogenicity; and E—Evidence of Noncarcinogenicity.
Adapted with permission from: USPHS. Toxicologic Profile for DDT, DDE, DDD. Agency for Toxic Substances and Disease Registry, US Public Health Service, 1989.

cord blood, and placental tissue (7–15). However, there is no correlation between the concentrations in human tissues and environmental concentrations. Higher ratios of DDD or DDT to DDE may indicate recent exposure, since DDT and DDD have shorter half-lives (16). Concentrations of DDT in fatty tissue are 300 times higher than those in blood (16). The partitioning of DDT among tissues as compared to blood (Fig. 102.4) demonstrates the high lipid solubility of the compound. Due to the fact that DDT and DDE are stored in fatty tissues and slowly released from these sites, it is difficult to make a correlation between concentrations in tissues and the time of exposure.

Environmental exposure concentrations are below any dose which will have identifiable health effects. There is evidence that a significant decline in human tissue concentrations of DDT has occurred over time (6). The estimated daily dietary intake of DDT declined from 0.24 mg/person/day in 1970 to 0.008 mg/person/day in 1973 (6). The World Health Organization (WHO) established an acceptable dietary intake (ADI) of DDT as 0.005 mg/kg/day and from 1965–1970, the dietary intake of DDT declined to 0.0007 mg/kg/day (6).

The metabolism of DDT, DDE, and DDD has been studied in humans and other animal species (Fig. 102.5). Chronic oral

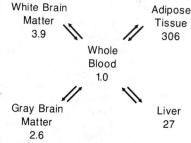

Figure 102.4. Relationship of the distribution of DDT and related chemicals between blood and certain tissues in humans. Reprinted from: de Vlieger, Robinson J, Crabtree A, van Dijk, M. The organochlorine insecticide content of human tissues. Arch Environ Health 1968;17:759–767.

ingestion of DDT induces the hepatic microsomal mixed function oxidase system (6, 16). Humans excrete DDT slower than animals. Also, it is estimated that if all human DDT exposure was terminated, it would take 10–20 years for all DDT to be removed from human tissue (6). However, DDE, with its longer half-life will persist much longer (6).

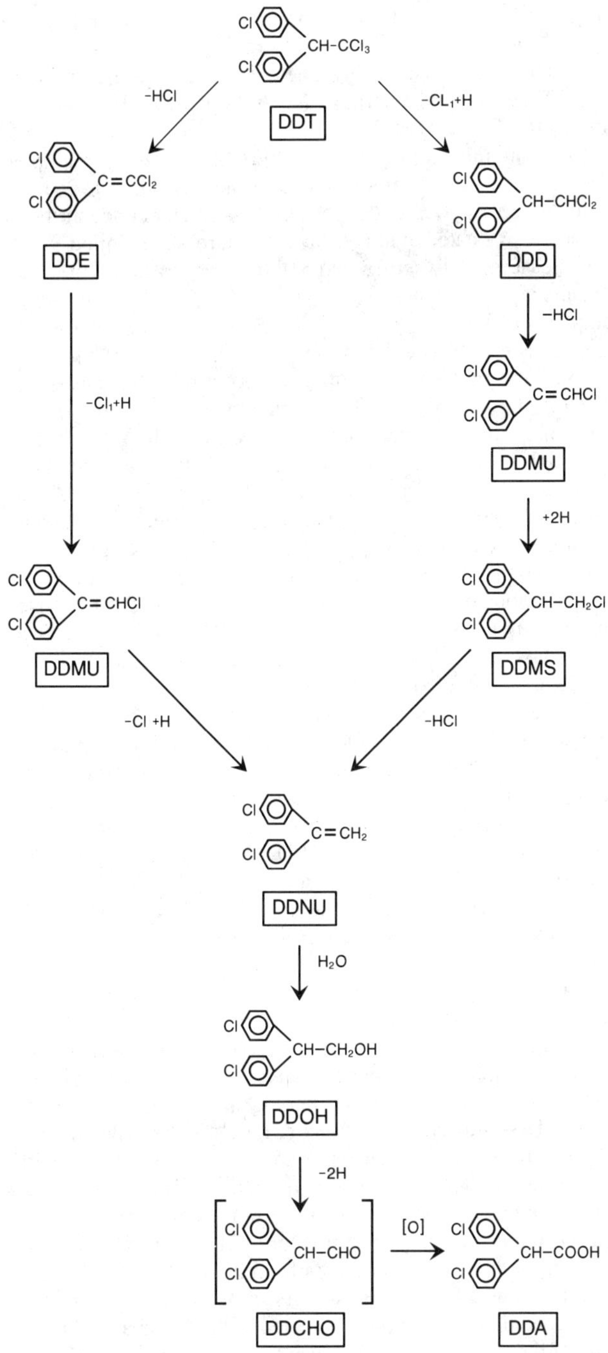

Figure 102.5. Metabolism of DDT. Reprinted from: USPHS. Toxicological profile for DDT, DDE, DDD. Agency for Toxic Substances & Disease Registry. U.S. Public Health Service, 1989.

Clinical Toxicity Associated with DDT Exposure

Volunteers given DDT orally have developed symptoms of gait disturbance, malaise, fatigue, headache, nausea, tremors, and vomiting, depending on the dose. Test doses were 750 mg, 1000 mg, or 1500 mg of DDT (16). All subjects recovered from their symptoms within 24 hours. Ingestion of DDT, either accidentally or intentionally, can result in similar symptoms. Exposure to large oral doses of DDT can result in excitability, tremors, and convulsions. This neurologic effect is probably a

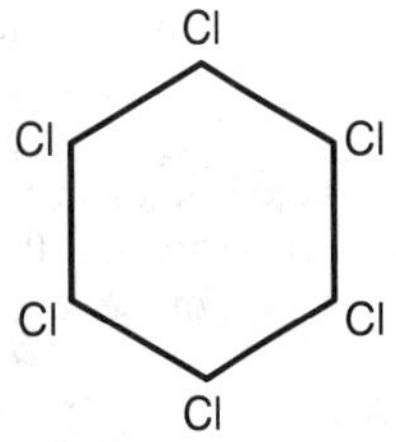

Figure 102.6.   Hexachlorocyclohexane (α, β, γ, δ isomers of HCH).

result of interference with sodium and potassium conductance across cell membranes.

Other known health effects at high exposure concentrations of DDT are irritation of the mucous membranes, nose, throat, and mouth, nausea, and headache.

Carcinogenesis and Immunotoxicity

There is no information on the immunotoxic effects of DDT or its metabolites in humans. Although immunologic effects in animals have been documented, it is difficult to extrapolate these findings to the human condition. Even though DDT has produced liver nodules in mice, several other studies in animals have not demonstrated carcinogenesis. There is no evidence that DDT or its metabolites are human carcinogens. Further, there is no information that establishes a causal relationship between DDT, DDE, and DDD concentrations in blood and fat or other tissues in relation to specific health effects.

The International Agency for Research on Cancer (IARC) has reviewed the literature on the carcinogenicity of these compounds and has found no convincing evidence of the carcinogenic risk of DDT and DDE in humans, although there was evidence of DDT carcinogenicity in the mouse model.

HEXACHLOROCYCLOHEXANE AND LINDANE

Hexachlorocyclohexane (HCH), sometimes misnamed benzene hexachloride, was prodigiously used as an insecticide through the 1960s and 1970s. HCH, discovered in 1825, was used as a smoke munition in World War I. The insecticide properties of HCH were discovered in 1942. Due to its chemical structure, various isomeric forms of HCH exist (Fig. 102.6), the best known of these being gamma-HCH or lindane. Technical grade lindane consists of several isomers: alpha, beta, gamma, delta. The toxicity of these isomers in terms of their effectiveness in controlling insects is as follows: Gamma > alpha > beta (17).

Chemical and Physical Properties

There are eight isomers of HCH, and all have the empirical formula of $C_6H_6Cl_6$ and a molecular weight of 290.8. The isomeric mixture of HCH is a brown off-white powder with a musty odor and is soluble in acetone, benzene, and chlorinated hydrocarbon solvents. HCH is almost insoluble in water (18). The gamma isomer or lindane is heat stable and can vaporize without decomposition.

Hexachlorocyclohexane is manufactured by ultraviolet photochlorination of benzene (17). Technical grade HCH consists of an isomeric mixture of alpha (70%), beta (7%), gamma (5%), delta (5%), and others (5%) (17). Fractional crystallization of the gamma-HCH isomer yields a 99.8% product of gamma-HCH called lindane (17). Production of lindane was terminated in 1976 in the United States. Lindane has been available as an emulsifiable concentrate, liquids, powders, gas, pressurized liquids, aerosol sprays, and granules. Besides its past use as an insecticide, lindane is still currently used as a scabicide for humans and animals. It has also been used on fruit and vegetable crops, for seed treatment, and animal treatment.

Environmental Regulations

Lindane is on the list of chemicals that appears in the Toxic Chemicals Substances Section, 313, of the Emergency Planning and Community Right to Know Act of 1986 (SARA Title III). The environmental regulations pertaining to lindane are summarized in Table 102.3.

Human Exposure Situations

Exposure to lindane and other HCH isomers occurs from occupational and environmental sources via dermal contact, inhalation, or ingestion.

Lindane and the other HCH isomers, can reach the environment through their use as pesticides and during the production of the product. HCH can be detected in air, soil, aquatic organisms, and water. Most human exposures occur through the ingestion of plants, animals, and dairy products. Alpha, beta, gamma, and delta HCH isomers have been detected at a number of hazardous waste sites. Lindane has been detected at waste sites in surface water at a mean concentration of 0.5 ppb and in the soil around these sites at a concentration of 11 ppb (19). The beta isomer of HCH has been found in surface water around hazardous waste sites at a mean concentration of 2.89 ppb and in soil at these sites at a mean concentration of 150 ppb. The delta isomer has been detected at hazardous waste sites at a mean concentration of 31 ppb and in the soil around these sites at a concentration of 6.6 ppb (19).

Release of lindane into the air has occurred through its application as a pesticide. Release of lindane into surface waters occurs from surface runoff or from deposition of the chemical through rain and other forms of precipitation. Low concentrations of lindane have been detected in samples of water runoff in a variety of cities around the United States. Lindane movement in the environment occurs via leaching from soil into ground water, adsorption to particles in the soil, and volatilization into the atmosphere. An important consideration pertaining to the release of lindane from soil into surface water is the relative content of the organic matter versus clay in the soil. Soil with a higher organic content will adsorb lindane and reduce leaching. Lindane in the soil is degraded primarily by microorganisms. Depending on the isomer, either anaerobic or aerobic conditions will be most conducive to biodegradation (18).

Lindane released into surface water can bioconcentrate in aquatic organisms. The other isomers of HCH, as well as lindane, bioconcentrate up through the food chain. Due to the lipophilic nature of lindane, it concentrates in adipose tissue. There is very little biodegradation of the HCH isomers.

Air monitoring lindane and other HCH isomers in ambient air in the United States over the period 1970–1972 has shown a mean concentration of 0.9 ng/m³ in a 10-state area (18). A maximum lindane concentration of 11.7 ng/m³ was reported in the same study (18). Other monitoring which has been performed at a variety of locations in the United States has shown

the gamma isomer of HCG to be present at concentrations of 0.1–7 ng/m³ (18). However, there were no detectable concentrations in rural areas. During a heavy period of pesticide usage in 1972–1974, atmospheric concentrations of lindane were as high as 9.3 ng/m³ (18).

Global monitoring of HCH isomers has shown air samples around the world in remote areas to range from 1.1–2.0 ng/m³ in air and 3.1–7.3 ng/L in water (18). Water concentrations of lindane evaluated at numerous areas across the United States have measured between 10 and 319 parts per trillion (ppt) (18). Lindane is detected in approximately 10% of urban water runoff samples in cities across the United States in concentrations ranging from 0.052–0.1 ppt (18).

Given the widespread, but low, environmental concentrations of HCH isomers, and their bioconcentration up the food chain, the most important human exposure at the present time is through ingestion of food products, mainly meats and dairy products. HCH isomers have been detected in dairy products, meats, fish, poultry, fruits, oils, fats, leafy vegetables, sugar, and other foods. To a lesser degree, other exposures to humans occur from the ingestion of drinking water which contains small concentrations of lindane. Previous estimates by the U.S. Department of Health, Education, and Welfare on the average daily intake of lindane have varied from 3 mcg/day to a low of 0.22 mcg/day (18).

Occupational exposure to HCH isomers has been studied extensively (17, 19–21). During the production of technical HCH and lindane, serum and adipose tissue concentrations of HCH isomers increase with exposure time. Human serum concentrations of HCH have been reported in the following ranges: alpha-HCH 10–273 µg/L, beta-HCH 17–760 µg/L, and gamma-HCH 5–188 µg/L (17). There appeared to be significant increase in beta-HCH concentrations in the serum of chronically exposed workers (17). Beta-HCH adipose concentrations were 300 times those of serum (17).

There have been no documented health effects of employees involved in lindane production when compared to control populations (19, 20). Serum concentrations of HCH are related the degree and duration of exposure, with beta-HCH accumulating more than the other isomers, making up around 30% of the total HCH serum concentrations (21). Workers who directly handled HCH, as well as exposed nonhandlers, had health complaints of headache, paresthesias, giddiness, malaise, tremors, apprehension, loss of sleep, confusion, vomiting, decreased libido, and impaired memory (21). The total HCH in the serum of those workers ranged from 0.143–1.152 µg/L (21).

Lindane and other HCH isomers as well as other organochlorine pesticides have been detected in the blood and adipose tissue of the general public in a variety of countries (7–15, 22–28). Lindane blood concentrations were found to be highest in people in the age group 41–60 years (19). The National Human Adipose Tissue Survey conducted in 1982 demonstrated that beta HCH was detected in 87% of samples collected, ranging in concentrations from 19–570 ng/g tissue (19). In autopsy surveys conducted between 1970 and 1975, beta HCH was present in more than 90% of human adipose tissue samples at a level of 300 ppb (19, 22). It has also been reported in a study by Mack in 1985 (19) that the median level of beta HCH in the United States has fallen from a level of 140 ppb–80 ppb in a study by Mack in 1985 (19). Even though the median concentration in human adipose tissue has declined, its still detected in nearly 100% of the general population (7–15, 22–28). Factors influencing the concentration of lindane in the

Table 102.3. Regulations and Guidelines Applicable to Hexachlorocyclohexane

Agency	Description	Value
	International	
Oral		
WHO	Acceptable Daily Intake	0.0–0.01 mg/kg
	Allowable Tolerances (gamma-HCH) Range	0.05 mg/kg (potatoes)–2 mg/kg (lettuce)
	Most fruits and vegetables	0.5 mg/kg
WHO	Guideline for drinking water	0.003 mg/L
Other		
IARC	Carcinogenic classification	Group 3
	alpha-HCH	
	beta-HCH	
	gamma-HCH	
Regulations	*National*	
Oral		
EPA	Tolerances (gamma-HCH) Range	0.01 ppm (pecans)–7 ppm (meat fat)
	Most fruits and vegetables	1 or 3 ppm
EPA	Maximum Contaminant Level (MCL) in drinking water (lindane)	0.004 mg/L
FDA	Permissible level in bottled water (lindane)	0.004 mg/L
	Action levels (lindane)	
	most fruit and vegetables	0.5 ppm
	cereals	0.1 ppm
	milk	0.3 ppm
Inhalation		
OSHA	Permissible Exposure Limit	
	Time Weighted Average (TWA)	
	lindane (skin)	0.5 mg/m^3
Other		
EPA	Reportable quantity lindane	1 lb
	Extremely Hazardous Substance	
	Threshold Planning Quantity	
	(TPQ) (lindane)	1,000/10,000 lb
	Listing as toxic waste: discarded commercial products, off-specification species, container residues, and spill residues of lindane. Listing as a Hazardous Waste Constituent. General Pretreatment Regulations for Existing and New Sources of Pollution.	
	Maximum Concentration of Contaminants for Characteristic of EP Toxicity (lindane)	0.4 mg/L
	TSCA Chemical Substance Inventory (all isomers)	
	General permits under the National Pollutant Discharge Elimination System (NPDES)	
Guidelines		
Oral		
EPA	Maximum contaminant Level Goal (MCLG) (proposed) (lindane)	0.0002 mg/L
	Health advisories (lindane)	
	1 day	1.2 mg/L
	10 day	1.2 mg/L
	Longer term	
	Adult	0.12 mg/L
	Child	0.033 mg/L
	Lifetime	0.2 µg/L
EPA	Ingestion of Water and Aquatic Organisms	
	alpha-HCH	0.92–92 ng/L
	beta-HCH	1.63–163 ng/L
		(risk 10^{-7}–10^{-5})
	gamma-HCH	1.86–186 ng/L
		(risk 10^{-7}–10^{-5})
	technical-HCH	1.23–23 ng/L
		(risk 10^{-7}–10^{-5})
	Ingestion of Aquatic Organisms Only	
	alpha-HCH	1–310 ng/L
		(risk 10^{-7}–10^{-5})
	beta-HCH	5.47–547 ng/L
		(risk 10^{-7}–10^{-5})
	gamma-HCH	6.25–625 ng/L
		(risk 10^{-7}–10^{-5})
	technical-HCH	4.14–414 ng/L
		(risk 10^{-7}–10^{-5})

continues

Table 102.3. *Continued*

Agency	Description	Value
NAS	Suggested No-Adverse-Effect Level (SNARL) (lindane)	
	7 day	0.5 mg/L
	24 hour	3.5 mg/L
Inhalation		
ACGIH	Threshold Limit Value	
	Time Weighted Average (TWA) for lindane (skin)	0.5 mg/m^3
NIOSH	Immediately Dangerous to Life or Health (IDLH) level (all isomers)	1000 mg/m^3
Other		
EPA	Carcinogenic classification	
	alpha-HCH	Group B2
	beta-HCH	Group C
	gamma-HCH	Group B2/C
	delta-HCH	Group D
	technical-HCH	Group B2
	RfD (oral) (gamma-HCH)	3×10^{-4} mg/kg/day
	q_1* (oral)	
	alpha-HCH	6.3 (mg/kg/day)$^{-1}$
	beta-HCH	1.8 (mg/kg/day)$^{-1}$
	gamma-HCH	1.3 (mg/kg/day)$^{-1}$
	technical-HCH	1.8 (mg/kg/day)$^{-1}$
	q_1* (inhalation)	
	alpha-HCH	6.3 (mg/kg/day)$^{-1}$
	beta-HCH	1.8 (mg/kg/day)$^{-1}$
	technical-HCH	1.8 (mg/kg/day)$^{-1}$

IARC weight of evidence classification scheme for carcinogens: Group 1—Carcinogenic to humans, sufficient evidence from human epidemiologic studies; Group 2A—Probably carcinogenic to humans, limited evidence from human epidemiologic studies; Group 2B—Probably carcinogenic to humans, inadequate data from human epidemiologic studies and sufficient evidence from animal studies; Group 3—Cannot be classified as to its carcinogenicity to humans.
EPA weight of evidence classification scheme for carcinogens: A—Human Carcinogen, sufficient evidence from human epidemiologic studies; B1—Probable Human Carcinogen, limited evidence from epidemiologic studies and adequate evidence from animal studies; B2—Probable Human Carcinogen, inadequate evidence from epidemiologic studies and adequate evidence from animal studies; C—Possible Human Carcinogen, limited evidence in animals in the absence of human data; D—Not Classified as to human carcinogenicity; and E—Evidence of Noncarcinogenicity.
The EPA Office of Drinking Water and the Office of Pesticide Programs are considering gamma-HCH (lindane) as Group C for regulatory purposes pending review.
Adapted with permission from: USPHS. Toxicologic Profile for DDT, DDE, DDD. Agency for Toxic Substances and Disease Registry, US Public Health Service, 1989.

body of exposed individuals include age, dietary habits, and location of the country in which the person lives (which would also be related to the pesticide spraying and occupational exposure). Higher levels of lindane and other HCH isomers are found in non-vegetarians. Studies of human breast milk have demonstrated HCH isomers in 82% of samples at a mean concentration of 81 ppb with a range from 0–480 parts per billion (ppb) (19, 24, 29, 30).

Gas chromatograph mass spectrometry methods are capable of detecting lindane and HCH isomers in the ppb level. Although methods are available that can detect and quantify concentrations of HCH isomers, it remains impossible to correlate these concentrations with environmental concentrations or toxic effects.

Despite the fact that HCH isomers can be detected in blood, serum, urine, and adipose tissue in the general population, the concentration in these tissues does not correlate with health effects. Mean serum concentrations of total HCH in these individuals were reported to be 0.27 ppm for those who did not handle the product and 0.6 ppm for those who directly handled the product. Sixty to 100% of total HCH assayed for in the serum of these individuals was in the form of the beta HCH isomer. The serum concentrations were reported as follows: 0.07–0.72 ppm of beta-HCH, 0.004–0.18 ppm alpha HCH, and 0–0.17 ppm for lindane, and 0–0.16 ppm for delta HCH (21). The investigators reported that handlers of this material, as well as those who were not directly exposed, had complained

of facial paresthesias, headaches, and dizziness, malaise, vomiting, tremors, confusion, and impaired memory (21). Serum levels were also measured on maintenance workers who periodically visited the worksite. Serum concentrations in these workers were much lower than in those occupationally exposed. The exposed workers had no statistically significant difference from controls in liver functions (31). Table 102.4 summarizes HCH serum and adipose tissue concentrations in occupational situations (17, 24, 32).

In one study, where exposure levels of alpha-HCH were 0.002–1.99 mg/m^3, beta-HCH 0.001–0.38 mg/m^3, and lindane or gamma-HCH 0.004–0.15 mg/m^3. The mean blood levels of 57 workers measured 0.5 μg/L of alpha-HCH, 0.9 μg/L beta-HCH, and 0.7 μg/L of gamma-HCH (17). The beta-HCH isomer accumulation has been demonstrated to increase in a linear fashion with duration of exposure. Adipose concentrations in samples from autopsies have ranged from 0.03–0.47 ppm for total HCH, and 0.04–0.57 ppm for beta-HCH (25).

Animal studies have indicated the various distribution patterns of hexachlorocyclohexane isomers. The gama- and beta-HCH isomers appear to be stored in the fatty tissues primarily (33). The distribution of lindane was also highest in the fatty tissue, followed by brain, kidney, muscle, lungs, heart, spleen, liver, and blood. Lindane has a propensity to accumulate in the brain more than the beta-HCH (34). Lindane also induces hepatic mixed function oxidase systems, increasing its own metabolism. This process may minimize or reduce the accu-

Table 102.4.   Summary of HCH Occupational Exposure

	Occupational Exposures Serum Concentrations (ppm)				
	Total-HCH	Beta-HCH	Alpha-HCH	Gamma-HCH	Delta-HCH
Control	0.05	0.029	0.022	0.0007	0
(mean)	(0–0.37)	(0–0.1)	(0–0.26)	(0–0.01)	
Handlers	0.60	0.41	0.10	0.06	0.04
(mean)	(0.20–1.15)	(0.16–0.72)	(0.024–0.18)	(0.01–0.17)	(0–0.16)
Nonhandlers	0.266	0.207	0.0412	0.016	0.0017
(mean)	(0.08–0.66)	(0.065–0.5)	(0.004–0.16)	(0–0.04)	(0–0.022)

	Occupational Exposure Adipose Tissue Concentrations (mg/kg)		
	Alpha-HCH	Beta-HCH	Gamma-HCH
Control	0.01–0.2	0.3–2.4	0.0.1
Workers	1–15	18–103	0–11
	(5.8 ± 5)	(45.6 ± 24.4)	(3.2 ± 3.1)

	Occupational Exposure Lindane (gamma-HCH/Blood Concs (ppb)	
	Lindane Blood Conc. ppb	Lindane Air Conc. (μg/m^3)
Non-production workers	0.93 (0.3–2.5)	9–49
Production workers with no skin contact Group I	4.6 (1.9–8.3)	31–1800
Production workers with no skin contact Group II	4.1 (1.0–8.9)	11–1170
Production workers with no skin contact Group III	30.6 (6.0–93)	11–1170

Adapted from: Baumann K, Angerer J, Heinrich R, Lehnert G. Occupational exposure to hexachlorocyclohexane, Part I. Int Arch Occup Environ Health 1980;47:119–127; Nigam SK, Karnik AB, Majumder SK, et al. Serum hexachlorocyclohexane residues in workers engaged at a HCH manufacturing plant. Int Arch Occup Environ Health 1986;57:315–320; Milby TH, Samuels AJ, Ottoboni F. Humane exposure to lindane: blood lindane levels as a function of exposure. J Occup Med 1968;10:584–587.

mulation of lindane in tissues (34). Lindane, has been detected in blood and central nervous system tissue of autopsies of infants that have died following total body application of a 1% lotion (35). Initial blood concentrations of lindane were 206 ppb and declined to 1.0 ppb in 25 days (35). Brain concentrations were three-fold that of blood in this case.

The accumulations of lindane in adipose tissue occurs through the passage of pesticides from mother to fetus across the placenta in pregnant women and to newborns through breast milk (36–38, 39). Concentrations of lindane in human breast milk are stated to be approximately 5–7 times higher than concentrations in the maternal blood or in umbilical cord blood. Older women tend to have higher lindane concentrations of HCH and lindane in placental and umbilical cord blood than younger women (36–38). It has also been noted that lindane concentrations increased in maternal blood during delivery and that during pregnancy higher concentrations have been found in fetal blood and fetal tissue as well as placenta and amniotic fluid compared to maternal fat tissue (36–38).

Metabolism of Lindane

The primary metabolites of lindane are chlorophenols and chlorobenzenes (Fig. 102.7) (34). Chlorinated metabolites in the urine have been found in lindane production workers. The major metabolite is trichlorophenol which accounted for approximately 58% of lindane metabolites identified in the urine (34). Other metabolites are dichlorophenols, tetrachlorophenols, hexachlorobenzene, tetrachlorocyclohexanol, and pentachlorocyclohexene. Pentachlorophenol has also been identified as a urinary metabolite in humans following occupational exposure (34).

CLINICAL TOXICITY AND HEALTH EFFECTS

Human exposure resulting in toxic health effects from hexachlorocyclohexane and isomers can occur by inhalation, dermal absorption, and through the gastrointestinal tract. Inhalational exposure to lindane vapor has occurred in the past through its use in home vaporizers (39). Most studies of acute lindane inhalational poisoning have come from anecdotal cases of home exposure from the use of vaporized lindane (39). Mucous membrane irritation, and irritation of the eye, throat, and upper airway may occur following short term exposure to lindane vapors. Further reports of effects secondary to inhalation of lindane have included blood dyscrasias such as anemia, leukopenia, leukocytosis, granulocytopenia, granulocytosis, eosinophilia, thrombocytopenia, increased bone marrow megakaryocytes, and decreased bone marrow megaloblastoid erythroid series (39, 40). Aplastic anemia and pancytopenia have also been reported following exposure to lindane (34, 39, 40).

Kashyap, 1986, reported statistically significant elevations in hepatic enzymes in 19 occupationally exposed individuals. These individuals were exposed to technical grade HCH for 10 years in a production plant (28). The same study also reported a significant increase in the concentrations of serum IgM. Other symptoms of exposed workers included facial paresthesias, headaches, and dizziness.

Ingestion of Lindane

Acute toxic effects from oral ingestion of lindane has been described in children. These reports are mainly from the 1950s and 1960s and involve children ingesting tablets of lindane meant to be used in vaporizers. Studies of acute oral toxicity

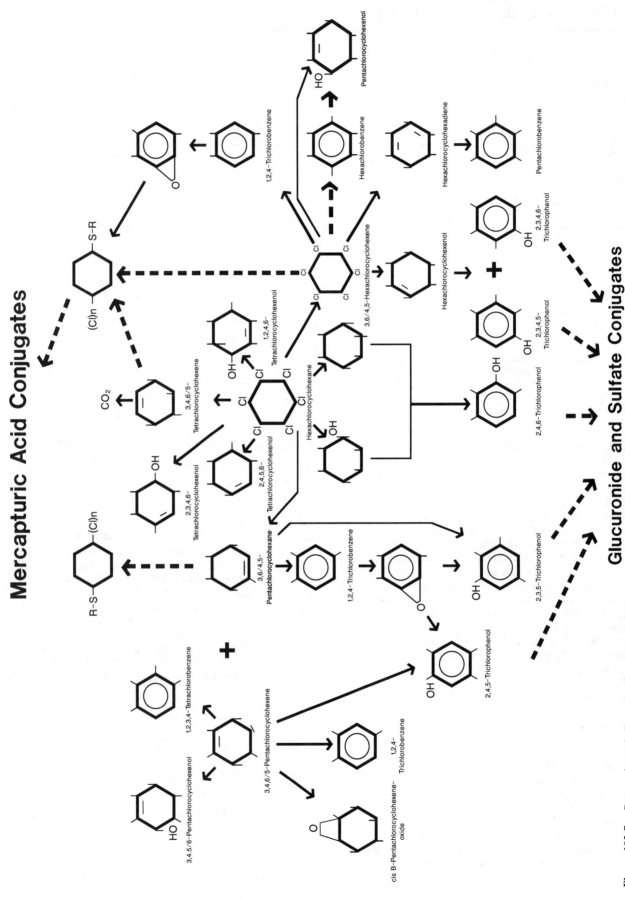

Figure 102.7. Proposed metabolism of γ-Hexachlorocyclohexane. Adapted with permission from: USPHS. toxicological profile for alpha-, beta-, gamma-, and delta- hexachorocyclohexane. Agency for Toxic Substances & Disease Registry. US Public Health Service, 1989.

in animals have reported ataxia, coma, and death. Clinical toxicity following an acute ingestion of lindane in humans consists of abdominal pain, nausea, vomiting, excitability, seizures, muscle tremors, hyper reflexia, and coma. Rhabdomyolysis, myoglobinuria, and leukocytosis have also been observed (41). Animal studies of oral dosing of lindane and technical grade HCH have been reported to cause fatty degeneration and necrosis of the liver (34). No immunotoxic effects of HCH isomers have been detected in humans. Nor have there been any studies of the reproductive effects or carcinogenicity of the isomers of HCH in humans. In animal studies, the isomers of HCH as well as technical grade HCH have been shown to produce liver cancer in rats and/or mice (34).

Dermal Absorption of Lindane

Most cases of lindane toxicity via dermal absorption have resulted from its use as a topical scabicide. Seizures and deaths in infants have been reported following topical application of 1% lindane lotion in large amounts (35, 40). Lindane blood concentrations 46 hours after application of a 1% topical lotion to treat scabies in an infant who developed seizures post application was $0.10 \mu g/L$ (42). This high concentration compares to a mean blood concentration of $0.005 \mu g/L$ in most children treated with the 1% lotion (42). Peak concentrations of lindane occur in 6 hours following dermal application (42). Inappropriate application of excessive amounts of lindane ointment to the skin can result in clinical symptoms including seizures, and should be avoided (35, 42). The dermal absorption of pesticides in general has been well-studied (43). Dermal absorption of organochlorine pesticide is dependent on the amount applied, surface area of application, breaks in the normal dermal barrier, and conditions which cause the compound to be removed from the skin, such as volatilization and dilution.

An important clinical concept involving delayed toxicity is the delayed absorption of some pesticides through the skin (43). Delayed and prolonged absorption of organochlorine pesticides such as lindane, dieldrin, and aldrin have been demonstrated by the prolonged urinary excretion of these compounds up to 120 hours post dermal application (43). The safety of lindane use as a 1% lotion for scabies has been reviewed (44).

Neurotoxic Effects of Lindane

The neurotoxic effects of HCH include seizures, headaches, dizziness, tremors, ataxia, facial and extremity paresthesias, giddiness, and coma. The mechanism of lindane and other HCH isomer neurotoxicity is thought to be due to inhibition of GABA-mediated neurotransmission (1, 2). In the limbic system, lindane acts directly to increase excitability of neurons (45). Also, lindane accelerates kindling seizures, which is the sequence of changes which results from repetitive stimulation (45).

CHLORDANE AND HEPTACHLOR

Chlordane has been extensively used the United States for years as a termiticide and has been heavily applied to soils in both urban and rural settings. Its persistency in the environment is one reason that chlordane has been successfully used as a termiticide. Chlordane is also a common indoor air contaminant and can be detected in the indoor air of homes 10–15 years after termite treatment (1). It is estimated that in the United States alone, approximately 50 million people have been ex-

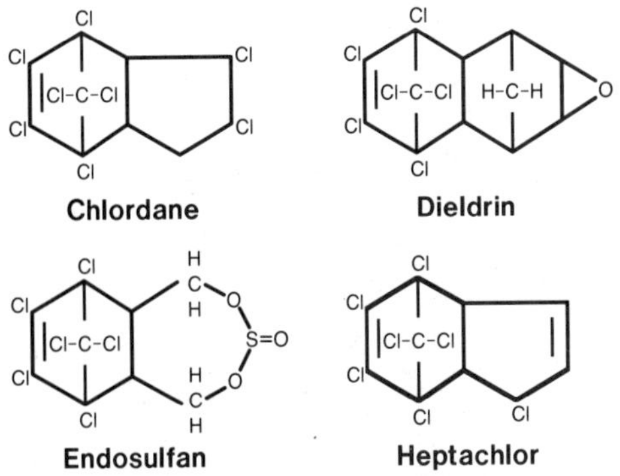

Figure 102.8. Cyclodienes.

posed to chlordane, principally in the home environment (46). Many foods also contain chlordane. Chlordane, along with heptachlor, endrin, aldrin, and dieldrin are members of the cyclodiene class of organochlorine compounds (Fig. 102.8).

Production and Use of Chlordane

Chlordane is produced by the chlorination of chlordene. Chlordene is the product of Diels-Alder reaction of hexochlorocyclopentadiene with cyclopentadiene (47). On April 14, 1988, the Environmental Protection Agency (EPA) cancelled the registration and use of chlordane for commercial production, delivery, and sale in the United States.

In addition to chlordane, heptachlor, a chlordane metabolite, was also used widely as a pesticide to control termites and other insects on a variety of crops, vegetation, and in home environments. In the United States, chlordane has been used almost exclusively as a termiticide by soil injection techniques in home environments (48). The volatilization of chlordane probably accounts for its presence in the air of some homes. Also, cracks in the foundation increase its release into indoor air. It is estimated that over 200 million pounds of chlordane has been applied to the soil in the United States alone (48).

Chlordane found in water due to runoff from soil, is a common chemical detected in the groundwater of hazardous waste sites. As a component of indoor air in the home environments, the chemical is usually present on dust particles and in a vapor phase. Following application to the soil, chlordane can continue to be released into the indoor air of the home for years. Generally, if this is occurring, air concentrations of chlordane may exceed the National Academy of Sciences standard of $5 \mu g/m^3$ (49, 50).

Chemical Structure and Physical Properties

Technical chlordane is a mixture of at least 50 different compounds with the major constituents being cis and trans chlordane, heptachlor, cis and trans nonachlor, alpha, beta, and gamma chlordane. Alpha and beta chlordane represent 70% of commercial preparations (51).

Chlordane is a viscous liquid that is a mixture of many different compounds. The individual components of the chlordane solution are usually solids. Pure chlordane has a molecular weight of 409.76, is brown in color, and is a viscous liquid as a technical product (51). The individual isomers have different melting points and boiling points. Chlordane is miscible with hydrocarbon solvents. Chlordane has two main isomers, trans and cis chlordane, the more abundant of which is cis chlordane

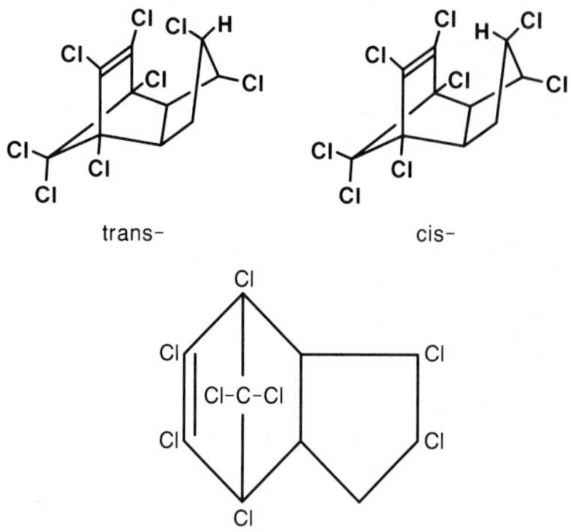

Chemical formula $C_{10}H_6Cl_{18}$

Chemical name 1,2,4,5,6,7,8,8-Octachloro-2,3 3a,4,7,7a-hexahydro-4,7-methano-1H-indene

Synonyms 1,2,4,5,6,7,8,8-Octachloro-3a,4,7,7a-tetrahydro-4,7-methanoindan

Trade name Chlordan; Velsicol 1068; Octachlor; Termicide C-100

Figure 102.9. Chlordane. Reprinted with permission from USPHS. Toxicological profile for chlordane. Agency for Toxic Substances and Disease Registry, U.S. Public Health Service, Government Printing Office, December 1989;1–8.

(Fig. 102.9). Other members of the cyclodiene class of insecticides are beta chlordane, heptachlor, aldrin, dieldrin, endrin, endosulfan, and isobenzan. In addition to the isomers of chlordane, technical chlordane solutions also contain heptachlor, nonachlor, and hexachlorocyclo-pentadiene (52).

Table 102.5. Drinking Water and Serum Concentrations of Organochlorine Pesticides and Metabolites in Samples from Individuals Who Use Well Water

Water (ppt)		Serum (ppb)				
HCH[a]	Dieldrin	HCB	B-HCH[b]	p,p'-DDE	Dieldrin	p,p'-DDT
ND[c]	<20	ND	ND	14.5	ND	<2.0
ND	<20	0.4	0.9	24.0	ND	2.0
ND	<20	0.3	<0.7	8.6	ND	ND
ND	<20	0.3	<0.7	17.0	<1.0	3.4
ND	<20	0.5	1.8	31.5	1.2	3.3
ND	<20	<0.2	0.8	22.0	ND	<2.0
ND	<20	<0.2	<0.7	6.8	<1.0	ND
ND	ND	0.3	<0.7	21.5	ND	<2.0
ND	ND	0.8	1.1	11.0	ND	ND
ND	<20	<0.2	0.9	17.2	<1.0	<2.0
		0.3	<0.7	32.0	<1.0	<2.0
		0.4	0.9	12.3	<1.0	<2.0
		0.3	0.6	11.5	ND	<2.0
		0.3	ND	7.0	ND	<2.0
		0.4	<0.7	18.0	ND	2.3
		0.3	<0.7	14.7	ND	<2.0
		<0.2	0.9	17.2	<1.0	<2.0
		0.3	0.7	9.7	ND	<2.0
		0.5	0.8	26.7	ND	2.3
		<0.2	<0.7	7.1	ND	ND
		0.7	1.2	31.6	1.4	4.6
		0.3	1.5	17.0	<1.0	<2.0
		0.4	0.7	20.8	ND	<2.0
		0.4	ND	10.8	<1.0	<2.0
		0.3	ND	3.4	ND	<2.0
		0.6	<0.7	12.9	ND	<2.0

Reprinted with permission from: Barquet A, Morgade C, Pfaffenberger CD. Determination of organochlorine pesticides and metabolites in drinking water, human blood serum, and adipose tissue. J Toxicol Environ Health 1981;7:469–479.
[a]HCH, hexachlorocyclohexane.
[b]B-HCH, B isomer of 1,2,3,4,5,6-hexachlorocyclohexane.
[c]ND, not detected.

Sites, Industries, and Locations Associated with Exposure

Chlordane was used to treat crops and other types of vegetation as well as to control termites. It has been intentionally applied to soils and agricultural urban settings for years. It is now found at 46 of 1117 hazardous waste sites on the National Priorities List in the United States (48). The majority of exposures to chlordane occur in the home environment due to the application of chlordane as a termiticide. Chlordane is detected in the indoor air of homes up to 15 years following treatment of the home for termites (48–50). It is estimated by the EPA that over 80 million people in the United States live in homes that have been treated with cyclodiene termiticide agents such as chlordane (48). This is probably an underestimation because foods and food sources also contain chlordane which bioaccumulates and produces further exposure in humans as they consume the food.

Chlordane and other organochlorines have been detected in surface groundwater (Table 102.5), in drinking water (Table 102.6) and in urban runoff water (48). Chlordane concentrations in surface water are generally in the low nanogram per liter range (parts per billion). Chlordane is also detected in soil, particularly around the outside walls of treated homes in concentrations ranging in less than 1 part per billion (ppb) to around 141 parts per million (ppm) (48–50). The major source of exposure to chlordane is living in homes treated with chlordane for termites. The majority

of the homes treated with chlordane have been in the Southeastern United States and the far Southwest where termites pose a significant problem. Other people with high exposure incidents include those involved in the manufacturing of chlordane.

Chlordane bioconcentrates in marine animals due to contamination of water. In soil, chlordane adsorbs to organic materials (48). Due to the fact that it does adsorb to organics and has a slow volatilization, it does not leach significantly from the soil. Depending on the type of soil, chlordane will be present to a lesser or greater extent. Sandy soils and soils that contain a small amount of organic materials retain chlordane less than soils that have a high organic content (48). Chlordane is degraded in air by photo-oxidation. Alpha chlordane is a photo byproduct of chlordane (48). Chlordane does not degrade rapidly in water.

Chlordane concentrations in air of homes in urban areas range from below the detection limit, which is less than 0.1 ng/m^3, all the way to 200 ng/m^3 (48–50). Rural air concentrations of chlordane are much less, ranging from less than $0.1–0.8 \text{ ng/m}^3$ (48). Compared to the outdoor air, chlordane concentrations in indoor air are much higher (49, 50). Chlordane has been used mainly for controlling termites in homes. One of the major routes of exposure to chlordane is living in treated houses. Indoor air concentrations in houses treated with chlordane range from 0.8–600,000 ng/m^3 (48–50). These concentrations can persist for years. Indoor air sampling in previously treated homes demon-

Table 102.6. Drinking Water and Serum Concentrations of Organochlorine Pesticides and Metabolites in Samples from Individuals Who Use City Water

Water (ppt)		Serum (ppb)				
HCH[a]	Dieldrin	HCB	B-HCH[b]	p,p'-DDE	Dieldrin	p,p'-DDT
30	<20	0.7	5.8	68.4	ND[c]	<2.0
68	<20	ND	ND	15.0	<1.0	ND
42	<20	0.7	0.9	7.4	ND	ND
<4	ND	<0.2	<0.7	ND	10.1	ND
ND	ND	ND	<0.7	10.9	ND	ND
ND	<20	0.4	0.8	16.8	ND	<2.0
ND	<20	0.4	1.0	20.0	0.9	<2.0
ND	<20	0.5	1.7	21.3	ND	ND
ND	<20	0.3	<0.7	17.6	ND	<2.0
ND	<20	0.9	1.1	36.1	<1.0	ND
		0.5	1.6	27.2	4.6	2.0
		0.7	1.7	22.0	1.9	4.7
		0.3	3.1	25.0	<1.0	3.0
		0.5	1.7	16.4	1.7	2.2
		0.3	0.8	14.2	<1.0	<2.0
		0.3	<0.7	23.9	<1.0	<2.0
		0.3	0.7	7.1	<1.0	<2.0
		<0.2	<0.7	3.9	ND	ND
		0.3	ND	24.3	<1.0	<2.0
		0.3	1.0	16.6	ND	<2.0
		0.4	<0.7	66.7	1.2	4.2
		0.3	ND	5.0	ND	ND
		0.2	ND	5.4	ND	ND
		0.7	0.8	21.0	ND	2.0
		0.4	<0.7	9.9	ND	<2.0
		0.4	0.8	19.0	<1.0	<2.0
		<0.2	<0.7	10.4	ND	<2.0
		<0.2	1.3	43.1	<1.0	3.4
		0.3	<0.7	12.6	ND	ND
		0.7	<0.7	20.7	ND	5.5
		1.1	1.0	20.6	1.3	3.5
		0.4	1.3	17.0	1.0	2.6
		0.5	0.8	10.6	ND	<2.0

Reprinted with permission from: Barquet A, Morgade C, Pfaffenberger CD. Determination of organochlorine pesticides and metabolites in drinking water, human blood serum, and adipose tissue. J Toxicol Environ Health 1981;7:469–479.
[a]HCH, hexachlorocyclohexane.
[b]B-HCH, B isomer of 1,2,3,4,5,6-hexachlorocyclohexane.
[c]ND, not detected.

strates concentrations of gamma chlordane, alpha chlordane, and trans-nonachlor (48–50). However, these concentrations were all below the 5 μg/m^3 guideline proposed by the National Academy of Sciences for indoor levels of chlordane.

Environmental Regulations of Chlordane

Chlordane is regulated by the Clean Water Act for certain industrial point sources such as electroplating, steam electric production, asbestos production, timber products processing, metal finishing, paving and roofing, paint formulating, ink formulating, gum and wood processing, pesticide production, and carbon black production (53). The International Agency for Research on Cancer (IARC) in 1987 was unable to determine that chlordane represented a human cancer risk. On March 6, 1978, registrations for all uses of chlordane on fruit products were cancelled (53). However, chlordane use was continued for treatment of homes for termite control. In 1988, the EPA cancelled registrations for chlordane-containing termiticide

products. Regulatory guidelines for chlordane are shown in Table 102.7.

CLINICAL TOXICOLOGY AND HEALTH EFFECTS OF CHLORDANE

Acute Toxicity

There are many reported cases in the literature of acute chlordane poisoning. Studies on laboratory animals have been extensive, and animals that have been given fatal doses of chlordane usually exhibited symptoms of dyspnea, depressed respirations, tremors, convulsions, and coma before death. In reported human cases of acute chlordane ingestion, convulsions, muscle tremors, increased excitability, confusion, and coma are common toxic manifestation (54–58). Following an acute ingestion, symptoms usually begin within an hour with manifestations of confusion followed by convulsions. Death has occurred following chlordane ingestion. Chlorinated hydrocarbons such as chlordane, are also absorbed through the skin, through inhalation, and through gastrointestinal routes. Once absorbed, most of these have a high distribution into adipose tissue. Other human cases of chlordane exposure have shown elevation of white blood cell count, pneumonias probably secondary to aspiration, and hepatic and renal damage. Some individuals have experienced nausea and vomiting following ingestion. However, it appears that central nervous system features of tremors and convulsions as well as coma, dominate the clinical picture. Treatment of acute ingestion as well as dermal absorption toxicity is symptomatic.

Subacute and Chronic Exposures to Chlordane

Retrospective cohort mortality studies of workers in chlordane and other organochlorine manufacturing industries as well as pesticide applicators have shown no increase in mortality rates and no increase in a specific cause of death that could be attributed to the exposure to chlordane (59–62).

One study that looked at cause-specific mortality among workers occupationally exposed to chlordane or heptachlor showed no overall excess of death from cancer even in workers who were followed 20 or more years after entry into the industry (61).

Another study which examined the mortality of a cohort of 3827 white males licensed to apply pesticides in Florida showed an excess mortality from lung cancer among pesticide applicators (63). However, his study did not account for other risk modifiers, such as smoking.

A retrospective mortality study of workers employed at organochlorine pesticide manufacturing plants looked at mortality of workers employed in the manufacture of several different organochlorine hydrocarbons for use as pesticides (62). This study concluded that the standardized mortality ratio (SMR) for all causes of death in each cohort was below the expected level (62).

Blood dyscrasias such as megaloblastic anemia and bone marrow depression have been associated with chlordane exposure in some instances (64, 65). However, these case reports identified other pesticide exposures besides chlordane, and no definitive study has indicated that chlordane is causative of blood dyscrasias. Investigations into the health status of people living in private residences previously treated with chlordane

Table 102.7. Regulations Applicable to Chlordane

Agency	Description	Value
WHO	Guidelines for drinking water	0.3 µg/L
WHO	Residue tolerances for sum of alpha- and gamma-isomers and oxychlordane	0.02–0.5 mg/kg
WHO	Acceptable daily intake (ADI)	0–0.001 mg/kg/bw
Regulations		
OSHA	Permissible exposure limit (PEL) (8-hour workday)	0.5 mg/m³
EPA	Reportable quantity (released to the environment)	1 pound
NAS	Recommended maximum indoor concentration in homes	5 µg/m³
	Threshold planning quantity (TPQ)	1000 pounds
Guidelines		
a. Air		
ACGIH	Threshold limit value (TWA-TLV) (8-hour workday)	0.5 mg/m³
STEL		2 mg/m³
NRC	Interm guideline for military housing	5 µg/m³
EPA	Inhalation	1.3 mg/kg/day
b. Water		
EPA	Health advisories	
	1-day (10 kg child)	0.06 mg/L
	10-day (10 kg child)	0.06 mg/L
	Longer term (10 kg child)	0.5 µg/L
	Longer term (70 kg adult)	2 µg/L
EPA	Maximum contaminant level goal (proposed)	0 mg/L
EPA	Ambient water quality criteria for the following lifetime increased cancer risk levels:	
	(with ingestion of water, fish, and shellfish)	
	10^{-5}	4.6 ng/L
	10^{-6}	0.46 ng/L
	10^{-7}	0.046 ng/L
	(with ingestion of fish and shell fish only)	
	10^{-5}	4.8 ng/L
	10^{-6}	0.48 ng/L
	10^{-7}	0.048 ng/L
c. Other		
EPA	q_1* (oral)	1.3 mg/kg/day
EPA	RfD (oral)	5×10^{-5} mg/kg/day
EPA	PADI (oral)	5.0×10^{-5} mg/kg/day
EPA	Group B2 (cancer ranking)	Probable human carcinogen
EPA	Designated as a hazardous waste	No. U036
State	Acceptable ambient air concentration	
Connecticut		2.5 µg/m³ (8 hr avg)
Kansas		1.19 µg/m³ (annual avg)
Kentucky		0.05 µg/m³ (8 hr avg)
Massachusetts		0.068 µg/m³ (24 hr avg)
Nevada		0.012 µg/m³ (8 hr avg)
New York		1.7 µg/m³ (1 yr avg)
Pennsylvania-Philadelphia		0.35 µg/m³ (1 yr avg)
Virginia		8.0 µg/m³ (24 hr avg)
State	Acceptable drinking water concentrations	
Arizona		0.5 µg/L
California		0.55 µg/L
Illinois		3 µg/L
Kansas		0.22 µg/L
Maine		0.55 µg/L
Minnesota		0.22 µg/L
New Jersey		0.5 µg/L

q_1* — The upper-bound estimate of the low-dose slope of the dose-response curve as determined by the multistage procedure. The q_1* can be used to calculate an estimate of carcinogenic potency, the incremental excess cancer risk per unit of exposure (usually µg/L for water, mg/kg/day for food, and g/m³ for air).
Reference dose (RfD) — An estimate (with uncertainty spanning perhaps an order of magnitude) of the daily exposure of the human population to a potential hazard that is likely to be without risk of deleterious effects during a lifetime. The RfD is operationally derived from the NOAEL (from animal and human studies) by a consistent application of uncertainty factors that reflect various types of data used to estimate RfDs and an additional modifying factor, which is based on a professional judgement of the entire database on the chemical. The RfDs are not applicable to nonthreshold effects such as cancer.
Adapted with permission from: Toxicological profile for chlordane. Agency for Toxic Substances and Disease Registry. (ATSDR), US Public Health Service. U.S. Government Printing Office, December 1989.

have been published (66). However, the study population in the investigation was self-selected. That is, individuals who were concerned about chlordane or who felt that they had experienced health problems with chlordane, were more prone to answer the survey (66).

Chlordane is one of the more common background chemicals found in indoor air sampling. Studies examining the amount of chlordane, heptachlor, and trans-nonachlor in the air of homes have been performed (49, 50). In the occupational environment, the threshold limit value of chlordane is 500 $\mu g/m^3$. However, the National Academy of Sciences, in 1979, felt that the occupational exposure limit of chlordane was unacceptable for the home environment and recommended a chlordane concentration of 5 $\mu g/m^3$ as acceptable in the home. Chlordane, when applied to a home for termite control is usually used in a diluted fashion and injected into the soil, into the wall void areas, and under slabs of homes, and in areas that might host termites.

Systemic effects of chlordane have included gastrointestinal complaints following exposure to high concentrations of chlordane either by the oral route or the inhalational route. Occupational exposure; however, is not associated with gastrointestinal effects. The overall occupational exposure to chlordane has not been associated with hepatotoxic effects, at least in terms of abnormal liver function tests. Neither were renal effects reported in occupational studies of chlordane production (59). Following acute inhalational exposure, neurological symptoms have included headache, dizziness, visual changes, incoordination, irritability, tremors, and seizures. These exposures have been either by gastrointestinal, dermal, or inhalational routes.

Most cases of death associated with chlordane exposure have been in children who have orally ingested the product. Animal studies on death following oral exposure have varied in terms of the amount, and there is much species variation and differences in the toxicity produced and the amount required to produce toxicity.

In individuals who have ingested chlordane, nausea, vomiting, abdominal pain, and diarrhea occur very early. Autopsies of individuals who have died following chlordane ingestion show inflammation of the mucosa of the upper gastrointestinal tract (59).

There are only scattered reports of bone marrow depression and of blood dyscrasias following chlordane exposure, and these are anecdotal reports (64, 65).

There is very little information regarding hepatotoxicity secondary to chlordane exposure, and in the studies that have been reported in human cases, there has been very little evidence of hepatotoxicity secondary to chlordane exposure. In animal studies following acute oral exposure to chlordane, there is evidence of hepatic microsomal enzyme induction and alteration in the activities of mitochondrial enzymes (59). There were also histochemical and morphological alterations in the liver of these animals.

Very few human renal health effects have been reported secondary to chlordane exposure.

Immunotoxicity, Carcinogenesis, and Reproductive Effects

There are currently no studies that suggest immunological effects in the human following exposure to chlordane.

There are no studies indicating reproductive toxicity secondary to chlordane exposure.

There is no evidence that chlordane is a human carcinogen, although it is ranked as a probable human carcinogen by the Environmental Protection Agency.

Absorption, Metabolism, and Excretion

Measurements of chlordane cis and trans isomers, heptachlor epoxide, oxychlordane, and trans-nonachlor in the blood of pest control operators and nonexposed workers in Japan were conducted by Kawano in 1982 (59). Concentrations in the blood of pest control operators ranged from 0.6–88 ppb, with an average of 13 ppb (59). Concentrations of heptachlor epoxide have been measured and sampled in the United States population by Kutz and were found to be 0.1 ppm in the adipose tissue samples collected (59). Kutz, in 1983, also reported mean values in human serum for chlordane components or metabolites of chlordane at less than 1 ppb (59). Human samples of adipose tissue (Tables 102.8 and 102.9) and plasma have been assayed on many occasions for the presence of organochlorine pesticides. Since these chemicals make up a background matrix in human adipose tissue and plasma, it is very difficult to associate their presence with a disease state, since they are commonly found in approximately 80% of the population in the United States. Chlordane and its metabolites can be detected in a variety of human biological tissues such as blood, brain (Table 102.10), adipose tissue, liver, breast milk (Table 102.11), kidneys, and urine. However, there is no information that correlates concentrations found in these tissues with environmental chlordane concentrations or with human health effects. In cases of intoxication, chlordane concentrations of the blood and other tissues have been found to be highly elevated. Blood chlordane concentrations of 3.4 $\mu g/L$ was associated with seizures in one child (55). The half-life of chlordane in this child was 8 days compared to other reports of 21 days. The urinary excretion of chlordane continued up to 130 days post ingestion (55). From this and other cases, it is thought that the seizure threshold for chlordane is between 2–4 $\mu g/L$ in serum (55).

Chlordane is well absorbed orally, dermally, and inhalationally. Blood and tissue concentrations of chlordane and chlordane metabolites will also increase with the duration of exposure. Information on the absorption and distribution of chlordane comes from acute oral exposures in humans from accidental or suicidal ingestions. Chlordane concentrates in the fatty tissues and has a very slow excretion rate. Following a massive ingestion which resulted in death of a 59-year-old male, concentrations of chlordane were measured in several tissues (58). In this case, fat tissue contained 22 $\mu g/g$ of chlordane, brain contained 23.3 $\mu g/g$, kidneys 14.1 $\mu g/g$, liver 59.9 $\mu g/g$, spleen 19.2 $\mu g/g$ (58). In a small child who drank technical grade chlordane, concentration in adipose tissue was measured. One half hour following the exposure, the chlordane concentration was approximately 3.1 mg/kg in the fat tissue. This peaked to 35 mg/kg of fat 8 days following the ingestion (67). Values for the concentration of the metabolite of chlordane, oxychlordane, in human adipose tissue has ranged from 0.03–0.5 mg/kg of fat tissue with an average concentration of 0.11 to 0.19 mg/kg of fat tissue (59, 68).

Chlordane has several metabolites (Fig. 102.10). The metabolites found in humans are usually heptachlor, oxychlordane, and heptachlor epoxide.

One excretion route of metabolites of chlordane is through

Table 102.8.   Residues of Organochlorine Compounds in Human Fat (mg/kg) in the United Kingdom, 1976–1977 (Results Obtained in 236 Subjects over 5-Years-Old)

	Beta-HCH	Total HCH	Heptachlor epoxide	Dieldrin (HEOD)	pp'-DDE	pp'-DDT	Total DDT*	Hexachlorobenzene	PCB
Arithmetic mean	0–31	0.33	0.03	0.11	2.1	0.21	2.6	0.19	0.7
Range #	T–1.2	T–1.2	T–0.12	T–0.49	0.03–15	T–2.4	0.04–17	0.02–3.2	T–10
Standard error of mean	0.01	0.01		0.01	0.12	0.01	0.15	0.01	0.05
Median value	0.29	0.31		0.09	1.7	0.17	2.1	0.15	0.7
Geometric mean	0.24	0.27		0.09	1.5	0.15	1.9	0.15	0.6
95% confidence	0.22–0.27	0.24–0.29		0.08–0.10	1.3–1.7	0.14–0.17	1.6–2.1	0.14–0.17	0.5–0.6

Reprinted with permission from: Abbott DC, Collins GB, Goulding R, Hoodless RA. Organochlorine pesticide residues in human fat in the United Kingdom 1976–7. Br Med J 1981;283:1425–1428.
*Total DDT was calculated by adding to the pp'-DDT found as such the pp'-DDT equivalent of the pp'-DDE and pp'-TDE.
#T is less than 0.01 (less than 0.1 for PCB).
HCH = Hexachlorocyclohexane. DDE = Derivative of DDT. PCB = Polychlorobiphenyls.

Table 102.9.   Concentration of Organochlorine Insecticides in Samples of Adipose Tissue and Liver

Lindane	Adipose						Liver		
	Heptachlor Epoxide	Dieldrin	p,p'-DDT	p,p'-DDE	Total Equiv DDT		Dieldrin	p,p'-DDE	Total Equiv DDT
0.12	0.008	0.16	0.36	2.18	2.79		0.030	0.16	0.18
0.21	0.014	0.25	0.28	1.88	2.38		0.050	0.16	0.18
0.05	0.005	0.14	0.14	0.36	0.54		0.040	0.05	0.06
0.11	0.008	0.18	0.42	2.50	3.21		0.026	0.15	0.17
0.06	0.006	0.13	0.19	1.15	1.47		0.024	0.12	0.13
0.07	0.009	0.25	0.35	1.95	2.52		0.025	0.08	0.10
0.12	0.009	0.21	0.44	2.10	2.78		0.035	0.19	0.21
0.10	0.004	0.05	0.10	0.08	0.19		0.007	0.01	0.01
0.13	0.030	0.50	0.35	2.66	3.31		0.081	0.12	0.13
0.16	0.013	0.23	0.58	2.32	3.17		0.041	0.13	0.14
0.09	0.005	0.10	0.35	1.51	2.03		0.014	0.20	0.22

Reprinted with permission from: de Vlieger M, Robinson J, Crabtree AN, van Dijk MC. The organochlorine insecticide content of human tissues. Arch Environ Health 1968;17:759–767.

Table 102.10.   Mean Concentrations of Organochlorine Insecticides in Human Brain Tissues

	Dieldrin (ppm)		Total Equiv DDT (ppm)	
	White Matter	Gray Matter	White Matter	Gray Matter
Arithmetic mean	0.009	0.006	0.033	0.025
SD	0.002	0.001	0.005	0.004
Geometric mean	0.0061	0.0047	0.0023	0.020
Confidence limits (p = 0.05)	0.0047–0.0080	0.0037–0.0059	0.018–0.031	0.015–0.026

Reprinted with permission from: de Vlieger M, Robinson J, Crabtree AN, van Dijk MC. The organochlorine insecticide content of human tissues. Arch Environ Health 1968;17:759–767.

the breast milk of nursing mothers. Oxychlordane trans-nonachlor and heptachlor epoxide have been identified in human breast milk (29). Trans-nonochlor has been reported to be present in human breast milk in concentrations of 0.027–0.210 µg/ml, heptachlor epoxide of 0.001–0.067 µg/ml, and oxychlordane of 0.011–0.160 µg/ml (29).

The biological half-life of chlordane and its metabolites have varied in clinical cases following human exposures. Most of these reports show that the elimination from plasma was biphasic. However, there were differences in the reported half-life of the beta elimination phase. The elimination half-life has been reported to be 21 days in one study, 34 days in another study, and 88 days (58, 67, 69). Only small amounts of chlordane are apparently excreted in the urine following ingestion. In animals models, the biliary excretion of chlordane and metabolites is significant (59). The fat serum-

partition ratio in exposed workers for chlordane was found to be 660:1 (70).

ALDRIN AND DIELDRIN

Aldrin and dieldrin are cyclodiene pesticides that are chemically related: aldrin is rapidly converted to dieldrin in the environment, and their toxicities are similar. Aldrin and dieldrin were used from the 1950s through the 1970s, but still manufactured through 1990. Both have been used in agricultural settings for control of disease vectors such as insects and as a soil insecticide. Dieldrin has also found use in the past as a veterinary dip for sheep. Their use was banned in 1975, and these compounds and manufacturing was terminated in 1987 for dieldrin and 1990 for aldrin. Aldrin is prepared by the Diels-Alder reaction using hexachlorocyclopentadiene. Dieldrin is prepared

Table 102.11. Mean Values of Samples Taken at Different Times During Breast Feeding (Pesticide Levels in ppm of Whole Milk)

Samples	Pre-Feed Mean ± SD (Range)	Post-Feed Mean ± SD (Range)	Random Mean ± SD (Range)
Urban			
No. Samples	43	42	45
% Lipid	2.7 ± 1.6 (0.3–9.7)	4.8 ± 1.8 (0.7–8.6)	3.3 ± 1.6 (0.8–7.9)
HCH	0.006 ± 0.004 (0.001–0.016)	0.010 ± 0.006 (0.002–0.025)	0.007 ± 0.005 (0.001–0.027)
gamma-HCH	0.001 ± 0.002 (0.000–0.007)	0.001 ± 0.002 (0.000–0.009)	0.001 ± 0.002 (0.000–0.006)
Dieldrin	0.010 ± 0.008 (0.002–0.038)	0.012 ± 0.008 (0.002–0.041)	0.007 ± 0.005 (0.002–0.024)
DDE	0.023 ± 0.013 (0.005–0.067)	0.039 ± 0.019 (0.011–0.077)	0.029 ± 0.022 (0.006–0.127)
DDT	0.011 ± 0.009 (0.002–0.033)	0.017 ± 0.011 (0.003–0.051)	0.010 ± 0.008 (0.002–0.037)
Total DDT	0.036 ± 0.020 (0.008–0.096)	0.060 ± 0.028 (0.015–0.136)	0.042 ± 0.030 (0.009–0.179)
Rural			
No. Samples	42	42	53*
% Lipid	2.8 ± 1.3 (0.3–5.9)	4.8 ± 1.5 (0.7–9.2)	2.6 ± 1.3 (0.3–6.2)
HCH	0.006 ± 0.003 (0.001–0.015)	0.009 ± 0.004 (0.002–0.024)	0.006 ± 0.003 (0.002–0.019)
gamma-HCH	0.000 ± 0.001 (0.000–0.003)	0.001 ± 0.002 (0.000–0.003)	0.000 ± 0.001 (0.000–0.002)
Dieldrin	0.006 ± 0.004	0.009 ± 0.006	0.008 ± 0.005

HCH = hexachlorocyclohexane.
Reprinted with permission from: Stacey CI, Perriman WS, Whitney S. Organochlorine pesticide residue levels in human milk: Western Australia, 1979–1980. Arch Environ Health 1985;40:102–108.

by the oxidation of aldrin with an organic acid or hydrogen peroxide and a tungsten oxide catalyst. The insecticide, dieldrin, contains 85% 1,2,3,4,10,10-hexachloro-6,7-epoxy-1,4, 4a,5,6,7,8,8a-octahydro-1,4-endo,exo-5,8-dimethanonaphthalene, termed HEOD for brevity (71).

Situations Producing Human and Environmental Exposure

Aldrin is readily converted to dieldrin in the environment. Dieldrin is very persistent and resists biodegradation. Therefore, dieldrin bioaccumulates throughout the food chain. Aldrin readily volatilizes from soil. Dieldrin, however, volatilizes more slowly because it adsorbs to soil. In soil, aldrin is converted to dieldrin by epoxidation. Aldrin and dieldrin do not leach to appreciable degrees into groundwater. Human exposure to aldrin and dieldrin have been mainly from dermal exposure and inhalation related to application as a pesticide. However, due to their persistence in the environment and the bioaccumulation of dieldrin, human exposure also occurs through the food chain. Environmental exposure to aldrin and dieldrin have occurred mainly through spraying in addition to soil volatilization of aldrin. With regard to human exposure, air and drinking water are minor sources. A study of U.S. drinking water samples revealed less than 17% contained dieldrin with very low concentrations of 4–10 ng/L of water (72).

Due to the conversion of aldrin to dieldrin, soil concentrations of dieldrin are higher. The contribution of diet Tables 102.12 through 102.16 to the exposure of aldrin and dieldrin in humans is the most significant source of exposure for the general population. Food is the main source of the human adipose tissue concentration of dieldrin in humans (72).

Occupational exposure to aldrin and dieldrin occurred mainly during its production. In 1974, the EPA suspended all use of aldrin and dieldrin, and all food uses were cancelled in 1975 (73). Specific precautions regarding the use of aldrin and dieldrin for termiticide use were instituted in 1981 and required label changes, precautions concerning the applications near water supplies, heating ducts, near intake ducts in dwellings, around structures with crawl spaces underneath, and also warned against yearly applications (73).

Populations who are at most risk from aldrin-dieldrin exposure in the diet include infants and toddlers. Transplacental transfer is possible, and concentrations in fetal tissue probably occurs. The concentration of dieldrin in breast milk is also a factor that places infants at risk of exposure. Breast milk is one of the major excretion routes for organochlorine compounds, and exposure to infants from human milk sources can be significant (29, 30). Dieldrin has been found in the breast milk of 80% of nursing mothers sampled (72). Placental-fetal transfer of aldrin/dieldrin has also been documented (36–38).

Homes treated for termite control with aldrin and dieldrin are another source of exposure. Indoor air in these homes contains aldrin in varying concentrations, depending on the sampling. In one study, the aldrin concentration ranged between 77 and 102 ng/m^3 within the first 7 days and fell to a low of 36 ng/m^3 by 1 year (72). The concentration in crawl spaces of treated homes was much higher.

Chemical and Physical Forms

The chemical structures of aldrin and dieldrin are shown in Figure 102.11. These compounds are in the organochlorine class of pesticides known as cyclodienes.

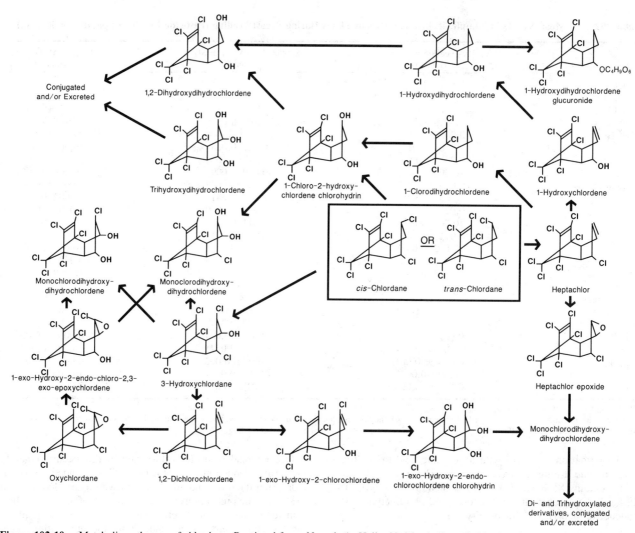

Figure 102.10.   Metabolic pathways of chlordane. Reprinted from: Nomeir A, Hajjar N. Metabolism of chlordane in mammals. Rev Environ Contam Toxicol 1987;100:1–22.

Absorption, Metabolism, and Excretion

Aldrin and dieldrin can be absorbed by inhalational, dermal, and gastrointestinal routes. There is a rapid conversion of aldrin to the dieldrin epoxide once absorption has occurred. Aldrin is rarely found in blood or tissue due to this rapid conversion. Dieldrin is stored in the fat and during periods of stress, such as weight loss and high fever, can be mobilized to the plasma where it can be metabolized. The half-life of dieldrin in humans is stated to be 266 days (74). There has been a correlation found between dieldrin concentrations in human breast milk and the pesticide treatment of homes. The distribution of dieldrin between blood and tissue of humans is shown in Figure 102.12. In human volunteers ingesting dieldrin, dieldrin concentrations in blood and fat tissue increased in a dose-related fashion with the fat tissue to blood ratio being 136:1 (74). In this same study, after dieldrin administration was terminated, the biological half-life decreased exponentially and was approximately 369 days with a range of 141–592 days (74). The biotransformation of aldrin is to the epoxide dieldrin, which occurs primarily in the liver (Fig. 102.13). Ackerman, in 1980, noted that the concentration of dieldrin in humans reaches a constant concentration and that the amount ingested and ab-

sorbed equals the amount metabolized and excreted after a period of time (75). With the increasing concentration of dieldrin in the liver, the rate of metabolism increases.

Another biological half-life of dieldrin in blood was estimated to be approximately 266 days, and this was found in workers who were followed for 3 years following an occupational exposure (76, 77). Hunter reported an estimated half-life of 369 days for dieldrin.

Clinical Toxicity and Health Effects

The clinical toxicology of aldrin and dieldrin can essentially be ascribed to dieldrin, since aldrin is rapidly metabolized to dieldrin after absorption in the human body. Once converted, dieldrin is distributed extensively into tissue spaces and accumulates in adipose tissue. Dieldrin is metabolized hepatically, and metabolites are excreted in bile and feces. Major toxicity involves the central nervous system. Toxic exposure produce tremors, giddiness, hyperexcitability, seizures, and coma (78). Dieldrin inhibits gamma amino butyric acid (GABA) neurotransmission similar to other cyclodiene pesticides.

In animal studies, LD50 values for species of all laboratory animals ranged from 40–70 mg/kg of aldrin and 40–90 mg/kg

Table 102.12.   Individual Donor Information (Urban)

HCH	gamma-HCH	Average Residue Levels (ppm) Dieldrin	DDE	DDT	Total DDT
0.003	0.002	0.013	0.012	0.021	0.034
0.002	0.003	0.011	0.010	0.013	0.024
0.002	Trace (TR)	0.008	0.009	0.017	0.027
0.002	0.001	0.009	0.017	0.011	0.030
0.009	Tr	0.013	0.033	0.020	0.057
0.005	0.005	0.017	0.026	0.019	0.048
0.010	0.002	0.024	0.026	0.007	0.036
0.009	0.007	0.011	0.019	0.021	0.042
0.009	0.001	0.008	0.024	0.007	0.034
0.002	Tr	0.005	0.023	0.005	0.031
0.015	0.001	0.015	0.055	0.029	0.090
0.008	Tr	0.009	0.020	0.004	0.026
0.012	0.001	0.009	0.046	0.022	0.073
0.016	0.001	0.024	0.057	0.028	0.092
0.007	Tr	0.005	0.014	0.005	0.021
0.012	0.003	0.015	0.041	0.013	0.059
0.011	0.003	0.011	0.044	0.037	0.086
0.004	Tr	0.007	0.026	0.008	0.037
0.006	Tr	0.010	0.047	0.015	0.067
0.006	Tr	0.012	0.029	0.007	0.039
0.007	0.002	0.012	0.050	0.012	0.068
0.010	Tr	0.005	0.039	0.014	0.057
0.005	0.002	0.008	0.034	0.027	0.065
0.006	Tr	0.003	0.023	0.006	0.032
0.003	0.001	0.024	0.024	0.014	0.041
0.010	0.001	0.007	0.029	0.009	0.041
0.004	0.001	0.003	0.012	0.003	0.016
0.005	0.001	0.007	0.036	0.013	0.053
0.004	Tr	0.007	0.034	0.010	0.048
0.003	0.001	0.002	0.011	0.004	0.016
0.017	Tr	0.012	0.073	0.027	0.108
0.006	Tr	0.004	0.025	0.006	0.034
0.012	Tr	0.007	0.039	0.011	0.054
0.011	Tr	0.009	0.041	0.009	0.055
0.007	Tr	0.003	0.016	0.005	0.023
0.007	Tr	0.003	0.037	0.006	0.047
0.010	Tr	0.008	0.034	0.012	0.050
0.011	Tr	0.005	0.025	0.007	0.035
0.013	Tr	0.007	0.043	0.009	0.057
0.007	0.004	0.005	0.024	0.006	0.033
0.006	Tr	0.003	0.022	0.004	0.029
0.010	Tr	0.005	0.034	0.009	0.047
0.008	0.001	0.008	0.022	0.007	0.032
0.008	Tr	0.021	0.028	0.008	0.039
0.004	Tr	0.006	0.013	0.004	0.018

Reprinted with permission from: Stacey CI, Perriman WS, Whitney S. Organochlorine pesticide residue levels in human milk: Western Australia, 1979–1980. Arch Environ Health 1985;40:102–108.

of dieldrin (74). In animal studies, it was also determined that weight loss resulted in immobilization of dieldrin from the fat stores, increased the blood levels peripherally, and produced toxic manifestations (74). There have been no deaths reported from human intoxication during the manufacture of aldrin or dieldrin. Most deaths are intentional or accidental exposures to concentrated amounts of the pesticides.

In occupational settings, aldrin and dieldrin have produced symptoms of headache, dizziness, ataxia, and muscle twitching (74). Occupational exposure to aldrin-dieldrin in pesticide workers was surveyed by Jager (77). In this survey, the average dieldrin blood level of those studied over a 4-year period was 0.035

µg/ml. Industrial and occupational surveys were also undertaken, and sprayers and pesticide applicators in India showed symptoms of intoxication which included headache, tremors, and seizures (74).

The mechanism of action of dieldrin in the CNS is at the level of the synapse, causing increased neuronal excitability. There is also evidence that dieldrin produces impairment of memory and emotional disturbances in humans. This may be due to the effect of the chemical on the limbic system. In general, the cyclodiene insecticides mimic the action of picrotoxin. It has been demonstrated that dieldrin binds to the picrotoxin receptor in rodent brain synaptosomes (79).

In exposed individuals manifesting serum concentrations of dieldrin, who had a range of 4–350 ppb, there was no evidence of hepatic injury (77). Hepatic enzyme activity levels were found to be normal in 233 pesticide applicators exposed occupationally to aldrin, dieldrin, endrin, and kelodrin for a period of 4–12 years (77). Studies have concluded that long-term exposure to aldrin and dieldrin do not produce liver disease detectable by enzyme elevation or hepatic enzyme induction (77). Blood concentrations of dieldrin are normally less than 10 ng/ml. Concentrations between 10–100 ng/ml probably are indicative of over-exposure (80). Dieldrin blood concentrations from 100–200 ng/ml indicate significant and potentially serious exposure. Concentrations above 200 ng/ml may be associated with toxic effects (80).

Carcinogenesis

The available data on aldrin and dieldrin are deemed to be inadequate to establish a clear relationship between these compounds and cancer in humans. However, malignant tumors of the liver were observed in animal studies (81). Mortality studies of workers engaged in the manufacturing of aldrin, dieldrin, and endrin revealed excess cancer (81).

Environmental Regulations of Aldrin and Dieldrin

The World Health Organization (WHO) recommended the following guideline levels for aldrin and dieldrin:

Food (extraneous residue limit): 0.02–0.2 mg/kg product
Food (maximum residue limit): 0.02–0.1 mg/kg
Drinking water: 0.03 µg/L

The WHO acceptable daily intake (ADI) is 0.1 µg/kg body weight (sum of aldrin and dieldrin).

The Occupational Safety and Health Administration (OSHA) established an 8-hour time-weighted average (TWA) atmospheric permissible exposure limit for aldrin of 0.25 mg/m^3 and for dieldrin of 0.25 mg/m^3 with the notation ''skin'' for each (OSHA 1985). In 1974, the EPA suspended nearly all uses of aldrin and dieldrin, and all food uses were cancelled in 1975. A Label Improvement Program (LIP) was initiated in 1981 to reduce potential risk due to the possibility of misapplication in termiticide use. Required label changes included precautions concerning application near domestic water supplies, near heating ducts, and around structures with subfloor crawl spaces and warnings against routine yearly retreatment of structures.

Effluent limitations of zero-discharge have been established by the EPA in 1986 under the National Pollutant Discharge Elimination System (NPDES) for both existing and new sources.

Table 102.13. Mean Levels of Organochlorine Pesticides in Milk of Individual Donors Exposed to Indoor Air Concentrations of Organochlorine Pesticides (Values Expressed in ng/g, Whole Milk Basis)

Donor No.	No. of Sample	HCH	gamma HCH	Chlordane	Heptachlor	Heptachlor Epoxide	Dieldrin	DDE	DDT	Total DDT
1	4	12	1	2	Tr	3	14	27	8	38
2	6	15	2	2	Tr	3	14	50	5	61
3	7	3	2	32	Tr	2	10	15	3	20
4	6	4	1	2	Tr	2	9	18	3	23
5	2	13	4	3	Tr	7	26	104	23	139
6	6	7	1	2	Tr	3	21	28	6	37
7	6	10	2	2	1	5	10	33	5	42
8	1	5	1	2	Tr	1	19	40	5	50
9	3	5	1	1	Tr	2	19	17	3	22
10	14	15	1	4	2	11	13	48	10	63
11	4	9	1	1	1	2	7	17	4	23
12	7	5	1	3	1	2	9	18	5	25
13	4	8	Tr	2	1	2	8	16	3	21
14	4	4	1	8	Tr	3	16	44	8	57

Reprinted with permission from: Stacey CI, Tatum T. House treatment with organochlorine pesticides and their levels in human milk—Perth, Western Australia. Bull Environ Contam Toxicol 1985;35:202–208.

Table 102.14. Dieldrin Levels in Donors Where Aldrin Was the Most Recent Pesticide Used in the Home. Note Decline in Concentration with Time (Values Expressed in ng/g, Whole Milk Basis)

Donor No.	Dieldrin levels in months after treatment							
	2 mths	3 mths	4 mths	5 mths	6 mths	7 mths	8 mths	9 mths
2	26	9	12	14	11	14		
6			19	21	26	31	21	8
9					16	24	16	

Reprinted with permission from: Stacey CI, Tatum T. House treatment with organochlorine pesticides and their levels in human milk—Perth, Western Australia. Bull Environ Contam Toxicol 1985;35:202–208.

Table 102.15. Chlordane Levels in One Breast Milk Donor Exposed to Home Pesticide Spraying (Values Expressed in ng/g Whole Milk Basis)

Sample No.	Sampling Time Relative to Treatment	Chlordane ng/g Whole Milk
1	3 days prior	Tr
2	1 week after	63
3	3 weeks after	66
4	7 weeks after	64
5	11 weeks after	26
6	15 weeks after	2
7	19 weeks after	2

Tr = trace less than 1 ng/g.
Reprinted with permission from: Stacey CI, Tatum T. House treatment with organochlorine pesticides and their levels in human milk—Perth, Western Australia. Bull Environ Contam Toxicol 1985;35:202–208.

Table 102.16. HBC, Heptachlor, and Heptachlor Epoxide Levels in Breast Milk of Individual Post Home Application of Pesticides (Values Expressed in ng/g, Whole Milk Basis)

Sample No.	Sampling Time Relative to Treatment	HCH	Heptachlor	Heptachlor Epoxide
1	3 months prior	3	—	1
2	2 months prior	8	Tr	4
3	1 month prior	7	Tr	3
4	1 day after	6	13	2
5	3 days after	22	2	4
6	1 week after	18	Tr	8
7	2 weeks after	17	Tr	8
8	3 weeks after	13	2	13
9	4 weeks after	22	3	29
10	5 weeks after	23	4	29
11	7 weeks after	21	2	21
12	9 weeks after	18	1	16
13	12 weeks after	17	Tr	7
14	15 weeks after	9	Tr	3

Reprinted with permission from: Stacey CI, Tatum T. House treatment with organochlorine pesticides and their levels in human milk—Perth, Western Australia. Bull Environ Contam Toxicol 1985;35:202–208.

Tolerances for residues of aldrin and dieldrin in or on various raw agricultural commodities are set at 0, 0.02, 0.05, or 0.1 ppm under section 408 of the Pesticide Residue Amendment to the Federal Food, Drug and Cosmetic Act as administered by the EPA. Aldrin (Waste Number P004) and dieldrin (Waste Number P037) are listed under the Resource Conservation and Recovery ACT (RCRA) as hazardous wastes.

Aldrin and dieldrin are listed under section 307 of the Federal Water Pollution Control Act as toxic pollutants. Aldrin and dieldrin are regulated as hazardous substances with a reportable quantity of 1 lb (0.454 kg) for each under section 102 of the Comprehensive Environmental Response, Compensation, and Liability Act (CERCLA) for releases from vessels and facilities.

The American Conference of Governmental Industrial Hygienists (ACGIH) has adopted TWA threshold limit values for exposure to aldrin and dieldrin of 0.25 mg/m³. The ACGIH recommendation includes a "skin" notation to indicate the potential for absorption of the compound by the dermal route, by airborne, or direct contact. The TWA limit for aldrin was chosen to prevent hepatic injury and in order for dieldrin to be sufficiently low to prevent systemic poisoning.

The National Institute for Occupational Safety and Health (NIOSH) has recommended a permissible exposure limit for both aldrin and dieldrin of 0.25 mg/m³ and has recommended

Aldrin

1,2,3,4,10,10-Hexachloro-
1,4,4a,5,8,8a-hexahydro-exo-
1,4-endo-5,8-dimethanoaph-
thalene, HHDN

Compound 118, Octalene,
Aldrec, Aldrex, Drinox

$C_{12}H_8Cl_6$

Dieldren

3,4,5,6,9,9-Hexachloro-
1a,2,2a,3,6,6a,7,7a-octa-
hydro 2,3:3,6-dimethano-
napth[2,3-b]-oxirene, HEOD

Compound 497, Octalox,
Panoram D-31, Alvit,
Dieldrex, Quintox

$C_{12}H_8Cl_6O$

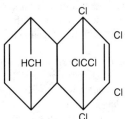
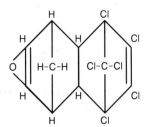

Figure 102.11. Chemical structures of aldrin and dieldrin. Reprinted with permission from: USPHS. Toxicological profile for aldrin/dieldrin. Agency for Toxic Substances & Disease Registry. US Public Health Service, 1989.

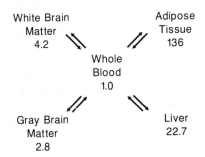

Figure 102.12. Relationship of the distribution of dieldrin between blood and certain tissues in humans. Reprinted from: de Vlieger, Robinson J, Crabtree A, van Dijk M. The organochlorine insecticide content of human tissues. Arch Environ Health 1968;17:759–767.

the designation of 100 mg/m³ for aldrin and 450 mg/m³ for dieldrin as that concentration which is immediately dangerous to life or health (IDLH).

The National Academy of Sciences has issued a health advisory for a level of 0.0031 ppb for chronic exposure in drinking water.

The Drinking Water Equivalent Level (DWEL) for dieldrin is 2 µg/L and the draft DWEL for aldrin is 0.9 µg/L. Based on estimates of carcinogenic potential, a level of 0.02 µg/liter of drinking water corresponds to a cancer risk level of 1 × 10⁻⁵. In 1980, the EPA established a National Ambient Water Quality Criterion (NAWQC) for aldrin of 0.074 µg/L and for dieldrin, 0.071 µg/L for human health (73). This was based on a 1:1,000,000 risk for cancer and was based on estimates for the ingestion of contaminated water and contaminated organisms in the water (73). The International Agency for Research on Cancer (IARC) in 1987 classified aldrin and dieldrin in group 3, a possible human carcinogen, based on limited evidence in animals in absence of human data (73). Aldrin is also listed as a probable human carcinogen on the weight of experimental evidence under the EPA Proposed Guidelines for Carcinogen Risk Assessment in 1984

Figure 102.13. Metabolism of aldrin and dieldrin. Reprinted with permission from: USPHS. Toxicological profile for aldrin/dieldrin. Agency for Toxic Substances & Disease Registry. US Public Health Service, 1989.

(73). The evidence of the carcinogenicity from animal studies appears sufficient, and human studies have been inadequate. Dieldrin is also classified by the EPA as a probable human carcinogen, with sufficient evidence in animals and inadequate evidence in humans (73).

ENDRIN

Endrin, a steroisomer of dieldrin, is a cyclodiene organochlorine pesticide with a formula of $C_{12}H_8Cl_6O$ and a molecular weight of 380.93 (52). The technical product is approximately 85% endrin. Endrin is a white crystalline solid. Endrin, introduced in 1951, is one of the most toxic of the cyclodiene compounds and produces dizziness, seizures, tremors, and confusion in acute toxicity. It has also been associated with hyperthermia followed by decerebrate rigidity (52). Endrin does not accumulate in human tissues following exposure and is rapidly metabolized. In animals, endrin is metabolized to water-soluble compounds and is excreted mainly in the feces. The threshold limit value of endrin is 0.1 mg/m³ and was set to prevent systemic toxicity. The short-term exposure limit for endrin is 0.3 mg/m³. Endrin is highly toxic to animals in oral overdose studies (80). Endrin is rapidly metabolized in animals and man with a half-life of 2–6 days. Endrin and a metabolite, anti-12-hydroxyendrin, can be found in the stool of humans (80). Anti-12-hydroxyendrin can also be found in the urine of occupationally exposed individuals and can be used as a biological monitoring marker. Endrin has not been found to be carcinogenic in animals studied, nor has it been found to be teratogenic nor cause reproductive effects in animals studied.

An outbreak of endrin poisoning from contaminated food in Pakistan in 1984 resulted in a 10% mortality rate from seizures (82). Seizures occurred within 2 hours following ingestion of contaminated food, and in some instances status epilepticus occurred. Endrin serum concentrations in these individuals ranged from 1.5–49.4 ppb. Nonfatal cases recovered in a few days (82).

Isobenzan

Isobenzan (telodrin) is a cyclodiene compound with a formula of $C_9H_4Cl_8O$ and a molecular weight of 411.79 (52). The technical product is greater than 95% isobenzan. The compound itself is a light brown crystalline powder (52). Isobenzan is soluble in other organic solvents. It is not soluble in water. It was produced between the years 1958–1965 and had limited agricultural use (80). Little human toxicology is known about isobenzan. The available human data indicate that clinical toxicology is related to CNS stimulation and seizures similar to other organochlorine compounds. Other symptoms associated with isobenzan include headaches, dizziness, irritability, parasthesias, and drowsiness (52).

Exposure of the general population to isobenzan has been limited. Clinical cases of seizures have been reported following serious exposure situations (80). Blood concentrations of isobenzan in nine workers who suffered intoxication showed a mean of 0.023 ng/ml (1.017–0.030 ng/ml) (80). Isobenzan is well absorbed by the gastrointestinal tract. It accumulates in adipose tissue and has one identified metabolite, telodrin lactane (80). Isobenzan crosses the placenta. Its biological half-life was reported to be 2.8 years (80).

Endosulfan

Endosulfan (Fig. 102.8) is a mixture of two isomers, alpha and beta endosulfan. Endosulfan was introduced in 1956. It has a formula of $C_9H_6Cl_6O_3S$ and molecular weight of 406.95 (52). Its common names include benzoepin, cyclodane, malix, thimul, thiosulfan, and thionex. The alpha isomer constitutes 70% of the mixture, the beta isomer approximately 30% of the mixture (52). Endosulfan is a brownish crystalline powder that smells like sulfur dioxide. It is soluble in organic solvents and insoluble in water.

The primary source of human exposure is through residues on food and residues on tobacco (83). Endosulfan contamination is not widespread in the environment. The beta isomer of endosulfan has a higher affinity for soil and thus a longer half-life in the environment. The soil half-life of alpha isomer is 60 days, and the half-life of the beta isomer is 900 days (83). Both isomers resist photodegradation.

Clinical toxicology has been described from cases of ingestion and occupational exposures. Following ingestion of endosulfan, symptomatology begins within a few hours, and death has been reported within 2 hours (83, 84). The clinical syndrome consists of vomiting, agitation, pulmonary edema, seizures, dyspnea, and cyanosis (84). Occupational exposure had

been associated with anxiety, headaches, dizziness, stupor, confusion, and seizures (83).

Chlordecone, Kelevan, and Mirex

Chemical formula for mirex is $C_{10}Cl_{12}$ with a molecular weight of 545.51 (Fig. 102.14) (85). Mirex is a crystalline white solid that melts at 485°C. It is insoluble in water, soluble in benzene, carbon tetrachloride, and xylene. Mirex, introduced in 1955, has been used extensively for the control of fire ants in the southern United States (85). Mirex has been found in fat samples collected in areas known to have been treated with the chemical (52). Mirex, also known as dechlorane, has also been used as a fire retardant (85).

Mirex is a very stable compound in the environment and bioaccumulates up the food chain. The Environmental Protection Agency began phasing out the use of mirex to control fire ants in the mid 1970s. Mirex has also been used as a fire retardant, under the name dechlorane, in plastics, rubber, paint, paper, and electrical products (85). Most of the mirex produced between 1959 and 1975 was used in the United States (85).

Human environmental exposures occurred from food ingestion and from contaminated soil. Mirex is excreted in human breast milk. Adipose tissue concentrations have been found in autopsy samples from persons residing in the southeastern United States ranging from 0.16 mg/kg of fat–6 mg/kg (85). Mean blood concentrations of mirex in pregnant women in Mississippi was 0.5 μg/L. Mirex resists metabolism in man and animals. Cases of human poisoning have not been reported. Mirex was not fetotoxic in animal studies and was not a teratogen. It crosses the placenta in animal studies. It is carcinogenic in mice and rats (85).

Chlordecone is also known as kepone (Fig. 102.15). It has a chemical formula of $C_{10}Cl_{10}O$ and a molecular weight of 490.61 (52). Chlordecone is soluble in acetone and less soluble in benzene and similar petroleum solvents. Chlordecone production began in 1965, but production was terminated in July

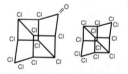

Chlordecone   Mirex
Figure 102.14.   Chlordecone and mirex.

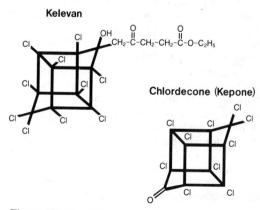

Figure 102.15.   Kelevan and chlordecone (Kepone).

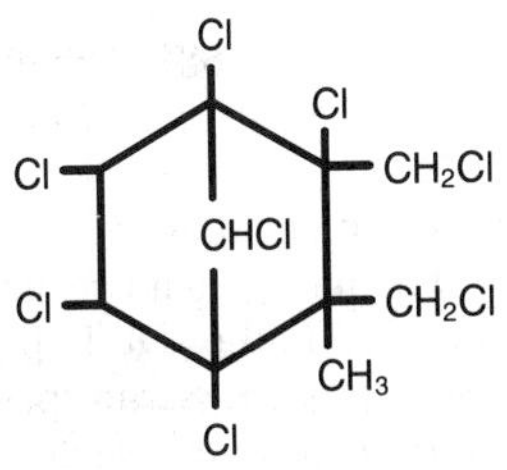

Figure 102.16. Toxaphene.

Figure 102.17. Methoxychlor (Marlate) and dicofol ((Kelthane).

of 1975 after the manufacturing plant had been in operation for 16 months (52). There was no effective occupational control of chlordecone exposure, and workers were being excessively contaminated. The clinical syndrome of chlordecone toxicity was insidious, and its onset involved some weight loss, tremor of the muscles of the upper extremity, muscle weakness, abnormal eye movements, slurring of speech, mental status changes, chest pain, arthralgias, dermatitis, and abnormality of liver function tests (52, 86). Following the manufacturing of chlordecone, blood levels in nearby residents of the community in close proximity to the plant were found to be as high as 0.033 ppm (52, 86, 87). Chlordecone is a known neurotoxin and can produce peripheral neuropathy.

Chlordecone is environmentally very stable. Human exposure to chlordecone occurred via food residues due to its bioaccumulation. It is excreted in human breast milk. Occupational exposure occurred in the production plant in 1975 with large amounts of chlordane contaminating the surrounding environment. Chlordecone blood concentrations in workers with health effects averaged 2.53 mg/L (87). Workers not ill had average blood concentrations of 0.60 mg/L (87). Chlordecone half-life has ranged from 63–148 days (87). Cholestyramine was found to enhance gastrointestinal elimination in exposed individuals.

Kelevan is a solid white powder with a molecular weight of 634.79 (Fig. 102.15). It is a condensation product of chlordecone and ethyl levulinate (88). Technical grade kelevan is 94–98% pure with minor contamination of chlordecone. Kelevan, once absorbed by animals or humans is metabolized to chlordecone (88). Chlordecone and kelevan are chemically related pesticides (86–88). Chlordecone is known under the trade name of Kepone. Kelevan has the trade names of Despirol and Elevat (88). Chlordecone is a tan to white solid which is soluble in organic solvents. Technical grade chlordecone is 88–99% pure with minor contamination by hexachlorocyclopentadiene (88).

Toxaphene

Toxaphene, introduced in 1948, is a mixture of chlorinated bicyclic terpenes (chlorinated camphenes) containing 67–69% chlorine. Toxaphene is a yellow waxy solid with a chemical formula of $C_{10}H_{10}Cl_{18}$ (Fig. 102.16). It is well absorbed dermally and via the gastrointestinal tract. Environmentally, toxaphene vaporizes from soil but can be adsorbed to soil with a half-life of up to 12 years. Toxaphene bioaccumulates in aquatic organisms (89). Toxaphene is soluble in organic solvents but insoluble in water. In the environment, toxaphene is photodegraded by ultraviolet light and in soil is degraded by the action of bacteria (89).

Clinical toxicity from toxaphene can occur from occupational exposures and ingestion of the product. Cases of poisoning have manifested seizures and respiratory depression (89). In occupational settings, inhalation of the product has been as-

sociated with decreased pulmonary functions and dyspnea (89). Toxaphene is considered to be a potential human carcinogen (89). Toxaphene is a carcinogen in mice and rats (89).

Toxaphene has resulted in death in some instances. Symptoms occur within 30 minutes to a few hours after ingestion. The main clinical manifestations of toxicity are convulsions, hyperthermia, tremors, and confusion (52). The TLV is 0.5 mg/m³ with a notation warning against dermal contact.

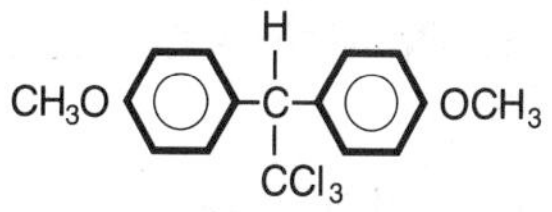

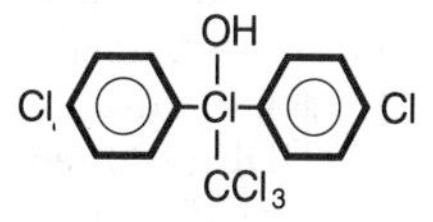

DICOFOL AND METHOXYCHLOR

Dicofol is a chlorinated hydrocarbon pesticide used mainly as an acaricide on grain crops (Fig. 102.17).

The chemical's generic name is 1,1-bis(p-chlorophenyl)-2,2,2-trichloroethanol. Its trade names are Kelthane, Acarin, and Mitigan. Dicofol has a molecular weight of 370.5 and is a white solid with a melting point of 79°C. The technical product is a light brown viscous oil with a density of 1.45. Dicofol is insoluble in water but soluble in most aliphatic and aromatic solvents. It is highly lipophilic. Dicofol is hydrolyzed by alkali to dichlorobenzophenone and chloroform (52).

Dicofol is manufactured by the chlorination of bis(4-chlorophenyl)carbinol. It is registered for use on vegetables, fruits, and a variety of field crops and is used widely in nurseries and greenhouses. It is relatively stable although when heated or in contact with strong acids it decomposes to hydrogen chloride, the vapors of which may cause acute health problems. The chemical is also structurally similar to DDT (52)).

Dicofol is stable in the environment after application; although residues decrease rapidly, traces can be found in soil up to a year later. Human toxicity information is limited. Animals given toxic doses have symptoms referable to central nervous system stimulation. Human exposures have demonstrated very little clinical toxicity.

Methoxychlor (1,1,1-trichloro-2,2-bis(p-methoxyphenyl) ethane) has a molecular weight of 345.65 with the chemical formula $C_{16}H_{15}C_{13}O_2$ (Fig. 102.17) (52). Methoxychlor's trade name is Marlate. The compound is a clear crystal in its pure state and a gray powder in its technical state (52). It was first introduced in 1945 as a wettable powder, dust, and concentrate. Methoxychlor, like dicofol, has a low order of animal toxicity, but in sufficient doses can produce seizures. Human volunteers ingesting up to 2 mg/kg/day for 8 weeks showed no health effects (52). In humans, dermatitis may occur from contact with either dicofol or methoxychlor. There are no reported cases of systemic intoxication from methoxychlor in humans.

Organochlorine Pesticide Concentrations in Human Tissues

The period from the 1950s to 1970s witnessed heavy use of many organochlorine pesticides. The concentration of DDT in human adipose tissue during this time was averaging around 5 ppm (25). At the same time, the adipose concentrations of DDT and DDE in combination averaged 15 ppm (25). Following the ban on DDT, a gradual reduction of adipose concentrations of both DDT and DDE occurred. By the late 1960s, the average concentration ranged from 1–2 ppm of DDT and approximately 9 ppm for all DDT- and DDE-related pesticides (25). Since pesticides had been extensively used throughout South Florida, the presence of organochlorine pesticides in the serum of 59 female residents in Dade County Florida was surveyed and compared with pesticide content in drinking water. Ten organochlorine pesticides and their metabolites were analyzed for in this monitoring program: hexachlorocyclohexane, β-HCH, heptachlor, oxychlordane, heptachlor epoxide, trans-nonachlor, DDE, dieldrin, o,p'-DDT, and p,p'-DDT (25). Drinking water concentrations of organochlorine pesticides were also determined in this study. In these individuals, HCH, β-HCD, p,p'-DDE, dieldrin, and p,p'-DDT were detected. Most of these organochlorine compounds ranged in the serum in concentrations of parts per billion (Table 102.6). Hexachlorocyclohexane concentrations ranged from nondetectable to 1.1 ppb, β-HCH ranged from nondetectable to 5.8 ppb, DDE ranged from nondetectable up to 68.4 ppb, dieldrin ranged from nondetectable to 10 ppb, and DDT ranged from nondetectable to 5.5 ppb (25). When these subjects were compared with individuals who consumed well water as opposed to city water, there was no significant difference in serum levels of organochlorine pesticides metabolites (Table 102.7).

Organochlorine pesticide residues were studied in human adipose tissue in the United Kingdom between the years of 1976 and 1977. These samples were taken from adipose tissue during autopsies on 236 individuals over 5 years of age (27). The range of these compounds in adipose tissue were as follows: β-HCH ranged from nondetectable to 1.2 mg/kg, heptachlor epoxide ranged from lower limits of detection to 0.12 mg/kg, dieldrin ranged from nondetectable to 0.49, DDE ranged from 0.03–15 mg/kg, DDT total ranged from 0.04–17 mg/kg, and total chlorinated byphenyls ranged from nondetectable to 10 mg/kg (27). The concentrations of these organochlorine compounds were similar to those observed in other studies carried out in the 1960s. A summary of the 1976 and 1977 study in the 236 subjects and the organochlorine pesticide residues found in human fat is summarized in Table 102.8.

Other studies performed in the 1960s in autopsy samples showed mean concentrations of dieldrin in the white matter of the brain being 0.0061 ppm, gray matter concentrations of 0.0047 ppm, liver concentrations of 0.03 ppm, and fatty tissue concentrations of 0.17 ppm (22). Figures 102.4 and 102.12 show the distribution of DDT and dieldrin between blood and other tissues in humans as prepared from this study (22). Dieldrin has a greater tendency to store in liver and brain tissue relative to adipose tissue as compared with DDT-related compounds. Concentrations of organochlorine pesticides typically found in adipose tissue, liver, and brain tissue are shown in Tables 102.9 and 102.10 (22).

Oxychlordane metabolites were assayed for in adipose tissues collected from postmortem examination and surgical procedures in the 1960s and 1970s (68). Oxychlordane in these specimens ranged from 0.03–0.40 ppm in 27 specimen samples (68).

Isomers and metabolites of a variety of organochlorines have been found in persons who have had no occupational exposure. These have included p,p'-DDT, o,p'-DDT, p,p'-DDE, β-HCH, dieldrin, and heptachlor epoxide. Serum pesticide concentrations in the parts per billion were detected by Morgan in a population studied between 1967–1973 (15). These concentrations were compared with various clinical chemistries in over 2600 subjects (15). DDT and DDE serum concentrations were found to be higher in these subjects living in the Southern United States. There was no evidence of abnormal hematology studies (15).

The presence of organochlorine pesticide residue concentrations in human breast milk was studied in Western Australia from 1979 to 1980 (Table 102.11) (30). In this study, 267 samples of human breast milk were supplied by 140 donors from urban and rural areas and analyzed for organochlorine pesticides. The organochlorine pesticides detected were aldrin, lindane, HCH, dieldrin, and DDT. Aldrin and lindane were found in trace amounts. DDT-related compounds were found ranging from 0.078–0.046 ppm. HCH compounds ranged from 0.025–0.008 ppm, and dieldrin ranged from 0.005–0.009 ppm. A previous study had been conducted during the 1970–1971 year. The results from this second study concluded that organochlorine pesticide concentrations in human breast milk were decreasing except for dieldrin, which showed an increase. The Australian government imposed controls on the use of organochlorine pesticides in Western Australia in 1971. During the years 1978–1979, there had been a documented decrease in the pesticide concentration in most countries where limitations were put on the use and application of chlorinated pesticides throughout the environment. Endeavors to correlate the pesticide concentrations in human tissues and the use of pesticides or the exposure to pesticides have been unsuccessful. The results of the 1979–1980 Australian study demonstrate that restricting the use of organochlorine pesticides reduces the human tissue content of these pesticides. Individual information on samples from the urban donors of human breast milk from this 1979–1980 study are shown in Table 102.12 (30).

It is now appreciated that indoor air concentrations of organochloride pesticides, particularly chlordane, contribute to the total body burden of the residues found in humans. Measurements of concentrations of chlordane in indoor air home environments are usually found to be higher compared with outdoor air concentrations (50). Since the average person spends up to 90% of his/her time inside the home, the quality of air in the home relates directly to human exposure to indoor air pollutants. Air sampling of indoor air environments and analysis for chlorinated pesticides has revealed low concentrations of chlordane and nonachlor (49, 50). Concentrations of γ-chlordane and α-chlordane along with trans-nonachlor were found in the various homes sampled (49, 50). In one study, 12 homes were sampled from November 1985 to October 1986 (50). The outdoor air concentration of chlordane and trans-nonochlor were very low and the average outdoor air concentration of γ-chlordane was 0.5 ng/m^3 (50). The indoor air concentration for γ-chlordane ranged from 29 ng/m^3 and averaged seven times higher than the outdoor air (50). It was interesting to note in this study that homes with windows closed versus windows opened did not show substantially different concentrations of indoor air (50). These homes had been treated with subsurface slab injection of chlordane for termites. Large cracks in the foundation were probably responsible for the high concentration of indoor air chlordane.

Another 1985 study correlated home treatment with organochlorine pesticides to their presence in human breast milk (24). Fourteen subjects supplied breast milk in this study and answered questions regarding treatment of their homes with organochlorine pesticides. The majority had applications of heptachlor and aldrin to their homes. This study concluded that there was a connection between the concentrations of the pesticides and other metabolites in human breast milk as a consequence of their use in spraying inside or outside of the home. The mean concentrations of the organochlorine pesticides in human breast milk from these individual donors are shown in Table 102.13. The subjects were chosen from those whose homes had been recently treated with organochlorine pesticides. Table 102.14 indicates the concentrations of dieldrin in breast milk donors and the decline in dieldrin concentrations months after the application of dieldrin in the home environment (24). Table 102.15 shows chlordane concentrations in one of the subjects expressed as nanograms per gram of whole breast milk correlating this with the time relative to chlordane treatment in the home. Table 102.16 shows concentrations of HCH, heptachlor, and heptachlor epoxide relative to treatment times in the home environment (24). These data demonstrate that home pesticide spraying with organochlorine pesticides is related to increased concentrations of pesticides in human breast milk (24).

The permissible occupational exposure limit to chlordane is 500 $\mu g/m^3$ for a 40-hour work week. The National Academy of Sciences (NAS) in 1979 considered this concentration to be unacceptable in the home environment because of continuous exposure 24 hours/day and recommended a concentration of chlordane of 5 $\mu g/m^3$ as acceptable in the home environment. The NAS also recommended a concentration of 2 $\mu g/m^3$ for heptachlor in homes (49). A variety of environmental home studies have been conducted throughout the years from 1970s through the early 1980s in which indoor air concentrations of chlordane have been measured. Concentrations of chlordane have varied widely in these home environments. Chlordane was measured in 474 family housing units at seven U.S. Air Force installations from the 1980–1981 (49). Chlordane had been used in these homes for treatment of termites by subsurface slab injection or exterior application and 86% of these homes had chlordane air concentrations below 3.5 $\mu g/m^3$, whereas 12% had concentrations between 3.5–6.5 $\mu g/m^3$, and 2% of these homes had concentrations in the indoor air above 6.5 $\mu g/m^3$ (49).

Human exposure to a variety of organochlorine pesticides is pervasive from environmental, occupational, food, and water sources. Assays of blood, adipose tissue, brain, liver, and breast milk indicate the widespread contamination of the human population throughout the world.

REFERENCES

1. Gant DB, Eldefrawi ME, Eldefrawi AT. Cyclodiene insecticides inhibit GABA receptor-regulated chloride transport. Toxicol Appl Pharmacol 1987;88:313–321.

2. Lawrence LJ, Casida JE. Interactions of lindane, toxaphene and cyclodienes with brain-specific t-butylbicyclophosphorothionate receptor. Life Sci 1984;35:171–178.

3. USPHS. Toxicological profile for p,p′-DDT, p,p′-DDE, p,p′-DDD. Agency for Toxic Substances and Disease Registry, US Public Health Service, Government Printing Office, December 1989:1.

4. USPHS. Toxicological profile for p,p′-DDT, p,p′-DDE, p,p′-DDD. gency for Toxic Substances and Disease Registry, US Public Health Service, Government Printing Office, December 1989:75.

5. USPHS. Toxicological profile for p,p′-DDT, p,p′-DDE, p,p′DDD. Agency for Toxic Substances and Disease Registry, US Public Health Service, Government Printing Office, December 1989:79

6. Coulston F. Reconsideration of the dilemma of DDT for the establishment of an acceptable daily intake. Regul Toxicol Pharmacol 1985;5:332–383.

7. Saxena MC, Siddiqui MKJ, Seth TD, Krishna Murti CR. Organochlorine pesticides in specimens from women undergoing spontaneous abortion, premature or full-term delivery. J Anal Toxicol 1981;5:6–9.

8. Mattison, DR. Pesticides in human breast milk: changing patterns and estimates of cancer risk. Graduate School of Public Health, University of Pittsburgh, Pittsburgh, PA, Presented at the 38th Annual Meeting, Mar 20–23, 1991, San Antonio, Texas.

9. Currie RA, Kadis VW, Breitkreitz WE, Cunningham GB, Bruns GW. Pesticide residues in human milk, Alberta, Canada—1966–70, 1977–78. Pestic Mon J 1979;133:52–55.

10. Griffith FD, Blanke RV. Pesticides in people: blood organochlorine pesticide levels in Virginia residents. Pesti Mon J 1975;8:219–224.

11. Polishuk ZW, Ron M, Wassermann M, Cucos S, Wassermann D, Lemesch C. Pesticides in people: organochlorine compounds in human blood plasma and milk. Pestic Mon J 1977;10:121–129.

12. Radomski JL, Deichmann WB, Rey AA, Merkin T. Human pesticide blood levels as a measure of body burden and pesticide exposure. Toxicol Appl Pharmacol 1971;20:175–185.

13. Radomski JL, Astolfi E, Deichmann WB, Rey AA. Blood levels of organochlorine pesticides in Argentina: occupationally and nonoccupationally exposed adults, children and newborn infants. Toxicol Appl Pharmacol 1971;20:186–193.

14. Dale WE, Curley A, Hayes WJ Jr. Determination of chlorinated insecticides in human blood. Ind Med Surg April, 1967:275–280.

15. Morgan DP, Lin LI. Blood organochlorine pesticide concentrations, clinical hematology and biochemistry in workers occupationally exposed to pesticides. Arch Environ Contam Toxicol 1978;7:423–447.

16. USPHS. Toxicological profile for p,p′-DDT, p,p′-DDE, p,p′-DDD. Agency for Toxic Substances and Disease Registry, US Public Health Service, Government Printing Office, December 1989:9–65.

17. Baumann K, Angerer J, Heinrich R, Lehnert G. Occupational exposure to hexachlorocyclohexane, Part I. Int Arch Occup Environ Health 1980;47:119–127.

18. USPHS. Toxicological profile for hexachlorocyclohexane. Agency for Toxic Substances and Disease Registry, US Public Health Service, Government Printing Office, December 1989:61–66.

19. USPHS. Toxicological profile for hexachlorocyclohexane. Agency for Toxic Substances and Disease Registry, US Public Health Service, Government Printing Office, December 1989:71–84.

20. Baumann K, Behling K, Brassow HL, Stapel K. Occupational exposure to hexachlorocyclohexane, Part III. Int Arch Occup Environ Health 1981;48:165–172.

21. Nigam SK, Karnik AB, Majumder SK, et al. Serum hexachlorocyclohexane residues in workers engaged at a HCH manufacturing plant. Int Arch Occup Environ Health 1986;57:315–320.

22. de Vlieger M, Robinson J, Crabtree AN, van Dijk MC. The organochlorine insecticide content of human tissues. Arch Environ Health 1968;17:759–767.

23. Pines A, Cucos S, Ever-Hadani P, Ron M. Some organochlorine insecticide and polychlorinated biphenyl blood residues in infertile males in the general Israeli population of the middle 1980s. Arch Environ Contam Toxicol 1987;16:587–597.

24. Stacey CI, Tatum T. House treatment with organochlorine pesticides and their levels in human milk—Perth, Western Australia. Bull Environ Contam Toxicol 1985;35:202–208.

25. Barquet A, Morgade C, Pfaffenberger CD. Determination of organochlorine pesticides and metabolites in drinking water, human blood serum, and adipose tissue. J Toxicol Environ Health 1981;7:469–479.

26. Dale WE, Curley A, Cueto C Jr. Hexane extractable chlorinated insecticides in human blood. Life Sci 1966;5:47–54.

27. Abbott DC, Collins GB, Goulding R, Hoodless RA. Organochlorine pesticide residues in human fat in the United Kingdom 1976–7. Br Med J 1981;283:1425–1428.

28. Kashyap SK. Health surveillance and biological monitoring of pesticide formulators in India. Toxicol Lett 1986;33:107–114.

29. Takahashi W, Saidin D, Takei G, Wong L. Organochloride pesticide residues in human milk in Hawaii, 1979–80. Bull Environ Contam Toxicol 1981;27:506–511.

30. Stacey CI, Perriman WS, Whitney S. Organochlorine pesticide residue levels in human milk: Western Australia, 1979–1980. Arch Environ Health 1985;40:102–108.

31. Brassow HL, Baumann K, Lehnert G. Occupational exposure to hexachlorocyclohexane, Part II. Int Arch Occup Environ Health 1981;48:81–87.

32. Milby TH, Samuels AJ, Ottoboni F. Humane exposure to lindane: blood lindane levels as a function of exposure. J Occup Med 1968;10:584–587.

33. Ramachandran M, Banerjee M, Grover A, Zaidi S. DDT and HCH residues in the body fat and blood samples from some Delhi hospitals. Ind J Med Res 1984;80:590–593.

34. USPHS. Toxicological profile for hexachlorocyclohexane. Agency for Toxic Substances and Disease Registry, US Public Health Service, Government Printing Office, December 1989:11–60.

35. Davies JE, Dedhia HV, Morgade C, Barquet A, Maibach HI. Lindane poisonings. Arch Dermatol 1983;119:142–144.

36. Saxena MC, Siddiqui MKJ, Bhargava AK, Krishna Murti CR, Kutty D. Placental transfer of pesticides in humans. Arch Toxicol 1981;48:127–134.

37. Saxena MC, Siddiqui MKJ. A comparison organochlorine insecticide contents in specimens of maternal blood, placenta, and umbilical cord blood from stillborn and live-born cases. J Toxicol Environ Health 1983;11:71–79.

38. Roncevic N, Pavkov S, Galetin-Smith R, et al. Serum concentrations of organochlorine compounds during pregnancy and the newborn. Bull Environ Contam Toxicol 1987;38:117–124.

39. Morgan DP, Stockdale EM, Roberts RJ, Walter AW. Anemia associated with exposure to lindane. Arch Environ Health 1980;35:307–310.

40. Berry DH, Brewster MA, Watson R, Neuberg RW. Untoward effects associated with lindane abuse (Letter). Am J Dis of Child 1987;14:125.

41. Jaeger U, Podczeck A, Haubenstock A, et al. Acute oral poisoning with lindane-solvent mixtures. Vet Hum Toxicol 1984;26:11–14.

42. Pramanik AK, Hansen RC. Transcutaneous gamma benzene hexachloride absorption and toxicity in infants and children. Arch Dermatol 1979;115:1224–1225.

43. Feldmann RJ, Maibach HI. Percutaneous penetration of some pesticides and herbicides in man. Toxicol Appl Pharmacol 1974;28:126–132.

44. Rasmussen JE. Lindane: a prudent approach (Editorial). Arch Dermatol 1987;123:1008–1010.

45. Joy RM, Albertson TE. Lindane and limbic system excitability. Neurol Toxicol 1985;2:193–214.

46. USPHS. Toxicological profile for chlordane. Agency for Toxic Substances and Disease Registry, US Public Health Service, Government Printing Office, December 1989:1–8.

47. USPHS. Toxicological profile for chlordane. Agency for Toxic Substances and Disease Registry, US Public Health Service, Government Printing Office, December 1989:67–68.

48. USPHS. Toxicological profile for chlordane. Agency for Toxic Substances and Disease Registry, US Public Health Service, Government Printing Office, December 1989:69–94.

49. Wright CG, Leidy RB. Chlordane and heptachlor in the ambient air of houses treated for termites. Bull Environ Contam Toxicol 1982;28:617–623.

50. Anderson DJ, Hites RA. Chlorinated pesticides in indoor air. Environ Sci Technol 1988;22:717–720.

51. USPHS. Toxicological profile for chlordane. Agency for Toxic Substances and Disease Registry, US Public Health Service, Government Printing Office, December 1989:63–65.

52. Hayes WJ. Chlorinated hydrocarbon insecticides. Chap 6 in: Pesticides studied in man. Baltimore, MD: Williams & Wilkins, 1982:172–283.

53. USPHS. Toxicological profile for chlordane. Agency for Toxic Substances and Disease Registry, US Public Health Service, Government Printing Office, December 1989;103–105.

54. Barnes R. Poisoning by the insecticide chlordane. Med J Aust May 13, 1967:972–973.

55. Aldrich FD, Holmes JH. Acute chlordane intoxication in a child. Arch Environ Health 1969;19:129–132.

56. Derbes VH, Dent JH, Forrest WW, Johnson MF. Fatal chlordane poisoning. Council on Pharmacy and Chemistry. JAMA 1955;158:1367–1369.

57. Dadey JL, Kammer AG. Chlordane intoxication. JAMA 1953;153:723–726.

58. Kutz FW, Strassman SC, Sperling JF, Cook BT. A fatal chlordane poisoning. J Toxicol Clin Toxicol 1983;20:167–174.

59. USPHS. Toxicological profile for chlordane. Agency for Toxic Substances and Disease Registry, US Public Health Service, Government Printing Office, December 1989:9–62.

60. Wang HH, MacMahon B. Mortality of pesticide applicators. J Occup Med 1979;21:741–744.

61. Wang HH, MacMahon B. Mortality of workers employed in the manufacture of chlordane and heptachlor. J Occup Med 1979;21:745–748.

62. Ditraglia D, Brown DP, Namekata T, Iverson N. Mortality study of workers employed at organochlorine pesticide manufacturing plants. Scand J Work Environ Health 1981;7:140–146.

63. Blair A, Grauman DJ, Lubin JH, Fraumeni JF. Lung cancer and other causes of death among licensed pesticide applicators. J Natl Cancer Inst 1983;71:31–37.

64. Furie B, Trubowitz S. Insecticides and blood dyscrasias: chlordane exposure and self-limited refractory megaloblastic anemia. JAMA 1976;235:1720–1722.

65. Mendeloff AI, Smith DE. Clinico-pathologic conference: exposure to insecticides, bone marrow failure, gastrointestinal bleeding, and uncontrollable infections. Am J Med August 1955:274–284.

66. Menconi S, Clark JM, Langenberg P, Hryhorczuk D. A preliminary study of potential human health effects in private residences following chlordane applications for termite control. Arch Environ Health 1988;43:349–352.

67. Curley A, Garretson L. Acute chlordane poisoning, clinical and chemical studies: Arch Environ Health 1969;18:211–215.

68. Biros FJ, Enos HF. Oxychlordane residues in human adipose tissue. Bull Environ Contam Toxicol 1973;10:257–260.

69. Olanoff L, Bristow W, Cololough J. Acute chlordane intoxication. J Toxicol Clin Toxicol 1983;20:291–306.

70. Garretson L, Guzelian PS, Blanke R. Subacute chlordane poisoning. J Toxicol Clin Toxicol 1984;22:565–571.

71. Hunter CG, Robinson J. Pharmacodynamics of dieldrin (HEOD): Part I. Arch Environ Health 1967;15:614–626.

72. USPHS. Toxicological profile for aldrin/dieldrin. Agency for Toxic Substances and Disease Registry, US Public Health Service, Government Printing Office, May 1989:71–76.

73. USPHS. Toxicological profile for aldrin/dieldrin. Agency for Toxic Substances and Disease Registry, US Public Health Service, Government Printing Office, May 1989;81–85.

74. USPHS. Toxicological profile for Aldrin/dieldrin. Agency for Toxic Substances and Disease Registry, US Public Health Service, Government Printing Office, May 1989:27–66.

75. Ackerman L. Humans—overview of human exposure to dieldrin residues in the environment and current trends of residue levels in tissue. Pestic Mon J 1980;14:64–69.

76. Hunter CG, Robinson J. Pharmacodynamics of dieldrin (HEOD): ingestion by human subjects for 18 to 24 months, and postexposure for eight months. Arch Environ Health 1969;18:12–21.

77. Jager K. Aldrin, dieldrin, endrin and telodrin—an epidemiological and toxicological study of long-term occupational exposure. New York, NY: Elsevier, 1970:121–131.

78. Patel TB, Hy B, Rao VN. Dieldrin poisoning in man: a report of 20 cases observed in Bombay State. Br Med J April 19, 1958:919–922.

79. Bloomquist JR, Soderlund DM. Neurotoxic insecticides inhibit GABA-dependent chloride uptake by mouse brain vesicles. Biochem Biophys Res Commun 1985;133:37–43.

80. Jong de G. Long-term health effects of aldrin and dieldrin. Toxicol Lett (Supp) 1991:1–206.

81. Ribbens PH. Mortality study of industrial workers exposed to aldrin, dieldrin and endrin. Int Arch Occup Environ Health 1985;56:75–79.

82. Rowley D, Rab M, Hardjotanojo W, Liddle J. Convulsions caused by endrin poisoning in Pakistan. Pediatrics 1987;79(6):928–934.

83. WHO. Environmental Health Criteria 40, Endosulfan, World Health Organization, Geneva, 1984.

84. Shemesh Y, Bourvine A, Gold D, Bracha P. Survival after acute endosulfan intoxication. J Toxicol Clin Toxicol 1988;26:265–268.

85. WHO. Environmental Health Criteria 44, Mirex, World Health Organization, Geneva, 1984.

86. Taylor J. Neurological manifestations in humans exposed to chlordecone: follow-up of results. Neurotoxicology 1985;6:231–236.

87. WHO. Environmental Health Criteria 43, Chlordecone, World Health Organization, Geneva, 1984.

88. WHO. Environmental Health Criteria 66, Kelevan, World Health Organization, Geneva, 1986.

89. WHO. Environmental Health Criteria 45, Camphechlor, World Health Organization, Geneva, 1984.

103

Fumigants

John Lowe, C.I.H.
John B. Sullivan, Jr., M.D.

INTRODUCTION

Fumigants are pesticides that exist as gases or vapors at specified temperatures and pressures (generally room temperature and ambient pressures). Fumigation is used to control a variety of pests including insect pests in stored grain products, wood-destroying insects, and nematodes or fungi in soil (1). The advantages of fumigation is that it is often the quickest method for controlling pests, it can kill pests in places where sprays cannot reach (i.e., within building materials or deep within soil), and in some cases may be less expensive than repeated spraying. Disadvantages to fumigation are the need for specialized equipment and training needed to safely use fumigants (2). Fumigants span several different classes of chemicals; however, nearly all of the chemicals used as fumigants are highly toxic, both to pest species and to nontarget organisms. Several chemicals that formerly were used as fumigants are poisons well known to toxicologists, such as carbon tetrachloride, carbon disulfide, and hydrogen cyanide. Other chemicals with important commercial uses as fumigants, such as 1,2-dibromo-3-chloropropane (DBCP), ethylene dibromide (EDB), 1,3-dichloropropene (1,3-D), methyl bromide, and aluminum phosphide, have been associated with significant chronic and acute health effects in humans and laboratory animals.

Many fumigants epitomize the balance of known economic benefits versus estimated health risks associated with chemical use. Classic examples of this balance include chemicals such as EDB and DBCP that have served vital roles in increasing crop yields by controlling soil-borne nematodes. Use of the compounds have resulted in potential widespread exposures of humans through ground water contamination in agricultural areas and, in the case of DBCP, adverse effects in workers. EDB and DBCP have been demonstrated to be carcinogens in laboratory animals, hence they represent a potential human cancer risk. The estimated cancer risk associated with these chemicals in ground water has significantly influenced decisions to no longer permit their use in agriculture.

Table 103.1 lists several chemicals used as fumigants and describes their uses, current status, and availability in the United States. The following describes further methods of fumigant use, the potential for human exposure to fumigants, and the toxic effects associated with fumigant exposure.

FUMIGATION METHODS

Fumigants afford a practical solution to control of insects and other pests within an enclosure. A good fumigant has several specific properties. The chemical must be volatile and be able to penetrate deeply into soil, stored products, or (in the case of structural fumigants) building materials where pests are located. The chemical must be toxic to pests but should not be corrosive or phytotoxic. The chemical must desorb readily from treated food products and not leave behind toxicologically significant or phytotoxic residues. Soil fumigants should also desorb or degrade readily prior to planting (1, 3).

Fumigation can be performed in almost any enclosed space. However, the principal classes of fumigant use are space fumigation of commodities or commodity-processing equipment, soil fumigation, and fumigation for structural pest control.

Space Fumigation

Space fumigation is often performed within standing fumigation chambers or by enclosing the commodity with "gas-proof" sheeting. A fumigation chamber consists of three elements:

Table 103.1. Selected Chemicals Used in Fumigation

Chemical	Uses	Status
Aluminum phosphide	Grain fumigant	Still in use
Calcium cyanide	Rodent control Beehive fumigant	Very limited uses
Carbon disulfide	Rodent control Soil fumigant	Early fumigant, no longer used
Carbon tetrachloride	Grain fumigant	Use suspended by EPA due to toxicity
Chloropicrin	Soil fumigant Warning agent	Still in use
Dibromochloro-propane (DBCP)	Soil fumigant	Use suspended by EPA due to toxicity and ground water contamination
1,3-Dichloropropene	Soil fumigant	Use suspended by EPA due to toxicity
Ethylene dibromide	Soil fumigant Grain fumigant Commodity fumigant "Spot" fumigant	Use suspended by EPA due to toxicity and ground water contamination
Ethylene dichloride	Grain fumigant	Use suspended by EPA due to toxicity
Ethylene oxide	Sterilant for medical instruments	Still in use
Methyl bromide	Soil fumigant Commodity fumigant Structural fumigant	Still in use
Sulfuryl fluoride	Structural fumigant	Still in use

(a) a system for introducing the fumigant into the chamber, (b) a chamber where the commodity to be fumigated is loaded, and (c) and exhaust ventilation system for removing the fumigant from the chamber. A great variety of fumigant delivery and ventilation systems are possible; these provide different levels of exposures and potential hazards to the fumigation workers. For example, liquid fumigants, such as ethylene dichloride or carbon tetrachloride, could be introduced into a space by volatilization from a heated pan. This method could result in inhalation exposures and dermal contact with the fumigant during pouring of the material. More sophisticated delivery systems include closed systems, where the fumigant is metered into the chamber from sealed containers or compressed gas cylinders. These systems serve to reduce potential exposures to fumigants. Phosphine, used as a grain fumigant is introduced into stockpiled grain as tablets of aluminum or magnesium phosphide. The tablets may be metered into the grain as it is poured into a silo, or are introduced into stockpiles that are then covered with polyethylene tarps. The moisture in the grain slowly hydrolyzes the solid compound, liberating phosphine gas over a period of several hours. The solid compound is relatively safe to handle, as long as it is kept dry, since the hydrolysis reaction is exothermic, and phosphine has a flash point at 100°C. Potential exposures to phosphine would occur by inhalation, most often following tarp removal or opening enclosures to ventilate the grain prior to transport.

Soil Fumigation

Soil fumigation normally involves injecting liquid fumigant into the soil to depth from 6 inches to 3 feet, depending upon the crop and pest being controlled, through tubing attached to a set of shanks that are pulled through the soil. The shanks are mounted on a tool bar attached either to a wheeled or track-laying tractor. The treated soil is then sealed by a roller or cultipacker drawn by the fumigant rig or a second tractor, in the case of low-volatile fumigants such as DBCP, EDB, or 1,3-dichloropropene. Application rates of these compounds range from 5–15 gallons/acre for row crops, and from 40–60 gallons/acre prior to establishing orchards or vineyards. Fumigation techniques differ when using methyl bromide. Methyl bromide is injected into the soil at rates of 200–325 pounds/acre. Immediately following fumigation with methyl bromide, the soil is sealed with a polyethylene sheet drawn over the soil by the fumigant rig. Employees shovel soil over the edges of the tarp to slow the dissipation of this highly volatile compound into the air.

DBCP, EDB, and 1,3-dichloropropene are liquids at ambient conditions and are loaded into tanks on the fumigant rig from a nurse truck stationed at the edge of the field. Loading is typically performed through closed systems using quick-disconnect, dry-break couplers and gasoline or electric pumps. The tractor tanks may be vented either to open air or into the shanks. Depending upon the number and capacity of tractor tanks and application rates, fumigant loads are performed every 45 minutes to 2 hours of application. The actual loading process requires from 5–15 minutes. Methyl bromide is a gas at ambient conditions, and is injected into the soil through a closed system from a compressed gas cylinder.

Structural Fumigation

Structural fumigations generally are performed using gas-proof tarpaulins which are not impermeable but hold the desired fu-

migant concentration inside the structure for a required period of time. Prior to tarping a structure, the fumigator determines the structure volume and calculates the required fumigant dose, inspects the structure and roof for possible leak points (attached buildings, tunnels, vents, or drains connecting to the outside or other buildings, roof vents, and television antennas), shuts off gas valves, removes furnishings, foods, and personal items as required, clears shrubbery away from the walls, pads sharp edges, corners, and projections to protect the tarps from tearing, and wets the soil around the perimeter of the structure to prevent migration of the gas. Tarpaulins are then carried up to the roof and draped over the structure. The tarpaulin edges are rolled and clamped together with steel clothespins. During tarping, the fumigant delivery hose and several fans are placed inside the structure. The tarpaulin edges are sealed at the bottom of the structure with sandsnakes (long canvas tubes filled with sand). Secondary locks, designed to enclose a doorknob and prevent it from being operated, are placed on all doors.

After inspecting the integrity of the tarpaulin and checking the location of all workers, the fumigant and warning agent are introduced into the structure. The fumigant, typically methyl bromide or sulfuryl fluoride, is dispensed from a compressed gas cyclinder through a heated manifold. The fumigant dose, in total pounds introduced, is measured by the loss of weight in the cylinder. Application rates of methyl bromide typically range from 1.5–3 pounds per 1,000 ft³ of structure volume, providing concentrations calculated to range from 6,000 to 12,000 ppm. Due to the hazards associated with such high concentrations, structural fumigants are used in conjunction with a warning agent, typically chloropicrin. Chloropicrin can be introduced by hand pouring into a shallow pan a few minutes prior to introduction of the fumigant. Many fumigants registered for structural use are formulated with 1–3% chloropicrin, which is then introduced along with the fumigant.

ASSESSMENT OF EXPOSURES TO FUMIGANTS

The potential pathways of human exposure for fumigants are inhalation exposure of workers and off-site individuals, skin and eye contact with liquids producing burns or irritation, and ingestion of ground water or treated commodities.

Space Fumigation

Studies of fumigant use on stored commodities, primarily with methyl bromide, indicate that large variations can exist in fumigation worker exposure. In studies performed by the California Department of Food and Agriculture that involved air monitoring of methyl bromide use in fumigation chambers, personal exposures ranged from 0.2–33.4 ppm based on sample durations of 3–20 minutes (sampling was performed only during work activities at the chamber). Area sampling performed during these studies indicated that methyl bromide concentrations in work areas located 50 feet or further from fumigation chambers were 1.0 ppm or less (4, 5).

Work activities that potentially bring workers into contact with fumigants include (a) introducing the fumigant into the chamber or tarped commodity, (b) ventilating the remaining fumigant from the commodity, and (c) opening the chamber door and removing the commodity from the fumigation chamber. Exposures could fluctuate depending upon several factors including chamber volume, number of fumigations performed per period of time, duration allowed for ventilation of the commodity, and fumigant dosage applied to the commodity. However, the highest exposures appeared to be associated with opening the chamber door after fumigation and removing the commodity (4, 5).

Soil Fumigation

Several studies have evaluated worker exposures associated with methyl bromide/chloropicrin used as soil fumigants. Several of these studies have been performed by the California Department of Food and Agriculture. Fumigant formulations used in the applications typically contained 67% methyl bromide and 33% chlorpicrin. Types of workers monitored were drivers and "co-pilots" on the fumigant rig and shovelers at the edge of the field sealing the tarp. Concentrations of methyl bromide as great as 8.3 ppm and chloropicrin as great as 0.18 ppm were found in air samples ranging from 30–45 minutes in duration. Most exposures to methyl bromide have not exceeded 5 ppm. Observation of work practices indicated that workers spent approximately half of a work day fumigating, with the balance spent driving to and from work sites or maintaining equipment. Exposures of tarp removal operations were not monitored in these studies (6–8). However, one case is reported in Connecticut in which nursery workers removing tarps days after fumigation with methyl bromide reported symptoms. Four field-workers developed fatigue and light-headedness, and three workers noted progressive respiratory, gastrointestinal (GI), and neurologic symptoms. The acute systemic symptoms improved over several days, but later-onset neuropsychiatric symptoms persisted over several weeks. Exposure monitoring data were not available to compare symptoms with methyl bromide concentrations in air. This incident raised the possibility of an increased risk of toxicity associated with methyl bromide fumigation during a cool season (9).

Studies of methyl bromide fumigation in greenhouses in Belgium indicate that peak exposures could range from 100–1,000 ppm (duration unspecified). Work practices were reported to be more primitive than in the United States, with workers pulling tarps over fumigated soil by hand, instead of the tarp being laid down automatically by the fumigation rig. Protective measures such as wetting the soil and better coordination of activities between the tractor driver and tarpers reduced concentrations to approximately 100 ppm. One study reported that tarp removal from the soil could result in peak exposures as high as 200 ppm and that tilling the soil several days after application produced concentrations up to 15 ppm (10, 11).

Another study reports an episode of acute symptoms in individuals residing near a field treated with methyl bromide and chloropicrin. These events appeared to occur during times of low wind, atmospheric inversions, and elevated air temperatures (which also possibly represented warmer soil temperatures). The most frequent symptoms reported included headache, eye and throat irritation, and dizziness. Reports of these symptoms dropped off rapidly with distance from the site. In field study of off-site movement of fumigants in Southern California, 30-minute air samples collected at the edge of the field showed concentrations of methyl bromide between 0.3 and 0.4 ppm, and concentrations of chloropicrin between 0.01 and 0.08 ppm immediately after fumigation. These concentrations typically declined over time. However, studies evaluated ambient concentrations under warm inversion conditions, as seen with the reported acute exposure incidents, have not been performed (12).

Factors that could affect volatilization of fumigants from soil include soil temperature, moisture and porosity, physical and chemical properties of the fumigant (such as vapor pressure, diffusion coefficient, and Henry's law constant), and the application rate. Some studies have reported that increasing the application rate also increases mobility of methyl bromide in soil. Higher application rates appear to result in increased methyl bromide concentrations in air. Soil porosity also influences fumigant mobility. Porosity in soil is reduced by soil moisture and clay content. Hence, fumigants have lower mobility in wet or clay soils. Soil temperature increases the volatility, hence the diffusivity of fumigants in soil (13–16). Emissions of fumigants from soil would then be highest under conditions of high application rates, high soil moisture, high clay content, and high soil temperatures.

Exposures to DBCP, EDB, and 1,3-D also have been evaluated in studies performed by the California Department of Food and Agriculture. Generally, inhalation exposures of EDB and 1,3-D were lower than methyl bromide, due to the lower vapor pressure of these compounds. Eight-hour time-weighted average (TWA) exposures of Telone (92% 1,3-D) and D-D (50% 1,3-D and 30% 1,2-D) soil fumigants were determined during application by 21 fumigators. The 1,3-D exposure concentrations ranged from 0.07 to 3.61 ppm, with a mean of 0.71 ppm. Eight-hour TWA exposures to 1,2-D ranged from 0.003 to 0.44 ppm with a mean of 0.17 ppm. Short-duration exposures during loading or repair operations were highly variable, ranging from 0.02 to 41.9 ppm (17). Eight-hour (TWA) exposures of 21 applicators applying EDB ranged from 0.001–4.3 ppm with a mean of 0.73 ppm. Short-duration exposures during loading or repair operations ranged from non-detected to 2 ppm (18).

Groundwater Contamination

Greater focus has been given to soil fumigants as contaminants of groundwater. In 1979, wells near a pesticide manufacturing facility near Lathrop, California were found to contain traces of DBCP at concentrations up to 68 ppb. An expanded study of water samples from 262 wells in several California counties detected concentrations of DBCP ranging from 0.1–39.2 ppb in 92 water samples (19). At this time, DBCP use had been suspended in California due to spermatotoxic effects observed in manufacturing workers and carcinogenicity in laboratory animals, and the California Department of Food and Agriculture was considering re-registration of this fumigant with special requirements for reducing exposures. However, following the finding of groundwater contamination, the state of California elected to suspend use of DBCP permanently. Suspension of all use nationwide by the EPA followed shortly.

Following the finding of DBCP in groundwater, attention turned to structurally similar compounds such as EDB; 1,2-D; and 1,3-D. In 1983, EDB was detected in concentrations up to 0.38 pb in 15 of 137 wells sampled in California, resulting in suspension of its use nationwide by EPA (20). In 1982, 1,2-D was detected in well water at concentrations ranging from 0.4–16 ppb (21). 1,3-D has not been detected in groundwater, probably due to its more rapid hydrolysis and degradation in soil (22). Methyl bromide has not been evaluated as a groundwater contaminant.

Structural Fumigation

Structural fumigation potentially poses greater worker and public health hazards than other fumigant uses. From 1977–1984,

16 persons have died in California from unauthorized entry into structures undergoing fumigation with methyl bromide (23, 24). Neurobehavioral evaluation of both soil and structural fumigators handling methyl bromide and sulfuryl fluoride indicate that even low levels of methyl bromide exposure could produce neurotoxic effects (25).

Monitoring of atmospheres inside structures undergoing fumigation with methyl bromide had shown that concentrations can range from 5,000–12,000 ppm. Exposures to such concentrations can be rapidly fatal, therefore chloropicrin is added as a warning agent. Chloropicrin concentrations during fumigation range from 1–10 ppm. Chloropicrin is a respiratory irritant, lacrimator, and skin irritant. A concentration of 15 ppm in air for 1 minute is considered intolerable, as is a concentration of 7.5 ppm for 10 minutes. The lowest concentration producing irritation reported is 1.3 ppm. An odor threshold of 1.1 ppm is reported. A concentration range of 0.3–3.7 ppm produced "closing of the eyelids according to individual sensitivity." Much of these data, still being cited currently, were produced during and following World War I. Also, it is not known how test concentration were verified analytically (23, 24).

Fatalities from unauthorized entry into structures fumigated with methyl bromide have occurred despite the apparent presence of odorous or irritating concentrations of chloropicrin. Some individuals may possess a greater tolerance to the effects of chloropicrin, and intoxication with drugs or alcohol may blunt an individual's perception of odor or irritation. Given the high toxicity of methyl bromide, the current use of chloropicrin may not be sufficiently irritating to deter an individual from remaining in the toxic atmosphere for a sufficient length of time to become incapacitated and unable to escape. Fumigators are reluctant to use increased dosage of chloropicrin as it may render a structure uninhabitable by creating objectionable odors or irritation to the occupants. Since chloropicrin is less volatile than methyl bromide, it can adsorb to interior surfaces, and later slowly desorb into the structure atmosphere once fumigation is completed (23, 24).

Worker exposure to methyl bromide, during removal of tarps following fumigation have ranged from 1.5–57 ppm, measured over durations of 10–53 minutes. These exposures periodically exceed occupational exposure standards. Peak exposures occurred during the first few moments during tarp removal; 500–2500 ppm methyl bromide can remain inside a structure 24 hour following injection. Concentrations exceeding 100 ppm can persist up to 20 minutes following tarp removal (23, 24).

FUMIGANT TOXICOLOGY
Halogenated Aliphatic Hydrocarbons

The chemicals 1,2-dibromo-3-chloropropane (DBCP); ethylene dibromide (EDB); and 1,3-dichloropropene (DCP) are grouped because they are halogenated short-chain aliphatic hydrocarbons and all have been used in the past as soil fumigants for the control of plant-parasitic nematodes (EDB has also had some use in fumigation of milling machinery). These chemicals are no longer used in fumigation due to carcinogenicity observed in laboratory animals. DBCP and EDB have also been shown to be spermatotoxic in laboratory animals, and DBCP has been shown to be spermatotoxic in humans.

DBCP

The effects of DBCP on male reproductive function observed in humans in the late 1970s were shown in laboratory animals

as early as 1961 (26), which created some controversy about the effectiveness at that time of pesticide regulatory programs in detecting and mitigating health hazards. Though all use in the United States was suspended in 1979, ground water contamination associated with DBCP use remains an environmental problem.

DBCP has been produced and used since the 1950s; however, the effects of this chemical on human health was not recognized until 1977, following studies of testicular function in DBCP production workers in California (27, 28). These studies had confirmed workers' concerns about apparent infertility by demonstrating azoospermia or severe oligospermia in 14 of 25 workers studied. Similar reductions in sperm count were observed in workers performing soil fumigations. These studies have shown a dose-response relationship for DBCP-induced spermatotoxicity. Reductions in sperm production are also accompanied by elevations in serum follicle stimulating and luetinizing hormones and reductions in spermatogenic cells in the seminiferous vesicles (29, 30). Follow-up studies of DBCP-exposed workers have shown that, after exposure ceases, recovery of sperm production does not occur, or is greatly impeded in cases where exposure has produced a complete absence of spermatogenesis. In cases where spermatogenesis was only partially inhibited, complete recovery appears to occur a few months after exposure ceases (28, 31, 32)). Exposure studies of pineapple workers performed by the National Institute for Occupational Safety and Health (NIOSH), involving monitoring both sperm counts and breathing-zone concentrations in air, indicated that sperm counts did not vary over exposures ranging from 0–1.8 ppm. NIOSH concluded that 1 ppm in air had no observable effects on male fertility (33).

Animal studies have shown that the kidneys and the testes are primary target organs of DBCP, in acute, subacute, and chronic exposure situations (26, 34). Studies of the mode of action have revealed conflicting results, with DBCP producing depletion of glutathione in different organs, but with toxicity not always being correlated with glutathione depletion (35, 36). The lowest-observed-effect-level in male rats from chronic oral exposure (for 8 months) in one study was reported to be 0.05 mg/kg, with 0.005 mg/kg a no-observed-effect-level. This same study reported that 0.5 and 5 mg/kg were both gonadotoxic and produced functional disturbances in the liver and kidneys (37). Dose-related histopathologic changes of the nasal turbinates, including focal hyperplasia, squamous metaplasia, and loss of cilia, were detected in male and female rats exposed to 0, 1, 5, and 25 ppm DBCP in air, 6 hours/day, 5 days/week for 13 weeks (38). Limited studies suggest that DBCP is not teratogenic in rats at doses up to 50 mg/kg but does produce some maternal toxicity (39).

DBCP is considered to be a potent mutagen with microsomal activation in the Ames assay. It had induced sister-chromatid exchanges in Chinese hamster ovary (CHO) cells and has produced increased frequency of chromosomal aberrations in sperm of exposed workers (37). In a cancer bioassay performed by the National Cancer Institute (NCI), technical grade DBCP (with 16 impurities) given by gavage to rats and mice produced squamous cell carcinoma of the forestomach in both species. The time-weighted average doses in rats were 0, 15, and 29 mg/kg/day; in male mice, 0, 114, and 219 mg/kg/day; and, in female mice 0, 110, and 209 mg/kg/day (40). The excess lifetime cancer risk based on the male rat data from this study is 7.8×10^{-6} per μg/l of DBCP in drinking water (37). In two different inhalation bioassays, mice or rats exposed to DBCP concentrations of 0, 0.6 or 3.0 ppm in air for 6 hours/day, 5 days/week over 103–104 weeks developed alveolar and bronchial adenomas and carcinomas and tumors of the nasal cavity (38, 41). DBCP is considered to be a complete carcinogen, producing tumors close to the site of administration (37).

EDB

EDB has been used extensively as a fumigant since 1948. Its volatility and versatility, based on chemical and biocidal properties, led to its use as a soil sterilant, as a spot fumigant of grain milling machinery, and as a control agent in grain, fruit, and vegetable infestations. In 1977 the EPA began a review of EDB's pesticidal uses which eventually led to its cancellation for most agricultural applications. Disposal of EDB and contamination of water supplies remain major environmental concerns (42)).

EDB is substantially more toxic than DBCP. Acute dermal exposure produces painful local inflammation, swelling, and blistering. The liver appears to be a principal target organ for EDB toxicity (37). The mechanism of action of EDB appears to involve its conversion to reactive metabolites that become irreversibly bound to macromolecules including DNA. Metabolism of EDB involves an oxidative pathway (cytochrome P-450) and a conjugation pathway (glutathione-S-transferase) (42). Oral administration of EDB to rats has been shown to deplete glutathione levels in the liver through this metabolic pathway and over time to decrease the activity of glutathione-S-transferase (43). When glutathione levels are sufficiently depleted, EDB reactive metabolites are apparently free to inhibit the transferases as well as to interact with other macromolecules.

EDB has been studied for mutagenic potential by a variety of in vitro and in vivo test systems. EDB has consistently mutagenic potential in both bacterial assays and in in vitro assays using eukaryotic cells. EDB caused an increase in unscheduled DNA synthesis in cultured mammalian cells (44–46) and single-strand DNA breaks in in vitro cultured cells (47) and in in vivo rat liver cells (48).

Numerous studies have shown that EDB is carcinogenic in laboratory animals. The NCI (1978) administered TWA doses of 27 and 29 mg/kg/day to male and 26 and 28 mg/kg/day to female rats by gavage for 49 and 61 weeks for the low- and high-dose groups, respectively. High treatment-related mortality prompted the early termination of the study (planned for 110 weeks) and alterations of the dosing regimen, resulting in similar TWA dosages for high- and low-treatment groups. Significant increased incidences of squamous cell carcinomas of the stomach (both sexes), hepatocellular carcinomas and neoplastic nodules of the liver (females), and hemangiosarcomas of the circulatory system (males) were observed upon histologic examination. The stomach tumors developed after a short latency period and were observed to metastasize to multiple sites. Male and female B6C3F1 mice received TWA doses of 44 or 77 mg/kg/day by gavage for 53 weeks and were observed for their lifetimes (49). The incidence of squamous cell carcinomas and alveolar/bronchiolar adenomas of the lung was significantly increased over the controls in all the mice. As in the rat bioassay, no tumors were observed in the controls, and high treatment-related mortality prompted dosing regimen alterations.

Fischer 344 rats and B6C3F1 mice of both sexes were exposed to EDB vapors at 0, 10, or 40 ppm, 6 hours/day, 5 days/week for their lifespans (50). The incidence of nasal cavity carcinomas and adenocarcinomas in the rats of both sexes and

alveolar/bronchiolar carcinomas in female rats and mice of both sexes was significantly increased over the controls. The chronic inhalation of EDB was also associated with circulatory system hemangiosarcomas in both sexes of rats (high-dose only), mammary gland fibroadenomas of female rats, mammary gland adenocarcinomas of female mice, subcutaneous fibrosarcomas of female mice, and tunica vaginalis mesotheliomas of male rats. Stinson et al. (1981), in a chronic inhalation study of experimental design identical to the NTP study (with B6C3F1 mice only), reported an elevated incidence of nasal cavity carcinomas in the female mice exposed to 40 ppm EDB. Both sexes had dose-related epithelial hyperplastic lesions of the nasal cavity. Histologic and pathologic exams were conducted only on the nasal cavity (51).

Wong et al. (1982) exposed Sprague-Dawley rats of both sexes by inhalation to 0 or 20 ppm EDB, 7 hours/day, 5 days/week for 18 months. Splenic hemangiosarcomas and adrenal gland tumors of both sexes, subcutaneous mesenchymal tumors in males, and mammary gland tumors in females were significantly increased over the controls. Histologic examination excluded the nasal cavity (52).

Epidemiologic investigation of exposed workers have not revealed increased cancer incidences associated with EDB. Mortality studies of workers occupationally exposed to EDB found neither total deaths nor total malignancies of individuals exposed to EDB exceeded the control rate (53). The studies are inconclusive due to their small cohort size; lack of, or poorly characterized, exposure concentrations; and/or concurrent exposure to other potential or known carcinogens (54).

1,2-D AND 1,3-D

Cis- and trans-1,3-dichloropropene (1,3-D) are components of the pre-plant soil fumigants Telone (Dow Chemical Company, 92 percent 1,3-dichloropropene) and D-D (Shell Chemical Company, 50 percent 1,3-D, 30 percent 1,2-dichloropropene or 1,2-D). 1,3-D is acknowledged as the nematocidal components of these pesticides, with dichloropropane representing an inactive impurity in the formulation (application rates for D-D were generally two-fold greater than application rates for Telone). Dichloropropane shares similarities in toxicity with the other halogenated aliphatic compounds, but generally is less toxic than either EDB or 1,3-D.

Exposures to 1,2-D results in injury to the liver and kidneys. The literature has reported a few cases of adverse effects from acute exposure; however, other data on human exposures to 1,2-D are very limited (37). Heppel et al. (1946) found that subacute inhalation exposures of 1,2-D at 1,000 ppm caused fatalities in dogs, rats, and guinea pigs. Severe liver damage was characteristic of the animals that had died. Exposures to 400 ppm for 7 hours/day, 5 days/week for 128–140 exposures produced no effects in rats, with the exception of a decrease in weight gain. However, this exposure to a group of CH-strain mice produce fatalities in some animals and hepatomas in others (55). More recent studies have been conducted on the subchronic toxicity of 1,2-D as it is formulated in D-D. Rats and mice were exposed to 5, 15, and 50 ppm for 6 hours/day, 5 days/week for up to 12 weeks. The only compound-related effect observed was slight enlargement of hepatocytes. The major cofounder to this study was the presence of 1,3-D, which produces similar toxicity at lower doses (56).

The National Toxicology Program (NTP) sponsored a 2-year cancer gavage bioassay in rats and mice. Male rats were administered 62 and 125 mg/kg, 5 days/week, female rats were administered 125 and 250 mg/kg, 5 days/week; and male and female mice were administered 125 and 250 mg/kg 5 days/week. Low survival was observed in the high-dose female rats and female mice groups. Dose-related hepatocellular adenomas were observed in male and female mice. Nonsignificant increases in hepatocellular adenocarcinomas were observed in both sexes. The incidence of benign tumors was combined with the incidence of carcinomas for purposes of judging carcinogenicity in mice. Dose-related mammary gland adenocarcinomas were observed in female rats; however, 1,2-D did not produce carcinogenicity in male rats. Carcinogenicity observed in female rats may have been associated with toxic doses of 1,2-D compromising metabolic or endocrine functions. The carcinomas in the female rats were observed to not be metastatic, anaplastic, or invasive and were judged by some pathologists as fibroadenomas. This study concluded that there was not evidence of carcinogenicity in male rats, equivocal evidence of carcinogenicity in female rats, and some evidence of carcinogenicity in mice (57).

1,2-D is considered to be weakly mutagenic in bacterial strains, compared with other halogenated hydrocarbons, such as 1,3-D. Mutagenicity is not greatly enhanced by metabolic activation (58).

Metabolism of 1,2-D in the rat results in the formation of a mercapturic acid conjugate excreted largely in the urine. Proposed reactive intermediates include 1,2-epoxopropane; this intermediate is suspected of being responsible for mutagenic effects of 1,2-D (59). Gluthathione pathways are seen as a detoxification mechanisms, and liver and kidney toxicity at high concentrations may be due to saturation of these pathways (56).

Few acute toxicity studies of 1,3-D are available; however, a study with D-D reported an oral LD$_{50}$ of 300 mg/kg in the mouse and 140 mg/kg in the rat. The animals exhibited hyperexcitability, followed by tremors, incoordination, depression, and respiratory distress. Other effects observed were fatty degeneration of the liver and hemorrhage of the lungs. The 4-hour lethal concentration of (LC$_{50}$) in the rat was estimated to be 1,000 ppm. The effects from acute inhalation exposure included severe pulmonary edema and alveolar hemorrhage (60). D-D was also shown to be a severe eye and skin irritant. Confirmation of this is found in reports of occupational exposures of agricultural workers that are maintained by the California Department of Food and Agriculture; these are predominantly eye and skin injuries.

Torkleson and Oyen (1977) investigated the effects of repeated inhalation exposure to 1,3-D. Initial subacute studies involving rats and guinea pigs exposed to 11 or 50 ppm produced gross evidence of liver and kidney injury. Subchronic studies were also performed with rats, rabbits, and guinea pigs, involving exposures to 1 or 3 ppm for 125–130 times over a period of 185 days. Male rats exposed to 3 ppm exhibited cloudy swelling of the renal tubular epithelium. Female rats exhibited slight but statistically significantly increases in liver-to-body weight ratio. The 1 ppm concentration appeared to be a no-observed-effect-level. This study is significant in that it was the basis for the Threshold Limit Value (TLV) recommended for 1,3-D by the American Conference for Governmental Industrial Hygienists (61).

One study has been conducted which exhibited a carcinogenic response with Telone in both rats and mice. F344 rats of each sex were gavaged with Telone in corn oil at doses of 0, 25, and 50 mg/kg/day 3 times/week. No increased mortality occurred in treated animals. Elevated incidence of the following tumors were observed at the highest dose tested: (a) forestomach squamous cell papillomas in males and females; (b) forestomach squamous cell papillomas and carcinomas combined in males; and (c) liver neoplastic nodules in males. The increased incidence of forestomach tumors was accompanied by a positive trend for forestomach basal cell hyperplasia in male and female rats of both treated groups (25 and 50 mg/kg/day). B6C3F1 mice of each sex were gavaged with Telone II in corn oil at doses of 0, 50, and 100 mg/kg/day 3 times/week for 104 weeks. A total of 50 mice/sex were used for each dose group. Due to excessive mortality in control male mice from myocardial inflammation approximately 1 year after the initiation of the study (a time when neoplastic lesions would not be expected to occur), conclusions pertaining to oncogenicity were based on both concurrent control data as well as on available NTP historical control data. Elevated incidence of the following tumors were observed either at the highest dose level tested or at both dose levels tested: (a) forestomach squamous cell papillomas or papillomas and carcinomas combined in males and females, and squamous cell carcinomas in females; (b) urinary bladder transitional cell carcinomas in males and females; and (c) lung adenomas, and adenomas and carcinomas combined in males and females (62).

Groups of 50 male and 50 female B6C3F1 mice and Fischer 344 rats were exposed to 0, 5, 20, or 60 ppm technical-grade 1,3-dichloropropene, i.e., Telone II (0, 21, 84, or 251 mg/cu.m assuming 25°C and 760 mmHg; 49.5% cis- and 42.6% trans-1,3-dichloropropene, 0.7% 1,2-dichloropropane, 2% epoxidized soybean oil, and a 5.2% mixture of hexanes and hexadienes), 6 hours/day, 5 days/week for 2 years. In the mice, exposure-related changes were observed in the urinary bladder and in the nasal tissue in both sexes exposed to 60 ppm and in the females exposed to 20 ppm after 2 years of treatment. The urinary bladders of both sexes of mice had hyperplasia characterized by diffuse, uniform thickening of the transitional epithelium. Both sexes of mice also had compound-related microscopic changes in the nasal tissue characterized by hypertrophy and hyperplasia of the respiratory epithelium and/or degeneration of the olfactory epithelium. Histopathologic examination revealed exposure-related effects in the nasal tissues of both male and female rats exposed to 60 ppm for 24 months. These effects included unilateral or bilateral decreased thickness of the olfactory epithelium due to degenerative changes, erosions of the olfactory epithelium, and fibrosis beneath the olfactory epithelium. No lesions of the respiratory tract were found after 6 or 12 months of treatment. In mice, the LOAEL is identified as 20 ppm for hypertrophy/hyperplasia of the nasal respiratory epithelium. The NOAEL in mice is 5 ppm for hypertrophy/hyperplasia of the nasal respiratory epithelium and for epithelial hyperplasia and inflammation of the urinary bladder. In rats, the LOAEL is 60 ppm and the NOAEL is 20 ppm for the effects on the nasal olfactory epithelium (63).

Evidence that the nasal region of the respiratory tract is the critical target organ in laboratory animals for 1,3-dichloropropene is provided by other studies (64). However, this effect has not been of primary concern for adverse effects to workers. 1,3-D is metabolized by conjugation with glutathione and is excreted primarily as a mecapturic acid conjugate (65). This urinary metabolite has been detected in workers exposed to 1,3-D vapor during fumigation. Applicator exposure was studied using personal air monitoring of 1,3-D, and monitoring of urinary excretion of the mercapturic acid metabolite and the excretion of the renal tubular enzyme, N-acetyl glucosaminidase (NAG). Urinary excretion of the metabolite correlated well with exposure to 1,3-D. Four workers (out of 15 studied) had clinically elevated activity of NAG in any of their urine collections after baseline. Nine workers showed greater than 25% increases in NAG excretion when compared to baseline. Dichloropropene air exposure products of greater than 700 mg min/m^3 or excretion of the metabolite greater than 1.5 mg/day distinguished abnormally high daily excretion of NAG. These data demonstrate a relationship between air exposure and dose, and a possible subclinical nephrotoxic effect in workers handling 1,3-D (66).

Methyl Bromide

Methyl bromide is particularly hazardous because it has practically no odor and causes no immediate irritation of the nose or respiratory tract, even at severely poisonous concentrations. Over 300 cases of systemic poisonings and 60 fatalities attributable to methyl bromide have been reported in the literature. Acute exposures to high concentrations produce rapid narcosis and death from respiratory failure. If death does not result, the most consistent response is lung irritation with congestion and edema. Neurotoxicity is the toxic effect of principal concern from exposure to methyl bromide. Early symptoms of exposure include headache, nausea, and vomiting, followed by tremors, twitching, and seizures. The onset of neurologic effects from acute exposure may be delayed from 1 to 36 hours, complicating the diagnosis of methyl bromide toxicity. The onset of neurologic effects shorten when acute exposure episodes are superimposed on chronic exposure. Signs and symptoms of chronic exposures include those from acute exposure plus visual and hearing disorders, numbness or tingling in the extremities, incoordination, ataxia, and loss of consciousness. Psychologic symptoms have been associated with chronic exposure, including loss of initiative, depressed libido, personality changes, hallucinations, and an intolerance to alcohol (67).

Studies with laboratory animals confirm the neurotoxicity observed in humans. In one study, rats and rabbits were exposed to 65 ppm methyl bromide for 7.5 hours/day, 4 days/week for 4 weeks. In rabbits, this exposure produced hindlimb paralysis, decreased nerve conduction velocity, and decreased magnitude of the eyeblink response (68). Neuropathic effects were not demonstrated in rats at these exposures. These studies confirm earlier studies demonstrating neurotoxicity in rabbits but not rats. Neurotoxic effects were investigated in rabbits exposed to lower concentrations for longer durations. An exposure concentration of 27 ppm for 7.5 hours/day, 4 days/week, for 8 months produced no neurologic impairments in rabbits (69). Neurobehavioral studies in soil and structural fumigators have shown slight neurotoxicity at low levels of exposure (approximately 2 ppm) (26). However, review of some of the air monitoring data used to assess fumigator exposure suggests that these exposures associated with the observed neurobehavioral effects may be slightly underestimated. Time-weighted average airborne concentrations may not be of great value in characterizing adverse effects from methyl bromide exposures in the workplace; these exposures appear to be intermittant and of relatively short duration.

Methyl bromide has been shown to produce mutations in Salmonella strains sensitive to alkylating agents and to *E. coli* both with and without the addition of a metabolic activation system (70–72). Methyl bromide was also mutagenic in a modification of the standard Salmonella assay employing vapor phase exposure (73–75).

Methyl bromide was evaluated for carcinogenicity in a subchronic gavage study in rats. Treatment of groups of 10 male and 10 female Wistar rats by gavage 5 days/week for 13 weeks with bromomethane at 0, 0.4, 2, 10, or 50 mg/kg resulted in severe hyperplasia of the stratified squamous epithelium in the forestomach at a dose of 50 mg/kg/day and slight epithelial hyperplasia in the forestomach at a dose of 10 mg/kg/day. No neurotoxic effects were observed at any dose level tested. Adverse effects were not observed at 0.4 or 2 mg/kg. There was an apparent dose-related increase in diffuse hyperplasia of the forestomach (76). These results were subsequently questioned (U.S. EPA, 1985; Schatzow, 1984). A panel of NTP scientists reevaluated the histologic slides and concluded that the lesions were hyperplasia and inflammation rather than neoplasia (77). An inhalation bioassay for evaluating chronic toxicity and carcinogenicity of methyl bromide is currently under way at the National Toxicology Program (NTP) (78).

Available epidemiologic data are inadequate for evaluating the carcinogenicity of methyl bromide in humans. A prospective mortality study was reported for a population of 3579 white male chemical workers, employed between 1935 and 1976, who were potentially exposed to 1,2-dibromo-3-chloropropane, 2,3-dibromopropyl phosphate, polybrominated biphenyls, DDT, and several brominated organic and inorganic compounds. Overall mortality for the cohort, as well as for several subgroups, was less than expected. Of the 665 men exposed to methyl bromides (the only common exposure to organic bromides), two died from testicular cancer, as compared with 0.11 expected. This finding may be noteworthy, as testicular cancer is usually associated with a low mortality rate. Hence, the incidence of this tumor could be greater than indicated from the mortality data. The authors noted that it was difficult to draw definitive conclusions as to causality because of the lack of exposure information and the likelihood that exposure was to many brominated compounds (79).

Methyl bromide is an odorless volatile liquid which rapidly disperses and penetrates rubber and clothes. It has a TLV of 5 ppm with a skin notation to indicate the potential of dermal absorption. The concentration immediately dangerous to life and health (IDLH) is 2000 ppm, and at this concentration, methyl bromide produces pulmonary edema, seizures, and death.

Acute toxic exposure to methyl bromide can result in initial symptoms of headache, nausea, vomiting, vertigo, myalgias, ataxia, diplopia, and decreased vision (80). These symptoms may be delayed for hours before onset and may not appear for up to 24 hours. Methyl bromide is a gas that is heavier than air and constitutes a hazard in confined spaces. Exposure to methyl bromide is mainly by inhalational and dermal routes. Dermal toxicity can range from local dermatitis to vesicle formation and serious burns, depending on the level of exposure. Prolonged skin contact may occur because of absorption by clothing, particularly leather.

Low level chronic exposure can result in neurologic symptoms consisting of weakness, tremors, parasthesias, ataxia, decreased reflexes, dysarthria, dysmetria, and disdiadochokinesia, seizures, and status epilepticus (80). Both acute and chronic exposure can result in behavioral toxicity manifested by psychosis, delerium, hallucinations, aggression, and mania (81). Cases of homicidal ideation and acute psychosis have been described following serious exposures (81). Reports of coma, seizures, and hepatic damage resembling Reyes syndrome have occurred (80).

Ophthalmologic toxicity consists of decreased vision, diploplia, lacrimation, disturbance of accommodation, and scotomatas. Optic nerve damage with optic neuropathy has been reported (81). The neurologic lesions and ophthalmologic changes may last weeks or be permanent.

The neurotoxicity of methyl bromide depends on the exposure concentration and duration. Short-term high exposures can produce abnormal reflexes, ataxis, visual changes, and muscle weakness (80, 81). Tremor, parasthesias, and peripheral neuropathy may occur following extended exposures (80, 81). Neurobehavioral evaluation of methyl bromide applicators indicated significant impairment in behavioral tests compared to controls (80, 81).

Sulfuryl Fluoride

Sulfuryl fluoride is a colorless and odorless gas with a TLV of 5 ppm and an IDLH level of 1000 ppm. The chemical is a strong irritant of the respiratory system, mucous membranes, eyes, and skin. Exposure routes are via inhalation and dermal contact, although skin absorption is minimal. Sulfuryl fluoride is also a neurotoxin and produce central nervous system depression and parasthesias (82). Symptoms following toxic exposure begin with nausea, vomiting, abdominal pain, and mucous membrane irritation. Serious exposure can result in bronchospasm and parasthesias. Fumigated foods may be left with a high residual fluoride content.

Chloropicrin

Chloropicrin (trichloronitromethane or nitrochloroform) is a colorless, oily liquid fumigant for cereals and grains with a TLV of 0.1 ppm and a very irritating odor that can produce lacrimation. The IDLH concentration is 4 ppm.

Exposure to chloropicrin can occur by the inhalation, dermal, or gastrointestinal routes. Due to the strong irritating properties of the chemical, exposure would produce eye irritation, pulmonary irritation, and dermatitis. More serious exposures can cause pulmonary edema, coma, hepatic necrosis, renal damage, and cardiac necrosis (83).

The irritantcy properties of chloropicrin have been studied in animals using the RD_{50} value, which is the air concentration of a chemical that elicits a 50% decrease in the respiratory rate of the animals studied. The RD_{50} of chloropicrin was 9 ppm compared to that of ammonia which was 303 ppm (83). Chloropicrin is one of the most irritating chemicals known, and exposure to vapors produces intense irritation and lacrimation. One report of a home treated with chloropicrin produced respiratory illness in the family and a pet dog (83). The dog developed bronchitis and pneumonia. The family members developed cough, sinus irritation, and inflammation of the oropharynx. Chloropicrin concentrations ranged up to 48 parts per billion in certain areas of the home.

In animal studies, chloropicrin vapors produced ulceration of the olfactory epithelium and necrosis of lung tissues (83). Human toxicity following inhalation of chloropicrin can be manifest by pulmonary irritation, mucous membrane irritation, and pulmonary edema.

Boron Trifluoride

Boron trifluoride (BF_3) is a colorless gas with a strong odor. It is a very reactive chemical used as a fumigant but finds its main use as a catalyst in the synthesis of other chemicals. The TLV as a ceiling is 1 ppm. It is stored and transported as a gas (84). BF_3 has fire-retardant and antioxidant properties and reacts with moist air to form a white misty fume.

Boron trifluoride is a severe irritant of the mucous membranes, skin, and lungs. Dermal contact can produce chemical burns. Exposure to the gas produces lacrimation, upper airway irritation, nasal discharge, and cough. Due to the fact that it forms a fuming mist in air, it has sufficient warning properties to help prevent exposure.

Aluminum and Zinc Phosphide

These compounds are used to produce phosphine gas and are extensively employed as grain fumigants. Phosphine (PH_3) is generated by the action of water or acid on aluminum or zinc phosphide. Phosphine gas is colorless and has a TLV of 0.3 ppm with a STEL of 1 ppm. The IDLH level is 200 ppm. Clinical toxicology of phosphine poisoning involves early symptoms of headache, dizziness, nausea, vomiting, dyspnea, and cough. Severe poisoning cases have resulted in pulmonary edema, ataxia, coma, and myocardial necrosis (84, 85). Phosphine has a garlic-like odor, and symptom onset may be delayed for hours.

1,2-Dichloropropane

1,2-Dichloropropane ($ClCH_2$-$CHClCH_3$) is a colorless liquid used as a fumigant as well as a chemical intermediate and as a lead scavenger for gasoline. It is also a solvent for oils, waxes, gums, and resins as well as for cellulose esters and ethers (84). It is incompatible with oxidizing agents and acids. It has a TLV of 75 ppm and an IDLH concentration of 2000 ppm (85). It is also known as propylene dichloride. The clinical toxicology of this compound is mainly that of an irritant. It can also produce central nervous system depression and hepatic damage following toxic exposure.

1,1-Dichloro-1-nitroethane

This fumigant is a colorless liquid with a formula of $CH_3CCl_2NO_2$ and a TLV of 2 ppm. It is an irritant of the skin and eyes. The IDLH level is 150 ppm. It is incompatible with stong oxidizers (84).

Miscellaneous Fumigants

Hydrogen cyanide (HCN) often generated from calcium cyanide has been used in vertebrate pest control (i.e., fumigation of rodent burrows) and in space fumigation. It has been used in fumigating mills, warehouses, greenhouses, and commodities under gas-proof sheets. Hydrogen cyanide toxicity in humans occurs by inhibition of the enzyme cytochrome oxidase, blocking the utilization of oxygen and producing respiratory arrest. HCN has an almond odor, but poor warning properties (i.e., it does not provide and indication of overexposure by the presence of odor). HCN now has only limited use as a fumigant.

Carbon disulfide (CS_2) has been used in soil fumigation and fumigation of rodent burrows. CS_2 vapor is explosive, igniting spontaneously on contact with sparks or at temperatures above 147°C. CS_2 is also highly neurotoxic in humans. It is no longer in use as a fumigant due to the toxicity and explosion hazards.

Aluminum phosphide, used to produce phosphine gas, is used extensively as a grain fumigant. Phosphine is a respiratory irritant at low concentrations in air. It provides some warning of overexposure with its distinctive garlic-like odor.

Carbon tetrachloride has been used in conjunction with EDB and ethylene dichloride (EDC) as a grain fumigant. EPA has suspended use of this compound due to severe hepatoxicity in humans and carcinogenicity in laboratory animals.

CONCLUSIONS

As stated previously, fumigants exemplify the balance between economic benefit and protection of public and worker health. Soil fumigants such as DBCP, EDB, and Telone/D-D have been seen as important elements in control of plant-parasitic nematodes. Historically, as use of one chemical was suspended, uses of the others have increased. Suspension of the use of all these chemicals has led to the use of very low volatile organophosphorus and carbamate compounds such as fenaminophos (Nemacur) and carbofuran (Furadan) for control of nematodes. Use of these chemicals, both of which are highly toxic cholinesterase inhibitors, results in an interesting trade-off in which potential long-term chronic health hazards such as carcinogenicity (found in laboratory animals) are replaced with known acute toxicity (and possible longterm neurotoxicity) hazards. Chemicals such as DBCP and EDB are no longer in use, not because of the significant hazards to workers, but because of the low and theoretical cancer risk posed from ingestion of ground water contaminated with part-per-billion concentrations. The utility of such trade-offs between long-term potential protection of public health, and short term worker risks and potential economic harm have not been analyzed sufficiently. Thus, at this time it is not known if regulatory actions to control carcinogenic or chronic exposure hazards from fumigants are being made appropriately. In some cases, such as with methyl bromide, the economic benefits and lack of suitable alternatives so outweigh the hazards that this highly toxic material remains in use while uses of other, less toxic compounds (i.e., DBCP, Telone) have been suspended. As further information on methyl bromide toxicology is obtained, and regulatory scrutiny of this chemical increases, we will be presented with an important case study of balancing the need for a highly toxic chemical with the need to protect public and worker safety and health.

REFERENCES

1. Wilbur DA, Mills RB. Stored grain insects. In: Pfadt RE, ed. Fundamentals of applied entomology. New York, NY: MacMillan Publishing Company, 1978.

2. Mallis A. Handbook of pest control. The behavior, life history, and control of household pests. 6th ed. Cleveland: Franzak & Foster, 1982.

3. Study guide for agricultural pest control advisers on nematodes and nematocides. University of California Davis, Division of Agricultural Sciences Publication No. 4045, 1976.

4. Maddy KT. Schneider F, Lowe J, Alcoser D, Fredrickson AS. Monitoring environmental levels of methyl bromide during commodity fumigation. California Department of Food and Agriculture Report No. HS-1078, 1983.

5. Maddy KT, Lowe J, Fredrickson AS. Inhalation exposure of commodity handlers to methyl bromide in Yolo County, California, October 1983. California Department of Food and Agriculture Report No. HS-1186, 1984.

6. Maddy KT, Richmond D, Lowe J, Fredrickson AS. A study of the inhalation exposure of workers to methyl bromide during preplant soil fumigations (shallow injections) in 1980 and 1981. California Department of Food and Agriculture Report No. HS-900, 1982.

7. Maddy KT, Gibbons D, Richmond DM, Fredrickson AS. A study of the inhalation exposure of workers to methyl bromide and chloropicrin during preplant soil fumigations (shallow injections) in 1982—a preliminary report. California Department of Food and Agriculture Report No. HS-1076, 1984.

8. Maddy KT, Gibbons D, Richmond DM, Fredrickson AS. Additional monitoring of the inhalation exposure of workers to methyl bromide and chloropicrin during preplant soil fumigation (shallow injection) in 1983. California Department of Food and Agriculture Report No. HS-1175, 1984.

9. Herzstein J, Cullen MR. Methyl bromide intoxication in four field-workers during removal of soil fumigation sheets. Am J Ind Med 1990;17:321–326.

10. Roosels D, Van Den Oever R, Lahaye D. Dangerous concentrations of methyl bromide used as a fumigant in Belgian greenhouses. Arch Occup Environ Health 1981;48:243–250.

11. Van Den Oever R, Roosels D, Lahaye D. Actual hazard of methyl bromide fumigation in soil disinfection. Br J Ind Med 1982;39:140–144.

12. Goldman LR, Mengle D, Epstein DM, Fredson D, Kelly K, Jackson RJ. Acute symptoms in persons residing near a field treated with the soil fumigants methyl bromide and chloropicrin. West J Med 1987;147:95–98.

13. Abdalla N, Raski D, Lear B, Schmitt RV. Distribution of methyl bromide in soils treated for nematode control in replant vineyards. Pestic Sci 1974;5:259–269.

14. Goring CA. Physical aspects of soil in relation to the action of soil fumigants. Annu Rev Phytopathol 1967;5:285–318.

15. Kolbezen MJ, Munnecke DE, Wilbur WD, Stolzy LH, Abu El-Haz FS, Szuszkiewics TE. Factors that affect deep penetration of field soils treated with methyl bromide. Hilgardia 1974;42:465–492.

16. Munnecke DE, Van Gundy SD. Movement of fumigants in soil: dosage, responses and differential effects. Annu Rev Phytopathol 1979;17:405–429.

17. Maddy KT, Edmiston S, Lowe J, Fredrickson AS. Exposures of agricultural employees to 1,2-dichloropropane and 1,3-dichloropropene (Telone and D-D) in California. California Department of Food and Agriculture Report No. HS-1161, 1984.

18. Maddy KT, Edmiston S, Meinders DD, Fredrickson AS, Margetich S. Potential exposure of loader/applications to ethylene dibromide (EDB) during pre-plant soil fumigation in California in 1983. California Department of Food and Agriculture Report No. HS-1148, 1984.

19. Peoples SA, Maddy KT, Cusick W, Jackson T, Cooper C, Fredrickson AS. A study of samples of well water collected from selected areas in California to determine the presence of DBCP and certain other pesticide residues. Bull Environ Contam Toxicol 1980;24:611–618.

20. Smith C, Margetich S, Fredrickson AS. A survey of well water in selected counties of California for contamination by EDB in 1983. California Department of Food and Agriculture Report No. HS-1123, 1983.

21. Cohen D, Bowes G. Water quality and pesticides: a California risk assessment program Vol I. Sacramento, CA: State Water Resources Control Board, 1984.

22. Maddy KT, Fong HR, Lowe JA, Conrad D, Fredrickson AS. A study of well water selected in California communities for residues of 1,3-dichloropropene, chloroallyl alcohol and 49 organophosphate or chlorinated hydrocarbon pesticides. Bull Environ Contam Toxicol 1982;29:354–359.

23. Maddy KT, Gibbons DB, Lowe JA. Evaluation of chloropicrin as a warning agent and employee exposure to methyl bromide and chloropicrin during structural fumigation. Abstract #181, presented at the American Industrial Hygiene Conference, Montreal, Quebec, Canada, May 31–June 5, 1987.

24. Maddy KT, Lowe JA, Gibbons DB, O'Connell LP, Richmond DM, Fredrickson AS. Studies of methyl bromide and chloropicrin used as structural fumigants in California. I. Evaluation of chloropicrin as a warning agent. II. Employee exposure to methyl bromide and chloropicrin. III. Penetration of methyl bromide in plastic food storage bags. California Department of Food and Agriculture Report No. HS-1352, 1984.

25. Anger WK, Moody L, Burg J, Brightwell WS, Taylor BJ, Russo JM, Dickerson N, Setzer JV, Johnson BL, and Hicks K. Neurobehavioral evaluation of soil and structural fumigators using methyl bromide and sulfuryl fluoride. Neurotoxicology 1986;7:137–156.

26. Torkleson TR, Sadek SE, Rowe VK, Kodama JK, Anderson HH, Loquvam GS, Hine CH. Toxicologic investigations of 1,2-dibromo-3-chloropropane. Toxicol Appl Pharmacol 1961;3:545–559.

27. Whorton D, Krauss RM, Marshall S, Milby TH. Infertility in male pesticide workers. Lancet 1977;2:1259–1261.

28. Whorton D, Milby TH, Krauss RM, Stubbs HA. Testicular function in DBCP exposed pesticide workers. J Occup Med 1979;21:161–166.

29. Biava CG, Smuckler EA, Whorton D. The testicular morphology of individuals exposed to dibromochloropropane. Exp Mol Pharmacol 1978;29:448–458.

30. Engnatz DG, Ott MG, Townsend JC, Olson RD, Johns DB. DBCP and testicular effects in chemical workers: an epidemiologic survey in Midland, Michigan. J Occup Med 1980;22:727–732.

31. Lantz GD, Cunningham GR, Huckins C, Lipshulz LI. Recovery from severe oligospermia after exposure to dibromochloropropane. Fertil Steril 1981;35:46–53.

32. Whorton MD, Milby TH. Recovery of testicular function among DBCP workers. J Occup Med 1980;22:177–179.

33. NIOSH. A recommended standard for occupational exposure to dibromochloropropane. DHEW (NIOSH) Publication No. 78-115. US Department of Health, Education and Welfare, National Institute for Occupational Safety and Health, 1978.

34. Kluwe WM. Acute toxicity of 1,2-dibromo-3-chloropropane in the F344 male rat. I. Dose-response relationships and differences in routes of exposure. Toxicol Appl Pharmacol 1981;59:71–83.

35. Kato K, Sato K, Matano O, Goto S. Alkylation of cellular macromolecules by reactive metabolite intermediates of DBCP. J Pestic Sci 1980;5:45–53.

36. Kluwe WM. Acute toxicity of 1,2-dibromo-3-chloropropane in the F344 rat. II. Development and repair of the renal, epididymal, testicular and hepatic lesions. Toxicol Appl Pharmacol 1981;59:84–95.

37. NRC. Drinking Water and Health Vol 6. Washington, DC: National Academy of Sciences Press, 1986:321.

38. NTP. Carcinogenesis bioassay of 1,2-dibromo-3-chloropropane (CAS No. 96-12-8) in F344 rats and B6C3F1 mice (inhalation study) NTP Technical Report Series No. 206. NTH Publication No. 82-1762. US Department of Health and Human Services, National Toxicology Program, 1982.

39. Ruddick JA, Newsome WH. A teratogenicity and tissue distribution study on dibromochloropropane in the rat. Bull Environ Contam Toxicol 1979;27:181–186.

40. NCI. Bioassay of dibromochloropropane for possible carcinogenicity. Technical Report Series No. 28. DHEW Publication No. (NIH) 78-828. US Department of Health, Education, and Welfare, National Cancer Institute, 1978.

41. Reznik G, Reznik-Schuller H, Ward JM, Stinson SF. Morphology of nasal cavity tumors in rats after chronic inhalation of 1,2-dibromo-3-chloropropane. Br J Cancer 1980;42:772–781.

42. Alexeeff GV, Kilgore WW, Li MY. Ethylene dibromide: toxicology and risk assessment. Rev Environ Contam Toxicol 1990;112:49–122.

43. Botti B, Moslen MT, Trieff NM, Reynolds ES. Transient decrease of liver cytosolic glutathione-*S*-transferase activity in rats given 1,2-dibromoethane or CCL$_4$. Chem Biol Interact 1982;42:259–270.

44. Meneghini R. Repair replication of opossum lymphocyte DNA: effect of compounds that bind to DNA. Chem Biol Interact 1974;8:113–126.

45. Perocco P, Prodi G. DNA damage by haloalkanes in human lymphocytes cultured in vitro. Cancer Lett 1981;13:213–218.

46. Williams GM, Laspia MF, Dunkel VC. Reliability of the hepatocyte primary culture/DNA repair test in testing of coded carcinogens and noncarcinogens. Mutat Res 1982;97:359–370.

47. Sina JF, Bean CL, Dysart GR, Taylor VI, Bradley MO. Evaluation of the alkaline elution/rat hepatocyte assay as a predictor of carcinogenic/mutagenic potential. Mutat Res 1983;113:357–391.

48. Nachtomi E, Sarma DSR. Repair of rat liver DNA in vivo damage by ethylene dibromide. Biochem Pharmacol 1977;26:1941–1945.

49. NCI. Bioassay of 1,2-dibromomethane for possible carcinogenicity. NCI Carcinogenicity Technical Report Series No. 86. Department of Health, Education and Welfare, National Cancer Institute, 1978.

50. NTP. Carcinogenesis bioassay of 1,2-dibromoethane in F344 rats and B6C3F1 mice (inhalation study), NTP-80-28. NIH Pub. No. 82-1766. US Department of Health and Human Services, National Toxicology Program, 1982.

51. Stinson SF, Reznik G, Ward JM. Characteristics of proliferative lesions in the nasal cavities of mice following chronic inhalation of 1,2-dibromoethane. Cancer Lett 1981;12:121.

52. Wong LCK, Winston JM, Hong CB, Plotnick H. Carcinogenicity and toxicity of 1,2-dibromoethane in the rat. Toxicol Appl Pharmacol 1982;63:155–165.

53. Ott MG, Scharnweber HC, Langer RR. Mortality experience of 161 employees exposed to ethylene dibromide in two production units. Br J Ind Med 1980;37:163–168.

54. EPA. Ethylene dibromide. Integrated Risk Information System, January 1, 1991. US Environmental Protection Agency, Environmental Criteria and Assessment Office, Cincinnati, OH, 1991.

55. Heppel LA, Neal PA, Highman B, Porterfield VT. Toxicology of 1,2-dichloropropane (propylene dichloride). I. Studies on effects of daily inhalations. J Ind Hyg Toxicol 1946;28:1–8.

56. Parker CM, Coate WB, Voelker RW. Subchronic inhalation toxicity of 1,3-dichloropropene/1,2-dichloropropane (D-D) in mice and rats. J Toxicol Environ Health 1982;9:899–910.

57. NTP. Toxicology and carcinogenesis studies of 1,2-dichloropropane (propylene dichloride) (CAS No. 78-87-5) in F344/N rats and B6C3F1 mice (gavage studies). NTP-TR 263, NIH Publication No. 86-2652. US Department of Health and Human Services, National Toxicology Program, 1986.

58. DeLorenzo I, Degl'Innocenti S, Ruocco A, Silengo L, Cortese R. Mutagenicity of pesticides containing 1,3-dichloropropene. Cancer Res 1977;37:1915–1917.

59. Jones AR, Gibson I. 1,2-dichloropropane: metabolism and fate in the rat. Xenobiotica 1980;10:835–846.

60. Hine CH, Anderson HH, Moon HD, Kodama JK, Morse M, Jacobson NW. Toxicology and safe handling of CBP-55 (technical 1-chloro-3-bromopropene-1). AMA Arch Ind Hyg Occup Med 1953;7:118–136.

61. Torkelson TR, Oyen F. The toxicity of 1,3-dichloropropene as determined by repeated exposure of laboratory animals. Am Ind Hyg Assoc J 1977;38:217–223.

62. NTP. Toxicology and carcinogenesis studies of Telone II in F344/N rats and B6C3F1 mice. Technical Report Series No. 269. US Department of Health and Human Services, National Toxicology Program, 1985.

63. Lomax LG, Stott WT, Johnson KA, Calhoun LL, Yano BL, Quast JF. The chronic toxicity and oncogenicity of inhaled technical grade 1,3-dichloropropene in rats and mice. Fundam Appl Toxicol 1989;12:418–431.

64. Stott WT, Young JT, Calhoun LL, Batties JF. Subchronic toxicity of inhaled technical grade 1,3-dichloropropene in rats and mice. Fundam Appl Toxicol 1988;11:207–220.

65. Hutson DH, Moss JA, Pickering BA. The excretion and retention of components of the soil fumigant D-D and their metabolites in the rat. Food Costmet Toxicol 1971;9:677–680.

66. Osterloh JD, Wang R, Schneider F, Maddy KT. Biological monitoring of dichloropropene: air concentrations, urinary metabolite, and renal enzyme excretion. Arch Environ Health 1984;44:207–213.

67. Alexeeff GV, Kilgore WW, Methyl bromide. Res Rev 1982;88:102–153.

68. Anger WK, Setzer JV, Russo JM, Brightwell WS, Wait RG, Johnson BL. Neurobehavioral effects of methyl bromide inhalation exposure. Scand J Work Environ Health 1981;7(suppl. 4):40–47.

69. Russo JM, Anger WK, Setzer JV, Brightwell WS. 1984. Neurobehavioral assessment of chronic low-level methyl bromide exposure in the rabbit. J Toxicol Environ Health 1984;14:247–255.

70. Voogd CE, Knaap AG, Vander Heijden CA, Kramers PG. Genotoxicity of methyl bromide in short-term assay systems. Mutat Res 1982;97:233.

71. Moriya M, Ohta T, Watanabe K, Miyazawa T, Kato K, Shirasu Y. Further mutagenicity studies on pesticides in bacterial reversion assay systems. Mutat Res 1983;116:185–216.

72. Kramers PG, Voogd CF, Knaap AG, vander Heijden CA. Mutagenicity of methyl bromide in a series of short-term tests. Mutat Res 1985;155:41–47.

73. Djalali-Behzad G, Hussain S, Osterman-Golker S, Segerback D. Estimation of genetic risks of alkylating agents. VI. Exposure of mice and bacteria to methyl bromide. Mutat Res 1981;84:1–10.

74. Simmon VF, Tardiff RG. The mutagenic activity of halogenated compounds found in chlorinated drinking water. Water Chlorination: Environ Impact Health Eff Proc Conf 1978;2:417–431.

75. Simmon VF. Structural correlations of carcinogenic and mutagenic alkyl halides. FDA (FDA-78-1046)), 1978:163–171.

76. Danse LH, van Velsen FL, vander Heijden CA. Methyl bromide: carcinogenic effects in th rat forestomach. Toxicol Appl Pharmacol 1984;72:262–271.

77. EPA. Chemical hazard information profile. Draft Report. Methyl Bromide. Rev Feb. 20, 1985. US EPA. Washington, DC: OTS, 1985.

78. EPA. Methyl bromide. Integrated Risk Information System. Cincinnati, OH: US Environmental Protection Agency, Environmental Criteria and Assessment Office, 1990.

79. Wong O, Brocker W, Davis HV, Nagle GS. Mortality of workers potentially exposed to organic and inorganic brominated chemicals, DBCP, TRIS, PBB, and DDT. Br J Ind Med 1984;41:15–24.

80. Shield L, Coleman T, Markesbery W. MB intoxication: neurologic features, including simulation of Reyes syndrome. Neurology 1977;27:959–962.

81. Chavez C, Hepler R, Straatsma B. Methyl bromide optic atrophy. Am J Ophthalmol 1985;99:715–719.

82. Taxay E. Vikane inhalation. J Occup Med 1966;8:425–426.

83. TeSlaa G, Kaiser M, Biederman L, Stowe C. Chloropicrin toxicity involving animal and human exposure. Vet Hum Toxicol 1986;28(4):323–324.

84. Proctor PN, Hughes J, Fischman M. Chemical hazards of the workplace. 2nd ed. New York, NY: J. Lippincott Co, 1988.

85. Sitting M. Handbook of toxic and hazardous chemicals. Park Ridge, NJ: Noyes Publications, 1981.

104

Herbicides, Fungicides, Biocides, and Pyrethrins

Alvin C. Bronstein, M.D.
John B. Sullivan, Jr., M.D.

HERBICIDES

Herbicides include a broad, diverse group of chemical compounds and are classified according to their mechanism of action on plants. The mechanisms of action of many herbicides remain unknown, and structure-activity relationships on plants of the better known herbicides are summarized in Table 104.1 (1). Commonly used herbicides are listed in Table 104.2.

Chlorophenoxy Herbicides

SOURCES AND PRODUCTION

Chlorophenoxy herbicides include 2,4-dichlorophenoxyacetic acid (2,4-D), 2,4,5-trichlorophenoxyacetic acid (2,4,5-T), 2-methyl, 4 chlorophenoxyacetic acid (MCPA), and others. The group members, organic acids, have similar biochemical properties (Fig. 104.1).

2,4-D ($Cl_2C_6H_3OCH_2COOH$), molecular weight 221.0 daltons, is a white to yellow crystalline odorless powder. Its melting point is 280°F (140.5°C) giving a slight phenolic odor. It is a noncombustible solid but may be found in flammable liquids. It was introduced as a plant growth regulator in 1942. 2,4-D is registered as a broadleaf weed herbicide and plant growth regulator. It is used extensively to control broadleaf weeds in cereal crops, sugarcane, turf pastures, and noncrop lands (2). Over 60 million pounds are used in the United States annually (2).

2,4,5-T ($Cl_3C_6H_2OCH_2COOH$), molecular weight 255.5 daltons, is a colorless to tan odorless solid with a melting point between 154–155°C.

2,4,5-T is synthesized from the intermediate compound 2,4,5-trichlorophenol (TCP). During the synthesis of TCP, it can react with itself to produce 2,3,7,8-tetrachlorodibenzo-p-dioxin (TCDD). TCDD is a contaminant of 2,4,5-T and other herbicide production such as hexachlorophene. TCDD has been associated in both animal and human epidemiologic studies with an increased risk of cancer and other symptoms such as chloracne (2, 3).

The most notable use of these compounds was the defoliant use of the 50:50 mixture of the *n*-butyl esters of 2,4,-D and 2,4,5-T known as "Agent Orange" (because of the orange stripe on the 55 gallon drums) during the Vietnam War from January, 1962–September, 1971. Agent White, 2,4-D was also used as well as Agent Blue, cacodylic acid. 2,4,5-T was banned in the United States by the Environmental Protection Agency in 1979. Millions of pounds of 2,4-D are still used in the United States annually.

SITES, INDUSTRIES AND BUSINESSES ASSOCIATED WITH EXPOSURES

The most common sources of exposure are individuals involved in the manufacture or application of these compounds. Dermal

Table 104.1. Herbicide Actions on Plants

Inhibitors of Photosynthesis

Anilides
Benzimidazoles
Biscarbamates
Pyridazinones
Triazinediones
Triazines
Triazinones
Uracils
Substituted ureas
Quinones
Hydroxybenzonitriles

Inhibitors of Amino Acid Synthesis

Glyphosate
Sulfonylureas
Imidazolinones
Bialophos
Glufosinate

Produce Photobleaching

Bipyridyliums (paraquat and diquat)
P-nitrodiphenyl ethers
Oxadiazoles
N-phenylimides

Inhibition of Lipid Synthesis

Aryloxphenoxy alkanoic acids
Cyclohexanediones

Inhibition of Cellulose Synthesis

Dichlorbenil

Inhibition of Cell Division

Phosphoric amides
Dinitroamilines

Inhibit Carotenoid Synthesis and Interferes with Protection against Photo-oxidation

Pyridazinones
Phenoxybenzamides
Fluoridone
Difunone
4-Hydroxypyridines
Amitrole

Inhibits Folate Synthesis

Asulam

Source: Adapted from Duke S. Overview of herbicide mechanisms of action. Environ Health Perspect 1990;87:263–271.

Table 104.2. Herbicides

Paraquat
Diquat
Nitrophenols (Dinosebs)
Substituted ureas (Diuron)
Tetradifon
Glyphosate (Roundup, Kleen-Up)
Propham
Barban
Terbutryne
Metachlor
Dicamba
2,4-Dichlorophenoxy acetic acid (2,4-D)
2,4,5-Trichlorophenoxy acetic acid (2,4,5-T)
Acrolein (Magnacide-H)

absorption is the major route of exposure for herbicide applicators with exposure levels being 4–50 times greater than the inhalation route (3). Potential exists for exposure of civilian populations near application sites.

CLINICAL TOXICOLOGY OF EXPOSURE

Chlorophenoxy herbicides appear to demonstrate similar pharmacokinetic profiles (4). 2,4-D and 2,4,5-T have been relatively intensively studied in animals and man. Rapid and almost complete absorption occurs after an oral dose (5, 6, 7, 8, 9). Differences exist between amine, salt, and ester formulations of 2,4-D and 2,4,5-T. The amine and salt compounds are rapidly hydrolyzed and absorbed (5, 7) while ester preparations of 2,4-D revealed lower plasma concentrations (6). Oral absorption follows first order kinetics (9, 10). This is estimated in humans to be between 1–27% per hour (7, 11). Almost all of a 2-4-D oral dose is absorbed in humans within 24 hours (12). Peak plasma concentrations are reached between 4–24 hours in humans (5–7, 12). Six human volunteers receiving 5 mg/kg (370 mg/70 mg) of 2,4-D orally. The average peak plasma concentration was 35 mg/L at 24 hours. The mean plasma half-life in this study was 33 hours (7). They are highly protein bound in plasma.

Elimination is rapid. 2,4-D metabolites other than conjugates have not been detected in human urine (7). During the 4 days following the ingestion by the six subjects above, 77% of the dose was eliminated unchanged in the urine (7). All remained asymptomatic. In another study five male human volunteers ingested a single oral dose of 5 mg/kg 2,4-D. No detectable clinical effects were noted. The average plasma $T_{1/2}$ was 11.6 hours with a mean urine $T_{1/2}$ of 17.7 hours. Eighty-three percent of the ingested oral dose was excreted as the parent compound, and 12.8% of the oral dose was excreted in the urine as an acid-labile conjugate (9, 12).

The chlorophenoxy herbicides first order elimination is dose-dependent, similar to that of salicylates (3, 13). Plasma half-lives range from 10–20 hours and may increase to 80–120 hours with large acute poisonings (3). No evidence has been found suggesting bioaccumulation (12).

Members of this herbicide group have small volumes of

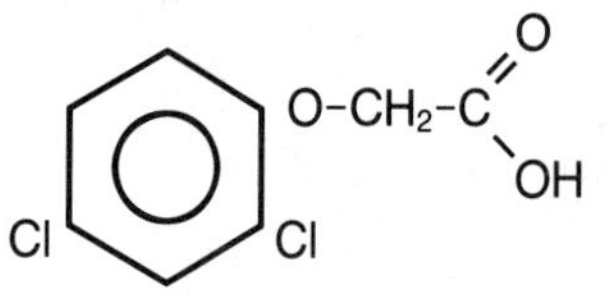

2,4-Dichlorophenoxyacetic Acid (2,4-D)

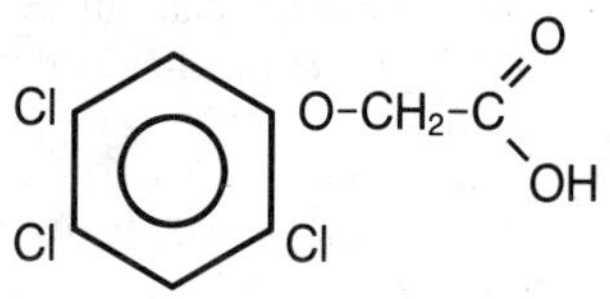

2,4,5-Trichlorophenoxyacetic Acid (2,4,5-T)

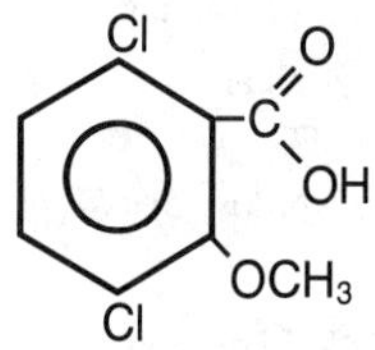

Dicamba

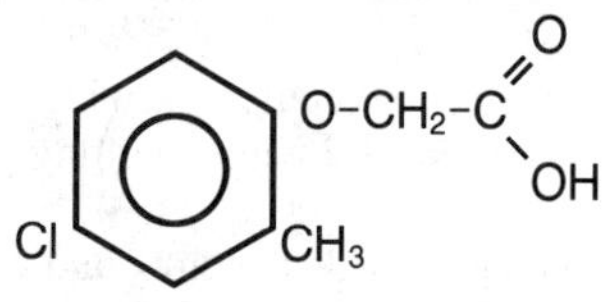

MCPA
2-Methyl-4-chlorophenoxyacetic Acid

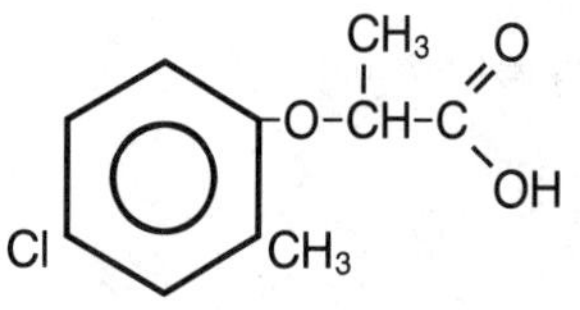

MCPP
2-(2-methyl-4-chlorophenoxy)proprionic Acid

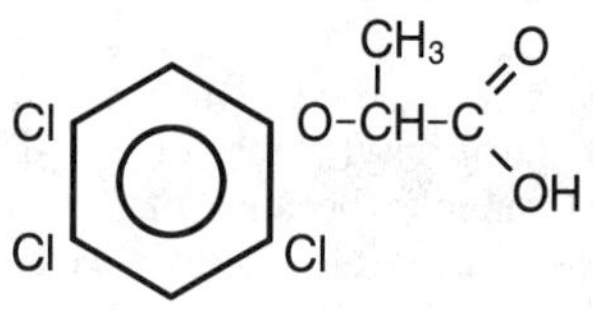

Silvex

Figure 104.1. Phenoxy acid herbicides.

distribution (3). The volume of distribution (Vd) of 2,4-D is 0.1 L/kg (13). The mean lethal human dose of 2,4-D is approximately 28 g (14).

Workers exposed to an air concentration of 2,4,-D at 0.1–0.2 mg/m^3 had urine concentrations ranging from 3–14 mg/L (15). The dose increases pharmacokinetic parameters. Various studies have found workers to have urinary 2,4-D concentrations ranging from 0.2–8.2 mg/L (14).

SIGNS, SYNDROMES, AND SYMPTOMS FROM TOXIC EXPOSURE

Acute Toxicity

Acute chlorophenoxy herbicide toxicity presents a clinical picture of gastroenteritis, skeletal muscle myotonia, myoglobinuria (15), cardiac dysrhythmias, and central nervous system depression. Peripheral neuropathy may be seen in survivors or in subacute cases (16, 17).

Major target organs are the central nervous and cardiovascular systems (18). EKG abnormalities flattening or inversion of the T-wave have been seen. Hervonen et al. found reversible damage to the endothelial cells of the blood brain barrier in rats exposed to 2,4-D (19). Dudley and Thapar reported autopsy findings in a 76-year-old white male with senile dementia who died 6 days after acute 2,4-D ingestion. Widespread plaques of acute perivascular demyelination and perivascular petechial hemorrhage without cellular infiltration were described (20). Single intraperitoneal doses of 200 mg/kg in rats produced reversible inhibition of cerebral electrical activity with direct attack on the reticular system. EEG changes were seen as early as 24 hours post dosing (21).

Goldstein was the first to report the development of peripheral neuropathy with electromyographic abnormalities in three cases following heavy 2,4-D ester dermal exposure (22). Symptomatology persisted, and recovery was incomplete even several years post exposure (22).

A 39-year-old male farmer who sustained excessive exposure to 2,4-D while spraying crops developed a primary sensory peripheral neuropathy 4 days after exposure (23). Electromyographic and peroneal nerve conduction studies were within normal limits. Symptoms improved, but the patient continued to complain of intermittent numbness of the hands after prolonged use.

Concentrated solutions of 2,4-D (greater than 12%) have been shown to cause severe skin burns in rats and rabbits (24, 25). Topical application of 24% solution of 2,4-D amine over a 3-week period produced ulcerative dermatitis, decreased body weight, and increased kidney size. A 12% solution of 2,4-D resulted in minimal skin changes. The dermal effect was thought to be due to a direct effect of the 2,4-D, as both the 12 or 24% solutions had a pH = 10. Additionally, these animals at necropsy revealed no neuropathologic changes (24, 25).

Various authors have reported fatal human poisonings with 2,4-D and its congeners (8, 24, 25). The mean adult estimated lethal dose of 2,4-D is 28 g (13). Two thousand milligrams of 2,4-D intravenously produced no symptoms in a patient terminally ill with coccidiomycosis (27). Three thousand, six hundred mg has caused serious side effects including fibrillary twitching of the mouth and both upper extremities and generalized hyporeflexia (27). Ingestion of 500 mg over 3 weeks

produced no definable symptoms (16). An intentional ingestion of 80 mg/kg caused death in a 23-year-old college student.

Postmortem 2,4-D blood concentrations of 720 mg/L were reported in a 64-year-old Caucasian woman found comatose, who died 12 hours after admission with pulmonary edema (29). In another report a 26-year-old male ingested 360 mL of Ortho Weed B-Gone M (dimethylamine salts of 2,4-D, 10.8% and MCPP (2-(2-methyl-4-chlorophenoxy)propionic acid, 11.6%; 77.6% inert ingredients); Dexol (chlorpyrifos, 6.7% in petroleum distillates, 76.8%) and a few granules of warfarin, 0.025%. The patient died approximately 30 hours after admission after four episodes of bradycardia, hypotension, and asystole. Other findings included hyperkalemia, thrombocytopenia, hypocalcemia, and hypophosphatemia (18). Postmortem concentration of 2,4-D was 389.5 μg/mL and MCPP 235.5 μg/mL (18).

Chronic Toxicity

Chronic neurologic toxicity is most likely due to a direct effect of the chlorophenoxy herbicides (21). TCDD (dioxin) contamination may be responsible for other longterm and neurologic problems as well.

Chloracne The most common finding in individuals exposed to TCDD has been chloracne (30). Chloracne can persist for years after exposure in severely contaminated individuals (31). Chloracne consists of comedones, cysts, pustules, and abscesses. Hepatic dysfunction, peripheral neuropathy, fat metabolism disorders, elevated serum cholesterol, and porphyria cutanea tarda are the other most frequent findings associated with TCDD exposure in industrial settings (32). Zack and Suskind followed 129 workers exposed to TCDD after an explosion at TCP plant in Nitro, West Virginia in 1949 (30). All 129 employees developed chloracne. No increased frequency of malignancies was found in this group after a 30-year follow-up (30). Symptoms reported following TCDD exposure included chloracne, severe pain in muscles of upper and lower extremities, shoulders, and thorax; fatigue; nervousness; vertigo; decreased libido; and cold intolerance. Liver impairment demonstrated by increased prothrombin times may be seen (30). Over time the symptom's may clear to some degree. Complaints of aches and pains in lower extremities and back, nervousness, fatigue, and dyspnea may continue (30). In a later study of 204 exposed and 163 nonexposed workers, chloracne persisted in 55.7% of the exposed group. A positive association was found with gastrointestinal tract ulcers, but no increased risk of cardiovascular disease, hepatic disease, renal disease, central or peripheral nervous system problems, or malignancies were found (33). In a related study focusing on workers with and without chloracne, the mean duration of chloracne was found to be 26 years. Increased GGT concentrations were found in the chloracne group. Abnormal sensory findings were also present in the chloracne group (34).

TCDD has been associated with soft-tissue sarcoma, Hodgkin's disease, non-Hodgkin's lymphoma, gastric cancer, nasal cancer, and liver cancer in various studies (35–46). Rats, mice, and hamsters exposed to TCDD have developed histiocytic lymphomas, fibrosarcomas, and tumors of liver, skin, lung, thyroid, tongue, hard palate, and nasal turbinates (46, 47). Initiating and/or promoting carcinogenesis may be functions of TCDD (48–53).

Fingerhut et al. (2) conducted a retrospective study of a cohort of 5172 workers occupationally exposed to TCDD during production of various chemicals contaminated with TCDD.

TCDD serum concentrations were measured in 253 workers. Mortality from all cancers was significantly increased in the cohort. Cancer mortality from stomach, liver, nasal, Hodgkin's disease, and non-Hodgkin's lymphoma was not significantly different from expected mortality rates in the overall cohort. A subcohort of 1520 workers with greater than 1 year of exposure and greater than 20 year latency since TCDD exposure mortality was significantly increased from all cancers specifically from soft-tissue sarcomas and respiratory tract cancers. Confounding variables such as smoking and exposure to other industrial chemicals could not be excluded as other potential causes of the cancer mortality rates. TCDD serum concentrations adjusted for lipids was 233 pg/g lipid (range 2:3000) This compared to 7 pg/g for unexposed individuals. The mean TCDD concentration for 119 workers with one year or more exposure was 418 pg/g with exposure being 15–37 years earlier (2).

Although this study had multiple potential pitfalls, the data indicate probable human risk from TCDD exposure (53). Based on this study, the life-time risk from TCDD-induced soft tissue sarcoma approximates 2 per 1000. This risk is far more than the commonly accepted lifetime risk of 1 per 100,000 or 1 per million from exposure by the general public to potential carcinogens (53).

Recent studies of Vietnam veterans, the so-called Operation Ranch Hand cohort, failed to show an increase risk of cancer (55, 56). The United States Air Force has been conducting a 20-year study to determine the health effects on Air Force veterans of Operation Ranch Hand (55). These veterans were responsible for the spraying of chlorophenoxy herbicides including Agent Orange during the Vietnam War. Most of the herbicides were sprayed from fixed wing aircraft, but herbicides were also applied from helicopters, trucks, riverboats, and hand applicators. The cohort studied consisted of 995 veterans who either flew application aircraft, maintained aircraft and spray equipment, or handled bulk quantities of TCDD-contaminated herbicides for a year or longer. This cohort was followed and compared to a group of 1200 Vietnam veterans who were not directly exposed. Several differences were found. The Ranch Hand group had alkaline phosphatase concentrations averaging 98 U/L with the control group having concentrations at 90 U/L (p<.01). No prevalence differences were found in verified skin or systemic malignancies. The Ranch Hand cohort had elevated serum TCDD concentrations compared to the comparison group. The median TCDD Ranch Hand TCDD concentration was 12.4 ppt compared to 4.2 ppt in the controls. In the Ranch Hand group nonflying enlisted personnel had the highest TCDD concentrations at 23.6 ppt compared to pilots at 7.3 ppt. No chloracne was found either in the Ranch Hands or the control group (55).

In a related study, the noncombat mortality in a group of 1261 Ranch Hand veterans was compared to that in a control of 19101 Air Force veterans primarily involved in cargo missions. There was no significant difference in the all-cause standardized mortality ratio after adjustment for age, rank, and occupation (56).

In 1971, sludge waste from a hexachlorophene manufacturing plant were mixed with waste oil and sprayed for dust control on dirt roads on residential, recreational, and commercial areas of eastern Missouri near St. Louis (57). By February 1986, 28 separate sites had been found to have TCDD soil concentrations of 1 ppb or more. Hoffman et al. studied 154 exposed mobile home park residents where the soil TCDD concentration ranged from 1–2200 ppb (57). 155 unexposed control subjects were used as controls. The exposed group demonstrated increased frequency of anergy, minor abnormalities in T-cell T_4/T_8 ratios of <1.0, and abnormal T-cell function, suggesting the possibility of longterm TCDD exposure being associated with alterations in cell mediated immunity. Peak urinary uroporphyrin levels were >13 μgm/gm creatinine in 16.3% of the exposed cohort compared to 7.5% of the controls. Mean urinary uroporphyrins were 9.6 μgm/gm creatinine versus 8.4 μgm/gm creatinine in the unexposed control group. The exposed group complained of parasthesias of the hands and feet and headaches more than the controls. Neuropsychologic testing failed to find significant differences between the two groups (57).

Serveso, Italy, about 20 miles north of Milan, was the site of a TCDD release in 1976. Large epidemiologic studies are continuing on the exposed populations. Chloracne appeared almost only in children and young people. Most cases spontaneously resolved. Transient lymphopenia and impaired liver function were observed. Studies are continuing longterm to determine any mutagenic or carcinogenic effects (58).

Management of Toxicity

Clinical Examination Acutely exposed patients should be removed from the source of the exposure and decontaminated as the exposure and condition warrants (59). Rescue personnel should wear appropriate gloves, boots, and goggles. Special attention should be directed to the respiratory system with monitoring of airway, breathing, and circulatory status. Begin supplemental oxygen and intravenous fluids as necessary.

Chronically exposed patients require a complete toxicologic history and physical examination with special attention to the neurologic system. A comprehensive occupational history should be obtained.

Alkaline diuresis has been proposed to enhance the elimination of 2,4-D (60). The patient should be monitored for the development of metabolic acidosis, hyperthermia, seizures, coma, hyperventilation, tachycardia, ECG abnormalities, vasodilation, diaphoresis, hypoxia, myotonia, hyperkalemia, myoglobinuria, hepatic dysfunction, or renal failure. Severe hypoxia associated with hyperventilation and normal pCO_2 may result from uncoupling of oxidative phosphorylation.

Treatment Supportive therapy is the mainstay of treatment for acute chlorophenoxy herbicide poisonings. Forced alkaline diuresis for acute poisoning has been advocated, since the chlorophenoxy herbicides are organic acids (60). Prescott reported the renal clearance of 2,4-D, with a measured pKa of 3.3, rising from 0.14 ml/min at a urine pH 5.1 to 5.1 ml/min at pH 8.3 (60). Flanagan et al. reported the effect of alkaline diuresis in a series of 41 acutely poisoned patients with chlorophenoxy herbicides and Ioxynil (3,5-diiodo-4-hydroxybenzonitrile). Plasma half-lives were reduced to less than 30 hours with alkaline diuresis. Alkaline diuresis is recommended in cases of severe poisoning with coma, acidemia, or total chlorophenoxy herbicide concentrations greater than 0.5g/L (61). 2,4-D pKa in this study was reported as 2.6 (61).

For adequate alkaline diuresis, urine pH should be maintained in the range of 7.6–8.8. Close attention to sufficient potassium replacement is required to obtain optimal urine alkalinity. Each liter of intravenous fluid should contain at least 20–40 mEq of KCl. Renal function and serum electrolytes need careful, frequent monitoring (62).

Laboratory Diagnosis Patients exposed to chlorophenoxy herbicides require a full biochemical profile including hepatic enzymes (AST, ALT, GGTP), electrolytes, glucose, blood urea nitrogen (BUN), and creatinine, serum aldolase, creatinine phosphokinase (CPK), complete blood count, and urinalysis. Baseline EKG and continuous monitoring should be done because of high probability of cardiac dysrhythmias. Treat cardiac dysrhythmia with standard advanced cardiac life support protocols.

Chronically exposed patients also require a thyroid profile and vitamin B_{12} and folate determinations to assist in the differential of other neurologic diseases. A computerized axial tomographic (CAT) or magnetic resonance imaging (MRI) scan of the brain and EEG may be necessary to rule out other possible CNS disease states. ENG/EMG studies should be done in cases or suspected cases of peripheral neuropathies. Serum or adipose tissue measurements for TCDD should be done to estimate exposure.

Special Diagnostic Tests   Concentrations of 2,4-D and other chlorophenoxy herbicides in various fluids may be measured with ultraviolet spectrophotometry, high performance liquid chromatography (14) (HPLC) (63) or flame-ionization or electron capture gas chromatography (63). The latter two methods appear to be more sensitive and specific (14). Chlorophenoxy concentrations in blood have ranged from 58–1220 mg/L in fatal acute overdoses (63). Dioxin, because of its extremely low concentrations in adipose tissue, is difficult to measure. It can be measured utilizing gas chromatography-mass spectrometry. It is usually measured as picograms per gram serum lipid.

Adipose tissue sampling or serum measurements for TCDD are the most reliable methods with which to estimate an individuals TCDD exposure. Adipose tissue sampling has been viewed as the most accurate index of TCDD body burden; recent use of TCDD determinations in the blood lipid component may prove as reliable (64). Preliminary data in Vietnam veterans reveals a TCDD blood concentration per gram of fat at 15 pg/g to be associated with heavy exposure and a correlation coefficient, r = +0.89, with adipose tissue sampling (61).

Thirty-nine of the Missouri residents exposed to either soil TCDD concentrations of 20–100 ppb for 20 or more years or exposed for 6 months or more to soil concentrations >100 ppb underwent adipose tissue sampling for TCDD. There values were compared to 57 unexposed controls with adipose tissue sampling obtained during surgical procedures. The mean TCDD concentration in the exposed group was 17.0 ppt (range: 2.8–750 ppt) compared with a median value of 6.4 (range: 1.4–20.2 ppt) in the controls (65). From this study the half-life of TCDD in humans was estimated to be between 5–8 years (65).

Environmental Monitoring

Air samples for 2,4-D air concentration determinations should be analyzed by the high pressure liquid chromatography with ultraviolet detection method as described in the NIOSH Manual of Analytical Methods, Vol III, (NIOSH 77-157-C).

Exposure Limits

The OSHA established permissible exposure limit (PEL) for inhalation exposure of 2,4-D is 10 mg/m³ (67). The PEL for 2,4,5-T is also 10 mg/m³.

The NIOSH recommended exposure limit (REL) for 2,4-D is 10 mg/m³. The immediately dangerous to life or health (IDLH) air concentration for 2,4-D is 500 mg/m³.

The American Conference of Governmental Industrial Hy-

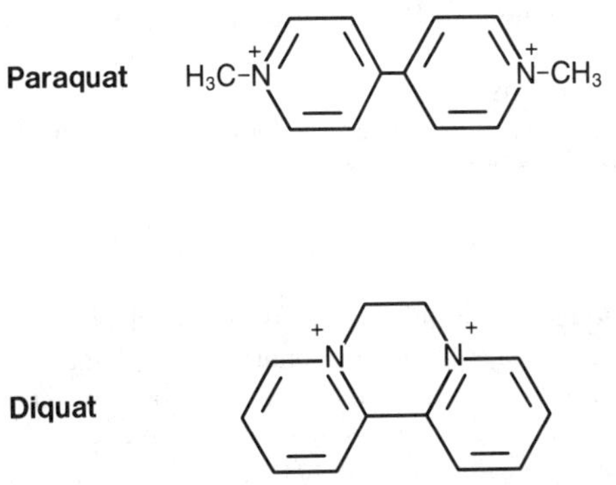

Figure 104.2.   Molecular structures for paraquat and diquat.

gienists (ACGIH) current threshold limit value-time weighted average (TLV-TWA) for 2,4-D 10 mg/m³. The ACGIH TLV-TWA for 2,4,5-T is 10 mg/m³. There is no ACGIH short term exposure limit (STEL) value.

Paraquat

SOURCES AND PRODUCTION

Paraquat (1,1'dimethyl-4,4'-dipyridyl) was first marketed in 1962 as a broad spectrum nonselective contact herbicide and desiccant (Fig. 104.2) after having been first described by Weidel and Rosso in 1882 (66). Paraquat's redox properties were published in 1933. It has been used as a redox indicator under the name of methyl viologen since 1933. It is a yellow solid with a faint ammonia-like odor. Its molecular weight is 257.2 daltons. The boiling point is 347–356°F. Paraquat is corrosive to metals and decomposes under ultraviolet light (66).

Diquat (6,7-Dihydrodipyrido[1,2-a:2',1'-c]pyrazidiinium dibromide) ($C_{12}H_{12}N_2Br_2$) is an analogue having similar properties to paraquat but causes a different human toxicologic presentation than paraquat and does not produce the pulmonary fibrosis seen in paraquat poisoning. Diquat forms a monohydrate which is a colorless to yellow crystal substance which decomposes above 300°C.

The most common paraquat formulation is a 20% solution (200 mg/100 cc). Manufacturers' directions usually recommend dilution about 40 times to a 0.5% w/v paraquat ion solution (66). Other application procedures suggest a 100–200 times dilution for a spray solution. Inhalation toxicity is thought to be minimal in normal use due to the nonrespirable size of the spray droplets. Inhalational poisonings may produce low toxicity because pulmonary absorption is low, as most of the aerosolized particles are greater than 5 μm in diameter and therefore do not reach the alveolar barrier (66, 67).

SITES, INDUSTRIES, AND BUSINESSES ASSOCIATED WITH EXPOSURES

Paraquat may be applied with hand-held or vehicle mounted sprayers. It may also be applied via aerial spraying (66). Skin exposure is thought to be the most significant route of occupation exposure (66). The most common sources of exposure are individuals involved in the manufacture or application of these compounds. Potential exists for exposure of civilian populations near application sites.

CLINICAL TOXICOLOGY OF EXPOSURE

After paraquat ingestion, edema, burns or ulceration may be seen in the mucosa of the mouth, pharynx, esophagus, stomach, and intestines (68). Centrizonal hepatic necrosis, proximal renal tubule damage, and myocardial muscle damage and skeletal muscle damage with focal necrosis may be seen. Pancreatic damage and CNS injury may occur. Pulmonary fibrosis usually begins in 2–14 days after poisoning. With large ingestions over 20 mg/kg, pulmonary edema may be seen. Paraquat oxidation produces superoxide (free radical oxygen) ions (O_2^-) which cause mucous membrane lesions and secondary necrosis of the gastrointestinal tract, liver, pancreas, renal tubules, and adrenal glands by lipid peroxidation. Paraquat ion is actively transported into pulmonary cells. Pulmonary edema and/or fibrosis is the sequelae of lung uptake (67, 68).

Paraquat is excreted unchanged in the urine. Paraquat renal elimination is greater that the GFR in individuals with normal creatinine clearance. Paraquat does not appear to bioaccumulate.

In animal models, low intravenous or subcutaneous doses are rapidly excreted in the urine (69–72). In the canine model, paraquat is not metabolized (73). Intravenous paraquat infusions at 30–50 μg/kg produced rapid urinary excretion at clearance rates in excess of the glomerular filtration rate signifying paraquat elimination by active secretion. Doses of 20 mg/kg produced renal failure. The kinetics could be described by a three compartment model with the lungs a slow uptake compartment with even paraquat doses high enough to cause renal failure not producing peak lung concentrations for 15 hours after ingestion. This means that initiation of removal of paraquat by hemoperfusion in the first 12–15 hours should be helpful. These authors proposed that within the first 24 hours, cases of human ingestion with urinary paraquat concentrations greater than 10 μg/ml and lower creatinine clearance values should receive hemodialysis or hemoperfusion. Other studies disagree.

Oral ingestion of paraquat (all dilutions) has an average mortality rate of 33–50%. Mortality from an ingestion of the 20% solution may approach 78% (67). Potential exists for fatality from as little as one mouthful of a 20% solution. This may either be from circulatory failure at 3 days post ingestion or progressive irreversible pulmonary fibrosis at 5–31 days post ingestion.

The minimum lethal human dose is approximately 35 mg/kg (67, 74). A mouthful (approximately 20 ml) produces a dose of 55 mg/kg in the average 70 kg adult. In a study of 28 paraquat oral poisoning victims, one mouthful produced 6/12 deaths (50%) from pulmonary fibrosis at 5–31 days post ingestion to 11/12 (92%) in the more than one gulp group from circulatory failure within 48 hours (67, 74).

The kinetics of paraquat poisoning in man are similar to the canine model with the peak plasma concentration being attained by two hours post ingestion (75, 76). Plasma concentrations decline quickly as the ion is distributed to the tissues. This fact obviously has implication in treatment, as any modality such as charcoal hemoperfusion must be initiated within this timeframe if it is to be effective.

Absorption of paraquat is believed to take place in the small intestine. In rats and dogs paraquat plasma concentrations are proportional to the amount of paraquat in the small intestine. Medications such as propantheline administered to dogs to decrease the gastric emptying time decrease paraquat plasma concentrations (73). Drugs which increase emptying time increase plasma concentrations. Food in the stomach or GI tract may decrease paraquat in plasma concentrations. Lung and kidney paraquat concentrations continue to rise even after plasma concentrations seem to stabilize. Lung paraquat accumulation is an energy dependent process which follows zero order (saturable) kinetics. This system can be blocked by metabolic inhibitors such as cyanide and iodoacetate.

Plasma paraquat concentrations have a predictive value with regard to survival. Plasma paraquat concentrations which do not exceed 2.0, 0.6, 0.3, 0.16, and 0.1 mg/L at 4, 6, 10, 16, and 24 hours respectively are likely to survive (77, 78).

SIGNS, SYNDROMES, AND SYMPTOMS FROM TOXIC EXPOSURE

Acute Toxicity

Paraquat poisoning symptoms depend on the dose consumed. Most human fatalities are the result of suicide. Individuals consuming large amounts of paraquat usually die within a few days from cardiovascular collapse, while those consuming less usually succumb many days to weeks later of irreversible pulmonary fibrosis (67, 74, 79).

Two phases of the pulmonary toxicity have been described. In Phase I, Type I and Type II epithelial cells are destroyed. An alveolitis may develop with extensive pulmonary destruction. Pulmonary edema may develop with the infiltration of polymorphonuclear leukocytes into the lung tissue. Phase II is marked with extensive intraalveolar and interalveolar fibrosis. Normal alveolar architecture is destroyed with the replacement by fibrous tissue. Gas exchange is severely impeded leading to hypoxia and death.

Paraquat ion exposure may cause injuries to the nails, skin, eyes, and nose. These result from exposure to the extremely irritating concentrated solutions prior to dilution. Paraquat produces a strong irritant action on various types of epithelial tissues. It can cause dryness, erythema, blistering, irritation, and ulceration and fissuring of the skin (80–82). Inhalation may cause epistaxis. Contact dermatitis has been reported following topical exposure. It is thought that paraquat diluted as the manufacturer recommends is unlikely to cause skin burns unless clothing soaked with spray is continued to be worn for prolonged periods.

Localized discolorations or a transverse white band of discoloration affecting the nail plate may be seen in spray operators (80–82). Transverse ridging and furrowing of the nail progressing to an irregular deformity of the nail and subsequent loss of the nail may occur. Once exposure stops normal nail growth usually returns.

Ocular exposure to paraquat concentrate may cause corneal and conjunctival inflammation. Inflammation may develop gradually and progress to maximal damage over a 12–24 hour period. Frank corneal ulceration and lachrymal duct stenosis has been reported (82). Sometimes the seriousness of these injuries go relatively unnoticed until symptoms have progressed to corneal scarring.

Paraquat can be absorbed through the skin. Local and systemic toxicity have been reported following dermal exposure. Dermal exposure may produce a local irritation, burn, and/or systemic effect.

Three stages of paraquat poisoning have been described (67, 68, 79):

Group 1—Mild Poisoning: Ingestion of less than 20 mg paraquat ion/kg body weight. Patients may be asymptomatic or have vomiting and diarrhea. Transient decrement in the carbon monoxide diffusing capacity (DLCO) and vital capacity may be seen. Complete recovery usually occurs.

Group 2—Moderate Poisoning: Ingestion of 20–40 mg/kg paraquat ion. Vomiting and diarrhea followed by generalized symptomatology of systemic toxicity. All patients will develop pulmonary fibrosis. Renal and hepatic failure may be present. Most patients will expire, but death may be delayed for 2–4 weeks.

Group 3—Severe Poisoning: Ingestion of greater than 40 mg/kg paraquat ion. Nausea, vomiting, and diarrhea with marked oropharynx and esophageal ulceration followed by multiple organ failure (cardiac, respiratory, hepatic, renal adrenal, pancreatic, and CNS). The mortality is usually 100% with death usually in the first 24 hours post ingestion.

Initial symptoms of paraquat ingestion include: burning of the mouth, throat, chest, and abdomen. Giddiness, headache, fever, myalgia, blood diarrhea, and abdominal pain may be present. Urinalysis may show proteinuria, hematuria or pyuria. Acute tubular necrosis may develop.

Management of Toxicity

Obtaining a clear history of the circumstances of the ingestion is vital in assessing victims of paraquat poisoning. Quantify the interval between ingestion and admission, circumstances of poisoning (accidental versus suicidal), exact name of paraquat or diquat compound and other ingredients such as solvent vehicles, amount ingested and route, vomiting after ingestion, time of last meal.

Clinical Examination Acutely exposed patients should be removed from the source of the exposure and decontaminated as the exposure and condition warrant. Rescue personnel should wear appropriate gloves, boots, and goggles (83).

Chronically exposed patients require a complete toxicologic history and physical examination with special attention to the pulmonary system. A comprehensive occupational history should be obtained. Areas of skin or eye exposure should be flushed copiously with water. Monitor for skin abrasions, inflammation, and the development of secondary infection.

Treatment Urinary paraquat excretion is 20–50 times greater than plasma concentrations (84). Patients with normal renal function post ingestion have a higher paraquat clearance than creatinine clearance. This is due to the fact that there is active tubular secretion and nonionic diffusion additive to the glomerular filtration rate. Paraquat is not reabsorbed from the renal tubules so that forced diuresis does not enhance the removal paraquat from the blood. Forced diuresis has still been advocated because it may reduce the concentration of paraquat in the renal tubules.

Gastrointestinal decontamination should be initiated as soon as possible after paraquat ingestion to maximize chances for paraquat removal. Institute if any suspicion of ingestion. Fuller's earth or Bentonite is usually used. If these are not available, then activated charcoal may be used. Activated charcoal has been shown to absorb paraquat almost as efficiently as Fuller's earth or Bentonite. Hypercalcemia may occur after Fuller's Earth use (85).

Bentonite (7.5% Suspension) Dose:

Adults:	100–150 g
Children under 12:	2 g/kg
Fuller's Earth (30%)	Same
Activated Charcoal	30–50 g initially

After gastric lavage using one of the above absorbents is performed initially, doses may be repeated at 2- to 4-hour intervals. Monitor bowel sounds and for signs of gastrointestinal perforation or ileus. Magnesium sulfate or sorbitol may be used as a cathartic with the absorbent (85).

Do not give supplemental oxygen, as this increases paraquat pulmonary toxicity. Late stages of poisoning may require oxygen as pulmonary fibrosis develops.

Hemodialysis is not effective in paraquat or diquat poisoning (86, 87). Charcoal hemoperfusion has not been shown to reduce paraquat morbidity or mortality. There is a theoretical benefit in clearing blood paraquat if hemoperfusion can be instituted during the first 2 hours following the poisoning. Hemoperfusion or hemodialysis have not been shown to effectively reduce paraquat or diquat body burden (86, 87).

Major prognostic indicators include route of administration (inhalation usually less severe than oral); ingested amount; time of last meal (food delays absorption and neutralizes paraquat); gastric lesions; renal failure; and plasma paraquat concentrations.

Diquat ingestion, like paraquat, damages multiple organ systems. The clinical pattern is different even though diquat and paraquat share common mechanisms of toxicity. Infarction and purpura of the brain stem appears to be specific to diquat poisoning (88, 89). Pontine purpura have been reported in 3/7 adults who died from diquat ingestion (88, 89). Potentially toxic diquat ion doses are in the range of 35–105 ml of the 20% solution. Diquat poisoning is characterized by gastrointestinal tract injury including burns to the oral mucosa, acute tubular necrosis, and bronchopneumonia. Paralytic ileus is seen more frequently in diquat than paraquat ion poisoning. Pulmonary fibrosis is not seen in diquat ion poisoning, as diquat is not actively transported by lung tissue. Inhalation may produce nonspecific respiratory distress presentations. Diquat produces cataracts in rats and dogs, but so far not in man. Treatment is similar to that of paraquat ion poisoning. Prompt initiation of charcoal hemoperfusion may be beneficial in minimizing tissue distribution and uptake by target organs.

Laboratory Diagnosis Patients exposed to paraquat or diquat require a full biochemical profile including hepatic enzymes (AST, ALT, GGTP), electrolytes, glucose, blood urea nitrogen (BUN), creatinine, serum aldolase, complete blood count, arterial blood gases, chest x-ray, and urinalysis. Chronically exposed patients also require a thyroid profile, vitamin B_{12} and folate determination to assist in the differential of other neurologic diseases.

Special Diagnostic Tests *Dithionite test* is a rapid semiquantitative colorimetric urine test that may be done to detect paraquat (90).

To one volume add 0.5 volume 1% sodium dithionite (sodium hydrosulfite) in one normal sodium hydroxide. Wait 1 minute and observe color change. A deep blue color reflects paraquat or diquat, urinary concentration less than 0.5 mg/L. Run positive or negative controls (90).

Urinary diquat is signified by a green color. In either case, the deeper the color, the higher relative paraquat or diquat concentration and worse prognosis.

Paraquat may be measured via spectrophotometric, gas chromograph, high performance liquid chromotography, or radioimmunoassay techniques. RIA is the sensitive and specific procedure.

Environmental Monitoring

Air samples for paraquat air concentration determinations should be analyzed by the high pressure liquid chromatography with ultraviolet detection method as described in the NIOSH Manual of Analytical Methods, Vol III, (NIOSH 77-157-C).

Paraquat Exposure Limits

The OSHA-established permissible exposure limit (PEL) for inhalation exposure to paraquat respirable dust is 0.5 mg/m^3 (91). To prevent skin absorption, an individual's skin exposure should be prevented or reduced to the extent necessary in the workplace through the use of gloves, coveralls, goggles, or other appropriate personal protective equipment, engineering controls, or work practices.

The NIOSH-recommended exposure limit (REL) for paraquat, either respiratory or skin exposure, is 0.1 mg/m^3. An immediately dangerous to life or health (IDLH) concentration has been established at 1.5 mg/m^3.

The American Conference of Governmental Industrial Hygienists (ACGIH) threshold limit value-time weighted average (TLV-TWA) for paraquat respirable sizes is 0.1 mg/m^3. There is no ACGIH STEL value (92).

The OSHA and ACGIH threshold limit value-time weighted average (TLV-TWA) for diquat is 0.5 mg/m^3.

Glyphosate

Glyphosate, a phosphorus-containing organic herbicide (Round-Up and Kleen-Up), inhibits plant amino acid synthesis and has a chemical formula as shown in Figure 104.3. The commercial product is formulated in water with a 15% concentration of the surfactant, polyoxyethlyeneamine (93). This surfactant aids in emulsifying the glyphosate. The toxicity of the Round-Up product has been attributed to both the glyphosate herbicide as well as the surfactant (93).

Clinical manifestations of ingestion of the product include pharyngitis, vomiting, diarrhea, abdominal pain, erosions of the esophagus as well as the oropharynx and stomach, hepatic damage, hypotension, and renal damage with oliguria (93). Ocular exposure can cause conjunctivitis. Inhalation of the mist of the product can cause respiratory irritation. Dermal contact has caused dermatitis and mild chemical burns. Glyphosate is not well absorbed from the gastrointestinal tract nor from the skin.

Since most poisoning cases from the product occur by ingestion, clinical management is directed at controlling the massive gastrointestinal fluid loss and renal failure. Since vomiting is common following ingestion, inducing emesis is unnecessary. Also, since the product is caustic to the esophagus, inducing emesis is not recommended. Administration of 30g of activated charcoal may aid in adsorption of glyphosate as well as the surfactant. Aspiration of the product can produce pulmonary injury with pulmonary edema, so the airway must be protected. Intravenous rehydration is crucial to maintaining blood pressure and urine output.

Round-Up contains 41% glyphosate, and Kleen-Up contains up to 5% of the base herbicide. There are no permissible exposure limits established for glyphosate.

The toxicity of the surfactant has been reviewed and includes vomiting, diarrhea, hemolysis of red blood cells, hypotension, altered mental status, and pulmonary edema (94).

FUNGICIDES AND BIOCIDES

Fungicides and biocides are commonly used in a variety of products to prevent the growth of microorganisms such as bacteria and fungi. Fungicides are used in a variety of paints and other products where the growth of bacteria and fungus is undesirable and on vegetables and fruits. Fungicides, as a group of compounds, are diverse (Table 104.3) and include inorganic compounds, organometals, nitrobenzene and phenol derivatives.

Pentachlorophenol

PRODUCTION, USES, AND SOURCES OF PENTACHLOROPHENOL

Pentachlorophenol has been used extensively as a preservative of wood and fungicide throughout the United States. Its most common use was as a wood preservative for telephone poles. The compound is produced by the chlorination of a phenol in the presence of a catalyst. Commercial grade pentachlorophenol is at least 86% pure and contains contaminants of other polychlorinated phenols such as polychlorinated dibenzodioxin and polychlorinated dibenzofurans (95). Eighty percent of the United States consumption of pentachlorophenol was as a wood preservative. It was registered for use as an insecticide, fungicide, acaricide, herbicide, and as a disinfectant. It was also formerly used as an antifouling agent in paint. Pentachlorophenol is now a restricted use compound and is no longer used as a wood preserving solution or as a fungicide available for home use.

Due to the extensive use of pentachlorophenol throughout the United States, it has been found in a variety of air, water, and soil. It is a very stable compound and is not easily hydrolyzed or oxidized. However, it does undergo photooxidation by sunlight and can be biotransformed by microorganisms in soil. Detection of pentachlorophenol in biological media from humans such as plasma, blood, and urine is common. Human exposure to pentachlorophenol is also common and occurs through ingestion of contaminated water and food as well as breathing contaminated air.

EXPOSURE TO PENTACHLOROPHENOL

Exposure to pentachlorophenol occurs in occupational settings and through environmental contamination sources. Some human exposure from indoor air pollution sources of pentachlorophenol occurs because the wood structure of the home may have been previously treated with the compound as a preservative. Pentachlorophenol is detected in adipose tissue, human milk, blood, and urine. On the average, the population in the United States has been shown to have urine concentrations of pentachlorophenol of approximately 5 parts per billion (ppb) (96). In those who are occupationally exposed to pentachlorophenol in its use as a wood preservative, urine concentrations approximate 120 ppb.

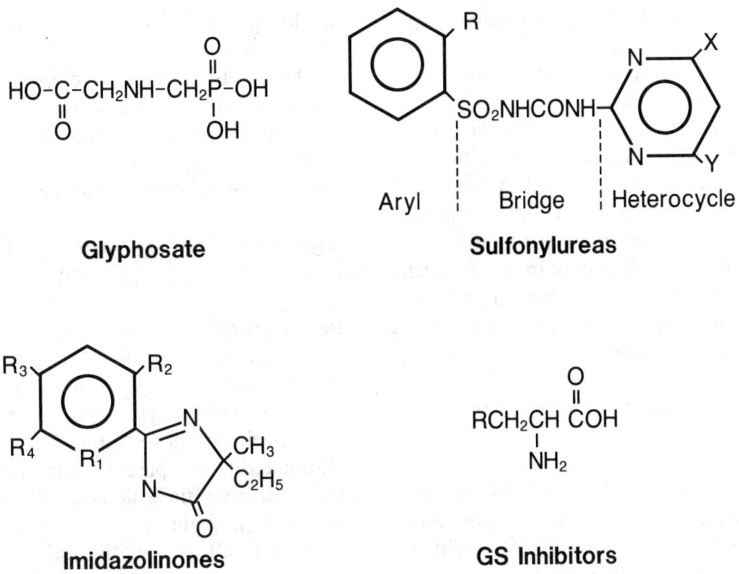

Glyphosate

Aryl ┆ Bridge ┆ Heterocycle

Sulfonylureas

Imidazolinones

GS Inhibitors

Figure 104.3. Herbicide classes that inhibit aminoacid biosynthesis. Sulfonylureas: R equals carboxymethyl,carboxyethyl,chloro, chloroethoxy. X + Y equals methoxy,chloro, methylethoxy. Imidizolinones: R_1 equals C or N; R_2 equals carboxy or carboxymethyl; R_3

equals H or phenylcarbon; R_4 equals H,ethyl,methyl or phenylcarbon. GH inhibitors: R equals $CH_3POOHCH_2$, $CH_3SONHCH_2$, cyclic $CH_2NHCOCOH$. From Duke S. Overview of herbicide mechanisms of action. Environ Health Perspect 199;263–271.

Table 104.3. Fungicides and Biocides

Inorganic metals
—copper sulfate

Organometals
—methylmercury
—cyclohexylhydrostannane (plictran)
—trimethyltin
—bis(tributyltin) oxide
—triphenyltin
—triethyltin

Acrolein
Formaldehyde
Pentachlorophenol
Pentachloronitrobenzene
Karathane (crotonic acid)
2,3-Dichloro-1,4-naphthaquinone

Thiabendazoles
—benomyl
—thiabendazole
—thiophanate methyl

Dithiocarbamates
—ferbam
—thiram
—ziram
—maneb
—zineb

Analyses of blood and urine samples from 6000 persons in 64 communities within the United States was conducted between 1976 and 1980 (96). Pentachlorophenol was one of the compounds detected in 79% of urine samples collected in this survey. The level of pentachlorophenol in these urine samples is between 6 and 193 ppb. Blood concentrations of pentachlorophenol also varied depending on the exposure. Individuals occupationally exposed to pentachlorophenol or using pentachlorophenol treated materials, have blood concentrations which

range from 83–57,600 ppb (96). Most of these individuals were involved in construction of log homes that were previously treated with pentachlorophenol. The adipose concentration of pentachlorophenol was shown in 1973 to be a mean of 26.3 μg/kg in the general U.S. population (96). Dietary intake of pentachlorophenol occurs through contaminated food products. Also, pentachlorophenol has been found in drinking water supplies in a 1976 survey at a mean concentration of 0.07 μg/L with a maximum concentration being 0.7 μg/L (96).

Another survey detected pentachlorophenol in drinking water supplies between the ranges of 1–12 μg/L in eight cities (96). The food and water supply are a common environmental source of human intake of pentachlorophenol.

Pentachlorophenol indoor air concentrations can be particularly high in log homes or older homes that have been pretreated with the compound as a preservative. In air samples taken in log homes, pentachlorophenol has been found in the range of 7–8 ppb. Pentachlorophenol treated wood products are the source of indoor air concentrations of pentachlorophenol. In older homes, pentachlorophenol has been found to range from 0.5–10 μg/m³ by the Environmental Protection Agency (EPA) (96). Higher concentrations of pentachlorophenol have been found in treated wood with these levels ranging from 34–104 μg/m³ (96).

Human exposure to pentachlorophenol occurs by the inhalational, dermal, and ingestion routes. Most occupational exposures have occurred to pest control applicators, carpenters, electrical power workers, and any of the trades or professions in contact with wood products. Other at risk populations include individuals living near pentachlorophenol manufacturing sites, waste disposal sites, and those who work in lumber mills.

REGULATORY ASPECTS

Pentachlorophenol is on the list of chemicals that appear in the "Toxic Chemicals Section 313 of the Emergency Planning and Community Right to Know Act of 1986." The Occupational

Safety and Health Administration (OSHA) permissible exposure limit (PEL) is 0.5 mg/m^3 as a time weighted average with a skin notation. The National Institute of Occupational Safety and Health (NIOSH) lists an immediately dangerous to life and health (IDLH) concentration as 150 mg/m^3. The American Conference of Governmental Industrial Hygienists (ACGIH) recommends a TLV of 0.5 mg/m^3. The National Academy of Sciences Safe Drinking Water Guide is 0.021 mg/L. The suggested no adverse effect level (SNARL) is 6 µg/L in a child, 7 µg/L of a technical grade pentachlorophenol in an adult, and 9 µg/L of commercial grade pentachlorophenol in an adult. Pentachlorophenol is listed as a hazardous waste by the EPA as well as being a priority toxic pollutant.

PHYSICAL AND CHEMICAL CHARACTERISTICS OF PENTACHLOROPHENOL

The molecular formula of pentachlorophenol is C_6Cl_5OH. It is a light brown solid and has a pungent odor, and a melting point of 187°C. Pentachlorophenol is also known as PCP (penchlorol and Dowicide EC-7). Pentachlorophenol is incompatible with strong oxidizers.

CLINICAL TOXICOLOGY AND HEALTH EFFECTS

In general, pentachlorophenol produces irritation of the eyes, nose, throat, and mucous membranes. Inhalational exposure to pentachlorophenol compounds is a common mode of exposure. Deaths have occurred following acute inhalation of pentachlorophenol (97). Inhalation of pentachlorophenol produces irritation of the upper respiratory tract as well as coughing and symptoms of bronchitis with chest tightness. Inhalational exposure can also produce cardiac effects of tachycardia. The ingestion of pentachlorophenol can result in abdominal pain, nausea, and vomiting with systemic absorption. Target organs for toxicity include the liver, kidneys, hematopoietic system, pulmonary system, and the central nervous system. Pulmonary inhalation of high concentrations can result in pulmonary edema and death (97).

Cases of aplastic anemia have been associated with pentachlorophenol exposure (97). Pentachlorophenol induced liver toxicity in humans has occurred in herbicide sprayers. Fatty infiltration of the liver and central lobular congestion with hepatocellular accumulation of fat has been noted. Also, elevation of liver enzymes has been seen following chronic dermal exposure to pentachlorophenol (97). Kidney effects secondary to exposure to pentachlorophenol have also been noted. Increased incidents of proteinuria and hematuria have been noted.

Ocular and dermal exposure to pentachlorophenol can produce serious damage. Corneal injury can occur from splashes to the eye. Also vapors of pentachlorophenol can produce ocular irritation. Pentachlorophenol can also induce dermatitis, inflammation of the skin, desclamation and hair loss (97).

The neurotoxicity of pentachlorophenol has also been recognized. Neurotoxicity of pentachlorophenol usually occurs only after massive exposure. Hyperthermia, probably due to uncoupling of oxidated phosphorylation, has been observed. There has been no report of peripheral neuropathy secondary to exposure. Lethargy and cerebral edema have occurred following short term, high level exposures to pentachlorophenol. This has also been accompanied by seizures, coma, delirium, and hyperthermia.

No evidence of immunotoxic effects in humans from pentachlorophenol has been documented. However, animal studies have shown immunotoxic effects. There is no evidence of reproductive toxicity or developmental effects secondary to human exposure to pentachlorophenol. However, there has been an increase in the frequency of chromosomal aberrations seen in the peripheral lymphocytes of workers occupationally exposed to pentachlorophenol (97).

ABSORPTION, METABOLISM, AND EXCRETION OF PENTACHLOROPHENOL

Pentachlorophenol is well absorbed by the inhalational, dermal, and gastrointestinal routes. The half-life of elimination of pentachlorophenol from plasma was found to be about 30 hours in human volunteers. Also, in the same study, 74% of pentachlorophenol dose administered to human volunteers was eliminated as the parent compound and 12% as a glucuronide metabolite within 168 hours (97). Pentachlorophenol elimination is thought to be first order with some enterohepatic recirculation following ingestion.

2,3,Dichloro-1,4-Naphthoquinone

2,3,Dichloro-1,4-naphthoquinone, also known as dichloronapthoquinone, this compound has a tradename of Compound 605, Phygon, and Algistat. It has a molecular formula of $C_{10}H_4Cl_2O_2$ and a molecular weight of 227.04. It is a fungicide that is used for foliage and textiles as well as seed disinfectant. This compound decomposes slowly in soil and water and may be stable enough to bioaccumulate up the food chain. It has a vapor density of 7.8 (air = 1.0). This compound is considered to be moderately toxic by ingestion and has irritancy properties to the skin, eyes, and mucous membranes. It can also produce central nervous system depression. It is a very irritating dust (98).

Thiabendazoles

The thiabendazole class of fungicides are heterocyclic derivatives of the parent thiabendazole (Fig. 104.4). These compounds include benomyl, thiabendazole, and thiophanatemethyl.

BENOMYL

Benomyl is a white, crystalline solid with a chemical formula of $C_{14}H_{18}N_4O_3$. It has been used widely as a fungicide for fruits and vegetables (99). Human health effects are related to its dermal irritancy effects. On contact with the skin it can produce erythema and edema (99).

THIABENDAZOLE

Thiabendazole has a formula of $C_{10}H_7N_3S$ and is a white odorless powder used as an antihelminthic and fungicide (99). Thiabendazole is used as an oral drug for treatment of nematodes such as hookworms, roundworms, pinworms, and threadworms. As a drug, it is rapidly absorbed via the gastrointestinal tract. It is also readily absorbed through the skin as a fungicidal agent. Thiabendazole orally has adverse effects of nausea, dizziness, diarrhea, abdominal discomfort, drowsiness, headache, and vertigo. Acute oral overdoses may result in seizures, hyperexcitability, hypotension, bradycardia, renal toxicity, and hepatic toxicity (100). Hypersensitivity reactions include rashes,

Thiabendazole

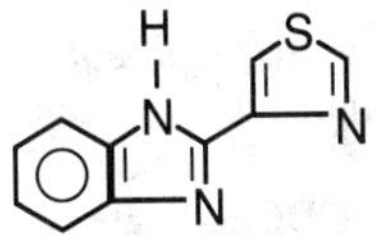

Thiophanate-methyl

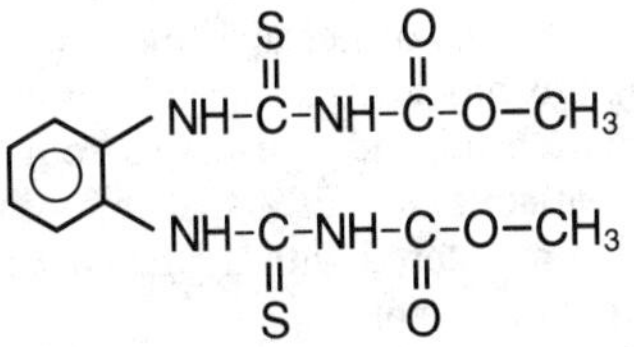

Benomyl

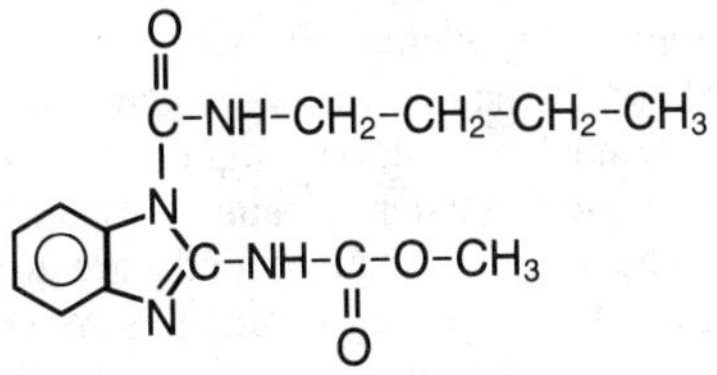

Figure 104.4. Thiabendazole fungicides.

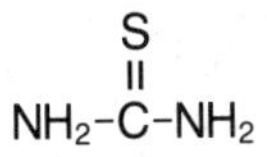

$$NH_2-\overset{\displaystyle S}{\overset{\displaystyle \|}{C}}-NH_2$$

Thiourea
(Thiocarbamide)

Figure 104.5. Thiocarbamate fungicides—general structure.

conjunctivitis, erythema multiforme, Stevens-Johnson syndrome, and angioedema (100).

THIOPHANATE-METHYL

Thiophanate-methyl is a colorless crystalline solid with a molecular formula of $C_{12}H_{14}N_4O_4S_2$ and is water soluble (99). This compound can cause dermatitis consisting of swelling, erythema, and itching upon contact (99).

Dithiocarbamates

Dithiocarbamates find use mainly as fungicides although some of these compounds are used as herbicides and nematocides (99). This class of fungicides includes ferbam, thiram, metham-sodium, ziram, sulfallate, anobam, maneb, nabam, and zineb (99). The well known drug, disulfiram (Antabuse), is in the class of dithiocarbamates. Dithiocarbamates have a general chemical formula as shown in Figure 104.5.

FERBAM

Ferbam is a dithiocarbamate fungicide with the tradename of Cormate or Fermacide. It has a molecular formula of $C_9H_{18}N_3S_6$. FE and a molecular weight of 416.5 (99). This fungicide does not tend to persist in the environment and is degraded by soil microbes. Toxicologic data on this compound is limited. However, it is an irritant chemical to the eyes, skin, and mucous membranes, and has a potential to produce kidney damage. The OSHA PEL for a time weighted average is 15 mg/m³. The ACGIH recommends a TLV of 10 mg/m³, with a STEL of 20 mg/m³ for 15 minutes (101).

THIRAM

Thiram (tetramethylthiuram disulfide) is a general use fungicide with a formula of $C_6H_{12}N_2S_4$ and molecular weight of 240.44 (99). It is in the form of colorless crystals and is formulated as a powder and dust for application as a seed treatment. The dithiocarbamates can produce systemic toxic reactions of a disulfiram-like reaction if absorbed concurrently with ethanol. Other systemic toxicity reported includes nausea, vomiting, abdominal pain, hyperexcitability, and weakness (99). Thiram can also produce contact dermatitis, but this is not very common. Thiram has been used in the rubber industry as a vulcanizing agent.

Thiram is insoluble in water but soluble in organic solvents. It is decomposed following exposure to acids (100). In addition to its use as a fungicide, it has been used as an accelerator in the rubber industry and as an antioxidant. Thiram is a degradation product of both ferbam and ziram (102).

Human exposure occurs via inhalation or skin exposure to dusts, sprays, mists, or aerosolized forms of the product. The workplace exposure limit is 5 mg/m³ as a TWA. Residue tolerance level as a fungicide on vegetables and fruits is 7 mg/kg (102).

Toxic exposure to thiram produces irritation of eyes and mucous membranes as well as the skin. Erythema and urticarial reactions can occur following dermal exposure to thiram. Allergic contact dermatitis can also occur (102).

Thiram is metabolized by the liver to carbon disulfide. Environmentally, thiram can be degraded to carbon disulfide, hydrogen sulfide, and dimethylamine which are all toxic by-products. Thiram may also produce hepatic toxicity once systemically absorbed (102). Other toxic manifestations of thiram include nausea, dizziness, headache, confusion, ataxia, vomiting, diarrhea, and flaccid paralysis (102). Death has occurred following ingestion. Thiram can produce gastrointestinal focal necrosis.

ZIRAM

Ziram (zinc dimethyldithiocarbamate) has a formula of $C_6H_{12}N_2S_4Zn$, and is an odorless powder with a molecular weight of 305.8 (99). Human toxic hazard is mainly due to airborne dust since it has negligible vapor pressure. Ziram is an irritant of the eyes, upper airway, and mucous membranes. Ingestion can produce localized necrosis of the gastrointestinal tract (99). Due to its irritant properties, ziram can produce respiratory irritation and distress on inhalation of dust.

Acrolein (Acrylaldehyde)

Acrolein (CH₂CHCHO) is a potent herbicide and biocide used to control weeds, algae, and plant growth in irrigation canals and water drainage areas. Acrolein is a clear to yellowish liquid with a pungent odor and is very irritating to the eyes, skin, and mucous membranes. Exposure occurs mainly by inhalation or contact of the liquid by accidental splash (103). Acrolein is contained in the product Magnacide-H. Human exposure can result in severe dermatitis and burns to the skin, eyes, and mucous membranes. The Environmental Protection Agency lists acrolein as a hazardous material and restricts its use as a pesticide. Acrolein is also used in the production of glycerine and in the synthesis of other chemicals. Acrolein is incompatible with oxidizers, ammonia, and alkalis.

Table 104.4. Health Effects Resulting from Vapor Concentrations of Acrolein

Vapor Concentration	Exposure	Effect
0.25 ppm	5 minutes	Moderate irritation
1 ppm	2–3 minutes	Ocular and nose irritation
5.5 ppm	1 minute	Intolerable
153 ppm	10 minutes	Can be fatal

The OSHA PEL is 0.1 ppm (0.25 mg/m^3), the STEL is 0.3 ppm, and the IDLH concentration is 5.0 ppm (103).

Routes of exposure to acrolein are by inhalation, dermal contact, and ingestion. It is a highly volatile liquid whose vapor is extremely irritating, flammable, and forms explosive mixtures in air. The basic product comes as 92% acrolein by weight in a cylinder connected to a nitrogen gas pressurized delivery system. Acrolein is a highly reactive aldehyde and readily polymerizes with generation of heat. Improper handling or storing of the product can create a hazard which can result in a polymerization reaction, release of heat, and rupturing of the container. Contamination with air, oxidizers, ammonia, or alkalis can initiate a violent polymerization reaction.

Acrolein products used as biocides contain nitrogen which excludes air and prevents polymerization reactions. Hydroquinone is added to help inhibit oxygen initiated polymerization.

Acrolein readily binds to sulfhydral groups and is a general cell poison. It will kill aquatic wildlife if the water concentration is not controlled. The permissible water concentration to protect aquatic life is 21 μg/L on a chronic basis and 68 μg/L on an acute basis (103). The product is forced from its container using pressurized oxygen free-N$_2$ and introduced directly into canal water to form a "wave" that slowly moves in the direction of water flow, killing all plant life as it comes into contact.

Acrolein vapor and liquid is a potent irritant and lachrymator and very toxic to all tissues. Due to its highly irritating vapor and lacrimating action, humans cannot tolerate vapor concentrations of 0.1–1 ppm for even short periods of time. Splash exposures to the liquid concentrate can produce ocular and skin damage rapidly. Skin injury from the concentrate can produce edema, erythema, and second degree burns. Inhalation of the vapor or liquid will produce respiratory irritation, mucous membrane irritation, difficulty breathing, and pulmonary edema. Any splash exposure should be immediately irrigated with water for 15–20 minutes.

The concentration of acrolein in water should not exceed 320 μg/L to protect human health (103). Vapor concentrations of acrolein produce health effects as shown in Table 104.4.

Personal protective equipment, including eye, skin, and respiratory protection, should be used when working with acrolein.

Organotin Compounds

Tributyltin oxide is used for mildew and fungicide control in paint. It is a fungicide manufactured for use in exterior paint and is a biocide in widely available commercial paint fungicides. Tributyltin oxide is both a solid and a liquid, and human exposures can occur from inhalation as well as skin absorption. In general, the organotin compounds produce irritation of the eyes, mucous membranes, throat, and skin. Some of the organotins are hepatotoxic. The trialkyltins are the most toxic (101, 103).

Exposure to tributyltin can produce irritation of the eyes, throat, conjunctivitis, and mucous membrane irritation. Dermal contact of a solution or a solid can produce chemical burns (101).

A report from the CDC indicates that a person who is exposed to tributyltin oxide as a biocide in paint developed health effects after the rooms of her apartment were painted with paint containing this biocide. Her symptoms included mucous membrane irritation, headache, epistaxis, cough, nausea, and vomiting. The paint contained 25% bistributyltin oxide (104). Tributyltin has been registered with the Environmental Protection Agency as a biocide in paint.

Animal studies indicate that tributyltin produces immunosuppression, anemia, and weight loss. Human health effects from tributyltin include mucous membrane irritation, irritation of the eyes, nose, and throat, and cough. Tributyltin as a fungicide is to be used in exterior paints only and not in interior paints.

The organotin compounds are used as additives in many products and processes that require preservation such as wood, leather, paper, paint, textiles, etc. The main use of organotin compounds is that of biocides. Tributyltin, triphenyltin, and tetraorganotin are incompatible with strong oxidizers. All of the organotin compounds, especially tributyl and dibutyltins, can produce severe dermal injury in chemical burns to the skin. Intense itching, inflammation, and erythema can occur upon exposure. The lesions that develop are generally diffuse, erythematous, and heal quickly after exposure is terminated. Exposure to the eyes can produce lacrimation, conjunctivitis, and conjunctival edema.

Trialkyl and tetra alkyltin compounds are neurotoxic and produce headache, dizziness, photophobia, vomiting, muscle weakness, and flaccid paralysis in severe cases (103). The alkyltins are also hepatotoxins. The typical organotins are triethyltin, dibutyltin, tributyltin, and triphenyltin. These compounds are in the form of triethyltin iodide, dibutyltin chloride, tributyltin chloride, triphenyltin acetate, and bistributyltin oxide.

Triethyltin can produce neurologic symptoms of severe headache, vertigo, photophobia, and other visual disturbances, abdominal pain and vomiting, urinary retention, paralysis, and psychic disturbances upon ingestion (101). Persistent neurologic sequelae include diminished visual acuity, focal anesthesia, flaccid paralysis, incontinence, and cerebral edema.

Triphenyltin is a hepatotoxin and in some occupational exposures has produced hepatic damage with hepatomegaly and elevated liver enzymes (101). Triphenyltin is also a dermal irritant and can produce other effects such as headache, nausea, vomiting, and blurred vision on toxic exposure (101).

Trimethyltin has produced hyperexcitability, neurologic and behavioral changes in animals, as well as seizures in some animal studies.

The organotin compounds are known to have immunotoxic properties in animals. Trimethyltin dichloride has shown histopathologic changes in the organ weight of the thymus and spleen of between 50 and 60%. Also, in animal studies, there was a decrease in T-cell dependent antibody response and B-cell lymphocyte proliferation of between 60 and 80%. In addition, trimethyltin affected cellular immunity and was shown to have an 80% decrease in T-lymphocyte proliferation from mitogen stimulation (105). Tributyltin oxide also has shown immunotoxic effects in animal species. Rats fed tributyltin oxide orally showed decreases in the lymphoid organ weight such as the thymus and spleen as well as decrease in white blood cell count and decreased lymphocyte counts. Animals fed triphenyltin also showed immunotoxic effects such as decreases in the weight of thymus,

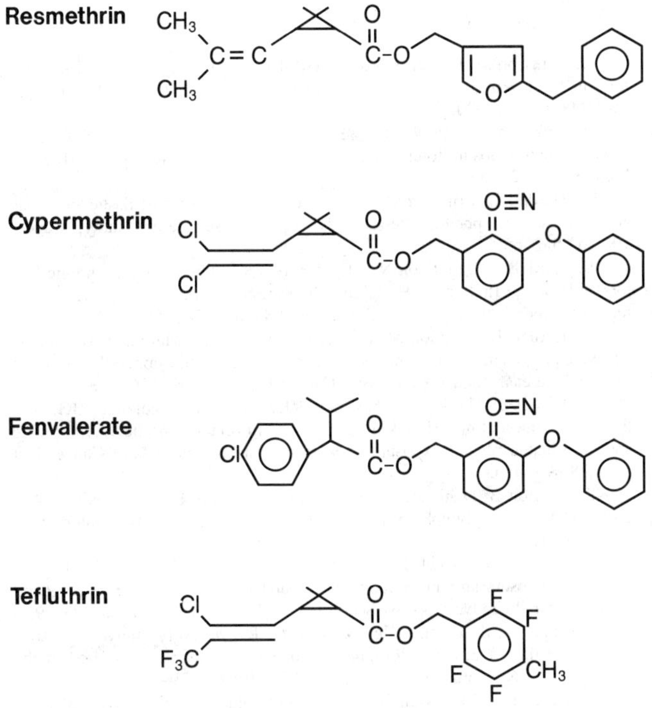

Resmethrin

Cypermethrin

Fenvalerate

Tefluthrin

Figure 104.6.   Synthetic pyrethroids.

Table 104.5.   Pyrethrins and Pyrethroids

Natural

Pyrethrin I
Pyrethrin II
Jasmolin I
Jasmolin II
Cinerin I
Cinerin II

Synthetic

Phenothrin
Resmethrin
Cypermethrin
Cyfluthrin
Deltamethrin
Cyhalothrin
Fenvalerate
Cyfluthrinate
Fluvalinate
Tralomethrin
Tralocythrin

---

spleen, and lymph nodes as well as a decrease in B-cell lymphocyte proliferation. Delayed hypersensitivity reactions and decrease in T-cell lymphocyte proliferation response to mitogen as well as decreased host resistance were also observed.

PYRETHRINS AND PYRETHROIDS

Pyrethrins are naturally occurring insecticides of the *chrysanthemum cinerariafolium*. As a class, pyrethrins are esters of chrysanthemic acid and pyrethric acid (Fig. 104.6) (106). There are six naturally occurring pyrethrins: pyrethrin I, pyrethrin II, jasmolin I, jasmolin II, cinerin I, cinerin II (106, 107). Pyrethrins are of low order of toxicity to humans but are highly insecticidal. Due to the photosensitivity of the naturally occurring pyrethrins, synthetic pyrethroids have been developed that are more stable when exposed to light (107). Pyrethrins and pyrethroids are listed in Table 104.5.

Synthetic pyrethroids include allethrin, resmethrin, and phenothrin (106). In order to increase compound stability, resmethrin has a phenyl ring incorporated into its structure. Phenothrin contains a stabilizing phenoxybenzyl group (106). Permethrin is a highly used commercial synthetic pyrethroid. The addition of a variety of chemical moieties to the pyrethroid molecular structure yields newer pyrethroids. Cypermethrin has the addition of a cyano (CEN) group. Adding chlorine or fluorine yields even more stable compounds (106, 107).

The synthetic pyrethroids are classed according to their chemical structure into: (a) those that contain the cyanogroup at the alpha carbon of the phenoxybenzyl moiety (type II) and (b) those that lack this cyano group (type I).

Clinical Toxicology of Pyrethroids

The cyano containing (type II) pyrethroids are the more toxic compounds to insects as well as to animals. Overall, the clinical toxicity of pyrethrins and pyrethroids are low. Both pyrethrins and pyrethroids are neurotoxins upon direct injection into the central nervous system of animals (106, 107). Direct toxic CNS effects in animals are tremor, choreoathetosis, hyperthermia, salivation, tachypnea, and seizures (106, 107). Symptoms may differ between type I and type II pyrethroids. Type I pyrethroids produce aggressive activity, hyperthermia, and tremors. Type II pyrethroids induce salivation, choreoathetosis, and seizures upon direct injection into the CNS (106). Pyrethroids are metabolized by ester hycholysis followed by hepatic oxidation.

The mechanism of pyrethroid toxicity is thought to be due to inhibition of normal chloride (Cl^-) channel function at the gamma aminobutyric acid (GABA) receptor site in the CNS (107). There is also evidence that pyrethroids can act on the nicotinic acetylcholine receptor sites (107). In addition, they can inhibit adenosine triphosphatase enzymes such as calcium-ATphase and interfere with sodium-calcium in exchange channels across all membranes (107).

The human clinical toxicity from exposure to pyrethrins and pyrethroids is mainly from the irritant and sensitivity properties of the chemicals. Toxicity is manifested by contact dermatitis with an erythematous rash and vesicle formation (99). Dermal effects of pyrethroids can be exacerbated by sunlight (99). The irritant and sensitizing effects can result in swelling of the face and asthma-like conditions. Pyrethrins can irritate the mucous membranes and upper airway. Allergic dermatitis may occur following repeated exposures. Toxicity in children has occurred following oral exposure with manifestations of seizures and vomiting (99).

REFERENCES

1. Duke S. Overview of herbicide mechanisms of action. Environ Health Perspect 1990;87:263–271.

2. Fingerhut MA, Halperin WE, Marlow BS, et al. Cancer mortality in workers exposed to 2,3,7,8-tetrachlorodibenzo-*p*-dioxin. N Engl J Med 1991;324:212–218.

3. Libich S. To JC, Frank R, Sirons GJ. Occupational exposure of herbicide applicators to herbicides used along electric power transmission line of right-of-way. Am Ind Hyg Assoc J 1984;45:56–62.

4. Arnold EK, Beasley VA. The pharmacokinetics of chlorinated phenoxy acid herbicides: a literature review. Vet Hum Toxicol 1989;31:121–125.

5. Erne K. Distribution and elimination of chlorinated phenoxyacetic acids in animals. ACTA Vet Scand 1966;7:240–256.

6. Bjorklund NE, Erne K. Toxicological studies of phenoxyacetic herbicides in animals. ACTA Vet Scand 1966;7:364–390.

7. Kohli JD, Khanna RN, Gupta BN, Dhar MM, Tandon JS, Sirca KP. Absorption and excretion of 2-4-dichlorophenoxyacetic acid in man. Xenobiotica 1974;4:97–100.

8. Gehring PJ, Betso JE. Phenoxy acids: effects and fate in mammals. Ecol Bull (Stockholm) 1978;27:122–133.

9. Sauerhoff MW, Braun WH, Blau GE, LeBeau JE. The fate of 2,4-dichlorophenoxyacetic acid (2,4-D) following oral administration. Toxicol Appl Pharmacol 1976;37:136–137.

10. Piper WN, Rose JQ, Leng ML, Gehring PJ. The fate of 2,4,5-trichlorophenoxyacetic acid (2,4,5-T) following oral administration to rats and dogs. Toxicol Appl Pharmacol 1973;26:339–351.

11. Gehring PJ, Kramer CG, Schweta BA, Rose JQ, Rowe VK. The fate of 2,4,5-trichlorophenoxyacetic acid (2,4,5-T) following oral administration to man. Toxicol Appl Pharmacol 1973;26:352–361.

12. Sauerhoff MW, Braun WH, Blau GE, Gehring PJ. Bergstrom R. The fate of 2,4-dichlorophenoxyacetic acid (2,4-D) following oral administration to man. Toxicology 1977;8:3–11.

13. Piper WN, Rose JQ, Leng ML, and Gehring PJ. The fat of 2,4,5-Trichlorophenoxyacetic acid (2,4,5-T following oral administration to rats and dogs. Toxicol Appl Pharmacol 1973;339–351.

14. Baselt RC, Cravey RH. Disposition of toxic drugs and chemicals in man. 3rd ed. Chicago, IL: Yearbook Medical Publishers, Inc, 1989:262–264.

15. Kolmodin-Hedman B, Akerblom M. Field application of phenoxy acid herbicides. In: Tordoir WF, van Heemstra EAH, eds. Field worker exposure during pesticide application. New York: Elsevier, 1980:73–77.

16. Berwick P. 2,4-Dichlorophenoxyacetic acid poisoning in man. JAMA. 214:1114–1117, 1970.

17. Wells WDE, Wright N, Yeoman WB. Clinical features and management of poisoning with 2,4-D and mecoprop. Clin Toxicol 1981;18:273–276.

18. Osterloh J. Lotti M. Pond SM. Toxicologic studies in a fatal overdose of 2,4-D, MCPP, and chlorpyrifos. J Anal Toxicol 7:125–129, 1983.

19. Hervonen H, Elo HA, Ylitalo P. Blood-brain barrier damage by 2-methyl-4-chlorophenoxyacetic acid herbicide in rats. Toxicol Appl Pharmacol 1982;65:23–31.

20. Dudley AW, Thapar NT. Fatal human ingestion of 2,4-D, a common herbicide. Arch Path 1972;94:270–275.

21. Desi I, Sos J, Olasz J, Sule F, Markus V. Nervous system effects of a chemical herbicide. Archiv Environ Health 1962;4:101–108.

22. Goldstein NP, Jones PH. Peripheral neuropathy after exposure to an ester of dichlorophenoxyacetic acid. JAMA 1959;171:1306–1309.

23. Berkley MC, Magee KR. Neuropathy following exposure to dimethylamine salt of 2,4-D. Arch Intern Med 1963;111:351–352.

24. Mattson JL, Johnson KA, Albee RR. Lack of neuropathologic consequences of repeated dermal exposure to 2,4-dichlorophenoxyacetic acid in rats. Fund Appl Toxicol 1986;6:175–181.

25. Kay JH, Plazzolo RJ, Calandra JC. Subacute dermal toxicity of 2,4-D. Arch Environ Health 1965;11:648–665.

26. Nielsen K, Kaempe B, Jenson-Holm J. Fatal poisoning in man by 2,4-dichlorophenoxyacetic acid (2,4-D): determination of the agent in forensic materials. Acta Pharmacol Toxicol 1965;22:224–234.

27. Seabury JH. Toxicity of 2,4 dichlorophenoxyacetic acid for man and dog. Arch Environ Health 1963;7:202–209.

28. Curry AS. Twenty-one uncommon cases of poisoning. Br Med J 1962;1:687–698.

29. Smith RA, Lewis D. Suicide by ingestion of 2,4-D: a case history demonstrating the prudence of using GC/MS as an investigative rather than a confirmatory tool. Vet Hum Toxicol 1987;29:259–261.

30. Zack JA, Suskinid RS. The mortality experience of workers exposed to tetrachlorobenzodioxin in a trichlorophenol process accident. J Occup Med 1980;22:11–14.

31. Mary G. Tetrachlorodibenzodioxin: a survey of subjects ten years after exposure. Br J Ind Med 1982;39:128–135.

32. Oliver RM. Toxic effects of 2,3,7,8-tetrachloro-1-4-dioxin in laboratory workers. Br J Ind Med 1975;32:49–53.

33. Suskind RR, Hertzberg VS. Human health effects of 2,4,5-T and its toxic contaminants. JAMA 1984;251:2372–2380.

34. Moses M, Lilis R, Crow KD, Thornton J, Fischbein A, Anderson HA, Selikoff IJ. Health status of workers with past exposure to 2,3,7,8-tetrachlorodibenzo-p-dioxin in the manufacture of 2,4,5-trichlorophenoxyacetic acid: comparison of findings with and without chloracne. Am J Ind Med 1984;5:161–182.

35. Hardell L, Sandstrom A. Case-control study: soft tissue sarcomas and

exposure to phenoxyacetic acids or chlorophenols. Br J Cancer 1979;39:711–7.

36. Eriksson M. Hardell L, Adami HP. Exposure to dioxins as a risk factor for soft tissue sarcoma: a population-based case-control study. J Natl Cancer Inst 1990;82:486–490.

37. Eriksson M, Hardell L, Berg N, Moller T, Axelson O. Soft-tissue sarcomas and exposure to chemical substances: a case referent study. Br J Ind Med 1981;38:27–33.

38. Hardell L, Eriksson M. The association between soft tissue sarcomas and exposure to phenoxyacetic acids: a new case-referent study. Cancer 1988;62:652–656.

39. Hardell L, Bengtsson NO. Epidemiologic study of socioeconomic factors and clinical findings in Hodgkin's disease, and reanalysis of previous data regarding chemical exposure. Br J Cancer 1983;48:217–225.

40. Hardell L, Eriksson M, Lenner P, Lundgren E. Malignant lymphoma and exposure to chemicals, especially organic solvents, chlorophenols and phenoxy acids: a case-control study. Br J Cancer 1981: 43:169–176.

41. Woods JS, Polissar L, Severson RK, Heuser LS, Kulander BG. Soft tissue sarcoma and non-Hodgkin's lymphoma in relation to phenoxyherbicide and chlorinated phenol exposure in western Washington. J Natl Cancer Inst 1987;78:899–910.

42. Persson B, Dahlander A, Fredriksson M, Brage HN, Ohlson CG, Axelson O. Malignant lymphomas and occupational exposures. Br J Intern Med 1989:516–520.

43. Axelson O, Sundell L, Andersson K, Edling C, Hogstedt C, Kling H. Herbicide exposure and tumor mortality: an updated epidemiologic investigation on Swedish railroad car workers. Scand J Work Environ Health 1980;6:73–79.

44. Thiess AM, Frentzel-Beyme R, Link R. Mortality study of persons exposed to dioxin in a trichlorophenol-process accident that occurred in the BASF AG on November 17, 1953. Am J Med 1982;3:179–189.

45. Hardell L, Johansson B, Axelson O. Epidemiological study of nasal and nasopharyngeal cancer and their relation to phenoxy acid or chlorophenol exposure. Am J Ind Med 1982;3:247–257.

46. Kociba R, Keyes D, Beyer J, et al. Results of a two-year chronic toxicity and oncogenicity study of 2,3,7,8-tetrachlorodibenzo-p-dioxin in rats. Toxicol Appl Pharmacol 1978;46:279–303.

47. Rao MS, Subbarao V, Prasad JD, Scarpelli DG. Carcinogenicity of 2,3,7,8-tetrachlorodibenzo-p-dioxin in the Syrian golden hamster. Carcinogenesis 1988;9:1677–1679.

48. Smith AH, Pearce NE, Fisher DO, Giles HJ, Teague CA, Howard JK. Soft tissue sarcoma and exposure to phenoxyherbicides and chlorophenols in New Zealand. J Natl Cancer Inst 1984;73:1111–1117.

49. Wiklund K, Holm L. Soft tissue sarcoma risk in Swedish agricultural and forestry workers. J Natl Cancer Inst 1986;76:229–234.

50. Pearce NE, Sheppard RA, Smith AH, Teague CA. Non-Hodgkin's lymphoma and farming: an expanded case-control study. Int J Cancer 1987;39:155–61.

51. Wiklund K, Dich J, Holm LE. Risk of malignant lymphoma in Swedish pesticide appliers. Br J Cancer 1987;56:505–8.

52. Olsen JH, Jensen OM. Nasal cancer and chlorophenols. Lancet 1984;2:47–8.

53. Hardell L, Bengtsson N, Jonsson V, Ericksson S, Larsson L. Aetiological aspects on primary liver cancer with special regard to alcohol, organic solvents and acute intermittent porphyria—an epidemiological investigation. Br J Cancer 1984;50:389–397.

54. Bailar JC. How dangerous is dioxin? N Engl J Med 1991;324:260–262.

55. Wolfe WH, Michalek JE, Miner JC, Rahe A, Silva J, Thomas WF, Grubbs WD, Lustik MB, Karrison TG, Roegner RH, Williams DE. Health status of Air Force veterans occupationally exposed to herbicides in Vietnam. I. Physical health. JAMA 1990;264:1824–1831.

56. Michalek JE, Wolfe WH, Miner JC. Health status of Air Force veterans occupationally exposed to herbicides in Vietnam. II. Mortality. JAMA 1990; 264:1832–1836.

57. Hoffman RE, Stehr-Green PA, Webb KB, et al. Health effects of long-term exposure to 2,3,7,8-tetrachlorodibenzo-p-dioxin. J Am Med Assoc 1986; 255:2031–2038.

58. Reggiani G. Medical problems raised by the TCDD contamination in Seveso, Italy. Arch Toxicol 1978;40:161–188.

59. Bronstein AC, Currance PL. Emergency Care for Hazardous Material Exposures. C.V. Mosby, St. Louis, MO: 1988:191–192.

60. Prescott LF, Park J. Darrien I. Treatment of severe 2,4-D and mecoprop intoxication with alkaline diuresis. Br J Clin Pharmacol 1979;7:111–116.

61. Flanagan RJ, Meredith TJ, Ruprah M, Onyon LJ, Liddle A. Alkaline diuresis for acute poisoning with chlorophenoxy herbicides and ioxynil. Lancet 1990;335;454:458.

62. Morgan DP. Recognition and management of pesticide poisonings. 4th

ed. Washington DC, US Environmental Protection Agency, US Government Printing Office, 1989:63:67.

63. Fraser AD, Isner IF, Perry RA. Toxicologic studies in a fatal overdose of 2,4-D, mecoprop, and dicamba. J Forensic Sci 1984;29:1237–1241.

64. Kahn PC, Gochfeld M, Nygren M, Hansson M, Rappe C, Velez H, Ghent-Guenther T, Wilson WP. Dioxins and dibenzofurans in blood and adipose tissue of agent orange—esposed Vietnam veterans and matched controls. JAMA 1988; 259:1661–1667.

65. Patterson DC, Hoffman RE, Needham LL, et al. 2,3,7,8-Tetrachlorodibenzo-p-dioxin levels in adipose tissue of exposed persons in Missouri. JAMA 1986, 256:2683–2686.

66. Hart TB. Paraquat—review of safety in agricultural and horticultural use. Hum Toxicol 1987;6:13–18.

67. Smith LL. Mechanism of paraquat toxicity in lung and its relevance to toxicity. Hum Toxicol 1987;6:31–36.

68. Vale JA, Meredith TJ, Buckley BM. Paraquat poisoning: clinical features and immediate general management. Hum Toxicol 1987;6:41–47.

69. Hawksworth GM, Bennett PN, Davies DS. Kinetics of paraquat elimination in the dog. Toxicol Appl Pharmacol 1981;57:139–145.

70. Kurisaki E, Sato E. Tissue distribution of paraquat and diquat after oral administration in rats. Forensic Sci Int 1979;14:165–170.

71. Daniel JW, Gage JC. Absorption and excretion of diquat and paraquat in rats. Br J Ind Med 1966;28:133–136

72. Murray RE, Gibson JE. Paraquat disposition in rats, guinea pigs and monkeys. Toxicol Appl Pharmacol 1974; 27:283–291.

73. Bennett PN, Davies DS, Hawkesworth GM. In vitro absorption studies with paraquat and diquat in the dog. Br J Pharmacol 1976;58:284.

74. Bismuth C, Garnier R, Dally S, Fournier PE. Prognosis and treatment of paraquat poisoning: a review of 28 cases. J Clin Toxicol 1982;19:461–474.

75. Rose MS, Lock EA, Smith LL, Wyatt I. Paraquat accumulation tissue and species specificity. Biochem Pharmacol 1976;25:419–423.

76. Rose MS, Smith LL. Tissue uptake of paraquat and diquat. Gen Pharmacol 1977;8:173–176.

77. Proudfoot AT, Stewart MS, Levitt T, Widdop B. Paraquat poisoning: significance of plasma-paraquat concentrations. Lancet 1979;2:330–332.

78. Scherrmann JM, Houze P, Bismuth C, Bourdon R. Prognostic value of plasma and urine paraquat concentration. Hum Toxicol 1987;6:91–93.

79. Pond SM. Manifestations and management of paraquat poisoning. Med J Aust 1990; 152:256–259.

80. Hearn CED, Keir W. Nail damage in spray operators exposed to paraquat. Br J Ind Med 1971;28:399–403.

81. Joyce M. Ocular damage caused by paraquat. Br J Ophthalmol 1969;53:688–690.

82. Karai I, Nakano H. Horiguchi S. A case of lacrimal duct stenosis due to a herbicide paraquat. Jpn J Ind Health 1981;23:552–553.

83. NIOSH pocket guide to chemical hazards, Cincinnati, OH: National Institute for Occupational Safety and Health; 1990. DHHS publication (PHS) 90–117:172.

84. Bismuth C, Scherrmann, Garnier R, Baud FJ, Pontal PG. Elimination of paraquat. Hum Toxicol 1987;6:63–67.

85. Meredith TJ, Vale JA. Treatment of paraquat poisoning in man: methods to prevent absorption. Hum Toxicol 1987;6;49–55.

86. Proudfoot AT, Prescott LF, Jarvie DR. Haemodialysis for paraquat poisoning. Hum Toxicol. 1987;6:69-74.

87. Edith CGM, Pond SM. Failure of haemoperfusion and haemodialysis to prevent death in paraquat poisoning. Med Toxicol 1988;3:64–71.

88. Powell D, Pond SM, Allen TB, Portale AA. Hemoperfusion in a child who ingested diquat and died from pontine infarction and hemorrhage. J Toxicol Clin Toxicol 1983;20(5):405–420.

89. Vanholder R, Colardyn F, DeReuck J, Praet M, Lameire N, Ringoir S. Diquat intoxication. Report of two cases and review of the literature. Am J Med 1981;70:1267–1271.

90. Braithwaite RA. Emergency analysis of paraquat in biological fluids. Hum Toxicol 1987;6:83–86.

91. Air contaminants—permissible exposure limits. Title 29 Code of Federal Regulations Part 1910.1000. US Department of Labor, Occupational Safety and Health Administration (OSHA 3112). 1989:57.

92. American Conference of Governmental and Industrial Hygienists. 1990–1991 Threshold limit values for chemical substances and physical agents and biological exposure indices. Cincinnati, OH: 1990:20,29.

93. Menkes D, Temple W, Edwards I. International self-poisoning with glyphosate-containing herbicides. Hum Exper Toxicol 1991;10:103–107.

94. Bartnik F, Kunstler K. Biological effects, toxicology, and human safety. In: Falbe ed. Surfactants in consumer products—theory, technology, and application. New York, NY: Springer-Verlag, 1987:475–499.

95. Toxicological profile for pentachlorophenol. Agency for Toxic Substances and Disease Registry, US Public Health Service, 1989:79–80.

96. Toxicological profile for pentachlorophenol. Agency for Toxic Substances and Disease Registry, US Public Health Service, 1989:81–96.

97. Toxicological profile for pentachlorophenol. Agency for Toxic Substances and Disease Registry, US Public Health Service, 1989:9–86.

98. (No author listed) Dangerous properties of industrials report, 1988;8:46–56.

99. Hayes W. Pesticides studies in man, Chap 2. Baltimore MD: Williams & Wilkins, 1982:75–111.

100. American hospital formulary service—drug information. American Society of Hospital Pharmacists, 1991. Bethesda, Maryland:

101. N Proctor, J Hughes, Fischman N. Chemical hazards of the workplace. 2nd ed. Philadelphia, PA: JB Lippincott, 1988.

102. Dalvi R. Toxicology of Thiram (tetramethylthiuram disulfide)—a review. Vet Hum Toxicol 1988;30:480–482.

103. Sittig M. Handbook of toxic and hazardous chemicals. Park Ridge, NJ: Noyes Publications, 1981.

104. Morbidity and Mortality Weekly Report, 1991;40:280–281.

105. Descotes J. Immunotoxicology of drugs and chemicals. New York, NJ: Elsevier, 1986.

106. Dorman D, Beasley V. Neurotoxicology of pyrethrin and the pyrethroid insecticides. Vet Hum Toxicol 1991;33:238–243.

107. Coats J. Mechanisms of toxic action of structure—activity relationships for organochlorine and synthetic pyrethroid insecticides. Environ Health Perspect 1990;87:255–262.

Ethylene Oxide

John B. Sullivan, Jr., M.D.

SOURCES, PRODUCTION, AND USES

Ethylene oxide (EtO), used widely as a gas sterilization agent, is a highly reactive biocide and fumigant. Due to its highly reactive nature, ethylene oxide is an ideal intermediate from which other chemicals are developed. It is estimated that the annual production of ethylene oxide is between 6 and 7 billion pounds, which makes it one of the most prolifically produced chemicals in the United States (1). Ethylene oxide has been produced commercially since the 1920s, and besides being a primary sterilization gas for medical equipment, it is also extensively used as an intermediate chemical in the production of other compounds such as ethylene glycol (2, 3). Over 99% of commercially produced ethylene oxide is used for manufacturing other products, and 70% is used to manufacture ethylene glycol. Ethylene oxide is also used in the production of nonionic surface active agents for detergents and industrial surfactants. Other uses include production of ethanolamines for cosmetics and detergents; glycol ethers used as coatings, fuel additives, brake fluids, inks, and coatings; diethylene and triethylene glycol used in manufacturing polyester resins, drying natural gas, emulsifiers, plasticizers, and lubricants; and polyethylene glycols (3, 4).

Less than 5% of ethylene oxide produced is used in the health care industry for sterilization purposes. For sterilization, ethylene oxide is sold in gas cylinders mixed with chlorofluorocarbons (freon) or carbon dioxide. It has also been used as a fumigant and a biocide in warehouses, granaries, and ship cargoes.

Ethylene oxide is very effective for sterilizing materials that are heat-sensitive. The vapor of ethylene oxide penetrates paper, cellophane, fabrics, rubber, polyethylene, and polyvinyl chloride and is used to sterilize surgical equipment. Ethylene oxide is used to sterilize a great variety of hospital products, including bronchoscopes, endoscopes, syringes, gloves, plastic goods such as catheters, tubing, surgical gloves, instruments, medications, implantable devices, and prosthetic devices.

Chemical Forms and Reactivity

Ethylene oxide (1,2-epoxyethane, oxirane, dihydrooxirene, dimethylene oxide) is the simplest epoxide (Fig. 105.1), C_2H_4O, with a molecular weight of 44.06. It is a clear, colorless liquid below its boiling point of 10°C, (51.3°F) and above this temperature it is a colorless gas. Ethylene oxide gas has an odor very similar to ether at around 700 ppm, which makes it easily

Ethylene Oxide

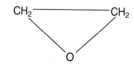

Figure 105.1. Ethylene oxide.

recognizable. It has a vapor density of 1.49 (air = 1.0), which makes it heavier than air. A 3% ethylene oxide vapor in air is combustible and can result in explosions in a confined space. It is also explosive when heated or in the presence of alkali metal hydroxides and catalytic surfaces. Dilution of ethylene oxide with 23 volumes of water renders it nonflammable. Due to the fact that it is heavier than air, ethylene oxide can disperse along the floor to ignition sources. To reduce the explosion hazard of ethylene oxide, it is mixed with inert gases such as carbon dioxide or halocarbons such as freon. Used as a sterilizing agent, it is prepared in mixtures of 10% ethylene oxide and 90% CO_2 or 12% ethylene oxide and 88% chlorofluorocarbon (freon). Ethylene oxide is readily mixable with water, alcohol, and organic solvents (3). Ethylene oxide is an alkylating agent and binds irreversibly with organic molecules such as amino acids, histidine, hemoglobin, and nucleoproteins (3). Due to its high degree of reactivity with organic molecules, it is a very effective fungicide for treatment of soil and plants (3). Ethylene oxide will violently polymerize if contaminated with aqueous alkalis, amines, mineral acids, metal oxides, and metal chlorides. Violent decomposition will occur at temperatures above 800°F. Hazardous products of decomposition are hydrochloric acid and carbon dioxide.

Ethylene oxide will also alkylate sulfhydryl groups, amino groups, carboxyl groups, and hydroxyl groups of proteins (4).

Sites, Industries, and Businesses Associated with Exposure

Persons at risk from ethylene oxide exposure are hospital sterilization workers and workers in the production and use of ethylene oxide in the chemical industry. The most commonly used mixture for cold sterilization purposes is 12% ethylene oxide and 88% freon in pressurized cylinders.

Due to the high solubility in porous plastics, residual amounts of ethylene oxide can degas from products after sterilization and constitute an exposure risk for hospital personnel (5). It is estimated that over 75,000 health care workers in the United States are exposed to ethylene oxide (1).

Given the fact that ethylene oxide is very well-controlled within the industrial environment and also due to its known flammability and explosive hazards, exposures to ethylene oxide are not that common. On the opposite extreme in the health care industry, since the use of pure ethylene oxide is not very common, exposures are probably more frequent. Exposures to health care workers occur during degassing from porous plastics as well as from residual gas from sterilization procedures (6). These exposures are usually low level, but bursts of higher ethylene oxide concentration exposures can occur upon opening sterilizer doors.

Hospital sterilization procedures require that the gas be retained in a pressurized sterilization unit long enough to penetrate all items present. The sterilization environment must be properly humidified to assist penetration of polyethylene plastic wrappings and to allow ethylene oxide gas to diffuse into small pores and cracks. Following the passage of an adequate sterilization time, the ethylene oxide gas is evacuated from the sterilizer chamber. Appropriate aeration time is necessary following sterilization procedures to allow degassing of ethylene oxide from plastic items. All plastic and rubber items must be allowed to aerate to safely release residual ethylene oxide. Removal of residual ethylene oxide from a sterilization chamber is also necessary in order to avoid exposure to workers.

Sterilizers using the 12% ethylene oxide (12/88) and 88% freon usually operate under a pressure of 10 pounds per square inch (7). Negative pressure sterilization uses 100% ethylene oxide and helps reduce risk of ethylene oxide exposure to workers (7). A negative pressure process reduces leaks around sterilizer seals, gaskets, and pressure-relief valves. Also, there is no connection valve for ethylene oxide gas to be introduced into the chamber, since the ethylene oxide cylinder is punctured once it is inside the closed unit. However, 100% ethylene oxide cylinders are a hazard, and their storage remains a problem. Also, negative pressure sterilizers do not have the capacity of the positive pressure sterilizer units. Since 100% ethylene oxide is an explosion and flammability hazard, most hospital sterilizers typically are pressurized and use the 12/88 mixture (7). The design of the sterilizer and appropriate engineering and administrative controls will determine exposure to personnel. Basic sterilizers operate through four phases (7):

1. Air evacuation, humidification, and introduction of ethylene oxide into the sterilizer chamber.
2. The dwell period in which sterilization occurs. This is usually at 130°F for 2.5 hours for non-heat-degree sensitive items and at 100°F for 5 hours for heat-degree sensitive items.
3. Evacuation of ethylene oxide from the chamber via a vacuum pump.
4. Aeration period of 12 hours to allow degassing of ethylene oxide residue from items sterilized. Depending on the sophistication of the sterilizer, some units have an aeration cycle that allows the articles to remain in the chamber, so transfer to a different area is unnecessary.

CLINICAL TOXICOLOGY OF EXPOSURE

Exposures may occur due to faulty ventilation, poor aeration of items, or faulty evacuation of ethylene oxide. Ethylene oxide is a recognized neurotoxin. Also, due to its highly reactive epoxide structure, it has mutagenic and carcinogenic potential. The health effects of ethylene oxide (Table 105.1) can be divided into the following broad categories:

1. Acute toxic effects
2. Chronic toxic effects
3. Mutagenic effects
4. Reproductive effects
5. Carcinogenic effects

Acute exposures to ethylene oxide of greater than 300 ppm in either the gas or liquid form have caused acute health effects (6). Acute exposure can result in ocular irritation, contact dermatitis, nausea, vomiting, dizziness, syncope, slurring of speech, seizures, ataxia, and acute pulmonary edema. In addition, ethylene oxide exposures of high intensity can result in neurologic manifestations. Chronic exposure can produce sensitization, which has been reported to result in type I IgE reactions (5).

Table 105.1. Ethylene Oxide Toxicity

Acute and chronic effects
  Ocular irritation and corneal injury
  Nausea
  Vomiting (periodic and prolonged)
  Dizziness
  Seizures
  Syncope
  Ataxia
  Urticaria (type I IgE)
  Contact dermatitis
  Pulmonary edema
  Pneumonitis
  Peripheral neuropathy
  Fatigue
  Nystagmus
Longterm sequelae
  Peripheral neuropathy
  Mutagenicity risk
  Carcinogenicity risk
  Hypersensitivity
  Reproductive effects
  Chromosomal aberrations
  Cataract formation
Neurotoxic effects
  Paresthesias
  Distal extremity weakness
  Peripheral neuropathy
  Neurobehavioral disturbances
  Ataxia
  Seizures

Manifestations of this include anaphylaxis, periorbital edema, facial erythema, and urticarial rashes. Dermatologic effects from ethylene oxide result from its vesicant action and ability to sensitize the skin.

Another health hazard of ethylene oxide results from the fact that it is highly explosive when mixed with air greater than 3% by volume (4). Ethylene oxide is unstable when mixed with acids or alkalis. Mixing ethylene oxide with an inert gas such as carbon dioxide or freon decreases its explosivity (4).

MANAGEMENT OF ACUTE EXPOSURE

Ethylene oxide in liquid form can produce eye injury and irritation following splash exposure. Injury to the cornea can occur. Chemical burn to the skin with blister formation can occur. Ingestion of the liquid can produce severe gastritis and hepatic damage. The liquid will easily penetrate rubber, leather, and other clothing.

Ocular Exposure Eyes should be flush immediately with copious amounts of water. Contact lenses should not be worn when working with ethylene oxide. Ocular exams should include evaluation of cornea and adjacent tissue for injury.

Dermal Exposure The site should be washed immediately with copious amounts of water. All contaminated clothing should be removed. Contaminated leather shoes or other leather articles must be discarded. Skin should be examined for burns, erythema, and blisters which may not be seen for 6–12 hours. Dermal exposure should be treated as a chemical burn. Bleb formation may occur with desquamation. Healing takes about 3–4 weeks. Injury areas may show residual brown pigmentation for weeks to months. Pure liquid ethylene oxide can produce frostbite.

Inhalation Exposure The patient should be moved to an area of fresh air and adequate ventilation. Medical management is symptomatic care. Syncope, seizures, pulmonary insult, and dermal and ocular injury should be considered. Seizures and pulmonary edema can occur. Clothing may be contaminated and should be removed.

Ingestion Ethylene oxide liquid ingestion will produce gastrointestinal distress with vomiting. Management is symptomatic.

The earliest effects of acute exposure are eye irritation, nausea, vomiting, and headache. The ether-like odor is not detectable until around 700 ppm, an extremely high exposure level. Thus, noticing the odor indicates a potentially serious toxic exposure. The next symptoms to appear are respiratory irritation, and if the exposure is high enough, pulmonary edema can follow. Syncope and seizures can also occur. Delayed symptoms include ataxia, fatigue, and weakness.

Neurotoxicity

Ethylene oxide is an established peripheral neurotoxin. Ethylene oxide impairs both sensory and motor function and can result in muscular atrophy. Human cases of peripheral neuropathy have been described.

Seizures, coma, respiratory failure, and vomiting were observed in animals as an effect of ethylene oxide in concentrations ranging from 200–700 ppm (8). Repeated exposures of animals to ethylene oxide also resulted in peripheral neuropathies affecting lumbosacral nerves (8). In most animal species studied, the range of ethylene oxide concentrations that produced neurotoxic effects was 100–200 ppm (8). Other neurologic manifestations include fatigue, dizziness, syncope, convulsions, and behavioral disturbances (8).

Vomiting may be periodic, occurring about every 30 minutes following an acute exposure (8). The vomiting and nausea can be prolonged and last for days. Following an acute exposure to ethylene oxide, coma and somnolence can occur. These symptoms can all occur from exposures to very high concentrations of the vapor or of the liquid in confined spaces (8). Ethylene oxide has a distinctive ether-like odor and can be detected in confined environments at around 700 ppm. The signs and symptoms that have been described would occur at concentrations of several hundred ppm (8).

Repeated exposures to ethylene oxide can result in symptoms similar to acute exposures: headache, dizziness, vomiting, nausea, ocular irritation, respiratory irritation, fatigue, nystagmus, ataxia, and slurred speech (8). Nerve biopsies on individuals with peripheral neuropathy following ethylene oxide exposure have demonstrated axonal degeneration (8). Exposure to ethylene oxide on a repeated basis can also produce certain behavioral effects such as disorientation, aggression, and some irrational behavior (8, 9). A report of cognitive changes associated with chronic ethylene oxide exposure to workers demonstrated impaired memory, increased irritability, clumsiness, and episodes of falling (9). Following cessation of exposure, these symptoms improved over a period of months but did not disappear. Environmental monitoring in this report indicated an ethylene oxide average concentration of 2.4 ppm (9). Ethylene oxide concentrations adjacent to the sterilizing area where the individual worked were 4.2 ppm (9).

Other studies of health care workers chronically exposed to ethylene oxide in normal sterilization operations indicate the occurrence of neuropsychologic effects and cognitive disorders (10, 11). These employees had detected the odor of ethylene oxide during operations of equipment, and ethylene oxide air concentrations had not been routinely monitored (10, 11). Sampling in breathing zones demonstrated concentrations of 15 ppm during these operations and up to 250 ppm in breathing zone areas for some locations during other monitoring periods (10, 11). These studies indicated that low level exposure to ethylene oxide can result in dysfunctional personality and cognitive disorders.

Peripheral neuropathy can occur following prolonged exposure to ethylene oxide and is associated with paresthesias of the distal extremities, weakness of the distal extremities, and fatigue (4). The peripheral neuropathy is also associated with decreased pinprick in fingers and toes and decreased vibratory sensation. Nerve conduction studies have been consistent with sensorimotor polyneuropathies (4). Neuropathies can occur following chronic exposure to ethylene oxide or after a one-time acute exposure. Due to its multiple health risk from ethylene oxide, the Occupational Safety and Health Administration (OSHA) in 1984 lowered the exposure standard from 50 to 1 ppm, with an action level of 0.5 ppm based on an 8-hour time-weighted average (TWA). In 1988, OSHA added an excursion limit of 5 ppm averaged over 15 minutes.

CHRONIC AND LONGTERM EFFECTS

The chronic and longterm effects of ethylene oxide are mainly neurologic manifestations. Mutagenicity, reproductive toxicity, and carcinogenicity are possible. The extreme reactivity of ethylene oxide with nucleoproteins and amino acids gives it carcinogenic and mutagenic potential (3).

Carcinogenicity

Animal studies have demonstrated that ethylene oxide is a carcinogen at levels below 50 ppm (1). Incidences of mononuclear cell leukemia were significantly increased in a dose-related fashion in female rats exposed to ethylene oxide (1). In male rats, the frequency of mononuclear cell leukemia, peritoneal mesothelioma, and cerebral glioma increased in a dose-related fashion (1).

Mortality studies in ethylene oxide production workers have not been able to conclude beyond doubt that ethylene oxide exposure was associated with human malignancies; however, it is considered a suspect as a cause of malignancies. A study of ethylene oxide production workers in Sweden was conducted from 1961 through 1977 (2). These workers had variable exposures to ethylene oxide depending on where they were employed in the production facility. It is important to realize that ethylene oxide wsas not the only potential exposure agent for these workers. Other chemical exposures occurred through the production of ethylene oxide by a chlorohydrin process which started with ethylene and produced ethylene chlorohydrin as a intermediate (2). Ethylene dichloride and bis(2-chloroethyl)ether were byproducts of the process and are carcinogens. Ethylene chlorohydrin is also a mutgen. This study found an excess of malignancies, which included leukemia and gastrointestinal tumors (2). However, multiple exposures to other chemicals were also occurring.

Another epidemiologic study from 1979 suggested that ethylene oxide was associated with an excess of hemopoietic cancers in Swedish workers (6). There were two incidences of leukemia reported out of 230 workers in this study and an earlier report of two incidences of leukemia out of 241 ethylene oxide production workers who were followed from 1960–1977 (6). A recent updating of this cohort included the reporting of a third group of 355 production workers in which a few more cases of leukemia were reported (6). In contrast to these Swedish reports, other studies in larger groups found no excess leukemia deaths among workers potentially exposed to ethylene oxide.

Due to the earlier reports that linked risk of leukemia with ethylene oxide exposure, another mortality study was published in 1981 which examined 767 men with a 5-year exposure history to ethylene oxide in a production plant from 1955–1977 (12). There were no deaths from leukemia observed, nor were there any significant excesses of mortality compared with the general population (12). This 1981 study did show an excess death rate from pancreatic cancer and Hodgkin's disease. In 1986, Hogstedt et al. published a mortality incidence of cancer in 733 ethylene oxide-exposed workers (13). They reported eight cases of leukemia that occurred among these workers and six cases of stomach cancer. They surmised that this study indicated a relationship between low level ethylene oxide exposure and cancer (12).

Animal studies have shown ethylene oxide to be a carcinogen by any route of administration and in multiple species of animals. Leukemia, brain cancer, and mesothelioma have been induced in animals in inhalational studies. When added to the human epidemiologic studies, ethylene oxide is suspected to have the potential to cause hemopoietic cancers as well as cancer in other organs in humans. The International Agency for Research on Cancer (IARC) has issued a statement that ethylene oxide is probably carcinogenic to humans.

Mutagenicity

Ethylene oxide is a mutagen for bacteria and human lymphocytes and produces chromosome damage in both experimental animals and humans (1). Unscheduled DNA synthesis, a measure of the repair of DNA damage, in germinal cells is increased with increasing doses of ethylene oxide in mice exposed to 300 or 500 ppm for 8 hours a day, 5 days a week, for 1 week (14). Studies of humans experiencing symptoms of ethylene oxide exposure have shown increased chromosomal aberrations. The frequency of sister chromatid exchanges and chromosomal aberrations has been studied in animals exposed to ethylene oxide as well as in humans (1). The frequency of sister chromatid exchanges is an indication of chromosomal damage and was found to increase in a dose-related fashion. In animals exposed to 50 ppm, this occurred 1.8 times more frequently than in the unexposed controls (1). In those animals exposed to 100 ppm, the sister chromatid exchange was 3.1 times more frequent than the controls (1). These studies have indicated that chromosomal changes from ethylene oxide exposure were dose-related. The frequency of sister chromatid exchange also has been found to increase with duration of exposure (2).

Due to the fact that ethylene oxide is a strong alkylating agent, mutagenicity and chromosomal damage studies have been conducted following human exposures (15, 16). Sister chromatid exchange (SCE) has been investigated as a tool to detect potential mutagenicity. SCE is the visual manifestation of a four-stranded exchange in the DNA. The number of such exchanges in chromosomes is a measure of exposure to an agent that produces damage to DNA through formation of covalent adducts or disturbing the bases. Increases in SCEs may

Table 105.2.   Reproductive and Mutagenic Toxicity of Ethylene Oxide

Unscheduled DNA synthesis
Sister chromatid exchange
Chromosomal aberrations
Functional sperm abnormalities
Spontaneous abortions

occur following exposure to mutagens and/or carcinogens SCEs are not accepted as absolute quantitations or predictors of health effects, but are a useful tool to probe potential health problems. Individuals working in sterilization areas of hospitals were monitored for SCE in lymphocytes cultured from individuals compared with controls (15). Environmental monitoring of the worksite of these individuals showed concentrations of ethylene oxide in the air of 36 ppm (15). Concentrations of ethylene oxide as low as 50 ppm in ambient air for 4 hours have been shown to produce mutagenic effects in mice (15, 16). For individuals who developed mild symptomatology secondary to ethylene oxide in the workplace, there was demonstrated chromosomal damage via increased SCE which persisted as long as 8 weeks after the last known exposure to ethylene oxide (15). In health care workers exposed to ethylene oxide, it has been observed that a statistically significant increase in SCEs occurred in workers in sterilizing areas who were most heavily exposed (15). These studies were controlled for age and smoking. In this study, subjects were divided into low and high exposure groups. The workers were exposed to ethylene oxide for brief periods, but those with the highest exposure had a significant increase in mean SCE per lymphocyte (15).

Another assessment of the mutagenicity of ethylene oxide was conducted in factory workers exposed to ethylene oxide at concentrations of 0.5–1 ppm (17). In this study, ethylene oxide was shown to significantly elevate unscheduled DNA synthesis as well as increase chromosomal aberrations in peripheral lymphocytes (17).

Reproductive Effects

Ethylene oxide has been shown to be a reproductive toxin in male and female animals (1). It induces dominant chromosomal lethal mutations in germinal cells. Experimental studies have indicated that ethylene oxide has had no adverse effects on reproduction in animals exposed to 100 ppm (3). Ethylene oxide exposure of hospital staff has also been related to an increased incidence of spontaneous abortions (1, 18). Compared with control subjects there was a 16.7% frequency for the exposed individuals and a 5.6% frequency for the nonexposed individuals in terms of spontaneous abortions. Animal and human studies demonstrating chromosomal mutations and spontaneous abortions corroborate the reproductive toxicity of ethylene oxide. Table 105.2 summarizes mutagenic and reproductive effects.

Dermatotoxicity

Dermal effects following ethylene oxide exposure include burns, blistering, vesicle formation, contact dermatitis, and allergic urticarial rashes.

Dermal contact with ethylene oxide has resulted in vesicular eruptions in workers who are exposed to 1% ethylene oxide in water (19). Patch testing with ethylene oxide demonstrated a delayed hypersensitivity reaction to approximately 100 ppm of ethylene oxide (19). The most common dermal reaction to ethylene oxide gas is a severe irritant reaction or burn with vesicular eruptions occurring in 6–12 hours.

Solutions of ethylene oxide have vesicant actions and can produce injury to the eye or skin on contact. Dermal irritation and burns occur most likely when the solution is in contact with the skin through clothing (20). Repeated exposures to ethylene oxide can result in a delayed allergic contact dermatitis (20).

Sterilized items can retain ethylene oxide residues that may produce effects via direct skin contact or from off gassing. Adequate aeration of sterilized items is imperative to ensure that residues of ethylene oxide do not come into human contact (20).

ENVIRONMENTAL MONITORING AND REGULATION

In 1984, OSHA established a permissible exposure limit (PEL) to ethylene oxide of 1 ppm for an 8-hour time-weighted average (TWA) and an action level of 0.5 ppm for an 8-hour TWA (14). This 1984 standard provided for methods of exposure control, monitoring of employee exposures, personal protrective measures, record keeping, signs and labels, medical surveillance, and emergency procedures (14). Reducing the exposure standard to 1 ppm decreased the risk to workers over the previous 50-ppm standard. The action level of 0.5 ppm was established as the level above which employers must initiate certain activities to protect and monitor workers as set forth in the OSHA ruling (14).

The reduction of the PEL from 50 to 1 ppm by OSHA was based on risk assessment studies which concluded that an excess cancer risk existed at the 50-ppm TWA for occupational exposures. By reducing the PEL to 1 ppm OSHA concluded that there would be a 98% reduction in cancer mortality risk (14).

In 1988, OSHA issued regulations adopting a short term exposure limit (STEL) of 5 ppm averaged over a sampling period of 15 minutes (21). This new regulation also established exposure monitoring and training programs for workers where exposure exceeded this 5-ppm STEL. The new ruling also required warning signs on products capable of releasing ethylene oxide to the extent that an employee may be exposed above the STEL as well as having those exposure areas identified as regulated (21). In the 1988 ruling, OSHA addressed the health effects of employees whose 8-hour TWA never exceeded 1 ppm but yet could be exposed to several short term releases of ethylene oxide which exceeded 5 ppm. Establishing such an excursion limit would further reduce the dose of ethylene oxide and consequently the cancer risk (14). Workers at risk for violation of this excursion limit are engaged in such activities as sterilizer loading and unloading, changing ethylene oxide tanks or sterilizer equipment, collecting samples from ethylene oxide processes, and disconnecting piping from a railroad tank car (21).

These types of activities might expose an employee to high shortterm concentrations of ethylene oxide. Due to this fact, OSHA requires monitoring of employees for potential shortterm exposure whose activities are associated with operations that are most likely to produce exposures above the 5-ppm excursion limit for each work shift, for each job classification in each work area (21). The final regulatory limits on ethylene oxide are summarized in Table 105.3.

OSHA also set forth required monitoring of ethylene oxide exposure to workers (Table 105.4). These monitoring requirements are based on the combination of scenarios involving the PEL based on an 8-hour TWA, the action level, and the excursion limit (21). According to OSHA, the action level of 0.5-ppm TWA largely determines monitoring requirements.

HUMAN EXPOSURE SITUATIONS

Exposure to ethylene oxide occurs mainly to health care workers who perform job-related sterilization procedures. Exposure scenarios include the following (7):

High level, acute exposure to several hundred or thousand ppm This could occur secondary to a sudden release from an ethylene oxide cylinder. Each cylinder may contain from 100 to several thousand grams of ethylene oxide. Releases can occur at cylinder connecting points or during the process of connecting to supply lines or from accidents. Ethylene oxide cylinders commonly used contain 12% ethylene oxide mixed with 88% freon. High level exposure to sterilizer workers may also occur from leaks around sterilizer gaskets in pressurized procedures or from faulty pressure relief valves during purging from sterilizer chambers.

Exposures that meet or exceed the excursion limit of 5 ppm Opening the sterilizer door at the completion of the sterilization process can expose a worker to air concentrations that meet or exceed the excursion limit of ethylene oxide. There

Table 105.3. OSHA Regulations Regarding Ethylene Oxide

1-ppm 8-hour TWA 0.5-ppm 8-hour TWA action level	OSHA 1984
5-ppm excursion limit determined as a 15-minute TWA	OSHA 1988

Table 105.4. Ethylene Oxide Monitoring Requirements of OSHA, 1988

Exposure	Required Monitoring
Below action level and at or below the excursion limit	No monitoring required
Below action level and above excursion limit	Monitor STEL 4 times per year; no TWA monitoring required
At or above level, at or below the TWA, and at or below the excursion limit	Monitor TWA exposures 2 times per year
At or above the action level, at or below the TWA, and above the excurstion limit	Monitor TWA exposures 2 times per year and monitor STEL 4 times per year
Above the TWA and at or below the excursion limit	Monitor TWA exposures 4 times per year
Above the TWA and above the excursion limit	Monitor TWA exposures 4 times per year; monitor excursion limit exposures 4 times per year

Adapted from Code of Federal Regulations. 29 CFR Part 1910. Fed Reg April 6, 1988; 53:66.

is normally an evacuation cycle that helps eliminate residual ethylene oxide; however, despite this cycle, some ethylene oxide usually remains (7). Escape of the hot gases into the room after the sterilization door is opened can diffuse ethylene oxide throughout the room. Local exhaust ventilation usually helps eliminate excess ethylene oxide gas. Normally, the residual ethylene oxide is removed from the sterilizer via a vacuum pump and release into a sewer drain. Plumbing codes require an air gap at this discharge point to prevent siphoning of liquid back up into the drainage system (7). This plumbing gap is a point of exposure of gas back into the atmosphere of the surrounding area (7). This can be a significant source of exposure. Residual ethylene oxide degasses from sterilized products, particularly plastics. Removal of these products from the sterilizer and transporting the load to the aerator is another source of exposure that can exceed or meet the excursion limit.

Exposure to a few parts per million that might meet or exceed the TWA This type of exposure scenario is the most common and results from opening sterilizer doors, transporting degassing sterilized items, and cleaning the inside of the sterilizer (7). Opening the sterilizer door is probably the source of greatest exposure risk.

EXPOSURE CONTROL

OSHA regulates occupational exposure of ethylene oxide using permissible exposure limits, required monitoring, engineering, and work practice controls (Tables 105.3 and 105.4). The OSHA PEL is 1-ppm (8-hour TWA) 0.5 action level (8-hour TWA) and a 5-ppm excursion limit.

All employees exposed to ethylene oxide must be monitored, and access to areas using ethylene oxide must be restricted to authorized personnel. In addition, an emergency warning system must be in place to warn employees of sudden ethylene oxide releases.

OSHA requires hazard warning signs and labels to be on an ethylene oxide cylinders and in areas where ethylene oxide exposure may occur. Regulated areas must be demarcated by posting a sign with the legend (14):

Danger
Ethylene Oxide
Cancer Hazard and Reproductive Hazard
Authorized Personnel Only
Respirators and Protective Clothing May Be
Required to Be Worn in This Area

The intent of OSHA is to warn employees who may not know that they are entering an area that is regulated and where exposure to ethylene oxide may exceed the permissible exposure limit. Warning signs are also necessary in area where there may be temporary exposure hazards, such as in times of maintenance or equipment repair where ethylene oxide leak could occur. OSHA also requires that ethylene oxide cylinders contain the warning label (14):

Caution
Contains Ethylene Oxide
Cancer and Reproductive Hazard

The use of personal protective devices such as respirators and special clothing is also required by OSHA to limit exposures for the following situations (14):

1. During intervals required to install or implement engineering and work practice controls;

2. In work operations such as maintenance and repair activities and chamber cleaning and in other situations where work practice controls are not feasible;
3. In situations where work practice controls are not sufficient to reduce exposures to or below permissible exposure limits or excursion limits;
4. In emergency situations.

Emergency warning alarms are required to alert employees when there is an unexpected, significant release of ethylene oxide into the environment. OSHA does not define such an emergency release beyond this. Presumably, such a release would be sudden and unexpected and would violate permissible exposure limits.

One of the primary methods to control ethylene oxide exposure is through ventilation. Local exhaust ventilation should be placed at certain points that best control releases of the gas into the work environment such as above sterilizer doors and at drain sites. Adequately functioning door and drain ventilations are critical to controlling employee exposure to gas releases during sterilizer operations. Cylinders should be stored under a ventilation hood.

Ethylene oxide odors are detected at air concentrations around 700 ppm, so odor detection indicates a high level exposure. Ten nonrecirculating air exchanges per hour is standard for ethylene oxide areas. Respiratory protection is required for cylinder or filter changing or in maintenance areas. The goal of OSHA's standard is to control emission sources and use respiratory protection as secondary protective means. OSHA requires employers to provide respirators to employees at no cost. Proper instruction and respirator fit testing are essential to provide maximum protection against ethylene oxide by the National Institute of Occupational Safety and Health (NIOSH) and the Mine Safety and Health Administration (MSHA).

Protective clothing is required in areas where eye or skin contact with gas or liquid might occur. A written emergency plan must also be developed for the workplace. Regulations regarding ethylene oxide control are detailed in 29 CFR part 1910, Occupational Exposure to Ethylene Oxide, Final Standard, Part II, *Federal Register* vol 49, No 122, June 22, 1984 (14).

Personal Protection

Ethylene oxide exposure is reduced by the use of technical and engineering controls. However, employers may be required to wear respirators at times and in certain exposure situations. Only air supplied positive pressure, full face piece respirators are approved for protection against ethylene oxide and then must have joint approval by NIOSH and MSHA (14).

Since ethylene oxide's odor is detectable at concentrations well above its permissible exposure limits, detecting the odor indicates a potentially high level exposure. Impermeable clothing may be required such as gloves, garments, and face shields. Splashproof eye protection is required in areas where ethylene oxide liquid is used or stored.

Ethylene oxide is a flammable liquid, and vapors can be explosive when mixed with air. Cylinders must be stored in cool, well-ventilated areas away from ignition sources, oxidizers, alkalis, acids, and acetylide-forming metals such as copper, silver, mercury, and their alloys. Protective clothing which becomes wet with liquid ethylene oxide may be a flammable hazard and ignite. Any clothes splashed with ethylene oxide should be immediately removed under a shower.

Medical Surveillance

Employers are required by OSHA standards to have a medical surveillance program for all employees who are or will be exposed to ethylene oxide at or above the action level (0.5 ppm TWA) for at least 30 days per year without regard to respirator use (OSHA, 1984). All medical evaluations must be performed by or under the supervision of a licensed physician. OSHA requires inclusion of the following in the medical surveillance program (14):

1. Medical and work histories with special emphasis directed to symptoms related to the pulmonary, hematologic, neurologic, and reproductive systems and to the eyes and skin;
2. Physical examination with particular emphasis given to the pulmonary, hematologic, neurologic, and reproductive systems and to the eyes and skin;
3. Complete blood count to include at least a white cell count (including differential cell count), red cell count, hematocrit, and hemoglobin;
4. Any laboratory or other test which the examining physician deems necessary by sound medical practice.

If requested by the employee, the medical examinations shall include pregnancy testing or laboratory evaluation of fertility as deemed appropriate by the physician.

In certain cases, to provide sound medical advice to the employer and the employee, the physician must evaluate situations not directly related to ethylene oxide. For example, employees with skin diseases may be unable to tolerate wearing protective clothing. In addition, those with chronic respiratory diseases may not tolerate the wearing of negative pressure (air-purifying) respirators. Additional tests and procedures that will help the physician determine which employees are medically unable to wear such respirators should include an evaluation of cardiovascular function; a baseline chest x-ray to be repeated at 5-year intervals and a pulmonary function test to be repeated every 3 years. The pulmonary function test should include measurement of the employee's forced vital capacity (FVC), forced expiratory volume at 1 second (FEV_1), as well as calculation of the ratios of FEV_1 to FVC, and measured FVC and measured FEV_1 to expected values corrected for variation due to age, sex, race, and height.

The employer is required to make the prescribed tests available at least annually to employees who are or will be exposed at or above the action level for 30 or more days per year, more often than specified if recommended by the examining physician, and upon the employee's termination of employment or reassignment to another work area. While little is known about the longterm consequences of high of high shortterm exposures, it appears prudent to monitor such affected employees closely in light of existing health data. The employer shall provide physician-recommended examinations to any employee exposed in emergency condition. Likewise, the employer shall make available medical consultations including physician-recommended exams to employees who believe they are suffering signs or symptoms of exposure to ethylene oxide.

The employer is required to provide the physician with the following information: a copy of this standard and its appendices; a description of the affected employee's duties as they relate to the employee exposure level; and information from the employee's previous medical examinations which is not readily available to the examining physician. Making this information available to the physician will aid in the evaluation of the employee's health in relation to assigned duties and fitness to wear personal protective equipment when required.

The employer is required to obtain a written opinion from the examining physician containing the results of the medical examinations; the physician's opinion as to whether the employee has any detected medical conditions which would place the employee at increased risk of material impairment of his or her health from exposure to ethylene oxide; any recommended restrictions upon the employee's exposure to ethylene oxide, or upon the use of protective clothing or equipment such as respirators; and a statement that the employee has been informed by the physician of the results of the medical examination and of any medical conditions which require further explanation or treatment. This written opinion must not reveal specific findings or diagnoses unrelated to occupational exposure to ethylene oxide, and a copy of the opinion must be provided to the affected employee.

The purpose in requiring the examining physician to supply the employer with a written opinion is to provide the employer with a medical basis to aid in the determination of initial placement of employees and to assess the employee's ability to use protective clothing and equipment.

OSHA requires that the hazards of ethylene oxide exposure be communicated to the employee. This is accomplished via (a) warning labels and warning signs in designated areas and attached to ethylene oxide cylinders, (b) material safety data sheets, and (c) training and information for employees exposed at or above the action level of 0.5 ppm TWA. This training and information must be provided annually and must include an explanation of the OSHA ethylene oxide standard as well as the health hazards of ethylene oxide.

The OSHA standard requires accurate records to be kept regarding employee exposures as well as the personal monitoring data, equipment used, and methods. These records must be accessible to employees upon request. Employees are required to retain employee medical records and exposure records for period of employment plus 30 years.

Personal Monitoring

Monitoring of employees' exposure to ethylene oxide is mandatory. Sampling frequencies are guided by the information in Table 105.4. Environmental monitoring must be performed initially to assess typical exposure concentrations for each work shift (7). Two types of monitoring are available: active sampling of air concentrations and personal passive dosimetry (7).

Active sampling includes charcoal tube adsorption, gas sampling bags, impingers, and detector tubes. There are also portable ethylene oxide gas analyzers. Descriptions of sampling methods are included in the OSHA standards (14).

The purpose of environmental monitoring is to accurately portray typical workplace exposures. This requires sampling workers with highest exposure risks (7). All monitoring, active and passive, must meet OSHA's accuracy requirements of ±25% at 1 ppm and ±35% below 1 ppm (7). Passive monitoring is performed by personal dosimetry badges worn by employees. These badges are designed to indicate the amount of ethylene oxide absorbed when they are developed. Personal dosimeters have an advantage over active sampling in terms of cost and reduced complexity (22). However, there have been conflicting data regarding the ability of passive dosimetry to accurately meet OSHA's regulations of 1-ppm PEL and 0.5-ppm action levels (23). Passive dosimeters that meet OSHA's monitoring standards have been developed (23). Errors in passive dosimetry monitoring can occur due to interference when the dosimetry is worn in direct sunlight. Dosimeters also must be worn for 8 hours before being analyzed to obtain accurate measurements (23). Also, the capacity of the dosimeter can be exceeded by concentrations of ethylene oxide greater than 9.9 ppm (23).

REFERENCES

1. Landrigan PJ, Meinhardt TJ, Gordon J, et al. Ethylene oxide: An overview of toxicologic and epidemiologic research. Am J Ind Med 1984;6:103–115.
2. Hogstedt C, Rohlen O, Berndtsson BS, Axelson O, Ehrenberg L. A cohort study of mortality and cancer incidence in ethylene oxide production workers. Br J Ind Med 1979;36:276–280.
3. Sheikh K. Adverse health effects of ethylene oxide and occupational exposure limits. Am J Ind Med 1984;6:117–127.
4. Gross JA, Haas ML, Swift TR. Ethylene oxide neurotoxicity: report of four cases and review of the literature. Neurology 1979;29:978–983.
5. Leitman SF, Boltansky H, Alter HJ, Pearson FC, Kaliner MA. Allergic reactions in healthy plateletpheresis donors caused by sensitization to ethylene oxide gas. N Engl J Med 1986;315:1192–1196.
6. Austin SG, Sielken RL. Issues in assessing the carcinogenic hazards of ethylene oxide. J Occ Med 1988;30:236–245.
7. Ethylene Oxide Control Technology I: Occupational Exposure. Healthcare Hazardous Materials Management, Plymouth Meeting, PA, Vol 3, September 1990.
8. Golberg L, Phil D. Neuropharmacologic and neurotoxic effects Chapt 5 in: Golberg, Phil D., eds. Hazard assessment of ethylene oxide. Boca Raton, FL: CRC Press.
9. Crystal HA, Schaumburg HH, Grober E, Fuld PA, Lipton RB. Cognitive impairment and sensory loss associated with chronic low-level ethylene oxide exposure. Neurology 1988;38:567–569.
10. Estrin WJ, Bowler RM, Lash A, Becker CE. Neurotoxicological evaluation of hospital sterilizer workers exposed to ethylene oxide. J Toxiol Clin Toxicol 1990;28:1–20.
11. Klees JE, Lash A, Bowler RM, Shore M, Becker CE. Neuropsychologic "impairment" in a cohort of hospital workers chronically exposed to ethylene oxide. J Toxicol Clin Toxicol 1990;28:21–28.
12. Morgan RW, Claxton KW, Divine BJ, Kaplan SD, Harris VB. Mortality among ethylene oxide workers. J Occup Med 1981;23:767–770
13. Hogstedt C, Aringer L, Gustavsson A. Epidemiologic support for ethylene oxide as a cancer-causing agent JAMA 1986;255:1575–1578.
14. Code of Federal Regulations. Occupational exposure to ethylene oxide; final standard. 29 CFR Part 1910. Fed Reg, June 22, 1984;49:122.
15. Yager J, Hines C, Spear R. Exposure to ethylene oxide at work increases sister chromatid exchanges in human peripheral lymphocytes. Science 1983;219:1221–1223.
16. Garry VF, Hozier J, Jacobs D, Wade RL, Gray DG. Ethylene oxide: evidence of human chromosomal effects. Environ Mol Mutagen 1979;1:375–382.
17. Pero RW, Widegren B, Hogstedt B, Mitelman F. In vivo and in vitro ethylene oxide exposure of human lymphocytes assessed by chemical stimulation of unscheduled DNA synthesis. Mutat Res 1981;83:271–289.
18. Hemminki K, Mutanen P, Saloniemi I, Niemi ML, Vainio H. Spontaneous abortions in hospital staff engaged in sterilizing instruments with chemical agents. Br Med J 1982;285:1461–1463.
19. Shupack JL, Anderson SR, Romano SJ. Human skin reactions to ethylene oxide. J Lab Clin Med 1981;98:723–729.
20. Taylor JS. Dermatologic hazards from ethylene oxide. Cutis 1977;19:189–192.
21. Code of Federal Regulations. Occupational exposure to ethylene oxide; final standard. 29 CFR Part 1910. Fed Reg, April 6, 1988;53:66.
22. Puskar MA, Hecker LH. Field validation of passive dosimeters for determination of employee exposures to ethylene oxide in hospital product sterilization facilities. Am Ind Hyg Assoc J 1989;50:30–36.
23. Puskar MA, Nowak JL, Hecker LH. Generation of ethylene oxide permissible exposuure limit data with on-site sample analysis using the EO self-scan passive monitor. Am Ind Hyg Assoc J 1990;51:273–279.

106

Alkylbenzene Solvents and Aromatic Compounds

John B. Sullivan, Jr., M.D.
Mark Van Ert, Ph.D., C.I.H.

CHARACTERISTICS OF SOLVENTS

Organic solvents are volatile compounds used to dissolve other materials. They are divided into two general classes: aromatic and aliphatic. Most aromatic solvents are benzene derivatives with attached alkyl or hydroxy groups. These compounds have low boiling points that increase with increasing molecular weight, are less dense than water, and are generally not very water soluble. They are used as starting chemicals or intermediate chemicals for synthesis of other compounds. Common aromatic solvents are: toluene, xylene, styrene, phenol, and ethylbenzene (Fig. 106.1). Other less commonly recognized aromatic compounds are alkyl derivatives of benzene, halogenated benzene, dihydroxy benzenes, and naphthalenes (Fig. 106.2). Exposure to solvents occurs through contact of vapor or liquid. The most common routes of absorption are dermal and pulmonary. Aromatic solvents are used in paints, chemical manufacturing, resins, pharmaceutical industry, printing glue and adhesives, metal degreasing, electronics, and rubber manufacturing. Large groups of workers are exposed to aromatic solvents.

Organic compounds with desirable solvent characteristics must also be inexpensive to produce, since they are so widely used. At atmospheric pressure they should have a boiling point not much lower than 0°C or higher than 200°C. If the boiling point of a solvent is too high and the vapor pressure too low, the solvent would be difficult to separate from the material it is dissolving. Most organic solvents are liquid at room temperature.

The aromatic solvents in general, as well as other hydrocarbon solvents, lack chemical reactivity as a prerequisite for their commercial and practical use. Solvents as a group include aromatic and aliphatic halogenated hydrocarbons, aliphatic hydrocarbons, oxygenated compounds such as alcohols, ketones, esters, ethers, and glycols. Solvent exposure occurs in a multiplicity of industries, particularly those that deal with painting, glueing, degreasing, cleaning, petroleum refining, and rubber and polymer manufacturing.

The alkylbenzenes, along with benzene, are the starting source of most other aromatic compounds. Basic aromatic compounds are derived from coal and petroleum. When coal is heated in the absence of air it is broken down into volatile compounds consisting of coal gas and coal tar. The residue of this process is termed coke. The distillation of coal tar results in the production of a number of aromatic compounds such as benzene, toluene, xylenes, phenols, cresols, and naphthalene. In addition, these aromatic compounds can be produced by catalytic reforming which employs aliphatic hydrocarbons at high temperatures and high pressures to dehydrogenate and form cyclic structures of the aromatic hydrocarbons.

The common aromatic solvents are generally characterized by nonpolarity and high lipid solubility. Organic solvents such as xylene and ethylbenzene are frequently used in combinations. Many of these solvent combinations contain toluene as well as other solvents such as ketones, glycols, and alcohols. Solvent mixtures are commonly used in the production of paints, varnishes, glues, and inks. Styrene is used in the production of styrene polymers and plastics (1). Naphthalene, not a solvent, is a white crystalline solid used as a repellant for moths and is a commonly used aromatic compound that easily volatilizes.

Solvent Vapor Pressure and Health Hazards

The concept of the vapor pressure of a solvent as it relates to hazards and toxic health effects is important. The vapor pressure of a solvent is directly related to its airborne concentration and to its toxic hazard and human exposure. Vapor pressure is the force per unit area exerted by molecules of a vapor that is in equilibrium with a liquid or solid (2). Vapor pressure is expressed in terms of mm Hg in relation to atmospheric pressure (1 ATM = 760 mm Hg). The vapor pressure of a solvent is also directly related to its economical use because of volatilization loss. The toxic hazard of an organic solvent is dependent on its vapor pressure and its intrinsic chemical properties. The vapor pressure directly relates to the concentration of solvent in the breathing zone of exposed individuals.

The vapor pressure of a solvents obeys the same physical laws as other gases:

$Pv = nRt/V$
$Pv =$ vapor pressure (mm Hg)

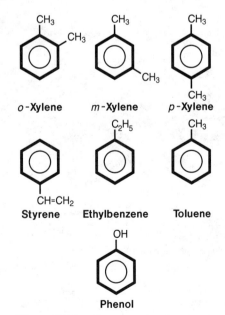

Figure 106.1. Common aromatic solvents.

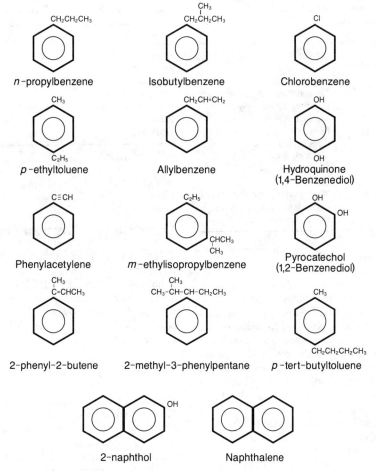

Figure 106.2.   Other alkylbenzenes and aromatic compounds.

n = moles
V = gas volume (M^3)
R = gas constant (6.236×10^{-5})
t = absolute gas temperature in K°

Rearrangement of this formula yields an equation that allows the calculation of the vapor concentration from the vapor pressure of a gas (vapor) that is in an equilibrium state:

Pv = nRt/V = CRt/Mw = (x)(ATM)(2×10^{-6})
C = concentration (mg/m^3)
Mw = molecular weight
X = concentration in ppm
ATM = 760 mm Hg

The vapor hazard ratio of solvents can be compared by this method in order to help determine potential of human exposure. The formula expresses the vapor pressure in terms of an equilibrium state, or worst case scenario, as would be achieved in a closed environment. Solvents or chemicals with the same threshold limit value (TLV) may present two distinctly different health hazards due to their different vapor pressures. An example of this hazard assessment with two related chemicals is as follows:

Chemical A   TLV = 0.02
              Vapor pressure = 0.00014 at 25°C

Chemical B   TLV = 0.02
              Vapor pressure = 0.00001 at 25°C

Rearranging this equation allows for a calculation of the vapor concentration in ppm of a vapor in an equilibrium state (Vpeq):

$$Vpeq = \frac{(pv) \times (1 \times 10^6)}{ATM}$$

The equilibrium vapor pressure, as calculated using the above formula, can be used to calculate a vapor hazard ratio (VHR):

$$VHR = \frac{Equilibrium\ vapor\ pressure\ (ppm)}{Threshold\ limit\ value\ (ppm)}$$

The greater the vapor hazard ratio, the greater the potential hazard for inhalation and dermal contact (1).

$$Vpeq\ (Chemical\ A) = \frac{(1.4 \times 10^{-4})\ (1 \times 10^6)}{760\ mm\ Hg} = 0.184\ ppm$$

$$Vpeq\ (Chemical\ B) = \frac{(1 \times 10^{-5})\ (1 \times 10^6)}{760\ mm\ Hg} = 0.0132\ ppm$$

$$Chemical\ A\ VHR = \frac{0.184\ ppm}{0.002\ ppm} = 92$$

$$Chemical\ B\ VHR = \frac{0.0132\ ppm}{0.002\ ppm} = 6.6$$

Chemical B would present much less of a hazard than chemical A in terms of vapor exposure. Also, chemical B would have a lower air concentration than its TLV.

Table 106.1.   Summary of Solvent Toxicity

Acute Exposure	Chronic Exposure
Dizziness	Fatigue
Euphoria	Headache
Confusion	Nausea
Agitation	Neurobehavioral disturbances
Syncope	Cerebral atrophy
Cardiac dysrhythmias	Confusion
Coma	Dementia
Ocular irritation	Cognitive decline
Respiratory irritation	Memory loss
Headache	Cerebellar signs
Liver damage	Ataxia
Renal damage	Neuropsychologic changes
	Liver damage
	Renal damage

Table 106.2.   Summary of Toluene Concentrations in Air

Sampling Location	Median Concentration ($\mu g/m^3$)
Remote	0.002
Rural	1.3
Suburban	0.7
Urban	10.9
Source-dominated	23.8
Indoor	31.7
Workplace	3.3

Source: EPA, 1988

General Toxicity of Aromatic and Alkylbenzene Solvents

The main target organs for toxicity are the central and peripheral nervous system, liver, kidneys, and skin. Most of these solvents are readily absorbed by lungs and skin (2). Irritation of the eyes, respiratory tract, mucous membranes, and skin occur from many of these solvents. Dermal absorption is a critical route that can produce toxicity. Both dilute aqueous solvent solutions and concentrated solvent solutions are readily absorbed across the dermal barrier. Thus skin contact should be avoided in order to prevent toxic exposure (2).

Phenol can produce dermal necrosis, is readily absorbed through the skin, and can cause seizures, renal and kidney damage, and cardiac dysrhythmias. Acute exposure to high vapor concentrations of aromatic solvents can produce dizziness, syncope, confusion, euphoria, respiratory irritation, and in some instances, coma (2). Chronic exposure to toxic amounts is associated with neurotoxicity manifested by neurobehavioral disturbances, cerebral atrophy, cerebellar dysfunction, and permanent neuropsychologic dysfunction (2). Table 106.1 summarizes the acute and chronic effects of solvent exposures.

TOLUENE

Production, Use, and Sources

Toluene is a widely used solvent present in many combinations of chemicals, gasoline, paints, and other solvent mixtures. Approximately 10–11% of the toluene produced in the United States is isolated as toluene (3), with the remaining 90% being used to formulate gasoline. Very little of the toluene produced yearly is used in solvents, paints, adhesives, cleaning agents, and other chemicals. Toluene also finds use as a starter chemical for the synthesis of other organic chemicals such as urethanes, polyurethane foams, and benzene. Toluene is regulated by the Resource Conservation and Recovery Act (RCRA) as a hazardous waste. Industrial wastes that contain solvents may not be disposed of on land if the extract of this waste contains more than 0.33 mg/L of toluene (3). Also, waste waters containing greater than 1.12 mg/L of toluene may not be land disposed (3). Toluene occurs naturally as a component of crude oil and is produced from petroleum refining as a byproduct of styrene production (4). It finds most of its use in the industry in the refinement of gasoline and the manufacture and production of paints, adhesives, printing materials, and general solvents.

Chemical and Physical Properties of Toluene

Toluene (methylbenzene) has the chemical structure as shown in Figure 106.1. It has a molecular formula of $C_6H_5CH_3$ and a molecular weight of 92.15. It is a clear, colorless liquid with a sweet odor. The boiling point of toluene is 110.6°C, its vapor pressure is 22 mm Hg at 20°C. It autoignites at 480°C. The odor threshold of toluene vapor is between 0.04 and 1 mg/L in water and 8 mg/m^3 in air.

Exposure to Toluene

Human exposure to toluene occurs from occupational use in the home environment, inhalational abuse of paints containing toluene, and by environmental exposure. The largest exposure source of toluene is in the production and use of gasoline, which contains up to 7% toluene by weight (5). Large amounts of toluene are introduced into the environment yearly through the use of gasoline and through its production and petroleum refinement processes. Other sources of toluene released into the environment include the disposal of solvents in home wastewater as well as industrial discharges, land disposal of solvents and petroleum wastes, and tobacco smoking. Toluene can volatilize from solvent mixtures, paints, and other products used in home of occupational settings. Concentrations of toluene in the air range from 5–25 $\mu g/m^3$ in suburban or urban areas (5). The source of toluene in the atmosphere comes mainly from the use of gasoline.

Toluene is also a common air contaminant arising from many sources (Table 106.2). Indoor air concentrations of toluene may average 32 $\mu g/m^3$, which is higher than outside air (5). Toluene degases from a variety of household products such as solvents, paints, plastics, and is a component of tobacco smoke. Toluene degrades very quickly in the atmosphere, and toluene released into water rapidly volatilizes into the air.

The presence of toluene in water supplies is generally, around 3 $\mu g/L$ (5). Toluene commonly contaminates both water and soil in the vicinity of waste sites or chemical and industrial sources that use or produce toluene. Concentrations in the water of such sites range up to 20 $\mu g/L$ and concentrations in soil may be around 70 $\mu g/kg$ (5).

Human exposure to toluene occurs from its presence in air, from indoor air contamination in home environments, from occupational uses of toluene or toluene containing products, from exposure to gasoline vapors or liquid gasoline, and from volatilization of toluene from a variety of products used both in the home as well as industrial settings. Calculations show that given an average concentration of toluene of 32 μg/m³ in the indoor air of homes with an inhalation rate of air at 20 m³ per day, a person can obsorb 320 μg/day if only 50% of the inhaled toluene is absorbed (5).

In terms of indoor air pollution, one of the most common sources of toluene exposure is tobacco smoke which may contribute 1,000 μg/day or more to the indoor environment.

The Occupational Safety and Health Administration has set a permissible exposure limit of 100 ppm as a time-weighted average (TWA) for toluene in the work environment. (OSHA 1989) This concentration of 100 ppm equals a dose of 3750 mg/day, typically in the occupational environment (5).

Toluene contamination or release in the water can be either by industrial discharge, home use of solvents which are discharged into residential waste water, or into the soil, or from spills or releases of gasoline. Since gasoline contains 5–7% toluene by weight, gasoline releases and spills into soil, water, or vaporization into the air are critical sources of toluene in the environment.

Release of toluene into water occurs by all the measures mentioned, and toluene concentration in industrial waste waters have been found to range from 1–2,000 μg/L (5). Toluene, although a liquid at room temperature, is very volatile and is therefore released into the air and vaporized from a variety of sources. Consequently, toluene needs to vaporize into air from surface water or soil. Following a spill or release of toluene into soil, depending on the environmental circumstances such as temperature and humidity and the type of soil, volatilization of more than 90% of a release usually occurs within 24 hours (5). Toluene is soluble in water and can also be removed from soil due to water runoff. Toluene will be retained more in soil which has excess organic matter and will be easily released from soils that have low organic matter content (5).

Toluene in the environment can accumulate in aquatic organisms due to its lipophilic properties.

Biodegradation is rapid both in the soil and in the atmosphere. Atmospheric toluene is degraded to cresol and benzaldehyde (5). It is estimated that the atmospheric half-life of toluene is about 13 hours (5). The primary degradation process in the atmosphere is reaction with hydroxyl radicals. Due to the moderate miscibility of toluene with water, the rate of biodegradation is somewhat slower than in the atmosphere. Degradation in water occurs mainly through the action of microorganisms. The biodegradation in shallow water may be 90% complete within seven days (5).

Concentrations of toluene in the air of remote areas is as low as 0.002 μg/m³. Concentrations in suburban and urban areas can range as high as 30 μg/m³. Again, the highest concentrations are found indoors in homes and are due to volatilization of toluene from paints, solvents, glues, adhesives, and other materials used within the home environment.

The most common means of exposure to toluene is via inhalation. Tobacco smoke is a significant source of toluene within the home environment with approximately 80–100 micrograms of toluene per cigarette (5). One pack of cigarettes per day would contribute approximately 1,000 μg/day of toluene.

The EPA has reported concentrations of toluene in surface water sources as high as 1.4 μg/L. The daily intake of toluene from drinking water is generally quite small and would be a negligible source of toluene absorption in most cases. Drinking water contamination by toluene is generally below 0.1 μg/L. However, EPA surveys have found levels greater than 0.1

Table 106.3.   Toluene Health Effects

Acute	Chronic
Central nervous system depression	Permanent central nervous system (CNS) impairment
Coma	Tremors
Agitation	Ataxia
Delerium	Cerebral atrophy
Euphoria	Cerebellar atrophy
	Brainstem atrophy
	Optic neuropathy
	Decreased visual acuity
	Severe cognitive impairment
	Oculomotor abnormalities
	Corticospinal tract dysfunction
	Deafness
	Hyposmia
	CNS demyelination
	Neurobehavioral abnormalities
	Renal tubular acidosis

μg/L. Assuming the ingestion of up to two liters per day, this would contribute up to only 0.2 μg/day total dose. Exposures to toluene also could occur near waste sites or from contaminated water or soil from hazardous waste sites. Calculating the human exposure to toluene secondary to such waste sites depends on the pathways of migration into air, water, and soil and the human intake of these materials. In situations such as this, exposure is via the inhalation route and dermal absorption routes mainly.

Calculating human exposure concentrations from air, soil, and water can be difficult. However, assessments of exposure developed from the Total Exposure Assessment Methodology (TEAM) study of the EPA in 1987 aimed at providing information on concentrations of toluene in human exposures. Typically, most people are exposed to toluene in the indoor home environment more than any other sources.

Clinical Toxicology and Health Effects from Toluene

Human health effects secondary to toluene exposure occur primarily by the inhalational and dermal routes (6–8). Toxicity is summarized in Table 106.3. Acute exposure produces central nervous system depression and coma. High level exposures can result in dizziness, giddiness, and euphoria. Chronic inhalational exposures are associated with more significant residual damage of the central nervous system (6–8).

Toluene Neurotoxicity

Ataxia, tremors, visual impairment, diffuse cerebral atrophy, cerebellar atrophy, and brainstem atrophy have been known to occur in chronic toluene exposure and in intentional abusers (9). Decreased vision and ataxia have been described in individuals chronically inhaling toluene-containing solvents (10). Optic neuropathy can be manifested as decreased visual acuity, normal pupillary reactions along with associated cerebellar signs. Improvement in vision has followed discontinuation of toluene exposure. Rosenberg has reported neurologic symptoms in chronic toluene abusers which has been characterized by severe cognitive impairment, cerebellar ataxia, corticospinal tract dysfunction, oculomotor abnormalities, tremor, deafness, and hyposmia (9). He has also described the results of magnetic resonance imaging studies (MRI) in toluene vapor abusers and has correlated this with neuropathologic findings. These MRIs have demonstrated multifocal central nervous system involvement and diffuse CNS demyelination (9). The clinical presentation of these individuals included neurobehavioral, cerebellar, brainstem, and pyramidal tract abnormalities (9). Severe and persistent neurotoxicity can be a result of chronic toluene inhalation and chronic toluene abuse. Optic neuropathy, hearing loss, cerebellar ataxia, and cognitive dysfunction have all been described. The MRI studies of Rosenberg suggest that central nervous system white matter changes from toluene appear to be irreversible. Autopsy findings of those who have died in this study revealed diffuse myelin pallor in the deep white matter of the cerebral hemispheres and the cerebellum (9). Also, in these autopsies, diffuse demyelination in the subcortical white matter and axonopathy of peripheral and central nervous systems were demonstrated (9). These MRI studies as well as other clinical evidence indicate that toluene abuse produces permanent central nervous system damage.

Acute exposure to high concentrations of toluene vapors are associated with neurologic symtoms such as CNS depression, syncope, euphoria, delusions, acute excitation, and dizziness. Chronic exposure to high toluene vapor concentrations can result in permanent neuropsychologic and central nervous system damage (6–8). In occupational studies, it has been very difficult to ascertain the precise contribution of toluene, due to the fact that exposures have been mixed, with many different solvents being involved. However, there are numerous studies of painters and others occupationally exposed for years to toluene as well as other solvents such as styrene and trichloroethylene that have demonstrated neurobehavioral and neurotoxicologic effects (11–14). Studies of individuals with chronic exposure or chronic abuse demonstrated cerebral atrophy, abnormal electroencephalograms, optic neuropathy, cerebellar dysfunction, increased cerebrospinal fluid, cerebrospinal fluid pleocytosis, and serious cognitive deterioration (6–9, 15–17).

Exposure Routes

Routes of absorption of toluene exposure are inhalational, dermal, and ingestion. Studies have shown that toluene is very well absorbed by the lungs (18). Toluene is also absorbed dermally, and rates of absorption have been studied and found to vary from 14–23 mg/cm^2/hr (18). Another effect of inhaled toluene is respiratory tract irritation. Humans exposed to concentrations of toluene of between 200–800 ppm may experience respiratory and ocular irritation (19).

Toluene Cardiac Toxicity

Toluene cardiotoxicity, such as cardiac dysrhythmias as seen with other solvents such as the chlorinated solvents, is not commonly observed in human exposures. Animal studies with chronic dosing of toluene intraperitoneally and subcutaneously have demonstrated atrial fibrillation and ventricular ectopy (6).

Toluene Hematotoxicity

There is documentation of a decreased leukocyte count observed in dogs exposed acutely to 700 ppm of toluene (19). Other hematologic effects such as decreased leukocyte count

and thrombocytopenia have been observed within other animal studies following exposure to toluene. The National Toxicology Program, in 1989, had reported that exposure to toluene concentrations up to 1200 ppm for up to 2 years had no hematopoietic system effects on mice or rats (19). Human occupational exposure studies have not demonstrated hematologic effects (19, 20). Previous investigations linking toluene to hematotoxicity failed to account for co-exposures to other solvents.

Toluene Hepatotoxicity

In most studies of human exposure to toluene, hepatic damage has not been observed (6–8, 20, 21). Also in animal studies, toluene has not been observed to be hepatotoxic. Studies were conducted in mice over a 2-year-period; the mice were exposed to 1200 ppm as a component of the National Toxicology Program exhibited no hepatotoxicity from toluene (19). However, there are some clinical reports of acute reversible liver damage following inhalational abuse of toluene (6–8, 21). Other clinical cases following single dose, massive exposure resulting in coma have not demonstrated liver injury. Occupational studies of exposed workers have failed to demonstrate a consistent pattern of liver injury or hepatic enzyme elevation (6–8, 20, 21). In most occupational studies, other solvents are involved and present a confounding factor.

Occupational studies of painters and others exposed to a wide variety of solvents, both aliphatic and aromatic, have demonstrated elevation of hepatic enzymes (22). Biopsies of affected individuals revealed liver histopathology of steatosis, enlarged portal tracts with fibrosis, and necrosis (22).

Toluene Renal Toxicity

Effects on the kidneys have been documented in chronic toluene abusers (6–8). These renal effects have included hematuria, protenuria, and Type 1 renal tubular acidosis (23–27). Animal studies, on the other hand, have been conflicting. In some studies, renal toxicity has been observed, and in other studies renal toxicity has not been observed. Workers exposed to over 100 ppm of toluene for 6½ hours demonstrated no significant increase in urinary excretion of beta-2-microglobulin, a sensitive indicator of renal damage (19). Other workers exposed to toluene between 80–107 ppm as well as other solvents have not had increased urinary excretion of beta-2-microglobulin (27).

Inhalant abusers of toluene intentionally expose themselves to up to 1000 ppm to achieve a euphoric effect. Chronic toluene inhalational abuse can result in a normal anion gap metabolic acidosis with hypokalemia, hypophosphatemia and hyperchloremia. This type of acidosis was first described in association with glue sniffing and is termed Type I renal tubular acidosis (24). Renal tubular acidosis is a derangement in the capacity of distal renal tubules to maintain a hydrogen ion gradient (23). This type of renal tubular acidosis is usually reversible in a few days once exposure to toluene occurs but may require several weeks. Treatment ranges from observation alone to administration of sodium bicarbonate and potassium, depending on the severity of the acidemia and electrolyte loss (23). Patients with metabolic acidosis following toluene inhalation abuse have also had associated muscular weakness and neuropsychiatric manifestations (28).

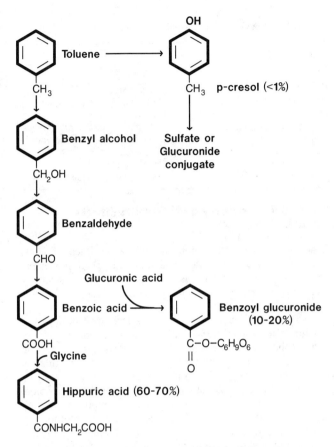

Figure 106.3. Metabolism of toluene in humans.

Absorption, Metabolism, and Excretion of Toluene

Toluene is absorbed from the respiratory tract, gastrointestinal tract, and through the skin. Due to the lipophilic nature of toluene, the concentration in adipose tissue can be high. The metabolism of toluene is shown in Fig. 106.3. The metabolic products of toluene are cresol (less than 1%) and the intermediate metabolite, benzaldehyde. Benzaldehyde is then metabolized to benzoic acid which is conjugated with glycine to form hippuric acid (29–34). In humans, up to 75% of inhaled toluene is metabolized to hippuric acid and excreted in the urine within 12 hours of exposure. The remainder of the toluene is mainly excreted unchanged with a small percent being excreted as a sulfate or glucuronide of cresol. The metabolism and excretion of toluene is rapid and occurs within 12 hours of exposure. The dermal absorption of toluene through human skin was found to range from 14–23 mg/cm²/hour (19). It has been estimated that the absorption of toluene through the skin at concentrations in water ranging from 0.005–0.5 mg/L would result in a daily absorption of 0.0001–0.03 mg/kg of body weight (35). Studies involving dermal absorption showed that toluene was easily detected in the blood after soaking of skin in volunteers. Toluene blood concentrations have been documented at autopsy following death from inhalational abuse. Toluene is distributed to adipose tissue in highly vascular tissues after absorption. These tissues include the brain, particularly the white matter, bone marrow, liver, kidneys, and nervous tissues.

Hippuric acid is a biological marker for occupational exposure to toluene (30). Minor toluene metabolites are o-

cresol, p-cresol, and phenol. The minor metabolites are conjugated with either sulfate or glucuronic acid and excreted in the urine (31–34).

The individual variations with respect to metabolism of toluene and the correlation of occupational exposure to toluene and urinary excretion of hippuric acid and cresol metabolites have been investigated (34, 36). However, due to the variability of metabolism in individuals, the biologic monitoring of hippuric acid and other metabolite excretions is ony a qualitative indication of exposure and not a quantitative indication of exposure to toluene. There is also ethnic variation in toluene metabolism (37). The half-life in fat tissue of humans has ranged from ½ day to 3 days. The excretion of hippuric acid has been studied in occupational environments as a marker for toluene exposure. Also, o-cresol is a biologic marker metabolite of toluene exposure. Studies performed in occupational settings have indicated that both hippuric acid and o-cresol excretion were related to environmental concentration of toluene and the worker exposure if excretion is corrected for creatinine and urine specific gravity (30). The correlation coefficient was stronger for hippuric acid (0.88 and 0.84) than it was for o-cresol (0.63–0.62) (30). The urinary excretion of hippuric acid can be a reliable biologic indicator of low level toluene exposure. At the exposure level below threshold limit values of toluene, urinary concentrations of hippuric acid and o-cresol may increase (30).

The presence of ethanol will decrease the metabolic clearance of toluene (38, 39). The drugs propranolol and cimetidine did not affect toluene metabolism (39). Blood concentrations of toluene have been shown to increase in exposed workers during shifts and correlate with the air concentrations (40).

A source of error in the biologic monitoring of solvents can be introduced by dermal absorption of a solvent (41).

Teratogenic, Genotoxic, and Reproductive Toxicity of Toluene

Animal studies have shown developmental effects secondary to toluene (19). Developmental effects have also been shown in pregnant women exposed occupationally to solvents of which toluene was one and in pregnant women as a result of solvent abuse (42, 43). However, it is difficult to say whether the toluene was actually causative, because these individuals were exposed to multiple solvents as well as to drugs and medications. Children with microcephaly, minor craniofacial and limb anomalies, central nervous system defects, attention disorders, developmental delay, learning disorders, and language deficits were born to mothers who abuse toluene by inhalation during pregnancy (42, 43). Whether these congenital defects and conditions are totally secondary to toluene alone remains unclear. However, exposure to organic solvents in general may have some embryotoxic effect (43). The recognition of this association has led to the adoption of the term "fetal solvent syndrome." In other animal studies, toluene was not shown to be a reproductive toxin (19).

Studies examining the incidence of sister chromatid exchange frequencies and chromosome aberrations in workers occupationally exposed to toluene have been reported (44–46). These studies indicated an increased frequency of sister chromatid exchange. The relevance of these findings is unclear. These workers had multiple other exposures to chemicals.

Toluene Carcinogenesis

Toluene is not considered to be carcinogenic. There has been no human epidemiologic study that has indicated that toluene exposure increases the risk of carcinogenesis. Retrospective mortality studies of workers exposed to toluene have also included exposures to other chemicals. Animal studies also have not demonstrated carcinogenic effects of toluene (19).

Immunotoxic Effects of Toluene

There are no human data to indicate that toluene is an immunotoxicant. Animal studies in mice exposed to toluene at concentrations of 2.5–500 ppm demonstrated decreased host defense to respiratory infections (19).

Effects of Low Level Toluene Exposure

Controlled exposure effects on volunteers were studied at toluene concentrations ranging from 40, 60, or 100 ppm. The exposed individuals experienced ocular and respiratory irritation along with a perceived deterioration of air quality, enhanced odor, headache, and dizziness at 100 ppm (47). Psychologic measurements indicated decrements in vigilance, visual perception, motor performance, and ability to carry out functions at 100 ppm (47).

Regulatory Aspects of Toluene

The OSHA permissible exposure limit for a time-weighted-average is 100 ppm with a short-term exposure limit (STEL) of 150 ppm. The American Conference of Governmental Industrial Hygienists (ACGIH) recommends a TLV of 100 ppm and a STEL of 150 ppm. The National Institute of Occupational Safety and Health (NIOSH) recommends a TLV of 100 ppm with a 10 minute ceiling of 200 ppm. The toluene vapor concentration that is immediately dangerous to life and health (IDLH) is 2000 ppm.

The 1980 National Academy of Sciences suggested no-adverse-response-level (SNARL) for chronic ingestion of drinking water with toluene is 0.34 mg/L on a chronic basis. The 7-day SNARL is 35 mg/L, and the 1-day SNARL is 420 mg/L. State drinking water guidelines vary as to ambient air concentration guidelines.

XYLENE

Uses and Sources

A mixture of xylene isomers (ortho, meta, and para xylenes) as well as ethylbenzene are widely used as solvents in a variety of commercial processes and sites (48). Xylene is heavily used in histology laboratories. Xylene is also used as the starting materials for manufacturing polymers (48). Xylene is also found in paints, varnishes, and glues. It has also been used as a solvent vehicle for pesticides.

Chemical and Physical Properties

Xylene is a dimethylbenzene compound with a molecular formula $C_6H_4(CH_3)_2$ and a chemical formula for its three isomeric forms as shown in Fig. 106.1 (ortho, meta, and para). Xylene is a clear liquid solvent whose vapors can be very irritating to eyes, nose, throat, skin, and mucous membranes.

Table 106.4. Xylene Vapor Health Effects

Acute	Chronic
Dizziness	Central nervous system
Fatigue	depression
Headache	Headache
Nausea	Fatigue
Ocular irritation	Irritation of mucous membranes
Mucous membrane irritation	Impairment of central nervous
Upper airway and respiratory	system
tract irritation	Cognitive changes
Syncope	Neurobehavioral changes

Clinical Toxicology and Health Effects from Xylene

Exposure to xylene is common since it is a constituent of paints and glues and is used as a general solvent in many processes. Most exposures to xylene as well as other solvents are by inhalation of the vapors or via skin contact. The OSHA PEL for xylene is 100 ppm.

Aromatic compounds are metabolized via the P-450 mixed function microsomal enzyme system in the endoplastic reticulum of the liver. The co-ingestion of ethanol has an effect on the metabolism of xylene (49). Ethanol inhibits the oxidation of the aromatic ring and also alkyl side chain oxidation. This is probably through a direct inhibitory effect on the microsomal oxidation by ethanol. Xylene blood concentrations increase up to two-fold following ethanol ingestion indicating inhibition of metabolism (49). It is appreciated that chronic or longterm exposure to organic solvents may have a role in the production of liver disease. Liver necrosis and steatosis after exposure to xylene has been reported (21). Steatosis hepatic cell necrosis and portal tract enlargement can be seen in a variety of medical conditions, one of which is the chronic ingestion of large amounts of alcohol. Other studies have shown no significant elevation in liver enzymes in workers exposed to a mixture of solvents including xylene (50).

Xylene and ethylbenzene are commonly used as aromatic solvents together. Xylene is used in histology laboratories in the isomeric form of m-xylene. The isomers of xylene are also used in polymer manufacturing, in paints, varnishes, and glues. Exposure to xylene can occur from dermal absorption as well as pulmonary absorption and ingestion. In concentrations above 5000 parts per million, xylene is an anesthetic (48). In concentrations in the few hundred parts per million, exposed workers will experience dizziness, fatigue, headache, and nausea. Acute high exposures to xylene vapors produces CNS symptoms of drowsiness, fatigue, and syncope. Xylene is also an irritant to mucous membranes and eyes. Studies have been performed showing that brief exposures to 300 ppm of xylene affected short term memory and prolonged the reaction time of subjects performing physical work (48). This effect on the central nervous system and task performance is of great concern since workers are exposed to xylene in occupational settings. Toxicity is summarized in Table 106.4.

Absorption, Metabolism, and Excretion

The kinetics of m-xylene have been studied in humans (48, 51). Physical exercise through increased rate of ventilation results in increased absorption of solvent vapors. One study looked at 18 healthy male volunteers and carried-out controlled vapor exposure studies of m-xylene (51). The study was designed to simulate a typical industrial exposure of xylene. The concentration of xylene in blood samples increased with physical activity. The biotransformation of xylene through side chain oxidation and aromatic oxidation resulted in metabolites of 2,4-xylenol and methyl hippuric acid (Fig. 106.4). The rate of methyl hippuric excretion increased concomitantly with the exposure through pulmonary absorption. The methyl benzoic acid which is produced as a metabolic byproduct of xylene metabolism is conjugated with glycine to form methyl hippuric acid. Methyl hippuric acid excretion is used as an index of exposure to xylene.

Despite the fact that ethanol decreases xylene metabolism by 50%, the urinary excretion of 2,4-xylenol, a minor xylene metabolite, was not decreased by ethanol (49). The ingestion of moderate doses of ethanol has increased blood xylene concentrations two-fold (49). Co-ingestion of ethanol and xylene also results in a decrease in methyl hippuric acid excretion in the urine. The ratio of 2,4-xylenol to methyl hippuric acid was significantly increased with the concomitant ingestion of alcohol and xylene exposure.

Dermal absorption of xylene liquid has been shown to be 4.5–9.6 mg/cm²/hr (19). The dermal route can be a significant cause of toxic effects.

PHENOL

Sources and Uses

Phenol, a monohydroxy benzene derivative also called carbolic acid, is obtained from petroleum as a naturally occurring compound as well as by the oxidation of toluene and by cumene hydroperoxidation (52). Phenol is used mainly for the production of phenolic resins such as phenol-formaldehyde resins. These resins are used in the plywood adhesive industry, construction industry, and the automotive and appliance industries (53). Phenol is used to manufacture bisphenol A as well as caprolactum. Bisphenol A is used to produce epoxy resins, and caprolactam is used in the manufacture of nylon. Phenol also finds use in the manufacture of numerous other organic compounds including herbicides (2,4-diphenoxy acetic acid), pharmaceuticals, cresols, xylenols, aniline, and alkylphenols. Phenol is used in the preparation of many medications such as ointments and lotions as a preservative (52, 53).

Phenol occurs naturally in animal wastes and is produced by decomposition of organic wastes (52, 53).

Chemical and Physical Characteristics

Phenol has a formula of C_6H_5OH and a molecular weight of 94.1 (Fig. 106.1). Pure phenol is a crystalline solid with a melting point of 43°C and boiling point of 182°C (52). It is soluble in water and most organic solvents. Phenol is an acidic compound with a pKa of 9.9 in aqueous solutions (52). The most important physiochemical characteristics of phenol are its acidity and reactivity. Both are due to the proximity of a hydroxy group with the resonance structure of an aromatic ring. This structure imparts a high electrophilic substitution reactivity property.

Phenol is not a very volatile compound. Consequently, most toxic effects occur from dermal and oral exposure. It has a distinctive odor which is somewhat acrid. The odor threshold of phenol is 7.9 part per million in water and 0.05 parts per

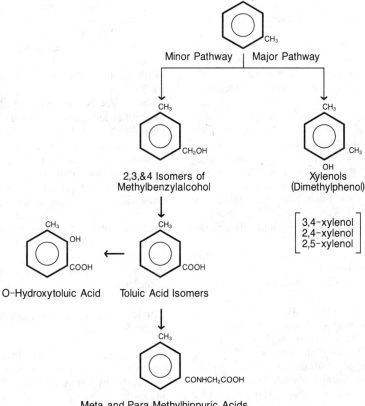

Figure 106.4. Metabolism of xylene.

million in air. Phenol is soluble in water as well as in organic solvents such as alcohol, carbon tetrachloride, acetic acid, benzene, and ether.

Exposure Sources of Phenol

Environmental contamination by phenol is principally due to its manufacturing and use in various chemical processes. Phenol is produced as a result of burning wood and automobile exhaustion. It is found in numerous hazardous waste sites on the National Priorities List (NPL). Phenol has a short half-life as a vapor phase in air which is approximately 12–15 hours, but persists in water much longer (52, 54). The biodegradation of phenol in water can range from 1 day to 9 days. Phenol is also photochemically oxidized, and its photo-oxidation half-life is approximately 19 hours (54). Peroxyl radicals are produced as a photodegradation of phenol. Phenol in soil generally degrades very quickly. Mean ambient air concentrations of phenol have been found to be 30 parts per trillion in urban and suburban atmospheres (52, 54).

Phenol enters the environment from natural sources such as coal tar as well as chemical wastes from industries which manufacture resin, plastics, adhesives, rubber, iron, steel, and aluminum (54). Phenol is also released from paper pulp mills and wood treatment facilities. Phenol finds use in general disinfectants and medicinal preparations. Other natural sources of phenol in water are animal wastes and decomposition of organic wastes. Phenol contamination of groundwater occurs secondary from leaching from contaminated soil after spills of phenol and hazardous releases. Phenol does not concentrate or bioconcentrate in aquatic organisms to any significant degree.

The transport and movement of phenol in the environment is affected by the pH of the environment or the medium in which phenol is present, since the pKa of phenol is 9.9 and it will, therefore, exist in a partially dissociated state in water and in moist soil (54). Phenol is biodegradable in water sources if the concentration is not high enough to produce significant inhibition of degradation by microorganisms. In fact, phenol may degrade in less than 1 day in surface waters (54). The degradation of phenol is slower in salt water as compared to fresh water.

Phenol is found in surface water, groundwater, drinking water, and rain water as well as urban runoff water and water in and around hazardous waste sites. The concentrations of phenol can be as high as one part per billion in uncontaminated groundwater (54). Phenol is found in higher concentration in bodies of water and water sources that receive discharge from industrial sites. Phenol has been detected in drinking water such as well water. Phenol has also been detected in water sources following spills and releases that have contaminated soil.

Another source of phenol is the mainstream smoke from tobacco products. The concentrations of phenol in this sidestream smoke ranges from 100–420 micrograms of phenol per cigarette which is released into the environment (52, 54).

Environmental exposure of humans to phenol occurs primarily in industrial settings or in areas that have a significant concentration of phenol in the environment. Human exposure from phenol occurs from ingestion of drinking water from contaminated sources, from ingestion of phenol-containing products, from the use of phenol-containing medicinals, and from sidestream tobacco smoke. Since phenol is used heavily within the pulpwood industry, this is one of the more common occupational exposure areas. Exposure and absorption of phenol is mainly via dermal or gastrointestinal pathways.

The industries and occupations associated with phenol exposure are iron and steel industries, leather tanning industry, aluminum forming industry, electrical industry, pharmaceuticals, organic and plastic manufacturing industries, paint and ink formulation industries, and rubber industry. Phenol-containing medicinal uses include mouthwashes, throat lozenges, phenol-containing ointments, nose and ear drops, analgesic rubs, and antiseptic lotions (54).

Regulations Regarding Phenol

The OSHA permissible exposure limit (PEL) for phenol is 5 ppm as a TWA for up to a 10-hour work shift. The ACGIH recommends a TLV of 5 ppm and a biologic exposure index (BEI) in urine for total phenol of 250 mg/g creatinine or 15 mg excreted in urine per hour.

Absorption, Metabolism, and Excretion of Phenol

Phenol is absorbed via the inhalational route, oral route, and dermal route. Due to its low volatility, the main routes of absorption are dermal and oral. Phenol is readily absorbed by the skin and gastrointestinal tract in humans. Phenol is also well absorbed by the lungs. Once absorbed from the gastrointestinal tract, phenol is rapidly excreted in the urine as free phenol or as a conjugate of phenol. In fact, phenol is normally found in human urine in subjects with no known exposure (52). A correlation exists between the urinary phenol concentrations and the exposure of humans to phenol and the amount that is absorbed (52). Due to the fact that phenol is rapidly excreted within 1 to 2 days following an exposure, the presence of phenol in the urine can be used as a marker of recent exposure. Phenol vapors and liquid are absorbed quickly and easily through the skin. Studies that measured the absorption of phenol through the skin in volunteers demonstrated that 13% of an applied dose of phenol in a solution was absorbed within 30 minutes (55). Eighty percent of this dose was recovered in the urine within 24 hours. As the concentration of phenol solution is increased, the dermal permeability of phenol increases. Concentrations of phenol may actually destroy the skin barrier for prevention of absorption, thus permitting increased absorption. The half-life of phenol is estimated to be 3.5 hours (52).

There are four major urinary metabolites of phenol (as well as the parent compound) which have been discovered in the urine (52). These metabolites are phenol glucuronide, phenol sulfate, 1,4-dihydroxybenzene glucuronide, and 1,4-dihydroxybenzene sulfate. Dehydroxylation of phenol is catalyzed by the P-450 microsomal cytochrome mono-oxygenate system. The sulfate and glucuronide conjugation of phenol varies depending on the animal. Phenol and its metabolites are excreted in the urine.

Clinical Toxicology and Human Health Effects from Phenol

Human health effects from phenol exposure can range from basic irritative symptoms to muscular weakness, convulsions, cardiac dysrhythmias, and coma, depending on exposure, dose, and route of absorption (Table 106.5).

Air concentrations of phenol vapors as found in occupational

Table 106.5. Phenol Health Effects

Tachycardia
Muscle tremors
Hypotension
Respiratory difficulty
Cardiac dysrhythmias
Syncope
Seizures
Coma
Gastrointestinal bleeding (oral ingestion)
Dermal necrosis
Nephritis
Metabolic acidosis
Increased levels of hepatic enzymes

settings below the PEL of 5 ppm are not associated with health effects, although the odor of phenol is noticeable. Air concentrations above the PEL of 5 ppm have been associated with irritation of mucous membranes (8 ppm) (52).

The clinical toxicity produced by phenol is the same no matter what route of absorption. Early signs of toxicity include tachycardia and increased blood pressure. This is followed by cardiac dysrhythmias, shortness of breath, and seizures. Due to its low odor threshold of 0.05 ppm in air, phenol can be detected long before it becomes a toxic hazard.

The ingestion of large amounts of phenol, particularly concentrated phenol, has been reported in clinical poisoning cases. Fatalities have occurred from dermal absorption of phenol in which death occurred within 10 minutes after 25% of an individual's body surface was exposed to liquid phenol (55). Death has occurred following intentional oral ingestion of phenol. Systemic effects from oral ingestion of phenol include gastrointestinal irritation, vomiting, diarrhea, gastrointestinal bleeding, and cardiac dysrhythmias. Application of concentrated solutions of phenol to the skin can result in skin necrosis and inflammation at the site of application (55).

Animal studies indicate that exposure to 0.5 ml/cm^2 is sufficient to cause skin irritation. The concentration of phenol is also very important in determining both dermal absorption, systemic toxicity, and the effects on the skin. Cardiac dysrhythmias are reported in clinical cases of individuals following both oral ingestion and dermal application of phenol solution, particularly concentrated solutions (55). Elevated liver enzymes have been demonstrated in individuals with phenol toxicity. Animal studies indicate neurologic toxicity such as tremors, convulsions, coma, and ataxia following either dermal or oral exposure to phenol.

Phenol is a denaturant, and skin exposure can result in severe burns and systemic toxicity, depending on the concentration. Acute phenol toxicity occurs following dermal absorption (56). Absorption of phenol is dependent on concentration, surface area of contact, duration of contact, and temperature of the skin (increased absorption with increased temperature), and condition of the skin (56). Phenol easily penetrates the human dermal barrier to be systemically absorbed and can produce serious toxicity via solutions that come into contact with the skin or by vapor contact (56). Urinary excretion of phenol occurs after 30 minutes of dermal contact.

Ventricular ectopy has occurred in clinical cases following application of solutions of 6 ml containing 40% phenol (2.4 g of phenol) to the skin (57, 58). High concentrations of phenol, such as 40% or more, denature the dermis and coagulate keratin

causing the underlying skin to become hyperemic. This results in an increased systemic absorption of phenol (56, 58).

Skin Decontamination

Dermal damage by concentrated phenol occurs in a minute and thus allows for increased systemic absorption that can result in serious toxicity. Management of dermal contamination by phenol with appropriate decontamination techniques is essential to prevent further tissue damage and toxicity.

Animal studies conducted using various skin decontamination procedures demonstrated that increased absorption of phenol occurred using water as a decontaminant (59, 60). The best decontaminant that prevented systemic toxicity was found to be glycerol or polyethylene glycol (PEG) (59). Another effective decontaminating solution studied is a combination of polyethylene glycol-400 and industrial methylated spirits (2:1 by volume) (60). Swabbing phenol contaminated skin with either PEG-300 or PEG-400 was found to be most effective at reducing dermal burns and systemic toxicity in all animal studies (59, 60).

Recommendations for managing a contaminated patient include removal of all clothes, swabbing the skin with cotton swabs soaked in glycerol or polyethylene glycol (PEG) for a minimum of 10–20 minutes and 24-hour medical observation for cardiac dysrhythmias and neurologic manifestations.

Speed of decontamination is essential in preventing dermal burns as well as systemic toxicity from phenol. The availability of an appropriate PEG decontamination solution can prevent morbidity and death following a phenol contamination of the skin.

The threshold concentration for human skin damage from phenol is 1.5% (61). Phenol chemically alters the stratum corneum and significantly impairs the capacity of the skin to prevent penetration. Increasing the concentration of phenol increases the permeability coefficient more than several fold (61). The permeability coefficient for a 5% phenol solution is 50-fold higher than for a 1% solution (61).

Phenol Immunotoxicity, Reproductive Effects, and Carcinogenicity

There are no known immunotoxic effects in humans secondary to phenol exposure. There are no developmental effects nor reproductive effects secondary to phenol in humans. There are no known genotoxic effects in humans secondary to phenol. Phenol is not a human carcinogen. The National Cancer Institute has reported cancer in laboratory animals secondary to phenol exposure. The National Cancer Institute testing of phenol for its carcinogen effects in animals has been equivocal. Phenol is a tumor promoter when applied to the skin and might be a complete carcinogen (initiator and promoter) in mice (55).

Phenol Renal Toxicity

Renal toxicity has been reported in laboratory animals. Phenol is nephrotoxic to humans and animals, especially following chronic exposure. Animal studies show a direct toxic effect on renal parenchyma. Humans have experienced nephritis following toxic dermal exposure (62).

Phenol Cardiotoxicity and Toxicity from Ingestion

One case report described in a 52-year-old female who was mistakenly administered 1 ounce of 89% phenol as a preoperative medication described her developing coma and respiratory arrest 30 minutes after the ingestion associated with hypotension and ventricular dysrhythmias, metabolic acidosis, and seizures. This patient also suffered esophageal erythema injury (57).

Environmental contamination of phenol leading to human health effects has occurred following spills or releases of phenol which contaminated drinking water (63). High drinking water concentrations of phenol were found within ½ km of a spill in Wisconsin.

STYRENE

Uses

Styrene is also known as cinnamene, vinylbenzene, ethenyl benzene, phenylethene, and phenylethylene. The structural formula for styrene is shown in Figure 106.1. Styrene has a molecular formula of C_8H_8 with a molecular weight of 104.1. Common uses of styrene are in production of polystyrene plastics, the production of styrene butadiene rubber, acrylonitrile butadiene-styrene polymers, and acrylonitrile copolymer resins. Styrene is also used to produce styrene-butadiene latex protective coatings and in formation of polyesters, and copolymer resins. Styrene is a 99% pure mixture of styrene monomers.

Regulatory Aspects of Styrene

The OSHA PEL standard for exposure to styrene monomers is 100 ppm TWA, with a ceiling value of 200 ppm, and an acceptable exposure of 600 ppm for 5 minutes in any 3-hour period (64). The ACGIH recommends a threshold limit value of 50 ppm and a short term exposure level of 100 ppm. In storage, styrene monomer vapors may form polymers. The Hazardous Materials Transportation Act designates styrene monomers in quantities of 1000 pounds and greater as a hazardous material for the purpose of transportation. Styrene monomer is considered to be a flammable liquid and requires labeling as such.

Chemical and Physical Properties of Styrene

Styrene monomer is a clear liquid, is flammable, and has a flash point between 73–141°F. Styrene has an odor threshold in air of 0.148 ppm and an odor threshold in water of 0.05 ml/ L. Styrene has a vapor density of 3.6. It has a sweet odor at low concentrations and a disagreeable odor at higher concentrations (64). It is an oily, colorless to yellow liquid. Styrene monomers are reactive in high temperatures and pressures and undergo polymerization on exposure to light and air and undergo oxidation with formation of peroxide. Polymerization of styrene monomers can occur if styrene is heated above 150°F. Metal salts and acids can also cause polymerization to occur. Styrene reacts violently with chlorosulfonic acids and sulfuric acids (64).

Absorption, Metabolism, and Excretion

Absorbed styrene is metabolized to styrene oxide (64). Styrene and styrene oxide are further metabolized hepatically as well as by the kidney, intestines, lungs, and skin. Styrene oxide is metabolized to styrene glycol and subsequently to mandelic acid, phenyl glyoxylic acid, and finally to hippuric acid (Fig. 106.5) (65). Styrene metabolism is suppressed by coexposure and absorption of toluene. Styrene absorption across the dermal barrier has been studied using the urinary excretion of mandelic acid. The rate of absorption of liquid styrene across the dermal barrier was 9–15 mg/cm²/hour, and the rate of aqueous solution absorption was 40–180 µg/cm²/hour and the absorption from solution was linear with the concentration (19).

Styrene is detectable in air at vapor concentrations of 0.148 ppm and has a disagreeable odor at higher concentrations. Aldehydes and peroxides can form from styrene when it is exposed to air, increasing the disagreeable odor. Vapors of styrene are very irritating. Styrene can be absorbed across the skin, inhalationally, and by gastrointestinal absorption.

Absorption of styrene by skin in the vapor stage is very small or negligible. Styrene is well-absorbed by the lungs. The metabolism of styrene is inhibited by ethanol as well as other solvents. The major metabolite of styrene found in the urine is mandelic acid. The excretion of mandelic acid in the urine appears to have a linear relationship between the exposure to styrene up to 150 ppm (65). Phenyl glyoxylic acid is a metabolite of mandelic acid. Investigations have shown that the summation of mandelic acid and phenyl glyoxylic acid in the urine correlates with total exposure to styrene (65). Other minor metabolites of styrene metabolism are 4-vinyl phenol, phenylethylene glycol, phenylethanol, and hippuric acid (65).

Clinical Toxicology and Exposure to Styrene

Styrene is very soluble in liquids and fully soluble in water. Occupational exposure to styrene occurs in the polyester glass fiber industry, paint industry, and in the production of styrene butadiene rubber. Styrene is a known neurologic toxin which has effects on both the central and peripheral nervous systems. Styrene is known to produce abnormal electroencephalograms in intoxicated individuals as well as impairment and peripheral nerve conduction velocities (65).

Mucous membrane, nasal, and skin irritation have been reported at 376 ppm in some individuals (64). Exposure to high vapor concentrations can also produce headache, nausea, and dizziness. Styrene vapors cause moderate irritation and burning of the skin. Prolonged dermal exposure can produce deeper degrees of chemical burn. Values that are immediately dangerous to life and health (IDLH) are 5000 ppm (64). Styrene vapors are heavier than air and can travel to distant ignition sources and produce flashback (64). In addition, polymerization can take place in closed containers leading to an explosion. Polymerization occurs if styrene is heated above 150°F which can rupture the container that it is encased in. Also metal salts, peroxides, and strong acids can cause polymerization (64).

Styrene is a solvent with known neurotoxic effects in humans for both peripheral and central nervous system. Occupational exposure to styrene has been associated with neurobehavioral toxicity (66, 67). Using the styrene metabolites of mandelic acid and phenyl glyoxylic acid, workers who were occupationally exposed to styrene were studied with neuropsycho-

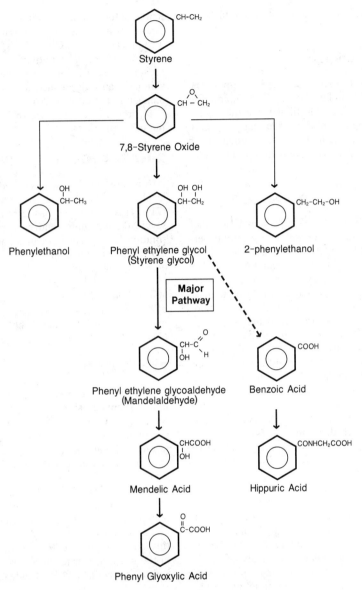

Figure 106.5.   Metabolism of styrene.

metric functions (67). It was demonstrated by such studies that certain cognitive skills were impaired by exposure to styrene concentrations in the air of more than 50 ppm on a chronic basis. Central nervous system effects included verbal learning skills, visuospatial skills, and memory (66, 67). Table 106.6 summarizes the toxicity from styrene exposure.

CHLOROBENZENE

Chlorobenzene has a molecular formula of C_6H_5Cl and a molecular weight of 112.56 (Fig. 106.2). It is also known as benzene chloride or monochlorobenzene. Chlorobenzene is an intermediate solvent used in production of phenols and analin compounds and has been used in production of DDT (68). It has a mild odor to somewhat sweet and aromatic and is a colorless liquid. Vapors of chlorobenzene can form dangerously explosive mixtures with air since the compound is highly reactive and the vapor pressure of chlorobenzene is heavier than

Table 106.6.   Styrene Health Effects

Acute	Chronic
Headache	Cognitive and Behavioral
Nausea	Changes
Dizziness	Personality Changes
Skin burns	Headache
Skin irritation	Fatigue
Mucous membrane irritation	Weakness
	Dizziness
	Depression
	Anxiety
	Emotional Lability
	Increased Irritability

air (68). Vapors can travel along the floor areas to ignition sources. The vapor density of chlorobenzene is 3.88 (air = 1). Chlorobenzene is a flammable liquid and reacts violently with oxidizers. When heated, toxic combustion products include chlorine (68).

Regulatory Considerations

The OSHA PEL as a TWA for chlorobenzene is 75 ppm. The NIOSH IDLH value for chlorobenzene is 2400 ppm. The ACGIH has recommended a threshold limit value for chlorobenzene as a TWA of 75 ppm. Chlorobenzene has a specific gravity (greater than water) equal to 1.107. Chlorobenzene is not easily biodegraded. The odor recognition threshold for chlorobenzene is 0.21 ppm (68).

Clinical Toxicity

The clinical toxicology of chlorobenzene is similar to other aromatic and chlorinated hydrocarbon solvents. Central nervous system depression and excitation with a possibility of seizures can occur. Inhalation of high concentrations of chlorobenzene can produce central nervous system depression, seizures, muscular twitching, cyanosis, and cardiac arrhythmias. The compound is toxic by inhalation and by skin contact absorption. Chlorobenzene is also an irritant to mucous membranes and respiratory tract. Repeated exposures of chlorobenzene to the skin can produce dermatitis. Inhalation of toxic concentrations of vapors or contact with the skin of sufficient concentrations can result in toxic health effects to the pulmonary system, kidneys, liver, and central nervous system.

Irritation of the eyes and mucous membranes in humans occurs at approximately 200 ppm, and at that level the odor threshold has been greatly exceeded; thus, the odor threshold and irritative phenomena are not sufficient to provide protective warning for exposure.

ETHYLBENZENE

Ethylbenzene has a molecular formula as shown in Figure 106.1 and a molecular formula of $C_6H_5(C_2H_5)$. Ethylbenzene, also known as phenylethane, is a colorless liquid solvent used as an intermediate chemical in the production of styrene as a general solvent. Ethyl-benzene is a known irritant of the skin, mucous membranes, and eyes. At high concentrations, it will produce central nervous depression in both humans and animals. The OSHA PEL for ethylbenzene is 100 ppm. Ethylbenzene is absorbed dermally, and studies have shown that dermal absorption is in the range of 22–33 mg/cm²/hour (69). Irritative effects from ethylbenzene occur at approximately 200 ppm.

Ethylbenzene is one of the more frequently used aromatic hydrocarbon solvents and is used as a paint thinner and a degreaser in paints, inks, and other chemical intermediate reaction processes. Ethylbenzene has a hepatotoxic potential and humans who are exposed to high concentrations should have monitoring of liver functions.

HYDROQUINONE

Hydroquinone, also known as 1,4-benzenediol, has a structure as shown in Figure 106.2, a molecular formula of $C_6H_3O_2$, and a molecular weight of 110.12. The compound has a specific gravity of 1.3. It is a white to light tan solid and is miscible with water. It is combustible, and dust concentrations of hydroquinone can explode in enclosed areas (70). The dust is

irritating to eyes, nose, and mucous membranes. The chemical is used as a reducer in photography, as an antioxidant, and as a chemical reagent. Clinical toxicity following acute ingestion consists of nausea, vomiting, muscular twitching, shortness of breath, cyanosis, confusion, and syncope. Contact with the skin can cause dermatitis, and contact with the eye can cause damage to the cornea (70).

Hydroquinone has a PEL of 2 mg/m³ and IDLH level of 200 mg/m3 (70).

2-NAPHTHOL

2-Naphthol, also known as 2-hydroxy naphthalene, has a molecular formula of $C_{10}H_8O$ and a molecular weight of 144.18 (71). This compound has a phenolic odor and can produce severe dermal injury and burn and eye irritation from a 1% solution (71). Ingestion can produce renal damage, vomiting, diarrhea, abdominal pain, syncope, convulsions, and hemolytic anemia. 2-naphthol is also absorbed dermally. The odor threshold of 2-naphthol ranges between 0.01 ppm–11.4 ppm. Flammability potential is slight. 2-Naphthol is used in the manufacture of other chemicals, dyes, manufacturing of perfumes, and the manufacture of synthetic rubber as well as pharmaceuticals (71).

PYROCATECHOL

Pyrocatechol is also known as 1,2-benzenediol, and its structural formula is shown in Figure 106.2. It has a molecular formula of $C_6H_6O_2$ and a molcular weight of 110.12. The common uses are in dyeing, chemical manufacturing, photography, and manufacturing of pharmaceuticals (72). Its general structure as a catechol gives it similar toxicity to other benzenediols. It is a white, odorless solid. The dust is an irritant. Toxicity from inhaled dust includes respiratory tract irritation, eye and mucous membrane irritation, coughing, and difficulty breathing (72). The solid material will cause chemical burns of the skin and eyes. Any contact with the eyes should be flushed out immediately with water for 15 minutes. Ingestion of the material can result in CNS stimulation and seizures as well as coma. The TLV of the compound is 5 ppm (72).

P-TERT-BUTYLTOLUENE

This solvent is a clear liquid used for chemical synthesis and as a solvent for resins. Its toxicity is mainly that of mucous membrane irritation, and there is some evidence of bone marrow depression as well (73). Concentrations up to 160 ppm produced mucous membrane irritation in volunteers. The odor threshold for butyltoluene is 5 ppm. High concentration exposures can produce central nervous system depression, confusion, and collapse. The structure is shown in Figure 106.2.

NAPHTHALENE

Naphthalene has a chemical formula of $C_{10}H_8$ and is shown in Figure 106.2. Naphthalene is a white crystalline solid used as a moth repellant and is also used in dye manufacturing. It has a PEL of 10 ppm and is a known cause of acute red blood cell hemolysis. It is also an irritant to the mucous membranes and the eyes. Clinical intoxication syndrome includes eye irritation, headache, confusion, excitement, diaphoresis, nausea, and vomiting which can progress to hemolytic anemia with jaundice

Table 106.7. Example of Compounds Identified in Creosote

Benzene
Toluene
Xylene
Trimethylbenzene
Methyl ethyl benzenes
Styrene
Phenol
Benzofuran and dibenzofuran
Benzonitrile and methyl benzonitrile
Methyl styrene
Cresols
Indenes and methyl indenes
Xylenols
Naphthalene and methyl naphthalene
Benzothiophenes
Quinoline and isoquinoline
Diphenyl
Dimethyl naphthalene
Ethyl napthalene
Acenaphthene
Fluorene
Dibenzothiophene
Acenaphthylene
Benzocalpyrene
Benzo(*ghi*)perylene
Anthracene
Pyrene
Penanthrene
Crysene
Benzo(*e*)pyrene
Dibenzo(*ah*)anthracene
Benzo(*k*)fluoranthrene
Benzo(*a*)fluorene

Reprinted with permission from: Heikkila PR, Hameila M, Pyy L, Raunu P: Exposure to creosote in the impregnation and handling of impregnated wood. Scand J Work Environ Health 1987;13:431–437.

and acute renal failure from myoglobinuria. Naphthalene itself is not a hemolytic agent. However, its metabolite, naphthol, is a hemolytic metabolite (73). Naphthalene vapor causes mucous membrane and eye irritation at 5 ppm. Contact with the skin can produce dermatitis. Ocular irritation and cataracts have been described in humans with prolonged exposure.

CREOSOTE

Creosote is a wood preservative that has been used worldwide for hundreds of years (74). Coal tar wood preservatives were first used in 1680 (74). Creosote is a black-brown, thick, oily liquid derived from distillation of coal tar, which is the by-product of destruction of coal to coke (74). Creosotes are actually complex mixtures of a variety of aromatic compounds (Table 106.7) of which only 100 have been identified (74).

Creosotes may contain 20 major compounds of which the main compounds are naphthalene and alkyl derivatives (74). Creosotes may also contain 15–21% polycyclic aromatic compounds and 0.03–0.12% benzo(*a*)pyrene (74).

The International Agency for Research on Cancer states that sufficient evidence exists to declare creosotes an animal carcinogen. There is only limited evidence of carcinogenicity in humans (74). Skin contact with creosote oils can cause photosensitivity in workers. Also, many of the aromatic compounds can be absorbed dermally to produce systemic toxicity.

Cresote vapors produce mucous membrane, ocular, and respiratory tract irritation.

NEUROTOXICOLOGY OF SOLVENT EXPOSURE

Due to the wide use of organic solvents, and in particular, the aromatic organic solvents such as toluene, xylene, ethylbenzene, and styrene, neurotoxicity secondary to exposure is important to appreciate. Human exposure can occur via solvent vapor as well as by liquid exposure to the skin and respiratory tract. Acute toxic neurologic effects of solvent exposure have been recognized since the nineteenth century and have manifestations of acute narcosis, dizziness, and syncope (12, 75).

Worker observations in the 1970s of occupational exposures to styrene began to identify that chronic solvent exposure could lead to neurologic impairment. This impairment has been identified as both subjective and objective in terms of neurologic function (12, 75–77). Due to dermal and pulmonary absorption, exposure is important to control. It has been shown that a 10–15 minute immersion of a person's hands in xylene produced blood concentrations similar to those following an 8-hour inhalational exposure of 100 ppm, which is at the threshold limit value of xylene (12). Thus, workers with chronic skin exposure are at high risk for neurotoxicity as well as for other manifestations of toxicity. Enhancement of solvent absorption can occur in work environment situations where temperatures may create increased blood flow to the skin as well as solvent contamination of clothing. Subjective effects of solvents on the central nervous system include transient changes in central nervous system function such as CNS depression, dizziness, loss of coordination, and confusion. Other more subtle changes actually have been described in terms of neuropsychologic parameters (78–81).

Solvent effects on the central nervous system can also be objective and include histologic changes in central nervous system tissue, cerebellar syndrome, alterations that are identifiable on computerized tomography scanning or magnetic resonance imaging of the brain.

Neurologic syndromes following solvent exposure have included loss of smell, loss of visual acuity, optic neuropathy, cerebral and cerebellar demyelination, cerebral atrophy, and dementia. Peripheral neuropathy with axonal degeneration has been described from a myriad of solvent exposures including hexane, methylbutyl ketone, and trichloroethylene. Worker protection from the toxic effects of solvents is based on air concentrations defined by threshold limit values to prevent subjective and objective complaints. The sources of these TLVs are shown in Table 106.8.

Neuropsychologic changes attributed to solvent exposure include alterations in psychomotor function, increased fatigue, difficulty concentrating, impairment of visuospatial coordination, impairment of visual motor performance, and impairment of memory. The term "solvent syndrome" has been applied to individuals with abnormal neuropsychologic functions following chronic longterm exposure to solvents (Table 106.9) (2, 9–16, 75–81).

Neuropsychologic deficits and neurobehavioral toxicity secondary to industrial solvents as well as other industrial toxins are recognized. The effects of inorganic lead, organic lead, other heavy metals, and carbon disulfide are appreciated. Studies of volunteer subjects demonstrated that brief exposures to styrene up to 7 hours to 375 ppm were associated with im-

Table 106.8.   Summary of Sources for 8-Hour TWA TLVs for Selected Solvents

100 ppm	Stoddard solvent	Prevention of irritation/narcotic effect
50 ppm	Styrene	One-tenth lowest concentration in rats causing hematopoietic tumors
100 ppm	Toluene	Experimental animal studies (change in weight and adrenal glands) and experimental human subjects showed prolongation of reaction time, decrease in pulse rate and systolic blood pressure
100 ppm	Methylene chloride	Human experience indicates no problem at this level, and COHb levels should not exceed 5% in nonsmokers
50 ppm	Methyl chloride	Human experience indicates no problem at this level but margin of safety small with respect to neurotoxic effects
50 ppm	Trichloroethylene	Prevent subjective complaints such as headaches, fatigue, instability, and other toxic effects
50 ppm	2-Ethoxyethanol	Avoidance of significant blood changes and by analogy with relative acute toxicity of other analogue (2-butoxyethanol)
300 ppm	Cyclohexane	Threshold of irritation effects (eyes/mucous membranes)
10 ppm	Carbon disulfide	Avoidance of cardiovascular and neurologic effects—human experience
200 ppm	MEK	Minimize complaints in odor and irritation
50 ppm	Cyclohexanol	Reduction of objectionable irritation
25 ppm	Cyclohexanone	Preclude throat irritation and avoidance of liver/kidney damage suggested by animal studies
25 ppm	Dioxane	Data on hepato- and nephrotoxic effects and this level can be achieved in practice
300 ppm	Gasoline	Based on probable compositions of gasoline vapor in relation to specific components, e.g., hexanes, pentane, butane, etc.
50 ppm	Perchloroethylene	Avoidance of neurologic effects, eye irritation and liver damage. The STEL will prevent anesthetic effects
1000 ppm	Trichlorofluoromethane	Absence of effects in animals at 1000 ppm and from human experience. Should prevent organic injury as well as cardiac sensitization
1000 ppm	1,1,2-Trichloro-1,2,2-trifluoroethane	Same as above
100 ppm	Turpentine	Prevention of nose and throat irritation
50 ppm	MIBK	Prevention of irritant effects and possible effects on kidney (animal study); also slightly higher levels reportedly produce headaches and nausea
50 ppm	n-Butanol (ceiling)	Avoidance of system effects are auditory nerves and vestibular function (from human experience)
200 ppm	n-Propanol	Analogy with butyl alcohols and eye, nose, and throat irritation
500 ppm	Hexane isomers	Analogy with pentane, heptane, and octane; absence of CNS effects; and metabolic differences with the n-isomer
50 ppm	n-Hexane	Avoidance of neurotoxicity (peripheral neuropathy)
750 ppm	Acetone	Avoidance of mild irritation and absence of serious ill effects at much higher concentrations
300 ppm	VM&P Naphtha	Analogy with rubber solvent (acute tox-animal study). Avoidance of irritation and nonspecific chronic effect
100 ppm	Xylene (o-, m-, p-)	Avoidance of irritant effects and prenarcosis effect
50 ppm	Halothane	Analogy with trichloroethylene and chloroform are relative toxicity to liver and CNS (anesthetic effects)
10 ppm	Vinyl acetate	Prevention of irritation and absence of acute or chronic effects observed after longterm exposure around this level

Reprinted with permission from: Cranmer J, Goldberg L. Neurobehavioral effects of solvents: Exposure Issues in the Evaluation of Solvent Effects.

pairment and manual dexterity as well as symptoms of light headedness and headache (76). Multiple studies have been performed demonstrating that chronic exposure to styrene is associated with neurobehavioral toxic effects. Testing of chronically exposed workers has demonstrated impaired psychomotor performance, impairment of vigilance, impairment of speed, and impairment of memory.

Acute intoxication with organic solvents produces dizziness, confusion, headache, CNS depression, lethargy, and incoor-

dination. Subacute and chronic exposure to solvents can result in a clinical syndrome of memory impairment, difficulty in concentration, alterations in attention, alterations in hand-eye coordination, dysfunction in reaction time in psychomotor function, and changes in personality. Neuropsychologic tests administered to individuals chronically exposed occupationally to a variety of organic solvents have demonstrated abnormal findings (9–16, 75–81). Abnormal electroencephalograms, intellectual deterioration, and impairment of visuospatial and

Table 106.9.   Solvent Syndrome

Subjective Symptoms	Objective Signs
Headache	Cerebellar signs
Nausea	Peripheral neuropathies
Dizziness	Gait disturbances
Fatigue	Tremor
Psychiatric disturbances	Nystagmus
Anxiety	Cognitive changes
Difficulty in concentration	Memory deficits
Emotional lability	Cerebral atrophy
	Gait disturbance
	Neuropsychologic deficits

visuoconstructive abilities. Psychomotor performance is usually the most affected as a consequence of longterm solvent exposure.

Other studies corroborate the chronic symptoms of intellectual and psychomotor impairment following prolonged exposure to solvents. Exposed workers were shown to have more dementia-like symptoms, poor performance on psychometric testing, and more neurobehavioral abnormalities (75–81). The testing of workers with histories of exposure to solvents show subtle changes in the Minnesota Multiphasic Personality Inventory (MMPI) in comparison with nonexposed workers of similar work class (78).

The "solvent syndrome" became recognized at the end of the nineteenth century in workers who were chronically exposed to solvents in the workplace (13). Controlled human experiments have shown that nerve conduction velocity is reduced following exposure to 200 ppm of styrene (76). Generally, the solvent exposure situations producing neurotoxicity have been documented by environmental monitoring which has demonstrated that these exposures were above known threshold limit values set to prevent health effects. In addition, in many work situations, mixtures of solvents are used. Neuropsychologic assessment and neuropsychometric testing have found a role in the evaluation of individuals exposed to solvents. Studies from the 1970s and 1980s have been duplicated in their findings of deficits in immediate memory, short term memory, learning, mental tracking, attention, concentration, and visuospatial abilities (82).

Evaluation of Solvent-Associated Neurotoxicity

The evaluation of an individual with neurobehavioral and neurologic toxicity and a history of solvent exposure can be difficult. Particularly in older individuals, the presence of cognitive changes and cognitive decay with a history of chronic exposure to organic solvents presents a difficult diagnostic workup. Neurologic tools for evaluation include CT, MRI, EEG, electromyography, nerve conduction velocities, evoked potentials, and neuropsychometrics. Individuals chronically exposed to solvents may have cerebral atrophy demonstrable on CT scanning or MRI. Objective neurologic findings may be present along with a clinical picture of dementia. Patients with Alzheimer's disease should be discerned from individuals who have solvent-induced neurotoxicity. Alzheimer's disease is associated with decline in language abilities, visuospatial skills, and memory function (83). However, patients with solvent neurotoxicity also demonstrate visuospatial difficulties and memory deficits. However, Alzheimer's disease is associated

with language dysfunction and solvent neurotoxicity is not. In addition, individuals with chronic neurotoxicity secondary to solvent exposure tend to remain the same or improve over time once the exposure has been terminated. Patients with Alzheimer's disease will generally show neuropsychologic decay over time (83). Patients with solvent-induced neurotoxicity may or may not have memory deficits. Solvent toxic individuals can have severe problems with attention and tracking as well as visuospatial processing and short term memory. This is also consistent with Alzheimer's diagnosis (83). However, retention of language, writing, and reading skills are more clearly indicative of solvent toxicity versus Alzheimer's disease (83). The IQ of an individual can be affected following both solvent toxic exposure and in Alzheimer's disease. However, with solvent exposure, IQ deterioration terminates following discontinuation of exposure, but in Alzheimer's disease, IQ deterioration can continue (83). Intact reading and writing abilities favor solvent-induced neurotoxicity. Progression of cognitive decline in the absence of exposure favors a diagnosis of dementia like Alzheimer's disease. Patients with solvent-induced neurotoxicity usually remain stable or improve in cognitive function once exposure is terminated (83). However, there have been some instances of further decline in abilities, but this is rare.

Individuals complaining of neurologic and neurobehavioral effects secondary to solvent exposure require evaluation. Many tests are insensitive to the more subtle effects produced by solvents. The general evaluation of a solvent exposed individual can be divided into (a) neurologic evaluation and (b) neuropsychologic evaluation. The neurologic evaluation involves careful history, physical examination with particular attention to neurologic functions. A complete neurologic examination is required. Ancillary tests that might be useful include CT scanning, evoked potentials, electromyography, and nerve conduction studies, and magnetic resonance imaging (MRI). In some situations, analysis of cerebrospinal fluid is also indicated to rule out other diseases.

Neuropsychologic evaluation is a relatively new tool used to assess solvent-exposed individuals. The World Health Organization Working Group in Copenhagen, in 1985, developed categories of solvent-related central nervous system toxicity. This categorization was based on the severity of condition: (a) minimal—inorganic affective syndrome; (b) moderate—a mild chronic toxic encephalopathy; or (c) pronounced—a severe toxic encephalography (84). The solvent syndrome can vary depending on the stage of neurotoxicity from mild neurobehavioral effects to mild encephalopathy or to severe encephalopathy and dementia. The time course for the development of neurobehavioral and neurologic toxicity secondary to solvent exposure may require years and has been noted to occur as early as 3 years following chronic exposure. It is also important to differentiate the acute effects of the solvent from chronic effects (Table 106.9). The acute effects generally occur quickly and are associated with central nervous system depression, dizziness, sometimes feeling of euphoria, and interference with coordination and mental thought processes. These symptoms generally clear once the exposure has terminated. The chronic effects of solvents are generally difficult to detect early on in the development of the syndrome because of the insensitivity and imprecision of testing methods currently available.

Electroencephalographic abnormalities may also be associated with chronic solvent exposure. One study demon-

Table 106.10.   Effects Occurring with Chemical Air Concentrations (89) in Studies in Table 106.9

None or Minimal Effect (ppm)		Definite Effect (ppm)
Toluene	34	338
Xylene	15	147
Styrene	6	59
Phenol	2	17
Ethylbenzene	14	143
Chlorobenzene	11	105

strated that abnormal EEGs were found in 17–67% of affected individuals (84). Also reductions in cerebral blood flow have been shown to exist in persons chronically exposed to solvents.

Evaluation of solvent-induced neurotoxicity should include clear definition of the exposure of the individual or individuals, focusing on the quality of exposure, duration, and intensity of the exposure. Confounding factors and other disease states must be ruled out first. The diagnosis of solvent neurotoxicity is one of probability and exclusion.

Many solvents have been implicated as causative of psycho-organic syndromes: jet fuel, toluene, xylene, styrene, trichloroethylene, gasoline, 1,1,1-trichloroethane, paint thinners, carbon disulfide, methylbutyl ketone, n-hexane, methyl n-butyl ketone, and perchloroethylene. Many subjects studied had exposure times of up to 20 years.

The prognosis of patients diagnosed as having solvent induced toxic encephalopathy has been reported (85, 86). One such study involved 26 individuals who had cerebral atrophy or intellectual impairment followed for a 2-year period post diagnosis and not exposed to solvents during this period of time. In general, their condition was unchanged as compared to their initial evaluation. However, there were some slight improvements with regard to some symptoms. In three of these patients, further deterioration was observed. However, in general, further progression of a syndrome is not expected once exposure to the solvent is discontinued (86).

The use of evoked potentials in assessing neurotoxicity to solvents is relatively new (87, 88). Evoked potentials are electrical manifestations of multisynaptic pathway activity within the central nervous system. Evoked potentials can be used to screen the integrity of the synapses in the central nervous system (87, 88). Evoked potentials can be auditory evoked potentials (AEPs) or visual evoked potentials (VEPs). At the present time, evoked potentials should be viewed as a screening tool for neurotoxicity. Evaluation of many other studies needs to be awaited in order to confirm their usefulness.

Irritancy Syndromes of Aromatic Solvents

Aromatic solvents are sensory irritants. Tests of sensory irritation have demonstrated this phenomenon with phenol, toluene, xylene, ethylbenzene, and styrene (89, 90). Concentration-response relationships were determined for these and many other chemicals to which humans are exposed by airborne vapors (Table 106.8). In these studies, minimal irritant effects occurred with chemical air concentrations (89) as shown in Table 106.10.

Even though these studies were performed in animals under controlled chamber conditions, a qualitative correlation from these studies exists for reported eye, nose, and throat irritation

Table 106.11.   Dermal Absorption of Solvents

Solvent	Rate	Reference
Toluene (liquid)	14–23 mg/cm²/hr	(19)
Xylene (liquid)	4.5–9.6 mg/cm²/hr	(19)
Styrene (liquid)	9–15 mg/cm²/hr	(19)
Aqueous styrene solution	40–180 µg/cm²/hr	
Ethylbenzene	20–33 mg/cm²/hr	(69)
Aqueous ethylbenzene solution	118–215 µg/cm²/hr	
Phenol (2.5 gm/L)	0.079–0.30 mg/cm²/hr	(56)
(5 gm/L)	0.181 ± 0.047 mg/cm²/hr	
(10 gm/L)	0.30 ± 0.048 mg/cm²/hr	

experienced by humans from vapors of these aromatic compounds (90).

Dermal Penetration of Alkybenzenes and Toxicity

The dermal absorption of alkylbenzenes has been extensively studied, since this can be a major route of toxicity. The absorption of toluene, styrene, xylene, phenol, and ethylbenzene across the human skin has been particularly studied (Table 106.11) (19, 56, 69). The absorption of toluene in solution was found to be proportional to the concentration of toluene in contact with the skin (19). Ethylbenzene also demonstrated very similar absorption rates across the skin being dependent on the concentration in contact with the skin (69). The dermal absorption rate of liquid toluene found to be 14–23 mg/cm²/hour in the subjects studied (19). The absorption of liquid styrene dermally was found to be 9–15 mg/cm²/hour. The dermal absorption of styrene was linear to the concentration of styrene. The rate of absorption of liquid xylene was from 4–10 mg/cm²/hour (19).

In the more realistic setting, the role of dermal absorption as a route of exposure to volatile solvents in water has been studied (35). The National Academy of Sciencies (NAS) has developed methodology to calculate acceptable concentrations of solvents in drinking water. This methodology is incorporated in the Environmental Protection Agency's Suggested No Adverse Response Level (SNARLS). The SNARL figures are the highest concentrations of the chemical that produce no observed adverse effect in chronic dosing in animals or humans. These figures are divided by a safety factor in order to obtain what is termed an Acceptable Daily Intake (ADI). In order to calculate the acceptable concentration of a chemical in water, the ADI is divided by the volume of water consumed by the average person, either adult or child. These calculations which involve ingestion of water containing organic solvents ignore the dermal absorption of these solvents (35). Absorption of the solvents from an aqueous solution has been demonstrated (19, 56, 69). Dermal absorption of a solvent is related to variables such as concentration of the solvent, duration of exposure, the condition of the skin, thickness and vascularity of the skin, and the surface area exposed. Other important variables which dictate absorption of volatile organic chemicals include the hydration status of the skin. The more hydrated the skin, as from perspiration or immersion in water, the more absorption is facilitated across the dermal barrier. Also, increased skin temperature will enhance skin absorption due to increased blood flow through the skin. Thus, immersion in an aqueous solution containing

Table 106.12.   Biologic Monitoring for Aromatic Solvents

Aromatic Solvent	Metabolites in Urine
Toluene	Hippuric acid
	Ortho-cresol
	Meta-cresol
	Para-cresol
Xylene	Methylhippuric acid
Phenol	Phenol (major)
	Phenol glucuronide
	Phenol sulfate
	1,4-dihydroxybenzene glucuronide and sulfate
Styrene	Mandelic acid
	Phenyl glyoxylic acid
Benzene	Phenol
	Catechol
	Hydroquinone
	Sulfate and glucuronide conjugates

volatile organics will enhance the absorption of those volatile organics. This can occur through bathing or swimming. The physical condition of the skin will also help dictate absorption of volatile organic chemicals. Injury, burn, or rashes will increase absorption. There are also variabilities in the absorption of solvents, depending on the anatomical location of the skin. The palms of the hands and soles of the feet, for instance, have more dermal barrier to absorption than do other parts of the body such as the scalp, neck, or abdomen and scrotal area. Other factors that affect the absorption of solvents include the solvent's chemical and physical properties. Studies have shown that combinations of solvents or multiple solvents in aqueous media have a greater chance of being more readily absorbed than a pure solvent (35).

Estimates of absorption across the skin have been made for alkylbenzenes such as toluene, styrene, and ethylbenzene. In environmental exposure situations, concentrations of alkylbenzenes may range in the low parts per billion to parts per million. Dermal absorption can represent a very significant exposure route for organic solvents, given the factors discussed. Dermal absorption may represent anywhere from 30–90 percent of the total daily intake of organic solvents from aqueous media (35). Thus, the dermal absorption of organic solvents from drinking water, swimming water, and other aqueous media can be a significant source of daily intake.

Biologic Markers of Solvent Exposure

Exposure to certain aromatic organic solvents can be verified by detection of metabolic products in urine (Table 106.12). These metabolites may also help quantify the exposure in some cases.

REFERENCES

1. Juntunen J. Occupational solvent poisoning: clinical aspects. In: V Riihimaki, U Ulfvarson, eds. Safety and health aspects of organic solvents. New York, NY: Alan R. Liss, Inc., 1986:265–279.
2. Popendorf W. Vapor pressure and solvent vapor hazards. Am Ind Hyg Assoc J 1984;45:719–726.
3. Agency for Toxic Substances and Disease Registry. US Public Health Service. Toxicological profile for toluene. Atlanta, GA: Clement Associates, Inc., Contract No. 205-88-0608, 1989:73–75.

4. Agency for Toxic Substances and Disease Registry. US Public Health Service. Toxicological profile for toluene. Atlanta, GA: Clement Associates, Inc., Contract No. 205-88-0608, 1989:1–8.
5. Agency for Toxic Substances and Disease Registry. US Public Health Service. Toxicological profile for toluene. Atlanta, GA: Clement Associates, Inc., Contract No. 205-88-0608, 1989:77–82.
6. Low LK, Meeds JR, Mackerer CR. Health effects of the alkylbenzenes. Toluene. Toxicol Ind Health 1984:49–75.
7. Hayden JW. Toxicology of toluene (methylbenzene): a review of current literature. Clin Toxicol 1977;11:549–559.
8. Cohr KH, Stokholm J. Toluene—a toxicologic review. Scand J Work Environ Health 1979;5:71–90.
9. Rosenberg NL, Kleinschmidt-DeMasters BK, Davis KA, Hormes JT. Toluene abuse causes diffuse central nervous system white matter changes. Ann Neurol 1988;23:611–614.
10. Keane JR. Toluene optic neuropathy. Ann Neurol 1978;4:390.
11. Maizlish NA, Langolf GD, Whitehead LW, et al. Behavioural evaluation of workers exposed to mixtures of organic solvents. Br J Ind Med 1985;42:579–590.
12. Baker EL, Smith TJ, Landrigan PJ. The neurotoxicity of industrial solvents: a review of the literature. Am J Ind Med 1985;8:207–217.
13. Grasso P, Sharbratt M, Davies DM, Irvine D. Neurophysiological and psychological disorders and occupational exposure to organic solvents. Food Chem Toxicol 1984;22:819–852.
14. Juntunen J, Hupli V, Hernberg S, Luisto M. Neurological picture of organic solvent poisoning in industry. Int Arch Occup Environ Health 1980;46:219–231.
15. King MD, Day RE, Oliver JS, Lush M, Watson JM. Br Med J 1981;283:663–665.
16. Flodin U, Edling C, Axelson O. Clinical studies of psychoorganic syndromes among workers with exposure to solvents. Am J Ind Med 1984;5:287–295.
17. Wikkelso C, Ekberg K, Lillienberg L, et al. Cerebrospinal fluid proteins and cells in men subjected to long-term exposure to organic solvents. Acta Neurol Scand 1984;70:113–119.
18. Carlsson A. Exposure to toluene uptake, distribution and elimination in man. Scand J Work Environ Health 1982;8:43–55.
19. Dutkiewicz T, Tyras H. Skin absorption of toluene, styrene, and xylene by man. Br J Ind Med 1968;25:243.
20. Tahti H. Karkkainen S, Pyykko K, et al. Chronic occupational exposure to toluene. Int Arch Occup Environ Health 1981;48:61–69.
21. Klockars M. Solvents and the liver. In: Riihimaki V, Ulfvarson U, eds. Safety and health aspects of organic solvents. New York, NY: Alan R. Liss, Inc., 1986:139–154.
22. Dossing M, Arlien-Soborg P, Petersen LM, Ranek L. Liver damage associated with occupational exposure to organic solvents in house painters. Eur J Clin Invest 1983;13:151–157.
23. Taher SM, Anderson RJ, McCartney R, Popovtzer MM, Schrier RW. Renal tubular acidosis associated with toluene "sniffing." N Engl J Med 1974;290:765–768.
24. Moss AH, Gabow PA, Kaehny WD, et al. Fanconi's syndrome and distal renal tubular acidosis after glue sniffing. Ann Intern Med 1980;92:69–70.
25. Voigts A, Kaufman CE. Acidosis and other metabolic abnormalities associated with paint sniffing. South Med J 1983;76:443–452.
26. Goodwin TM. Toluene abuse and renal tubular acidosis in pregnancy. Obstet Gynecol 1988;71:715–718.
27. Nielsen HK, Krusell L, Baelum J, et al. Renal effects of acute exposure to toluene. Acta Med Scand 1985;218:317–321.
28. Bennett RH, Forman HR. Hypokalemic periodic paralysis in chronic toluene exposure. Arch Neurol 1980;37:673.
29. Toftgard R, Gustafsson JA. Biotransformation of organic solvents. Scand J Work Environ Health 1980;6:1–8.
30. De Rosa E, Bartolucci GB, Sigon M, et al. Hippuric acid and ortho-cresol as biological indicators of occupational exposure to toluene. Am J Ind Med 1987;11:529–537.
31. Hasegawa K, Shiojima S, Koizumi A, Ikeda M. Hippuric acid and o-cresol in the urine of workers exposed to toluene. Int Arch Occup Environ Health 1983;52:197–208.
32. Angerer J. Occupational chronic exposure to organic solvents. XII. o-cresol excretion after toluene exposure. Int Arch Occup Environ Health 1985;56:323–328.
33. De Rosa E, Brugnone F, Bartolucci GB, et al. The validity of urinary metabolites as indicators of low exposures to toluene. Int Arch Occup Environ Health 1985;56:135–145.
34. Andersson R, Carlsson A, Nordqvist MB, Sollenberg J. Urinary excre-

tion of hippuric acid and *o*-cresol after laboratory exposure of humans to toluene. Int Arch Occup Environ Health 1983;53:101–108.

35. Brown HS, Bishop DR, Rowan CA. The role of skin absorption as a route of exposure for volatile organic compounds (VOCs) in drinking water. Am J Public Health 1984;74:479–484.

36. Baelum J, Anderson IB, Lundqvist GR, et al. Response of solvent-exposed printers and unexposed controls to six-hour toluene exposure. Scand J Work Environ Health 1985;11:271–280.

37. Inoue O, Seiji K, Watanabe T, et al. Possible ethnic difference in toluene metabolism: a comparative study among Chinese, Turkish, and Japanese solvent workers. Toxicol Lett 1986;34:167–174.

38. Wallen M, Naslund H, Nordqvist B. The effects of ethanol on the kinetics of toluene in man. Toxicol Appl Pharmacol 1984;76:414–419.

39. Dossing M, Baelum J, Hansen SH, Lundqvist GR. Effect of ethanol, cimetidine and propranolol on toluene metabolism in man. Int Arch Occup Environ Health 1984;54:309–315.

40. Konietzko H, Keilbach J, Drysch K. Cumulative effects of daily toluene exposure. Int Arch Occup Environ Health 1980;46:53–58.

41. Aitio A, Pekari K, Jarvisalo J. Skin absorption as a source of error in biological monitoring. Scan J Work Environ Health 1984;10:317–320.

42. Hersh JH, Podruch PE, Rogers G, Weisskopf B. Toluene embryopathy. J Pediatr 1985;106:922–927.

43. Holmberg PC. Central nervous system defects in children born to mothers exposed to organic solvents during pregnancy. Lancet July 28, 1979:177–179.

44. Maki-Paakkanen J, Husgafvel-Pursiainen K, Kalliomak PL, Tuominen J, Sorsa M. Toluene-exposed workers and chromosome aberrations.

45. Haglund U, Lundberg I, Zech L. Chromosome aberrations and sister chromatid exchanges in Swedish paint industry workers. Scand J Work Environ Health 1980;6:291–298.

46. Forni A, Pacifico E, Limonta A. Chromosome studies in workers exposed to benzene or toluene or both. Arch Environ Health 1971;22:373–378.

47. Andersen I, Lundqvist GR, Molhave L, et al. Human response to controlled levels of toluene in six-hour exposures. Scand J Work Environ Health 1983;9:405–418.

48. Riihimaki V, Savolainen K. Human exposure to *m*-xylene kinetics and acute effects on the central nervous system. Ann Occup Hyg 1980;23:411–422.

49. Riihimaki V, Savolainen K, Pfaffli P, Pekari K, Sippel HW, Laine A. Metabolic interaction between *m*-xylene and ethanol. Arch Toxicol 1982;49:253–263.

50. Lundberg I, Hakansson M. Normal serum activities of liver enzymes in Swedish paint industry workers with heavy exposure to organic solvents. Br Med J 1985;42:596–600.

51. Riihimaki V, Pfaffli P, Savolainen K. Kinetics of *m*-xylene in man. Scand J Work Environ Health 1979;5:232–248.

52. Bruce RM, Santodonato J, Neal MW. Summary review of the health effects associated with phenol. Toxicol Ind Health 1987;3:535–569.

53. Agency for Toxic Substances and Disease Registry. Production, import, use, and disposal. Toxicological profile for phenol. Agency for Toxic Substances and Disease Registry. US Health Service. Atlanta, GA: 1989:59–62.

54. Agency for Toxic Substances and Disease Registry. Potential for human exposure. Toxicological profile for phenol. Agency for Toxic Substances and Disease Registry. US Health Service. Atlanta, GA: 1989:63–74.

55. Agency for Toxic Substances and Disease Registry. Health effects. Toxicological profile for phenol. Agency for Toxic Substances and Disease Registry. US Health Service. Atlanta, GA: 1989:11–54.

56. Baranowska-Dutkiewicz B. Skin absorption of phenol from aqueous solutions in men. Int Arch Occup Environ Health 1981;49:99–104.

57. Haddad LM, Dimond KA, Schweistris JE. Phenol poisoning. J Am Coll Emergency Phys 1979;8:267–269.

58. Warner MA, Harper JV. Cardiac dysrhythmias associated with chemical peeling with phenol. Anesthesiology 1985;62:366–367.

59. Conning DM, Hayes JM. The dermal toxicity of phenol: an investigation of the most effective first-aid measures. Br J Ind Med 1970;27:155–159.

60. Brown VKH, Box VL, Simpson BJ. Decontamination procedures for skin exposed to phenolic substancs. Arch Environ Health 1975;30:1–6.

61. Behl CR, Linn EE, Flynn GL, et al. Permeation of skin and eschar by antiseptics. I: Baseline studies with phenol. J Pharm Sci 1983;72:391–397.

62. Coan ML, Baggs RB, Bosmann HB. Demonstration of direct toxicity of phenol on kidney. Res Commun Chem Pathol Pharmacol 1982;36:229–239.

63. Baker EL, Landrigan PJ, Bertozzi PE, Field PH, Skinner HG. Phenol poisoning due to contaminated drinking water. Arch Environ Health March/April 1978:89–94.

64. Chemical review: styrene. Dangerous Properties of Industrial Materials Report 1988;8:10–44.

65. Guillemin MP, Berode M. Biological monitoring of styrene: a review. Am Ind Hyg Assoc J 1988;49:497–505.

66. Lindstrom K, Harkonen H, Hernberg S. Disturbances in psychological functions of workers occupationally exposed to styrene. Scand J Work Environ Health 1976;3:129–139.

67. Mutti A, Mazzucchi A, Rustichelli P, Frigeri G, Arfini G, Franchini I. Exposure-effect and exposure-response relationships between occupational exposure to styrene and neuropsychological functions. Am J Ind Med 1984;5:275–286.

68. (No author listed). Chlorobenzene. Dangerous Properties of Industrial Materials Report 1990;10:66–77.

69. Dutkiewicz T, Tyras H. A study of skin absorption of ethylbenzene in man. Br J Ind Med 1967;24:330–332.

70. (No author listed). Hydroquinone. Dangerous Properties of Industrial Materials Report. 1988;8:51–60.

71. (No author listed). 2-Naphthol. Dangerous Properties of Industrial Materials Report 1988;8:79–86.

72. (No author listed). Pyrocatechol. Dangerous Properties of Industrial Materials Report 1988;8:87–94.

73. Proctor NH, Hughes JP. Chemical hazards of the workplace. Philadelphia, PA: Lippincott, 1978.

74. Heikkila PR, Hameila M, Pyy L, Raunu P. Exposure to creosote in the impregnation and handling of impregnated wood. Scand J Work Environ Health 1987;13:431–437.

75. Gregersen P, Angelso B, Nielson TE, Norgaard B, Uldal C. Neurotoxic effects of organic solvents in exposed workers: an occupational, neuropsychological, and neurological investigation. Am J Ind Med 1984;5:201–225.

76. Feldman RG, Ricks NL, Baker EL. Neuropsychological effects of industrial toxins: a review. Am J Ind Med 1980;1:211–227.

77. Seppalainen AM, Lindstrom K, Martelin T. Neurophysiological and psychological picture of solvent poisoning. Am J Ind Med 1980;1:31–42.

78. Morrow LA, Ryan CM, Goldstein G, Hodgson MJ. A distinct pattern of personality disturbance following exposure to mixtures of organic solvents. J Occup Med 1989;31:743–746.

79. Seppalainen AM. Neurophysiological aspects of the toxicity of organic solvents. Sand J Work Environ Health 1985;11:61–64.

80. Valciukas JA, Lilis R, Singer RM, Glickman L, Nicholson WJ. Neurobehavioral changes among shipyard painters exposed to solvents. Arch Environ Health 1985;40:47–52.

81. Gregersen P, Stigsby B. Reaction time of industrial workers exposed to organic solvents: relationship to degree of exposure and psychological performance. Am J Ind Med 1981;2:313–321.

82. Crossen JR, Wiens AN. Wechsler memory scale-revised: deficits in performance associated with neurotoxic solvent exposure. The Clin Neuropsychol 1988;2:181–187.

83. White RF. Differential diagnosis of probable Alzheimer's disease and solvent encephalopathy in older workers. The Clin Neuropsychol 1987;1:153–160.

84. Neuropsychological toxicology of solvents. Chapt IV in: Hartman DE, ed. Neuropsychological toxicology identification and assessment of human neurotoxic syndromes. New York, NY: Pergamon Press, 1988.

85. Antti-Poika M. Overall prognosis of patients with diagnosed chronic organic solvent intoxication. Int Arch Occup Environ Health 1982;51:127–138.

86. Bruhn P, Arlien-Soborg P, Gyldensted C, Christensen EL. Prognosis in chronic toxic encephalopathy. Acta Neurol Scand 1981;64:259–272.

87. Arezzo JC, Simson R, Brennan NE. Evoked potentials in the assessment of neurotoxicity in humans. Neurobehav Toxicol Teratol 1985;7:299–304.

88. Pakalnis A, Drake ME, Dadmehr N, Weiss K. Evoked potentials and EEG in multiple sclerosis. Electroencephalogr Clin Neurophysiol 1987;67:333–336.

89. De Ceaurriz JC, Micillino JC, Bonnet P, Guenier JP. Sensory irritation caused by various industrial airborne chemicals. Toxicol Lett 1981;9:137–143.

90. Hellquist H, Irander K, Edling C, Odkvist L. Nasal symptoms and histopathology in a group of spray-painters. Acta Otolaryngol 1983;96:495–500.

107

Oxygenated Compounds: Alcohols, Glycols, Ketones, and Esters

Daniel A. Spyker
John B. Sullivan, Jr., M.D.

INTRODUCTION

Alcohols, glycols, ketones, ethers, and esters are oxygenated compounds primarily used as solvents or intermediate chemicals in the synthesis of other compounds. Summary listing of many of the more toxicologically important compounds can be found in Tables 107.1–107.4.

ALCOHOLS

Alcohols have the general formula R–OH, where R is an alkyl or substituted alkyl group. The R group can be a variety of structures. Alcohols contain a hydroxyl (–OH) group. An exception to this are phenols, where the alcohol group is attached directly to the benzene ring. Alcohols and phenols have very diverse chemical and toxicologic characteristics. Table 107.1 summarizes many of the health hazards of alcohols.

Alcohols are used in a variety of industrial and commercial situations. They are frequently used as solvents and chemical intermediates. The toxicity of alcohols varies as a function of their metabolites, systemic absorption, and volatility.

Three of the more commonly recognized toxic alcohols are ethyl alcohol, isopropyl alcohol, and methyl alcohol.

Ethyl Alcohol (Ethanol)

Ethanol is completely and rapidly absorbed, distributed in total body water (60% for men, 48% for women), and eliminated by saturable hepatic metabolism. This maximum rate of ethanol metabolism (V_{max}) is about 24 mg/dl/hr, and the process is half saturated (K_m) at a blood level of 9 mg/dl. Most states consider operating a motor vehicle with a blood alcohol concentration (BAC) of 100 mg/dl (0.1 g%) to be illegal *per se*. A BAC of 100 mg/dl (about four drinks) increases the likelihood of a motor vehicle accident by sevenfold, and of 150 mg/dl increases the likelihood 25-fold (3).

Isopropyl Alcohol (Isopropanol)

This clear, colorless aliphatic alcohol has chemical, physical, and toxicologic properties similar to ethanol. Isopropanol has been widely substituted for ethanol in industrial processes including food processing and generally has a reputation as a relatively safe solvent. Isopropanol is widely available to the general public as rubbing alcohol (usually, though not always, 70% isopropanol). It is also an inconstant ingredient in paint thinners, medications, racing fuels, fuel line deicer, paint removers, cleaners, and disinfectants.

Like ethanol, isopropanol is rapidly absorbed from the gastrointestinal (GI) tract and distributes in total body water (0.5–0.7 l/kg). The kidney excretes 25–50% unchanged, and the balance is metabolized (by alcohol dehydrogenase) to acetone. Acetone is more slowly eliminated than isopropanol, and acetone levels typically exceed isopropanol levels a few hours after absorption. Although acetone may contribute to central nervous system (CNS) depression, longterm sequelae are not generally attributed to either isopropanol or acetone toxicity. Ingestion studies in experimental animals showed isopropanol to be twice as lethal as ethanol on a ml/kg basis (4). While the factor of 2 may not find uniform acceptance, toxicity in humans seems to follow this pattern.

Although ingestion is generally considered to represent the greatest hazard, the use of isopropanol, with or without water, in a "sponge bath" to lower fever has led to coma in a number of infants and adults. A review of these cases and a study of the relative contribution of the two routes in a rabbit model suggested that dermal absorption probably contributes more to isopropanol poisoning than inhalation in these cases (5).

Methyl Alcohol

Methyl alcohol (wood alcohol, Manhattan spirit, colonial spirit, methanol) is in wide use as an industrial and household solvent. Methanol has caused poisonings by inhalation and skin absorption as well as by ingestion. Due in part to the variation in methanol toxicity among species, the human toxicity was not fully recognized until the 1920s. This lack of appreciation of methanol toxicity provided several opportunities to study the variability of human methanol poisoning following substitution of methanol for ethanol in beverages.

Methanol itself has about one third of the intoxicating effect of ethanol, but hepatic metabolism via alcohol dehydrogenase produces (12–48 hours later) highly toxic formic acid (formate). Methanol is slowly metabolized to formaldehyde, but the conversion to formic acid follows rapidly, and formic acid concentrations correlate well with the acidemia. Thus **formic acid** appears to be the principal toxic metabolite accounting for the metabolic acidemia (6) and the ocular toxicity (7). The large anion gap metabolic acidosis is the hallmark of methanol toxicity.

In 1978, 372 patients were poisoned by ingesting 82% methanol and 18% isopropanol mistakenly substituted for their methylated spirits. Visual disturbance was noted by 27% (102 of 372 patients), four patients ended up totally blind, and mortality was 5% (18 of 372). Of the 102 patients with visual disturbances, 29 were blind, 65 reported blurring of vision (44 with pupil or fundus changes), and 10 had dilated pupils (two nonreactive).

Toxicity may occur following doses of 0.21 ml/kg (15 ml/kg) methanol, and 70 ml/70 kg is the maximum dose survived.

Table 107.1. Alcohols

Chemical Name	Chemical Formula	Toxicity
Allyl alcohol	CH_2OH	Colorless flammable liquid incompatible with oxidizers. It has been used as a fungicide and a herbicide in the past and in preparation of acrolein and glycerol. It is an eye, skin, and respiratory tract irritant. Allyl alcohol can cause dermal and ocular burns on contact and any contact with the skin or eye should immediately be decontaminated with water. It can be absorbed through the skin or inhaled. OSHA PEL = 2 ppm, and IDLH level = 150 ppm.
n-Butyl alcohol (n-butanol)	C_4H_9OH	Colorless flammable, liquid with a very strong disagreeable odor. It has been used as a solvent for lacquers and also in the manufacturing of plastics and cement. It is incompatible with oxidizing agents. It is a strong irritant of the mucous membranes, eyes, skin and respiratory tract. In high concentrations in the air it can cause CNS depression. OSHA PEL = 100 ppm, ACGIH TLV (ceiling) = 50 ppm, and IDLH level = 8000 ppm.
sec-Butyl alcohol	$CH_3CH_2CHOHCH_3$	Colorless flammable liquid with a strong disagreeable odor. Also known as 2-butynol. Used as a solvent for paint removing and in polishing and cleaning materials. It is also used in the synthesis of methyl ethyl ketone. It is incompatible with strong oxidizing agents. At high concentrations in the air sec-butyl alcohol can cause narcosis and CNS depression. It is a strong irritant of the mucous membrane, eyes, and respiratory tract. OSHA PEL = 150 ppm, ACGIH TLV = 100 ppm, and IDLH level = 10,000 ppm.
tert-Butyl alcohol (n-propanol)	$(CH_3)_3COH$	Colorless flammable liquid with a disagreeable odor. It is used in the manufacturing of plastics and esters and as an intermediate in the formulation of other chemicals. High concentrations in the area can cause CNS depression and are irritating to the eyes, throat, and mucous membranes. Contact to the skin of the liquid can cause mild chemical burns. OSHA PEL = 100 ppm, ACGIH PLV = 100 ppm, and IDLH level = 8000 ppm.
Isobutyl alcohol	$(CH_3)_2CH_2OH$	Colorless flammable liquid used in paint removers and as a general solvent. It is also used in the manufacture of esters. Isobutyl alcohol is an irritant to the skin, eyes, and mucous membranes. OSHA PEL = 100 ppm, ACGIH TLV = 50 ppm, and IDLH level = 8000 ppm.
Cyclohexanol	$C_6H_{11}OH$	Colorless thick liquid with odor of camphor. It is used as a solvent for ethyl cellulose and other resins, in the manufacture of soap, and in the manufacture of adipic acid, which is used in nylon production. It is also used in plastic manufacturing. It is incompatible with strong oxidizers. It is an irritant of the eyes, skin, and mucous membranes. It can produce CNS depression at high air concentrations. OSHA PEL = 50 ppm, IDLH level = 3500 ppm, and ACGIH TLV = 50 ppm.
Diacetone alcohol	$(CH_3)_2C(OH)CH_2COCH_3$	Flammable liquid used as a solvent for cellulose esters, pigments, oils, and fats. It is also used in hydraulic brake fluids and as an antifreeze. It is incompatible with strong oxidizers and alkaline substances. On exposure it produces skin irritation and irritation of the eyes, mucous membranes and respiratory tract. At higher concentrations in the air it can also produce CNS depression. OSHA PEL = 50 ppm, IDLH level = 2100 ppm, and ACGIH TLV = 50 ppm.
Dibutylaminoethanol	$(C_4H_9)_2NCH_2OH$	Colorless flammable liquid. It is an irritant to eyes, skin, and mucous membrane. There is no OSHA PEL. ACGIH TLV-TWA = 2 ppm with a skin notation.
Diethylaminoethanol	$(C_2H_5)_2NCH_2CH_2OH$	Colorless flammable liquid used as a chemical intermediate in the production of numerous compounds and products such as detergents, cosmetics, textile finishing agents, and pharmaceuticals. It is incompatible with strong oxidizing agents and acids. It is an irritant to the eyes, mucous membranes, skin, and respiratory tract. It can also produce nausea and vomiting. OSHA PEL = 10 ppm, ACGIH TLV = 10 ppm, and IDLH level = 500 ppm.
Ethyl alcohol (ethanol)	C_2H_5OH	Colorless, very volatile, flammable liquid used in grain alcohol, wines, and other alcoholic consumption beverages. It is also used in the chemical synthesis of many other compounds. It is a general solvent used in many processes such as the manufacturing of pharmaceutical agents. It is used also as a general solvent in perfumes, cosmetics, adhesives, inks, and preservatives. It is used as a fuel and an antifreeze. Ingestion of ethyl alcohol can result in common intoxication states that are well known. The OSHA PEL = 1000 ppm.

continues

Table 107.1. *Continued*

Chemical Name	Chemical Formula	Toxicity
β-Chloroethyl alcohol (ethylene chlorohydrin)		Flammable colorless liquid that has an odor like ether. It is used in the production of ethylene glycol and ethylene oxide. It also is used as a solvent for cellulose acetates and esters, resins, waxes, and ethers. It is used in chemical reactions where hydroxyethyl groups have to be introduced into organic compounds. In the cleaning industry it is used to remove tar from clothing. It is also used as a general solvent and for fabric dying. It is incompatible with strong oxidizing agents and alkaline substances. Ethylene chlorohydrin is an irritant to the skin, eyes, and mucous membranes. It is also a hepatotoxin and its metabolites are chloroacetaldehyde and chloroacetic acid. It is also a renal toxin. Toxic exposure to the vapors can produce irritation to the eyes, mucous membranes, and respiratory tract along with nausea and vomiting. Low level exposure can produce headache, hypotension, cardiovascular collapse, and coma. OSHA PEL = 5 ppm, ACGIH TLV = 1 ppm, IDLH level = 10 ppm, and ACGIH ceiling value is 1 ppm with a skin notation.
Furfuryl alcohol (furfural alcohol, 2-furanmethanol)	$C_4H_3OCH_2OH$	Colorless liquid used as a starting monomer in the production of furan resins or furan polymers. It is incompatible with strong acids and strong oxidizing agents, which can lead to rapid polymerization. The liquid also turns dark in air. It is also used as a solvent for cellulose ethers, esters, resins, and dyes, as well as in the manufacturing of resin compounds. It is an irritant of the respiratory tract, mucous membranes, and eyes and high concentrations in the air can produce CNS depression. OSHA PEL = 50 ppm, ACGIH TLV = 10 ppm with a skin notation, and IDLH level = 250 ppm.
Isoamyl alcohol (fusel oil, 3-methyl-1-butanol)	$(C_2H_5)_2CHOH$	Colorless flammable liquid. Amyl alcohol is used in the manufacture of lacquers, paint, varnishes, paint removers, cements, perfumes, pharmaceuticals, rubber, and plastic. It is also used in the production of isobutyl esters. Exposure to the skin and eyes can produce irritation. Amyl alcohol is a mild irritant to the mucous membranes and respiratory tract as well as the skin. At high air concentrations it can produce CNS depression; upon ingestion it can produce narcosis, headache, vomiting, weakness, and CNS depression. OSHA PEL = 100 ppm, ACGIH TLV = 100 ppm, and IDLH concentration = 8000 ppm.
Isopropyl alcohol (isopropanol)	$CH_3CHOHCH_3$	Colorless flammable liquid. It can be an irritant of the eyes, mucous membranes, and respiratory tract. At high concentrations it can produce CNS depression on inhalation. On ingestion it can produce GI bleeding as well as CNS depression and hypotension. Isopropyl alcohol is widely used in cosmetics and as a solvent in perfumes and many other commercial processes. It is incompatible with strong oxidizing agents. OSHA PEL = 400 ppm, ACGIH TLV = 400 ppm, and the IDLH level = 20,000 ppm.
Isooctyl alcohol (isooctanol)	$C_7H_{15}CH_2OH$	Clear liquid. It is used as a raw material for surfactants, as an antifoaming agent, and as a solvent. It is used in the formation of phthalate esters, maleate esters, and adipate esters, which are used in the formation of plastics. The ACGIH TLV as a TWA = 50 ppm with a skin notation.
Methyl alcohol (methanal)	CH_3OH	Colorless flammable liquid used in many organic syntheses such as the formation of formaldehyde, ethylene glycol, ethyl amines, pesticides, and methacrylates. It is also used as an antifreeze. The most common toxic manifestation of methyl alcohol is a metabolic acidosis with an anion gap due to the ingestion of methanol with formation of toxic metabolites of formaldehyde and formic acid. OSHA PEL = 200 ppm, ACGIH TLV = 200 ppm with a skin notation, and IDLH level = 25,000 ppm.
Methyl cyclohexanol	$CH_3C_6H_{10}OH$	Slightly yellow-colored flammable liquid with a slight odor of coconuts. It is used as a solvent for lacquers and as an antioxidant in lubricants. It is incompatible with strong oxidizing agents. Exposure to vapors can produce irritation to the eyes, skin, and mucous membranes. Methyl cyclohexanol is easily detected at airborne concentrations of 500 ppm, a concentration that can produce irritant effects. OSHA PEL = 100 ppm, ACGIH TVL = 50 ppm, and IDLH level = 10,000 ppm.
Methyl amyl alcohol (methyl isobutyl carbinol)	$CH_3CHOHCH_2CH(CH_3)_2$	Colorless flammable liquid. It is used as a solvent and in the manufacturing and formulation of brake fluid as well as an intermediate in the synthesis of other organic compounds. This alcohol is an irritant of eyes and mucous membranes at high concentrations and also can produce CNS depression. OSHA PEL = 25 ppm, ACGIH TLV = 25 ppm, and IDLH level = 2000 ppm.

continues

Table 107.1. *Continued*

Chemical Name	Chemical Formula	Toxicity
N-Propyl alcohol (1-propanol)	CH_3CH_2OH	Clear flammable liquid used in lacquers, cosmetics, cleaners, polishers, polishing agents, and pharmaceuticals and is also used as an antiseptic agent. It is incompatible with strong oxidizing agents. N-Propyl alcohol is an irritant of the eyes, skin, and mucous membranes and in high concentrations in air can produce CNS depression. Following ingestion, it can also produce CNS depression and is thought to be more toxic than isopropyl alcohol. N-Propanol is not very irritating to the skin. OSHA PEL = 200 ppm, ACGIH TLV = 200 ppm, and IDLH level = 4000 ppm.

Since a typical swallow is 0.33–0.5 ml/kg, this potency places methanol-rich solutions among the most toxic substances routinely found in our environment.

Although methanol-poisoned patients who are many hours postingestion and in coma usually die, both the severe acid-base disturbances and the toxic levels of formic acid are effectively managed with hemodialysis and supportive measures. The lethal synthesis of formic acid by the liver is readily blocked by "therapeutic levels" (100 mg/dl) of ethanol. Thus the profound toxicity of methanol is readily prevented by an easily administered and widely available beverage (8).

GLYCOLS

Glycols are alcohols containing two hydroxyl (–OH) groups and include such compounds as ethylene glycol, diethylene glycol, propylene glycol, and glycerol.

Ethylene Glycol

This clear, colorless liquid has a pleasant, warm, sweet taste. An exploratory taste by a child or pet all too frequently leads to a serious poisoning. Ethylene glycol's water solubility, high boiling point, and low vapor pressure have led to wide use as a solvent, coolant, and antifreeze. As with methanol, even a single swallow of permanent automotive antifreeze (typically 95% ethylene glycol) can result in serious toxicity.

The parent compound, approximately equitoxic with ethanol, is metabolized via alcohol dehydrogenase (ADH) to several more toxic metabolites which, in turn, produce metabolic acidosis, CNS and cardiopulmonary toxicity, and renal injury. **Glycolic acid** accounts for 96% of the free acid (9) and will thus be considered the principal toxic metabolite. Although oxalic acid was previously considered a principal toxic metabolite, only about 1% of ethylene glycol winds up as oxalate and provides the crystalluria associated with ethylene glycol ingestion.

Ethylene glycol toxicity develops in three phases. During the **glycol phase** (1–12 hours) the clinical effects reflect the direct CNS effects, which approximate those of ethanol. Absorption from the GI tract is somewhat slower than ethanol, it has a slightly larger volume of distribution, and metabolism proceeds in a linear (proportional to plasma level) manner. Half-life is about 3 hours and increases to about 15 hours when concomitant ethanol competes for the ADH.

The toxic effects of the principal toxic metabolite mark the **glycolate phase** (4–24 hours). Glycolic acid levels peak between 4 and 8 hours in the absence of ethanol and may peak at 12 or more hours when ethanol is present. We believe that the glycolate is directly responsible for the profound acidemia, neurologic toxicity (10), and cardiopulmonary injury including noncardiogenic pulmonary edema (11). Finally, the development of renal injury (usually reversible) defines the **nephropathy phase** ((24–72 hours). The relative contribution of the glycolate versus the calcium oxalate or other metabolites to this injury is not known.

As with methanol, the toxicity of ethylene glycol is probably completely prevented by early and adequate ADH blockade with ethanol. A potent, relatively nontoxic inhibitor of ADH, 4-methylpyrazole is currently undergoing human trials (12). If human trials demonstrate the expected efficacy and safety, it should prove useful in the treatment of methanol and glycol poisoning.

Diethylene Glycol

In 1937, 76 people died following ingestion of a newly marketed sulfanilamide elixir (dissolved in alcohol) medication containing 72% diethylene glycol. Animal experiments showed that the diethylene glycol was the responsible toxin in the "Massingale Disaster" (13). This disaster helped initiate the passage of the Food, Drug and Cosmetics Act of 1937 (under development from 1930 to 1935) which, for the first time, required manufacturers to demonstrate **safety** of their products prior to marketing. A similarly unfortunate substitution of diethylene glycol for propylene glycol in a pediatric sedatives (Pronap and Plaxim) resulted in fatal poisoning of seven children in Cape Town, South Africa, in 1967 (14). These events echo the prophetic words of Dr. Leake in 1929 who observed, "There is no short cut from the laboratory to clinic, except one that passes too close to the morgue" (15).

The presentation and clinical courses of these patients ingesting diethylene glycol appear to have been little different from what would be expected to result from ethylene glycol exposure. Thus, it seems most appropriate to manage a diethylene poisoning similar to ethylene glycol and monitor for metabolic acidosis.

ESTERS

Esters are compounds that are prepared by the reaction of an alcohol or phenol with acids or derivatives of acids. The most common esters are those prepared by carboxycilic acids and the reactions of alcohols. An example is the reaction of acetic acid with benzyl alcohol to produce benzyl acetate. Table 107.2 summarizes toxicological properties of acetate esters.

Table 107.2.   Esters

Chemical Name	Chemical Formula	Toxicity
n-Amyl acetate	$CH_3COOC_5H_{11}$	Clear flammable liquid with a banana-like odor. Exposure to n-amyl acetate vapors can produce irritation of the mucous membranes, eyes, and throat. n-Amyl acetate can also produce CNS depression. OSHA PEL = 100 ppm, ACGIH TLV = 100 ppm, and IDLH level = 4,000 ppm.
Sec-amyl acetate (α-methylbutyl acetate, banana oil)	$C_7H_{14}O_2$	Clear flammable liquid and an irritant of mucous membranes, eyes, and skin and in high concentrations can produce CNS depression. OSHA PEL = 125 ppm, ACGIH TLV = 125 ppm, and IDLH level = 9000 ppm.
Isoamyl acetate (amyl acetate, banana oil, pear oil)	$CH_3C(O)CH_2(CH_3)C_2H_5$	Colorless flammable liquid that is an irritant to the mucous membranes, eyes, and throat and at high concentrations can produce CNS depression. OSHA PEL = 100 ppm, ACGIH TLV = 100 ppm, and IDLH level = 3000 ppm.
Iso-n-butyl acetate	$CH_3CH_2CH_2CH_2OCOCH_3$	Clear flammable liquid with a pleasant fruity odor. One of four isomers of the butyl acetates. n-Butyl acetate is used as a solvent for nitrocellulose, resins, waxes, fats, and oils and in the manufacture of lacquer, plastics, and perfumes. It is irritating to the mucous membranes and eyes and in high concentrations can produce CNS depression. OSHA PEL = 100 ppm, ACGIH TLV = 150 ppm, and IDLH level = 10,000 ppm.
sec-Butyl acetate (2-butanol acetate)	$CH_3CH_2CH(CH_3)OCH_3$	Clear flammable liquid with a fruity odor. It is used as a solvent for lacquers and paper coatings. At high air concentrations it is a CNS depressant and can produce irritation of the mucous membranes, eyes, and respiratory tract. Sec-butyl acetate is also used as a solvent for nitrocellulose and nail enamels. OSHA PEL = 200 ppm, ACGIH TLV = 200 ppm, and IDLH level = 10,000 ppm.
Isobutyl acetate	$(CH_3)_2CHCH_2OCOCH_3$	Colorless flammable liquid used as a solvent and a flavoring agent. It is also used as a solvent for nitrocellulose and as a solvent in perfumes. It can produce CNS depression in high air concentrations as well as mucous membrane and eye irritation. OSHA PEL = 150 ppm, ACGIH TLV = 150 ppm, and IDLH level = 7,500 ppm.
tert-Butyl acetate	$(CH_3)_3COCOCH_3$	Colorless flammable liquid with a pleasant odor used as a gasoline additive and as a solvent. It is an irritant to the eyes and mucous membranes and can be a CNS depressant. OSHA PEL = 200 ppm, ACGIH TLV = 200 ppm, and IDLH level = 8000 ppm.
n-Butyl acrylate (butyl ester)	$CH_2{=}CHCOOC_4H_9$	Colorless flammable liquid. It is a monomer used in the production of polymers for solvent coatings, adhesive, paints, and binders. It is an irritant to the mucous membranes and the eyes. On eye exposure in animals it can produce corneal damage and necrosis. It is also an irritant of the respiratory tract. ACGIH TLV = 10 ppm.
2-Ethoxyethyl acetate (cellosolve acetate, glycol monoethyl ether acetate)	$C_2H_5OCH_2OCOCH_3$	Colorless flammable liquid. It is used as a solvent for nitrocellulose and resins. In high concentrations it can produce CNS depression and is an irritant to the eyes and mucous membranes. ACGIH TLV = 5 ppm.

continues

Table 107.2. *Continued*

Chemical Name	Chemical Formula	Toxicity
Ethyl acetate	$CH_3COOC_2H_5$	Clear flammable liquid with a pleasant odor that is used as a solvent for lacquers and as an artificial perfume agent. Ethyl acetate can produce irritation of the eyes and mucous membranes as well as the respiratory tract. In high concentrations it can produce CNS depression. OSHA PEL = 400 ppm, ACGIH TLV = 400 ppm, and IDLH level = 10,000 ppm.
Ethyl acrylate	$CH_2{=}CHCOOC_2H_5$	Clear flammable liquid used as a monomer in the manufacture of polymer resins and also in the production of paints and plastics. It is an irritant to the eyes, mucous membranes, and skin and may produce skin sensitization. The vapor of ethyl acrylates can be very irritating at 4–5 ppm. The odor of the compound is detectable at concentrations in the air below 1 ppm. ACGIH TLV = 5 ppm.
Ethyl formate (formic acid ethyl ester)	$HCOOC_2H_5$	Colorless flammable liquid with a fruity odor. It is used as a solvent for cellulose nitrate and acetate. It is also used as a solvent for oils and greases and as a fumigant. it is an irritant of the eyes, mucous membranes, and can cause CNS depression. It is incompatible with nitrates, strong oxidizers, and strong acids. OSHA PEL = 100 ppm, ACGIH TLV = 100 ppm, and IDLH level = 8000 ppm.
2-Ethylhexyl acrylate	$H_2C{=}CHC(O)OCH_2CH(C_2H_5)(CH_2)_3$	Colorless flammable liquid used to produce latex paint, plastics, and protective coatings. It is an irritant to the skin and mucous membranes and can produce skin sensitization. No TLV is set for this compound.
Ethyl methacrylate [Plexiglas (when in polymeric form)]	$CH_2{=}C(CH_3)COOC_2H_5$	Clear flammable liquid. The compound is used to make polymers of Plexiglas and in polymerized form is nontoxic; however, the ethyl methacrylate monomers are irritants to skin, eyes, mucous membranes, and lungs.
sec-Hexyl acetate	$CH_{15}O_2$	Clear flammable liquid with a pleasant fruity odor and is used as a solvent in spray lacquers and solvent for cellulose esters and resins. It has incompatibilities with strong alkalis, acids, and oxidizing agents. It is an irritant of the mucous membranes and respiratory tract and eyes. ACGIH TLV = 50 ppm, OSHA PEL = 50 ppm, and IDLH level = 4000 ppm.
Isopropyl acetate (2-propyl acetate)	$CH_3COOCH(CH_3)_2$	Flammable liquid solvent. It is an irritant to the eyes, mucous membranes, and lungs and in high air concentrations can produce CNS depression. It is incompatible with strong oxidizing agents, strong alkalis, and acids. OSHA PEL = 250 ppm, ACGIH TLV = 250 ppm, IDLH level = 16,000 ppm.
2-Methoxyethyl acetate		Clear flammable liquid used in lacquer industry, printing, and photographic film and in coatings and adhesives. It is a mild irritant of mucous membranes and eyes and can produce CNS depression in high concentrations. ACGIH TLV = 5 ppm.

Table 107.3.   Principal Hazard, Target Organ(s), and Toxicity Syndrome(s)

Category Solvent CAS number[a]	Principal Toxic Hazard (route(s) of exposure)	Target Organ/Principal Toxicity
Alcohols and glycols		
Ethyl alcohol 64-17-5	Ingestion	CNS: intoxication[b] (acute), alcoholism (chronic)
Isopropyl alcohol 67-63-0	Ingestion, skin absorption	CNS: intoxication; GI: gastritis[c]
Methyl alcohol 67-56-1	Ingestion, inhalation	CNS: intoxication, blindness Metabolic: acidosis[d]
Ethylene glycol 107-21-1	Ingestion	Metabolic: acidosis, hypocalcemia, renal toxicity
Diethylene glycol 111-46-6	Ingestion	Metabolic: acidosis, hypocalcemia, renal toxicity
Ketones		
Acetone 67-64-1	Inhalation	CNS: intoxication (mild)
Methyl n-butyl ketone (MnBK) 591-78-6	Inhalation, skin absorption	Hexacarbon polyneuropathy[e], motor and sensory
Glycol ethers		
EG methyl ether (EGME) 1-9-86-4	Ingestion, inhalation, skin absorption	Metabolic: acidosis, hypocalcemia, renal toxicity
EG ethyl ether (EGEE) 110-80-5	Ingestion, skin absorption	Metabolic: acidosis, hypocalcemia, renal toxicity
EG butyl ether (EGBE) 111-76-2	Ingestion	Metabolic: acidosis, hypocalcemia, renal toxicity

[a]CAS number, Chemical Abstract Services identification number.
[b]CNS intoxication, the dose and time related CNS depression which generally progresses from higher to lower brain function (in a cranial-to-caudal fashion) including decreased inhibition, euphoria, increased confidence, altered judgement, loquaciousness, decreased attention, ataxia, tremor, slurring of speech, decreased motor skills, altered perception, diplopia, coma, respiratory depression, through death.
[c]Gastritis, the dose-related irritation of the GI mucosae, particularly of the stomach, including asymptomatic erythema, abdominal burning/pain, minor through major blood loss.
[d]Metabolic acidosis, the dose-related injury resulting from the metabolism of the parent compound to a free acid. The salient features include initial osmolar gap, acidemia, nausea, vomiting, coma, convulsions, myoclonic jerks, neurotoxicity, and death.
[e]Hexacarbon polyneuropathy, a characteristic "dying back neuropathy" progressing from distal to proximal with a distal motor and sensory neuropathy (weakness and loss of sensitivity to pinprick, touch, and temperature) in both upper and lower extremities. The deficit is usually symmetric and insidious in onset and may progress after exposure ceases. Recovery is slow and may take several years. CNS changes (e.g., spasticity, confusion, changes in color vision) tend to be permanent.

Table 107.4.   Physical Properties and Skin Absorption

Category Solvent	Molecular Weight[a]	Boiling Point[b] (°C)	Vapor Density	Vapor Pressure (mmHg at °C)	Skin Absorption[c] (mg/cm^2/hr)
Alcohols/glycols					
Ethyl alcohol	46.07	78.3	1.59	59 at 20°	0.57
Isopropyl alcohol	60.09	82.5	1.06	44 at 25°	
Methyl alcohol	32.04	64.8	1.11	100 at 21°	8.4
Ethylene glycol	62.07	197.5	2.14	0.05 at 20°	
Diethylene glycol	106.12	245.8	3.66	1 at 92°	
Ketones					
Acetone	58.08	56.4	2.00	185 at 20°	
Methyl n-butyl ketone	100.16	126.	3.5	3.8 at 25°	
Glycol ethers					
EG methyl ether	76.09	124.5	2.62	0.09 at 16°	2.82
EG ethyl ether	90.12	135.1	3.10	3.8 at 20°	0.80
EG butyl ether	118.17	168.4	4.1	0.76 at 20°	0.20

[a]Molecular weight: Budaveri S, O'Neil MJ, Smith A, Heckelman PE. The Merck Index. 11th ed. Rathway, NJ: Merck & Co, 1989.
[b]Boiling point, vapor density and vapor pressure. Walsh D. Chemical safety data sheets—Vol 1: Solvents. Cambridge, England: The Royal Society of Chemistry, 1989.
[c]Skin absorption: Duggard PH, Walker M, Mawdsley SJ, Scott RC. Absorption of some glycol ethers through human skin in vitro. Environ Health Perspect 1984;57:193–197.

The following compounds are esters of carboxylic acids:

Methyl acetate
Ethyl acetate
n-Propyl acetate
n-Butyl acetate
n-Pentyl acetate
Isopentyl acetate
Benzyl acetate
Phenyl acetate
Ethyl formate
Ethyl acetate
Ethyl propionate
Ethyl n-butyrate
Ethyl n-valerate
Ethyl stearate
Ethyl phenyl acetate
Ethyl benzoate

Esters are compounds that are used in a multiplicity of industries and commercial processes.

Ethyl acetate is formed by the reaction of ethyl alcohol with acetic acid. It is also known as ethyl ester or acidic ether. Ethyl acetate is a flammable colorless liquid with a very fruity odor. Ethyl acetate is used as a lacquer solvent and as an artificial perfume agent. Ethyl acetate is an irritant of the mucous membranes and the respiratory tract and in higher concentrations can produce central nervous system depression in humans and in animals. The Occupational Safety and Health Administration (OSHA) Permissible Exposure Limit (PEL) of ethyl acetate is 400 ppm with a concentration that is immediately dangerous to life and health (IDLH) of 400 ppm. Another common ester is 2-ethoxyethyl acetate. This is also known as ethylene glycol monoethyl acetate or cellosolve acetate. 2-Ethoxyethyl acetate

is a flammable colorless liquid. It is used as a solvent for nitrocellulose and resins and is incompatible with oxidizing agents, alkalis, and nitrates. It is a very irritating compound to the mucous membranes, eyes, and respiratory system. In high air concentrations it can produce CNS depression and respiratory depression. The American Conference of Governmental Industrial Hygienists (ACGIH) has recommended a Threshold Limit Value (TLV) of 5 ppm with a skin notation due to potential skin absorption of the compound.

Amyl acetates are clear colorless flammable liquids with banana-like odors. There are three isomers of amyl acetate: n-amyl acetate, sec-amyl acetate, and isoamyl acetate. The amyl acetates in general are used as solvents and as flavoring. The amyl acetates are incompatible with strong oxidizing agents, alkalis, and nitrates. In general, amyl acetates are irritants to the eyes and mucous membranes. In high air concentrations the amyl acetates can produce CNS depression. The amyl acetates are used in the manufacturing of furniture polish, photographic film, celluloid, lacquers, and artificial leathers.

KETONES

Organic compounds containing a carbonyl (C=O) group attached to two carbon atoms (R–CO–R′) belong to the ketone family of chemicals. Several billion pounds are produced annually in the United States and comprise mainly acetone, methyl ethyl ketone, methyl isobutyl ketone, cyclohexanone, and isophorone. Their extensive industrial use reflects low production costs, excellent solvent properties, moderate vapor pressure, and miscibility with other liquids. We will discuss in some detail acetone (the simplest) and methyl n-butyl ketone (a representative neurotoxic hexacarbon).

Table 107.5.   Odor Threshold and Exposure Guidelines

Category Solvent	Odor Threshold (ppm)	OSHA 8-hour TWA (ppm)	NIOSH 8-hour TWA (ppm)	NIOSH 15-min TWA (ppm)	Health Effects Considered	Special Comments
Alcohols/glycols						
Ethyl alcohol	5100	1000				
Isopropyl alcohol	40–200	400	400	800	Mucous membrane irritation	Stringent work practices and medical surveillence
Methyl alcohol	5900	200	200	800	Blindness, metabolic acidosis	None
Ethylene glycol	0.08	50				
Diethylene glycol		23[a]				
Ketones						
Acetone	.2–1.5	750	250		Irritation, hepatic, renal, NS	
Methyl n-butyl ketone		5	1		Peripheral neuropathy	U/A required; Workers must be warned of NS toxicity
Glycol ethers						
EG methyl ether		5	LFL[b]		Reproductive, teratogenicity	Prevent skin contact
EG ethyl ether		5	LFL		Reproductive, teratogenicity	Prevent skin contact
EG butyl ether		25	25	75[c]	Reproductive, teratogenicity	Prevent skin contact

[a]UK exposure limits, 8-hr TWA, USA TWA not available.
[b]LFL, lowest feasible level.
[c]ACGIH recommended TLVs.

Table 107.6. Laboratory Tests and Principal Toxic Metabolites

Category Solvent Trade names	Principal Metabolites Principal enzyme system	Laboratory Tests
Alcohols/glycols		
Ethyl alcohol	Acetaldehyde, acetic acid ADH[a]	Blood or breath alcohol concentration, serum glucose, hepatic enzymes
Isopropyl alcohol	Acetone	Serum and urine acetone, osmolar gap, gastric and stool for hemoglobin
Methyl alcohol	Formic acid ADH	Osmolar gap, serum bicarbonate and blood pH, serum methanol, serum glucose
Ethylene glycol	Glycolic acid ADH	Osmolar gap, serum bicarbonate and blood pH, serum calcium, serum ethylene glycol, urine for crystals
Diethylene glycol	Glycolic acid (probable) ADH (probable)	Osmolar gap, serum bicarbonate and blood pH, serum calcium, serum ethylene glycol, urine for crystals
Ketones		
Acetone	None	Serum and urine acetone, osmolar gap
Methyl n-butyl ketone	2,5-Hexanedione	Neurological exam (weakness and numbness), EMG (denervation, conduction velocity), sural nerve biopsy
Glycol ethers		
EG methyl ether	Glycolic acid (probable) ADH (probable)	Osmolar gap, serum bicarbonate and blood pH, serum calcium, serum ethylene glycol (probable)
EG ethyl ether	Glycolic acid (probable) ADH (probable)	Osmolar gap, serum bicarbonate and blood pH, serum calcium, serum ethylene glycol (possible)
EG butyl ether	Glycolic acid (probable) ADH (probable)	

[a]ADH, alcohol dehydrogenase.

Acetone

The simplest aliphatic ketone (CH_3COCH_3), acetone, is a clear liquid with a characteristic pungent odor and a sweet taste. Acetone and the other ketones are widely used as solvents in the production of lubricating oils, in the dyeing and celluloid industries, and as chemical intermediates in a number of synthetic processes.

The metabolism of fat in vivo produces acetone with levels reaching 10–70 mg/dl in diabetic ketoacidosis. At levels of <100 mg/dl, the half-life is about 4 hours, with the kidneys excreting about 30% and respiration accounting for about 20%, with the balance being metabolized. At higher blood levels, elimination half-life increases to about 30 hours.

Acetone exhibits a relatively low toxicity with no fatal exposures reported in the industrial setting. CNS effects are roughly equivalent to those of ethanol, with a somewhat greater anesthetic effect. Acetone is a defatting agent, and vapor causes eye and mucous membrane irritation.

Methyl n-Butyl Ketone

Although most of the commercially important ketones are of low toxicity, methyl n-butyl ketone (MnBK) poses a distinct neurotoxic hazard. MnBK (propyl acetone, 2-hexanone) is a clear, colorless liquid with an acetone-like odor used in painting and plastic coating.

MnBK, acrylamide, and n-hexane share a wide industrial use, a 6-carbon structure, and a demonstrated ability to cause severe central and peripheral neurotoxicity. Such epidemic outbreaks have been reported in many countries including Italy, Austria, France, Japan, and the United States. Toxic metabolites, principally 2,5-hexanedione, inhibit gluteraldehyde-3-phosphate dehydrogenase and disable the rapid axon protein transport system, producing the characteristic dying-back (distal-to-proximal) neuropathy. Long distal myelinated nerves are most vulnerable. The neuropathy is associated with a retraction of the myelin sheath, axonal enlargement, and neurofilament accumulation. Since the larger myelinated fibers are involved, the hexacarbons produce primarily a distal motor and sensory neuropathy (weakness and loss of sensitivity to pinprick, touch, and temperature) in both upper and lower extremities. The deficit is usually symmetric and insidious in onset and may progress after exposure ceases. Recovery is slow and may take several years (16). CNS changes (e.g., spasticity, confusion, changes in color vision) tend to be permanent.

The toxicity shared by the hexacarbons seems to reflect their common metabolism to the 2,5-hexanedione, the putative neurotoxin. This metabolite also causes profound immunologic impairment in mice prior to the onset of the neuropathy (17). Although relatively nonneurotoxic themselves, concomitant exposure to methyl ethyl ketone, and probably other solvents, potentiates the toxicity of the hexacarbons (18).

GLYCOL ETHERS

Glycol ethers are general solvents, also known as cellosolves, with low vapor pressure and a high potential for dermal absorption. The following glycol ethers are important in occupational and environmental exposure:

Ethylene glycol monomethyl ether—$CH_3OCH_2CH_2OH$ (EGME, 2-methoxyethanol, methyl cellosolve)

Ethylene glycol monoethyl ether—$CH_3CH_2OCH_2CH_2OH$ (EGEE, 2-ethoxyethanol, cellosolve)

Ethylene glycol monobutyl ether—$CH_3(CH_2)_3OCH_2CH_2OH$ (EGBE, 2-butoxyethanol, butyl cellosolve)

Propylene glycol monomethyl ether—$CH_3OCH_2CHOHCH_3$ (PGME, 1-methoxy-2-propanol)

Table 107.7. Treatment Summary

Category Solvent Specific gravity Volume of distribution	Criterion	Triage Recommendations		Treatment Recommendations
		Dose[a]		
		ml/kg	ml/70	Blood Level[b] mg/dl	

Category/Solvent/SG/Vd	Criterion	ml/kg	ml/70	mg/dl	Treatment Recommendations
Alcohol/glycols					
Ethyl alcohol	EC_{50}[c]	0.8	53	100	Symptomatic measures
SG 0.789	LD_{50}[d]	3.4	240	450	Support, respiratory
Vd 0.55 l/kg	MDS[e]	11.5	804	1510	Support, respiratory
Isopropyl alcohol	Sxs	0.4	29	50	Symptomatic measures
SG 0.787	MLD[f]	1.2	87	150	Support, respiratory
Vd 0.65 l/kg	MDS	3.6	254	440	Support, respiratory
Methyl alcohol	Action	0.2	14	25	EtOH + support (E + S)
SG 0.79	Dialysis	0.4	27	50	Hemodialysis + E + S
Vd 0.61 l/kg	MDS	1.0	73	135	Hemodialysis + E + max S + Folic acid 10 mg IV Q dy
Ethylene glycol	Action	0.2	13	25	EtOH + support (E + S)
SG 1.113	Dialysis	0.4	26	50	Hemodialysis + E + S
Vd 0.83 l/kg	MLD	1.5	104	200	Hemodialysis + E + max S + Thiamine 100 mg
	LD_{50} GP[g]	5.9	416	796	IV Q dy + Pyridoxine 100 mg IV Q d
Diethylene glycol	Action	0.2	11	25[i]	EtOH + support (E + S)
SG 1.118	Dialysis	0.3	22	50	Hemodialysis + E + S
Vd 0.83 l/kg[h]	MLD	1.3	89	200	Hemodialysis + E + max S
Ketones					
Acetone	8 h TWA[j]	0.07	5		
SG 0.797	Tol × dys[k]	0.3	20	28	None
Vd 0.82 l/kg	LD_{50} Rab[l]	6.6	465	646	Supportive measures
MnBK					
SG 0.83	8 h TWA[j]	0.0014	0.1		
Vd 0.82 l/kg[m]	LD_{50} Mse[n]	1.2	84	122	Supportive measures
Glycol ethers					
EG methyl ether	Action	0.5	37	50[q]	EtOH[r] + support (E + S)
SG 0.966	LD_{50} Rab[l]	0.9	64	87	
Vd 0.83 l/kg[h]	Dialysis	1.1	74	100	Hemodialysis + E + S
	OD Surv[o]	1.4	100	136	Hemodialysis + E + max S
	OD Fatal[p]	3.4	240	326	
EG ethyl ether	Action	0.4	27	30	EtOH + support (E + S)
SG 0.931	Dialysis	0.8	54	60	Hemodialysis + E + S
Vd 0.83 l/kg[h]	LD_{50} GP[g]	1.5	105	116	Hemodialysis + E + max S
EG butyl ether	LD_{50} Rab[l]	0.4	25	20	EtOH + support (E + S)
SG 0.901	OD Surv[o]	0.4	30	24	
Vd 0.83 l/kg[h]	Dialysis	0.7	49	40	Hemodialysis + E + S

[a]Dose calculated from blood level based on Vd and specific gravity, i.e., neglecting absorption.

[b]Blood level is the primary assumption in most cases, i.e., is based on literature and clinical experience. The relation to dose neglects absorption and elimination.

[c]EC_{50} means concentration at which 50% of people would be expected to show the effect. In this case the effect is gross intoxication (speech and/or gait impaired). This is also the usual target concentration for therapeutic use of ethanol (EtOH).

[d]LD_{50} means concentration (dose) likely lethal to 50% of people. In this case the lethal effect is respiratory depression.

[e]MDS, maximum dose (concentration) survived.

[f]MLD, minimum lethal dose (concentration).

[g]LD_{50}GP means lethal dose (concentration) to 50% of guinea pigs. The lowest animal LD_{50} was generally chosen from a secondary source, e.g., Patty (246), for comparison in this table.

[h]In the absence of Vd data for this solvent, the Vd for ethylene glycol was used.

[i]Blood level was "corrected" for the presumed metabolism of diethylene glycol to two ethylene glycol molecules by the molecular weight ratio (2 × 62.07/106.12) to give blood levels of ethylene glycol.

[j]For the purposes of comparison only, a dose calculated from OSHA 8-hour TWA assuming a ventilation of 720 l/hr (twice resting ventilation) for 8 hour and assuming 100% of inspired solvent (1 mg/l for acetone, 0.02 mg/L for MnBK) absorbed.

[k]A daily dose of 15–20 ml was tolerated for several days without apparent effect.

[l]LD_{50} Rab means lethal dose (concentration) to 50% of rabbits, the most sensitive animal in this case.

[m]In the absence of Vd data for this solvent, the Vd for acetone was used.

[n]LD_{50} Mse means lethal dose (concentration) to 50% of mice, the most sensitive animal in this case.

[o]Approximate dose consumed by two patient(s) who survived the mishap.

[p]Approximate dose (240 ml) consumed by a patient who did not survive the mishap.

[q]Blood levels for all glycol ethers were "corrected" by the molecular weight ratio for each. Thus (62.07/76.09) for EGME, (62.07/90.12) for EGEE, and (62.07/118.17) for EGBE.

[r]Although not yet verified in humans, the clinical similarity to ethylene glycol poisoning and animal studies (24) suggest the efficacy of ethanol therapy.

The alkyl ether derivatives of ethylene, diethylene, and triethylene glycol represent a widely used class of solvents the hazard of which has been increasingly appreciated in the last decade. The glycol ethers find application in surface coatings (lacquers, paints, varnishes), fingernail polishes and removers, dyes, writing inks, cleaners, and degreasers. These agents appear to share the toxicity of ethylene glycol, but exhibit significant absorption by both inhalation and skin exposure.

In addition to the neurotoxicity and metabolic hazards, a cross-sectional study of lithographers exposed to glycol ethers showed bone marrow toxicity, even in workers with a normal peripheral blood picture (19). A survey of shipyard painters showed some suggestive hematologic changes related to glycol ether exposure (20). Thus, although not irrefutably established, it would seem prudent to consider the glycol ethers as possibly hemotoxic.

Ethylene Glycol Monomethyl Ether

Ethylene glycol monomethyl ether (EGME, 2-methoxyethanol, methyl cellosolve), finds wide use as a solvent (cellulose esters, dyes, resins, lacquers, varnishes, enamels) and as an additive (deicer in jet engine fuel, wood stains). EGME appears to be the most hazardous of the glycol ethers, probably due to its greater volatility and skin absorption (21).

Ethylene Glycol Monoethyl Ether

Ethylene glycol monoethyl ether (EGEE, 2-ethoxyethanol, cellosolve) is used as a solvent (nitrocellulose, certain insecticides, synthetic and natural resins), as an additive (lacquers, printing inks, textile dyes, varnish removers, aviation fuel), and as a diluent in hydraulic brake fluids. It is probably intermediate in toxicity of the three here considered.

Ethylene Glycol Monobutyl Ether

Ethylene glycol monobutyl ether (EGBE, 2-butoxyethanol, butyl cellosolve) finds wide use in industry as a solvent (cellulose, paints, lacquers, enamels, stains, inks) and as a dry cleaning solvent. EGBE is probably the least toxic of the three, although clearly hazardous.

CHRONIC EXPOSURE AND LONGTERM EFFECTS

The physical properties of the solvent and extent of exposure are major determinants of the hazard. Table 107.4 lists the physical properties and data for the skin absorption characteristics where available.

Table 107.5 presents the odor thresholds and exposure guidelines including PELs as Time-Weighted Averages (TWAs) for 8 hours and for 15 minutes (where available).

Although the odor threshold might offer some protection for isopropyl alcohol and acetone, such does not seem to be the case for the other solvents for which data are available. The toxic hazards, physical properties, and skin absorption of common solvents are summarized in Tables 107.4 and 107.5.

MANAGEMENT OF TOXICITY

The most important aspect of toxicity management is prevention. Interventions which are "passive" by nature, that is, require no action on the part of the employee, are much more likely to succeed. Thus reduction in the amount of solvent vaporization is more likely to reduce exposure than requiring the employee to wear protective breathing apparatus. A logical extension of this important concept is to simply avoid use of particularly hazardous solvents when substitution or redesign is possible. Most solvents have a CNS depressant effect. Acute exposure to most of these types of solvents produces drowsiness and irritation of the mucous membranes, eyes, and respiratory tract. Chronic exposure to certain solvents is associated with neurotoxicity, either peripheral or central. Ingestion of ethylene glycol or methanol can result in severe metabolic acidosis. A summary of relevant laboratory tests is presented in Table 107.6 and a summary of treatment is presented in Table 107.7.

Eye exposures are generally handled in the same manner. Flush as soon as possible with Large volumes of Low pressure water for a Long time. Long time should be at least 5 minutes. If symptoms or signs of injury persist after a 5-minute postflush recovery, the patient should be evaluated by a physician.

REFERENCES

1. Pendleton CS. Drugs in the workplace—management options and considerations. Constructor 1986;(May):46–47.

2. Levin-Epstein M, Sala S. Alcohol and drugs in the workplace: costs, controls and controversies. Washington, DC: 1986.

3. AMA Council On Scientific Affairs. Alcohol and the driver. JAMA 1986;255:522–527.

4. Lehman AJ, Chase HF. The acute and chronic toxicity of isopropyl alcohol. J Lab Clin Med 1944;29:561–567.

5. Martinez TT, Jaeger RW, De Castro FJ, et al. A comparison of the absorption and metabolism of isopropyl alcohol by oral, dermal, and inhalation routes. Vet Hum Toxicol 1986;28:233–236.

6. McMartin KE, Ambre JJ, Tephly TR. Methanol poisoning in human subjects. Am J Med 1980;68:414–418.

7. Osterloh JD, Pond SM, Grady S, Becker CE. Serum formate concentrations in methanol intoxication as a criterion for hemodialysis. Ann Intern Med 1986;104:200–203.

8. Bergerdon R, Cardinal J, Geadah D. Prevention of methanol toxicity by ethanol therapy. N Engl J Med 1982;9:1528.

9. Jacobsen D, Ovrebo S, Ostborg J, Sejersted O. Glycolate causes the acidosis in ethylene glycol poisoning and is effectively removed by hemodialysis. Acta Med Scand 1984;216:409–416.

10. Berger JR, Ayyar DR. Neurological complications of ethylene glycol intoxication—report of a case. Arch Neurol 1981;38:724–726.

11. Catchings TT, Beamer WC, Lundy L, Prough DS. Adult respiratory distress syndrome secondary to ethylene glycol ingestion. An Emerg Med 1985;14:594–596.

12. McMartin KE, Dies DF, Sebastian CD, Barron SK, Smith RL, Spann EG. Effects of intravenous 4-methylpyrazole in healthy human subjects. Vet Hum Toxicol 1989;31:365.

13. Geiling EMK, Cannon PR. Pathological effects of elixir of sulfanilamide (diethylene glycol) poisoning. JAMA 1938;111:919–926.

14. Bowie MD, McKenzie D. Diethylene glycol poisoning in children. S Afr Med J 1972;46:931–934.

15. Leake CD. The pharmacologic evaluation of new drugs. JAMA 1929;93:1632–1634.

16. Spencer PS, Schaumberg HH, Sabri MF, Veronise B. The enlarging view of hexacarbon neuropathy. CRC Crit Rev Toxicol 1980;7:279–356.

17. Upreti RK, Shanker R. 2,5-Hexanedione-induced immunomodulatory effect in mice. Environ Res 1987;43:48–59.

18. Altenkirch H, Wagner HM, Stoltenburg-Didinger G, Steppat R. Poten-

tiation of hexacarbon-neurotoxicity by methyl-ethyl-ketone (MEK) and other substances: clinical and experimental aspects. Neurobehav Toxicol Teratol 1982;4:623–627.

19. Cullen MR, Raldo T, Waldron JA, Sparer J, Welch LS. Bone marrow injury in lithographers exposed to glycol ethers and organic solvents used in multicolor offset and ultraviolet curing printing processes. Arch Environ Health 1983;38:347–354.

20. Welch LS, Cullen MR. Effect of exposure to ethylene glycol ethers on shipyard painters. III. Hematologic effects. Am J Ind Med 1988;14:527–536.

21. Duggard PH, Walker M, Mawdsley SJ, Scott RC. Absorption of some glycol ethers through human skin in vitro. Environ Health Perspect 1984;57:193–197.

22. Budavari S, O'Neil MJ, Smith A, Heckelman PE. The Merck index. 11th ed. Rahway, NJ: Merck & Co., 1989.

23. Walsh D. Chemical safety data sheets—Vol 1: solvents. Cambridge, England: The Royal Society of Chemistry, 1989.

24. Romer KG, Balge F, Freundt KJ. Ethanol-induced accumulation of ethylene glycol monoalkyl ethers in rats. Drug Chem Toxicol 1985;8:255–264.

108

Carbon Disulfide and Select Miscellaneous Solvents

Donald B. Kunkel, M.D.
John B. Sullivan, Jr., M.D.

INTRODUCTION

Many solvents are commonly used in industrial and commercial processes. Some solvents are used commonly in select processes and it is important to have some understanding of their toxicity. These solvents include carbon disulfide, nitromethane, dioxane, 2-nitropropane, pyridine, dimethylformamide, butyl-mercaptan, isophorone, and the common petroleum solvents, turpentine, Stoddard solvent, coal naphtha, and petroleum naphtha (Table 108.1, Fig. 108.1).

Solvents that have great importance in organic reactions due to their strong ionizing power are termed aprotic solvents. This type of solvent is able to dissolve ionic reagents, which are often inorganic chemicals, and also promote dissociation of organic molecules. Solvents like water and alcohol are called protic solvents because they contain hydrogen that is attached to oxygen or nitrogen and are acidic in nature. Typical aprotic solvents are dimethylformamide and dimethyl sulfoxide (DMSO). Aprotic solvents dissolve both organic and inorganic compounds, but during the dissolution of these compounds they leave the anionic portions unencumbered and highly reactive for chemical reactions.

Protic solvents solvate anions strongly, and the anions as bases or nucleophiles are usually the important component of an ionic reagent. Thus protic solvents can drastically lower the reactivity of compounds (1). There are other types of commonly used miscellaneous solvents such as turpentine, naphtha, and Stoddard solvent. These solvents compose a wide variety of organic compounds to which humans are widely exposed (Table 108.1) and have some unique toxic properties.

CARBON DISULFIDE

Carbon disulfide (CS_2; carbon disulphide; carbon bisulphide; carbon sulfide; dithiocarbonic anhydride; CAS 75-15-0) was

accidentally discovered in 1796 by the German chemist, W. A. Lampadius, while studying the action of pyrites on carbon. In the first half century after its discovery, the compound was used in medicine in the treatment of a variety of diseases and was used experimentally as an anesthetic agent before the onset of chloroform.

Recognizing the remarkable organic solvent properties of carbon disulfide (gums, resins, waxes, sulfur, phosphorus, iodine, bromine, camphor), industry began the use of CS_2 in 1851 as a phosphorus solvent in the manufacture of matches, and its utilization rapidly spread to such endeavors as the refining of paraffins and petroleum and the extraction of plant and animal oils. Major use of CS_2 began in Europe in the middle and latter 19th century with, first, the discovery of the

Table 108.1. Miscellaneous Solvents

Carbon disulfide
Nitromethane
Dioxane
Pyridine
Dimethylformamide
Turpentine
Stoddard solvent
Butyl mercaptan
Isophorone
Dimethyl sulfoxide (DMSO)
1-Nitropropane
2-Nitropropane
Naphtha—coal tar
Naphtha—petroleum

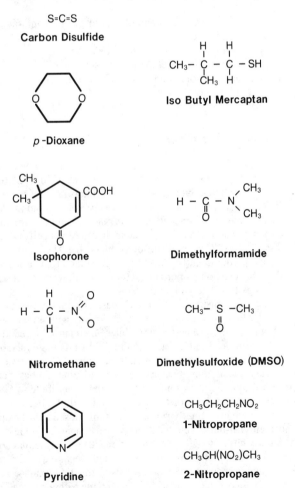

Figure 108.1. Commonly used solvents used in industry and commercial processes.

"cold" vulcanization process for rubber manufacture and, second, the development of the viscose rayon industry.

The "cold" vulcanization of rubber involved the dipping of thin strips of rubber into a solution of sulfur monochloride and carbon disulfide. This process softened the rubber and made the manufacture of thin sheets of rubber possible. This material was used in the production of surgical gloves, balloons, and contraceptives. "Cold" vulcanization was often done in small, poorly ventilated workshops. This process was abandoned after several decades following unequivocal evidence of severe toxic effects of CS_2 in this work environment. "Cold" vulcanization was not used in the United States to any great extent.

Uses

The United States Department of Labor in 1989 (2) reported the following uses for carbon disulfide in the United States:

—Chemical intermediate for rayon, cellophane, carbon tetrachloride, xanthogenates, soil disinfectants and herbicides, carbonyl sulfide, adhesives, and other compounds
—Solvent for phosphorus, selenium, bromine, iodine, fats, and resins
—Manufacture of electronic vacuum tubes
—Fumigant for commodities and space fumigation (insecticide)
—Agent in metal treatment and plating (e.g., gold and nickel)
—Corrosion inhibitor
—Polymerization inhibitor for vinyl chloride
—Agent in removal of metals from waste water
—Regenerator for transition metal sulfide catalysts
—Instant color photography
—Veterinary antihelminthic

Exposure Situations

Carbon disulfide is efficiently absorbed by vapor inhalation, ingestion, or by skin contact [thereby rating a "skin" notation by the Occupational Safety and Health Administration (OSHA)]. Following absorption via inhalation, free CS_2 in animal models reaches steady state concentrations in plasma within 15 minutes of exposure and approaches a plateau in red blood cells (RBC) within 2 hours. Carbon disulfide in blood has been shown to be bound predominantly (90%) to RBC (3), and RBC transport is thought to be an important factor in the movement of CS_2 from lungs to tissue and vice versa.

Toxic mechanisms of action may basically follow two pathways (4). First, CS_2 is known to react directly with amines and thiols and to interfere with their cellular functions. This reaction may, in turn, lead to the formation of dithiocarbamate metabolites capable of inactivating metalloenzymes by chelation of necessary metal ions such as copper and zinc. It has been proposed that the thiol/amine pathway may contribute to CS_2-induced neurotoxicity of the "filamentous, dying-back" category, which is distinctly similar to lesions caused by n-hexane and methyl n-butyl ketone. A second mechanism, related to hepatotoxicity, is the formation of reactive intermediates of CS_2 caused by metabolism of CS_2 through hepatic cytochrome P-450 and associated microsomal mixed function oxidase systems. CS_2 may directly damage liver enzyme pathways, leading to alterations in lipid metabolism, which may have an impact on cardiovascular function (5).

Table 108.2. Symptoms of 27 Patients Acutely Exposed to Airborne Carbon Disulfide

Symptom	Subjects No.	%
Headache	16	59
Slight	8	30
Moderate	6	21
Severe	2	7
Nausea	14	52
Vomiting	1	4
Burning of throat, lips, or skin	11	40
Dizziness	16	59
Shortness of breath or chest pain	4	15
Impotence	2	7

From: Spyker DA, Gallanosa AG, Suratt PM. Health effects of acute carbon disulfide exposure. J Toxicol Clin Toxicol 1982;19:87–93.

Approximately 8–20% of an absorbed dose of CS_2 is eliminated unchanged in breath, with only about 0.5% being excreted in urine. Of absorbed CS_2, 50%–90% is metabolized in the body. The half-life in blood is less than 1 hour. Metabolized CS_2 appears in urine as inorganic sulfates, thiourea, 2-mercapto-2-thiazolin and 2-thiothiazolidine-4-carboxylic acid (6). The latter metabolite is considered a reliable marker of CS_2 exposure, and its direct measurement appears far superior to the older, nonspecific iodine-azide test for urinary metabolites of CS_2 in the workplace (7).

It is of some interest to this discussion that the drug disulfiram (Antabuse) is partially metabolized to carbon disulfide, and that neurotoxic effects of disulfiram use and overdose may reflect CS_2 toxicity (8).

Acute Toxicity

Following dermal contact with CS_2, erythema and pain may be experienced with lesser exposures, but more significant skin contact may result in full thickness burns. CS_2 is considered one of the strongest skin irritants known due to its potent defatting activity. Skin absorption may cause headache, nausea, vomiting, dizziness, cardiac dysrhythmias, and coma (2). Eye exposures may result in immediate discomfort and conjunctional inflammation.

Ingestion of CS_2 in a volume of 15 ml has been fatal in adults. Victims have exhibited a variety of neurologic (spasmodic tremor, convulsions, coma), cardiovascular (cyanosis, cardiovascular collapse), and pulmonary (dyspnea, respiratory failure) signs following significant ingestions (9). Ingestions have been rarely reported and are usually suicidal in nature.

Inhalation of CS_2 vapors in a concentration of 4800 ppm for 1 hour may be fatal (9). An Immediately Dangerous to Life or Health (IDLH) level of 500 ppm has been established (10). Inhalation of high levels of CS_2 may result in delirium, hallucinations, convulsions, and coma. Spyker et al. (11) have reported on the acute toxic effects of CS_2 in air following a massive leak from a railroad tank car, resulting in airborne CS_2 concentrations of 20 ppm at a site distant from the incident. The symptoms of 27 patients, mostly police and firefighters, are summarized in Table 108.2. In addition, pulmonary function tests revealed acute changes at the time of the incident as compared with subsequent studies.

Chronic Toxicity

NEUROTOXICITY

Numerous hypotheses concerning the mode of action of CS_2 on nerve tissue have been put forth to explain the widespread effects of this solvent on central and peripheral systems. In addition to basic concepts mentioned above, various authors have debated the effects of CS_2 on catecholaminergic and dopaminergic systems, its possible interference with vitamin B_6 (pyridoxine) metabolism, the possible effects of free sulfur and free radical formation in the metabolism of CS_2, and, interestingly, whether neurotoxic effects might only reflect vascular damage caused by this agent (12).

The focus of earlier reports of CS_2 toxicity among workers was the observation of bizarre behavioral patterns, with many unfortunate victims of CS_2 relegated to European insane asylums in the 19th century. Among the more noticeable symptoms recorded were: (a) extreme irritability and uncontrollable anger with rapid mood changes, including mania and suicidal tendencies, (b) memory defects of a rather marked degree, (c) severe insomnia and constant bad dreams, and (d) interference with sexual functions in individuals who were below the normal age group for loss of libido (13).

Although behavioral and cognitive dysfunctions accounted for the great majority of reports of chronic and subacute exposure-related findings in earlier reports, later reports and studies involving perhaps lesser exposure levels have tended to focus on extrapyramidal, cerebellar, and peripheral nerve dysfunction. An excellent (and unfortunately recent) study (13) of 21 workers in the United States who were exposed to CS_2 as a fumigant for grain revealed evidence of atypical parkinsonism, cerebellar signs, hearing loss, and sensory changes. Of the group studied, 80% exhibited cogwheel rigidity, 71% displayed decreased movement, 48% had resting tremors, and 52% had intention tremors. Peripheral sensory shading was detected in 62%, and 44% had abnormal nerve conduction studies.

Although better hygienic practices have markedly reduced reports of neurotoxicity in the workplace, concern has been expressed over prolonged exposures at even low levels of CS_2 in workplace air, with evidence that ambient CS_2 concentrations below 20 ppm may cause subtle peripheral neuropathic changes over several years of worker exposure (15).

OCULAR TOXICITY

Severe acute CS_2 intoxication and significant chronic CS_2 exposure are both known to result in optic nerve damage resembling optic neuritis. Chronic CS_2 exposure also affects choroidal microvascular circulation, and the observation of delayed choroidal filling has been considered essential for the diagnosis of chronic CS_2 intoxication. Microvascular aneurysms may be found but seem to follow ethnic boundaries (e.g., Japanese workers). Additionally, discrete pigmentary changes of the posterior pole have been described (16).

In severe poisonings, a central scotoma with an impaired red-green discrimination may be detected, suggesting an impairment in the receptiveness of the ganglion cells or demyelination of optic nerve fibers (17).

CARDIOVASCULAR EFFECTS

Numerous cohort studies have shown increased incidence of cardiovascular disease among CS_2 workers, and a recent epidemiologic critique of literature has concluded that there is no good reason to doubt this association (18). An increased incidence of atherosclerosis in workers has been suggested, but the mechanisms of causation are not well understood (19). One extensive study of exposed workers suggests that the increased risk of cardiac death in CS_2 workers may not be due to atherosclerotic disease, rather it may possibly be due to a direct cardiotoxic or thrombotic effect (20).

REPRODUCTIVE EFFECTS

Numerous worldwide studies of the potential effects of CS_2 on reproductive function have been conducted using such endpoints as spermatogenesis, serum follicle-stimulating hormone and luteinizing hormone levels, and libido. A 1981 study of U.S. CS_2 workers failed to document impaired semen quality, but this report has been criticized because of relatively short durations of exposure (21, 22).

MISCELLANEOUS FINDINGS

As noted earlier, CS_2 can alter hepatic microsomal enzyme systems, with the potential of interfering with drug metabolism. Other toxic hepatic effects have not been demonstrated. Scant data exist to implicate CS_2 with renal toxicity. Chronic cough has been described in viscose rayon workers, but the presence of other irritants in the work setting makes pulmonary disease questionable. Effects on endocrine systems, in addition to those above, include corticosteroidal effects, impairment of thyroid function, and possible diabetogenic changes (12). CS_2 is not classified as a carcinogen by authoritative agencies.

Treatment

Treatment of acute CS_2 exposures consists of decontamination of eye, skin, or gastrointestinal tract and supportive care. There is no known "antidote" for this compound.

Regulatory Considerations

OSHA has recently established a Permissible Exposure Limit (PEL) in air of 4 ppm (12 mg/m^3), determined as an 8-hour Time-Weighted Average (TWA) with a Short-Term Exposure Limit (STEL) of 12 ppm (36 mg/m^3). NIOSH has recommended an 8-hour TWA of 1 ppm (3 mg/m^3) with a STEL of 10 ppm (30 mg/m^3). Both OSHA and NIOSH have added the "skin" notation. As noted earlier, IDLH level is 500 ppm (10). "Occupational exposure" to CS_2 is defined as exposure above an action level of 1.5 mg/m^3. CS_2 is considered both a hazardous substance and hazardous waste by the U.S. Environmental Protection Agency (EPA) (23).

NITROMETHANE

Nitromethane, also known as nitrocarbol (Fig. 108.1), has a chemical formula of CH_3NO_2 and Threshold Limit Value (TLV) of 100 ppm on a TWA (24). Nitromethane is an oily, liquid solvent used in the electronics industry and also as a rocket fuel. Nitromethane is used in production of chloropicrin, a fumigant, and as a fuel in racing cars. It is incompatible with amines, strong acids, oxidizers, metallic oxides, and other combustible materials (24). The IDLH level is 1000 ppm. In animal studies, nitromethane produces central nervous system (CNS) excitation as well as CNS depression, both of which can lead to convulsion and coma. Nitromethane toxicity includes irritancy to mucous membranes, skin, and the lungs. Nitromethane is a hepatotoxin. Nitromethane in contact with the skin can produce a dermatitis. Skin and eye contact should be immediately decontaminated with water.

DIOXANE

Dioxane (*p*-dioxane or 1,4-dioxane) is also known as diethylene dioxide, diethylene ether, or diethylene oxide (Fig. 108.1). It has a molecular formula of $C_4H_8O_2$ and a molecular weight of 88.12. It is commonly used as a solvent for resins and oils. Dioxane is very flammable and can be an explosion hazard when exposed to heat or flame. Due to its high degree of reactivity, vapors of dioxane can form explosive mixtures with air. Dioxane can also form explosive peroxides under certain conditions (25). Dioxane has a vapor density equal to 3.0 (air = 1.0) that of air. It persists in the environment and does not biodegrade readily, but may be subject to some photochemical oxidation.

Dioxane is a colorless liquid with a slight faint alcohol odor. It is heavier than water and thus sinks when mixed with water. It is flammable and produces an irritating vapor. Workers should avoid contact with both the liquid and vapor. Workers should have appropriate personal protective equipment when working with dioxane. Due to the flammability of dioxane, it may explode if ignited in an enclosed area. Also flashback along a vapor trail can occur.

The IDLH inhalational concentration of dioxane is 200 ppm. OSHA has set PELs with a skin notation for dioxane of 100 ppm. The National Institute of Occupational Safety and Health (NIOSH) has suggested a ceiling of 1 ppm for 30 minutes. The TLV for dioxane is 25 ppm with a shortterm inhalation limit of 100 ppm for 16 minutes (25). The American Conference of Governmental and Industrial Hygienists (ACGIH) suggests a TLV of 25 ppm. The ACGIH also recommends a STEL of 100 ppm.

Dioxane is a mucous membrane irritant and produces ocular, nasal, and pulmonary irritation. It has a pleasant odor with an air threshold recognition odor of 170 ppm. This threshold recognition odor allows for dioxane to be detected before acute toxic effects occur. However, chronic exposure can result in serious health effects. Irritation from dioxane vapors occurs somewhere between 0.1% and 3% vapor concentration, which can produce CNS depression and, if the exposure continues, pulmonary edema and death.

Renal and hepatic injury can occur following toxic exposure to dioxane. Dioxane is an acute health hazard and is highly toxic by inhalational and dermal routes as well as ingestion. Lethal concentrations for humans can occur at 470 ppm.

Carcinogenicity testing conducted shows that dioxane can produce hepatocellular carcinomas or adenomas of the liver in animals as well as squamous cell carcinoma of the nasal passages of certain animals (25).

Workers exposed to high vapor concentrations of dioxane experience mucous membrane irritation, pulmonary irritation, drowsiness, headache, nausea, vomiting, and hepatic and renal damage. Acute exposure to dioxane can result in confusion, ataxia, drowsiness, convulsions, and renal and hepatic damage as well as pulmonary edema. Skin contact with vapor or liquid can result in dermatitis. Due to its mild odor, which serves as a warning to exposure at the odor threshold level, workers may be exposed to chronically high concentrations without knowing that they are being exposed.

Due to its flammability and explosive hazards, any spill or release of dioxane must be handled with caution. Any ignition sources can create a serious hazard due to the flammability and explosive nature of dioxane vapors.

Persons exposed to high concentrations of the vapor experience irritation of the eyes, nose, throat, and pulmonary system and may develop pulmonary edema. Liquid dioxane is an irritant to the skin and is a defatting agent and can produce dermatitis. It is absorbed dermally. Exposures to the eye must be flushed immediately with water. Exposures to the skin should also be flushed with water. Because of the poor warning properties of the vapor threshold of dioxane, illness in exposed individuals may be delayed. Exposure of the eyes can lead to corneal damage.

Any clothing contaminated with dioxane should be removed and contaminated skin irrigated with soap and water. The flammability limits in air of dioxane range from 1.97–22.5% by volume. When heated, toxic vapors are generated. Dioxane vapors are heavier than air and consequently travel along lower areas to ignition sources and produce dangerous flashback or explosion. Also, due to the fact that dioxane has a vapor pressure three times that of air, the chemical may reside in confined spaces below surface level. Dioxane mixes with water with no reaction and is a liquid at 1°C in one atmosphere with a boiling point of 101.3°C (214.3°F).

PYRIDINE

Pyridine is a colorless liquid solvent also known as azine or azabenzene. Pyridine is used in the synthesis of many organic compounds and agriculture chemicals. It has a molecular formula of C_5H_5N and a molecular structure as seen in Fig. 108.1. Pyridine is a flammable liquid used in manufacturing dyes, rubber, paints, explosives, and pharmaceuticals (24). The IDLH level is 3600 ppm, and the PEL is 5 ppm. Exposure occurs via vapor inhalation and skin absorption. Pyridine produces dermal and ocular irritation as well as irritation of the upper respiratory tract (24). Skin sensitization may occur following dermal exposure. Clinically, pyridine produces central nervous system depressant effects following inhalation of vapors or ingestion of the liquid. Acute ingestion can also produce hepatic and renal toxic damage (24, 26). Due to its very unpleasant odor, which is detectable at 1 ppm, the presence of pyridine vapors are readily noted in the environment. However, olfactory fatigue may occur following chronic exposure to pyridine, and thus the odor warning properties are not sufficient to help prevent injury.

Clinical symptoms following exposure include dizziness, headache, irritability, irritation of mucous membranes, confusion, syncope, coma, and hepatic and renal toxicity (24, 26).

ISOPHORONE

Isophorone is a solvent used for natural and synthetic polymers, resins, fats, and oils. It is also specifically used as a solvent for vinyl chloride-acetate-based coating systems, for metal cans, metal paints, nitrocellulose finishes, inks used for plastics, pesticide formulations, and adhesives for plastics and polystyrene materials (27). Most of the isophorone that is produced is used in vinyl coatings and inks. The next largest amount is used for agricultural products. The chemical structure for isophorone is shown in Fig. 108.1. It has a chemical formula of $C_9H_{14}O$ and is also known as isoacetophorone or isoforon. Isophorone has a molecular weight of 138.2. It is a clear liquid with a boiling point of 215°C and a mild odor threshold in water of 5.4 ppm and in air of 0.2 ppm. Isophorone is soluble in organic solvents such as ether, acetone, and alcohol. It has a flash point of 184°F, and its flammability limits vary from 0.8–3.5 volume percent.

The regulations pertaining to isophorone include OSHA, permissible limits in air of 4 ppm. Ambient water quality standards set by the EPA are 5.2 ml/L. The ACGIH has recommended a ceiling limit for isophorone of 5 ppm. NIOSH has recommended an exposure limit of 4 ppm for occupational exposures as a TWA for up to a 10-hour work day. Isophorone is also regulated by the Clean Water Effluent Guidelines for certain industrial point sources such as electroplating, metal finishing, paint formulating, ink formulating, and electrical and electronic components (28).

Respiratory and skin irritation health effects were common complaints of workers exposed to isophorone in printing plants (29). There have been no clinical reports of hepatic, renal, or hematologic toxic effects secondary to isophorone exposure. Animal studies have not indicated that isophorone is a hepatotoxin.

The main health effects noted from exposure to isophorone in humans appear to be irritation of the eyes and mucous membranes. Studies have indicated that exposure duration of 10 ppm for 15 minutes was tolerated by humans, but 25 ppm produced irritation of the upper airway and the eyes (29). It is thought that the threshold for eye and nose irritation falls between 35 and 55 ppm.

Neurologic effects secondary to occupational exposure to isophorone have been reported (29). Employees exposed to isophorone concentrations between 5 and 8 ppm had health complaints of fatigue and malaise. These complaints abated when the exposure concentrations in the work area were decreased below 5 ppm (29). This report helped form the basis for the ACGIH ceiling limit of 5 ppm. CNS depression and ataxia have been demonstrated in animals exposed to high concentrations of isophorone for 6–24 hours (29).

The National Toxicology Program (NTP) concluded that there was some evidence of carcinogenicity in male rats and an increase in the incidence of renal tubular cell adenomas and adenocarcinomas in the animals studied (29).

In animals studied for neurologic toxic effects of isophorone, no pathotoxicology has been found in either the brain or nerves. However, animal studies have indicated that, at high inhalational concentrations, isophorone is a CNS depressant and produces ataxia, lethargy, and coma. Humans in occupational environments have experienced lethargy, fatigue, malaise, headache, and some CNS depression at concentrations of 5–8 ppm (29).

Isophorone is one of a few chemicals that have been found to cause renal tubular tumors in male rats but not female rats (29).

The known health effects secondary to isophorone exposure in humans are mucous membrane and eye irritation, fatigue, and malaise.

Isophorone is released into the environment mainly from volatilization from solvents containing the chemical. Isopho-

rone also enters the environment from industrial and commercial discharges as well as runoff from soils at hazardous waste sites or other contaminated areas. In the air, isophorone has a half-life of less than 5 hours but may persist in water for several days up to a month (27). Isophorone is found in a few of the hazardous waste sites on the National Priorities List (NPL) in the United States. The occupational exposures to isophorone occur by inhalation or dermal contact and mainly occur in the printing industry.

Isophorone is used as a solvent which volatilizes or evaporates during or after use. Populations with high exposure to isophorone are screen print workers, some adhesive formulators, and coating manufacturing workers.

BUTYL MERCAPTAN

n-Butyl mercaptan, also known as thiobutyl alcohol, is a colorless flammable liquid solvent with a chemical formula of C_4H_9SH and a TLV of 0.5 ppm as recommended by the ACGIH. The OSHA PEL is 10 ppm. *n*-Butyl mercaptan is a mucous membrane and ocular irritant. It has a very objectionable odor; thus humans are not likely to be exposed to high concentrations. The odor threshold for butyl mercaptan is 0.001–0.001 ppm and the chemical has a typical sulfhydryl type smell of rotten eggs. The IDLH level is 2500 ppm (24, 26). It is used as an odorant added to gas and as an intermediate chemical in the production of insecticides.

DIMETHYLFORMAMIDE

Dimethylformamide has a chemical formula of $(CH_3)_2NCHO$ and is a colorless liquid solvent whose exposure hazards are mainly inhalational and dermal absorption. The PEL for dimethylformamide is 10 ppm TWA. The IDLH level is 3500 ppm. Dimethylformamide is a hepatotoxin (30). In addition, contact with the skin can result in dermatitis and systemic absorption, which can produce toxicity. Dimethylformamide has been used since the 1950s in the manufacturing of polyurethane products as well as in the pharmaceutical industry. It is well-absorbed by the skin and also by inhalation of vapors and is metabolized by the liver. Clinical hepatotoxicity associated with occupational exposure to dimethylformamide has been described (30).

Animal experiments have also documented the hepatotoxic properties of dimethylformamide. Acute or subchronic exposure of dimethylformamide results in hepatic necrosis in the central lobular area with fatty degeneration (30). Histologic findings on biopsy of patients with occupational exposure to dimethylformamide, as well as to other solvents, showed hepatocellular injury (30). Reports of workers in industries where dimethylformamide is used have complained of symptoms of anorexia, abdominal pain, and disulfiram-like reactions after ingesting alcohol. In addition, aminotransferase enzymes were elevated with the ratio of alanine aminotransferase to aspartate aminotransferase ratio always greater than one (30). In these workers, chronic exposure to dimethylformamide resulted in mildly increased hepatic enzymes, steatosis, without inflammation or fibrosis on biopsy of the liver. Following removal from exposure, the symptoms of these individuals resolved within 16 months (30).

NITROPROPANE

Nitropropane (1-nitropropane) is a liquid solvent used for organic materials, propellants, and solvent for organic cellulose esters, resins, waxes, fats, and dyes. Nitropropane has a chemical formula $CH_3CH_2CH_2NO_2$ (1-nitropropane) and $CH_3CHNO_2CH_3$ (2-nitropropane). 1-nitropropane has a TLV of 25 ppm and 2-nitropropane has a TLV of 10 ppm (24, 26). Nitropropane vapors of either solvent are mucous membrane, ocular, and pulmonary irritants. 2-Nitropropane, besides being a respiratory irritant, is a hepatotoxin. Workers exposed to 2-nitropropane vapors have developed headache, anorexia, nausea, and vomiting. Fulminant liver failure has been reported following occupational exposure to 2-nitropropane (31).

2-Nitropropane has been used since 1940 as a solvent for resins, waxes, water-resistant coatings, dyes, inks, and adhesives. It has also been used as a rocket propellant. Exposures to 2-nitropropane occur in highway maintenance, shipbuilding and plastic production and in the construction industry due to its use as a solvent for water-resistant coatings and in resins (31). Fatalities from massive hepatic failure have been previously reported following toxic exposure to 2-nitropropane (31). Its use in confined spaces is a health hazard. One report reviewed a fatality which occurred when a 45-year-old man applied a resin sealer to water pipes in a confined space. The resin system contained 2-nitropropane in addition to cyclohexane and toluene. The patient developed symptoms of headache, dizziness, nausea, vomiting, and anorexia during the application process. He was admitted to the hospital with elevated liver functions and died from massive hepatic necrosis 10 days after last exposure (31). His admission blood contained a 2-nitropropane concentration of 13 mg/l. Autopsy confirmed massive hepatocellular necrosis. His blood contained no other organic chemical compounds.

Another man was also exposed to the same resin sealer and developed headache, nausea, and dizziness. He had elevated liver functions and a blood nitropropane concentration of 8.5 mg/l. He eventually improved, but his liver functions remained elevated for 12 months (31).

There have been at least nine deaths reported from 2-nitropropane exposure involving coating applications in enclosed, poorly ventilated spaces (31). Liver necrosis and hepatic failure was the cause of death in each case. Chemical workers exposed to 2-nitropropane at the TLV of 25 ppm did not show evidence of liver function abnormalities (31).

2-Nitropropane is very volatile and is absorbed via the skin and lungs. It is a documented animal hepatotoxin. NIOSH recommends that the chemical be handled as a potential human carcinogen. In animal studies, 2-nitropropane had a half-life of 48 minutes at blood concentrations of 8–10 mg/l produced at an air concentration of 154 after 6 hours exposure ppm (31).

NAPHTHA

Naphtha is a general hydrocarbon solvent produced in two forms: petroleum distillate or coal tar. Petroleum naphtha contains aliphatic hydrocarbons, and coal tar naphtha contains mainly aromatic hydrocarbons. Petroleum naphtha is a colorless liquid solvent which also contains benzene as well as numerous other hydrocarbons. It is used as a solvent for oils, lacquers, paints, rubber cement, dry cleaning, and degreasing. Petroleum naphtha vapor is a CNS depressant as well as an irritant of the mucous membranes and respiratory tract. Exposure to high concentrations of the vapor can produce headache, dizziness, nausea, and shortness of breath. Dermal contact to vapor or liquid can produce dermatitis. The PEL for petroleum naphtha is 500 ppm (24, 26).

Coal tar naphtha is a light yellow liquid solvent which boils between 110–190°C. It is a general solvent for a variety of uses and is a CNS depressant. Coal tar naphtha is a mixture of aromatic hydrocarbons including toluene, xylene, cumene, and benzene (24, 26).

The PEL for coal tar naphtha is 100 ppm. Exposure to coal tar naphtha vapors or liquid produces symptoms similar to other aromatic hydrocarbons such as CNS depression, dermal irritation, potential hepatotoxicity, and renal toxicity (24, 26). The presence of benzene in coal tar naphtha can result in bone marrow depression and other toxic effects secondary to benzene. Clinical toxicity consists of dizziness, irritation of mucous membranes and eyes, and dermatitis following exposure. The overall toxicity of coal tar naphtha is similar to its individual aromatic hydrocarbon components. The IDLH level for both naphthas is 10,000 ppm.

STODDARD SOLVENT

Stoddard solvent is also known as white spirits or mineral spirits and is a colorless liquid used in paint thinner and degreasing operations. Stoddard solvent consists of 15–20% aromatic hydrocarbons and 80–85% paraffin and naphthenic hydrocarbons (24, 26). The TLV for Stoddard solvent is 100 ppm as a TWA. Due to its chemical makeup, Stoddard solvent exposure produces toxicity of CNS depression. It is also an irritant of the mucous membrane, eyes, and skin. The toxicity of Stoddard solvent is related to the aromatic and aliphatic hydrocarbon content. The odor threshold of Stoddard solvent is 0.9 ppm, and the irritative properties and odor are not sufficient to provide adequate warning to prevent dangerous concentrations and thus serious exposures (24, 26).

TURPENTINE

Turpentine is also known as oil of turpentine or spirit of turpentine. It is a colorless or slightly yellow volatile solvent which may vary in its composition depending on method of production. It has an approximate formula of $C_{10}H_{16}$ and is derived from the *Pinus pinacea* tree as an oleoresin (24). Turpentine is a flammable general solvent and has been used as an insecticide in the past. Exposure occurs by inhalation, skin absorption, or ingestion. Turpentine is an irritant of the mucous membranes and eyes and is a CNS depressant. Irritant phenomena secondary to turpentine exposure occur at air concentrations of 75 ppm (24, 26).

Chemical analysis of turpentine shows that it consists of 83% α-pinene; approximately 9% camphene; 2% β-pinene, and 7% other terpenes (37). It is a skin irritant, and dermal exposure should be avoided. Turpentine can be absorbed via the dermal route as well as mucous membranes, and intoxication by these routes has been reported (24, 26). The PEL is 100 ppm with an IDLH level of 1900 ppm (24, 26).

ISOBUTYL MERCAPTAN

Isobutyl mercaptan has a chemical formula of $C_4H_{10}S$ and a molecular weight of 90.2. It has a recognition odor of 0.00097 ppm in air and has a very disagreeable "skunk-like" odor. Isobutyl mercaptan is highly reactive with oxidizing materials and has moderate flammability. It is an irritant, has moderate toxicity by ingestion or inhalation, and emits toxic vapors when heated to decomposition or when it comes into contact with an acid. Isobutyl mercaptan has an OSHA PEL and a TWA of 10 ppm. NIOSH has given isobutyl mercaptan an IDLH value of 2500 ppm. The ACGIH have listed TLVs of a TWA of 0.5 ppm.

DIMETHYL SULFOXIDE (DMSO)

DMSO is a highly polar solvent and is termed a universal solvent (Fig. 108.1). DMSO alters the stratum corneum barrier of the skin, allowing dermal absorption of many substances. Ocular toxicity with cataract formation in animals has been reported following dermal or ocular application (34). However, human studies have not shown any lenticular changes or changes in visual acuity in the eyes of scleroderma patients receiving DMSO therapy. As a therapeutic agent, DMSO is used only in the treatment of interstitial cystitis.

Exposure to DMSO will result in absorption of chemicals in which it is used as a solvent. Thus toxicity assessment should be directed toward the agents dissolved by DMSO. There are no TLVs or OSHA PELs.

REFERENCES

1. Morrison R, Boyd R. Organic chemistry. 2nd ed. Boston: Allyn and Bacon, 1967:492–497.

2. United States Department of Labor (OSHA). Industrial exposure and control technologies for OSHA regulated hazardous substances (part 1 of 4): carbon disulfide. Document PB89-210199, 1989:366–369.

3. Lam CW, Di Stefano V. Characteristics of carbon disulfide binding in blood and to other biological substances. Toxicol Appl Pharmacol 1986;86:235–242.

4. Bus JS. The relationship of carbon disulfide metabolism to development of toxicity. Neurotoxicology 1985;6:73–80.

5. Rojas MM, Oehme FW. A review of the acute effects of carbon disulphide on lipid liver metabolism. Vet Hum Toxicol 1982;24:337–342.

6. Baselt RC, Cravey RH, eds. Disposition of toxic drugs and chemicals in man. 3rd ed. Chicago: Year Book Medical Publishers, 1989.

7. Campbell L, Jones AH, Wilson HK. Evaluations of occupational exposure to carbon disulphide by blood, exhaled air and urine analysis. Am J Ind Med 1985;8:143–153.

8. Rainey JM. Disulfiram toxicity and carbon disulphide poisoning. Am J Psychiatry 1977;134:371–378.

9. Gosselin RE, Smith RP, Hodge HC. Clinical toxicology of commercial products. 5th ed. Baltimore: Williams & Wilkins, 1984.

10. United States Department of Health and Human Services (National Institute for Occupational Safety and Health). NIOSH pocket guide to chemical hazards. DHHS (NIOSH) publication number 90-117, 1990:60.

11. Spyker DA, Gallanosa AG, Suratt PM. Health effects of acute carbon disulfide exposure. J Toxicol Clin Toxicol 1982;19:87–93.

12. Seppalainen AM, Haltia M. Carbon disulfide. In: Spencer PS, Schaumburg HH, eds. Experimental and clinical neurotoxicology. Baltimore: Williams & Wilkins 1980:356–373.

13. Davidson M, Feinleib M. Carbon disulfide poisoning: a review. Am Heart J 1972;83:100–114.

14. Peters HA, Levine RL, Matthews CG, Chapman LJ. Extrapyramidal and other neurologic manifestations associated with carbon disulfide fumigant exposure. Arch Neurol 1988;45:537–540.

15. Johnson BL, Boyd J, Burg JR, Lee ST, Xintaras C, Albright BE. Effects on the peripheral nervous system of workers' exposure to carbon disulfide. Neurotoxicology 1983;4:53–66.

16. De Laey JJ, De Rouck A, Priem H, Vanhoorne M. Ophthalmological aspects of chronic CS_2 intoxication. Int Ophthalmol 1980;3:51–56.

17. Raitta CR, Teir H, Tolonen M, Nerminen M, Helpio E, Malmstrom S. Impaired color discrimination among viscose rayon workers exposed to carbon disulfide. J Occup Med 1981;23:189–192.

18. Kristensen TS. Cardiovascular diseases and the work environment. Scand J Work Environ Health 1989;15:245–264.

19. Kruppa K, Hietanen E, Klockars M, et al. Chemical exposures at work and cardiovascular morbidity. Scand J Work Environ Health 1984;10:381–388.

20. Sweetnam PM, Taylor SWC, Elwood PC. Exposure to carbon disulphide and ischaemic heart disease in a viscose rayon factory. Br J Ind Med 1987;44:220–227.

21. Meyer CR. Semen quality in workers exposed to carbon disulfide compared to a control group from the same plant. J Occup Med 1981;23:435–439.

22. Schrag SD, Dixon RL. Occupational exposures associated with male reproductive dysfunction. Am Rev Pharmacol Toxicol 1985;25:567–592.

23. Sittig M. Handbook of toxic and hazardous chemicals and carcinogens. 2nd ed. Park Ridge, NJ: Noyes Publications, 1985.

24. Sittig M. Handbook of toxic and hazardous chemicals. Park Ridge, NJ: Noyes Publications, 1981.

25. (No author listed) Dangerous properties of industrial material report 1988;8:32–42.

26. Proctor N, Hughes J, Fischman M. Chemical hazards of the workplace. 2nd ed. New York: JB Lippincott, 1988.

27. Toxicological Profile for Isophorone, Agency for Toxic Substances and Disease Registry, US Public Health Service, 1989:61–62.

28. Toxicological Profile for Isophorone, Agency for Toxic Substances and Disease Registry, US Public Health Service, 1989:83–86.

29. Toxicological Profile for Isophorone, Agency for Toxic Substances and Disease Registry, US Public Health Service, 1989:9–56.

30. Redlich C, West A, Fleming L. Clinical and pathological characteristics of hepatotoxicity associated with occupational exposure to dimethylformamide. Gastroenterology 1990;99:748–757.

31. Harrison R, Letz G, Pasternak G. Fulminant hepatic failure after occupational exposure to 2-nitropropane, Ann Intern Med 1987;107:466–468.

32. (No author listed) Dangerous properties of industrial materials report 1988;8:61–67.

n-Hexane and 2-Hexanone

Lorne K. Garrettson, M.D.

INTRODUCTION

The two common, six-carbon, aliphatic compounds, n-hexane and 2-hexanone, have the same neurotoxic metabolite, 2,5-hexanedione. n-Hexane is used as a solvent in glues, adhesives, and cements. 2-Hexanone (methyl n-butyl ketone, MBK) is also a commonly used solvent (Table 109.1).

CHEMICAL AND PHYSICAL FORM

Both compounds are nonionized, flammable, volatile liquids at ambient temperature and pressure. n-Hexane has a chemical formula of C_6H_{14} and a molecular weight of 86.20. Its vapor density is 2.97 (air = 1.0). Hexane is flammable and explosive when exposed to heat. Hexane vapor is flammable in air at concentrations between 1.2–7.7%. 2-Hexanone is a colorless liquid solvent, also flammable, with a chemical formula of $C_6H_{12}O$ and a molecular weight of 100.16 (Figure 109.1, Table 109.2). 2-Hexanone has a vapor density of 3 (air = 1.0).

n-Hexane is a component of crude oil and is manufactured from distillation.

MECHANISMS AND PROCESSES LEADING TO EXPOSURE

Exposure has primarily been from the inhalation of these compounds such as during volatilization from products in which they are used as solvents. Worker exposure to n-hexane occurs during the production of glues and adhesives. Others are exposed during the application of glues and adhesives containing n-hexane as it volatilizes. Reports from Japan and the United States have linked peripheral neuropathy with n-hexane used in shoe and furniture manufacture where it was used for dissolving glue (1, 2). An epidemic of weakness due to exposure to 2-hexanone (MBK) was seminal in initiating the studies that identified the putative toxic metabolite. Cases came from an Ohio plant making coated fabrics (3, 4). A similar cluster of cases of polyneuropathy was reported in spray painters repainting a dam (5). These epidemics involved two compounds, but there was no difference in the clinical findings. The saga of discovery of the relationship of these compounds to a common disease with a common metabolite responsible for toxicity has

Table 109.1. Uses and Users

Uses	Users
Glues, rubber glues	Shoemakers
Cleaners	Furniture makers
Paint and lacquer solvents	Industrial painters
Seed oil extraction (soy, flax, safflower)	Hobbyist using rubber glues
Grinding with diamond dust	Precision industrial grinding
	Adhesive tape manufacturers
	Glue sniffers

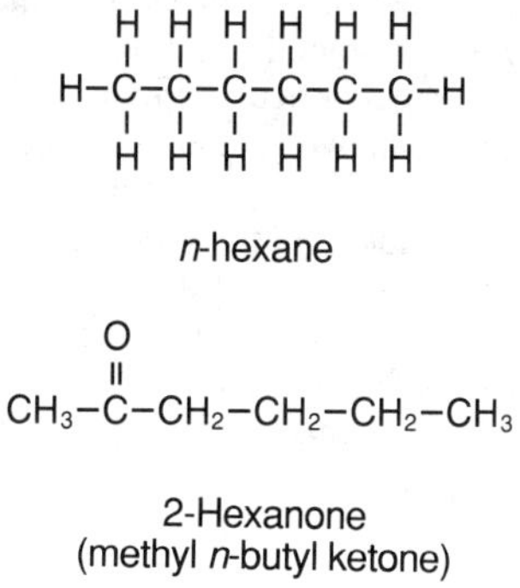

Figure 109.1. Chemical formulas for n-hexane and 2-hexanone.

been reviewed (Fig. 109.2) (6). The neurotoxic metabolite is 2,5-hexanedione (7). Exposures are worse in enclosed places due to the high vapor density and high vapor pressures of both n-hexane and 2-hexanone.

CLINICAL TOXICOLOGY OF EXPOSURE

Routes of Exposure

Inhalation is the primary route of exposure; however, dermatologic exposure can lead to skin irritation and this absorption may contribute to chronic exposure and polyneuropathy. Ingestion has rarely been reported.

Absorption

Both compounds are readily absorbed from the lungs. Systemic absorption from dermal exposure has not been well studied.

Metabolism

Both compounds are metabolized by the liver to a common toxic metabolite, 2,5-hexanedione (Fig. 109.2) (8, 9). This compound is a direct neurotoxin. There seems to be a high degree of specificity for the toxic effect of this compound, as related metabolites of similar solvents have no similar toxicity. 2,5-Hexanedione is a γ-diketone. Other diketones (α, β, δ) do not produce neurotoxicity. The metabolite is reduced to the corresponding 2,5-hexanediol or to 5-hydroxy-2-hexanone. Compounds with a hydroxyl group are conjugated with glucuronide and eliminated in the urine. 2,5-Hexanedione can be found in the urine of workers as a marker of occupational exposure to n-hexane.

Elimination

Renal clearance of n-hexane has been measured and found to be 2 l/min (10). Elimination of the parent compounds is primarily

Table 109.2. Common Names and Chemical Names

Chemical Name	Common Names
n-Hexane (CAS #110-54-3)	Dipropyl Hexane Hexyl hydride Skellysolve B
2-Hexanone (CAS #591-78-6)	Methyl butyl ketone (MBK) 2-oxohexane Ketone, butyl methyl Methyl *n*-butyl ketone (MNBK or MnBK) Propylacetone Hexan-2-one

by metabolism, and very little is exhaled unchanged. The toxic metabolite, 2,5-hexanedione is the principal metabolite. There are other minor metabolites, but none has been found to be toxic.

SIGNS, SYMPTOMS, AND SYNDROMES

Acute Toxicity

Acute exposure to *n*-hexane vapor produces upper airway irritation, drowsiness, central nervous system depression, confusion, and giddiness. 2-Hexanone vapor produces ocular and upper airway irritation. Brief exposures to high vapor concentrations of around 5000 ppm can produce drowsiness and central nervous system depression.

Chronic Toxicity

After chronic exposure to large amounts of these solvents, a syndrome of sensorimotor polyneuropathy may occur. Maculopathy and diminished color discrimination were common among workers in one study of an *n*-hexane-exposed group (11). Evidence for central nervous system effects are also reported. Memory loss after solvent abuse with *n*-hexane has been reported (4). More recently, parkinsonism has been suggested as a result of exposure to *n*-hexane (13). Loss of memory or other cognitive effects of these compounds have not been reported following industrial exposure. However, the potential for central nervous system effects is supported by the finding of alteration in evoked potentials in workers. There is no known teratogenic or carcinogenic potential known for these compounds.

CLINICAL EVALUATION

An accurate history is essential to determine if the person has been exposed to one of the offending agents. Proof of the exposure may require the review of the products used at a worksite and may require the assessment of the work environment by an industrial hygienist. Patients may complain of weakness, muscle cramps, numbness, and paresthesias such as the feeling of tingling, burning, and freezing. Impotence may occur (Table 109.3).

The physical examination should examine all muscle groups for weakness. Peripheral muscles are affected first, with more proximal weakness following after more prolonged exposure. Muscle stretch reflexes are absent distally where there is weakness. Atrophy of the hand muscles has been reported. Hyperhidrosis may occur. All sensory modalities may be affected on examination, including sensation and proprioception. Patients should be assessed for cerebellar signs and tremor. Visual acuity and peripheral vision changes have not been reported. Blurred vision has been reported. Tinnitus may occur, and parkinsonism has been reported. Studies of evoked potentials suggest that there may be central nervous system involvement not noted in the clinical exam. Recovery is slow, requiring the regeneration of axon fibers. Complete recovery of strength may not occur.

The differential diagnosis of weakness in workers includes exposure to triocresyl phosphate, although patients with this intoxication are less likely to show sensory loss, and muscle stretch reflexes remain normal even with debilitating weakness. Other compounds causing peripheral nerve injury include carbon disulfide, lead, arsenic, acute or chronic exposure to organophosphates, acrylamide, toluene, and ethylene oxide.

TREATMENT

The patient must be removed from all future exposure. Physical therapy should be initiated to maintain full range of motion until renervation occurs.

LABORATORY DIAGNOSIS

n-Hexane and 2-hexanedione can be assayed for levels in blood in some laboratories, but this has little utility since the clearance of the compound is rapid (10). Determination of 2,5-hexanedione in the urine documents the level of exposure (14). Normal values for 2,5-hexanedione are below 10 µg/l, the current limit of detection.

Urine from exposed workers can have concentrations of 2,5-hexanedione over 200 µg/l.

SPECIAL DIAGNOSTIC STUDIES

Nerve conduction studies will be abnormal after clinical weakness has become apparent. Fast fibers are affected at lower levels of exposure than slow fibers (15, 16). Nerve conduction velocity is correlated with clinical severity. Studies of evoked potential in exposed workers have shown abnormalities (17). There is depression in the amplitude of several peaks in the visual evoked response. Auditory evoked potentials show prolongation of peak V latency and in the central conduction time. Sensory evoked potentials show delayed conduction times (16). The amplitude of the electroretinogram has been found to be reduced in *n*-hexane workers (17). Documentation that these compounds are the cause of the peripheral neuropathy requires a biopsy of a peripheral nerve (sural). The findings expected are of paranodal axonal swellings which consist of neurofilaments. Retraction of the myelin sheaths and focal demyelination may be seen (18, 19).

BIOLOGIC MONITORING

The measurement of 2,5-hexanedione in the urine after 8 hours of environmental exposure correlates well with the active air sampling of the workplace (20). The TLV on a time-weighted average is 50 ppm for *n*-hexane and 100 ppm for 2-hexanedione (Table 109.4). The urine concentration of 2,5-hexanedione in exposed workers should not exceed 5 mg/l (21).

ENVIRONMENTAL MONITORING

Passive dosimeters are as effective as active air sampling and may be used for assessment of the exposure of the workers (20).

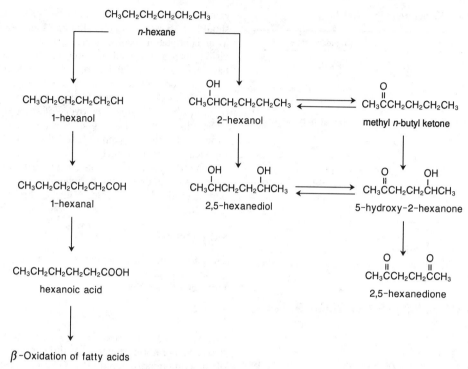

Figure 109.2. Metabolism of *n*-hexane.

Table 109.3   Clinical Presentation of *n*-Hexane Neurotoxicity

Extremity paresthesias
Muscle cramping
Distal muscle weakness
Blurred vision
Tinnitus
Fatigue
Loss of muscle stretch reflexes
Sensory impairment
Muscle atrophy
Parkinsonism

REFERENCES

1. Yamamura Y. *n*-Hexane polyneuropathy. Folia Psychiatr Neurol Jpn 1969;23:45–50.
2. Herskowitz A, Ishii N, Schaumburg H. *n*-Hexane neuropathy: a syndrome occurring as a result of industrial exposure. N Engl J Med 1971;285:82–85.
3. Billmaier D, Yee HT, Allen N, Craft B, Williams N, Epstein S, Fontaine R. Peripheral neuropathy in a coated fabrics plant. J Occup Med 1974;16:665-671.
4. Allen N, Mendell JM, Billmaier DJ, Fontaine RE, O'Neil J. Toxic polyneuropathy due to methyl *n*-butyl ketone. Arch Neurol 1975;32:209–218.

5. Mallov JS. MBK neuropathy among spray painters. JAMA 1976;235:1455–1457.
6. Couri D, Milks MM. Hexacarbon neuropathy: tracking a toxin. Neurol Toxicol 1985;6:65–72.
7. DeCaprio AP. Molecular mechanisms of diketone neurotoxicity. Chem-Biol Interact 1985;54:257–270.
8. DiVincenzo GD, Kaplan CJ, Dedinas J. Characterization of the metabolites of methyl *n*-butyl ketone, methyl isobutyl ketone, and methyl ethyl ketone in guinea pig serum and their clearance. Toxicol Appl Pharmacol 1976;36:511–522.
9. Spencer PS, Schaumburg HH. Feline nervous system response to chronic intoxication with commercial grades of methyl *n*-butyl ketone, methyl isobutyl ketone, and methyl ethyl ketone. Toxicol Appl Pharmacol 1976;37:301–311.
10. Filser JG, Peter H, Bolt HM, Fedtke N. Pharmacokinetics of the neurotoxin *n*-hexane in rat and man. Arch Toxicol 1987;60:77–80.
11. Raitta CH, Seppalainen AM, Huuskonen MS. *n*-Hexane maculopathy in industrial workers. Albrecht V, Graefes Arch Klin Exp Ophthalmol 1979;209:99–110.
12. Towfighi J, Gonatas N, Pleasure D, Cooper H, McCrea L. Glue sniffer's neuropathy. Neurology 1976;26:238–243.
13. Pezzolii G, Barbieri S, Ferrante C, Zecchinelli A, Foa V. Parkinsonism due to *n*-hexane (Letter). Lancet 1989;2:874.
14. Dawai T, Mizunuma K, Yasugi T, Uchida Y, Ikeda M. The method of choice for the determination of 2,5-hexanedione as an indicator of occupational exposure to *n*-hexane. Int Arch Occup Environ Health 1990;62:403–408.
15. Yokoyama K, Feldman RG, Sax DS, Salzsider BT, Kucera J. Relation of distribution of conduction velocities to nerve biopsy findings in *n*-hexane poisoning. Muscle Nerve 1990;13:314–320.
16. Huang C-C, Chu N-S. Evoked potentials in chronic *n*-hexane intoxication. Clin Electroencephalogr 1989;20:162–168.
17. Seppalainen AM, Raitta C, Huuskonen MS. Hexane induced changes in visual evoked potentials and electroretinograms of industrial users. Electroencephalogr Clin Neurophysiol 1979;47:492–498.
18. Saida K, Mendell Jr, Weiss HS. Peripheral nerve changes induced by methyl *n*-butyl ketone and potentiation by methyl ethyl ketone. J Neuropathol Exp Neurol 1976;35:207–225.
19. Krobkin R, Asbury AK, Sumner A, Nielsen SL. Glue-sniffing neuropathy. Arch Neurol 1975;32:158–162.
20. Bartolucci GB, Perbellini L, Gori GP, Brugnone F, Chiesura-Corona P, DeRosa E. Occupational exposure to solvents: field comparison of active and passive samplers and biologic monitoring of exposed workers. Ann Occup Hyg 1986;30:295–306.
21. American Conference of Governmental Environmental Hygienist. The 1990–1991 TLV and BEI indices. Cincinnati, OH: ACGIH, 1990.

Table 109.4.   Threshold Limit Values from ACGIH (21)

Compounds	Threshold Limit Values Time-Weighted Averages
n-Hexane	50 ppm (8 hr) excursion limit: <5 TLV for <30 min
2-Hexanedione	100 ppm (8 hr) excursion limit: <5 TLV for <30 min

John P. Holland, M.D., M.P.H.

SOURCES AND PRODUCTION

Common Names and Chemical Forms

Asbestos is the commercial designation given collectively to a group of six distinct types of natural mineral fibers. It is subdivided into two groups, serpentine and amphibole. The only fiber in the serpentine group is chrysotile (commonly known as white asbestos). The five amphibole fibers are crocidolite (blue asbestos), amosite (brown asbestos), tremolite, actinolite, and anthophyllite.

Chemical Forms

All types of asbestos are hydrated magnesium silicates. Each fiber type has its own general chemical form and crystalline structure, but even for fibers of a specific type there is variability in the percentages of major chemical components. Differing amounts of metals may also be found with asbestos including iron, chromium, cobalt, manganese, and nickel. These are either incorporated into the crystalline structure or are contaminants from surrounding minerals which cannot easily be removed.

Chrysotile contains about 40% each of magnesium oxide and silica but very little iron oxide (1%). Crocidolite and amosite contain more iron oxides (20–44%) and silica (49–53%) but have little magnesium oxide (0–7%). Tremolite, actinolite, and anthophyllite also have large amounts of silica (51–60%) but are intermediate in their content of magnesium oxide (15–34%) and iron oxides (0–15%) (1, 2).

The general chemical formula of chrysotile is $(Mg_3Si_2O_5(OH)_4)$ which makes it chemically similar to micas and kaolinites. However, chrysotile has a fibrous structure which is not found in these other minerals.

General chemical formulas for the amphibole fibers are: crocidolite $[Na_2(MgFe^{+++}Fe^{++})Si_8O_{22}(OH)]$, amosite $[MgFe^{++}{}_7Si_8O_{22}(OH)_4]$, tremolite $[(Ca_2(MgFe^{++})_5Si_8O_{22}]$, actinolite $[Ca_2(MgFe^{++})_5Si_8O_{22}(OH)_2]$, and anthophyllite $[(MgFe^{++})_7Si_8O_{22}(OH)_2]$ (3).

Although they are relatively resistant to degradation by chemicals and heat, asbestos fibers dissolve to various degrees in strong acid and alkali solutions. Asbestos fibers are not flammable, but when heated above 800°F (427°C) amphiboles tend to lose the water incorporated in their crystalline structure and become very brittle, while chrysotile keeps its flexibility at this temperature (1–3).

Physical Forms

Asbestos particles found in natural mineral deposits do not have fixed dimensions but form as parallel aggregations of long crystalline fibrils or fibers. In natural mineral formations these fibers can be up to several centimeters long. They are quite brittle and when stressed break easily into shorter lengths. In preparing it for commercial use, asbestos-containing rock is crushed mechanically and cleaned in a process called milling. This results in an infinite variety of sizes for commercial asbestos fibers; most are less than 50 microns long, and many are shorter than 1 micron (1).

SERPENTINE GROUP

Chrysotile is the only fiber type in the serpentine group. It is also the only asbestos fiber that is curly and is often found in intertwined bundles. The crystalline structure of chrysotile consists of parallel sheets of silica and magnesium hydroxide (i.e., brucite), which give the appearance of overlapping scrolls in cross-section (Fig. 110.1).

The basic structural unit of chrysotile is the fibril, which is a curved sheet of this material that forms into a scroll or tube. Chrysotile fibrils have a fixed diameter of 0.02–0.04 microns, which make them the thinnest fiber found in nature (in comparison the diameters of a cotton fiber and a human hair are 10 and 40 microns, respectively). In nature, these chrysotile fibrils are usually found bunched together to form a chrysotile fiber with a typical diameter of 0.75–1.5 microns.

Serpentine fibers derive their name from serpentine rocks where they are found. Asbestos forms when very hot liquid supersaturated with minerals invades fissures in serpentine rock and then slowly cools and crystallizes into veins. In natural formations chrysotile is often found with quartz micas, fosterite, brucite, and feldspar, so commercial formulations can be contaminated with these materials (1, 3).

AMPHIBOLE GROUP

All the amphiboles have a straight, needle-like shape and are found in nature stacked in parallel rows. In crystalline structure the amphiboles are parallel chains of silica tetrahedras which have incorporated in them varying amounts of different metal ions, giving each type its unique chemical form (Figs. 110.2 and 110.3).

Amphiboles do not have a true fibril structure but are formed as parallel plates of crystalline material which can shear apart to form fibers with a variety of diameters. The thinnest amphibole fibers are 0.1–0.2 microns, but more typical diameters are 1.5–4.0 microns.

Amphibole asbestos is formed by forces of heat and pressure rearranging and recrystallizing materials in existing mineral formations. Crocidolite and amosite are found in sedimentary rocks called banded ironstones. Tremolite, actinolite, and anthophyllite deposits are found as pockets in igneous, metamorphic, or sedimentary rocks. In natural mineral formations the amphibole fiber types are often mixed with iron oxides and quartz, so commercial formulations can be contaminated with these materials (1, 3). Asbestos is found in numerous common locations (Table 110.1) and sites.

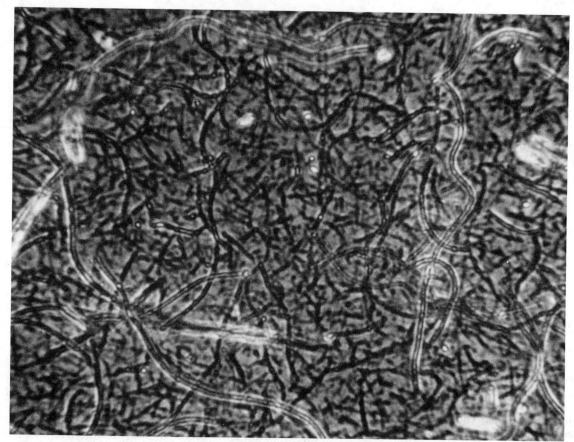

Figure 110.1.   Chrysotile fibers (magnified 300×).

EXPOSURE TO ASBESTOS

Production of Asbestos

Commercial asbestos is obtained from asbestos-bearing rocks mined in open-pit or underground mines. The rock is then crushed and asbestos fibers separated and washed in a process known as milling. The commercial asbestos fibers are then shipped in bags; in the past these bags were often woven jute, which allowed fibers to escape, but today they are made of impervious paper or plastic.

The Soviet Union is the largest producer of asbestos, with most of this being used in the Eastern Bloc countries. Historically, most of the asbestos mined in North America has been chrysotile; 90% of this has come from Canada, especially from large mines in Quebec. In the past, chrysotile was mined in smaller amounts in the United States. South Africa has been the third largest producer of asbestos worldwide, and has produced most of the crocidolite and amosite used in the United States; some crocidolite from Australia was also used in this country.

In worldwide consumption of commercial asbestos peaked in the early 1970s with six million tons a year, and the annual U.S. consumption then was about 1.6 million tons. Commercial use has dropped since then, but it is estimated that over 30 million tons of asbestos have been used in the United States over the past century, and much of this is still in existing structures and manufactured items.

About 95% of all asbestos used in the United States has been chrysotile, and over 90% of this has come from mines in Que-

bec. In the United States chrysotile has been mined in Arizona, California, Vermont, and other states, but is no longer produced in significant quantities.

The only other fiber types used in large quantities in the United States have been crocidolite and amosite, which were imported primarily from South Africa, although some came from Australia. Tremolite and actinolite have little commercial importance but may be found as contaminants in other types of commercially used asbestos. Tremolite is also sometimes found in small amounts in industrial talc, vermiculite, and sandstone. Anthophyllite has little commercial importance in North America but is found in exposed natural deposits in Finland (1, 3).

Commercial Uses of Asbestos

The physical properties of asbestos make it a unique and commercially useful material. These include resistance to degradation by heat and chemicals, strength, durability, and a fibrous structure (which allows it to be made into cloth or felt and to act as a good binder in ceramic materials).

Asbestos has been used extensively in the industrialized world since the exploitation of large commercial deposits in Quebec in the 1860s and South Africa in the 1890s. Asbestos has over 3000 commercial uses, the most important of which are listed in Table 110.1. The majority of asbestos used commercially has been in the construction of buildings, ships, power plants, chemical plants, and other industrial facilities.

The largest single use of asbestos has been as a binder in cement pipes and cement panels. Asbestos has also been used

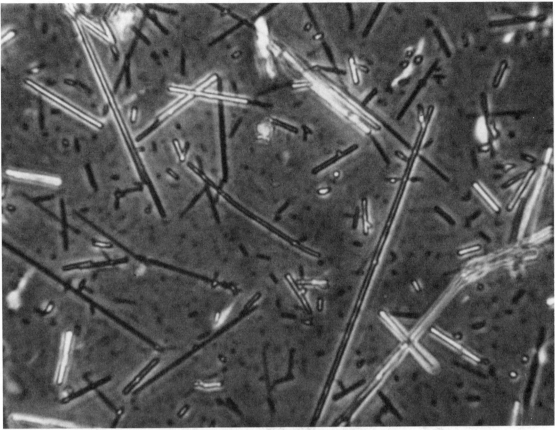

Figure 110.2. Amosite fibers (magnified 300×).

extensively in all types of insulation and fireproofing including pipe and boiler insulation (where loose asbestos fibers mixed with water were often applied as a ''mud'') and spray-on fire-proofing on ceilings and exposed structural beams. Asbestos has been incorporated into a variety of building products including house siding, wall board, and floor and ceiling tiles.

Asbestos cloth has been used in fire-resistant clothing and fire and welding blankets. When pressed into a felt, asbestos is used in pipe gaskets, and it is also used as a binder in plastics and paper. As a filtering material asbestos has been used in gas masks and a variety of chemical processes, such as in the membranes of hydrolytic cells in chlorine production plants. Finally, asbestos has been used extensively in friction products such as auto brake shoes (1, 4).

Sources of Occupational and Environmental Exposures

OCCUPATIONAL EXPOSURES

In the United States millions of individuals have had significant workplace exposures to asbestos since the beginning of this century, with the most extensive exposures occurring in the three decades during and after World War II. Limited information is available on historical levels of asbestos exposure for U.S. workers prior to 1970, but in many industries airborne asbestos levels were over 100 fibers/ml (this is 500 times higher than the current Occupational Safety and Health Administration (OSHA) Permissible Exposure Level (PEL) of 0.2 fibers/ml) (1, 5, 6).

Historically, workers in the United States who had the highest asbestos exposures were in mining and milling, primary manufacturing (i.e., use of asbestos as a raw material to make products such as concrete pipe or floor tiles) and insulation trades (including those in both general construction and shipbuilding). The next highest exposures were for workers in secondary manufacturing (i.e., incorporating asbestos-containing materials into manufactured items), and construction and shipbuilding workers who were not insulators.

In the United States the shipbuilding and construction industries have had the largest cohorts of workers with heavy asbestos exposures (it is estimated that in shipyards alone more than one million workers have had significant exposure). In both these industries, insulators have had twice the rate of asbestos-related diseases compared with workers in other trades.

At the other end of the spectrum, workers whose only exposure to asbestos was in changing auto brake shoes containing asbestos have shown no increased incidence of any asbestos-related disease. The reason for this is unclear, although one theory suggests that high heat from friction on the brake shoe transforms the asbestos into a nontoxic material that does not cause disease. In spite of this, the same OSHA standards apply for asbestos exposures in all types of industries (1).

By the mid-1960s it was apparent that asbestos was a serious health hazard which could cause asbestosis, lung cancer, and mesothelioma. Workplace regulation of asbestos exposure has become increasingly more stringent in the United States since passage of the OSHA Act of 1970. In 1986 OSHA lowered

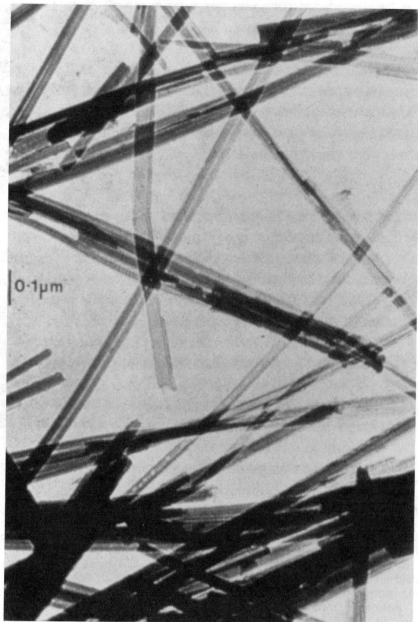

0·1μm

Figure 110.3. Amosite asbestos fibers magnified 400×. Fibers by definition are 5 microns in length with length to width aspect ratio of 3:1 respectively.

the PEL for asbestos in workplace air to its current level of 0.2 fiber/ml. Spray-on applications of asbestos for insulation or fireproofing have been completely banned, and the Environmental Protection Agency (EPA) has proposed a complete ban on asbestos use in industry although this has not been approved (7).

During the past two decades there has been a steady decline in the commercial use of asbestos, along with increased use of industrial respirators and changes in production processes, all of which resulted in markedly reduced worker exposures. Heavy unprotected asbestos exposures are now rare in the United States and most developed countries. Since most epidemiologic studies of asbestos-related disease are based on occupational groups who had heavy exposures prior to 1970, the risk estimates

derived from these studies may not reflect the health risks for similar jobs today.

However, because diseases caused by asbestos often have latency periods of 10–40 years, many workers who were heavily exposed in the past will continue to develop asbestos-related diseases in the coming decades. Asbestos present in existing structures, plants, ships, and equipment will also remain a potential hazard for workers who demolish, repair, or refurbish these items. In addition, asbestosis and other asbestos-related diseases may continue to be significant problems in many rapidly industrializing Third World countries where occupational exposures are not well controlled (4, 5).

Epidemiologic studies of asbestos have generally focused on cumulative lifetime exposure as the most important risk factor

Table 110.1   Sites and Businesses Linked with Asbestos Exposures[a]

Mining and milling asbestos
Manufacture of:
    Cement pipe
    Cement panels and flooring
    Pipe and boiler insulation
    Electrical insulation
    Gaskets and fittings
    Roofing, wall board, and siding materials
    Composite floor and ceiling tiles
    Friction products
    Fireproof clothing
    Chemical filters
    Paper and plastics
    Insulation work
    General construction
    Shipbuilding and shipwrecking
    Locomotive repair
    Building demolition
    Power plants
    Marine engine rooms
    Chemical plants
    Automobile repair
    Building maintenance

[a]Selikoff IJ, Lee DH. Asbestos and disease. New York: Academic Press, 1978:34–50.

for asbestos-related diseases. These exposures estimated for individuals are based on either: (a) years worked in specific job categories multiplied times estimated exposures for these jobs or (b) asbestos fiber counts from lung tissue specimens. Both types of estimates have significant limitations.

Exposure estimates based on work history can be inaccurate since historical data on exposure levels and fiber mix are seldom known and probably vary greatly over the working life of an individual. Retrospective studies also often lack good work histories. Basing exposure estimates on fiber counts of lung tissue specimens also has limitations (see *Deposition and Clearance of Fibers* below) (5).

The differential toxic effects of specific fiber types have been investigated in many studies. These have looked at groups whose lifetime exposures appeared to be predominantly from a single fiber type, such as chrysotile miners in Quebec, gas mask assemblers in England (who worked primarily with crocidolite), and those living near anthophyllite outcroppings in Finland. Typically these studies have found crocidolite to be most toxic in causing asbestos-related diseases; amosite has intermediate toxicity, and chrysotile is least toxic.

However, recent studies suggest that the supposedly "pure" forms of asbestos seem to be contaminated with small amounts of other fiber types. This makes it difficult to draw conclusions about unique effects of a specific fiber type. For example, chrysotile from one mine in Quebec, which was previously thought to be pure, was found to contain small amounts of tremolite which may be the major cause of toxicity for this material (5).

ASBESTOS EXPOSURES TO BUILDING OCCUPANTS

In the past decade there has been public concern about health risk from exposures to low levels of airborne asbestos among occupants in schools and other public buildings. Asbestos has

been used extensively in these buildings since World War II for boiler and pipe insulation, spray-on insulation, and fireproofing for ceilings and structural beams, and as a component in wall board and floor or ceiling tiles. It is estimated 20% of all building in the United States have some asbestos-containing material (8).

The EPA regulates the disposal of asbestos as a hazardous waste and its release into the atmosphere as an air pollutant. Although it can issue advisory statements, the EPA does not have legal authority to regulate asbestos exposures to students in schools or other occupants of public buildings. No government agency regulates asbestos exposures to individuals inside their own homes.

Since 1984, the EPA has required all school districts to survey their buildings for asbestos, and many purchasers of commercial and residential real estate are requiring similar inspections. This has resulted in a sizable effort to remove or encapsulate asbestos materials in these buildings. Although the EPA has not set a PEL or required any remedial action, many school districts that found asbestos have removed it or encapsulated it in place (i.e., covered it was a plastic coating).

Surveys of airborne asbestos fibers in public buildings and schools known to contain asbestos found mean levels of .0004–0.0010 fibers/ml even when damaged asbestos-containing material was present. These levels of exposure are 200–500 times lower than the OSHA PEL and 10,000 times lower than the heavy exposures prior to 1970 experienced by those workers who have been the subjects of most epidemiologic studies of asbestos-related disease. In addition, recent studies have shown that levels of airborne asbestos fibers in school buildings are sometimes actually higher after asbestos containing-materials have been removed.

ASBESTOS EXPOSURES IN OUTDOOR AMBIENT AIR

Asbestos fibers can be found in the outdoor ambient air in all industrialized and urban areas. These fibers come from a variety of sources including worn or damaged asbestos-containing building materials, demolished buildings, worn auto brake shoes, and improper disposal of asbestos wastes. In some areas asbestos also enters the atmosphere from weathering of natural rock formations or surface wastes of mines. Levels of asbestos found in ambient atmosphere in industrialized areas in the United States are very low and not considered significant health risks (9).

ASBESTOS IN DRINKING WATER AND FOOD

Asbestos is found in very low concentrations as a normal contaminant in drinking water in many areas of the United States. Much of this comes from water passing over natural formations of asbestos-containing rock, and some may come from asbestos cement pipes. Asbestos fibers are also found in trace amounts as a contaminant in some processed foods. These exposures to asbestos fibers in drinking water and food are not considered significant health hazards (10).

CLINICAL TOXICOLOGY OF EXPOSURE

Routes of Exposure

INHALATION

Inhalation of asbestos fibers is the only significant route of exposure leading to adverse health effects. Asbestos appears to exert its effect either by direct contact with lung tissue (as a basis for carcinogenesis) or by stimulating an acute and chronic inflammatory reaction in lung tissue (as in asbestosis). Asbestos in the lungs does not become absorbed into the blood, so there is no true systemic effect, although the fibers that can mechanically penetrate into lung tissue also find their way into the lymphatics.

INGESTION

The primary source of ingestion of asbestos fibers is from inhaled asbestos which is captured in respiratory mucus and then swallowed. Trace amounts of asbestos are also ingested in drinking water and food. Most authorities believe that ingestion of asbestos fibers does not lead to adverse health effects. Asbestos fibers in the gut have been found to penetrate the gastrointestinal mucosa, especially about the cecum. However, there is no systemic absorption of these asbestos fibers, and they do not appear to stimulate an inflammatory reaction, cancer, or any other adverse effect.

SKIN CONTACT AND OTHER ROUTES OF EXPOSURE

Asbestos fibers have no adverse effects on contact with the eyes, intact skin, or wounds, and asbestos is not absorbed through the skin. Proper safety practices for working with asbestos do include protective clothing to keep asbestos fibers off the skin and clothes, but this is to avoid carrying fibers out of the workplace where they may later be reintrained in the air and inhaled. Other than inhalation, there are no other routes of exposure for asbestos which appear to cause adverse health effects.

Deposition and Clearance of Asbestos Fibers

DEPOSITION IN THE LUNG

As with any inhaled particles, the pattern of initial deposition of asbestos fibers in the lungs is determined by particle size and shape, the principles of aerodynamics (i.e., the settling time of fibers and air flow dynamics), and the physical structure and protective mechanisms of the respiratory system.

A fiber is defined as a particle with a length to diameter ratio of over 3:1. The settling time of fibers is inversely related to the square of its diameter. For atypical asbestos fiber 5 microns long and 1 micron in diameter, the settling time in still air is about 4 hours. Air turbulence from a person walking into a room can reintrain settled asbestos fibers into the air, so that free asbestos particles in an area should be assumed to be airborne by persons entering that space.

When asbestos is inhaled, fibers over 10–20 microns long tend to be filtered out in the upper airways or collide with the walls of the conducting airway walls in the lungs where they are captured in the respiratory mucus. These fibers are then removed from the lung by the mucociliary elevator and swallowed. Occasionally fibers up to 50 microns long are seen in the lungs, especially if they are draped over a branch point of conducting airways in a saddle-like effect. Asbestos fibers less than 10 microns long are more likely to stay in the center of the air stream and eventually reach the alveoli.

Fibers captured in respiratory mucus are then coughed up or swallowed (11, 12).

CLEARANCE AND PERSISTENCE OF FIBERS IN THE LUNGS

Autopsy specimens suggest that amphiboles tend to persist in the alveoli, while chrysotile fibers are less prominent even though this was the most common type of asbestos used in the United States. This suggests chrysotile fibers are more easily removed from the alveolar spaces by respiratory macrophages. Asbestos fibers can be found in bronchial washing obtained by bronchoscopy, but it is difficult to estimate the amount of asbestos deposited in the lung using this technique.

Asbestos fibers deposited in the alveoli can undergo a variety of fates. They can remain in place in the aveoli, penetrate the alveolar walls, enter the interstitial fluid, or be cleared by the lymphatic drainage and deposited in the perihilar nodes. Other fibers, especially amphiboles, may penetrate the lung parenchyma and enter the pleural place or peritoneal space via the diaphragm.

Some asbestos fibers in the alveoli are engulfed by respiratory macrophages with varying results. Chrysotile appears to be susceptible to degradation by macrophages, which may explain why this is the least toxic of the fiber types and is found in smaller amounts in autopsy specimens.

Amphibole fibers over 10 microns are not easily degraded by macrophages and tend to persist in the alveoli. Some of these larger fibers become partially engulfed by macrophages but are not degraded. Instead the macrophage dies, leaving a brown proteinaceous coating about the fiber; this is known as an asbestos body and can be seen in light microscopy of lung tissue or sputum. Although asbestos bodies in the sputum do indicate prior exposure, they do not signify disease and cannot be reliably used to determine the extent of exposure or screen for asbestos-related disease.

The number, size, and type of asbestos fibers deposited in the lung have been studied extensively in specimens from autopsy and open lung biopsy. This involves treating the specimen with a chemical that dissolves the tissue but leaves the asbestos fibers intact. Fibers are then counted using standard techniques, with results reported as the number and type of fibers per gram of dried lung.

Asbestos fiber counts can be done on lung tissue specimens obtained by biopsy or at autopsy. This involves treating a weighed amount of dried lung with weak acid to dissolve the tissue; the asbestos fibers remain intact. The number and types of asbestos fibers present can be used as a rough estimate of cumulative asbestos exposure. This technique has been used extensively to study dose-response relationships for asbestos-related diseases.

There appears to be a background level of asbestos in the lungs in the general population in the United States of less than 30,000 fibers per gram of dried lung. Individuals with a history of some type of occupational asbestos exposure had at least three times this number of fibers in the lungs, while those with asbestosis had over 100 times the background level. This method for estimating exposure suggests the dose-response relationship between asbestos exposure and disease is strong for lung cancer but less strong for mesothelioma (some persons with these tumors had as few as 100,000 fibers per gram of dried lung).

However, relying on fiber counts in lung tissue to estimate exposures presents some problems, since amphiboles are more persistent in the lung than chrysotile fibers. Chrysotile fibers in the alveoli have a greater tendency to either dissolve or be removed by macrophages, possibly because with time magnesium leaches out of the fibers, which may make them more susceptible to degradation. In addition, it is unknown to what extent asbestos is related to acute reactions to chrysotile fibers which are then cleared versus chronic reactions to persistent amphibole fibers (4, 5, 12, 13).

SIGNS, SYMPTOMS, AND SYNDROMES FROM EXPOSURE

Target Organ Toxicity

The only target organ affected acutely by asbestos is the lungs, but no clinical effects are noted from acute asbestos exposures. However, recent research suggest that, within weeks after asbestos fibers are inhaled into the lungs, an asymptomatic inflammatory reaction occurs at the level of the terminal bronchioles and alveoli. This is the first stage of a reaction that may lead to asbestosis (see *Syndromes* below) (5).

All chronic adverse health effects from asbestos are related to fibers being inhaled in the lungs. The target organs affected chronically are the lungs (asbestosis and lung cancer), pleura (malignant mesothelioma, benign pleural effusion, pleural plaques, pleural thickening), pericardium (benign effusion), and peritoneum (mesothelioma). There may also be a slightly increased incidence of laryngeal cancer in asbestos-exposed individuals.

There has been a recent controversy among some researchers as to whether asbestos can be a causative factor for chronic obstructive pulmonary disease (COPD). This issue is difficult to study since workers with asbestos-related diseases also have a history of being heavy smokers, and smoking is a well-known cause of COPD. However, several recent well-controlled studies have not found any evidence that asbestos contributes to COPD.

There is no convincing evidence that asbestos has any adverse effects on other target organs, even though it has been implicated as a cause of other types of cancers (see *Carcinogenesis* below) (4, 5, 13).

Asbestosis

EPIDEMIOLOGY

All types of asbestos fibers can cause asbestosis, but the amphiboles, especially crocidolite, are more potent or toxic than chrysotile. The exact nature of the dose-response relationship and differences in toxicity by fiber type are difficult to determine because of inherent problems in both epidemiologic and pathology studies of the issue. Smoking does not increase the risk of developing asbestosis (5, 13).

PATHOPHYSIOLOGY

Asbestosis is an interstitial fibrosis of the lung parenchyma due to asbestos exposure; it is a form of pneumoconiosis along with silicosis and coalworkers' pneumoconiosis. This is a nonmalignant disease that occurs only after heavy and prolonged asbestos exposures. The typical latency period between first exposure to asbestos and diagnosis is over 20 years.

The primary lesion of asbestosis is fibrosis about the terminal bronchiole which then extends to the adjacent alveoli. This appears to be caused by an inflammatory response to asbestos fibers deposited in the alveoli and is probably mediated by respiratory macrophages.

Asbestos fibers in the alveolar spaces stimulate both acute and chronic inflammatory responses. Within several weeks after deposition of asbestos fibers in the alveoli, an acute inflammatory response occurs where respiratory macrophages attempt to digest the fibers with varying results. In this process macrophages release various chemical mediators which stimulate an infiltrate of neutrophils and eosinophils and also induce formation of fibrous tissue (14–16).

Fibers less than 5 microns long, and especially chrysotile, are readily digested by the macrophages. However, larger amphibole fibers are not as easily dissolved or readily digested; they tend to persist in the alveoli and apparently stimulate a chronic antiinflammatory response.

As fibrous tissue forms about the alveoli, passive diffusion of oxygen from the alveolar space into the pulmonary capillaries is inhibited. As fibrosis becomes more extensive, the lung contracts and loses elasticity. However, asbestos does not appear to cause obstructive lung disease.

In about one third of those who develop asbestosis, the disease progresses to massive pulmonary fibrosis (MPF). In these cases the diffuse fibrosis and contraction of lung tissue causes constriction of the pulmonary vasculature, leading to pulmonary hypertension, often leading to death from right-sided heart failure.

The two thirds of asbestos cases that do not develop MPF may experience very little limitation in their daily activities, since they tend to be an older age group that has already cut back on vigorous physical activities. Those with milder exposures to asbestos are not likely to progress. There are no effective preventive measures or treatments for asbestosis (17).

Those with asbestosis are more susceptible to pulmonary infections for reasons that are not clear. Lung cancer is the most common cause of death for those with asbestosis. However, there is no direct connection between these diseases, other than sharing the common etiologic factor of heavy asbestosis exposure (4, 5, 13).

CLINICAL PRESENTATION

The first symptoms of asbestosis are dyspnea with exertion and reduced exercise tolerance. These early effects may be overlooked or interpreted as normal aging changes, since they usually occur when individuals are in their 50s or 60s and may no longer be doing vigorous physical exertion. Other manifestations include cough and inspiratory rales in the lung bases.

For the two thirds of those with asbestosis who do not progress to MPF, there may be little practical limitation on normal activities. For those whose disease does progress, dyspnea with exertion worsens and may lead to dyspnea at rest, clubbing of the fingers, and cyanosis. If MPF develops, signs of pulmonary hypertension and right-sided heart failure are seen (18).

Sputum production is not a manifestation of asbestosis itself, but is frequently seen since many with asbestosis also have chronic obstructive pulmonary disease due to smoking and are more susceptible to lung infections. Finally, chest pain is not common due to asbestosis but may be related to lung cancer or mesothelioma, which are significant risks for those with asbestos exposures heavy enough to have caused asbestosis (14).

DIAGNOSTIC TESTS

With asbestosis the earliest physiologic change to be detected is decreased oxygen saturation of arterial blood with maximal exercise (diagnosed by taking arterial blood gases from an indwelling arterial catheter during an exercise stress test). As the disease progresses oxygen saturation of arterial blood can be seen at rest, and tests of diffusing capacity, such as the DLco, become abnormal.

Lung function abnormalities are also noted, including decreases in vital capacity, residual volume, functional residual capacity, and lung compliance. Asbestos does not appear to cause obstructive lung disease, so the FEV_1/FVC ratio may remain normal unless other disease processes are present.

Chest x-ray abnormalities consistent with asbestosis may be seen either before or after abnormalities in lung function tests are noted. Typical findings are evidence of parenchymal interstitial fibrosis, first noted as small opacities in the periphery of the lung, especially in the lung bases. This may progress to a more diffuse opacification of the lung parenchyma. Asbestos-related pleural changes may also be seen on x-ray, but these are disease processes separate from asbestosis.

A standard rating system has been developed by the International Labor Organization (ILO) for interpreting chest x-ray changes of asbestosis and other pneumoconioses. This uses standardized scales to rate the extent of parenchymal fibrosis as well as asbestos-related pleural changes (18).

The National Institute of Occupational Safety and Health (NIOSH) certifies physicians who interpret chest x-rays using the ILO criteria. They are designated as B-readers. Interpretation of chest x-rays by a B-reader is required for OSHA-mandated screening exams for asbestos workers and is considered the standard of care for diagnosing asbestos-related diseases (7).

Although the intent of the ILO criteria is to promote consistency in interpreting chest x-rays, there is a great deal of variation between B-readers in interpreting normal versus mild changes of asbestosis on chest x-rays. Interpretation of these borderline cases presents a major problem in evaluating the validity and significance of epidemiologic and clinical studies and is also often a contentious issue in litigation.

TREATMENT AND PREVENTION

There is no effective treatment for asbestosis once it has developed. The only effective preventive measure is to keep large quantities of asbestos fibers out of the lungs; individuals with low cumulative exposures do not develop this disease. Cigarette smoking does not appear to increase the risk for asbestosis.

It is controversial as to whether those with objective evidence of asbestosis should be restricted from working around asbestos. Some studies suggest that once asbestosis has started, further inhalation of asbestos fibers causes acute inflammatory reactions which can worsen the disease. However, in the United States individuals with asbestosis probably do not need to be removed from work with asbestos as long as proper protective equipment and work practices are used, since these measures should effectively prevent workers from inhaling asbestos fibers (4, 19).

Lung Cancer

EPIDEMIOLOGY

Several studies have shown an increased incidence of lung cancer, or bronchogenic carcinoma, in groups of workers with moderate to heavy asbestos exposure. All fiber types are associated with this disease, but crocidolite is most toxic, followed by amosite and chrysotile. About 130,000 persons die of lung cancer in the United States annually, and about 5% of these cases are attributed at least partially to asbestos exposure, while cigarette smoking accounts for 75%. A dose-response relationship appears to exist for cumulative asbestos exposures which are moderate and heavy, but this may not hold true at very low doses (20).

Previous theories said that very low cumulative exposure to asbestos presented a real, although small, risk for developing lung cancer. However, recent studies suggest that there may be a lower threshold effect, so that those currently exposed below the OSHA PEL of 0.1 fibers/ml may not be at any real increased risk for lung cancer (21–26).

Cigarette smokers who have also had heavy cumulative asbestos exposure have a combined lung cancer risk greater than expected for each exposure alone. One large study of insulators who had 20 years of heavy asbestos exposure found relative risks for lung cancer of 5.0 for nonsmokers and 50–84 for cigarette smokers, while those without asbestos exposure had relative risks for lung cancer of 1.0 for nonsmokers and 11.0 for cigarette smokers.

Some recent studies have questioned whether asbestos alone can cause lung cancer. Other studies suggest lung cancer after asbestos exposure only occurs in the presence of asbestosis, suggesting that this may be a type of scar cancer. These theories remain controversial (20, 27, 28).

In addition, a study of textile workers in a factory where there was exposure to both organic solvent mists and asbestos found a risk of lung cancer greater than expected for either exposure alone, suggesting an additive effect (15).

PATHOPHYSIOLOGY

Lung cancer related to asbestos exposure appears the same histologically as lung cancer caused by cigarette smoking, radiation, or chemical carcinogens. The latency period for lung cancer is 20–30 years.

Fibers longer than 20 microns are thought most likely to initiate lung cancer, especially those that become caught at branch points of the conducting airways in a saddle effect. The tumor starts in the airway walls and invades locally, often blocking airways and eroding into blood vessels leading to hemoptysis. Metastatic spread also occurs throughout the lung and to other parts of the body, especially to the spine or brain.

The reasons that combined exposure to asbestos and cigarette smoking appears to greatly increase the risk for lung cancer are not clear. Smoking itself is the most common cause of lung cancer. Cigarette smoke also inhibits ciliary function in the lung epithelium, inhibiting clearance of asbestos from the lung and possibly increasing the risk of lung cancer from asbestos.

In the period during and after World War II when many U.S. workers had their heaviest asbestos exposures, the prevalence of cigarette smoking among blue collar workers was about 80%. Since lung cancer caused by asbestos and cigarette smoking look the same histologically, attribution of the cause of lung cancer is often a contentious issue in litigation in the United States. In Germany and the United Kingdom, lung cancer is legally attributed to asbestos if asbestosis is also present (5, 29).

CLINICAL PRESENTATION

The presenting symptoms of lung cancer can vary. Chest pain, chronic cough, hemoptysis, and decreased exercise tolerance may reflect local extension about the airways. In some cases subtle neurologic symptoms may be the presenting sign due to metastases to the brain.

DIAGNOSTIC TESTS

The diagnosis is usually first suspected based on an abnormal chest x-ray. No effective screening tests exist to effectively diagnose lung cancer at an early enough stage to cause improved survival. Neither periodic chest x-rays nor sputum cytology testing has been useful in screening high risk populations.

Computed tomography (CT) and magnetic resonance imaging (MRI) scans can sometimes detect small lesions not seen on chest x-rays; these tests can be useful in establishing the diagnosis but have not been evaluated as screening tools. Tissue biopsy via bronchoscopy or thoracotomy is usually obtained to confirm the diagnosis. The presenting finding may also be a pleural effusion which may or may not contain malignant cells.

TREATMENT AND PREVENTION

At the time of diagnosis lung cancer is usually too advanced for successful treatment, although palliative treatment is often started. There have been improvements in the treatment of lung cancer in recent years, but longterm survival rates are still low following surgical resection and treatment with chemotherapy or radiation therapy. The only proven preventive measures are to keep asbestos fibers out of the lungs and avoid cigarette smoking.

Mesothelioma

Mesothelioma is the second type of malignancy associated with asbestos exposure. Asbestos is the only known cause for this tumor, and a history of significant asbestos exposure is found in 80% of cases, while the causative agent in the other 20% is unknown. The latency period for mesothelioma is 35–40 years since first asbestos exposure. Smokers have no increased risk for this tumor compared with nonsmokers. All fiber types except anthophyllite have been associated with mesothelioma. As with asbestosis and lung cancer, crocidolite is most toxic followed by amosite and chrysotile (30).

The strength of the dose-response relationship between the cumulative asbestos exposure and mesothelioma has been shown (37).

Studies of worker groups with heavy asbestos exposure found an increased risk for mesothelioma. Groups of workers exposed to mixed fiber types have had 7–10% death rates from mesothelioma. However, those with moderately low exposures have also developed this tumor. Mesothelioma has been seen in family members of asbestos workers whose primary exposure was apparently asbestos fibers carried home on the workers'

clothes, as well as in those living near crocidolite mines in South Africa whose exposures were from windborne fibers in the environment. However, studies have not shown increased risk for mesothelioma in those groups with extremely low dose asbestos exposures in the general urban environment or as occupants of buildings containing asbestos (7, 13).

PATHOPHYSIOLOGY

Mesotheliomas appear to be initiated by asbestos fibers that have migrated through the lung parenchyma to the pleural surfaces or through the diaphragm to the peritoneum. Presumably a chronic irritation from these fibers stimulates malignant cell growth. Experiments with rodents show that when asbestos is injected into the pleural space, it is a complete carcinogen with both initiating and promoting properties (4, 31).

As the tumor grows, it further expands in the pleural and peritoneal spaces but does not metastasize. Portions of the lung parenchyma and pulmonary vasculature may become significantly compressed or entrapped in the tumor, leading to reduced air exchange and pulmonary hypertension. Death may be due to respiratory or cardiac failure or general debilitation due to the tumor. Survival is usually less than 1 year after diagnosis (30).

CLINICAL PRESENTATION

The first symptoms of mesothelioma are those associated with pleural irritation, such as cough and chest pain. In contrast to lung cancer, hemoptysis is not common, since airways are not eroded. The diagnosis is often first suggested by a chest x-ray showing a pleural effusion or mass (half of these show calcifications). Evidence of interstitial fibrosis on chest x-ray, indicating asbestosis, or pleural thickening is seen in about 20% of cases at diagnosis.

Pleural effusions due to mesothelioma may not be initially attributed to this disease, since malignant cells are not always seen in pleurocentesis fluid. CT and MRI scans may be useful in establishing the presence of a mass. A biopsy obtained by thoracotomy or laparotomy is usually necessary to confirm the diagnosis, since needle biopsy specimens are often inadequate. Even after adequate tissue is obtained, the histologic interpretation is often difficult and may be confused with inflammatory reactions, exuberant mesothelial hyperplasia, or metastatic cancer (30, 32, 33).

TREATMENT AND PREVENTION

There is no effective treatment for mesothelioma, and death usually occurs within 1 year after diagnosis. Radiation therapy and chemotherapy may prolong survival, but surgical resection does not. The only effective preventive measure is avoidance of significant asbestos exposure (30).

Nonmalignant Pleural Diseases

EPIDEMIOLOGY

Nonmalignant pleural changes are the fourth major type of health effect caused by asbestos; these include benign pleural effusions, pleural thickening, pleural plaques, and rounded atelectasis.

The dose-response relationships and the relative toxicity of fiber types are not as well defined for these nonmalignant pleural conditions as for other asbestos-related diseases. It is not clear whether smokers are at increased risk for these problems.

PATHOPHYSIOLOGY

The cause of these changes is not clear but is presumed to be related to irritation effects from asbestos fibers which migrate through the lung parenchyma to lodge in the pleura.

Benign pleural effusions are seen in a small number of workers; diagnosis is made if all other causes of effusion are ruled out and if there is no history of asbestos exposure. Symptoms seen only in one third of cases might include dyspnea and pleuritic pain. Most effusions resolve spontaneously on their own (34).

Pleural thickening related to asbestos can be unilateral or bilateral and is most often seen in the lower lobes. Histologically, asbestos-related pleural thickening may not be distinguishable from pleural thickening due to other causes such as lung infections. Rounded atelectasis occurs when pleural fibrosis entraps adjacent lung parenchyma; on chest x-ray this is sometimes mistaken for a tumor (35).

Pleural plaques form as discrete confluent patches of fibrohyaline tissue on the pleural surfaces of the chest wall or diaphragm, and occasionally the pericardium. They may become calcified. Pleural plaques are considered pathognomonic signs of asbestos exposure and are the most common objective test finding related to asbestos exposure (35).

CLINICAL PRESENTATION

In the past all of these pleural changes were regarded as markers of asbestos exposure that probably had no clinical significance. However, recent studies suggest that extensive pleural thickening and/or plaques can produce significant restrictive lung disease leading to dyspnea with exertion or even at rest and reduced exercise capacity, even in those with significant asbestosis. Few other clinical manifestations may be seen.

DIAGNOSTIC TESTS

Nonmalignant pleural diseases are usually first suspected based on chest x-ray findings. Pleural plaques noted on chest x-ray may be subtle and can be confused with old rib fractures or pleural fat pads. With standard PA view a plaque covering the anterior of the chest, known as an en face plaque, may not be identified easily and can be mistaken for a parenchymal infiltrate or tumor. Oblique and lateral x-ray views often reveal such plaques well and are done routinely by some clinicians evaluating asbestos-related disease. CT or MRI scans can more accurately differentiate plaques from fat pads and lesions in the lung parenchyma (5, 18).

Depending on the extent of involvement, lung function tests may show restrictive disease with decreased FVC, residual capacity, and measurements of lung compliance. However, diffusing capacity should be normal unless there is concomitant parenchymal fibrosis due to asbestosis. Exercise testing may also be useful in determining to what extent restrictive impairment is due to pleural disease versus parenchymal fibrosis related to asbestosis (5).

TREATMENT AND PREVENTION

There are no effective treatments for these nonmalignant pleural diseases. There are no known preventive measures other than keeping asbestos fibers out of the lungs.

Teratogenesis

Asbestos has not been implicated as a teratogen. Asbestos fibers are not absorbed into the blood, and they do not cross the placenta.

Carcinogenesis

Asbestos does cause lung cancer and malignant mesothelioma (see *Syndromes* above). Some studies have suggested that asbestos exposure is also associated with cancers of the larynx, colon, kidney, pancreas, ovary, and eye, as well as lymphomas. However, there is no convincing evidence that asbestos is associated with increased rates of any of these cancers, except for a slightly increased risk of cancer of the larynx.

From a practical point of view, the slight increase in risk of laryngeal cancer after asbestos exposure is insignificant when compared with the much larger attributed risks for this disease from alcohol consumption and smoking (19, 36). More than 30 epidemiology studies have looked at the risk of colon cancer from asbestos exposure; most have shown no increased risk, and the few positive studies have found a SMR of about 2, which is not convincing evidence for causation (37).

Biologic Monitoring

Biologic monitoring is not done for asbestos. Blood and urine tests are not useful since asbestos is not absorbed systemically, and there is no good biochemical marker of acute or chronic exposure.

Environmental Monitoring

SAMPLING METHODS

Asbestos fibers are measured in ambient air using standardized monitoring methods specified by OSHA and the EPA. This involves pumping a measured volume of air through a piece of filter paper fixed in a container worn by an individual workers (personnel monitoring) or placed in a specific area (area monitoring). Asbestos surveys of buildings involve bulk samples taken from materials that might contain asbestos or wipe samples of settled dust (7).

FIBER COUNTING AND IDENTIFICATION

The number of fibers captured on a filter or in a bulk sample can be counted under a phase-contrast light microscope using standardized techniques approved by OSHA. Fibers are counted only if they are over 5 microns and have a length to diameter ratio greater than 3:1. Individuals doing asbestos fiber counts to meet OSHA regulations must undergo a formal training course and become certified.

The limit of resolution of light microscopes is about 0.1 micron. Electron microscopes can identify much smaller fibers, and some researches suggest 90% of all asbestos fibers are of this smaller size. However, the health effects of these very small asbestos fibers are not clear, and almost all epidemiology studies and government regulations deal with asbestos counts by light microscopy.

Fiber type can be determined by specialized techniques such as electron microscopy or x-ray dispersion analysis of samples. This is not required by OSHA but is important in epidemiologic research. Airborne concentrations of asbestos are either reported as of "mixed fiber types" or by the percentages of each type of fiber. Since both types of reporting are found in the research literature, comparison of findings between studies can often be difficult.

Exposure Limits (PELs, TLVs)

The OSHA PEL for asbestos is 0.2 fiber/ml of air. The Threshold Limit Value (TLV) for asbestos established by the American Conference of Governmental Industrial Hygienists (ACGIH) is also 0.2 fibers/ml for crocidolite, 0.5 fibers/ml for amosite, and 2.0 fibers/ml for chrysotile (38).

OSHA requires that workers be in a medical surveillance program of regular medical examination if they are exposed above the action level of 0.1 fibers/ml of asbestos for more than 30 days per year, or if they must wear a negative pressure respirator when working around asbestos. These exams must include a standardized medical history form, physical exam, spirometry (FVC and FEV_1), and PA chest x-ray with B-reader interpretation. Baseline, annual, and exit exams are required, although chest x-rays are not always done annually. Reporting of results and record-keeping are specified by the standard, which should be referred to before carrying out these exams (7).

LOW LEVEL ASBESTOS EXPOSURES AND PUBLIC POLICY

There is great public concern about risks to building occupants from very small exposures, but recent studies suggest that the health risks from such exposures are minimal (39). Asbestos fibers are only a health hazard if they become airborne and are inhaled. Sources of these fibers in the environment include settled dust and loose fibers in worn or damaged asbestos-containing materials (i.e., friable asbestos). Asbestos that is well bound in building materials does not pose an immediate hazard, although this could be potentially hazardous if damaged or worn.

Since 1984 the EPA has required that school buildings be surveyed to see if they have asbestos-containing materials, but until recently that agency issued no guidelines regarding what should be done once this material was found. School districts and other building owners have been left on their own to decide whether asbestos-containing materials should be removed or encapsulated using plastic coating. Some left it in place if undamaged. It is estimated that removing asbestos from U.S. schools could cost as much as $160 billion over the next decade. However, there is controversy as to whether this will result in any meaningful reduction in health risk for the public (39).

Most epidemiologic studies on the health effects of asbestos are based on worker cohorts with the heavy historical exposures, and these are the basis for most dose-response calculations. Risk assessment techniques allow extrapolation of these risk estimates to much lower levels of exposure using various mathematical models. However, the assumptions upon which risk assessments are based can be open to question. For example, the commonly used assumption that health risks will

decrease linearly with dose would be invalid at low doses if there were a lower threshold for health effects.

Risk assessments based on the levels of airborne asbestos typically found in schools (i.e., 0.00024 fibers/ml) found very small health risks for these exposures when compared with risks most individuals commonly accept in everyday life. This study estimated that the death from lung cancer or mesothelioma from such exposures would be 0.005–0.093 per million students, compared with 6 deaths from aircraft accidents, 10 from high school football, and 27 from drowning per million students (40).

In addition, the assumptions used in developing risk assessments have been seriously questioned by many scientists. Some studies have found evidence for a threshold effect for cancers caused by asbestos. If correct, this suggests that very low level asbestos exposures may pose no real health risk for society even if millions of persons are exposed (39).

These types of considerations have significant economic and policy implications for U.S. society, which may be spending billions of dollars to remove asbestos from public schools over the next decade for questionable improvements in public health. In reaction to these concerns, the EPA issued a statement in 1990 recommending that asbestos-containing materials in schools and public buildings should be left in place if they are undamaged. The agency also recommended that the material be repaired, encapsulated in place, or removed if it is damaged so that fibers are potentially friable.

Those wishing to remove asbestos materials from a building should be aware that strict OSHA guidelines exist for removal and repair of asbestos in the workplace. Such tasks should be done only be specially trained workers in a manner that prevents contamination of the surrounding area and prevents worker exposures. OSHA, the EPA, and equivalent local agencies should be consulted for details.

Individuals wishing to remove asbestos themselves from their own homes are not covered by OSHA requirements; however, to protect their own health they should consult with their local health department or EPA office before handling these materials. Asbestos-containing wastes must be disposed of following EPA guidelines.

REFERENCES

1. Selikoff IJ, Lee DH. Asbestos and disease. New York: Academic Press, 1978:34–50.
2. Pooley FD. Asbestos mineralogy. In: Antman K, Aisner J, eds. Asbestos-related malignancy. Orlando, FL: Grune & Stratton, 1987:3–27.
3. Morgan WK, Seaton A, eds. Occupational lung diseases. 2nd ed. Philadelphia: WB Saunders, 1984:323–376.
4. Mossman BT, Gee JB. Asbestos-related diseases. N Engl J Med 1989;320:1721–1730.
5. Becklake MR. Asbestos-related fibrosis of the lungs (asbestosis) and pleura. In: Update Pulmonary Diseases and Disorders.
6. Davis JM, McDonald C. Low level exposure to asbestos: is there a cancer risk? Fr J Ind Med 1988;45:505.
7. United States Occupational Safety and Health Administration. Occupational Health Standard for Asbestos. Fed Reg 1986;51:22753–22790.
8. EPA Report to Congress. Study of asbestos-containing materials in public buildings. Washington, DC: U.S. Environmental Protection Agency, 1988:5.
9. McDonald JC. Health implications of environmental exposure to asbestos. Environ Health Perspect 1985;62:319–328.
10. National Research Council, Committee on Nonoccupational Health Risks of Asbestiform Fibers. Asbestiform fibers: nonoccupational health risks. Washington, DC: National Academy Press, 1984.
11. Wright GW. The pulmonary effects of inhaled inorganic dust. In: Clayton GD, Clayton EC, eds. Patty's industrial hygiene and toxicology. 3rd Ed. New York: John Wiley and Sons, 1981:165–202.

12. Timbrell V, et al. Hollow casts of lungs for experimental purposes. Nature 1970;225:9708.

13. Bignon J, Jaurand MC. Asbestos fiber toxicity and lung disease. In: Gee JB, ed. Occupational lung disease. New York: Churchill Livingstone, 1984:51–71.

14. Craighead JE, et al. The pathology of asbestos-associated diseases of the lungs and pleural cavities: diagnostic criteria and proposed grading schema. Arch Pathol Lab Med 1982;106:544–596.

15. Rom WN, et al. Characterization of the lower respiratory tract inflammation of nonsmoking individuals with interstitial lung disease associated with chronic inhalation of inorganic dusts. Am Rev Respir Dis 1987;136:1429–1434.

16. Robinson BW, et al. Alveolitis of pulmonary asbestosis: bronchoalveolar lavage studies in crocidolite- and chrysotile-exposed individuals. Chest 1986;90:396–402.

17. Gaensler EA, et al. Progression of asbestos. (Abstract.) Chest 1987;91:305.

18. American Thoracic Society. Medical Section of the American Lung Association: the diagnosis of nonmalignant diseases related to asbestos. Am Rev Respir Dis 1986;134:363–368.

19. Chan CK, Gee JB. Asbestos exposure and laryngeal cancer: an analysis of the epidemiologic evidence. J Occup Med 1988;30:34–27.

20. McDonald JC, McDonald AD. Epidemiology of asbestos-related lung cancer. In: Antman K, Aisner J, eds. Asbestos-related malignancy. Orlando, FL: Grune & Stratton, 1987:57–79.

21. Berry G. Newhouse ML. Mortality of workers manufacturing friction materials using asbestos. Br J Ind Med 1983;40:1–7.

22. Gardner JM, et al. Follow-up study of workers manufacturing chrysotile asbestos cement products. Br J Ind Med 1986;43:726–732.

23. Ohlson CG, Hogstedt C. Lung cancer among asbestos cement workers: a Swedish cohort study and a review. Br J Ind Med 1985;43:397–402.

24. Thomas HF, et al. Further follow-up of workers from an asbestos cement factory. Br J Ind Med 1982;39:273–276.

25. Churg A. Lung asbestos content in long-term residents of a chrysotile mining town. Am Rev Respir Dis 1987;134:125–127.

26. Cordier S, et al. Epidemiologic investigation of respiratory effects related to environmental exposure to asbestos inside insulated buildings. Arch Environ Health 1987;42:303–309.

27. Kuschner M. The effects of MMMF on animal systems: some reflections on their pathogenesis. Ann Occup Hyg 1987;31:791–797.

28. Kipen HM, Lilis R, Suzuki Y, Valciukas JA, Selikoff IJ. Pulmonary fibrosis in asbestos insulation workers with lung cancer: a radiological and histopathological evaluation. Br J Ind Med 1987;44:96–100.

29. United States Surgeon General. The health consequences of smoking: cancer and chronic lung disease in the workplace. Washington, DC: U.S. Dept of Health and Human Services, 1985;19–96.

30. Antman KH, Corson JM. Benign and malignant pleural mesothelioma. Clin Chest Med 1985;6:127–140.

31. Stanton MF, Wrench C. Mechanisms of mesothelioma induction with asbestos and fibrous glass. Natl Cancer Inst 1972;48:797–821.

32. Grant DC, Seltzer SE, Antman KH, Finberg HJ, Koster K. Computed tomography of malignant pleural mesothelioma. J Comput Assist Tomogr 1983;7:626–632.

33. Craighead JE. Current pathogenetic concepts of diffuse malignant mesothelioma. Hum Pathol 1987;18:544–557.

34. Robinson BW, Musk AW. Benign asbestos pleural effusion: diagnosis and course. Thorax 1981;36:896–900.

35. Stephens M, et al. Asbestos induced diffuse pleural fibrosis: Pathology and mineralogy. Thorax 1987;42:583–588.

36. Churg A. Lung cancer cell type and asbestos exposure. JAMA 1985;253:2984–2985.

37. Edelman DA. Exposure to asbestos and the risk of gastrointestinal cancer: a reassessment. Br J Ind Med 1988;45:75–82.

38. TLVs-Threshold Limit Values and Biological Exposure Indices for 1990–91. Cincinnati, OH. American Conference of Governmental Industrial Hygienists (ACGIH), 1990.

39. Mossman BT, et al. Asbestos: scientific developments and implications for public policy. Science 1990;247:294–301.

40. Weill H, Hughes JM. Asbestos as a public health risk: disease and policy. Annu Rev Public Health 1986;7:171–192.

111

Manmade Mineral Fibers

William B. Bun III, M.D., J.D., M.P.H.
Gerald R. Chase, Ph.D.
Thomas W. Hesterberg, Ph.D.
Richard A. Versen, M.P.H., C.I.H.
Robert Anderson, M.D., M.P.H.

INTRODUCTION

Manmade mineral fibers (MMMF) are a class of insulating materials which have found widespread applications in both residential and industrial settings. MMMF is a generic expression for fibrous inorganic substances made primarily from rock, clay, slag, or glass. Most MMMF are also referred to as manmade vitreous fibers (MMVF) due to their synthetic, amorphous, glassy nature. The information presented in this chapter will deal with three subgroupings of MMMF—fibrous glass, mineral wool, and refractory ceramic fibers.

Since the initial development of some of these fibers in the late 1800s, large numbers of individuals in various occupational settings have been exposed to these materials. There is a natural concern about the safety of any material which has the potential to give off particles or vapors which can be inhaled and/or ingested. There is a heightened awareness for all such fiber materials, and, for that reason, there have been and continue to be many studies dealing with MMMF. There have also been reviews of those studies and other pertinent information, such as exposure levels, by various national and international agencies and organizations.

In assessing the risks of exposure to any possible occupational hazard, research is pursued through several different scientific techniques. Studies of morbidity (analysis of impairment) and studies of mortality (analysis of death rates) are used to evaluate the potential adverse health effects associated with direct human exposure. Animal exposure studies are used to not only evaluate the potential health effects but also to investigate the mechanisms of disease development.

MMMF TYPES

The three general types of MMMF (Fig. 111.1) are fibrous glass, mineral wool, and refractory ceramic fibers (RCFs) (1).

Production of fibrous glass began in the 1930s, with materials generally supplied in two basic forms: wool-type fibers and textile fibers.

Wool-type glass fibers are produced by spinning or blowing molten glass, consisting of silicon, aluminum, boron, calcium, sodium, and/or other metal oxides (2). For thermal and acoustical applications, the nominal diameter of the fiber ranges from 3–8 micrometers. Where weight and volume are important in thermal and acoustical insulation, fibers ranging from 1–3 micrometers in nominal diameter are used. In addition, the range of fiber from 1 through 5 micrometers in diameter is used in filter media for heating, ventilating, and air conditioning systems.

Glass wool fibers are also manufactured in the submicrometer diameter range (less than 1 micrometer). This fine diameter material, or glass Microfiber, is produced in the United States in limited quantities comprising less than 1% of total fibrous glass production. It is usually limited to use in fine particulate filtration, battery components, specialty paper, and sophisticated aerospace insulations.

Textile glass fibers differ from the wool type in that they are drawn or extruded from holes in the base of a platinum container in a continuous process, rather than being spun or blown. The process results in continuous strands or filaments and a distribution of diameters, ranging from 3.5–25 micrometers. Textile fibers are used to reinforce other materials, especially plastics, and in woven and nonwoven fabrics.

A second type of MMMF is mineral wool, composed of two subgroups: rockwool and slagwool. These mineral wools were first produced in Europe in 1840 (3). The first commercial operation in the United States began in 1897. The number of mineral wool production facilities peaked between 80 and 90 in the 1950s, at which time the production of glass wools began to acquire more market share for insulating applications.

Both rock wool and slag wool are produced by melting raw materials and centrifuging, drawing, or blowing the molten matter into the desired fibrous form. Because the fibers are cooled quickly after formation, the fibers remain noncrystalline. Due to this processing, these mineral wools contain a very high nonfibrous particle, or shot, ratio. Shot particles have little insulating capacity and do not add to the product's utility. After formation, the materials are sprayed with lubricating oils and binders to reduce dustiness and product breakage. Typical materials used fall into three classes: water-based emulsion of mineral oil; straight mineral oil; or polyethylene glycol or related compound.

Rock wool is typically produced from the melting of igneous rock containing high levels of calcium and magnesium. Most of the mineral wool produced in Europe is rock wool.

Slag wool is produced from the byproducts of metal smelting. The composition of the fibers varies with the source of the slag used. It is essentially a calcium aluminum silicate with varying amounts of iron and magnesium. The majority of the mineral wool produced in the United States is slag wool.

Refractory ceramic fiber is the third broad classification of MMMF. A variety of fiber types are produced depending on the intended application. All types are blends of alumina and silica, with other refractory oxides added, including chromous and zirconia oxides, depending on service requirements (4).

There are three general categories of RCF: (a) kaolin clay-based products, where the clay is obtained by mining; (b) blends

MAN-MADE MINERAL FIBER FAMILY

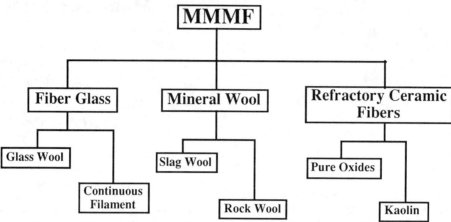

Figure 111.1. Three classifications of humanmade vitreous fibers (MMVF). Fibrous glass is further classified into glass wool and continuous filament. Mineral wool is further classified into rock wool and slag wool.

of alumina, silica, and refractory metal oxide (e.g., chromous and zirconia oxides); and (c) high purity products that are a blend of alumina and silica processed to control the levels of impurities found in other RCF products.

The fibers are produced by spinning molten mixtures. The nominal diameter of the fibers produced in this manner is in the 1.2–3.5-micrometer range. Fiber length can be varied in steps from long fibers down to micron-sized (2).

MATERIAL CHARACTERISTICS

MMMF do not burn, rot, or absorb moisture or odors. Under normal conditions, they do not support the growth of mildew, mold, or bacteria. However, there are conditions, such as when insulating materials become dirty and remain wet for a prolonged period of time, where such growth may naturally occur. In addition, MMMF are dimensionally stable and have high tensile strength. These fibers can absorb acoustical energy, help control heat flow, remove impurities from gases and liquids, and, with a vapor barrier, help control condensation. In fact, due to fiber configuration, fibrous glass is a highly efficient filter medium with substantial particle-holding capacity. Mineral wool is used primarily for thermal and acoustical insulation applications. RCF is formulated to help control heat flow in high temperature areas. Because of these characteristics, these materials have become some of the world's most useful and beneficial humanmade materials. In addition, they reduce the need for energy for heating and the accompanying air pollution caused from burning fossil fuels to provide this energy (5).

An especially important characteristic for health study is that glass fibers do not split longitudinally. They break horizontally into shorter fibers which can be more readily cleared from the lung.

MAJOR APPLICATIONS

Fibrous glass was originally developed in the early 1930s for use in home panel filters and home insulation. Textile fibers appeared commercially in the late 1930s, followed by glass microfibers in the late 1940s.

Today, the wool-like form of glass fiber is widely used to control temperature and sound. Its major applications are in commercial and residential insulation, acoustical control products, air-handling ducts, pipe insulation, air filters, roof insulation, and insulation for automobiles, aircraft, mobile homes, refrigerators, domestic cooking appliances, and a wide variety of other appliances and equipment.

Textile glass fibers are most commonly used in curtains and draperies, screening, electrical yarns, built-up roofing, shingles, and industrial fabrics and as reinforcement for plastics, papers, rubber, and other materials.

The fine diameter glass wool fibers are generally utilized in high technology products, such as specialty filter papers, battery components, and aerospace insulation.

Mineral wool applications are very similar to those of glass wool—thermal, acoustical, and fire protection. Much of the mineral wool produced is used for blown-in insulation in attics and side walls. In addition, decorative and acoustical ceiling tiles are widely commercialized.

Applications vary for RCFs, but all are high temperature environments. Blankets are used primarily as furnace and kiln wall liners, as backup insulation to refractory brick, as soaking pit covers, and in annealing welds. The loose fiber is used as a filler in packing voids and in expansion joints. Custom-molded shapes are widely used in the metal molding area and as furnace combustion chamber liners (2, 6).

MMMF: HEALTH EFFECTS

Skin Irritation

MMMF may irritate the skin of some workers in manufacturing facilities as well as some people who fabricate or install MMMF-containing materials. This skin irritation and possible inflammation is a mechanical reaction due to sharp, broken ends of fiber that rub or become embedded in the outer layer of the skin. Skin reactions vary directly with the size and the stiffness of the fiber handled, with fibers of large diameter (greater than 5 micrometers) being more likely to cause irritation and itching. Fine diameter fibers usually do not cause skin irritation. Irritation normally does not persist and can be relieved by washing exposed skin areas gently in warm water with mild soap.

Some individuals may be more sensitive to irritation from MMMF than are others, and a relatively small number of these unusually sensitive individuals may be forced to seek other types of employment. The vast majority of workers, however, can control skin irritation by following appropriate work practices and utilizing proper personal protective equipment (7).

Upper Respiratory Irritation

It is possible that some workers may experience temporary upper respiratory irritation (that is, scratchiness or burning of the nose or throat) if large amounts of airborne MMMF are released during manufacture or handling of MMMF-containing products and improper work practices permit inhalation of the fibers. Like skin irritation, upper respiratory irritation is a mechanical reaction to sharp, broken fibers. It is not an allergic reaction, and the irritation does not persist.

Unprotected exposures to high concentrations of airborne MMMF may produce a nonspecific, transitory lung condition, usually manifested by coughing or wheezing. The effects subside soon after the worker is removed from exposure and should have no further impact on the health and well-being of the worker exposed.

Whenever practicable, the use of engineering controls should be the primary means of controlling the airborne release of dust from MMMF-containing products. In addition, careful attention to housekeeping and proper work practices, including the use of approved respiratory protection, can effectively control airborne MMMF concentrations and exposures to prevent upper respiratory irritation (8, 9).

EPIDEMIOLOGIC STUDIES

Tens of thousands of workers have been employed in manufacturing MMMF since their initial development almost 120 years ago. There have been a number of epidemiologic studies, which look for unusual occurrences or unexpected patterns of diseases or their signs and symptoms, that have been performed on various groups of those workers. As with all mortality studies, all causes of death are reviewed. However, investigations involving potential exposure to fibers pay particular attention to lung cancer, mesothelioma, and nonmalignant respiratory diseases. Two major studies conducted on large groups of workers in MMMF manufacturing have been determinative in epidemiologic reviews.

The mortality of almost 25,000 workers (2836 deaths) employed in thirteen European factories engaged in the production of MMMF (including 11,852 fibrous glass production workers and 10,115 mineral wool production workers) has been studied by Saracci et al. and updated by Simonato et al. in 1986. The mortality has been followed through 1982. A historical environmental investigation was conducted in parallel to collect information on past working conditions in the plants included in the study in relation to exposure to fibers and to other potential contaminants. An overall mortality excess was found, mainly due to deaths from violent causes, with the excess concentrated among shortterm employees. Lung cancer increased with time since first exposure in both mineral wool and glass wool productions. For glass wool production, there was no overall excess mortality from lung cancer compared to regional rates. However, the authors reported an "excess of lung cancer among rock-wool/slag wool workers employed during an early technological phase before the introduction of dust

suppressing agents," and concluded that "fiber exposure, either alone or in combination with other exposures, may have contributed to the elevated risk." The authors also reported that "no excess of the same magnitude was evident for glass-wool production, and the follow-up of the continuous filament cohort was too short to allow for an evaluation of possible long-term effects." It was also noted that "there was no evidence of an increased risk for pleural tumors or nonmalignant respiratory diseases." "No consistent mortality excess was found for other cancer sites nor for non-malignant respiratory diseases" (10).

Enterline's (11) comprehensive mortality review of almost 17,000 workers, many with longterm exposure up to 40 years, was undertaken at 17 U.S. fibrous glass and mineral wool manufacturing plants (including 14,800 fibrous glass workers in 11 plants and 1846 mineral wool workers in six plants). The original report, given in 1982, covered the mortality experience from the 1940s to the end of 1977. The same group of workers was followed through 1982 (reported in October 1986, with additional analyses available in June 1987). The June 1987 report contained, for the first time, local area mortality statistics for each of the plants as the primary basis for studying the mortality experience. Some comparisons with national mortality statistics were also given. As with the European study, there was an overall mortality excess compared with both local and national mortality patterns. Using local statistics, while there was an excess of observed mortality over expected, there were no statistically significant excess malignant respiratory disease deaths reported for any of the 11 fibrous glass plants, or any grouping of those plants by glass wool or textile production for total deaths or by interval from onset of exposure. There were also no significant findings in support of a dose relationship for respiratory cancer. The authors did discuss the respiratory cancer experience of a subgroup of workers classified as having worked with finer diameter fibers in the 1987 update. There were no statistically significant findings relating to the 22 respiratory cancer deaths in that subgroup; they were considered noteworthy not so much from the results of the analyses as from the way "they relate to probable fiber exposure." The overall relative excess in respiratory cancer was greatest for the mineral wool production workers. Although there were some statistically significant findings for the mineral wool workers, there were also several features that were not consistent with a casual relationship. While the authors regarded the respiratory cancer findings for continuous filament workers and glass wool workers as "essentially negative," it is generally agreed that the overall relationship between work in the humanmade mineral fiber industry and health should continue to be investigated. There were no other noteworthy mortality groupings, including nonmalignant respiratory disease deaths, for fibrous glass workers. An excess of nonmalignant respiratory disease was noted for mineral wool workers, but there does not appear to be much evidence in support of a dose-response relationship. Deaths from mesothelioma in the cohort are considered to be within the expected range. The study has been further updated through 1985, with publication in 1990. In the 1985 update, a small excess in respiratory cancer deaths is statistically significant for workers employed in glass wool and mineral wool plants. The experience of the group of workers classified as having worked with finer diameter fibers is not distinguishable in this update. Looking at the cumulative evidence for respiratory cancer of all factors that might support a relationship in the 1985 update, the researchers concluded that the evidence of an association appeared "somewhat weaker" than in the 1982 update (11, 11a).

In addition, a more limited mortality study of 2557 male workers at a Canadian fibrous glass wool plant has been studied through 1977 (Shannon et al., 1984) and updated (Shannon et al., 1987) to extend the follow-up to the end of 1984. In the updated study the authors reported a statistically significant excess of lung cancer. In discussing the excess of lung cancer, the authors concluded that the interpretation of the information was difficult since there was no relationship between the excess of lung cancer and length of time since first exposure to the fibrous glass manufacturing environment (11b, 12).

Morbidity studies, which study the disease occurrence among living workers, are extremely useful in assessing the potential risk of nonmalignant disease. In the most widely cited morbidity study, Weill (13, 14) reported on the respiratory health assessment of 1089 workers who were currently employed in 1979–1980 at five fibrous glass and two mineral wool plants in the United States. Reporting on the respiratory questionnaire and lung function assessments, the researchers noted that the study population was found to be generally healthy, with respiratory symptoms not related to the fiber exposure and with no detected adverse lung function consequences of that exposure. Regarding the readings of chest x-rays, a low level of profusion of small opacities (i.e., opaque appearances that are looked for on the x-rays of workers who are employed in potentially "dusty" trades) was reported and discussed. In summarizing their findings, Weil noted that, in general, "the minimal evidence of respiratory effects detected in the investigation, which cannot, at present, be considered clinically significant, is encouraging concerning the question of potential health effects of exposure to MMVF" (13, 14).

The European and U.S. studies continue to be updated. The U.S. study will incorporate new data on potential confounders (e.g., smoking and other occupational exposures).

Although many studies have been conducted on fibrous glass and mineral wool exposed workers, RCF is a relatively new material, commercialized in the early 1960s, with relatively small numbers of workers exposed. There are no known published reports in medical literature dealing with the health experience of people who work with RCFs. Two investigations, one in Europe and the other in the United States, are studying the health of workers involved in the manufacture of RCFs. These studies address the respiratory morbidity of RCF using pulmonary function tests, chest x-rays, and questionnaires. Although the feasibility of performing a mortality study has been considered, the limited number of exposed workers, short total length of production, and confounding with past asbestos exposure present significant challenges for investigators (15).

EXPERIMENTAL STUDIES

The toxicologic studies of MMMF have been conducted in both in vitro (in glass, not in the whole animal) and in vivo (in animal) systems. In addition, studies of the physical and chemical characteristics thought to correlate with toxicity have been conducted. The in vitro studies have been conducted in cells from the lungs of animals as well as bacterial and cell lines. Two categories of whole animal studies have been reported—studies using artificial methods to implant high concentrations of fibers in the abdomen, pleura, or trachea of animals, and inhalation studies of maximum tolerated doses and multiple dose levels of fibers.

Cell Culture Studies

A number of studies have shown that fiber length and diameter are important in determining the toxicity of mineral fibers of various chemical compositions to cells grown in culture (16–18). Chemical composition has also been shown to be critical to the toxicity of fibers (19). MMMFs have also been shown to induce neoplastic transformation (18, 20) and genetic damage to cells in culture (21, 22). These cell culture models could be used as part of a battery of shortterm screening tests to assess the toxic and tumorigenic potential of mineral fibers. Further validation and correlation with inhalation studies may also lead to these cell culture studies as predictors of relative toxicity.

Implantation Studies

Using various types and dimensions of fibers, researchers have studied the effects of "artificially" exposed animals by surgically implanting fibrous material in the pleural (chest) and abdominal cavities of laboratory animals and by injecting fibers directly into the trachea (23–25). Those studies have shown that high levels of virtually all durable fibrous materials of certain dimensions, regardless of their physical or chemical makeup, can have adverse biologic effects in laboratory animals. From these study results, scientists have also hypothesized that biologic activity correlates with fiber length and diameter, since "long, thin" fibers are the most active. The actual physicochemical makeup appears to play only a minor role, if any, in such "artificial exposure" experiments (25).

For example, glass fibers with diameters less than 1.5 micrometers have produced tissue changes, including cancer and scarring of the lung, in such experiments (25). While these studies are felt to generate data for further evaluation by inhalation tests and generate mechanistic data, they are not commonly used for risk determination and assessment. Intraperitoneal studies have not been consistent predictors of the results of inhalation studies, however.

In a recent study conducted at the Los Alamos National Laboratories, Smith (26, 27) performed intraperitoneal injections of RCF using both hamsters and rats. Half of the hamsters did not tolerate the initial injection of the fiber into their abdomens and died immediately after injection. Seven of the 36 hamsters that survived the initial injections were found to have abdominal mesotheliomas. Nineteen of 23 rats developed tumors (primarily mesotheliomas) after intraperitoneal injection of RCF.

Another study using intraperitoneal injections of RCF was conducted in Edinburgh, Scotland (28, 29). In that study, three of 32 animals developed primary abdominal tumors (including one mesothelioma which was not statistically significant). This result was very different from the results obtained at Los Alamos.

In contrast to the intraperitoneal studies, the inhalation portions of the study were negative in the Smith study and positive in the Davis study.

Even though these experiments are of value in studying mechanisms of tissue reactions, they are based on introducing large amounts of fiber into the animals by artificial means that bypassed normal body defense mechanisms. Since the circumstances of actual exposure are totally different in humans, the studies cannot be used for risk assessment or to conclude that inhalation of glass fiber or RCF is hazardous to workers. For that reason, several animal inhalation studies have been initiated at independent research centers, using both commercially available fiber and specially prepared fiber with well-defined length and diameter distributions.

Animal Inhalation Studies

Animal inhalation studies are more relevant than intracavity administration studies for risk assessment because the exposure conditions of inhalation experiments more closely approach the circumstances of human exposure.

FIBROUS GLASS

A number of studies of fibrous glass have been used for risk assessment in man (27, 30–35), and virtually all of these studies have demonstrated a lack of tumor induction by fibrous glass. Gross et al. (30) exposed rats and hamsters for 2 years to high concentrations (135 mg/m^3) of relatively long, thin fibrous glass. Although no tumors were reported, the authors note the small number of animals exposed and poor survival of exposed animals.

In 1981, Lee et al. (31) showed that no significant increase in tumorigenesis was observed in rats, hamsters, or guinea pigs exposed to high concentrations of inhaled fibrous glass (400 mg/m^3). LeBouffant et al. (34) demonstrated no significant increase in tumor incidence in rats exposed to 5 mg/m^3 of two different types of fibrous glass (including JM100) for 12 or 24 months. A similar mass concentration of chrysotile asbestos produced a 19% incidence of lung tumors.

In 1987, Muhle et al. (35) exposed rats for one year to 3 mg/m^3 of fibrous glass (JM104) in which 90% of the fibers in the aerosol were less than 12.4 μm long. Although no tumors were observed in the fibrous glass-treated groups, neither were they observed in the "positive control" groups treated with chrysotile or crocidolite asbestos.

Two important studies for use in human risk assessment of fibrous glass exposure were reported by Wagner et al. (32) and McConnell et al. (33). In parallel studies using the same lot of JM100 fibrous glass these two groups of researchers demonstrated that inhalation exposure of rats to 10 mg/m^3 of the fibrous glass for 12 months resulted in no significant increase in lung tumors during the lifetime of the animals. As noted by the authors, exposure to a similar mass concentration of chrysotile, based on mass asbestos, resulted in a significant increase in lung tumors.

Another important study that suggests that fibrous glass is not tumorigenic in animals was reported by Smith et al. (27). In that study, no tumors were observed in rats or hamsters after inhalation exposure to between 3 and 12 mg/m^3 of several different compositions of fibrous glass. The negative tumor finding with JM100 fibrous glass is especially compelling since the small diameter of this fiber would have allowed significant deposition in the deep lung.

Recently, another chronic inhalation toxicity study of fibrous glass was initiated. Rats are being exposed using nose-only inhalation chambers, 6 hrs/day, 5 days/week, for 24 months to three concentrations (3, 16, and 30 mg/m^3) of two different compositions of fibrous glass, or to filtered air (negative control). This is a lifetime study, and animals will be held until 20% survival occurs. The fibrous glasses used in this study were presized to have an average diameter of approximately 1 μm and an average length of approximately 20 μm so that they

would be comparable to the dimensions of fibers found in workplace air and also rat respirable. Interim sacrifices are scheduled at 3 or 6 month intervals to monitor the progression of pulmonary changes during the study. Exposure for 18 months resulted in a dose- and time-dependent increase in cellularity, characterized by an influx of pulmonary macrophages in the proximal alveoli, minimal microgranuloma formation, and some bronchiolization. These minimal or mild increases in cellularity are thought to be reversible and occur to some extent when any particulate gains entry into the deep lung regions. No lung or pleural fibrosis was observed in any of the treatment groups. In a parallel study using the same test system, 10 mg/m^3 of chrysotile asbestos resulted in pulmonary fibrosis as early as 3 months after the exposure was initiated.

MINERAL WOOL

There have been three inhalation studies conducted with mineral wool. As was seen with fibrous glass, all of these studies have shown that mineral wool is not tumorigenic by this route of exposure.

In the first study, reported by Wagner et al. (32), rats were exposed for 12 months to 10 mg/m^3 of mineral wool fibers having diameters in the 1-μm range and lengths in the 8-μm range. No significant increase in tumor incidence was observed in the mineral wool-exposed animals, while a 25% incidence of tumors was observed in animals treated with a similar mass concentration of chrysotile asbestos.

In another inhalation study, reported by LeBouffant et al. in 1984 (34), rats were exposed to 5 mg/m^3 of mineral wool for 24 months. No tumors were observed in the mineral wool-treated group compared to a 19% incidence in the chrysotile asbestos-treated group.

Smith et al. (27) reported that 10 mg/m^3 mineral wool exposure of rats and hamsters for 24 months resulted in no tumors. The incidence of tumors in the control group exposed to short crocidolite asbestos was not statistically increased. Additional dose-response studies of two different compositions of mineral wool have been initiated at RCC, Geneva.

REFRACTORY CERAMIC FIBERS

There are three known investigations of RCF which have included experiments that studied the effects of exposing the animals more naturally by having them breathe high concentrations of RCFs. Two investigations have been completed and published: one by Davis et al. in Edinburgh, Scotland (28), and the other by Smith et al. at the Los Alamos National Laboratories (27). The third study that should be completed in 1991 is being conducted by Bernstein et al., at Research and Consulting Company (RCC), Geneva, Switzerland (36–38).

Davis exposed 48 rats to RCF by inhalation for 7 hours/day, 5 days/week, over a period of 224 days. The airborne dose of fibers longer than 5 microns was reported to be 95 fibers/ml. Animals sacrificed at the end of the study were reported to have an average of 5% pulmonary fibrosis. At the end of the study, eight of the rats were found to have pulmonary tumors with three animals demonstrating lung carcinomas. There was also one peritoneal mesothelioma reported (28).

In 1979, a large scale animal exposure experiment was begun at the Los Alamos National Laboratories involving several types of humanmade fibers, including RCF, using both rats and hamsters. The experiments involving rats showed no cancer and little pulmonary fibrosis; this conflicts sharply with the Davis study. Inhalation experiments on hamsters showed one cancer (mesothelioma) in 50 animals, but no fibrosis was observed. One of 157 control animals developed a spontaneous tumor without exposure to fibers. The exposures were conducted at 200 fibers/ml, 6 hours/day, 5 days/week, for 24 months (27).

In the RCC study specially sized fibers 1 by 25 microns were used to represent a fiber cloud that was almost completely rat respirable. Groups of rats were exposed for 6 hours/day, 5 days/week to 30 mg/m³ (between 200 and 250 fibers/ml of four different types of RCF. Hamsters were exposed to only kaolin RCF fibers. Positive controls (chrysotile asbestos) and negative controls (filtered air) were included in both the rat and the hamster studies.

Interim sacrifices have revealed lung fibrosis beginning at 9 months and development of malignant mesothelioma in 36 of 102 hamsters (35%) exposed to RCF (38a). In the rat inhalation study, similar levels of lung fibrosis were observed and in addition lung tumors and pleural mesothelioma were observed (38b).

Although these results are preliminary, the fibrosis and early mesothelioma in the hamster suggest that RCF may have significantly different effects from other MMMF (36, 38).

STUDIES OF PHYSICAL CHARACTERISTICS OF FIBERS

In addition to data on health effects, evidence from animal experiments indicates that glass fibers are attacked by fluids normally present in the lung. This can cause fragmentation to shorter fibers that are biologically less active and are more readily removed from the lungs by clearance mechanisms, or can even lead to the total dissolution of fine fibers. In fact, fine fibers which have the potential to be the most biologically active are the fibers most readily attacked by body fluids because of their relatively large surface area. It is therefore thought that some glass fibers may be less toxic and less likely to cause lung tumors in the animals because they are more soluble and do not remain in the lung long enough to cause damage.

The lack of durability of glass fibers has also been demonstrated in the laboratory using physiologic solutions that simulate the natural lung environment. The dissolution rate of mineral fibers has been shown to be dependent on chemical composition and can differ between fiber types by several orders of magnitude.

In Fig. 111.2, scanning electron micrographs of two types of fibrous glass fibers before and after incubation in Gamble's solution (a physiologic solution) for 180 days are shown. Note the pitting and etching of the surface of the fibers after incubation in Gamble's solution. At 180 days, 87% of the silica content has been leached from these fibers, and the length and diameter of the fibers had decreased.

If fiber solubility is a factor in determining the toxicity of fibers to the animal lung, then one might expect to find a range of toxicities of mineral fibers in the lung, which is dependent on their chemical composition. Future studies will focus on correlating the solubilities of mineral fibers of various chemical compositions in Gamble's solution with their durabilities and toxicities to the lung (39–42).

MECHANISMS OF ACTION FOR FIBER TOXICITY AND CARCINOGENICITY

The mechanisms whereby inhaled fibers result in pathologic changes in the respiratory tract and lining surfaces of the chest and abdominal cavities are not completely understood. Nevertheless, certain principles of biologic activity have been elucidated which appear to explain the differing responses to fibers on the basis of size, geometry, durability, and, to a lesser extent, chemical composition.

Fiber size and geometry are the determinants of host entry and intrapulmonic distribution. The essential determinant of entry is aerodynamic diameter. The aerodynamic diameter of a fiber is determined by the formula:

$$D_A = 1.3p^{1/2}d^{5/6}L^{1/6}$$

where

D_A = aerodynamic diameter
p = density
d = diameter
L = length

Fibers of an aerodynamic diameter greater than 12 microns are not likely to reach the target areas (bronchioles and alveoli). Therefore, while both aspects of size (length and width) are important, the diameter of fibers appears to be of greater significance in relation to initial deposition and also their translocation within the lung and their extension to the pleural and peritoneal surfaces. The length of the fiber does have an impact on the ability of the lung to clear the fiber once it reaches the target area (longer fibers = reduced clearance). Fibers greater than 5 microns in length and less than 1–1.5 microns in diameter have the greatest potential to reach the target areas of the lung and pleura (43).

Although dimension controls the entry and final site of deposition in the lung, durability is the critical basis for the accumulation of a lung burden of fibers. Numerous investigators have shown that, in the case of asbestos, the amphibole, the more durable fiber type, accumulates in human lungs in quantities that correlate with cumulative exposure; while chrysotile, a less durable fiber, does not. Other factors that may affect the intrapulmonic anatomic fate are the rigidity of fibers, surface properties, and fiber end architecture (smooth, grainy, spiculed edges, etc.) (44).

The primary site of response of the lungs to fiber inhalation is at the level of respiratory bronchioles, alveolar ducts, and alveoli.

Inflammatory Response

The initial response to deposition of fiber in the alveoli is an alveolitis with fluid exudation, and inflammatory cell infiltration. Aggregation of macrophages in bronchioloalveolar regions is accompanied by the ingestion of fibers. Short fibers and, to a certain degree, long fibers are engulfed by macrophages, the latter often fusing to engulf longer fibers. These fibers then can be coated with an iron-protein complex forming ferruginous bodies. Fibers of sizes that frustrate complete ingestion by single or groups of macrophages result in the liberation of a variety of proteins and proteases from the macrophages.

Fibrosis

Incomplete ingestion of fibers results in the liberation of endogenous mediators of fibrosis and proliferation of epithelial cells. It is currently believed that the most important of these is platelet-derived growth factor (PDGF). Concom-

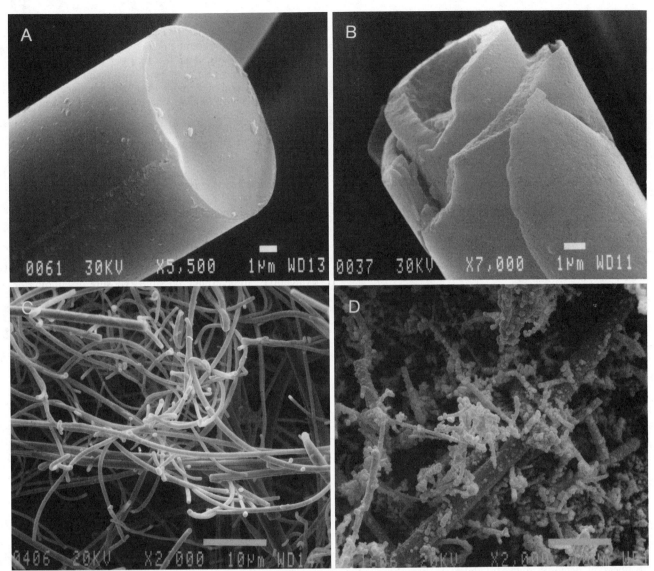

Fig. 111.2.   Scanning electron micrographs of two types of borosilicate glasses. Top micrographs show glass BG2 before (A) and after (B) incubation for 180 days in Gamble's fluid (a physiological solution).

Note the pitting and etching of the surface of the fibers in B. Lower micrographs show glass BG4 before (C) and after (D) incubation for 180 days in Gamble's fluid.

mitantly released proteases attack duct and septal walls resulting in tissue necrosis. Recent studies suggest a possible role in fiber toxicity for active oxygen species (AOS) liberated by phagocytic cells (45).

The fibrogenic process originates in the bronchioloalveolar region, with fibrosis initially becoming manifest in the peribronchiolar regions. Progression of fibrosis occurs interstitially along the scaffolding provided by alveolar duct and alveolar septal walls. Further advance of the process is characterized by the coalescence of microfibrotic areas into larger areas with ultimate replacement of parenchymal zones by larger scars.

Tissue Response—Neoplastic

The ability of fibers to induce malignant neoplasms following inhalation has been amply demonstrated for asbestos and erionite in humans and experimental animals. While asbestos fibers do in fact vary significantly in their neoplasm-producing

potential, it is clear that dose, dimension, and durability are crucial but not exclusive determinants of oncogenicity. Two sites of oncogenic effect have been verified, the lung and the pleura surrounding the lung (bronchogenic carcinoma and mesothelioma) (46, 47).

Lung Cancer Pulmonary

One potential mechanism of action is the fibrosis that is the result of the release of endogenous mediators of fibrosis and epithelial proliferation. The theoretical mechanism of development for bronchogenic carcinoma is the replacement of the normal architecture of the peripheral lung parenchyma by scar, leading to anatomic deformity, and epithelial proliferation that provides a milieu similar to that reported in studies of scar cancer in the past. The sequestered or entrapped pulmonary epithelium is more susceptible to malignant transformation and carcinoma development. The paucity of lung cancer occurrence in authenticated nonsmokers implicates cigarette smoking as a crucial factor in the enhanced lung cancer risk observed in workers exposed to asbestos. Any etiologic role for asbestos in the pathogenesis of lung cancer in the absence of a history of cigarette smoking would appear to be limited to bronchioloalveolar type of cancer in the presence of advanced fibrosis.

In contrast to asbestos, it should be noted that, until the current study of RCF, fibrosis has not been reported with any humanmade fiber. This lack of fibrosis despite multiple studies of sometimes massive doses of fibers suggests that this mechanism of tumorigenicity may not be applicable to many fibers and that individual scrutiny should be given to each fiber.

A second possible mechanism of action is a direct genotoxic effect as suggested by cell culture studies. Several studies have shown that concentrations of asbestos and MMMFs which induce neoplastic transformation of cells in culture also induce mutations at the chromosomal level, including chromosomal aberrations and numerical changes. These findings suggest that mineral fibers may act by a direct genotoxic mechanism to induce neoplasms (22, 48).

Mesothelioma

Malignant neoplasms arising from mesothelial surfaces have been described in the pleura, pericardium, and peritoneum with asbestos and erionite. The initial step in the development of malignant mesothelioma is the translocation of fibers to the pleura, peritoneum, or pericardium. The induction of fibrosis has been theorized to be a required antecedent for mesothelioma development much in the manner of malignant neoplasms following the subcutaneous implantation of solid state materials—plastics, metal, etc. Solid state carcinogenesis studies have shown that the pattern of fibrosis with implants is similar to the fibrosis seen in the pleura exposed to fibers. The potential genotoxicity of the fibers deposited in the pleural space is a second potential mechanism of action. Lechner and coworkers have shown that chromosomal aberrations are associated with asbestos-induced transformation of human mesothelial cells in culture (48).

To summarize the mechanistic potentials, the biologic effect of fibers is determined by (a) ability to gain host entry, (b) anatomic distribution, (c) translocation within the lung, (d) clearance from the respiratory tract, (e) natural and cellular components of the acute inflammatory response, (f) initiation of fibrosis and epithelial proliferation, and (g) capability of the fiber to induce neoplastic change. The mechanism of action for fibrosis and tumorigenicity of fibers has not been clearly developed.

However, the foregoing are in turn critically related to the exposure dose (amount × time), fiber size, geometry, durability, surface area and charge, and possible co-factor effects of exposure to toxic inhalants or the presence of antecedent or concurrent disease.

INDUSTRIAL HYGIENE STUDIES

In order to determine concentrations of airborne MMMF during manufacture and field application, industrial hygiene surveys have been undertaken. For example, in 20 MMMF manufacturing plants in North America and Europe, over 1000 occupational exposure samples are taken by industrial hygienists annually. Sampling and analysis is conducted in accordance with the National Institute for Occupational Safety and Health's

(NIOSH) methods for "Fibers in Air," "Nuisance Dust, Total," and "Nuisance Dust, Respirable" (51).

Airborne fiber concentrations are typically less than 0.2 fiber/ml, with the majority being less than 0.1 fiber/ml. Particulate mass sampling has also conducted in 20 manufacturing plants and results of total mass monitoring indicate, once again, extremely low concentrations. Concentrations are typically less than 1.0 mg/m^3 (52).

Studies evaluating occupational exposures during the installation of MMMF products also have been conducted. Typically, fibrous glass exposures determined optically averaged less than 0.5 fiber/ml, with a range of 0–20 fibers/ml. At the same time, total particulate mass concentrations averaged 4.2 mg/m^3, with a range of 0.04–113.6 mg/m^3.

In addition to manufacturing and field use surveys, release of fibrous glass during actual use of products, particularly fiber released from air filter media, has been monitored.

Ambient air was sampled in a number of public buildings in which fibrous glass products had been installed. These evaluations, to determine possible exposure of building occupants to fibrous glass, showed no significant erosion of fibers (53, 54).

To evaluate the efficiency of fibrous glass filter blankets, several high volume air samples were collected at various points in the ductwork of a large office complex at the intake and the exhaust prior to changing the filter media, and at the exhaust 23 days after installation of the new filter. Analyses of the samples using electron microscopy indicate little initial fiber release which decreases rapidly thereafter to the limit of detection (55).

Airborne concentrations of dust and fibers reported from U.S. mineral wool plants is generally higher than in U.S. glass wool facilities. This includes both airborne fibers and total particulate matter. Fiber levels reported ranged from 0.01–1.4 fibers/ml compared with 0.1–0.3 fiber/ml for glass wool. Total particulate matter sample results ranged from 0.05–23.6 mg/m^3 in the mineral wool facilities and 0.09–8.48 mg/m^3 for glass wool (56).

Exposures incurred in the actual application or installation of mineral wool products are also typically higher than those found in similar glass wool applications. These levels are directly related to the methods of application and the engineering controls or work practices instituted to limit exposure.

Industrial hygiene monitoring data obtained on a regular basis at locations where RCF products are manufactured show that exposures are generally below 1.0 fiber/ml, typically below 0.2 fiber/ml. End-user studies have indicated that RCF exposures can exceed 1.0 fiber/ml, 5 fibers/ml, or higher if appropriate engineering controls and work practices are not followed (52).

ANALYTICAL METHODS FOR AIRBORNE PARTICLES

Exposure to airborne MMMF is generally assessed by drawing air through a suitable filter and analyzing the materials collected. One method established by NIOSH for total particulate matter uses a filter which is weighed before and after the sample has been collected. The difference in weight is reported as the number of milligrams of particles per cubic meter of air sampled. This type of measurement does not allow determination of the physical structure of the particles captured, and it is believed to be less useful in assessing any possible risk associated with exposure to fibrous materials. In the United States this method is referred to as NIOSH method 0500 (51).

In order to assess any possible risk posed by inhalation of fibrous materials, a method that allows for particle discrimination and respirability is needed. Only those fibers that are small enough to penetrate into the lower regions of the lung are considered biologically active. Such methods as the NIOSH 7400, and the World Health Organization's (WHO) reference method for MMMF, utilize microscopic analysis of samples to report the number of respirable fibers per cubic centimeter of air sampled. Although the MMMF product being handled may contain varying percentages of respirable fiber due to the nature of the manufacturing process, the size distribution of the fibers in the air is much different. Larger, nonrespirable-sized fibers do not remain airborne as readily as the smaller fibers. Microscopic analyses allow for this size discrimination, and an adequate picture of the fiber exposure to be developed (51, 57).

OCCUPATIONAL EXPOSURE LIMITS

Currently, there are no specific regulations which govern exposure to MMMF. In the United States, the Occupational Safety and Health Administration (OSHA) considers these fibers to be nuisance dusts. Permissible exposure limits (PELs) for respirable and total nuisance dusts have been established at 5.0 and 15.0 mg/m^3, respectively. NIOSH has recommended a fiber-based exposure limit of 3.0 fibers/ml, fibers <3.5 μm diameter and >10 μm in length. Several MMMF manufacturers have recommended exposure limits of 1.0–2.0 fibers/ml for fibrous glass, mineral wool, and RCF.

Because of the added concern associated with exposure to RCF, one manufacturer is not utilizing an exposure limit concept. Exposure is to be controlled to the lowest practicable level, and respiratory protection required, until additional information is received which will allow for adequate risk assessments to be conducted (5, 8).

EXPOSURE TO COMPOUNDS OTHER THAN MMMF IN PRODUCTION

It is important to consider all substances that are present in the work environment when assessing the relative toxicologic potential of any substance. Many of the various MMMF products are produced by adding chemical binders and lubricating oils. Exposure to formaldehyde, phenol, ammonia, urea, crystalline silica, asbestos, polycyclic aromatic hydrocarbons, and asphalt have been reported. The potential cumulative effects of exposure to some or all of these materials must be considered in any operation to develop a sound employee and environmental health and safety plan.

REVIEWS OF MMMF

The Overall IARC Evaluation

In 1971, IARC initiated a program on the evaluation of the carcinogenic risk of chemicals to humans, involving the production of critically evaluated monographs on individual chemicals. In 1980, the program was expanded to include the evaluation of carcinogenic risks associated with exposures in specific occupations and, more recently, exposures to complex mixtures have been considered. Almost 700 individual chem-

icals, groups of chemicals, or complex mixtures have been evaluated under the program to date.

Under the 1980 expanded program, IARC convened from June 16–23, 1987, a working group on chemical carcinogenesis to evaluate the carcinogenic risk to humans of exposures to humanmade mineral fibers (MMMF). This working group also considered an unrelated topic, radon and its decay products. Volume 43 of the IARC Monographs on the Evaluation of Carcinogenic Risks to Humans, "Man-Made Mineral Fibres and Radon," was published by IARC in 1988 (58).

Under IARC procedures, any agent under study as a potential carcinogen may be classified under one of the following categories:

Group 1—sufficient evidence of human carcinogenicity;
Group 2A—probably carcinogenic to humans;
Group 2B—possibly carcinogenic to humans;
Group 3—not classifiable as to human carcinogenicity;
Group 4—probably not carcinogenic to humans.

The data for each agent under study are reviewed in detail before the meeting by selected members of the group. Animal studies and shortterm test results (e.g., tests done with living cells in test tubes and requiring at most only a few months to complete) are evaluated by experimentalists, and human studies are reviewed by epidemiologists. During the June 1987 meeting, the 20 participants first met as subgroups to classify the animal studies and human studies separately. Subsequently, the entire working group assigned one of the classifications listed above to each of the MMMF reviewed.

In that review, even though the data from extensive human studies were judged "inadequate" for carcinogenicity, IARC designated glass wool as a group 2B, "possibly carcinogenic to humans." This was substantially based on evidence that artificial implantation of fibers caused tumors in laboratory animals. Continuous filament was designated as IARC group 3, "not classifiable as to human carcinogenicity."

Based on "limited" evidence in experimental animals and "limited" evidence in humans, IARC designated rock wool as a group 2B, "possibly carcinogenic to humans." Slag wool was also designated as a Group 2B, based on "inadequate" evidence in animals and "limited" evidence in humans.

It was noted earlier that there are no data from human studies to evaluate RCF for carcinogenicity. IARC designated RCF as a group 2B, "possibly carcinogenic to humans." This was based on studies using laboratory animals.

IPCS Evaluation of Human Health Risks

In 1977, the 30th World Health Assembly requested the Director-General of WHO to devise longterm strategies to control and limit the impact of chemicals on human health and the environment. This concern was reiterated by the 1978 Assembly, and in January 1979 the 63rd session of the WHO Executive Board endorsed a plan of action. The IPCS became operational in April 1980.

IPCS is a joint venture of the United Nations Environment Program, the International Labor Organization, and WHO. The main objective is to carry out and disseminate evaluations of the effects of chemicals on human health and the quality of the environment. Supporting activities include the development of epidemiologic, experimental laboratory, and risk-assessment methods that could produce internationally comparable results (including extrapolating experimental data to effects on human subjects). Evaluations are published in a WHO monograph series.

Under the IPCS Program, a task group was assembled in London from September 14–18, 1987, to finalize the Environmental Health Criteria document on manmade mineral fibers. During the early part of the meeting, subgroups were formed to separately discuss the human epidemiologic data and the animal experimental data. Both occupational and general population health risks, including risks such as nonneoplastic lung disease and dermatitis, in addition to possible carcinogenic disease were considered. On the basis of available data (no epidemiologic data were available for RCF), no quantitative risks were given in the report. The possibility of effects such as skin and upper respiratory irritation, mentioned earlier in this bulletin, were noted in the IPCS report.

The task group then met in plenary session for final consideration of the document. Environmental Health Criteria 77, ''Man-Made Mineral Fibres,'' was published by WHO in 1988 (59).

Considering the results of the animal studies, in toto, the IPCS panel concluded that an increased risk of lung cancer in some sectors of the MMMF industry is ''biologically plausible.'' Protective equipment was recommended to guard against a potential elevation in lung cancer risk for workers engaged in activities where higher airborne exposure levels are possible.

For MMMF in general, the IPCS report stated that ''the overall picture indicates that the possible risk of lung cancer among the general public is very low, if there is any at all, and should not be a cause for concern if the current low levels of exposure continue'' (59).

PROTECTIVE MEASURES

Where exposure to any substance occurs, it is prudent to minimize the extent of exposure to its lowest practicable levels. Engineering modification of the process to minimize the amount of dust generated and appropriate location of local exhaust ventilation to remove dusts from their point of generation are the preferred methods of control. Appropriate work practices limit the amount of dust generated—e.g., vacuum cleaning instead of dry sweeping or using compressed air lines for cleaning.

It may also be prudent in many instances to augment the engineering controls and work practices with appropriate personal protective equipment. For example, when exposed to MMMF, the use of safety glass or goggles to prevent fibers from irritating the eyes, long-sleeved shirts to minimize the potential for skin irritation, and respiratory protection to minimize the potential risk of inhalation are recommended. Careful evaluation of the workplace and the existing conditions of exposure will identify the appropriate devices to be used in an individual situation (5, 8).

EXPOSURE MONITORING AND MEDICAL SURVEILLANCE PROGRAMS

Programs to routinely assess the exposure of employees and monitor their health are implemented whenever employees are exposed to potentially harmful substances. Exposure monitoring of each operation to establish baseline levels of exposure enable the development of appropriate engineering controls and the selection of personal protective equipment. Once the baseline has been established and confidence in the range of ex-

posures has been gained, then additional monitoring is recommended on a regular basis (e.g., yearly), or whenever processes or practices change.

Medical surveillance programs should include a review of general health, occupational history, physical examination, clinical chemistries and blood count, pulmonary function testing, and a baseline chest x-ray. The history and physical examination should focus on the respiratory and dermatologic findings. Other testing should be performed as indicated by the occupational history. The examination should be repeated on a regular basis (e.g., yearly), and testing repeated after review of the individual health history and exposure history. The results of these tests should be reviewed individually and as a group on a regular basis (5, 8).

SUMMARY

Studies concerning MMMF, whether epidemiologic, industrial hygiene, or experimental, have yielded significant data. MMMFs are among the world's most studied commercial products. Large epidemiologic studies of MMMF have been conducted, and updated studies will be completed. The two largest studies are the Marsh/Enterline in the United States and the Saracci study in Europe. Neither study has associated increased pulmonary morbidity or mortality with exposure to fibrous glass. A small excess exists for mineral wool, but there is no dose-response correlation, and it does not correlate with length of employment.

Laboratory studies, using animal models as well as other experimental techniques, have been valuable in understanding the mechanisms by which glass fibers may interact with living tissue.

Much of this information has been obtained through techniques that purposely bypass normal animal defense systems. In such cases, it has been demonstrated that surgically implanted long, thin MMMF are capable of producing fibrosis and malignant tumors. However, when laboratory animals have been exposed for years to high concentrations of long, thin glass fibers by the normal route of inhalation, no permanent changes in lung tissue have been observed throughout the animals' entire life spans. These results are encouraging since they demonstrate that glass fiber differs in important ways from natural mineral fibers such as asbestos. In addition, toxicologic studies show a spectrum of response to fibers, suggesting that MMMF groups should be considered independently. Conflicting results of earlier studies and interim results of an ongoing study of RCF suggest further risk evaluation may be necessary for this fiber type.

Another important result of laboratory studies is the indication that glass fibers are considerably less durable in the presence of body fluids than asbestos fibers.

Industrial hygiene studies conducted in the MMMF manufacturing plants typically demonstrate low exposures to both fiber and particulate. However, industrial hygiene studies conducted during the field application of MMMF products indicate that there are some individual field installations that can result in high occupational exposures to both fiber and particulate. Based on these results, respiratory protection, enhanced work practices, and/or applied engineering controls are appropriate and prudent in some field applications, such as blowing, of MMMF products.

The potential health effects of MMMFs have been reviewed by scientific panels. The IARC designation of group 2B for glass fiber wool, and RCF resulted from a finding of sufficient evidence of cancer from animal studies based largely on implantation studies but inadequate evidence of cancer in studies of humans. The data on cancer in studies of both humans and animals were found to be inadequate evidence for carcinogenicity for glass filament, and continuous filament fibrous glass was therefore designated IARC group 3.

As discussed in the IPCS review and risk assessment of MMMF, the absence of disease in the vast majority of workers exposed to fibrous glass during the last 50 years suggests that fibrous glass products pose ''little, if any, health risk to humans.'' This risk assessment, based on environmental studies, demonstrates very low concentrations of ambient glass fiber during normal manufacture and use.

However, the critical reviews of studies point to the need for more research to better understand the questions that have been raised. New research is being planned. Future, broadened updates of the U.S. (March/Enterline) mortality study including further review of potential confounders are already under way. In addition to an update of Weill's morbidity study, which is in progress, the industry initiated in 1984 the largest respiratory health surveillance program for production workers in the world, and initial study of that database has begun. Additional animal studies are also under way for MMMF. A dose-response study of RCF has been initiated and a study of glass fibers using the protocol developed at RCC—Geneva has been initiated. Further solubility testing in cell culture and extracellular systems is also being conducted. The combination of these studies should advance the knowledge of the potential mechanisms of action for fibers and promote more accurate risk determination and assessment.

REFERENCES

1. Pundsack FL. Fibrous glass—manufacture, use, and physical properties. In: LeVee WN, Schulte PA, eds. Occupational exposure to fibrous glass (DHEW [NIOSH] Publ. NO. 76-151; NTIS Publ. No. PB-258869), Cincinnati, OH: National Institute for Occupational Safety and Health, 1976:11–18.

2. Boyd DC, Thompson DA. Glass. In: Grayson M, Mark HF, Othmer DF, Overberger CG, Seaborg GT, eds. Kirk-Othmer encyclopedia of chemical technology. 3rd ed. Vol 11. New York: John Wiley & Sons, 1980:807–880.

3. Mohr JG, Rowe WP. Fiber glass, New York: Van Nostrand Reinhold, 1978.

4. Arledter HF, Knowles SE. Ceramic fibers. In: Battista OA, ed. Synthetic fibers in papermaking. New York: Interscience, 1964:185–244.

5. Chase G, Anderson R. Health and safety aspects of fiber glass. Manville Corp., 1986:22.

6. Dement JM. Environmental aspects of fibrous glass production and utilization. Environ 1975;9:295–312.

7. Possick PA, Gillin GA, Key MM. Fibrous glass dermatitis, Am Ind Hyg Assoc J 1970;31(1):12–15.

8. Chase G, Anderson R. Health and safety aspects of refractory ceramic fibers. Manville Corp, 1988.

9. Parmeggiani L, ed. Encyclopedia of occupational health and safety. 3rd ed. Vol 1. Geneva: International Labor Office.

10. Simonato L, Fletcher AC, Cherrie J, et al. International Agency for Research on Cancer. Historical cohort study of MMMF production workers in seven European countries, extension of the follow-up. Ann Occup Hyg 1987;31:603–623.

11. Enterline PE, Marsh GM, Henderson V, Callahan C. Mortality update of a cohort of US man-made mineral fibre workers. Ann Occup Hyg 1987;31:625–656.

11a. Marsh GM, Enterline PE, Stone RA, Henderson MS. Mortality among a cohort of US man-made mineral fiber workers. 1985 follow-up. J Occup Med 1990;32:594–604.

11b. Shannon HS, Hayes M, Julian JA, Muir DCF, Walsh C. Mortality experience of glass fibre workers. Br J Ind Med 1984;41:35–38.

12. Shannon HS, Hayes M, Julian JA, Muir DCF. Mortality experience of Ontario glass fibre workers—extended follow-up. Ann Occup Hyg 1987;31:657–662.

13. Weill H, Hughes JM, Hammad YY, Glindmeyer HW III, Sharon G, Jones RN. Respiratory health in workers exposed to man-made vitreous fibers. Am Rev Respir Dis 1983;128:104–122.

14. Weill H, Hughes JM, Hammad YY, Glindmeyer HW III, Sharon G, Jones RN. Respiratory health of workers exposed to MMMF. In: Biological effects of man-made mineral fibres (Proceedings of a WHO/IARC Conference), Vol 1. Copenhagen: World Health Organization, 1984:387–412.

15. Bunn WB, Hesterberg T, Versen R. The health effects of fibrous glass and refractory ceramic fiber. Glass Technology, 1989.

16. Chamberlain M, Brown RC, Davies R, Griffiths DM. In vitro prediction of the pathogenicity of mineral dusts. Br J Exp Pathol 1979;60:320–327.

17. Tilkes F, Beck EG. Comparison of length-dependent cytotoxicity of inhalable asbestos and man-made mineral fibres. In: Wagner JC, ed. Biological effects of mineral fibres (IARC Scientific Publications No. 30). Lyon: International Agency for Research on Cancer, 1980:475–483.

18. Hesterberg TW, Barrett JC. Dependence of asbestos- and mineral dust-induced transformation of mammalian cells in culture on fiber dimension. Cancer Res 1984;44:2170–2180.

19. Ririe DG, Hesterberg TW, Barrett JC, Nettesheim P. Toxicity of asbestos and glass fibers for rat tracheal epithelial cells in culture. In: Beck EG, Bignon J, eds. In vitro effects of mineral dusts. NATO ASI Series, Vol G3. Berlin: Springer, 1985:177–184.

20. Poole A, Brown RC, Rood AP. The in vitro activities of a highly carcinogenic mineral fibre—potassium octatitanate. Br J Exp Pathol 1986;67:289–296.

21. Sincock A, Seabright M. Induction of chromosome changes in Chinese hamster cells by exposure to asbestos fibres. Nature 1925;257:56–58.

22. Oshimura M, Hesterberg TW, Tsutsui T, Barrett CJ. Correlation of asbestos-induced cytogenetic effects with cell transformation of Syrian hamster embryo cells in culture. Cancer Res 1984;44:5017–5022.

23. Pott F, Ziem U, Mohr U. Lung carcinomas and mesotheliomas following intratracheal instillation of glass fibres and asbestos. In: Proceedings of the VIth International Pneumoconiosis Conference, Bochum: Federal Republic of Germany, 20–23 September 1983. Vol 2. Geneva: International Labour Office, 1984:746–756.

24. Pott F, Schlipkoter HW, Ziem U, Spurny K, Huth F. New results from implantation experiments with mineral fibres. In: Biological effects of man-made mineral fibres (Proceedings of a WHO/IARC Conference). Vol 2. Copenhagen: World Health Organization, 1984:286–302.

25. Stanton JF, Layard M, Tegeris A, Miller E, May M, Morgan E, Smith A. Relation of particle dimension to carcinogenicity in amphibole asbestoses and other fibrous minerals. J Natl Cancer Inst 1981;67:965–975.

26. Smith DM, Ortiz LW, Archuleta RF. Long-term exposure of Syrian hamsters and Osborne-Medel rats to aerosolized 0.45 μm mean diameter glass. In: Biological effects of man-made mineral fibres (Proceedings of a WHO/IARC Conference). Vol 2. Copenhagen: World Health Organization, 253–272.

27. Smith DM, Ortiz LW, Archuleta RF, Johnson NF. Long-term health effects in hamsters and rats exposed chronically to man-made vitreous fibers. Ann Occup Hyg 1987;31:731–754.

28. Davis JMG, Addison J, Bolton RE, Donaldson K, Jones AD, Wright A. The pathogenic effects of fibrous ceramic aluminum silicate glass administered to rats by inhalation or peritoneal injection. In: Biological effects of man-made mineral fibres (Proceedings of a WHO/IARC Conference). Vol 2. Copenhagen: World Health Organization, 1984:303–322.

29. Davis JMG. A review of experimental evidence for the carcinogenicity of man-made vitreous fibers. Scand J Work Environ Health 1986;12 (suppl 1) 12–17.

30. Gross P, de Treville RTP, Cralley LJ, Granquist WT, Pundsack FL. The pulmonary response to fibrous dusts of diverse compositions. Am Ind Hyg Assoc J 1970;31:125–132.

31. Lee KP, Barras CE, Griffith FD, Waritz RS, Lapin CA. Comparative pulmonary responses to inhaled inorganic fibers with asbestos and fiberglass. Environ Res 1981;24:167–191.

32. Wagner JC, Berry GB, Hill RJ, Munday DE, Skidmore JW. Animal experiments with MMM(V)F—effects of inhalation and intrapleural inoculation in rats. In: Biological effects of manmade mineral fibres (Proceedings of a WHO/IARC Conference). Vol 2. Copenhagen: World Health Organization. 1984:209–233.

33. McConnell EE, Wagner JC, Skidmore JW, Moore JA. A comparative study of the fibrogenic and carcinogenic effects of UICC Canadian chrysotile B asbestos and glass microfibre (JM 100). In: Biological effects of man-made mineral fibres (Proceedings of a WHO/IARC Conference). Vol 2. Copenhagen: World Health Organization, 1984:234–252.

34. LeBouffant L, Daniel H, Henin JP, Martin JC, Normand C, Thichoux G, Trolard F. Experimental study on long-term effects of inhaled MMMF on the lung of rats. Ann Occup Hyg 1987;31:765–790.

35. Muhle H, Pott F, Bellmann B, Takenaka S, Ziem U. Inhalation and

injection experiments in rats to test the carcinogenicity of MMMF. Ann Occup Hyg 1987;31:755–764.

35a. Hesterberg TW, Bunn WB, Hadley J, Bernstein DM, Anderson R. Chronic inhalation toxicity of fibrous glass in rats. Proceedings of the Fourth International Conference on Environmental Lung Disease (Abstract), 1991, In Press.

36. Bernstein DM, Fleisner H, Bouvier C, Vogel O, Chevalier J, Mast R, Anderson R. (Carouge-Geneva, Switzerland; Cleveland and Denver, USA) Refractory ceramic fibers (RCF): experimental design and interim results from inhalation oncogenicity studies in rats comparing 4 RCFs with chrysotile asbestos. V International Congress of Toxicology (in press).

37. Imamura T, Vogel O, Chevalier J, Mast R, Hesterberg T, Anderson R, Bernstein D. Evaluation of pulmonary functions during chronic inhalation studies with refractory ceramic fibers (RCF) and an experimental fiber in rats. Toxicologist (in press).

38. Bunn WB, Chase G, Versen R. The health and safety aspects of manmande mineral fibers. (Abstract). Glass Proceedings, 1989.

38a. Hesterberg TW, Mast R, McConnell EE, Chevalier J, Bernstein DM, Bunn WB, Anderson R. Chronic inhalation toxicity of refractory ceramic fibers in Syrian hamsters. In: Proceedings of International Workshop on Mechanisms of Fibre Carcinogenesis (in press).

38b. Hesterberg TW, Mast R, McConnell EE, Vogel O, Chevalier J, Bernstein DM, Anderson R. Chronic inhalation toxicity and oncogenicity study of refractory ceramic fibers in Fisher 344 rats. Toxicologist 1991;11(1), No. 254:85.

39. Klingholz R, Steinkopf B. The reactions of MMMF in a physiological model fluid and in water. In: Biological effects of man-made mineral fibres (Proceedings of a WHO/IARC Conference). Vol 2. Copenhagen: World Health Organization, 1984:60–86.

40. Leineweber JP. Solubility of fibres in vitro and in vivo. In: Biological effects of man-made mineral fibres (Proceedings of a WHO/IARC Conference). Vol 2. Copenhagen: World Health Organization, 1984:87–101.

41. Law B, Hesterberg T. Solubility of natural and man-made mineral fibers in Karnovsky's fixative. Toxicologist (in press).

42. Law B, Hesterberg T, Bunn W. Solubility of organic and borosilicate fibers in physiological fluid (in preparation).

43. Stober W. Dynamic shape factors of nonspherical aerosol particles. In: Mercer TT, Morrow PE, Stober W, eds. Assessment of airborne particles. Springfield, IL: Charles C Thomas, 1972.

44. Lippman Morton. Review Asbestos Exposure Indices. Environ Res 1988;46:86–106.

45. Hansen L, Mossman BT. Generation of superoxide (O2) from alveolar macrophages exposed to asbestiform and nonfibrous particles. Cancer Res 1987;47:1681–1686.

46. Demy NG, Adler H. Asbestos and malignancy. Am J Roentgenol 1967;100:597.

47. McDonald JC, Becklake MR, Gibbs GW, McDonald AD, Rossiter DE. The health of chrysotile asbestos mine and mill workers of Quebec. Arch Environ Health 1974;38:61.

48. Lechner JF, Tokiwa T, Yeager Jr, H, Harris CC. Asbestos-associated chromosomal changes in human mesothelial cells. In: Beck EG, Bignon J, eds. In vitro effects of mineral dusts. Berlin: Springer-Verlag, 1985.

49. Wagner JC, Sleggs CA, Marchand P. Diffuse pleural mesothelioma and asbestos exposure in the North Western Cape Province. Br J Ind Med 1960;17:260.

50. Seilikoff IJ, Churg J, Hammond EC. The occurrence of asbestosis among insulation workers in the United States. Ann NY Acad Sci 1965;132:139.

51. NIOSH manual of analytical methods. 3rd ed. U.S. Dept. of Health and Human Services. Public Health Service, Centers for Disease Control.

52. Unpublished data from industrial hygiene surveys conducted by Manville Corporation, 1985–1988.

53. Balzer JL, Cooper WC, Fowler DP. Fibrous glass-lined air transmission systems: an assessment of their environmental effects. Am Ind Hyg Assoc J 1971;32:512–518.

54. Cholak J, Schafer L. Erosion of fibers from installed fibrous glass ducts. Arch Environ Health 1971;22:220–229.

55. Unpublished data from industrial hygiene surveys conducted by Manville Corporation, 1987.

56. Esmen N, et al. Estimation of employee exposures to total suspended particulate matter and airborne fibers in insulation installation operations. Pittsburgh: University of Pittsburgh, 1980.

57. WHO. Reference methods for measuring airborne man-made mineral fibres. WHO/EURO Technical Committee for Monitoring and Evaluating Airborne MMMF. Copenhagen: World Health Organization, 1985.

58. WHO. IARC Monographs on the evaluation of carcinogenic risks to humans. Vol 43. World Health Organization International Agency for Research on Cancer. Man-made mineral fibres. Environmental Health Criteria 77. Geneva: WHO, 1988.

59. WHO. IARC Monographs on the evaluation of carcinogenic risks to humans. Vol 43. World Health Organization International Agency for Research on Cancer. Man-made mineral fibres. Environmental Health Criteria 77. Geneva: WHO, 1988.

112

Polycyclic Aromatic Hydrocarbons

Steven Pike, M.D.

Polycyclic aromatic hydrocarbons (PAHs) belong to a class of chemicals characterized by molecules containing three or more fused unsaturated carbon rings. PAHs are ubiquitous in the environment and are formed during the process of incomplete combustion or pyrolysis of organic matter. The burning of oil, gas, and other fossil fuels constitutes the main sources of PAHs emitted in the atmosphere. Hundreds of different PAHs are formed in this way as well as heterocyclic or polynuclear aromatic hydrocarbons (PNAs), which are PAHs containing elements other than carbon in their ring structure, such as sulfur, oxygen, or nitrogen. Those compounds containing four to six rings present in PAH mixtures may be carcinogenic.

These compounds have relatively high molecular weights and exist in solid form at room temperature most commonly as condensates on particles or surfaces. They are practically insoluble in water but are soluble in organic solvents. PAHs entering the atmosphere condense when hot combustion gases cool, and form very small particles that can be adsorbed onto existing particles. In addition, PAHs can be formed on surfaces or deep inside organic matter undergoing incomplete pyrolysis. PAH aerosols may be transported great distances by winds. PAHs are found in soot, coal, charcoal, automobile exhaust, tobacco smoke, tar, oil, smoked foods, sewage sludge, flue gases, etc. Atmospheric levels vary but are typically higher in urban regions compared with rural, restaurants compared with general office environments, and winter compared with summer. The composition of PAH emissions varies with the source and location, so comparisons are often made by reference to concentrations of benzo(a)pyrene (BaP), which is used as a surrogate or index compound for all the other PAHs contained in the mixture.

Benzo(a)pyrene is not a consistently reliable surrogate for comparing PAH mixtures because the relative concentrations of BaP to other constituents in different mixtures from different sources can vary widely. For example, in cigarette smoke condensate, BaP comprises approximately 1% of the carcinogenic effect, but in extracts of sewage sludge BaP accounts for nearly 23%.

ENVIRONMENTAL SOURCES

Over 97% of the estimated BaP emissions are attributed to stationary fuel combustion—refuse fires, residential furnaces, and coke ovens contributing the largest share, over 87% of the total. A review of PAHs in the environment has been published by Edwards (1983) (1). Tables 112.1 and 112.2 list some common sources of airborne PAH emissions. PAH concentrations in air range from 0.1 ng/m³ (detection limit) to about 100 ng/m³ (2, 3). Average urban PAH concentrations in selected cities have been reported as approximately 2.17 ng/m³ (4). Sawicki (1960) (5) reported BaP air concentrations in urban centers to range from 0.1–61.0 ng/m³, and in nonurban regions to range from 0.01–1.9 ng/m³. Using BaP as a rough index of exposure, generally heavily polluted air (6) contains approximately 100 ng/m³, drinking water (7) contains approximately 27 ng/l, and smoked foods (8) contain 100 µg/kg.

Large concentrations of PAHs exist as waste deposits throughout developed countries where manufactured gas plants produced gas for lighting and heating from coal or oil. These plants were in common operation from the mid 1800s until the early 1950s, when they were phased out by the introduction of interstate natural gas pipelines. It is estimated that there were over 1000 such plants throughout the United States prior to World War II, with most concentrated in the Midwest and East (9). The major classes of chemicals associated with gas plant wastes are PAHs, phenolics, volatile organic hydrocarbons (VOCs), various inorganic sulfur and nitrogen species, and, to a lesser extent, trace metals. Table 112.3 lists some published concentrations of BaP detected in soil and water in various geographic locations. Surface water concentrations are reported to range from 0.6–114 ng/l (10).

PAHs are present in foods as a result of biosynthesis, adsorption of particulates on leafy surfaces from atmospheric

Table 112.1. Emission Sources (Tons/y)

Source	BaP Emissions	% of total
Wood burning fireplaces, etc.	25	2.8
Coal refuse fires	310	34.7
Residential furnaces	300	33.6
Coke production	170	19.0
Mobile sources, gasoline	11	1.2
Forest and agricultural refuse burning	11	1.2
Open refuse burning	11	1.2
Vehicle disposal open burning	25	2.8

Source: U.S. Environmental Protection Agency. Preferred Standards Path Report for Polycyclic Organic Matter. Durham, N.C.: U.S. Environ. Prot. Agency, Office Air Qual. Plan. Stand., Strategies Air Stand. Div., 1974. Adapted from adaptation by: Baum EJ. Occurrence and surveillance of polycyclic aromatic hydrocarbons. Polycyclic hydrocarbons and cancer. Vol 1. Orlando, FL: Academic Press 1978.

Table 112.2. Environmental Sources

Exposure Category	BaP (µg/m³)
Cigarettes unfiltered (1 pack/day)	0.7 µg/day
Cigarettes filtered (1 pack/day)	0.4 µg/day
Airline cockpits (prior to nonsmoking regulations)	
Transatlantic	0.093 (8-hr TWA)
Domestic	0.138 (8-hr TWA)
Coke oven workers	
Topside	18 (8-hr TWA)
Side and bench	7 (8-hr TWA)
Roof tarring	14
Sidewalk tarring	78
Restaurant	0.8 µg/day
	0.03–0.14

Adapted from: Bridbord K, Finlea JF, Wagoner JK, Moran JB, Caplan P. Human exposure to polynuclear aromatic hydrocarbons. Freudenthal RI, Jones PW, ed. Carcinogenesis. Vol 1. Polynuclear aromatic hydrocarbons: chemistry, metabolism, and carcinogenesis. New York: Raven Press, 1976.

Table 112.3.   Soil and Water BaP Concentrations (μg/kg)

Source	BaP (μg/kg)
Forest	up to 1300[4]
Nonindustrial sites	up to 127
Towns and vicinities	up to 939
Soils near traffic	up to 2000
Near oil refinery	200,000
Near airport	785
Contaminated by coal tar pitch	685,000
Remote areas	10 to 20

Source: World Health Organization. Monograph on the evaluation of carcinogenic risks of the chemical to man. Certain polycyclic aromatic hydrocarbons and heterocyclic compounds. Vol. 3. Geneva: International Agency Research on Cancer, WHO, 1973. As adapted by: Baum EJ. Occurrence and surveillance of polycyclic aromatic hydrocarbons. Polycyclic hydrocarbons and cancer. Vol. 1. Orlando, FL: Academic Press, 1978.
[4]Seldom exceeding 10–20 μg/kg in remote areas.

Table 112.4.   PAH in Food (μg/kg dried material)

Source	BaP	Chrysene	Benzanthracene
Cereals	0.25–0.84	0.8–14.5	0.4–6.8
Salad	2.8–5.3	5.7–26.5	4.6–15.4
Spinach	7.4	28.0	16.1
Tomatoes	0.22	0.5	0.3
Refined oils/fats	0.9–15	0.5–129	0.5–13.5
Broiled meat/fish	0.2–162	0.5–25.4	0.2–31
Smoked meat/fish	0.2–107	0.3–123	0.02–189
Roasted coffee	0.1–4	0.6–19.1	0.5–14.2
Tea	3.9–21.3	4.6–6.3	

Source: Grimmer G. Carcinogenic hydrocarbons in the human environment. Dtsch. Aptoth. Ztg. 108:529, 1968. Shabad LM, Cohan YL. Contents of benzo(a)pyrene in some crops. Arch. Geschwulstforsch. 40:237, 1972. World Health Organization. Monograph on the evaluation of carcinogenic risks of the chemical to man. Certain polycyclic aromatic hydrocarbons and heterocyclic compounds. Vol 3. Geneva: International Agency for Research in Cancer, WHO. As adapted by: Baum EJ. Occurrence and surveillance of polycyclic aromatic hydrocarbons. Polycyclic hydrocarbons and cancer. Vol 1. Orlando, FL: Academic Press, 1978.

fallout, or more significantly as a result of the processing or cooking of foods prior to consumption. Concentrations are higher on plant surfaces compared with internal tissue, and above ground plants have much higher concentrations than below ground plants. Broad-leafed plants contain more PAHs than thin-leafed, and, while most of this PAH in plants is from atmospheric deposition, washing plants with water is not an effective method for removing PAH contamination from vegetables. Concentrations of BaP in vegetation range from 0.1–150 μg/kg. Wang and Meresz (1981) (11) reported vegetation: soil BaP ratios to range from 0.0001–0.085, while Shabad (1971) (12) and Fritz (1971) (13) reported soil concentrations worldwide to range from 100–1000 μg/kg, with total PAH to typically be 10 times the BaP concentration. Their vegetation:soil ratios were reported to range from 0.002–0.33 for BaP and 0.001–0.183 for total PAH. Some terrestrial plants can take up and translocate PAHs through roots and leaves. The rate of uptake is dependent on physical factors of PAH deposition, soil type and condition, and plant species. Plants can synthesize BaP, and this has been reported to occur during germination of beech, oak, tobacco, wheat, rye, and lentils with concentrations ranging from 10–20 μg/kg of dried material (14). Solid residues from water and sewage treatment plants are also high in PAH content (15–17). Table 112.4 lists some common foods and the reported concentrations of benzo(a)pyrene, chrysene, and benzanthracene in μg/kg of dried material.

METABOLISM

PAHs are metabolized by the cytochrome P450/448-dependent microsomal enzyme system, aryl hydrocarbon hydroxylase (AHS), to form epoxides. The epoxides formed are then converted by epoxide hydrolases to dihydrodiols and diol-epoxides. For BaP metabolism by AHH, the 7,8-epoxide is mainly formed which is considered to be a proximate carcinogen (18). BaP 7,8-epoxide can then be converted to BaP 7,8-dihydrodiol, which can itself be oxidatively metabolized by AHH to the BaP 7,8-diol-9,10-epoxide. Several enantiomeric diol-epoxides are possible, demonstrating wide variations in tumorigenic potency. The wide variability in potency of the enantiomeric forms of diol-epoxides led to Jarina et al. proposing the "bay region" theory to assist in understanding the carcinogenicity of PAHs (19, 20). The "bay region" theory predicted that

epoxides located on saturated angular rings in the bay region of a PAH should be highly reactive.

In addition to epoxidation and epoxide conversion to dihydrodiols, a number of other metabolic pathways for PAHs have been observed. Phenols, quinones, sulfates, glucuronates, and reactions with DNA, proteins, and glutathione have been reported (21).

TOXICITY

There are few published reports regarding the acute toxicity of PAHs in animals. Some reports do exist concerning the acute toxicity of specific compounds, but there is little to no information regarding the acute toxicity of PAH mixtures. In general the acute toxicity of PAHs increases as the molecular weight increases and with increasing side chain alkyl substitution on the aromatic nucleus. In animals the acute toxicity of oral or dermal exposure is relatively low, based on experiments on mice and rats. However, repeated exposure to some low dose PAHs resulted in carcinogenicity to these animals. As little as a few micromoles of benzo(a)pyrene were sufficient to cause cancer in less than 6 months in mice repeatedly dosed (22). Chronic exposure to low concentrations of PAHs in water can result in decreased survival, behavioral changes, reproductive effects, and cancer in some sensitive aquatic species (23). The proportionate concentrations of specific compounds in PAH mixtures vary considerably by source, which compounds the problem of evaluating acute toxicity of PAH mixtures. PAHs appear to be mildly to moderately toxic to humans and animals by acute exposure, but in animals chronic exposures to certain PAHs result in cancer. Air pollution studies demonstrating an excess in lung cancer among workers exposed to PAHs from coal gas, tar, coke oven emissions, and soot strongly suggest that PAHs are carcinogenic to humans (24–33). Published reports of acute toxicity studies for the various PAHs are limited.

PAHs produced systemic toxicity manifested by inhibition of growth in mice and rats at doses above 150 mg/kg (34). Rapidly proliferating tissues such as bone marrow, intestinal epithelium, lymphoid tissues, and reproductive organs appear

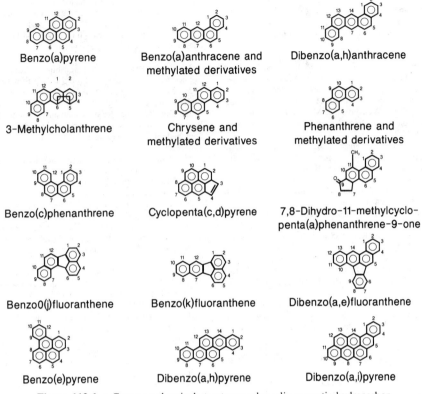

Figure 112.1. Common chemical structures polycyclic aromatic hydrocarbon.

to be most susceptible to PAH toxicity. Specific effects that have been observed in rats fed dimethylbenzanthracene at doses between 50 and 300 mg/kg include: agranulocytosis, anemia, lymphopenia, pancytopenia, and testicular degeneration (35). In mice, thymic degeneration, impaired thyroid development, general wasting, and immunosuppression have been observed at doses of 3-methylcholanthrene (3MC) over 150 mg/kg (36, 37). Some of the PAHs have also been shown to be mutagenic and teratogenic in in vitro test systems and in rodents, respectively. Examination of Table 112.5, which presents the LD_{50} values for several PAH compounds, reveals the lack of acute toxicity data for many of these compounds.

REGULATIONS AND STANDARDS

The 1990–91 American Conference of Governmental Industrial Hygienists' (ACGIH) threshold limit value (TLV) for coal tar pitch volatiles is 0.2 mg/m³. In the early 1970s the USSR issued a maximum allowable concentration (MAC) for benzo(a)pyrene of 0.15 μg/m³. The USSR has proposed a 1-ng/m³ BaP standard for ambient air and a 150-ng/m³ limit for work environments (38). Sweden issued a TLV of 10 μg/m³ in 1978 for benzo(a)pyrene and lowered it to 5 μg/m³ in 1982. Limits for PAH concentrations in drinking water have been recommended by the World Health Organization (WHO) as 7.5 ng/l for BaP and 30 ng/l for total carcinogenic PAHs. The Safe Drinking Water Committee of the National Academy of Sciences was unable to determine a Suggested No Adverse Effect Level (SNARL) for PAHs because of their proven carcinogenicity in animals and their suspected carcinogenicity in humans. Insuf-

Table 112.5. Acute Toxicity LD_{50} mg/kg[a]

PAH	ORL Rat	ORL Mouse	SQ Rat	SQ Mouse	IVN Rat	IVN Mouse
7,12-Dimethylbenzanthracene	327	340	—	—	54	—
Benzanthracene	—	—	—	—	—	10[b]
Chrysene	—	—	—	—	—	—
Benzo(a)pyrene	—	—	50	—	—	—
Phenanthrene	—	700	—	—	—	56
Anthracene	—	—	—	—	—	—
Pyrene	—	—	—	—	—	—
Naphthalene[c]	1780	—	—	969	—	100
Acenaphthylene	—	—	—	—	—	—
Benzo(j)fluoranthene	—	—	—	—	—	—
Benzo(k)fluoranthene	—	—	—	—	—	—
Benzo(b)fluoranthane	—	—	—	—	—	—
Benzo(ghi)perylene	—	—	—	—	—	—
Benzo(c)phenanthrene	—	—	—	—	—	—

[a]Source: NIOSH Registry of Toxic Effects of Chemical Substances. Tatken RL, Lewis Sr. RJ, eds. Cincinnati, OH: U.S. Department of Health and Human Services, Public Health Service, Centers for Disease Control, National Institute for Occupational Safety and Health, 1983.
[b]LD_{LO}.
[c]Oral-child LD_{LO}, 100 mg/kg; unk, man LD_{LO} − 74 mg/kg.

ficient data were cited for their inability to set 7-day and 24-hour PAH exposure limits for humans (39).

REFERENCES

1. Edwards NT. Polycyclic aromatic hydrocarbons (PAH's) in the terrestrial environment—a review. J Environ Qual 1983;12(4):427–441.

2. Sawicki E, Elbert WC, Hauser TR, Fox FT, Stanley TW. Benzo(a)pyrene content of the air of American communities. J Am Ind Hyg Assoc 1960;21:443.

3. Sawicki E, Hauser TR, Elbert WC, Fox FT, Meeker JE. Polynuclear aromatic hydrocarbon composition of the atmosphere in some large American cities. J Am Ind Hyg Assoc 23:137.

4. United States Environmental Protection Agency. Preferred standards path report for polycyclic organic matter. Durham, North Carolina: U.S. Environ. Prot. Agency, Office Air Qual. Plan. Stand., Strategies Air Stand. Div, 1974.

5. Sawicki E, Elbert WC, Hauser TR, Fox FT, Stanley TW. Benzo(a)pyrene content of the air of American communities. J Am Ind Hyg Assoc 1960;21:443.

6. Sawicki E, Houser TR, Elbert WC, Fox FT, Meeker JE. Polynuclear aromatic hydrocarbon composition of the atmosphere in some large American cities. J Am Ind Hyg Assoc 1962;23:137.

7. Sawicki E, Corey RC, Dooley AE, Giselard JB, Monkman JL, Neliganund RE, Ripperton LA. Tentative method of spectrophotometric analysis for benzo(a)pyrene in atmospheric particulate matter. Health Lab Sci 7 (suppl 68) (1970).

8. Wierzchowski J, Gajewska R. Determination of 3,4-benzopyrene in smoked fish. Bromatol Chem Toksykol 1972;5:481.

9. Handbook on manufactured gas plant sites. Prepared for: Utility Solid Waste Activities Group, Superfund Committee, Washington, DC by Environmental Research and Technology, Inc. and Koppers Company, Inc., Pittsburgh, PA: Edison Electric Institute, 1984.

10. Sawicki E, Corey RC, Dooley AE, Giselard JB, Monkman JL, Nehgamund RE, Ripperton LA. Tentative method for spectrophometric analysis for benzo(a)pyrene in atmospheric particulate matter. Health Lab Sci 1970; 7 (suppl 68).

11. Wang DT, Meresz O. Occurrence and potential uptake of polynuclear aromatic hydrocarbons of highway traffic origin by proximally grown food crops. (Abstract). Sixth Int. Symp. on PAH. Columbus, OH: Battelle Columbus Laboratory, 1981.

12. Shabad LM, Cohan YL, Ilnitsky AP, Khesina AYA, Shcherbak NP, Smirnov GA. The carcinogenic hydrocarbon benzo(a)pyrene in the soil. J Natl Cancer Inst 1971;47:1179–1191.

13. Fritz W. Extent and sources of contamination of our food with carcinogenic hydrocarbons. Ernaehrungsforschung 1971;16:547–557.

14. Graef W, Diehl H. The natural normal levels of carcinogenic polycyclic aromatic hydrocarbons and the reasons therefore. Arch Hyg Bakteriol 1966;150:49.

15. Borneff J, Fischer R. Carcinogenic substances in water and soil. IX. Investigations on filter mud of a lake water (treatment) plant for PAH. Arch Hyg Bakteriol 1962;146:183.

16. Borneff J, Fischer R. Carcinogenic substances in water and soil. XII. PAH in surface waters. Arch Hyg Bakteriol 1963;146:572.

17. Borneff J, Kunte H. Carcinogenic substances in water and soil. XVII. About the origin and evaluation of PAH in water. Arch Hyg Bakteriol 1965;149:226.

18. Levin W, Wood AW, Yagi H, Dansette PM, Jerina DM, Conney AH. Carcinogenicity of benzo[a]pyrene 4,5-, 7,8-, and 9,10-oxides on mouse skin. Proc Natl Acad Sci USA 1976;73:243.

19. Jerina DM, Daly JW. Oxidation at carbon. In: Parke DV, Smith RL, eds. Drug metabolism. London: Taylor and Francis, Ltd., 1976.

20. Jerina DM, Lehr RE, Yagi H, et al. Mutagenicity of benzo(a)pyrene derivatives and the description of a quantum mechanical model which predicts the ease of carbonium ion formation from diol epoxides. In: DeSerres FJ, Fouts JR, Bend JR, Philpot RM, eds. Vitro metabolic activation and mutagenesis testing. Amsterdam: Elsevier/North-Holland Biomedical, 1976.

21. Pott F, Oberdorster G. Intake and distribution of PAH, In: Grimmer G, ed. Environmental carcinogens: polycyclic aromatic hydrocarbons. Boca Raton, FL: CRC Press, 1983.

22. Rigdon RH, Neal J. Relationship of leukemia to lung and stomach tumors in mice fed benzo(a)pyrene. Proc Soc Exp Biol 1969;130:146.

23. Neff JM. Polycyclic aromatic hydrocarbons in the aquatic environment: sources, fates and biological effects. London: Applied Science Publishers, 1979.

24. Doll R, Fisher REW, Gammon EJ, Gunn W, Hughes GO, Tyrer FH, Wilson W. Mortality of gasworkers with special reference to cancers of the lung and bladder, chronic bronchitis, and pneumoconiosis. Br J Ind Med 1965;22:1–12.

25. Doll R, Vessey MP, Beasley RWR, et al. Mortality of gasworkers—final report of a prospective study. Br J Ind Med 1972;29:394–406.

26. Hammond EC, Selikoff IJ, Lawther PL, Seidman H. Inhalation of benzpyrene and cancer in man. Ann NY Acad Sci 1976;271:116–124.

27. Henry SA, Kennaway NM, Kennaway EL. The incidence of cancer of the bladder and prostate in certain occupations. J Hyg 1931;31:125–137.

28. Kawai M, Amamoto H, Harada K. Epidemiologic study of occupational lung cancer. Arch Environ Health 1967;14:859–864.

29. Kuroda S. Occupational pulmonary cancer of generator gas workers. Ind Med 1937;6:304–306.

30. Mazumdar S, Redmond C, Sollecito W, and Sussman N. An epidemiological study of exposure to coal tar pitch volatiles among coke oven workers. J Air Pollut Cont Assoc 1975;25:382–389.

31. Redmond CK, Ciocco A, Lloyd JW, Rush HW. Long term mortality study of steelworkers. VI. Mortality from malignant neoplasms among coke oven workers. J Occup Med 1972;14:621–629.

32. Redmond CK, Strobino BR, Cypress RH. Cancer experience among coke by-product workers. Ann NY Acad Sci 1976;271:102–115.

33. Reid DD, Buck C. Cancer in coking plant workers. Br J Ind Med 1956;13:265–269.

34. Haddow A, Scott CM, Scott JD. The influence of certain carcinogenic and other hydrocarbons on body growth in the rat. Proc R Soc Lond Ser B 1937;122:477–507.

35. Philips FS, Sternberg SS, Marquardt H. In vivo cytotoxicity of polycyclic hydrocarbons. In: Loomis TA, ed. Pharmacology and the future of man, toxicological problems. Proceedings of the Fifth International Congress on pharmacology, San Francisco, CA, July 23–28, 1972. 1973;2:75–88.

36. Malmgren RA, Bennison BE, McKinley Jr, TW. Reduced antibody titers in mice treated with carcinogenic and cancer chemotherapeutic agents. Proc Soc Exp Biol Med 1952;79:484–488.

37. Yasuhira K. Damage to the thymus and other lymphoid tissues from 3-methylcholanthrene, and subsequent thymoma production, in mice. Cancer Res 1964;24:558–569.

38. Shabad LM. On the so-called MAC (maximal allowable concentrations) for carcinogenic hydrocarbons. Neoplasma 1972;22:459.

39. National Academy of Sciences. Drinking Water and Health. Vol 4. Safe Drinking Water Committee, Board on Toxicology and Environmental Health Hazards, Assembly of Life Sciences, National Research Council. Washington, DC: National Academy Press, 1982.

SOURCES AND FORMS OF URANIUM

Uranium as found in nature, U_{nat}, is a radioactive element that contains three isotopes: 99.27% by weight ^{238}U, 0.72% ^{235}U, and less than 0.01% ^{234}U. U_{nat} is widely distributed in small quantities throughout the earth's crust, in water, and in a variety of minerals. The ^{238}U is the long-lived parent (half-life = 4.5 billion years) of the uranium series (Table 113.1). Minerals and ores of U_{nat} contain daughter products such as thorium-230, radium-226, and many nuclides with shorter half-lives, formed during radioactive decay throughout the series. In the natural state, these nuclides are often present by weight in proportion to their radioactive half-life, a condition termed radioactive equilibrium. Because of its long half-life, ^{238}U itself has a very low level of radioactivity, and its principal hazard comes from chemical toxicity rather than radiation.

A wide variety of chemical forms of uranium may be encountered in industry. Two of the more common ones in the uranium-processing industry are uranium oxide (U_3O_8) and uranium hexafluoride (UF_6). Yellowcake is the semirefined product that comes from milling of uranium ore. It contains over 80% uranium in the form of uranium oxide.

For understanding potential toxic effects, it is useful to classify uranium compounds according to their solubility and transportability between organs of the body and excretion from the body (Table 113.2). Scott divided uranium compounds into three classes: highly transportable (biologic half time of days), moderately (weeks to months), and slightly (months to years) (1). Highly transportable uranium compounds include UF_6, $UO_2(NO_3)_2$, sulfates, and carbonates. In the moderately transportable class are UO_3, UF_4, UCl_4, and nitrates. The slightly transportable compounds are UO_2, U_3O_8, oxides, hydrides, and carbides. Scott also noted that subjecting some compounds to high temperatures tends to decrease their rate of transportability.

Table 113.1. Isotopes Present in Natural Uranium

Isotope	Abundance (%)	Half-Life (Years)
^{238}U	99.3	45×10^8
^{235}U	0.7	8×10^8
^{234}U	0.005	2×10^5

Table 113.2. Transportability of Uranium Compounds

Highly Transportable	Moderately Transportable	Slightly Transportable
UF_6	UF_4	UO_2
UO_3	UO_3	U_3O_8
$UO_2(NO_3)_2$	UO_2	Uranium oxides
UF_4	U_3O_8	Uranium hydrides
Uranium sulfates	Uranium nitrates	Uranium carbides
Uranium carbonates		

URANIUM INDUSTRY

The principal use of uranium is as fuel for the 410 nuclear power reactors in the world (2) and nuclear-powered submarines. The ^{235}U atom fissions into two or three parts, called fission products, when an extra neutron enters its nucleus. This reaction gives off a large amount of energy. Most reactors require a higher content of ^{235}U in the uranium fuel rods than is found in U_{nat}. The uranium industry processes U_{nat} so as to provide appropriate fuel rods. Uranium production is about 43 million kilograms per year (3).

Other industrial uses of uranium are limited. It is used as an intensifier in photography, in dry copying ink, as a colorant in ceramics, and as ballast. Uranium is also used as an additive to dental porcelain to provide a more natural fluorescent appearance. In the past two decades, depleted uranium has been used in armor-piercing bullets for conventional armaments. The term depleted uranium signifies it is essentially all ^{238}U, much of the ^{235}U having been removed.

Because nuclear fuel is the major product of uranium, the uranium fuel manufacturing process is of interest (Fig. 113.1). It consists of mining uranium ore, milling ore to yellowcake, converting yellowcake to UF_6, enriching the ^{235}U in the UF_6, and then fabricating uranium oxide fuel pellets (4). Each of these steps is done at different plant facilities and locations. The process thus involves packaging and shipping of the intermediate products to the next facility.

Uranium ore is mined by normal open-pit and underground mining methods. Raw ores contain from 0.1–1% of U_{nat}. The radiation hazard in uranium mining is principally the inhalation of radon and radon daughter products. Increased incidence of lung cancer in miners has been associated with radiation from radon and radon daughters in the series and not uranium itself. Likewise, most external gamma radiation in uranium mines comes from the various radionuclides associated with the uranium series rather than uranium itself. Dust hazard in uranium mines is about the same as in other hard rock mines.

Inhalation of airborne uranium compounds is the main pathway for occupational exposure in milling. The materials inhaled are ore dust in crushing operations and yellowcake dust in drying and packaging.

Production of the volatile UF_6 involves sampling and preparing the yellowcake feed, converting it to fluoride, and purifying the product. Inhalation of dusts occur mainly in emptying and refilling yellowcake drums, removing ash waste after the purification phase, and performing maintenance jobs throughout the facilities. The dust may contain yellowcake, uranium daughters, UF_4, UO_2, UO_3, and uranyl fluoride (UO_2F_2). The product, UF_6, if released in air reacts with moisture to form UO_2F_2 and hydrofluoric acid (HF). Inhalation of HF has been a major toxic hazard in accidental exposures.

In the United States, enrichment of the ^{235}U in UF_6 has been done by a gaseous diffusion process at one of three Department of Energy facilities. The final product contains from 0.9% up

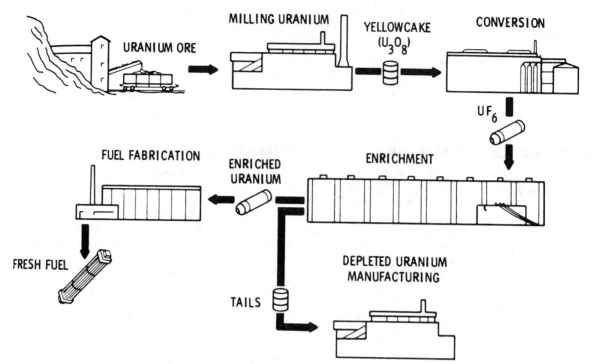

Figure 113.1. Uranium fuel manufacturing.

to about 5% ^{235}U for commercial use and greater than 90% for military reactors and research uses. Exposures may occur during sampling operations, during maintenance procedures, or when loading UF$_6$ in or taking product out of the process.

Uranium fuel fabrication consists of converting enriched UF$_6$ to uranium dioxide powder, which is used to produce U pellets. The pellets are placed into the fuel pins or rods used in nuclear reactors. Inhalation of gases or dusts is the major exposure potential in fuel fabrication.

ABSORPTION AND METABOLISM

As described above, inhalation of uranium particles is the most common route of occupational exposure. Uptake can occur by ingestion, but the uptake via the human gastrointestinal tract is low; the best value for drinking water is judged to be 1.4% of the soluble uranium present (5). Soluble uranium compounds are also absorbed through skin. In experimental animals, sufficient amounts could be absorbed through skin to cause severe uranium poisoning and death (6). Some uranium compounds cause mild to moderate skin irritation.

Particle size and chemical solubility in body fluids determine the absorption rate of uranium particles from the lung. A general idea of this uptake rate, redistribution to other organs, and excretion in urine can be obtained from the compound classification by transportability described above. Longterm inhalation experiments with UO$_2$ in dogs showed a lung clearance half-time of 340 days (6). In humans, biologic half-times for uranium oxide exposures have been estimated to be as long as 1470 days (7). On average, however, an overall biologic half-time of about 15 days is commonly cited (8), but this value obviously varies with different compounds. For example, after inhaling UF$_6$ particles, humans during the first day excrete in urine about 73% of the solubilized uranium from the lung with a biological half-time of about four hours and another 10%

with a half-time of 1.3 days (9). In a second stage of slower excretion, a biologic half-time of about 6 days is estimated by the second day or later.

Uranium once absorbed into the blood is principally passed through the kidney. From 50% to over 80% of intravenously administered U was excreted in urine within 24 hours in most people (10). From excretion data after an accidental inhalation exposure of soluble uranium particles, Chalabreysse (11) estimated that about 80% of the absorbed uranium was excreted during the first 24 hours. In reviewing the literature, Durbin (12) concludes that about 70% of uranium taken up in the blood is excreted in the urine during the first day. A significant percentage of uranium retained in the body is deposited in the kidney. Dog and rat experiments indicate about 5–10% of the absorbed dose is present in the kidneys is eliminated with a half-time of 2.2 days, and the rest is eliminated with a half-time of 103 days (14).

Very little U is present in feces, less than 0.1% to about 0.3% of intravenous doses administered in humans (10). After inhalation, particles brought out of the lung by mucociliary clearance will be swallowed to add to the quantity of uranium found in feces.

Deposition in bone is the most important longterm storage site in the body for uranium introduced in soluble form. The process of deposition by ionic exchange processes and involving the entire bone volume rather than surfaces was described by Neuman in 1953 (15). Donoghue et al. (16) estimated that uranium deposited in bone accounted for about 85% of that absorbed and metabolized. Some portion of this deposition has a very long biologic half time; the International Commission on Radiological Protection (17) describes a biokinetic model for uranium in bone in which fractions of 0.2 and 0.023 are transferred to mineral bone and retained there with half-times of 20 and 5000 days, respectively.

For further details on metabolic models, the reader is referred to Durbin's comprehensive review (12), which describes the pathways and transfer rates of soluble uranium in the body.

HEALTH EFFECTS AND CLINICAL MANAGEMENT

Acute Toxicity

Biologic hazard from uranium exposures may occur from chemical toxicity, radiation dose, or both. This fact, together with the complex chemical forms, isotopic mixtures, and metabolic pathways, gives rise to an interesting toxicologic puzzle, but it can be greatly simplified for clinical management. For acute toxicity, chemical toxicity of the kidney is clearly the most important effect from soluble forms of uranium (18).

About 60% of uranium absorbed into the blood is transported in the form of a bicarbonate complex and 40% is bound to plasma proteins. The uranyl-bicarbonate complex is filtered out of the blood by the renal glomerulus and passed into the tubules. The pH of urine decreases in the tubules, resulting in dissociation of the complex and release of the reactive uranyl ion. Nephrotoxicity results primarily from damage to the tubular epithelium, which allows leakage of glucose, protein, amino acids, and enzymes into the urine. In high doses, above 6 milligrams uranium per kilogram, glomerular damage may also occur with decreased renal blood flow and a decreased glomerular filtration rate.

The kidney responds to toxic levels of uranium within 24–48 hours after exposure. The changes become progressively more severe over about a 5-day period. The damaged tubular epithelium regenerates quickly as the uranium concentration is reduced.

Large accidental intakes of U_{nat} in industrial accidents are summarized by Hursh and Spoor (10). In more than 40 workers with acute U exposures, the estimated systemic uptakes of uranium were mostly from about 1–3 milligrams total. One case had an estimated uptake in excess of 15 milligrams. Initial uranium excretion rates in urine ranged from about 0.15 to over 6 mg/l. None of the workers apparently sustained permanent injury resulting from internal exposure to uranium.

Effects of UF_6 exposures were impressively displayed in a 1944 accident involving 21 workers (19). One individual died in 15 minutes due to severe steam burns and the effects of UF_6 and its degradation products, hydrogen fluoride and uranium oxyfluoride. Another worker died 70 minutes after exposure due to progressive respiratory distress. Most of the other 14 persons requiring hospitalization had corrosive irritation of the eyes, skin, and respiratory tract, but were well enough to be released in 48 hours. Three more seriously exposed individuals were retained for observation from 10–14 days due to pulmonary edema and nephrotoxicity. The peak urine uranium excretion values ranged from 0.15–0.5 mg/l. All three persons had some urine volume suppression for 3 days and had albumin, red cells, and casts in their urine. One individual had mild elevation of blood urea and nonprotein nitrogen for 3 weeks after the accident. Two of the three persons with acute toxicity were examined 38 years later (20). No physical changes related to their exposure and no uranium deposition were detected. An observation from these cases and other exposed workers suggests that the pulmonary edema may have slowed the absorption of uranium from the lungs and lengthened its biologic half-life (9, 20). Human data on acute poisoning from uranium are not adequate enough to estimate an LD_{50} dose. System dose of 0.1–0.3 mg/kg of soluble uranium have not produced human mortality. The animal (dog, rat) LD_{50} dose is about 1–2 mg/kg (21).

Chronic and Longterm Toxic Effects

The search for acute and chronic effects from uranium in animals and humans spans a long history starting in 1824. This history is brilliantly recorded by Hodge (22). The early studies of humans were made from about 1860 into the early 1900s, during which time uranium was administered as a therapeutic agent for diabetes and other diseases. Toxic effects recorded were neither consistent nor specific.

Exposure conditions in uranium work areas during the early 1940s were dusty and dirty. Stannard (23) indicates that they were "some of the worst conditions of exposure with the largest number of persons exposed of any section of the Atomic Bomb Project." For a decade after World War II, potential occupational exposures increased markedly with expansion of the industry. Fortunately, industrial hygiene controls also improved. Now, after some 40 years of operations of the nuclear industry, the evidence for chronic effects in workers is still not consistent or specific. The chief potential effects are considered to be chronic effects on the kidney for soluble compounds and radiogenic lung cancer for inhaled particles with low solubility in body fluids. Radiogenic bone cancer is also a concern for soluble compounds of enriched uranium.

The uranium toxicity in the kidney is the basis for the limits for occupational exposure to soluble unenriched uranium (24). Only a few studies on renal tubular dysfunction in chronically exposed workers have been performed. Dounce et al (25) reported increased tubular enzyme catalase in urine of 46 exposed chemical workers, but the results were not controlled for differences in urine concentration. Clarkson and Kench (26) measured increased excretion of total amino-nitrogen and some individual amino acids in 18 exposed workers. Thun et al (27) found low level beta-2-microglobulinuria and aminoaciduria in 39 uranium mill workers. The clinical significance of these findings, if any, is unclear. The potent uranium nephrotoxicity demonstrated in animal experiments has not resulted in identified clinical problems in workers with chronic occupational exposures.

Inhalation of poorly solubilized uranium particles results in a radiologic risk to the lung. Other target organs for radiation effects are tracheobronchial lymph nodes, bone, bone marrow, and kidney. It has generally been estimated that the radiation risk does not exceed the chemical nephrotoxicity for soluble uranium until the enrichment is 5–8% by weight ^{235}U, but the relative risk between chemical and radiation risks continues an open question (23, 24, 28).

Results of epidemiologic studies of workers (29–37) have been variable and have not resolved the issue between chemical and radiation risk. Checkoway et al. found a slight excess of lung cancer in white male employees from a facility that produces enriched uranium (35). A radiation dose-response relationship was found for lung cancer, but the rate ratios were imprecise due to the small number of cases in the analysis. Also the influence of smoking could not be taken into account. Cookfair et al. found increased relative risk for lung cancer in workers with a cumulative lung dose of 20 rads or more from inhaled uranium, but only for those workers who were over the age of 45 when first exposed (33). The other studies have not demonstrated increased risks of lung cancer due to uranium.

Waxweiler et al. (34) found a significant excess risk for non-malignant respiratory disease in uranium mill workers.

Archer (30, 32) found a significant excess of lymphatic and hematopoietic tissue cancers other than leukemia (four cases observed, one expected) in a preliminary study of uranium mill workers. Thus far, this finding has not been confirmed by other studies.

None of these studies has reported a significant excess risk of kidney disease. Waxweiler et al. (34) observed six cases of chronic nephritis deaths compared with an expected 3.6 cases, which was not a statistically significant increase.

In an excellent review of human studies, the BIER IV Committee of the National Academy of Sciences, National Research Council, found that "there is little convincing epidemiological evidence that serious renal disease has occurred in human populations as a result of chronic low-level exposure nor of increased rates of malignant tumors (21)." Considering the exposure conditions in the industry during and after World War II, one might consider this conclusion as reassuring that the hazards of uranium have not been underestimated. Under current industrial hygiene and radiation protection standards and practice, the health risks from uranium in industry should be extremely low.

MANAGEMENT OF TOXICITY

No specific clinical findings are ordinarily associated with uranium exposure. In the exceptional accidental inhalation of high concentrations of uranium hexaflouride, signs and symptoms of pulmonary edema from hydrogen fluoride will predominate the clinical course. Significant irritation of the eyes and skin from the fluoride ion may also be present after such exposure.

Monitoring of accidental uranium exposures and its effects on the kidney are done by measurement of the uranium excreted in the urine and abnormalities in the clinical urinalyses. Glucose and albumin in urine are among the most sensitive indicators of kidney damage (18). Henge-Napoli et al. have found urinary excretion of gamma-glutamyltransferase to be the most sensitive indicator (38). These various indicators of renal injury occur in a few hours after dose levels at and above 0.1 milligram of uranium per kilogram (18).

Daily urine samples should be collected after large accidental exposures (18, 39) and continued for at least 2 weeks. It is advantageous to collect 24-hour urine samples whenever possible. These samples will be used for measuring uranium excretion and for clinical urinalysis. Bacterial degradation of glucose and other constituents of urine can be prevented by the addition of sodium azide to the sample or by immediate cooling of the sample to 5°C. If analysis for amino acids or enzymes are to be done later, freezing the sample at −40°C is advisable. Quantitative measurement of glucose and protein in the urine are preferable to the usual qualitative analyses. Quantitative measurement of glucose and protein in the serum should also be performed. Serum creatinine and creatinine clearance studies are needed to assess glomerular function. Clearance tests may underestimate filtration rate if tubular injury is present.

The many methods used to measure uranium in urine and other sample matrices were extensively reviewed recently by Wessman (40). Fluorometry is the most widely used method in monitoring and bioassay, but it is the most inaccurate and least reliable method due to interferences. Mass spectrometry and alpha spectrometry are the most accurate and reliable methods and produce the most isotopic information.

Direct or in vivo measurements over the chest are often superior to urine excretion data in evaluating depositions and this is the best method available to assess the inhalation of insoluble material. Palmer (41) described the performance of high purity germanium planar detectors used in chest counting. The sensitivity for a 1-hour count is about 1.6 milligrams of U_{nat} at 99% confidence level. Sensitivity for phoswich detectors is about 4 milligrams and for NaI(Tl) detectors is somewhat less, about 8 milligrams. The sensitivity will vary with the isotopic mixture of uranium to be counted, being better with material enriched with ^{235}U and ^{234}U.

For acute uranium nephrotoxicity, oral doses or infusions of sodium bicarbonate are administered to maintain an alkaline urine (39, 42), which should be monitored frequently with pH measurements. Alkaline urine prevents dissociation of the uranium-bicarbonate complex and thus protects the renal tubular epithelium from exposure to the reactive uranyl ion. Forcing fluids to increase urinary output is desirable.

The use of chelation drugs for acute uranium exposures, an area of controversy in the literature, was recently reviewed by Lincoln and Voelz (39). Limited animal research indicates that the LD_{50} can be raised by a factor of two to three through the immediate administration of chelating drugs, such as calcium disodium ethylenediaminetetraacetic acid ($CaNa_2$ EDTA) and diethylenetriamine pentaacetic acid (DTPA) (44, 45). Chelation must begin within 4 hours of the exposure to be effective and is most effective if given within a few minutes of the exposure. Others have advised against the use of chelation because precipitation of uranium in the kidney may cause additional damage, although support for this concern has not been presented. Recent Soviet research (46) indicates that chelating agents can significantly reduce the risk of acute uranium injury to kidneys. A Soviet drug preparation, called trimephacin, was found to be more effective than DTPA in their studies and is adopted in the Soviet Union as an antidote for uranium intoxication. No cases of uranium exposure have been reported as being treated with chelation in the western world. The current Investigational New Drug agreement with the U.S. Food and Drug Administration for the use of DTPA does not include uranium on the list of radionuclides approved for treatment. The use of chelating agents seems quite improbable for acute uranium exposures, especially given the need for immediate administration. Its place, if there is one, is in the event of an exposure so high that it is judged to be life-threatening.

EXPOSURE STANDARDS

Current threshold limit values for U_{nat} exposures to insoluble compounds is 0.2 mg/m^3 for an 8-hour time weighted average (TWA) and 0.6 mg/m^3 for a 15-minute shortterm exposure limit. For soluble uranium compounds, the 8-hour TWA limit is 0.05 mg/m^3. For occupational emergency use, a recent review in the United Kingdom (24) recommended emergency standards of 1, 2, and 3 mg/m^3 for 10, 30, and 60-minute exposures respectively.

REFERENCES

1. Scott LM. Environmental monitoring and personnel protection in uranium processing. In: Hodge HC, Stannard JN, Hursh JB, eds. Uranium-plutonium-transplutonic elements. New York: Springer-Verlag, 1973:271–306.
2. Anonymous. World list of nuclear power plants. Nuclear News 1988;69–88.

3. Walton H. Uranium industry annual 1987 preliminary data. Presentation to the U.S. Council for Energy Awareness Fuel cycle 88 conference, April 1988.

4. Stoetzel GA, Moore RH, Fisher DR, Quilici DG, McCormack WD, Hoenes GR. Occupational exposures to uranium: processes, hazards and regulations. Report PNL-3341 USUR-01, Springfield, VA: National and Technical Information Service, 1981.

5. Wrenn ME, Durbin PW, Howard B, et al. Metabolism of ingested U and RA. Health Phys, 1985;48:601–633.

6. Yulie CL. Animal experiments. In: Hodge HC, Stannard JN, Hursh JB, eds. Uranium-plutonium-transplutonic elements. New York: Springer-Verlag, 1973:165–196.

7. West CM, Scott LM. Uranium cases showing long chest burden retention—an update. Health Phys 1969;17:781.

8. National Council on Radiation Protection and Measurements. Management of persons accidentally contaminated with radionuclides. NCRP Report 65. Washington, DC: NCRP Publications, 1980.

9. Beau PG, Chalabreysse J. Knowledge gained from bioassay data on some metabolic and toxicological features of uranium hexafluoride and of its degradation products. Radiat Protect Dos 1989;26:107–112.

10. Hursh JB, Spoor NL. Data on man. In: Hodge HC, Stannard JN, Hursh JB, eds. Uranium-plutonium-transplutonic elements. New York: Springer-Verlag, 1973:197–239.

11. Chalabreysse J. Etudes et resultats d'examens effectues a la suite d'une inhalaton de composess dits solubles d-uranium naturel. Radioprot 1970;5:305–310.

12. Durbin PW. Metabolic models for uranium. In: Biokinetics and analysis of uranium in man. F1-F65. US Uranium Registry report USUR-05-HEHF-47. Springfield, VA: National Technical Information Service, 1984.

13. Morrow PE, Leach LJ, Smith FA, et al. Acute effects of inhalation exposure to uranium hexafluoride and patterns of deposition. Report NUREG/CR-1045. Springfield, VA: National Technical Information Service, 1980.

14. Wrenn ME, Lipsztein J, Bertelli L. Pharmacokinetic models relevant to toxicity and metabolism for uranium in humans and animals. Radiat Protect Dos 1989;26:243–248.

15. Neuman WF, Tishkoff GH. The deposition of uranium in bone. Chapt 24 in: Voegtlin C, Hodge HC. Pharmacology and toxicology of uranium compounds. National Nuclear Energy Series. New York: McGraw-Hill, 1953:1911–1991.

16. Donoghue JK, Dyson ED, Hislop JS, Leach AM, Spoor NL. Human exposure to natural uranium: a case history and analytical results from some postmortem tissues. Br J Ind Med 1972;29:81–89.

17. International Commission on Radiological Protection. Individual monitoring for intakes of radionuclides by workers: design and interpretation. ICRP Publication 54. Annals of ICRP 1988;19:209–236.

18. Diamond GL. Biological consequences of exposure to soluble forms of natural uranium. Radiat Protect Dos 1989;26:23–33.

19. Howland JW. Studies in human exposure to uranium compounds. In: Pharmacology and toxicology of uranium compounds. Vol 2. New York: McGraw-Hill 1949:993–1017.

20. Moore RH, Kathren RL. A World War II uranium hexafluoride inhalation event with pulmonary implications for today. J Occup Med 1985;27:753–756.

21. National Academy of Science/National Research Council. Uranium. Chapter 6 In: Health risks of radon and other internally deposited alpha-emitters. BEIR-IV, Committee on the Biological Effects of Ionizing Radiation. Washington, DC: National Academy Press, 1988:276–302, at 297.

22. Hodge HC. A history of uranium poisoning (1824–1942). Chap 1 in: Hodge HC, Stannard JN, Hursh JB, eds. Uranium-plutonium-transplutonic elements. New York: Springer-Verlag, 1973:5–68.

23. Stannard JN. Uranium and man. In: Biokinetics and analysis of uranium in man. D1-D26. US Uranium Registry report USUR-05 HEHF-47. Springfield, Va: National Technical Information Service, 1984, at D3.

24. Spoor NL, Harrison NT. Emergency exposure levels for natural uranium. National Radiographical Protection Board report NRPB-R1111, Harwell, England, NRPB, 1980. 15 p.

25. Dounce AL, Roberts E, Wills JH. Catalasuria as a sensitive test for uranium poisoning. In: Voegtlin C, Hodge HC, ed. Pharmacology and toxicology of uranium compounds. Vol 1. New York: McGraw-Hill, 1949:889–950.

26. Clarkson TW, Kench JE. Urinary excretion of amino acids by men absorbinig heavy metals. Biochem J 1952;62:361–271.

27. Thun MJ, Baker DB, Steenland K, Smith AB, Halperin W, Berl T. Renal toxicity in uranium mill workers. Scand J Work Environ Health 1985;11:83–90.

28. Morrow PE. Biokinetics and toxicology of uranium. In Biokinetics and analysis of uranium in man. D1-E27. US Uranium Registry report USUR-05 HEHF-47. Springfield, VA: National Technical Information Service, 1984.

29. Wagoner JK, Archer VE, Carroll BE, et al. Cancer mortality patterns amongst U.S. uranium miners and millers, 1950 through 1962. J Natl Cancer Inst 1964;32:787–801.

30. Archer VE, Wagoner JK, Lundin FE. Cancer mortality among uranium mill workers. J Occup Med 1973;15;11–14.

31. Poledak AP, Frome EL. Mortality among men employed between 1943 and 1947 at a uranium processing plant. J Occup Med 1981;23;169–178.

32. Archer VE. Health concerns in uranium mining and milling. J Occup Med 1981;23:502–505.

33. Cookfair DL, Beck WL, Shy C, Lushbaugh CC, Sowder CL. Lung cancer among workers at a uranium processing plant. In: Epidemiology applied to health physics. CONF-830101. Springfield, VA: National Technical Information Service, 1983:398–406.

34. Waxweiler JK, Archer VE, Roscoe RJ, Watanabe A, Thun MJ. Mortality patterns among a retrospective cohort of uranium mill workers. In: Epidemiology applied to health physics. CONF-830101. Springfield, VA: National Technical Information Service, 1983:428–435.

35. Checkoway H, Pearce N, Crawford-Brown DJ, Cragle DL. Radiation doses and cause-specific mortality among workers at a nuclear materials fabrication plant. Am J Epidemiol 1988;127:255–266.

36. Dupree EA, Cragle DL, McLain RW, et al. Mortality among workers at a uranium processing facility, the Linde Air Products Company ceramics plant, 1943–1949. Scand J Work Environ Health 1987;13:100–107.

37. Burr WW. Human experience and epidemiology. In: Biokinetics and analysis of uranium in man. H1-H21. US Uranium Registry report USUR-05 HEHF-47. Springfield VA: National Technical Information Service, 1984.

38. Henge-Napoli MH, Rongier E, Ansoborlo E, Chalabreysse J. Comparison of the in vitro and in vivo dissolution rates of two diuranates and research on an early urinary indicator of renal failure in humans and animals poisoned with uranium. Radiat Protect Dos 1989;26:113–117.

39. Lincoln TA, Voelz GL. Management of persons accidentally exposed to uranium compounds. In: The medical basis for radiation preparedness II. Clinical experience and follow-up since 1979. Ricks R.C, Fry, S.A, eds. New York, NY: Elsevier, 1990:221–230.

40. Wessman RA. An overview of the radiochemical analysis of uranium. In: Biokinetics and analysis of uranium in man. JA-J57. US Uranium Registry report USUR-05 HEHF-47. Springfield, VA: National Technical Information Service, 1984.

41. Palmer HE. In vivo counting of uranium. In: Biokinetics and analysis of uranium in man. I1-I29. US Uranium Registry report USUR-05 HEHF-47. Springfield, VA: National Technical Information Service, 1984.

42. MacNider WDB. The inhibition of the toxicity of uranium nitrate by sodium carbonate, and the protection of the kidney acutely nephropathic from uranium from the toxic action of an anesthetic by sodium carbonate. J Exp Med 1916;23:171–187.

43. Catsch A. Die Wirkung einger Chelatbidner auf die akute Toxicitat von Uranylnitrat. Klin Wachr 1959;37:657–666.

44. Catsch A. Radioactive metal mobilization in medicine. Springfield, IL: Charles C Thomas, 1964:9,57,105–106.

45. Ivannikov AT. On medicative application of complexing agents in the case of uranium intoxication. Central Scientific Inst. of Information and Technical Research on Nuclear Science and Technology. Moscow: TsNIIatominform. 1987:3–15.

Carbon Monoxide

Donna L. Seger, M.D.
Larry Welch, Ed.D.

SOURCES OF EXPOSURE

The optimal setting for carbon monoxide (CO) exposure is a place where fuel is being burned and ventilation is insufficient. Fires with associated smoke inhalation and motor vehicle exhaust are the two most common sources of CO poisonings that result in fatalities. CO or asphyxia causes 80% of the deaths due to smoke inhalation. Due to the difficulty in diagnosing CO intoxication, the number of deaths caused by CO is probably grossly underestimated (1–3).

Atmospheric CO varies in urban areas and depends on weather conditions and individual activity. Concentrations may vary from 1 ppm in rural areas to 140 ppm in urban areas with heavy traffic. The majority of atmospheric CO (approximately 60%) comes from vehicular fuel combustion (diesel fumes produce very little CO). U.S. emission standards are met when automobile exhaust contains as much as 8% CO. Automobiles currently produce 0.37 kilograms of CO for each mile traveled. Other vehicles, such as ice-surfacing machines and propane-powered vehicles such as trucks and forklifts, also produce CO. Lesser amounts come from industrial processes such as coke ovens and solid waste incineration. Smoke from both humanmade and forest fires can contain up to 10% CO. Fuels for home use, such as oil-powered furnaces and natural gas used in furnaces, space heaters, ovens, and fireplaces, add minimally to atmospheric CO but may be a major risk for CO poisoning in the event of a malfunction. Atmospheric CO is removed by migration to the upper atmosphere, oxidation to carbon dioxide, and reduction to methane by microorganisms (2, 4—6).

Workers in the steel industry, miners, auto mechanics, and those in warehouse storage and loading facilities may be exposed to high concentrations of CO. Ventilation of these areas may be the determining factor in toxicity. Malfunctioning equipment may also be responsible for exposure to high levels of CO. Occupational Safety and Health Administration (OSHA) guidelines limit exposure to no more than 50 ppm over an 8-hour time-weighted average. Firefighters also run the occupational hazard of CO exposure (5, 7).

People in houses with furnaces that do not have adequate venting or use fuels that involve carbon combustion (e.g., indoor burning of charcoal briquettes or Sterno) may be poisoned by CO. Proper oxygenation is required to prevent incomplete combustion of natural gas. A danger of natural gas is that irritating vapors do not occur when combustion is incomplete and high levels of CO are present (5, 7).

CO fatalities associated with suicide are likely to be linked to exposure to automobile exhaust. In a closed garage, lethal CO concentrations may be present in less than 10 minutes. Passengers in motor vehicles may be exposed to CO fumes entering the driving cabin through rusted floor boards (5, 7).

Physiologic CO occurs from endogenous degradation of hemoglobin and nonhemoglobin heme leading to carboxyhemoglobin levels of 0.5% in normal individuals. These levels may be elevated to 4–6% in patients with acute hemolytic anemia. Cigarette smoking may also lead to levels of 10–18%. Secondary smoke to which nonsmokers are exposed contains more than twice the amount of CO as directly inhaled smoke (2, 5).

Methylene chloride (dichloromethane), a simple halogenated hydrocarbon, is found in industrial products such as paint strippers, insecticides and other fumigants, aerosol propellants, and Christmas tree bubble lights. It is inhaled by persons using products containing the ingredient, with up to 75% of the vapor absorbed through normal respiration. It is then slowly metabolized to carbon dioxide (70%) and CO (30%). It is highly lipid soluble and concentrates in the liver and kidneys. Slow release from adipose results in prolonged availability to the liver and kidneys (1). Individuals with daily exposure may be symptomatic initially, but become asymptomatic as exposure continues. The National Institute of Occupational Safety and Health (NIOSH) recommendation is 100 ppm for methylene chloride. Uncontrolled exposures by individuals working with paint strippers may be fatal (7, 8).

MECHANISM OF TOXICITY

Carbon monoxide is a tasteless, colorless, odorless gas that is rapidly absorbed by the lungs. This gas rapidly diffuses across alveolar-capillary membranes and attaches to hemoglobin with an affinity 250 times greater than that of oxygen. As CO concentrations increase, the number of hemoglobin sites available for oxygen binding decrease. Normally, a decreased number of oxygen-hemoglobin binding sites (e.g., simple anemia) causes oxygen to be released more freely in an attempt to maintain tissue oxygenation. The oxyhemoglobin curve is shifted to the right. Although CO causes a functional anemia, an allosteric change in the oxyhemoglobin complex causes an increased affinity of oxygen, and the oxyhemoglobin dissociation curve is shifted to the left. Tissue oxygenation is decreased and tissue hypoxia results in anaerobic metabolism and lactic acidosis. Anaerobic metabolism yields acidosis, which shifts the oxyhemoglobin dissociation curve back to the right in an attempt to maintain tissue oxygenation.

CO uptake is determined by the concentration of CO in the inspired air, the ventilatory rate, and the duration of the CO exposure. CO is excreted by the lungs at a rate dependent on the patient's minute volume. CO elimination is complex, and elimination time appears to depend on length of exposure, and whether the exposure was continuous or discontinuous.

The half-life of carboxyhemoglobin (Cohgb) is about 4.5 hours with room air oxygen concentrations (21%) at 1 atmosphere of pressure. Increasing the atmospheric pressure with 100% oxygen will reduce the half-life. If 100% oxygen is delivered at 3 atmospheres of pressure, the half-life is reduced to 23 minutes. These values have individual variation.

Approximately 10–115% of total body CO is bound to extravascular proteins such as myoglobin, cytochrome oxidase, cytochrome P-450, catalases, and peroxidases. CO competes with oxygen for enzyme binding sites on the cytochrome chain. CO inhibits cytochrome oxidase in vitro and may block the respiratory chain in vivo, prolonging cellular hypoxia. However, the affinity of CO for cytochrome oxidase is much lower than the affinity of oxygen for cytochrome oxidase. In fact, oxygen's affinity for cytochrome A3 is nine times that of CO. CO may not compete with oxygen for cytochrome oxidase at high Cohgb concentrations. However, under hypoxic conditions, CO binding to proteins increases. When PaO_2 drops below 40 torr, up to 40% of intravascular CO shifts into muscle, and binding of CO to cytochrome oxidase increases. The rates of dissociation from cytochrome oxidase is slow, raising the possibility that CO may cause a prolonged adverse effect despite transient hypoxia. Cellular compensations may include reducing electron flow via uninhibited cytochrome molecules (9, 11).

The physiologic significance of this extravascular protein binding and cellular impairment has led to much controversy regarding the etiology of CO toxicity, i.e., is CO toxicity simply due to hypoxia or is there also a direct cellular toxicity?

Cytochrome binding by CO causing cellular toxicity has been proposed as the primary mechanism of CO toxicity. Opposing opinions contend that CO toxicity can be explained by hypoxia, hypotension induced by hypoxia, and CO binding to cardiac myoglobin which depresses myocardium. Lack of correlation between Cohgb levels and clinical course may be due to postanoxic encephalopathy (10, 12).

As early as 1926, research data suggested that oxygenation under hyperbaric conditions did not prevent CO toxicity. Further support for cellular toxicity was presented in 1944 when changes in pyruvate and lactate metabolism were demonstrated in dogs chronically poisoned with low levels of CO. Conflicting data were presented in 1951 by the discovery that the cytochrome A3 oxidase system has nine times the affinity for oxygen as opposed to CO in isolated beef heart. Toxic concentrations of CO would not result in CO preferentially combining with cytochrome oxidase. In 1976, Goldbaum transfused dogs with red cells highly saturated with CO to produce Cohgb levels of 60% to 70%. This high level produced no symptoms. Direct inhalation of CO in control animals resulted in death with Cohgb levels of 57% to 64%. Goldbaum concluded that dissolved CO which freely enters tissues was the primary mechanism of toxicity. However, vital signs and arterial blood gases were not monitored and autopsies were not performed. Therefore, tissue hypoxia and hypotension secondary to CO binding with cardiac myoglobin may explain the results. Goldbaum's conclusions were refuted when a study in which animals whose blood was replaced by perfluorocarbon emulsions (capable of carrying large quantities of oxygen) survived indefinitely despite CO administration (12–14).

Neuropathologic changes that occur as a result of CO exposure add support to the theory that hypoxia, hypotension, and decreased myocardial performance are the primary causes of toxicity.

Neuropathologically, CO induces parenchymal necrosis in vulnerable areas of cerebral gray matter. Bilateral necrosis of the globus pallidus is the hallmark of CO poisoning, but it should be noted that this lesion occurs in other hypoxic-is-

chemic settings as well. The globus pallidus lies within an arterial border zone territory which is susceptible to hypoxia and ischemia during inadequate perfusion. Other areas that may be affected are cerebral cortex, hippocampus, cerebellum, and substantia nigra (1, 10).

Lesions of the cerebral white matter are frequently found in patients who suffer a delayed neuropsychiatric syndrome. Research data reveal that white matter pathology occurs when ischemia is superimposed on hypoxia and does not occur due to hypoxia alone. Usually, hypoxia induces cerebral vasodilatation, which increases cerebral perfusion. However, if hypotension occurs concurrently, the increase in cerebral perfusion is prevented. Additionally, oligemia hinders delivery of glucose and interferes with the removal of metabolic waste. Ischemia is far more damaging to the central nervous system (CNS) than pure hypoxia (1, 10). The controversy will continue until further research delineates the role of hypoxia versus cellular toxicity.

DIAGNOSIS AND EVALUATION OF POISONING

Originally, diagnosis was based on the presence of elevated Cohgb which quantitates the percentage of hemoglobin in the blood that is bound to CO. The presumption prevailed that Cohgb levels correlated with clinical severity of intoxication. Although an elevated Cohgb provides and unequivocal diagnosis of exposure, it does not correlate with tissue level of CO and is not always a reliable indicator of the severity of intoxication. Although an elevated Cohgb provides an unequivocal diagnosis of exposure, it does not correlate with tissue level of CO and is not always a reliable indicator of the severity of the poisoning. Conversely, an insignificant Cohgb level may be present in severe poisoning. Carboxyhemoglobin levels may be misleading for a number of reasons. Carboxyhemoglobin levels do not reflect the length of time of exposure or the peak Cohgb level, both of which may be a factor in outcome. Nor do these serum levels reflect delay between CO exposure and blood sampling or the interim use of supplemental oxygen, both of which will yield a falsely reassuring decreased Cohgb serum level. Age, metabolic rate, pulmonary function, and physical activity also affect the Cohgb level. Various tables have related Cohgb serum levels to signs and symptoms of presentation. Most tables report that patients with Cohgb levels up to 20% may develop headache and dyspnea on exertion. At levels of 30–40%, ataxia and dizziness may develop, and at levels greater than 50%, syncope, seizures, and coma may occur. However, recent reports have clearly determined that serum Cohgb levels may have no correlation with the severity of the acute poisoning or the potential for delayed contraindications. Therefore, the diagnosis of CO poisoning cannot be made based solely on CO levels. In patients with initial high Cohgb levels, levels should be obtained every 1–2 hours to determine progressive decreases. These blood samples may be nonclotted venous blood, thus eliminating the need for arterial punctures. Decreasing levels do not reflect prognosis or outcome (6, 7, 14–16).

Laboratory findings may be deceptively normal even in severe CO intoxications. Since arterial oxygen pressure (P_aO_2) is a measure of oxygen dissolved in plasma, it is not affected by changes in hemoglobin saturation. Therefore P_aO_2 may be normal, while hemoglobin saturation is decreased. Lactic acid levels should be obtained as metabolic acidosis due to the presence of lactic acid may be present in severe poisonings. Other tests that may be elevated include creatine kinase, lactate dehydrogenase, alanine transferase, aspartate transferase, and glucose (6, 7, 14–16).

Computerized tomography (CT) of the brain, electroencephalogram (EEG), and magnetic resonance imaging (MRI) may show abnormalities in the early stages of the poisoning. The hallmark of CO target organ toxicity is bilateral low density lesions of the globus pallidus demonstrated on the CT scan. This lesion is seen in 50% of patients with severe poisonings—a fact that may be related to the lack of sensitivity of the CT. Patients with changes in the gray matter (e.g., basal ganglia) may have good recovery, whereas lesions in the white matter are prognostic for the development of the delayed neuropsychiatric syndrome. MRI of the brain is superior to CT, but may not be as readily available. Visual evoked potentials may be more sensitive than EEG. There may be a lag period of 2–3 days before either CT or MRI are positive (2, 7, 9, 10, 17–19). Due to myocardial sensitivity to CO, an electrocardiogram should be obtained in any potentially significant poisoning and in all patients with a history of coronary artery disease (1, 7).

Infants, the elderly, and patients with coronary artery disease, anemia, and lung disease are at the greatest risk of toxicity from exposure to CO. Unfortunately, a wide spectrum of clinical abnormalities arises from CO intoxication, none of which are pathognomonic for this poisoning. Therefore, diagnosis is difficult for this insidious poisoning which can mimic a variety of illnesses (20).

The diagnosis may be suggested by the circumstances that caused the patient to seek medical attention. CO poisoning must be considered in patients with smoke inhalation or who were in a closed space during a fire, as well as patients who present with flu-like illness during the winter (especially if multiple members of the same family have similar complaints). A thorough environmental history with special attention to home heating materials and recreational activity (such as ice skating) is mandatory to make the diagnosis (15, 16, 20).

The acute and chronic effects of CO can mimic virtually any neurologic or psychiatric illness. Symptoms resembling multiple sclerosis, parkinsonism, Korsakoff's amnestic syndrome, bipolar disorder, schizophrenia, and hysterical conversion reaction have been reported. Headache, fatigue, malaise, nausea, vomiting, or diarrhea may be the only complaints on presentation. Patients may complain of chest pain, and although tachycardia and tachypnea are frequently present, patients rarely complain of respiratory distress (9, 21).

Although the person with severe CO intoxication may have a completely normal physical exam, abnormalities of basal ganglia function are characteristic of CO neurotoxicity. Basal ganglia function includes planning, staging, and execution of movements. Insults to this area cause tremor, decreases in motor speed, slowed reaction time, poor manual dexterity, decreased eye-hand coordination, and poor sequencing of complex motor movements. These physical findings may not be found on routine physical examination, but require more detailed psychometric testing (22).

Routine physical exam is frequently unremarkable. Skin color is more likely to be cyanotic or pale, not the tauted "cherry red" coloration that is usually a postmortem finding. Although papilledema and retinal hemorrhages are rarely found, when present they suggest the diagnosis of CO poisoning. Special attention should be paid to signs of smoke inhalation in order to address associated problems such as airway obstruction from thermal and chemical injury, pulmonary edema, and chemical pneumonitis. Singed nasal hairs, singed eyebrows, and soot in the oral cavity and sputum are indicative of smoke inhalation.

The nervous system and heart are the tissues with the highest metabolic rate and are most susceptible to oxygen deprivation (12, 23). Tachycardia occurs in an attempt to compensate for tissue hypoxia. In healthy individuals, dilatation of the coronary vessels caused by CO meets the increased cardiac oxygen requirements. However, in patients with coronary artery disease (CAD), exacerbation of angina can occur at Cohgb levels less than 10%. Patients with CAD are at increased risk for myocardial infarction. Myocardial infarction has been reported up to five days after CO exposure in a young patient with no cardiac risk factors and no clinical or electrocardiographic evidence of earlier cardiac dysfunction (13, 24). Myocardial ischemia may occur immediately after exposure or several days after exposure (5, 7, 23, 25).

Ventricular fibrillation threshold is lowered by CO. Cardiac arrhythmias are the most frequent cause of death in the acute poisoning (23, 25). Headache, dizziness, visual disturbances, muscle weakness, fatigue, and confusion are the most commonly described neurologic symptoms. Initially, neurologic findings are usually symmetric. Seizures and coma may occur with severe intoxication. Prognosis is poor when coma is prolonged more than 48 hours after poisoning (5, 23, 24).

NEUROLOGIC, COGNITIVE, AND BEHAVIORAL TOXICITY

CO can induce a delayed neuropsychiatric syndrome which consists of a pseudorecovery period of up to several weeks that is followed by an abrupt onset of neurologic and psychiatric deterioration. Manifestations include gross neurologic impairment such as parkinsonism, apraxia, and psychosis, as well as more subtle deficits such as intellectual deterioration, memory impairment, and personality changes. The first case was described in 1926. A 58-year-old woman had an apparently normal recovery from a suicide attempt in which she had suffered a CO-induced coma. One month later, she became disoriented, mute, and parkinsonian and subsequently died. Autopsy revealed bilateral necrosis of the globus pallidus and widespread demyelination of the entire subcortical white matter (1, 20).

The incidence of delayed neurotoxicity is reported to range from 2–30%. Unfortunately, the only prognostic indicators for the occurrence of this syndrome are extremes of age or loss of consciousness. However, not all young or elderly patients who suffer loss of consciousness demonstrate this complication. Abnormal CT and/or EEG, as well as metabolic acidosis, have been associated with the delayed syndrome, but incidence is unknown. Neuroradiologic findings are frequently normal in patients who develop delayed complications. High Cohgb levels are not predictive of the occurrence of this syndrome (26).

Cognitive function deficits may be the only consistent predictor of delayed neurologic or psychiatric complications. Psychometric testing may be the only way to reveal these deficits, as routine physical exam does not include the necessary testing. Standardized, quantifiable batteries, however brief, are more reliable than bedside qualitative testing. Defects in attention and concentration, eye-hand coordination, manual dexterity, pure motor speed, reaction time, memory, and reasoning can be revealed by psychometric tests which should be performed as soon as possible after the exposure. Hyperbaric oxygen therapy may prevent this syndrome (22, 27).

It is difficult to evaluate the effect of low Cohgb levels on cognitive function. Slowed reaction time has been reported at Cohgb levels as low as 4.5%, but motor slowing was not demonstrated at levels of 20%. Overall impairment at lower Cohgb levels appears to be correlated with task complexity and vigilance required to detect subtle changes in the environment (22, 28).

Low dose CO exposure over an extended period of time (as in toll booth operators) reduces visual attention, simultaneous processing tasks, and peripheral vision. Deficits occur in the recovery phase and residual deficits in spatial memory have been reported months later. It should be noted that neuropsychologic outcome may vary greatly with exposure parameters such as age, severity of poisoning, and preexisting physical conditions (22, 28).

Behavioral disturbances, often subtle or transient, occur in most neurotoxin exposure, including CO. Because these changes may occur in the absence of cognitive or sensori-motor changes, they may be misdiagnosed as a reactive or preexisting condition. Additionally, these severe psychiatric disturbances may occur after a cogent period lasting from several days to weeks.

A longterm sequela of CO poisoning is depression. However, the more time that has elapsed from the exposure, the more difficult it is to determine reactive depression from depression induced by the neurochemical or structural CNS changes caused by the poisoning (22). The causes of anxiety, agitation, and other stress-related reactions are also difficult to discern after CO exposure. It is sometimes difficult to discern whether anxiety and preoccupation are stress related or a sequela of the poisoning.

MANAGEMENT

Initial treatment of CO poisoning involves removal from the source and institution of basic life support measures. 100% oxygen should be administered to facilitate dissociation of CO from the hemoglobin molecule. Plastic rebreather masks are typically administered to deliver ''100% oxygen.'' However, due to lack of a tight seal, these masks deliver only 55–60% oxygen. Endotracheal intubation and mechanical ventilation with 100% oxygen should be initiated if the patient is unconscious. Relative tissue hypoxia leads to lactic acidosis. Acidosis shifts the oxyhemoglobin dissociation curve to the right in an attempt to increase tissue oxygen delivery. Administration of bicarbonate will shift the oxyhemoglobin curve back to the left and aggravate tissue hypoxia. Bicarbonate administration should be withheld except in cases of life-threatening acidosis (15, 20, 29).

The treatment controversy is the value of hyperbaric oxygen (HBO). HBO causes a high oxygen tension which displaces CO from the blood and tissues rapidly and dissolves enough oxygen in the plasma to meet the body's metabolic needs, even in the absence of functioning hemoglobin. HBO may also be of benefit if cerebral edema is present. HBO will shorten the length of symptoms in the acute poisoning and may prevent the delayed neurologic sequelae (provided structural brain damage has not occurred). However, there is no conclusive evidence that shortening the duration of symptoms will diminish the severity of delayed sequelae as there have been no controlled trials. Nor have there been any controlled studies which included appropriate psy-

chometric testing on follow-up that compared the effectiveness of HBO with 100% oxygen administration. Evidence indicates that systematic examination with psychometric testing of patients exposed to CO will indicate which patients require aggressive therapy with HBO. One of the problems is the lack of clinical or laboratory prognostic indicators to determine which patients will develop late neuropsychiatric sequelae. Irrefutably, prognosis and indications for HBO are not dependent on Cohgb level. The value of delayed HBO is prone to subjective controversy. Proponents of HBO feel it may be useful for weeks after CO poisoning (27, 30, 31).

There is agreement that any patient with a Cohgb level greater than 25% should be treated with HBO, although some authorities may disagree with this cutoff number. Other indications for HBO include: any neurologic deficit (other than headache), including disorientation and focal neurologic signs, history of loss of consciousness or syncope, cardiac ischemia, dysrhythmia, or electrocardiographic evidence of ischemia after CO exposure, seizures or history of seizures, metabolic acidosis, pulmonary edema, or pregnancy in women who are symptomatic. There is no agreement on whether the following patients need HBO: patients with a headache after CO exposure, children, or asymptomatic patients with levels greater than 10%.

Infants and children have an increased susceptibility to CO toxicity due to their higher metabolic rate and higher tissue oxygen demand. They seem to have an increased incidence of lethargy and syncope at lower Cohgb levels than adults. Delayed neurologic sequelae have been reported. Children who have been exposed to CO should be treated aggressively with HBO (22, 33).

The fetus is extremely susceptible to CO toxicity. The fetal oxyhemoglobin dissociation curve is to the left of the adult curve, so oxygen does not dissociate easily from fetal hemoglobin. The curve is further shifted to the left by CO. The half-life of fetal Cohgb is 15 hours. It takes 5 times longer to reduce fetal Cohgb to normal than maternal Cohgb. HBO therapy is considered safe in pregnancy and should be administered in all exposures (6, 34).

There are a number of recommended diving schedules. Schedules vary from three atmospheres to 46 minutes repeated every 6 hours, dependent on the clinical picture, to two atmospheres for 90 minutes repeated six hourly, dependent on the clinical picture. There is currently no proof that repeated sessions are better than single sessions or that three atmospheres are preferable to two atmospheres. In fact, pressures over 2.5 atmospheres may cause cerebral capillary leakage and perivascular edema (6).

Complications of HBO are minimal. Ear barotrauma and ear pain, sinus pain, and tooth pain are common complaints. Oxygen toxicity seizures infrequently occur. Patients with obstructive lung disease may lose their hypoxic drive. Patients may complain of claustrophobia, but this does not have life-threatening consequences. Emesis may occur. Resources should be available to treat cardiac dysrhythmias, hypotension, and seizures (6, 35).

Most states now have a hyperbaric facility either within the state or nearby. The Divers Alert Network at Duke University (919/684–8111) provides emergency consultation and maintains a list of all available chambers. Cost is a consideration, and the decision to refer a patient to a chamber is made by the individual clinician. A consultation to the physician of the nearest chamber may be of benefit (7, 15, 29).

REFERENCES

1. Ginsberg M. Carbon monoxide. In: Spencer P, Schaumberg, eds. Experimental and clinical neurotoxicology. Baltimore: Williams & Wilkins, 1980:374–394.

2. Kunkel DB, The toxic emergency. J Emerg Med 1988; 20, 150–155.

3. Caplan Y, Thompson B, Levine B, et al. Accidental poisoning involving carbon monoxide, heating systems, and confined spaces. J Forensic Sci 1986;1:117–121.

4. Myers R, Goldman B. Planning an effective strategy for carbon monoxide poisoning. Emerg Med Rep 1987;25:193–200.

5. Ilano AL, Raffin TA. Management of carbon monoxide poisoning. Chest 1990;97:165–169.

6. Lowe-Ponsfort FL, Henry JA. Clinical aspects of carbon monoxide poisoning. Adverse Drug React 1989;4:217–235.

7. Myers R. Carbon monoxide poisoning. In: Haddad LM, Winchester JF, eds. Clinical management of poisoning and drug overdose. Philadelphia: WB Saunders, 1990: 1139–1152.

8. Horowitz BZ. Carboxyhemoglobinemia caused by inhalation of methylene chloride. Am J Emerg Med 1986;1:48–51.

9. Thom S, Keim L. Carbon monoxide poisoning: a review epidemiology, pathophysiology, clinical findings and treatment options including hyperbaric oxygen therapy. Clin Toxicol 1989;13:141–156.

10. Ginsberg MD. Carbon monoxide intoxication: clinical features, neuropathology, and mechanisms of injury. Clin Toxicol 1985;4–6:281–288.

11. Ball E, Stritmatter C, Cooper O. The reaction of cytochrome oxidase with carbon monoxide. J Biol Chem 1951;193:635–647.

12. Goldbaum LR, Ramirez RG, Absalon KB. What is the mechanism of carbon monoxide toxicity? Aviat Space Environ Med 1975;46:1289–1291.

13. Yokoyama K. Effect of perfluorochemical (PFC) emulsion on acute carbon monoxide poisoning in rats. Jpn J Surg 1978;4:342–352.

14. Davis SM, Levy RC. High carboxyhemoglobin level without acute or chronic findings. J Emerg Med 1984;1:539–541.

15. Zimmerman S, Truxal B. Carbon monoxide poisoning. Pediatrics 1981;68:215–224.

16. Crocker P. Carbon monoxide poisoning, the clinical entity and its treatment: a review. Milit Med 1984;149:257–259.

17. Horowitz AL, Kaplan R, Sarpel G. Carbon monoxide toxicity: MR imaging in the brain. Radiology 1987;162:787–788.

18. Sawanda Y, Sakamoto T, Nishide K, et al. Correlation of pathological findings with computed tomographic findings after acute carbon monoxide poisoning. N Eng J Med 1983;308:1296.

19. Miura T, Mitomo M, Kawai R, et al. CT of the brain in acuite carbon monoxide intoxication: characteristic features and prognosis. AJNR 1985;6:739–741.

20. Meredith T, Vale A. Carbon monoxide poisoning. Br Med J 1988;6615:77–79.

21. O'Donoghue J. Carbon monoxide, inorganic nitrogenous compounds and phosphorus. In: O'Donoghue J, ed. Neurotoxicity of industrial and commercial chemicals. Vol I. Boca Raton, FL: CRC Press, 1985:193–203.

22. Hartman D. Neuropsychological toxicology: identification and assessment of human neurotoxic syndrome. New York, NY: Pergam Press, 1988:244–253.

23. Anderson RF, Allensworth DC, DeGroot WJ. Myocardial toxicity from carbon monoxide poisoning. Ann Intern Med 1967;6:1172–1181.

24. Winter A, Shatin L. Hyperbaric oxygen in reversing carbon monoxide coma: neurologic and psychological study. J Med 1970;70:880–884.

25. Ebisuno S, Yasuno M, Yamada Y, et al. Myocardial infarction after acute monoxide poisoning: case Report. J Vasc Dis 1986;Aug:621–624.

26. Choi I. Delayed neurologic sequelae in carbon monoxide intoxication. Arch Neurol 1986;40:433–435.

27. Meyers R, Mitchell J. Cowley R. Psychometric testing and carbon monoxide poisoning. Disaster Med 1983;1:279–281.

28. Mihevic P, Gliner J, Horvath S. Carbon monoxide exposure and information processing during perceptual motor performance. Int Arch Occup Environ Health 1983;51:355–363.

29. Kindwall EP. Hyperbaric treatment of carbon monoxide poisoning. Ann Emerg Med 1985;14:139–140.

30. Meyers R, Snyder S, Emhoff T. Subacute sequelae of carbon monoxide poisoning. Ann Emerg Med 1985;14:59–63.

31. Raphael J, Elkharrat D, Jars-Guincestre M, et al. Trial of normobaric and hyperbaric oxygen for acute carbon monoxide intoxication. Lancet 1989;2:414–419.

32. Parish R. Smoke inhalation and carbon monoxide poisoning in children. Pediatr Emerg Care 1986;1:36–39.

33. Crocker PJ, Walker JS. Pediatric carbon monoxide toxicity. J Emerg Med 1986;3:443–448.

34. Longo LD. The biological effects of carbon monoxide on the pregnant woman, fetus, and newborn infant. Am J Obstet Gynecol 1977;129:69–99.

35. Sloan E, Murphy D, Hart R, et al. Complications and protocol considerations in carbon monoxide poisoned patients who require hyperbaric oxygen therapy: report from a ten-year experience. Ann Emerg Med 1989;18:629–634.

Gary R. Krieger, M.D., M.P.H.
Jan A. Larson

INTRODUCTION

Basic Physics

In 1960, the world was introduced to a new type of high technology instrument: the laser. Initially viewed as a research tool, laser technology has been applied to an astounding range of applications from consumer electronics (compact disc players) to sophisticated medical-surgical devices.

The term "laser" is an acronym for "Light Amplification by Stimulated Emission of Radiation." The basic physics of light related stimulated emissions derives from theoretical investigations by two famous physicists, Niels Bohr in 1913 and Albert Einstein in 1917.

Bohr postulated that the atom consisted of a nucleus composed of protons and neutrons surrounded by electrons in orbit around the nucleus (Fig. 115.1). Utilizing this model, Bohr developed a mathematical theory of atomic spectra in order to explain the experimentally observed fact that atoms emit or absorb only specific characteristic frequencies of light. When an electron jumped from one allowed orbit to another, a photon of energy was either absorbed or emitted. Thus, an electron could either be excited to a higher energy level by the *absorption* of energy (in the form of a photon) or it could return to a lower energy state by the *emission* of a photon. Significantly, the frequency of the emitted radiation was proportioned to the difference between the two energy levels.

Overall, there are three main types of energy transitions which can occur in atoms or molecules: (a) absorption, (b) spontaneous emission, and (c) stimulated emission. Einstein's 1917 work demonstrated that the spontaneous emission process could be accelerated if the excited state atom was struck by a photon of exactly the same energy as the spontaneously emitted photon. This accelerated process yields two photons of the same energy level which leave the atom in the exact same direction and phase. Thus, *stimulated emissions* of photons could be produced from a variety of external sources.

Based on this process, laser devices utilize two main approaches: (a) optical pumping and (b) electrical discharge. Op-

tical pumping occurs when a material is illuminated by a high energy optical source. This source can be a broad-based light device such as a flash lamp or a device that produces a specific light spectrum such as another laser. Atoms can also be excited by an electrical discharge. This technique stimulates atoms as a result of collisions with electrons.

The probability of stimulated emission increases as more electrons enter an excited state. This condition is called *population inversion* and is a requirement for all potential lasing mediums (Fig. 115.2). Thus, a prototypical laser instrument consists of four generic components: (a) energy input source, (b) an active medium—atoms capable of undergoing stimulated emissions, (c) feedback mechanism—total and partial reflecting mirrors and (d) standard optical devices to focus the electromagnetic energy (Fig. 115.3). When more than 50% of the active medium's ions are energized, lasing begins. This process produces an intense beam of coherent electromagnetic radiation. All lasers, regardless of type of active medium, follow these fundamental principles.

Laser Operational Concepts

The selection of the active lasing medium has rapidly expanded over the last 30 years and may be a solid, liquid, or gas. The choice of an active medium is a direct function of the output power and wavelength required for a given application. Output may be delivered as a continuous level of power (CW: continuous wave) in a single pulse or as a series of pulses. With CW lasers, the amplitude of the output beam is expressed in terms of power (watts), while in a pulsed laser both power and time are critical and the output is measured in terms of energy (joules). If the output beam is continuously pulsed, the output is expressed in terms of average power (watts), pulse repetition (pps), and single pulse duration (sec). One additional variant of lasing is known as *Q-switching*. Q-switching is an operational mode in which energy is stored in the laser during pumping and is suddenly released in a single powerful short burst. This mode generates an extremely high peak power output pulse in the range of 100 million to over one billion watts. The associated electromagnetic field strengths are high enough to ionize air and water.

To illustrate these concepts, a variety of prototypical mediums are analyzed and specific performance criteria are listed (Tables 115.1, 2, 3) (1–5).

Solid—The active medium consists of a lasing element suspended in a host compound. The ruby crystal was the first operational lasing material. The ruby laser is a rod-shaped solid form of aluminum oxide with approximately 0.05% trivalent chromium as an impurity. The chromium is the active lasing material and emits photons of red light at 695.3 μm, while the aluminum oxide serves as the host material. The ruby laser uses an optical pumping technique consisting

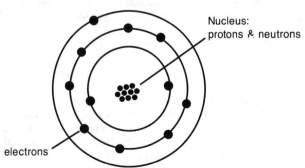

Figure 115.1. Conceptual Bohr atom.

Nucleus:
protons & neutrons

electrons

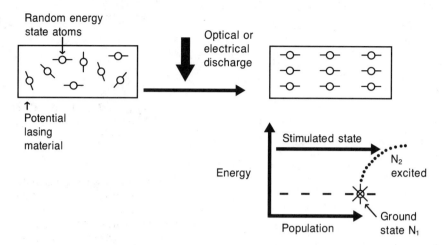

Figure 115.2.   Basic laser concepts: population inversion.

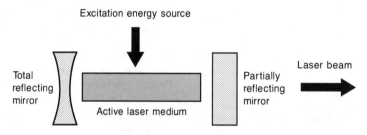

Figure 115.3.   Prototypical laser configuration.

Table 115.1.   Spectral Domains

Ultraviolet C	200 nm–280 nm
Ultraviolet B	280 nm–315 nm
Ultraviolet A	315 nm–400 nm
Visible	400 nm–780 nm
Infrared A	780 nm–1400 nm
Infrared B	1.4 μm–3.0 μm
Infrared C	3.0 μm–1000 μm

nm = nanometers
μm = micrometers

of a xenon flash lamp. The chromium atoms absorb photons and are stimulated to a higher energy state such that a population inversion occurs and stimulated emission begins. The ruby laser is operated in a pulse mode only and is limited to 100 pulses per second (1–5).

One of the most widely used solid sources for moderate to high power applications consists of a single crystal of yttrium-aluminum-garnet (YAG) doped with 1–3% neodymium (Nd) ions. The lasing material is optically pumped by a broad band of incoherent light obtained from xenon, krypton flash or CW lamps. The Nd:YAG system is capable of CW output approaching 500 watts at the 1.06 μm wavelength.

Gas—The most widely used gas lasers are helium-neon (HeNe), carbon dioxide (CO_2) and argon-ion. A large variety of other gas lasers have also been formulated: krypton, helium-cadmium, nitrogen, hydrogen fluoride, carbon monoxide, water vapor, and hydrogen cyanide. While gas lasers are capable of pulsed operation, they typically operate in the CW mode. The gas lasers have a tremendous range of applications, and the three most commonly employed mediums will be discussed in detail.

Helium-Neon (HeNe)—The He-Ne laser is the dominant laser in use today and has wide industrial applications. Currently available He-Ne gas lasers use direct current excitation and produce power levels from a fraction of a milliwatt to approximately 100 milliwatts. The power output is a function of the laser tube length. The He-Ne laser is a CW system and typically operates at the orange 0.633 μm transition.

Ion Lasers—The ion lasers are based upon the noble gases: argon, krypton, xenon, and neon. This family of gases provides a source for over 35 different laser frequencies ranging from near-ultraviolet (neon—0.322 μm) to near-infrared (krypton—0.799 μm). These gases are used both singly and in combination. For example, argon and krypton can be combined to produce simultaneous emissions at ten different wavelengths. The ion lasers are very stable and can be operated in both the pulsed and CW modes. The most common commercial models use both argon and krypton while simultaneously employing high current densities (15–40 amps) through the discharge tube. The discharge current is forced through a small bore tube, and current densities can be generated as high as 1000 amps/cm². This intense current density generates considerable heat and requires both heat stable refracting materials and a continuous source of cooling. Typically, most argon ion laser tubes are water cooled; however, if the water does not flow at a sufficient rate, boiling can occur along the tube generating amplitude and frequency instabilities (1–5).

CO_2 Lasers—The CO_2 laser is known as a molecular laser because the energy structure of its molecules is more complicated than that of atomic or ion lasing mediums. Molecular laser energy structures originate from electronic, vibrational, and rotational motions. Thus, the energy level structure of the CO_2 molecule is substantially more complex than the energy structure of an ion because of the existence of additional energy-

Table 115.2. Typical Laser Characteristics

Laser Media	Predominant Wavelengths (nm)	Active Media	Common Method of Operation	Continuous Power (W)	Peak Power (MW)
Ruby	694.3	Solid	Pulsed	1.0	1–1000
Neodymium-YAG	1,060	Solid	CW	1–100	1–10
Helium-neon	632.8 1,150 3,390	Gas	CW	0.001–0.100	
Argon ion	476.5 488.0 514.5	Gas	CW	1–20	10^{-4}
Krypton ion	647.1 568.2 520.8 476.2	Gas	CW	0.5–2.0	
Tunable dye	360–650	Liquid	CW normal pulsed	variable	variable
Gallium arsenide	904	Semiconductor	repeatively pulsed	1–20	
Carbon dioxide	10.6×10^3	Gas	CW normal pulse	variable	10^{-2}

exchange mechanisms. Therefore, CO_2 lasers are capable of producing extremely high output power in either the pulsed or CW mode. Gigawatts of peak power (one billion watts) have been obtained in short nanosecond (10^{-9}) duration pulses. The CO_2 laser typically uses a mixture of CO_2 (9%), nitrogen (15%), and helium (76%). Nitrogen acts as an aid in the transfer of energy to the upper excitation level for the CO_2 molecule. After lasing, the CO_2 molecule is left at an energy level above the ground state. Helium is added to the mixture in order to empty this energy to the ground level.

CO_2 lasers can be coupled to surgical microscopes and have become relatively common surgical instruments because of their ability to convert solid tissue (tumors) to smoke. The power of CO_2 lasers is sufficient to bypass any significant liquid phase intervening between the solid tissue and the smoke (6, 7).

Liquid Tunable Dye Lasers—In 1966, the first multiwavelength dye laser was introduced. This device used three different organic dyes and was capable of producing red, green, and yellow laser emissions. Liquid lasers are optically pumped by very fast optical pulses from another laser. The dye is typically rhodamine-6G and is mixed with water. This solution continuously flows through a cell in order to prevent dye fading and to provide system cooling. The liquid dye lasers are "tunable" across most of the visible spectrum by varying the choice of dye solution (e.g., coumarin versus rhodamine). Tunable dye lasers operate in the CW mode and are commonly used in high resolution atomic and molecular spectroscopy (1). Tables 115.4 and 115.5 list common dyes and solvents employed in laser operations.

Semiconductor Lasers—The active medium of a semiconductor laser is the junction between two types of semiconductor materials. A semiconductor is a material with an intermediate ability to conduct electricity greater than an insulator (glass or plastic) but less than copper or silver. The photo-typical semiconductor laser employs gallium arsenide (Ga As). Semiconductor material can exist in two forms: (a) p-type—deficiency of negatively charged free electrons in the crystal structure,

and (b) n-type—surplus of electrons that act as current carriers. If p-type and n-type materials are joined, a pn junction is created. When current flows across a pn junction, energy is released because free electrons from the n-type material combine with holes in the p-type material. Semiconductor lasers usually have outputs in the infrared wavelength, although models that emit in the visible region are available (1, 3).

Excimer Lasers—Excimers employ a lasing medium that consists of an atom of an inert gas and an atom of a highly reactive halogen gas such as fluorine, chlorine, or bromide. These excited pairs are known as dimers. These lasers have extremely high peak powers (10^9 W) at ultraviolet ranges and can be used for a variety of novel medical applications: (a) laser coronary angioplasty and (b) corneal sculpting for the correction of visual defects (1, 3, 13).

Chemical Lasers—Populations inversion can also be achieved by utilizing a chemical reaction as the active medium. These lasers have four common elements: (a) gas mixing system, (b) method initiating the chemical reaction, (c) optical cavity, and (d) exhaust system for removal of spent reactant gases. Hydrogen fluoride and/or deuterium fluoride are typically used as the active molecules. These lasers can produce a peak output of 35 W with a 1-μsec pulse duration. Fluorine is a highly reactive and corrosive substance, and these lasers pose significant safety problems. Tables 115.2 and 115.3 summarize many of the important characteristics of each of the previously discussed lasers (1, 3–5).

LASER APPLICATIONS

Exposure Demographics

It is difficult to accurately estimate the number of individuals potentially exposed to laser energy. Initially, lasers were primarily confined to research and engineering applications so that the potentially exposed population was relatively restricted.

Table 115.3.   Laser Types for Current Applications

Laser Media	Wavelength μm	Major Applications
Ruby laser	0.6943	Satellite ranging Medical Drilling holes in aircraft engine parts
Neodymium-YAG	1.06	Various laser metal processing, welding Medical (surgery, eye) Military (ranging)
Carbon Dioxide	10.6	High powers metals treatments Surgery Laser fusion research
Argon	0.488–0.514	Laser eye treatments
Ion Gas	0.351 & 0.363	Photoetching Laser entertainment Medical: cell counters and other medical diagnostics
Helium neon	0.6328	UPC checkout systems Alignment Construction Videodisc
Gallium arsenide diode	0.840	Communications Infrared beacons (in array formats)
Krypton	0.4762 & 0.5280	Entertainment
Ion Gas	0.5682 & 0.8471	Holography Diagnostics
Dye lasers such as: Rhodamine 6-G	Tunable: 0.400–0.600	Spectroscopy IC circuit etching Special photography
Excimer	0.175–0.351	Research & development High peak power uses at UV wavelengths, laser angioplasty, corneal sculpting
Chemical	10–11	Research & development (experimental) High output, high efficiency

Table 115.4.   Laser Dyes

Dye	Non-Laser Application
Rhodamine	Drug products, cosmetics, fabrics, printing inks, tracing agent
Fluorescein	Cosmetics, household products, detection of corneal defect
Polymethine	Photographic developing processes
Coumarins	Whitening agents, drugs
Stilbenes	Scintillation counting dye

Table 115.5.   Dye Solvents

Cyclohexane	Dimethyl sulfoxide (DMSO)
Toluene	1,2-Dichloroethane
Chlorobenzene	1,1,1-Trichloroethane
Ethylene glycol	o-Dichlorobenzene
Glycerol	Dichloromethane
Chloroform	N,N-Dimethylformamide
N,N-Dipropylacetamide	Tetrahydrofuran
Trifluoroethanol	Triethylamine
p-Dioxane	Benzonitrile
Ethyl alcohol	Hexafluoroisopropanol
Methyl alcohol	1-Methl-2-pyrrolidinone
Benzyl alcohol	Tetrahydrothiophene oxide

Based upon a 1980 National Institutes of Occupational Safety and Health (NIOSH) report and using 20–25% yearly increases, Rockwell estimated that up to six million workers could be potentially exposed to lasers by the early 1990s (1). The spectacular growth in laser applications in increasingly shifting potential exposures, from the research realm to the general workforce. Table 115.6, based upon Rockwell's work, illustrates the wide variety of laser applications, while Table 115.2 lists many of the most common laser types and current applications (1).

Manufacturing Applications

The laser is a well-controlled and focused heat source which can be precisely directed. Therefore, it is not surprising that lasers have wide applications in the area of materials processing. Specifically, lasers are used to drill, weld, and cut a wide variety of materials including cloth, paper, metals, and plastics. CO_2 and Nd-YAG lasers are commonly used to thermally etch parts during manufacturing for coding and identification. Ultraviolet and short wave visible spectra laser applications are employed in the photoetching processes for the manufacturing of multi-layer integrated circuits. Low power (>10 mW) CW He-Ne or gallium arsenide diode lasers are frequently used for precision alignment and machine control applications. These CW low power lasers are also ideal for diagnostic or measurement applications involving trenching and digging. The depth

Table 115.6. Major Categories of Laser Uses

Alignment	*Information handling (cont.)*
Annealing	Reading
Balancing (dynamic)	Recording
Biomedical	Scanning
Cellular research	Typesetting
Dental	Videodisc
Diagnostics	Compact disc
Dermatology	Marking
Ophthalmology	Laboratory instruments
Surgical	Interferometry
Communication	Metrology
Construction	Plasma diagnostics
Alignment	Spectroscopy
Ranging	Velocimetry
Surveying	Lidar
Cutting	Special photography
Displays	Scanning microscopy
Drilling	Military
Entertainment	Distance ranging
Heat treating	Rifle simulation
Holographic	Weaponry
Information handling	Nondestructive testing
Copying	Scanning
Displays	Sealing
Plate making	Scribing
Printing	Soldering
	Welding

Adapted from Laser Safety Training Manual. 6th ed. Cincinnati, OH: Rockwell Associates, 1984; Lazan. Laser Hazard Analysis Program. 1st ed. Cincinnati, OH: Rockwell Associates, 1988; Safety of Lasers and Other Optical Radiation Sources, Cincinnati, OH: Rockwell Associates, 1986.

of the excavation is continuously monitored and controlled by the laser beam as the laser light strikes a detector fixed to the grading or digging equipment. Laser beams can also be used as a reference line for the installation of acoustical ceiling tiles or other types of paneling.

Medical Applications

Laser applications for medicine and surgery have experienced tremendous growth over the last decade. Technical details and specific applications have been extensively and well reviewed by a variety of authors (6–8, 13). Surgical applications are based on both thermal and nonthermal effects including the ability of laser beams to drive chemical reactions, break atomic bonds, and create shock waves (13). The dominant non-ophthalmologic surgical laser is the 50–100 watt CO_2 laser. The CO_2 laser is a common tool for both neurologic and on-cologic surgery. The CO_2 laser has multiple properties that make it an ideal surgical instrument: (a) vaporization of dis-eased tissue, (b) controlled cutting in a thin precise line, (c) hemostasis via direct heat sealing of vessels, and (d) speed combined with gentleness (6–8).

While the CO_2 laser dominates most general and neurosurgical applications, the Nd:YAG, argon, and excimer lasers all have specific and unique surgical applications. Due to their specific wavelength, argon lasers are used for a large number of ophthal-mologic procedures. Nd:YAG lasers have been employed during bronchoscopy to vaporize lung tumors that were pretreated with specific fluorescent dyes and they are used extensively for ocular surgery involving the posterior capsule. Excimer lasers are used for coronary angioplasties and corneal sculpting (13).

Surgical applications generally require high output devices

with beams that are open to the environment. Rockwell pos-tulates that the medical use of lasers may generate the greatest potential for daily routine exposure (1). The health and safety standards and monitoring programs required by law will be discussed in the final section of this chapter.

Information Storage and Playback

The late 1980s and certainly the 1990s have become the in-formation age. Laser technology has played an extremely prom-inent role in the recording and retrieval of information. The compact disc player, laser videodisc, laser printers, and product code scanning systems all represent novel applications based upon precision laser scanning devices. Usually, low power, CW, He-Ne lasers are used by these devices. The potential hazards of these lasers are quite low.

Arts and Entertainment

Since the early 1990s, the live entertainment media, including such events as half-time spectaculars, rock concerts, and dis-cotheque lighting, have become dominated by complex com-binations of lasers and other ancillary electro-optic equipment. The lasers are usually ion gas types (argon, krypton), although tunable dye lasers are occasionally used. Laser emission levels for most indoor projection effects are usually less than 240 mW, while outdoor "sky scans" generally require at least 5–20 watts power. The potential for significant hazards exists with the more powerful lasers; therefore, adequate planning and safeguards must be initiated (1, 3–5).

THIN FILM SUPER-CONDUCTOR APPLICATIONS

Pulsed laser evaporation (PLE) is a powerful technique capable of depositing a wide variety of materials in thin film form (12). This technique has been used to deposit thin films of barium-copper-oxygen ($Ba_2Cu_3O_x$). These materials are used as high temperature superconductors. Other superconducting materials including bismuth and yttrium combinations can also be de-posited via PLE. Both Nd:YAG (1.06 µm) and CO_2 (10.6 µm) lasers have been used for this technique (12).

LASER SAFETY AND HEALTH STANDARDS

Background

The development of laser safety standards began during the mid-1960s. By 1972, two primary groups in the United States were developing laser standards: (a) a consortium of industry, university, and governmental experts and (b) the Bureau of Radiological Health within the Food and Drug Administration (FDA). The nonregulatory consortium developed standard Z-136.1 (1973) under the auspices of the American National Standards Institute (ANSI) (9). This committee classified lasers by a graded system of four basic classes of risk ranging from Class I (least hazardous) to Class IV (greatest hazard). Control measures were also graded in a similar fashion.

Concomitantly, the FDA created a National Center of De-vices and Radiological Health (NCDRH) which developed per-formance requirements that applied to manufacturers but not to users. The standard did not contain specific design speci-fications, but rather was directed towards performance criteria that a designer should consider. The NCDRH laser standard has undergone several revisions during the 1980s, although change has been a slow and tedious process.

By contrast, the ANSI standard was revised initially in 1972 and again in 1980. The 1980 revision is compatible with the NCDRH standard and was released in February 1981 (ANSI-Z-136.1-1980) (9). The ANSI standard has been adopted by both laser producers and users and is the basis for all U.S. and many international standards.

Interestingly, the Occupational Safety and Health Administration (OSHA) does not have an all-inclusive laser standard. OSHA does have a very limited standard that applies to the use of lasers at construction sites. Under this regulation, the use of any laser at a construction site with a power greater than 5 mW requires eye protection. Non-construction laser applications are addressed by OSHA via the General Duty Clause. This clause requires that an employer must provide a safe work place for all employees. In general, OSHA requires that companies follow ANSI-Z-136 Standard.

Laser Classification

Under the ANSI standard, laser hazard classes are used to help define the severity of potential injury (1, 3–5, 9). There are four basic classes with several sub-groups ranging from Class I (least hazard) to Class IV (greatest hazard). Manufacturers are required to inform users of the hazard class by placing a warning label in clear view of the user (Fig. 115.4). Knowledge of hazard class is an important prerequisite for determining the nature, extent of danger, and the subsequent control requirements.

These classes relate to laser beam hazards only:

Class I— Not able to cause injury to skin or eye during a 1-day maximum exposure. These lasers do not pose a hazard even if collecting optics are used. Class I lasers are exempt from all control requirements unless there is a more dangerous laser contained within the enclosure. If a second laser is present, suitable warning labels must be placed on the laser access panel.

Class II— Low power lasers that emit visible laser radiation and may be an ocular hazard for chronic viewing if a person continuously stares into the light source. The upper limit of total emitted power is 1.0 mW collected within an 80-mm aperture.

Class IIa— Similar to Class II (i.e., visible, not intended for viewing) but the accessible radiation cannot exceed the Class I Allowable Exposure Limit (AEL) for more than 1000 seconds. The concept of AELs will be further discussed in the section on eye and skin hazards.

Class IIIa—Medium power systems; these lasers can pose a hazard for chronic viewing when the beam is collected and viewed through collecting optics. These lasers emit visible radiation; they do not exceed the Class II AEL when collected in a 7-mm aperture.

Class IIIb—These moderately powered lasers pose an ocular and skin hazard for direct exposure. Nonvisible laser radiation can be emitted.

Class IV— Relatively high powered lasers that pose ocular and skin hazards from both direct and scattered radiation. These lasers also pose a fire danger if flammables are in the beam path. UV and IR systems can emit radiant power in excess of 0.5 W

for greater than 0.25 seconds or a radiant exposure of 10 J/cm^2 for 0.25 seconds or less.

Overall, lasers operating in the lower hazard classifications (Class I, II, and IIIa) do not typically generate significant ocular or skin hazards. Class IIIb and IV systems are frequently used in manufacturing processes and do present the potential for significant eye and skin exposure. Usually, higher class systems are totally enclosed during standard operation and functionally perform in a Class I fashion. Finally, many of the lasers found in many research and development environments may not have been purchased from a manufacturer and would require classification by the institution's health and safety organization.

LASER HAZARDS

Non-Skin/Eye

Non-skin/eye dangers associated with laser work are generally from electrical and chemical sources (10, 11).

Industrial lasers such as the CO_2 and Nd:YAG present a variety of safety hazards. The risk of electrical shock is significant, and several deaths from this source have occurred (1). Shock hazards include high energy capacitors in pulsed laser systems, high voltage in CW power supplies, and hot mirror mounts.

Although not unique to lasers, metal fumes released from the material being processed can also present a serious health hazard. As in the case with standard industrial operations such as welding, cutting, and brazing, good ventilation and/or personal protection equipment are needed to minimize employee exposures.

Collateral radiation is an often overlooked hazard. Sources of this radiation include intense light from pulsed laser flash lamps, CW arc lamps, and ultraviolet radiation from both electrical discharge tubes and optical pumping systems. The result of this type of exposure is not immediately apparent; however, it may present several hours after exposure as painful photokeratitis.

Laboratories and research and development environments may pose greater hazards due to the presence of high powered and unusual lasing media; in addition, unique or unusual setups/configurations are common.

Eye and Skin

SKIN

Laser radiation can inflict irreversible skin and eye damage. The cause of this damage is thermal. Tissue proteins are denatured secondary to the temperature rise in tissues generated by the absorption of laser energy of sufficient intensity. Thermal damage is more commonly associated with lasers operating at exposure time greater than 10 microseconds and in wavelengths from the near ultraviolet to the far infrared (0.315–10^3 μm).

Other specific wavelength ranges and or exposure times are capable of producing other types of damage mechanisms. For example, photochemical reactions can occur following exposures to UV radiation in the 0.200–0.315 μm range. Short-wave visible radiation (0.4–0.55 μm) exposures for greater than 10 seconds can produce similar photochemical reactions. Tissue damage can also be thermally induced by the acoustic-shock waves associated with very short-time (sub-microsecond) laser exposure.

The skin presents a large available surface area for potential laser exposure. Laser sources in the 0.3–1.0-μm range will

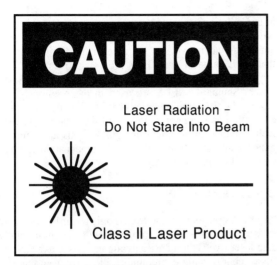
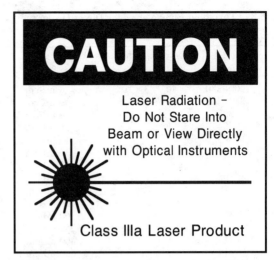
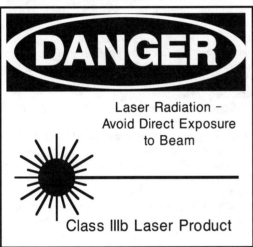
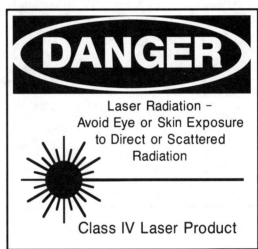

Figure 115.4. Laser safety signs and labels (based on ANSI-Z-136.1).

Table 115.7. Minimal Skin Reaction Levels (14)

Laser Type	Radiant Exposure (J/cm^2)	Exposure Time (sec.)
Ruby (unpigmented skin)	11–20	2.5×10^{-3}
(pigmented skin)	2.2–6.9	
Q-switched ruby	0.25–0.24	75×10^{-9}
Argon	4.0–8.2	1.0
Carbon dioxide	2.8	1.0
Neodymium glass Q-switched	2.5–5.7	75×10^{-9}
Neodymium-YAG	46–78	1.0

generate radiation capable of penetrating at least the outer 4 mm of tissue. Table 115.7 presents the minimal skin reaction levels from radiant exposure. The mechanism of injury is a thermal coagulation necrosis. Rockwell has classified the principle thermal effects of laser exposure based upon these five factors (1):

1. Absorption and scattering coefficients of the tissue at the laser wavelength
2. Irridance or radiant exposure of the laser beam
3. Duration of the exposure
4. Extent of the local vascular flow
5. Size of the area irradiated.

The medical examiner should always keep in mind that preexisting phototoxic and photosensitizing chemicals in the skin may potentiate the effects of the delivered dose of laser radiation. In general, the internal organs of humans have not been associated with biologic effects under normal nonsurgical conditions.

EYE

The eye is the prime exposure point associated with laser radiation. The dominant spectral regions of exposure are the visible and near-infrared regions (0.400–1.400 μm), although other serious hazards can occur in different spectral regions.

Due to the geometry and structure within the eye, optical energy can be transmitted, reflected, and absorbed. The retina is the light-absorbing structure within the eye and is the critical target structure for laser radiation. Retinal effects due to laser exposure are influenced by the transmission losses which occur within the ocular media. Typically, retinal effects are generated only for laser wavelengths between 0.400 and 1.41 μm. Outside of this range, thermal injury can cause damage to other eye structures. In addition to wavelength, both the size of the

Table 115.8. Threshold Limit Values for Direct Ocular Exposure (Intrabeam Viewing) from a Laser Beam

Spectral region	Wavelength (nm)	Exposure time (t) (sec)	TLV
UVC	200–280	10^{-9}–3×10^4	3 mJ/cm²
UVB	280–302	10^{-9}–3×10^4	3 mJ/cm²
	303		4 mJ/cm²
	304		6 mJ/cm²
	305		10 mJ/cm²
	306		16 mJ/cm²
	307		25 mJ/cm²
	308		40 mJ/cm²
	309		63 mJ/cm²
	310		100 mJ/cm²
	311		160 mJ/cm²
	312		250 mJ/cm²
	313		400 mJ/cm²
	314		630 mJ/cm²
UVA	315–400	10^{-9}–10	$0.56t^{1/4}$ J/cm²
		10–10^3	1.0 J/cm²
		10^3–3×10^4	1.0 mW/cm²
Light	400–700	10^{-9}–1.8×10^{-5}	5×10^{-7} J/cm²
	400–700	1.8×10^{-5}–10	$1.8(1/t^{0.75})$ mJ/cm²
	400–549	10–10^4	10 mJ/cm²
	550–700	10–T_1	$1.8(1/t^{0.75})$ mJ/cm²
	550–700	T_1–10^4	$10C_B$ mJ/cm²
	400–700	10^4–3×10^4	C_B µW/cm²
IR-A	700–1049	10^{-9}–1.8×10^{-5}	$5C_A \times 10^{-7}$ J/cm²
	700–1049	1.8×10^{-5}–10^3	$1.8CA(1/t^{0.75})$ mJ/cm²
	1050–1400	10^{-9}–10^{-4}	5×10^{-6} J/cm²
	1050–1400	10^{-3}–3×10^4	$320\,C_A$ µW/cm²
IR-B and C	1.4–10^3 µm	10^{-9}–10^{-7}	10^{-2} J/cm²
		10^{-7}–10	$0.56\, t^{0.75}$
		10–3×10^4	J/cm²

With permission from American Conference of Governmental Industrial Hygienists. Threshold Limit Values. 1990–1991. Cincinnati, OH.

retinal image, the time duration of the exposure, and the location of the exposure are critical factors. The fovea (the central two degrees of the visual field) is the region maximally sensitive to the laser radiation while the peripheral structure (such as the parafovea) are less functionally critical.

The ocular hazards depend upon which structure absorbs the most radiant energy per unit volume of tissue. Excessive irradiance, measured in watts/cm², can cause significant retinal damage even though corneal exposure levels are quite modest.

Maximum permissible exposure (MPE) limits for direct ocular exposure have been set. Simplistically, these limits are a function of wavelength, exposure duration, limiting aperture, pulse duration, repetitiveness, and source (14).

Limiting aperture is 7 mm for visible lasers. This figure is approximately the size of the "worst case" pupil diameter under conditions of a well-lighted environment. When visible lasers are viewed using collecting optics (binoculars, etc.) an 80-mm limiting aperture is used for all calculations (14).

Sources can be either specular or diffuse. Specular sources are materials with mirror-like surfaces capable of producing reflections which preserve the point source nature of the original beam. These reflections can be as hazardous as the original beam. Diffuse reflections follow an inverse squared law such that irradiance (radiant exposure) decreases in proportion to the inverse of the square of the distance. Table 115.8 lists the threshold limit values for direct ocular exposure (14).

The amount of radiant power or energy in the limiting aperture is defined as the Allowable Exposure Levels (AEL). The AELs for Class I lasers are the product of two factors: MPE and ALA where ALA is the area of the limiting aperture for that MPE value in cm². Thus AEL = MPE × ALA. Values for MPE levels are provided in the ANSI-Z-136.1 Safe Use of Lasers Standard. AELS are used in the previously discussed hazard classification scheme (Class I–IV) and allow the proper evaluation and categorization of different laser systems. Rockwell provides an excellent indepth analysis and computer program for the calculation of the various input parameters associated with AEL concepts (1, 2).

Dye Toxicity

Laser dyes present unique toxicologic hazards. In general, toxicity information on the approximately 100 commercially available laser dyes is not easily available. Laser dyes are complex fluorescent organic compounds which, when in the proper organic solvent solution, form a lasing medium. These lasers are "tunable" because the wavelength of a dye laser's output can vary with different dyes, concentrations, and solvents. This tunability has increased the popularity of these lasers and has generated increasing concern with the potential hazards associated with dye handling, solution preparation, and overall laser operation.

The dyes can be categorized as a function of their central chemical structures: (a) xanthenes—rhodamines and fluoresceins, (b) polymethine—cyanines and carbocyanines, (c) coumarines, (d) stilbens, and (e) miscellaneous dyes (1). Table 115.4 lists these chemicals and their typical non-laser uses.

Standard laser dye solutions are very dilute, and dye concentrations range from 10^{-2}–10^{-5} molar. Although the total dye constituent quantity is low, dyes have been dissolved in a large variety of hazardous solvents. Many of these solvents are highly toxic and are discussed in greater detail in other chapters in this book.

Laser dye exposures can occur under a multitude of circumstances: (a) solution preparation, (b) failure of the laser's pressure system, and (c) planned or unplanned maintenance or repair. Standard chemical hygiene procedures should always be in effect when using these lasing materials.

Given the myriad of laser types and potential hazards, source control measures offer the best line of defense for the prevention of accidents and injuries.

LASER CONTROL MEASURES (10, 11)

Laser safety measures are designed to reduce the possibility of personnel exposure to the various hazards associated with laser operation (e.g., eye, skin, electrical, etc.). The laser safety officer (LSO) has the specific responsibility of deciding which controls are appropriate for a specific laser system during a given operation. The LSO must also communicate the safety requirements to all users and must monitor compliance.

Control measures fall into these three general categories:

1. *Engineering controls*—designed into the laser system or area of use in order to reduce or eliminate laser exposure.
2. *Administrative controls*—designed to prevent unsafe acts by personnel.
3. *Personal protective devices*—designed to prevent injury should an exposure occur.

Engineering Controls

These strategies may be required or at least desirable to prevent exposures above the maximum permissible exposure (MPE) level. Engineering controls are preferable from a safety standpoint because they represent primary prevention:

—Enclosures or protective housings that prevent access to laser radiation. This type of protection may also be used to protect personnel from collateral radiation, such as x-rays emitted by the laser.
—Interlocks provided for protective housings that disconnect power if the housing is removed.
—Interlocks that shut down the laser if unintentional or unauthorized access to the laser area occurs. This often takes the form of an entry door interlock.
—Key controls that prevent unauthorized use of the laser system.
—Emission indicators such as lights or audible alarms that warn personnel of laser radiation. These devices are positioned so they are seen prior to personnel exposure to the laser radiation.
—Beam stops or alternators that reduce accessible laser radiation levels to the appropriate maximum permissible exposure (MPE).
—Viewing optics must limit accessible laser and other radiation levels to not greater than Class I limits. Filters or interlocks may be required to accomplish the required level of radiation.
—Service panel access should be limited through the use of interlocks or tools required. Warning labels should be affixed to the laser so that service personnel are aware of accessible emission levels above the MPE.
—Elimination of reflective hazards by removing or covering reflective materials in Class III and Class IV laser areas. Use less reflective paints in the laser laboratory.
—Windows allowing viewing access into a Class III or IV laser area should be covered or a protective coating applied to prevent unintended exposure.
—Whenever possible, the use of remote firing and monitoring systems should be encouraged. This type of setup is particularly advantageous in manufacturing facilities where isolation from an untrained workforce is often needed.
—Engineering controls are critical for the safe operation of laser systems for the general public. Specific outdoor control measures that prevent unprotected and unauthorized people from exposure to the beam path are essential. Tracking the nontarget aircraft or vehicles should be prohibited. Beam path elevation limits are established for laser demonstrations depending on the level of technical supervision. An evaluation of hazardous reflections from atmospheric conditions such as fog, rain, snow, etc., must be made by a qualified person throughout the duration of the public display.
—The general public should not be exposed to laser radiation outside the visible range (400–700 mm) at levels exceeding the applicable MPE.

Administrative Controls

—Warning labels or signs placed on housing, control panels, entry doors to laser laboratories. These are designed to prevent exposure to otherwise uninformed personnel.
—Restricted access areas may be established which allow only a limited number of trained personnel to enter the laser area.
—Ambient light levels must be sufficient to allow visibility where

personnel are wearing laser eyewear. Full spectrum fluorescent tubes can be a help in improving visibility for argon lasers operating in the blue-green wavelengths. The laser filters will of course block similar blue-green frequencies from the standard fluorescent tube. However, using a broad band tube allows more visible light to reach the operator.
—Establish beam paths either above or below normal eye height whenever possible. The type of chairs, stools, etc., in the laser facility should be such that personnel are above the beam height when working with bench top lasers.
—Establish and enforce standard operating procedures that reduce or eliminate hazards. This is particularly critical during alignment procedures when many of the other controls and protective devices are not in effect. For example, a written procedure requiring the use of a low power visible laser to align the optical path of a Class IV invisible laser would be extremely helpful.

PERSONAL PROTECTIVE EQUIPMENT

Protective equipment usually consists of laser safety glasses but may also include special shielding or protective clothing. In all cases, the use of personal protective equipment (PPE) as the primary means of laser radiation exposure protection should be discouraged. Engineering and/or administrative controls should be used whenever possible. Laser eyewear should be used as an additional protective measure along with other preventive strategies.

In selecting laser eyewear, great care must be taken to ensure its adequacy and use in a given situation. These factors should be considered by the laser safety officer during this evaluation:

—Ability to cover all potential exposure wavelengths. The laser eyewear must have sufficient optical density (prevent exposure above the MPE) for the range of wavelengths propagated by the laser system.
—Visible light transmission should be maximized so as not to inhibit the operation or work process. Eyewear will probably not be used if it is too difficult to see with it on.
—The need for prescription lenses can be critical. Laser eyewear can be fitted with specially made prescription lenses. This can be accomplished by fitting the prescription lenses inside a pair of laser goggles.
—Comfort often plays a major role in how laser safety glasses or goggles are consistently used.
—The need for peripheral adequate vision can be a factor that determines whether laser glasses or goggles are selected.
—Experience has shown that laser eyewear is seldom, if ever, inspected. This can be very important, as over time the laser glasses/goggles can be damaged. Careful inspection for filter adequacy should be accomplished at least annually and following any known laser hit.

The overall impact of engineering, administrative, and PPE controls should dramatically reduce the likelihood and severity of any exposures. These preventive strategies can be summarized in the form of a site-operating procedure (SOP) for each Class IIIb and IV laser. An example of a SOP for laser operations is illustrated in Table 115.9 (1, 10, 11).

MEDICAL SURVEILLANCE

Laser medical surveillance programs are used to document the absence of exposure effects prior to laser work and to determine

Table 115.9. Laser Site Operating Procedures

1. Introduction
    a. Location of laser (site, building, room)
    b. Description of laser (beam characteristics, divergence, aperture diameter, and maximum output)
    c. Purpose/application of beam
    d. ANSI-Z-136.1 Classification
    e. Other (if applicable, include proposed use at the site, arrival date, pulse length, and repetition rate)

2. Hazards
    a. Identification of the hazard (beam, electrical, chemical)
    b. Analysis of hazards (include target area, absorbing media)

3. Controls
    a. Access controls (door interlocks, signs, signals)
    b. Beam controls (key-lock, enclosures, shutters, stops)
    c. Electrical controls (light on power supply, HV signs)
    d. Eye protection (eye examination, type of eyewear, optical density for beam)
    e. Other

4. Operation procedures
    a. Initial preparation of laboratory environment (key position, warning lights on, interlock activated, identification of personnel)
    b. Personnel protection (eyewear, isolation, barriers)
    c. Target preparations
    d. Countdown procedures
    e. Shut down procedures

5. Emergency procedures
    a. List potential emergencies and corresponding procedures
    b. Describe specific rescue or evacuation procedures

6. Training
    a. Indoctrination of operating personnel
    b. Training of on-site laser safety officer

7. Responsibilities
    a. Supervisory (include emergency contact)
    b. Support personnel

if known adverse biologic effects have occurred secondary to acute or chronic laser exposure.

The focus of the medical surveillance program should be directed toward the target organs of concern: eye and skin. A prelaser eye examination usually by an ophthalmologist is required. Nonexposure periodic examinations have minimal value *if* proper engineering, administrative, and PPE controls are in place. An eye examination **is** required following a suspected overexposure to laser radiation; in addition, sequential follow-up evaluations may also be indicated. While a variety of sophisticated ophthalmological examinations can be performed, the basic visual acuity test is highly sensitive and specific for the existence of retinal pathology (1, 3). Visual acuity should always be carefully documented by an accurate and reproducible method.

The ANSI-Z-136 standard provides general guidelines and recommendations for the medical surveillance program (9):

—Medical surveillance is **not** required for Class I and II lasers;
—The laser safety office should designate potentially exposed workers;
—Medical history is directed toward the ocular and dermato-

logic systems; in addition, a drug history should be obtained in order to evaluate the potential for photosensitization;
—Visual acuity determinations;
—Examination of various structures of the eye depending upon the wavelength of the laser system;
—Prelaser visual examination;
—Visual examination following any suspected laser injury;
—Periodic examinations are not required;
—Optional termination visual examination;
—Skin examination for employees with a history of photosensitivity or those working with UV lasers.

Various specific examinations including external ocular (<350 nm or >1400 nm exposure), slit lamp (<420 nm or >750 nm) and fundoscopic evaluations (0.390–1.4 nm and any aphakic worker) are required as a function of the type of potential laser exposure. Tonometry and fundoscopic photographs are not required but may be useful in specific circumstances or for employees with previous laser eye problems.

The use of an outside ophthalmology consultant may be required in accident investigations or as part of the ongoing program. While important, medical surveillance programs are *not* a substitute for adequate institutional controls or safety programs.

SUMMARY AND CONCLUSION

Lasers represent a relatively new form of toxicologic and occupational hazard. There are a myriad of health and safety issues associated with the establishment of an adequate laser health and safety program. The ability to access a wide variety of health and safety professionals is required. The expansion of laser technology and applications will inevitably lead toward greater human exposure and the discovery of new medical and safety hazards.

REFERENCES

Note:
A variety of medical (ophthalmology) textbooks are available for specific consultation. *Laser Safety Training Manual* and *Laser Hazard Analysis Program* from Rockwell Associates probably present the most readable and detailed discussions currently available.
1. Laser Safety Training Manual. 6th ed. Cincinnati, OH: Rockwell Associates, 1984.
2. Lazan. Laser Hazard Analysis Program. 1st ed. Cincinnati, OH: Rockwell Associates, 1988.
3. Sliney DH, Wolborst ML. Safety with lasers and other sources. New York, NY: Plenum Press, 1980.
4. Safety of Lasers and Other Optical Radiation Sources. Cincinnati, OH: Rockwell Associates, 1986.
5. Laser safety guide. Toledo, OH: Laser Institute of America, 1986.
6. Stellar S. The carbon dioxide surgical laser in neurological surgery, decubitous ulcers, and burns. Lasers Surg Med 1980;1:15–33.
7. Fuller TA. The physics of surgical lasers. Lasers Surg Med 1980;1:5–14.
8. Rockwell RJ, Jr, ed. Laser safety in surgery and medicine. 2nd ed. Cincinnati, OH: Rockwell Associates, 1985.
9. ANSI. American national standard for the safe use of lasers, ANSI Z-136.1. New York: American National Standards Institute, 1986.
10. Rockwell RJ, Jr. Controlling laser hazards. Lasers Applic September 1986:93–99.
11. Rockwell RJ, Jr. Analyzing laser hazards. Lasers Applic May 1986:97–103.
12. Liou SH, Ianno NJ. Pulsed laser evaporation of Tl-Ba-Ca-Cu-O films in science and technology of thin film superconductors. McConnell RD, Wolf SA, eds. New York: Plenum Press, 1989.
13. Berns MW. Laser surgery. Sci Am 1991;264:84–90.
14. American Conference of Governmental Industrial Hygienists. Threshold Limit Values. 1990–1991. Cincinnati, OH.

116

Nonionizing Electromagnetic Radiation

Gary R. Krieger, M.D., M.P.H.
Richard Irms Ph.D.

INTRODUCTION AND BACKGROUND

The electromagnetic (EM) spectrum is a general term that encompasses energy over an enormous range of wavelengths. These wavelengths extend from less than 10^{-12} centimeters for cosmic and x-rays to 10^{+10} centimeters for microwave and electrical power generation energy. Electromagnetic energy is described by Planck's law $E = hV$, where E equals energy in electron volts, V equals the frequency of oscillation, and h equals Planck's constant (Table 116.1).

The relationship of these variables is such that, as wavelength decreases, frequency and energy increase. Therefore, the higher energies are associated with x-ray and gamma-radiation (10^8 electron volts) while the lower energies (e.g., 10^{-6} eV) are associated with radio frequency and microwave emissions.

Figure 116.1 displays the full electromagnetic spectrum as a function of frequency and wavelength. This figure divides the EM spectrum into two broad categories: ionizing and nonionizing radiation. The ability to ionize atoms is at the heart of the distinction between the two broad forms of radiation. The lower limit for ionization in biological systems is 10–12 eV (Table 116.2) where one million (10^6) electron volts represent the ability to lift a 1-milligram weight to a height of 10 nanometers. EM radiation less than the 10–12 eV level is considered insufficient to ionize biologically significant atoms. Nonradiant energy is absorbed into a molecule and either affects the electronic energy levels of its atoms or changes the transitional, rotational, or vibrational energies of the specific molecule. It is important to realize that the term nonionizing radiation is generic and, in fact, does not accurately describe the interaction of electric and magnetic fields. This interaction does not involve radiation; therefore, the term "nonionizing radiation" is a misnomer when applied to direct current (DC) and extremely low frequency (ELF) forms of energy. Nevertheless, as illustrated in Figure 116.1, nonionizing radiation has become the general descriptive term of choice for a wide variety of energy forms: radio frequency (RF), microwave (MW), infrared (IR), visible, and part of the ultraviolet (UV) spectrum.

A basic description of the IR, visible, and UV energies will be presented; however, these energies are more fully covered in the chapter on lasers. Microwave and radio frequency energy will be discussed separately with special emphasis on the controversy surrounding the potential toxicity associated with the interaction of electric and magnetic fields. The constants, prefixes, units of measure, and conversion factors associated with the discussion of nonionizing radiation are particularly critical and are listed in Tables 116.1 and 116.2.

UV, visible, and IR energies will be initially discussed, followed by separate sections on microwave and radio frequency energies.

Ultraviolet Spectrum

Exposure to the UV spectrum of radiation is a universal experience. The sun represents the most common source of UV radiation and accounts for the greatest source of overexposure (e.g., sunburning) (1). The UV spectrum and its associated target organs and effects are shown in Table 116.3.

While solar radiation is the dominant source of UV exposure, there are a variety of industrial UV sources: lasers, arc welding, hot-metal operation, and plasma-torch operations. Significant exposures to these sources can also produce target organ morbidity.

UV energies produce photochemical reactions or fluorescence. These effects are a function of the absorption spectrum of the molecule and the efficiency of specific wavelength energies in producing a particular effect. In certain circumstances, such as those associated with high energy lasers, a high rate of energy delivery coupled with sufficient absorption will produce thermal rather than photochemical effects.

UV — Health Effects and Toxicity

The skin and eyes are the two main target organs associated with UV exposure. UV radiation causes vasodilation and a concomitant increase in the volume of blood in the dermis (1). These effects can be produced by either solar or artificially generated UV radiation. Skin effects are quantified and classified both by visual production of erythema and by the quantity of specific wavelength energy delivered per square centimeter (Table 116.4). The minimal erythema dose (MED) is quite variable and is a function of an individual's skin type, skin thickness, quantity of melanin in the skin, and wavelength of the delivered UV radiation (1). Tables 116.3 and 116.4 correlate specific UV wavelength with maximal erythemal effect.

Photodamage, regardless of source, can produce significant longterm cutaneous changes. Histologically, these changes are dominated by the development of large quantities of thickened,

Table 116.1. Constants and Prefixes

Constants		
Planck's constant	h	6.63×10^{-34} J/H
Speed of light in vacuum	c	3×10^{10} cm/sec
Electron volt	eV	1.6×10^{-19} J
Prefixes		
p pico = 10^{-12}		
n nano = 10^{-9}		
μ micro = 10^{-6}		
m milli = 10^{-3}		
c (as in cm) centi = 10^{-2}		
k (as in kg) kilo = 10^3		
M mega = 10^6		
G giga = 10^9		

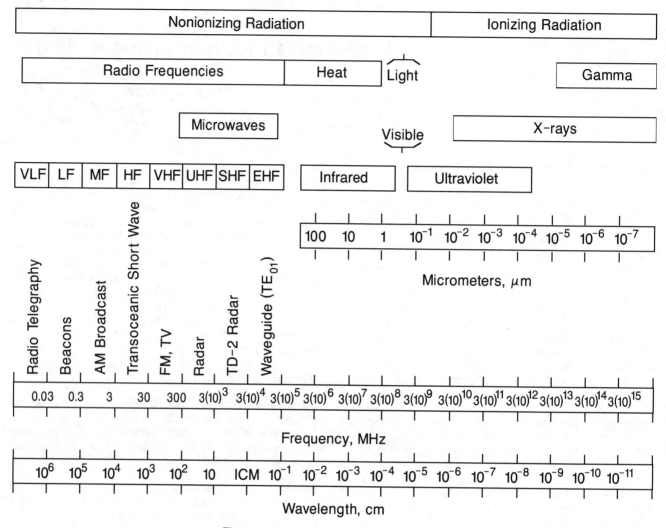

Figure 116.1.   The electromagnetic spectrum.

tangled elastic fibers (2). Typically, these changes have been considered irreversible; however, work in animals demonstrates that further avoidance of significant UV exposure coupled with sunscreen application will allow normal repair mechanisms an opportunity to reverse some of the damage (3). In addition, wrinkling, roughness, and mottling skin changes are positively affected by the longterm application of 0.1% tretinoin cream (4). While noncarcinogenic UV skin effects are quite common, the carcinogenic potential of UV-B radiation poses a significant source of both morbidity and mortality (1). Both cutaneous malignant melanoma and nonmelanoma skin cancers are highly related to solar UV-B exposure; however, the shorter UV-B and the UV-A ranges appear to be less injurious to the skin (5–10). Equivalent industrial UV-B source exposures are infrequent, but mechanistically can produce both photodamage and carcinogenesis (11). UV exposures in the range of 320–400 nanometers are capable of producing phototoxic skin reactions. These reactions are not immunologically mediated and occur on first exposure to UV radiation and the potentially offending material (1). A wide variety of chemicals and drugs are capable of phototoxicity (Table 116.5) (12).

Unlike the skin, ocular structures are particularly sensitive to UV radiation because of the thinness of the conjunctival

epithelium and the lack of protective stratum cornea and melanin granules. Repeated UV exposure can cause thickening and hypervascularity of the conjunctiva. The cornea is sensitive to UV wavelengths below 295 nanometers because nucleic and amino acids in the cornea act as chromophores and absorb these wavelengths (13). Fortunately, the corneal epithelium is highly regenerative, and clinical keratitis is usually transient with resolution in 24–48 hours. Figure 116.2, from the National Institute for Occupational Safety and Health (NIOSH), illustrates the general absorption properties of the eye for EM radiation (11).

The differences between short and long wavelength UV are very significant and produce different ocular pathology. Intense UV radiation of wavelengths between 295 and 325 nanometers can photochemically induce cataracts within 24 hours (14, 15). These types of lesions are often produced by discrete laser exposures (14).

In addition to photochemical cataracts, thermally induced lesions can be immediately produced by lens absorption to 365 nanometers radiation (16). Energy in the 365-namometer wavelength range can excite the lens or cause the aqueous or vitreous humor to fluoresce and produce a temporary diffuse impairment of visual acuity. While immediate high intensity exposure can

Table 116.2.   Units of Measure

Term	Symbol	Description	Unit and Abbreviation	
Radiant energy	O	Capacity of electromagnetic waves to perform work	Joule (J)	
Radiant power	P	Time rate at which energy is emitted	Watt (W) 1 W = 1 J/s	
Irradiance or radiant flux density	E	Radiant flux density	Watt per square	
Radiant intensity	I	Radiant flux or power emitted per solid angle (steradian)	Watt per steradian	
Radiant exposure (dose in photobiology)	H	Total energy incident on unit area in a given time interval	Joule per square meter	
Beam divergence		Unit of angular measure. One radian = 57.3°, two radians = 360°	Radian	
Standard SI unit				
Length		1 m = 100 cm = 1000 mm	Meter	(m)
Area		$1\ m^2 = 10^4\ cm^2$	Square Meter	(m^2)
Mass		$1\ kg = 10^3\ g$	Kilogram	(kg)
Energy		$1\ J = 10^7\ erg = 2.389$ (10^{-4}) kcal	Joule	(J)
Power		1 W = 1 Joule/sec	Watt	(W)
Force		$1\ N = 1\ kg\ m/sec^2$	Newton	(N)
Electrical potential		1 V = 1 J/C where C = coulomb	Volt	
Power per unit mass		1 W/kg = 1 mW/g	1 Watt/kilogram	(1 W/kg)
Power per unit area		$1\ W/m^2 = 0.1\ mW/cm^2$	Watt/square meter	(W/m^2)
Frequency (symbol f)		1 Hz = 1 cycle per second	Hertz	(Hz)
Electric resistance		1 Ohm = 1 V/A	Ohm	
Electric potential difference			Volt	(V)
Electric current			Ampere	(A)
Electric current density			$Ampere/m^2$	(A/m^2)
Electric field intensity			Volt per meter	(V/m)
Flux of magnetic induction		1 Wb = 1 V/sec	Weber	(Wb)
Magnetic field intensity H			Ampere per meter	(A/m)
Magnetic flux density		$1\ T = 10^4\ Gauss = 10^7 mG$ $1\ T = 1\ Wb/m^2$	Telsa	(T)

Table 116.3.   UV Spectrum: Target Organs and Effects

Spectral Domain	Eye	Skin	Description
UV-C 200–280			Ozone production 170–230 nm Germicidal 220–280 nm
UV-B 280 nm–315 nm	Photokeratitis Cataracts 295 nm–325 nm	Erythema skin cancer photoaging	Maximal erythema effect 290–310 nm
UV-A 315 nm–400 nm	Photochemical cataract	Pigment darkening	"Blacklight" region

Table 116.4.   Visible and Infrared Spectrum

	Wavelength	Eye Effects	Skin
Visible	400–780 nm	Photochemical and thermal retinal injury	Photosensitive
Infrared A	780–1400 nm	Cataract retinal burn	Burn
Infrared B	1.4–3.0 μm	Corneal burn aqueous flare cataract	Burn
Infrared C	3.0–1000 μm	Corneal burn	Burn

produce cataracts, there is increasing evidence that repeated exposure to longer UV wavelengths (greater than 324 nm) can also produce cataracts. Thus, UV radiation has been implicated as an etiologic agent in the development of posterior cataracts (17, 18).

Retinal damage from UV radiation is also possible, although

Table 116.5. Systemic Photosensitizers

Compound	Action Wavelength
Antibiotics	320–400
Tetracyclines and derivatives	
Griseofulvin	
Nalidixic acid	
Sulfonamides	
Chlorothiazides	290–400
Estrogens and progesterones	290–320
Furocoumarins	320–400
Psoralen and derivatives	
Psychoactive drugs	
Phenothiazines	290–400
Chlordiazepoxide	290–360

Contact Photosensitizers	
Compound	Use
Dyes	Cosmetics and dye industry
Coal tar and derivatives	Hair shampoos, therapy for psoriasis
Cadmium sulfide	Tattoos
Hexachlorophene	Antiseptic
Halogenated salicylanilides	Bacteriostatic agents in soaps
Essential oils	Cosmetics and beauty aids

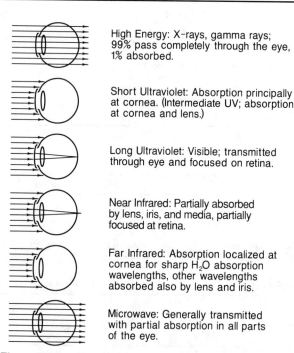

High Energy: X-rays, gamma rays; 99% pass completely through the eye, 1% absorbed.

Short Ultraviolet: Absorption principally at cornea. (Intermediate UV; absorption at cornea and lens.)

Long Ultraviolet: Visible; transmitted through eye and focused on retina.

Near Infrared: Partially absorbed by lens, iris, and media, partially focused at retina.

Far Infrared: Absorption localized at cornea for sharp H_2O absorption wavelengths, other wavelengths absorbed also by lens and iris.

Microwave: Generally transmitted with partial absorption in all parts of the eye.

Figure 116.2.   General absorption properties of the eye for electromagnetic radiation. Source: National Institute of Occupational Safety and Health.

the effects are usually limited because of the absorptive characteristics of the cornea and lens. Aphakic or pseudoaphakic conditions enhance the likelihood of retinal damage and would lower exposure thresholds. The UV spectrum where retinal damage may occur is between 325 and 441 nanometers (19).

UV — Exposure and Photoprotection

Threshold Limit Values (TLVs) have been developed for nonlaser UV exposures. TLVs represent conditions under which it is believed that nearly all workers may be repeatedly exposed without adverse health effects (20). These TLVs are values for exposures to the eye and skin from various nonlaser sources: arcs, gas and vapor discharge, fluorescent and incandescent sources, and solar radiation. UV lasers are covered by a separate set of TLVs and are discussed in the chapter on lasers. Three groups not covered by the American Conference of Governmental Industrial Hygienists (ACGIH) TLVs are: (a) photosensitive individuals, (b) individuals exposed to photosensitizing agents, and (c) aphakics. Table 116.5 lists one variety of common systemic and contact photosensitizers (12). The UV TLVs for occupational exposure are keyed to two variables: (a) irradiance values are known and (b) exposure time is controlled. The most current ACGIH TLVs should be consulted for further details and explanations.

In addition to the TLV guidance, a variety of protective measures are available: (a) chemical sunscreens that provide protection by absorbing UV radiation and (b) physical barriers that block UV radiation from reaching the skin or eye. Protection goggles containing special glass lenses can absorb all UV-A, UV-B, and visible light up to 500 nanometers. Simply closing the eyes and using regular sunglasses are not sufficient for full ocular protection (1).

Visible Spectrum

The visible radiation spectrum is a narrow band between 400 and 780 nanometers (Fig. 116.1 and Table 116.4). There are a large variety of sources for visible radiation: sunlight, lighting fixtures, lasers, and arcs. Vision is a complex photochemical and physiologic process; however, exposure to nonlaser-generated visable radiation spectrum does not typically produce significant morbidity. Flash blindness can be produced by exposure to visible wavelength and is caused by the temporary depletion of visual pigments. If the intensity and exposure are sufficient, an outer image or temporary scotoma will be produced in the visual field. Normally, serious injuries are avoided due to a variety of indigenous protective mechanisms: (a) pupil size changes, (b) eyelids, and (c) aversion response within 0.25 seconds of exposure. These mechanisms are protective under most circumstances; however, thermal injury can occur if source intensity and exposure times are high. In addition, some individuals may be highly photosensitive or may be concomitantly exposed to photosensitizing agents.

High-powered pulsed visible wavelength lasers can produce both thermal damage and structural damage to the retinal and choroidal tissue from acute pressure differentials known as acoustic transients. Lasers and the beneficial uses of laser-induced shock waves are discussed in a previous chapter.

TLVs are available for visible radiation and are a function of the spectral and total irradiance of the source as measured at the position(s) of the worker's eyes. The most current ACGIH handbook should be consulted for further detail (20).

Infrared Spectrum

As shown in Table 116.4, infrared radiation covers wavelengths from 780 nanometers (0.78 micrometers) to 10^6 nanometers (1000 micrometers). Within this broad range, infrared radiation is divided into three regions: A, B, and C. In general, biologic materials are opaque to energies within the infrared B and C regions. Radiation in the infrared B and C region is almost

Table 116.6. Microwave Band Designations

Band	Wavelength	Frequency	Typical Uses
Very high frequency (VHF)	10–1.0 m	30–300 MHz	FM radio Television Air traffic control
Ultra high frequency (UHF)	1.0–0.1 m	0.3–3 GHz	Television CB radios Microwave ovens
Super high frequency (SHF)	10–0.01 m	3–30 GHz	Satellite communication Weather radar
Extra high frequency (EHF)	0.01–0.001 m	30–300 GHz	Radio astronomy Cloud detection radar

completely absorbed by water; therefore, these energies produce a thermal response.

Infrared wavelengths are produced in a large variety of industrial and domestic sources: metal and glass fabrication and heating, baking and drying operations for paints and coatings, hot furnaces, arc processes, and even with incandescent bulbs. While the dominant effect of IR irradiation is thermal, the vibrational modes of large molecules can also be affected and produce fluorescent UV emissions. Thus, both UV and IR radiation can be generated by a given source (11).

IR — Health Effects

IR-A (780–1400 nanometers) can produce direct skin effects including acute skin burn and persistent increases in skin pigmentation (21). Ocular effects can be quite prominent and damaging. Figure 116.2 illustrates the differential ocular effects associated with various wavelengths of infrared radiation. The iris is particularly sensitive to IR-A. In addition, small retinal lesions can also occur. The lens is more susceptible to IR-B, and thermally generated opacities can be produced. As previously discussed in the section on UV radiation, glassblower's cataracts are probably due to both IR and UV radiation (22–24).

ACGIH TLVs are available for IR exposures and are directed toward the prevention of cataractogenesis. IR exposures to wavelengths over 780 nanometers should be limited to 10 mW/cm^2. Where IR exposures occur without a concomitant visible light stimulus, radiation is limited by a calculation based on spectral radiance, viewing angle, and a 7-millimeter pupil diameter. Detailed calculations and tables are available in the current ACGIH TLV handbook (20).

Microwave Spectrum

Microwave (MW) radiation is energy in the EM spectrum with frequencies between 300 MHz (million) and 300 GHz (billion) (Fig. 116.1, Table 116.6). The unit of frequency for MW radiation is the hertz (Hz). One hertz is equal to one cycle per second. Wavelengths for MW frequencies are usually measured in meters (Table 116.2). While microwaves are part of the board radio frequency (RF) spectrum, the increasing controversy over low power frequency fields necessitates separate evaluation and discussion for these energies.

As shown in Table 116.6, microwave energy is divided into four general bands. There are a wide variety of uses and applications for these frequencies, and the potential for exposure has significantly increased (25).

The principal mechanism of action for MW frequencies is the conversion of electromagnetic energy into thermal energy. This process occurs secondary to the linear rotational vibration of ions and polar molecules. These thermal effects do not result in uniform heating patterns because the MW strikes different materials (e.g., bone, fat, muscle), producing a nonuniform combination of reflected and standing waves. The spatial distribution of the absorbed energy is dependent on a variety of parameters: (a) frequency of initial radiation, (b) electrical properties of the target material, (c) recipient material thickness, (d) geometrical shape and size of the receiving object, and (e) orientation of the object relative to the direction of the electric field of the incident wave (26). The increasing use of stealth (e.g., radar absorbing) technology for radar evasion is based on many of these parameters. Stealth aircraft are uniquely shaped and fabricated with a variety of nonreflective and highly absorbent materials.

The rate at which energy is absorbed per unit mass of absorbing material is known as the Specific Absorption Rate (SAR). SAR is described in watts per kilogram. The calculation of SARs for a variety of shapes and materials is possible and, when coupled with knowledge of the parameters of the incident field, is quite useful. For example, the irradiation of the human body with a power density of 10 mW/cm^2 will produce an absorption of approximately 58 watts (27). This absorption will result in an overall increase in body temperature of 1°C.

A 1°C elevation is considered acceptable and should be viewed within the context of other standard physiologic parameters. By way of comparison, the resting human basal metabolic rate is approximately 80 watts (approximately 1.1–1.3 W/kg) while moderate work produces 290 watts (28).

Microwave — Health Effects

The potential health effects of MW in humans and animals has been the subject of a number of extensive reviews (25, 26, 29–35). Over the last decade, the health effects focus has switched from microwave frequencies to extremely low power frequency fields. However, there is still an extensive body of older microwave-specific literature.

Microwave wavelengths penetrate the skin and internal organs of humans and animals as a function of wavelength. Wavelengths less than 0.03 meter (3 centimeters) are absorbed in the outer skin surface, while 0.03–0.1 m (3–10 cm) wavelengths can penetrate 1 millimeter to 1 centimeter into the skin. Internal organ penetration is associated with wavelengths from 0.25–2 meters (25–200 centimeters). The human body is essentially transparent to wavelengths greater than 2 meters (200 centimeters) (11).

In 1982, the American National Standards Institute (ANSI) C95 Committee conducted an extensive review of the microwave health effects literature (36). This committee was organized in order to update and revise the ANSI 1974 microwave and radio frequency exposure guide. An enormous number of papers were reviewed according to a four-part criteria: (a) positive findings, (b) relevance, (c) reproducibility, and (d) dosimetric quantifiability. Approximately 30 papers were chosen, and 15 categories of bioeffects were selected (Table 116.7) (36).

Selected studies within each of these bioeffects categories were well reviewed by Petersen in 1983, Aldrich and Easterly in 1987, Office of Technology Assessment in 1989, and by the EPA in 1990 (25, 26, 37). (The 1990 EPA Draft Review, "Evaluation of the Potential Carcinogenicity of Electromag-

Table 116.7. Microwave Bioeffects

Environmental factors
Behavior and physiology
Immunology
Teratology
CNS/blood-brain barrier
Cataracts
Genetics
Human studies
Thermoregulation and metabolism
Circadian
Endocrinology
Development
Evoked auditory response
Hematology
Cardiovascular

Sources: Petersen RC. Bioeffects of microwaves: a review of current knowledge. J Occup Med 1983;25:103–110 and American National Standards Institute (ANSI). American National Standards Institute safety levels with respect to human exposure to radio frequency electromagnetic fields, 300 kHz to 100 GHz. New York, NY: Institute of Electrical and Electronics Engineers, Inc. ANSI C95.1-1982.

netic Fields,'' EPA/600/6-90/0058, has not been released in final form for official citation.) While many of these studies were focused on extremely low frequency fields (ELF), microwave frequencies were utilized in many test systems and animal studies. Table 116.8 summarizes many of the bioeffects specifically associated with microwave energies (38–51); however, the possible association of cataracts and MW exposure in humans requires a detailed discussion. (ELF bioeffects are reviewed in a separate section of this chapter.)

Ocular effects, particularly those associated with the lens, have been investigated in both animals and humans (26, 52–63). Overall, the severity of ocular damage associated with MW is a function of intensity, wavelength, and direction of exposure. The human exposure data are controversial, and standards are based on extrapolation from animal studies (53). Animal data demonstrate a threshold effect for microwave cataractogenesis. The rabbit eye requires a minimum exposure level of 100 mW/cm². The application of a 10-fold safety factor for animal to human extrapolation results in a maximal permissible exposure level of 10 mW/cm². This number was incorporated into the 1982 ANSI standard and current 1990/91 ACGIH TLVs (30, 36).

Recently, Paz et al. reported the potential for significant exposures to MW energy under operating room conditions (53). These authors raised the specter of substantial exposures in the spectral range associated with cataractogenesis to surgeons and other operating room personnel. The MW sources in this situation are electrosurgical units (ESUs). ESUs are capable of MW emissions exceeding 150 mW/cm² (53). Clearly, this potential exposure source requires further investigation and monitoring since 150 mW/cm² exposures for 100 minutes can thermally produce cataracts in animals (26).

Microwave Exposure Criteria and Control Measures

The current 1990/91 ACGIH TLVs were selected in order to limit the average whole body SAR to 0.4 W/kg in any 6-minute (0.1 hour) period over frequencies 3 MHz–300 GHz. International standards vary from country to country and have been extensively reviewed by Polk and Postow (65). U.S. standards

are generally based on two factors: (a) the amount of heat resulting from MW absorption and (b) the ability of the exposed organism to dissipate the heat. In the USSR, Soviet health standards for MW exposure are based on both thermal and nonthermal effects.

Soviet investigators have published a number of papers that report a variety of nonthermal effects: (a) central nervous system/behavioral, (b) decreases in cholinesterase levels, (c) changes in RNA, and (d) disturbances of the menstrual cycle (66–70). These reports are controversial and have met with considerable skepticism (26). Nevertheless, the Soviet standards for radiation power density and field strength are significantly lower than equivalent U.S. standards. Table 116.9 illustrates a variety of U.S., Soviet, and other international standards.

In general, engineering controls are usually the most satisfactory technique for minimizing exposures to MW radiation. Personal protective devices have been developed but are less useful than engineering controls.

ELECTROMAGNETIC FIELDS

Background

Electric power systems produce electric and magnetic fields. These fields are associated with power lines, wiring, and lighting in the home and workplace and all non-battery-dependent electrical appliances. Electric fields represent the forces or strength that electric charges exert on other charges at a distance, while magnetic fields are produced by the motion of the charge. The combination of the electric and magnetic effects is known as an electromagnetic field (EMF). Power systems produce an oscillating EMF at 50–60 times per second. These EMFs are known as 50–60 hertz power. In North America, 60 hertz is the standard, while in Europe 50 hertz is commonly found.

EMF did not emerge as a potential health and environmental issue until the late 1960s. As power companies utilized extra high voltage (EHV) transmission lines, a variety of environmental effects were raised: (a) aesthetics, (b) right-of-way issues, (c) nuisance effects such as TV/radio interference and audio noise, and (d) induced shocks that can occur when an individual located beneath an EHV line touches an ungrounded metal object.

In the late 1960s, Soviet investigators published a series of papers describing the potential adverse biologic effects of various wavelength microwave and radio frequency energy (66–70). These reports were further amplified by Korobkova's 1972 report of adverse health impacts on Soviet EHV switch yard workers (70). When this undercurrent of potential harmful human health effects was coupled with a voluminous experimental body of biologic effects data, the issue was brought center stage. While there are numerous papers associated with potential biologic effects of broad spectrum radio frequency/microwave emissions, there has been considerable skepticism surrounding the claims of adverse biologic health effects of electromagnetic fields (25, 37, 65, 71–88). There are three sources of this skepticism: (a) there is no significant transfer of energy from power-frequency fields to biologic systems; (b) 50–60 Hz EMFs do not break chemical bonds and cannot cause significant thermal effects in tissue; and (c) in humans, all cells maintain large natural electric fields across their outer membranes. Naturally occurring fields are at least 100 times more intense than those typically associated with 50–60 Hz

Table 116.8.   Bioeffects—Microwave Energy

Bioeffect	Species	SAR	Power/Frequency	Result
Environmental (34, 46)	Male CFI mice	0.06–64 w/kg		Threshold of the animal for mw varies inversely with temp.
Behavior and physiology (47)	Female Sprague-Dawley rats		Pulsed/continuous wave	Pulsed energy is more effective than CW in evoking a response
Cytogenetics (48)	Chinese hamsters	0–20.7 w/kg	2.45 GHz (-cw)	No chromosomal abnormalities nor ONA damage Positive lymphocyte transformation
Teratology (49)	Pregnant CD-1 mice	2–8.1 w/kg	2.45 GHz (-cw)	Positive observed effects noted for mean fetal weight. No difference with live, dead, total fetuses per litter
CNS/blood brain (50, 51)	Killed neonatal chicks	0.003 w/kg	147 MHz	Positive possible power density window for calcium efflux
Cataracts	See text			
Thermoregulation metabolism (38, 39)	Squirrel monkeys	0.15–3.25 w/kg	1–22 mw/kg 2.45 GHz	Positive ? via internal thermoreceptors
Circadian (40)	Male Long-Evans rats	0.36–36 w/kg	1–10 mW/cm²	Positive effect on timing of rectal temperature rise, positive effects on corticosteroid
Development (41)	Neonatal rats	13 w/kg	0–40 mw/cm² 2.45 GHz	Positive increased adrenal responsiveness
Evoked auditory response (42)	Cats, humans	10–16 mJ/kg 16 mJ/kg	Positive exposure to pulse-modulated fields, procedure checking or buzzing sensation if the modulation rate is within the normal frequency rate	
Hematologic (43, 48)	Mice, rats, rabbits	1.8 w/kg	2 mw/cm² 3.105 GHz	Positive, increase in protein synthesis in the liver, thymus, spleen
Cardiovascular (30, 31)	Rat	1.5–2.5 w/kg	960 MHz	Negative

Sources: References 25, 26, 37, 65.

EMF exposure. Specifically, the earth has an electric field of approximately 130 V/m. This field is static, vertically directed, and caused by the separation of charges between the earth and the ionosphere.

Nevertheless, in a variety of laboratory studies involving animal cells and tissues, diverse and potentially significant biologic effects have been reported (25, 37, 89–92):

1. Modulation of ion flows (93–99)
2. Interference with DNA synthesis and RNA transcription (100, 101)
3. Interaction with the response of normal cells to various agents and biochemicals (102–107)
4. Interaction with the biochemical kinetics of cancer cells (108–113)

Despite these observations, it is crucial to recognize that isolated test system effects may not be directly translated into adverse effects on the total organism. Furthermore, there has been a lack of any large scale and obvious public health effects despite decades of increasing electrification (37).

While large scale public health effects have not been reliably reproduced, the last decade (1980–1990) has generated intense public concern over low power EMF exposure in two specific areas:

1. The potential reproductive effects of exposure to very low frequency EMFs associated with video display terminals (VDTs)
2. Potential carcinogenicity of EMFs based on human epidemiologic studies

Before these issues are discussed, several terms, units, and basic physics concepts will be reviewed.

Fundamentals — Electric Fields

The electric field on a charged object describes the electric force that the object is capable of exerting on other charged particles brought into close proximity. The intensity of the electric field is proportional to the magnitude of this force. Electric field intensity is measured in volts per meter (Table 116.2). The fields produced by alternating current (AC) electric generators are dynamic rather than static. For example, bat-

Table 116.9. Microwave Exposure Standards and Recommendations

Standard	Frequency Range/Duration	Exposure Limit where f = frequency in MHz
ANSI–1982	300–1500 MHz continuous	4000 (F/300) V²/m² 0.025 (F/300) A²/m² F/30 W/m²
	1.5–100 GHz continuous	2 (10⁴) V²/m² 0.125 A²/m² 50 W/m²
ACGIH–1990/ 1991	100–1000 MHz 8-hour work day	F/100 (mW/cm²) 3770 (F/100) V²/m² f/(37.7 × 100) A²/m²
	1–300 GHz 8-hour work day	10 mW/cm² 37,700 V2/m² 0.265 A²/m²
OSHA–1983	10 MHz–100 GHz 8-hour work day	100 W/m²
France	0.03–300 GHz Greater than 1 hour	10 W/m²
USSR–1984	0.3–300 GHz 24 hours	0.1 W/m²

Table 116.10. Magnetic Flux Densities of Common Appliances (mG)

Appliance	Distance		
	1 cm	5 cm	15 cm
Hair dryer	60–20,000	1–70	0.1–3
Electric razor	150–15,000	1–90	0.4–3
Microwave oven	750–2,000	40–80	3–8
Electric range	60–2,000	4–40	0.1–1
Television	25–500	0.4–20	0.1–2

Adapted from: Business Week: April 15, 1991:72–72 and Edison Electric Institute, Carniege Mellon University.

teries produce DC or direct, nonalternating current. Electric fields also change as a function of distance from the primary source. Simplistically, the strength or magnitude of an electric field (E) between two conductive plates is given by the equation $E = v/d$ where v equals the potential difference and d equals distance. Electric fields are also *vector* fields. This means that the field specifies a magnitude and a direction for each point in space. This is important because in environmental exposure the direction of the electric field can vary for each point in space.

Humans and several other mammals can perceive electric fields at approximately 15 kV/m. To place this number in perspective, directly beneath a 500 kV transmission line, maximum electric fields are approximately 5 kV/m. At the edge of a typical EHV transmission line, fields are typically 1–2 kV/m.

Fundamentals — Magnetic Fields

Magnetic fields are produced when charges are in motion, for example, by an alternating current generator. Magnetic fields can exert a force on both electric charges and on ions or electrolytes moving through the bloodstream. The magnitude of the magnetic field (H) (see Table 116.2) can be represented by the simple equation: $H = I/2\pi d$ where I equals current and d equals distance. Similar to an electric field, the direction of a magnetic field can also vary for each point in space. Magnetic fields are measured in amperes (current) per meter.

Both electric and magnetic fields can act on certain materials. These materials can be described by their conductivity, δ, permittivity, E, and permeability, μ. When exposed to an electric field, certain materials demonstrate charge separation or the ability to provide insulation. Insulators are also known as dielectrics. Although there are no perfect insulators, the insulating ability of fused quartz is about 10^{25} times as great as that of copper. The electric displacement or electric flux density, D, can be used when dielectrics are present such that $D = eE$.

The permittivity or dielectric constant, E, of air is close to that of a vacuum so that for air exposures, a fixed relationship exists between E and D. In most bioeffect experiments, the exposure field, E, is described before the subject is placed in the field.

Analogously to electric fields, magnetic materials have induced magnetic movements when exposed to a magnetic field. The magnetic flux density, B, is related to the magnetic field by the equation $B = \mu H$. Unlike the variability of dielectric constants, the permeability of most biologic materials is very close to that of air or a vacuum. Therefore, B and H are basically interchangeable. As Table 116.2 illustrates, the magnetic flux density B, is measured in the System Internationale (SI) system in teslas (7). B can also be measured in the older nomenclature of the centimeter-gram-second (CGS) system. In the CGS system, B is quantified in gauss. There are 10,000 gauss in 1 tesla. Gauss units are further subdivided into thousandths of a gauss or milligauss. The preferred unit of measure is the tesla; however, many older papers and popular descriptions still employ the CGS units of gauss and milligauss.

To illustrate these units, consider the previously discussed 500 kV transmission line. This line has a right-of-way electric field of 1–2 kV/m and a magnetic flux density of approximately 10 mG. To further place these numbers in perspective and understand why there is considerable skepticism associated with EMF exposure, it is necessary to consider the earth's natural magnetic field. The naturally occurring magnetic field is static and has a flux density of 500–670 mG in the vertical direction. In the horizontal direction, flux densities are approximately 300 mG at the equator and zero at the magnetic poles. By way of comparison, Table 116.10 illustrates the magnetic flux density in milligauss of several common household appliances.

General Discussion — Electric and Magnetic Fields

Electric and magnetic fields can vary according to the frequency or number of times that the field oscillates per second. In addition, the dielectric properties of biologic substances vary with the frequency of the applied electric field exposure. For extremely low frequency (ELF) fields (3–300 Hz) the two fields are virtually independent and are unrelated to concepts of radiation. Therefore, the term extremely low frequency electromagnetic radiation is inappropriate.

As previously discussed in the section on microwaves, power density can be described in W/m², although radio frequency bioeffects exposures are commonly reported in mW/cm² (Table 116.2). Power density is a useful concept because many bioeffects studies consider the amount of energy input to the biologic system from the electromagnetic field. Unfortunately, the relationship between field strength, power density, and biologic systems is quite complex such that power density units can be inaccurate. A more useful quantity is the specific absorption rate (SAR) (See previous discussion of SAR under microwave section.) SAR is a measure in W/kg of the power absorbed per unit mass of the biologic specimen under consideration. The measurement of the SAR is more useful than the individual specification of external field strength or power density. This is illustrated by the observed phenomena of biologic specimens absorbing energy from reactive fields when power density calculations are extremely low (37).

Overall, the coupling of ELF fields to the body is complicated by a number of factors:

1. Body orientation
2. Field polarization
3. Grounding condition
4. Contact with other conductors
5. Body geometry

For example, the internal electric fields and current densities in a human and a rat exposed to the same external ELF electric field are significantly different. Thus, the extrapolation of animal to human exposure is quite complex and fraught with methodologic problems and illustrates the difficulty of isolating and detecting potentially deleterious effects in living systems that are constantly exposed to high levels of background energy (37).

Biologic Effects

A variety of biologic effects for ELF fields have been reported (25, 37, 71–113, 114–150):

—Time-varying fields do not cause DNA breaks, gene mutations, or sister chromatid exchanges. This result should be expected since ELF fields do not have sufficient energy to break chemical bonds (100, 101, 118, 123, 124).
—ELF magnetic fields have been reported to cause an enhancement of DNA synthesis within a very limited range of frequency and intensity windows (120–122, 131, 137).
—Chromosomal aberrations are inconsistently found. The frequency of ELF exposure appears to be a significant variable (119, 126, 127, 134, 142).
—Pulsed versus sinusoidal waveforms are major experimental variables. Transcription synthesis of mRNA experiments illustrate this observation (119–123).
—ELF electric and combined electric and magnetic fields have delayed the cell cycle and caused transient reductions in the rate of cell division (77).
—The release of calcium ions from chick brain tissue into the medium surrounding the tissue has been affected by ELF electric and crossed ELF electric and magnetic fields. The conditions under which this phenomenon has been observed are very precise and unexplainable by current theory. The biologic significance of this phenomenon is unclear (94–99).
—Pulsed magnetic ELF fields have been reported to alter the chemical signaling process between an exogenous hormone (parathyroid hormone) and the cellular activity induced by the hormone. To date, nonpulsed fields have not been tested (143–145).
—The intracellular enzyme ornithine decarboxylase (ODC) is induced by specific frequency ELF electric fields in a variety of cell lines. ODC is induced by a variety of substances including chemical promoting agents (112, 113, 146).
—Selective ELF field exposure has been reported to cause an inhibition of the nocturnal synthesis of melatonin by the pineal gland. Melatonin has a variety of significant circadian and oncostatic properties (103, 104, 107, 116, 132, 133, 136, 138–141).
—ELF fields are reported to cause small, but inconsistent, changes in white blood cells in one human and three animal studies. In vivo and in vitro studies are *not* consistent and the ability to make predictions from cell culture experiments to whole animal responses is uncertain (114, 115, 125, 128).
—A variety of morphologic effects in developing animal brain cells has been described. The central nervous system (CNS) may be a sensor for ELF magnetic fields; however, this research is very preliminary (93, 102, 105, 130, 135).

Despite the variety and potential significance of these findings, there are important reasons for skeptically reviewing these studies. The overwhelming majority of experiments employ field strengths many times higher than that seen in ambient residential exposures. Only three phenomena have been reported under ambient residential exposure conditions (10 V/m and 2 mG or 0.2 μT): (a) calcium efflux from chick brain tissue induced by crossed electric and magnetic fields (95–97); (b) calcium efflux from chick brain tissue after exposure of the developing embryo to electric fields (95–97); and (c) inhibition of nocturnal melatonin synthesis by small changes in the orientation of static magnetic fields (128–141).

A further complicating observation is the existence of intensity "windows." A variety of effects are reported *only* within a specific and occasionally unique frequency. Not only is classical dose-response not observed but nonlinearity is seen within the observed frequency dependence. In addition, the intermittency of field application appears to be a significant observation, implying that the timing and fluctuations in exposure are more significant than the magnitude of exposure.

Overall, biologic effects have been demonstrated under a variety of experiment dependent conditions. The theoretical basis and implication for adverse health effects is at best uncertain (147–149).

Human Studies — Reproductive Effects

Beginning in the early 1980s, a variety of reports raised concerns about the potential reproductive effects of VDT-generated ELF (45–60 Hz) and VLF (15 kHz) electromagnetic fields (150–154). Unfortunately, none of these studies and several subsequent reports measured the actual EMFs produced by the VDTs. Schnorr et al. in a well-designed and controlled study, compared a cohort of female telephone operators who used VDTs at work with a cohort of similarly matched operators who did not use VDTs (155). Careful measurements of both the VDTs electric and magnetic fields were made for the exposed group. Non-VDT field exposures were also obtained. ELF measures for frontal emissions ranged from 1.8–1.9 V/m for E fields and 236–314 mA/m for H fields. When the operators were present, abdominal exposures were 0.4–0.8 V/m (E field) and 58–62 mA/m for H fields. Overall, no excess risk of spontaneous abortion during the first trimester of pregnancy was observed. Additionally, a dose-response relationship between first trimester pregnancy outcome and hours of VDT use was not found (155).

HUMAN EPIDEMIOLOGIC STUDIES

Over the last 10–15 years, more than 40 studies have been published that studied the possible relationship between EM fields and cancer (156–214). These studies have been well reviewed by Ahlbom in 1987 and 1988 (156, 157). In addition, the EPA review is exhaustive but, unfortunately, cannot be officially cited and referenced at this time.

The human epidemiologic studies can be divided into four categories: (a) studies of children exposed residentially to 50 or 60 Hz magnetic fields (158–167), (b) adult exposure studies to radio frequency emissions (168–176), (c) residential adult exposures to 50 or 60 Hz EM fields (165, 177–182), and (d) adult occupational exposure studies (182–214). Overall, these retrospective studies are inconsistent with respect to both the diseases associated with exposure and the quality of study design. The results have ranged from those indicating a positive relationship between EMF and cancer to those demonstrating inconsequential or no positive results.

Residential Exposure and Childhood Cancer

In 1979, Wertheimer and Leeper published the results of a case-control study conducted in Denver which indicated a 2–4-fold increased incidence of childhood leukemia associated with exposure to EMF (159). The study suffers from critical design shortcomings and a very controversial dosimetry model. Exposures were ranked according to a wire code configuration (WCC) constructed for the study purpose and were not blindly coded. Wertheimer and Leeper developed a novel exposure scheme utilizing maps of the electrical wires and transformers in the vicinity of birth and death addresses for cases and controls. Primary wires were classified as ''large-gauge'' or ''thin gauge.'' Large-gauge wires were designed to carry high currents. Based upon their maps, the authors classified homes as either having ''high current configuration (HCC)'' or ''low current configuration (LCC).'' The WCC was a surrogate for presumed EMF exposures. Correlations between actual EMF exposures were not obtained, multivariant analysis was not performed and, in many cases, birth and death addresses were summed, resulting in double counting. Interestingly, the results of this study triggered a flurry of news media coverage and launched several new and more sophisticated experimental designs.

Since Wertheimer and Leeper's 1979 paper, the issue of surrogate exposure measures has received extensive investigation. In order to understand the controversy associated with many of the residential exposure papers, the concept of wire code configurations requires further explanation. Originally, Wertheimer and Leeper took 558 magnetic field measurements under or in close proximity to power distribution facilities (159). These measurements were used to correlate magnetic field levels and study subject residences. Based on these initial data, study homes were classified as either ''low current configuration'' (LCC) or HCC. Despite multiple methodologic problems, this classification system was expanded in their 1982 paper and included four wiring configuration categories (177):

1. Very high current configuration (VHCC)
2. Ordinary high current configuration (OHCC)
3. Ordinary low current configuration (OLCC)
4. Endpole

Again, magnetic measurements were made outside of 417 homes and the authors reported a correlation between high magnetic field levels and HCCs.

The wire code configuration scheme is based on four general assumptions:

1. High average current flow is associated with high amp conductors.
2. Distance from conductors is linearly related to magnetic field strength.
3. A high magnetic field is associated with the first span from a secondary distribution transformer. Spans further downstream have commensurately lower magnetic fields.
4. The magnetic field associated with a given distribution line remains constant over time.

This classification scheme is a two-part process. First, overhead transmission and distribution lines are classified by the number and size of conductors and proximity (within 45 meters) to transformers. Second, the target home(s) are classified as either VHCC, OHCC, OLCC, or endpole, based on the wiring configuration and distance from the previously described lines.

Fulton conducted a similar study of childhood leukemia in Rhode Island using Wertheimer's wire code configuration scheme (160). This study was negative but is statistically flawed. In 1986, Tomenius conducted a case-control study in which he combined ''measured fields'' with line-of-sight determinations, arbitrarily ranking fields plus or minus 3kV (161). The dosimetry is however clearly problematic. Although the author reports an overall positive relationship, a review of his tables reveals a *protective* effect. There was an inverse relationship between CA and distance from transmission lines. In 1988, Savitz conducted a well-executed case-control study in Denver (163). This study combined in-home measurements and the Wertheimer-Leeper wire codes. This study found a variety of statistically insignificant odds ratios; however, the odds ratio compared with wire code configuration (OHCC and VHCC) was positive. The odds ratio (1.53) was significantly smaller than Wertheimer's original 2–4-fold increase. The study is complicated by a number of confounding variables including a differential in mobility and incidence between cases and controls.

Socioeconomic status is an extremely important potential confounding variable. Childhood cancer rates, in particular leukemia rates, are associated with socioeconomic status. It is possible that control subjects could have higher socioeconomic status than cases *and* are less likely to live in VHCC-OHCC-coded-homes. Thus, modestly elevated odds ratios could be explained by this source of study bias. Significantly, Peters et al. presented prepublication findings of an Electric Power Research Institute EMF-leukemia study on February 6 and 7, 1991 (personal communication). This study was based on 232 cases of childhood leukemia among children aged 10 and under and diagnosed during the 1980–1987 time period in Los Angeles County. Controls and cases were matched for geographic area, gender, age, and race. Wire code configuration was assessed and actual magnetic fields were measured for 24–72 hours in the child's sleeping area.

The authors reported an odds ratios of 2.5 for exposure to VHCC-and OHCC-coded homes. In addition, an odds ratio of 1.5 for homes with background 60 Hz magnetic fields greater than 2 mG. Interestingly, no association was found between measured electric field exposure and leukemia risk, while only minimal support was rated for a relationship between magnetic field exposure and leukemia risk.

Based on these findings, there remains an unexplained ob-

Table 116.11. EMF and Childhood Cancer

Study	Odds Ratio*
Wertheimer and Leeper, 1979 (159)	3.09
Fulton, 1980 (160)	1.2
Myers, 1985 (162)	>1.2
Tomenius, 1988 (161)	1.3
Savitz, 1988 (163)	1.35
Lin, 1989 (164)	1.3
Coleman, 1989 (165)	0.7–1.6

*Odds ratios vary for magnetic versus electric fields and as a function of wire code configuration and distance from presumed primary exposure source.

servation that wire code configuration correlates with leukemia risk *better* than *measured* exposures.

CHILDHOOD CANCER — SUMMARY

A relatively small number of studies examining the relationship between childhood cancer (leukemia) and EMF exposure have been published (159–163). These studies are all fraught with a number of serious methodologic and dose-response problems. As the studies have improved in experimental design and sophistication, the reported positive odds ratio has substantially declined (Table 116.11). These elevated odds ratios were associated with exposure to magnetic fields, which were estimated by the types of wires near their homes. Magnetic field measurements of 2 mG (0.2 μT) have been reported. Unfortunately, while no other agents have been identified that explain the reported association, there are contradictory results within the same studies, and dose-response relationships were not confirmed except in very limited circumstances (163). In addition, there is limited information on personal exposure, length of residency in EM exposed areas, and socioeconomic status.

Overall, since 1979 there is a persistent unexplained association between wire code configuration and leukemia risk. This risk does not correlate with actual measured electric and magnetic fields. Therefore, the source and significance of this risk are at best unclear. It is apparent, however, that wire code configuration is not a surrogate for actual exposure but may be covariate with other non-EMF-related variables.

Adult Residential Studies

As previously mentioned, Wertheimer and Leeper published results in 1982 of another case-control study relating adult CA to distance from power distribution facilities (177). The number of confounding variables were large and the case-control design was never validated. In 1988, Severson reported on a case-control study in Washington state of acute nonlymphocytic leukemia (ANLL) versus EMF (180). Exposure was assessed using both measured fields and the wire code configuration. Results of this well-designed study were negative.

In 1986, McDowell published a cancer mortality study of 8000 subjects using distance from an electrical substation or overhead line as surrogate for exposure (179). The results were positive when stratified by distance from electrical installations; however, there were a large number of methodologic problems. No exposure measurements were obtained. In 1988, a case-control study of the relationship between acute myelocytic and chronic myelocytic leukemia (AML/CML) and electric blanket

use was negative; however, no exposure estimates were obtained (182).

The adult residential and radiofrequency (RF) papers consist of a variety of case-control and cohort studies (168–176). RF studies examined special populations in the United States (169, 170–175), Moscow (168), and Poland (176). These studies all suffer from a variety of methodologic problems and present inconsistent and inconclusive results. A variety of hematologic malignancies (leukemia, Hodgkin's disease, lymphoma) were reported.

Residential adult studies also present weak and mixed results. (177–181). One 1982 study (177) was significantly positive; however, as previously discussed, it is unclear whether these authors' wire code configuration was an adequate surrogate for exposure. Furthermore, occupational confounding is a serious possibility. Whether there is a true association between exposure to EMF and certain forms of adult site-specific cancer will require further investigations.

Occupational Studies

A large number of studies (183–214) and reviews (215–220) have evaluated the possible relationship between cancer incidence or mortality and workers in areas with a high potential for exposure to EM fields (183–214). EM field exposure typically involved ELFs including 50–60 Hz power fields.

A variety of occupational studies reported significantly elevated risks of leukemia associated with jobs having a high potential for EM field exposure: (a) New Zealand—electronic equipment assemblers and radio/television repairmen (196); (b) underground miners with 25 years exposure (198); (c) Sweden—electrical workers (201); (d) United States—electricians and welders at naval nuclear shipyards (190, 191); and (e) New Zealand—electrical workers (204). However, a 16-state National Center for Health Statistics Survey of industries and occupations was negative for excess risk of leukemia (203). Matanoski's 1989 study of 50,000 active male telephone company employees is the most rigorous of these studies. In this study, three preliminary conclusions can be drawn (190):

1. There may be increased leukemia risk for some active linemen.
2. The group with the *presumed* highest EMF exposure, cable splicers, had generally high incidence rates for almost all types of cancer.
3. Two cases of breast cancer were found in male technicians who worked in central office switching equipment. Male breast cancer is a very unusual and low incidence disease.

CNS concerns have also been significantly elevated in several studies of electrical workers (203, 205–208); however, no measurements of actual exposures were obtained. There was, however, evidence of increased risk associated with employment in job categories where there was likelihood of EMF exposures.

Overall, while an excess risk has been reported with certain jobs and the potential for EMF exposure, the net effect is uncertain because of serious confounding exposures to other carcinogens. In addition, information about occupations can be incomplete, and misclassification bias is a significant problem.

Overall — Epidemiologic Studies and Cancer

When viewed in total, the EMF epidemiology studies of the last 15 years may reveal more about the problems and limitations of epidemiology than about an associative link between EMF exposure and cancer. A dose-response relationship with magnetic field strengths has not been firmly established, and there are multiple confounding and methodologic problems. Actual measurements have infrequently correlated with exposure surrogates. While further investigation is ongoing and clearly warranted, a compelling case that EMF exposures represent a serious environmental problem is lacking.

REGULATORY AND LEGAL ISSUES OF EMF EXPOSURE

While the scientific arguments over EMF are unsettled, the political, regulatory, and legal processes have gathered increasing momentum and produced a wide variety of decisions. These decisions can be divided into five categories (221): (a) siting cases, (b) zoning cases, (c) condemnation cases, (d) tort cases, and (e) state and regulatory actions.

Siting Cases

Typically, a variety of local, state, and federal approvals are required for the construction and operation of major transmission line projects. Over the last 15 years, the issue of EMF health effects has been raised to have an impact on these projects. Based on the premise of potentially widespread adverse health effects, a variety of alternatives have been proposed: (a) avoiding residential areas, (b) widening proposed rights-of-way, (c) buying proposed power lines, (d) engineering alternatives to minimize field levels, and (e) modifying existing rights-of-way to minimize or avoid further EMF exposure.

The engineering required to implement these alternatives is complex, costly, and occasionally problematic. Electric fields are generally managed by two techniques: (a) cancellation and (b) shielding. Cancellation of the electric field can be achieved when two conductors are placed in close spatial proximity. Cancellation is not always practical and is more difficult to apply than shielding. Shielding is an effective strategy and can be directly applied to devices such as pad-mounted transformers (221).

Similar to electric fields, magnetic fields can be managed by cancellation and shielding strategies; however, both tasks can be quite complex. Cancellation is an effective technique if the range of reduction is less than two orders of magnitude. If greater reductions are required, shielding strategies may be required.

Shielding of magnetic fields requires either diversion of the magnetic field from potentially affected receptors or source containment. Source containment is difficult to achieve because of the enormous number of devices which produce magnetic fields. The drive to reduce magnetic fields is based on an assumption of either a no adverse effects level or a general notion that any magnetic field exposure is unhealthy and that no or minimal exposure must be health protective. As previously discussed, the current scientific database has not reliably generated a dose-response curve; therefore, siting arguments frequently end in stalemate over the inability of the applicant to prove a negative. Several key cases illustrate this problem.

- New York Public Service Commission (NYPSC) hearing over the health and safety aspects of two 750-kV lines. On June 19, 1978, the NYPSC found that the scientific evidence did not demonstrate endangering human health and safety impacts; however, the commission approved operation of the line provided that the utilities contributed to a research program for the study of biologic effects of transmission line electric and magnetic fields.
- Potomac Electric Power Company (PEPCO) proposed Brighton-High Ridge 500 kV line. After a protracted series of hearings and appeals, a hearing officer found on December 21, 1989, no scientific basis that power line fields caused adverse health effects and rejected proposals for wider rights-of-way, redesign, rerouting, and field limits in adjacent homes.

Condemnation Cases

- *San Diego Gas & Electric Company (SDG&E) v Donald L. Daly.* In condemnation cases, the central issue is the amount of compensation payable to a landowner as a result of utilities' exercise of eminent domain authority. A landowner is entitled to just compensation for the lost property plus damages, if any, to the remainder of the property. On November 14, 1985, a jury awarded $1 million to Daly because of the perception that the value of his land, near SDG&E's 500 kV transmission line, was reduced because of public fear of EMF health effects. This decision was upheld on November 17, 1988, by the Fourth Appellate District Court of Appeal of California because controversy existed and caused calculated decrease in the market value of the property secondary to the public's fear of EMF.
- *Donald Zappavigna v State of New York and Power Authority of the State of New York.* This case mirrored the Daly situation; however, on September 24, 1989, the State Court of Claims denied the claimants argument that the scientific data indicated an adverse health effect from EMF exposure and that a general fear of EMF existed among potential real estate buyers. Furthermore, the court rejected the *SDG&E v Daly* as a precedent.

Tort Cases

Over the last 6 years, increasing numbers of wrongful and product liability cases have involved EMF issues. Several of these cases have involved school districts and transmission lines (*Houston Lighting and Power Company v Klein Independent School District* and *Raush v The School Board of Palm Beach County, Florida*). The fear of adverse health effects in school-children has been a prominent issue; in addition, right-of-way considerations have also been quite prominent.

A recent case, *Robert Strom v Boeing*, was settled out of court in favor of the plaintiff on August 14, 1990. This case revolved around the casual relationship between chronic granulocytic leukemia and exposure to electromagnetic pulse energy. Finally, in April 1991, two former Petaluma, California, police officers filed suit alleging that microwaves and EMF from portable traffic radar guns caused the to contract non-Hodgkin's lymphoma. The manufacturers of the radar equipment were named as defendants (*Bendure v Kuston Signals, Inc.*, D.C., N Calif, No. C 91-1173, 4/18/91; *Hutchinson v Kuston Signals Inc.*, D.C., N Calif, No. C 91/1174, 4/18/91).

Table 116.12. Right-of-Way Field Limits

Location	Field Limit
Florida	10 kV/m for 500 kV 8 kV/m for 230 kV 2 kV/m at edge of row for all new lines
Florida	200 mG for 500 kV single 250 mG for 500 kV double 150 mG for 230 kV maximum at edge of row
Montana	1 kV/m residential row
Minnesota	8 kV/m maximum
New Jersey	3 kV/m
New York	1.6 kV/m
Oregon	9 kV/m
USSR	10 kV/m publicly accessible 2 kV/m occupied areas
International Radiation	5 kV/m continuous exp

Adapted from: Polk C, Postow E. CRC handbook of biological effects of electromagnetic fields. Boca Raton, FL: CRC Press, 1987.

State Regulatory Actions

Seven states have passed regulations that place limits on the field associated with transmission lines (65). Table 116.12 lists these and other international right-of-way (ROW) limits. Interestingly, there is no consistency among the various ROW limits. The variation seen in ROW limits is not surprising since there are no clear scientific reasons for selecting one limit versus another. Given the lack of a dose-response curve coupled with the possible window effect, it is obvious that legal and political arguments are the main decision drivers. Unfortunately, there is no evidence that lower field limits will mitigate any biologic or health effects. While a number of strategies are available for reducing field levels, cost considerations are significant. In the light of scientific uncertainty, the cost-benefit ratio is very tenuous. Further research may clarify the scientific issues and provide rationale and prudent societal choices.

SUMMARY

EMF health effects will continue to be major environmental issues for the next decade. Health professionals will be increasingly asked by both individual patients and the regulatory/legal system for advice and opinions. The current scientific database is not consistent with a general widespread environmental hazard. Therefore, at this time, stringent exposure avoidance and minimization efforts may not be warranted.

REFERENCES

1. AMA Council on Scientific Affairs. Harmful effects of ultraviolet radiation. JAMA 1989;262:380–384.
2. Kligman AM. Early destructive effects of sunlight on human skin. JAMA 1969;210:2377–2380.
3. Kligman LH, Atkin FJ, Kligman AM. Sunscreens promote repair of ultraviolet-induced dermal damage. J Invest Dermatol 1983;81:98–102.
4. Weiss JS, Ellis CN, Headington JT, Tincoff T, Hamilton TA, Voorhees JJ. Topical tretinoin improves photodamaged skin: a double-blind vehicle-controlled study. JAMA 1988;259:527–532.
5. Epstein JH. Photocarcinogenesis, skin cancer and aging. J Am Acad Dermatol 1983;9:487–502.
6. Urbach F, Rose DB, Bonnem M. Genetic and environmental interactions in skin carcinogenesis. In: Environment and cancer. Baltimore, MD: Williams & Wilkins, 1972:356–371. M. D. Anderson Hospital Conference Proceedings.
7. Horm JW, Asire AJ, Young JL Jr, Pollack ES. SEER program: cancer incidence mortality in the United States, 1973–1981. Bethesda, MD: National Cancer Institute, 1984. Dept of Health and Human Services publication (NIH) 85-1837.
8. Kopf AW, Kripke ML, Stern RS. Sun and malignant melanoma. J Am Acad Dermatol 1984;11:674–684.
9. Rhodes AR, Weinstock MA, Fitzpatrick TB, Mihm MC, Sober AJ. Risk factors for cutaneous melanoma: a practical method of recognizing predisposed individuals. JAMA 1987;258:3146–3153.
10. Forbes PD. Experimental photocarcinogenesis: an overview. J Invest Dermatol 1981;77:139–143.
11. Wilkening GM. Nonionizing radiation. In: The industrial environment—its evaluation & control. NIOSH. U.S. DHEW, 1973.
12. Pathak MA, Fitzpatrick TB, Parrish JA. Photosensitivity and other reactions to light. In: Harrison's principles of internal medicine. 10th ed. New York: McGraw Hill, 1983.
13. Anderson RR. Tissue optics in photoimmunology. In: Parrisk JA, Kripke ML, Morison WL, eds. Photoimmunology. New York: Plenum Press, 1983.
14. Sliney DH. Safety with lasers and other optical sources. New York: Plenum, 1980.
15. Zuclich JA. Hazards of the eye from UV, non-ionizing radiation. Proceedings of a Topical Symposium, American Conference of Governmental Industrial Hygienists, Washington, DC: November 26–28, 1980:129–144.
16. Cooper GF, Robson JG. The yellow colour of the lens of man and other primates. J Physiol (Lond) 1969;230:411.
17. Parrish JA, Anderson RR, Urbach F, et al. UV-A: biological effects of ultraviolet radiation with emphasis on human responses to long-wave ultraviolet. New York: Plenum, 1978.
18. Zuclich JA. Cumulative effects of near-ultraviolet induced corneal damage. Health Phys 1980;38:833.
19. Ham WT, Ruffolo JJ, Mueller HA, Guerry D III. The nature of retinal radiation damage: dependence on wavelength power level and exposure time. Vision Res 1980;20:1105–111.
20. American Conference of Governmental Industrial Hygienists. 1990–1991 Threshold Limit Values for chemical substances and physical agents. Cincinnati, OH: ACGIH, 1990.
21. Emmett EA, Buncher CR, Suskind RB, Rowe KW. Skin and eye diseases among arc welders and those exposed to welding operations. J Occup Med 1981;23:85–90.
22. Pollak VA, Romanchuk KG. The risk of retina damage from high intensity light sources. Am Ind Hyg Assoc 1980;41:322–327.
23. Lövsund P, Nilsson SEG, Lindh H, Oberg RA. Temperature changes in contact lenses in connection with radiation from welding arcs. Scand J Work Environ Health 1979;5:271–279.
24. Pitts DG, Cullen AP, Dayhaw-Barker P. Determination of ocular threshold levels for infrared radiation cataractogenesis. DHHS (NIOSH) publication No. 80-121. National Institute for Occupational Safety and Health, Cincinnati, OH: NIOSH, 1980.
25. Aldrich TE, Easterly CE. Electromagnetic fields and public health. Environ Health Perspect 1987;75:159–171.
26. Petersen RC. Bioeffects of microwaves: a review of current knowledge. J Occup Med 1983;25:103–110.
27. Mumford WW. Heat stress due to R. F. radiation. Proc IEEE 1969;57:171–178.
28. Gandhi OP. Dosimetry—The absorption properties of man and experimental animals. Bull NY Acad Med 1979;55:1016.
29. Ghandi OP. State of knowledge for electromagnetic absorbed dose in man and animals. Proc IEEE 1980;68:24–32.
30. Durney CH. Electromagnetic dosimetry for models of humans and animals: a review of theoretical and numerical techniques. Proc IEEE 1980;68:33–40.
31. Radiofrequency electromagnetic fields—properties, quantities and units, biophysical interaction, and measurements. National Council on Radiation Protection Report No. 67;1981:52.
32. Glaser ZR. Bibliography of reported biological phenomena ("effects"), on clinical manifestations attributed to microwave and radio-frequency radiation, Naval Medical Research Institute Research Report, project MF 12-524-015-004 B, report No. 2, 1971.
33. Schwan HP. Biological effects and health implications of microwave radiation. Washington, DC: US Govt. Printing Office, 1970.
34. Monahan JC, Ho HS. The effect of ambient temperature on the reduction of microwave energy absorption by mice. Radio Sci 1980;12:257–262.
35. Stuchly MS. Interaction of radiofrequency and microwave radiation with living systems: a review of mechanisms. Radiat Environ Biophys 1979;16:1.
36. American National Standards Institute (ANSI). American National

Standards Institute safety levels with respect to human exposure to radio frequency electromagnetic fields, 300 kHz to 100 GHz. New York: Institute of Electrical and Electronics Engineers, Inc., 1982. ANSI C95.1-1982.

37. U.S. Congress, Office of Technology Assessment. Biological effects of power frequency electric and magnetic fields—background paper, prepared by I. Nair, M.G. Morgan, H.K. Florig, of the Department of Engineering and Public Policy, Carnegie Mellon University, OTA-BP-E-53. Washington, DC: US Government Printing Office, 1989.

38. Adair ER, Adams BW. Microwaves, modify thermoregulatory behavior in squirrel monkeys. Bioelectromag 1980;1:1–20.

39. Stern S, Margolin L, Weiss B, et al. Microwaves: effect on thermoregulatory behavior in rats. Science 1979;206:1198–1201.

40. Lu ST, Lebda N, Michaelson SM, et al. Thermal and endocrinological effects of protracted irradiation of rats by 2,450-MHz microwaves. Radio Sci 1977;12:147–156.

41. Guillet R, Michaelson SM. The effect of repeated microwave exposure on neonatal rats. Radio Sci 1977;12:125–129.

42. Guy AW, Chou CK, Lin JC, et al. Microwave-induced acoustic effect in mammalian auditory systems and physical materials. Ann NY Acad Sci 1975;247:194–215.

43. Miro L, Loubierre R, Fister AP. Effects of microwaves on the cell metabolism of the reticulo-histocytic system. In: Czerski P (ed. Biologic effects and health hazards of microwave radiation. Warsaw: Polish Medical Publishers, 1974:89–97.

44. Reed JR, Lords JL, Durney CH. Microwave irradiation of the isolated rat heart after treatment with ANS blocking agents. Radio Sci 1979;12:161–165.

45. Tinney CE, Lords JL, Durney CH. Rate effects in isolated turtle hearts induced by microwave radiation. IEEE Trans Microwave Theory Tech 1976;MTT-24:18–24.

46. Ghandi OP. State of the knowledge for electromagnetic absorbed dose in man and animals. Proc IEEE 1980;68:24–32.

47. Frey AH, Feld SR, Frey B. Neural function and behavior: defining the relationship. Ann NY Acad Sci 1975;247:433–428.

48. Huang AT, Engle ME, Elder JA, et al. The effects of microwave radiation (2,450 MHz) on the morphology and chromosomes of lymphocytes. Radio Sci 1977;12:173–177.

49. Berman E, Kinn JB, Carter HB. Observations of mouse fetuses after irradiation with 2.45-GHz microwaves. Health Physics 1978;35:791–801.

50. Bawin SM, Kaczmarete LK, Adey WR. Effects of modulated VHF fields on the central nervous system. Ann NY Acad Sci 1975;247:74–80.

51. Blackman CF, Elder JA, Weil CM, et al. Induction of calcium-ion efflux from brain tissue by radio-frequency radiation: effects at modulation and field strength, Radio Sci 1979;14:93–98.

52. Silverman O. Epidemiological studies of microwave effects. Proc IEEE 1980;68:78–84.

53. Paz, JD, Milliken R, Ingram WT, Frank A, Atkin A. Potential ocular damage from microwave exposure during electrosurgery: dosimetric survey. J Occup Med 1987;29:580–583.

54. Birenbaum L, Kaplan LT, Metaly W, et al. Effect of microwave on the rabbit eye. J Microwave Power 1969;4:232–243.

55. Michaelson SM. Microwave biological overview. Proc IEEE 1980;68:40–49.

56. Carpenter RL, Van Ummerson CA. The effects of 2.45 GHz radiation. J Microwave Power 1968;3:3–19.

57. Cleary S. Microwave cataractogenesis. Proc IEEE 1980;68:49–55.

58. Silverman C. Epidemiologic approach to the study of microwave effects. Bull NY Acad Med 1979;55:1166–1181.

59. Cleary SF, Pasternak BS. Lenticular changes in microwave workers: a statistical study. Arch Environ Health 1966;12:23–29.

60. Odland LT. Observation on microwave hazards to USAF personnel. J Occup Med 1972;14:544–547.

61. Shacklett DE, Tredici TJ, Epstein DL. Evaluation of possible microwave-induced lens changes in the United States Air Force. Aviat Space Environ Med 1975;46:1403–1406.

62. Hollows FC, Douglas JB. Microwave cataract in radiolinemen and controls. Lancet 1984;2:406–407.

63. Czerski P, Siekierzynski M, Gidynski A. Health surveillance of personnel occupationally exposed to microwaves. Aerospace Med 1974;45:1137–1147.

64. Guy AW, Lin JC Kramer PO, et al. The effects of 2450-MHz radiation on rabbit eye. IEEE Trans Microwave Theory Tech MTT-23 1975;6:492–498.

65. Polk C, Postow E. CRC handbook of biological effects of electromagnetic fields. Boca Raton, FL: CRC Press, 1987.

66. Tolgskaya MS, Gordon, ZV. Trans Inst Labor Hyg Occup Dis Acad Med Sci 1960:99.

67. Orlova AA. Proceedings on labor hygiene and the biological effects of electromagnetic radio frequency waves. 1959:25.

68. Presman AS, Levitina, NA. Bull, Exp, Biol Med (Moscow) 1962;1:41.

69. Kholodov Yu A. Proc. on problems of the biological effects of superhigh frequency fields. 1962:58.

70. Korobkva VP, Morozov YA, Stolarov MD, and Yakub YA. Influence of the electric field in 500 and 750 kV switchyards on maintenance staff & means for its protection. Technical Report 23-06, CIGRE paper, 1972.

71. Barnes FS, Seyed-Madani M. Some possible limits on the minimum electrical signals of biological significance. In: Blank M, Findl E, eds. Mechanistic approaches to interactions of electric and electromagnetic fields with living systems. New York NY: Plenum Press, 1987.

72. Adey WR, Lawrence AF. Nonlinear dynamics in biological systems. New York: Plenum Press, 1984.

73. Adey WR, Lawrence AF, eds. Nonlinear electrodynamics in biological systems. New York: Plenum Press, 1984.

74. Adey WR. Electromagnetic fields, cell membrane amplification, and cancer promotion, in extremely low frequency electromagnetic fields. In: Wilson BW, Stevens RG, Anderson LE. The question of cancer. Columbus, OH: Batelle Press, 1990:211–240.

75. Blank M, Findl E. Mechanistic approaches to interactions of electric and electromagnetic fields with living systems. New York: Plenum Press, 1987.

76. Guy AW. Dosimetry associated with exposure to non-ionizing radiation: very low frequency to microwaves. Health Phys 1987;53:569–584.

77. Chiabrera A, Nicolini C. Schwan HP, eds. Interactions between electromagnetic fields and cells. New York: Plenum Press, 1985.

78. Chen JY, Gandhi OP. RF currents induced in an anatomically-based model of a human for plane-wave exposures (20-100 MHz). Health Phys 1989;57:89–98.

79. International Radiation Protection Association (IRPA). Interim guidelines on limits of exposure to 50/60 Hz electric and magnetic fields. Health Phys 1979;58:113–122.

80. New York Power Lines Project. Biological effects of power line fields. Scientific Advisory Panel final report. Ahlbom A, Albert EN, Fraser-Smith AC, Grodzinsky AJ, Marron MJ, Martin AO, Persinger MA, Shelamski ML, Wolpow EE. Albany, NY: Wadsworth Center for Laboratories and Research, 1987.

81. Polk C. Nuclear precessional magnetic resonance as a cause for biological effects of time-varying electric or magnetic fields in the presence of an earth strength static magnetic field. Bioelectromagnetics Society, Eleventh Annual Meeting Abstracts, 1989.

82. Tenforde TS. Biological interactions and human health effects of extremely low frequency magnetic fields. In: Wilson BW, Stevens RG, Anderson LE, eds. Extremely low frequency electromagnetic fields: the question of cancer. Columbus, OH: Batelle Press, 1990;291–315.

83. Tenforde TS, Kaune WT. Interaction of extremely low frequency electric and magnetic fields with humans. Health Phys 1987;53:585–606.

84. US Environmental Protection Agency (US EPA). The radiofrequency radiation environment: environmental exposure levels and RF radiation emitting sources. Washington, DC: Office of Air and Radiation. EPA 521/1-85-014, 1986.

85. Weaver JC, Astumian RD. The response of living cells to very weak electric fields: the thermal noise limit. Science 1990; 247:459–462.

86. Wilson BW, Stevens RG, Anderson LE. Extremely low frequency electromagnetic fields: the question of cancer. Columbus, OH: Batelle Press, 1990.

87. World Health Organization (WHO). Magnetic fields. Environmental Health Criteria 69. Geneva, Switzerland: WHO, 1987.

88. World Health Organization (WHO). Extremely low frequency fields. Environmental Health Criteria 35. Geneva, Switzerland: WHO, 1984.

89. Elder JA. Radiofrequency radiation activities and issues: a 1986 perspective. Health Phys 1987a;53:607–612.

90. Elder JA. A reassessment of the biological effects of radiofrequency radiation: non-cancer effects. Research Triangle Park, NC: Health Effects Research Laboratory, U.S. Environmental Protection Agency. Unpublished.

91. Elder JA, Cahill DF, eds. Biological effects of radiofrequency radiation. Washington, DC: US Environmental Protection Agency, 1984. EPA-600/8-83-026F. Available from: NTIS, Springfield, VA; PB-85/20848.

92. US Environmental Protection Agency (US EPA) Biological effects of radiofrequency radiation. Office of Research and Development, 1984. EPA-600/8-83/026F.

93. Bawin SM, Gavalas-Medici RJ, Adey WR. Effect of modulated very high frequency fields on specific brain rhythms in cats. Brain Res 1973;58:365.

94. Blackman CF, Elder JA, Weil CM, Benane SG, Eichinger DC, House DE. Induction of calcium ion efflux from brain tissue by radiofrequency radiation: effects of modulation frequency and field stength. Radio Sci 1979;14(6S):93–98.

95. Blackman CF, Benane SG, House DE, Jones WT. Effects of ELF (1-120 Hz) and modulated (50 Hz) fields on the efflux of calcium ions from brain tissue in vitro. Bioelectromagnetics 1985;6:1–11.

96. Blackman CF, Benane SG, Elliot DJ, House DE, Pollock MM. Influence of electromagnetic fields on the efflux of calcium ions from brain tissue in vitro: a three-model analysis consistent with the frequency response up to 510 Hz. Bioelectromagnetics 1988;9:215–227.

97. Blank M, Blank JN. Concentration changes at ion channels due to oscillating electric fields. J Electro Chem Soc 1986;133:237–238.

98. Barnes FS, Hu CL. Model for some non-thermal effects of radio and microwave fields on biological membranes. IEEE Trans. Microwave Theory Technol. 1977;25:742.

99. Findl E. Membrane transduction of low energy level fields and the Ca^{++} hypothesis. In: Blank M, Findl E, eds. Mechanistic approaches to interactions of electric and electromagnetic fields with living systems. New York: Plenum Press, 1987.

100. Bauchinger M, Hauf R, Schmid E, Dresp J. Analysis of structural chromosome changes and SCE after occupational long-term exposure to electric and magnetic fields from 380 kV-systems. Radiat Environ Biophys 1981;19:235–238.

101. Baum JW, Nauman CH. Influence of strong magnetic fields on genetic endpoints in Tradescantia tetrads and stamen hairs. Environ Mutagen 1984;6:49–58.

102. Barnothy MF, Sumegi I. Abnormalities in organs of mice induced by a magnetic field. Nature 1969; 221:270–271.

103. Bartsch C, Bartsch H, Fluechter S, et al. Evidence for modulation of melatonin secretion in men with benign and malignant tumors of the prostate. J Pineal Res 1985;21:121–132.

104. Bassett CAL. Low energy pulsing electromagnetic fields modify biomedical processes. Bioessays 1987;6:36–42.

105. Blackman CF, House DE, Benane SG, Joines WT, Spiegel RJ. Effect of ambient levels of power-line-frequency electric fields on a developing vertebrate Bioelectromagnetics 1988;9:129–140.

106. Blackman CR. Effects of modulated RFR. In: Elder J., ed. A reassessment of the biological effects of radiofrequency radiation: non-cancer effects. Research Triangle Park, NC: Health Effects Research Laboratory, U.S. EPA, 1987.

107. Wilson BW, Chess EK, Anderson LE. 60-Hz electric field effects on pineal melatonin rhythms: time course for onset and recovery. Bioelectromagnetics 1986;7:239–242.

108. Adey WR. Cell membranes: the electromagnetic environment and cancer promotion. Neurochem Res 1988;13:671–677.

109. Akamine T, Muramatsu H, Sakou T. Effects of pulsed electromagnetic field on growth and differentiation of embryonal carcinoma cells. J Cell Physiol 1985;124:247–254.

110. Balcer-Kubiczek EK, Harrison GH. Evidence for microwave carcinogenesis in vitro. Carcinogenesis 1985;6:859–864.

111. Balcer-Kubiczek EK, Harrison GH. Induction of neoplastic transformation in C3H/10T1/2 cells by 2.45 GHz microwaves and phorbol ester. Radiat Res 1989;117:531–537.

112. Byus CV, Pieper SE, Adey WR. The effects of low-energy 60-Hz environmental electromagnetic fields upon the growth-related enzyme ornithine decarboxylase. Carcinogenesis 1987;8:1385–1389.

113. Byus CV, Dartun K, Pieper S, Adey WR. Increased ornithine decarboxylase activity in cultured cells exposed to low energy modulated microwave fields and phorbol ester tumor promoters. Cancer Res 1988;48:4222–4226.

114. Cohen MM, Kunska A, Astemborski JA, McCulloch D, Paskewitz DA. Effect of low level, 60-Hz electromagnetic fields on human lymphoid cells: I. Mitotic rate and chromosome breakage in human peripheral lymphocytes. Bioelectromagnetics 1986;7:415–423.

115. Cohen MM, Kunska A, Astemborski JA, McCulloch D. The effect of low-level 60-Hz electromagnetic fields on human lymphoid cells: II. sister-chromatid exchanges in peripheral lymphocytes and lymphoblastoid cell lines. Mutat Res 1986;172:177–184.

116. Cohen M, Lippman M, Chabner B. Role of pineal gland in aetiology and treatment of breast cancer. Lancet 1978;2:814–816.

117. Druker BJ, Marmon HJ, Roberts TM. Oncogenes, growth factors, and signal transduction. N Engl J Med 1989;321:1383–1391.

118. Frazier ME, Samuel JE, Kaune WT. Viabilities and mutation frequencies of CHO-K1 cells following exposure to 60-Hz electric fields. In: Anderson LE, Kelman BJ, Weigle RJ, eds. Interactions of biological systems with static and ELF electric and magnetic fields: proceedings of the 23rd Hanford Life Sciences Symposium; October 2-4, 1984. Richland, WA: Pacific Northwest Laboratory, 1987:255–267.

119. Goodman EM, Greenebaum B, Marron MT, Carrick K. Effects of intermittent electromagnetic fields on mitosis and respiration. J Bioelectricity 1984;3:57–66.

120. Goodman R, Henderson AS. Sine waves enhance cellular transcription. Bioelectromagnetics 1986;7:23–29.

121. Goodman R, Henderson AS. Exposure of salivary gland cells to low-frequency electromagnetic fields alters polypeptide synthesis. Proc Natl Acad Sci USA 85: 1988:3928–3932.

122. Goodman R, Bassett CAL, Henderson AS. Pulsing electromagnetic fields include cellular transcription. Science 1983;220:1283–1285.

123. Goodman R, Abbott I, Henderson AS. Transcriptional patterns in the x chromosome of Sciara coprophila following exposure to magnetic fields. Bioelectromagnetics 1987;8:1–7.

124. Portnov FG, Shakarnis VF, Maiore DYa. Study of the mutagenic effect of static electric fields on Drosophila melanogaster females. Sov Genet 1975;11:797–799.

125. Ragan HA, Buschbom RL, Pipes MF, Phillips RD, Kaune WT. Hematologic and serum chemistry studies in rats exposed to 60-Hz electric fields. Bioelectromagnetics 1983;4:79–90.

126. Ramaiya LK, Pomerantseva MD, Vilkina GA, Tikhonchuk VS. Study of the action of UHF microwaves on mammalian germ and somatic cells. Cytol Genet 1980;14(6):1–5.

127. Reese JA, Jostes RF, Frazier ME. Exposure of mammalian cells to 60-Hz magnetic or electric fields: analysis for DNA single-strand breaks. Bioelectromagnetics 1988;9:237–247.

128. Szmigielski S. Effect of 10-cm (3-GHz) electromagnetic radiation (microwaves) on granulocytes in vitro. Ann NY Acad Sci 1975;247:275–280.

129. Stevens RG. Electric power use and breast cancer: a hypothesis. Am J Epidemiol 1987;125:556–561.

130. Takashima S, Onaral B, Schwan HP. Effects of modulated RF energy on the EEG of mammalian brains. Radiat Environ Biophys 1979;16:15–27.

131. Takahashi K, Kaneko I, Date M, Fukada E. Effect of pulsing electromagnetic fields of DNA synthesis in mammalian cells in culture. Experientia 1986;42:185–186.

132. Tamarkin L, Baird CJ, Almeida OF. Melatonin: a coordinating signal for mammalian reproduction. Science 1985;227:714–720.

133. Tamarkin L, Cohen M, Roselle D, Reichert C, Lippman M, Chabner B. Melatonin inhibition and pinealectomy enhancement of 7,12-dimethyl-benz(a)anthracene-induced mammary tumors in the rat. Cancer Res 1981;41:4432–4436.

134. Tsoneva MT, Penchev PR, Karev GB, Gishin SS. Effect of magnetic fields on the chromosome set and cell division. Sov Gene 1975;11:398–401.

135. Webber MM, Barnes FS, Seltzer LA, Bouldin TR, Prasad KN. Short microwave pulses cause ultrastructural membrane damage in neuroblastoma cells. J Ultrastruct Res 1980;71:321–330.

136. Welker HA, Semm P, Willig RP, Commenty JC, Wiltschko W, Volbrath L. Effects of an artificial magnetic field on serotonin N-acetyltransferase activity and melatonin content of the rat pineal gland. Exp Brain Res 1983;50:426–432.

137. Whitson GL, Carrier WL, Francis AA, et al. Effects of extremely low frequency (ELF) electric fields on cell growth and DNA repair in human skin fibroblasts. Cell Tissue Kinet 1986;19:39–47.

138. Wilson BW, Anderson LE, Hilton DI, Phillips RD. Chronic exposure to 60-Hz electric fields: effects on pineal function in the rat. Bioelectromagnetics 1981;2:371–380.

139. Wilson BW, Anderson LE, Hilton DI, Phillips RD. Chronic exposure to 60-Hz electric fields: effects on pineal function in the rat. Bioelectromagnetics 1983;4:293.

140. Wilson BW, Chess EK, Anderson LE. 60-Hz electric-field effects on pineal melatonin rhythms: time course for onset and recovery. Bioelectromagnetics 1986;7:239–242.

141. Wilson BW, Lueng F, Buschbom R, Stevens RG, Anderson LE, Reiter RJ. Electric fields, the pineal gland, and cancer. In: Gupta D, Attanasio A, Reiter RJ, eds. The pineal gland and cancer. Tubingen, Germany: Brain Research Promotion, 1988:245–259.

142. Wolff S, James TL, Young GB, Margulis AR, Bodycote J, Afzal V. Magnetic resonance imaging: absence of in vitro cytogenetic damage. Radiology 1985;155:163–165.

143. Rosen DM, Luben RA. Multiple hormonal mechanisms for the control of collagen synthesis in an osteoblast-like cell line, MMB-1. Endocrinology 1983;112:992–999.

144. Luben RA, Cain CD, Chen MC, Rosen DM, Adey WR. Effects of electromagnetic stimuli on bone and bone cells in vitro: inhibition of responses to parathyroid hormone by low-energy low-frequency fields. Proc Natl Acad Sci USA 1982;79:4180–4184.

145. Cain CD, Luben RA. Pulsed electromagnetic field effects on PTH-stimulated cAMP accumulation and bone resorption in mouse calvaria. In: Anderson LE, Kelman BJ, Weigel RJ, eds. Interaction of biological systems with static and ELF electric and magnetic fields: proceedings of the 23rd Hanford Life Sciences Symposium; October 2-4, 1984. Richland, WA: Pacific Northwest Laboratory, 1987:269–278.

146. Cain CD, Malto MC, Jones RA, Adey WR. Effects of 60 Hz-fields on oxinithine decarboxylase activity in bone cells and fibroblasts. Technical Report. Contractors' Review Meeting. US Dept. of Energy. Office of Energy Storage

and Distribution and the EPRI Health Studios Program. New York State Department of Health. November 1986.

147. Florida Electric and Magnetic Fields Science Advisory Commission. Biological effects of 60-Hz power transmission lines. Technical Report. Florida Department of Environmental Regulation, Tallahassee, FL, March 1985.

148. Florig HK, Nair F, Morgon MG. Briefing Paper 1: Sources and dosimetry of power-frequency fields. Florida Department of Environmental Regulation. DER Contract SP117, March 1987.

149. Pool R. Electromagnetic fields: the biologic evidence. Science 1990;249:1378–1381.

150. Bergqvist UO. Video display terminals and health: a technical and medical appraisal of the state of the art. Scand J Work Environ Health 1984;10:Suppl 2:62–7.

151. Schnorr TM. Video display terminals and pregnancy. New York State Department of Health Occupational Medicine. Current concepts. Vol. 8, No. 3. Albany, NY: New York State Department of Health, Division of Health Risk Control, 1985.

152. National Institute for Occupational Safety and Health. Health hazard evaluation 84-297-1609. General Telephone Company of Michigan, Alma, Michigan. Cincinnati, OH: National Institute for Occupational Safety and Health, 1984. (DHHS (NIOSH) publication no. 893-329-1498.)

153. National Institute for Occupational Safety and Health. Health hazard evaluation 83-329-1498, Southern Bell, Atlanta, Georgia. Cincinnati, GA: National Institute for Occupational Safety and Health, 1983. (DHHS (NIOSH) publication no. 83-329-1498.)

154. National Institute for Occupational Safety and Health. Health hazard evaluation 84-191, United Airlines, San Francisco, California. Cincinnati, OH: National Institute for Occupational Safety and Health, 1984.

155. Schnorr TM, Grajewskf BA, Hornung RW, et al. Video display terminals and the risk of spontaneous abortion. N Engl J Med 1991;324:727–733.

156. Ahlbom A. Biological effects of power line fields, New York State Power Lines Project, Scientific Advisory Panel Final Report; July 1, 1987.

157. Ahlbom A. A review of the epidemiologic literature on magnetic fields and cancer. Scand J Work Environ Healgh 1988;14:337–343.

158. Aldrich TE, Glorieux A, Castro S. Florida cluster of five children with endodermal sinus tumors. Oncology 1984;41:233–238.

159. Wertheimer N, Leeper E. Electrical wiring configurations and childhood cancer. Am J Epidemiol 1979;109:273–284.

160. Fulton JP. Electrical wiring configurations and childhood leukemia in Rhode Island. Am J Epidemiol 1980;111:292–296.

161. Tomenius L. 50-Hz electromagnetic environment and the incidence of childhood tumors in Stockholm County. Bioelectromagnetics 1986;7:191–207.

162. Myers A, Cartwright RA, Bonnell JA, Male JC, Cartwright SC. Overhead power lines and pediatric cancer. IEE International Conference in Medicine and Biology. IEE Conference Pub. 257. Hertz, England, 1985;122–125.

163. Savitz DA, Wachtel HA, Burns F. Case-control study of childhood cancer and exposure to 60-Hertz magnetic fields. Am J Epidemiol 1988;128:21–38.

164. Lin R, Lu P. Abstract of presentation at the annual Department of Energy (DOE)/EPRI Contractors review on biological effects from electric and magnetic fields, Portland, Oregon 1989. Available through DOE, Washington, DC.

165. Coleman MP, Bell CMJ, Taylor H-L, Primig-Zakel, M. Leukemia and residence near electricity transmission equipment: a case-control study. Br J Cancer 1989;60:793–798.

166. Spitz M, Johnson C. Neuroblastoma and paternal occupation. A case-control analysis. Am J Epidemiol 1989;121:924–929.

167. Wilkins JR, Koutras RA. Paternal occupation and brain cancer in offspring: a mortality-based case-control study. Am J Ind Med 1988;14:299–318.

168. Lilienfeld AM. Foreign Service health status study—evaluation of health status of foreign service and other employees from selected eastern European posts. Final Report, Contract No. 6025-619073. Dept. of State, Washington, DC 1978. Available from: NTIS, Springfield, VA, PB-288163.

169. Robinette CD, Silverman C. Causes of death following occupational exposure to microwave radiation (radar) 1950-1974. In: Hazzard DG, ed. Symposium on biological effects and measurements of radiofrequency/microwaves. Food and Drug Administration, Rockville, MD 1977. HEW Publication (FDA) 77-8026:338-334.

170. Robinette CD, Silverman C, Jablon S. Effects upon health of occupational exposure to microwave radiation (radar). Am J Epidemiol 1980;112:39–53.

171. Milham S, Jr. Silent keys: leukemia mortality in amateur radio operators. Lancet 1985;1:812.

172. Milham S, Jr. Increased mortality in amateur radio operators due to lymphatic and hematopoietic malignancies. Am J Epidemiol 1988;127:50–54.

173. Milham S Jr. Mortality by license class in amateur radio operators. Am J Epidemiol 1988;128:1175–1176.

174. Environmental Epidemiology Program, State of Hawaii Department of Health. Cancer incidence in census tracts with broadcasting towers in Honolulu, Hawaii. Report to the City Council, City and County of Honolulu, Hawaii, 1986.

175. Hill D. A longitudinal study of a cohort with past exposure to radar: the MIT Radiation Laboratory follow-up study [dissertation]. Ann Arbor, MI: University of Michigan Dissertation Service, 1988.

176. Szmigielski S. Immunological and cancer-related aspects of exposure to low-level microwave and radiofrequency fields. In: Marino A, ed. Modern electricity. Marcel Dekker, 1988.

177. Wertheimer N, Leeper E. Adult cancer related to electrical wire near the home. Int J Epidemiol 1982;11:345–355.

178. Coleman M, Bell CMJ, Taylor H-L, Thornton-Jones H. Leukemia and electromagnetic fields: a case-control study. In: Electric and magnetic fields in medicine and biology. London: IEE Conf. Pub. No. 257, 1985:122–123.

179. McDowall MN. Mortality of persons resident in the vicinity of electricity transmission facilities. Br J Cancer 1986;53:271–279.

180. Severson RK, Stevens RG, Kaune WT. Acute nonlymphocytic leukemia and residential exposure to power frequency magnetic fields. Am J Epidemiol 1988;128:10–20.

181. Kaune WT, Stevens RG, Callahan NJ. Residential magnetic and electric fields. Bioelectromagnetics 1987;8:315–335.

182. Preston-Martin S, Peters SM, Yu MC. Myelogenous leukemia and electric blanket use. Bioelectromagnetics 1988;9:207–213.

183. Wiklund K, Einhorn J, Eklund G. An application of the Swedish Cancer-Environment Registry. Leukaemia among telephone operators at the Telecommunications Administration in Sweden. Int J Epidemiol 1981;10:373–376.

184. Howe GR, Lindsay JP. A follow-up study of a ten-percent sample of the Canadian Labour Force. 1. Cancer mortality in males. 1965-73. J Natl Cancer Inst 1983;70:37–44.

185. Olin R, Vagero DS, Ahlbon S. Mortality experience of electrical engineers. Br J Ind Med 1985;42:211–212.

186. Vagero D, Allbom A, Olin R. Cancer morbidity among workers in the telecommunications industry. Br J Ind Med 1985;42:191–195.

187. Barregård L, Järvholm B, Ungethüm E. Cancer among workers exposed to strong static magnetic fields. Lancet 1985;2:892.

188. Obrams G Iris. Leukemia in telephone linemen [dissertation]. Ann Arbor, MI: University of Michigan Dissertation Service, 1988.

189. Guberán E, Usel M, Raymond L, et al., Disability, mortality, and incidence of cancer among Geneva painters and electricians. Br J Ind Med 1989;46:16–23.

190. Matanoski G, Elliott E, Breysse P. Poster presented at the annual Department of Energy (DOE)/EPRI Contractors review on biological effects from electric and magnetic fields. Portland, OR, 1989.

191. Milham S Jr. Mortality from leukemia in workers exposed to electrical and magnetic fields. N Engl J Med 1982;307:249.

192. Milham S Jr. Mortality in workers exposed to electromagnetic fields. Environ Health Perspec 1985;62:297–300.

193. Wright W, Peters J, Mack T. Leukemia in workers exposed to electric and magnetic fields. Lancet 1982;1160:61.

194. McDowall MN. Leukemia mortality in electrical workers in England and Wales. Lancet 1983;1:246.

195. Coleman M, Bell J, Skeet R. Leukemia incidence in electrical workers. Lancet 1983;982–983.

196. Pearce N, Reif J, Fraser J. Case-control studies of cancer in New Zealand electrical workers. Int J Epidemiol 1984;18:55–59.

197. Calle E, Savitz DA. Leukemia in occupational groups with presumed exposure to electrical and magnetic fields. N Engl J Med 1985;313:1476–1477.

198. Gilman PA, Ames RG, McCawley MA. Leukemia risk among U.S. white male coal miners. J Occup Med 1985;27:669–671.

199. Flodin U, Anderson L, Ansou C. Background radiation, electrical work, and some other exposures associated with acute myeloid leukemia in a case-referent study. Arch Environ Health 1986;41:77–84.

200. Stern FB, Waxweiler RA, Beaument JJ, et al. A case-control study of leukemia at a naval nuclear shipyard. Am J Epidemiol 1986;123:980–992.

201. Linet MS. Leukemias and occupation in Sweden: a registry-based analysis. Am J Ind Med 1988;14:319–330.

202. Juutilainen J, Pukkala E, Laara E. Results of an epidemiological cancer study among electrical workers in Finland. J Bioelectrics 1988;7(1):119–121.

203. Loomis DP, Savitz DA. Brain cancer and leukemia mortality among electrical workers. Am J Epidemiol 1989;130:814 (abstract).

204. Pearce NE, Sheppard RA, Howard JK, et al. Leukemia in electrical workers in New Zealand. Lancet 1985;1:811–812.

205. Preston-Martin S, Henderson BE, Peters JM. Descriptive epidemiology of central nervous system neoplasms in Los Angeles County. In: Selikoff IJ,

Hammond, EC, eds. Brain tumors in the chemical industry, Ann NY Acad Sci 1982;381:202–208.

206. Lin R, Diselinger PC, Conde J, et al. Occupational exposure to electromagnetic fields and the occurrence of brain tumors. J Occup Med 1985;27:413–419.

207. Thomas TL, Stolley PD, Stemhagen A, et al. Brain tumor mortality risk among men with electrical and electronic jobs: a case-control study. Natl Cancer Inst 1987;79:233–238.

208. Speers MA, Dobbins JG, Miller VS. Occupational exposures and brain cancer mortality: a preliminary study of East Texas residents. Am J Ind Med 1988;13:629–638.

209. Reif JS, Pearce N, Fraser J. Occupational risks for brain cancer: a New Zealand cancer registry-based study. J Occup Med 1989;31:863–867.

210. Swerdlow AJ. Epidemiology of eye cancer in adults in England and Wales, 1962–77. Am J Epidemiol 1983;118:294–300.

211. De Guire L. Increased malignant melanoma of the skin in workers in a telecommunications industry. Br J Ind Med 1988;45:824–828.

212. Bonnell J. Leukemia and electrical workers. Lancet 1988;1:1168.

213. Broadbent D. Health of workers exposed to electric fields. Br J Ind Med 1985;42:75–84.

214. Hoar SK, Morrison AS, Cole P, et al. An occupation and exposure linkage system for the study of occupational carcinogenesis. J Occup Med 1980;22:722–726.

215. Brown HD, Chattopadhyay SK. Electromagnetic-field exposure and cancer. Cancer Biochem Biophys 1988;9:295–342.

216. Coleman M, Beral V. A review of epidemiological studies of the health effects of living near or working with electricity generation and transmission equipment. Int J. Epidemiol 1988;17:1–13.

217. Modan, B. Exposure to electromagnetic fields and brain malignancy: a newly discovered menace? Am J Med 1988;13:625–627.

218. Savitz DA, Calle E. Leukemia and occupational exposure to electromagnetic fields: review of epidemiological surveys. J Occup Med 1987;29:47–51.

219. Sheikh K. Exposure to electromagnetic fields and the risk of leukemia. Arch Environ Health 1986;41:56–63.

220. US Environmental Protection Agency (US EPA). Biological effects of radiofrequency radiation. Elder JA, Cahill, DF, eds. EPA 600/8-83-026F, 1984. Available from: NTIS, Springfield, VA; PB 85-120-848.

221. Tennessee Valley Public Power Association. Communicating with customers about electric and magnetic fields (EMF). Research and Development Department Project EMF-1, May 1991.

117

Cryogenics, Oxidizers, Reducing Agents, and Explosives

John B. Sullivan, Jr., M.D.

INTRODUCTION

Many substances and chemicals transported on the highway and rail, as well as used in the workplace, are potentially explosive and flammable and have a high degree of reactivity with other substances. These highly reactive substances increase the danger of personnel responding to releases and spills and have special hazard labels or placards warning of their dangerous properties. Such hazards include: (a) explosives, (b) oxidizers, (c) reducing agents, and (d) cryogenics such as liquefied gases.

The Department of Transportation (DOT) lists three classes of explosives:

Class A Explosives—Materials that can detonate by flame, spark, or shock—recognized as high explosives.
Class B Explosives—Rapidly combustible materials which can explode under extreme temperatures—recognized as low explosives.
Class C Explosives—Minimum explosion hazard.

These categories of explosives must be properly labeled according to the DOT for transport. Some explosive materials are forbidden to be transported due to their extreme degree of reactivity.

Oxidizers are chemically reactive materials that can stimulate or enhance the combustion of materials. Oxidizing materials require specific DOT warning labels, since they can be explosive and produce violent reactions. Reducing agents give up electrons. Some reducing agents can react violently, depending on the rapidity of their reaction.

Cryogenics are liquefied gases under extreme pressures and low temperatures. Some of these gases such as oxygen, hydrogen, liquefied petroleum gas, and liquefied natural gas are flammable, and a vapor-air combination of these gases can explode. The *Emergency Response Guidebook* of the DOT should be consulted for emergency response to these hazards.

EXPLOSIVE MATERIALS

An explosive material is a solid or a liquid which can undergo rapid decomposition producing a large volume of rapidly expanding gas and intense heat (1). Explosives are categorized as high or low explosives. High explosive materials detonate, that is, they react very quickly, while low explosive materials react much slower. Detonation causes a rapid release of large amounts of gases and heat, whereas low explosives burn rapidly instead of detonating. Most of these gases consist of carbon monoxide, carbon dioxide, nitrogen, and oxygen. A tremendous release of heat and very high pressure is also produced by the detonation. A listing of such explosives include: nitroglycerin, dynamite, trinitrotoluene, cyclonite, tetryl, PETN, mercuric fulminate, lead azide, lead styphnate, and picric acid (Fig. 117.1). High explosives have detonation rates as fast as 4 miles per second. Low explosives

have detonation rates of 900 feet per second (2). Explosives that detonate can also be divided into primary and secondary explosives. Many explosives develop a detonation wave in very short periods of time and are very sensitive to heat, physical trauma, and friction. Common primary explosives are lead azide and mercury fulminate. Secondary explosives require a booster or a form of detonation to explode. Secondary explosives are sensitive to heat and friction and include tetryl and cyclonite (2).

Explosives can be further classified according to the type of oxidation reduction reaction which occurs (2). Examples of internal oxidation-reduction explosives are nitroglycerin and picric acid. Internal oxidation reduction explosive compounds contain an active chemical group which aids in the detonation of the explosives called an "explosophore" (2).

The DOT defines an explosive as "any materials whose function is destruction by detonation" (2). The Department of Transportation has three DOT classes of explosives according to sensitivity, shock, and heat. Table 117.1 lists common explosives, their classification, and characteristics. Some materials are forbidden for transport because of their highly explosive nature. An example of these are: mercuric fulminate, lead azide, and lead styphnate. These materials are not in a "wetted" state, that is, they are dry and unstable. The transportation of these materials is forbidden.

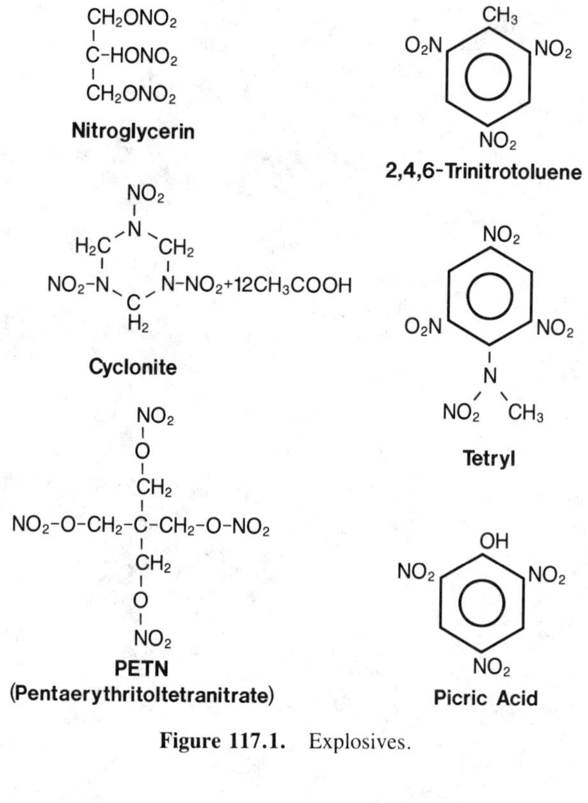

Figure 117.1. Explosives.

Table 117.1.

Chemical Name	Explosivity	Physical Characteristics
Nitroglycerin (NTG)	High explosive DOT Class A explosive	Oily liquid, clear to yellow color, sensitive to shocks, jarring, and impacts on hard surfaces
Dynamite	High explosive Straight form DOT Class A explosive	20–60% NTG Sodium Nitrate Carbonaceous material moisture antacid
Dynamite	High explosive Ammonia form DOT Class A explosive	20–60% NTG Ammonium Nitrate Sulfur Carbonaceous material antacid moisture
Dynamite	High explosive Gelatin form DOT Class A explosive	20–90% NTG Nitro-cellulose gel
Trinitrotoluene (TNT)	High explosive DOT Class A explosive	Yellow, solid when pure. Commercial product is yellow to dark brown
Cyclonite (RDX, hexogen)	High explosive DOT Class A explosives in all forms	Stable when mixed with beeswax. Main content of "plastic explosives." Not sensitive to normal shocks. May be molded into shapes
Tetryl	High explosive DOT Class A explosive	Yellow solid, sensitive to friction and shock
PETN	High explosive DOT Class A explosive	White solid, used in detonation fuses
Picric acid (trinitrophenol)	High explosive DOT Class A explosive	Yellow solid
Mercuric fulminate* Hg (CNO₂)	High explosive DOT Class A explosive	Used in percussion caps, cartridges, shells, detonators to produce deterioration
Lead azide* Pb (N₃)₂	Primary explosive DOT Class A explosive	Used in detonators and fuses to produce deterioration
Lead styphnate* (lead trinitroresorcinate)	Primary explosive DOT Class A explosive	Sensitive to sparks and static electricity

*Transport of these three when dry is prohibited.

Primary Explosives

Primary explosives are used as detonators and fuses to initiate detonations. The three more common ones are mercuric ful-

minate, lead azide, and lead styphnate. None of these three primary explosives can be transported when dry, since they are so sensitive to sparks and to friction and will decompose explosively (2).

Trinitrotoluene (TNT)

TNT was discovered in 1902. When pure, it is a pale yellow solid. In a commercial grade it may be yellow to dark brown (2). TNT is not susceptible to spontaneous decomposition. As a consequence, it may be stored for years and has a high degree of stability. TNT is also flammable and burns when contacted to flames. The more common form of TNT is 2,4,6-trinitrotoluene. Since it is a high explosive, it should be kept from other initiator explosives and protected from trauma and physical damage and also separated from oxidizing materials, combustibles, and other sources of heat (3). This material is highly explosive and reactive to high temperatures or pressures and will detonate under strong shock conditions. It has a Threshold Limit Value (TLV) recommended by the American Conference of Governmental Industrial Hygienists (ACGIH) of 1.5 mg/m³ with a skin notation. It produces toxic combustion products of nitrogen oxides. Toxicity of trinitrotoluene is similar to other nitrates, and it can produce weakness, headache, dizziness, methemoglobinemia, and hypotension upon absorption. Trinitrotoluene can be absorbed dermally, can produce dermatitis and eczema, and forms an irritant vapor. Trinitrotoluene can also produce hepatitis and has been associated with aplastic anemia. Individuals working with trinitrotoluene can be at risk for cataract formation (3). Trinitrotoluene is very dangerous, and upon impact or any form of physical shock can explode. It detonates around 240°C. Trinitrotoluene can also burn and as such is one of the more stable explosive compounds.

Tetryl

Tetryl (2,4,6-trinitrophenylmethylnitramine) is made from 2,4-nitrochlorobenzene and methylamine with nitration of the aromatic ring. It has a TLV of 1.5 mg/m³ with a skin notation. Tetryl is also known as tetralite, pyrenite, and nitramine. Tetryl is a yellow crystal. The toxic exposure routes are skin absorption or inhalation. Tetryl is known to produce contact dermatitis and is an irritant of the upper respiratory tract (4). Skin contact with tetryl produces yellow staining. Workers exposed to tetryl may experience headaches, increased fatigue, malaise, nausea, and vomiting. Bone marrow depression with anemia has occurred. Chemical conjunctivitis may occur following eye contact. Monitoring of the workplace is important in order to keep the concentration of dust below the 1.5-mg/m³ TLV. Fatal liver disease has occurred from tetryl toxicity. Contact sensitization from tetryl may present as an erythema and itching of the skin. This may progress to vesicular rash with edema. Workers developing such a rash require removal from the workplace and from the exposure (4).

Nitroglycerin and Dynamite

Nitroglycerin is an oily liquid, clear and yellow in color. It is very sensitive to shock, trauma, and impact which will cause it to detonate. Nitroglycerin is an ester of glycerol (glycerol trinitrate) and is used to form dynamite. To form dynamite, nitroglycerin is mixed with a substance such as sawdust or pulpwood to reduce the sensitivity of the compound to detonation. Dynamite may also have an oxidant mixed with it such as ammonium nitrate or sodium nitrate. Dynamite may also be mixed with a nitrocellulose gel to thicken the compound. The TLV for nitroglycerin is 0.05 ppm of the vapor with a skin notation warning indicating the potential for dermal absorption. Typical human exposure develops through inhalation of the vapor or skin absorption of the liquid. Nitroglycerin exposure can cause peripheral vasodilation, hypotension, syncope, headache, and methemoglobinemia. Worker protection from inhalation of vapors or skin contact is required. Clinical symptomatology of nitroglycerin exposure includes: dizziness, vomiting, hypotension, palpitation, tachycardia, low levels of methemoglobinemia, and angina pectoris. Some workers may be susceptible to arrhythmia and sudden death secondary to nitroglycerin exposure (4).

Picric Acid

Picric acid (trinitrophenol) is a yellow, crystalline solid explosive which detonates following rapid heating or physical trauma. Picric acid is used in the manufacture of rocket fuel explosives and fireworks. It is also used in the pharmaceutical industry. The Permissible Exposure Limit (PEL) of picric acid is 0.1 per mg/m^3 with a skin notation. The level Immediately Dangerous to Life and Health (IDLH) is 100 mg/m^3. Picric acid as a crystalline solid and as a solution can produce skin irritation and sensitization. The inhalation of picric acid can produce weakness, headache, coma, nausea, vomiting, diarrhea, and myalgia. Hemolysis can also occur as well as renal damage and liver damage. Exposure to picric acid will cause tissues, particularly in the skin and eyes, to turn yellow (5). It can also cause dermatitis and skin sensitization. Eye injury is possible following exposure to acid dust with corneal injury.

Cyclonite

Cyclonite (cyclotrimethylenetrinitramine) is a white crystalline compound and a secondary high explosive. It is also known as hexogen HMX-RDX and RDX. Cyclonite is incompatible with oxidizing materials as well as combustibles. It can be detonated by sudden heat or shock. The ACGIH in 1980 set a TLV for cyclonite of 1.5 mg/m^3 with a skin notation to indicate dermal toxicity. The ACGIH also set a Short Term Exposure Limit (STEL) of 3.0 mg/m^3. Cyclonite dust can produce ocular and skin irritations as well as irritations of the respiratory tract. Worker exposure can produce headaches, irritability, seizures, and coma.

PETN

PETN (pentaerythritoltetranitrate) is a white crystalline solid high explosive. It is also used to manufacture alkyld resins and plasticizers (5). The ACGIH in 1980 recommended a TLV for PETN as 10 mg/m^3 and a STEL of 20 mg/m^3. There is no documented toxic effect secondary to PETN exposure, and 85% of the compound is excreted in the urine unchanged within 30 hours (5).

OXIDIZERS AND OXIDIZING AGENTS

Oxidizing agents can be very hazardous and react violently with organic materials by contributing oxygen to further combustion. An oxidation reaction is one in which an atom gives

Table 117.2. Oxidizers

Perchloryl fluoride	ClO_3F
Hexachlorodiphenyl oxide	$C_{12}H_4Cl_6O$
Sodium chlorate	$NaClO_3$
Sodium chlorite	$NaClO_2$
Sodium hypochlorite	$NaClO$
Perchloric acid	$HClO_4$
Chloric acid	$HClO_3$
Chlorous acid	$HClO_2$
Hypochlorous acid	$HClO$
Chlorine	Cl_2
Fluorine	F_2
Bromine	Br_2
Iodine	I_2
Bromine pentafluoride	BrF_5
Chlorine trifluoride	ClF_3
Chlorine dioxide	ClO_2
Oxygen difluoride	OF_2
Nitrogen trifluoride	NF_3
Hydrogen peroxide	H_2O_2
Benzoyl peroxide	$(C_6H_5CO)_2O_2$
Peracetic acid	$CH_3CO—O—O—COCH_3$
Methylethyl ketone peroxide	
Oxygen	O_2
Concentrated sulfuric acid	H_2SO_4
Concentrated nitric acid	HNO_3
Osmium tetroxide	OSO_4
Quinone	$C_6H_4O_2$
Tetranitromethane	$C(NO_2)_4$
Permanganates	MnO_4^-
Dichromates	$Cr_2O_7^-$
Ozone	O_3
Stannic salts	

up its electrons; the atom that accepts the electrons is reduced. The substance that gains the electrons is called the oxidizing agent. The substance losing the electron is termed the reducing agent (6). The chemical characteristics of oxidizers allow them to react with a large number of other substances.

When oxidizing agents react they can release large amounts of heat. They can cause the ignition of many other materials, particularly organic materials. Oxidizing agents that contain oxygen are unstable when exposed to heat and can help propagate a fire (6). Probably the most recognized oxidizers are ammonium nitrate, organic peroxides, and hydrogen peroxide. Organic peroxides are extremely hazardous materials. Other oxidizing agents are halogen gases, perchlorates, chlorates, chlorites, hypochlorites, ammonium compounds, nitrates, nitrites, chromium oxidizers, permanganates, and hydrazine. Tables 117.2 and 117.3 list a variety of common oxidizing agents. In general, oxidizing agents can produce toxicity consisting of methemoglobinemia, hemolysis, dermal injury, and pulmonary injury.

Hydrogen Peroxide (H_2O_2)

Pure hydrogen peroxide is a colorless liquid. It is used as a bleaching agent for paper and textiles, as a rocket fuel, and as a general disinfectant (6). Hydrogen peroxide has a TLV of 1 ppm. Human toxicology occurs through inhalation and dermal contact as well as ingestion. Hydrogen peroxide is completely miscible with water and is sold commercially in concentrations of 3%, 35%, 50%, 70%, and 90% solutions. The DOT designates hydrogen peroxide as a detonator, oxidizer, and corrosive material. Potential exposures to hydrogen peroxide occur in industrial settings in the manufacturing of various chemicals such as acetone, antiseptics, benzoyl peroxide, disinfectants, and pharmaceuticals. Hydrogen peroxide is incompatible with several metals: iron, copper, brass, bronze, bromium, zinc, lead, manganese, and silver (5). The IDLH level is 75 ppm, and the STEL is 2 ppm (3 mg/m^3).

Exposure to hydrogen peroxide can occur from inhalation of vapors of aerosolized mist, ingestion of a liquid, and skin and eye contact from splashes. Hydrogen peroxide is an irritant of the skin, eyes, and mucous membranes from direct contact of all solutions or as a concentrated vapor or aerosolized mist. Burning sensations of the skin and eyes will occur following contact with solutions of hydrogen peroxide. Concentrations higher than 30% can result in dermal burns and blisters. The ingestion of hydrogen peroxide can result in erythema and irritation of the oropharynx and esophagus as well as potentially rupturing the stomach through production of gases. Exposure to high mist concentrations of hydrogen peroxide can result in pulmonary edema, coma, convulsions, and seizures. Dermal

Table 117.3. Ammonium and Nitrate Oxidizer Compounds

Ammonium nitrate
Ammonium nitrite
Ammonium chlorate
Ammonium perchlorate
Ammonium permanganate
Ammonium dichromate
Ammonium peroxydisulfate
Ammonium picrate
Sodium nitrate
Ethylene glycol dinitrate
n-Propyl nitrate

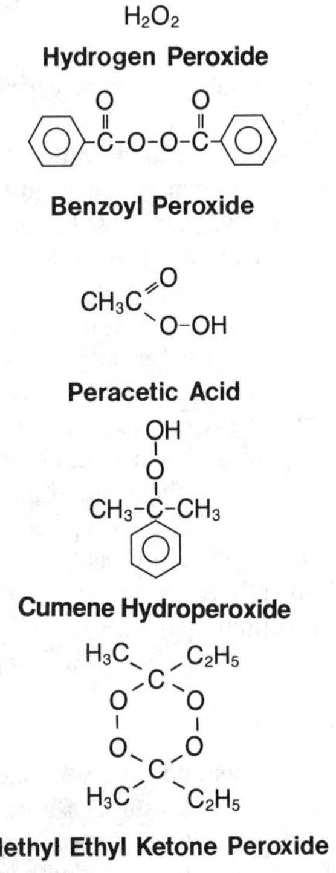

Figure 117.2. Peroxides.

contact will produce a bleaching effect, and if the hydrogen peroxide is not sufficiently diluted it can result in dermal burns, vesicular eruption, and skin edema.

Hydrogen peroxide can undergo explosion and violent decomposition if it is contaminated by incompatible metals. Hydrogen peroxide can accelerate combustion of other materials due to its oxidizing effect. Hydrogen peroxide is also an explosive hazard when mixed with organic compounds (4). Hydrogen peroxide solutions greater than 30% have the ability to spontaneously decompose and thus present an explosion hazard. Hydrogen peroxide concentrations less than 30% undergo spontaneous decomposition but not in a violent manner. Stabilizers, such as sodium pyrophosphate, are added to hydrogen peroxide solution to help prevent decomposition. The heating of hydrogen peroxide to 144°C (291°F) causes violent decomposition (6). Since hydrogen peroxide is a source of oxygen, solutions of 30% and 50% or more can cause combustible materials to be ignited without other ignition sources. Hydrogen peroxide is one of the strongest oxidizing agents known. Most organic materials will immediately combust on contact with hydrogen peroxide (6). This combustion can release toxic byproducts. The physical and toxic hazard of hydrogen peroxide increases as the percentage of the concentrate increases. Concentrations of hydrogen peroxide greater than 30% or equal to or greater than 30% are corrosive on the skin and can produce burns on contact.

Organic Peroxides

Organic peroxides are the most hazardous of the oxidizing agents. Organic peroxides are used in the production and processing of reinforced plastics, plastic film, and synthetic rubber. They are also used in other processes requiring bleaching such as in the textile, printing, and pharmaceutical industries. Organic peroxides are very reactive and are explosion hazards. They are sensitive to thermal and physical trauma which can cause a combustion and violent composition to the point of detonation. The common ones are:

—benzoyl peroxide
—peracetic acid
—cumene hydroperoxide
—methyl ethyl ketone peroxide

Organic peroxides contain the peroxo group (—O—O—) and are much more hazardous than inorganic peroxides. Organic peroxides are synthesized by chemical reactions of organic agents and hydrogen peroxides. The decomposition of organic peroxide produces free radicals.

Benzoyl Peroxide

This is a crystalline solid which can explode when heated. The molecular formula of benzoyl peroxide is C_6H_5CO—O—COC_6H_5. Benzoyl peroxide is explosive at high temperatures (5). It has a TLV of 5 mg/m^3. Benzoyl peroxide is an irritant of the mucous membrane and eyes and can cause irritation of the respiratory tract as well as skin sensitization. The major health hazards from benzoyl peroxide are respiratory, ocular, and dermal injury. Benzoyl peroxide produces intense irritation of eyes, skin, and mucous membranes as well as dermatitis. Benzoyl peroxide will explode when suddenly contacted with heat.

Peracetic Acid

Peracetic acid, also known as acetyl hydroperoxide, is used as a bactericide, fungicide, and sterilizing agent and is extremely explosive at temperatures of 100°C (230°F).

Cumene Hydroperoxide

Cumene hydroperoxide is used in the plastic industry and for the production of phenol.

Methyl Ethyl Ketone Peroxide

Methyl ethyl ketone peroxide is a colorless liquid and is used in polymerization reactions and as a curing agent for polyester resins. It is a severe irritant of eyes, lungs, and mucous membranes. Animal data show that methyl ethyl ketone peroxide can produce pulmonary hemorrhage on surface contact with the lungs as well as gastrointestinal tract chemical burns (5).

HALOGENATED OXIDIZERS AND HALOGEN GASES

Perchloryl Fluoride

Perchloryl fluoride has a TLV of 3 ppm and a chemical formula of ClO_3F. It is a gas used in organic synthesis to produce fluorinated organic compounds. It is also a strong oxidizing agent and is used in rocket fuels and as an insulator (4). Perchloryl fluoride is a strong irritant of the eyes, mucous membranes, and lungs. In high concentrations it can produce pulmonary edema as well as methemoglobinemia. Exposure to toxic concentrations can produce weakness, syncope, and headache as well as severe respiratory tract irritation and pulmonary edema. Skin contact from the liquid form can produce burns. Clinical symptomatology includes dizziness, headache, cyanosis, and syncope. Perchloryl fluoride is incompatible with compounds that are combustible, strong bases, amines, and metal particulates, as well as other oxidizable materials. The IDLH level is 385 ppm (5).

Oxychlorinated Compounds

These include hypochlorous acid, chlorous acid, chloric acid, and perchlorates. Sodium hypochlorite is contained in commercial bleaches in strengths of 3–5%. Hypochlorites can react with organic materials and produce spontaneous combustion. Hypochlorites should not be mixed with organic materials.

Chlorates

Potassium, sodium, and ammonium chlorates (ClO_3^-) are strong oxidizing agents that are found in fireworks, gunpowder, matches, flares, and fuses. The combination of organic material and chlorates form a combustible combination that can burst into flames (2). When chlorates are mixed with sulfur and charcoal, spontaneous combustion can occur. Chlorates also spontaneously explode and ignite when mixed with finely ground-up metal. Toxic exposure can produce hemolysis, methemoglobinemia, and renal and kidney damage.

Perchlorates

Perchlorates (ClO_4^-) are more stable than hypochlorites, chlorites, and chlorates. They have slower chemical reactivity and are less hazardous to store and transport (2). Perchlorates react with organic matter to produce an ignition process. Perchloric acid ($HClO_4$) is both an oxidizer and a corrosive material. Perchlorates can cause methemoglobinemia following exposure.

Halogen Gases

Halogen gases (Cl_2, F_2, Br_2, and I_2) are strong oxidizing agents and corrosive agents. Chlorine and fluorine exist in a gaseous state. Bromine is a liquid, and iodine is a solid.

Bromine (Br₂)

Bromine is a reddish-brown, dark, volatile liquid and is very corrosive as well as being a strong oxidizing material. Bromine is used in the manufacturing of gasoline antiknock compounds such as 1,2-dibromomethane, fire retardants, pharmaceuticals, and pesticides (5). Bromine reacts with aqueous ammonium, organics, aluminum, titanium, mercury, potassium, and other metals to produce combustible hazards. The TLV of bromine is 0.1 ppm with a STEL of 0.3 ppm. The IDLH concentration is 10 ppm. Human toxicity of bromine is due to its effects on lungs, eyes, mucous membranes, and skin. Ten ppm bromine gas is a severe irritant and cannot be tolerated. High bromine concentrations produce dizziness, headache, nosebleeds, and severe irritation of the eyes and throat. Bromine is such a strong irritant that it can produce edema of the upper airway as well as pulmonary edema on inhalation of high concentrates. Skin burns can occur from liquid bromine spills. Bromine initially causes a cooling effect on the skin and after a delay will produce a burning sensation that can progress to deep chemical burns as well as a brown discoloration of the skin (4).

Chlorine

Chlorine is a green-yellow gas and is very irritating. It has a TLV of 1 ppm with a STEL of 3 ppm. Chlorine is a very powerful irritant of the eyes, skin, mucous membranes, and lungs. Chlorine inhalation can produce burning of the throat, chest, and eyes, difficulty breathing, bronchospasm, and pulmonary edema. A concentration of 1000 ppm can be rapidly fatal (7). Chlorine gas is used in a variety of chemical processes and as a bleaching agent. It is also commonly used in swimming pools as a disinfectant. Chlorine is only slightly soluble in water and very soluble in alkaline solutions. Chlorine is a nonflammable gas but a strong oxidizer. Chlorine as a bleaching agent is often used in the pulp and paper industry as well as textile industries. It is also used in the formation of a variety of inorganic and organic chlorinated compounds. Chlorine is incompatible with other combustible substances as well as fine particulates of metals. NIOSH has recommended a ceiling limit of 0.5 ppm for a 15-minute period.

Fluorine (F₂)

Fluorine is a yellowish gas and a very strong oxidizing agent. Fluorine is used in the production of fluorinated organic and inorganic compounds. It is a strong oxidizer and is used in rocket fuel. Fluorine is incompatible with water, nitric acid, and other oxidizing materials. The TLV of fluorine is 0.1 ppm.

It has an IDLH level of 5 ppm. The ACGIH recommends a TLV of 1 ppm and a STEL of 2 ppm.

Fluorine is a very severe irritant of the lungs, mucous membranes, skin, and eyes. Fluorine in high concentrations can produce laryngospasm as well as pulmonary edema. Exposure to lower concentrations around 25 ppm can result in sore throat, difficulty breathing, chest pain, and cough. Dermal and eye burns can occur secondary to fluorine skin exposure.

Iodine

Iodine (I_2) is a purple solid with a sharp odor. Iodine is used in the manufacture of organic materials and pharmaceuticals. Iodine has threshold limit value of 0.1 ppm. It is also used in the photography industry. Iodine is a strong irritant of the mucous membrane, respiratory tract, eyes, and skin. Ocular exposure can result in intense pain and blepharitis. Ingestion of 2–3 grams of iodine is said to be possibly fatal and can result in a syndrome of tachychardia, parotitis, bronchitis, and difficulty sleeping (4). Iodine is incompatible with gaseous or aqueous ammonium, acetylene, acetylhyde, powdered aluminum, and other active metals (5). Iodine in contact with the skin can produce hypersensitivity as well as burns.

Bromine Pentafluoride

Bromine pentafluoride (BrF_5) is a dense colorless liquid with a boiling point of 40°C. It is a strong oxidizer and corrosive material. It is used as an oxidizer in liquid rocket propellants (5). Bromine pentafluoride is a strong irritant of the eyes, skin, and other mucous membranes. The ACGIH has recommended a TLV of 0.1 ppm and a STEL of 0.3 ppm.

Chlorine Trifluoride

Chlorine trifluoride (ClF_3) is a green-yellow liquid and can also be a gas. It has a sweet irritating odor, and it has a boiling point of 11°C. It is a strong oxidizing agent and a corrosive agent. The TLV is 0.1 ppm, and the IDLH level is 20 ppm (5). Chlorine trifluoride is used in rocket fuel, in nuclear reactor fuel processing, and as an incendiary agent. Human exposure occurs mainly from skin contact and inhalation. It is a very strong irritant of the eyes, respiratory system, and mucous membrane. The hydrolysis of chlorine trifluoride produces chlorine and hydrogen fluoride and chlorine dioxide. Human toxic effects are also related to these hydrolysis products.

Chlorine Dioxide

Chlorine dioxide (ClO_2) is yellow to slightly yellow gas and has a very sharp pungent odor. Chlorine dioxide is used as a bleach in water purification, and also as a disinfectant and fungicide; it is a strong oxidizing agent. It is incompatible with other combustible materials, organic matters, materials, and solvents. The chlorine dioxide TLV is 0.1 ppm, and the ACGIH recommended STEL of 0.3 ppm. The IDLH level is 10 ppm (5). Chlorine dioxide is a severe ocular, mucous membrane, and respiratory irritant. Exposure to concentrations up to 1 ppm has been fatal.

Oxygen Difluoride

Oxygen difluoride (OF_2) is a rocket propellant and oxidizing agent. It is a colorless gas with a TLV of 0.05 ppm. It is a potent irritant of mucous membranes and the respiratory tract.

Ammonium Nitrate and Nitrite

The ammonium compounds are represented by ammonium nitrate and ammonium nitrite. Ammonium nitrate is a synthetic fertilizer. Ammonium nitrate has also been used in formulations of dynamite since 1933. There are two grades of ammonium nitrate: the fertilizer grade and an explosive grade. Both of these pose different hazards relative to their decomposition and explosivity. The ammonium agents which are oxidizers are shown in Table 117.3. Ammonium nitrate is found in a variety of forms such as fertilizer and explosives (4). The decomposition of ammonium salt oxidizing agents is explosive. When these compounds are exposed to heat they can explode or detonate. The heating of ammonium nitrate produces decomposition into a variety of chemical products. At low temperatures ammonium nitrate decomposes to nitrous oxide and water. When exposed to high temperatures, it becomes explosive. Ammonium nitrate is also incompatible with powered metals, charcoal, and sulfur (6).

When ammonium nitrate is heated in an enclosed area which can retain the products of decomposition, a dangerous explosion can occur (6).

Ammonium Picrate

This is a picric acid ammonium derivative used in explosives, fireworks, and rocket propellants. It is also known as ammonium picrate. It is considered to be a high explosive and reacts with metal and sodium nitrite. The compound has a bitter taste and has the same properties as picric acid. It can be absorbed through the skin and can produce nausea, vomiting, diarrhea, staining of the skin, dermatitis, circular eruptions of the skin, coma, and seizures. On decomposition it emits nitrogen oxide (8).

CHROMATES, CHROMIUM METALS, AND CHROMIUM SALTS

Chromium with a 6+ oxidation state (hexavalent) includes 4 compounds: metallic chromates, metallic dichromates, chromium trioxide, and chromyl chloride (2). The hexavalent chromium compounds are severe irritants of the lungs, eyes, mucous membranes, nose, and throat. The hexavalent chromium compounds are also the most toxic of the chromium compounds. Exposure to chromate dusts can produce nasal ulcerations and perforations, epistaxis, respiratory irritation, bronchospasm, renal failure, dermatitis, skin sensitization, skin discoloration, and skin ulceration. Prolonged exposure can also result in dental erosions (4, 5, 9).

Chromic Acid

Chromic acid (H_2CrO_4) is a strong hexavalent oxidizing agent. Chromic acid and the chromates are incompatible with other combustible materials, organic materials, or readily oxidizable materials such as paper, sulfur, and aluminum. Chromic acid and chromates have an IDLH level of 30 mg/m³. NIOSH has recommended a threshold limit value of chromic acid of 0.05 mg/m³. The federal TLV for hexavalent chromium compound is 0.05 mg/m³. Chromic acid is used as a metal and glass cleaner prior to electroplating. Chromic acid is a highly toxic compound that can produce dermal burns resulting in systemic absorption with acute renal failure. Dermal burns less than 3%

can produce renal failure. Contact with the eyes can produce severe corneal injury. Dermatitis from chromic acid can vary from erythematous rash to eczematous lesions (4, 5, 9).

Chromyl Chloride

Chromyl chloride (CrO_2Cl_2) is a red liquid produced by addition of concentrated hydrochloric acid and sulfuric acid to potassium dichromate (4, 5).

Ammonium Dichromate

Ammonium dichromate [$(NH_4)_2Cr_2O_7$] can undergo thermal decomposition producing a violent conflagration (4, 5). It is a strong oxidizing agent and flammable solid.

Chromium Trioxide

Also known as chromium anhydride (CrO_3), chromium trioxide is a solid which may also be produced as a red liquid (4, 5).

Permanganates

Permanganate is the manganese atom in the 7 + oxidation state (MnO_4^-. Ammonium permanganate (NH_4MnO_4) is a very strong oxidizing agent which upon exposure to heat can explode violently. Permanganates salts are very strong oxidizing agents. Permanganate solutions are used as coating on magnesium alloys to protect from corrosion (4–6).

Potassium Persulfate

Potassium persulfate ($K_2S_2O_8$) is a crystalline white material which decomposes below 100°C. It is a very strong oxidizing agent and is used as a bleaching agent and as a polymerization catalyst. It is incompatible with combustible materials, organic materials and other oxidizable materials, sulfur, metallic dust, aluminum dust, chlorates, and percholates (4, 5). The ACGIH has recommended a TLV of 2 mg/m³. The potassium persulfate reacts with moisture to produce ozone and sulfuric acid, which can produce an explosion in a closed container (5).

REACTIVE REDUCING CHEMICALS

Reducing agents are chemicals that lose electrons in oxidation-reduction reactions. The rapidity with which a chemical undergoes an oxidation-reduction reaction also determines its hazard. Several reducing agents are known to be hazardous materials, due to their extreme reactivity as well as due to their clinical toxicity. These compounds include:

Hydrazine
Monomethylhydrazine
Hydroxylamine
Decaborane
Pentaborane
Boron trifluoride
Boron tribromide
Lithium hydride

Many of these are used as rocket propellants and in fuels as well as in a variety of other industrial processes requiring strong reducing chemical properties.

Hydrazine

Hydrazine (H_2N—NH_2) is commonly used as rocket fuel and a reducing agent. It is a colorless, oily liquid which fumes in the air (4, 5). It is a flammable liquid with a strong reducing capacity. It is used in the preparation of anticorrosive materials and pesticides and as a scavenging agent for oxygen in boiler water (5). It is used as a rocket fuel as well as in the pharmaceutical industry. Hydrazine is incompatible with oxidizing agents, hydrogen peroxide, nitric acid, metal oxides, and strong acids. The IDLH level is 80 ppm. Hydrazine is used in manufacturing insecticides, plastics, rubber compounds, textile treating agents, dyes, and pharmaceuticals and is an antioxidant. It carries a hazard warning label as a corrosive material.

Hydrazine should be stored in order to avoid any contact with oxidizing material such as perchlorates, peroxides, permanganates, chlorates, nitrates, and strong acids as well as hydrogen peroxide and metal oxides, since a violent reaction can occur upon contact with these materials. Hydrazine is a flammable liquid and should be stored away from ignition sources. On decomposition, it gives off toxic nitrogen oxide combustion products. It is toxic by inhalational routes and can also be absorbed through the skin. It is a suspected human carcinogen. Hydrazine is also very corrosive and can cause chemical burns of the skin. Its vapors may cause irritation of the mucous membrane, eyes, nose, and throat. Inhaling vapors can produce coughing, shortness of breath, and pulmonary edema (10). Clinical toxicity includes methemoglobinemia, vomiting, tremors, seizures, liver necrosis, and hemolysis.

The vapor density of hydrazine is 1.1 (air = 1). It reacts exothermically and very violently with metal oxides as well as oxidizing agents due to the fact that it is a powerful reducing agent. Vapors are very irritating to the mucous membranes, nose, throat, and upper respiratory tract. Exposure to the eyes can produce temporary blindness. Liquid splashes to the eyes can produce corneal injury and burns. Liquid splashes to the skin can also produce severe burns. Hydrazine can also produce dermatitis and skin sensitization. The odor threshold of hydrozene is 3.7 ppm and serves as a warning of exposure. Acutely breathing the vapors will cause intense irritation of the mucous membrane and lungs as well as causing nausea, vomiting, and dizziness. Higher vapor concentrations can produce tremors, seizures, and comas with hemolysis. Hydrazine is a probable human carcinogen and has been shown to produce lung and liver cancers and leukemia in animals (10). Workers who are to be in contact with hydrazine should have medical surveillance, including a complete blood count, liver and kidney function tests, pulmonary function tests, and neurologic evaluation prior to placement.

The OSHA permissible exposure limit with a skin notation is 0.1 ppm. NIOSH recommends a ceiling limit of 0.04 mg/m³ over a 2-hour period of time. NIOSH also recommends an IDLH concentration of 80 ppm. Hydrazine has an odor that resembles ammonia gas (10). A person who swallowed a mouthful of hydrazine exhibited rapid coma and dilated pupils but recovered with residual ataxia, nystagmus, and lost vibratory sensations. Hydrazine concentrations greater than 25% can produce severe burns and eye injury. It can readily penetrate the skin and eye, and contact should be diluted immediately with water if skin or eye exposure occur. Skin contact can result in itching and suppurative eczema after exposure (4, 5, 10).

Hydroxylamine

Hydroxylamine is a reducing agent used in organic synthesis and in the production of acrylonitrile. Hydroxylamine is flammable and produces toxic combustion byproducts of nitrous oxides. Hydroxylamine may explode when exposed to heat or flames. It is corrosive to the skin and mucous membranes on contact (11).

Hydroxylamine is a colorless crystalline substance. It finds use as a reducing agent in synthetic rubbers and graphic developing solutions. Its TLV has not been established. Hydroxylamine is irritating to the skin, eyes, and mucous membrane and can cause dermatitis. It also produces methemoglobinemia.

Monomethylhydrazine

Monomethylhydrazine (CH_3NHNH_2) is a fuming, colorless liquid that has an ammonia odor and boils at 88°C. It is a flammable liquid and is also known as methylhydrazine. Monomethylhydrazine has been used as rocket propellant and as a solvent. It is incompatible with metal oxides and oxidizing materials such as hydrogen peroxide. The ceiling limit value of monomethylhydrazine is 0.2 ppm. The IDLH level is 5 ppm (4, 5). Monomethylhydrazine is strong eye, mucous membrane, and upper respiratory irritant. It can produce symptoms of vomiting, respiratory irritation, and neurologic symptoms of tremors, ataxia, and seizures as well as methemoglobinemia on systemic absorption.

Boron Hydride

Boron hydride (B_2H_6) is also known as diborane. Boron hydride is a strong reducing agent and is used in rubber manufacturing, for high energy fuels, and is also used for rocket fuel. Diborane has a TLV of 0.1 ppm and is a very strong pulmonary irritant (4, 5). The odor detection theshold for diborane is 3.3 ppm. It has a sickening odor of rotten eggs. Diborane is very flammable as a gas and should be protected against physical damage and stored in a refrigerated area that is well-ventilated. Diborane should not be allowed to come into contact with oxidizing agents such as halogens, hydrogen peroxide, or oxygen (4, 5). It is very flammable and produces highly toxic combustion products. The boron hydrides as a class are very corrosive to synthetic rubbers and natural rubbers. The IDLH inhalation limit is 40 ppm. The OSHA PEL is 0.1 mg/m^3 (0.1 ppm as a time weighted average). The ACGIH recommends a TLV of 0.1 ppm. The NIOSH IDLH value is 40 ppm. Diborane is a colorless gas and has a very nauseating odor (4, 5, 12, 13).

Clinical toxicity on exposure presents with chest tightness, cough, and difficulty in breathing. Its recognition odor at 3.3 ppm helps avoid further injury. However, chronic exposure to diborane may produce olfactory fatigue. High concentrations can produce severe pulmonary irritation and pulmonary edema (12, 13).

Decaborane

Decaborane ($B_{10}H_{14}$) is a colorless crystalline solid reducing agent with a strong pungent odor. It is used in rocket propellants. It is a flammable solid and is also used as a vulcanizing agent in rubber manufacturing. It is incompatible with oxidizers, water, and halogenated hydrocarbons (4, 5, 12). The TLV for decaborane is 0.05 ppm with a dermal absorption warning. The IDLH level is 20 ppm. Clinical toxicity is manifested by central nervous system stimulation, hyperexcitability, headaches, muscle tremors, and seizures. Decaborane can be absorbed via the skin. Early symptoms consist of dizziness, nausea, headaches, muscle tremors; seizures occur with more severe intoxication. Symptoms usually subside in 24–48 hours, but fatigue may remain for days (12–14). Neurobehavioral changes may also occur following exposures (13).

Pentaborane

Pentaborane (B_5H_9) is a colorless volatile liquid that ignites spontaneously in air. It hydrolyzes in water and decomposes at 150°C. Its TLV is 0.005 ppm with a IDLH value of 3 ppm. Pentaborane is a strong reducing agent used in rocket fuel and as a gasoline additive. It is incompatible with oxidizers, halogenated hydrocarbons, and halogens. It can spontaneously ignite. It can be absorbed by inhalation and dermal routes. Pentaborane is the most toxic of the boron hydrides and can produce central nervous system excitation, muscle tremors, seizures, and hiccups. Early symptoms of toxicity consist of dizziness, headache, confusion, hiccups, ataxia, and tremors. Symptoms may be delayed 24–48 hours. Severe symptoms include coma, seizures, and neurobehavioral changes (12–14). Convulsions can occur rapidly following toxic exposure and present as opisthotonos and tonic contractions of facial muscles, neck muscles, abdomen, and extremities (12–14). Liver necrosis has also been noted.

Lithium Hydride

Lithium hydride (LiH) is a reducing agent and a severe irritant of the skin, eyes, and mucous membranes. It is in the form of white crystals and has a TLV of 0.025 mg/m^3. Lithium hydride is a flammable solid and is dangerous when wet. It can be used as a dessicant. Lithium hydride is incompatible with other oxidizing agents, halogenated hydrocarbons, acids, and water. The IDLH value is 15 mg/m^3 (4, 5). Lithium hydride can cause severe burns on skin and ocular contact. Systemic absorption can produce muscular tremors, nausea, and confusion. On ingestion, it can also produce burns of the esophagus and mouth. Powdered lithium hydride can ignite spontaneously in humid air or on contact with mucous membrane surfaces or moist skin surfaces and result in thermal and alkaline burns (4, 5).

Boron Tribromide

Boron tribromide (BBr_3) is a fuming liquid which boils at 90°C (4, 5). It is a highly corrosive reducing agent used as a catalyst in organic chemical synthesis. The ACGIH recommends a TLV of 1 ppm. Hydrolysis produces hydrogen bromide and the toxicity of BBr_3 is that of hydrogen bromide. Hydrogen bromide (HBr) has a ceiling limit of 5 ppm. It is a gas and strong irritant of the eyes, lungs, and mucous membranes and may cause chemical burns by contact with vapors of the gas.

Boron Trifluoride

Boron trifluoride (BF_3) is a colorless nonflammable gas used as a fumigant and a catalyst. It is a highly reactive gas with

Table 117.4.   Liquefied Cryogenic Gases

Oxygen
Nitrogen
Argon
Ammonia
Helium
Hydrogen
Liquefied natural gas
Liquefied petroleum gas
    Propane
    Propylene
    Butane
    Butylene

fire-retardant and antioxidant properties. When exposed to air, BF_3 forms a white fume (4, 5). It is highly reactive with alkalis and moist air. Clinical toxicity consists of severe irritant effects of the eyes, lungs, and mucous membranes. It can produce epistaxis. BF_3 has a ceiling limit of exposure of 1 ppm.

COMPRESSED FLAMMABLE GASES AND CRYOGENIC GASES

The DOT defines four classes of flammable products: flammable gases, flammable liquids, combustible liquids, and flammable solids. Compressed liquefied gases and compressed gases include: liquid hydrogen, liquid helium, liquid oxygen, liquid nitrogen, and liquid argon, liquefied natural gas (LNG), and liquefied petroleum gas (LPG) (Table 117.4). An understanding of liquefied gases must be accompanied by an understanding of the cryogenic process which helps to make these gases liquid. In the conversion of a liquid to a gas, two factors are critical: the gas is under extreme pressure and extremely low temperature. Both the increased pressure and the low temperature are responsible for liquefication of the gas. There is a certain temperature, no matter what pressure is applied, that the gas will not liquefy; this is termed the "critical temperature." The pressure that is required to produce a liquefied gas at its critical temperature is also termed "critical pressure" (1, 2). These liquefied gases are also referred to as cryogenics. Cryogenic compounds are liquid and gases at temperatures between $-150°C$ ($-238°F$) and absolute zero. The lower limit of freezing is absolute zero. The upper limit of cryogenic liquid gases is set at $-101°C$, which is $-150°F$ or $123°K$ (Kelvin) (1–3). Liquefied gases are very cold and can be used as coolants. Dermal exposure can produce serious thermal injury with deep tissue necrosis from the extremely low temperatures and high pressures.

Liquid Hydrogen

Liquid hydrogen rapidly expands its volume 850 times when released into the air. It is a highly flammable gas with a flammability range from 4–75% (1, 2). Liquid hydrogen spills can be very hazardous for responding emergency personnel because of its extreme flammability. Once it unites with oxygen in the air, ignition can occur. A release of spilled or liquefied hydrogen results in a potentially explosive vapor cloud in the vicinity of the spill. Once this vapor cloud is ignited, it can produce a large fireball and produce explosions and combustion of other flammable materials when they are within the area of the explosion.

Liquid hydrogen should never be exposed to the air. Human contact with liquid hydrogen may produce a cryogenic burn of the skin. This is due to the extreme low temperature required to liquefy the hydrogen (1, 2).

Liquefied Oxygen

The temperature of liquid oxygen is $-297.3°F$ ($-182.9°C$). Liquid oxygen has a pale blue color and a density similar to that of water. A small quantity of liquefied oxygen and other liquefied gases can expand to tremendous volumes of gases at atmospheric pressure (1, 2). Liquid oxygen and other liquefied gases such as nitrogen, argon, and helium will produce cryogenic burns of the skin on contact due to the extremely cold temperatures they are stored under. A small amount of heat can cause an explosion of liquid oxygen. Any foreign material, when combined with liquid oxygen and another substance with which oxygen will combine chemically, can produce an explosion in a liquid oxygen system.

Liquefied Helium

Liquefied helium is extremely cold and has a boiling point of $-452.1°F$ ($-268.95°C$), $7.6°F$ above absolute zero. Liquid helium is a colorless fluid with a density of approximately one-eighth that of water (1, 2). Liquid helium is extremely easy to vaporize, and all sources of heat must be insulated away from liquid helium. Liquefied helium, similar to other liquefied gases, can produce cryogenic burns to the skin on contact.

Liquefied Natural Gas (LNG)

Liquefied natural gas is a liquid fuel that readily vaporizes and can ignite and burn when mixed with air. It is typically stored at temperatures of $-2600°F$ ($-162.2°C$).

Liquefied Ammonia Gas (NH_3)

Liquefied ammonia freezes at $-108°F$ ($-77.8°C$) and boils at $-28°F$ ($-33.3°C$) (1, 2). Anhydrous ammonia will autoignite if exposed to heat during a release. Following its release from pressurized storage containers, liquid ammonia will vaporize and expand very rapidly and occupy approximately 850 times its liquid volume (1, 2). Due to this, it creates water vapor in the air and a white cloud. Ammonia gas can produce pulmonary, ocular, and skin irritation. Its odor is detectable at 50 ppm, and its TLV is 25 ppm. Exposure to high concentrations can result from accidental spills of liquefied ammonia gas. Inhalation of 2000–7000 ppm can produce severe bronchospasm, dyspnea, chest pain, and pulmonary edema, and can be fatal (1, 2). Individuals exposed to 100–200 ppm can experience intense irritation of mucous membranes, eyes, and respiratory tract. The ignition temperature of anhydrous ammonia is 1562°F (850°C). Ammonia vapor created on spill or by accident of a pressurized container will release vapor concentrations that can be as high as 10,000 ppm. Ammonia vapor at 50 ppm is detectable by both people and is an irritating, pungent odor. At 400–700 ppm, it is a severe irritant of the eye and mucous membranes, producing lacrimation. Up to 3000 ppm, it can produce severe eye irritation, difficulty breathing, and between 5000–10,000 ppm, can produce bronchospasm, pulmonary edema, and death.

Cryogenic burns can occur from liquefied ammonia. Also,

the formation of ammonium hydroxide on mucous membranes or skin can result in chemical burns.

Liquefied Petroleum Gas (LPG)

Liquefied petroleum gas can be used to describe any of the following: propane, butane, propylene, and butylene. Liquefied petroleum can be one of these gases or a mixture and combination of these gases. One of the main hazards of these gases is that they displace oxygen and produce asphyxiant hazards in confined spaces. All of these gases are flammable hazards. These gases are shipped and stored under pressure as a liquid and also have cryogenic potential in terms of producing dermal injury on contact. The TLV for liquefied petroleum gas is 1000 ppm.

REFERENCES

1. Isman W, Carlson G. Hazardous materials. Chapt 4 in: Explosives, oxidizers and radioactive materials. Encino, CA: Glenco Publishing, 1980: 61–88.
2. Myer E. Chemistry of hazardous materials—twelve chemical explosives. Englewood Cliffs, NJ: Tintus-Hall, 1977:306–327.
3. (No author listed.) Dangerous properties of industrial materials reports July–August, 1988;8:75–80.
4. Proctor N., Hughes J, Fischman M. Chemical hazards of the work place. 2nd ed. New York, NY: JB Lippincott, 1988.
5. Sittig M. Handbook of toxic and hazardous chemicals. Park Ridge, NJ: Noyes Publications, 1981.
6. Myer E. Chemistry of hazardous materials. Chapt 9 in: Oxidation-reduction phenomena. Englewood Cliffs, NJ: Prentice Hall, 1977:216–230.
7. Hedges J, Morrissey W. Acute chlorine gas exposure. J Am Coll Emerg Phys 1979;8:59–63.
8. (No author listed.) Dangerous properties of industrial materials reports. March–April, 1988;8:43–44.
9. Sawyer JH. Chromium and its compounds. In: Zenz C, ed, Occupational medicine: principles and practical applications. Chicago: Year Book Medical Publishers, 1988.
10. (No author listed.) Dangerous properties of industrial materials reports 1990;10:21–58.
11. (No author listed.) Dangerous properties of industrial materials reports 1988;8:34–39.
12. Naeger L, Leibman K. Mechanisms of decaborane toxicity. Toxicol Appl Pharmacol 1972;22:517–527.
13. Rousch G. The toxicology of the boranes. J Occup Med 1959;1:46–52.
14. Hart R, Silverman J, Garretson L. Neuropsychological function following mild exposure to pentaborane. Am J Ind Med 1984;6:37–44.
15. Isman W, Carlson G. Explosives, oxidizers and radioactive materials. Chapt 5 in: Hazardous materials. Encino, CA: Glenco Publishing, 1980: 89–130.

Page numbers in *italics* denote figures; those followed by "t" denote tables.